TOP DRUG LIST (Continued)

Brand	Generic	Brand	Generic
Cortisporin Otic	Neomycin/polymyxin/ hydrocortisone	Flonase	Fluticasone propionate
Cosopt	Dorzolamide/Timolol	Flovent HFA or Diskus	Fluticasone propionate
Coumadin, Jantoven	Warfarin Sodium	Focalin (XR)	Dexmethylphenidate
Cozaar, Hyzaar	Losartan, Los/HCTZ	Foradil	Formoterol
Crestor	Rosuvastatin	Fosamax	Alendronate
Cymbalta	Duloxetine	Geodon	Ziprasidone
Delta D3	Cholecalciferol	Glucophage (XR), Fortamet	Metformin
Deltasone	Prednisone	Glucotrol (XL)	Glipizide
Depakote (ER)	Divalproex	Humalog	Insulin Lispro
Depo-Provera	Medroxyprogesterone	Humulin N	Insulin - NPH
Desyrel	Trazodone	Humulin R	Insulin - regular
Detrol (LA)	Tolterodine	Hytrin	Terazosin
Differin	Adapalene	Imdur, ISMO	Isosorbide Mononitrate
Diflucan	Fluconazole	Imitrex	Sumatriptan
Dilantin Kapseals	Phenytoin Sodium	Imodium	Loperamide
Diovan, Diovan HCT	Valsartan, Val/HCTZ	Incruse Ellipta	Umeclidinium
Ditropan (XL)	Oxybutynin	Inderal, Inderal LA, Innopran, Innopran XL	Propranolol
Dulera	Mometasone/ Formoterol		
Duragesic	Fentanyl	Indocin	Indomethacin
Dyazide capsules or Maxzide tablets	Triamterene + HCTZ	Januvia, Janumet (XR)	Sitagliptin, Sit+Metformin
		Kariva, Ortho-Cept, Mircette, Desogen or Apri	Ethinyl Estradiol / Desogestrel
Ecotrin	Aspirin		
Effexor (XR)	Venlafaxine	Keflex	Cephalexin
Elavil	Amitriptyline	Kenalog	Triamcinolone
Elidel	Pimecrolimus	Keppra	Levetiracetam
Eliquis	Apixaban	Klonopin	Clonazepam
Elocon	Mometasone	Klor-Con	Potassium Chloride
Enablex	Darifenacin	Lamictal	Lamotrigine
Eskalith or Lithobid	Lithium Carbonate	Lamisil	Terbinafine
Estratest (HS)	Estrogen/ Methyltestosterone	Lanoxin	Digoxin
Evista	Raloxifene	Lantus	Insulin Glargine
Exelon, Exelon Patch	Rivastigmine	Lasix	Furosemide
Exforge, Exforge HCT	Amlodipine+Valsartan, amlo/ val/HCTZ	Levaquin	Levofloxacin
		Levemir	Insulin Detemir
Feldene	Piroxicam	Levitra	Vardenafil
Fioricet, Fioricet with codeine	Butalbital + acetaminophen + caffeine (sometimes called B-A-C), available with or without codeine	Levsin/Levbid/Levsinex	Hyoscyamine
		Lexapro	Escitalopram
		Lidex, Lidex-E, Vanos	Fluocinonide topical
Fiorinal, Fiorinal with codeine	Butalbital + aspirin + caffeine, available with or without codeine	Lidoderm Patches	Lidocaine
		Lipitor	Atorvastatin
Flagyl, Flagyl ER	Metronidazole	Lodine (XL)	Etodolac
Flexeril	Cyclobenzaprine	Loestrin FE	Norethindrone/Ethinyl Estradiol, Fe+
Flomax	Tamsulosin		

(Continued)

Brand	Generic	Brand	Generic
Lomotil	Diphenoxylate/Atropine	Novolog Mix 70/30, Humalog Mix 75/25	Insulin 70% protamine/ 30% rapid acting
Lopid	Gemfibrozil	NuvaRing	Ethinyl Estradiol / Etonogestrel
Lopressor	Metoprolol Tartrate	Omnicef	Cefdinir
Lotensin, Lotensin HCT	Benazepril, Ben/HCTZ	Onglyza	Saxagliptin
Lotrel	Amlodipine + Benazepril	Oretic, Microzide	Hydrochlorothiazide (aka HCTZ)
Lotrisone	Clotrimazole/ Betamethasone Dipropionate	Ortho Evra	Ethinyl Estradiol / Norelgestromin
Lovenox	Enoxaparin	Ortho Tri-Cyclen (Lo)	Norgestimate/Ethinyl Estradiol
Lozol	Indapamide	Oxycontin, Roxicodone	Oxycodone
Lumigan	Bimatoprost	Pataday or Patanol	Olopatadine
Lunesta	Eszopiclone	Paxil (CR), Brisdelle	Paroxetine
Lyrica	Pregabalin	Pepcid	Famotidine
Macrobid, Macrodantin, Furadantin	Nitrofurantoin	Percocet or Roxicet	Oxycodone/APAP
		Peridex, PerioGard	Chlorhexidine Gluconate
Maxalt, Maxalt MLT	Rizatriptan	Phenergan	Promethazine
Medrol	Methylprednisolone	Phenobarbital	Phenobarbital
Metrogel, Metrogel-Vaginal, Metrocream, Metrolotion	Metronidazole	Plavix	Clopidogrel
		Pradaxa	Dabigatran
Mevacor, Altoprev ER	Lovastatin	Pravachol	Pravastatin
Micronase, Glucovance	Glyburide, Glyburide/Metformin	Premarin	Conjugated Estrogens
Miralax, Glycolax	Polyethylene Glycol	Prempro or Premphase	Conjugated Estrogens with medroxyprogesterone
Mirapex	Pramipexole		
Mobic	Meloxicam	Prevacid	Lansoprazole
Motrin or Advil	Ibuprofen	Prilosec	Omeprazole
MS Contin, MSIR	Morphine Sulfate	Pristiq	Desvenlafaxine
Mucinex (D)	Guaifenesin	Proair HFA or Ventolin HFA or Proventil HFA	Albuterol
Mycolog II	Nystatin + Triamcinolone		
Mycostatin, Nystop	Nystatin	Procardia, Procardia XL, Adalat CC	Nifedipine
Namenda	Memantine	Propecia or Proscar	Finasteride
Naprosyn, Anaprox/Aleve	Naproxen and Naproxen sodium	Protonix	Pantoprazole
Nasonex	Mometasone	Provera	Medroxyprogesterone Acetate
Neurontin	Gabapentin	Provigil	Modafinil
Nexium	Esomeprazole	Prozac or Sarafem	Fluoxetine
Niaspan ER	Niacin	Pulmicort Respules, Flexhaler	Budesonide Inhalation
Nitro-Dur	Topical Nitroglycerin	Pyridium	Phenazopyridine
Nitrostat	Nitroglycerin SL	QVAR	Beclomethasone
Nizoral	Ketoconazole	Reglan	Metoclopramide
Norco, Vicodin	Hydrocodone/APAP	Relafen	Nabumetone
Normodyne or Trandate	Labetalol	Relpax	Eletriptan
Norvasc	Amlodipine	Remeron	Mirtazapine
Novolin 70/30, Humulin 70/30	Insulin 70% NPH/ 30% Regular	Requip	Ropinirole
		Restasis	Cyclosporine
Novolog	Insulin Aspart	Restoril	Temazepam

(Continued)

Brand	Generic	Brand	Generic
Retin-A	Tretinoin	Uroxatral	Alfuzosin
Rhinocort Aqua	Budesonide Nasal Spray	Vagifem	Estradiol
Risperdal	Risperidone	Valium	Diazepam
Serevent	Salmeterol	Valtrex	Valacyclovir
Seroquel (XR)	Quetiapine	Vasotec	Enalapril
Sinemet (CR)	Levodopa/Carbidopa	Veetids, Pen-Vee K	Penicillin V Potassium
Singulair	Montelukast	Viagra	Sildenafil
Skelaxin	Metaxalone	Vibramycin, Doryx, Adoxa, Monodox, Oracea, Periostat	Doxycycline
Soma	Carisoprodol		
Sonata	Zaleplon	Vicoprofen	Hydrocodone/Ibuprofen
Spiriva HandiHaler or Respimat	Tiotropium	Victoza	Liraglutide
Strattera	Atomoxetine	Vigamox	Moxifloxacin
Stribild	elvitegravir + cobicistat + tenofovir disoproxil fumarate + emtricitabine	Vistaril	Hydroxyzine pamoate
		Vivelle-Dot, Estraderm	Estradiol
Striverdi Respimat	Olodaterol	Voltaren, Cataflam	Enteric Diclofenac sodium, Diclofenac potassium (non-enteric coated formulation)
Symbicort	Budesonide/ Formoterol		
Synthroid, Levoxyl	Levothyroxine	Vytorin	Simvastatin/ezetimibe
Tamiflu	Oseltamivir	Vyvanse	Lisdexamfetamine
Tegretol (XR)	Carbamazepine	Wellbutrin (SR) (XL)	Bupropion
Tenoretic	Atenolol/chlorthalidone	Xalatan	Latanoprost
Tenormin	Atenolol	Xanax (XR)	Alprazolam
Thalidone, Hygroton	Chlorthalidone	Xarelto	Rivaroxaban
Timoptic (XE)	Timolol	Xenical	Orlistat
Tobradex	Tobramycin/ Dexamethasone	Xopenex (HFA)	Levalbuterol
Tofranil (PM)	Imipramine	Yasmin, Ocella, Yaz	Ethinyl Estradiol/ Drospirenone
Topamax	Topiramate	Zantac	Ranitidine
Toprol XL	Metoprolol Succinate	Zaroxolyn	Metolazone
Toradol	Ketorolac Tromethamine	Zebeta, Ziac	Bisoprolol, Bisoprolol + HCTZ
Transderm-Scop	Scopolamine	Zegerid	Omeprazole/sodium bicarbonate
Travatan	Travoprost	Zestril or Prinivil, Zestoretic	Lisinopril, Lis/HCTZ
Tricor, Trilipix	Fenofibrate	Zithromax, Zmax, Azasite	Azithromycin
Trileptal	Oxcarbazepine	Zocor	Simvastatin
TriNessa, Tri-Sprintec	Norgestimate & Ethinyl Estradiol	Zofran, Zofran ODT	Ondansetron
Tudorza Pressair	Aclidinium	Zoloft	Sertraline
Tussionex	Hydrocodone / Chlorpheniramine Polistirex	Zovirax	Acyclovir
Tylenol	Acetaminophen	Zyban	Bupropion
Tylenol with Codeine	Acetaminophen/ Codeine	Zyloprim	Allopurinol
Uloric	Febuxostat	Zymar	Gatifloxacin
Ultracet	Tramadol + acetaminophen	Zyprexa	Olanzapine
Ultram, Ultram ER	Tramadol	Zyrtec	Cetirizine

McGraw-Hill's
NAPLEX®
Review Guide
Third Edition

Editor

S. Scott Sutton, PharmD

Professor and Chair
Department of Clinical Pharmacy
   and Outcomes Sciences
University of South Carolina College
   of Pharmacy
Columbia, South Carolina

New York   Chicago   San Francisco   Athens   London   Madrid
Mexico City   Milan   New Delhi   Singapore   Sydney   Toronto

1 2 3 4 5 6 7 8 9   LOV   23 22 21 20 19 18

ISBN: 978-1-260-13592-3
MHID: 1-260-13592-6

This book was set in Minion Pro by Cenveo® Publisher Services.
The editors were Michael Weitz and Christina M. Thomas.
The production supervisor was Richard Ruzycka.
Project management was provided by Radhika Jolly, Cenveo Publisher Services.
The cover designer was W2 Design.

Notice

Medicine is an ever-changing science. As new research and clinical experience broaden our knowledge, changes in treatment and drug therapy are required. The authors and the publisher of this work have checked with sources believed to be reliable in their efforts to provide information that is complete and generally in accord with the standards accepted at the time of publication. However, in view of the possibility of human error or changes in medical sciences, neither the authors nor the publisher nor any other party who has been involved in the preparation or publication of this work warrants that the information contained herein is in every respect accurate or complete, and they disclaim all responsibility for any errors or omissions or for the results obtained from use of the information contained in this work. Readers are encouraged to confirm the information contained herein with other sources. For example, and in particular, readers are advised to check the product information sheet included in the package of each drug they plan to administer to be certain that the information contained in this work is accurate and that changes have not been made in the recommended dose or in the contraindications for administration. This recommendation is of particular importance in connection with new or infrequently used drugs.

Library of Congress Cataloging-in-Publication Data

Names: Sutton, S. Scott (Shawn Scott), editor.
Title: Mcgraw-Hill's NAPLEX review guide/editor, S. Scott Sutton, PharmD.
Other titles: NAPLEX review guide
Description: Third edition. | New York : McGraw-Hill, [2018] | Includes index.
Identifiers: LCCN 2018033390| ISBN 9781260135923 (paperback : alk. paper) |
    ISBN 1260135926 | ISBN 9781260135930 (ebook) | ISBN 1260135934 (ebook)
Subjects: LCSH: Pharmacy—Outlines, syllabi, etc. | Pharmacy—Examinations,
    questions, etc.
Classification: LCC RS98. M37 2018 | DDC 615.1076—dc23

McGraw-Hill Education books are available at special quantity discounts to use as premiums and sales promotions, or for use in corporate training programs. To contact a representative please visit the Contact Us pages at www.mhprofessional.com.

To my students

You have inspired and challenged me for years;
therefore, I have developed and dedicated this book
for you. My desire is that this textbook will inspire and
challenge you to be the best pharmacist you can be and
to serve others; and I hope you ace the NAPLEX®.

About the Editor

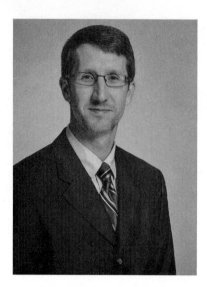

S. Scott Sutton, PharmD, is a Professor and Chair in the Department of Clinical Pharmacy and Outcomes Sciences at the University of South Carolina College of Pharmacy (USC COP). He received his Bachelor of Science and Doctor of Pharmacy degrees from the University of South Carolina and completed a clinical pharmacy residency in medicine and infectious diseases at the W.J.B. Dorn Veterans Affairs Medical Center in Columbia, South Carolina. He teaches in Pharmacotherapy, Pharmacokinetics, Clinical Applications, Infectious Diseases Pharmacotherapy, and Clinical Research. He is also a clinical researcher at the Dorn Research Institute, Veterans Affairs Medical Center. His research areas include pharmacoepidemiology and drug repurposing. He has received Teacher and Researcher of the Year awards from the University of South Carolina and has served as sports medicine pharmacist for the Department of Athletics. He is an educational consultant and professor for WA Associates, LLC, for which he teaches a national NAPLEX® Review course. He has taught thousands of students in this review course and continues teaching the course every spring and available on-line at https://rxexamcoach.com/. Dr. Sutton also has several products on McGraw Hill's access pharmacy including a Naplex Central tab. He is a husband, father, gamecock sports fan, golfer, and guitarist.

Contents

Contributors viii | Associate Editor xiii | Assistant Editors xiv | Peer Reviewers xv | Preface xvii | Acknowledgments xviii

To access your complimentary online question exams, visit https://accesspharmacy.mhmedical.com/NAPLEX.aspx

Contributors

Michaela M. Almgren, PharmD, MS
Clinical Assistant Professor
Department of Clinical Pharmacy and
Outcomes Sciences
University of South Carolina
College of Pharmacy
Columbia, South Carolina

**Miranda R. Andrus, PharmD,
FCCP, BCPS**
Associate Clinical Professor of
Pharmacy Practice
Auburn University Harrison School
of Pharmacy
University of Alabama at Birmingham
Huntsville Regional Medical Campus
Family Medicine Center
Huntsville, Alabama

Elizabeth W. Blake, PharmD, BCPS
Clinical Association Professor and
Director of Interprofessional Education
University of South Carolina College
of Pharmacy
Columbia, South Carolina

**Christopher M. Bland, PharmD,
FCCP, FIDSA, BCPS**
Clinical Associate Professor
Clinical and Administrative Pharmacy
University of Georgia College
of Pharmacy
Clinical Pharmacy Specialist
St. Joseph's/Candler Health System
Savannah, Georgia

**P. Brandon Bookstaver, PharmD,
FCCP, FIDSA, BCPS, AAHIVP**
Associate Professor and Director of
Residency and Fellowship Training
Department of Clinical Pharmacy and
Outcomes Sciences
University of South Carolina College
of Pharmacy
Infectious Diseases PGY2 and Clinical
Fellowship Director
USC/Palmetto Health
Columbia, South Carolina

Nancy Borja-Hart, PharmD, BCPS
Associate Professor
University of Tennessee Health
Science Center
College of Pharmacy—Nashville
Campus
Department of Clinical Pharmacy and
Translational Science
Nashville, Tennessee

**Michelle M. Bottenberg, PharmD,
BCPS**
Associate Professor of Pharmacy Practice
Director of the Pharmacy Skills and
Applications Course Series
Drake University College of Pharmacy
and Health Sciences
Des Moines, Iowa

Trisha N. Branan, PharmD, BCCCP
Clinical Assistant Professor
University of Georgia College
of Pharmacy
Critical Care Clinical Pharmacist
Piedmont Athens Regional
Athens, Georgia

Wendy Brown, PharmD, PA-C, AE-C
Primary Care Telemedicine Provider
Fargo VA Health Care System
Fargo, North Dakota

**Melinda (Mindy) J. Burnworth,
PharmD, FASHP, FAzPA, BCPS**
Professor
Department of Pharmacy Practice
Adult Internal Medicine Clinical
Pharmacy Specialist
Midwestern University College of
Pharmacy
Glendale, Arizona

**Joshua Caballero, PharmD,
BCPP, FCCP**
Professor and Chair
Department of Clinical and
Administrative Sciences
Larkin University College of Pharmacy
Miami, Florida

Matthew A. Cantrell, PharmD, BCPS
Associate Professor (Clinical)
University of Iowa College
of Pharmacy
Iowa City VA Health Care System
Iowa City, Iowa

Betty M. Chan, PharmD, BCOP
Assistant Professor of Clinical Pharmacy
University of Southern California
School of Pharmacy
Clinical Pharmacist, Ambulatory
Pharmacy Manager
USC/Norris Comprehensive Cancer
Center and Hospital
Los Angeles, California

Daniel B. Chastain, PharmD, AAHIVP
Clinical Assistant Professor
University of Georgia College of
Pharmacy, SWGA Clinical Campus
Infectious Diseases Pharmacist, Phoebe
Putney Memorial Hospital
Albany, Georgia

**Steven W. Chen, PharmD, FASHP,
FCSHP, FNAP**
Associate Professor and Chair
Department of Clinical Pharmacy and
Pharmaceutical Economics and Policy
Hygeia Centennial Chair in
Clinical Pharmacy
University of Southern California
School of Pharmacy
Los Angeles, California

**Jennifer N. Clements, PharmD,
BCPS, CDE, BCACP**
Associate Professor, Pharmacy Practice
Coordinator, Postgraduate Education
Presbyterian College School
of Pharmacy
Clinton, South Carolina

Kristen Cook, PharmD, BCPS
Clinical Assistant Professor
University of Nebraska Medical Center
College of Pharmacy
Omaha, Nebraska

Tammy Cummings, PhD
Biostatistician
Dorn Research Institute
WJB Dorn Veterans Affairs
Medical Center
Columbia, South Carolina

Quang Dam, PharmD
Pharmacist
Long Beach Memorial Hospital
and Miller Children's and Women's
Hospital of Long Beach
Long Beach, California

**David L. DeRemer, PharmD,
FCCP, BCOP**
Clinical Associate Professor
University of Florida College
of Pharmacy
Department of Pharmacotherapy and
Translational Research
Gainesville, Florida

Brianne L. Dunn, PharmD
Associate Dean for Outcomes
Assessment and Accreditation
Clinical Associate Professor
University of South Carolina College
of Pharmacy
Columbia, South Carolina

David Eagerton, PhD, F-ABFT
Chair and Associate Professor
Department of Pharmaceutical
Sciences
Campbell University College of
Pharmacy and Health Sciences
Buies Creek, North Carolina

Darla Klug Eastman, PharmD, BCPS
Associate Professor of Clinical Sciences
Drake University College of Pharmacy
and Health Sciences
Des Moines, Iowa

**Rebecca F. Edwards, PharmD, BCPS,
BCACP, CDE**
Clinical Pharmacy Specialist
Salisbury VA Health Care System
(SVAHCS)
Program Manager, Kernersville VA
Health Care Center
Kernersville, North Carolina

**Shareen El-Ibiary, PharmD,
FCCP, BCPS**
Professor
Midwestern University College of
Pharmacy
Glendale, Arizona

Rickey A. Evans, PharmD, BCPS
Assistant Professor
Department of Clinical Pharmacy and
Outcomes Sciences
Clinical Pharmacist-Critical Care,
Palmetto Health Richland
University of South Carolina College
of Pharmacy
Columbia, South Carolina

Patricia H. Fabel, PharmD, BCPS
Clinical Associate Professor
University of South Carolina College
of Pharmacy
Columbia, South Carolina

Michele A. Faulkner, PharmD, FASHP
Professor of Pharmacy Practice
and Neurology
Creighton University Schools
of Pharmacy and Medicine
Omaha, Nebraska

**McKenzie C. Ferguson, PharmD,
BCPS**
Associate Professor Pharmacy Practice
Director
Drug Information and Wellness Center
Southern Illinois University
Edwardsville School of Pharmacy
Edwardsville, Illinois

Anisa Fornoff, PharmD
Associate Professor of Clinical Sciences
Drake University College of Pharmacy
and Health Sciences
Des Moines, Iowa

Howell R. Foster, PharmD, DABAT
Director
Arkansas Poison and Drug Information
Center
Associate Professor
Department of Pharmacy Practice
University of Arkansas for
Medical Sciences
College of Pharmacy
Little Rock, Arkansas

**W. Anthony Hawkins, PharmD,
BCCCP**
Clinical Assistant Professor
University of Georgia College
of Pharmacy
Assistant Professor
Medical College of Georgia at Augusta
University
Albany, Georgia

Keith A. Hecht, PharmD, BCOP
Associate Professor, Pharmacy Practice
Southern Illinois University
Edwardsville School of Pharmacy
Edwardsville, Illinois

Hansen Ho, PharmD, BCOP
Health Sciences Assistant
Clinical Professor
University of California, San Francisco,
School of Pharmacy
Clinical Pharmacist, UCSF Medical
Center
San Francisco, California

Natalia M. Jasiak, PharmD, BCPS
Solid Organ Transplant Pharamcist
Ann and Robert H. Lurie Children's
Hospital of Chicago
Chicago, Illinois

Caitlin Jenkins, PharmD
PGY-2 Critical Care Pharmacy
Resident
Florida Hospital Orlando
Orlando, Florida

Kendrea Jones, PharmD, BCPS
Associate Professor
University of Arkansas for Medical
Sciences College of Pharmacy
Little Rock, Arkansas

**Julie Ann Justo, PharmD, MS, BCPS
(AQ ID)**
Clinical Assistant Professor
University of South Carolina College
of Pharmacy
Infectious Diseases Clinical Pharmacy
Specialist
Palmetto Health Richland Hospital
Columbia, South Carolina

Michael W. Kelly, PharmD, MS
Associate Dean for Professional
Education and Professor (Clinical)
University of Iowa College
of Pharmacy
Iowa City, Iowa

Jessica L. Kerr, PharmD, CDE
Assistant Chair and Professor
Department of Pharmacy Practice
Southern Illinois University
Edwardsville School of Pharmacy
Edwardsville, Illinois

Minou Khazan, PharmD, PhD
Clinical Assistant Professor
University of South Carolina College
of Pharmacy
Columbia, South Carolina

Carrie Koenigsfeld, PharmD, FAPhA
Professor of Clinical Sciences
Drake University College of Pharmacy
and Health Sciences
Des Moines, Iowa

Catherine H. Kuhn, PharmD
Clinical Pharmacist
Nationwide Children's Hospital
Columbus, Ohio

Justin Kullgren, PharmD, CPE
Palliative Medicine Clinical Pharmacy
Specialist
The Ohio State University Wexner
Medical Center, James Cancer Center
Dublin, Ohio

Kyle J. LaPorte, PharmD
Assistant Professor
Department of Pharmacy Practice
South Dakota State University College
of Pharmacy
Clinical Pharmacy Specialist
Avera Cancer Institute
Sioux Falls, South Dakota

**Jennifer Le, PharmD, MAS, BCPS-ID,
FIDSA, FCCP, FCSHP**
Professor of Clinical Pharmacy
University of California San Diego
Skaggs School of Pharmacy and
Pharmaceutical Sciences
La Jolla, California

**Kelly C. Lee, PharmD, MAS,
FCCP, BCPP**
Professor of Clinical Pharmacy
University of California San Diego
Skaggs School of Pharmacy and
Pharmaceutical Sciences
La Jolla, California

Daniel S. Longyhore, PharmD, BCPS
Associate Professor
Department of Pharmacy Practice
Nesbitt College of Pharmacy
Wilkes University
Wilkes-Barre, Pennsylvania

Bryan L. Love, PharmD, BCPS (AQ ID)
Associate Professor
University of South Carolina College of
Pharmacy
Columbia, South Carolina

Caitlin Mardis, PharmD, BCPS
Director of Continuing Education
and Professional Development
Clinical Assistant Professor
Clinical Pharmacy and Outcomes Sciences
University of South Carolina
College of Pharmacy
Columbia, South Carolina

Keith R. McCain, PharmD, DABAT
Clinical Toxicologist
Arkansas Poison and Drug Information
Center
Associate Professor
Department of Pharmacy Practice
University of Arkansas for Medical
Sciences
College of Pharmacy
Little Rock, Arkansas

Sean McConachie, PharmD
PGY2 Pharmacotherapy Resident
Harper University Hospital
Detroit, Michigan

Karen H. McGee, PharmD, CDE, CGP
Clinical Faculty
South Carolina College of Pharmacy
University of South Carolina
Columbia, South Carolina

Cydney E. McQueen, PharmD
Clinical Associate Professor
University of Missouri-Kansas City
School of Pharmacy
Kansas City, Missouri

Sarah J. Miller, PharmD, BCNSP
Professor, Pharmacy Practice
University of Montana Skaggs School
of Pharmacy
Clinical Pharmacy Coordinator
Saint Patrick Hospital
Missoula, Montana

**Anne Misher, PharmD, CDE,
BC-ADM**
Clinical Assistant Professor
University of Georgia
Savannah, Georgia

Lisa Narveson, PharmD
Assistant Professor
Department of Pharmacy Practice
College of Health Professions
North Dakota State University
Fargo, North Dakota

**LeAnn B. Norris, PharmD, FCCP,
BCPS, BCOP**
Clinical Associate Professor
Department of Clinical Pharmacy and
Outcomes Sciences
University of South Carolina College
of Pharmacy
Columbia, South Carolina

Kelly K. Nystrom, PharmD, BCOP
Associate Professor of Pharmacy
Practice
Creighton University School of
Pharmacy and Health Professions
Omaha, Nebraska

Rory O'Callaghan, PharmD
Assistant Professor
Department of Clinical Pharmacy and
Pharmaceutical Economics and Policy
University of Southern California
School of Pharmacy
Los Angeles, California

**Kathleen Packard, PharmD, MS,
BCPS, AACC**
Professor
Creighton University
Omaha, Nebraska

Jeong M. Park, MS, PharmD, BCPS
Clinical Associate Professor
Department of Clinical Pharmacy,
College of Pharmacy, University
of Michigan
Clinical Transplant Specialist
Department of Pharmacy Services,
Michigan Medicine, University of
Michigan College of Pharmacy
Ann Arbor, Michigan

**Susie H. Park, PharmD,
BCPP, FCSHP**
Associate Professor of
Clinical Pharmacy
University of Southern California
School of Pharmacy
Los Angeles, California

Krina H. Patel, PharmD, BCPP
Clinical Assistant Professor
Rutgers, The State University of
New Jersey
New Brunswick, New Jersey

Patricia A. Pepa, PharmD, MS
PGY2 Psychiatric Pharmacy Resident
University of California San Diego Health
San Diego, California

**Beth B. Phillips, PharmD, FASHP,
FCCP, BCPS, BCACP**
Rite Aid Professor
University of Georgia College
of Pharmacy
Athens, Georgia

Cynthia Phillips, PharmD
Clinical Assistant Professor
University of South Carolina College
of Pharmacy
Columbia, South Carolina

Nathan A. Pinner, PharmD, BCPS
Associate Clinical Professor
Auburn University Harrison School
of Pharmacy
Birmingham, Alabama

Andrea J. Potter, PharmD
Drug Information Fellow
University of Missouri-Kansas City
School of Pharmacy
Kansas City, Missouri

**April M. Quidley, PharmD, BCCCP,
BCPS, FCCM, FCCP**
PGY2 Critical Care Residency Program
Director/Critical Care Pharmacist
Vidant Medical Center
Greenville, North Carolina

Hana Rac, PharmD
Clinical Instructor and Antimicrobial
Stewardship Collaborative of South
Carolina Lead Pharmacist
University of South Carolina College
of Pharmacy
Columbia, South Carolina

**Brent N. Reed, PharmD, BCPS
(AQ Cardiology), FAHA**
Associate Professor, Pharmacy Practice
and Science
University of Maryland School
of Pharmacy
Baltimore, Maryland

Alison M. Reta, PharmD, CDE
Clinical Pharmacist
Adjunct Assistant Professor of
Pharmacy Practice
University of Southern California
School of Pharmacy
Los Angeles, California

**Jo E. Rodgers, PharmD, BCPS (AQ
Cardiology), FCCP, FHFSA, FAHA**
Clinical Associate Professor
Eshelman School of Pharmacy
University of North Carolina
Chapel Hill, North Carolina

Renee Rose, PharmD, BCPS
Development and Training Coordinator
Florida Hospital Orlando
Orlando, Florida

**Jennifer Rosselli, PharmD,
BCPS, BCACP**
Clinical Associate Professor
Southern Illinois University
Edwardsville School of Pharmacy
Edwardsville, Illinois

Brea Rowan, PharmD, BCPS
Clinical Pharmacy Specialist
Princeton Baptist Medical Center
Affiliate Clinical Professor
Auburn University
Birmingham, Alabama

Nicholas C. Schwier, PharmD, BCPS
Assistant Professor
The University of Oklahoma Health
Sciences Center College of Pharmacy
Oklahoma City, Oklahoma

**Julie Sease, PharmD, FCCP, BCPS,
CDE, BCACP**
Associate Dean for Academic Affairs
and Professor of Pharmacy Practice
Presbyterian College School
of Pharmacy
Clinton, South Carolina

Samantha Y. Shi, PharmD
Oncology Clinical Pharmacist
USC/Norris Comprehensive Cancer
Center and Hospital
Los Angeles, California

**Marintha R. Short, PharmD, BCPS
(AQ Cardiology)**
Clinical Pharmacy Specialist—
Cardiology/Critical care
KentuckyOne Health—Saint Joseph
Hospital
Lexington, Kentucky

**Douglas Slain, PharmD, BCPS,
FCCP, FASHP**
Professor and Infectious Diseases
Clinical Specialist
West Virginia University
Morgantown, West Virginia

Jessica Starr, PharmD, BCPS
Associate Clinical Professor of
Pharmacy Practice, Auburn University
Birmingham, Alabama

S. Scott Sutton, PharmD
Professor and Chair
Department of Clinical Pharmacy and
Outcomes Sciences
University of South Carolina College
of Pharmacy
Columbia, South Carolina

Robert K. Sylvester, PharmD
Professor Emeritus
Department of Pharmacy Practice
North Dakota State University
College of Health Sciences
Fargo, North Dakota

Robyn Teply, PharmD, BCACP, MBA
Associate Professor
Creighton University
Omaha, Nebraska

Jennifer E. Thomas, PharmD, AAHIVP
Assistant Professor
Department of Pharmacy Practice
Husson University School of Pharmacy
Bangor, Maine

Scott M. Vouri, PharmD, MSCI, BCPS, BCGP, FASCP
Associate Professor
Department of Pharmacy Practice
Assistant Director
Center for Health Outcomes Research and Education
St. Louis College of Pharmacy
St. Louis, Missouri

Ted Walton, PharmD, BCPS
PGY-2 Adult Internal Medicine
Residency Director
Nephrology Clinical Pharmacy Specialist
Grady Health System
Atlanta, Georgia

Kenric Ware, PharmD, MBA, AAHIVP
Assistant Professor of Pharmacy Practice
South University School of Pharmacy
Columbia, South Carolina

Kurt A. Wargo, PharmD, FCCP, BCPS
Regional Dean and Associate Professor
Wingate University
Hendersonville, North Carolina

Kirby Welston, PharmD, BCPS
Clinical Pharmacy Specialist—Primary Care
Charlie Norwood VA Medical Center
Augusta, Georgia

Karen Whalen, PharmD, BCPS, CDE, FAPhA
Clinical Professor
University of Florida College of Pharmacy
Department of Pharmacotherapy and Translational Research
Gainesville, Florida

Sheila M. Wilhelm, PharmD, FCCP, BCPS
Clinical Associate Professor
Wayne State University Eugene Applebaum College of Pharmacy and Health Sciences
Clinical Pharmacy Specialist
Harper University Hospital
Detroit, Michigan

Associate Editor

Christopher M. Bland, PharmD, FCCP, FIDSA, BCPS
Clinical Associate Professor
Clinical and Administrative Pharmacy
University of Georgia College of
Pharmacy
Clinical Pharmacy Specialist
St. Joseph's/Candler Health System
Savannah, Georgia

Assistant Editors

Keith A. Hecht, PharmD, BCOP
Associate Professor, Pharmacy Practice
Southern Illinois University
Edwardsville School of Pharmacy
Edwardsville, Illinois

Shareen El-Ibiary, PharmD, FCCP, BCPS
Professor
Midwestern University College of
Pharmacy
Glendale, Arizona

Peer Reviewers

Michaela M. Almgren, PharmD, MS
Clinical Assistant Professor
Department of Clinical Pharmacy and
Outcomes Sciences
University of South Carolina College
of Pharmacy
Columbia, South Carolina

Miranda R. Andrus, PharmD, FCCP, BCPS
Associate Clinical Professor of Pharmacy
Practice
Auburn University Harrison School
of Pharmacy
University of Alabama at Birmingham
Huntsville Regional Medical Campus, Family
Medicine Center
Huntsville, Alabama

Kylie Barnes, PharmD, BCPS
Clinical Assistant Professor
University of Missouri-Kansas City School
of Pharmacy
Kansas City, Missouri

Elizabeth W. Blake, PharmD, BCPS
Clinical Association Professor and Director
of Interprofessional Education
University of South Carolina College of
Pharmacy
Columbia, South Carolina

**Christopher M. Bland, PharmD, FCCP,
FIDSA, BCPS**
Clinical Associate Professor
Clinical and Administrative Pharmacy
University of Georgia College of Pharmacy
Clinical Pharmacy Specialist
St. Joseph's/Candler Health System
Savannah, Georgia

**P. Brandon Bookstaver, PharmD, FCCP,
FIDSA, BCPS, AAHIVP**
Associate Professor and Director of Residency
and Fellowship Training
Department of Clinical Pharmacy and
Outcomes Sciences
University of South Carolina College
of Pharmacy
Infectious Diseases PGY2 and Clinical
Fellowship Director
USC/Palmetto Health
Columbia, South Carolina

Michelle M. Bottenberg, PharmD, BCPS
Associate Professor of Pharmacy Practice
Director of the Pharmacy Skills and
Applications Course Series
Drake University College of Pharmacy
and Health Sciences
Des Moines, Iowa

Wendy Brown, PharmD, PA-C, AE-C
Primary Care Telemedicine Provider
Fargo VA Health Care System
Fargo, North Dakota

**Melinda (Mindy) J. Burnworth, PharmD,
FASHP, FAzPA, BCPS**
Professor
Department of Pharmacy Practice
Adult Internal Medicine Clinical Pharmacy
Specialist
Midwestern University College of Pharmacy
Glendale, Arizona

Joshua Caballero, PharmD, BCPP, FCCP
Professor and Chair
Department of Clinical and Administrative
Sciences
Larkin University College of Pharmacy
Miami, Florida

Matthew A. Cantrell, PharmD, BCPS
Associate Professor (Clinical)
University of Iowa College of Pharmacy
Iowa City VA Health Care System
Iowa City, Iowa

Cara Coffelt, PharmD
PGY2 Critical Care Pharmacy Resident
St. Joseph's/Candler Health System
University of Georgia College of Pharmacy
Savannah, Georgia

Kristen Cook, PharmD, BCPS
Clinical Assistant Professor
University of Nebraska Medical Center
College of Pharmacy
Omaha, Nebraska

Quang Dam, PharmD
Pharmacist
Long Beach Memorial Hospital and Miller
Children's and Women's Hospital of Long Beach
Long Beach, California

Darla Klug Eastman, PharmD, BCPS
Associate Professor of Clinical Sciences
Drake University College of Pharmacy and
Health Sciences
Des Moines, Iowa

**Rebecca F. Edwards, PharmD, BCPS,
BCACP, CDE**
Clinical Pharmacy Specialist
Salisbury VA Health Care System (SVAHCS)
Program Manager, Kernersville VA Health
Care Center
Kernersville, North Carolina

Shareen El-Ibiary, PharmD, FCCP, BCPS
Professor
Midwestern University College of Pharmacy
Glendale, Arizona

Rickey A. Evans, PharmD, BCPS
Assistant Professor
Department of Clinical Pharmacy and
Outcomes Sciences
Clinical Pharmacist-Critical Care, Palmetto
Health Richland
University of South Carolina College
of Pharmacy
Columbia, South Carolina

Patricia H. Fabel, PharmD, BCPS
Clinical Associate Professor
University of South Carolina College
of Pharmacy
Columbia, South Carolina

Michele Faulkner, PharmD, FASHP
Professor of Pharmacy Practice and
Neurology
Creighton University Schools of Pharmacy
and Medicine
Omaha, Nebraska

McKenzie C. Ferguson, PharmD, BCPS
Associate Professor Pharmacy Practice
Director
Drug Information and Wellness Center
Southern Illinois University Edwardsville
School of Pharmacy
Edwardsville, Illinois

Anisa Fornoff, PharmD
Associate Professor of Clinical Sciences
Drake University College of Pharmacy and
Health Sciences
Des Moines, Iowa

Keith A. Hecht, PharmD, BCOP
Associate Professor, Pharmacy Practice
Southern Illinois University Edwardsville
School of Pharmacy
Edwardsville, Illinois

Caitlin Jenkins, PharmD
PGY-2 Critical Care Pharmacy Resident
Florida Hospital
Orlando, Florida

Michael W. Kelly, PharmD, MS
Associate Dean for Professional Education
and Professor (Clinical)
University of Iowa College of Pharmacy
Iowa City, Iowa

Jessica L. Kerr, PharmD, CDE
Assistant Chair and Professor
Department of Pharmacy Practice
Southern Illinois University Edwardsville
School of Pharmacy
Edwardsville, Illinois

Carrie Koenigsfeld, PharmD, FAPhA
Professor of Clinical Sciences
Drake University College of Pharmacy and
Health Sciences
Des Moines, Iowa

Catherine H. Kuhn, PharmD
Clinical Pharmacist
Nationwide Children's Hospital
Columbus, Ohio

**Jennifer Le, PharmD, MAS, BCPS-ID,
FIDSA, FCCP, FCSHP**
Professor of Clinical Pharmacy
University of California San Diego
Skaggs School of Pharmacy and
Pharmaceutical Sciences
La Jolla, California

Anne Marie Liles, PharmD, BCPS
Director
Clinical Services—Student Health Center
Pharmacy
Clinical Associate Professor of
Pharmacy Practice
The University of Mississippi School
of Pharmacy
Oxford, Mississippi

Bryan L. Love, PharmD, BCPS (AQ ID)
Associate Professor
University of South Carolina College of Pharmacy
Columbia, South Carolina

Anne Misher, PharmD, CDE, BC-ADM
Clinical Assistant Professor
University of Georgia
Savannah, Georgia

Kathleen Packard, PharmD, MS, BCPS, AACC
Professor
Creighton University
Omaha, Nebraska

Alyssa M. Peckham, PharmD, BCPP
Clinical Assistant Professor
Midwestern University College of Pharmacy
Glendale, Arizona

Nathan A. Pinner, PharmD, BCPS
Associate Clinical Professor
Auburn University Harrison School of Pharmacy
Birmingham, Alabama

Talia Puzantian, PharmD, BCPP
Associate Professor
Keck Graduate Institute School of Pharmacy
Claremont, California

Hana Rac, PharmD
Clinical Instructor and Antimicrobial
Stewardship Collaborative of South Carolina
Lead Pharmacist
University of South Carolina College of
Pharmacy
Columbia, South Carolina

Jennifer Rosselli, PharmD, BCPS, BCACP
Clinical Associate Professor
Southern Illinois University Edwardsville
School of Pharmacy
Edwardsville, Illinois

Kelly Scolaro, BSPharm, PharmD
Associate Professor
Lake Erie College of Osteopathic Medicine
(LECOM) School of Pharmacy
Bradenton, Florida

Gregory Seagraves, PharmD
Academic Professional
University of Georgia College of Pharmacy
Athens, Georgia

S. Scott Sutton, PharmD
Professor and Chair
Department of Clinical Pharmacy and
Outcomes Sciences
University of South Carolina College of Pharmacy
Columbia, South Carolina

Robyn Teply, PharmD, BCACP, MBA
Associate Professor
Creighton University
Omaha, Nebraska

Jennifer E. Thomas, PharmD, AAHIVP
Assistant Professor
Department of Pharmacy Practice
Husson University School of Pharmacy
Bangor, Maine

**Scott M. Vouri, PharmD, MSCI, BCPS,
BCGP, FASCP**
Associate Professor
Department of Pharmacy Practice
Assistant Director
Center for Health Outcomes Research and
Education
St. Louis College of Pharmacy
St. Louis, Missouri

Robin Wackernah, PharmD, BCPP
Clinical Associate Professor
Regis University School of Pharmacy
Denver, Colorado

Kenric B. Ware, PharmD, MBA, AAHIVP
Assistant Professor of Pharmacy Practice
South University School of Pharmacy
Columbia, South Carloina

Stephanie Weisberg, PharmD
PGY-2 Infectious Diseases Pharmacy Resident
Novant Health Presbyterian Medical Center
Charlotte, North Carolina

Andrew Williams, PharmD, BCPP, BCGP
Clinical Pharmacist, Psychiatry
Riverside University Health System
Riverside, California
Assistant Clinical Professor of Pharmacy
Practice
Loma Linda University School of Pharmacy
Loma Linda, California
Adjunct Assistant Professor of Pharmacy
Practice
University of Southern California School
of Pharmacy
Los Angeles, California
Adjunct Assistant Clinical Professor
University of the Pacific Thomas J. Long
School of Pharmacy
Stockton, California

Preface

The North American Pharmacist Licensure Examination (NAPLEX®) measures a candidate's knowledge of pharmacy practice. The examination is used by Boards of Pharmacy as part of the assessment of a candidate's competency to practice pharmacy. The National Association of Boards of Pharmacy (NABP) publishes a competency statement that provides a blueprint of the topics covered in the examination. The blueprint offers important information about the knowledge and skills that are expected for an entry-level pharmacist. The NAPLEX® competency statement may be viewed at www.napb.net. The three areas of competency include:

- Assess pharmacotherapy to ensure safe and effective therapeutic outcomes (56% of exam)
- Assess safe and accurate preparation and dispensing of medications (33% of exam)
- Assess, recommend, and provide health care information that promotes public health (11% of exam)

The *NAPLEX® Review Guide* published by McGraw-Hill has been organized around the NABP competencies and is designed to assist students in their preparation of the exam, stimulate critical thinking, consolidate key information, advance knowledge, and improve exam-taking ability.

The textbook was developed and reviewed by pharmacists, faculty, students, recent graduates, and education consultants with a priority focus on the NABP competency statements.

I have taught a NAPLEX® review course for Morris Cody and Associates since 2005 and have instructed thousands of students representing over 70 schools of pharmacy. I have been in a unique position to be able to talk with students and new graduates from across the country and discuss with them what they need to be successful when taking the exam and as a practicing pharmacist. The input given by the students and the faculty, pharmacists, and educational consultants was instrumental in the organization, development, and content of this textbook. As there are many ways to assess knowledge,

there are equally as many ways to prepare for an exam. People are different and thrive in different preparatory methods. The development of this textbook was tailored to various learning and studying styles.

Each chapter within the textbook contains the following sections: Foundation Overview, Prevention or Treatment, Case Application questions, and Takeaway Points. The Foundation Overview consists of a general overview of the topic, pathophysiology, clinical presentation, and diagnosis. The Prevention or Treatment section provides a general overview and goals of prevention or treatment, followed by a focus on specific agents including indication, route of administration, rationale for use, and adverse reactions. Several chapters have incorporated and developed tables and figures for enhancement of the material in the chapter. The Case Application section is extremely unique and will provide students and graduates ample opportunity to apply their knowledge in each of the 76 chapters. Each chapter contains at least 20 Case Application questions (more than 1540 questions within the textbook). The Case Application questions are based on the material within the chapter with a focus on the NABP competency statements. Numerous students discussed with me their need and desire to have a lot of questions, especially questions that can serve as teaching points. Therefore, each Case Application question is provided with a detailed answer section at the end of the book. For each question, there is an explanation of why one answer is correct and why the other choices are incorrect. This is a valuable tool that you can tailor to your specific learning or studying style. At the end of each chapter, the Case Application questions are followed by the Takeaway Points section. This section summarizes the key concepts within the text to bring together all the information you have studied and reviewed.

S. Scott Sutton
December 2018

Acknowledgments

I would like to acknowledge the commitment and dedication of the contributing authors and peer reviewers of the chapters contained within this text. I am very grateful to the staff of McGraw-Hill, especially Michael Weitz, Christina Thomas, and Laura Libretti, for the opportunity to develop this textbook and for their dedication to this project. Finally, I would like to thank the students, graduates, faculty, pharmacists, and educational consultants who provided feedback for the development and design of this textbook.

Cardiovascular Disorders

1

Chronic Heart Failure

Brent N. Reed and Jo E. Rodgers

FOUNDATION OVERVIEW

Heart failure (HF) is a syndrome of reduced cardiac output (CO) resulting from impaired ventricular ejection, impaired filling, or components of both. HF with reduced ejection fraction (HFrEF) was formerly known as systolic dysfunction whereas HF with impaired filling or HF with preserved ejection fraction (HFpEF) was formerly known as diastolic dysfunction. Although half of HF cases are due to HFpEF, the majority of studies enrolled patients with HFrEF. Chronic HFrEF management includes lifestyle modifications, medications, and implantable devices. However, there are few therapeutic approaches for HFpEF management.

Etiology and Pathophysiology

The etiology of HF is often classified as being ischemic or nonischemic. Ischemic causes are more common, and may result from a sudden event such as a myocardial infarction (MI) or from longstanding coronary artery disease. Nonischemic etiologies include uncontrolled hypertension (HTN), viral diseases, sarcoidosis, peripartum cardiomyopathy, uncorrected valvular heart disease, alcohol, or thyroid disease.

The pathophysiology of HFrEF is characterized by compensatory mechanisms intended to maintain systemic perfusion in response to a decline in CO (Figure 1-1). The sympathetic nervous system (SNS) and renin-angiotensin-aldosterone system (RAAS) are primarily responsible for this compensatory response (although vasopressin and nitric oxide are also involved). Norepinephrine is released from the SNS in an effort to maintain CO by increasing contractility and heart rate (HR). Renal hypoperfusion results in RAAS activation with a resultant rise in serum angiotensin II and aldosterone concentrations. As potent vasoconstrictors, norepinephrine and angiotensin II compromise CO by increasing afterload while aldosterone increases preload via enhanced sodium and fluid retention. Increased preload and afterload initially improve organ perfusion but ultimately result in a decline in CO as a consequence of ventricular remodeling and hypertrophy. This cycle is propagated as further declines in CO produce additional release of compensatory neurohormones.

The pathophysiology of HFpEF has not been well elucidated, although impaired diastolic function is thought to play a major role. Therapies aimed at disrupting the neurohormonal systems responsible for HFrEF have not substantially improved outcomes in HFpEF, suggesting different pathophysiologic features are involved.

Clinical Presentation

HF patients present with signs and symptoms of volume overload, low CO, or both. Patients with volume overload present with signs and symptoms of pulmonary congestion (eg, dyspnea, orthopnea, crackles on auscultation) or peripheral congestion (eg, ascites, jugular venous distension, lower extremity edema). Weight gain can be a helpful marker of volume status for patients to self-monitor, as it often precedes signs and symptoms. Signs and symptoms of low CO are more challenging to identify and may be subjective. Vague symptoms such as fatigue or nausea and vomiting are common. Worsening renal function is a common objective measure of low CO, whereas exercise intolerance and early satiety may be present with either volume overload or low CO.

Diagnosis

HF is a clinical diagnosis and no single test establishes its presence or absence. The most frequent clinical findings in HF are related to decreased exercise tolerance or fluid retention. Decreased exercise tolerance typically presents as dyspnea or fatigue on exertion. Fluid retention results in orthopnea, crackles, elevated jugular venous pressure, dependent edema, and radiographic findings of cardiomegaly, pulmonary edema, and pleural effusion.

A comprehensive patient history should be obtained to elucidate causes of HF. Both MI and HTN are common causes, thus cardiovascular risk factors should be addressed. Detailed medication histories should be completed to assure dietary and medication adherence and avoidance of substance abuse. Presence of medications known to exacerbate fluid retention (eg, nonsteroidal anti-inflammatory drugs [NSAIDs]), alter left ventricular function (eg, certain antineoplastic agents), and those with negative inotropic effects (nondihydropyridine calcium channel blockers) should also be assessed (Table 1-1). Measurement of B-type natriuretic peptide (BNP) may be helpful in differentiating HF from other disease states associated with similar symptoms. An echocardiogram to evaluate ventricular function should be performed to determine

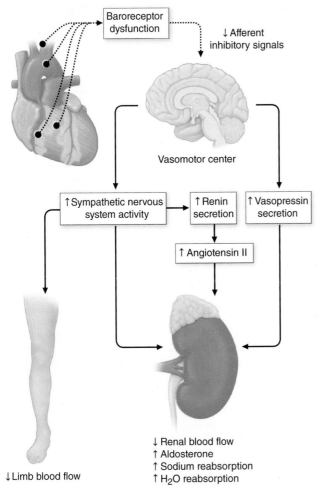

FIGURE 1-1 Activation of neurohormonal system in heart failure. Reproduced with permission from Longo DL, Fauci AS, Kasper DL, et al: *Harrison's Principles of Internal Medicine,* 18th ed. New York, NY: McGraw-Hill; 2012.

TABLE 1-1	Drugs That May Precipitate or Exacerbate Heart Failure
Negative Inotropic Effect	
Antiarrhythmics (eg, disopyramide, flecainide, propafenone)	
β-Blockers (eg, propranolol, metoprolol, atenolol)	
Nondihydropyridine calcium channel blockers (eg, verapamil, diltiazem)	
Itraconazole	
Dronedarone	
Cardiotoxic	
Cocaine	
Doxorubicin	
Daunorubicin	
Epirubicin	
Cyclophosphamide	
Propofol (high doses)	
Trastuzumab	
Imatinib	
Ethanol	
Amphetamines (eg, cocaine, methamphetamine)	
Sodium and Water Retention	
Nonsteroidal anti-inflammatory drugs	
Thiazolidinediones (eg, rosiglitazone)	
Glucocorticoids	
Androgens and estrogens	
Salicylates (high dose)	
Sodium-containing drugs (eg, piperacillin sodium)	
Uncertain mechanism	
Infliximab	
Etanercept	
Dipeptidyl peptidase-4 inhibitors (eg, sitagliptin)	
Bezlotoxumab	

Adapted with permission from DiPiro JT, Talbert RL, Yee GC, et al: *Pharmacotherapy: A Pathophysiologic Approach,* 9th ed. New York, NY: McGraw-Hill; 2014.

etiology and severity of HF. An ejection fraction (EF) of less than or equal to 40% is considered the threshold for HFrEF classification.

Classification/Staging

HF severity is classified according to disease state progression (American College of Cardiology/American Heart Association [ACC/AHA]) or functional class (New York Heart Association [NYHA]). The ACC/AHA system stages patients based upon risk for developing HF (stage A), having asymptomatic structural heart disease (stage B), HF signs and symptoms (stage C), or end-stage disease despite maximal medical therapy (stage D). The NYHA functional classification system is a subjective measure of exercise tolerance and ability to perform activities of daily living. Patients are classified as having no symptoms limiting activity (class I), symptoms with mild or moderate physical activity (class II and III, respectively), or symptoms at rest (class IV). A patient may shift between NYHA functional classes as HF status improves or declines, but cannot regress from an advanced ACC/AHA stage.

PREVENTION

General Considerations

Patients without structural heart disease (ACC/AHA stage A) should have comorbidities managed according to established practice guidelines (eg, HTN, dyslipidemia). Patients with asymptomatic left ventricular dysfunction (stage B) are at a high risk for developing HF and should receive an angiotensin-converting enzyme (ACE) inhibitor or angiotensin receptor blocker (ARB) and a β-blocker to reduce mortality and risk of HF progression. Because most of the studies evaluating these therapies have enrolled patients with symptomatic HF, they are discussed in detail in the sections to follow.

TABLE 1-2	Dosing and Monitoring for Neurohormonal Blocking Agents		
Drug	**Initial Dose**	**Target or Maximum Dose**	**Monitoring**
ACE Inhibitors			
Captopril	6.25 mg three times daily	50 mg three times daily	BP
Enalapril	2.5 mg twice daily	10-20 mg twice daily	Electrolytes (K+), BUN, SCr at baseline, 2 wk, and after dose
Fosinopril	5-10 mg once daily	40 mg once daily	titration, CBC periodically
Lisinopril	2.5-5 mg once daily	20-40 mg once daily	Adverse effects: rash (captopril), hyperkalemia, hypotension,
Perindopril	2 mg once daily	8-16 mg once daily	acute kidney injury, cough, angioedema
Quinapril	5 mg twice daily	20 mg twice daily	
Ramipril	1.25-2.5 mg once daily	10 mg once daily	
Trandolapril	1 mg once daily	4 mg once daily	
Angiotensin Receptor Blockers			
Candesartan	4-8 mg once daily	32 mg once daily	BP
Losartan	25-50 mg once daily	100-150 mg once daily	Electrolytes (K+), BUN, SCr at baseline, 2 wk, and after dose titration, CBC periodically
Valsartan	20-40 mg twice daily	160 mg twice daily	Adverse effects: hyperkalemia, hypotension, acute kidney injury
Aldosterone Antagonists			
Spironolactone	12.5-25 mg once daily	25 mg once daily	BP
Eplerenone	25 mg once daily	50 mg once daily	Electrolytes (K+) at baseline and within 1 wk of initiation and dose titration
			Adverse effects: gynecomastia or breast tenderness (primarily spironolactone), menstrual changes, hirsutism, hyperkalemia
β-Blockers			
Bisoprolol	1.25 mg once daily	10 mg once daily	BP, HR baseline and after each dose titration, ECG
Carvedilol	3.125 mg twice daily	25 mg bid (50 mg twice daily for patients >85 kg)	
Metoprolol succinate	12.5-25 mg once daily	200 mg once daily	Adverse effects: worsening HF symptoms (edema, SOB, fatigue), depression, sexual dysfunction, bradycardia, hypotension
Miscellaneous Agents			
Sacubitril/valsartan	24 mg/26 mg-49 mg/ 51 mg twice daily	97 mg/103 mg twice daily	BP
			Electrolytes (K+), BUN, SCr at baseline, 2 wk, and after dose titration
			Adverse effects: hyperkalemia, hypotension, acute kidney injury, angioedema
Isosorbide dinitrate/ hydralazine	20 mg/37.5 mg three times daily	40 mg/75 mg three times daily	BP, HR
			Adverse effects: headache, flushing, hypotension, dizziness
Ivabradine	2.5-5 mg twice daily	7.5 mg twice daily	BP, HR baseline and after each dose titration, ECG
			Adverse effects: bradycardia, hypotension, atrial fibrillation, visual disturbances
Digoxin	125-250 mcg once daily	Target serum concentration of 0.5-0.9 ng/mL	HR, ECG, SDC
			Adverse effects (usually concentration-related): neurologic changes, visual disturbances, nausea/vomiting, arrhythmias

Abbreviations: BP, blood pressure; BUN, blood urea nitrogen; CBC, complete blood cell count; ECG, electrocardiogram; HF, heart failure; HR, heart rate; K+, potassium; SCr, serum creatinine; SDC, serum digoxin concentrations; SOB, shortness of breath.

Adapted with permission from Chisholm-Burns MA, Wells BG, Schwinghammer TL, et al: *Pharmacotherapy Principles & Practice.* New York, NY: McGraw-Hill; 2008.

TREATMENT

General Considerations

The goals of HF management are to maximize quality of life (QOL), minimize symptoms, prevent hospitalizations, slow disease progression, and prolong survival. It is important to identify and treat reversible, underlying causes of HF. Patients should be educated on fluid and sodium restrictions and encouraged to weigh themselves daily to detect changes in volume status. Drug therapy is the cornerstone of treatment and

focuses on inhibiting the neurohormonal cascade described above (Table 1-2 and Figure 1-2 for mechanism, dosing, and monitoring of neurohormonal blocking agents).

Pharmacologic Therapy

Loop Diuretics

Sodium and fluid retention is common in HF and loop diuretics are frequently used to assist in fluid elimination. Loop diuretics (furosemide, bumetanide, torsemide, and ethacrynic

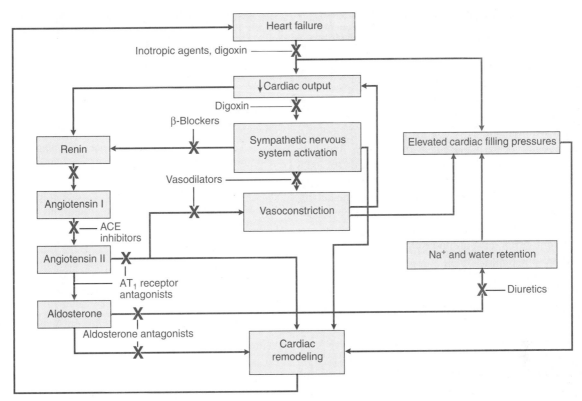

FIGURE 1-2 Pharmacotherapy of heart failure. Reproduced with permission from Brunton LL, Chabner BA, Knollmann BC: *Goodman & Gilman's The Pharmacological Basis of Therapeutics,* 12th ed. New York, NY: McGraw-Hill; 2011.

acid) block sodium reabsorption in the ascending loop of Henle. Loop diuretics provide symptomatic relief of volume overload, improve exercise tolerance, and prevent hospitalization; however, they do not confer a mortality benefit. Patients can develop resistance to loop diuretics requiring escalation of dose or addition of thiazide diuretics. Common adverse effects include hypokalemia, hypomagnesemia, hypotension, and renal dysfunction. Weight should be monitored daily to prevent over-diuresis.

Angiotensin-Converting Enzyme Inhibitors

ACE inhibitors prevent the conversion of angiotensin I to angiotensin II and have demonstrated reductions in mortality, HF progression, hospitalizations, and improvement in symptoms. Unless contraindicated, ACE inhibitors are recommended for all patients with a reduced EF, regardless of symptoms. ACE inhibitors should be titrated as tolerated to target doses achieved in clinical trials (see Table 1-2), although this is not required prior to the addition of β-blocker therapy. Patients should be monitored for hypotension, hyperkalemia, renal dysfunction, cough, and angioedema. Absolute contraindications include a history of angioedema, bilateral renal artery stenosis, and pregnancy.

Angiotensin Receptor Blockers

ARBs competitively inhibit angiotensin II receptors. ACE inhibitors remain first-line because comparable improvements with ARBs have not been observed across all HF outcomes.

ARBs may be considered in patients who are intolerant of ACE inhibitors, such as those who experience cough and angioedema, as these adverse effects are thought to be due to bradykinin accumulation. Patients who develop renal dysfunction, hyperkalemia, or hypotension with an ACE inhibitor are likely to experience these adverse effects with an ARB.

β-Adrenergic Blockers

Historically, β-blockers were not used to manage HF because of their negative inotropic effects. However, long-term inhibition of the SNS with β-blocker therapy is associated with improvements in mortality, even in advanced disease. These benefits do not appear to be class-related, as only bisoprolol, carvedilol, and metoprolol succinate (controlled or extended-release) have demonstrated mortality improvements in HF. β-Blockers should be started at low doses once patients are euvolemic and titrated as tolerated to the doses achieved in clinical trials (see Table 1-2). When adjusted under optimal conditions, symptoms may transiently worsen until a new equilibrium is established. Patients with volume overload should not have doses increased until excess fluid is removed. Patients should be monitored for hypotension, bradycardia, fluid retention, and fatigue. Comorbidities such as diabetes mellitus, chronic obstructive pulmonary disease, asthma, and peripheral vascular disease should not be considered absolute contraindications to β-blocker therapy. A β_1-selective agent (eg, metoprolol succinate, bisoprolol) is preferred in patients with asthma.

Neprilysin Inhibitor/Angiotensin Receptor Blocker

Neprilysin degrades natriuretic peptides and other circulating mediators responsible for counteracting the compensatory neurohormonal response in patients with HF. A combination of the neprilysin inhibitor sacubitril and the ARB valsartan demonstrated reductions in mortality, hospitalizations, and HF symptoms compared to an ACE inhibitor. Thus, in patients who remain symptomatic despite receiving an ACE inhibitor or ARB and a β-blocker, replacement of the ACE inhibitor or ARB with sacubitril/valsartan is recommended. Patients previously receiving an ACE inhibitor should have therapy withdrawn for at least 36 hours prior to initiating sacubitril/valsartan due to an increased risk of angioedema with overlapping therapy. Monitoring parameters are similar to those for ACE inhibitors. Absolute contraindications include a history of angioedema and pregnancy.

Aldosterone Antagonists

Although ACE inhibitors and ARBs reduce the amount of aldosterone release in the short term, further suppression of aldosterone can be achieved with the addition of an aldosterone receptor antagonist (ARA), such as spironolactone or eplerenone. Reductions in mortality and hospitalizations have been observed with the addition of an ARA to ACE inhibitor and β-blocker therapy in patients with symptomatic HF (NYHA Classes II-IV). Strict serum potassium and creatinine monitoring is necessary and therapy should be avoided if serum potassium is more than 5 mEq/L or creatinine clearance is less than 30 mL/min. Eplerenone is more selective for aldosterone receptors, resulting in less gynecomastia than spironolactone.

Isosorbide Dinitrate and Hydralazine

Several proposed mechanisms support the combined use of isosorbide dinitrate (ISDN) and hydralazine for HF. While ISDN is a venous vasodilator and hydralazine is an arterial vasodilator, ISDN also increases nitric oxide, which may be deficient in HF. Hydralazine also possesses antioxidant properties which eliminate the need for a nitrate-free interval with ISDN. Combination therapy is associated with a reduction in mortality among African Americans who remain symptomatic despite background therapy with an ACE inhibitor and β-blocker. The combination may also be used in patients of any race who cannot tolerate an ACE inhibitor or ARB. Dizziness and headache are the most common adverse effects with ISDN and hydralazine therapy, although temporary dose-reductions often improve tolerability.

Ivabradine

Elevated HR has been associated with poor outcomes in HF, and some patients may be unable to tolerate target doses of β-blocker therapy. Ivabradine is an inhibitor of I_f current in the sinoatrial node, leading to reductions in HR without an effect on contractility. A reduction in hospitalizations for HF was observed with ivabradine in patients with resting HR more than or equal to 70 beats/min in normal sinus rhythm who remained symptomatic despite maximally tolerated β-blocker therapy. Therapy should be adjusted to a maximum of 7.5 mg twice daily to maintain HR between 50 and 60 beats/min. Ivabradine increases the risk of atrial fibrillation and should be avoided (or discontinued) in patients with atrial fibrillation. Bradycardia and visual disturbances are the most common adverse effects of ivabradine.

Digoxin

Digoxin may have neurohormone modulating effects that confer benefit in patients with advanced HF. Digoxin improves symptoms and reduces hospitalizations, but does not impact mortality. Its use should be reserved for advanced disease (ie, symptomatic HF despite standard therapy). Low doses (eg, 125-250 mcg/d) are recommended and serum digoxin concentrations should be maintained in the range of 0.5 to 0.9 ng/mL. Dose reductions may be required in older patients, impaired renal function, or low body weight. Common adverse effects include bradycardia, altered mental status, gastrointestinal upset, and visual disturbances.

Nonpharmacologic Therapy

Ventricular arrhythmias and sudden cardiac death are major causes of mortality in HF patients. Placement of an implantable cardioverter defibrillator (ICD) is recommended to reduce mortality in patients with an EF less than or equal to 35% despite standard HF therapy. Ventricular dyssynchrony may compromise CO and use of a biventricular pacemaker with cardiac resynchronization therapy (CRT) is associated with a reduction in hospitalizations and improved QOL. Patients with symptomatic HF and EF less than or equal to 35% and a QRS interval more than or equal to 150 ms are eligible for CRT. An ICD and/or CRT may be considered in select patients with less severe HF and other electrocardiographic findings but a discussion of these indications is beyond the scope of this review.

Heart Failure With Preserved Ejection Fraction

Drug therapies associated with clinical improvement in patients with HFrEF have mostly failed to produce similar outcomes in patients with HFpEF. Use of ARBs and aldosterone antagonists has been associated with improvements in hospitalizations whereas other therapies have had no impact on clinical endpoints or have produced conflicting results. As a result, recommendations for the treatment of HFpEF focus on symptomatic relief and management of common comorbidities, such as HTN and coronary artery disease. Diuretics should be considered for those with HFpEF and volume overload while comorbidities should be managed according to established practice guidelines for each specific condition.

CASE Application

1. MM is a 58-year-old woman with cardiomyopathy (left ventricular ejection fraction [LVEF] 25%) following an acute MI. Immediately following her MI, she developed signs and symptoms of HF including shortness of breath

(SOB) at rest. Which of the following best characterizes MM's current ACC/AHA HF stage and NYHA class?

   a. Stage A, NYHA class not applicable
   b. Stage B, NYHA class I
   c. Stage C, NYHA class II
   d. Stage C, NYHA class IV

2. Which of the following therapies decreases HR via inhibition of the I_f current in the sinoatrial node?

   a. Metoprolol succinate
   b. Carvedilol
   c. Digoxin
   d. Ivabradine

3. Which of the following laboratory values may be helpful in differentiating HF from other disease states that cause similar symptoms?

   a. Serum sodium
   b. Serum creatinine
   c. BNP
   d. Norepinephrine

4. KW is a 53-year-old man with HF (NYHA class I) receiving furosemide 40 mg twice daily, lisinopril 10 mg daily, metoprolol succinate 50 mg daily, digoxin 0.125 mg daily, and spironolactone 25 mg daily. During a routine clinic visit today, pertinent findings include: BP 120/80 mm Hg, HR 70 beats/min, RR 14, K^+ 5.1 mmol/L, BUN 35 mg/dL, and creatinine 1.2 mg/dL (baseline). Which of the following is the most appropriate change to optimize KW's medical regimen? Select all that apply.

   a. Increase ACE inhibitor dose
   b. Increase β-blocker dose
   c. Add ivabradine
   d. Increase spironolactone dose

Questions 5 through 8 pertain to the following case.

JC is a 64-year-old African American man with HFrEF presenting with a 2-week history of SOB which limits his normal daily activities and increased lower extremity edema. His weight has recently increased by 10 lb. His physical examination is notable for BP 148/72 mm Hg, HR 68 beats/min, RR 24, rales, and 3+ lower extremity edema. Pertinent laboratory values include: sodium 138 mmol/L, potassium 5.4 mmol/L, BUN 35 mg/dL, creatinine 0.9 mg/dL, and digoxin 2.1 ng/mL. Past medical history is significant for HTN, gout, and chronic obstructive pulmonary disease (COPD). Current medications include lisinopril 20 mg daily, diltiazem CD 120 mg daily, digoxin 0.250 mg daily, and salmeterol/fluticasone 250/50 two puffs bid. JC recently began taking naproxen 220 mg tid for gout pain.

5. In addition to counseling on salt and fluid restriction, which of the following pharmacologic options is most appropriate for managing JC's fluid overload?

   a. Initiate hydrochlorothiazide 50 mg daily.
   b. Initiate furosemide 40 mg twice daily.

   c. Initiate metolazone 2.5 mg daily.
   d. Initiate spironolactone 25 mg daily.

6. Within the following 24 hours, JC experiences a brisk diuresis with considerable improvement in HF signs and symptoms. What additional medication changes should be considered?

   a. Continue current regimen and initiate hydrochlorothiazide 50 mg daily.
   b. Continue current regimen and initiate spironolactone 25 mg daily.
   c. Discontinue lisinopril and initiate combination hydralazine 25 mg and ISDN 20 mg three times daily.
   d. Discontinue over-the-counter naproxen and initiate colchicine 0.6 mg bid until gout pain resolves.

7. Once optimal fluid status has been achieved, which of the following represents the best option to manage JC's HTN?

   a. Initiate amlodipine 5 mg daily.
   b. Initiate carvedilol 3.125 mg twice daily.
   c. Initiate hydrochlorothiazide 25 mg daily.
   d. Initiate prazosin 2 mg daily.

8. What additional medication change should be considered to optimize JC's medical regimen? Select all that apply.

   a. Discontinue diltiazem.
   b. Reduce digoxin to 0.125 mg daily.
   c. Initiate spironolactone 25 mg daily.
   d. Initiate candesartan 4 mg daily.
   e. Initiate ivabradine 5 mg twice daily.

Questions 9 and 10 pertain to the following case.

RJ is a 61-year-old woman with a history of ischemic cardiomyopathy who presents to clinic with symptoms consistent with NYHA class IV HF. Past medical history includes hyperlipidemia, diabetes mellitus, MI, and hypothyroidism. RJ complains of progressive weight gain (~6 lb increase since visit 3 months ago), SOB at rest, 2 pillow orthopnea, and occasional paroxysmal nocturnal dyspnea (PND). Her physical examination is positive for 1+ pitting edema in her ankles and minimal jugular vein distention (JVD). Vital signs include BP 105/70 mm Hg and HR 91 beats/min. Laboratory results include: potassium 3.6 mmol/L, BUN 39 mg/dL, and creatinine 1.4 mg/dL (baseline creatinine 1.2-1.6 mg/dL). RJ's current medications are levothyroxine 0.05 mg daily, furosemide 40 mg twice daily, lisinopril 20 mg daily, atorvastatin 40 mg daily, aspirin 81 mg daily, insulin glargine 46 units at bedtime, and insulin as part 6 units before meals.

9. Which of the following is the best treatment option to manage RJ's hypokalemia and fluid overload? Select all that apply.

   a. Continue furosemide 40 mg twice daily.
   b. Increase furosemide to 80 mg twice daily.
   c. Initiate spironolactone 25 mg once daily.
   d. Initiate hydrochlorothiazide 25 mg daily.

10. Which of the following represents the next best option to manage RJ's HF?

    a. Initiate metoprolol succinate 25 mg daily immediately.
    b. Initiate metoprolol succinate 25 mg daily once euvolemia is achieved.
    c. Initiate metoprolol tartrate 12.5 mg bid immediately.
    d. Initiate digoxin 0.25 mg daily.

11. Which of the following are absolute contraindications to the use of β-blockers? Select all that apply.

    a. Asthma with active bronchospasm
    b. Diabetes
    c. Chronic obstructive pulmonary disease
    d. Peripheral vascular disease
    e. Complete heart block

Questions 12 and 13 pertain to the following case.

SD is a 54-year-old man with NYHA class III HF due to non-ischemic cardiomyopathy. His past medical history is notable for moderate asthma since childhood and HTN. Current medications include salmeterol, one inhalation twice daily; fluticasone 88 mcg, inhaled twice daily; furosemide 80 mg twice daily; enalapril 20 mg twice daily; and spironolactone 25 mg daily.

12. Which of the following β-blockers is the best option to treat SD's HF and minimize aggravating his asthma?

    a. Carvedilol
    b. Metoprolol succinate
    c. Propranolol
    d. Atenolol

13. Which of the following medication changes may provide further mortality benefit for SD once stabilized on β-blocker therapy?

    a. Addition of digoxin 0.125 mg daily.
    b. Substitution of sacubitril/valsartan 49 mg/51 mg for enalapril 20 mg twice daily.
    c. Addition of valsartan 160 mg twice daily.
    d. Addition of amlodipine 5 mg daily.

14. Which of the following is appropriate rationale for switching an ACE inhibitor to an ARB? Select all that apply.

    a. Hypotension
    b. Renal dysfunction
    c. Hyperkalemia
    d. Cough
    e. Angioedema

15. IH is a 44-year-old African American man presenting with dizziness and orthostatic hypotension. His laboratory values reveal the following: potassium 5.8 mmol/L, BUN 60 mg/dL (baseline 18), and serum creatinine 2.0 mg/dL (baseline 0.9). IH's medications include furosemide 80 mg twice daily, ramipril 5 mg twice daily, and metoprolol XL 50 mg daily. Which of the following immediate medication adjustments are appropriate? Select all that apply.

    a. Temporarily hold furosemide.
    b. Temporarily hold metoprolol XL.
    c. Temporarily hold ramipril.
    d. Continue current regimen with no changes.
    e. Increase metoprolol XL to 100 mg daily.

16. Which of the following β-blocker regimens would represent target therapy for most HF patients?

    a. Toprol XL 150 mg once daily
    b. Coreg 25 mg twice daily
    c. Tenormin 100 mg once daily
    d. Zebeta 2.5 mg once daily

17. Which of the following are important to consider when initiating combination hydralazine and ISDN in an African American patient with HF? Select all that apply.

    a. Initiate hydralazine 37.5 mg and ISDN 20 mg one tablet three times daily.
    b. Discontinue background ACE inhibitor therapy.
    c. Utilize a nitrate-free interval.
    d. Lower doses may be used in patients who develop a headache with therapy.
    e. Discontinue background β-blocker therapy.

18. Patients should be counseled to monitor for which of the following when initiating β-blocker therapy?

    a. Tachycardia
    b. Dehydration
    c. Fatigue
    d. Hypokalemia

19. In which HF patients should aldosterone antagonists be avoided? Select all that apply.

    a. Serum potassium <3.5 mmol/L
    b. Creatinine clearance <30 mL/min
    c. Concomitant sacubitril/valsartan therapy
    d. NYHA class III to IV despite standard HF therapy
    e. Serum potassium >5 mmol/L

20. Select the brand name of torsemide.

    a. Lasix
    b. Bumex
    c. Toprol XL
    d. Demadex

TAKEAWAY POINTS »

- Common causes of HF are coronary artery disease and uncontrolled HTN.

- HF may result from impaired ventricular ejection (HFrEF), impaired filling/HF with preserved EF (HFpEF), or both.

- HF is categorized by two classification systems. The ACC/AHA staging system classifies patients according to the progression of HF as being at risk for HF (stage A), having structural heart disease without symptoms (stage B), having HF signs and symptoms (stage C), or end-stage HF (stage D). The NYHA functional classification system categorizes patients as being asymptomatic (class I), symptomatic with mild or moderate physical activity (class II or III, respectively), or symptomatic at rest (class IV).

- Patients with HF often present with signs and symptoms of volume overload such as dyspnea on exertion and lower extremity edema. Signs and symptoms of low CO (eg, fatigue) are less common.

- Activation of neurohormonal pathways such as the SNS and RAAS occur in HF, resulting in vasoconstriction, sodium and fluid retention, and cardiac remodeling. Treatment strategies in HFrEF target these systems.

- The goals of HF drug therapy include a reduction in mortality, prevention of disease progression, reduction in hospitalizations, and improvement in QOL.

- Lifestyle modifications such as fluid and sodium restriction are important for maintaining fluid balance, although loop diuretic therapy is often required. Addition of a thiazide diuretic may be considered in diuretic-refractory patients.

- Both ACE inhibitors and β-blockers reduce mortality in HF patients and are considered cornerstones of therapy.

- An ARB should be considered in patients with intolerable cough or angioedema with an ACE inhibitor.

- Substitution of sacubitril/valsartan for ACE inhibitor or ARB therapy should be considered in patients who remain symptomatic despite receiving an ACE inhibitor or ARB and a β-blocker.

- Addition of an ARA to an ACE inhibitor and β-blocker reduces mortality and hospitalizations in symptomatic HF patients. Close monitoring of serum potassium and renal function is imperative, and ARA therapy should be avoided in the setting of hyperkalemia or renal dysfunction.

- The combination of ISDN and hydralazine reduces mortality in African Americans symptomatic despite standard HF therapy. Therapy should also be considered for patients of any race who are intolerant to ACE inhibitors and ARBs.

- Ivabradine may be considered for reducing the risk of hospitalization in patients with resting HR more than or equal to 70 beats/min in normal sinus rhythm who remain symptomatic despite maximally tolerated doses of β-blocker therapy.

- Digoxin reduces hospitalizations and improves HF symptoms. It may be considered for patients symptomatic despite standard HF therapy. Digoxin concentrations should be maintained at less than 1 ng/mL.

- Implantation of an ICD significantly reduces sudden cardiac death and should be considered in eligible patients. Biventricular pacing with CRT provides symptomatic improvement and reduces hospitalizations, but has not been shown to reduce mortality.

- Few therapies have been shown to improve clinical outcomes in patients with HFpEF. Recommendations for treatment focus on symptomatic relief and adequate control of common comorbidities, such as HTN and coronary artery disease.

BIBLIOGRAPHY

Katzung BG. Drugs used in heart failure. In: Katzung BG, Masters SB, Trevor AJ, eds. *Basic & Clinical Pharmacology*. 12th ed. New York, NY: McGraw-Hill; 2012:chap 13.

Lindenfeld J, Albert NM, Walsh MN, et al; for the Heart Failure Society of America. HFSA 2010 Comprehensive Heart Failure Practice Guideline. *J Card Fail*. 2010 Jun;16(6): e1-e194.

Mann DL, Chakinala M. Heart failure and cor pulmonale. In: Longo DL, Fauci AS, Kasper DL, Hauser SL, Jameson J, Loscalzo J, eds. *Harrison's Principles of Internal Medicine*. 18th ed. New York, NY: McGraw-Hill; 2012:chap 234.

Maron BA, Rocco TP. Pharmacotherapy of congestive heart failure. In: Brunton LL, Chabner BA, Knollmann BC, eds. *Goodman & Gilman's The Pharmacological Basis of Therapeutics*. 12th ed. New York, NY: McGraw-Hill; 2011:chap 28.

Parker RB, Nappi JM, Cavallari LH. Chronic heart failure. In: DiPiro JT, Talbert RL, Yee GC, Matzke GR, Wells BG, Posey L, eds. *Pharmacotherapy: A Pathophysiologic Approach*. 9th ed. New York, NY: McGraw-Hill; 2014:chap 4.

Yancy CW, Jessup M, Wilkoff BL, et al; for the American College of Cardiology Foundation; American Heart Association Task Force on Practice Guidelines. 2013 ACCF/AHA guideline for the management of heart failure: a report of the American College of Cardiology Foundation/American Heart Association Task Force on Practice Guidelines. *J Am Coll Cardiol*. 2013 Oct 15;62(16):e147-e239.

KEY ABBREVIATIONS

ACC = American College of Cardiology
ACE = angiotensin-converting enzyme
AHA = American Heart Association
ARA = aldosterone receptor antagonist
ARB = angiotensin receptor blocker
BNP = B-type natriuretic peptide
CO = cardiac output
COPD = chronic obstructive pulmonary disease
CRT = cardiac resynchronization therapy
EF = ejection fraction
HF = heart failure
HFpEF = heart failure with preserved ejection fraction
HFrEF = heart failure with reduced ejection fraction
HR = heart rate

HTN = hypertension
ICD = implantable cardioverter defibrillator
ISDN = isosorbide dinitrate
JVD = jugular vein distention
LVEF = left ventricular ejection fraction
MI = myocardial infarction
NSAIDs = nonsteroidal anti-inflammatory drugs
NYHA = New York Heart Association
PND = paroxysmal nocturnal dyspnea
QOL = quality of life
RAAS = renin-angiotensin-aldosterone system
SNS = sympathetic nervous system
SOB = shortness of breath

2 Acute Decompensated Heart Failure

Brent N. Reed and Jo E. Rodgers

FOUNDATION OVERVIEW

Heart failure (HF) is a progressive syndrome resulting from abnormal cardiac structure or function impairing the ability of the ventricle to fill with or eject blood. Acute decompensated heart failure (ADHF) characterizes patients with worsening HF, often requiring hospitalization. Patients with persistent symptoms or refractory HF despite optimal oral therapies are classified as stage D by the American College of Cardiology/American Heart Association staging system. Additionally, ADHF patients have symptoms with minimal activity or at rest and thus are most commonly classified as New York Heart Association class III or IV.

Etiology and Pathophysiology

ADHF is characterized by a rapid decline in condition due to fluid retention and/or compromised cardiac function. Acute decompensation is frequently a consequence of disease progression or stems from medication or lifestyle nonadherence. Alternatively, ADHF may occur abruptly as a result of an acute insult (eg, atrial fibrillation, acute coronary syndrome).

While the sympathetic nervous system (SNS) and renin-angiotensin-aldosterone system (RAAS) are initially activated to maintain cardiac output and vital organ perfusion, activation of these systems ultimately deteriorate cardiac function. The SNS increases systemic vascular resistance (SVR, afterload) causing pump dysfunction. The RAAS results in vasoconstriction and sodium and water retention leading to increased intravascular fluid volume (preload). Furthermore, arginine vasopressin is secreted causing vasoconstriction, free water retention, and hyponatremia.

B-type natriuretic peptide (BNP) is secreted from ventricular tissue in response to fluid overload and ventricular wall stretch. The physiologic effect of BNP is to induce natriuresis as well as venous and arterial vasodilation. However, the release of endogenous BNP only mildly attenuates the negative compensatory neurohormonal cascade.

Diagnosis

HF is a clinical diagnosis and no single test establishes its presence or absence. Nearly all patients with HF present with dyspnea. The absence of dyspnea makes HF highly unlikely and other explanations for the patient's symptoms should be sought first.

When used in conjunction with patient history and physical examination, BNP can be helpful in distinguishing ADHF from other conditions. A BNP concentration below 100 pg/mL is highly predictive for the *absence* of fluid overload. Unfortunately, BNP concentrations may be *falsely* elevated due to non-HF causes such as pneumonia or pulmonary embolism.

Placement of a pulmonary artery catheter (PAC, also known as a Swan-Ganz catheter) may be helpful in distinguishing a patient's hemodynamic profile in ADHF. While hemodynamic parameters may assist in the development of a pharmacotherapy plan, use of a PAC does not improve outcomes. Consequently, a PAC should only be employed in patients: (1) not responding to initial therapy, (2) whose volume status cannot be determined by history and physical examination, or (3) who experience hemodynamic instability during treatment.

PAC Measurements

Patients with low cardiac index (CI) less than 2.2 L/min/m^2 are referred to as "cold" because of reduced perfusion. Patients with a CI more than 2.2 L/min/m^2 are termed "warm." Another useful PAC measurement is the pulmonary capillary wedge pressure (PCWP). The PCWP is a marker of intravascular fluid status and ventricular filling pressures. Normal, healthy individuals have a PCWP of 6 to 12 mm Hg, but those with HF may require a PCWP of 15 to 18 to optimize cardiac output. Patients with a PCWP more than 18 mm Hg are generally considered "wet" as a consequence of fluid overload, whereas those with a PCWP of 15 to 18 mm Hg or less are considered "dry" (euvolemic). Using PAC measurements, patients are classified as "warm and wet," "cold and wet," "warm and dry," or "cold and dry." Additionally, the degree of arterial vasoconstriction or SVR can also be measured using a PAC. A normal SVR is 800 to 1200 dyne·sec·cm^5. Values of SVR greater than 1200 dyne·sec·cm^5 represent a state of vasoconstriction, whereas values less than 800 dyne·sec·cm^5 represent a state of vasodilation.

Clinical Presentation

The presenting signs and symptoms of ADHF vary with the degree of underlying disease. Signs and symptoms are predominantly associated with fluid accumulation. Pulmonary edema presents as dyspnea, orthopnea, crackles, and hypoxemia and is associated with an elevated PCWP. Peripheral edema, ascites, and hepatomegaly/hepatojugular reflux are signs of systemic fluid overload. "Congested" patients may also present with systemic hypertension. Additional signs of ADHF are consistent with hypoperfusion and include increased serum creatinine (SCr) and hepatic transaminases, altered mental status, and cool extremities. Additionally, gut ischemia can occur leading to pain or vomiting with eating.

TREATMENT

Goals of Therapy/Prognosis

The immediate goals of treatment for ADHF are restoration of hemodynamic stability and correction of fluid overload. Additionally, attempts should also be made to identify and manage treatable underlying causes. Hospital admissions represent an important opportunity to educate patients about their disease, enact lifestyle modifications and optimize chronic HF medication regimens.

Pharmacologic Treatment

Initial Management of Chronic Heart Failure Medications

Chronic HF medications may need to be temporarily modified upon admission for ADHF. If patients present with hypotension (systolic blood pressure [BP] <90 mm Hg) a dose reduction or discontinuation may be required for medications that affect BP. If β-blocker initiation or uptitration is the cause of ADHF, a reduction to the previously tolerated dose should occur. Discontinuation of β-blocker therapy should only be considered in the setting of overt cardiogenic shock or clinically significant hypotension.

Therapies affecting the RAAS and digoxin may be held or discontinued if a patient presents with acute kidney injury. Digoxin undergoes primarily renal clearance, making accumulation and toxicity a possibility. Measuring a serum digoxin concentration may be useful to determine if it is safe to continue treatment. Additionally, angiotensin-converting enzyme (ACE) inhibitors, angiotensin receptor blockers, and aldosterone receptor antagonists cause hyperkalemia. These medications may need to be held since patients with hyperkalemia upon admission may be worsened in the setting of decreased

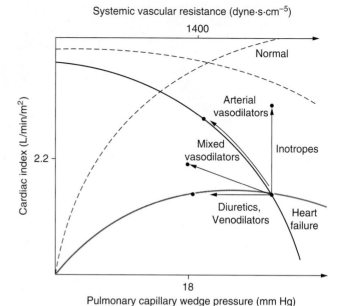

FIGURE 2-1 Hemodynamic response to pharmacologic interventions. Reproduced with permission from DiPiro JT, Talbert RL, Yee GC, et al: *Pharmacotherapy: A Pathophysiologic Approach,* 10th ed. New York, NY: McGraw-Hill; 2017.

urine output. In the absence of the above situations, it is reasonable to continue chronic HF medications during ADHF.

Intravenous Diuretics

Treatment of ADHF in patients with fluid overload includes intravenous (IV) loop diuretics. Loop diuretics rapidly reduce ventricular filling pressures and decrease PCWP by blocking sodium and chloride reabsorption in the Loop of Henle leading to fluid excretion (Figure 2-1). Given intravenously, furosemide, bumetanide, and torsemide are equally effective at equipotent doses. Patients with inadequate urine output *after* initial intermittent bolus doses may require an increased dose or addition of thiazide-type diuretic (oral hydrochlorothiazide, oral metolazone, or IV chlorothiazide). Another alternative for diuretic resistance is use of a continuous infusion loop diuretic. Table 2-1 lists commonly used IV diuretics. Those who respond to loop diuretics should experience a net fluid loss of at least 1 to 2 L every 24 hours. This represents a 1 to 2 kg weight loss each day. At the initiation of treatment, it is useful to ascertain the goal weight for a patient.

TABLE 2-1	Intravenous Diuretics Used to Treat Heart Failure-Related Fluid Retention				
	Onset of Action (min)	Duration of Action (h)	Relative Oral Potency (mg)	Intermittent Bolus Dosing (mg)	Continuous Infusion Dosing (Bolus [mg]/Infusion) (mg/h)
Furosemide	2-5	6	40	20-200+	80-120/10-40
Torsemide	<10	6-12	20	N/A[a]	N/A
Bumetanide	2-3	4-6	0.5-1	1-10	1-4/0.5-2
Ethacrynic acid	5-15	2-7	50	0.5-1 mg/kg/dose up to 100 mg/dose	N/A

[a] Torsemide no longer available intravenously in the United States.

Adapted with permission from Chisholm-Burns MA, Wells BG, Schwinghammer TL, et al: *Pharmacotherapy Principles & Practice,* 3rd ed. New York, NY: McGraw-Hill; 2013.

TABLE 2-2	Hemodynamic Effects of Commonly Used Intravenous Agents for Treatment of Acute or Severe Heart Failure				
Drug	**CO**	**PCWP**	**SVR**	**BP**	**HR**
Diuretics	↑/↓/0	↓↓ – ↓↓↓		↓	0
Nitroglycerin	↑	↓↓	↓	↓↓	↑/0
Nitroprusside	↑	↓↓↓	↓↓↓	↓↓↓	↑
Nesiritide	↑	↓↓	↓↓	↓↓	0
Dobutamine	↑↑	↓/0	↓/0	↓/0	↑↑
Milrinone	↑↑	↓↓	↓	↓	↑

Abbreviations: BP, blood pressure; CO, cardiac output; HR, heart rate; PCWP, pulmonary capillary wedge pressure; SVR, systemic vascular resistance; ↑, increase; ↓, decrease; 0, no or little change.

Adapted with permission from Chisholm-Burns MA, Wells BG, Schwinghammer TL, et al: *Pharmacotherapy Principles & Practice,* 3rd ed. New York, NY: McGraw-Hill; 2013.

TABLE 2-3	Doses and Monitoring of Commonly Used Hemodynamic Medications	
Drug	**Dose**	**Monitoring Variables**[a]
Dobutamine	2.5-20 mcg/kg/min	BP, HR urinary output and function, ECG
Milrinone	0.1-0.75 mcg/kg/min	BP, HR, urinary output and function, ECG, changes in ischemic symptoms (eg, chest pain), electrolytes
Nitroprusside	0.25-3 mcg/kg/min	BP, HR, liver and kidney function, blood cyanide and/or thiocyanate concentrations if toxicity suspected (nausea, vomiting, altered mental function)
Nitroglycerin	5-200 mcg/min	BP, HR, ECG, changes in ischemic symptoms
Nesiritide	Bolus: 2 mcg/kg; Infusion: 0.01 mcg/kg/min	BP, HR, urinary output and kidney function

[a]In addition to pulmonary capillary wedge pressure and cardiac output.
Abbreviations: BNP, B-type natriuretic peptide; BP, blood pressure; ECG, electrocardiogram; HR, heart rate.

Adapted with permission from Chisholm-Burns MA, Wells BG, Schwinghammer TL, et al: *Pharmacotherapy Principles & Practice,* 3rd ed. New York, NY: McGraw-Hill; 2013.

Monitoring of loop diuretics includes vital signs, strict input/output, patient weight, physical examination, renal function, and electrolytes. Hypotension results from intravascular volume depletion because mobilization of extravascular fluid into the intravascular space may lag behind urinary fluid elimination. Monitoring of BP including orthostasis should occur at frequent intervals. Decreased renal function and electrolyte abnormalities (hypokalemia, hypomagnesemia) are common with high doses of loop diuretics. Addition of a thiazide-type diuretic to loop diuretics potentiates diuresis as well as hypotension and electrolyte abnormalities.

Intravenous Vasodilators

Intravenous vasodilators are considered for persistent ADHF despite aggressive treatment with diuretics in the absence of low BP (SBP <90 mm Hg). Vasodilators may be useful for quickly improving symptoms of pulmonary congestion in ADHF patients. They assist in relieving pulmonary edema through increased venous capacitance and decreasing venous pressures. They also may decrease SVR leading to increased cardiac output and subsequent renal perfusion and urine output. It is important, however, to understand that the use of IV vasodilators, like other ADHF therapies, has not been shown to exert a beneficial effect on mortality. The three commonly used IV vasodilators for ADHF are nitroglycerin, nesiritide, and nitroprusside (Figure 2-1; Tables 2-2 and 2-3).

Nitroglycerin is a nitric oxide donor causing vasodilation by relaxing vascular smooth muscle. Nitroglycerin reduces preload through dilation of venous blood vessels leading to a reduction in ventricular filling pressures and pulmonary artery pressures. Nitroglycerin is initiated at 5 to 10 mcg/min and titrated based on response. At higher doses (>100 mcg/min), nitroglycerin also dilates the arterial vasculature, decreasing afterload and SVR and increasing CO. Continuous BP monitoring is important with nitroglycerin, as hypotension is common. As with any nitrate, patients may experience a headache. If nitroglycerin is administered for longer than 12 hours, tolerance may develop, necessitating increased doses to maintain similar pharmacologic effects.

Nesiritide is a recombinant BNP molecule that promotes natriuresis, venodilation, and arterial vasodilation. When administered as a continuous infusion, nesiritide decreases PCWP and SVR (indirectly increasing CO), and assists in diuresis when coadministered with loop diuretics. As with other vasodilators, frequent BP monitoring is required, and the use of nesiritide in patients with low BP (eg, systolic BP <90 mm Hg) should be avoided.

Nitroprusside is a nitric oxide donor with potent vasodilatory effects on venous and arterial vasculature. Nitroprusside decreases pulmonary artery pressures, preload, and afterload, resulting in a net increase in CO. Caution should be exercised in patients with hepatic and/or renal dysfunction, as nitroprusside is metabolized into cyanide. Hepatic or renal dysfunction as well as use of prolonged high doses of nitroprusside can lead to accumulation of cyanide byproducts.

Intravenous Inotropes

Intravenous inotropes are utilized in diuretic refractory patients with low cardiac output. Examples of IV inotropes are dobutamine and milrinone (Figure 2-1; Tables 2-2 and 2-3). Dobutamine is a nonselective β-adrenergic receptor agonist with α_1-adrenergic agonist effects. Milrinone is a phosphodiesterase type III (PDE$_3$) inhibitor. Dobutamine and milrinone are useful agents for the acute management of ADHF; however, they may cause arrhythmias, including sinus tachycardia, atrial fibrillation, and ventricular tachycardia. Milrinone may cause hypotension especially with bolus doses or renal dysfunction where accumulation may occur.

Administration of inotropes may worsen long-term prognosis. Therefore, when feasible (eg, adequate BP), IV vasodilators are preferred over inotropes for patients with low cardiac output. Inotrope therapy should be reserved for short-term use in patients with low BP refractory to other ADHF therapies, bridging patients to surgical devices or heart transplant, or for palliative care of end-stage patients.

Transition to Chronic Heart Failure Medications

Once patients are euvolemic and successfully weaned from IV medications, attention turns to implementing chronic, oral HF medications. Certain steps should also be taken prior to assure compliance with the American College of Cardiology/American Heart Association HF performance measures, such as documentation of ejection fraction (EF) and a prescription for an ACE inhibitor or ARB as well as a β-blocker at discharge for those with HF and a reduced EF. Additionally, discharge counseling and smoking cessation education should also be completed. Adherence to these measures helps to ensure that HF care is optimized.

Nonpharmacologic Treatment

Pharmacologic treatment of ADHF can be augmented by mechanical support. Short-term options such as intra-aortic balloon pumps (IABPs) assist with acute management and permanent options such as left ventricular assist devices (LVADs) and heart transplantation can prolong survival and improve quality of life. An in-depth discussion of these nonpharmacologic treatment modalities is beyond the scope of this review.

CASE Application

Questions 1 through 3 pertain to the following case.

RF is a 62-year-old man with nonischemic cardiomyopathy (LVEF 30%-35%) presenting to the emergency department (ED) with an acute HF exacerbation. His vital signs include BP 155/90 mm Hg, heart rate (HR) 85 beats/min, RR 20, and O_2 sat 94% on 4 L/min of oxygen by nasal cannula (NC). Physical examination reveals jugular venous distension (JVD), regular rate and rhythm (RRR), crackles bilaterally at bases, and 2+ bilateral lower extremity edema. He admits to a 12-lb weight gain in the past 2 weeks since his carvedilol dose was increased and reports strict adherence to both dietary restrictions and medications. In the ED, he has already received furosemide 80 mg IV ×1 dose with minimal response in urine output. Pertinent laboratory results include potassium 3.9 mmol/L, BNP 1550 pg/mL, BUN 37 mg/dL, and SCr 1.3 mg/dL (baseline). RF's home medications include lisinopril 10 mg daily, carvedilol 25 mg twice daily, digoxin 0.125 mg/d, and furosemide 80 mg orally twice daily.

1. Based on the BNP value, RF is experiencing which one of the following?

   a. Active myocardial ischemia
   b. Shortness of breath due to a noncardiac etiology
   c. Significant volume overload and ventricular wall stretch
   d. Renal insufficiency

2. Which of the following interventions is best for RF on arrival to the intensive care unit (ICU)?

   a. Dobutamine 2.5 mcg/kg/min infusion
   b. Milrinone 0.375 mcg/kg/min infusion
   c. Metolazone 10 mg po now and then daily
   d. Furosemide 120 mg IV twice daily

3. Select the appropriate management of RF's β-blocker based upon his history and clinical presentation?

   a. Continue carvedilol 25 mg twice daily.
   b. Increase carvedilol to 50 mg twice daily.
   c. Decrease carvedilol to 12.5 mg twice daily.
   d. Discontinue carvedilol.

4. Which of the following should be closely monitored during initial intravenous diuretic administration?

   a. Hypokalemia
   b. Hypernatremia
   c. Hypertension
   d. Hypouricemia

Questions 5 through 7 pertain to the following case.

BG is a 72-year-old woman complaining of being "extremely tired all the time." Her exercise tolerance is significantly less than it was 2 months ago; she now has to rest during daily activities. This has come on gradually. She has a history of hypertensive cardiomyopathy (LVEF 25%-30% by ECHO 1 year ago). She is strictly adherent with both diet restrictions and medications. Vital signs include BP 92/63 mm Hg, HR 105 beats/min with symptomatic orthostasis upon standing, and RR 14. BG does complain of recent dizziness; however, she denies palpitations and her electrocardiogram (ECG) is normal. On physical examination, her lungs are clear and she has no jugular venous distention, ascites or lower extremity edema. Laboratory analysis reveals sodium 129 mmol/L, potassium 4.2 mmol/L, BUN 65 mg/dL, and SCr 2.1 mg/dL (baseline BUN/SCr 32/0.9). BG has been stable on the following oral regimen for several months: valsartan 80 mg twice daily, metoprolol XL 50 mg/d, furosemide 40 mg twice daily, amiodarone 200 mg/d, and digoxin 0.125 mg/d.

5. Which one of the following clinical categories best describes BG?

   a. Warm and dry
   b. Warm and wet
   c. Cold and dry
   d. Cold and wet

6. Which one of the following is the optimal initial intervention for BG?

   a. Change furosemide to 80 mg intravenously twice daily.
   b. Hold furosemide and begin cautious hydration with IV fluids.
   c. Hold metoprolol and begin dobutamine at 2 mcg/kg/min.
   d. Increase metoprolol XL to 100 mg/d.

7. After your intervention, BG feels much better. Her vital signs today include BP 132/76 mm Hg, HR 78 beats/min, and RR 14, and her orthostasis has resolved. An echocardiogram (performed today) reveals LVEF of 15% to 20% with increasing ventricular dilation. Her relevant laboratory values are sodium 129 mmol/L, potassium 5.1 mmol/L, BUN 40 mg/dL, and SCr 1.2 mg/dL.

   Which one of the following most likely explains BG's change in EF?

   a. Acute arrhythmia
   b. Dietary nonadherence
   c. Renal insufficiency
   d. Progression of heart failure

Questions 8 through 12 pertain to the following case.

JF is a 57-year-old woman who presents to the hospital with ADHF. Vital signs include BP 105/67 mm Hg, HR 83 beats/min, and RR 21. Physical examination reveals 12 cm JVD elevated, $+S_3$, bilateral rales on auscultation, abdominal ascites, and 4+ bilateral edema extending to her thighs. Chest radiograph reveals pulmonary edema and pleural effusions. Hemodynamic measurements obtained by PAC include PCWP 29 mm Hg, CI 1.7 L/min/m², and SVR 700. Her laboratory values are all normal, except sodium 132 mmol/L, BUN 49 mg/dL, and SCr 2.1 mg/dL (baseline BUN/SCr 32 and 0.9). Her drugs on admission include enalapril 10 mg twice daily, carvedilol 12.5 mg twice daily, bumetanide 2 mg twice daily, hydralazine 50 mg three times daily, isosorbide dinitrate 40 mg three times daily, and aspirin 81 mg/d.

8. Which of the following is a reasonable choice for diuretic therapy in JF?

   a. JF should not receive diuretic therapy because she is volume-depleted.
   b. Intravenous loop diuretic therapy should be given to provide a net fluid loss of 500 to 2000 mL/d.
   c. Metolazone should be considered a first-line option because of JF's impaired renal function.
   d. Nesiritide therapy should be used as a replacement for diuretic therapy because JF is volume overloaded.

9. Which of the following best describes what PCWP represents in JF? Select all that apply.

   a. Fluid status
   b. Inotropy
   c. Afterload
   d. Chronotropy

10. What is the desired PCWP for JF? Select all that apply.

   a. Less than 2.2 L/min/m²
   b. Greater than 2.2 L/min/m²
   c. Between 6 and 12 mm Hg
   d. Between 15 and 18 mm Hg

11. Once JF has undergone successful diuresis and returned to her euvolemic weight, her CI and SVR do not change substantially. Her vital signs and oral HF medications remain unchanged with the exception of her diuretic dose. Her renal function has improved to baseline. Which of the following therapies are now appropriate to manage JF's ADHF?

   a. Nitroprusside
   b. Nesiritide
   c. Dopamine
   d. Milrinone

12. Discharge for JF is planned with outpatient inotropic therapy based on your recommendations. According to the American College of Cardiology/American Heart Association (ACC/AHA) HF performance measures, which one of the following should be completed prior to JF's discharge?

   a. BNP measurement
   b. Written documentation of her EF
   c. Care of her IV access site
   d. Advance directives

13. Which of the following should be assured prior to administering intravenous inotropes and vasodilators?

   a. Adequate filling pressures with a PCWP 6 to 12 mm Hg
   b. Adequate filling pressures with a PCWP >15 mm Hg
   c. Adequate filling pressure with an SVR >1200 dyne/s/cm⁵
   d. Adequate filling pressure with an SVR >1500 dyne/s/cm⁵

14. Which of the following would be an absolute contraindication to intravenous vasodilators?

   a. Heart rate >90 beats/min
   b. Heart rate >110 beats/min
   c. Systolic blood pressure <90 mm Hg
   d. Systolic blood pressure <110 mm Hg

15. Which of the following are adverse effects of dobutamine? Select all that apply.

   a. Hyponatremia
   b. Renal dysfunction
   c. Hypokalemia
   d. Arrhythmia
   e. Thrombocytopenia

16. Which of the following is referred to as an "inodilator," having both inotropic and vasodilatory properties?

   a. Milrinone
   b. Dobutamine
   c. Nesiritide
   d. Nitroprusside

17. JT is an 81-year-old man (70 kg) admitted for ADHF refractory to outpatient titration of oral diuretics, including torsemide and metolazone. He is now receiving intravenous furosemide 20 mg/h and chlorothiazide 500 mg intravenously twice daily. While JT's vital signs

and renal function appear stable (BP 127/65 mm Hg, HR 90 beats/min, SCr 1.2 mg/dL), his urine output is unchanged despite over 24 hours of the above regimen. Additionally, review of continuous telemetry demonstrates multiple 10-beat runs of ventricular tachycardia. Which of the following is an appropriate next step in therapy?

a. Initiate milrinone 0.1 mcg/kg/min
b. Initiate dobutamine 2.5 mcg/kg/min
c. Initiate nesiritide 0.01 mcg/kg/min
d. Increase furosemide to 60 mg/h

18. Which of the following is associated with the use of IV nitroglycerin in ADHF?

a. Natriuresis
b. Increased risk of ventricular arrhythmias
c. Accumulation of toxic metabolites in hepatic or renal impairment
d. Primarily venous dilation at lower doses (ie, <100 mcg/min)

19. Place the following diuretics in order of potency. Start with the least potent agent. Select all that are in the correct order.

a. Torsemide, furosemide, bumetanide
b. Furosemide, torsemide, bumetanide
c. Bumetanide, furosemide, torsemide
d. Lasix, demadex, bumex
e. Bumex, lasix, demadex

20. Select the intravenous agent(s) utilized for ADHF that has a neutral effect on heart rate (no change when utilized at recommended doses). Select all that apply.

a. Loop diuretics
b. Nitroprusside
c. Nesiritide
d. Dobutamine
e. Milrinone

TAKEAWAY POINTS »

- The sympathetic nervous system (SNS) and renin-angiotensin-aldosterone system (RAAS) are beneficial in maintaining cardiac output and vital organ perfusion; however, persistent activation of these systems ultimately deteriorate cardiac function.
- B-type natriuretic peptide (BNP) is secreted from ventricular tissue in response to fluid overload and ventricular wall stretch.
- Obtaining BNP can be helpful in distinguishing ADHF from other noncardiac disease states.
- Pulmonary artery catheter placement may assist in the management of complex ADHF patients, but should only be used in patients who do not respond to initial treatment, whose volume status is uncertain, or who are hemodynamically unstable.
- The presenting signs and symptoms of ADHF vary with the degree of underlying disease. Signs and symptoms are predominantly associated with fluid accumulation.

- Immediate goals of treatment for ADHF are restoration of hemodynamic stability and correction of fluid overload. Additionally, attempts should also be made to identify and manage treatable underlying causes.
- Chronic HF medications may need to be dose-reduced or discontinued at admission for ADHF, with attempts to reinitiate prior to discharge.
- Fluid overloaded patients should be treated initially with IV loop diuretics.
- Loop diuretics rapidly reduce ventricular filling pressures and decrease PCWP.
- Intravenous vasodilators are considered for persistent ADHF despite aggressive treatment with diuretics. Patients with adequate filling pressure and blood pressure may benefit from the addition of nitroglycerin, nitroprusside, or nesiritide.
- Intravenous inotropes are utilized in diuretic refractory patients with signs or symptoms of hypoperfusion or low cardiac output.

BIBLIOGRAPHY

Katzung BG. Drugs used in heart failure. In: Katzung BG, Masters SB, Trevor AJ, eds. *Basic & Clinical Pharmacology.* 12th ed. New York, NY: McGraw-Hill; 2012:chap 13.

Lindenfeld J, Albert NM, Boehmer JP, et al. HFSA 2010 Comprehensive Heart Failure Practice Guideline. *J Card Fail.* 2010 Jun;16(6):e1-e194.

Maron BA, Rocco TP. Pharmacotherapy of congestive heart failure. In: Brunton LL, Chabner BA, Knollmann BC, eds. *Goodman & Gilman's The Pharmacological Basis of Therapeutics.* 12th ed. New York, NY: McGraw-Hill; 2011: chap 28.

Rodgers JE, Reed BN. Acute decompensated heart failure. In: DiPiro JT, Talbert RL, Yee GC, Matzke GR, Wells BG, Posey L, eds. *Pharmacotherapy: A Pathophysiologic Approach.* 10th ed. New York, NY: McGraw-Hill; 2017:chap 15.

Yancy CW, Jessup M, Wilkoff BL, et al; for the American College of Cardiology Foundation; American Heart Association Task Force on Practice Guidelines. 2013 ACCF/AHA guideline for the management of heart failure: a report of the American College of Cardiology Foundation/American Heart Association Task Force on Practice Guidelines. *J Am Coll Cardiol.* 2013 Oct 15;62(16):e147-e239.

KEY ABBREVIATIONS

ACE inhibitor = angiotensin-converting enzyme inhibitor
ADHF = acute decompensated heart failure
ARA = aldosterone receptor antagonist
ARB = angiotensin receptor blocker
BP = blood pressure
BNP = B-type natriuretic peptide
CI = cardiac index
CO = cardiac output
EF = ejection fraction
HF = heart failure

HR = heart rate
IABPs = intra-aortic balloon pumps
LVADs = left ventricular assist devices
PAC = pulmonary artery catheter
PCWP = pulmonary capillary wedge pressure
RAAS = renin-angiotensin-aldosterone system
SCr = serum creatinine
SNS = sympathetic nervous system
SV = stroke volume
SVR = systemic vascular resistance

FOUNDATION OVERVIEW

Hypertension is defined as persistently elevated arterial blood pressure (BP). BP is the mathematical product of peripheral vascular resistance (PVR) and cardiac output (CO) and hypertension is the result of increased PVR or CO. Aberrations in the normal function of neurohormonal systems, such as the renin-angiotensin-aldosterone system (RAAS), sympathetic nervous system (SNS), and disturbances in sodium, calcium, and natriuretic hormones, have been implicated in the pathophysiology of hypertension (Table 3-1). Hypertension is usually multifactorial; consequently, multiple antihypertensive drugs are often necessary to control BP. Cardiovascular risk reduction can occur with lower BP. A reduction in systolic blood pressure (SBP) as small as 2 mm Hg reduces the risk of death from ischemic heart disease or other vascular causes by 7% and from stroke by 10%. The majority of patients with hypertension have essential hypertension because their BP is elevated for unknown reasons. Secondary hypertension accounts for less than 10% of patients (Table 3-2).

Diagnosis

Hypertension is diagnosed when the average of two or three BP measurements are elevated at two or three separate clinical encounters. The 2017 Guideline for the Prevention, Detection, Evaluation, and Management of High Blood Pressure in Adults, provide specific details for appropriate blood pressure measurement. Common errors in practice can occur by not following blood pressure technique recommendations leading to an inaccurate diagnosis or assessment of elevated blood pressure. Patients should be relaxed, sitting in a chair for at least 5 minutes. Refraining from caffeine, exercise and smoking is advised for at least 30 minutes prior to measurement. To ensure proper assessment of the blood pressure, the patient's bladder should be emptied and neither the patient nor the clinician should talk during the rest period or during the assessment. All patients should have their arm supported and at heart level. Using the correct cuff size is critical that allows for the cuff's bladder to encircle 80% of the arm. During the first visit, the clinician should record the blood pressure in both arms and use the arm that gives the higher reading for subsequent readings. A repeat blood pressure should be done

after waiting one to two minutes from the previous measurement. Documentation of the blood pressure result is critical, and it is of importance to know when the patient had their previous dose of blood pressure medication if applicable. Table 3-3 provides guideline recommendations for diagnosis and staging of hypertension.

Evaluation

Assessment of hypertensive patients should identify cardiovascular risk factors and concomitant disorders that may affect prognosis and guide treatment. This can be accomplished by obtaining a thorough medical history, physical examination, routine laboratory tests, and diagnostic procedures.

TREATMENT

Lifestyle Modification

Lifestyle factors are associated with the development of hypertension and include excess body weight, excess sodium intake, alcohol intake, reduced physical activity, inadequate intake of fruits, vegetables, and potassium, and smoking. Lifestyle modifications stall the development and progression of hypertension, enhance antihypertensive drug efficacy and decrease cardiovascular risk. Despite irrefutable evidence supporting the relationship between lifestyle choices and cardiovascular risk, there remains considerable resistance on the part of patients to implement these changes and non-adherence is high. Table 3-4 lists lifestyle modifications that lower BP; the focus is centered on diet, exercise, quitting smoking, and moderation of alcohol.

Diet

The Dietary Approaches to Stop Hypertension (DASH) eating plan was developed to aid in the prevention and treatment of hypertension. Recommendations include a high intake of fruits, vegetables, and low-fat dairy products along with a reduced content of dietary cholesterol, saturated fat, and total fat. The diet is rich in potassium and calcium and low in sodium. The preferred intake of dietary sodium is less than 2.4 g of sodium per day.

TABLE 3-1 Pathophysiology of Hypertension

BP = PVR × CO	
CO = HR × SV	
Peripheral Vascular Resistance	**Increased Cardiac Output**
Excess stimulation of the RAAS	Increased intravascular volume from excess sodium intake
SNS overactivity	SNS overactivity
Genetic alterations of cell membranes	Increased intravascular volume from renal sodium retention Excess stimulation of the RAAS
Endothelial-derived factors	
Hyperinsulinemia resulting from obesity or the metabolic syndrome	

Abbreviations: BP, blood pressure; CO, cardiac output; HR, heart rate; PVR, peripheral vascular resistance; RAAS, renin-angiotensin-aldosterone system; SNS, sympathetic nervous system; SV, stroke volume.

Exercise

Lack of physical activity is an important cardiovascular risk factor because excess weight and obesity increase the risk for hypertension, hyperlipidemia, and diabetes. A weight loss of 10 lb may reduce BP and prevents hypertension in a large proportion of overweight persons. Patients should be encouraged to achieve normal body weight. In the absence of contraindications or disability, hypertensive patients should participate in regular, aerobic physical activity most days of the week (eg, brisk walking at least 30 min/d).

Alcohol

Excessive consumption of alcohol can increase BP. Alcohol intake should be limited to 1 oz (30 mL) or less of ethanol, the equivalent of two drinks per day in most men and one drink (0.5 oz) per day in women and lighter weight persons.

Treatment Goals

The goal of hypertension management is to reduce morbidity and mortality. Most hypertensive patients will reach the DBP goal once the SBP goal is achieved. Adults with confirmed

TABLE 3-2 Secondary Causes of Hypertension

Identifiable Causes

Chronic kidney disease

Coarctation of the aorta

Cushing syndrome and other glucocorticoid excess states including chronic steroid therapy

Drug induced or drug related

Obstructive uropathy

Obstructive sleep apnea

Pheochromocytoma

Primary aldosteronism and other mineralocorticoid excess states

Renovascular hypertension

Thyroid or parathyroid disease

Associated Conditions

Anxiety

Chronic pain

Excessive ethanol intake

Hyperinsulinemia

Obesity

Obstructive sleep apnea

Smoking

Medications

Antidepressants (MOAIs, SNRIs, TCAs)

β-blockers or centrally acting alpha agonists (when abruptly discontinued)

Cyclosporine

Erythropoietin

Licorice

Nonsteroidal anti-inflammatory drugs (NSAIDs)

Oral contraceptives

Sympathomimetics

Steroids

Illicit Drug Use

Abbreviations: MAOIs, monoamine oxidase inhibitors; SNRIs, serotonin and norepinephrine reuptake inhibitors; TCAs, tricyclic antidepressants.

hypertension and known cardiovascular disease or 10-year ASCVD event risk of at least 10% should attain a blood pressure goal of less than 130/80 mm Hg. Patients with comorbidities such as ischemic heart disease, heart failure with reduced ejection fraction and preferred ejection fraction,

TABLE 3-3 Blood Pressure Classification

BP Classification	SBP (mm Hg)	DBP (mm Hg)	Intervention	Threshold for starting therapy
Normal	<120	And ≤80	Lifestyle modification	N/A
Elevated	120-129	And <80	Lifestyle modification	N/A
Stage 1	130-139	Or 80-90	Lifestyle modification if clinical ASCVD calculation is <10%	Lifestyle modification and pharmacotherapy if clinical ASCVD calculation is ≥10%
Stage 2	≥140	Or ≥90	Lifestyle modification and pharmacotherapy. Combination therapy is recommended for Stage 2 or those with BP >160/100 mm Hg. Prompt treatment, careful monitoring and medication titration is needed.	

TABLE 3-4	Lifestyle Modifications to Prevent and Manage Hypertension[a]	
Modification	**Recommendation**	**Approximate SBP Reduction (Range)[b]**
Weight reduction	Maintain normal body weight (body mass index 18.5-24.9 kg/m²)	5-20 mm Hg/10 kg
Adopt DASH eating plan	Consume a diet rich in fruits, vegetables, and low-fat dairy products with a reduced content of saturated and total fat	8-14 mm Hg
Dietary sodium reduction	Reduce dietary sodium intake to no more than 2.4 g sodium or 6 g sodium chloride	2-8 mm Hg
Physical activity	Engage in regular aerobic physical activity such as brisk walking (at least 30 min/d, most days of the week)	4-9 mm Hg
Moderation of alcohol consumption	Limit consumption to no more than two drinks (eg, 24 oz beer, 10 oz wine, or 3 oz 80-proof whiskey) per day in most men, and to no more than one drink per day in women and lighter weight persons	2-4 mm Hg

[a]For overall cardiovascular risk reduction, stop smoking.

[b]The effects of implementing these modifications are dose and time dependent, and could be greater for some individuals.

Abbreviations: DASH, dietary approaches to stop hypertension; SBP, systolic blood pressure.

chronic kidney disease (including renal transplant), cerebrovascular disease, atrial fibrillation, peripheral artery disease, diabetes and metabolic syndrome should also attain a goal of less than 130/80 mm Hg. Guidelines indicate that primary prevention patients without additional markers of increased cardiovascular risk can attain a reasonable goal of less than 130/80 mm Hg. Although guidelines support clinical trial evidence with the strongest recommendation for these primary prevention patients to attain a target BP of <140/90 mm Hg it is suggested through observational studies that these individuals often have a high lifetime risk that could benefit from earlier BP control.

Pharmacotherapy

Several antihypertensive medications are available for the management of BP and should be used to combat the mechanism of hypertension pathophysiology. Table 3-5 provides key drug knowledge while Table 3-6 provides lists of the antihypertensive agents. In the nonblack population (including patients with diabetes), initial treatment should include a thiazide type diuretic, calcium channel blocker (CCB), angiotensin-converting enzyme inhibitor (ACEI), or angiotensin receptor blocker (ARB). In the black population (including patients with diabetes), initial treatment should include a thiazide-type diuretic or CCB. Patients with CKD and greater than 18 years of age, initial treatment should include an ACEI or ARB. β-Blockers are generally no longer recommended as initial therapy except for patients with a compelling indication (eg, coronary artery disease or left ventricular dysfunction). Guidelines recommend combination therapy when the SBP is 20 mm Hg above goal or the DBP is 10 mm Hg above goal.

Individual Classes

Thiazide-Type Diuretic

Thiazide diuretics are especially effective in the elderly and blacks where volume and heightened PVR are major

contributors to elevated BP. In patients with renal insufficiency, thiazide diuretics are less effective. Thiazide diuretics become ineffective in the management of BP when creatinine clearance approaches 30 mL/min and below. At this point it becomes necessary to switch to (or add) a loop diuretic. Diuretics are well tolerated at doses equivalent to 25 mg of hydrochlorothiazide or 12.5 to 25 mg of chlorthalidone. Higher doses have demonstrated little additional antihypertensive efficacy and are associated with increased adverse effects. Side effects of thiazides include dysglycemia, dyslipidemia, hyperuricemia, sexual dysfunction, and nephrolithiasis may occur. Unlike loop diuretics, thiazides increase renal tubular reabsorption of calcium. Routine laboratory monitoring is required with thiazide-type diuretics to ensure that electrolytes, uric acid, lipids, and blood glucose remain within the normal range (Table 3-5).

Other Diuretics

Loop diuretics can also cause lipid, glucose, and electrolyte abnormalities; therefore, laboratory monitoring may be required to observe this transient effect. An important distinction, however, is that loops increase calcium excretion while thiazides decrease calcium excretion.

Potassium-sparing diuretics, such as amiloride or triamterene, can be used in combination with other agents in order to offset hypokalemia. These agents are not used as monotherapy for BP management.

Aldosterone antagonists are reserved for treating patients with resistant hypertension, hyperaldosteronism, or compelling indications (such as HF or post-MI). They can cause life-threatening hyperkalemia, especially when potassium is elevated at baseline, in patients with CKD, or when concomitant medications predispose patients to hyperkalemia.

Angiotensin-Converting Enzyme Inhibitors

ACEIs compete with angiotensin I for the angiotensin-converting enzyme and reduce the conversion of angiotensin I to angiotensin II (Table 3-5). Additionally, ACEIs

TABLE 3-5 Details of Oral Antihypertensive Agents

Class	Mechanism of Action	Adverse Reactions	Contraindications	Monitoring Parameters[a]
Thiazide diuretics	Increase the excretion of Na^+, Cl^-, and H_2O by inhibiting Na^+/Cl^- ion exchange in the early part of the distal tubule; lower blood pressure by decreasing extracellular fluid volume which decreases peripheral vascular resistance	Glucose disturbance Negative effects on lipids Electrolyte abnormalities ($\downarrow K^+$, Mg^{2+}, Cl^-, and HCO_3^-; $\uparrow UA$, Ca^{2+})	Anuria Thiazide or sulfonamide hypersensitivity	Blood glucose Lipids Electrolytes (Ca^{2+}, Mg^{2+}, K^+) BUN/SrCr UA
Loop diuretics	Inhibit the reabsorption of Na^+ and Cl^- in the ascending limb of the loop of Henle by interfering with the Cl^- binding of the $Na^+/K^+/2Cl^-$ cotransport system; renal vasodilation occurs, decreasing renal vascular resistance; reduce peripheral vascular resistance; the subsequent decrease in left ventricular filling pressure may contribute to the drug's beneficial effect in patients with congestive heart failure	Glucose disturbance Increase cholesterol and triglycerides Electrolyte abnormalities ($\downarrow Na^+$, Cl^-, K^+, Ca^{2+}, Mg^{2+}, and HCO_3^-; $\uparrow UA$)	Anuria	Audiometry Blood glucose BUN/SrCr Serum electrolytes UA Lipids
Potassium-sparing diuretics	Inhibit the Na^+/K^+ ion exchange in the distal renal tubule; inhibit sodium transport mechanisms directly, thereby setting up an electrical-potential difference across the membrane that blocks the passive distal tubular secretion of potassium; increase in urinary excretion of electrolytes and H_2O leads to a slight diuresis	Glucose disturbance Negative effects on lipids Electrolyte abnormalities ($\downarrow Na^+$, HCO_3^-, Ca^{2+}, and Cl^-; $\uparrow K^+$) Note: triamterene decreases Mg^{2+}, amiloride increases Mg^{2+}	Anuria Hepatic disease Renal failure Hyperkalemia	Blood glucose Lipids Serum electrolytes BUN/SrCr UA
Aldosterone antagonists	Inhibit effects of aldosterone on the distal renal tubules; enhance Na^+, Cl^-, and H_2O excretion; reduce the excretion of K^+, ammonium, and phosphate	Electrolyte abnormalities Gynecomastia and breast pain with spironolactone	Anuria Hyperkalemia Renal failure	BUN/SrCr Serum electrolytes
β-Blockers	Reduce both resting and exercise heart rate, cardiac output, and both systolic and diastolic blood pressure; reduce sympathetic outflow from the CNS and suppress renin release from the kidneys; agents with ISA stimulate β-receptors when sympathetic tone is low; agents that also block α-receptors or increase nitric oxide reduce peripheral vascular resistance	Exercise intolerance Fatigue Bradycardia Sexual dysfunction Depression Cold extremities Exacerbate reactive airway disease Exacerbate peripheral vascular disease Glucose disturbance $\uparrow$Triglycerides $\downarrow$HDL	AV block Cardiogenic shock Heart failure Hypotension	None
Angiotensin-converting enzyme inhibitors	Block the conversion of angiotensin I to angiotensin II by interfering with ACE activity; BP is also lowered through arterial dilation, lowering total peripheral vascular resistance; also inhibit kininase II (identical to ACE), an enzyme that degrades bradykinin, a potent vasodilator	Cough Angioedema Hyperkalemia Worsening renal function	Angioedema Hypersensitivity to ACE inhibitors Pregnancy	BUN/SrCr Electrolytes (K^+, Na^+)
Angiotensin receptor blockers	Antagonize angiotensin II at the AT_1 receptor subtype, which decreases systemic vascular resistance	Angioedema Hyperkalemia Worsening renal function	Pregnancy	BUN/SrCr Electrolytes (K^+, Na^+)

(Continued)

TABLE 3-5 | **Details of Oral Antihypertensive Agents (Continued)**

Class	Mechanism of Action	Adverse Reactions	Contraindications	Monitoring Parameters[a]
Calcium channel blockers: non-dihydropyridines	Inhibit the influx of extracellular Ca^{2+} across the myocardial and vascular smooth muscle cell membranes; decrease in intracellular calcium inhibits the contractile processes of the myocardial smooth muscle cells, resulting in dilation of the coronary and systemic arteries	Bradycardia Constipation Gingival hyperplasia Worsening of heart failure due to negative inotropic effect	Acute myocardial infarction AV block Cardiogenic shock Heart failure Hypotension Lown-Ganong-Levine syndrome Sick sinus syndrome Ventricular dysfunction Ventricular tachycardia Wolff-Parkinson-White syndrome	ECG ECHO LFTs
Calcium channel blockers: dihydropyridines	Inhibit the influx of extracellular Ca^{2+} across the vascular smooth muscle cell membranes; decrease in intracellular calcium inhibits the contractile processes of smooth muscle cells, resulting primarily in dilation of arteries	Dose dependent peripheral edema Headache Flushing	Dihydropyridine sensitivity	None
α_1-blockers	Cause peripheral vasodilation by selective, competitive inhibition of vascular postsynaptic α_1-adrenergic receptors, thereby reducing peripheral vascular resistance	Mild sexual dysfunction Nasal stuffiness Postural hypotension	None	None
Central α_2 agonists	Agonize presynaptic α_2-receptors in the medulla, inhibiting sympathetic outflow and tone; suppression of efferent sympathetic pathways decreases vascular tone in the heart, kidneys, and peripheral vasculature; lowers peripheral resistance	Bradycardia Dry mouth Orthostatic hypotension Rash (transdermal patch) Rebound hypertension	None	None
Direct vasodilators	Direct vasodilatory effect on arterial smooth muscle, reducing peripheral resistance; all direct vasodilators produce a compensatory sympathetic response including an increase in heart rate, stroke volume, and cardiac output, and a marked increase in plasma renin activity, which, in turn, leads to increased sodium and water retention	Orthostatic hypotension Reflex tachycardia (can abate with BB) Rebound Na^+ retention (abate with a loop diuretic) Minoxidil: hirsutism Hydralazine: drug-induced lupus	Minoxidil: pheochromocytoma Hydralazine: coronary heart disease, rheumatic heart disease	BUN/SrCr ANA with hydralazine

[a]With all antihypertensive medications, the response to therapy should be evaluated with careful monitoring of blood pressure and heart rate.

Abbreviations: ACE, angiotensin-converting enzyme; ACEIs, angiotensin-converting enzyme inhibitors; BBs, β-blockers; BUN, blood urea nitrogen; Ca^{2+}, calcium; CCBs, calcium channel blockers; Cl^-, chloride; ECG, electrocardiogram; ECHO, echocardiogram; HCO_3, bicarbonate; H_2O, water; ISA, intrinsic sympathomimetic activity; K^+, potassium; Mg^{2+}, magnesium; Na^+, sodium; SrCr, serum creatinine; UA, uric acid.

inhibit kininase II degrading the potent vasodilator brady-kinin to inactive peptides. Bradykinin-induced vasodilation is thought to contribute to the blood pressure lowering and cardiovascular protection afforded by ACEIs. Bradykinin has been implicated as the cause of ACEI-induced cough and angioedema. Compelling indications for the use of ACEIs are listed in Table 3-7.

Angiotensin Receptor Blockers

ARBs selectively block the effects of angiotensin II by binding to the AT_1 receptor subtype. Two angiotensin II receptors,

AT_1 and AT_2, have been identified. By selectively blocking the AT_1 receptor in tissues such as vascular smooth muscle and the adrenal gland, ARBs block the vasoconstrictor, inflammatory, and aldosterone-secreting effects of angiotensin II. ARBs do not influence bradykinin metabolism and therefore do not cause cough. In patients who experience a cough during treatment with an ACEI, an ARB can safely be substituted. ARBs can cause angioedema but the incidence is less than ACEIs.

While ACEIs initially suppress angiotensin II levels, other enzymes eventually restore angiotensin II production. These non-ACE pathways for angiotensin II formation have been

TABLE 3-6 **Oral Antihypertensive Drugs for Adults for HTN Indication[a]**

Class	Drug (Trade Name)	Dosage Range [Max Daily Dose (mg/d)][b]	Dose Frequency[b]	Most Common Routes of Administration
Thiazide diuretics[c]	Chlorothiazide (Diuril)	125-500[2000]	1-2	po, IV
	Chlorthalidone (generic)	12.5-25[50]	1	po
	Hydrochlorothiazide (Microzide, HydroDIURIL)	12.5-50[50]	1	po
	Indapamide (Lozol)	1.25-2.5[5]	1	po
	Metolazone (Zaroxolyn)	2.5-5[5]	1	po
Loop diuretics	Bumetanide (Bumex),	0.5-2[10]	2	po, IV
	Furosemide (Lasix),	20-80[600]	2	po, IV
	Torsemide (Demadex)	2.5-10[10]	1	po, IV
Potassium-sparing diuretics[c]	Amiloride (Midamor)	5-10[20]	1-2	po
	Triamterene (Dyrenium)	50-100[300]	1-2	po
Aldosterone antagonists[c]	Eplerenone (Inspra)	50-100[100]	1	po
	Spironolactone (Aldactone)	25-50[100]	1	po
BBs[c]	Atenolol (Tenormin)	25-100[100]	1-2	po, IV
	Betaxolol (Kerlone)	5-20[20]	1	po
	Bisoprolol (Zebeta)	2.5-10[20]	1	po
	Metoprolol (Lopressor)	50-100[450]	1-2	po, IV
	Metoprolol extended release (Toprol XL)	50-100[400]	1	po
	Nadolol (Corgard)	40-120[320]	1	po
	Propranolol (Inderal)	40-160[640]	2	po, IV
	Propranolol extended release (Inderal LA,)	60-180[160]	1	po
	Propranolol long acting (InnoPran XL/ Inderal XL)	80-120[120]	1	po
	Timolol (Blocadren)	20-40[60]	2	po
BBs with ISA	Acebutolol (Sectral)	200-800[1200]	2	po
	Penbutolol (Levatol)	80	1	po
	Pindolol (generic)	10-400[60]	2	po
Combination alpha-and β-blockers[c]	Carvedilol (Coreg)	12.5-50[100]	2	po
	Carvedilol extended release (Coreg CR)	20-40[80]	1	po
	Labetalol (Normodyne, Trandate)	200-800[2400]	2-3	po, IV
BB with NO activity	Nebivolol (Bystolic)	5-40[40]	1	po
ACE inhibitors[c]	Benazepril (Lotensin)	10-40[80]	1	po
	Captopril (Capoten)	25-100[450]	2-3	po
	Enalapril (Vasotec)	2.5-40[40]	1-2	po, IV
	Fosinopril (Monopril)	10-40[80]	1	po
	Lisinopril (Prinivil, Zestril)	10-40[80]	1	po
	Moexipril (Univasc)	7.5-30[30]	1	po
	Perindopril (Aceon)	4-8[16]	1	po
	Quinapril (Accupril)	10-40[80]	1	po
	Ramipril (Altace)	2.5-20[20]	1	po
	Trandolapril (Mavik)	1-4[8]	1	po
Angiotensin II receptor blockers[c] (ARB)	Candesartan (Atacand)	8-32[32]	1-2	po
	Edarbi (Azilsartan)	40-80[80]	1	po
	Eprosartan (Teveten)	400-800[900]	1-2	po
	Irbesartan (Avapro)	150-300[300]	1	po
	Losartan (Cozaar)	25-100[100]	1-2	po
	Olmesartan (Benicar)	20-40[40]	1	po
	Telmisartan (Micardis)	20-80[80]	1	po
	Valsartan (Diovan)	80-320[320]	1-2	po
Direct Renin Inhibitor[c]	Aliskiren (Tekturna)	150-300[300]	1	po

(Continued)

TABLE 3-6	Oral Antihypertensive Drugs for Adults for HTN Indication[a] (*Continued*)

Class	Drug (Trade Name)	Dosage Range [Max Daily Dose (mg/d)][b]	Dose Frequency[b]	Most Common Routes of Administration
CCBs: non-dihydropyridines[c]	Diltiazem (Cardizem)	30-180[480]	1	po, IV[d]
	Diltiazem extended release (Cardizem CD, Dilacor XR, Diltia XT, Tiazac, Tiazac XT)	240-360[540]		
	Diltiazem extended release (Cardizem LA)	120-540	1	
	Verapamil immediate release (Calan, Isoptin)	80-320[480]	2-3	po, IV
	Verapamil long acting, extended release, controlled acting(Calan SR, Covera HS, Isoptin SR[c], Verelan ER)	120-360[480]	1	po
	Verapamil long acting, extended release, controlled acting (Verelan PM)	120-360[400]	1	po
CCBs: dihydropyridines[c]	Amlodipine (Norvasc)	2.5-10[10]	1	po
	Felodipine extended release (Plendil)	2.5-10[10]	1	po
	Isradipine extended release (Dynacirc CR)	2.5-10[20]	1	po
	Nicardipine regular release	60-120[120]	3	po, IV
	Nicardipine sustained release (Cardene SR)	60-120[120]	2	po
	Nifedipine extended release (Adalat CC)	30-90[90]	1	po
	Nifedipine extended release (Procardia XL)	30-90[120]	1	po
	Nisoldipine extended release (Sular)	17-34[34]	1	po
α$_1$-blockers	Doxazosin (Cardura)	1-16[16]	1	po
	Prazosin (Minipress)	2-20[20]	2-3	po
	Terazosin (Hytrin)	1-20[20]	1-2	po
Central α$_2$ agonists[c]	Clonidine (Catapres)	0.1-0.8[2.4]	2	po, IV
	Clonidine patch (Catapres-TTS)	0.1-0.3[0.6]	1/wk	Transdermal
	Methyldopa (Aldomet)	250-1000[3000]	2-3	po, IV
	Reserpine (generic)	0.05-0.25[0.5]	1	po
	Guanfacine (Tenex)	0.5-2[3]	1	po
Direct vasodilators	Hydralazine (Apresoline)	25-100[300]	2-4	po, IV
	Minoxidil (Loniten)	2.5-80[100]	1-2	Po

[a]In some patients treated once daily, the antihypertensive effect may diminish toward the end of the dosing interval (trough effect).

[b]Dosage and frequency are for oral dosage forms.

[c]Drug class may be available in combination product.

[d]Diltiazem is also available as a powder for injection.

BP should be measured just prior to dosing to determine if satisfactory BP control is obtained. Accordingly, an increase in dosage or frequency may need to be considered. These dosages may vary from those listed in online drug resources of clinical pharmacology and package inserts.

Abbreviations: ACEIs, angiotensin-converting enzyme inhibitors; BBs, β-blockers; CCBs, calcium channel blockers; ISA, intrinsic sympathomimetic activity; NO, nitric oxide.

TABLE 3-7	Compelling Indications for the Use of Select Antihypertensive Classes

	Diuretic	BB	ACEI	ARB	CCB	AA
Heart failure	√	√	√	√		√
Post-MI		√	√	√		√
CAD risk	√	√	√		√	
DM	√	√	√	√	√	
Renal disease			√	√		
Recurrent stroke prevention	√		√	√		

Abbreviations: AA, aldosterone antagonist; ACEI, angiotensin-converting enzyme inhibitor; ARB, angiotensin II receptor blocker; BB, β-blocker; CCB, calcium channel blocker; DM, diabetes mellitus; post-MI, post-myocardial infarction.

deemed "ACE escape" and prompted the design of studies evaluating the benefit of combining an ACEI with an ARB. However, the combination of an ACEI and ARB is not recommended for the treatment of uncomplicated hypertension.

Calcium Channel Blockers

Dihydropyridine (DHP) and non-dihydropyridine (NDHP) CCBs have demonstrated efficacy in lowering BP and reducing cardiovascular events equal to that of other classes of blood-pressure medications. CCBs cause vasodilation and decrease total peripheral resistance. NDHPs slow heart rate, atrioventricular conduction, and should be used with caution in patients who are taking a β-blocker. DHPs can cause an initial reflex tachycardia; however, this is minimally seen with sustained release nifedipine and amlodipine. Short-acting CCBs (immediate release nifedipine) should be avoided due to the potential for rapid and profound BP changes and the risk of cardiovascular events. Side effects vary among CCBs because of the location of calcium antagonism (peripheral versus cardiac). See Tables 3-6 and 3-8 for key characteristics about CCBs.

β-Blockers

There are several types of β-blockers (BBs) and they include nonselective, cardioselective, intrinsic sympathomimetic activity, alpha blocking activity, and nitric-oxide activity

TABLE 3-8 | Causes of Resistant Hypertension

Improper blood pressure measurement
Volume overload
Excess sodium intake
Volume retention from kidney disease
Inadequate diuretic therapy
Drug-induced or other causes
Nonadherence
Inadequate doses
Inappropriate combinations
Nonsteroidal anti-inflammatory drugs; cyclooxygenase 2 inhibitors
Cocaine, amphetamines, other illicit drugs
Sympathomimetics (decongestants, anorectics)
Oral contraceptive hormones
Adrenal steroid hormones
Cyclosporine and tacrolimus
Erythropoietin
Licorice (including some chewing tobacco)
Selected over-the-counter dietary supplements and medicines (eg, Ephedra, ma huang, bitter orange)
Associated conditions
Obesity
Excess alcohol intake

(Table 3-5). BBs may be considered for the treatment of hypertension in patients with a compelling indication such as migraine headaches, cardiac arrhythmias, angina, MI, or heart failure. BBs are inferior to other classes of antihypertensive medications as first-line therapy in the absence of compelling indications. See Tables 3-6 and 3-8 for key characteristics about BBs.

Other Classes of Medications

- α₁ Blockers, such as doxazosin, terazosin, and prazosin, are reserved for patients with benign prostatic hypertrophy (BPH).
- Centrally-acting medications (eg, clonidine) and direct vasodilators (eg, minoxidil, hydralazine) should be reserved for resistant hypertension after spironolactone has been considered or ruled out due to contraindications or past adverse drug reaction or allergy.
- When direct-acting vasodilators are used for resistant hypertension, BBs and diuretics are often required to offset the reflex tachycardia and fluid retention that occurs with these agents.
- Aliskiren blocks the enzymatic activity of renin thereby interrupting the conversion of angiotensinogen to angiotensin I. It is as effective as other antihypertensives (eg, ACE inhibitors and ARBs) and works well with diuretics and CCBs. Preliminary studies suggest that the addition of aliskiren to an ACE inhibitor or ARB is associated with favorable changes in surrogate markers in patients with heart failure, proteinuria, and left ventricular hypertrophy.

Follow-up and Monitoring

After the initiation of antihypertensive therapy, patients should return for follow-up at monthly intervals until the BP goal is reached. More frequent visits are necessary for patients with stage 2 hypertension or complicating comorbid conditions or those with concerning laboratory levels that may be affected by therapy. Once BP goal is reached, follow-up visits can be at 3 to 6 month intervals. Serum creatinine and electrolytes should be monitored one to two times per year, perhaps more often in patients with CKD. Comorbidities such as heart failure, diabetes, and the need for laboratory testing influence the frequency of visits. Other cardiovascular risk factors should be monitored and treated to their respective goals, especially the cessation of tobacco use.

Special Populations

Diabetes

Hypertension and diabetes frequently coexist and together they significantly increase the risk of cardiovascular disease including stroke, progression of renal disease, and retinopathy. Patients with diabetes manifest hypertension at a disproportionate rate and the converse is also true such that patients with elevated BP are 2.5 times more likely to develop diabetes within 5 years. Consequently, persons with hypertension and diabetes warrant a tailored approach to BP control. Several classes of medications including diuretics, ACEIs, BBs, ARBs, and CCBs have been proven effective for reducing risk in patients with type 1 and type 2 diabetes. Each of these medications can be considered to treat elevated BP in persons with diabetes; however, an ACEI or ARB is considered first line. The majority of patients with diabetes will need two or more medications to control their BP. The most rationale combinations include either an ACEI or ARB combined with a diuretic or CCB.

Chronic Kidney Disease

More than 70% of patients with CKD, defined as a glomerular filtration rate (GFR) less than 60 mL/min/1.73 m^2 or the presence of albuminuria (>300 mg/d or 200 mg/g creatinine), have comorbid hypertension. Age-related deterioration of renal function is closely linked to BP, making aggressive BP control an important consideration in the prevention of end-stage renal disease, dialysis, and renal transplant. Treatment should consist of either an ACEI or ARB and diuretic in most patients. A loop diuretic should be substituted for a thiazide agent when GFR is markedly reduced (<30 mL/min/1.73 m^2).

While ACEIs and ARBs are recommended to control BP in patients with CKD, the GFR may decrease shortly after starting treatment. Angiotensin II is responsible for maintaining efferent arteriolar tone. Consequently, treatment with an ACEI or ARB will transiently reduce efferent arteriolar tone and lower GFR; this is a hemodynamic decline in GFR and does not represent kidney damage. In patients who experience a transient reduction in GFR, serum creatinine should not increase more than 30% and typically stabilizes or normalizes after 4 weeks. Treatment should continue in these patients. If creatinine increases by more than 30% or fails to stabilize after 4 weeks, other causes like NSAID use or volume depletion should be sought and corrected. Rarely, bilateral renal artery stenosis might be the culprit.

Heart Failure

Hypertension doubles the risk of developing HF and 90% of patients with HF have a history of hypertension. Both the sympathetic and renin-angiotensin systems are overactive in the setting of HF and contribute to disease progression. For these reasons, ACEIs, ARBs, and BBs are the cornerstone of treatment. These agents should be used routinely in patients with HF, in the absence of contraindications, because they reduce morbidity and mortality. Because volume retention is a hallmark of HF, loop diuretics are often necessary to control volume; however, these agents do not improve survival and thus should be used for symptomatic purposes. The aldosterone antagonists, spironolactone and eplerenone, reduce morbidity and mortality in advanced stages of HF (New York Heart Association class III and IV).

Spironolactone and eplerenone must be used cautiously in the setting of renal insufficiency due to the risk of hyperkalemia. While there are no authoritative recommendations for target BP in HF, there is evidence to suggest that BP lowering is beneficial.

Ischemic Heart Disease

The presence of hypertension increases the risk of coronary events and progression of atherosclerosis. Correspondingly, lowering BP reduces ischemic events and retards the progression of atherothrombotic disease in patients with ischemic heart disease. While lower BP generally improves outcomes, efforts should be made to maintain DBP above 55 to 60 mm Hg. Levels below have been shown to increase the risk for coronary vascular disease events due to the impairment of coronary artery filling during diastole. This J-shaped phenomenon has not been detected with systolic BP.

In patients with angina, BBs should be used to lower heart rate and BP, alleviate angina symptoms, and improve survival. If a BB is not appropriate due to bradycardia, AV block or severe reactive airway or peripheral arterial disease, DHP or NDHP CCBs may be considered.

Cerebrovascular Disease

The risk for ischemic stroke, hemorrhagic stroke, and dementia increases as a function of BP. BP control is the most important factor in the prevention of cerebrovascular disease. No specific agent or class of agents has been identified as the preferred method for BP control though preference should be given to diuretics, ACEIs, and ARBs.

In the setting of an acute stroke, the ideal strategy for BP control has not been elucidated. After an acute stroke, if systolic BP is above 220 mm Hg or DBP is between 120 and 140 mm Hg, it should be lowered cautiously by 10% to 15%. Simultaneously, neurological function should be vigilantly monitored for deterioration.

Resistant Hypertension

Resistant hypertension is defined as failure to achieve BP goal with full doses of an appropriate three-drug regimen that includes a diuretic. Implied within this definition is that patients are adherent to drug and lifestyle therapies and that a diuretic appropriate for renal function is being used. The causes of resistant hypertension are multifactorial and include drug and non-drug factors (Table 3-8). Improper measurement of BP is a common cause of falsely elevated BP. For example, use of a BP cuff that is too small in patients with obesity can result in an overestimation of BP. In patients with advanced atherosclerotic vascular disease, the brachial artery may not be easily compressible due to calcification and this may cause an overestimation of BP.

A transient rise in BP that occurs in the health-care setting, also known as white coat hypertension, can produce elevated BP readings in clinic settings but normal readings at home; this phenomenon can be documented with ambulatory

BP monitoring or home BP measurements. Volume overload is a common cause of resistant hypertension. Fortunately, diuretic therapy can easily palliate this type of BP.

Drug interactions are frequent causes of resistant hypertension. NSAIDs, steroids, sympathomimetic agents (eg, cold medications), and nontraditional remedies may increase BP or interfere with antihypertensive drugs. When remediable causes of secondary hypertension are unclear, secondary causes for hypertension should be explored. Of the secondary forms of hypertension, renal parenchymal disease is the most common secondary cause.

Other options in patients with resistant hypertension include the addition of spironolactone, direct-acting vasodilators, or referral to a specialist.

Hypertensive Crises

A hypertensive emergency is defined by a BP above 180/120 mm Hg with evidence of impending or progressive target organ dysfunction. These patients are susceptible to developing hypertensive encephalopathy, intracerebral hemorrhage, acute MI, acute left ventricular failure with pulmonary edema, unstable angina pectoris, dissecting aortic aneurysm, or eclampsia. Immediate BP lowering is warranted but the extent and timing of BP lowering is not clearly defined. When target organ damage is *absent* but BP is severely elevated, the event is deemed hypertensive urgency.

Hypertensive emergencies should be treated with a parenteral antihypertensive agent administered in an intensive care setting with continuous monitoring of BP. The goals of therapy are to avoid cardiovascular events and reduce mean arterial BP by up to 25% within the first hour, then, if stable, to 160/100 to 110 mm Hg within the next 2 to 6 hours. Gradual lowering of BP is necessary to avoid precipitating ischemic events. Normal BP should be achieved by 24 to 48 hours. In hypertensive urgency, immediate BP lowering is less urgent and rapid-acting *oral* agents such as captopril, labetalol, or clonidine can be considered; however, there is no evidence that these agents improve outcomes. When these therapies are used, it is important that patients have a follow-up visit within several days to ensure that BP has responded and that hypotension is not an issue. Alternatively, it is appropriate to adjust or titrate medications in treated patients and to encourage adherence.

Women

In women who are pregnant or are attempting to conceive, ACEIs and ARBs are contraindicated because of the risk of fetal developmental abnormalities. Lifestyle modifications are the mainstay of treating hypertension in pregnant women. When drug therapy is warranted, methyldopa is the drug of choice based on reports of stable uteroplacental blood flow and fetal hemodynamics and the absence of long-term adverse effects on development of children exposed to methyldopa in utero. BBs, especially labetalol, are considered alternatives to methyldopa.

Minorities

Hypertension is more common, more severe, develops at an earlier age, and leads to more clinical sequelae in blacks compared with persons of other descent. Mexican Americans and Native Americans also exhibit poor BP control rates. Minorities may respond well to weight reduction and sodium restriction and these interventions should be encouraged. Drugs that block the renin–aldosterone system, such as ACEIs, ARBs, and BBs, lower BP less in blacks compared with whites.

Other Special Considerations

In patients experiencing urinary outflow obstruction due to BPH, α_1 receptor antagonists may be used because they lower BP and dilate prostatic and urinary sphincter smooth muscle. α-blockers may cause stress incontinence in women and postural hypotension in elderly patients.

CASE Application

1. According to the 2017 guidelines for hypertension, what is the BP goal for a 58-year-old African American male with diabetes and chronic kidney disease?

   a. <130/80 mm Hg
   b. <140/90 mm Hg
   c. <150/90 mm Hg
   d. <160/100 mm Hg

2. Which of the following recommendations for lifestyle modification is correct?

   a. A minimum weight loss of 15 lb
   b. Sodium restriction of 4 g or less per day
   c. Reduce alcohol intake to no more than two drinks a day for a woman, one for a man
   d. Exercise for at least 30 minutes most days of the week
   e. Adopt an eating plan low in potassium and carbohydrates

3. JD is a 55-year-old African American woman with newly diagnosed hypertension. Her average BP is 164/91 mm Hg. Which of the following is the best recommendation for JD?

   a. Begin hydrochlorothiazide and return to clinic in 3 months.
   b. Begin metoprolol and prescribe monitoring blood pressure at home.
   c. Begin two medications since most patients with stage 2 hypertension will not reach goal with one agent alone.
   d. Prescribe lifestyle modifications first, and return to clinic in 1 month to determine if pharmacotherapy is warranted.
   e. Begin clonidine patch since a once weekly patch increases patient compliance.

4. TM was started on a new medication for her blood pressure. About a week later she noticed a persistent cough. Which of the following medications could be the cause?

   a. Maxzide
   b. Bystolic
   c. Vasotec
   d. Aldactone
   e. Catapres

5. You have identified the cause of the cough. At the next visit, TM wants to change the medication as she cannot tolerate the cough. Unfortunately, she missed her follow-up and returns to you in 6 months. In between appointments, she was admitted to the hospital and diagnosed with type 2 diabetes. Which of the following recommendations is best for TM assuming no insurance or cost issues?

   a. Switch to Lopressor
   b. Switch to Atacand
   c. Switch to Altace
   d. Switch to Cardizem
   e. Continue her current medication as this side effect usually resolves in a couple of months.

6. FS is a 50-year-old woman diagnosed with osteoporosis and hypertension. Which of the following antihypertensives is likely to help the FS's osteoporosis in addition to lowering her BP?

   a. Demadex
   b. Microzide
   c. Capoten
   d. Toprol XL

7. Which of the following statements is true regarding lifestyle modifications (LSM)? Select all that apply.

   a. LSM decreases the risk for cardiovascular disease.
   b. LSM decreases the risk for renal disease.
   c. LSM decreases morbidity.
   d. LSM is critical for the prevention of hypertension but not the treatment.

8. A patient presents to the emergency department with signs and symptoms of hyperkalemia. Electrolyte testing reveals serum potassium of 6.7 mmol/L. Which agents could cause or exacerbate the electrolyte abnormality? Select all that apply.

   a. Bumex
   b. Mavik
   c. Dyrenium
   d. Aldactone
   e. Cozaar

9. Which of the following is *true* regarding the use of combination treatment with an ACEI and an ARB for the treatment of hypertension?

   a. The combination significantly reduces the risk of cardiovascular events.
   b. The combination increases the risk of hyperkalemia.
   c. The combination is more effective for controlling blood pressure than monotherapy.
   d. This combination is recommended because it does not reduce cardiovascular events in this setting.

10. DL is a 35-year-old man recently diagnosed with type 2 diabetes, hypertension, hyperlipidemia, and sexual dysfunction induced by diabetic neuropathy. Which of the following two-drug regimens is most appropriate to initiate in DL for antihypertensive therapy?

    a. Amlodipine + lisinopril
    b. Short-acting nifedipine + trandolapril
    c. Doxazosin + HCTZ
    d. Pindolol + losartan
    e. HCTZ + lisinopril

11. ER is a 72-year-old male who presents to clinic. He is currently on lisinopril 40 mg daily, HCTZ 25 mg daily, and Amlodipine 10 mg daily. His blood pressure in clinic supports his elevated home readings, providing an average BP of 162/89 mm Hg. He is open to going adding therapy in addition to altering his diet with reduced sodium intake (however, in discussion his diet seemed appropriate). You have agreed to start spironolactone 25 mg daily. What side effects do you educate the patient about regarding the addition of spirlonlactone?

    a. Retrograde ejaculation
    b. Rebound hypertension if immediate discontinuation occurs
    c. Hypokalemia
    d. Gynecomastia

12. Which of the following is correct regarding the pathophysiology of hypertension?

    a. Most patients with hypertension have an identifiable secondary cause such as hyperaldosteronism.
    b. Cardiac output and peripheral vascular resistance are the two key factors that determine blood pressure.
    c. Stroke volume and heart rate are the two key factors that determine blood pressure.
    d. In the elderly, cardiac output rises, increasing the risk of hypertension, especially diastolic hypertension.

13. AC is a 46-year-old white man with a medical history significant for type 2 diabetes obesity, and new-onset hypertension. His current HA1c is 7.2%. He was started on lisinopril 10 mg daily 6 weeks ago and the dose was increased after 2 weeks to 20 mg daily. It has been 4 weeks since any alterations in therapy and in clinic his BP is 146/94 mm Hg and his heart rate is 67 beats/min. Which of the following is the most appropriate recommendation for AC?

a. Continue current regimen.
b. Discontinue lisinopril and start diltiazem.
c. Discontinue lisinopril and start HCTZ.
d. Add atenolol.
e. Add amlodipine.

14. TJ is a 64-year-old man with long-standing hypertension. He has recently been diagnosed with chronic kidney disease and his estimated glomerular filtration rate (eGFR) is 24 mL/min. He is currently taking ramipril 10 mg daily. His blood pressure is 148/86 mm Hg, heart rate is 58 beats/min, and electrolytes notable for a potassium of 5.1 mEq/L. Upon physical examination, the patient is noted to have slight peripheral edema; however, ECHO was without evidence of systolic heart failure (ejection fraction estimated at 60%) however noted left ventricular dysfunction. Which of the following would be the most appropriate recommendation at this time?

a. Continue current therapy and monitor BP regularly.
b. Add HCTZ 12.5 mg daily.
c. Add furosemide 20 mg daily.
d. Start verapamil ER to 360 mg daily.
e. Add spironolactone 25 mg daily.

15. RH is a 47-year-old white woman who has been seen by her family physician twice in the last 2 weeks, and her BP (measured properly) was similar at both visits, averaging 138/88 mm Hg. RH has no significant medical history or risk factors for cardiovascular disease; she is relatively active and likes to exercise. Which of the following would be the most appropriate recommendation for RH?

a. She should be seen again by her physician within 3 months to see if she has hypertension, but in the meantime work with recommended lifestyle modifications listed within this chapter.
b. She should be counseled to undertake an intensive weight reduction program, with follow-up in 2 years.
c. Initiate treatment with ramipril.
d. Initiate treatment with atenolol.
e. Initiate treatment with clonidine.

16. In a patient with risk factors for hyperkalemia and history of hyperkalemia, which of the following agents would be acceptable treatment to avoid hyperkalemia risk?

a. Amiloride
b. Amlodipine
c. Enalapril
d. Spironolactone
e. Valsartan

17. Which of the following agents is likely to increase blood glucose? Select all that apply.

a. Chlorthalidone
b. Furosemide
c. Hydrochlorothiazide
d. Lisinopril
e. Propranolol

18. FS is a 56-year-old man with diabetes mellitus and newly diagnosed hypertension. His mean blood pressure in clinic today after three proper measurements is 158/101 mm Hg. He is not currently on treatment. Which of the following drug regimens would be the most appropriate to treat FS?

a. Chlorthalidone
b. Quinapril
c. Benazepril + amlodipine
d. Benazepril + losartan
e. Atenolol + HCTZ

19. What diagnostic classification is an average blood pressure of 158/104 mm Hg on June 1st and an average blood pressure of 150/110 mm Hg on June 4th (both blood pressure averages were taken on two separate clinic dates as the patient refused to go to the emergency department)?

a. Normal
b. Elevated
c. Stage 1 hypertension
d. Stage 2 hypertension

20. Which of the following requires monitoring in a patient on HCTZ? Select all that apply.

a. Renal function
b. Hepatic function
c. Electrolytes
d. Uric acid
e. Blood glucose

21. Which of the following should be considered in patients with resistant hypertension? Select all that apply.

a. Volume overload is a common cause.
b. Spironolactone might be effective.
c. Minoxidil might be effective.
d. A loop diuretic might be necessary.

22. Which of the following blood pressure classifications would include lifestyle modifications as a recommended intervention? Select all that apply.

a. Blood pressure 130/84
b. Elevated
c. Stage 1 hypertension
d. Stage 2 hypertension
e. Blood pressure 149/92

23. Place the lifestyle modifications of weight reduction, moderation of alcohol consumption, and physical activity in order of the decrease in expected/approximate systolic blood pressure reduction. Start with the lowest expected decrease in SBP.

    a. Moderation of alcohol consumption, physical activity, weight reduction
    b. Weight reduction, physical activity, moderation of alcohol consumption
    c. Physical activity, moderation of alcohol consumption, weight reduction

24. Which of the following lifestyle recommendation would have the potential to decrease the SBP the greatest in a 58-year-old patient with chronic kidney disease, diabetes, atrial fibrillation, and hypertension. The patient currently has stage 2 hypertension and is not receiving pharmacologic therapy.

    a. Physical activity
    b. Moderation of alcohol consumption
    c. Adopting the DASH eating plan
    d. Initiating an ACEI + chlorthalidone

TAKEAWAY POINTS ≫

- Hypertension is common, asymptomatic, and results in increased morbidity and mortality.
- Essential hypertension is the most common type of hypertension.
- Medications such as NSAIDs, hormonal therapy, and corticosteroids can be a cause of secondary hypertension.
- Lifestyle modification is the cornerstone of effective treatment. Limiting sodium intake and increasing intake of calcium and potassium, increasing physical activity, and avoiding smoking and alcohol are important lifestyle changes.
- Diuretic therapy should be considered for most patients as the initial treatment.
- Certain comorbidities, such as CKD, diabetes, and heart failure, should be considered in order to customize drug therapy.

- ACEIs and ARBs are mainstays in the treatment of diabetes, heart failure, and post-MI.
- BBs are important in patients with ischemic heart disease, HF, post-MI, angina, and arrhythmias, however, they are no longer recommended as first-line agents in the general population.
- Renal function and serum electrolytes should be monitored in patients treated with diuretics and antagonists of the renin-angiotensin system.
- RAAS blockers are contraindicated in pregnant women.
- Common side effects with antihypertensive medications include exercise intolerance and fatigue (BBs), bradycardia (BBs and NDHP CCBs), dose-dependent peripheral edema (DHP CCBs), electrolyte abnormalities (diuretics and RAS blockers), cough (ACEIs), and glucose and lipid disturbances (diuretics and BBs).

BIBLIOGRAPHY

Benowitz NL. Antihypertensive agents. In: Katzung BG, Masters SB, Trevor AJ, eds. *Basic & Clinical Pharmacology*. 12th ed. New York, NY: McGraw-Hill; 2012:chap 11.

Go AS, Bauman MA, Coleman King SM, et al. An effective approach to high blood pressure control: a science advisory from the American Heart Association, the American College of Cardiology and the Centers for Disease Control and Prevention. *Hypertension*. 2014;63:878-885.

National Institute for Health and Clinical Excellence. Hypertension: clinical management of primary hypertension in adults. National Institute for Health and Clinical Excellence 2011. Available at: http://www.nice.org.uk/. Accessed March 3, 2018.

Saseen JJ, MacLaughlin EJ. Hypertension. In: DiPiro JT, Talbert RL, Yee GC, Matzke GR, Wells BG, Posey L, eds. *Pharmacotherapy: A Pathophysiologic Approach*. 10th ed. New York, NY: McGraw-Hill.

Weber MA, Schiffrin EL, White WB, et al. Clinical practice guidelines for the management of hypertension in the community a statement by the American Society of Hypertension

and the International Society of Hypertension. *J Hypertens*. 2014;32(1):3-15.

Whelton PK, et al. 2017 High Blood Pressure Clinical Practice Guideline 2017 ACC/AHA/AAPA/ABC/ACPM/AGS/APhA/ASH/ASPC/NMA/PCNA Guideline for the Prevention, Detection, Evaluation, and Management of High Blood Pressure in Adults. file:///C:/Users/Jessica/AppData/Local/Packages/Microsoft.MicrosoftEdge_8wekyb3d8bbwe/TempState/Downloads/HYP.0000000000000065.full%20(2).pdf. Accessed March 3, 2018.

WS Aronow et al. ACCF/AHA 2011 expert consensus document on hypertension in the elderly: a report of the American College of Cardiology Foundation Task Force on Clinical Expert Consensus documents developed in collaboration with the American Academy of Neurology, American Geriatrics Society, American Society for Preventive Cardiology, American Society of Hypertension, American Society of Nephrology, Association of Black Cardiologists, and European Society of Hypertension. *J Am Coll Cardiol*. 2011;57:2037.

KEY ABBREVIATIONS

ACEI = angiotensin-converting enzyme inhibitor
AHA = American Heart Association
ASH = American Society of Hypertension
BBs = β-Blockers
BP = blood pressure
BPH = benign prostatic hypertrophy
CCB = calcium channel blocker
CKD = chronic kidney disease
CO = cardiac output
DASH = dietary approaches to stop hypertension
DBP = diastolic blood pressure

DHP = dihydropyridine
GFR = glomerular filtration rate
HF = heart failure
ISH =International Society of Hypertension
MI = myocardial infarction
NDHP = non-dihydropyridine
PVR = peripheral vascular resistance
RAAS = renin-angiotensin-aldosterone system
SBP = systolic blood pressure
SNS = sympathetic nervous system

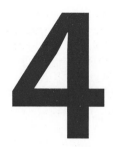

4 Acute Coronary Syndromes

Marintha R. Short, Nicholas C. Schwier, and
W. Anthony Hawkins

FOUNDATION OVERVIEW

Acute coronary syndrome (ACS) is a set of cardiovascular diagnoses that have similar pathophysiology, which involves atherosclerosis of the coronary arterial system. Atherosclerotic plaque may become unstable and lead to the development of a thrombus. Depending on the degree of coronary artery occlusion from the thrombus, the patient may experience ischemia and/or infarction of the neighboring tissue supplied by the occluded coronary artery or arteries. Diagnosis of the ACS subtype is important to guide life-saving interventions such as percutaneous coronary interventions (PCI), which include percutaneous transluminal coronary angioplasty (PTCA), as well as stent implantation into the inflicted coronary arteries. Both types of PCI facilitate unobstructed or improved flow of the coronary circulation distally from a thrombus. The first step in the recognition of ACS is to understand the classic clinical presentation. As the word "acute" implies, all subtypes of ACS have a sudden onset, differentiating them from stable angina. A patient presenting with ACS typically describes crushing chest pressure with radiation to the jaw, arm, and shoulder. Patients may also have a combination of nonspecific symptoms including diaphoresis, nausea, vomiting, and a sense of illness (Table 4-1). The diagnosis of ACS is confirmed with electrocardiography (ECG), which differentiates T-wave changes, and/or ST-segment depressions seen with unstable angina (UA) and non-ST segment elevation myocardial infarctions (NSTEMI), from the ST-segment elevation observed with ST-segment elevation myocardial infarction (STEMI). Additionally, cardiac biomarkers (troponin, creatine kinase-MB) are used to further differentiate UA (negative troponins) from myocardial infarction (positive troponins) (Figure 4-1).

PRIMARY PREVENTION

An estimated 16.5 million Americans more than or equal to 20 years of age has coronary artery disease (CAD), with a total prevalence of a 6.3%. The prevalence of MI (including both NSTEMI and STEMI) is 3%. Men have a higher prevalence with 7.4% compared to women at 5.3%. Due to the vast number of people afflicted with ACS each year, there is great interest in the prevention of ACS, as every 40 seconds, an American will suffer an MI. Large cohort studies have been performed to identify characteristics that put individuals at increased risk of developing CAD. The current risk calculator promoted by the American College of Cardiology (ACC), which is used to predict atherosclerotic cardiovascular disease (ASCVD), assesses gender, age, race, high total cholesterol measurement (or treatment with cholesterol-lowering medications), low HDL measurement, hypertension (or current treatment for hypertension), current cigarette smoking, and history of diabetes. Initiation of high or moderate intensity statin is recommended to reduce ASCVD based on risk score. Modifiable risk factors that are not incorporated in the risk calculator include abdominal obesity, low fruit and vegetable consumption, and lack of physical activity. If these risk factors are prevented or aggressively treated, the prevalence of ACS would likely decrease. The US Preventive Services Task Force recommends initiating low-dose aspirin use for the primary prevention of cardiovascular disease in adults aged 50 to 59 years who have a 10% or greater 10-year CVD risk, are not at increased risk for bleeding, have a life expectancy of at least 10 years, and are willing to take low-dose aspirin daily for at least 10 years. Once ACS events occur, initial treatments, medical management, and secondary prevention become vitally important.

TREATMENT

Overview and Treatment Goals

In the treatment of ACS, a clear delineation must be made between the emergency of treating STEMI and the urgency of treating NSTEMI and UA, now collectively referred to as NSTE-ACS. In patients experiencing STEMI, complete occlusion of a coronary artery results in elimination of blood flow to the distal heart muscle. It is vital that this vessel be revascularized in the shortest time possible from the onset of symptoms, in order to decrease morbidity and mortality. Therefore, patients with STEMI should proceed emergently to the cardiac catheterization lab, where they will undergo revascularization of the occluded coronary artery. Beyond 24 hours, it is likely that even if blood flow were restored, lack of oxygen would result in permanent muscle damage. Whereas, patients with NSTE-ACS may undergo early PCI or be managed more conservatively with medical therapy alone, due to the fact that NSTE-ACS usually represents a partial occlusion of coronary artery or arteries.

To access your complimentary online question exams, visit https://accesspharmacy.mhmedical.com/NAPLEX.aspx

TABLE 4-1	**Signs and Symptoms of Acute Coronary Syndrome**[a]

Signs of Acute Coronary Syndrome

- Elevated cardiac biomarkers
  - Troponin I or T
  - Creatine kinase-MB (CK-MB)
- Other potentially abnormal laboratory values
  - Elevated white blood count
  - Increased aspartate transaminase (AST)
  - Elevated lactate dehydrogenase (LDH)
- Electrocardiography (ECG) findings
  - ST-segment elevation myocardial infarction (STEMI)
  - New left bundle branch block (STEMI)
  - ST-segment depressions (NSTE-ACS)
  - T-wave changes (NSTE-ACS)

Symptoms of Acute Coronary Syndrome

- Chest pain (angina)
- Chest tightness/pressure (angina)
- Pain radiation to the left arm and/or jaw
- Diaphoresis (sweating)
- Nausea
- Vomiting
- Shortness of breath
- Palpitations
- Anxiety or sense of doom

[a]ACS presentation can be clinically silent, particularly in women and diabetes patients.

Symptomatic Therapies

Several therapies can be administered that are potentially life-saving and improve symptoms while the processes of diagnosing the ACS subtype and while early treatment strategies are being decided. These therapies include nitroglycerin (NTG), analgesia, oxygen, oral β-adrenergic receptor blockade, and antiplatelet therapies.

Because nitric oxide is an endogenous vasodilator that is decreased in patients with CAD, NTG can be given as an exogenous source of nitric oxide. In patients experiencing ACS, it is recommended to give NTG as a sublingual tablet or spray to relieve the acute symptoms associated with myocardial ischemia (MI) (ie, angina-like chest pain). The oral formulations of NTG are preferentially venodilators, thus decreasing preload and subsequently myocardial oxygen demand. Intravenous NTG may reduce ischemia via coronary vasodilation, increasing myocardial oxygen supply. NTG does not reduce mortality in the management of ACS. For patients with home NTG prescriptions, they may take one sublingual tablet or spray, and if there is no chest pain relief, emergency medical system (EMS) should be notified. The patient can continue taking NTG every 5 minutes (maximum of three doses in 15 minutes) until EMS arrives. Upon arrival to the hospital, intravenous NTG may be initiated and continued for the first

48 hours to treat ischemia that is refractory to SL or NTG spray, concomitant heart failure, or hypertension. Due to the risk of hypotension, NTG should be avoided in patients with evidence of right heart failure, systolic blood pressure (SBP) less than 90 (or ≥30 mm Hg below baseline), or received sildenafil/vardenafil in last 24 hours (tadalafil in last 48 hours).

In patients with chest pain, refractory to NTG, or present with contraindications to NTG, morphine 2 to 4 mg intravenously every 5 to 15 minutes may be given to aid in pain control but it does not provide survival benefit. In addition to opiate-mediated analgesia, morphine causes vasodilation of both veins (preload) and arteries (afterload), which decreases myocardial oxygen demand and increases myocardial oxygen supply, respectively. The pain felt is from MI. Morphine related vasodilation may also cause hypotension, limiting its usefulness in certain patients and requires blood pressure monitoring in all recipients. Although morphine is the analgesic of choice in patients experiencing STEMI, studies have brought into question the safety of use in NSTE-ACS, due to serious adverse effects such as respiratory depression. This has resulted in a downgrading of guideline recommendations regarding morphine use. Moreover, some data suggest that morphine may delay and diminish ticagrelor exposure and effect in patients suffering an MI.

In patients experiencing ACS, supplemental oxygen (delivered by nasal cannula or face mask) should be provided to maintain oxygen saturation greater than 90%. Adequate oxygenation ensures that blood reaching ischemic tissue has the maximum oxygen content available for delivery.

Initial Treatment

Antiplatelet Agents (Figure 4-2)

Oral Antiplatelet Agents (Table 4-2) ASA irreversibly inhibits formation of thromboxane A2 through cyclooxygenase inhibition, thus inhibiting vasoconstriction, platelet aggregation, and activation. At the onset of chest pain, patients should chew and swallow ASA 162 to 325 mg (two to four 81 mg chewable tablets are preferred). It is imperative that patients avoid simply swallowing ASA, especially enteric-coated formulations, as this may delay absorption. If not taken at home (or unknown), ASA should immediately be administered by EMS or upon arrival to the emergency department (ED). The benefit of ASA in patients with ACS has been clearly established and is strongly recommended in American Heart Association and the American College of Cardiology's (AHA/ACC) guidelines as antiplatelet agents, in general, limit the infarct size, reduce recurrent ischemia/infarction, and improve survival. Clopidogrel can be considered as an alternative to ASA, if a patient has a true ASA allergy.

In addition to ASA, it is recommended that patients with ACS be "loaded" on a P2Y$_{12}$ receptor antagonist (clopidogrel, prasugrel, or ticagrelor) unless the patient is known to already have CAD requiring surgery, and then the shorter-acting, intravenous, P2Y$_{12}$ receptor antagonist, cangrelor, may be considered. The thienopyridine class of P2Y$_{12}$ receptor antagonists (clopidogrel and prasugrel) inhibit platelet activation

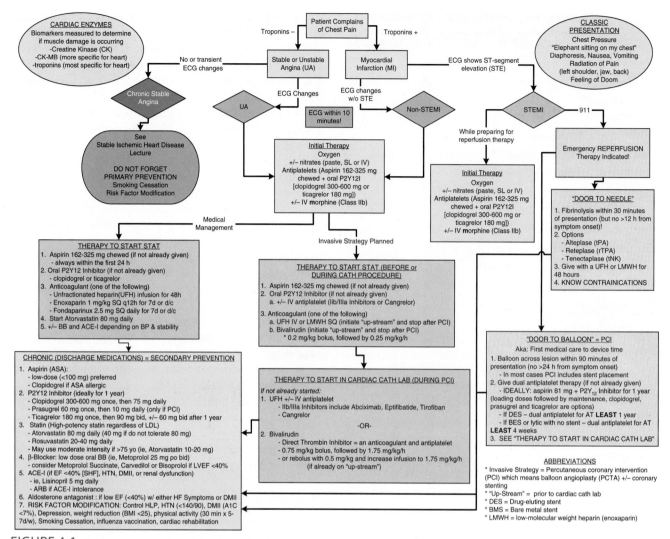

FIGURE 4-1   Acute coronary syndromes treatment flowchart.

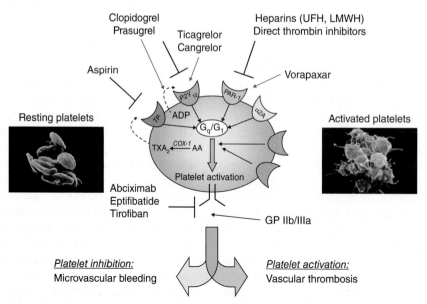

FIGURE 4-2   Overview of platelet activation and targeted inhibition.

TABLE 4-2   Oral Antiplatelet Therapies for Acute Coronary Syndrome

Drug	Aspirin	Ticagrelor	Clopidogrel	Prasugrel
MOA	Block production of thromboxane A2	Antagonists to adenosine diphosphate	Antagonists to adenosine diphosphate	Antagonists to adenosine diphosphate
Initial dose (pre-PCI)	162-325 mg	LD: 180 mg MD: 90 mg bid (Note: If given with ASA dose must be <100 mg daily)	LD: 300-600 mg MD: 75 mg daily	LD: 60 mg MD: 10 mg daily
PCI dose timing	Ideally, give at least 1 h before PCI	Load 6 h before PCI or up to PCI	Load 6 h before PCI or up to PCI	Load 30 min before PCI or up to 1 h after
Metabolism	Hepatic esterases	Transformed to active metabolite by CYP 3A4 (parent drug active as well) Hepatic and biliary	Transformed to active metabolite by mainly CYP-2C19	Multiple CYP450 isoenzymes
Elimination half-life	15-20 min parent drug; 3 h for metabolites	7-9 h	7-8 h	7 h (range 2-15 h)
Onset of antiplatelet effect	1-2 h	1-2 h	2-6 h	30 min
Offset of antiplatelet effects	7 d	5-7 d	5-7 d	5-7 d
CI	Severe thrombocytopenia (TTP/ITP), hematologic disorders, active bleeding, recent major surgery, hypersensitivity reactions	Active PUD or ICH, severe liver dysfunction, hematopoietic disorders	High risk for bleeding or severe HF, taking OAC, revascularization in previous 3 mo, received IIB/IIIa inhibitors within 3 d; PUD, ICH	FDA blackbox warning: history of ischemic or hemorrhagic stroke. Caution if weight ≤60 kg (lower dose). Not recommend if ≥75 unless STEMI or DM
ADE	Bleeding, GI ulcers	Dyspnea, increased cholesterol and triglycerides, TTP, diarrhea, life-threatening hematologic reactions, liver injury	GI: abdominal pain, vomiting dyspepsia, bleeding	Bleeding

Abbreviations: ADE, adverse drug effects; CI, contraindications; DM, diabetes mellitus; GI, gastrointestinal; ICH, intracranial hemorrhage; LD, Loading dose; MD, Maintenance Dose; MOA, mechanism of action; OAC, oral anticoagulant; PCI, percutaneous coronary intervention; PUD, peptic ulcer disease; TIA, transient ischemic attack; TTP/ITP, thrombotic thrombocytopenic purpura/idiopathic thrombocytopenic purpura.

by irreversibly blocking the $P2Y_{12}$ component of adenosine diphosphate (ADP) receptors. The nonthienopyridines (ticagrelor and cangrelor) reversibly inhibit the $P2Y_{12}$ receptor at an allosteric site. Dual antiplatelet therapy (DAPT) with a $P2Y_{12}$ receptor antagonist plus ASA is recommended over ASA monotherapy, both in the medical management of ACS and following PCI with coronary stent placement (bare metal or drug-eluting) because it decreases post-PCI re-thrombosis and recurrent MI. Historically, the thienopyridine most utilized in the United States is clopidogrel, as severe toxicities associated with ticlopidine, including hematologic side effects, limit its use. Clopidogrel is administered as a 300 mg or 600 mg oral loading dose and is available generically, but it does have multiple drug interactions that must be considered since it is a prodrug, metabolized to its active form by CYP 2C19. Therefore, it is recommended to avoid using clopidogrel with "potent CYP2C19 inhibitors" such as omeprazole, although the data are conflicting. Additionally, clopidogrel can possess variable effectiveness based on the patient due to a potential polymorphism through CYP 2C19. Because of this, the AHA/ACC guidelines initially recommended ticagrelor over clopidogrel. Ticagrelor should be administered as a 180 mg loading dose. Whether clopidogrel or ticagrelor is used, they should both be given as soon as possible or at the time of PCI. Due to the fact that ticagrelor is a nonthienopyridine, it may be used in patients with allergy to clopidogrel or prasugrel, as it is structurally unrelated. Prasugrel 60 mg should be administered as soon as possible or up to 1 hour after PCI. Prasugrel may infer increased antiplatelet benefits compared to clopidogrel, with the trade-off of increased bleeding. Prasugrel can be used in PCI-treated patients but is not recommended in patients who do not receive PCI with stenting and is contraindicated in patients with history of stroke or transient ischemic attack (TIA). An important pharmacodynamic difference in clopidogrel and prasugrel/ticagrelor is the onset of full antiplatelet activity; following clopidogrel loading, antiplatelet onset takes 1 to 6 hours (depending on the dose), while prasugrel and ticagrelor's antiplatelet onset is 30 minutes. Following discontinuation, it takes 5 to 7 days with clopidogrel and ticagrelor and 7 to 10 days with prasugrel for restoration of normal platelet function. Clopidogrel/ticagrelor and prasugrel should be stopped 5 to 7 days prior to coronary artery bypass surgery (CABG), respectively, in order to reduce bleeding risk. If surgery is performed in this platelet restoration window,

TABLE 4-3 Intravenous Antiplatelet Therapies for Acute Coronary Syndrome

Drug	Eptifibitide[a]	Tirofiban[a]	Abciximab	Cangrelor
MOA	Cyclic heptapeptide: blocks GPIIb/IIIa receptor	Nonpeptide inhibitor of GPIIb/IIIa	Antibody Fab fragment GPIIb/IIIa	Nonthienopyridine adenosine triphosphate analog (P2Y12) blocks ADP-induced platelet activation and aggregation
Initial dose (pre-PCI)	180 mcg/kg IV bolus followed by 1-2 mcg/kg/min for 12-96 h	Rapid infusion of 0.4 mcg/kg/min for 30 min, then 0.1 mcg/kg/min for 12-24 h	Not recommended prior to PCI	30 mcg/kg bolus prior to PCI
PCI dose	180 mcg/kg IV bolus over 1-2 min, times 10 min apart with an infusion of 1-2 mcg/kg/min for 18 h	25 mcg/kg over 3 min, then 0.15 mcg/kg/min for 24-48 h	0.25 mg/kg IV bolus; 0.125 mcg/kg/min (max 10 mcg/min) for 12 h	4 mcg/kg/min for 2 h or duration of PCI
Metabolism	Nonhepatic, renal	Metabolism unknown; 65% renally excreted	Unknown	Rapidly inactivated in the circulation by dephosphorylation to its primary metabolite
Elimination half-life	150 min	90-180 min	Phase 1 = 10 min Phase 2 = 30 min	3-6 min
Onset of antiplatelet effect	Within 20 min	Within 20 min	Within 20 min	2 min
Offset of antiplatelet effects	5-10 h	4-8 h	Usual 12 h, up to 24-48 h	1 h
CI	Hypersensitivity, major surgery within 6 wk, uncontrolled hypertension, history of hemorrhagic stroke, recent ischemic stroke within 30 days	Hypersensitivity, active bleeding, history of thrombocytopenia with prior exposure, major surgical procedure or severe physical trauma within past 30 days	Hypersensitivity, active bleeding or recent (within 6 wk), history of stroke within 2 y, bleeding diathesis, administration of oral anticoagulant within 7 d, thrombocytopenia (<100 K), major surgery or trauma within past 6 wk, intracranial neoplasm, arteriovenous malformation, aneurysm, severe uncontrolled hypertension, history of vasculitis, use of dextran before PCI or intent to use dextran with PCI	Allergy, significant bleeding, can't give clopidogrel or prasugrel until after discontinuing cangrelor. Ticagrelor can be administered during or after infusion.
ADE	Severe bleeding, hypotension (6%), thrombocytopenia (rare)	Major bleeding (1.4%), minor bleeding (10.5%), thrombocytopenia	Bleeding, GI hemorrhage, severe thrombocytopenia, hypotension (14.4%), bradycardia, GI intolerance	Hemorrhage, renal insufficiency, dyspnea

[a]Require renal adjustment.

Abbreviations: ADP, adenosine diphosphate; ADE, adverse drug effects; CI, contraindications; DM, diabetes mellitus; GI, gastrointestinal; ICH, intracranial hemorrhage; MOA, mechanism of action; PCI, percutaneous coronary intervention.

increased bleeding is likely. A thienopyridine alone may be given, if the patient has an ASA allergy.

Intravenous Antiplatelet Agents (Table 4-3) Glycoprotein IIb/IIIa inhibitors (GPI) block the final step of platelet aggregation. These medications have an established role *during* PCI in STEMI patients, to prevent early in-stent thrombosis following stent deployment, but their use is diminishing as more potent oral P2Y12 inhibitors come to market. They are reasonable for potential add-on therapy, up-front when DAPT is not used or the full loading dose of a P2Y12 receptor antagonist is not administered. The contemporary use of GP IIb/IIIa receptor antagonists is comprised of high-risk patients and use for

"bail-out" therapy. High-risk patients are those with complex lesions, large thrombi, and relatively high troponin levels. Patients considered for "bail-out therapy," are those who may present with coronary thrombus formation, vessel closure, dissection, and those patients who undergo complex PCI. However, several of these medications have also demonstrated benefit when started before PCI and in the medically managed patient. Eptifibatide and tirofiban can be used in addition to anticoagulants and oral antiplatelets in patients who will be medically managed or if delayed-PCI is anticipated. Abciximab should be reserved for patients who are managed with PCI only. Utility of GPI for medical management and as adjunctive treatment with PCI should be balanced with

TABLE 4-4	Anticoagulants for Treatment of Acute Coronary Syndrome			
Parameter	Unfractioned Heparin	Enoxaparin[a]	Fondaparinux	Bivalirudin
Mechanism	Inactivates IIa, IX, X, XI, XII, and plasmin	Inactivates Xa, IIa	Xa inhibitor	Direct thrombin inhibitor
Excretion	Hepatic (reticuloendothelial system)	Primarily renal	Renal	<20% renal
Half-life	1.5 h	4.5-7 h	17-21 h	25-57 min
Dose[b]	60 units/kg IVP (maximum of 4000 units), then 12 units/kg/h (maximum 1000 units/h) to target aPTT 50-70 s (or 1.5-2 times control)	NSTEMI/UA: 1 mg/kg every 12 h STEMI with thrombolytics: 30 mg IV bolus, followed by 1 mg/kg every 12 h (0.75 mg/kg every 12 h in patients >75 y)	2.5 mg subcutaneously daily (for medical management only, if given before PCI change to UFH for antithrombotic during procedure)	0.1 mg/kg IVP then 0.25 mg/kg/h with extra 0.5 mg/kg upon arrival to cath lab and increase infusion to 1.75 mg/kg/h. If started in cath lab, 0.75 mg/kg bolus, followed by 1.75 mg/kg/h
Contraindications	History of heparin-induced thrombocytopenia	Active heparin-induced thrombocytopenia	CrCl <30 mL/min	Active bleeding; Hypersensitivity
Monitoring	aPTT and ACT during PCI	None required, anti-Xa available if needed (obesity or renal insufficiency)	None	aPTT
Reversibility	Protamine	66% by protamine, FFP	FFP (No true antidote)	None

[a]Dose during PCI dependent on the timing of the last subcutaneous dose and concomitant IIb/IIIa use.

[b]Doses are based on normal renal function.

Abbreviations: ACT, activated clotting time; aPTT, activated partial thromboplastin time; CrCl, creatinine clearance; FFP, fresh frozen plasma; NSTEMI, non-ST segment elevation myocardial infarction; PCI, percutaneous coronary interventions; STEMI, ST-segment elevation myocardial infarction; UA, unstable angina; UFH, unfractionated heparin.

an increased bleeding risk and contraindications should be strictly observed. There is no readily available monitoring assay. If bivalirudin is chosen as the anticoagulant, it is reasonable not to use a GPI or heparin during PCI. The goal during PCI is 90% platelet inhibition, if stents are placed.

Currently, there is one available intravenous P2Y$_{12}$ receptor antagonist, cangrelor. Its use in ACS has not been fully established, but it has a quick onset/offset, is reversible, and was primarily used in patients that received PCI. This characteristic makes it a reasonable option for a patient that has coronary vessels that are more amenable for surgical bypass as opposed to stent placement for reperfusion (left main disease or multiple occlusions).

While STEMI patients must receive timely revascularization, patients with NTE-ACS may be treated in a variety of ways upon presenting to the ED. Some patients may proceed to early invasive therapy (PCI with stenting or CABG) while others will be managed conservatively with ischemia-guided therapy alone or as a bridge to delayed invasive therapy. Medical regimens within ischemia-guided therapy involve several acceptable anticoagulant schemes, with a gold standard of unfractionated heparin (UFH), given as an IV loading dose and then a continuous maintenance infusion adjusted to maintain an activated partial thromboplastin time (aPTT) 1.5 to 2 times baseline or 50 to 70 seconds (Table 4-4). Institutional nomograms will differ depending on the reagent used for testing. Although aPTT is the gold standard for UFH monitoring, an increasing number of institutions are utilizing anti-factor Xa for adjusting heparin across a variety of clinical scenarios. Determination of the appropriate anti-factor Xa level in ACS requires further study. Additional anticoagulation options include low molecular weight heparin (LMWH),

fondaparinux, or bivalirudin. Advantages of LMWH include ease of administration and usually do not require routine monitoring. Fondaparinux is preferred if the patient is at an increased risk of bleeding or has a history of heparin-induced thrombocytopenia (HIT), but only if PCI is not planned. Caution should be utilized with LMWH or fondaparinux in kidney disease which may impair elimination and increase the risk of bleeding. Finally, bivalirudin is recommended if PCI is planned, as a bridge to PCI. When bivalirudin is initiated prior to PCI, a small bolus (0.1 mg/kg) and low infusion rate are utilized (0.25 mg/kg/h). If bivalirudin is chosen when the patient arrives in the cardiac path lab for PCI, they receive a second larger bolus and the infusion rate is increased. Higher doses used during PCI are potent inhibitors of platelet activity. Bivalirudin may also be considered in patients with a history of HIT and dose adjustment may be warranted in patients with renal impairment. For patients that are medically managed, UFH may been continued 2 to 5 days. Fondaparinux and enoxaparin have been continued for the duration of hospitalization up to a total of 8 days.

Revascularization Therapy

If STEMI is diagnosed, the primary goal is to open occluded coronary vasculature in the shortest time possible with fibrinolysis and/or PCI but the latter is preferred in most areas of the country with access to an institution that is PCI-capable. Fibrinolytics (Table 4-5) catalyze the conversion of endogenous plasminogen to plasmin, which degrades fibrin and results in lysis of the thrombus. Although fibrinolysis may be administered up to 12 hours after the onset of chest pain, accrediting bodies have developed standards to guide how

TABLE 4-5	**Thrombolytics for Treatment of STEMI**
Drug[a]	**Dose**
Alteplase (tPA)	15 mg IV bolus followed by 0.75 mg/kg IV over 30 min (max 50 mg) followed by 0.5 mg/kg (max 35 mg) over 60 min (Maximum total dose: 100 mg)
Reteplase (rPA, Retevase)	10 units IV bolus over 10 min 2 times, 30 min apart
Tenecteplase (TNK)	<60 kg give 30 mg IV bolus over 5 sec 60-69.9 kg give 35 mg IV bolus over 5 sec 70-79.9 kg give 40 mg IV bolus over 5 sec 80-89.9 kg give 45 mg IV bolus over 5 sec >90 kg give 50 mg IV bolus over 5 sec

[a]Administer with UFH or LMWH for at least 48 h.

Abbreviation: IV, intravenous.

rapidly this emergency should be handled. The standard for fibrinolysis is a goal "door to needle time" of less than 30 minutes. Prior to administration of these potentially deleterious medications, it is always important to ensure that the patient does not have contraindications to fibrinolysis (Table 4-6). Because fibrinolytic therapy is unsuccessful in approximately 25% of patients, PCI with balloon angioplasty followed by coronary stenting is the preferred method of reperfusion. First medical contact (FMC) to device (PCI), is defined as the time between when the EMS provider arrives at the patient's side and when the patient receives some sort of PCI. The change in nomenclature (door-balloon) now accounts for the time the patient is experiencing ischemia, before they arrive to

TABLE 4-6	**Thrombolytic Absolute and Relative Contraindications**

Absolute Contraindications
▪ Any history of intracranial hemorrhage (ICH)
▪ Known malignant intracranial neoplasm (primary or metastatic)
▪ Ischemic stroke within 3 mo
▪ Suspected aortic dissection
▪ Active bleeding or bleeding diathesis (excluding menses)
▪ Significant closed-head or facial trauma within 3 mo
▪ Major surgery within 14 d
▪ Severe uncontrolled hypertension (SBP >180 mm Hg)
Relative Contraindications
▪ Chronic, severe, poorly controlled hypertension
▪ Traumatic or prolonged (>10 min) cardiopulmonary resuscitation (CPR)
▪ Major surgery within 14-21 d
▪ Internal bleeding within 2-4 wk
▪ Noncompressible vascular punctures
▪ Pregnancy
▪ Active peptic ulcer
▪ Concurrent use with oral anticoagulant (correct INR [international normalized ratio] first with fresh frozen plasma)

the hospital. The goal FMC to device is less than 90 minutes. Unfortunately PCI is not always possible, making fibrinolytics a viable option for hospitals that do not have cardiac catheterization services. If the patient can be transferred to a hospital with PCI capabilities and the stent deployed in less than or equal to 120 minutes, they should be transferred instead of using fibrinolytics. To prevent recurrent coronary thrombosis, anticoagulants (UFH, LMWH) should be used as adjunct with fibrinolytics for a minimum of 48 hours and recommended for the duration of the index visit up to 8 days. DAPT (ASA with clopidogrel and prasugrel) should be continued at least 14 days and ideally 12 months.

SECONDARY PREVENTION

The prevention of re-infarction and other complications from ACS should begin immediately. Prevention of re-thrombosis is not only aided by the previously mentioned antiplatelet therapies and short-term anticoagulation, but with other medications as well. These include hydroxy-methylglutaryl (HMG) coenzyme A reductase inhibitors (statins), β-adrenergic receptor blockers, and in certain patients, angiotensin-converting enzyme inhibitors (ACE-I) or angiotensin receptor blockers (ARB), as well as aldosterone receptor antagonists.

ASA should be given initially (325 mg) and then continued indefinitely in all patients with CAD, without contraindications. To minimize bleeding complications, it is preferred to give low dose ASA (75-81 mg) daily. Continuation of a $P2Y_{12}$ receptor antagonist is indicated for at least 12 months following the index event, and may be considered longer in patients who receive drug eluting stents. The ticagrelor dose after 12 months decreases to 60 mg twice daily, in certain patients. If the patient was medically managed using ischemia-guided therapy without stenting, prasugrel is not recommended for secondary prevention. Patients receiving ticagrelor therapy should not receive more than 100 mg of ASA daily as this may decrease the effect of ticagrelor therapy. If cangrelor is used, clopidogrel and prasugrel should be started after cangrelor is stopped while ticagrelor can be started during the cangrelor infusion. If there is a high bleed risk (eg, on anticoagulant) or developed significant overt bleeding, it is reasonable to stop the $P2Y_{12}$ receptor antagonist at 6 months. Vorapaxar 2.08 mg oral daily is a protease-activated receptor-1 antagonist that can be given with ASA and/or plavix for secondary myocardial infarction, stroke, or thrombosis prophylaxis for reduction of thrombotic cardiovascular events in patients with a history of myocardial infarction. Vorapaxar is contraindicated in patients with active pathological bleeding including intracranial bleeding or gastrointestinal (GI) bleeding and in patients with a history of stroke, TIA, or intracranial bleeding due to an increased risk of intracranial hemorrhage in such patients. This medication is a new addition to the armamentarium for secondary prevention for ACS and its niche or utility is yet to be determined.

HMG-coenzyme A reductase is the rate-limiting step in synthesis of atherogenic low density lipoproteins (LDL). The pharmacologic class of HMG-CoA reductase inhibitors

TABLE 4-7 High/Moderate Intensity Statin Dosing

High-Intensity Statin Dosing	
Atorvastatin	40-80 mg
Rosuvastatin	20-40 mg
Moderate-Intensity Statin	
Atorvastatin	10-20 mg
Rosuvastatin	5-10 mg
Simvastatin	20-40 mg
Pravastatin	40-80 mg
Lovastatin	40 mg
Fluvastatin XL	80 mg
Fluvastatin	40 mg bid
Pitavastatin	2-4 mg

(statins) that target this process have become an essential part of secondary prevention of ACS. Data support early and ongoing treatment with high-intensity statin therapy following ACS (Table 4-7). Benefits of statin therapy include slower progression of CAD, reduction of mortality if used more than 5 years, reduction of future cardiac events as well as prevention of plaque rupture leading to ACS, reduction of inflammation in coronary plaques, and inhibition of local platelet aggregation at the site of plaque rupture. This is why guidelines recommend use in patients whose cholesterol levels are unknown at the time of their event. The LDL goals have been a moving target over the past decade. The 2013 ACC/AHA guidelines for treatment of cholesterol to control ASCVD defined as coronary heart disease, stroke, and peripheral arterial disease in adults do not target LDL goals. Treatment with high-potency statin therapy should be initiated in anyone with an ACS event. If more than 75 years old, it is reasonable to use moderate intensity (Table 4-7). Secondary goals include LDL-C less than 100 mg/dL or LDL-C less than 70 mg/dL for very high risk patients (anyone with an ACS event).

β-Adrenergic receptor blockers are a diverse class of medications that are used in ACS to antagonize β_1-receptors in the heart with various other effects (Table 4-8). The preferred β-blocker would be void of intrinsic sympathomimetic activity. In the setting of ACS, β-adrenergic receptor blockers decrease heart rate which decreases myocardial oxygen demand, and also allow for increased perfusion of coronary arteries by augmenting time in diastole. Other benefits of β-blockers following an MI include decreasing arrhythmias and preventing recurrent events. It was previously recommended to give metoprolol 5 mg IV every 5 minutes; however, recent studies have demonstrated that early IV β-blockers increase the risk of cardiogenic shock. It is now recommended that early oral β-blockers are reasonable for patients that have high-risk characteristics (eg, high blood pressure), and are hemodynamically stable without evidence of heart failure, cardiogenic shock, or bradycardia. In the first 48 hours following MI, patients are at an increased risk of ventricular arrhythmias, sudden cardiac death, and are at the highest

risk for recurrent ischemia. The current goal is to initiate oral therapy within 24 hours of an MI. If there are contraindications, the patient should be re-evaluated at a later time for use as secondary prevention. Use of long-term β-blocker therapy (at least 3 years and indefinitely if left ventricular ejection fraction ≤40%) is recommended in patients without absolute contraindications. Long-term benefits of β-blockers are well established, particularly in patients with impaired ventricular function (heart failure). However, initiation should be with low doses and slow titration in these patients. Individual differences in the medications help guide which β-adrenergic receptor blocker to choose (Table 4-8). For example, patients with asthma should receive a β_1-selective β-blocker, while heart failure (HF) patients should receive metoprolol succinate, carvedilol, or bisoprolol.

Several studies have evaluated the use of ACE-I in patients who post-ACS have shown decreased mortality and incidence in recurrent MI. According to ACC/AHA guidelines, ACE-I therapy should be considered in all patients post-ACS indefinitely due to their ability to decrease sympathetic activity and improve baroreceptor sensitivity leading to increased vagal tone as well as slowing the rate of left ventricular dilatation and remodeling. ACE-I therapy is particularly useful in patients with the highest risk of recurrent MI (smokers, diabetes, multiple vessel disease, hypertension, renal dysfunction) and in those with heart failure. Absolute contraindications include allergy (history of angioedema to ACE-I), bilateral renal artery stenosis, and pregnancy. During initiation of ACE-I therapy, serum creatinine, potassium, and blood pressure should be monitored. In patients who experience bradykinin-mediated cough, ARBs are a reasonable alternative. Finally, the aldosterone receptor antagonist eplerenone showed mortality benefit when evaluated in post-MI patients with an ejection fraction less than or equal to 40% and either symptoms of HF or diabetes. Eplerenone should optimally be initiated within 3 to 14 days of the MI.

In addition to using medications to decrease remodeling of the heart tissue and decreasing plaque burden, there are several medications that can increase cardiac risk and should be avoided in patients who have a cardiac history. Hormone therapy with estrogen plus progestin, or estrogen alone, can increase coronary heart disease and thromboembolic events and should not be continued in previous users unless the benefits outweigh the estimated risks. Nonsteroidal anti-inflammatory drugs (NSAIDs) should not be administered to patients with ACS and chronic musculoskeletal discomfort unless acetaminophen, nonacetylated salicylates, tramadol, or small doses of narcotics are not effective or tolerated. If NSAIDs are used, it is important that the ASA dose is given at least 1 hour prior to the NSAID so that the ASA can reach its site of action on the platelet before the NSAID is administered and blocks ASA's access to its active site.

Similar to primary prevention, aggressively treating modifiable risk factors for CAD is essential to secondary prevention as well. These goals include: blood pressure reduction, depression, influenza vaccination, smoking cessation, heart healthy diet, exercise (at least 30 min/d, 5-7 days per week),

TABLE 4-8 β-Blockers

Generic Name	Brand Names	Pharmacology	Dose (po)	Dose (IV)	A	D	M	E	Role in Therapy
Propranolol	Inderal, Inderal LA	β_1- and β_2-blocker	80-320 mg divided 2-4 times daily (LA dosed once daily)	1 mg/dose over 5 min (max 10 mg)	Almost complete	Extensive	Hepatic	$t_{1/2}$ = 4 h LA: $t_{1/2}$ = 10 h	Angina, thyroid storm, migraine prophylaxis
Atenolol	Tenormin	β_1-selective	50-100 mg once or twice daily	5 mg IV every 10 min	F = 0.5	6%-16% protein bound	None	>50% renal, 50% unchanged $t_{1/2}$ = 6-7 h	Tachyarrhythmias, post-ACS/MI; dose adjust in patients with renal dysfunction
Metoprolol	Lopressor (metoprolol tartrate) Toprol XL (metoprolol succinate)	β_1-selective	100-400 mg daily (divided 2-3 times daily unless Toprol XL which is once daily). May be initially given every 6 h in initial management of ACS.	5 mg IV every 5 min 3 times	Tartrate: rapid and complete Succinate: F = 0.77	12% protein bound	Hepatic, >50% first-pass	<5% renal Tartrate: $t_{1/2}$ = 3-7 h Succinate: $t_{1/2}$ = 4-10 h	Consider metoprolol succinate in patients with decreased LVEF
Carvedilol	Coreg, Coreg CR	α_1-, β_1-, β_2-blocker	3.125-25 mg twice daily (50 mg twice daily if ≥85 kg); 10-80 mg daily (CR)	n/a	F = 0.25-0.3	98% protein bound	Hepatic via CYP2D6	$t_{1/2}$ = 7-10 h	Consider using carvedilol in patients with decreased LVEF
Bisoprolol	Zebeta	β_1-selective	2.5-20 mg daily	n/a	F = 0.8	30% protein bound	Hepatic (not P450 2D6)	Renal and nonrenal, 50% unchanged $t_{1/2}$ = 9-12 h	Consider using carvedilol in patients with decreased LVEF
Labetalol	Normodyne Trandate	α_1-, β_1-, β_2-blocker	200-400 mg bid or tid	0.25 mg/kg (20 mg) every 10 min	F = 0.25	50% protein bound	Hepatic conjugation	Fecal, renal (55%-60%) $t_{1/2}$ = 6-8 h (po), 5.5 h IV	Treatment of emergent hypertension
Esmolol	Brevibloc	β_1	n/a	500 mcg/kg IV bolus, 50 mcg/kg/min	n/a	55% protein bound	Esterases, hydrolysis	73%-88% renal $t_{1/2}$ = 9 min	Hypertensive emergency, aortic aneurysm, tachyarrhythmias
Nebivolol	Bystolic	β_1-selective vasodilatory properties	5-40 mg once daily	n/a	F = 0.12-0.96	98% protein bound	Hepatic, CYP2D6	Fecal 44%, renal 38%-67% $t_{1/2}$ = 12-19 h	Hypertension

Abbreviations: A, absorption; ACS, acute coronary syndrome; D, distribution; E, elimination; F, bioavailability; IV, intravenous; ISMA, intrinsic sympathomimetic activity; LVEF, left ventricular ejection fraction; M, metabolism; MI, myocardial ischemia; n/a, not available; po, oral.

weight reduction (body mass index to 18.5-24.9 kg/m²), and goal-directed treatment of diabetes (HbA1C <7%). Recently, the AHA/ACC, and American Society of Hypertension released a statement regarding blood pressure control in patients with CAD and hypertension. A target blood pressure of less than 140/90 mm Hg may be considered in most patients with CAD and hypertension. A target of less than 130/80 mm Hg is also reasonable in selected patients with CAD, including those with previous MI, stroke, or CAD risk equivalents. Since the coronary arteries are filled with blood during diastole, it is recommended that diastolic blood pressure not fall below 60 mm Hg, in order to maximize perfusion of the coronary arteries.

CASE Application

Questions 1 to 3 refer to the following patient case.

LC is a 76-year-old woman who presents to ED via EMS to a large academic medical center (with a coronary catheterization laboratory) complaining of sudden onset of diaphoresis and nausea. She states, "About 5 hours ago my chest started hurting and I just don't feel well." LC's weight is 65 kg.

Past medical history: CAD and arthritis

Family history: Father died of acute myocardial infarction at 76 years of age and mother passed away at age 70 from pneumonia

Social history: Does not drink alcohol; smokes 1 pack of cigarettes per week

Medications: ASA 81 mg orally once daily, atorvastatin 40 mg orally at bedtime, conjugated estrogens 0.625 mg orally daily, and celecoxib 200 mg orally daily

Laboratory data: Serum creatinine (SCr) = 1.9 mg/dL, total cholesterol 250 mg/dL, triglycerides 150 mg/dL, high-density lipoprotein (HDL) 40 mg/dL, LDL 130 mg/dL, troponin I = 5.7 ng/mL

Electrocardiogram: ST-segment elevation

1. Which one of the following is the preferred approach to reperfuse this patient?

   a. Chew ASA 81 mg, clopidogrel 75 mg, UFH for 48 hours
   b. Reteplase 10 units IV for two doses 30 minutes apart and UFH for 48 hours
   c. Chew ASA 325 mg, administer ticagrelor 180 mg orally once, abciximab 16.25 mcg IV bolus and percutaneous intervention with coronary stent placement
   d. Streptokinase 1,500,000 units IV over 30 minutes, ASA 81 mg, clopidogrel 300 mg

2. The physicians are debating on whether LC should receive early oral β-blockers after receiving ASA, ticagrelor, oxygen, nitrates, and morphine. Which of the following vital signs for TS would be conducive for early β-blocker use?

   a. Heart rate 110 beats/min; SBP 85 mm Hg
   b. Heart rate 50 beats/min; SBP 120 mm Hg
   c. Heart rate 120 beats/min; SBP 120 mm Hg
   d. Heart rate 120 beats/min; SBP 120 mm Hg with rales and rhonchi on physical examination

3. Which one of the following statements would you suggest to the attending physician prior to patient discharge regarding her home medication regimen? Select all that apply.

   a. Discontinue conjugated estrogens
   b. Continue ASA
   c. Discontinue celecoxib
   d. Start a β-blocker
   e. Start prasugrel

4. A patient experiencing chest pain for a few hours decides to take an SL tablet of NTG. The first tablet provides no pain relief, so EMS is contacted. The patient continued to take the NTG every 5 minutes. The third tablet she took provided relief. How do oral nitrates decrease chest pain?

   a. Vasoconstriction of venous vasculature
   b. Vasoconstriction of arterial vasculature
   c. Vasodilation of venous vasculature
   d. Decreased cardiac output

5. What is the mechanism of ticagrelor's benefit in a STEMI patient that has already received ASA, oxygen, nitrates, and morphine?

   a. Ticagrelor improves myocardial oxygen supply.
   b. Ticagrelor opens up the infarct-related artery.
   c. Ticagrelor reduces myocardial oxygen demand.
   d. Ticagrelor prevents myocardial reinfarction.

Questions 6 to 8 refer to the following patient case.

SK is a 68-year-old man who presents to his local physician's office after eating lunch at a local fast food restaurant. He complains of chest pain with radiation to his jaw. His physician has him chew ASA 325 mg and calls 911. He is transported to the local hospital where electrocardiogram shows ST-segment elevation.

Past medical history: Hypertension, CAD, chronic obstructive pulmonary disease (COPD), stage IV chronic kidney disease, cerebrovascular accident 2 months ago

Family history: Mother died of a stroke at 85 years and father passed away at 75 years in a car accident.

Social history: Smokes 1.5 packs of cigarette per day for 50 years; no alcohol history

Medications: Hydrochlorothiazide 25 mg orally daily, metoprolol tartrate 25 mg orally bid, tiotropium 18 mcg inhaled once daily, albuterol inhaler 1 puff every 6 hours as needed, fluticasone/salmeterol 250/50 mcg inhaled bid

Vital signs: Blood pressure 185/90 mm Hg, heart rate 98 beats/min, respiratory rate 22, O₂ saturation 88%, weight 100 kg

Laboratory data: Unavailable

Allergies: Heparin

6. SK presents at a hospital that does not have a cardiac catheterization laboratory; therefore, they have 30 minutes to verify his candidacy for fibrinolytic therapy. Which of the following is a contraindication (relative or absolute) to SK receiving a fibrinolytic? Select all that apply.

   a. SK already received ASA and clopidogrel.
   b. SK's blood pressure is 185/90 mm Hg.
   c. SK had a recent cerebrovascular accident.
   d. SK has an allergy to heparin.
   e. SK has a respiratory rate of 22.

7. Given SK's contraindication to fibrinolytic therapy, he was life-flighted to a hospital with 24 hour cardiac catheterization capabilities. The plan is for emergent PCI on arrival. Rank the anticoagulants in the order of shortest half-life to longest half-life.

Unordered Options	Ordered Response
Heparin	
Enoxaparin	
Fondaparinux	
Bivalirudin	

8. Which anticoagulant is the treatment of choice in a STEMI patient that is also dialysis dependent?

   a. Enoxaparin
   b. Dalteparin
   c. Fondaparinux
   d. Heparin

9. What laboratory value may be used to monitor the level of anticoagulation achieved with UFH?

   a. International normalized ratio (INR)
   b. Prothrombin time (PT)
   c. Anti-Xa level
   d. aPTT

10. Which of the following antiplatelet/anticoagulant regimens would be recommended for treatment of an NSTEMI patient with a heparin allergy? The patient is going to receive PCI later in the day.

    a. Bivalirudin
    b. Eptifibatide and LMWH
    c. Abciximab and UFH
    d. Fondaparinux

11. Which of the following agents is indicated in the setting of NSTEMI? Select all that apply.

    a. Eptifibatide
    b. UFH
    c. ASA
    d. Reteplase
    e. Clopidogrel

12. Once the acute phase of myocardial infarction has passed, which of the following therapies is most likely to slow the development of heart failure?

    a. Clopidogrel
    b. Atenolol
    c. Ramipril
    d. Amiodarone

13. PR is an 82-year-old woman who is status post drug-eluting stent placement following presentations with a STEMI. She has a past medical history significant for hypertension, dyslipidemia, and hypothyroidism. She has no known drug allergies. Which of the following is the best choice of long-term antiplatelet therapy?

    a. ASA 325 mg orally daily
    b. ASA 325 mg plus Ticagrelor 90 mg orally twice daily
    c. Ticagrelor 180 mg orally twice daily
    d. ASA 81 mg plus clopidogrel 75 mg orally daily

14. A patient with recent NSTEMI with an LDL of 150 mg/dL, total cholesterol (TC) of 192 mg/dL, triglycerides (TG) of 140 mg/dL, and HDL of 47 mg/dL and needs to be on a statin. Rank the following statins in order of lowest to highest potency.

Unordered Options	Ordered Responses
Pravastatin 20 mg po daily	
Simvastatin 20 mg po daily	
Atorvastatin 20 mg po daily	
Rosuvastatin 20 mg po daily	

15. Which of the following therapies requires routine monitoring of serum creatinine and potassium?

    a. Carvedilol
    b. Spironolactone
    c. Atenolol
    d. Pravastatin

16. Which of the following is an appropriate fibrinolytic dosing regimen for a 78-kg person with STEMI?

    a. Streptase 1 million units intravenously over 20 minutes
    b. Reteplase or rPA 10 units IV bolus twice 30 minutes apart
    c. Tenecteplase or TNK 80 mg IV bolus once
    d. Alteplase 100 mg IV over 2 hours

17. KE presents with chest pain, nausea, vomiting, and diaphoresis. He is diagnosed with an NSTEMI. Current blood pressure is 92/56 mm Hg and HR is 105 beats/min. Which of these medications should be given to this patient?

    a. ASA EC 325 mg orally once
    b. ASA 81 mg two tablets chewed once
    c. NTG IV drip at 20 mcg/min
    d. IV metoprolol 5 mg IV once

18. PR is a 62-year-old woman who presents to the ED with an NSTEMI. She has no significant past medical history. Pertinent data include: blood pressure 125/79 mm Hg, heart rate 75 beats/min, SCr 1.2 mg/dL, platelet count 142 k/uL, weight 94 kg. She has allergies to penicillin, sulfa, and ASA. Which of the following regimens are okay to give PR while she waits for her PCI? Select all that apply.

    a. ASA 324 mg once, then 81 mg daily
    b. Clopidogrel 300 mg once, then 75 mg daily
    c. ASA 162 mg once, then 81 mg daily plus clopidogrel 600 mg once, then 75 mg daily
    d. Prasugrel 60 mg once then 10 mg daily

19. Which of the following β-blockers are available in both oral and IV formulations? Select all that apply.

    a. Atenolol
    b. Esmolol
    c. Metoprolol
    d. Carvedilol
    e. Labetalol

20. Secondary prevention of an ACS in a patient with resulting HF (EF 35%) should include which of the following therapies assuming normal blood pressure? Select all that apply.

    a. HMG-CoA reductase inhibitors
    b. ASA
    c. Calcium channel blockers
    d. Fenofibrates
    e. ACE-I

TAKEAWAY POINTS »

- Hyperlipidemia, hypertension, tobacco abuse, and diabetes are major risk factors for the development of ACS.
- Reperfusion with fibrinolysis or PCI, in order to restore blood flow to the heart muscle, is the primary goal for treatment of STEMI.
- Home medications that increase risk for coronary events should be discontinued at the time of ACS event (eg, hormone replacement therapy [HRT] and NSAIDs).
- ASA should be chewed at the onset of chest pain to prevent thrombosis extension and continued for life for prevention of future cardiovascular events.
- When added to ASA, P2Y$_{12}$ receptor antagonists have been shown to decrease recurrent ischemic events. This benefit has to be balanced with the increased risk of bleeding.
- Morphine is the analgesic of choice for pain related to ACS; however, morphine should be used cautiously in patients who are hypotensive and those without planned PCI.
- Nitrates should be given at onset of chest pain as long as patient is not hypotensive or have used phosphodiesterase inhibitors within the last 24 hours (sildenafil or vardenafil) or 48 hours (tadalafil).
- Secondary prevention of ACS begins immediately with antiplatelet medications, HMG-CoA reductase inhibitors, β-adrenergic receptor blockers, and ACE-I. Eplerenone may be considered in patients with an EF ≤40% with either HF symptoms or diabetes mellitus (DM), after myocardial infarction.
- Secondary prevention includes aggressive treatment of modifiable risk factors (smoking, hypertension, dyslipidemia, diabetes, obesity, diet, and physical inactivity).
- GPI or direct thrombin inhibitors should be considered for management of patients with NSTE-ACS, reserving abciximab and bivalirudin for patients with planned (within 24 hours) PCI.

BIBLIOGRAPHY

Amsterdam EA, Wenger NK, Brindis RG, et al. 2014 AHA/ACC Guideline for the management of patients with non-st-elevation acute coronary syndromes: executive summary. *Circulation*. 2014;130:2354-2394.

Benjamin EJ, Blaha MJ, Chiuve SE, et al. Heart disease and stroke statistics 2017 update. *Circulation*. 2017;135:e1-e458.

Bibbins-Domingo K. Aspirin use to prevent cardiovascular disease and colorectal cancer: U.S. Preventive Services Task Force Recommendation Statement. *Annals of Internal Medicine*. 2016;164(12):836-845.

Katzung BG. Vasodilators and the treatment of angina pectoris. In: Katzung BG, Masters SB, Trevor AJ, eds. *Basic & Clinical Pharmacology*. 12th ed. New York, NY: McGraw-Hill; 2012:chap 12.

Kushner FG, Ascheim DD, Casey DE, et al. 2013 ACCF/AHA guideline for the management of ST-elevation myocardial infarction: Executive Summary. A report of the American College of Cardiology Foundation/American Heart Association Task Force on Practice Guidelines: developed in collaboration with the American College of Emergency Physicians and Society for Cardiovascular Angiography and Interventions. *Circulation*. 2013;127:529-555.

Michel T, Hoffman BB. Treatment of myocardial ischemia and hypertension. In: Brunton LL, Chabner BA, Knollmann BC, eds. *Goodman & Gilman's The Pharmacological Basis of Therapeutics*. 12th ed. New York, NY: McGraw-Hill; 2011:chap 27.

Rosendorff C, Lackland DT, Allison M. American Heart Association, American College of Cardiology, and American Society of Hypertension, et al. Treatment of hypertension in patients with coronary artery disease: a scientific statement from the American Heart Association, American College of Cardiology, and American Society of Hypertension. *J Am Coll Cardiol.* 2015;65:1998-2038.

Spinler SA, de Denus S. Acute coronary syndromes. In: DiPiro JT, Talbert RL, Yee GC, Matzke GR, Wells BG, Posey L, eds. *Pharmacotherapy: A Pathophysiologic Approach.* 9th ed. New York, NY: McGraw-Hill; 2014:chap 7.

Stone NJ, Robinson J, Lichtenstein AH, et al. ACC/AHA Blood Cholesterol Guideline to Reduce Atherosclerotic Cardiovascular Risk in Adults. *J Am Coll Cardiol.* 2013;25:2889-2934.

KEY ABBREVIATIONS

ACS = acute coronary syndrome
ACC = American College of Cardiology
ACE-I = angiotensin-converting enzyme inhibitor
ADP = adenosine diphosphate
AHA = American Heart Association
aPTT = activated partial thromboplastin time
ARB = angiotensin receptor blocker
ASA = aspirin
ASCVD = atherosclerotic cardiovascular disease
CABG = coronary artery bypass surgery
COPD = chronic obstructive pulmonary disease
DAPT = dual antiplatelet therapy
DM = diabetes mellitus
ECG = electrocardiography
EMS = emergency medical system

FMC = first medical contact
GI = gastrointestinal
GPI = glycoprotein IIb/IIIa inhibitor
HF = heart failure
HMG = hydroxy-methylglutaryl
LDL = low density lipoprotein
MI = myocardial ischemia
NSTEMI = non-ST segment elevation myocardial infarction
PCI = percutaneous coronary interventions
PTCA = percutaneous transluminal coronary angioplasty
STEMI = ST-segment elevation myocardial infarction
TIA = transient ischemic attack
UA = unstable angina
UFH = unfractionated heparin

5

Dyslipidemia

Rebecca F. Edwards

FOUNDATION OVERVIEW

General Overview

Dyslipidemia is defined as elevated total cholesterol (TC), low density lipoprotein cholesterol (LDL-C), triglycerides (TG), or high density lipoprotein cholesterol (HDL-C). LDL-C incites the atherosclerotic inflammatory response promoting unstable lesions concentrated with lipid-laden macrophages. The degree of LDL-elevation is proportionally linked with risk of developing atherosclerotic cardiovascular disease (ASCVD) (1 mg/dL: 1% change). Elevated TG have indirect atherosclerotic effects from procoagulant properties and an adverse impact on endothelial function. In contrast, HDL-C is an inverse predictor for ASCVD risk (1 mg/dL: 2% change) due to reverse cholesterol transport (delivering cholesterol from the cell wall to the liver for disposal). Additionally, HDL-C inhibits LDL-C oxidation and platelet aggregation and activation.

Dyslipidemia is a risk factor for clinical ASCVD, defined as coronary heart disease (CHD), cerebrovascular disease, or peripheral artery disease. Dyslipidemia is asymptomatic until vascular disease develops. Patients may present with pain or cramping with walking, cold extremities, shortness of breath, chest pain, sweating, difficulty with speech or movement, and sudden death. Severe hypertriglyceridemia (TG >1000 mg/dL) can lead to abdominal pain, nausea, vomiting, and other symptoms of pancreatitis.

Diagnosis

For adults 20 years of age or older, a lipid profile is recommended once every 5 years after a 12-hour overnight fast. The National Cholesterol Education Program (NCEP) ATP III classifies optimal and abnormal findings (Table 5-1). If testing is nonfasting, only HDL-C and TC will be accurate, and follow-up fasting lipid panel (FLP) is required for TC more than or equal to 200 or HDL-C less than 40 mg/dL. The LDL-C can be measured directly or calculated using the Friedewald equation (LDL-C = TC − HDL-C − TG/5). The calculation is less accurate when TG are more than 200 and inaccurate when more than 400 mg/dL.

Secondary causes of dyslipidemia such as obesity, obstructive liver disease, Cushing syndrome, tobacco use, alcohol overuse, hypothyroidism, anorexia nervosa, nephrotic syndrome, and undiagnosed or uncontrolled diabetes should

be considered. TG level can be lowered by improving glucose control. Many medications also increase cholesterol (eg, β-blockers, estrogens, androgens, thiazide diuretics, glucocorticoids, isotretinoin, protease inhibitors, mirtazapine, and cyclosporine). Conversely, acutely ill patients or those with recent cerebrovascular events may have significant drops in LDL-C within 24 to 48 hours of the event and falsely low levels for weeks.

PREVENTION

Dyslipidemia is associated with sedentary lifestyle, poor dietary choices, and obesity. Therapeutic lifestyle changes are strongly encouraged for all individuals with dyslipidemia and can prevent ASCVD. Individuals should be advised to exercise regularly if no precautions, follow a heart healthy diet, achieve and maintain a healthy weight, and stop smoking.

TREATMENT

General Overview and Goals of Treatment

The primary goal of dyslipidemia management is to reduce morbidity and mortality. The foundation of management is lifestyle modification. Although many efficacious lipid-lowering drugs exist, none is effective in all lipoprotein disorders, and all such agents are associated with some adverse effects. Lipid-lowering drugs can be broadly divided into agents that decrease the synthesis of very low density lipoprotein (VLDL) and LDL, agents that enhance VLDL clearance, agents that enhance LDL catabolism, agents that decrease cholesterol absorption, agents that elevate HDL, or some combination of these characteristics (Table 5-2). However, statins are usually recommended first-line when pharmacotherapy is indicated. Numerous randomized controlled trials demonstrate that statins reduce nonfatal and fatal ASCVD events, and all-cause mortality. Although pre-statin era studies support improved cardiovascular outcomes with niacin, fibrate, and bile acid sequestrant (BAS) monotherapy, the potential for harm from combining therapy with statins usually appears to outweigh benefits. As one example, women in the Action to Control Cardiovascular Risk in Diabetes (ACCORD) study taking fenofibrate with simvastatin had

TABLE 5-1 Classification of Total-, LDL-, HDL-C, and TG

Total cholesterol

<200 mg/dL (<5.17 mmol/L)	Desirable
200-239 mg/dL (5.17-6.20 mmol/L)	Borderline high
≥240 mg/dL (≥6.21 mmol/L)	High

LDL cholesterol

<100 mg/dL (<2.59 mmol/L)	Optimal
100-129 mg/dL (2.59-3.35 mmol/L)	Near or above optimal
130-159 mg/dL (3.36-4.13 mmol/L)	Borderline high
160-189 mg/dL (4.14-4.90 mmol/L)	High
≥190 mg/dL (≥4.91 mmol/L)	Very high

HDL cholesterol

<40 mg/dL (<1.03 mmol/L)	Low
≥60 mg/dL (≥1.55 mmol/L)	High

Triglycerides

<150 mg/dL (<1.70 mmol/L)	Normal
150-199 mg/dL (1.70-2.25 mmol/L)	Borderline high
200-499 mg/dL (2.26-5.64 mmol/L)	High
≥500 mg/dL (≥5.65 mmol/L)	Very high

Reproduced with permission from DiPiro JT, Talbert RL, Yee GC, et al: *Pharmacotherapy: A Pathophysiologic Approach*, 10th ed. New York, NY: McGraw-Hill; 2017

increased cardiovascular events compared to those on statin monotherapy. Therefore, nonstatin drugs are more reasonably selected for high-risk individuals unresponsive or unable to tolerate statins.

NCEP ATP III 2001 guidelines and a 2004 update recommended specific LDL-C goals based on the presence of CHD or equivalents, the number of heart disease risk factors, and Framingham risk scoring. LDL-C was endorsed as the primary target with aggressive reductions of less than 100 or less than 70 mg/dL for high-risk patients. The exception to targeting LDL-C is when TG are more than or equal to 500 mg/dL, when clinicians were advised to first consider use of fibrates, fish oil, or nicotinic acid to lower pancreatitis risk. Once LDL-C is at goal, the guidelines then suggested non-HDL-C (if TG remain ≥200 mg/dL) and metabolic syndrome as secondary targets, and HDL-C as a tertiary target.

However, the 2013 American College of Cardiology/ American Heart Association (ACC/AHA) guidelines advocate a new ASCVD risk-based treatment paradigm. The panel identified four groups of patients who would benefit from statin treatment with an acceptable margin of safety (Figure 5-1). The Pooled Cohort Equations for ASCVD risk prediction can be used to identify individuals in the fourth group. This prediction tool better estimates risk in black and white women and men. Clinicians may also elect to prescribe

TABLE 5-2 Effects of Drug Therapy on Lipids and Lipoproteins

Drug	Mechanism of Action	Effects on Lipids	Effects on Lipoproteins	Comment
Cholestyramine, colestipol, and colesevelam	↑ LDL catabolism Cholesterol ↓ absorption	↓ Cholesterol	↓ LDL ↑ VLDL	Problem with compliance; binds many coadministered acidic drugs
Niacin	↓ LDL and VLDL ↓ synthesis	↓ Triglyceride and ↓ cholesterol	↓ VLDL, ↓ LDL, ↑ HDL	Problems with patient acceptance; good in combination with bile acid resins; extended-release niacin causes less flushing and is less hepatotoxic than sustained release
Gemfibrozil, fenofibrate, clofibrate	↑ VLDL clearance ↓ VLDL synthesis	↓ Triglyceride and cholesterol	↓ VLDL, ↓ LDL, ↑ HDL	Clofibrate causes cholesterol gall stones; modest LDL lowering; raises HDL; gemfibrozil inhibits glucuronidation of simvastatin, lovastatin, and atorvastatin
Lovastatin, pravastatin, simvastatin, fluvastatin, atorvastatin, rosuvastatin	↑ LDL catabolism; inhibit LDL synthesis	↓ Cholesterol	↓ LDL	Highly effective in heterozygous familial hypercholesterolemia and in combination with other agents
Ezetimibe	Blocks cholesterol absorption across the intestinal border	↓ Cholesterol	↓ LDL	Few adverse effects; effects additive to other drugs
Mipomersen	Inhibitor of apolipoprotein B-100	↓ Cholesterol, LDL, non-HDL	↓ LDL, non-HDL	Increase in transaminases, risk of hepatosteatosis and hepatotoxicity; must be given by SQ injection. Only indicated for familial hypercholesterolemia. To be used along with other lipid-lowering therapies (statins)
Lomitapide	Microsomal triglyceride transfer protein inhibitor	↓ Cholesterol	↓ LDL, non-HDL	Hepatotoxicity must be monitored via Juxtapid Risk Evaluation and Mitigation Strategy program. Only indicated for familial hypercholesterolemia. To be used along with other lipid-lowering therapies (statins)
Alirocumab	PCSK9 inhibitor	↓ Cholesterol, ↓ Lpa	↓ Cholesterol and LDL	Given by SQ injection, injection site pain, low risk of hepatoxicity
Evolocumab	PCSK9 inhibitor	↓ Cholesterol, ↓ Lpa	↓ Cholesterol and LDL	Given by SQ injection, injection site pain, low risk of hepatoxicity

Reproduced with permission from DiPiro JT, Talbert RL, Yee GC, et al: *Pharmacotherapy: A Pathophysiologic Approach*, 10th ed. New York, NY: McGraw-Hill; 2017.

FIGURE 5-1 Four major statin benefit groups.

Four major groups of patients who would benefit most from statin treatment with an acceptable margin of safety, as defined by the 2013 ACC/AHA Guideline on the Treatment of Blood Cholesterol to Reduce Atherosclerotic Cardiovascular Risk in Adults.

Abbreviations: ASCVD, atherosclerotic cardiovascular disease; LDL-C, low density lipoprotein cholesterol

statins when 10-year risk is less than 7.5% considering other risk factors (eg, family history of premature ASCVD, high coronary calcium scores, ankle-brachial index <0.9%, LDL-C >160 mg/dL, or elevated lifetime ASCVD risk).

Moderate or high-intensity statin therapy is recommended depending on group classification (Table 5-3). High-intensity statin is preferred for most patients with clinical ASCVD, LDL-C more than or equal to 190 mg/dL, or diabetes with estimated 10-year risk more than or equal to 7.5%. Moderate-intensity statin is preferred for patients with clinical ASCVD over 75 years of age (although reasonable to continue high-intensity if tolerable), diabetes and 10-year risk less than 7.5%, or who are otherwise not candidates for high-intensity therapy. Either high- or moderate-intensity statin therapy is reasonable for patients without clinical ASCVD or diabetes

TABLE 5-3	High, Moderate, and Low Intensity Statin Therapy	
High	↓ LDL-C ≥50%	**Atorvastatin 40-80 mg** **Rosuvastatin 20**-*(40)* mg
Moderate	↓ LDL-C 30 to <50%	**Atorvastatin 10** *(20)* mg **Rosuvastatin** *(5)* **10 mg** **Simvastatin 20-40 mg** **Pravastatin 40** *(80)* mg **Lovastatin 40 mg** *Fluvastatin XL 80 mg* **Fluvastatin 40 mg bid** *Pitavastatin 2-4 mg*
Low	↓ LDL-C <30%	*Simvastatin 10 mg* **Pravastatin 10-20 mg** **Lovastatin 20 mg** *Fluvastatin 20-40 mg* *Pitavastatin 1 mg*

Bold indicates statins and doses studied in randomized controlled trials (RCTs) reviewed by the 2013 ACC/AHA expert panel, while those in italics are FDA-approved but were not evaluated in the reviewed RCTs. Simvastatin 80 mg was evaluated in RCTs but is not recommended due to higher risk of myopathy, including rhabdomyolysis.

who have estimated 10-year risk more than or equal to 7.5%. Patients with New York Heart Association (NYHA) class II-IV heart failure or receiving maintenance hemodialysis may not benefit from statins. In the setting of primary prevention where potential benefit is not as strong, clinician judgment, patient preference, and statin safety concerns guide treatment decisions. For patients not prescribed medication, the 10-year risk should be recalculated every 4 to 6 years.

If medication is started, a repeat FLP after 4 to 12 weeks with subsequent monitoring every 3 to 12 months is recommended. Follow-up testing can confirm an appropriate LDL-C decrease, which is sometimes not achieved due to either nonadherence or variability in statin response. If two consecutive LDL-C measurements are less than 40 mg/dL, consider decreasing the statin dose.

Specific Agents

HMG-CoA Reductase Inhibitors (Statins)

Statins competitively inhibit 3-hydroxy-3-methylglutaryl coenzyme A (HMG-CoA) reductase and reduce the biosynthesis of a cholesterol precursor mevalonate. Additionally, LDL-C clearance is enhanced by an increased expression of LDL receptors. Statins are the most effective class of drugs at reducing LDL-C (20%-55%). A 6% decrease in LDL-C can be expected for every doubling of the statin dose. Additionally, statins raise HDL-C (5%-15%) and lower TG to varying degrees. Statins also have pleiotropic effects including reduced inflammation, coronary plaque stabilization, improved endothelial cell function, reduced viscosity and fibrinogen levels, reduced uptake of aggregated LDL-C by vascular smooth muscle cells, reduced platelet aggregation, suppressed release of tissue factor, and activation of endothelial nitric oxide synthase.

Statins are well tolerated and side effects include dyspepsia, headache, insomnia, constipation, and diarrhea (<5% of patients). Statins have been associated with a small increased risk of diabetes (0.1-0.3 excess case per 100 individuals treated for 1 year) and hemorrhagic stroke (~0.01 excess case per 100). Additionally, patients rarely report rash, arthralgia, peripheral neuropathy, joint pain, and memory problems.

Myalgias occur in 5% to 10% of patients and are usually mild and tolerable. The myalgias are symmetrical and involve large proximal muscle groups. Myopathy describes all statin effects on muscle including symptomatic myopathy (myalgias, weakness, and cramps), creatine kinase (CK) elevations, and rhabdomyolysis. Mild CK elevation is less than 10 times the upper limit of normal (ULN), moderate more than or equal to 10 but less than 50 times ULN, and severe more than or equal to 50 times ULN. Moderate to severe CK elevations occurred in 0.17% of statin-treated and 0.13% of placebo-treated patients in clinical trials. Rhabdomyolysis refers to muscle cell destruction (regardless of CK level) that causes renal function changes. Rhabdomyolysis risk is increased with statin drug interactions (fibrate or CYP-3A4 inhibitors). Awareness of pharmacokinetic differences can help avoid these interactions (Table 5-4).

TABLE 5-4	**Pharmacokinetics of the Statins**						
Parameter	Lovastatin	Simvastatin	Pravastatin	Fluvastatin	Atorvastatin	Rosuvastatin	Pitavastatin
Isoenzyme	3A4	3A4	None	2C9	3A4	2C9/2C19	UGT1A3/UGT2B7
Lipophilic	Yes	Yes	No	Yes	Yes	No	Yes
Protein binding (%)	>95	95-98	~50	>90	96	88	99
Active metabolites	Yes	Yes	No	No	Yes	Yes	No
Elimination half-life (h)	3	2	1.8	1.2	7-14	13-20	12

Isoenzyme refers to the specific isoenzyme in the cytochrom P450 system which is responsible for the metabolism of each drug. Pharmacokinetic parameters in this table are based on studies and reviews presented in the literature.

Reproduced with permission from DiPiro JT, Talbert RL, Yee GC, et al: *Pharmacotherapy: A Pathophysiologic Approach*, 10th ed. New York, NY: McGraw-Hill; 2017.

Statin contraindications include pregnancy and active liver disease. However, studies support safety of statin therapy in patients with nonalcoholic fatty liver, and hepatitis B and C. Liver function tests (LFTs) have been historically recommended at baseline, 12 weeks after starting therapy, 12 weeks after any dose increase, and periodically thereafter. However, practice guidelines more recently advise LFT monitoring based upon clinical indication (symptoms). LFT elevations are usually transient and mild to moderate. Baseline CK levels are recommended in high-risk individuals. The CK is not routinely monitored but advisable in cases of unexplained muscle pain.

Niacin/Nicotinic Acid

Niacin is a B-complex vitamin that inhibits hepatic production of VLDL-C by reducing mobilization of free fatty acids from adipose tissues. It also increases the rate of TG removal from plasma, resulting in 20% to 50% decrease in TG. Niacin lowers LDL-C 20% to 30% by reducing hepatic synthesis and causes a shift to larger, less atherogenic particles. Niacin is the most potent medication at increasing HDL-C (15%-35%) and also reduces lipoprotein(a).

Prostaglandin-mediated flushing is a common adverse effect that mitigates over time. Paresthesias, headaches, pruritus, and syncope may also be reported with niacin. Niacin can cause gastrointestinal (GI) effects such as dyspepsia, nausea, anorexia, diarrhea, and peptic ulcer disease. Other side effects include maculopathy and hyperpigmentation (acanthosis nigricans), atrial fibrillation, increased LFTs, and severe hepatic toxicity.

LFTs, uric acid, and glucose/hemoglobin A1c should be assessed at baseline, during titration of therapy, and every 6 months (especially for doses >1500 mg/d). Absolute contraindications include active liver disease, unexplained LFT elevations, active peptic ulcer disease, arterial bleeding, and known hypersensitivity. Precautious include unstable angina or acute phase of myocardial infarction, use of concomitant anticoagulants, concomitant vasodilators, renal disease, substantial alcohol consumption, and history of liver disease. Niacin should also be used with caution in patients with gout and diabetes due to potential uric acid and glucose increases.

Bile Acid Sequestrants

BAS bind to cholesterol-containing bile acids in the intestinal lumen preventing their reabsorption. The liver then uses cholesterol to make more bile, which further lowers cholesterol. BAS reduce LDL-C (up to 25%), increase HDL-C (4%-5%) and either have no effect or can increase TG. Additionally, BAS lower apo B, C-reactive protein, and in combination with a statin or niacin, reduce small, dense LDL-C particles. BAS also lower fasting glucose and hemoglobin A1c (colesevelam is approved for type 2 diabetes).

Primary side effects of BAS include GI (eg, constipation, nausea, vomiting, dyspepsia, bloating, flatulence, and aggravation of hemorrhoids). BAS interfere with absorption of fat and fat-soluble vitamins (A, D, E, and K). BAS contraindications include history of hypersensitivity, elevated TG more than 500 mg/dL (colesevelam) or hyperlipidemia types III, IV, or V (cholestyramine), history of bowel or biliary obstruction, and history of hypertriglyceridemia-induced pancreatitis. BAS should be avoided for patients at risk for bowel obstruction secondary to gastroparesis, GI motility disorders, and history of major GI surgery. Caution should be used for patients with TG more than 300 mg/dL, susceptibility to fat-soluble vitamin deficiencies, preexisting constipation, and dysphagia (colesevelam).

Omega-3 Fatty Acids

The active lipid-lowering components of fish oil are eicosapentaenoic acid (EPA) and docosahexaenoic acid (DHA). EPA and DHA increase lipoprotein lipase activity, lower TG biosynthesis, and reduce hepatic lipogenesis. Additionally, they have cardioprotective effects (reduce platelet aggregation, decrease inflammation and blood pressure, reduce arrhythmias, improved endothelial function). The AHA recommends patients with CHD consume 1 g of EPA and DHA per day (preferably from diet) for potential cardiovascular benefits. Higher intake of 3 to 4 g/d of EPA and DHA is utilized for TG reduction (25%-30%) and HDL increases (3%). LDL-C can increase with higher doses, secondary to a shift to larger, less atherogenic particles.

Fish oil supplements are well tolerated even at higher doses. Dose-dependent eructation, dyspepsia, taste perversion, and GI disturbances are the most common adverse effects, occurring in 5% to 20% of patients. Clinical trials using standard dosing have shown no significant increase in bleeding risk. High doses may increase infection risk due to suppression of T- and B-cell function. Alanine aminotransferase and

LDL-C should be monitored periodically due to occasional increases. Clinically significant drug interactions are unlikely, with the exception of orlistat reducing absorption. Two prescription products, omega-3-acid ethyl esters (Lovaza®) and icosapent ethyl (Vascepa®) are approved for treatment of high TG (≥500 mg/dL) in adults. They are contraindicated in patients with past hypersensitivity (eg, anaphylaxis) to product ingredients.

Fibric Acid Derivatives (Fibrates)

Fibrates activate peroxisome proliferator–activated receptors (PPARs) to stimulate lipoprotein lipase accelerating lipoprotein degradation. Fibrates reduce hepatic apoprotein synthesis, resulting in lower TG (20%-50%) and higher HDL-C (10%-20%). Additionally, fibrates lower LDL-C (up to 20%) and cause a beneficial shift in particle size.

GI side effects are generally transient and occur in 5% of patients (less often with fenofibrate). Fibrates increase creatinine and LFTs and may cause gallstones and myopathy. Anemia and leukopenia have been observed and usually stabilize with long-term administration. Additional side effects include urticaria, increased homocysteine, acute hypersensitivity reactions, and venous thromboembolism (rare). Patients on warfarin should be closely monitored since fibrates can increase prothrombin time.

Contraindications to fibrates include gallbladder disease, history of hypersensitivity reactions, hepatic dysfunction, and severe renal impairment (creatinine clearance <30 mL/min for fenofibrate and <10 mL/min for gemfibrozil). Fibrates require renal adjustment in patients with mild to moderate renal impairment. Fenofibrate is also contraindicated in nursing mothers, and gemfibrozil is contraindicated in patients taking repaglinide (due to increased risk of hypoglycemia). Monitor complete blood count periodically during the first year of therapy, CK in patients with muscle pain or taking other myopathy-associated medications, LFTs every 3 months during the first year of gemfibrozil and then periodically thereafter, and LFTs periodically throughout therapy with fenofibrate. ACC/AHA guidelines also recommend renal function monitoring at baseline, within 3 months, and every 6 months for patients on fenofibrate.

Cholesterol Absorption Inhibitors

Ezetimibe inhibits dietary cholesterol absorption at the brush border of the small intestine. Ezetimibe also increases cholesterol clearance from the plasma, reduces formation of LDL-C, and decreases hepatic cholesterol stores. LDL-C is reduced by 15%-20%. Ezetimibe is approved as monotherapy and in combination with a statin or fenofibrate, but concomitant gemfibrozil should be avoided because of increased cholelithiasis risk. No dose adjustments are necessary in renal or hepatic impairment, but ezetimibe should be avoided in patients with moderate to severe hepatic disease.

Ezetimibe is well tolerated. Adverse reactions include diarrhea, fatigue, upper respiratory infection, arthralgia, fatigue, and myalgias. There are rare case reports of myopathy and rhabdomyolysis (usually when combined with a statin or fibrate). There are rare reports of angioedema and allergic reactions, and ezetimibe is contraindicated in patients with past hypersensitivity reactions. Patients on ezetimibe with statins are more likely to have elevated LFTs compared to statin monotherapy; therefore, LFTs should be monitored as clinically indicated.

Special Populations

Despite higher ASCVD risk, elderly patients with dyslipidemia are often undertreated. Studies support the safety and efficacy of statins and other medications in this population, but lower doses may be required to prevent adverse effects (eg, orthostatic hypotension with niacin). Fertile women on statins must use appropriate contraception and stop therapy 1 to 3 months prior to attempts to conceive. With the exception of BAS and LDL-C apheresis, other lipid-lowering treatments should also be avoided in pregnancy and during breastfeeding. Although high cholesterol in children is associated with premature CHD risk, there are limited outcomes data to support dyslipidemia treatment in this population. If diet changes are ineffective, the American Academy of Pediatrics recommends consideration of drug therapy in:

- Children 8 years of age or older with an LDL-C more than or equal to 190 mg/dL,
- Family history of early CHD,
- Two or more additional risk factors with LDL-C more than or equal to 160 mg/dL, and
- Those with diabetes when LDL-C is more than or equal to 130 mg/dL.

For children younger than 8 years of age, pharmacologic interventions are considered only for severe LDL-C elevations (>500 mg/dL). Both statins and BAS are FDA-approved for use in children.

Reducing ASCVD risk in patients unable to tolerate statins or very high LDL-C (eg, familial hypercholesterolemia) despite optimized statin therapy can be uniquely challenging. In infrequent cases of statin intolerance, first-line options include switching to another statin, intermittent-dosage regimens, and nonstatin lipid-lowering medications. Proprotein convertase subtilisin kexin type 9 (PCSK9) inhibitors alirocumab and evolocumab, FDA approved in 2015, may also be considered in carefully selected patients. PCSK9 is a hepatically produced serine protease implicated in LDL receptor degradation and subsequently increased LDL-C levels. Studies have demonstrated a 55% to 60% reduction in LDL-C, reduced atheroma volume, induction of plaque regression, favorable safety profile, and improved cardiovascular outcomes in patients taking maximally tolerate statin therapy. The limited long-term experience, requirement for injections, and expense (with need for prior authorization) currently compel use in only the highest risk patients. Lomitapide, a microsomal triglyceride transfer protein inhibitor, and mipomersen, an apo B production inhibitor, have significant safety limitations and are used only rarely to treat homozygous FH.

CASE Application

1. CX is a 62-year-old patient that presents to your pharmacy seeking guidance on an appropriate diet to reduce heart disease risk in a patient with high cholesterol. Which of the following lifestyle changes should be recommended to patients with dyslipidemia?

    a. Increase intake of animal products and low carbohydrate vegetables, and limit grains and fruit
    b. Reduce trans fat and limit saturated fat to <10% of calories
    c. Engage in regular physical activity
    d. Eat one serving per week of fatty fish

2. RR is a 56-year-old Asian man with an LDL-C of 180 mg/dL, HDL-C 28 mg/dL, and TG 140 mg/dL. His fasting glucose is 96 mg/dL, waist circumference 41 inches, and BP 128/82 mm Hg. Medications include hydrochlorothiazide and gemfibrozil. Which of the following indicates a risk for metabolic syndrome? Select all that apply.

    a. HDL-C
    b. TG
    c. Fasting glucose
    d. Waist circumference
    e. BP

3. MM is a 54-year-old woman with a past medical history of unstable angina, hypertension, and diabetes. She smokes two packs of cigarettes daily. Her LDL-C is 120 mg/dL, HDL-C 48 mg/dL, and TG 220 mg/dL. Which of the following therapy is recommended?

    a. Simvastatin 80 mg daily
    b. Atorvastatin 80 mg daily
    c. Pravastatin 20 mg daily
    d. Lovastatin 40 mg daily

4. CE is a 72-year-old man with no clinical ASCVD, no diabetes, and a 10-year ASCVD risk of 12%. Which of the following is recommended for this patient?

    a. Simvastatin 10 mg daily
    b. Fluvastatin 40 mg daily
    c. Pitavastatin 1 mg daily
    d. Rosuvastatin 10 mg daily

5. KW is a 53-year-old Asian woman with an LDL-C of 210 mg/dL, HDL-C 56 mg/dL, and TG 182 mg/dL. Her PMH is notable for hypertension with a recent BP of 118/70 mm Hg on lisinopril monotherapy. She is a non-smoker. Her father died of a myocardial infarction at 58 years of age. Her physician elects to use rosuvastatin and requests a dosing recommendation. Although a high-intensity statin is preferred for most patients with LDL-C >190 mg/dL, what is the most appropriate starting dose for KW considering genetic factors?

    a. 5 mg daily
    b. 10 mg daily
    c. 20 mg daily
    d. 40 mg daily

6. MJ has a history of subtherapeutic anticoagulation on warfarin (due to poor adherence) until the administration time was changed from evening to morning. The patient also frequently skips meals and takes antacids for reflux. Which of the following statins is optimal for this patient?

    a. Pravastatin
    b. Atorvastatin
    c. Lovastatin
    d. Rosuvastatin

7. CE is a 74-year-old man with a PMH of CHD, stroke, and hypothyroidism. He currently takes aspirin, levothyroxine, and simvastatin and has now been prescribed cholestyramine. What will you discuss with the patient?

    a. Take on an empty stomach once daily.
    b. Mix each dose with at least 12 ounces of juice or soda.
    c. Sip slowly to reduce side effects.
    d. Take other medications at least 1 to 2 hours before or 4 to 6 hours after taking cholestyramine.

8. Select the brand name for fenofibrate. Select all that apply.

    a. Fenoglide®
    b. Tricor®
    c. Triglide®
    d. Lipofen®
    e. Lopid®

9. What medication or combination is safest to use for a patient with advanced hepatic disease?

    a. Colesevelam
    b. Ezetimibe/simvastatin
    c. Niacin
    d. Gemfibrozil

10. JM is a 64-year-old woman with a PMH of pancreatitis (when TG 2200 mg/dL), uncontrolled gout, severe psoriasis, recurrent infections requiring hospitalization, and lovastatin-associated myopathy. Her current medications include rosuvastatin, prednisone, and allopurinol. Colchicine was also added a few days ago for a gout exacerbation. She reports an anaphylactic reaction after eating seafood in college. Her LDL-C is 96 mg/dL, HDL-C 42 mg/dL, and TG 640 mg/dL. Which of the following is the safest addition to her therapy?

    a. Niacin
    b. Colesevelam
    c. Fish oil
    d. Fenofibrate

11. Select the brand name for lovastatin.

    a. Lescol®
    b. Crestor®
    c. Mevacor®
    d. Zocor®

12. Which of the following statin(s) should be temporarily discontinued for a patient starting a short course of clarithromycin? Select all that apply.

    a. Simvastatin
    b. Pravastatin
    c. Lovastatin
    d. Atorvastatin
    e. Rosuvastatin

13. Which of the following statin doses may be dispensed to a patient also taking gemfibrozil? Select all that apply.

    a. Rosuvastatin 20 mg
    b. Simvastatin 20 mg
    c. Lovastatin 40 mg
    d. Fluvastatin 40 mg

14. LR is a 54-year-old woman with elevated TG who wants to substitute over-the-counter (OTC) fish oil instead of omega-3-acid ethyl esters (Lovaza®) to save money. Her physician approves this change. She mentions past gastrointestinal problems with dietary fish. What should you advise the patient regarding a product with 180 mg of EPA and 120 mg of DHA per capsule? Select all that apply.

    a. Change to the more concentrated cod liver oil
    b. Six capsules a day will equal the dose of the prescription product
    c. Take with meals to improve tolerability
    d. Eleven capsules a day will equal the dose of the prescription product
    e. Have your mercury levels tested periodically

15. Select a patient risk factor for development of myopathy on statin therapy. Select all that apply.

    a. Larger body size
    b. Hyperthyroidism
    c. Female sex
    d. Vitamin D deficiency
    e. Young age

16. What lipid-lowering medication(s) should be adjusted in a patient with renal impairment?

    a. Atorvastatin
    b. Gemfibrozil
    c. Ezetimibe
    d. Cholestyramine
    e. Niacin

17. A patient on simvastatin complains of muscle pain, weakness, and cramps since running a marathon this past weekend. His CK is 1760 U/L today (normal range, 50-160) and 280 U/L when checked 3 months ago. His Cr is 1.0 mg/dL. How should you manage this patient?

    a. Continue therapy and closely monitor the CK.
    b. Stop simvastatin until symptoms and CK improve, then try another statin.
    c. Add coenzyme Q10.
    d. Change simvastatin to ezetimibe.

18. JT is a 62-year-old woman with low HDL-C who was prescribed niacin. She did not fill her prescription because of the expense and instead took five 100-mg immediate-release crystalline niacin tablets at bedtime. She complains of flushing and dizziness after the first dose that almost caused her to fall. What is the best recommendation to improve overall tolerability?

    a. Change to a "no-flush" formulation and take 81 mg of aspirin 30 to 60 minutes before each dose.
    b. Start with 100 mg bid after breakfast and supper.
    c. Take with food and a hot liquid.
    d. Change to sustained-release OTC formulation.

19. LE is a 33-year-old woman currently attempting to become pregnant. Her physician decides that benefits of dyslipidemia treatment outweigh fetal risks. Her LDL-C is 240 mg/dL, HDL-C 64 mg/dL, and TG 132 mg/dL. Her PMH includes recent cholelithiasis. What is the most appropriate medication for LE?

    a. Rosuvastatin
    b. Niacin
    c. Colesevelam
    d. Gemfibrozil
    e. Omega-3-acid ethyl esters

20. CL is a 10-year-old boy with familial hyperlipidemia (FH). His physician wishes to use drug therapy since lifestyle changes have failed. His LDL-C is 320 mg/dL. Which of the following medications would you recommend?

    a. Atorvastatin
    b. Colesevelam
    c. Ezetimibe
    d. Niacin
    e. Fenofibrate

TAKEAWAY POINTS »

- Dyslipidemia, particularly elevated LDL-C, is strongly associated with ASCVD.
- TC less than 200, LDL-C less than 100, HDL-C more than or equal to 60, and TG less than 150 mg/dL are considered optimal.
- Adults over 20 years of age should have cholesterol screening every 5 years.
- Therapeutic lifestyle changes are the foundation of care for dyslipidemia.

- Statins are first-line drug therapy for dyslipidemia, reducing both cardiovascular and all-cause mortality.
- Niacin, fish oil, or gemfibrozil may be considered for patients with TG more than 500 mg/dL.
- Combining statins with other lipid-lowering medications increase risk for adverse effects.
- Four major groups of patients benefit from statin therapy with an acceptable margin of safety.

- High-intensity statin therapy is preferred for most patients with clinical ASCVD or with higher ASCVD risk.
- Fatal rhabdomyolysis with statins is rare. Myopathy is usually associated with preventable drug interactions or underlying patient risk factors.
- Statins and BAS are approved for treatment of hyperlipidemia in children.
- PCSK9 inhibitors may be considered in high-risk patients intolerant of statins or with very high LDL-C on maximally tolerated therapy.

BIBLIOGRAPHY

Baum SJ, Toth PP, Underberg JA, et al. PCSK9 inhibitor access barriers—issues and recommendations: improving the access process for patients, clinicians and payers. *Clin Cardiol*. 2017;40:243-254.

Bersot TP. Drug therapy for hypercholesterolemia and dyslipidemia. In: Brunton LL, Chabner BA, Knollmann BC, eds. *Goodman & Gilman's The Pharmacological Basis of Therapeutics*. 12th ed. New York, NY: McGraw-Hill; 2011:chap 31.

Daniels SR, Greer FR, and the Committee on Nutrition. American Academy of Pediatrics Clinical Report. Lipid screening and cardiovascular health in children. *Pediatrics*. 2008;122:198-208.

Eckel RH, Jakicic JM, Ard JD, et al. 2013 AHA/ACC Guideline on Lifestyle Management to Reduce Cardiovascular Risk: A Report of the American College of Cardiology/American Heart Association Task Force on Practice Guidelines. *J Am Coll Cardiol*. 2013;doi:10.1016/j.jacc.2013.11.003.

Expert Panel on Detection, Evaluation, and Treatment of High Blood Cholesterol in Adults. Executive Summary of the Third Report of the National Cholesterol Education Program (NCEP) Expert Panel on Detection, Evaluation, and Treatment of High Blood Cholesterol in Adults (Adult Treatment Panel III). *JAMA*. 2001;285(19):2486-2497.

Joy TR, Hegele RA. Narrative review: statin-related myopathy. *Ann Intern Med*. 2009;150:858-868.

Orringer CE, Jacobson TA, Saseen JJ, et al. Update on the use of PCSK9 inhibitors in adults: recommendations from an Expert Panel of the National Lipid Association. *J Clin Lipidology*. 2017;11:880-890.

Rader DJ, Hobbs HH. Disorders of lipoprotein metabolism. In: Longo DL, Fauci AS, Kasper DL, Hauser SL, Jameson J, Loscalzo J, eds. *Harrison's Principles of Internal Medicine*. 18th ed. New York, NY: McGraw-Hill; 2012:chap 356.

Stone NJ, Robinson J, Lichtenstein AH, et al. 2013 ACC/AHA Guideline on the Treatment of Blood Cholesterol to Reduce Atherosclerotic Cardiovascular Risk in Adults: A Report of the American College of Cardiology/American Heart Association Task Force on Practice Guidelines. *J Am Coll Cardiol*. 2013; doi:10.1016/j.jacc.2013.11.002.

Talbert RL. Hyperlipidemia. In: DiPiro JT, Talbert RL, Yee GC, Matzke GR, Wells BG, Posey L, eds. *Pharmacotherapy: A Pathophysiologic Approach*. 9th ed. New York, NY: McGraw-Hill; 2014:chap 11.

KEY ABBREVIATIONS

ACC = American College of Cardiology
ACCORD = Action to Control Cardiovascular Risk in Diabetes
AHA = American Heart Association
ASCVD = atherosclerotic cardiovascular disease
BAS = bile acid sequestrants
CHD = coronary heart disease
CK = creatine kinase
DHA = docosahexaenoic acid
EPA = eicosapentaenoic acid
FH = familial hyperlipidemia
FLP = fasting lipid panel
GI = gastrointestinal
HDL = high density lipoprotein
HDL-C = high density lipoprotein cholesterol
LDL = low density lipoprotein

LDL-C = low density lipoprotein cholesterol
LFT = liver function test
NCEP ATP III = National Cholesterol Education Program Adult Treatment Panel III
NYHA = New York Heart Association
OTC = over-the-counter
PCSK9 = proprotein convertase subtilisin kexin type 9
PMH = past medical history
PPAR = peroxisome proliferator–activated receptor
RCT = randomized controlled trial
TC = total cholesterol
TG = triglycerides
ULN = upper limit of normal
VLDL = very low density lipoprotein

CHAPTER 6

Stroke

Jessica Starr and Brea Rowan

FOUNDATION OVERVIEW

Ischemic stroke is an acute onset of focal neurological deficit that involves permanent infarction of central nervous system tissue. A transient ischemic attack (TIA) is similar to ischemic stroke but is caused by focal brain, spinal cord, or retinal ischemia without acute infarction. Cranial occlusions result from an embolus formed in the carotid arteries or the ventricles of the heart. Atherosclerosis of the carotid arteries leads to plaque formation and if plaque ruptures, collagen is exposed resulting in platelet aggregation and thrombus formation. The clot may break off and cause cranial vessel occlusion (decreased blood flow to the brain region it supplies) resulting in ischemia. Strokes originating from a cardioembolic source are presumed to originate from thrombus formation in the left ventricle. Clinical presentation includes weakness on one side of the body, visual impairment, and inability to speak. Diagnosis is confirmed via computed tomography (CT) scanning and magnetic resonance imaging (MRI). Risk factors for an ischemic stroke include hypertension, dyslipidemia, diabetes, cigarette smoking, and atrial fibrillation (Table 6-1).

PREVENTION

Primary prevention against ischemic stroke focuses on the reduction of modifiable risk factors (Table 6-1).

TREATMENT

The immediate goal of therapy is to reduce neurologic injury and long-term disability. Once the patient is through the hyperacute period, the goal of therapy is to prevent reoccurrence and decrease mortality.

ACUTE TREATMENT

The treatment for acute ischemic stroke has a narrow therapeutic window; therefore, a timely evaluation and diagnosis is essential. There are two pharmacologic agents recommended by the American Heart Association Stroke Council for acute stroke treatment (recombinant tissue plasminogen activator [rtPA/Activase®]) and aspirin.

rtPA is a fibrinolytic agent able to achieve early reperfusion and improve neurological outcomes. rtPA exerts its effects via the initiation of local fibrinolysis. It binds directly to fibrin thereby causing plasminogen to convert to plasmin. Plasmin is the enzyme responsible for clot dissolution. rtPA is administered intravenously at a dose of 0.9 mg/kg (10% of the total dose given as an intravenous bolus over 1 minute and the remainder of the dose given over 1 hour). The maximum dose is 90 mg in patients weighing more than 100 kg. rtPA should be administered within 3 hours of symptom onset and if the time of onset is unknown, patients are ineligible to receive rtPA. The benefit of rtPA up to 4.5 hours after symptom onset has been established in specific patients. As a result, the American Heart Association Stroke Council now recommends the use of rtPA out to 4.5 hours in most patients. Because certain patient populations were not studied in the extended 3 to 4.5 hour window, guidelines list the following as relative exclusion criteria for rtPA use 3 to 4.5 hours after symptom onset: (1) age over 80 years, (2) oral anticoagulation regardless of the international normalized ratio (INR) value, (3) score greater than 25 on National Institutes of Health Stroke Scale, and (4) history of diabetes *and* stroke. Patients falling into these four exclusion criteria may be considered for rtPA, if they present within 3 hours of symptom onset.

Due to its effects on fibrin, rtPA puts patients at risk for major bleeding. Therefore, there are multiple exclusion criteria including platelets less than 100,000 mm^3, history of intracranial hemorrhage, elevated aPTT, and recent head trauma or stroke in previous 3 months. The American Heart Association Stroke Council differentiates several relative exclusions for which the benefits and risks of giving rtPA must be carefully weighed. Some of these relative exclusions are pregnancy, recent major surgery, and recent acute myocardial infarction (Table 6-2).

The other pharmacologic agent approved for acute stroke is aspirin. Aspirin decreases morbidity and mortality when administered within 24 to 48 hours of stroke onset. The recommended initial dose is 325 mg. Aspirin does not alter the neurological outcomes of stroke; aspirin prevents recurrent strokes. If a patient receives rtPA, aspirin and other antithrombotic agents should be held for at least 24 hours after rtPA is administered.

TABLE 6-1	**Risk Factors for Ischemic Stroke**
Nonmodifiable	
Age	Younger age groups (25-44 y) are at lower risk
Low birth weight	Low birth weight patients have a higher mortality rate
Race/ethnicity	Blacks and some Hispanic/Latino Americans are at higher risk
Genetics	Positive family history increases risk
Gender	Men have a greater risk than women
Modifiable	
Hypertension	Most important modifiable risk factor Treat to a goal of <140/90 mmHg
Dyslipidemia	Use of statin therapy in addition to lifestyle changes decreases risk in high-risk patients (coronary heart disease or diabetes)
Diabetes	There is no correlation with glycemic control; however, risk is reduced when blood pressure is controlled
Cigarette smoking	Abstention from cigarette smoking by nonsmokers and smoking cessation by current smokers decreases risk
Atrial fibrillation	Risk is decreased with concomitant use of antithrombotic therapy

Neurological deterioration occurs with low and high blood pressures. Blood pressure treatment should be withheld unless systolic blood pressure is above 220 mm Hg or diastolic blood pressure is above 120 mm Hg. However, if a patient meets all other criteria for rtPA, except elevated blood pressure, the recommendation is to decrease the blood pressure to less than 185/110 mm Hg before rtPA administration. Frequent blood pressure monitoring should occur during rtPA administration and during the subsequent 24 hours. Several antihypertensive agents are recommended for use during acute stroke. These include labetalol, nicardipine, and sodium nitroprusside. Sodium nitroprusside is reserved for blood pressure not controlled by labetalol and nicardipine, and should be used with caution in patients with renal insufficiency due to the risk of cyanide toxicity with prolonged use. If antihypertensive therapy is necessary, the blood pressure should be decreased by approximately 15% within the first day.

SECONDARY PREVENTION

Patients with a history of an ischemic stroke are at significantly increased risk of having another stroke. The American Heart Association Stroke Council recommends several different pharmacotherapy options for secondary prevention. The mainstay of therapy is long-term treatment with an antiplatelet agent; however, blood pressure and cholesterol lowering are also important. Currently, aspirin, clopidogrel, and extended-release dipyridamole plus aspirin are acceptable antiplatelet options for initial therapy. The American Heart Association Stroke Council does not give preference for one agent over another (Table 6-3). Ticlopidine is not recommended for

TABLE 6-2	**Exclusion Criteria for rtPA**

Exclusion Criteria

- Symptom onset >4.5 h
- Significant head trauma or prior stroke in previous 3 mo
- Symptoms suggest subarachnoid hemorrhage
- Arterial puncture at a noncompressible site within the previous 7 d
- History of previous intracranial hemorrhage
- Intracranial neoplasm, arteriovenous malformation, or aneurysm
- Recent intracranial or intraspinal surgery
- Elevated blood pressure (systolic >185 or diastolic >110 mm Hg)
- Active internal bleeding
- Acute bleeding diathesis
- Platelets <100,000 mm^3
- Heparin therapy within previous 48 h *and* aPTT above upper limit of normal
- Oral anticoagulation *and* INR >1.7 or PT >15 s
- Current use of direct thrombin inhibitors or direct factor Xa inhibitors with elevated sensitivity lab tests
- Blood glucose <50 mg/dL
- CT with multilobar infarction

Relative Exclusion Criteria

- Only minor or rapidly improving stroke symptoms (clearing spontaneously)
- Pregnancy
- Seizure at onset with postictal residual neurological impairments
- Major surgery or serious trauma within the previous 14 d
- Recent gastrointestinal or urinary tract hemorrhage within the previous 21 d

Relative Exclusion Criteria for Extended Window (3-4.5 h)

- Age >80 years
- National Institute of Health Stroke Scale (NIHSS) score >25
- Taking oral anticoagulants *regardless* of INR value
- History of *both* diabetes and previous stroke together

Abbreviations: aPTT, activated partial thromboplastin time; INR, international normalized ratio; NIHSS, National Institute of Health Stroke Scale; PT, prothrombin time; rtPA, recombinant tissue plasminogen activator.

TABLE 6-3	**Antiplatelet Therapy Recommendations for the Secondary Prevention of Ischemic Stroke**

Antiplatelet Therapy	**Recommendation**
Aspirin 50-325 mg po daily	Acceptable initial therapy
Clopidogrel 75 mg po daily	Acceptable initial therapy Alternative to aspirin-allergic patients Do not use in combination with aspirin
Extended-release dipyridamole 200 mg plus aspirin 25 mg po twice daily	Acceptable initial therapy

use. Patients with a cardioembolic source (atrial fibrillation) should be treated with antithrombotic therapy including warfarin, dabigatran, apixaban, rivaroxaban, or aspirin.

Patients with a TIA or acute minor stroke may benefit from dual antiplatelet therapy with aspirin and clopidogrel for 21 days followed by clopidogrel therapy for days 22 through 90.

Aspirin is the most well-studied antiplatelet agent used in the secondary prevention of stroke. Aspirin's antithrombotic effects occur by irreversible inhibition of platelet cyclooxygenase ultimately leading to a reduction in platelet aggregation. The current dosing recommendation varies from 50 to 325 mg/d. Most studies have shown that high and low dose aspirin prevent the reoccurrence of stroke with higher doses associated with a greater risk of gastrointestinal hemorrhage. Adverse reactions include gastrointestinal ulcerations and duodenal ulcers.

Clopidogrel works through selective, irreversible inhibition of adenosine diphosphate–induced platelet aggregation. It is given as a 75-mg tablet once daily. The safety of clopidogrel is comparable to aspirin and the incidence of neutropenia and thrombotic thrombocytopenic purpura are low. Clopidogrel is an alternative to aspirin in those patients who are allergic to aspirin. The combination of clopidogrel with aspirin is not recommended as there is an increased risk of hemorrhage.

Dipyridamole inhibits phosphodiesterase resulting in accumulation of adenosine and cyclic-3′,5′-adenosine monophosphate and platelet aggregation inhibition. The combination of aspirin and dipyridamole is given as a capsule that contains dipyridamole extended-release pellets in 200 mg and immediate-release aspirin in 25 mg. The combination capsule is taken twice daily. Adverse effects include headache, dyspepsia, and abdominal pain.

Ticlopidine is not recommended by the American Heart Association Stroke Council due to side effects. Ticlopidine causes severe gastrointestinal effects, neutropenia, agranulocytosis, aplastic anemia, and thrombotic thrombocytopenic purpura.

Oral anticoagulants including warfarin, dabigatran, apixaban, and rivaroxaban are effective treatment options for the prevention of stroke in patients with a cardioembolic source (atrial fibrillation). The selection of an antithrombotic agent should be individualized based on risk factors for stroke, bleeding, cost, and preference. Aspirin is recommended as an alternative to anticoagulation therapy in patients at low risk for stroke or with contraindications to anticoagulant therapy. In high-risk patients who have contraindications to anticoagulation that are not related to bleeding, dual-antiplatelet therapy with clopidogrel and aspirin may be considered.

Antihypertensive treatment is recommended for patients with a history of ischemic stroke who are beyond the first 24 hours, regardless of whether or not the patient has a history of hypertension. The optimal medication regimen remains unknown; however, there are data to support a thiazide-type diuretic or an angiotensin-converting enzyme inhibitor plus a thiazide-type diuretic.

Ischemic stroke patients should receive hydroxymethylglutaryl-coenzyme A (HMG-CoA) reductase inhibitors (statins) with intensive lipid-lowering effects to reduce the risk of recurrent events.

CASE Application

1. A 38-year-old white man with a past medical history. (PMH) significant for hypertension, diabetes, and chronic alcoholism comes to your clinic for routine follow-up. His social history is significant for alcohol and tobacco abuse. He currently drinks one case of beer per night and smokes two packs per day. Pertinent laboratory findings are as follows: total cholesterol (TC) 182 mg/dL, TG 218 mg/dL, low density lipoprotein (LDL) 96 mg/dL, high density lipoprotein (HDL) 52 mg/dL, glucose 146 mg/dL. Current blood pressure is 158/94 mm Hg and heart rate (HR) is 92 beats/min. He is 69 in tall and weighs 232 lb. Which of the following are risk factors for ischemic stroke in this patient? Select ALL that apply.

   a. Hypertension
   b. Tobacco abuse
   c. Diabetes
   d. African-American race
   e. Age

2. Which of the following statements accurately describes the acute presentation of ischemic stroke?

   a. Acute infarction of the central nervous system tissue, one-sided weakness, systolic blood pressure >200 mm Hg
   b. Neurologic dysfunction without infarction, one-sided weakness, visual impairment
   c. Acute infarction of the central nervous system tissue, one-sided weakness, visual impairment
   d. Neurologic dysfunction without infarction, one-sided weakness, blood glucose >200 mg/dL

3. JS is a 78-year-old white woman with a PMH significant for atrial fibrillation, systolic heart failure with an ejection fraction of 35%, and hypertension. She presents to the emergency department with symptoms of right-sided paralysis. She is not able to communicate, but her family member states that the symptoms began approximately 5 hours ago. MRI of the brain confirms the patient has had an ischemic stroke. At home she takes metoprolol 100 mg po bid, lisinopril 40 mg po daily, and furosemide 20 mg po daily. Which of the following medications would be the most appropriate for secondary stroke prevention in JS?

   a. Ticlopidine
   b. Clopidogrel
   c. Warfarin
   d. Extended-release dipyridamole plus aspirin

4. HB is a 54-year-old African American man who presents to the emergency department with symptoms of left-sided paralysis and visual impairment. He has a

PMH significant for hypertension, dyslipidemia, and benign prostatic hyperplasia. MRI of the brain confirms the patient has had an ischemic stroke. Which of the following medications would be the most appropriate for secondary stroke prevention in HB?

a. Ticlopidine
b. Dipyridamole
c. Aspirin
d. Clopidogrel plus aspirin

5. Which of the following is a common side effect of extended-release dipyridamole plus aspirin?

a. Agranulocytosis
b. Visual disturbances
c. Pancreatitis
d. Headache

6. A 63-year-old African American man with a PMH significant for dyslipidemia presented to the emergency department several days ago with symptoms of an acute stroke. The physician you are working with wants your recommendations on what to send this patient home on for blood pressure control. Current vitals are as follows: BP 138/88 mm Hg, HR 86 beats/min What do you recommend?

a. β-Blocker
b. Nondihydropyridine calcium channel blocker
c. Angiotensin-converting enzyme inhibitor plus a diuretic
d. No blood pressure medication. The patient's blood pressure is at goal.

7. What is the brand name of extended-release dipyridamole 200 mg plus aspirin 25 mg?

a. Angiomax
b. Aggrastat
c. Aggrenox
d. Abraxane

8. A 49-year-old white man with a PMH significant only for osteoarthritis was diagnosed with an ischemic stroke due to an atherosclerotic process several days ago. The patient drinks one to two beers per day and denies smoking. Family history is unremarkable. His current lipid panel is as follows: TC 168 mg/dL, TG 88 mg/dL, HDL 44 mg/dL, LDL 116 mg/dL. Vitals: BP 136/84 mm Hg, HR 78 beats/min. The physician you are working with wants to know if this patient needs to be placed on statin therapy. What do you recommend?

a. This patient's only major risk factor for coronary heart disease is his age. He does not need to be placed on statin therapy.
b. This patient's only major risk factors for coronary heart disease are his age and history of previous ischemic stroke. He does not need to be placed on statin therapy.

c. This patient's only major risk factors for coronary heart disease are his age and history of previous ischemic stroke. He does not need to be placed on statin therapy, but therapeutic lifestyle recommendation should be initiated.
d. Statin therapy is recommended for all patients with an atherosclerotic ischemic stroke. He should be put on statin therapy.

9. Which of the following medications inhibit platelet activity? Select all that apply.

a. Clopidogrel
b. Aspirin
c. Dipyridamole
d. Warfarin
e. Ticlopidine

10. Which of the following is an appropriate way to counsel patients on taking extended-release dipyridamole plus aspirin therapy?

a. Extended-release dipyridamole 200 mg plus aspirin 25 mg po daily
b. Extended-release dipyridamole 25 mg plus aspirin 200 mg po daily
c. Extended-release dipyridamole 200 mg plus aspirin 25 mg po bid
d. Extended-release dipyridamole 25 mg plus aspirin 200 mg po bid

11. CS is a 61-year-old white woman who has a PMH significant for hypertension and diabetes mellitus. She presented to the emergency department yesterday with signs and symptoms of an ischemic stroke. CT of the brain confirmed this diagnosis. Which of the following medications would be the most appropriate for secondary stroke prevention in CS?

a. Extended-release dipyridamole 200 mg plus aspirin 25 mg two capsules po bid
b. Aspirin 81 mg po daily
c. Clopidogrel 75 mg po bid
d. Warfarin 5 mg po daily

12. Which of the following describes the mechanism of action of clopidogrel?

a. Irreversible inhibition of adenosine diphosphate–induced platelet aggregation
b. Irreversible inhibition of platelet cyclooxygenase
c. Reversible inhibition of adenosine diphosphate–induced platelet aggregation
d. Reversible inhibition of platelet cyclooxygenase

13. Which of the following medications works by binding to fibrin and subsequently converting plasminogen to plasmin?

a. Plavix
b. Aggrenox

c. Argatroban

d. Activase

14. Which of the following is the correct dose of aspirin for use during an acute stroke? Select all that apply.

    a. Aspirin 81 mg within 24 hours
    b. Aspirin 81 mg within 48 hours
    c. Aspirin 325 mg within 24 hours
    d. Aspirin 325 mg within 48 hours
    e. Aspirin 162 mg within 24 hours

15. A 68-year-old man with a PMH significant for diabetes mellitus, DVT 5 years ago, and GI bleed 2 weeks ago presents with right-sided weakness and right facial droop that began 2 hours ago. CT of the head confirms ischemic stroke. Home medications include: warfarin 5 mg po daily, pantoprazole 40 mg po daily, and metformin 1000 mg po bid. Pertinent laboratory values on admission include INR 1.4, hemoglobin 14, hematocrit 41, platelets 175,000, and glucose 200 mg/dL. Blood pressure on admission is 160/90 mm Hg. Which of the following is a relative exclusion criterion for this patient to receive rtPA?

    a. Elevated INR
    b. Low platelets
    c. Recent GI bleed
    d. Elevated blood pressure on admission

16. A 72-year-old woman (68 in, 111 kg) is admitted for acute ischemic stroke confirmed by CT of the head. She presents within 1.5 hours of symptom onset and meets all criteria to receive rtPA. The physician asks you what the appropriate dose is for this patient and how to administer it. Your response is:

    a. Give 10 mg over 1 minute and then 90 mg over an hour
    b. Give 9 mg over 1 minute and then 81 mg over an hour
    c. Give 10 mg over 10 minutes and then 90 mg over an hour
    d. Give 9 mg over 10 minutes and then 81 mg over an hour

17. Current guidelines recommend the use of rtPA up to 4.5 hours after symptom onset in many patients. Patients who are candidates to receive rtPA in this extended time window include: Select all that apply.

    a. Age younger than 80 years
    b. Patients taking oral anticoagulants regardless of INR
    c. Score of less than 25 on the National Institutes of Health Stroke Scale (NIHSS)
    d. History of both previous stroke and diabetes together
    e. History of intracranial hemorrhage

18. An 81-year-old man with a PMH significant for diabetes, hypertension, and ischemic stroke 3 years ago presents with slurred speech and left-sided weakness that began 3.5 hours ago. NIH stroke score is calculated to be 15.

Home medications include lisinopril 40 mg po daily and glipizide 5 mg po bid. Laboratory values are within normal limits and blood pressure is 150/84 mm Hg. The patient weighs 80 kg. Which of the following may be used as initial treatment for ischemic stroke in this patient?

    a. rtPA 72 mg (10% IV bolus over 1 minute and the remainder over 1 hour)
    b. Aspirin 325 mg po
    c. Aspirin 162 mg po
    d. Lovenox 1 mg/kg SQ q12h

19. Which of the following may be used to treat elevated blood pressure in acute stroke patients who have concomitant renal dysfunction? Select all that apply.

    a. Labetalol
    b. Nicardipine
    c. Sodium nitroprusside
    d. Perindopril
    e. Indapamide

20. A 62-year-old woman is admitted 2 hours after onset of acute stroke symptoms including blurred vision, slurred speech, and right facial droop. CT of the head confirms ischemic stroke. Past medical history is nonsignificant, and the patient takes no medications at home. All laboratory values are within normal limits. Blood pressure is 200/110 mm Hg. Patient meets all other inclusion criteria for rtPA use. Which of the following is the best option for blood pressure control in this patient?

    a. No treatment should be given since the systolic blood pressure is <220 mm Hg and the diastolic blood pressure is <120 mm Hg.
    b. Since the patient meets all other inclusion criteria for rtPA, labetalol should be given to lower blood pressure to <185/110 mm Hg so that the patient can receive rtPA.
    c. Since the patient meets all other inclusion criteria for rtPA, nicardipine infusion should be initiated to lower blood pressure to <140/90 mm Hg.
    d. Since the patient meets all other inclusion criteria for rtPA, sodium nitroprusside should be initiated to lower the blood pressure by 15% within the first day.

21. TP is a 62-year-old patient presenting at 8 pm to the emergency department. The patient has symptoms of weakness to the left side and inability to speak. A CT scan was ordered and revealed an ischemic stroke. The time is now 10:30 pm and the physician wants to treat the patient with rt-PA. Which of the following would be exclusion criteria that would prevent TP from receiving rt-PA? Select all that apply.

    a. Platelets <100,000 mm^3
    b. Oral anticoagulation *and* INR >1.7 or PT >15 seconds
    c. Active internal bleeding
    d. Blood pressure of 156/92 mm Hg

TAKEAWAY POINTS ❯❯

- Ischemic stroke presents as an acute onset of focal neurological deficit and is associated with infarction of central nervous system tissue.
- Risk factors for ischemic stroke include hypertension, diabetes, dyslipidemia, atrial fibrillation, and cigarette smoking.
- Intravenous rtPA and aspirin are the two pharmacologic agents recommended for treatment of acute ischemic stroke.
- rtPA is recommended within 3 hours of symptom onset due to its ability to achieve early reperfusion and improve neurological outcomes. Select patients may receive rtPA with 4.5 hours of symptom onset.

- Aspirin, clopidogrel, and extended-release dipyridamole plus aspirin are the antiplatelet options for the secondary prevention of ischemic stroke.
- Oral anticoagulants are preferred for the secondary prevention of ischemic stroke in patients with a cardioembolic source.
- Antihypertensive treatment is recommended for ischemic stroke patients regardless of whether or not the patient has a history of hypertension.
- Patients with atherosclerotic, ischemic stroke should receive HMG-CoA reductase inhibitors to reduce the risk of recurrent events.

BIBLIOGRAPHY

Easton JD, Saver JL, Albers GW, et al. Definition and evaluation of transient ischemic attack: a scientific statement for healthcare professionals from the American Heart Association/American Stroke Association Stroke Council; Council on Cardiovascular Surgery and Anesthesia; Council on Cardiovascular Radiology and Intervention; Council on Cardiovascular Nursing; and the Interdisciplinary Council on Peripheral Vascular Disease. *Stroke.* 2009;40:2276-2293.

Fagan SC, Hess DC. Stroke. In: DiPiro JT, Talbert RL, Yee GC, Matzke GR, Wells BG, Posey L, eds. *Pharmacotherapy: A Pathophysiologic Approach.* 10th ed. New York, NY: McGraw-Hill; 2017.

Furie, K, Goldstein L, Albers, G, et al. Oral antithrombotic agents for the prevention of stroke in nonvalvular atrial fibrillation: A Science Advisory for Healthcare Professionals From the American Heart Association/American Stroke Association. *Stroke.* 2012;43:3442-3453.

Goldstein L, Bushnell C, Adams R, et al. Guidelines for the primary prevention of stroke: A Guideline for healthcare professionals from the American Heart Association/American Stroke Association. *Stroke.* 2011;42:517-584.

Jauch EC, Saver JL, Adams HP Jr, et al.; on behalf of the American Heart Association Stroke Council, Council on Cardiovascular Nursing, Council on Peripheral Vascular Disease, and Council on Clinical Cardiology. Guidelines for the early management of patients with acute ischemic stroke: a guideline for healthcare professionals from the American Heart Association/American Stroke Association. *Stroke.* 2013;44:870-947.

Weitz JI. Blood coagulation and anticoagulant, fibrinolytic, and antiplatelet drugs. In: Brunton LL, Chabner BA, Knollmann BC, eds. *Goodman & Gilman's The Pharmacological Basis of Therapeutics.* 12th ed. New York, NY: McGraw-Hill; 2011:chap 30.

KEY ABBREVIATIONS

CT = computed tomography
INA = international normalized ratio
MRI = magnetic resonance imaging

PMH = past medical history
rtPA = recombinant tissue plasminogen activator
TIA = transient ischemic attack

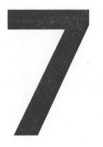

7 Anticoagulation/Venous Thromboembolism

Beth B. Phillips and Kirby Welston

FOUNDATION OVERVIEW

Venous thromboembolism (VTE) is a common and serious disorder that includes deep venous thrombosis (DVT) and pulmonary embolism (PE). Patients presenting with VTE often have one or more risk factors for thromboembolism. Classic symptoms of a DVT include unilateral pain, swelling, erythema, and tenderness usually of the lower extremity; although some patients may be symptom free. Compression ultrasound is typically used to diagnose a DVT. The symptoms of a PE are nonspecific and may include chest pain, shortness of breath, tachypnea, dyspnea, and hemoptysis. Most PEs originate from a DVT. The diagnosis of a PE is made by the presence of symptoms in conjunction with findings on ventilation-perfusion (V/Q) and computerized tomography (CT) scans. Medical work-up of patients presenting with VTE include determination of risk factors for VTE. Certain risk factors are reversible (eg, estrogen use, recent orthopedic surgery, smoking, prolonged immobility) and may be eliminated over time. The presence of irreversible or continuing risk factors (eg, cancer, thrombophilia, previous history of VTE) requires longer or an extended duration of therapy.

Key Definitions

Anticoagulation—the process of preventing blood clot formation

Deep venous thrombosis (DVT)—blood clot formation in a deep vein, usually in the leg (eg, iliac vein)

Postphlebitic syndrome—chronic condition occurring after DVT characterized by venous insufficiency, pain, edema, stasis dermatitis, varicose veins, and ulceration

Pulmonary embolism (PE)—blockage of a pulmonary artery, usually from a thrombus that has traveled from another site, such as the deep vein of the leg

Thromboembolism—occlusion of a blood vessel due to a blood clot that has broken away and traveled from its place of origin

Thrombophilia—genetic or acquired predisposition to thrombosis

Thrombosis—pathologic blood clot formation

TREATMENT OPTIONS

The goals of treatment in the management of VTE include preventing complications, such as thrombus extension, PE formation, VTE recurrence, mortality, and postphlebitic syndrome. Anticoagulants are the primary drug therapy used to achieve these goals and may be classified by basic mechanism of action into three groups: (1) indirect thrombin inhibitors, (2) direct thrombin inhibitors (DTIs), and (3) vitamin K antagonists. Both parenteral and some oral indirect thrombin inhibitors may be used for initial treatment of VTE. In most cases, patients receiving initial treatment with parenteral agents are transitioned to an oral anticoagulant for extended or indefinite therapy. In addition to treatment of VTE, anticoagulants are also used short and long term to prevent thromboembolic events, including those associated with cardiac valve replacement and myocardial infarction; thromboembolic stroke prevention related to atrial fibrillation, and VTE prevention in hospitalized or surgical patients at increased risk of thrombosis.

Treatment

Indirect Thrombin Inhibitors

Heparin, low molecular weight heparins (LMWH), and factor Xa inhibitors comprise the commercially available indirect thrombin inhibitors (Table 7-1). These agents mediate their anticoagulant effect by activating antithrombin, an inhibitor of activated clotting factors, or directly inhibiting factor Xa.

Heparin and LMWH bind to antithrombin to exert their pharmacologic effects. The heparin–antithrombin complex inactivates factors IIa (thrombin), Xa, IXa, XIa, and XIIa. Both factor IIa and Xa, the main components responsible for the anticoagulant activity, are inactivated to an equal extent by heparin. The LMWH have a higher affinity for binding to factor Xa and inhibit its activity two to four times more than activity of factor IIa. Additionally, heparin binds to platelets, osteoblasts, macrophages, and a number of plasma proteins. LMWH bind to these other targets to a lesser extent. Both heparin and LMWH have a short onset of anticoagulant effect, making them good choices for initial treatment of DVT.

Heparin may be administered by the intravenous (IV) or subcutaneous route. In the treatment of VTE, an initial IV weight-based bolus dose is given followed by a weight-based continuous infusion. Heparin must be monitored closely by the activated partial thromboplastin time (aPTT) or anti-Xa concentrations for efficacy and risk of bleeding. For the prevention of VTE, heparin is generally administered

---

To access your complimentary online question exams, visit https://accesspharmacy.mhmedical.com/NAPLEX.aspx

TABLE 7-1   **Properties of Parenteral Anticoagulants**

Properties	Indirect Thrombin Inhibitors		Factor Xa Inhibitor	Direct Thrombin Inhibitors
	Heparin	**LMWH**		
Available agents	Heparin	Enoxaparin (Lovenox®) Dalteparin (Fragmin®)	Fondaparinux (Arixtra®)	Argatroban Bivalirudin (Angiomax®)
Mechanism of action	Inhibits IIa, Xa, IXa, and XIIa through AT-III–binding complex	Inhibits Xa to greater extent through AT-III–binding complex	Selective factor Xa inhibitor through AT-binding complex	Binds to and inactivates thrombin
Thrombin binding	N/A	N/A	N/A	Reversible
Anti-Xa/Anti-IIa ratio	1	Dalteparin 2.7 Enoxaparin 3.8	Anti-Xa only	Anti-IIa only
Plasma half-life	30-90 min	110-234 min	15-18 h	10-80 min
Elimination	Multifactorial	Renal	Renal	Hepatic: argatroban Renal: bivalirudin
Monitoring	aPTT or anti-Xa (rarely) levels; monitor closely	Not routinely done; anti-Xa activity in select patients	Not routinely done	aPTT; monitor closely
Protamine Reversal	Yes	Yes (incomplete)	No	No
Interaction with platelets	High	Low	No	No
May be used in HIT	No	No	Yes	Yes

subcutaneously at lower fixed doses. The LMWH are administered subcutaneously on a weight-based regimen once or twice daily for the treatment of VTE. Like heparin, lower fixed doses are used in the prevention of VTE, varying according to indication and patient characteristics. Unlike heparin, the LMWH exhibit a predictable dose–response relationship and routine monitoring is not needed, but may be considered in select patient populations. LMWH product formulation should be taken into consideration when dosing and dispensing the various products.

Bleeding is the most common adverse effect associated with heparin and LMWH therapies, ranging from minor to severe and life threatening. The bleeding risk increases in heparin patients with advanced age and those receiving higher doses. In many cases, bleeding may be managed by suspending the continuous infusion for a few hours. For more severe cases, protamine sulfate may be administered to reverse the effects of heparin. Protamine may also be used to reverse the effects of LMWH administered within the previous 8 hours and should equal the dose of enoxaparin administered, but the reversal provided is incomplete.

One of the most serious complications associated with heparin is an antibody-mediated drop in platelets known as heparin-induced thrombocytopenia (HIT). This is a serious and potentially fatal condition that can be associated with a paradoxical increase in thrombosis. HIT is suspected if the platelet count decreases 50% or more within 5 to 14 days after initiation of therapy. In some cases, a rapid decline in platelet count may be seen after 24 hours of initiation of therapy if a patient was previously exposed to heparin within 100 days prior to therapy. This phenomenon is known as "rapid-onset HIT." Heparin should be discontinued immediately in patients with HIT. When HIT develops in a patient receiving

treatment with heparin or LMWH, alternative anticoagulation with a parenteral DTI must be administered to treat or prevent thrombosis until the platelet count has recovered (see Table 7-1). Fondaparinux may also be used, but there is not enough evidence to support the use of other newer oral factor Xa or DTIs. LMWH have a much lower incidence of HIT due to a reduced affinity to platelets. However, cross-reactivity can occur and LMWH should be avoided in suspected HIT. If indicated, the initiation of warfarin therapy should be delayed until the platelet count has recovered. For patients with a history of HIT in whom circulating antibodies are no longer present (usually 80-100 days after initial diagnosis), heparin and LMWH may theoretically be used with caution. However, many clinicians and patients are reluctant to do so due to the serious nature of HIT.

Other adverse effects associated with heparin therapy include osteoporosis, skin necrosis, hyperkalemia, hypersensitivity, and an elevation in hepatic transaminases. The LMWH are associated with a lower risk of osteoporosis when compared to heparin. Contraindications to heparin and LMWH include active bleeding, hypersensitivity, and HIT. Heparin should be used over LMWH in patients with creatinine clearance (CrCl) less than 30 mL/min in the treatment of VTE. In the prevention of VTE, lower LMWH doses are generally recommended when CrCl is less than 30 mL/min. Additionally, the LMWH carry a black box warning regarding the use of these agents in patients undergoing epidural anesthesia due to the potential for development of spinal hematoma and long-term or permanent paralysis. The use of platelet inhibitors, other anticoagulants, or nonsteroidal anti-inflammatory drugs concomitantly increases this risk.

Factor Xa inhibitors include both oral and parenteral treatment options (Tables 7-1 and 7-2). Fondaparinux (Arixtra®) is an injectable agent that exerts its anticoagulant

TABLE 7-2 Properties of Oral Anticoagulants

Properties	Warfarin	Dabigatran (Pradaxa®)	Rivaroxaban (Xarelto®)	Apixaban (Eliquis®)	Edoxaban (Savaysa®)
Mechanism of action	Inhibits vitamin K epoxide reductase inhibiting factors II, VII, IX, X, proteins C and S	Directly inhibits both free and clot-bound thrombin	Selective, direct factor Xa inhibitor		
Thrombin binding	N/A	Reversible inhibitor of free and clot-bound thrombin	N/A	N/A	N/A
Platelet inhibition	No	Yes	No	No	No
Monitoring	PT/INR	Not routinely done	Not routinely done	Not routinely done	Not routinely done
DVT/PE Dose	Individualized	150 mg bid (after 5-10 d parenteral anticoagulant)	15 mg bid × 21 d, then 20 mg once daily	10 mg bid × 7 d then 5 mg bid	60 mg once daily (after 5-10 d parenteral anticoagulant)
Nonvalvular atrial fibrillation dose	Individualized	150 mg bid	20 mg once daily	5 mg bid	60 mg once daily
Renal dose adjustment (DVT/PE)	No	No; Patients with CrCl ≤30 mL/min were excluded from clinical trials	Avoid CrCl <30 mL/min	None recommended; Patients with SCr >2.5 or CrCl 25 mL/min excluded from trials	Avoid CrCl <15 mL/min. 30 mg daily for CrCl 15-50 mL/min
Renal dose adjustment (Nonvalvular atrial fibrillation)	No	Avoid CrCl <15 mL/min; renal dose of 75 mg bid for CrCl 15-30 mL/min not validated in clinical trials	CrCl 15-50 mL/min: 15 mg once daily	Reduce dose to 2.5 mg bid if 2 of these factors present: SCr ≥1.5 mg/dL, age ≥80, or weight ≤60 kg	Use not recommended if CrCl >95 mL/min or <15 mL/min CrCl 15-50 mL/min: 30 mg once daily
Hepatic dose adjustment	Caution due to decreased clotting factor synthesis	None recommended	Avoid in moderate to severe impairment	Not recommended in severe impairment	Not recommended in moderate to severe impairment
Age-based dose adjustment	Consideration warranted	Caution ≥80 y of age	None	Age ≥80 y + SCr ≥1.5 mg/dL OR weight <60 kg (atrial fibrillation only)	None
Weight-based dose adjustment	Consideration warranted	None	None	Body weight ≤60 kg + SCr ≥1.5 mg/dL OR age ≥80 y (atrial fibrillation only)	≤60 kg 30 mg once daily
		International Society on Thrombosis and Haemostasis recommend avoiding use in patients with BMI >40 kg/m² or weight >120 kg due to lack of clinical data			
Elimination half-life	1 wk	12-17 h	5-9 h	11.1-12 h	10-14 h
Elimination	Renal	Renal	Renal, fecal	Renal, fecal	Renal
Reversal agent	Vitamin K	Idarucizumab; Hemodialysis removes approximately 60% after 4-h session	No	No	No
Drug interactions	CYP-2C9, 3A4, 1A2 inhibitors or inducers	P-gp inhibitors or inducers	Strong inhibitors or inducers of CYP-3A4 and P-gp	Strong inhibitors or inducers of CYP-3A4 and P-gp	Strong P-gp inhibitors (reduce dose to 30 mg once daily)

effect by binding to antithrombin and inactivating factor Xa. Fondaparinux is administered subcutaneously once daily and may be used in the treatment or prevention of VTE. It has a rapid onset of anticoagulation and a long half-life. Rivaroxaban (Xarelto®), apixaban (Eliquis®), betrixaban (Bevyxxa™), and edoxaban (Savaysa®) are oral direct factor Xa inhibitors that do not require antithrombin to mediate their anticoagulant effect. All of the agents are approved for treatment of DVT and PE, although edoxaban may not be used for initial treatment of DVT/PE. Apixaban and rivaroxaban carry additional indications including the reduction in the risk of recurrent DVT or PE after an initial 6 months of treatment and postoperative DVT prophylaxis. Apixaban is administered orally twice daily while rivaroxaban is administered orally once daily, except during the initiation of treatment when for a period of time it is administered twice daily. Rivaroxaban, apixaban, and edoxaban may also be used for prevention of stroke and systemic embolism in patients with atrial fibrillation.

Like LMWH, factor Xa inhibitors have a predictable dose–response relationship and routine laboratory monitoring is not necessary. Bleeding is the most common adverse effect and the anticoagulant effects may not be reversed with protamine. These agents are not associated with HIT due to the lack of significant platelet binding seen with heparin. Use should be avoided in severe renal impairment (CrCl <30 mL/min for fondaparinux and rivaroxaban). Normal doses of apixaban may be given in ESRD patients for DVT/PE treatment; however, should be reduced by 50% in nonvalvular atrial fibrillation patients who have a serum creatinine more than 1.5 mg/dL and who are older than or equal to 80 years or less than or equal to 60 kg. Significant drug interactions may occur when used in combination with drugs that are strong inhibitors or inducers of cytochrome P-450 (CYP) 3A4 and/or p-glycoprotein (P-gp) (Table 7-3). Additionally, the benefits and risks should be evaluated in patients with renal insufficiency (CrCl 15-50 mL/min) who are taking weak to moderate CYP-3A4 and P-gp inhibitors.

Direct Thrombin Inhibitors

DTIs prevent clot formation by binding directly to thrombin leading to inactivation. Argatroban and bivalirudin are administered as continuous IV infusions and their effects are monitored by the aPTT. Parenteral DTIs are the preferred agents to prevent and treat thrombosis associated with HIT. When used for HIT, they should be continued until the platelet count has completely recovered. Bleeding is the most common adverse effect associated with DTIs. No specific agents exist that can reverse the anticoagulant effects. When used in combination with warfarin therapy, DTIs increase the international normalized ratio (INR). Argatroban has the most effect on the INR when compared to the other DTIs. Argatroban should be avoided in patients with hepatic dysfunction. Bivalirudin is used primarily in patients undergoing cardiac procedures.

Dabigatran etexilate mesylate (Pradaxa®) is currently the only oral DTI and is indicated for prevention of stroke in nonvalvular atrial fibrillation, postoperative thromboprophylaxis as well as treatment of DVT/PE after 5 to 10 days of a parenteral anticoagulant (Table 7-2). Dabigatran is a prodrug that is orally absorbed and is a selective, reversible DTI. Dabigatran is administered orally twice daily and requires no routine laboratory monitoring. Dose reduction is indicated in patients with renal impairment using dabigatran for nonvalvular atrial fibrillation with a creatinine clearance of 15 to 30 mL/min; however, no dose adjustment is recommended for DVT/PE treatment. The most clinically significant adverse effect is bleeding; however, dyspepsia is also common and limits tolerability. Dabigatran is the first new oral anticoagulant to have a reversal agent, idarucizumab (Praxbind®). Idarucizumab is a humanized monoclonal antibody fragment that binds specifically to dabigatran and its metabolites and is administered IV. Drug interactions include P-gp inhibitors or inducers. P-gp inducers should not be given concomitantly with dabigatran and P-gp inhibitors are of even greater concern in patients with renal dysfunction.

Vitamin K Antagonist

Warfarin is consistently among the top 200 most commonly dispensed drugs in the United States each year. Warfarin reduces thrombus formation by inhibiting the activation of the vitamin K-dependent clotting factors, II, VII, IX, and X. Warfarin also inhibits the anticoagulant proteins C and S which in theory produces an initial increased risk of thrombosis but data are lacking. The anticoagulant effect produced by warfarin is delayed and it takes several days to achieve a steady state anticoagulant effect due to its dependence on the depletion of these activated clotting factors. Warfarin is a racemic mixture of R and S enantiomers, each metabolized by a different cytochrome P (CYP)-450 pathway. S-warfarin, the more potent enantiomer, is metabolized by CYP-2C9, and R-warfarin is metabolized by CYP-3A4 and CYP-1A2.

In the treatment of VTE, warfarin therapy is used in combination with a parenteral anticoagulant with close monitoring of INR until therapeutic levels are achieved. The maintenance dose required to maintain a therapeutic INR must be individualized and adjusted as needed. The target INR is 2.5 (range 2.0-3.0) for most patients. A higher target INR of 3.0 (range 2.5-3.5) is recommended for patients with mitral mechanical cardiac valve replacements and patients who failed therapy with the lower target INR. Genetic variants may alter individual maintenance warfarin doses. Patients with CYP2C9 polymorphisms or vitamin K epoxide reductase

TABLE 7-3	Inhibitors and Inducers of CYP-3A4 and P-gp
	Responsible Drugs
Strong Inhibition of CYP-3A4 and P-gp	Ketoconazole
	Itraconazole
	Ritonavir
	Indinavir
	Clarithromycin
	Conivaptan
Strong Induction of CYP-3A4 and P-gp	Carbamazepine
	Rifampin
	Phenytoin
	St. John's Wort

complex 1 (VKORC1) mutation often require lower warfarin doses. Current guidelines do not support the use of genetic testing to determine initial warfarin dosing.

Warfarin has a narrow therapeutic index, exhibits variability in individual dose requirements, and is subject to a number of drug–drug, drug–food, and drug–disease interactions, all of which necessitate close patient monitoring preferably by a specialized anticoagulation monitoring service. Warfarin therapy is adjusted to a target INR range generally in 5% to 15% increments. Patients with subtherapeutic INRs are at higher risk of thromboembolic complications and patients with supratherapeutic INRs are at higher risk of bleeding. Bleeding is the most significant adverse effect associated with warfarin and may range from minor epistaxis to life-threatening intracranial hemorrhage. One of the most important risk factors for bleeding is intensity of anticoagulation. Other risk factors include concomitant use of other drugs increasing bleeding risk (eg, antiplatelet or nonsteroidal anti-inflammatory drugs), advanced age, history of previous gastrointestinal bleed, and concomitant disease states. Patients with genetic polymorphisms in CYP2C9 may also have a higher risk of bleeding. The effects of warfarin may be reversed by administration of vitamin K. Oral vitamin K is preferred but IV vitamin K may be administered when urgent reversal is needed. More rapid reversal may be achieved with fresh frozen plasma (FFP) or prothrombin complex concentrate (PCC). These therapies are short acting and should generally be followed with vitamin K supplementation for reversal. Other uncommon adverse effects associated with warfarin include skin necrosis and purple toe syndrome.

Warfarin is perhaps one of the best known agents with many drug–drug interactions. Drugs may interact with warfarin based on a number of different mechanisms, including stereoselective interactions (eg, CYP2C9/3A4/1A2), impaired absorption (eg, bile acid sequestrants), degradation of clotting factors (eg, levothyroxine), inhibition of cyclic conversion of vitamin K (eg, 2nd and 3rd generation cephalosporins), and potentiation of bleeding. Drugs that interact with warfarin by inhibiting or inducing CYP2C9, which metabolizes S-warfarin, have the greatest and most consistent effect on the INR

TABLE 7-5	Select Drugs Increasing the Bleeding Risk with Warfarin
Antiplatelets	
Nonsteroidal anti-inflammatory drugs (NSAIDs)	
Cyclooxygenase-2 (COX-2) inhibitors	
Aspirin	
High-dose penicillins	

(Table 7-4). Drugs inhibiting or inducing CYP3A4 or CYP1A2, which metabolize the less potent R-warfarin, have a less consistent effect on the INR. Table 7-5 lists several drugs that increase the risk of bleeding when used in combination with warfarin.

Another important interaction unique to warfarin is the drug–food interaction with vitamin-K–containing foods. Achieving a therapeutic warfarin dose is a fine balance with the vitamin K-dependent clotting factors. Introducing more or less vitamin K to the system upsets this balance and changes the INR. Common foods/drinks high in vitamin K content include dark green, leafy vegetables, green cabbage, beef liver, and many green teas. Patients should be aware of this interaction and make an effort to keep their diet consistent in vitamin K. Patients and clinicians should also be aware of other sources of vitamin K, such as multivitamins and dietary supplements, which can alter the INR.

In addition to drug–drug and drug–food interactions, several other factors can affect the INR and therapeutic anticoagulation. An exacerbation of heart failure can increase the INR, while hypothyroidism can decrease warfarin sensitivity. Nonadherence to therapy can cause a decrease in the INR. Warfarin tablets are uniquely colored by strength and can be of assistance when determining the dose the patient has been taking (Table 7-6). Acute and chronic alcohol use can alter warfarin response as well with chronic low-level alcohol use "inducing" warfarin metabolism while binge drinking may inhibit warfarin metabolism. For these reasons, thorough and frequent patient education is essential for all patients receiving chronic warfarin therapy.

Guideline Approach to Treatment

The 2016 CHEST Guidelines for Antithrombotic Therapy for VTE Disease recommend that initial therapy for patients

TABLE 7-4	Stereoselective CYP-2C9 Warfarin Drug–Drug Interactions	
Mechanism of Interaction	Effect on INR	Responsible Drugs
Inhibition of CYP-2C9 (S warfarin)	Increase	Amiodarone
		Azole antifungals
		Imatinib
		Metronidazole
		Sulfamethoxazole/ Trimethoprim
Induction of CYP-2C9 (S warfarin)	Decrease	Carbamazepine
		Rifampin
		Dicloxacillin
		Nafcillin
		Phenytoin
		Phenobarbital

TABLE 7-6	Available Warfarin Tablets
Tablet Strength	Tablet Color
1	Pink
2	Lavender
2.5	Green
3	Tan
4	Blue
5	Peach
6	Teal
7.5	Yellow
10	White (Dye-Free)

with a DVT of the leg or PE be treated with anticoagulant therapy including apixaban, dabigatran, edoxaban, and rivaroxaban. Warfarin may be indicated for some patient-related factors (eg, renal disease, history of gastrointestinal bleed, adherence). Treatment with anticoagulation should be carried out for at least 3 months and possibly longer depending upon the patient's risk of bleeding. After patients who experienced an unprovoked DVT or PE have been treated for at least 3 months and are not electing to continue anticoagulation therapy, aspirin can be used for prevention of recurrent VTE.

CASE Application

1. A 59-year-old man with past medical history significant for diabetes, hypertension, hyperlipidemia, seizure disorder, and depression presents to the anticoagulation clinic for management of his warfarin. His current medication list includes metformin, lisinopril, cholestyramine, phenytoin, levetiracetam, and mirtazapine. His physician asks you which of his current medications could interact with his warfarin. Select all that apply.

   a. Metformin
   b. Cholestyramine
   c. Phenytoin
   d. Levetiracetam
   e. Mirtazapine

2. KP is 72-year-old woman who presents to the emergency department and reports hematuria for the past 2 days. The patient's INR is 7.2 and KP reports she may have accidentally taken old 10 mg warfarin tablets instead of her currently prescribed 5 mg tablets for the past week. Which agent is the most appropriate reversal agent to be used in the case of warfarin overdose?

   a. Phenprocoumon
   b. Protamine sulfate
   c. Vitamin K
   d. Idarucizumab

3. Which adverse reaction(s) may be associated with vitamin K antagonist use? Select all that apply.

   a. Melena
   b. Cardiac arrhythmias (QT prolongation)
   c. Bleeding
   d. Purple toe syndrome
   e. Anemia

4. JC is a 36-year-old pregnant woman with an active DVT. She takes no other medications and has no significant past medical history. Which agent is the best choice for the initial treatment of her DVT?

   a. Enoxaparin
   b. Aspirin
   c. Warfarin
   d. Dabigatran

5. A 55-year-old woman is diagnosed with a new DVT. She weighs 80 kg and her SCr is 1.0 and CrCl is 89 mL/min. Her past medical history includes type 2 diabetes and hypertension. Which is an appropriate initial treatment recommendation?

   a. Xarelto® 20 mg once daily with the evening meal
   b. Eliquis® 10 mg bid for 7 days then 5 mg bid
   c. Lovenox® 120 mg bid
   d. Pradaxa® 150 mg bid

6. Which drug can be used safely in a Heparin-induced thrombocytopenia (HIT) patient with a creatinine clearance of 25 mL/min?

   a. Enoxaparin
   b. Dalteparin
   c. Fondaparinux
   d. Argatroban

7. Which agent has a delayed onset of anticoagulant effect?

   a. Arixtra®
   b. Coumadin®
   c. Fragmin®
   d. Lovenox®

Questions 8 and 9 refer to the following case.

A 64-year-old woman (70 kg) followed in your anticoagulation clinic presents for routine monitoring of her warfarin. Her past medical history is significant for recurrent DVT, hypertension, and osteoarthritis. She currently takes warfarin 5 mg daily, lisinopril 10 mg daily, and acetaminophen 1000 mg four times daily as needed. Her current laboratory values are INR 2.0, SCr 1.1 mg/dL, K⁺ 4.5 meq/L, and TSH 10.5 µIU/mL. The primary care provider plans to initiate levothyroxine today due to her symptoms of hypothyroidism.

8. Initiation of levothyroxine for this patient's hypothyroidism is most likely going to result in which effect?

   a. Decreased INR
   b. Increased INR
   c. Increased TSH
   d. Increased SCr

9. The patient returns to clinic and her primary care provider has decided to transition the patient from warfarin to a direct oral anticoagulant (DOAC) today. Her INR is 2.7. Which DOAC can be safely initiated today?

   a. Xarelto®
   b. Eliquis®
   c. Pradaxa®
   d. Savaysa®

10. Select all of the factors that could result in a supratherapeutic INR.

   a. Binge alcohol use
   b. Diarrhea
   c. Missed doses

    d. Increased dietary vitamin K

    e. Initiation of azole antifungal agents

11. A 57-year-old woman (65 kg, BMI 28) was just admitted to the hospital for treatment of a pulmonary embolism. An order was written for heparin IV bolus 80 units/kg followed by a continuous infusion of 18 units/kg/h. What are respective heparin bolus dose and continuous infusion rate for this patient?

    a. 5000 units IV bolus; 1200 units/h infusion

    b. 4000 units IV bolus; 800 units/h infusion

    c. 6000 units IV bolus; 1150 units/h infusion

    d. 4000 units IV bolus; 1150 units/h infusion

12. Select the appropriate routes of administration for unfractionated heparin. Select all that apply.

    a. Intravenous

    b. Subcutaneous

    c. Intramuscular

    d. Oral

    e. Intrathecal

Questions 13 and 14 pertain to the following patient case.

JT is a 62-year-old woman with a history of atrial fibrillation, coronary heart disease, hypertension, and diabetes mellitus. Her current medications include warfarin 5 mg daily, amlodipine 5 mg daily, clopidogrel 75 mg daily, lisinopril 10 mg daily, metformin XR 1000 mg daily, and ibuprofen 600 mg three times daily.

13. Which of her medications increases the risk of bleeding with warfarin? Select all that apply.

    a. Clopidogrel

    b. Amlodipine

    c. Metformin

    d. Ibuprofen

    e. Lisinopril

14. JT presents to her PCP with polyuria and pain on urination and is diagnosed with a urinary tract infection. Which antibiotic would be expected to have the least effect on her warfarin therapy?

    a. Sulfamethoxazole-trimethoprim

    b. Nitrofurantoin

    c. Ciprofloxacin

    d. Fluconazole

15. A patient returns to the anticoagulation clinic for routine monitoring of her INR, which is below the goal range of 2 to 3 today. The patient stated she has recently started a multivitamin. Which ingredient in the patient's multivitamin is likely to have contributed to a decrease in the INR?

    a. Zinc

    b. Riboflavin

    c. Phytonadione

    d. Selenium

16. A middle-aged woman presents a new prescription for her husband to your pharmacy for enoxaparin (Lovenox®) 240 mg subcutaneously once daily for 7 days for deep venous thrombosis. The patient's weight is 150 kg. What is the most appropriate action for dispensing the medication?

    a. Dispense 21 80-mg syringes with instructions to inject three 80-mg syringes daily.

    b. Repackage the 240-mg dose in one syringe and dispense seven 220-mg syringes.

    c. Call the prescriber and recommend changing the dose to 150 mg twice daily.

    d. Call the prescriber and recommend changing the dose to 200 mg daily.

17. An 87-year-old man presents to the anticoagulation clinic for follow-up after recent initiation of warfarin for treatment of a PE. You ask the patient what dose he is currently taking but the patient cannot remember. You then ask him what color tablets the patient has and how many he takes per day. The patient responds that he takes 1 blue tablet every day. Based upon this information, what is the patient's current warfarin dose?

    a. 2.5 mg daily

    b. 4 mg daily

    c. 5 mg daily

    d. 7.5 mg daily

18. A patient comes to your pharmacy asking for Boost® dietary supplement. In your discussion, she tells you that she is also taking warfarin for recurrent DVT. Which of the following is a likely consequence of starting this dietary supplement in someone who is receiving chronic warfarin therapy?

    a. Increased risk of bleeding

    b. Increase in the INR

    c. Decrease in the INR

    d. Decrease in warfarin dose

Questions 19 to 21 correspond to the following patient case.

TS is a 46-year-old man who was admitted to your hospital with an acute DVT. The patient has no other significant medical history and this is the first episode of DVT in this patient. Warfarin was initiated 2 days ago and a therapeutic INR has not yet been achieved. The patient is being discharged today with discharge prescriptions for warfarin and Lovenox.

19. What counseling information should be provided to TS upon discharge from the hospital? Select all that apply.

    a. Rotate injection site to minimize bruising and pain.

    b. Inject at least 2 inches from your belly button and out toward your sides.

    c. Prior to injection, gently press the plunger to remove the air bubble from the syringe.

    d. Avoid rubbing site of injection after administration to minimize risk of bruising.

    e. Store unused syringes in the refrigerator until just before use.

20. TS presents to the anticoagulation clinic for his initial visit, what counseling information is appropriate for educating TS about taking chronic warfarin therapy? Select all that apply.

    a. All herbal therapies are safe in combination with warfarin therapy.
    b. Report any missed warfarin doses to your physician or clinic.
    c. Over-the-counter analgesics are safe in combination with warfarin therapy.
    d. Avoid wide fluctuations in the consumption of foods high in vitamin K content.
    e. Alcohol consumption does not affect warfarin therapy.

21. Which agent would be the best pain management option for TS to utilize while on chronic warfarin therapy?

    a. Celebrex®
    b. Excedrin®
    c. Aspirin
    d. Acetaminophen

22. In which procedure should Lovenox® use be avoided?

    a. Computed tomography (CT) scan
    b. Magnetic resonance imaging (MRI) scan
    c. Epidural anesthesia
    d. Liver biopsy

23. The effects of which anticoagulant(s) can be reversed by idarucizumab? Select all that apply.

    a. Rivaroxaban
    b. Dabigatran etexilate mesylate
    c. Warfarin
    d. Apixaban
    e. Heparin

24. Dose adjustment or avoidance may be necessary in a patient with renal dysfunction for which of the following agents? Select all that apply.

    a. Argatroban
    b. Warfarin
    c. Dabigatran etexilate
    d. Rivaroxaban
    e. Enoxaparin sodium

25. A 62-year-old female patient presents with acute PE and is initially managed with enoxaparin sodium. The patient has a past medical history significant only for hypertension. The patient has no history of renal or hepatic dysfunction. Which of the following would be appropriate for continued treatment? Select all that apply.

    a. Warfarin
    b. Dabigatran etexilate
    c. Apixaban
    d. Aspirin
    e. Rivaroxaban

26. Rank the following anticoagulants in order from shortest to longest half-life. (ALL options must be used.)

Unordered Options	Ordered Response
Enoxaparin	
Warfarin	
Heparin	
Fondaparinux	
Rivaroxaban	

27. A 76-year-old woman with atrial fibrillation, hypertension, and diabetes mellitus presents to the clinic with complaints of indigestion, bloating, and nausea. Her current medications include dabigatran 150 mg bid, lisinopril 20 mg daily, chlorthalidone 25 mg daily, metformin 1000 mg bid, and glipizide 10 mg bid. Which medication is the likely cause?

    a. Dabigatran
    b. Lisinopril
    c. Chlorthalidone
    d. Glipizide

28. A patient tells you she has recently started a new diet that has given her more energy and an optimistic outlook on life. You see from her medication list she is currently taking warfarin. You ask her about her new diet and she tells you she eats protein smoothies for breakfast (bananas, strawberries, spinach, kale, protein powder), onion broth soup for lunch, and baked chicken, collard greens, and an apple at dinner. What foods in her new diet can affect her INR? Select all that apply.

    a. Strawberries
    b. Spinach
    c. Kale
    d. Chicken
    e. Protein powder

29. A 42-year-old male patient presents with new onset nonvalvular atrial fibrillation. The patient's past medical history is significant for simple partial seizures, hypertension, and type 2 diabetes. Current medications include Tegretol-XR® 400 mg bid, Januvia® 100 mg daily, metformin 500 mg bid, and lisinopril 20 mg daily. The patient's physician would like to initiate rivaroxaban for treatment of atrial fibrillation. Which medication the patient is currently receiving presents the most significant interaction with rivaroxaban?

    a. Lisinopril
    b. Januvia®

c. Tegretol-XR®
d. Metformin

30. A 45-year-old man on lifelong therapy with warfarin for recurrent DVT has been prescribed metronidazole for *Clostridium difficile* infection. Addition of metronidazole to this patient's warfarin will likely have what effect on the INR and by what mechanism?

a. Increase INR due to CYP2C9 inhibition
b. Decrease INR due to CYP2D6 inhibition
c. Increase INR due to CYP1A2 inhibition
d. Decrease INR due to CYP3A4 inhibition

TAKEAWAY POINTS »

- Anticoagulants are frequently used drugs for the treatment of VTE and prevention of thromboembolic events associated with a variety of disorders, such as recurrent VTE, atrial fibrillation, mechanical cardiac valve placement, and myocardial infarction.

- VTE encompasses both DVT and PE. Complications of DVT include PE and development of the postphlebitic syndrome. PEs are potentially fatal and are often not preceded by a symptomatic DVT.

- The duration of VTE treatment is determined by the presence of a reversible risk factor, presence of a continuing risk factor, or absence of an identifiable risk factor.

- Bleeding is the most common adverse effect of oral and parenteral anticoagulants.

- Heparin and warfarin therapies are monitored by the aPTT and INR, respectively. Routine laboratory monitoring of LWMH, factor Xa inhibitors and oral DTIs is not needed.

- Protamine sulfate may be used to reverse heparin therapy and may partially reverse LMWH. Vitamin K may be used to reverse the effects of warfarin, and idarucizumab can reverse the effects of dabigatran. At this time, there are no reversal agents available for factor Xa inhibitors.

- Heparin may cause an immune-mediated thrombocytopenia, known as HIT. This significant complication may also occur with LMWH but it is less common. Heparin and LMWH are contraindicated in patients who have developed HIT.

- No dose adjustments are needed when unfractionated heparin or warfarin are used in patients with renal impairment.

- Drugs inhibiting or inducing cytochrome P-450 2C9 are expected to have the greatest effect on INR values when used in combination with warfarin therapy. Significant drug interactions can occur when oral factor Xa inhibitors are used concomitantly with drugs that are strong inhibitors or inducers of CYP-3A4 and P-gp or when oral DTIs are used with strong P-gp inhibitors or inducers.

- The anticoagulant effect of warfarin is delayed with steady state anticoagulation occurring only at a minimum of several days of therapy.

- Warfarin has a significant drug–food interaction with vitamin K–containing foods and supplements. Foods with high vitamin K content typically include dark green, leafy vegetables. Patients should be educated to keep their diet consistent with respect to vitamin K–containing foods.

- Warfarin therapy should be avoided in pregnant women (pregnancy category X). Heparin or LMWH are preferred treatments in pregnancy.

BIBLIOGRAPHY

Ageno W, Gallus AS, Wittowsky A, et al. Oral anticoagulant therapy. Antithrombotic Therapy and Prevention of Thrombosis, 9th ed: American College of Chest Physicians Evidence-Based Clinical Practice Guidelines. *Chest.* 2012;141(2)(Suppl):e44S-e88S.

Garcia DA, Baglin TP, Weitz JI, et al. Parenteral anticoagulants. Antithrombotic Therapy and Prevention of Thrombosis, 9th ed: American College of Chest Physicians Evidence-Based Clinical Practice Guidelines. *Chest.* 2012;141(2)(Suppl):e24S-e43S.

Guyatt GH, Akl EA, Crowther M, et al. Executive summary. Antithrombotic Therapy and Prevention of Thrombosis, 9th ed: American College of Chest Physicians Evidence-Based Clinical Practice Guidelines. *Chest.* 2012;141(2)(Suppl):7S-47S.

Kearon C, Akl EA, Ornelas J, et al. Antithrombotic therapy for VTE disease: CHEST guideline and expert panel report. *Chest.* 2016;149(2):315-352.

Linkins LA, Dans AL, Moores LK, et al. Treatment and prevention of heparin-induced thrombocytopenia. Antithrombotic Therapy and Prevention of Thrombosis, 9th ed: *Chest.* 2012;141(2)(Suppl):e495S-e530S.

Weitz JI. Blood coagulation and anticoagulant, fibrinolytic, and antiplatelet drugs. In: Brunton LL, Chabner BA, Knollmann BC., eds. *Goodman & Gilman's The Pharmacological Basis of Therapeutics.* 12th ed. New York, NY: McGraw-Hill; 2011:chap 30.

Witt DM, Clark NP, Vazquez SR. Venous thromboembolism. In: DiPiro JT, Talbert RL, Yee GC, Matzke GR, Wells BG, Posey L, eds. *Pharmacotherapy: A Pathophysiologic Approach.* 10th ed. New York, NY: McGraw-Hill; 2017:chap 16.

KEY ABBREVIATIONS

aPTT = activated partial thromboplastin time
CrCl = creatinine clearance
CT = computerized tomography
DTIs = direct thrombin inhibitors
DVT = deep venous thrombosis
FFP = fresh frozen plasma
HIT = heparin-induced thrombocytopenia

INR = international normalized ratio
IV = intravenous
LMWH = low molecular weight heparins
PCC = prothrombin complex concentrate
PE = pulmonary embolism
VTE = Venous thromboembolism

8

Peripheral Arterial Disease

Jennifer Rosselli

FOUNDATION OVERVIEW

Peripheral arterial disease (PAD) encompasses noncardiac systemic atherosclerosis. PAD most commonly manifests in arteries of the lower extremities and may also be present in the carotid, mesenteric, renal, brachiocephalic, and subclavian vasculature. The incidence of PAD increases with age beginning at 40 years. Additional factors identified by the Framingham Heart Study to increase the risk for developing PAD include diabetes, hypercholesterolemia, cigarette smoking, and hypertension (Table 8-1). Patients with PAD have a fourfold increase in coronary artery disease and death compared to individuals without PAD.

Clinical manifestations of PAD vary based on disease severity and can range from asymptomatic disease to limbs in jeopardy of amputation. Atherosclerotic lesions in the peripheral vessels that impair lower extremity arterial circulation result in intermittent claudication (IC) or symptoms during exercise. IC is characterized by fatigue, pain, discomfort, cramping, or numbness in the buttock, thigh, or calf upon exertion and typically relieved within 10 minutes by rest. Resting pain, limb ischemia, nonhealing wounds, or gangrene can manifest from severe disease. PAD is stratified based on presentation: asymptomatic, atypical leg pain, classic claudication, and critical limb ischemia.

Clinical history and physical examination findings suggestive of PAD warrant diagnostic testing with a resting ankle-brachial index (ABI). An ABI of less than or equal to 0.90 indicates PAD, borderline PAD is recognized by an ABI 0.91-0.99, normal is 1.00-1.40. Additional testing may include exercise treadmill ABI, duplex ultrasound, toe-brachial index, and angiography. Table 8-2 lists key factors associated with the clinical presentation and risk assessment of PAD.

TREATMENT

Several of the treatment goals for these patients involve the reduction of confounding variables that attribute to the disease process, progress, and eventual outcome. Specific goals should include increasing maximal walking distance, duration, and pain-free walking, improving control of comorbid conditions (hypertension, hyperlipidemia, and diabetes), protecting lower extremities from tissue loss, improving overall quality of life, and reducing cardiovascular complications and death.

First-line treatment of mild to moderate PAD symptoms includes exercise therapy, while risk factor modification should be implemented at all severity levels. These first steps of PAD treatment include:

1. Exercise rehabilitation through supervised exercise programs or structured community- or home-based programs.
2. Control of comorbid conditions and risk factors:
   a. Smoking cessation and avoid passive tobacco smoke exposure
   b. Diabetes management
   c. Antihypertensive therapy for presence of hypertension and PAD
   d. Lipid control with statin therapy
   e. Annual influenza vaccination

Nonpharmacologic Treatment

Structured exercise therapy can decrease leg symptoms associated with IC and improve the patient's functional status and quality of life. This treatment modality uses intermittent walking in a setting supervised by a qualified health care provider or can be self-guided to take place in a personal setting of the patient with guidance from the health care provider. Exercise therapy lasts a minimum of 30 minutes per session, occurs at least 3 days per week and requires a minimum treatment duration of 12 weeks.

Counsel on self-foot examinations and healthy foot behaviors to minimize tissue loss in patients with PAD. Patients should be encouraged to perform daily inspection of feet, to wear shoes and socks, avoid walking barefoot, select proper footwear, and advised to seek medical attention for new foot concerns.

Revascularization and surgical treatments are reserved for patients in the following situations:

a. Limb-threatening ischemia manifested as rest pain, ischemic ulcers, or gangrene.
b. Inadequate response or predicted inadequate response to exercise rehabilitation and pharmacologic therapy.
c. Significant disability due to IC manifested by inability to perform normal work or other activities.

TABLE 8-1 | Factors that Increase Risk for Lower Extremity Peripheral Arterial Disease (PAD)

- Age <50 y with diabetes plus one additional factor for atherosclerosis (history of smoking, hypertension, hyperlipidemia)
- Age 50-64 y plus family history of PAD or personal risk factors for atherosclerosis
- Age ≥65 y
- Individuals of any age with known atherosclerotic disease (eg, coronary, carotid, subclavian, abdominal, or renal artery disease)

Patients may require palliative analgesic medications and anticoagulants while awaiting invasive intervention.

Pharmacologic Treatment

Pharmacologic interventions for PAD involve antiplatelet drug therapies, statins, diabetes medications, and antihypertensives as necessary, and cilostazol. Antiplatelet therapy with aspirin or clopidogrel is indicated to reduce the risk of myocardial infarction, stroke, or vascular death in individuals with atherosclerotic lower extremity PAD. Angiotensin-converting enzyme inhibitors can reduce the risk of ischemic cardiovascular events in patients with hypertension and PAD. Cilostazol is an effective therapy for improving leg and walking symptoms in IC. Anticoagulation with heparin should be given to those with acute limb ischemia. Table 8-3 lists key medication properties.

Aspirin

Aspirin, at doses of 75 to 325 mg/d, is recommended for PAD and is the drug of choice because of low cost and the high concomitant incidence of coronary atherosclerosis among PAD patients. Enteric-coated products should be swallowed intact and not be chewed or crushed. Aspirin is a more potent inhibitor of both prostaglandin synthesis and platelet aggregation compared to other salicylic derivatives due to the acetyl group on the aspirin molecule. Aspirin inhibits platelet aggregation by irreversibly inhibiting platelet cyclooxygenase; therefore, it prevents the production of thromboxane A2, a powerful inducer of platelet aggregation and vasoconstriction.

Common adverse effects with aspirin use are gastrointestinal (indigestion, nausea, and vomiting). Serious adverse effects are gastrointestinal (peptic ulcer disease, bleeding), hematologic (thrombocytopenia, anemia), otic (tinnitus), and respiratory (bronchospasm). Angioedema and Reye syndrome are also potential serious adverse effects associated with aspirin use. The range of toxicity for salicylates is: acute ingestions greater than 150 mg/kg are toxic and should be referred to a health care facility; chronic ingestions of greater than 100 mg/kg/d for 2 days may cause toxicity.

Precautions for the utilization of aspirin include alcohol use (three or more standard servings per day), gastrointestinal symptoms, peptic ulcer disease, renal failure, and severe hepatic insufficiency.

Contraindications to the use of aspirin include:

- Hypersensitivity to nonsteroidal anti-inflammatory drugs or salicylates
- Use in children and teenagers (<16 years of age) with chickenpox or flu symptoms because of the risk of Reye syndrome
- Use in individuals with asthma, rhinitis, and nasal polyps

The pregnancy rating of aspirin is that fetal risk cannot be ruled out. Aspirin should be avoided in the third trimester, and used with caution during the first and second trimesters.

Clopidogrel

Clopidogrel (Plavix) 75 mg by mouth daily is an alternative antiplatelet therapy to aspirin for PAD. Clopidogrel requires *in vivo* biotransformation to an active metabolite. The clopidogrel active metabolite inhibits platelet aggregation by selectively and irreversibly inhibiting the binding of adenosine diphosphate (ADP) to its platelet receptor and the subsequent activation of ADP-mediated glycoprotein GPIIb/IIIa complex.

Common adverse effects of clopidogrel include chest pain, hypertension, rash, constipation, diarrhea, gastritis, bleeding, and headache. Serious adverse effects include gastrointestinal hemorrhage, gastrointestinal ulcer, agranulocytosis, and abnormal liver function tests (rare).

Precautions for the use of clopidogrel are:

- Concomitant use with omeprazole or esomeprazole (may reduce clopidogrel efficacy due to lack of conversion to active metabolite)
- Patients scheduled for elective surgery (clopidogrel should be discontinued 5 days prior)
- Premature discontinuation (increases risk of cardiovascular events)
- Thrombotic thrombocytopenic purpura (TTP) which can be life threatening

TABLE 8-2 | Clinical Presentation of Peripheral Arterial Disease

Signs and Symptoms

Asymptomatic	Abnormal pedal pulses
Intermittent claudication	Femoral artery bruit
Resting pain	Cool skin temperature
Nonhealing wounds	Gangrene
Lack of hair on calves, feet, or toes	Toenail dystrophy
Critical limb ischemia (at least 2 wk of ischemic rest pain, nonhealing wound, gangrene)	Acute limb ischemia (<2 wk with pain, pulselessness, pallor, paresthesias, or paralysis)

Laboratory Tests

- None specific to PAD

Other Diagnostic Tests

- An ABI is a simple, noninvasive, quantitative test that has been proven to be highly sensitive and specific in the diagnosis of PAD.
  - Normal: 1-1.40
  - Borderline: 0.91-0.99
  - PAD: <0.9

Abbreviations: ABI, ankle-brachial index; average ankle systolic pressure divided by average brachial systolic; PAD, peripheral arterial disease.

TABLE 8-3 Pharmacotherapy Options for Patients with Peripheral Arterial Disease

Medication	Normal Dose	Side Effects	Contraindications	Mechanism of Action	Miscellaneous
Aspirin (Bayer, Bufferin, numerous others)	75 - 325 mg daily	Common: Indigestion/gastritis; Serious: Stomach ulcer, bleeding, tinnitus, bronchospasm, Reye syndrome, angioedema	Hypersensitivity to NSAIDs; children <16 y with chickenpox or flu-like symptoms; syndrome of asthma, rhinitis, nasal polyps; active bleeding, thrombocytopenia	Irreversibly inhibits prostaglandin cyclooxygenase in platelets, preventing formation of thromboxane A2, which inhibits platelet aggregation	Take with food or large volume of water to minimize GI upset; do not crush sustained release or enteric coated
Clopidogrel (Plavix)	75 mg daily	Common: Headache, hypertension, purpura, rash, gastrointestinal; Serious: Gastrointestinal bleeding, thrombotic thrombocytopenic purpura chest pain	Hypersensitivity to clopidogrel or any component of the formulation, active bleeding, intracranial hemorrhage	Selectively and irreversibly inhibits ADP binding to its platelet receptor and subsequently activates the ADP-mediated glycoprotein GPIIb/IIIa complex	CYP 450 substrate: CYP 2C19 (minor), 3A4 (minor); 1A2 (minor); CYP 450 inhibitor: 2C9 (weak)
Ticlopidine (Ticlid)	250 mg bid	Common: Rash, dizziness, diarrhea, nausea; Serious: Bleeding, bone marrow suppression	Active bleeding, severe hepatic impairment, neutropenia, thrombocytopenia	Irreversibly alters platelet membrane function resulting in platelet aggregation inhibition	Take with food; a complete blood count should be obtained every 2 wk starting the second week through the third month of treatment; more frequent monitoring is recommended for patients whose neutrophils have been decreasing or are less than 30% of baseline; ticlopidine is a substrate of CYP 3A4 (major) and inhibits 1A2 (weak), 2C9 (weak), 2C19 (strong), 2D6 (moderate), 2E1 (weak), 3A4 (weak)
Cilostazol (Pletal)	100 mg bid	Common: Palpitations, tachycardia, edema, headache, diarrhea, dizziness, infection, cough, rhinitis; Serious: Heart failure, leukopenia, aplastic anemia, thrombocytopenia, fever from infection	All degrees of HF, active bleeding	Inhibit phosphodiesterase and suppresses cAMP degradation resulting in increased cAMP in platelets and blood vessels; reversible inhibitor of platelet aggregation; produces vasodilation, but not in renal arteries	High-fat food increases absorption; take 30 min before or 2 h after a meal; substrate of CYP 1A2 (minor), 2C19 (minor), 2D6 (minor), 3A4 (major)
Pentoxifylline (Trental)	400 mg tid	Common: Nausea, vomiting, dizziness, headache; Serious: Angioedema, anemia, blurred vision, bone marrow suppression, and purpura	Recent cerebral or retinal hemorrhage, active bleeding	Reduces blood viscosity and improves erythrocyte flexibility, inhibits platelet aggregation, decreases fibrinogen concentrations	Take with food; inhibits CYP 450 1A2 (weak); tablets should be swallowed whole

Abbreviations: ADP, adenine di-phosphate; cAMP, cyclic adenosine monophosphate; bid, twice daily; CYP 450, cytochrome p450; GI, gastrointestinal; GPIIb/IIIa, glycoprotein IIb/IIIa; HF, heart failure; NSAIDs, nonsteroidal anti-inflammatory drugs; tid, three times daily.

Contraindications for the use of clopidogrel are active bleeding (such as peptic ulcer or intracranial hemorrhage) and/or hypersensitivity to clopidogrel or any component of the product. Clopidogrel is category B in pregnancy, but reports state that the use of clopidogrel in breast-feeding women may pose infant risk.

Ticlopidine

Ticlopidine (Ticlid) is a thienopyridine antiplatelet drug structurally similar to clopidogrel. Hematologic effect of ticlopidine limits its utilization in patients with PAD and is not a recommended therapy. Ticlopidine has a black box warning—may cause life-threatening hematologic reactions, including neutropenia, agranulocytosis, TTP, and aplastic anemia.

Cilostazol

Cilostazol (Pletal) is a phosphodiesterase inhibitor indicated for patients with IC to improve pain-free walking and increase maximal walking distance. The dose of cilostazol is 100 mg orally twice daily. Cilostazol dosing adjustments are required for concomitant use with diltiazem, ketoconazole, erythromycin, omeprazole, and other cytochrome P450 3A4 or 2C19 inhibitors (decrease dose to 50 mg orally bid). As a result, cyclic adenosine monophosphate is increased leading to reversible inhibition of platelet aggregation, vasodilation, and inhibition of vascular smooth muscle cell proliferation.

Common side effects associated with cilostazol include: headache, dizziness, palpitations, abnormal stools, diarrhea, rhinitis, and infection. Other side effects include: edema, nausea, and abdominal pain. Rare life-threatening reactions include agranulocytosis, anemia, heart failure, and hemorrhage.

Precautions associated with the use of cilostazol include concomitant therapy with platelet-aggregation inhibitors, or in patients with thrombocytopenia, renal impairment (creatinine clearance <25 mL/min) or hepatic impairment. Hematologic events, such as thrombocytopenia or leukopenia progressing to agranulocytosis, have been reported with the use of this drug. Contraindications to the use of cilostazol include heart failure of any severity (black box warning), hemostatic disorders or active pathological bleeding (bleeding peptic ulcer or intracranial bleeding), and hypersensitivity to cilostazol or any of its components. Cilostazol is category C risk in pregnancy and should be avoided in breastfeeding female patients.

Pentoxifylline

Pentoxifylline (Trental) has been evaluated for claudication symptom management; however, it is not an effective treatment for PAD. Pentoxifylline was not better than placebo in randomized controlled trials aimed to improve walking distance. Pentoxifylline reduces blood viscosity via increased leukocyte and erythrocyte deformability and decreased neutrophil activation. It improves tissue oxygenation presumably through enhanced blood flow. Pentoxifylline is dosed 400 mg by mouth three times daily with meals (may reduce dose to 400 mg twice daily if gastrointestinal or central nervous system side effects occur). Tablets should be swallowed whole; not chewed, broken, or crushed.

Side effects associated with pentoxifylline include gastrointestinal problems (nausea and vomiting). Rare life-threatening reactions include angioedema, anemia, blurred vision, bone marrow suppression, and purpura. Contraindications for pentoxifylline include hypersensitivity to pentoxifylline, xanthines (eg, caffeine, theophylline), and recent cerebral and/or retinal hemorrhage. Pentoxifylline is category C risk in pregnancy and should be avoided in breast-feeding female patients.

CASE Application

1. A 42-year-old smoker with hypertension, diabetes, hypercholesterolemia, and PAD complains of pain in his calves when he walks two to three blocks. What therapy might offer him the greatest benefit in symptom reduction and in overall mortality?

   a. Limb revascularization procedure
   b. Cilostazol
   c. Smoking cessation
   d. Pravastatin

2. Which of the following are contraindications to the use of aspirin? Select all that apply.

   a. Asthma
   b. Hypersensitivity to NSAIDS
   c. Nasal polyps
   d. 30-year-old man with influenza

3. Which of the following is recommended as an alternative antiplatelet therapy for patients with PAD who do not tolerate aspirin?

   a. Pentoxifylline 400 mg twice daily
   b. Clopidogrel 225 mg daily
   c. Clopidogrel 75 mg daily
   d. Pentoxifylline 400 mg three times daily

4. Which of the following pharmacologic interventions may achieve a reduction in cardiovascular events for a patient with established peripheral arterial disease? Select all that apply.

   a. Aspirin
   b. Clopidogrel
   c. Statin therapy
   d. Pentoxifylline

5. Which of the following antiplatelet agents is not generally used in the treatment of PAD and should be monitored with periodic complete blood count testing related to potential hematologic complications that include agranulocytosis and aplastic anemia?

   a. Aspirin
   b. Simvastatin
   c. Ticlopidine
   d. Dipyridamole plus aspirin

6. Which of the following patients would have a contraindication for receiving cilostazol as treatment for peripheral arterial disease?

    a. A 49-year-old woman with hypertension
    b. A 60-year-old man with a history of benign prostatic hypertrophy
    c. A 48-year-old man with congestive heart failure
    d. A 52-year-old woman with hypothyroidism

7. A 58-year-old male patient with heart failure, erectile dysfunction, and CAD with stable angina underwent testing for PAD after having findings suggestive of PAD on physical examination at his last primary care office visit. Which of the following diagnostic tests is most appropriate to confirm a PAD diagnosis in this patient?

    a. Fecal occult blood test
    b. Toe-brachial index
    c. Cardiac catheterization
    d. Ankle-brachial index

8. The 58-year-old male patient with heart failure and CAD was diagnosed with PAD after recent testing. Current medications: carvedilol 25 mg po bid, lisinopril 40 mg po daily, aspirin 81 mg po daily. The patient describes his lower extremity pain as cramping up and down the backs of his legs, worse during busy times at the restaurant and resolves with rest. Which of the following therapies would be the best treatment for his leg symptoms?

    a. Cilostazol 100 mg po twice daily
    b. Structured walking exercise therapy
    c. Pentoxifylline 400 mg po three times daily
    d. Clopidogrel 75 mg po daily

9. Select the treatment goal(s) for PAD in patients with intermittent claudication. Select all that apply.

    a. Increase maximal walking distance
    b. Increase duration of walking
    c. Increase amount of pain-free walking
    d. Decrease preload
    e. Decrease afterload

10. Select the risk factors (comorbidities) that should be controlled in a patient with PAD. Select all that apply.

    a. Blood pressure
    b. Cholesterol
    c. Blood glucose
    d. International normalized ratio (INR)

11. Select the primary pharmacologic management for PAD.

    a. Anticoagulants
    b. Antiplatelet agents
    c. Antihypertensive agents
    d. Sympatholytic agents

12. A 28-year-old mother with no significant medical history asks her pharmacist if she can start taking low-dose aspirin herself and also thinks it is a good idea to keep a bottle in the house in case anyone in her family gets a headache or has some mild pain. Which of the following counseling points should be discussed with the patient? Select all that apply.

    a. Low-dose aspirin is perfectly fine to have around the house. Many people find it works well for mild pains and headache and it is safe for anyone over the age of 12.
    b. You should discuss this with your physician. Some of the common side effects include indigestion and nausea and some of the serious side effects include bleeding, ringing in the ears, and peptic ulcer disease.
    c. Should you decide to become pregnant while you are taking aspirin, let your doctor know right away because aspirin may not be safe while pregnant, especially during the third trimester.
    d. Do not give aspirin to anyone who has asthma or breathing problems without discussing with their physician because aspirin may cause bronchospasm.

13. Select the dose(s) of aspirin utilized in the management of PAD. Select all that apply.

    a. 81 mg
    b. 162 mg
    c. 50 mg
    d. 325 mg

14. Clopidogrel works by which of the following mechanisms?

    a. Selectively and irreversibly inhibits ADP-induced platelet aggregation.
    b. Reversibly inhibits platelet aggregation.
    c. Reduces blood viscosity by inhibiting phosphodiesterase.
    d. Suppresses cyclic adenosine monophosphate (cAMP) degradation, which produces vasodilation.

15. Which of the following medications is contraindicated in patients with hypersensitivity to xanthines?

    a. Aspirin
    b. Plavix
    c. Trental
    d. Pletal

16. Which of the following medications require dosage reduction when administered with strong CYP3A4 inhibitors?

    a. Aspirin
    b. Cilostazol
    c. Pentoxifylline
    d. Clopidogrel

17. Which of the following immunizations is recommended for patients with PAD?

    a. Pneumococcal PPSV-23
    b. Pneumococcal PCV-13
    c. Annual influenza vaccine
    d. Zoster vaccine

18. Which of the following symptoms suggest limb-threatening ischemia and should prompt immediate referral for further evaluation? Select all that apply.

    a. Toenail dystrophy
    b. Gangrene
    c. Paralysis
    d. Severe lower extremity pain at rest

19. Which of the following treatments are recommended as standard therapy for all patients with PAD? Select all that apply.

    a. Aspirin or clopidogrel
    b. Cilostazol
    c. Statin
    d. Ticlopidine
    e. Pentoxifylline

20. A 66-year-old female patient with PAD and exertional pain in her lower extremities is currently taking cilostazol, aspirin, atorvastatin, and lisinopril. Which of the following is the most common adverse effect of taking cilostazol and aspirin in combination?

    a. Heart failure hospitalizations
    b. Subtherapeutic effects of cilostazol
    c. Skeletal muscle soreness
    d. Increased bleeding risk

TAKEAWAY POINTS »

- Peripheral arterial disease (PAD) commonly involves atherosclerotic occlusion of the lower extremities and is one of many potential manifestations of systemic atherosclerosis.
- A higher prevalence of PAD is associated with increased age, tobacco abuse, diabetes mellitus, hypertension, and hyperlipidemia.
- Patients with PAD have approximately the same relative risk of death from cardiovascular disease as patients with a history of coronary or cerebrovascular disease, and PAD should be considered a surrogate marker of subclinical coronary artery disease.
- Specific treatment goals should include:
  - Increasing maximal walking distance, duration of walking, and amount of pain-free walking
  - Risk factor modification focused on reducing overall cardiovascular risk (smoking cessation, optimal management of hypertension, hyperlipidemia, and diabetes). Improving control of comorbid conditions can result in improvement in overall quality of life and reduction in cardiovascular complications and death
  - Limb preservation
- Structured exercise rehabilitation programs are effective for claudication symptoms.
- Primary pharmacologic interventions for PAD involve antiplatelet drug therapies and statins to reduce the risk of myocardial infarction, stroke, or vascular death in individuals with atherosclerotic lower extremity PAD.
- Cilostazol is an effective pharmacologic agent for claudication to improve pain-free walking and increase maximal walking distance.

BIBLIOGRAPHY

Aspirin. Micromedex Solutions. Truven Health Analytics, Inc. Ann Arbor, MI. Available at: http://www.micromedexsolutions.com. Accessed April 10, 2018.

Chow SL, Hoeben BJ. Peripheral arterial disease. In: DiPiro JT, Talbert RL, Yee GC, Matzke GR, Wells BG, Posey L, eds. *Pharmacotherapy: A Pathophysiologic Approach.* 10th ed. New York, NY: McGraw-Hill. http://accesspharmacy .mhmedical.com.libproxy.siue.edu/content.aspx?bookid=1861 &sectionid=146078809. Accessed September 28, 2017.

Gerhard-Herman MD, Gornik HL, Barrett C, et al. 2016 AHA/ACC Guideline on the Management of Patients With Lower Extremity Peripheral ArteryDisease: A Report of the American College of Cardiology/American Heart Association Task Force on Clinical Practice Guidelines. *Circulation.* 2017;135:e726-e779.

Michel T, Hoffman BB. Treatment of myocardial ischemia and hypertension. In: Brunton LL, Chabner BA, Knollmann BC, eds. *Goodman & Gilman's: The Pharmacological Basis of Therapeutics.* 12th ed. New York, NY: McGraw-Hill. http://accesspharmacy.mhmedical.com.libproxy.siue.edu/content .aspx?bookid=1613&sectionid=102160058. Accessed September 28, 2017.

Weitz JI. Blood coagulation and anticoagulant, fibrinolytic, and antiplatelet drugs. In: Brunton LL, Chabner BA, Knollmann BC, eds. *Goodman & Gilman's The Pharmacological Basis of Therapeutics.* 12th ed. New York, NY: McGraw-Hill; 2011:chap 30.

Zehnder JL. Drugs used in disorders of coagulation. In: Katzung BG, Trevor AJ, eds. *Basic & Clinical Pharmacology.* 13th ed. New York, NY: McGraw-Hill; 2015. http://accesspharmacy .mhmedical.com.libproxy.siue.edu/content.aspx?bookid=1193 &sectionid=69108955. Accessed September 28, 2017.

KEY ABBREVIATIONS

ABI = ankle-brachial index
ADP = adenosine diphosphate
IC = intermittent claudication

PAD = peripheral arterial disease
TTP = thrombotic thrombocytopenic purpura

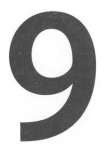

CHAPTER 9

Arrhythmias

Robyn Teply and Kathleen Packard

FOUNDATION OVERVIEW

Cardiac arrhythmia is an abnormality of impulse generation, impulse propagation, or a combination of both. *Normal* conduction and cardiac rhythm are initiated by the sinoatrial (SA) node. The electrical current then travels through the conduction network and enters the ventricle via the atrioventricular (AV) node and bundle of His. From the bundle of His, the electrical activity moves into the branch-like system called the Purkinje system. As the current flows through the myocardium, the excitation coordinates the contraction of the atria and ventricles. After stimulation, each group of cells experiences a refractory period in which it cannot be excited. As the electrical current meets refractory tissue, the stimulation ceases allowing for the process to begin again.

Conduction of electrical impulses through the myocardium is represented on an electrocardiogram (ECG) as waves of depolarization and repolarization. As depolarization occurs, the heart's myocytes become positive and contract. Recovery immediately follows as the myocytes return to their resting negative charge during repolarization. The initial p wave on an ECG represents depolarization leading to contraction of the atria, or top chambers of the heart. The QRS complex on an ECG represents depolarization of the ventricles and subsequent ventricular contraction. Finally, the T wave represents ventricular repolarization. One cardiac cycle consists of atrial systole, then ventricular systole, and finally a resting phase (Figure 9-1).

Atrial Fibrillation

Atrial fibrillation (AF) is disorganized atrial activation and subsequent uncoordinated atrial contraction. AF can be symptomatic, lead to hemodynamic compromise and result in increased morbidity and mortality. AF is characterized as recurrent (having presented with two or more episodes), paroxysmal (if the recurrent AF terminates spontaneously), persistent (if it is sustained for at least 7 days), or permanent (in which attempts to convert to sinus rhythm have failed). It is the most common cardiac arrhythmia and the onset is associated with increasing age, male sex, and presence of cardiovascular disease. AF can be asymptomatic or symptomatic (palpitations, shortness of breath [SOB], and fatigue). The ECG of AF is an irregularly, irregular supraventricular rhythm, with no discernable p waves, and a variable ventricular rate often between 120 and 180 beats/min.

Paroxysmal Supraventricular Tachycardia

Paroxysmal supraventricular tachycardia (PSVT) is a tachyarrhythmia with an abrupt onset and termination which results from an arrhythmia originating or involving supraventricular tissue. Many patients with PSVT are asymptomatic while others have symptoms including palpitations, fatigue, light-headedness, chest discomfort, and dyspnea.

Premature Ventricular Complexes

Premature ventricular complexes (PVCs) are a common, most often benign, arrhythmia originating from the ventricular tissue. In the general population, PVCs are present in people with and without structural heart disease. For patients with a previous myocardial infarction or who have structural heart disease, PVCs have greater prognostic value and are associated with an increased risk of sudden death. Many patients are asymptomatic and PVCs are found incidentally on ECG. When symptomatic, patients present with palpitations, dyspnea, chest pain, syncope, or presyncope.

Ventricular Tachycardia and Ventricular Fibrillation

Ventricular tachycardia (VT) is characterized as nonsustained VT (three or more beats in duration which terminate in less than 30 seconds) or sustained VT (VT lasting greater than 30 seconds in duration and/or involving hemodynamic compromise in less than 30 seconds). Torsade de pointes (TdP) is a rapid form of VT seen when the QTc interval is prolonged greater than 500 milliseconds and is diagnosed by an undulating party-streamer appearance on the ECG. VT results from fibrous scar tissue formed after an acute myocardial infarction or from nonischemic cardiomyopathy.

Ventricular fibrillation (VF) is a rapid (300 beats/min), irregular ventricular rhythm leading to asynchronous contraction of the left ventricle and rapid hemodynamic compromise. Sudden cardiac death occurs rapidly if medical intervention is not performed. In hemodynamically stable patients with VT, symptoms include palpitations and in those that are unstable,

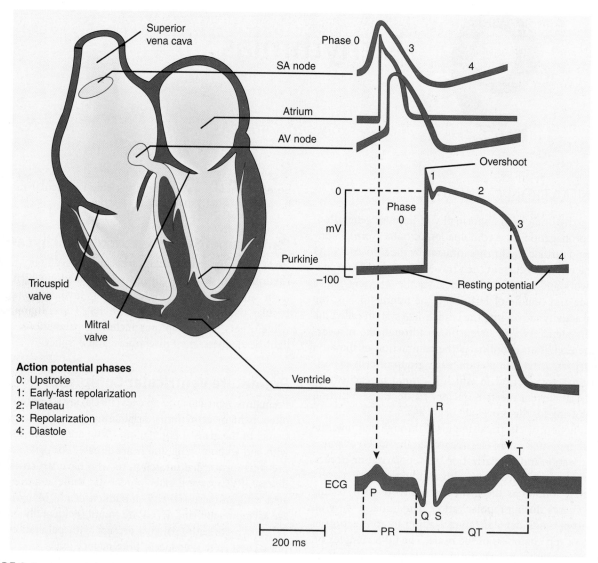

Action potential phases
0: Upstroke
1: Early-fast repolarization
2: Plateau
3: Repolarization
4: Diastole

FIGURE 9-1 Agents used in cardiac arrhythmias. Reproduced with permission from Katzung BG, Masters SB, Trevor AJ: *Basic & Clinical Pharmacology*, 12th ed. New York, NY: McGraw-Hill; 2012.

patients can experience light-headedness, dizziness, loss of consciousness, and potentially sudden cardiac death.

Sinus Bradycardia

Sinus bradycardia is described as a regular rhythm with a heart rate (HR) of less than 60 beats/min. It can be asymptomatic in young, active individuals or symptomatic in patients with etiologies such as sinus node dysfunction. The resulting decrease in cardiac output causes hypotension leading to dizziness, syncope, fatigue, and/or confusion.

TREATMENT

Classification of the antiarrhythmic drugs including mechanism of action, side effects, and contraindications can be found in Table 9-1. Table 9-2 lists specific monitoring recommendations for amiodarone.

Atrial Fibrillation

AF management involves evaluating the need for immediate treatment, assessing the need for rate and/or rhythm control, and evaluating the need for anticoagulation for the prevention of thromboembolic complications. Acute treatment is warranted if the patient is hemodynamically unstable with direct current cardioversion (DCC) indicated. If the patient has been in AF for less than 48 hours, DCC can proceed without a transesophageal echocardiogram (TEE), but the patient should be anticoagulated. Anticoagulation options include treatment dose unfractionated heparin (80 units/kg intravenous [IV] bolus followed by 18 units/kg/h IV continuous infusion) or treatment dose low molecular weight heparin such as enoxaparin (1 mg/kg subcutaneous [SQ] every 12 hours with normal renal function). Parenteral anticoagulation is not required if a patient has been adherent to a direct-acting oral anticoagulant (DOAC) or warfarin with a therapeutic international normalized ratio (INR) (2-3). If the AF duration is unknown

TABLE 9-1   Antiarrhythmic Drugs

Type	Generic Name/Route of Administration	Brand Name	Mechanism of Action	Adverse Effects	Contraindications
Ia	Quinidine IV, IM, po	Quinidex, Quinaglute	Slow depolarization through Na$^+$ channel blockade	N/V/D, cinchonism, TdP	
	Procainamide IV, IM	Pronestyl, Procan, Procanbid		Lupus-like-syndrome, N/V/D, hypotension, TdP	LVEF <40%
	Disopyramide po	Norpace		Anticholinergic symptoms, N, anorexia, TdP, HF	Glaucoma
Ib	Lidocaine IV, IO, ET	Xylocaine		CNS including slurred speech, blurry vision, tinnitus, seizures	Third-degree AV heart block
	Mexiletine po	Mexitil		CNS including tremors, dizziness, confusion	Third-degree AV heart block
Ic	Flecainide po	Tambocor		Blurry vision, dizziness, tremor, HF	HF, CAD, valvular disease, LVH
	Propafenone po	Rhythmol		Taste disturbances, dizziness, HF, bronchospasm, bradycardia	HF (NHYA III-IV), liver disease, valvular disease
II	Metoprolol IV, po	Toprol XL, Lopressor	Slow AV nodal conduction through β-blockade	Hypotension, bradycardia, dizziness, mask hypoglycemia symptoms except sweating	Severe COPD/asthma, severe bradycardia, heart block, severe hypotension, decompensated HF
	Esmolol IV	Brevibloc			
	Atenolol IV, po	Tenormin			
III	Amiodarone IV, po	Cordarone	Slow repolarization through K$^+$ channel blockade	QT prolongation, bradycardia, pulmonary fibrosis, hypothyroidism, hyperthyroidism, CNS toxicity, photosensitivity, corneal deposits, macular degeneration, hepatitis, blue-gray skin, heart block	Iodine hypersensitivity, third-degree heart block
	Dofetilide po	Tikosyn		TdP, dizziness, diarrhea	Baseline QTc >440 ms, CrCl <20 mL/min
	Sotalol IV, po	Betapace, Betapace AF, Sorine		HF, bradycardia, TdP, bronchospasm, dizziness, fatigue, N/V/D	Baseline QTc >440 ms, CrCl <40 mL/min
	Ibutilide IV	Covert		TdP, heart block, hypotension	Baseline QTc >440 ms, concomitant antiarrhythmics, LVEF <30%
	Dronedarone po	Multaq		QT prolongation, increased SCr, hepatic toxicity	NYHA Class IV HF or recent decompensation, QTc ≥500
IV	Verapamil IV, po	Calan, Covera, Isoptin, Verelan	Slow AV nodal conduction through Ca$^+$ channel blockade	Gingival hyperplasia, constipation	LV dysfunction, SBP <90 mm Hg, sick sinus syndrome, AV block
	Diltiazem IV, po	Cardizem, -CD, -LA, Cartia XT, Dilacor XR, Dilt-XR,-CD, Diltia XT, Diltzac, Taztia XT, Tiazac		Edema, headache	Sick sinus syndrome, AV block, SBP <90 mm Hg, pulmonary congestion

Abbreviations: AF, atrial fibrillation; AV, atrioventricular; CAD, coronary artery disease; COPD, chronic obstructive pulmonary disease; CNS, central nervous system; CrCl, creatinine clearance; D, diarrhea; ET, endotracheal; HF, heart failure; IM, intramuscular; IO, intraosseous; IV, intravenous; LV, left ventricular; LVH, left ventricular hypertrophy; LVEF, left ventricular ejection fraction; N, nausea; NYHA, New York Heart Association Classification; po, oral; QTc, corrected QT interval; SBP, systolic blood pressure; SCr, serum creatinine; TdP, torsade de pointes; V, vomiting.

or greater than 48 hours, a TEE is recommended along with the above-mentioned anticoagulation prior to the DCC. If the patient is stable in an outpatient setting, the therapy should be rate control and anticoagulation leading up to DCC. With no comorbid conditions, initial therapy choices for rate control are β-blockers or nondihydropyridine calcium channel blockers (diltiazem, verapamil). In patients with decreased left ventricular (LV) function (ejection fraction [EF] ≤40%),

digoxin or amiodarone are recommended for initial rate control. Stable patients who do not require an urgent TEE and DCC can be conservatively managed and anticoagulated on an outpatient basis for 3 to 4 weeks prior to DCC. All patients that undergo DCC (stable and unstable) should be anticoagulated for 4 weeks following the cardioversion. Decisions about anticoagulation thereafter should be based on thrombotic risk. Sinus rhythm can be restored through DCC or pharmacologic

TABLE 9-2 Amiodarone Monitoring

Side Effect	Monitoring Recommendations	Management of Side Effect
Pulmonary fibrosis	Chest radiograph (baseline, and then every 12 mo) Pulmonary function tests (baseline, and then if symptoms develop) High-resolution CT (if symptoms develop)	Discontinue amiodarone immediately; may consider corticosteroid therapy
Hypothyroidism	TFTs (baseline, and then every 6 mo)	Thyroid hormone supplementation (eg, levothyroxine)
Hyperthyroidism	TFTs (baseline, and then every 6 mo)	Antithyroid drugs (eg, methimazole, propylthiouracil) or corticosteroids; may need to discontinue amiodarone
Optic neuritis/neuropathy	Ophthalmologic examination (baseline [only if visual impairment present], and then if symptoms develop)	Discontinue amiodarone immediately
Corneal microdeposits	Slit-lamp examination (routine monitoring not necessary)	No treatment necessary
Hepatotoxicity	LFTs (baseline, and then every 6 mo)	Lower the dose or discontinue amiodarone if LFTs >2 times the upper limit of normal
Bradycardia/heart block	ECG (baseline, and then every 3-6 mo)	Lower the dose, if possible, or discontinue amiodarone if severe (or continue amiodarone and implant permanent pacemaker)
Tremor, ataxia, peripheral neuropathy	History/physical examination (each office visit)	Lower the dose, if possible, or discontinue amiodarone if severe
Photosensitivity/blue-gray skin discoloration	History/physical examination (each office visit)	Lower the dose; advise patients to wear sunblock while outdoors

Abbreviations: CT, computed tomography; ECG, electrocardiogram; LFTs, liver function tests; TFTs, thyroid function tests.
Reproduced with permission from DiPiro JT, Talbert RL, Yee GC, et al: *Pharmacotherapy: A Pathophysiologic Approach*, 10th ed. New York, NY: McGraw-Hill; 2017.

cardioversion. In patients without structural heart disease, flecainide, propafenone, amiodarone, dofetilide, or ibutilide can be used. In patients with structural heart disease, amiodarone or dofetilide are the drugs of choice for pharmacologic cardioversion.

For the chronic management of patients with AF, there is ongoing debate on controlling HR or maintaining sinus rhythm. There is no difference in mortality between rate or rhythm control. If patients are symptomatic despite rate control, rhythm control can be attempted. The antiarrhythmic should be selected based upon the patients past medical history.

- Dofetilide, dronederone, flecainide, propafenone, and sotalol can be used if the patient has no structural heart disease.
  - Alternatively, amiodarone is a second-choice therapy.
- If coronary artery disease is present, dofetilide, dronederone, or sotalol are the first-choice agents and amiodarone is a second-choice therapy.
- If the patient has heart failure (HF), amiodarone or dofetilide are the drugs of choice.

Long-term oral anticoagulation is recommended to prevent thromboembolic complications in most AF patients. The CHA_2DS_2-VASc score is used to assess stroke risk in nonvalvular AF as follows:

C = Congestive HF 1 point

H = Hypertension 1 point

A = Age more than or equal to 75 years 2 points

D = DM 1 point

S = Stroke, transient ischemic attack (TIA), or thromboembolism 2 points

V = Vascular disease (prior MI, peripheral arterial disease [PAD], or aortic plaque) 1 point

A = Age 65 to 74 years 1 point

Sc = Sex category, female = 1 point

If prior stroke, TIA, or CHA_2DS_2-VASc score is more than or equal to 2, long-term oral anticoagulation is recommended with either a DOAC or warfarin. If the CHA_2DS_2-VASc score is equal to 1, no antithrombotic therapy or therapy with aspirin or an oral anticoagulant are reasonable.

If the CHA_2DS_2-VASc score is 0, antithrombotic therapy can be omitted.

Paroxysmal Supraventricular Tachycardia

DCC is recommended in the acute management of PSVT, if the symptoms are severe (syncope, angina, severe HF). For mild symptoms, vasovagal maneuvers (unilateral carotid sinus massage, Valsalva maneuver, ice water facial immersion, or induced retching) are recommended. If vasovagal maneuvers are unsuccessful, acute treatment is based on ECG findings and includes:

1. narrow QRS interval and regular rhythm, drugs of choice are adenosine, β-blockers, verapamil, or diltiazem;
2. wide QRS interval and regular rhythm, drugs of choice are adenosine or procainamide; and
3. wide QRS interval and irregular rhythm, drugs of choice are procainamide or amiodarone.

After a definitive diagnosis is made, the treatment of choice for those with severe and frequent symptoms is catheter ablation and if symptoms are mild and infrequent, antiarrhythmics can be used as needed.

Premature Ventricular Complexes

Many patients with PVCs do not require intervention. Treatment of symptomatic patients with PVCs should be limited to the use of β-blockers. Class Ic agents should be avoided due to the increased risk of mortality postmyocardial infarction.

Ventricular Tachycardia

For stable patients with monomorphic VT, first-line therapy is a loading dose of adenosine 6 mg followed by a second dose of 12 mg, if necessary. If adenosine is unsuccessful, the next step is amiodarone (150 mg) over 10 minutes followed by an amiodarone drip. After the drip has been started, prepare for DCC. If the patient is unstable, perform immediate DCC. If the patient is experiencing polymorphic VT (torsades de pointes), discontinue any potential offending agents (Class Ia or III antiarrhythmics, erythromycin, clarithromycin, fluoroquinolones, pentamidine, fluconazole, haloperidol, phenothiazines, tricyclic antidepressants, diuretics, or other agents causing electrolyte disturbances). If the patient is unstable, DCC is indicated and magnesium 1 to 2 g IV push is recommended regardless of serum electrolyte concentrations. If the patient is stable, administer 1 to 2 g IV push of magnesium.

Ventricular Fibrillation or Pulseless Ventricular Tachycardia

If a patient is found to be in VF or pulseless VT, begin advanced cardiopulmonary life support. After the primary CABs (compression, airway, and breathing) have been enacted and a shockable rhythm has been detected, initiate DCC. Following cardiopulmonary resuscitation (CPR) and DCC, give epinephrine 1 mg IV every 3 to 5 minutes (no maximum). Repeat DCC and resume CPR immediately. Antiarrhythmics can be considered at this time, amiodarone 300 mg IV one time and repeated at a dose of 150 mg IV or lidocaine 1 to 1.5 mg/kg IV and repeated at a dose of 0.5 to 0.75 mg/kg IV every 5 to 10 minutes (maximum dose of 3 mg/kg). If the rhythm is not shockable (pulseless electrical activity or asystole), begin CPR. Give epinephrine 1 mg IV every 3 to 5 minutes.

Sinus Bradycardia

If the patient is stable, observe and monitor the patient. If the patient is hemodynamically unstable, begin transcutaneous pacing and consider atropine 0.5 mg IV which can be repeated up to 3 mg total. If the patient does not respond, an infusion of epinephrine at 2 to 10 mcg/min or dopamine at 2 to 10 mcg/kg/min can be initiated. The long-term therapy of choice in patients with symptomatic bradycardia is the implantation of a permanent pacemaker.

CASE Application

1. The onset of AF is associated with which patient characteristics? Select ALL that apply.

   a. Hepatitis
   b. Increasing age
   c. Female sex
   d. Cardiovascular disease

2. A 68-year-old woman weighing 60 kg presents to the emergency room in AF and is hemodynamically unstable. It is decided to proceed with DCC. Which of the following would be appropriate anticoagulation therapy to administer prior to DCC? Select ALL that apply.

   a. Enoxaparin 60 mg
   b. Unfractionated heparin 4800 unit bolus followed by 1100 units/h by continuous infusion
   c. Enoxaparin 40 mg
   d. Enoxaparin 30 mg

3. Which of the following is/are available in oral and IV preparations? Select ALL that apply.

   a. Diltiazem
   b. Dofetilide
   c. Dronedarone
   d. Amiodarone

4. A patient with an HR of 53 beats/min is complaining of SOB, light-headedness, and has a blood pressure (BP) of 80/58 mm Hg. Transcutaneous pacing is being prepared. What is the first drug and dose that should be administered?

   a. Epinephrine 1 mg IV
   b. Atropine 0.5 mg IV
   c. Atropine 1 mg IV
   d. Dopamine 1-5 mcg/kg/min IV

5. You respond with the code team to a patient that is in cardiac arrest. High-quality chest compressions are being given. The patient is intubated and an IV has been started. ECG reveals that the patient is in asystole. The first IV drug and dose to administer is:

   a. Amiodarone 300 mg IV
   b. Epinephrine 1 mg IV
   c. Dopamine 1 to 5 mcg/kg/min
   d. Lidocaine 1 to 1.5 mg/kg IV

6. Which of the following antiarrhythmic drugs is *likely* to cause TdP? Select ALL that apply.

   a. Quinidine
   b. Sotalol
   c. Lidocaine
   d. Dofetilide

7. A nonresponsive patient in ventricular fibrillation has received multiple appropriate defibrillations and

epinephrine 1 mg IV twice. Which antiarrhythmic drug can be used next?

a. Cordarone
b. Isoptin
c. Brevibloc
d. Quinidex

8. A 79-year-old man weighing 80 kg presents to your hospital emergency room with newly discovered AF with rapid ventricular response and is symptomatic with little rate control achieved after initiation of a diltiazem drip. It is decided by the attending physician to proceed with electrical cardioversion. The patient's wife reports that he underwent a cardiac workup the day before for routine knee replacement surgery. The ECG from that workup is retrieved and shows normal sinus rhythm. What is the next appropriate step in this patient's care?

a. Proceed with synchronized direct cardioversion after receiving enoxaparin 80 mg.
b. Anticoagulate with warfarin for 3 weeks, target INR 2.0 to 3.0, then cardioversion.
c. Obtain transesophageal ECHO to rule out thrombus then cardioversion.
d. Proceed with synchronized direct current cardioversion without anticoagulation.

9. A 65-year-old patient presents with AF and HF. Which of the following is the best choice for pharmacologic cardioversion of AF in this patient?

a. Flecainide
b. Sotalol
c. Dofetilide
d. Dronedarone

10. Amiodarone requires substantial safety monitoring during long-term therapy due to its numerous side effects. Which of the following is required to be routinely performed in a patient on long-term amiodarone therapy?

a. Hepatic function panel
b. Renal function panel
c. Erythrocyte sedimentation rate
d. B-type natriuretic peptide (BNP) levels

11. Dofetilide is indicated in which of the following?

a. A patient initiated in an outpatient setting
b. A patient with creatinine clearance (CrCl) <20 mL/min
c. A baseline QTc 510 millisecond
d. A patient with LV hypertrophy

12. Which antiarrhythmic drug is safer to use for maintenance of sinus rhythm in a patient with AF, HF, and an ejection fraction of 15%?

a. Sotalol
b. Flecainide
c. Amiodarone
d. Procainamide

13. RT is a 65-year-old woman who presents with PSVT with a regular rhythm. RT is experiencing mild symptoms and was given unilateral carotid sinus massage with no success. If the patient has a narrow QRS interval, what medication(s) is(are) first-line agent(s) to treat this patient? Select ALL that apply.

a. Adenosine
b. Verapamil
c. Procainamide
d. Amiodarone

14. Which antiarrhythmic drug has the potential for causing taste disturbances?

a. Norpace
b. Mexitil
c. Betapace
d. Rythmol

15. KG is a 55-year-old man who presents with recurrent complaints of SOB and describes feeling like his heart is racing. An ECG is performed and it is determined that he is in AF with a ventricular rate of 160 beats/min. An evaluation of his LV function concluded that his ejection fraction is 35%. While the patient was still in the examination room, he reports that his symptoms have subsided and a repeat ECG was completed and it was found that the patient was in normal sinus rhythm. What medication should be prescribed to KG to control his rate?

a. Flecainide
b. Amiodarone
c. Diltiazem
d. Verapamil

16. Potential side effect(s) of dronedarone is (are): (select ALL that apply)

a. Gingival hyperplasia
b. Increased serum creatinine
c. QT prolongation
d. Hypothyroidism

17. CB is a 56-year-old woman who presents with palpitations, dyspnea, and presyncope. An ECG is performed and PVCs are found. CB has a past medical history of hypertension, hyperlipidemia, and postmyocardial infarction 2 years ago. What is the treatment of choice for CB?

a. Flecainide
b. Propafenone
c. Metoprolol succinate
d. Amiodarone

18. What is the initial step in therapy for a stable patient presenting with monomorphic VT?

a. Epinephrine
b. Adenosine
c. Lidocaine
d. Immediate DCC

19. Which of the following medications given during the treatment of VF or pulseless VT has no dose maximum?

    a. Vasopressin
    b. Epinephrine
    c. Lidocaine
    d. Amiodarone

20. JL is a 47-year-old man with new onset AF and seasonal allergies. After cardioversion and 4 weeks of anticoagulation, which of the following would be appropriate therapy to prevent thromboembolic complications in JL long-term?

    a. No therapy necessary
    b. Warfarin with a target INR 2.5
    c. Aspirin 325 mg daily
    d. Rivaroxaban 20 mg once daily

21. Which of the following medications slows depolarization through sodium channel blockade?

    a. Brevibloc
    b. Tambocor
    c. Tiazac
    d. Covert

22. TG is an 85-year-old woman who is currently hospitalized for pneumonia. Her current medications include levofloxacin, albuterol via nebulization, zolpidem, and acetaminophen. On the second day of her hospitalization, her ECG reveals that she is experiencing polymorphic VT. If TG remains stable, what would be the first step of treatment?

    a. Immediate DCC
    b. Epinephrine 1 mg IV
    c. Discontinue levofloxacin
    d. Amiodarone 150 mg over 10 minutes

23. Place the following Class I antiarrhythmics in order based upon classification. Start with Class Ia.

Unordered Response	Ordered Response
Lidocaine	
Procainamide	
Flecainide	

24. Place the following antiarrhythmics in order based upon classification. Start with Class I.

Unordered Response	Ordered Response
Esmolol	
Sotalol	
Verapamil	
Mexiletine	

TAKEAWAY POINTS »

- Arrhythmias can occur in a variety of patient populations with AF being the most common type.
- Arrhythmias can be asymptomatic and incidentally discovered on an ECG.
- Potential symptoms associated with arrhythmias are palpitations, SOB, fatigue, and in more serious situations loss of consciousness.
- Immediate cardioversion for AF is necessary, if the patient is hemodynamically unstable.
- The focus of AF therapy in stable patients is rate control and prevention of thromboembolic complications reserving rhythm control for symptomatic patients.
- Most AF patients should receive anticoagulation with either warfarin or DOAC unless no known risk factors for stroke are present and in this case, aspirin may be appropriate.
- If symptoms are severe, the acute management of a patient with PSVT is DCC.
- If symptoms are mild in a patient with PSVT, vasovagal maneuvers should initially be attempted. If unsuccessful, pharmacologic therapy should be based on the ECG findings.
- Treatment of symptomatic patients with PVCs should be limited to the use of β-blockers.
- In unstable patients with monomorphic VT, immediate DCC should be performed.
- In addition to pharmacologic measures used to treat a patient with VT, discontinue any agent that has the potential for inducing the arrhythmia.
- If a patient is found to be in VF or pulseless VT, initiate advanced cardiopulmonary life support with shockable rhythms receiving DCC.
- If the patient has been shocked or if the rhythm is not shockable, proceed with pharmacologic measures in addition to CPR.
- If a patient presents with symptomatic bradycardia, begin transcutaneous pacing and start atropine.

BIBLIOGRAPHY

Goldberger AL. Atlas of cardiac arrhythmias. In: Longo DL, Fauci AS, Kasper DL, Hauser SL, Jameson J, Loscalzo J, eds. *Harrison's Principles of Internal Medicine*. 18th ed. New York, NY: McGraw-Hill; 2012:chap e30.

Hume JR, Grant AO. Agents used in cardiac arrhythmias. In: Katzung BG, Masters SB, Trevor AJ, eds. *Basic & Clinical Pharmacology*. 12th ed. New York, NY: McGraw-Hill; 2012:chap 14.

January CT, Wann LS, Alpert JS, et al. 2014 AHA/ACC/HRS guideline for the management of patients with atrial fibrillation: A report of the American College of Cardiology/American Heart Association Task Force on Practice Guidelines and the Heart Rhythm Society. *J Am Coll Cardiol.* 2014;64:e1-e76.

Sampson KJ, Kass RS. Anti-arrhythmic drugs. In: Brunton LL, Chabner BA, Knollmann BC, eds. *Goodman & Gilman's The Pharmacological Basis of Therapeutics.* 12th ed. New York, NY: McGraw-Hill; 2011:chap 29.

Sanoski CA, Bauman JL. The arrhythmias. In: DiPiro JT, Talbert RL, Yee GC, Matzke GR, Wells BG, Posey L, eds. *Pharmacotherapy: A Pathophysiologic Approach.* 10th ed. New York, NY: McGraw-Hill; 2017.

You JJ, Singer DE, Howard PA, et al. Antithrombotic therapy for atrial fibrillation: Antithrombotic Therapy and Prevention of Thrombosis, 9th ed: American College of Chest Physicians Evidence-Based Clinical Practice Guidelines. *Chest.* 2012;141:e531S-e575S.

KEY ABBREVIATIONS

AF = atrial fibrillation
AV = atrioventricular node
BNP = B-type natriuretic peptide
BP = blood pressure
CABs = compressions, airway, breathing
CAD = coronary artery disease
CPR = cardiopulmonary resuscitation
CrCl = creatinine clearance
D = diarrhea
DCC = direct current cardioversion
DM = diabetes
DOAC = direct-acting oral anticoagulant
ECG = electrocardiogram
EF = ejection fraction
ET = endotracheal
HF = heart failure
HR = heart rate
IM = intramuscular
INR = international normalized ratio
IO = intraosseous
IV = intravenous
LFT = liver function test
LMWH = low molecular weight heparin
LV = left ventricular

LVEF = left ventricular ejection fraction
MI = myocardial infarction
N = nausea
NOAC = new oral anticoagulant
NYHA = New York Heart Association classification
PAD = peripheral arterial disease
po = oral
PSVT = paroxysmal supraventricular tachycardia
PVCs = premature ventricular complexes
QTc = corrected QT interval
SA = sinoatrial node
SBP = systolic blood pressure
SCr = serum creatinine
SOB = shortness of breath
SQ = subcutaneous
TdP = torsade de pointes
TEE = transesophageal echocardiogram
TIA = transient ischemic attack
UFH = unfractionated heparin
V = vomiting
VF = ventricular fibrillation
VT = ventricular tachycardia
VTE = venous thromboembolism

Immunologic, Hematologic, and Oncologic Disorders

10

Oncology Overview and Supportive Care

Keith A. Hecht

FOUNDATION OVERVIEW

Modern medical science has led to significant improvement in survival and quality of life for individuals with neoplastic (*neoplasm*) conditions. Neoplasm (**tumor** or cancer) is an abnormal mass of tissue, the growth of which exceeds and is uncoordinated with that of normal tissues and persists after cessation of the stimuli which evoked the change. The key feature of cancer is unregulated cell division and growth, secondary to the loss of normal control mechanisms that govern cell survival, proliferation, and differentiation. Benign tumors are limited to the tissue of origin and do not invade surrounding tissue. Their dangerous counterpart, malignant tumors can invade local tissues and undergo distant spread (*metastasis*). Malignant tumors (often referred to as cancer) are predominantly of two types, solid tumors and hematologic malignancies. Solid tumors include various types of cancer, typically arising from a specific organ or site. They are characterized by their initial location as well as their cell of origin, including carcinomas (of epithelial origin) and the sarcomas (of connective tissue origin, mesenchymal origin). Hematologic malignancies include cancers that arise from cells in the hematopoietic cascade and are most commonly categorized as leukemias, lymphomas, or myeloma.

The impact of a particular cancer on a population can be assessed by calculating the lifetime risk of developing that cancer, the median age at diagnosis, and 5-year probability of survival after diagnosis (Table 10-1). The 5-year probability of survival for an individual with prostate cancer is nearly 100%, while the 5-year survival probability for pancreatic cancer and lung cancers are 9.1% and 18.7%, respectively. Several internal (eg, genetic predisposition, race, sex) and external (eg, environmental exposures like ionizing radiation, chemical carcinogens, viral infections) factors have been implicated as the cause of various types of cancer and are beyond the scope of this chapter. Screening can be used to detect cancer at an earlier, more treatable stage. Current recommendations for cancer screening are summarized in Table 10-2.

Cancer may present with a number of different signs and symptoms. After the initial visit with the provider, a variety of tests will be performed. These tests are dependent upon the initial differential diagnosis. Appropriate tests include:

- Blood work
- Radiologic scans
- Tissue sample

The tissue sample may be obtained by a biopsy, fine-needle aspiration, or exfoliative cytology and should be done before treatment is initiated. It is important to obtain accurate tissue diagnosis prior to initiation of therapy. Once the pathology of the cancer is established, cancer staging is conducted. Cancer stage is the single best predictor of survival from cancer. The stage of the disease is a compilation of the primary tumor size, lymph node involvement, and distant metastases and is generally referred to as stages I through IV, with higher stages representing more advanced disease. Some cancers (eg, leukemia) cannot be measured by size, so biopsy of the bone marrow provides a cellular indication of the extent of disease.

Chemotherapy may be given to cure cancers that are curable (curative intent) or to help control symptoms of an incurable cancer (palliative intent). The response to chemotherapy is generally described as complete response (CR), partial response (PR), stable disease (SD), or progressive disease (PD).

- CR is complete disappearance of all cancer for 1 month after treatment.
- PR is 50% or greater decrease in tumor diameter.
- SD is a tumor that has not changed in size to a degree to be classified as PR or PD.
- PD refers to tumor that has spread or the primary tumor that has increased in size by at least 20% while receiving treatment.

Antineoplastic treatment plans require a complex interdisciplinary approach that involves shared decision making between individuals and their health care providers. It is important to take into account social, cultural, and emotional outlook. Once the diagnosis is confirmed (almost always requiring a tissue sample from the cancer site and having that sample examined by a pathologist), a detailed evaluation to estimate the stage and extent of the disease (*staging*) is undertaken. Treatment is customized based on

TABLE 10-1 | **Top 10 United States Invasive Cancer Statistics**

Invasive Cancer by Site (All Races)	Lifetime Risk for Cancer (Male, Female, Both)	Median Age (in years) at Diagnosis (Male, Female, Both)	5-y Relative Survival for Those Diagnosed in 2007 (Male, Female, Both)
Prostate	11.6% /—/—	66 /—/—	98.5% /—/—
Breast	—/ 12.41% /—	—/ 62 /—	—/ 89.7% /—
Lung and bronchus	6.85% / 6.4% / 5.95%	70 / 71 / 70	15.6% / 22.2% / 18.7%
Colon and rectum	4.5% / 4.2% / 4.3%	66 / 69 / 67	64.7% / 65.7% / 65.2%
Uterine corpus	—/ 2.9% /—	—/ 62 /—	—/ 81.4% /—
Non-Hodgkin lymphoma	2.4% / 1.9% / 2.1%	66 / 68 / 67	69.8% / 73.3% / 71.4%
Melanoma of the skin	2.8% / 1.7% / 2.2%	66 / 59 / 64	89.9% / 94.2% / 91.8%
Kidney and renal pelvis	2.1% / 1.2% / 1.6%	64 / 65 / 64	68.2% / 69.9% / 74.6%
Pancreas	1.6% / 1.5% / 1.6%	68 / 73 / 70	9.2% / 9.0% / 9.1%
Leukemia	1.8% / 1.3% / 1.51%	66 / 67 / 66	62.8% / 60.4% / 61.8%
All sites	39.7% / 37.7% /38.5%	66 / 65 / 66	66.5% / 67.8% / 67.2%

tumor burden, concurrent medical problems, assessment of the patient's performance status (such as Karnofsky performance status score [Table 10-3]), organ function (eg, kidney, liver, cardiac function), and patient expected treatment outcomes. The effectiveness of antineoplastic treatments are measured by reduction of tumor size, decrease or reversal in tumor progression, reduction of tumor-related symptoms, improvement in quality of life, and prolongation of survival. Multiple organizations publish free updated guidelines for the management of various types of cancer and supportive care of cancer patients. The National Comprehensive Cancer Network (NCCN) (www.nccn.org) and the American Society of Clinical Oncology (ASCO) (www.asco.org) are two sources for cancer guidelines. In this chapter, you will receive an overview of select pharmacological drugs used in antineoplastic therapy.

PHARMAGOLOGIC PROPERTIES OF ANTINEOPLASTIC DRUGS

Nomenclature The term antineoplastic *chemotherapy* describes a type of antineoplastic therapy that uses pharmacological agents to treat cancer. Other modalities of antineoplastic therapy include surgery and radiotherapy. Surgery and radiation may be used alone or in combination with chemotherapy. The key difference between surgery, radiation, and chemotherapy is that surgery and radiation therapy is almost always *localized* therapy, while chemotherapy is *systemic* therapy. If a cancer is detected early and is localized to a specific area of the body, the main treatment will generally be local nonpharmacological modalities (surgery or radiotherapy). However, if the cancer is detected later or is suspected to have

TABLE 10-2 | **Cancer Detection and Screening Recommendations for Average Risk Asymptomatic Individuals**

Cancer Site	Population	Test or Procedure	Special Note
Breast	Women, aged 40-44y[a] Women aged 45+y	Annual mammography up to age 54 then every 2 y	Recommended to continue as long as life expectancy ≥10 y
Colorectal	Men and women, aged 50+ y	Annual high sensitivity guaiac-based fecal occult blood test or fecal immunochemical test	Routine screening to be continued at least till 75 y, optional after
		Colonoscopy or flexible sigmoidoscopy or double-contrast barium enema or computed tomography colonography	Colonoscopy every 10 y, other tests to be performed every 5 y
Prostate	Men, aged 50+ y	Digital rectal examination and prostate-specific antigen test[a]	Annual
Cervix	Women, aged ≥21 y	Papanicolaou (Pap) test	Routine screening to be continued at least till 65 y, optional after. National organizations vary in their recommendations about the frequency of screening, with recommendations for annual to triennial screening
Lung	Men and women aged 55-80 y who have a 30-pack-year or more smoking history	Low-dose (helical) computed tomography	Not recommended for patients who have stopped smoking more than 15 y ago

[a]Optional and not routine screening, based on informed shared decision making between client and clinician.

TABLE 10-3 **Karnofsky Performance Status Scale**

Value	Level of Functional Capacity
100	Normal, no complaints, no evidence of disease
90	Able to carry on normal activity, minor signs or symptoms of disease
80	Normal activity with effort, some signs or symptoms of disease
70	Cares for self, unable to carry on normal activity or to do active work
60	Requires occasional assistance, but is able to care for most needs
50	Requires considerable assistance and frequent medical care
40	Disabled, requires special care and assistance
30	Severely disabled, hospitalization is indicated although death is not imminent
20	Hospitalization is necessary, very sick, active supportive treatment necessary
10	Moribund, fatal processes progressing rapidly
0	Dead

spread, then systemic chemotherapy is utilized, either alone or as adjuvant to surgery and radiotherapy.

Antineoplastic chemotherapy can be classified into three major groups:

- *Adjuvant chemotherapy:* Chemotherapy given after local treatment (eg, surgery or radiotherapy) because of concern of residual disease not removed by the local treatment.

- *Neoadjuvant chemotherapy:* Chemotherapy given prior to main treatment, with an aim to reduce the size or extent of local cancer thus improving success of local main treatment.

- *Primary induction chemotherapy:* Chemotherapy is the main modality of treatment and is used in patients with advanced or metastasized disease that do not have suitable local treatment options.

Goals of Therapy The goal of chemotherapy is to selectively kill or suppress cancer cells and to achieve this with minimal or no damage to normal cells. All modalities of treatment damage cells (normal and neoplastic) and damage to normal cells leads to adverse effects. The cardinal feature of the cancer cells is to proliferate (divide or reproduce) and chemotherapeutic agents act by damaging proliferating cells. As chemotherapeutic agents damage proliferating cancer cells, they may cause collateral damage to normal noncancerous proliferating cells in the body such as in the hair follicles, intestinal epithelial lining, or bone marrow.

Cell Cycle As our body grows from an early embryonic stage to adult stage, our embryonic stem cells undergo controlled and regulated cell cycle division with proliferation to ultimately form differentiated cells that have lost their ability to divide. However, certain cells called committed adult stem cells lie dormant in various tissues and activate their ability to divide in response to bodily demands. These committed stem cells serve the physiological function of cell replenishment and repair. In the presence of a cancer causing condition, such as **carcinogens** that induced genetic **mutation**, such stem cells (and rarely an adult cell) may enter cell division cycle in an uncontrolled fashion leading to cancer. The stages of cell division cycle and common chemotherapeutic agents active in those cycles are shown in Figure 10-1. The chemotherapeutic agents that specifically target cells that are moving through the various stages of cell division are called *cell cycle specific drugs*, while those chemotherapeutic agents that target cancer cells regardless of cell cycle phase are referred to as *cell cycle nonspecific drugs*. Generally, it is easier to kill cells when they are metabolically active, that is when they are cycling through cell cycle.

CHEMOTHERAPY REGIMEN PRINCIPLES

Principles of chemotherapy regimen are similar to the principles of antimicrobial therapy. In both, the goal is to achieve suppression/eradication of disease using optimal dosing and scheduling. Another goal is to minimize host toxicity, adverse events, and prevent the development of drug resistance.

Dosing Optimal chemotherapy dosing and schedule is based on knowledge of mechanism of action and detailed experimental evidence. Most chemotherapeutic agents have a narrow therapeutic range and it is critical to ensure that the dose is within the recommended therapeutic window to ensure damage to cancer cells and minimal effects to normal cells. Achieving subtherapeutic dosage may not kill cancer cells and lead to development of resistance, while achieving supratherapeutic dosage may cause unacceptable collateral damage to normal cells. Most chemotherapy doses are measured per meters squared of body surface area, or in some cases, per kilogram of body weight. Other factors that influence dosing include the patient's ability to metabolize and/or excrete drug (eg, kidney or liver disease), age, comorbidities, and drug interactions.

Cycles and Intermittent Chemotherapy Administration Cancer cells originate from normal host cells and share metabolic and biologic components of normal cells. Damage to shared components will lead to collateral damage to normal cells. Thus it is important to identify differentiating factors that provide selective survival benefit to normal cells over cancer cells. One such differentiating factor is that, in most cases, normal cells such as bone marrow tend to recover faster after a chemotherapeutic insult compared to cancer cells. If chemotherapy is provided intermittently, the interval between cycles may allow selective survival benefit to normal cells compared to cancer cells. Duration between the cycles must be long enough to allow recovery of the most sensitive normal cells, but not long enough to allow growth of cancer cells. The duration and frequency of the cycles are dependent on

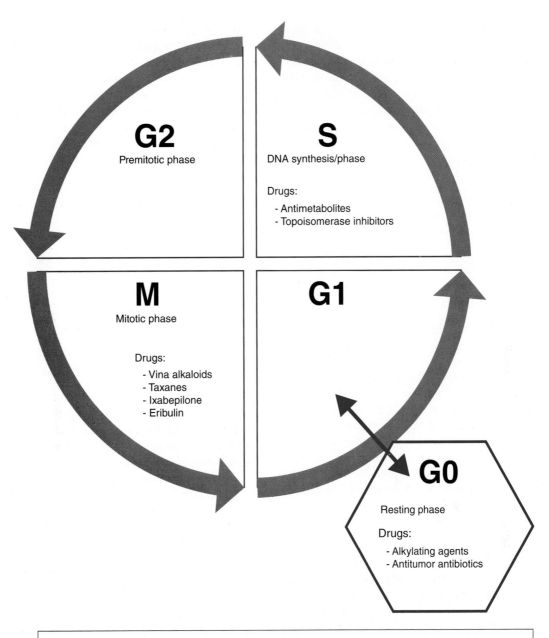

During G1 phase (Growth 1 phase) the cell prepares for cell division. Here the cells start assembling essential components for DNA synthesis and is generally accompanied by increase in cell mass. S phase (Synthetic phase) is the period of DNA synthesis. G2 (Growth 2 phase) follows immediately after S-phase and involves organization of newly formed DNA. During M-phase (Mitotic phase) the cell divides into two daughter cells, both of which will now be in G1 phase.

Immediately after G1 phase, a new daughter cell may continue in cell cycle or go into G0 resting phase. The G0 cells may either stay dormant in G0 for prolonged period of time with a future potential to re-enter cell cycle or may undergo differentiation producing various stages of mature nondividing functional adult cells.

Drugs that act on G1, S, G2, or M-phase are called cell-cycle specific drugs, while those that can act on G0 with or without additional actions on other phases are called cell-cycle nonspecific drugs.

FIGURE 10-1 Cell cycle and site of action of various antineoplastic agents.

type of drug or cancer and are based on expert consensus and evidence from observational and experimental science. Some regimens may use a single dose followed by several days or weeks without treatment. Others may involve several day dosing, or intermittent day dosing followed by treatment-free periods. Rarely, there may be regimens that have protracted duration of treatment without interruption.

Multidrug Regimens Use of combination chemotherapy provides similar benefits in antineoplastic chemotherapy as in antimicrobial chemotherapy. Using multiple drugs will lead to maximum focused damage at lower doses of individual drugs without compromising therapeutic efficacy. This will reduce the adverse event profile of individual drugs. Secondly, combination drugs may work synergistically achieving higher kill rate then otherwise expected. Further, development of resistance to multidrug regimens is far more difficult compared to individual drug therapy. This is especially true if the individual drugs target cells differently and do not have overlapping toxicity profiles. There are numerous multidrug chemotherapy regimens that are clinically utilized. These regimens are typically referred to by their acronyms. Select examples of evidence-based multidrug regimens include:

- Colorectal cancer: FOLFOX—5-fluorouracil, leucovorin, oxaliplatin
- Diffuse large B-cell lymphoma: CHOP—cyclophosphamide, doxorubicin (hydroxy-daunorubicin), vincristine (Oncovin™), and prednisone
- Breast cancer: AC—doxorubicin (Adriamycin™) and cyclophosphamide
- Hodgkin lymphoma: ABVD—doxorubicin (Adriamycin™), bleomycin, vinblastine, dacarbazine

Drug Resistance   Drug resistance is a common problem in antineoplastic chemotherapy. It can be classified into two types. First is the *primary drug resistance*, where the cancer cells are intrinsically resistant to the chemotherapeutic agent even prior to first exposure. This could be because of gene mutation in the cancer cells that provide the cancer cells survival benefits. Second is the *acquired drug resistance*, where the cancer cells were initially susceptible to the chemotherapeutic agent but over time became resistant, presumably because of increased expression of genes that promote resistance by increased cellular metabolism of the drug. Just like antimicrobial therapy, ensuring optimal dosing and using multidrug regimens are ideal methods to avoid development of drug resistance.

Routes of Administration   Chemotherapy can be administered enterally (orally) or parenterally (intravenous, subcutaneous, intramuscular). Since most chemotherapeutic agents may damage skin and muscle tissue, subcutaneous and intramuscular administration is almost never done. Although intravenous administration can be done through smaller veins in the arms and hands, access to larger more central veins through central venous catheter, such as peripherally inserted central catheter (PICC) or implantable venous access port (Port-A-Cath) are preferred as they allow administration of multiple drugs simultaneously, reduce the number of needle sticks by allowing long-term access, allow for frequent and longer duration of continuous infusions, and avoid damage to skin and muscle tissues from unintended accidental leakage (extravasation) from smaller veins into subcutaneous tissue. Oral administration although possible, is not preferred because of irritation caused to gut mucosa by the drugs.

Alternatively, local administration of chemotherapeutic agents can be performed for specific types of cancers that are located at certain regions of the body. Intravesicular chemotherapy is administration of chemotherapeutic agent directly into the urinary bladder for treatment of bladder cancer, while intraperitoneal chemotherapy is administration into the peritoneal cavity of the abdomen for cancer such as ovarian

cancer. The most commonly performed local administration is intrathecal administration for cancers that affect the central nervous system. Here, the chemotherapeutic agent is administered directly into the cerebrospinal fluid surrounding the brain and spinal cord after performing a lumbar puncture procedure. The rationale for intrathecal therapy is that chemotherapeutic agents administered via veins may not enter the intrathecal compartment because of restriction to flow of drug imposed by normal blood brain barrier.

CHEMOTHERAPEUTIC AGENTS
Cell Cycle Specific Agents

Antimetabolites   Antimetabolites interfere with cellular metabolism required for deoxyribonucleic acid (DNA) and ribonucleic acid (RNA) synthesis during cell cycle, preventing progression in cell division and slowing down cell replication. They have molecular structures that are similar to normal metabolites such as folic acid and nucleotides, and thus get inserted into the DNA causing loss of function and damage. Common antimetabolites include 5-flurouracil, pemetrexed, cytarabine, and gemcitabine.

Antimitotic Agents   Antimitotic agents affect cell division, specifically in the M phase of the cell cycle. They work by inhibiting microtubule assembly (vinca alkaloids and eribulin) or stabilizing the microtubules preventing shortening and disassembly (taxanes and ixabepilone). Important examples of this group include paclitaxel (taxane) and vincristine (vinca).

Topoisomerase Inhibitors   Topoisomerase I and II provide DNA strand breaks during replication allowing for the relief of torsional strain. Topoisomerase I cleaves the DNA in one location while topoisomerase II cleaves both strands of DNA. The topoisomerase I inhibitors, irinotecan and topotecan, prevent the cleaving of the DNA. The topoisomerase II inhibitors, etoposide and teniposide, prevent the reattachment of the cleaved DNA. These agents are most active during DNA replication during the S phase of the cell cycle

Cell Cycle Nonspecific Agents

Alkylating Agents   Alkylating agents are most effective in the G1 and S phase of cell cycles but because of its action on G0 resting phase cells are classified as cell cycle nonspecific drugs. Drugs of this class transfer their alkyl- group into cellular components especially in the cell's nucleus and interfere with DNA replication process. Cyclophosphamide is the most commonly used chemotherapeutic agent in this group with some other common drugs being the platinum analogues (cisplatin, carboplatin, oxaliplatin), temozolomide and dacarbazine.

Antineoplastic Antibiotics   These are compounds that were found to have anticancer activity originally discovered during research for antibiotics against infection. As a class, they have multiple mechanisms of action including intercalation of nucleotides, inhibition of topoisomerase II, and production of oxygen free radicals. Drugs in this group include bleomycin, mitomycin, and anthracyclines such as doxorubicin.

Other Therapies

Hormones Certain types of cancer, such as prostate cancer and breast cancer, are sensitive to stimulation by naturally occurring body hormones such as testosterone or estrogen. Such hormone sensitive tumors can be suppressed by using hormone antagonists or by reducing circulating levels of endogenous hormones. Examples of hormone antagonists include bicalutamide (testosterone antagonist) and tamoxifen (select estrogen receptor modulator, antagonizing estrogen receptors in the breast). Suppression of circulating endogenous hormones can be achieved by interfering with the feedback mechanism involved with estrogen and testosterone production (luteinizing hormone-releasing hormone [LHRH] agonists such as leuprolide) or through direct inhibition of their production (aromatase inhibitors such as letrozole).

Monoclonal Antibodies

Monoclonal antibodies (MABs) are specifically targeted antibodies produced by recombinant DNA technology. There are numerous MABs used in the treatment of various cancers. Most MABs used in the treatment of cancer target specific cell surface markers found on malignant cells. MABs can cause cell death through multiple mechanisms, such as complement-mediated cytotoxicity, localized delivery of chemotherapy, and targeted delivery of radiation. Unlike the other MABs used in the treatment of cancer, bevacizumab binds to a circulating cytokine, vascular endothelial growth factor. As a class, the MABs are associated with a risk of an allergic-type reaction. The immunogenicity of individual MABs can be predicted by evaluating the syllable of the drug name immediately prior to the suffix –mab. In order of least immunogenic to most immunogenic, the MABs with a "-u-" or "-mu-" are human protein and least immunogenic, "-zu-" indicates humanized, "-xi-" chimeric, and "-mo-" mouse. Patients should be carefully monitored during the infusion of the MAB, especially if they are chimeric (-xi-) or mouse (-mo-) in origin. Examples of MABs include rituximab, trastuzumab, and atezolizumab.

Kinase Inhibitors

Kinase inhibitors are a rapidly expanding class of anticancer agents. These drugs are frequently referred to as "small molecules" in reference to their actual size. Unlike most anticancer medications, the agents in this class are administered orally. Kinase inhibitors have their effect on cells through inhibition of various kinases (such as tyrosine kinases or serine kinases) that are important for intracellular communication. Many of the agents in this class are associated with significant drug/drug interactions through activity in the CYP450 system. Examples of kinase inhibitors include imatinib, erlotinib, sunitinib, and ibrutinib.

Immune Therapies

One strategy for treating cancer involves stimulating the immune system with the intent that it will induce immune-system mediated cell death. This strategy has been used against cancers such as melanoma, renal cell carcinoma, and prostate cancer. This has been accomplished with the administration of cytokines (such as interferon alfa and interleukin-2 [IL-2]), through autologous cellular immunotherapy (Sipuleucel-T), frequently referred to as an anticancer vaccine and MABs that promote T-lymphocyte activity (ipilimumab, nivolumab, pembrolizumab).

See Table 10-4 for an overview of select anticancer medications.

SUPPORTIVE CARE

The treatment of cancer is complicated by the toxicities associated with the use of antineoplastic agents (Table 10-5). Certain toxicities may be life threatening and require aggressive monitoring with early interventions to minimize complications, while others such as mucositis, nausea, and vomiting, although may not be life threatening may be prevented or minimized leading to improved patient satisfaction and compliance. Table 10-6 lists key parameters for agents used to manage these toxicities.

Myelosuppression Myelosuppression or bone marrow suppression is the most common dose-limiting side effect of cytotoxic agents. This includes anemia, neutropenia, and thrombocytopenia. Neutrophils (a white blood cell) are affected more than red blood cells or platelets because they have shorter life span and proliferate rapidly. Myelosuppression, especially neutropenia usually occur within 7 to 14 days after starting chemotherapy administration. It begins to recover by about 2 weeks after the last chemotherapy dose. With some chemotherapy regimens this may be delayed or prolonged, lasting for about 4 to 6 weeks.

Anemia Anemia is the most common symptomatic hematologic complication of cancer chemotherapy, with the common symptoms reported being fatigue and shortness of breath. The presence of fatigue in cancer patients correlates well with the severity of the anemia. Treatment of the anemia results in improvement in fatigue and quality of life. The initial step in the management of anemia includes identifying the cause of the anemia and starting appropriate therapy (eg, patients with low iron should receive iron supplementation). Recombinant human erythropoietic products (epoetin alfa and darbepoetin alfa) are useful in the management of anemia. They increase hemoglobin and hematocrit levels, decrease transfusion requirements, and improve quality of life. However, clinical trials have shown that using these agents in patients whose cancer is being treated with curative intent may decrease the likelihood of cure. Patients should only receive these agents if they have chemotherapy-induced anemia and if their cancer is considered to be incurable. Blood transfusions are appropriate for patients with severe symptomatic anemia.

TABLE 10-4 Select Antineoplastic Agents

Antineoplastic	Mechanism of Action	Uses	Contraindications (C); Warnings/ Precautions (W/P)	Adverse Effects (A) and Interactions (I)	Dosing	Administration
Alkylating Agents						
Cyclophosphamide (Cytoxan)	Prevents cell division by cross-linking DNA strands and decreasing DNA synthesis. Cell cycle nonspecific	Hodgkin and non-Hodgkin lymphoma; chronic and acute leukemia; breast, testicular, endometrial, ovarian, and lung cancers	C: Hypersensitivity to cyclophosphamide, pregnancy W/P: Hazardous agent—use precautions for handling and disposal. Dosage adjustment may be needed for hepatic or renal dysfunction, may cause cardiotoxicity (high dose) and may potentiate anthracycline cardiac toxicity	A: Myelosuppression; gastrointestinal; dermatologic; genitourinary; endocrine (sterility, syndrome of inappropriate antidiuretic hormone secretion [SIADH]) I: Substrate, inhibitor, and inducer of CYP450	400-800 mg/m² per treatment course may be repeated at 2-4 wk intervals	To minimize bladder toxicity, increase normal fluid intake during and for 1-2 d after dosing. Most adults require at least 2 L/d. High-dose regimens should be accompanied by hydration and mesna
Temozolomide (Temodar)	Prevents cell division by cross-linking DNA strands and decreasing DNA synthesis. Cell cycle nonspecific	Anaplastic astrocytoma of the brain (AA) Glioblastoma multiformens of the brain (GBM) Melanoma	C: Hypersensitivity to temozolomide W/P: Hazardous agent—use precautions for handling and disposal, myelosuppression, secondary malignancies, *Pneumocystis* pneumonia (patients should receive prophylaxis when receiving temozolomide daily with radiation), hepatotoxicity	A: Alopecia, fatigue, nausea, vomiting, headache, constipation, rash, diarrhea, anorexia, fever, dizziness, myelosuppression, infections I: Valproic acid decreases oral clearance of temozolomide by approximately 5%	GBM: 75 mg/m² daily for 42 d with radiation followed by 150 mg/m² daily on days 1-5 of 28-d cycle AA: 150 mg/m² daily on days 1-5 of 28-d cycle Melanoma: 200 mg/ m² daily on days 1-5 of 28-d cycle	Available for oral or intravenous administration. Oral administration is most commonly used
Cisplatin (Platinol)	Inhibits DNA synthesis by the formation of DNA cross-links; covalently binds to DNA bases and disrupts DNA function	Bladder, testicular, ovarian, and lung cancers Has many other indications as well	C: Hypersensitivity to platinum containing products; preexisting renal dysfunction, myelosuppression, or hearing impairment; pregnancy W/P: Hazardous agent—use precautions for handling and disposal, **cumulative renal toxicity may be severe**, dose-related toxicities include myelosuppression, nausea, and vomiting; **ototoxicity is manifested by tinnitus or loss of high-frequency hearing; anaphylactic-like reactions have been reported and may be managed with epinephrine, corticosteroids, and/or antihistamines**	A: Neurotoxicity (peripheral neuropathy), dermatologic (alopecia), gastrointestinal (nausea and vomiting—highly emetogenic), myelosuppression, hepatic (increased liver function tests); nephro- and ototoxicity	Advanced bladder cancer: 50-70 mg/ m² every 3-4 wk Metastatic ovarian cancer: 75-100 mg/ m² every 3-4 wk	Patients should receive adequate hydration prior to and for 24 h after administration; maintain urine output (>100 mL/h) for 24 h; maximum rate of infusion for patients with heart failure is 1 mg/min

Antimetabolites

Methotrexate (Rheumatrex, Trexall)	Irreversibly binds to dihydrofolate reductase resulting in inhibition of purine and thymidylic acid synthesis (inhibits DNA synthesis). Methotrexate (MTX) is cell cycle specific of the S phase	Leukemias; breast, head, and neck cancers; osteosarcoma; soft-tissue sarcomas; lymphomas	C: Hypersensitivity to methotrexate; severe renal or hepatic dysfunction; AIDS; preexisting myelosuppression W/P: Hazardous agent—use precautions for handling and disposal; **MTX has been associated with acute and potentially fatal hepatotoxicity; MTX elimination is reduced in patients with ascites and may require dose modification; may cause renal damage; tumor lysis syndrome may occur in patients with high tumor burden; may cause life-threatening pneumonitis; may cause myelosuppression; low-dose MTX has been associated with development of malignant lymphomas; diarrhea and ulcerative stomatitis may require interruption of therapy; may cause seizures; may cause severe and fatal dermatologic reactions; concomitant administration with NSAIDs may cause severe myelosuppression or gastrointestinal toxicity**	A: Central nervous system (headache, nuchal rigidity, vomiting, fever, seizure, motor paralysis); dermatologic; endocrine (hyperuricemia); gastrointestinal (ulcerative stomatitis, nausea, vomiting, diarrhea, mucositis); myelosuppression; renal failure; hepatotoxicity	Head and neck cancer: 25-50 mg/m² once weekly; Lymphoma: 1 g/m² every 3 wk or 1.5 g/m² every 4 wk	Specific dosing schemes vary for methotrexate, but high dose should be followed by leucovorin to prevent toxicity
5-Fluorouracil (Adrucil)	A pyrimidine antimetabolite that interferes with DNA synthesis by blocking the methylation of deoxyuridylic acid	Carcinomas of breast, colon, head and neck, pancreas, rectum, or stomach	C: Hypersensitivity to fluorouracil, dihydropyrimidine dehydrogenase deficiency, pregnancy W/P: Hazardous agent—use appropriate precautions for handling and disposal; discontinue use in patients with intractable vomiting, precipitous fall in blood counts, stomatitis, hemorrhage, or myocardial ischemia occurs	A: Central nervous system (cerebellar syndrome—confusion, disorientation, headache); dermatologic (alopecia, rash); cardiovascular (angina, myocardial ischemia); gastrointestinal (anorexia, diarrhea, stomatitis); myelosuppression; allergic reaction	500-600 mg/m² every 3-4 wk (there are numerous dosing regimens)	Intravenous bolus as a slow push or short (5-15 min) bolus infusion, or as a continuous infusion; doses greater than 1000 mg/m² are usually administered as a 24-h infusion; toxicity may be reduced by giving the drug as a constant infusion Frequently given with leucovorin as leucovorin enhances its toxicity
Cytarabine/Ara-C (Cytosar)	Inhibits DNA synthesis. Cytarabine is specific for the S phase of the cell cycle	Leukemias and lymphomas	C: Hypersensitivity to cytarabine W/P: Hazardous agent—use appropriate precautions for handling and disposal; **potent myelosuppressive agent**; use caution in patients with renal or hepatic dysfunction	A: Central nervous system (neurotoxicity); conjunctivitis; myelosuppression; gastrointestinal	75-200 mg/m²/d for 5-10 d	When administering via intravenous infusion, infuse over 1-3 h or as a continuous infusion. Intravenous doses greater than 1.5 g/m² may produce conjunctivitis, dexamethasone eye drops should be administered at 1-2 drops every 6 h during and for 2-7 d after cytarabine is done. Can also be given intrathecally

(Continued)

TABLE 10-4   Select Antineoplastic Agents (Continued)

Antineoplastic	Mechanism of Action	Uses	Contraindications (C); Warnings/ Precautions (W/P)	Adverse Effects (A) and Interactions (I)	Dosing	Administration
Anthracycline/Antibiotic						
Doxorubicin (Adriamycin)	Inhibition of DNA and RNA synthesis by intercalation between DNA base pairs by inhibition of topoisomerase II	Leukemias, lymphomas, multiple myeloma, and carcinoma of the head and neck, thyroid, lung, breast, stomach, pancreas, liver, ovary, bladder, prostate, and uterus	C: Hypersensitivity to doxorubicin or other anthracyclines; recent myocardial infarction, severe arrhythmia, exceeding cumulative dose of anthracyclines; Baseline neutrophil count less than 1500/mm³; severe hepatic impairment W/P: Hazardous agent—use appropriate precautions for handling and disposal; **Reduce dose in patients with impaired hepatic function; dose-limiting myelosuppression may occur; leukemia has been reported following treatment; potent vesicant, if extravasation occurs; severe tissue damage leading to ulceration, necrosis, and pain may occur**	A: Cardiotoxicity; dermatologic; endocrine (infertility, hyperuricemia); gastrointestinal; myelosuppression I: Substrate and inhibitor of CYP450	60-75 mg/m²/dose every 21 d	Administer intravenous push over at least 3-5 min, intravenous piggyback over 15-60 min, or continuous infusion Only given in central IV line to decrease risk of extravasation
Bleomycin (Blenoxane)	Inhibits synthesis of DNA; binds to DNA leading to single and double-strand breaks	Squamous cell carcinoma, melanomas, sarcomas, lymphoma	C: Hypersensitivity to bleomycin, severe pulmonary disease, pregnancy W/P: Hazardous agent—use appropriate precautions for handling and disposal; **occurrence of pulmonary fibrosis is higher in elderly patients, smokers, and patients with prior radiation or concurrent oxygen; idiosyncratic reactions consisting of chills, hypotension, fever, wheezing has been reported in lymphoma patients**	A: Dermatologic (rash, peeling of skin, hyperpigmentation, alopecia); gastrointestinal (stomatitis); pulmonary (pulmonary fibrosis, cough)	0.25-0.5 units/kg 1-2 times per week	
Vinca Alkaloids						
Vincristine (Vincasar)	Binds to tubulin and inhibits microtubule formation	Leukemias, lymphomas	C: Hypersensitivity to vincristine; for intravenous use only (fatal if given intrathecally); pregnancy W/P: Hazardous agent—use appropriate precautions for handling and disposal; **vincristine is a vesicant—avoid extravasation;** dosage modification required for those with hepatic dysfunction or neuromuscular disease	A: Dermatologic (alopecia, rash); cardiovascular (orthostatic hypotension); central nervous system (headache, confusion); gastrointestinal I: Substrate of CYP 450 system and weak CYP 450 inhibitor	0.25-0.5 mg/m² for 5 d every 4 wk	Fatal if given intrathecally; intravenously administered as short (10-15 min) infusion, slow IV push (1-2 min), or 24-h continuous infusion. Administration of vincristine with itraconazole has been reported to cause paralytic ileus, neurogenic bladder, absence of deep reflexes, and severe paralysis of lower extremities within 10 d of starting itraconazole

Taxanes

Drug	Mechanism	Indication	Dose	Adverse/Warnings/Interactions	Administration
Paclitaxel (Taxol)	Promotes microtubule assembly inhibiting cell replication	Breast, nonsmall cell lung, head and neck cancers	Nonsmall cell lung cancer: 135 mg/m² over 24 h every 3 wk	C: Hypersensitivity to paclitaxel W/P: Hazardous agent—use appropriate precautions for handling and disposal; **severe hypersensitivity reactions reported;** stop infusion and do not re-challenge for severe hypotension requiring treatment or if angioedema occurs; **myelosuppression is dose-limiting toxicity, do not administer if baseline absolute neutrophil count is less than 1500 cells/mm³**; caution in patients with hepatic dysfunction; peripheral neuropathy may occur, reduce dose by 20% for severe neuropathy; infusion related reactions may occur (monitor vital signs during infusion) A: Myelosuppression; dermatologic (flushing, alopecia); neuropathy I: Substrate of the CYP 450 system and a weak CYP 450 inducer	When administered as sequential infusions, taxane derivatives should be administered before platinum derivatives to limit myelosuppression; premedication with dexamethasone, diphenhydramine, and H2 receptor antagonist (such as ranitidine) is recommended

Monoclonal Antibodies

Drug	Mechanism	Indication	Dose	Adverse/Warnings/Interactions	Administration
Rituximab (Rituxan)	Binds to CD20 antigen found on B-lymphocytes inducing antibody dependent cell cytotoxicity and complement dependent cytotoxicity	Non-Hodgkin lymphoma (NHL) Chronic lymphocytic leukemia (CLL)	NHL: 375 mg/m² every 28 d CLL: 375 mg/m² for first dose then 500 mg/m² every 28 d	C: None W/P: Potentially fatal infusion reactions, tumor lysis syndrome, infections, cardiac arrhythmias, angina, myelosuppression A: Fever, chills, infection I: Risk of increased nephrotoxicity when administered with cisplatin	Administered as slow intravenous infusion. Rate is dependent on cycle: First dose: Initiate at 50 mg/h then titrate by 50 mg/h every 30 min to a maximum of 400 mg/h Subsequent doses: Initiate at 100 mg/h then titrate by 100 mg/h every 30 min to a maximum of 400 mg/h Premedicate patients with acetaminophen and an antihistamine (such as diphenhydramine). Premedication with a glucocorticoid is also used
Trastuzumab (Herceptin)	Binds to HER-2 protein inducing antibody dependent cell cytotoxicity	HER-2 positive breast cancer HER-2 positive gastric cancer	4 mg/kg loading dose then 2 mg/kg weekly 8 mg/kg loading dose then 6 mg/kg every 3 wk	C: None W/P: Cardiomyopathy, infusion reactions, pulmonary toxicity A: Headache, diarrhea, nausea, chills, fever, insomnia, cough, rash I: Cardiomyopathy is worsened when administered concurrently with anthracyclines	Administered intravenously over 30 (2 mg/kg) to 90 (4-8 mg/kg) min Decrease rate of infusion for moderate infusion reactions. Interrupt infusion for dyspnea or hypotension. Discontinue for severe infusion reactions

(Continued)

TABLE 10-4 **Select Antineoplastic Agents (Continued)**

Antineoplastic	Mechanism of Action	Uses	Contraindications (C); Warnings/Precautions (W/P)	Adverse Effects (A) and Interactions (I)	Dosing	Administration
Kinase Inhibitors						
Imatinib (Gleevec)	Inhibits tyrosine kinase resulting from bcr-abl translocation mutation (Philadelphia chromosome) and also inhibits tyrosine kinases c-kit mutation	CML ALL with Philadelphia chromosome Gastrointestinal stromal tumor (GIST)	C: None W/P: Edema and severe fluid retention, myelosuppression, hepatotoxicity, hypothyroidism, tumor lysis syndrome	A: Edema, nausea, vomiting, muscle cramps, diarrhea, rash, fatigue I: Is a substrate and inhibitor of CYP450 3A4. Also inhibits CYP450 2D6	CML: Chronic phase: 400 mg/d Accelerated phase or blast crisis: 600 mg/d ALL: 600 mg/d GIST: 400 mg/d	Orally administered, best taken with a meal and full glass of water. Therapy is continued until disease progression or intolerable side effects
Erlotinib (Tarceva)	Inhibits the kinase activity of the epidermal growth factor receptor (EGFR)	Nonsmall cell lung cancer (NSCLC) Pancreatic cancer	C: None W/P: Interstitial lung disease, renal failure, hepatotoxicity, GI perforation, myocardial infarction, cerebrovascular accident	A: Rash, diarrhea, anorexia, fatigue, dyspnea, cough, nausea, vomiting I: Is a substrate of CYP450 3A4. Drugs affecting gastric pH decrease erlotinib absorption; cigarette smoking decreases erlotinib plasma concentrations	NSCLC: 150 mg/d Pancreatic cancer: 100 mg/d	Administer orally on an empty stomach. Therapy is continued until disease progression or intolerable side effects
Miscellaneous Antineoplastics						
Asparaginase (Elspar)	Inhibits protein synthesis by hydrolyzing asparaginase to aspartic acid and ammonia	Leukemia	C: History of serious allergic reaction to asparaginase or any E. coli derived asparaginase; history of serious thrombosis, pancreatitis, or hemorrhagic events with prior asparaginase treatment W/P: Hazardous agent—use appropriate precautions for handling and disposal; may alter hepatic function; monitor for allergic reactions; use caution with pre-existing hepatic dysfunction		6000 units/m²/dose 3 times per week for 6-9 doses	May be administered intramuscularly, intravenously, or intradermal (skin test only for allergic reaction); intravenous administration increases the risk of allergic reactions; manufacturer recommends a test dose prior to initial administration and when given after an interval of 7 d or more; the skin test site should be observed for at least 1 h for a wheal or erythema; a negative skin test does not preclude the possibility of an allergic reaction; desensitization may be performed in allergic patients

Drug	Mechanism of action	Uses	Contraindications (C)/Warnings and precautions (W/P)	Adverse effects (A)/Interactions (I)	Dosage	Administration
Hydroxyurea (Hydrea)	Interferes with synthesis of DNA during S phase of cell division	Melanoma, leukemia, ovarian, head and neck cancer	C: Hypersensitivity to hydroxyurea; severe anemia; severe myelosuppression; pregnancy W/P: Hazardous agent—use appropriate precautions for handling and disposal; hydroxyurea is mutagenic and clastogenic. Treatment of myeloproliferative disorders with long-term hydroxyurea is associated with leukemia	A: Myelosuppression; gastrointestinal; dermatologic (rash)	Dose should be titrated to patient response and white blood cell counts; usual oral doses range from 10-30 mg/kg/d; if white blood cell count falls to less than 2500 cells/mm^3 or platelet count to less than 10,000 cells/mm^3 therapy should be stopped for at least 3 d and resumed when values rise toward normal	Capsules may be opened and emptied into water (will not dissolve completely)
(Tretinoin (Vesanoid)	Binds to nuclear receptors and inhibits clonal proliferation and granulocyte proliferation	Leukemia	C: Sensitivity to parabens, vitamin A, retinoids; pregnancy W/P: Hazardous agent—use appropriate precautions for handling and disposal; about 25% of patients with acute promyelocytic leukemia experience a syndrome characterized by fever, dyspnea, acute respiratory distress, weight gain, pulmonary infiltrates, edema, and multiorgan failure; during treatment, 40% develop rapidly evolving leukocytosis; high risk of teratogenicity—not to be used in women of childbearing potential	A: Retinoic acid syndrome; gastrointestinal; cardiovascular; hematologic I: Substrate of CYP 450 system; weak inhibitor and inducer of CYP 450 system	45 mg/m^2/d in 2-3 divided doses for up to 30 d	Administer with meals; do not crush capsules

TABLE 10-5	Adverse Effects Associated With Antineoplastic Agents

General: Chemotherapy agents are toxic not only to cancer cells but also to various host tissues and organs. Toxicities generally occur as a result of inhibition of host cell division. Host tissues most susceptible to chemotherapy include tissues with renewal cell populations (eg, bone marrow and epithelium of gastrointestinal tract and skin). The toxicities of antineoplastic agents are the most important factors limiting the use of potentially curative doses.

Myelosuppression (Bone Marrow Suppression): Although not seen with all antineoplastics, myelosuppression is the most common dose-limiting side effect of antineoplastic agents. Antineoplastics can affect any cell line, including red blood cells, neutrophils (a white blood cell), and platelets. Decreased red blood cells can cause anemia and patients present with fatigue. Low neutrophil counts (neutropenia) increase the risk of infections. Reduced platelets (thrombocytopenia) increases the risk of bleeding. There are numerous antineoplastic agents and regimens that cause myelosuppression. Most targeted agents are not associated with myelosuppression.

Gastrointestinal: Gastrointestinal toxicities include nausea and vomiting (N&V), oral complications, and lower bowel disturbances. N&V are common serious toxicities associated with most chemotherapy agents. While the emetogenic potential of antineoplastic agents varies, emesis commonly occurs on the first day of treatment and may persist for several days. Complications of the oral cavity include mucositis/stomatitis, xerostomia (dry mouth), infection, and bleeding. Approximately 40% of patients treated with antineoplastic develop oral complications. Chemotherapy may also damage the lining of the esophagus leading to esophagitis. Lower gastrointestinal complications include malabsorption, diarrhea, or constipation.

Dermatologic: Dermatologic toxicities associated with antineoplastic agents include alopecia (hair loss), hypersensitivity reaction including rash, extravasation (passage/leakage of agent into tissue), and hyperpigmentation (pigment changes in skin, hair, or nails). Numerous antineoplastic agents are associated with dermatologic reactions.

Specific Organ Toxicities: Specific organ adverse effects (eg, neurotoxicity, nephrotoxicity, hepatotoxicity) are attributed to a unique uptake of the antineoplastic agent by the organ or a select toxicity of the agent to the organ. While there are numerous antineoplastic agents that cause specific organ toxicities, they are not as wide spread as the general toxicities (myelosuppression, gastrointestinal, and dermatologic).

Neurotoxicity: Neurotoxicity as a central nervous system toxicity is manifested by a generalized encephalopathy with symptoms of confusion, seizures, and/or coma. Cerebral dysfunction (ataxia, coordination difficulties) and leukoencephalopathy (change in personality, dementia) may also be seen. The antineoplastic agents most commonly associated with neurotoxicity include cytarabine and L-asparaginase. Other agents that produce central nervous system toxicities include: methotrexate (encephalopathy, leukoencephalopathy), fluorouracil (cerebral dysfunction), interferon (encephalopathy), fludarabine (altered mental status, blindness), and alkylating agents (encephalopathy).
Peripheral nerve toxicity: Paresthesia is numbness and tingling involving the feet, hands, or both. This nerve toxicity is associated with agents that affect microtubules (vinca alkaloids and taxanes) and the heavy metal alkylating agents (cisplatin, carboplatin, oxaliplatin). Oxaliplatin associated peripheral neuropathy is exacerbated by cold temperatures.
Cranial nerve toxicity: Cranial nerve toxicity may cause trigeminal neuralgia, facial palsy, depressed corneal reflexes, and vocal cord paralysis. Agents associated with cranial nerve toxicity include the vinca alkaloids, ifosfamide, and cisplatin. Cisplatin may also cause ototoxicity.
Autonomic neuropathy: Autonomic neuropathy is abdominal pain with or without constipation and may lead to ileus (small bowel obstruction). The vinca alkaloids as associated with autonomic neuropathy.

Pulmonary: Pulmonary edema (fluid in the lungs) is associated with docetaxel, cytarabine, aldesleukin (interleukin), and gemcitabine. Pulmonary fibrosis is a scarring/thickening of the lungs and may cause shortness of breath, chest pain, and coughing. Pulmonary fibrosis is associated with bleomycin and busulfan.

Cardiovascular: The anthracycline antibiotics (eg, doxorubicin) cause a dose-dependent cardiac toxicity (cardiomyopathy). Patients will experience heart failure symptoms (shortness of breath and tachycardia). Electrocardiographic (EKG) changes may be seen with anthracyclines, cisplatin, etoposide, paclitaxel, and cyclophosphamide. The EKG changes (ST segment changes, T wave flattening) may lead to arrhythmias. Fluorouracil is associated with causing angina.

Nephrotoxicity: Platinum analogs (cisplatin and carboplatin) may damage the kidney function leading to nephrotoxicity (decrease in kidney filtration and urine output). Oxaliplatin is not associated with nephrotoxicity.

Hepatotoxicity: Hepatotoxicity is destruction of the liver leading to jaundice, nausea, vomiting, abdominal pain, encephalopathy, and cirrhosis. Antineoplastic agents associated with hepatotoxicity are vinca alkaloids, anthracyclines, L-asparaginase, carmustine, etoposide, mercaptopurine, and methotrexate.

Genitourinary (GU): Cyclophosphamide and ifosfamide produce a metabolite, acrolein, that can cause a cystitis characterized by tissue edema and ulceration followed by sloughing of epithelial cells leading to hemorrhage. Mesna is a protective agent used with these drugs to bind to acrolein.

Neutropenia Neutropenia increases the risk for infection and is defined as absolute neutrophil count (ANC) less than 500/mm³. The ANC is calculated by multiplying the percentage of neutrophils (segmented plus banded neutrophils) by the total white blood cell count. The diagnosis of infection in neutropenic patients is difficult because usual signs and symptoms are often absent. Clinicians must treat fever in such a patient as a medical emergency and initiate antibiotics for suspected infection unless proven otherwise. Colony stimulating factors (CSFs) are naturally occurring proteins used to increase the neutrophils. Granulocyte colony stimulating factor (G-CSF, filgrastim) and granulocyte-macrophage colony stimulating factor (GM-CSF, sargramostim) are examples of agents used to increase the neutrophils. CSFs stimulate the production of neutrophils and promotes proliferation of granulocytes and monocytes/macrophages. The CSFs reduce the incidence, magnitude, and duration of neutropenia as well as prevent febrile neutropenia when used as preventive therapy following myelosuppressive chemotherapy regimens. These agents are recommended if the risk of febrile neutropenia from chemotherapy is at least 20%. CSFs should be initiated 24 to 72 hours after the last dose of chemotherapy.

Thrombocytopenia Chemotherapy-induced thrombocytopenia may lead to significant bleeding and are often managed by platelet transfusions. Platelet transfusions are typically reserved

TABLE 10-6   **Agents use for supportive care of patients with cancer**

Agent	Mechanism of Action	Use	Contraindications (C)/Warnings & Precautions (W/P)	Adverse Effects (AE) & Interactions (I)	Formulation (F), Dosing (D) & Administration (A)	Comments
Epoetin alfa (Epogen/Procrit)	Induces erythropoiesis by stimulating the division and differentiation of committed erythroid progenitor cells; induces the release of reticulocytes from the bone marrow into the bloodstream	Treatment of chemotherapy-induced anemia in patients receiving chemotherapy for palliative care only (decrease need for transfusions)	C: Hypersensitivity to albumin or mammalian cell-derived products; uncontrolled hypertension W/P: **Erythropoiesis-stimulating agents (ESA) increase the risk of serious cardiovascular events, mortality, and/or tumor progression; a shortened overall survival and/or increased risk of tumor progression or recurrence has been reported in studies with breast, cervical, head and neck, lymphoid, and nonsmall cell lung cancer patients; use lowest dose needed to avoid red blood cell transfusions to decrease risk of cardiovascular and thrombovascular events, dosing should be individualized to maintain hemoglobin levels within 10-12 g/dL;** use caution in patients with hypertension or with a history of seizures; prior to treatment with ESAs, correct or exclude deficiencies of iron, vitamin B12, and/or folate	Cardiovascular (hypertension, thrombotic/vascular events); central nervous system (fever, dizziness, insomnia, headache, seizure); dermatologic (pruritus, skin pain, rash); neuromuscular (arthralgia)	F: injection D: Initial dose—150 units/kg 3 times per week or 40,000 units once weekly A: Hemoglobin levels should not exceed 12g/dL and should not rise greater than 1 g/dL per 2-wk time period	Darbepoetin alfa (Aranesp) is also an erythropoiesis-stimulating agent with a longer half-life. Darbepoetin dosing interval may be as long as 3 wk
Filgrastim (Neupogen)—also referred to as granulocyte-colony stimulating factor (G-CSF)	Stimulates the production, maturation, and activation of neutrophils	Prevention of febrile neutropenia in patients receiving chemotherapy that puts them at an increased risk of infection	C: Hypersensitivity to filgrastim or E. coli derived products W/P: Administer no earlier than 24 h after chemotherapy because of the potential sensitivity of rapidly dividing myeloid cells; allergic-type reactions (rash, urticaria, wheezing, dyspnea, tachycardia, and/or hypotension) have occurred	AE: Bone pain	F: Injection D: Dosing should be based on actual body weight, even in obese patients; 5 µg/kg/d— doses may be increased by 5 µg/kg according to the duration and severity of neutropenia A: Continue for 14 d or the absolute neutrophil count reaches 10,000/mm³; may be administered undiluted by subcutaneous injection; may be administered by intravenous bolus over 15-30 min in D₅W	Pegfilgrastim (Neulasta) is a pegylated form of filgrastim—this increases the effect of the medication allowing for one time dosing given one day after chemotherapy Sargramostim (leukine) is a granulocyte-macrophage colony stimulating factor (GM-CSF). GM-CSF is used to shorten the time to neutrophil recovery and to reduce the incidence of severe and life-threatening infections

(Continued)

TABLE 10-6 Agents use for supportive care of patients with cancer (Continued)

Agent	Mechanism of Action	Use	Contraindications (C)/Warnings & Precautions (W/P)	Adverse Effects (AE) & Interactions (I)	Formulation (F), Dosing (D) & Administration (A)	Comments
Oprelvekin (Neumega)	Growth factor which stimulates thrombopoiesis—increased platelet production	Prevention of severe thrombocytopenia; reduce the need for platelet transfusions following myelosuppressive chemotherapy	C: Hypersensitivity to oprelvekin W/P: **Allergic reactions including anaphylaxis have been reported. Permanently discontinue in any patient developing an allergic reaction;** may cause fluid retention—use caution in heart failure and hypertension patients; arrhythmia, pulmonary edema, and cardiac arrest have been reported; use caution in patients with renal or hepatic dysfunction	AE: Cardiovascular (tachycardia, edema, syncope, arrhythmia); central nervous system (headache, dizziness); endocrine/metabolic (fluid retention)	F: Injection D: 50 μg/kg once daily for 10–21 d (until post-nadir platelet count is greater than 50,000 cells/mcL A: Administer subcutaneously in the abdomen, thigh, hip, or upper arm	Administer first dose 6–24 h after the end of chemotherapy. Discontinue at least 48 h before beginning the next cycle of chemotherapy
Amifostine (Ethyol)	Prodrug that is metabolized to free thiol. The free thiol binds and detoxifies reactive metabolites of cisplatin; also acts as a scavenger of free radicals generated by cisplatin or radiation therapy in tissues	Reduce the cumulative renal toxicity associated with repeated administration of cisplatin; reduce the incidence of moderate to severe xerostomia in patients undergoing postoperative radiation treatment for head and neck cancer	C: Hypersensitivity to aminothiol compounds W/P: Patients who are hypotensive or dehydrated should not receive amifostine; interrupt hypertensive therapy for 24 h before treatment; adequately hydrate prior to treatment and keep in a supine position during infusion; monitor blood pressure every 5 min during infusion; serious cutaneous reactions including Stevens-Johnson syndrome have been reported; it is recommended that antiemetic medication be administered prior to and in conjunction with amifostine; hypersensitivity reactions have been reported; reports of clinically-relevant hypocalcemia are rare, but serum calcium levels should be monitored in patients at risk of hypocalcemia	AE: Hypotension; gastrointestinal (nausea/vomiting); endocrine/metabolic (hypocalcemia)	F: Injection D: 910 mg/m² over 15 min once daily 30 min prior to cisplatin Xerostomia dosing: 200 mg/m² over 3 min once daily for 15–30 min prior to radiation A: Refer to dosing recommendations for blood pressure. There are specific recommendations for dosing dependent upon the patient's blood pressure	Administer over 3 min (prior to radiation therapy) or 15 min (prior to cisplatin); administration as a longer infusion is associated with a higher incidence of side effects; antiemetic medication, including dexamethasone 20 mg intravenous and a serotonin receptor antagonist is recommended prior to and in conjunction with amifostine
Palifermin (Kepivance)	Recombinant keratinocyte growth factor that leads to proliferation, differentiation, and migration of epithelial cells in multiple tissues including the tongue, buccal mucosa, esophagus, and salivary gland	Decrease the incidence and severity of oral mucositis associated with hematologic malignancies in patients receiving myelotoxic therapy	C: Hypersensitivity to palifermin or E. coli derived proteins W/P: Edema, erythema, pruritus, rash, taste alteration, tongue discoloration/thickening may occur	AE: Edema, dysesthesia, rash, pruritus, mouth/ tongue discoloration/ thickness, cough	F: Injection D: 60 μg/kg/d for 3 consecutive days before and after myelotoxic therapy; total of 6 doses A: Administer by intravenous bolus; do not administer during or within 24 h of chemotherapy (before or after); allow solution to reach room temperature before administration; do not use if at room temperature for more than 1 h	Administer first 3 doses prior to myelotoxic therapy, with the 3rd dose given 24–48 h before therapy begins; the last 3 doses should be administered after myelotoxic therapy, with the first of these doses after but on the same day as stem cell infusion and at least 4 d after the most recent dose of palifermin

Drug	Mechanism	Indication	Contraindications/Warnings	AE/Interactions	Formulation/Dosing/Administration	Notes
Dexamethasone (Decadron)	Mechanism of antiemetic activity in unknown; decreases inflammation by suppression of neutrophil migration and decreased production of inflammatory mediators; suppresses normal immune response	Antiemetic and many other indications	C: Hypersensitivity to dexamethasone; systemic fungal infections W/P: Use with caution in patients with thyroid, hepatic, or renal impairment, cardiovascular disease, diabetes, glaucoma, cataracts, myasthenia gravis, patients at risk for osteoporosis, patients at risk for seizures, or gastrointestinal diseases	AE: Cardiovascular (edema, heart failure); central nervous system (euphoria, headache, insomnia, mood swings, psychic disorder); dermatologic (acne, alopecia, hyper/hypopigmentation, wound healing impaired); endocrine/metabolic (adrenal suppression, Cushing syndrome, diabetes, sodium retention); neuromuscular (arthropathy, myopathy, osteoporosis, weakness); ocular (cataracts, glaucoma); miscellaneous (moon face, abnormal fat distribution) I: Substrate of the CYP 450 system; inducer of the CYP450 system	F: Elixir, injection, solution, tablet D: 10-20 mg 15-30 min before treatment on each treatment day; numerous dosage regimens exist A: Administer oral formulation with meals to decrease gastrointestinal upset	May cause adrenal suppression, particularly in younger children or in patients receiving high doses for prolonged periods; Withdrawal and discontinuation should be done slowly and carefully
Ondansetron (Zofran)	Selective 5-HT₃ receptor antagonist, both peripherally on vagal nerve terminals and centrally in the chemoreceptor trigger zone	Prevention of nausea and vomiting associated with moderately to highly emetogenic cancer chemotherapy	C: Hypersensitivity to ondansetron or 5-HT₃ receptor antagonist W/P: Ondansetron should be used on a scheduled basis, not on an as needed (prn) basis; use caution in patients with congenital long QTc syndrome or risk factors for QTc prolongation (eg, medications known to prolong QTc interval, electrolyte abnormalities)	AE: Central nervous system (headache, drowsiness); gastrointestinal (constipation); dermatologic (rash) I: Substrate of the CYP450 system; weak inhibitor of the CYP 450 system	F: Injection; solution; tablet; oral disintegrating tablet D: Highly emetogenic agents: 24 mg given 30 min prior to start of therapy; moderately emetogenic agents: 8 mg every 12 h beginning 30 min before chemotherapy A: Oral disintegrating tablets—do not remove from blister until needed; peel backing off blister, do not push tablet through; using dry hands, place tablet on tongue and allow to dissolve. Swallow with saliva	Several 5-HT₃ receptor antagonists are available: Dolasetron (Anzemet); Granisetron (Kytril), patch (Sancuso), long acting injection (Sustol); Palonosetron (Aloxi) also available in a tablet formulation combined with netupitant (Akynzeo)

(Continued)

TABLE 10-6 Agents use for supportive care of patients with cancer (Continued)

Agent	Mechanism of Action	Use	Contraindications (C)/Warnings & Precautions (W/P)	Adverse Effects (AE) & Interactions (I)	Formulation (F), Dosing (D) & Administration (A)	Comments
Aprepitant, fosaprepitant (Emend)	Inhibits substance p/ neurokinin 1(NK₁) receptor; augments the activity of 5-HT₃ receptor antagonist and corticosteroid activity	Prevention of acute and delayed nausea and vomiting associated with moderately and highly emetogenic chemotherapy (in combination with other antiemetics)	C: Hypersensitivity to aprepitant W/P: Use caution with agents primarily metabolized via CYP450 3A4; use caution with hepatic impairment; not intended for treatment of existing nausea and vomiting or for chronic continuous therapy	AE: Central nervous system (fatigue, dizziness); gastrointestinal (nausea, constipation, diarrhea); neuromuscular (weakness) I: Substrate of CYP450 system; inhibitor and inducer of CYP450 system	F: Capsule (aprepitant); injection (fosaprepitant) D: 125 mg on day 1, followed by 80 mg on days 2 and 3 in combination with other antiemetics; alternatively, may use IV fosaprepitant 150 mg IV on day 1 only A: First dose should be given 1 h prior to antineoplastic therapy; subsequent doses should be given in the morning	Aprepitant serum concentration may be increased when taking with grapefruit juice – avoid concurrent use; Other NK₁ receptor antagonists include: Netupitant (combination product with palonosetron (Akynzeo) Rolapitant (Varubi)
Mesna (Mesnex)	In blood, mesna is oxidized to dimesna which in turn is reduced in the kidney back to mesna, supplying a free thiol group which binds to and inactivates acrolein, the urotoxic metabolite of ifosfamide and cyclophosphamide	Reduce the incidence of drug-induced hemorrhagic cystitis	C: Hypersensitivity to mesna or other thiol compounds W/P: Examine morning urine specimen for hematuria prior to ifosfamide or cyclophosphamide treatment; if hematuria (greater than 50 RBC/HPF) develops, reduce dose or discontinue drug; allergic reactions have been reported; patients should receive adequate hydration	AE: Cardiovascular (flushing); central nervous system (dizziness, headache, fever); dermatologic (rash); gastrointestinal (taste alteration)	F: Injection, tablet D: Short infusion—mesna dose is equal to 60% of the ifosfamide dose given in 3 divided doses (0,4, 8 h after the start of ifosfamide) Continuous infusion: Mesna dose is equal to 20%(bolus) of the ifosfamide dose, followed by a continuous infusion of mesna at 40% of the ifosfamide dose A: Oral: Administer orally in tablet formulation or parenteral solution diluted in water, milk, juice, or carbonated beverage; patients who vomit within 2 h after taking oral mesna should repeat the dose or receive intravenous mesna; intravenous: administer by short (15-30 min) infusion or continuous infusion)	Mesna dosing schedule should be repeated each day ifosfamide is received. If ifosfamide dose is adjusted, then mesna dose should also be modified to maintain the mesna-to-ifosfamide ratio

Drug	Mechanism	Indications	Contraindications/Warnings	Adverse Effects	Forms/Dosing/Administration	Notes
Dexrazoxane (Zinecard, Totect)	Chelating agent that interferes with free radical generation	Reduction of the incidence and severity of cardiomyopathy associated with anthracyclines who have received a cumulative dose of 300 mg/m² and who would benefit from receiving additional therapy anthracyclines; treatment of anthracycline extravasation	C: Hypersensitivity to dexrazoxane W/P: May add to myelosuppression of anthracyclines; adjust does for renal insufficiency	AE: Myelosuppression; dermatologic; gastrointestinal	F: Injection D: Cardiotoxicity: 10:1 ratio of dexrazoxane:doxorubicin (eg, 500 mg/m² dexrazoxane: 50 mg/m² doxorubicin); extravasation: 1000 mg/m² (max 2g) day 1, 2 then 500 mg/m² (max 1g) day 3 A: Cardiotoxicity: Doxorubicin should be given within 30 min after beginning the infusion of dexrazoxane, infuse over 30 min Extravasation: Initiate as soon as possible after extravasation of anthracycline occurs, infuse over 1-2 h	Cardiac monitoring should continue during dexrazoxane therapy Reduce dose by 50% in patients with CrCl <40 mL/min
Leucovorin (Folinic Acid)	A reduced form of folic acid, leucovorin supplies the cofactor blocked by methotrexate	Antidote for folic acid antagonists (methotrexate) and rescue therapy following high-dose methotrexate	C: Pernicious anemia or vitamin B_{12} deficient megaloblastic anemias W/P: When used for treatment of overdose administer as soon as possible; when used for methotrexate rescue therapy methotrexate serum concentrations should be monitored to determine dose and duration of leucovorin therapy	AE: Dermatologic (rash)	F: Injection, tablet D: Treatment of overdose—oral 5-15 mg/d High-dose methotrexate therapy—10mg/m²—start 24 h after beginning of methotrexate infusion—continue every 6 h for 10 doses until methotrexate level is less than 0.05 micromole/L A: Due to calcium content do not administer intravenous solutions at a rate greater than 160 mg/min	Leucovorin should not be administered concurrently with methotrexate. It is usually initiated 24 h after the start of methotrexate; Toxicity to normal tissues may be irreversible if leucovorin is not initiated by 40 h after the start of methotrexate infusion; Leucovorin also used to enhance toxicity of 5-flurouracil. Refer to colorectal cancer chapter for more information on this use.

for patients with a platelet count less than 10,000 cells/mm³ unless they are actively bleeding or are planned to undergo a surgical procedure. Patients with nonmyeloid malignancies who experienced thrombocytopenia with a prior chemotherapy cycle may receive oprelvekin (IL-11). Oprelvekin decreases the need for platelet transfusions and the numbers of platelets required for transfusions. Unfortunately, oprelvekin is associated with significant adverse reactions.

Mucositis The gastrointestinal mucosa is composed of epithelial cells with a rapid turnover. Cells with rapid turnover are the common sites for chemotherapy-induced toxicity. Mucositis of the oral cavity (also called stomatitis) can lead to painful ulcerations, infection, and inability to eat, drink, or swallow. The most effective means of preventing stomatitis is through good oral hygiene. Pharmacologic management of mucositis includes:

- Amifostine for mucositis caused by radiation.
- Cryotherapy (eg, ice chips) as a prophylactic measure for standard and high-dose chemotherapy regimens.
- Antimicrobial lozenges, sucralfate and chlorhexidine rinses, "salt and soda"—a solution of sodium bicarbonate and sodium chloride, and magic mouthwash compound rinses are sometimes used in clinical practices although not advocated by clinical guidelines.
- Palifermin for prevention and treatment of mucositis in patients receiving high-dose chemotherapy for stem cell transplant or leukemia induction.

Chemotherapy-Induced Nausea and Vomiting (CINV) Nausea and vomiting are the toxicities that are the most feared by patients who are undergoing chemotherapy. The rate of emesis varies depending upon the patient risk factors and the drug therapy regimen. Cancer treatments are stratified into high, moderate, low, and minimal emetogenic potential. In general, chemotherapy that is cell cycle nonspecific, such as alkylating agents and anthracyclines, have a higher emetogenic potential than cell cycle specific chemotherapy. High emetogenic antineoplastics cause emesis in 90% of cases (if no antiemetic prophylaxis is given). The rates of emesis among moderate, low, and minimal emetogenic antineoplastics are 30% to 90%, 10% to 30%, and less than 10%, respectively. With proper prophylaxis using antiemetics, the rate of emesis when receiving a highly emetogenic regimen can be reduced to about 30%. The optimal method of managing CINV is to provide adequate pharmacologic prophylaxis given a patient's risk level for emesis. CINV regimens should include a prophylactic regimen and a breakthrough antiemetic drug as needed. Management of CINV includes:

- Behavior therapy (eg, relaxation, guided imagery, and music therapy)
- Antisecretory agents can be helpful in reducing gastroesophageal reflux that may trigger or exacerbate CINV.
- Antiemesis guidelines recommend corticosteroids (dexamethasone), serotonin receptor antagonists, and NK_1 receptor antagonist.

Pharmacotherapy principles regarding the management of CINV include:

- High emetogenic regimens should be managed with a triple-drug combination consisting of dexamethasone, aprepitant, and serotonin antagonist to prevent both acute and delayed emesis.
- Moderate emetogenic regimens should be managed with dexamethasone and a serotonin antagonist.
- Low emetogenic regimens may be managed with a single antiemetic such as dexamethasone.
- Minimal emetogenic regimens may be managed with as needed antiemetics.

Hemorrhagic Cystitis Hemorrhagic cystitis is acute bleeding from the lining of the bladder caused by cyclophosphamide and ifosfamide. Cyclophosphamide and ifosfamide are metabolized to acrolein leading to the bladder toxicity. Patients receiving ifosfamide or high-dose cyclophosphamide (≥ 1 g/m²) are at highest risk for hemorrhagic cystitis. The use of preventive strategies can significantly reduce the incidence of hemorrhagic cystitis. Management of hemorrhagic cystitis includes:

- Administration of mesna: Mesna binds to acrolein preventing the bladder toxicity
- Hydration
- Bladder irrigation

Anthracycline Cardiotoxicity Anthracyclines may form free radicals and the free radicals combine with oxygen to form superoxide which can make hydrogen peroxide. Oxygen free radical formation is a cause of cardiac damage and may be prevented by the use of dexrazoxane.

Methotrexate Bone Marrow and Gastrointestinal Toxicity High-dose methotrexate administration is associated with the development of irreversible myelosuppression and gastrointestinal mucosa damage. Leucovorin (tetrahydrofolate) is administered to bypass the methotrexate inhibition of dihydrofolate reductase of normal cells.

Platinum Nephrotoxicity Cisplatin and carboplatin may cause nephrotoxicity and can be prevented by the administration of fluids and in some cases, amifostine. Oxaliplatin is not known to cause nephrotoxicity.

ADMINISTRATION

Administration of antineoplastic chemotherapy is a complex process and is mostly performed on an outpatient basis. Because of increasing reports of errors in the administration of chemotherapeutic agents, the ASCO and the Oncology Nursing Society (ONS) published nursing safety practices that promote standardization of care, increase efficiency, and provide a framework for best practice with the overarching goal of reducing risk to subject from human errors. It is important for an oncology nurse to be appropriately credentialed and privileged along with detailed understanding of local institutional/governmental policies and guidelines through ongoing continuing medical education before getting involved with the practice of oncology.

Assessment Initial assessment prior to drug administration should include verification of chart documentation, verification of patient identity, up-to-date information on allergies, and verification of cancer diagnosis (eg, reviewing a copy of the pathological report). A review of the chemotherapy treatment should include chemotherapy drugs, doses, duration, and goals of therapy. Additionally, up-to-date information on baseline measurements such as weight, height, vital signs, and organ-specific functional status (such as liver function test, renal function tests) should be evaluated. Health care practitioners administering chemotherapy should check the dosage calculation for the body size and the five Rs of administering medication (right patient, right medication, right dose, right route, right time). Providers should perform a through medication review and this review should include herbal and supplements. For example, St. John's Wort has significant drug interactions and may severely interact with chemotherapy regimens.

Chemotherapy Administration Local institutional policies regarding obtaining and documenting informed consent process should be followed, and documentation of informed consent process should be verified prior to chemotherapy administration. Drug preparation should be performed under the supervision of a licensed pharmacist and be labeled immediately on preparation. Labeling should include at least two patient identifiers, drug and prescription information and detailed instructions. Prior to administration of chemotherapy, at least two approved personnel should reconfirm the identity of the patient using at the minimum two methods of identification, should cross check the labeling of the drug and verify if it matches that prescribed for the patient and document such verification.

- Evaluate the chemotherapy regimen to ensure the correct dose and route of administration.
- Check patient laboratory values to ensure that the complete blood count and blood chemistries are as expected prior to administering chemotherapy.
- If a patient has renal or hepatic dysfunction, check to see if chemotherapy dose has been adjusted appropriately.
- Ensure appropriate antiemetic therapy was provided for the expected degree of emetogenicity.
- Assess the regimen to determine if white blood cell support with CSFs is needed.
- Assess the patient's concurrent medications for the possibility of drug interactions.
- Employ safe handling and disposal methods of antineoplastic agents.

Monitoring Efficacy: Monitor imaging or other studies and categorize patient into either a CR, PR, SD, or PD. Toxicity:

Monitor complete blood count and other blood chemistries (eg, basic metabolic panel); monitor patient for known toxicities of the chemotherapy regimen (eg, hemorrhagic cystitis) and modify the dose or discontinue if necessary.

CASE Application

1. Which of the following is the correct route of administration for vincristine administration?

   a. Intramuscular
   b. Intrathecal
   c. Intravenous
   d. Subcutaneous

2. Select the supportive care medication that is associated with fluid retention.

   a. Darbepoetin
   b. Peg-filgrastim
   c. Amifostine
   d. Oprelvekin

Use the following scenario to answer questions 3 to 8.

WF is a 70-year-old man with a recent diagnosis of stage IV colorectal cancer with the primary tumor in the sigmoid colon and multiple metastases found in his liver. The oncologist indicated that cure is not a realistic goal of treatment for WF because of his advanced disease. He is scheduled to begin chemotherapy with the regimen FOLFOXIRI, which contains 5-fluorouracil, leucovorin, oxaliplatin, and irinotecan. In addition, the patient is to receive bevacizumab.

3. What is the term for chemotherapy that is being used with the intention of prolonging life and improving quality of life but not of curing the patient?

   a. Curative intent
   b. Stabilization intent
   c. Palliative intent
   d. Hospice intent

4. Which of the medications that WF is to receive as part of his treatment regimen is not chemotherapy?

   a. 5-Fluorouracil
   b. Leucovorin
   c. Oxaliplatin
   d. Irinotecan

5. Which of the medication(s) in WF's treatment regimen is a cell cycle specific drug? Select all that apply.

   a. 5-Fluorouracil
   b. Oxaliplatin
   c. Irinotecan
   d. Bevacizumab

6. Shortly after receiving his first dose of chemotherapy, WF begins to experience numbness and painful tingling that is exacerbated by cold. Which of the medications in

his treatment regimen is most likely causing these new symptoms?

a. 5-Fluorouracil
b. Leucovorin
c. Oxaliplatin
d. Irinotecan

7. Approximately 8 weeks after the beginning of his chemotherapy, WF begins complaining about feeling more tired and weak lately. He also mentions that he becomes short of breath after even moderate physical activity. Blood tests showed a hemoglobin level of 8.6 g/dL. Which of the following is correct regarding WF's anemia?

a. He should begin treatment with erythropoietin to treat chemotherapy-induced anemia.
b. He should receive a blood transfusion to treat severe anemia from blood loss.
c. He should begin treatment with darbepoetin once his hemoglobin level fall below 8 g/dL.
d. He is not a candidate for treatment with an erythropoiesis stimulating agent since his cancer is being treated with curative intent.

8. After the completions for 4 cycles of his chemotherapy, WF undergoes imaging scans to determine the cancer's response to therapy. The imaging tests reveal that the patient's total tumor burden has decreased by approximately 65%. Which of the following best describes WF's response to his treatment?

a. Progressive disease
b. Stable disease
c. Partial Response
d. Complete Response

9. Rank the following MABs in order for lowest immunogenicity to highest immunogenicity.

Unordered options	Ordered response
Ibritumomab	
Rituximab	
Pertuzumab	
Denosumab	

10. A patient is newly initiated on erlotinib for the treatment of nonsmall cell lung cancer. Which of the following medications may pose a drug/drug interaction with his new medication?

a. Phenytoin
b. Pregabalin
c. Heparin
d. Sulfamethoxazole/trimethoprim

Use the following scenario to answer questions 11 to 15.

YM is a 62-year-old woman with a recent diagnosis of stage III diffuse large B-cell lymphoma. Her disease is characterized by multiple areas of involvement including the spleen, pelvic lymph nodes, and mediastinal lymph nodes. She is scheduled to begin chemotherapy with the regimen EPOCH-R, which includes etoposide, prednisone, vincristine, cyclophosphamide, doxorubicin, and rituximab.

11. Oncovin is the brand name of which of the medications in YM's treatment regimen?

a. Etoposide
b. Vincristine
c. Doxorubicin
d. Rituximab

12. The medical team asks the pharmacists if YM needs to receive any medications to prevent allergic reactions from her treatment regimen. Which of the medications in her treatment regimen is most likely to cause an infusion reaction and could benefit from premedication with acetaminophen and diphenhydramine?

a. Cyclophosphamide
b. Vincristine
c. Doxorubicin
d. Rituximab

13. The EPOCH-R regimen that YM is receiving is considered to be a high risk of developing febrile neutropenia. Which of the following is a medication that could be used to help YM's white blood cell count recover faster and decrease her risk of developing febrile neutropenia? Select all that apply.

a. Peg-filgrastim
b. Oprelvekin
c. Sargramostim
d. Darbepoetin

14. Approximately 4 hours after the infusion of the first cycle of chemotherapy, YM begins experience severe nausea and has episodes of vomiting. Which of the medications in her treatment regimen is the most likely to be causing her nausea and vomiting?

a. Etoposide
b. Prednisone
c. Cyclophosphamide
d. Vincristine

15. On her second cycle, during the infusion of the doxorubicin YM begins experiencing extreme pain at the injection site. The nurse observes new onset redness and swelling around the infusion site and is concerned that extravasation has occurred. Which of the following agents is the most appropriate to treat this extravasation injury?

a. Hyaluronidase
b. Dexrazoxane
c. Sodium thiosulfate
d. Silver sulfadiazine

16. Select the chemoprotectant that supplies a free thiol that binds to acrolein preventing a major antineoplastic adverse reaction.

a. Mesna
b. Leucovorin
c. Dexrazoxane
d. Hydroxyurea

Use the following scenario to answer questions 17 to 21.

JH is a 56-year-old woman who was recently diagnosed with stage IIIa adenocarcinoma of the lung. She has an extensive smoking history, smoking one and a half packs of cigarettes per day for 30 years. Her oncologist indicated that the cancer is too large to operate on and she will receive chemotherapy first to shrink the tumor, followed later by surgery. She is to receive chemotherapy with cisplatin and pemetrexed.

17. Prior to her diagnosis of lung cancer, would JH have been an appropriate candidate for lung cancer screening?

    a. Yes, she would have been a good candidate for lung cancer screening.
    b. No, she would not have been a good candidate for lung cancer screening because she is too old.
    c. No, she would not have been a good candidate for lung cancer because she smoked too much.
    d. No, she would not have been a good candidate for lung cancer screening because she does not have chronic obstructive pulmonary disease (COPD).

18. What is the term that best describes the timing of JH's chemotherapy in relation to her surgery?

    a. Adjuvant
    b. Adjunct
    c. Neoadjuvant
    d. Neoadjunct

19. Which of the following organ toxicities is most likely to occur as a result of the patient receiving cisplatin?

    a. Hepatotoxicity
    b. Nephrotoxicity
    c. Pulmonary toxicity
    d. Cardiotoxicity

20. Which of the following medications should the patient receive to decrease toxicity from pemetrexed? Select all that apply.

    a. Folic acid
    b. Cyanocobalamin
    c. Thiamine
    d. Dexamethasone

21. Two year after her initial lung cancer diagnosis, JH has achieved a complete remission and has been cancer free for over a year following the completion of all her therapy. She is interested in early detection of other types of cancer. Which of the following types of cancer should JH be screened for? Select all that apply.

    a. Breast cancer
    b. Colorectal cancer
    c. Melanoma
    d. Uterine cancer

Use the following scenario to answer questions 22 to 26.

HM is a 51-year-old postmenopausal woman with a recent diagnosis of stage II ductal carcinoma of the breast.

Pathology reports revealed her tumor is estrogen/progesterone receptor positive and HER2 negative. She undergoes a bilateral mastectomy and is scheduled to begin chemotherapy with the regimen AC → T. This regimen contains doxorubicin and cyclophosphamide followed by paclitaxel.

22. Which of the following toxicities may occur as the result of administration of paclitaxel in HM?

    a. Ototoxicity
    b. Nephrotoxicity
    c. Cerebellar toxicity
    d. Peripheral neuropathy

23. Which of the following is a long-term toxicity that may occur in HM as a result of the administration of doxorubicin?

    a. Cardiotoxicity
    b. Nephrotoxicity
    c. Colitis
    d. Pulmonary toxicity

24. After the completion of her chemotherapy, the oncologist plans to initiate hormonal therapy. Which of the following hormonal therapies is an appropriate choice to treat HM's breast cancer?

    a. Degarelix
    b. Bicalutamide
    c. Letrozole
    d. Raloxifene

25. HM is concerned about her daughter developing breast cancer and is asking about early detection recommendations for her. Her daughter is 29. Which of the following is the most appropriate breast cancer screening recommendation for HM's 29-year-old daughter?

    a. Breast cancer screening is not recommended for the general population.
    b. She should begin screening for breast cancer now.
    c. She should begin screening for breast cancer when she turns 50 years old.
    d. She should begin screening for breast cancer when she turns 55 years old.

26. Three years after the completion of her chemotherapy, HM presents to her primary care provider with abdominal pain and increased yellowing of the skin. Laboratory evaluation showed increased bilirubin and markedly elevated liver function tests. Imaging scans showed breast cancer recurrence with widespread metastases to the liver. Which of the following chemotherapy agents used in the treatment of relapsed breast cancer should be used with caution in HM due to her liver disease?

    a. Eribulin
    b. Docetaxel
    c. Gemcitabine
    d. Ixabepilone

TAKEAWAY POINTS »

- Neoplasm (sometimes called **tumor** or cancer) is an abnormal mass of tissue, the growth of which exceeds and is uncoordinated with that of normal tissues and persists after cessation of the stimuli which evoked the change.

- Antineoplastic treatment plans require a complex interdisciplinary approach that involves shared decision making between individual client and their health care providers.

- The term antineoplastic **chemotherapy** describes a type of antineoplastic therapy that uses pharmacological agents to treat cancer. Other modalities of antineoplastic therapy include surgery and radiotherapy.

- Antineoplastic chemotherapy can be classified into three major groups: *adjuvant chemotherapy*, *neoadjuvant chemotherapy*, and *primary induction chemotherapy*.

- The goal of chemotherapy is to selectively kill or suppress cancer cells and to achieve this with minimal or no damage to normal cells.

- Optimal chemotherapy dosing and schedule is based on knowledge of mechanism of action and detailed experimental evidence. Most chemotherapeutic agents have a narrow therapeutic range and it is critical to ensure that the dose is within the recommended therapeutic window to ensure damage to cancer cells and minimal effects to normal cells.

- Use of combination therapy provides similar benefits in antineoplastic chemotherapy as in antimicrobial chemotherapy. Using multiple drugs will lead to maximum focused damage at lower doses of individual drugs without compromising therapeutic efficacy.

- Chemotherapy can be administered enterally (orally) or parenterally (intravenous, subcutaneous, intramuscular).

- Antineoplastic classes consist of alkylating agents, antimetabolites, antibiotics, hormones, antimitotic, and miscellaneous agents.

- Chemoprotectants protect organs or cells from toxic effects of the antineoplastic agents.

BIBLIOGRAPHY

American Cancer Society. Cancer screening guidelines. https://www.cancer.org/healthy/find-cancer-early/cancer-screening-guidelines.html. Accessed July 2017.

Chabner BA, Bertino J, Cleary J, et al. Cytotoxic agents. In: Brunton LL, Chabner BA, Knollmann BC, eds. *Goodman & Gilman's The Pharmacological Basis of Therapeutics.* 12th ed. New York, NY: McGraw-Hill; 2011:chap 61.

Chabner BA. General principles of cancer chemotherapy. In: Brunton LL, Chabner BA, Knollmann BC, eds. *Goodman & Gilman's The Pharmacological Basis of Therapeutics.* 12th ed. New York, NY: McGraw-Hill; 2011:chap 60.

Chu E, Sartorelli AC. Cancer chemotherapy. In: Katzung BG, Trevor AJ, eds. *Basic & Clinical Pharmacology.* 13th ed. New York, NY: McGraw-Hill; 2015:chap 54.

Howlader N, Noone AM, Krapcho M, Miller D, Bishop K, Kosary CL, Yu M, Ruhl J, Tatalovich Z, Mariotto A, Lewis DR, Chen HS, Feuer EJ, Cronin KA, et al. (eds). SEER Cancer Statistics Review, 1975-2014, National Cancer Institute. Bethesda, MD. https://seer.cancer.gov/csr/1975_2014/, based on November 2016 SEER data submission, posted to the SEER web site, April 2017.

Sausville EA, Longo DL. Principles of cancer treatment. In: Kasper DL, Fauci AS, Hauser SL, Longo DL, Jameson J, Loscalzo J, et al. (eds). *Harrison's Principles of Internal Medicine.* 19th ed. New York, NY: McGraw-Hill; 2015:chap 103e.

Shord SS, Cordes LM. Cancer treatment and chemotherapy. In: DiPiro JT, Talbert RL, Yee GC, Matzke GR, Wells BG, Posey L, eds. *Pharmacotherapy: A Pathophysiologic Approach.* 10th ed. New York, NY: McGraw-Hill; 2017:chap 127.

KEY ABBREVIATIONS

ANC = absolute neutrophil count
ASCO = American Society of Clinical Oncology
CINV = chemotherapy-induced nausea and vomiting
COPD = chronic obstructive pulmonary disease
CR = complete response
DNA = deoxyribonucleic acid
G-CSF = granulocyte colony stimulating factor
GM-CSF = granulocyte-macrophage colony stimulating factor
IL-2 = interleukin-2

LHRH = luteinizing hormone-releasing hormone
NCCN = National Comprehensive Cancer Network
ONS = Oncology Nursing Society
PD = progressive disease
PICC = peripherally inserted central catheter
PR = partial response
RNA = ribonucleic acid
SD = stable disease

11 Immune System

S. Scott Sutton

FOUNDATION OVERVIEW

The immune system protects the body from invading pathogens and has an amazing ability to evolve and adapt based upon environmental exposure. The immune system is designed to attack and destroy foreign antigens/pathogens; however, the immune system must be able to distinguish self from nonself. Failure to differentiate self from nonself may lead to autoimmune diseases (see Table 11-1 for a list of autoimmune diseases). The immune system includes two functional divisions: (1) innate or nonspecific and (2) adaptive or specific. The body uses the innate and adaptive immune responses to kill foreign pathogens. The greatest differences between the responses are in specificity and memory. The adaptive immune response can evolve with each subsequent infection, whereas the innate immune response stays the same with each infection. Awareness of immune systems components and consequences of disrupting homeostasis must be understood in order to appropriately dose, administer, and monitor effects of medications given to manipulate immune responses.

INNATE IMMUNE SYSTEM

Physical and chemical defenses compose the innate immune system and are the first line of defense against pathogens.

Physical Defense

The skin is the primary method of physical defense. Alterations in the skin allow for an easy portal of entry for pathogens. Burns and abrasions are common examples that alter the physical defense of the skin; however, medications can also alter this nonspecific system (drug-associated Stevens Johnson syndrome [SJS]—see Table 11-2). The low pH of the stomach serves as a major defense to pathogen entry through the gastrointestinal system. Medications that alter the pH of the stomach may change the gastrointestinal bacterial flora and increase risk of infections. Antisecretory agents such as proton pump inhibitors have been associated with pH changes in the stomach and subsequent development of bacterial infections. The rapid turnover of gastrointestinal cells also limits systemic infection, as cells are frequently sloughed. Cell-cycle antineoplastics that disrupt the sloughing process may leave the patient at increased risk for infections. The respiratory

tract has forms of physical defense such as coughing, mucous coating the epithelial cells, and the cilia lining the epithelium of the lungs. The combination of coughing, cilia, and mucus provide a barrier to invasion of the respiratory tract. Disruption of the respiratory physical defense through mechanical ventilation can increase the risk for penetration by a pathogenic organism (pneumonia) or anti-infectives that alter gastrointestinal flora leaving the patient at an increased risk of infection (eg, *Clostridium difficile* infection). Other examples of nonspecific defenses include: normal urine flow, lysozymes in tears and saliva, and the normal flora in the throat, gastrointestinal tract, and genitourinary tract.

Cellular Components Defense

If a pathogen invades and is able to infiltrate through a host's physical defense system, innate immunity (cellular) is used to halt progression of the pathogen. Innate immunity cells include the leukocytes or white blood cells (WBCs) (monocytes, neutrophils, basophils, and eosinophils). Other WBCs (lymphocytes) are involved in adaptive immunity. The innate cells are one of the most widely monitored clinical laboratory tests. Innate cells may be evaluated by ordering a complete blood count (CBC). When a CBC is ordered, part of the laboratory test reports a tally of the total WBCs in a given volume of blood plus the relative percentages that each cell type contributes to the total. Table 11-3 provides a breakdown of the different types of WBCs and their usual cell counts in peripheral blood for an adult.

Granulocytes

Granulocytes are phagocytes (engulfing cells) and derive their name from the presence of granules within the cytoplasm. The granules store lysozymes and other chemicals needed to produce the oxidative and nonoxidative burst to lyse the pathogen. Granulocytic leukocytes include neutrophils, eosinophils, basophils, and monocytes. Granulocytes are formed in large numbers in the bone marrow, undergo numerous steps in the marrow, and are usually released into the peripheral blood in their mature form. Neutrophils, eosinophils, and basophils die in the course of destroying pathogens, yielding pus. In contrast, monocytes do not die when destroying pathogens because they play a critical role in activating the adaptive immune response via antigen presentation.

TABLE 11-1	Autoimmune Diseases

An autoimmune disorder is a condition that occurs when the immune system mistakenly attacks and destroys healthy body tissue. A person may have more than one autoimmune disorder at the same time. Examples of autoimmune disorders include:

Addison disease

Hashimoto thyroiditis

Rheumatoid arthritis

Systemic lupus erythematosus

Sjogren syndrome

Multiple sclerosis

Myasthenia gravis

Insulin-dependent diabetes mellitus

Graves disease

Idiopathic thrombocytopenia purpura

Sarcoidosis

Scleroderma

TABLE 11-3	Normal White Blood Cell Count and Differential in Adults

Cell Type	Normal Range
Total white blood cell count	4.4-11.3 × 10³ cells/mm³
Polymorphonuclear neutrophils (polys, segs, PMN)	2.3-7.7 × 10³ cells/mm³
Band neutrophils (immature neutrophils, bands, stabs)	0-10 × 10³ cells/mm³
Eosinophils	0.0-0.7 × 10³ cells/mm³
Basophils	0.0-0.2 × 10³ cells/mm³
Monocytes	0.3-0.8 × 10³ cells/mm³
Lymphocytes	1.6-2.4 × 10³ cells/mm³

Neutrophils Neutrophils represent the majority of granulocytes and leukocytes and serve as the primary defense against bacterial infections. Neutrophils, also termed segs or polymorphonuclear cells, migrate from the bloodstream into infected or inflamed tissue. In this migration process known as chemotaxis, neutrophils reach the desired site and adhere to, recognize, and phagocytose pathogens. During phagocytosis, the pathogen is internalized within the phagocyte. The neutrophil releases its granular contents which lead to destruction of the engulfed pathogen. The less mature form of a neutrophil is a band. During an acute infection, there is an increase in the percentage of neutrophils as they are released from the bone marrow. Less mature band forms may also be released. These immature neutrophils are still considered active. The appearance of band cells is called a shift to the left. The actions of cytokine medications such as

TABLE 11-2	Stevens Johnson Syndrome

Stevens Johnsons Syndrome (SJS) is a rare, serious disorder in which the skin and mucous membranes react severely to a medication or infection. Often SJS begins with flu-like symptoms, followed by a painful red or purplish rash that spreads and blisters, eventually causing the top layer of skin to die and shed. Examples of drug-induced SJS are:

Allopurinol

Nonsteroidal anti-inflammatory drugs (NSAID)

Sulfonamides

Penicillins

Phenytoin

Carbamazepine

Valproic acid

Lamotrigine

Phenobarbital

granulocyte colony-stimulating factor (G-CSF) and granulocyte-macrophage colony-stimulating factor (GM-CSF) may intensify neutrophil activity. G-CSF (filgrastim [Neupogen]) and long-acting G-CSF (pegylated filgrastim [Neulasta]) are G-CSFs licensed to prevent chemotherapy-induced neutropenia or to stimulate granulocyte production among patients with severe chronic neutropenia. GM-CSF (sargramostim [Leukine]) is a GM-CSF licensed to shorten the time to neutrophil recovery in acute myelogenous leukemia and stem cell transplantation.

Eosinophils and Basophils The major role of eosinophils is in host defense against parasitic infections; however, eosinophils can phagocytize, kill, and digest bacteria and yeast, but not as efficiently as neutrophils. Eosinophils account for less than 7% of circulating leukocytes and are present in the intestinal mucosa and lungs, two locations where foreign proteins enter the body. Elevations of eosinophil counts are highly suggestive of parasitic infections. Along with mast cells, eosinophils play an important role in allergies and allergic asthma.

Basophils are the least common granulocyte, accounting for 0.1% to 0.3% of granulocytes. They contain heparin, histamine, and leukotriene B_4. Along with eosinophils and mast cells, basophils play a role in allergies and allergic asthma. Basophils may also be associated with immediate hypersensitivity and delayed hypersensitivity reactions, and increased chronic inflammation and leukemia.

Monocytes Functions of monocytes include removal of necrotic apoptotic tissues, lysis of cancer cells, and antigen presentation. They account for 1% to 10% of circulating leukocytes. Monocytes migrate to tissues (lymph nodes, spleen, liver, lung), where they mature into macrophages. After engulfing pathogens, monocytes/macrophages are transformed into antigen-presenting cells (APC). These transformed macrophages present antigen (lysed pathogens) to CD4(+) helper T lymphocytes; therefore, macrophages and other antigen presenting cells (eg, dendritic cells) activate the adaptive immune response (Figure 11-1). Dendritic cells are the most potent antigen presenting cell; however, they make up less than 1% of circulating leukocytes. Dendritic cells, like macrophages,

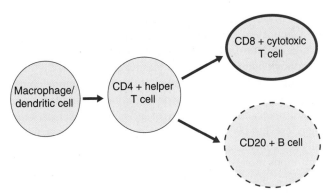

FIGURE 11-1 Activation of the adaptive immune response. Macrophage and/or dendritic cells present antigen to the CD4+ helper T cell. If the CD4+ T cell recognizes the antigen by its T cell receptor (TCR), the CD4+ helper T cell becomes activated to secrete cytokines to stimulate either a CD8+ cytotoxic T cell response or a CD20+ B cell response to produce antibody. Reproduced with permission from Sutton S, ed. *McGraw-Hill's NAPLEX® Review Guide*. New York, NY: McGraw-Hill; 2011.

TABLE 11-4	Subtypes of T Lymphocytes	
Surface Marker	Common Name	Comment
CD4(+)	Helper	Plays critical role in upregulating immune response
CD8(+)	Cytotoxic or suppressor	Cytotoxic: Plays critical role in lysing cells, particularly viral cells Suppressor: Plays critical role in downregulating the immune response

are found more commonly in tissues (eg, spleen, liver). Tissue macrophages also salvage iron from hemoglobin of old erythrocytes and return iron to transferrin for delivery to bone marrow.

ADAPTIVE IMMUNE SYSTEM

The adaptive immune response consists of two parts, humoral and cell-mediated. The B lymphocytes compose the humoral part, and the T lymphocytes compose the cell-mediated part. T lymphocytes are tailored to defend against infections that are intracellular (viral infections), whereas B lymphocytes secrete antibodies that neutralize pathogens prior to their entry into host cells. However, there is cross talking and interplay between humoral and the cell-mediated immune responses.

Lymphocytes

Lymphocytes make up the second major group of leukocytes. They are characterized by a less granular cytoplasm and large, smooth nuclei. These cells give specificity and memory to the body's defense against foreign invaders. A lymphocyte that has never encountered an antigen it recognizes is referred to as naive. Lymphocytes are not phagocytic, but the T-cells are cytotoxic. Morphologic differentiation of lymphocytes is difficult; visual inspection of a blood smear cannot distinguish between T and B cells. Fortunately, lymphocytes can be distinguished by the presence of lineage-specific membrane proteins, termed clusters of differentiation (CD). Mature T cells express CD4 or CD8, while B lymphocytes express CD20. Identification of the subtype of lymphocyte is not a routine clinical hematology test; they are reported as a total lymphocyte count on the CBC. An exception is the reporting/monitoring of CD4 cells for patients with human immunodeficiency virus (HIV), as low CD4 cell counts are associated with increased risks of opportunistic infections.

T Lymphocytes

T lymphocytes are responsible for cell-mediated immunity and are the predominant lymphocyte in circulation and tissue. There are two major subtypes of T lymphocytes: helper and cytotoxic/suppressor (Table 11-4). To activate the adaptive immune response, APCs must present antigen to be recognized by helper T lymphocytes which then activate either cytotoxic T cells or B cell. The role of the T cell is to search and destroy pathogens that infect and replicate intracellularly. When these pathogens enter a cell, they are no longer vulnerable to innate host defenses. Therefore, it is critical that T cells be able to distinguish which cells are infected and which cells are not. In addition to identifying infections, T cells play a prominent role in delayed hypersensitivity reactions (eg, skin reaction to poison ivy, skin tests for tuberculosis, mumps, and *Candida*) and rejection of transplanted organs. In order for a foreign antigen to be recognized by a CD4(+) T lymphocyte, the antigen must be presented by macrophages/dendritic cells in major histocompatibility complex (MHC) II. In contrast, CD8(+) T lymphocytes recognize antigen presented in MHC class I molecules. MHC molecules are often referred to as human leukocyte antigens (HLA).

B lymphocytes

A B lymphocyte recognizes antigen via its antibody or immunoglobulin located on its cell surface. The antibody on the surface can recognize an intact pathogen, such as bacteria, and then present antigen to T cells (ie, acts as an APC). However, the major function of B cells is to produce antibodies to bind to the invading pathogen, a process that first entails activation of the B cell. B cells, once activated by CD4(+) helper T lymphocytes, become a plasma cell that will produce one of five immunoglobulin types: IgA, IgD, IgE, IgG, or IgM. The two antibodies most commonly associated with the development of immunity to foreign proteins, viruses, and bacteria are IgM and IgG. A fraction of the B cells do not differentiate into plasma cells but rather form a pool of memory cells. Memory cells will respond to subsequent encounters with the pathogen, generating a quicker and more vigorous response to the pathogen.

One of the most important functions of the adaptive immune response is to produce antibodies or immunoglobulins. IgG is the prevalent immunoglobulin in the serum, and IgG concentrations less than 600 mg/dL (hypogammaglobulinemia) are associated with bacterial infections. IgA is the

TABLE 11-5   Quantitative Leukocyte Disorders[a]

WBC Abnormality	Cell Count (cells/mm³)	Potential Causes
Neutrophilia	>12,000	Acute bacterial infection Trauma Myocardial infarction Chronic bacterial infection Epinephrine Lithium G-CSF GM-CSF Glucocorticosteroids
Neutropenia	<1500	Antineoplastic agents Captopril Cephalosporins Chloramphenicol Ganciclovir Methimazole Penicillin Phenothiazines Procainamide Ticlopidine Tricyclic antidepressants Vancomycin Zidovudine Radiation exposure Overwhelming bacterial infection
Eosinophilia	>350	Allergic disorders Asthma Parasitic infections Leukemia ACE inhibitors Antibiotics (allergic reaction)
Basophilia	>300	Chronic inflammation Leukemia
Monocytosis	>800	Tuberculosis Endocarditis Protozoal infection Leukemia
Lymphocytosis	>4000	Mononucleosis Viral infections Rubella Varicella Mumps CMV Pertussis Tuberculosis Syphilis Lymphoma
Lymphopenia	<1000	HIV Radiation Glucocorticosteroids Lymphoma Aplastic anemia

[a]White blood cell counts are sensitive, not specific markers. For example, if a patient has a lymphocyte count <1000 (lymphopenia), the patient may or may not have HIV or radiation exposure. There are numerous things that may cause a lymphopenia; those listed in the above chart serve as examples.

Abbreviations: ACE, angiotensin converting enzyme; CMV, cytomegalovirus; HIV, human immunodeficiency virus; G-CSF, granulocyte colony stimulating factor; GM-CSF, granulocyte-macrophage colony-stimulating factor; WBC, white blood cell.

second most prevalent concentration in the serum, but IgA's most important role relates to its secretion in the respiratory, gastrointestinal, and genitourinary tract. IgM is the first immunoglobulin secreted by a plasma cell, and it is the most efficient activator of complement of the five immunoglobulin subtypes. There are very low concentrations of circulating IgE in serum because the majority of IgE is bound to mast cells. Therefore, IgE plays a critical role in allergic disorders. Clinically, IgE concentrations are measured in IU/mL, and IgE concentrations more than 200 IU/mL are associated with allergic disorders. IgD is one of the surface immunoglobulins on B cells, but the function of circulating IgD is unknown. Serum concentrations of the immunoglobulins are:

Isotype	Serum concentration (mg/dL)
IgG	600-1200
IgA	140-260
IgM	70-120

Clinically, only IgG, IgA, and IgM isotypes are determined. IgE concentrations must be ordered separately, usually as IU/mL.

LEUKOCYTE DISORDERS

Patients can suffer from disorders of the WBCs. Leukocyte disorders can be classified into three major classes: (1) functional, (2) quantitative, and (3) myeloproliferative.

Functional Leukocyte Disorders

Functional WBC disorders consist of recognition, signaling, and cytotoxic effects. Examples include hypogammaglobulinemia and chronic granulomatous disease.

Quantitative Leukocyte Disorders

Quantitative leukocyte disorders involve too few or too many WBCs, however, several terms are used to refer to low numbers of WBCs. Examples are listed in Table 11-5. Key definitions for quantitative disorders include: neutropenia, leukopenia, granulocytopenia, and agranulocytosis.

- Neutropenia is the presence of abnormally low numbers of neutrophils in circulating blood. Neutropenia is a neutrophil count less than 1500 cells/mm³, but one clinically becomes concerned when the neutrophil count falls below 500 cells/mm³.

- Leukopenia is a total WBC less than 3000 cells/mm³. Leukopenia maybe from any cause (neutrophils, lymphocytes, etc.), but almost all leukopenia patients are neutropenic since the neutrophils comprise the majority of circulating leukocytes.

- Granulocytopenia is a granulocyte count less than 1500 granulocytes/mm³. Granulocytes consist of neutrophils, eosinophils, and basophils. Because neutrophils comprise the vast majority of circulating granulocytes, granulocytopenia is generally caused by neutropenia.

- Agranulocytosis is defined as a severe form of neutropenia with a total granulocyte count less than 500 cells/mm³. Unfortunately, clinicians use variable definitions when reporting WBC dyscrasias. The term agranulocytosis has been used to describe granulocyte counts ranging from less than 100 cells/mm³ to less than 1000 cells/mm³.

Myeloproliferative Leukocyte Disorders

Myeloproliferative disorders involve an abnormal proliferation of bone marrow cells. Neoplasms of the myeloproliferative stem cells may involve a leukocyte progenitor line. Leukemias are classified as myeloblastic (granulocytic lineage) or lymphoblastic (lymphocytic lineage) and according to whether they primarily affect the very early progenitor cells (acute) or more mature cells (chronic).

- Acute myelogenous leukemia (AML)
- Acute lymphocytic leukemia (ALL)
- Chronic myelogenous leukemia (CML)
- Chronic lymphocytic leukemia (CLL)

A lymphoma is a neoplasm of lymphocytic origin but predominates in the lymph nodes rather than the bone marrow. Therefore, patients with lymphomas present with lymphadenopathy. Lymphomas are categorized as Hodgkin and non-Hodgkin lymphoma. Lymphomas can evolve from either T- or B-lymphocyte precursors, and many express CD markers characteristic of mature lymphocytes. Identification of the CD20 marker on B-cell lymphomas provides an opportunity to treat these patients with recombinant antibodies specific to this surface marker (eg, rituximab).

SPECIAL CONSIDERATIONS

The complement system, mannose-binding lectin, and C-reactive protein (CRP) are also mediators of innate immunity. The complement system consists of more than 30 circulating proteins that play a key role in immune defense. The complement system serves as an adjunct or "complement" to humoral immunity. The four major functions of the complement system include:

1. Direct lysis of pathogens and cells
2. Stimulate chemotaxis
3. Opsonize foreign pathogens for recognition by neutrophils, macrophages, and dendritic cells
4. Clear immune complexes

Complement factors (C3a, C5a) act as chemotactic factors for phagocytic cells. Patients with hereditary deficiencies of complement may have recurrent bacterial infections or autoimmune syndromes. Both mannan-binding lectin and CRP are acute phase reactants produced by the liver during early stages of infection or inflammation. Acute phase reactants or proteins increase in response to inflammatory stimuli such as tissue injury or infection. CRP is a plasma protein that can increase up to 1000 times its baseline concentration in inflammatory conditions (eg, infections, autoimmune disorders). Recent clinical evidence suggests that CRP is also released in response to inflammatory markers present within atherosclerotic plaques that lead to cardiovascular disease. Cholesterol medications (hydroxymethylglutaryl-coenzyme A [HMG-CoA] reductase inhibitors/statins) decrease CRP levels, and rosuvastatin was found to decrease cardiovascular disease in patients with elevated CRP levels.

Chemokines play an essential role in linking the innate and adaptive immune response by orchestrating traffic. The chemokine system consists of a group of small polypeptides and their receptors. Chemokines possess four cysteines. Based upon the positions of the cysteines, almost all chemokines fall into one of two categories: (1) CC group or (2) CXC group. The CC group has cysteines that are contiguous and the CXC group has cysteines separated by another amino acid (X). A cell can only respond to a chemokine if the cell possesses a receptor that recognizes the chemokine. An example is maraviroc (Selzentry) used for treatment of CCR5-tropic HIV-1 infection. Maraviroc selectively and reversibly binds to the chemokine receptor (C-C motif receptor 5 [CCR5]) co-receptors located on CD4 cells. CCR5 antagonism prevents interaction between the human CCR5 co-receptor and the gp120 sub unit of the viral envelope glycoprotein, thereby inhibiting gp120 conformational change required for fusion of CCR5 HIV fusion with the CD4 cell and subsequent entry.

CASE Application

1. The immune system is designed to attack and destroy foreign antigens and should be able to differentiate self from nonself. Failure to differentiate self from nonself may lead to which of the following? Select all that apply.

   a. Addison disease
   b. Rheumatoid arthritis (RA)
   c. Systemic lupus erythematosus (SLE)
   d. Multiple sclerosis (MS)

2. Select the nonspecific functional division of the immune system.

   a. Innate
   b. Adaptive
   c. Granulocytes
   d. Lymphocytes

3. The difference between the innate and adaptive immune system is described by which of the following? Select all that apply.

   a. Specificity
   b. Memory
   c. Strength
   d. Size

4. Physical and chemical defenses compose the innate immune system and consist of which of the following? Select all that apply.

   a. Skin
   b. Lymphocytes
   c. Granulocytes
   d. Normal urine flow

5. Examples of physical defense innate immunity include which of the following? Select all that apply.

   a. Skin
   b. Stomach pH
   c. Normal flora of gastrointestinal tract
   d. Coughing

6. Select the medication that may cause SJS and in turn alter the skin, leading to an easy portal of entry for bacterial pathogens. Select all that apply.

   a. Carbamazepine
   b. Lamotrigine
   c. Loratadine
   d. Levothyroxine

7. Select the agent(s) that may cause pneumonia by altering the pH of the stomach. Select all that apply.

   a. Omeprazole
   b. Ranitidine
   c. Ceftriaxone
   d. Sucralfate

8. Select the medication that may alter the normal flora of the gastrointestinal tract leading to infection. Select all that apply.

   a. Lansoprazole
   b. Clindamycin
   c. Pantoprazole
   d. Levofloxacin

9. Select the chemical cell(s) of the innate immune system. Select all that apply.

   a. Neutrophils
   b. Eosinophils
   c. Basophils
   d. Granulocytes

10. Innate cells may be evaluated clinically by ordering which laboratory test? Select all that apply.

    a. CRP
    b. Chemokines
    c. Complete blood cell count
    d. CD4 count

11. Select the innate cell that represents the majority of granulocytes and serves as the primary defense against bacterial infections.

    a. Lymphocytes
    b. Neutrophils
    c. Monocytes
    d. Eosinophils
    e. Basophils

12. Select the innate cell that is immature.

    a. Basophil
    b. Eosinophil
    c. Band
    d. Neutrophil
    e. Macrophage

13. Select the cell that is part of cell-mediated immunity.

    a. B lymphocyte
    b. Neutrophil
    c. Macrophage
    d. T lymphocyte
    e. Complement

14. B and T lymphocytes may be distinguished from each other by the presence of lineage specific membrane markers termed:

    a. CD
    b. Complement
    c. CRP
    d. Chemokines
    e. CCR5 coreceptor

15. A neutrophil count greater than 12,000 cells/mm³ is termed which of the following?

    a. Neutrophilia
    b. Bandemia
    c. Lymphocytosis
    d. Agranulocytosis

16. Select the cause(s) of neutrophilia. Select all that apply.

    a. Acute bacterial infections
    b. G-CSF
    c. Glucocorticoids
    d. Lithium

17. Select the drug-induced cause of a neutrophil count less than 1500 cells/mm³. Select all that apply.

    a. Zidovudine
    b. β-Lactam antibiotics
    c. Angiotensin-converting enzyme (ACE) inhibitors
    d. Ticlopidine

18. Select the cause(s) of an eosinophil count greater than 350 cells/mm³. Select all that apply.

    a. Asthma
    b. Parasitic infections
    c. Antibiotics (allergic reaction)
    d. Lymphoma

19. HIV is most likely to cause which of the following?

    a. Neutrophilia
    b. Eosinophilia

c. Monocytosis

d. Lymphocytosis

e. Lymphopenia

20. A patient that is found to have a granulocyte count less than 500 cells/mm³ would be classified as which of the following?

a. Lymphopenia

b. Basophilia

c. Agranulocytosis

d. Eosinophilia

21. Which of the following functions is performed by neutrophils?

a. Antigen presentation to T lymphocytes

b. Engulfing pathogens

c. Lysing virally infected cells

d. Secreting antibody

22. Which of the following cell types can present peptide fragments from an engulfed pathogen in association with MHC class II to T lymphocytes?

a. Neutrophils

b. Basophils

c. Dendritic cell

d. Eosinophils

23. Which of the following cell types plays a critical role in parasitic infections?

a. Basophil

b. Macrophage

c. Plasma cell

d. Eosinophil

TAKEAWAY POINTS »

- The immune system protects the body from invading pathogens and has an amazing ability to evolve and adapt based upon environmental exposure.

- The immune system is designed to attack and destroy foreign antigens/pathogens; however, the immune system must be able to distinguish self from nonself. Failure to differentiate self from nonself may lead to an autoimmune disease.

- The immune system includes two functional divisions: (1) innate or nonspecific and (2) adaptive or specific.

- Physical and chemical defenses compose the innate immune system and are the first line of defense against pathogens.

- The skin is the primary method of physical defense.

- Innate immunity cells include the leukocytes or WBCs (monocytes, neutrophils, basophils, and eosinophils).

- Granulocytes are phagocytes (engulfing cells) and derive their name from the presence of granules within the cytoplasm.

- Granulocytic leukocytes include neutrophils, eosinophils, and basophils.

- Neutrophils represent the majority of granulocytes and leukocytes and serve as the primary defense against bacterial infections.

- Eosinophils can phagocytize, kill, and digest bacteria and yeast. Elevations of eosinophils counts are highly suggestive of parasitic infections. Along with mast cells, eosinophils control mechanisms associated with allergies and asthma.

- Basophils may be associated with immediate hypersensitivity and delayed hypersensitivity reactions, and increased chronic inflammation and leukemia.

- Monocytes migrate to tissues (lymph nodes, spleen, liver, lung), where they mature into macrophages. Macrophages play a critical role in the adaptive immune response in the eradication of pathogens.

- Macrophages not only engulf and destroy pathogens, but also present antigens from the engulfed pathogen to helper T lymphocytes.

- The adaptive immune response consists of two parts, humoral (B cells) and cell-mediated (T cells).

- CD4(+) helper T lymphocytes upregulate the immune response by activating either CD8(+) cytotoxic T lymphocytes or CD20(+) B lymphocytes.

- CD8(+) T lymphocytes destroy cells within intracellular infections (eg, viruses).

- B lymphocytes secrete antibodies that neutralize pathogens prior to their entry into host cells.

- Leukocyte disorders can be classified into three major classes: (1) functional, (2) quantitative, and (3) myeloproliferative.

- Patients with neutropenia (neutrophil count less than 1500 cells/mm³) are particularly vulnerable to bacterial infections.

BIBLIOGRAPHY

Baird SM. Morphology of lymphocytes and plasma cells. In: Beutler E, Coller BS, Lichtman MA, et al. eds. *Williams Hematology.* 6th ed. New York, NY: McGraw Hill; 1999:911-919.

Chaplin DD. Overview of the human immune response. *J Allergy Clin Immunol.* 2006;117:S430-S435.

Dale DC. Neutropenia and neutrophilia. In: Beutler E, Coller BS, Lichtman MA, et al. eds. *Williams Hematology.* 6th ed. New York, NY: McGraw Hill; 1999:823-834.

Delves PJ, Roitt IM. The immune system, second of two parts. *N Engl J Med.* 2000;343:108-117.

Ganz T, Lehrer RI. Production, distribution, and fate of monocytes and macrophages. In: Beutler E, Coller BS, Lichtman MA, et al. eds. *Williams Hematology.* 6th ed. New York, NY: McGraw Hill; 1999:873-876.

Toutman WG. Drug induced diseases. In: Anderson PO, Knoben JE, Troutman WG, eds. *Handbook of Clinical Drug Data.* 10th ed. New York, NY: McGraw Hill; 2002:817-829.

KEY ABBREVIATIONS

ACE = angiotensin-converting enzyme
ALL = acute lymphocytic leukemia
AML = acute myelogenous leukemia
APC = antigen-presenting cell
CBC = complete blood count
CCR5 = C-C motif receptor 5
CD = clusters of differentiation
CLL = chronic lymphocytic leukemia
CML = chronic myelogenous leukemia
G-CSF = granulocyte colony-stimulating factor

GM-CSF = granulocyte-macrophage colony-stimulating factor
HLA = human leukocyte antigen
HMG-CoA = hydroxymethylglutaryl-coenzyme A
MCV = mean corpuscular volume
MHC = major histocompatibility complex
RA = rheumatoid arthritis
SLE = systemic lupus erythematosus
WBC = white blood cell

12

Anemia

Keith A. Hecht

FOUNDATION OVERVIEW

Anemia is a decline in the concentration of hemoglobin resulting in a reduction of the oxygen-carrying capacity of the blood. Patients with anemia may be asymptomatic initially, but the lack of oxygen eventually results in fatigue, lethargy, shortness of breath, headache, edema, and tachycardia. Clinical complications of anemia arise when the hemoglobin concentration falls below 7 to 7.9 g/dL (70-79 g/L or 4.34-4.9 mmol/L) and include cardiovascular sequelae and hypoxia. Common causes of anemia include blood loss, decreased production of red blood cells (RBCs), increased destruction of RBCs, or a combination of these factors. Comorbid conditions increase the risk of anemia, particularly in cancer patients receiving chemotherapy and chronic kidney disease (CKD) patients. Factors leading to hypoproductive anemia are: nutritional (such as iron, vitamin B_{12}, and folic acid), cancer, and CKD. Patients with immune-related diseases (such as rheumatoid arthritis and systemic lupus erythematosus) can develop anemia as a complication of their disease. Anemia related to these chronic inflammatory conditions is termed anemia of chronic disease (ACD). Management of the anemia is determined by the underlying cause. Drug therapy is key in the management of anemia secondary to decreased production of RBCs and will be the focus of this chapter.

Erythropoiesis is a process that starts with a pluripotent stem cell in the bone marrow that eventually differentiates into an erythroid colony-forming unit (CFU-E). The development of these cells depends on stimulation from appropriate growth factors, primarily erythropoietin. Other cytokines involved include granulocyte-monocyte colony-stimulating factor (GM-CSF) and interleukin-3. Eventually, the CFU-Es differentiate into reticulocytes and cross from the bone marrow in the peripheral blood. Finally, these reticulocytes mature into erythrocytes after 1 to 2 days in the bloodstream. Throughout this process, the cells gradually accumulate more hemoglobin and lose their nuclei. The following are areas that disrupt this process:

- Deficiencies in nutrients such as folic acid and vitamin B_{12} hinder the process of erythrocyte maturation. Folic acid and vitamin B_{12} are required for the formation of DNA. Poor diet can be a contributor to the vitamin deficiencies. Patients with pernicious anemia are not able to absorb vitamin B_{12} from the gastrointestinal tract.

- Iron is another vital nutrient in the development of erythrocytes. Iron deficiency decreases hemoglobin synthesis and ultimately RBCs production. Iron deficiency may result from inadequate dietary intake or overutilization of iron.

- Patients with cancer may suffer from anemia caused by chemotherapy, radiation therapy, or tumor effects. Chemotherapy may cause destruction of proliferating stem cells, thereby decreasing erythrocyte production and decreasing the life span of RBCs. Radiation fields including bone marrow may decrease RBC production. Tumors can cause anemia via hemorrhage, replacing normal bone marrow with malignant cells, and/or releasing cytokines that decrease erythropoietin production or decrease the body's ability to respond to erythropoietin.

- CKD patients develop anemia because of deficiency of erythropoietin, which is primarily produced in the kidneys.

- ACD patients has a diminished production of erythropoietin and also has a blunted response to the limited supply that is made. ACD also affects iron homeostasis via iron sequestration, thereby decreasing the amount available to the rest of the body.

Functionally, anemia can be described as a disorder of decreased RBC production (hypoproliferative), impaired RBC maturation, or blood loss from hemorrhage or hemolysis (Figure 12-1). Characteristic changes in the size of RBCs seen in erythrocyte indices can be the first step in the morphologic classification and understanding of anemia. Anemias are classified by RBC size as macrocytic, normocytic, or microcytic. Anemias secondary to deficiencies in vitamin B_{12} or folic acid are macrocytic, iron-deficiency anemia is microcytic, and normocytic anemias are associated with recent blood loss or chronic disease. Multiple anemias and etiologies can occur concurrently. Laboratory evaluation of anemia includes a complete blood count, reticulocyte count, and examination of stool for occult blood. Table 12-1 lists and defines normal hematologic values, although these values may differ in certain populations, such as individuals living at high altitudes or endurance athletes. Figure 12-2 is an algorithm for the diagnosis of anemias based upon laboratory data. The algorithm is less useful in the presence of more than one cause of anemia.

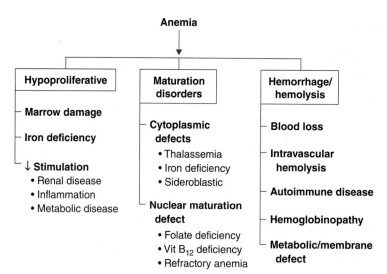

FIGURE 12-1 Functional classification of anemia. Reproduced with permission from DiPiro JT, Talbert RL, Yee GC, et al: *Pharmacotherapy: A Pathophysiologic Approach,* 10th ed. New York, NY: McGraw-Hill; 2017

TABLE 12-1   Laboratory Tests in the Evaluation of Anemia

Test Name	Normal Range	Description/Significance
CBC		
Hgb	Males: 14.0-17.5 g/dL (140-175 g/L or 8.69-10.9 mmol/L) Females: 12.3-15.3 g/dL (123-153 g/L or 7.63-9.50 mmol/L)	Amount of Hgb in the blood; signifies oxygen-carrying capacity of the blood and determines whether a patient is anemic
Hct	Males: 40.7%-50.3% (0.407-0.503) Females: 36.1%-44.3% (0.361-0.44.3)	The percent of blood that the erythrocytes encompass; also indicates anemia; the Hgb is measured, and the Hct is calculated
RBC	Males: 4.5-5.9 × 10⁶ cells/μL (4.5-5.9 × 10¹² cells/L) Females: 4.1-5.1 × 10⁶ cells/μL (4.1-5.1 × 10¹² cells/L)	The number of erythrocytes in a volume of blood; also indicates anemia, but seldom used
RBC Indices		
MCV	80-97.6 μm³/cell (80-97.6 fL/cell)	A widely used laboratory value to measure RBC "size"; higher values indicate macrocytosis and lower values indicate microcytosis
MCH	27-33 pg/cell	Amount of Hgb per RBC; may be decreased in IDA
MCHC	32-36 g/dL (320-360 g/L)	Hgb divided by the Hct; also low in IDA
Iron Studies		
Serum iron	Males: 45–160 μg/dL (8.1-28.6 μmol/L) Females: 30-160 μg/dL (5.4-28.6 μmol/L)	Measures amount of iron bound to transferrin; low in IDA
Serum ferritin	Males: 20-250 ng/mL (20-250 μg/L; 45-562 pmol/L) Females: 10-150 ng/mL (10-150 μg/L; 22-337 pmol/L)	Ferritin is the protein–iron complex found in macrophages used for iron storage; low in IDA
TIBC	220-420 μg/dL (39.4-75.2 μmol/L)	Measures the capacity of transferrin to bind iron; high in IDA
TSAT	15%-50% (0.15-0.50)	TSAT (%) = (serum iron/TIBC) × 100; a saturation of less than 15% (0.15) is common in IDA
Other Tests		
RBC distribution width (RDW)	11.5%-14.5% (0.115-0.145)	A higher value means the presence of many different sizes of RBCs; the MCV is, therefore, less reliable
Reticulocyte count	Males: 0.5%-1.5% of RBCs (0.005-0.015) Females: 0.5%-2.5% of RBCs (0.005-0.025)	Should be elevated in patients who are responding to treatment
Folic acid (plasma)	3.1-12.4 ng/mL or μg/L (7.0-28.1 nmol/L)	Used to determine folic acid deficiency
Folic acid (RBC)	125-600 ng/mL (283-1360 nmol/L)	Used to determine folic acid deficiency
Vitamin B₁₂	180-1000 pg/mL (133-738 pmol/L)	Used to determine vitamin B₁₂ deficiency
EPO level	2-25 mIU/mL (2-25 IU/L)	Patients may benefit from EPO therapy if they are anemic and EPO levels are normal or mildly elevated

Reproduced with permission from Chisholm-Burns MA, Schwinghammer TL, Wells BG, et al: *Pharmacotherapy Principles and Practice,* 4th ed. New York, NY: McGraw-Hill; 2016

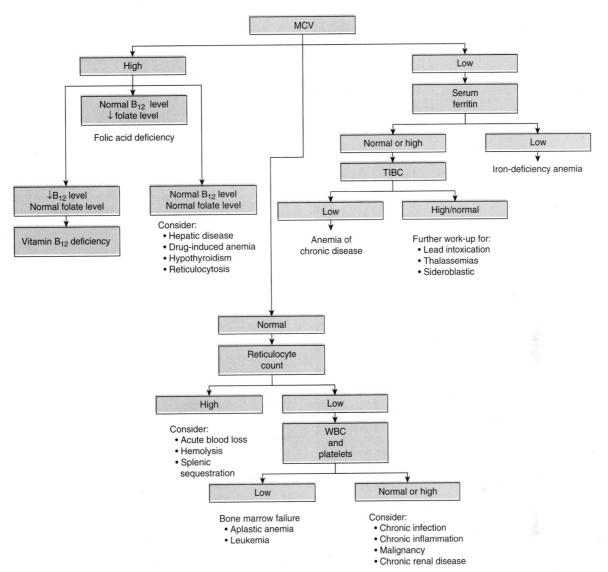

FIGURE 12-2   Algorithm for diagnosis of anemia.   Reproduced with permission from DiPiro JT, Talbert RL, Yee GC, et al: *Pharmacotherapy: A Pathophysiologic Approach,* 10th ed. New York, NY: McGraw-Hill; 2017.

TREATMENT

The goal of anemia therapy is to increase the hemoglobin level, which will improve the red cell oxygen-carrying capacity, alleviate symptoms, and prevent anemia complications. The underlying cause of anemia must be determined to guide therapy.

Nonpharmacologic Therapy

Nonpharmacologic therapy plays a limited role in the management of anemia. Diets lacking key nutrients are rarely the sole cause of anemia in the United States. Therefore, ingesting a diet rich in iron, folic acid, or vitamin B_{12} should not be the only modality of treatment. Symptomatic anemia patients with a hemoglobin concentration less than 7 g/dL (70 g/L or 4.34 mmol/L) are candidates for transfusion of RBCs. Because of the risk of infection, immunosuppression, and microcirculatory complications, the threshold for transfusion has been debated. Generally, only patients requiring immediate correction receive blood transfusions.

Pharmacologic Therapy

Iron-Deficiency Anemia

The preferred treatment of iron-deficiency anemia is oral iron therapy with 200 mg of elemental iron daily. There are different iron products and salt forms available (Table 12-2), with different amounts of elemental iron in each product. Iron supplementation resolves anemia by replacing iron stores in the body that are necessary for RBC production and maturation. A response (presence of reticulocytosis) should be seen in 7 to 10 days and the hemoglobin values should rise by approximately 1 g/dL (10 g/L or 0.62 mmol/L) per week. Patients should be reassessed if hemoglobin values do not increase by 2 g/dL (20 g/L or 1.24 mmol/L) in 3 weeks. Hemoglobin levels should normalize in 6 to 8 weeks, but iron therapy may continue for 6 to 12 months in order to fully replenish iron stores. Iron dosing should be divided into two to three daily doses, depending upon the oral formulation utilized. Maximal absorption is achieved on an empty stomach (1 hour before

TABLE 12-2 | **Iron Products (Oral and Intravenous) and Elemental Iron Content**

Salt Form	Brand Name	Elemental Iron Content per Dose Form
Oral		
Ferrous sulfate	Feosol	65 mg/325 mg tablet 60 mg/300 mg tablet
Ferrous sulfate, anhydrous	N/A	65 mg/200 mg tablet
Ferrous gluconate	Fergon	39 mg/325 mg tablet 37 mg/300 mg tablet
Ferrous fumarate	Feostat	33 mg/100 mg capsule
Polysaccharide-iron complex	Niferex	150 mg/capsule 50 mg/tablet
Intravenous		
Iron dextran[a]	InFED	50 mg/mL
Iron sucrose	Venofer	20 mg/mL
Sodium ferric gluconate	Ferrlecit	62.5 mg/5 mL
Ferumoxytol	Feraheme	30 mg/mL
Ferric carboxymaltose	Injectafer	50 mg/mL

[a]Dose of iron dextran can be calculated by: Dose (mL) = 0.0442 (Desired Hb − Observed Hb) × LBW + (0.26 × LBW)

Note: Lean body weight should be used for adults and children weighing more than 15 kg. Actual body weight should be used for children weighing 5 to 15 kg. The dose in milligrams can be calculated based on a standard concentration of 50 mg elemental iron per milliliter. A test dose (0.5 mL over 30 seconds) must be administered to patients receiving their first dose of iron dextran because of an anaphylaxis risk. Patients should be monitored for signs of anaphylaxis for at least 1 hour after the test dose before administering the total dose.

or 2 hours after a meal); however, patients who cannot tolerate iron on an empty stomach may take it with food. Side effects for oral iron include: dark/discolored stools, abdominal pain, nausea, constipation, and heartburn. Iron may bind to medications causing a decreased absorption of the interacting drug; examples include fluoroquinolones, tetracyclines, and phenytoin. This interaction is avoided if the administration of iron and the interacting drug are separated by 2 to 4 hours.

Parenteral iron therapy is for patients unable to tolerate the oral formulation, noncompliance, or nonresponders (malabsorption). Table 12-2 lists the parenteral formulations of iron. Iron dextran is Food and Drug Administration (FDA) approved for the treatment of iron deficiency in patients unable to tolerate the oral formulation. Sodium ferric gluconate is indicated to treat anemia associated with CKD in patient undergoing hemodialysis and receiving an erythropoiesis stimulating agent (ESA). Ferric carboxymaltose is indicated for the treatment of iron-deficiency anemia in patients with CKD not receiving dialysis, regardless of ESA use. Iron sucrose and ferumoxytol are indicated to treat anemia associated with CKD, regardless of hemodialysis or use of ESAs. Side effects associated with parenteral products are: anaphylaxis (dextran only), arthralgias, arrhythmias, hypotension, flushing, and pruritus. A test dose of iron dextran should be given on the first day of therapy and patients should be observed for 1 hour for the hypersensitivity reaction. The remaining iron dextran dose (dose minus test dose) should be given if patients tolerate the test dose.

Vitamin B₁₂ and Folic Acid Anemia

Vitamin B_{12} and folic acid anemias are treated by replacing the missing nutrient. Both vitamin B_{12} and folic acid are essential for erythrocyte production and maturation. Replacing these factors allows for normal DNA synthesis and erythropoiesis.

Vitamin B₁₂ Anemia The goals of treatment for vitamin B_{12} deficiency include reversal of hematologic manifestations, replacement of body stores, and prevention or resolution of neurologic manifestations. Early treatment is paramount because neurologic damage may be irreversible if the deficiency is not detected and corrected within months. Permanent disabilities range from mild paresthesias and numbness to memory loss and psychosis.

Vitamin B_{12} (cyanocobalamin) administered orally or parenterally is effective in treating vitamin B_{12} anemia. Parenteral use is more common because absorption is higher and more predictable. Subcutaneous or intramuscular administration may be given. A common oral dosing regimen is 1000 to 2000 mcg/d. Parenteral regimens consist of daily injections of 1000 mcg for 1 week to saturate vitamin B_{12} stores in the body and resolve clinical manifestations. Parenteral administration can be given weekly for 1 month and monthly thereafter for maintenance. Vitamin B_{12} nasal spray is available for patients in remission following intravenous (IV) vitamin B_{12} who have no nervous system involvement. The response to therapy is quick, neurologic symptoms and megaloblastic cells disappear within days and hemoglobin levels increase after a week of therapy. Vitamin B_{12} is well tolerated and has minimal adverse effects. Injection site pain, pruritus, fluid retention, rash, and diarrhea have been reported. Drug interactions with omeprazole and ascorbic acid may decrease oral absorption.

Folic Acid Anemia Folic acid deficiency is a common cause of vitamin anemia, largely resulting with pregnancy and excessive alcohol intake. An initial daily dose of oral folic acid 1 mg/d is effective. Resolution of symptoms is prompt, occurring within days of starting therapy. Hemoglobin levels will start to rise after 2 weeks and may take 2 to 4 weeks to resolve the anemia completely. If the underlying deficiency is corrected, folic acid replacement can be discontinued. Folic acid is well tolerated. Nonspecific adverse effects are: allergic reactions, flushing, malaise, and rash.

Anemia of Chronic Disease

ACD is a term describing anemia caused by underlying chronic conditions. These chronic conditions include cancer, CKD, and inflammatory disorders such as rheumatoid arthritis. Treatment of ACD is less specific than treatment of other anemias. In patients with anemia from chemotherapy or CKD, therapy with the ESAs epoetin or darbepoetin can increase hemoglobin, decrease transfusions, and improve quality of life.

Chemotherapy Induced Anemia The National Comprehensive Cancer Network (NCCN) recommends an anemia work-up for patients with hemoglobin levels less than 11 g/dL (110 g/L or 6.8 mmol/L). Cancer patients with chemotherapy-related anemia who are symptomatic or asymptomatic with risk factors (extensive transfusion history or myelosuppressive therapy) qualify for treatment with ESAs such as epoetin-alfa or darbepoetin. Epoetin is recombinant human erythropoietin and darbepoetin is structurally similar to endogenous erythropoietin. Both bind to the same receptor to simulate RBC production. Darbepoetin differs from epoetin in that it has a longer half-life due to additional N-linked carbohydrate side chains. The response to ESAs must be monitored closely to prevent adverse effects. Adverse events include hypertension, thrombosis, and increased risk of tumor progression. Concomitant drugs with the same adverse-event profile may increase a patient's risk for side effects. Patient survival may be decreased if the hemoglobin level is titrated above 11 to 12 g/dL (110-120 g/L or 6.82-7.44 mmol/L). Hemoglobin values should be monitored at least every 2 weeks. The following are recommendations for modification of the ESA:

- If hemoglobin levels rise above 1 g/dL (10 g/L or 0.62 mmol/L) or greater in 2 weeks, decrease the dose by 25%.

- If hemoglobin levels rise above 12 g/dL (120 g/L or 7.44 mmol/L), hold dose until hemoglobin levels fall below 12 g/dL. Therapy can be restarted after hemoglobin levels fall, but decrease the dose by 25%.

- Increase dose by 50% in nonresponding patients. Nonresponding is defined as patients who do not exhibit at least a 1 g/dL (10 g/L or 0.62 mmol/L) increase in hemoglobin after 4 to 6 weeks. In addition, if their hemoglobin has not increased by 1 g/dL after 8 weeks of therapy, the drug should be discontinued.

Table 12-3 provides dosing recommendations for chemotherapy-related anemia.

Cancer patients may have concurrent iron-deficiency anemia secondary to cancer. It is imperative that these patients have iron studies performed to assess adequate iron stores needed to drive hematopoiesis.

Chronic Kidney Disease Patients with CKD progress through five stages of disease based upon glomerular filtration rate (GFR). Anemia is a common development in patients with CKD, and evaluation and treatment should be initiated in patients with stage 3 CKD (GFR less than 60). CKD anemia typically is a normocytic, normochromic anemia that is due to erythropoietin deficiency. Therefore, therapy with ESAs is effective in treating CKD anemia. Using ESAs to target a hemoglobin level greater than 11 g/dL in patients with CKD is associated with an increased risk of serious cardiovascular reactions, stroke, and death. Because anemia in CKD is due to a deficiency in erythropoietin, the required doses of ESA is lower than for chemotherapy-induced anemia (Table 12-3). ESA doses should be:

- Decreased by 25% if Hgb increases by greater than 1 g/dL in 2 weeks

- Increased by 25% if Hgb increases by less than 1 g/dL in 4 weeks

It can take up to 6 to 12 weeks to see the maximal effects, so doses should not be changed more frequently than once every 4 weeks.

Iron stores in patients with CKD should be maintained. If iron stores are not maintained, epoetin and darbepoetin will not be effective. Oral iron therapy can be used, but is often ineffective, particularly in dialysis patients. Therefore, IV iron therapy (see Table 12-2) is used extensively in these patients.

Special Considerations

Erythropoiesis Stimulating Agents Epoetin-alfa (Epogen, Procrit) and Darbepoetin-alfa (Aranesp) are effective agents in the treatment of anemia. Epoetin-alfa is used in the treatment of anemia associated with human immunodeficiency virus (zidovudine therapy), chronic renal failure, and concurrent chemotherapy in patients with metastatic cancer. Darbepoetin-alfa is used in the treatment of anemia associated with chronic renal failure and treatment of anemia due to concurrent chemotherapy in patients with metastatic cancer. ESAs are *not* indicated for use in cancer patients under the following conditions:

1. Receiving hormonal therapy, therapeutic biologic products, or radiation therapy unless the patient is also receiving concurrent myelosuppressive chemotherapy.
2. Receiving myelosuppressive therapy when the expected outcome is curative.
3. Anemia due to other factors (eg, iron deficiency, folate deficiency, gastrointestinal bleed).

ESAs have a pregnancy category C. There are no adequate and well-controlled studies in pregnant women. Contraindications for ESAs are hypersensitivity to the agent, uncontrolled hypertension, and hypersensitivity to albumin or mammalian cell-derived products (epoetin-alfa only). There are several

TABLE 12-3	Erythropoietin Products and Doses for Anemia for Chemotherapy and CKD	
	Epoetin-Alfa (Epogen, Procrit)	**Darbepoetin-Alfa (Aranesp)**
Cancer/ chemotherapy dosing regimens	150 units/kg subcutaneously three times per week 40,000 units subcutaneously once every week	2.25 mcg/kg subcutaneously once every week, may increase to 4.5 mcg/kg; 500 mcg every 3 wk
CKD dosing regimens[a]	50-100 units/kg subcutaneously three times per week	0.45 mcg/kg subcutaneously once every week; 0.75 mcg/kg subcutaneously once every 2 wk

[a]According to National Kidney Foundation guidelines for the use of epoetin in patients with anemia owing to kidney disease, the subcutaneous route is preferred. However, the intravenous route is used commonly in clinical practice.

Reproduced with permission from Chisholm-Burns MA, Wells BG, Schwinghammer TL, et al: *Pharmacotherapy Principles and Practice,* 3rd ed. New York, NY: McGraw-Hill; 2013.

black box warnings for erythropoietin products and they include:

- Increased risk of serious cardiovascular events, thromboembolic events, mortality, and/or tumor progression. A rapid rise in hemoglobin (>1 g/dL over 2 weeks) or maintaining higher hemoglobin levels may contribute to these risks.

- A shortened overall survival and/or increased risk of tumor progression or recurrence has been reported in studies with breast, cervical, head and neck, lymphoid, and non–small-cell lung cancer patients.

- To decrease the risk of cardiovascular and thromboembolic events, use erythropoietin products in cancer patients only for the treatment of anemia related to concurrent chemotherapy and use the lowest dose needed to avoid RBC transfusions. Discontinue erythropoietin products following completion of the chemotherapy course. Erythropoietin products are not indicated for patients receiving myelosuppressive therapy when the anticipated outcome is curative.

- An increased risk of death and serious cardiovascular events was reported in chronic renal failure patients administered erythropoietin products to target higher versus lower hemoglobin levels (13.5 vs 11.3 g/dL; 14 vs 10 g/dL) in two clinical studies. Dosing should be individualized to achieve and maintain hemoglobin levels within 10 to 11 g/dL range. Hemoglobin rising greater than 1 g/dL in a 2-week period may contribute to the risk.

CASE Application

1. JM is a 43-year-old man with metastatic small-cell lung cancer that is currently receiving chemotherapy. He was recently diagnosed with chemotherapy-induced anemia with a hemoglobin level of 7.7 g/dL and was initiated on erythropoietin therapy. Two weeks after initiating erythropoietin, his hemoglobin level is 9.5 g/dL. Which of the following represents the most appropriate course of action for JMs erythropoietin?

    a. Continue erythropoietin at the same dose
    b. Decrease the dose of erythropoietin by 25%
    c. Increase the dose of erythropoietin by 50%
    d. Discontinue the erythropoietin

The following case pertains to questions 2 and 3:

MG is a 62-year-old woman with a prior medical history of CKD, hypertension, and stage II colon cancer. Her social history is significant for a long standing history of alcoholism. She underwent surgical resection of her primary cancer 6 months ago and is currently undergoing chemotherapy with the intent to cure her cancer. Routine laboratory monitoring revealed the patient has a hemoglobin level of 8.8 g/dL.

2. MG's nephrologist wants to start him on an ESA. Which of the following is true regarding the use of ESAs in MG?

    a. Darbepoetin can be used in MG at a dose of 500 mcg every 3 weeks
    b. Epoetin can be used in MG at a dose of 40,000 units every week
    c. Darbepoetin can be used in MG at a dose of 0.45 mcg/kg every week
    d. ESAs should not be used in MG

3. Due to her social history, MG should be evaluated for his anemia being complicated by deficiency in:

    a. Vitamin B_{12}
    b. Iron
    c. Vitamin D
    d. Thiamine

4. Most flour in the United States is fortified with which of the following?

    a. Folic acid
    b. Potassium
    c. Vitamin B_{12}
    d. Vitamin C

5. SL is a 57-year-old man who is admitted to the hospital for pneumonia. During his clinical and laboratory evaluation, he was found to have a microcytic anemia. Which of the following additional diagnostic tests would be most useful in determining if SL has anemia as a result of iron deficiency?

    a. Ferritin
    b. Red cell distribution width
    c. Transferrin saturation
    d. Reticulocyte count

6. Which of the following iron preparations requires a prescription?

    a. Ferrous fumarate
    b. Polysaccharide-iron complex
    c. Ferrous sulfate
    d. Ferrous gluconate

The following case pertains to questions 7 through 9:

DE is a 49-year-old woman with a diagnosis of breast cancer that is currently being treated with chemotherapy. Her prior medical history is significant for allergic rhinitis and chronic heartburn. Her home medications include cetirizine, pantoprazole, and transdermal norelgestromin/ethinyl estradiol. The patient was recently diagnosed with chemotherapy-induced anemia with a hemoglobin level of 8.8 g/dL. She was prescribed darbepoetin to treat her anemia.

7. DE may require supplementation with which of the following agents to optimize the effectiveness of darbepoetin?

    a. Folic acid
    b. Iron
    c. Vitamin B_{12}
    d. Thiamine

8. Six weeks after initiating darbepoetin, DEs hemoglobin level is 9.6 g/dL. Which of the following represents the most appropriate course of action for DEs darbepoetin?

    a. Continue darbepoetin at the same dose
    b. Decrease the dose of darbepoetin by 25%
    c. Increase the dose of darbepoetin by 50%
    d. Discontinue the darbepoetin

9. Four months after the patient began treatment with darbepoetin, she began experiencing edema and warmth of her left lower extremity. She was diagnosed with a deep vein thrombosis (DVT). Which of her medications contributed to her increased risk of DVT? Select all that apply.

    a. Cetirizine
    b. Darbepoetin
    c. Pantoprazole
    d. Norelgestromin/ethinyl estradiol

10. Vitamin B_{12} supplementation is available by which of the following routes? Select all that apply.

    a. Oral
    b. Transdermal
    c. Injectable
    d. Intranasal

11. Rank the following oral iron salts in order from highest percentage of elemental iron to lowest percentage of elemental iron.

Unordered options	Ordered response
Ferrous fumarate	
Ferrous gluconate	
Ferrous sulfate anhydrous	
Ferrous sulfate	

The following case pertains to questions 12 and 13:

JS is an 18-year-old woman who presents to urgent care with a chief complaint of increasing fatigue that has gotten progressively worse over the last 2 months. Physical examination is notable for diffuse pallor and tachycardia. Her prior medical history is significant only for occasional reflux disease that she manages with OTC omeprazole and calcium carbonate. She also notes she has a history of heavy menstrual blood flow. Laboratory examination reveals a hemoglobin level of 9.4 g/dL and a mean corpuscular volume (MCV) of 73 fL.

12. Based on the information provided, JS most likely has anemia as a result in deficiency of:

    a. Iron
    b. Vitamin B_{12}
    c. Folic acid
    d. Erythropoietin

13. The decision is made to treat JS's anemia with medication instead of blood transfusion. Which of the following medications used in the treatment of anemia may have a drug interaction with JS's current medications?

    a. Ferrous sulfate
    b. Cyanocobalamin
    c. Folic acid
    d. Epoetin

The following case pertains to questions 14 and 15:

LJ is a 38-year-old woman who recently underwent gastric resection for the management of extreme obesity that was complicated by hypertension and type 2 diabetes. Twelve weeks after her surgery, she is complaining of fatigue and become short of breath when climbing steps. Laboratory evaluation revealed a hemoglobin level of 10.2 g/dL and an MCV of 120 fL.

14. LJs anemia is best described as:

    a. Normocytic
    b. Macrocytic
    c. Hypochromic
    d. Normochromic

15. Which of the following deficiencies is most likely responsible for LJs anemia?

    a. Erythropoietin
    b. Iron
    c. Vitamin B_{12}
    d. Folic acid

16. JR is a 37-year-old woman patient who was previously diagnosed with iron-deficiency anemia. She has been taking oral iron supplementation as directed for 16 weeks without achieving her goal hemoglobin of 12 g/dL. Her most recent hemoglobin level was 9.8 g/dL. The decision has been made to administer IV iron dextran. She is 5'4" tall and weighs 150 lb. What is the correct dose of iron dextran for CR?

    a. 19.5 mL
    b. 21.1 mL
    c. 24.4 mL
    d. 29.2 mL

17. Which of the following types of deficiencies typically results in a macrocytic anemia? Select all that apply.

    a. Erythropoietin
    b. Iron
    c. Vitamin B_{12}
    d. Folic acid

18. Venofer is the brand name for which of the following iron preparations?

    a. Iron sucrose
    b. Ferumoxytol
    c. Ferric sodium gluconate
    d. Polysaccharide-iron complex

19. Deficiency in which of the following can result in severe neurologic complications?

    a. Erythropoietin
    b. Iron

c. Vitamin B$_{12}$
d. Folic acid

20. GC is a 72-year-old man with stage 4 CKD, not receiving dialysis. He was recently diagnosed with anemia. He is currently not receiving any medications to treat his anemia. Assessment of iron stores revealed the patient to be iron deficient. Which of the following is an IV iron preparation that is indicated for CF? Select all that apply.

a. Iron dextran
b. Iron sucrose
c. Sodium ferric gluconate
d. Ferumoxytol

TAKEAWAY POINTS »

- Anemia is a decline in the concentration of hemoglobin resulting in a reduction of the oxygen-carrying capacity of the blood.
- Lack of oxygen may result in fatigue, lethargy, shortness of breath, headache, edema, and tachycardia. Complications arise when the hemoglobin concentration is below 7 to 7.9 g/dL and include cardiovascular sequelae and hypoxia.
- Drug therapy is a key component to decreased production. Factors leading to hypoproductive anemia are: nutritional (iron, vitamin B$_{12}$, and folic acid), cancer, and CKD.
- Deficiencies in nutrients such as folic acid and vitamin B$_{12}$ hinder the process of erythrocyte maturation.
- Iron deficiency decreases hemoglobin synthesis and ultimately RBCs.
- Chemotherapy may cause destruction of proliferating stem cells, thereby decreasing erythrocyte production.
- CKD patients develop anemia because erythropoietin is produced in the kidneys.
- Anemias are classified by RBC size as macrocytic, normocytic, or microcytic. Vitamin B$_{12}$ and folic acid deficiency are macrocytic anemias, iron deficiency is a microcytic anemia, and normocytic anemia is associated with recent blood loss or chronic disease.

- The goal of anemia therapy is to increase the hemoglobin level, which will improve the red cell oxygen-carrying capacity, alleviate symptoms, and prevent anemia complications.
- Treatment of iron-deficiency anemia is oral iron therapy with 200 mg of elemental iron daily.
- Parenteral iron therapy is for patients unable to tolerate the oral formulation, noncompliance, or nonresponders (malabsorption).
- Vitamin B$_{12}$ or folic acid anemias are treated by replacing the missing nutrient.
- ACD is a term describing anemia caused by underlying chronic conditions. These chronic conditions include cancer, CKD, and other inflammatory disorders.
- In patients with anemia from cancer or CKD, therapy with epoetin or darbepoetin can increase hemoglobin, decrease transfusions, and improve quality of life.
- Contraindications for erythropoietin products are hypersensitivity to the agent, uncontrolled hypertension, and hypersensitivity to albumin or mammalian cell-derived products (epoetin-alfa only).
- There are several black box warnings for erythropoietin products related to cardiovascular, thromboembolic, and tumor progression risks.

BIBLIOGRAPHY

Cook K. Anemias. In: DiPiro JT, Talbert RL, Yee GC, Matzke GR, Wells BG, Posey L, eds. *Pharmacotherapy: A Pathophysiologic Approach.* 10th ed. New York, NY: McGraw-Hill; 2017:chap 100.

Kidney disease: improving global outcomes (KDIGO) anemia work group. KDIGO clinical practice guideline for anemia in chronic kidney disease. *Kidney Inter Suppl.* 2012;2:279-335.

Kliger AS, Foley RN, Goldfarb DS, et al. KDOQI US commentary on the 2012 KDIGO Clinical Practice Guideline for Anemia in CKD. *Am J Kidney Dis.* 2013;62(5):849-859.

Rizzo JD, Brouwers M, Hurley P, et al. American Society of Clinical Oncology/American Society of Hematology clinical practice guideline update on the use of epoetin and

darbepoetin in adult patients with cancer. *J Clin Oncol.* 2010;28:4996-5010.

Ryan L. Anemia. In: Attridge RL, Miller ML, Moote R, Ryan L, eds. *Internal Medicine: A Guide to Clinical Therapeutics.* New York, NY: McGraw-Hill; 2013:chap 21.

Sylvester RK. Anemias. In: Chisholm-Burns MA, Schwinghammer TL, Wells BG, Malone PM, Kolesar JM, DiPiro JT, eds. *Pharmacotherapy Principles and Practice.* 4th ed. New York, NY: McGraw-Hill; 2016:chap 66.

The NCCN Cancer-and Chemotherapy-Induced Anemia Clinical Practice Guidelines in Oncology (version 1.2016). National Comprehensive Cancer Network, Inc. 2016. http://www.nccn.org/professionals/physician_gls/pdf/anemia.pdf.

KEY ABBREVIATIONS

CFU-E = erythroid colony-forming unit
FDA = Food and Drug Administration
GFR = glomerular filtration rate
GM-CSF = granulocyte-monocyte colony-stimulating factor

IV = intravenous
MCV = mean corpuscular volume
NCCN = National Comprehensive Cancer Network
RBC = red blood cell

13

Lung Cancer

Keith A. Hecht

FOUNDATION OVERVIEW

Lung carcinomas arise from normal bronchial cells that have acquired multiple genetic lesions and are capable of expressing a variety of phenotypes. There are four major subtypes of lung cancer: small cell, squamous cell, adenocarcinoma, and large cell. Squamous cell, adenocarcinoma, and large cell are collectively referred to as non–small-cell lung cancer (NSCLC). NSCLC represents 85% of the lung cancer diagnoses while the aggressive histology small-cell lung cancer (SCLC) represents 15% of lung cancer diagnoses. Adenocarcinoma is the most common histology of NSCLC (50% of all lung cancer) and is associated with a high incidence of distant metastasis at diagnosis. Squamous cell is the second most common histology of NSCLC (30% of all lung cancer) followed by large cell. Adenocarcinoma and large-cell lung cancer generally present as peripheral lesions in the lung, whereas squamous cell and small-cell histologies commonly present as central lesions, often causing hemoptysis or postobstructive pneumonia.

Smoking is the primary risk factor for development of lung cancer. The risk of lung cancer increases with the amount and duration of smoking. Smoking history is defined by packs per day (amount) and duration (eg, 2 packs per day × 20 years = 40 pack years). The risk of lung cancer decreases after smoke cessation but remains above the risk of a nonsmoker. Additionally, asbestos exposure increases the risk of lung cancer by five-fold and is synergistic with smoking for causing lung cancer. Although the most common lung cancer associated with asbestos exposure is NSCLC; patients with mesothelioma almost always have a history of asbestos exposure. Other risk factors associated with lung cancer include radon exposure, ionizing radiation, a diet low in fruit, vegetables, β-carotene, and vitamin E, a family history of lung cancer, and occupational exposures (eg, coal, arsenic, nickel, and other mining jobs).

Signs and symptoms of lung cancer include cough, increased sputum production, pleuritic chest pain, dyspnea, wheezing, and stridor. However, these symptoms are also common in smokers in general. A suspicion of lung cancer should increase if the patient experiences hemoptysis. Extrapulmonary symptoms associated with lung cancer include bone pain and/or fracture from bone metastasis, neurologic deficits secondary to brain metastasis, and spinal cord compression secondary to bone metastasis in the spinal vertebrae.

Multiple paraneoplastic syndromes can occur in lung cancer. Paraneoplastic syndromes are caused by proteins secreted by the malignancy (Table 13-1).

Evaluating a patient with suspected lung cancer begins with a complete medical history, physical examination, and diagnostic imaging of the lung. A diagnostic biopsy is recommended if the physical examination or lung imaging is suspicious. A diagnosis is established by a bronchoscopy for medial lesions, image-guided biopsy for peripheral lesions, or thoracentesis for pleural effusions. Because of the importance of lymphatic spread to prognosis, the patient's lymph nodes must be assessed for staging.

In addition to histological type determination, additional pathologic review must be performed to evaluate patients for targeted therapies. These therapies used in the treatment of NSCLC target epidermal growth factor receptor (EGFR) pathway, anablastic lymphoma kinase (ALK), ROS1, the V600E mutation in BRAF, and the programmed-death receptor 1 (PD-1) pathway. Activating mutations in EGFR include exon 19 deletion and mutations in exons 18 (G719X, G719), 20 (S768I), and 21 (L858R, L861). EGFR mutations are found in approximately 10% of patients with NSCLC. Mutations in Kirsten-Rous sarcoma virus (KRAS) are associated with resistance to EGFR targeting medications. ALK gene rearrangements are present in 1% to 2% of patients with NSCLC and frequently coexists with ROS1 expression, although each may occur independently. V600E is an activating mutation in the BRAF mutation that is found in 1% to 2% of patients with lung cancer. PD-1 stimulation on T-lymphocytes by its ligand, programmed-death ligand 1 (PDL-1), leads to decreased T-lymphocyte activity and proliferation. Inhibition of this pathway can lead to a more active immune system response against the cancer.

Key predictors of survival in lung cancer are staging at presentation and performance status. Accurate staging of patients with lung cancer is critical because it determines appropriate treatment and predicts survival. SCLC is staged as limited (confined to one lung and able to fit in a radiation field) or extensive stage (distant metastases or the disease that cannot fit into a radiation field). Extensive-stage SCLC has a worse prognosis than limited-stage SCLC. In contrast, NSCLC is staged based upon the TNM (tumor, node, and metastasis) staging (Table 13-2). Unfortunately, the majority of patients

TABLE 13-1 | Paraneoplastic Syndromes Associated With Lung Cancer

Paraneoplastic Syndrome	Comments
Cachexia	Extreme muscle wasting and malnutrition
SIADH	Hyponatremia due to ADH secretion
Hypercalcemia	Caused by PTH-rp secretion; associated with squamous cell histology
Cushing syndrome	Caused by the tumor secreting ACTH
Pulmonary hypertrophic osteoarthropathy	Associated with clubbing of the fingers and toes, and painful swollen joints
Hypercoagulable state	Increased risk of DVTs and PE
Eaton-Lambert syndrome	Upper extremity weakness and diminished reflexes

Abbreviations: ACTH, adrenal corticotropin hormone; DVT, deep vein thrombosis; PE, pulmonary embolus; PTH-rp, parathyroid hormone-related peptide; SIADH, syndrome of antidiuretic hormone.

TABLE 13-3 | ECOG Performance Status

Grade	Description
0	Fully active, no restrictions in predisease activities
1	Ambulatory, able to carry out most sedentary work
2	Ambulatory, out of bed <50% of the day, unable to work
3	In bed <50% of the day, capable of limited self-care
4	Totally confined to the bed, unable to perform self-care

with lung cancer present with unresectable, advanced disease. Performance status is used to quantify the functional status of patients with cancer. One commonly used tool is the Eastern Cooperative Group (ECOG) scale. The ECOG scale delineates ranges from fully active to confinement to bed (Table 13-3). Generally, patients with a performance status of 4 do not receive benefit from aggressive therapy and are managed with best supportive care.

SCREENING AND PREVENTION

To reduce the morbidity and mortality of lung cancer, several studies have evaluated various screening methodologies to detect lung cancer at an early stage. The first early detection studies investigated annual or semiannual chest radiography (x-rays) with or without sputum cytology. Unfortunately, the trials failed to demonstrate a reduction in lung cancer mortality. Recently, the National Lung Screening Trial (NLST)

TABLE 13-2 | Lung Cancer Staging

- Lung cancer is staged from I to IV with worsening prognosis as the stage increases.
- NSCLC stages I, II, and resectable stage IIIA are considered early-stage.
- Unresectable stage IIIB and stage IV are referred to as advanced disease.
- Stage I has no evident lymph node involvement or distant metastasis.
- Stages II and III involve lymph nodes with exception of tumors invading the chest wall, diaphragm, mediastinal pleura, pericardium, or tumors within 2 cm of the carina and no lymph node involvement are stage II.
- The primary differences between stages II and III include the size of the primary tumor with larger masses in stage III and different intrathoracic lymph node chains involved.
- Stage IIIA disease involves ipsilateral lymph nodes while stage IIIB involves contralateral lymph nodes.
- Stage IV disease involves distant metastasis.
- The most common sites for distant metastasis for either NSCLC or SCLC include lymph nodes, bone, bone marrow, liver, brain, and the adrenal glands.

compared the effectiveness of annual low-dose computed tomography (CT) scan, also known as helical CT, to annual chest x-rays for the early detection of lung cancer in subjects aged 55 to 74 with at least a 30 pack year smoking history. Results of the NLST showed that annual helical CT reduced the risk of lung cancer-related mortality by 20%. Based on these results, the American Cancer Society recommends annual helical CT scans in patients who met the NLST criteria (age 55-74, at least 30-pack year history). The term chemoprevention refers to the use of prophylactic medications to prevent the development of cancer. Several chemoprevention studies have been conducted evaluating non-steroidal anti-inflammatory agents (NSAIDs), retinoids, inhaled glucocorticoids, vitamin E, and green tea extracts. Unfortunately, the chemoprevention trials have not been successful.

Because the benefit of screening is being defined and chemoprevention trials have not demonstrated a survival benefit, the current recommendation is to avoid smoking and maintain a healthy diet with high amounts of fruits and vegetables.

TREATMENT

Non–Small-Cell Lung Cancer

Initial treatment for early stage (I, II, and III) NSCLC involves surgery, radiation, and pharmacotherapy. For stage I disease, resection of the mass offers the best chance for cure. Radiation therapy is utilized for patients that are not candidates for surgery in stage I NSCLC and in patients with positive surgical margins. The use of adjuvant chemotherapy in stage I NSCLC is controversial. Stage I NSCLC can be divided into stage IA (mass is ≤3 cm) or stage IB (tumor is <3 cm, the mass involves the main stem bronchus, or close to the carina). Adjuvant chemotherapy has not demonstrated survival benefits in stage IA NSCLC; therefore, chemotherapy does not have a role in stage IA disease. Stage IB patients appear to benefit from adjuvant cisplatin-based chemotherapy. For patients with stage II disease (lymph node positive disease), the combination of surgery followed by adjuvant chemotherapy provides the best survival. For stage IIIA, surgery followed by adjuvant chemotherapy offers the greatest benefit. Stage IIIB patients are typically not resectable. For unresectable stage III patients, concurrent chemotherapy and radiation therapy (termed chemoradiation) is recommended. In some cases of large masses (<5 cm) or a specific location (superior sulcus masses), neoadjuvant chemotherapy may be utilized to shrink the tumor and potentially makes the patient a surgical candidate. Chemotherapy used

TABLE 13-4 Adjuvant Regimens in NSCLC

Recommended based upon clinical trials
Cisplatin plus vinorelbine × 4 cycles
Cisplatin plus etoposide × 4 cycles
Cisplatin plus vinblastine × 4 cycles
Cisplatin plus pemetrexed × 4 cycles
Potential alternative regimens
Carboplatin plus paclitaxel × 4 cycles
Cisplatin plus gemcitabine × 4 cycles
Cisplatin plus docetaxel × 4 cycles

in the treatment of non-metastatic chemotherapy is platinum-based. Cisplatin or carboplatin can be combined with various agents such as pemetrexed (in patients with non-squamous disease), vinblastine, or etoposide (Table 13-4). However, carboplatin plus paclitaxel is an alternative for patients unable to tolerate other regimens.

For patients with stage IV (metastatic) or recurrent disease after primary therapy (eg, surgery and/or chemotherapy), therapy is based on the presence or absence of specific genetic or molecular features as well as tumor type (squamous vs non-squamous).

Patients who are ALK or ROS1 positive should receive system therapy with crizotinib, an oral ALK inhibitor. ALK positivity only occurs in 2% to 7% of patients with NSCLC; ROS1 prevalence is only 1%. In a clinical trial of crizotinib versus chemotherapy in patients with advanced disease who have received one prior chemotherapy regimen, patients receiving crizotinib had a progression-free survival of 7.7 months vs 3.1 months. The most common toxicities associated with crizotinib are vision disorders, nausea, vomiting, diarrhea, constipation, edema, fatigue, and elevated liver transaminases. Ceritinib and alectinib are both approved in patients who progress following crizotinib therapy.

Approximately 10% of patients with lung cancer will have activating mutations in EGFR. These patients should receive therapy with anti-EGFR kinase inhibitors (erlotinib, gefitinib, or afatinib) should be used. Clinical trials with each agent have shown improved progression-free survival when compared to chemotherapy as first-line therapy for advanced disease or salvage therapy in patients who progress after adjuvant chemotherapy. Mutation in KRAS have been shown to be predictive or resistance to EGFR-targeting kinase inhibitors, thus when KRAS mutation is detected, these agents should not be used. The most common toxicities associated with erlotinib are acneiform rash, dry skin, and diarrhea. The most common toxicities associated with afatinib are acneiform rash, dry skin, diarrhea, and stomatitis. Patients who progress on EGFR targeted kinase inhibitors should be tested for the T790M mutation, which is responsible for treatment failure in 2/3 of these patients. Osimertinib is an EGFR-targeting kinase that is active in the presence of the T790M mutation and could be considered as next-line therapy. Genetic mutations in ALK and EGFR are generally considered mutually exclusive. Because of

this, patients who progress on crizotinib therapy should not receive erlotinib, gefitinib, or afatinib. Because these agents are not chemotherapeutic, they are not associated with causing myelosuppression.

The significance of mutation in BRAF, specifically the V600E mutation, is newly recognized in NSCLC. Combined inhibition of this pathway with dabrafenib and trametinib has shown to be an effective treatment for patients who are BRAF V600E mutation positive. Dabrafenib inhibits the kinase resulting from this mutation while trametinib is an inhibitor of mitogen-activated extracellular signal regulated kinase (MEK), an enzyme system responsible for downstream signaling from BRAF. In early results of a small clinical trial, these agents combined resulted in a response rate exceeding 60% with a median duration of response of at least 12 months. This was seen in both newly diagnosed and relapsed metastatic NSCLC.

In patients who do not have activating mutations in EGFR and are negative for ALK mutation, combination chemotherapy is typically utilized. Chemotherapy regimens are typically platinum-based (eg, carboplatin or cisplatin) as they offer the most benefit, and two-drug regimens offer superior response rates compared to single-agent therapy. A meta-analysis comparing the outcomes between the platinums found a survival benefit, although small (11%), in those receiving cisplatin rather than carboplatin. The platinum agents are commonly combined with paclitaxel, docetaxel, gemcitabine, vinorelbine, etoposide, and pemetrexed (non-squamous only) as first-line regimens in metastatic NSCLC (Table 13-5). No regimen has been proven to be superior to another; therefore, decisions about regimens are based upon adverse events (Table 13-6). In patients with non-squamous cell NSCLC (eg, adenocarcinoma, large-cell carcinoma), cisplatin plus pemetrexed demonstrates benefit over cisplatin plus gemcitabine. In contrast, patient with squamous cell histology had a significant improvement in survival if they received cisplatin plus gemcitabine as compared to cisplatin plus pemetrexed.

The addition of a bevacizumab (non-squamous NSCLC) or necitumumab (squamous NSCLC) to combination chemotherapy has been shown to improve median overall survival. Bevacizumab is a monoclonal antibody that binds circulating vascular endothelial growth factor (VEGF). VEGF promotes new blood vessel formation. Carboplatin/paclitaxel plus bevacizumab demonstrated a 2-month improvement in median survival compared to chemotherapy alone. However, bevacizumab should not be used in squamous cell carcinoma because it is associated with pulmonary hemorrhage in these patients. Other toxicities associated with bevacizumab include gastrointestinal perforation, wound dehiscence, impaired wound healing, hypertension, thromboembolic events, and proteinuria. Because of its effects on wound healing, one should not administer bevacizumab for 42 to 48 days before surgery or 28 days after surgery. Necitumumab is a monoclonal antibody targeting EGFR. The combination of necitumumab, cisplatin/gemcitabine prolonged median survival by 1.6 months compared to chemotherapy alone in patient with squamous NSCLC. Unlike the EGFR specific kinase inhibitors, patients

TABLE 13-5   Common Agents Utilized in Lung Cancer

	Mechanism of Action	Route of Administration	Usual Doses
Cisplatin (Platinol)	Alkylating agent	IV over 60 min	50-100 mg/m² every 3 wk
Carboplatin (Paraplatin)	Alkylating agent	IV over 30 min	AUC of 5-7 every 3 wk
Gemcitabine (Gemzar)	Antimetabolite	IV over 30 min	1000 mg/m² on days 1, 8, and 15 every 28 d or 1250 mg/m² on days 1 and 8 every 21 d
Pemetrexed (Alimta)	Antimetabolite (inhibitor of thymidylate synthase)	IV over 10 min	500 mg/m² every 21 d
Docetaxel (Taxotere)	Antimicrotubule	IV over 60 min	75 mg/m² every 21 d
Paclitaxel (Taxol)	Antimicrotubule	IV over 180 min	175 mg/m² every 21 d
Vinorelbine (Navelbine)	Antimicrotubule	IV over 10 min	30 mg/m² on days 1, 8, and 15 every 28 d
Topotecan (Hycamtin)	Topoisomerase I inhibitor	IV over 30 min or oral	IV: 1.5 mg/m² on days 1-5 every 21 d Oral: 2.3 mg/m² daily × 5 d every 3 wk
Etoposide (Toposar, Vepesid)	Topoisomerase II inhibitor	IV over 30-60 min or oral	IV: 80-100 mg/m² on days 1-3 Oral: 50 mg/m² daily × 3 wk every 4 wk
Erlotinib (Tarceva)	EGFR kinase inhibitor	Oral	150 mg daily
Gefitinib (Iressa)	EGFR kinase inhibitor	Oral	250 mg daily
Afatinib (Gilotrif)	EGFR kinase inhibitor	Oral	40 mg daily
Osimertinib (Tagrisso)	EGFR kinase inhibitor	Oral	80 mg daily
Crizotinib (Xalkori)	ALK, ROS1 kinase inhibitor	Oral	250 mg twice daily
Ceritinib (Zykadia)	ALK kinase inhibitor	Oral	750 mg daily
Alectinib (Alecensa)	ALK kinase inhibitor	Oral	600 mg twice daily
Brigatinib (Alunbrig)	ALK kinase inhibitor	Oral	90 mg daily for 7 d then 180 mg daily
Dabrafenib (Tafinlar)	BRAF V600 E inhibitor	Oral	150 mg twice daily
Trametinib (Mekinist)	MEK inhibitor	Oral	2 mg daily
Bevacizumab (Avastin)	Anti-VEGF antibody	IV First dose: 90 min Second dose: 60 min Third dose: 30 min	15 mg/kg every 3 wk
Ramucirumab (Cyramza)	Anti-VEGF antibody	IV over 60 min	10 mg/kg every 3 wk
Necitumumab (Portrazza)	EGFR antibody	IV over 60 min	800 mg days 1 and 8 of 3 wk cycle
Pembrolizumab (Keytruda)	PD-1 receptor antibody	IV over 30 min	200 mg every 3 wk
Nivolumab (Opdivo)	PD-1 receptor antibody	IV over 60 min	240 mg every 2 wk
Atezolizumab (Tecentriq)	PDL-1 antibody	IV over 60 min (first dose), may shorten to 30 min if tolerated	1200 mg every 3 wk

Abbreviations: AUC, area-under-the-curve; IV, intravenous.

do not have to test positive for activating EGFR mutations to benefit from necitumumab. In the clinical trial, there was an increased risk of cardiopulmonary arrest in patients receiving necitumumab (3% of necitumumab patients). Patients with heart disease should be carefully screened before initiating this agent. Like other EGFR targeting antibodies (cetuximab, panitumumab), necitumumab is associated with electrolyte wasting. Patients should be carefully monitored for hypomagnesemia, hypokalemia, and hypocalcemia during therapy. Other toxicities associated with necitumumab include acne-like rash, thromboembolic events and changes to the nails (paronychia). Necitumumab should not be used in patients with non-squamous NSCLC due to lack of efficacy and increased toxicity.

The PD-1 pathway represents another therapeutic area in patients with advanced NSCLC. Pembrolizumab and nivolumab bind the PD-1 receptor and are referred to as PD-1 inhibitors, while atezolizumab binds to the ligand and is referred to as a

PDL-1 inhibitor. These agents are used in patients with metastatic, or recurrent NSCLC who are not candidates for kinase inhibitor therapy (EGFR, ALK, and ROS1 negative). All three agents are indicated as second-line therapy expression. Pembrolizumab is the only agent of the three that is indicated as first-line treatment for metastatic NSCLC. Pembrolizumab is indicated as a single agent for the treatment of metastatic NSCLC. Additionally, emerging evidence has shown that pembrolizumab added to carboplatin/pemetrexed in the treatment of non-squamous NSCLC improved response rates and progression free survival compared to chemotherapy alone. Pembrolizumab is now approved for this indication as well. The most common side effects associated with these medications include fatigue, muscle/joint pain, and rash. Immune-mediated serious side effects may occur including pneumonitis, colitis, hepatitis, nephritis, endocrinopathies, and encephalitis.

For patients with NSCLC who progress after initial chemotherapy, single agent docetaxel, pemetrexed, and erlotinib

TABLE 13-6	Common Toxicities of Chemotherapy Utilized in Lung Cancer			
Agent	**Acute[a]**	**Delayed[b]**	**Long Term[c]**	**Comments**
Cisplatin	Severe N/V acute and delayed	Anemia; thrombocytopenia	Mg^{++} and K^+ wasting; nephrotoxicity (cumulative); neurotoxicity (cumulative); ototoxicity	Requires hydration with normal saline to reduce risk of nephrotoxicity
Carboplatin	Mild to moderate acute and delayed N/V	Myelosuppression (particularly platelets)	Alopecia	Dosed based on AUC
Vinorelbine	Mild N/V	Mild myelosuppression	Mild neurotoxicity	
Vinblastine	Mild N/V	Severe myelosuppression; mucositis		
Docetaxel	Mild N/V	Severe myelosuppression; mucositis	Alopecia; mild neurotoxicity	Must receive dexamethasone premedication to reduce the risk of fluid retention
Paclitaxel	Mild N/V	Severe myelosuppression; arthralgias/myalgias	Neurotoxicity (cumulative); alopecia	Must receive premedication to reduce the risk of hypersensitivity reaction (eg, dexamethasone, antihistamine)
Gemcitabine	Mild N/V; fever and chills	Elevated transaminases; mild myelosuppression	Alopecia	May cause radiation recall in patients who have received prior radiation therapy
Pemetrexed	Mild N/V; rash	Mild myelosuppression		Must receive folate and vitamin B_{12} supplementation to minimize myelosuppression; give dexamethasone 4 mg po bid the day before, the day of, and day after pemetrexed to prevent rash
Topotecan	Mild N/V	Severe myelosuppression; mucositis	Alopecia	
Etoposide	Mild N/V; IV infusion reactions (fever, chills, hypotension, bronchospasm)	Severe myelosuppression; mucositis	Alopecia	Infusion reactions related to diluent in IV formulation

[a]Occurs during the infusion of the drug or within 1-3 d of administration.
[b]Occurs 1-2 wk after administration of the agent.
[c]Occurs after multiple cycles of the agent.
Abbreviations: AUC, area-under-the-curve; NS, normal saline; N/V, nausea and vomiting; RBC, red blood cell.

are alternatives. However, docetaxel is associated with an increased risk of neutropenia, febrile neutropenia, hospitalizations, infections, and alopecia compared to pemetrexed. Ramucirumab is a monoclonal antibody with a similar mechanism of action as bevacizumab; however, it binds to the VEGF receptor. In combination with docetaxel, ramucirumab has been shown to increase median overall survival compared to docetaxel alone in the treatment of relapsed NSCLC. Unlike bevacizumab, it can be used in patients with squamous cell pathology. As mentioned previously, drugs inhibiting the PD-1 pathway are beneficial in the treatment of relapsed disease as well.

Small-Cell Lung Cancer

SCLC is initially very sensitive to chemotherapy with response rates up to 90%. The treatment of choice for limited stage SCLC is chemotherapy with concurrent thoracic radiation therapy. The most common chemotherapy regimen utilized is cisplatin plus etoposide (see Tables 13-5 and 13-6) for four cycles, although carboplatin/etoposide is used as well. If the patient

achieves a complete remission from concurrent chest radiation and chemotherapy, prophylactic cranial irradiation (PCI) is recommended because the development of brain metastases is greater than 30%. For extensive stage SCLC, chemotherapy with cisplatin or carboplatin plus etoposide or irinotecan is recommended. Complete response in patients with extensive stage disease is rare; however, if the patient achieves a complete remission with the chemotherapy regimen, the patient should receive PCI to decrease the incidence of brain metastases and to potentially improve survival. Surgery has a minimal role in SCLC.

SCLC patients who relapse or progress after first-line therapy have a median survival of 4 to 5 months. If the SCLC is refractory (relapsed <3 months since completing first-line therapy), the patient is unlikely to benefit from further therapy; so best supportive care or a clinical trial is recommended in these patients. A patient in whom SCLC relapsed greater than 3 months since completing first-line therapy may benefit from second-line therapy. Options in this patient population include a clinical trial, topotecan (an FDA-approved indication), gemcitabine, or taxanes (eg, paclitaxel, docetaxel).

SPECIAL CONSIDERATIONS

Generally, cycles of chemotherapy are given every 3 or 4 weeks. In lung cancer, cycles are commonly given for a total of four to six cycles. Patients are restaged after every two to three cycles to determine response to the chemotherapy. Chemotherapy is continued if the restaging demonstrates tumor shrinkage or stable disease and the patient is tolerating the treatment. A change in the regimen is considered if the tumor has progressed.

CASE Application

1. What is the brand name of crizotinib?

   a. Xalkori
   b. Opdivo
   c. Cyramza
   d. Iressa

2. A 59-year-old man with recently diagnosed limited-stage small-cell lung cancer comes to clinic for treatment. Which of the following would be the most appropriate treatment for him?

   a. Cisplatin plus vinorelbine
   b. Surgery followed by adjuvant cisplatin plus etoposide
   c. Carboplatin, paclitaxel, and bevacizumab
   d. Cisplatin and etoposide along with concurrent thoracic radiation therapy

3. A 60-year-old woman comes into your pharmacy to pick up her usual prescription for her maintenance medications. She asks you about taking vitamin supplements to decrease her risk of lung cancer. Her social history is significant for smoking a pack of cigarettes a day for 25 years, but she stopped 3 years ago. Based upon this information, you should recommend which of the following?

   a. β-Carotene
   b. Vitamin E plus β-carotene
   c. β-Carotene plus retinyl palmitate
   d. No supplement is recommended

4. A 62-year-old woman who quit smoking 15 years ago comes to clinic asking, "Should I undergo screening for lung cancer?" Her past medical history is significant for hypertension and chronic obstructive pulmonary disease. Her social history is significant for a 31-pack year history of smoking and drinks a beer or two a day. Which of the following represent appropriate lung cancer screening recommendations for this patient?

   a. Annual chest MRI
   b. Annual chest x-ray
   c. Annual sputum cytology
   d. Annual helical CT scan

Use the following scenario to answer questions 5 to 8.

SM is a 52-year-old man with a new diagnosis of metastatic adenocarcinoma of the lung. Complete pathologic review revealed the following profile: ALK negative, EGFR negative, BRAF V600E negative. The oncologist has recommended to start chemotherapy with carboplatin/pemetrexed.

5. The carboplatin for SM should be dosed based on:

   a. Body surface area
   b. Target area under the curve
   c. Ideal body weight
   d. Actual body weight

6. Which of the following monoclonal antibodies could be added to SM's chemotherapy regimen to help improve efficacy?

   a. Necitumumab
   b. Atezolizumab
   c. Cetuximab
   d. Pembrolizumab

7. Which of the following should the patient receive to lessen the severity of side effects from pemetrexed? Select all that apply.

   a. Dexamethasone
   b. Vitamin B_{12}
   c. Pyridoxine
   d. Folic acid

8. SM continued on his prior treatment for 14 months with stable disease. Unfortunately his lung cancer has now progressed and he is to begin a new lung cancer treatment. Which of the following would be most appropriate for him at this time?

   a. Cisplatin/gemcitabine
   b. Docetaxel/ramucirumab
   c. Carboplatin/paclitaxel
   d. Paclitaxel/erlotinib

9. Rank the following chemotherapy agents used in the treatment of lung cancer in order of their emetogenicity, from least emetogenic to most emetogenic.

Unordered options	Ordered response
Cisplatin	
Bevacizumab	
Docetaxel	
Carboplatin	

10. A 68-year-old man with recently diagnosed adenocarcinoma of the lung is found to have stage IV disease (liver metastases). He tests negative for ALK and EGFR mutations. At home, he is bedridden due to severe chronic obstructive pulmonary disease that requires home oxygen. His social history is significant for an 80-pack

year history. Which of the following chemotherapy regimens would be rational?

a. Best supportive care
b. Crizotinib
c. Carboplatin, pemetrexed, and pembrolizumab
d. Cisplatin plus gemcitabine and necitumumab

11. What is the best treatment option for a 61-year-old man who is chemotherapy naïve and was recently diagnosed with extensive-stage small-cell lung cancer?

a. Carboplatin, pemetrexed, plus pembrolizumab
b. Cisplatin plus gemcitabine
c. Carboplatin plus paclitaxel
d. Cisplatin plus etoposide

Use the following scenario to answer questions 12 to 14.

MK is a 62-year-old woman with a recent diagnosis of stage II squamous NSCLC. Complete pathological evaluation showed ALK positive, EGFR negative, BRAF V600E negative. She has a prior medical history of hypertension, type 2 diabetes, stage 3b chronic kidney disease (last estimated glomerular filtration rate 35 mL/min), and gastroesophageal reflux disease. She underwent surgery and is ready to receive chemotherapy.

12. Which of the following therapies is most appropriate for MK at this time?

a. Carboplatin and pemetrexed
b. Carboplatin, pemetrexed, and bevacizumab
c. Cisplatin and etoposide
d. Cisplatin, etoposide, and bevacizumab

13. Which of the problems in the patient's prior medical history is most likely to be worsened by her receiving platinum-based chemotherapy?

a. Hypertension
b. Type 2 diabetes
c. Chronic kidney disease
d. Gastroesophageal reflux disease

14. Four years after completing chemotherapy, MK presents to her primary care physician with new onset coughing with hemoptysis. Complete evaluation revealed the patient's lung cancer has relapsed, now with multiple tumors in the original lung as well as several suspicious tumors in the liver. The pathologic evaluation reveals the same genetic features as her original tumor. Which of the following is the most appropriate treatment for MK at this time?

a. Docetaxel and ramucirumab
b. Atezolizumab
c. Crizotinib
d. Erlotinib

15. Which of the following patients with small-cell lung cancer should receive prophylactic cranial irradiation?

a. Patients with limited-stage SCLC who achieve a complete response to their initial therapy.

b. Patients with extensive-stage SCLC who do not respond to their initial therapy.
c. All patients with limited-stage SCLC.
d. All patients with extensive-stage SCLC.

16. A 64-year-old man with a performance status of 1 returns to clinic with relapsed small-cell lung cancer (SCLC), new bone and liver metastases. He completed his previous chemotherapy of carboplatin and etoposide 5 months ago and reports no other medical problems. He and his wife request further treatment if it is reasonable. Based upon this information, which of the following treatments would be rational?

a. Topotecan
b. Osimertinib
c. Pembrolizumab
d. Best supportive care

17. HM is a 54-year-old man with a recent diagnosis of metastatic squamous NSCLC. He is scheduled to receive chemotherapy with cisplatin and gemcitabine. Which monoclonal antibody should be added to HM's chemotherapy to improve the efficacy of his chemotherapy?

a. Bevacizumab
b. Necitumumab
c. Pembrolizumab
d. Ramucirumab

18. Which of the following kinase inhibitors should be used in the treatment of metastatic NSCLC that tests positive for the BRAF V600E mutation? Choose all that apply.

a. Afatinib
b. Trametinib
c. Ceritinib
d. Dabrafenib

19. Which of the following chemotherapy agents should be added to carboplatin for the adjuvant treatment of stage III adenocarcinoma of the lung?

a. Pemetrexed
b. Etoposide
c. Vinorelbine
d. Cisplatin

20. Rank the following histologies of lung cancer in order of prevalence, from least prevalent to most prevalent.

Unordered Options	Ordered Response
Small-cell carcinoma	
Adenocarcinoma	
Large-cell carcinoma	
Squamous cell carcinoma	

TAKEAWAY POINTS ❱❱

- The leading causes of lung cancer include smoking and asbestos exposure.
- There are four major subtypes of lung cancer: adenocarcinoma, large-cell carcinoma, squamous cell, and small cell.
- Adenocarcinoma, large-cell carcinoma, and squamous cell carcinoma are referred to as NSCLC.
- Lung cancer prevention involves avoiding smoking and maintaining a healthy diet.
- Screening for lung cancer using low-dose helical CT is recommended for patients 55 to 74 years old with at least a 30-pack year smoking history.
- The treatment of choice for NSCLC is surgery. For inoperable patients radiation therapy may be utilized.
- For advanced or recurrent NSCLC, therapy is based on genetic features. Patients who are ALK positive should receive crizotinib. Patients who are EGFR positive should receive erlotinib or afatinib. Patients who are BRAF V600E positive should receive dabrafenib/ trametinib. All other patients should receive chemotherapy or pembrolizumab.

- Platinum-based (cisplatin, carboplatin) therapy is recommended as the front-line chemotherapy for NSCLC. The platinum is usually combined with a taxane (eg, paclitaxel, docetaxel), gemcitabine, or vinorelbine. Pemetrexed may be added to platinum therapy if the patients does not have squamous cell histology.
- Bevacizumab (non squamous), necitumumab (squamous), or pembrolizumab may be added to front-line therapy of metastatic NSCLC.
- Second-line therapy for NSCLC includes single-agent chemotherapy or erlotinib. Ramucirumab can be added to single-agent chemotherapy.
- The best predictor of response to erlotinib is EGFR mutation status.
- Because of its high propensity to metastasize early, the front-line treatment of either stage of SCLC includes systemic chemotherapy with cisplatin plus etoposide.
- Most patients with SCLC initially respond to chemotherapy but relapse.

BIBLIOGRAPHY

Adams VR, Scarpace Peters S. Lung cancer. In: DiPiro JT, Talbert RL, Yee GC, Matzke GR, Wells BG, Posey L, eds. *Pharmacotherapy: A Pathophysiologic Approach.* 10th ed. New York, NY: McGraw-Hill; 2017:chap 129.

Chabner BA, Bertino J, Cleary J, Ortiz T, Lane A, Supko JG, Ryan D. Cytotoxic agents. In: Brunton LL, Chabner BA, Knollmann BC, eds. *Goodman & Gilman's The Pharmacological Basis of Therapeutics.* 12th ed. New York, NY: McGraw-Hill; 2011:chap 61.

Chu E, Sartorelli AC. Cancer chemotherapy. In: Katzung BG, Trevor AJ, eds. *Basic & Clinical Pharmacology.* 13th ed. New York, NY: McGraw-Hill; 2015:chap 54.

Horn L, Lovly CM, Johnson DH. Neoplasms of the lung. In: Kasper DL, Fauci AS, Hauser SL, Longo DL, Jameson J, Loscalzo J, eds. *Harrison's Principles of Internal Medicine.* 19th ed. New York, NY: McGraw-Hill; 2015:chap 107.

National Comprehensive Cancer Network. Non-Small Cell Lung Cancer (Version 8.2017). https://www.nccn.org/professionals/physician_gls/pdf/nscl.pdf. Accessed July, 2017.

National Comprehensive Cancer Network. Small Cell Lung Cancer (Version 3.2017). https://www.nccn.org/professionals/physician_gls/pdf/sclc.pdf. Accessed May, 2017.

KEY ABBREVIATIONS

ALK = anablastic lymphoma kinase
EGFR = epidermal growth factor receptor
KRAS = Kirsten-Rous sarcoma virus
MEK = mitogen-activated extracellular signal regulated kinase
NLST = National Lung Screening Trial
NSAIDs = anti-inflammatory agents

NSCLC = non–small-cell lung cancer
PCI = prophylactic cranial irradiation
PD-1 = programmed-death receptor 1
PDL-1 = programmed-death ligand 1
SCLC = small-cell lung cancer
TNM = tumor, node, and metastasis
VEGF = vascular endothelial growth factor

14

Prostate Cancer

LeAnn B. Norris

FOUNDATION OVERVIEW

Prostate cancer is the most common cancer in men. Most prostate cancers are adenocarcinomas, and occur when normal semen-secreting cells mutate into cancer cells and grow uncontrollably. Normal growth and differentiation of the prostate depends on the presence of androgens, specifically dihydrotestosterone (DHT). Hormonal regulation of androgen synthesis is mediated by a negative feedback loop involving the hypothalamus, pituitary, adrenal glands, and testes. Luteinizing hormone–releasing hormone (LH-RH) released from the hypothalamus stimulates the release of luteinizing hormone (LH) and follicle-stimulating hormone (FSH) from the anterior pituitary gland. LH stimulates the production of testosterone and small amounts of estrogen. FSH acts on the Sertoli cells within the testes to promote the maturation of LH receptors and to produce an androgen-binding protein. Circulating testosterone and estradiol influence the synthesis of the hormones involved in the negative feedback. Testosterone, the major androgenic hormone, accounts for 95% of the androgen concentration. The primary source of testosterone is the testes; however, 3% to 5% of the testosterone concentration is derived from direct adrenal cortical secretion of testosterone or steroids such as androstenedione.

Prostate cancer presentation may be without symptoms, but is curable if diagnosed as localized disease. Prostate cancers may be identified prior to the development of symptoms because of screening. On presentation, most patients with localized disease are asymptomatic. Ureteral dysfunction, frequency, hesitancy, dribbling, and impotence are common symptoms in patients with locally invasive disease. Advanced disease is accompanied with a variety of symptoms including back pain, spinal cord compression, lower extremity edema, pathologic fractures, anemia, and weight loss. Metastatic spread of prostate cancer occurs by lymphatic drainage, hematogenous dissemination, or local extension. The pelvic and abdominal lymph node groups are the most common sites of lymph node involvement. Bone metastases from hematogenous spread are the most common sites of distant spread. The lung, liver, brain, and adrenal glands are the most common sites of visceral involvement.

After a biopsy where two samples are taken, prostate cancer is graded according to the histologic appearance of the malignant cell and grouped into well, moderately, or poorly differentiated grades. Gland architecture is examined in two separate specimens and rated on a scale of 1 (well differentiated) to 5 (poorly differentiated). The grades of each specimen are added together to determine the Gleason score. Groupings for total Gleason score are 2 to 4 for well-differentiated, 5 or 6 for moderately differentiated, and 7 to 10 for poorly differentiated tumors. Poorly differentiated tumors grow rapidly (poor prognosis), while well-differentiated tumors grow slowly (better prognosis).

The information obtained from the diagnostic tests is used to stage the patient. There are two commonly recognized staging classification systems: the International Classification System (tumor, node, metastases; TNM) and the American Urologic System (AUS Stages A-D). The AUS classification is the most commonly used staging system in the United States. Patients are assigned to stages A through D and corresponding subcategories based on size of the tumor (T), local or regional extension, presence of involved lymph node groups (N), and presence of metastases (M).

Prevention

The benefits of prostate cancer screening remain controversial. Detecting prostate cancer in those not needing therapy not only increases the cost of care through unnecessary screening and workup, but also increases harm by subjecting some patients to unnecessary therapy. The United States Preventive Services Task Force (USPSTF) now recommends against screening for prostate cancer (grade D recommendation), due to high certainty that screening has no benefit or that harms outweigh the benefits. The American Urologic Association (AUA) does not recommend routine screening for any man with a life expectancy less than 10 to 15 years, men under 40, men between 40 and 54 years at average risk, or men over the age of 70. Shared decision making is recommended for men age 55 to 69 years who are considering screening based on patients' values and preferences. If the decision is made to screen, a digital rectal examination (DRE) is recommended for the detection of an abnormal shaped prostate. However, DRE has poor compliance and minimal effect on preventing metastatic prostate cancer. Prostate specific antigen (PSA) is used for prostate cancer screening. However, PSA may be elevated in men with acute urinary retention, acute prostatitis, prostatic ischemia or infarction, and benign prostatic hyperplasia (BPH). PSA elevations between 4.1 and 10 ng/mL (10 mcg/L) cannot distinguish between BPH and prostate cancer, limiting the utility of PSA

TABLE 14-1	**5-α Reductase Inhibitors**	
Drug	**Trade Name**	**Dose**
Finasteride	Proscar	5 mg daily
Dutasteride	Avodart	0.5 mg daily

TABLE 14-2	**LH-RH Agonists and GnRH Antagonists**	
Drug	**Trade Name**	**Dose**
LH-RH Agonists		
Leuprolide depot	Lupron	7.5 mg IM monthly 22.5 mg IM every 3 mo 30 mg IM every 4 mo
Leuprolide implant	Viadur	72 mg SQ in abdomen every 12 mo
Goserelin implant	Zoladex	3.6 mg SQ mo 10.8 mg SQ every 3 mo
Triptorelin depot	Trelstar Depot	3.75 mg every 28 d
Triptorelin LA depot	Trelstar LA	11.25 mg every 84 d
GnRH Antagonists		
Degarelix depot	Firmagon	Initial dose: 240 mg SQ × 1 dose (two separate 120 mg injections) Maintenance dose: 80 mg SQ every 28 d

Abbreviations: IM, intramuscular; LH-RH, luteinizing hormone–releasing hormone; SQ, subcutaneous.

alone for the early detection of prostate cancer. PSA velocity (change in PSA over time) is used to monitor patients over an extended period. Neither DRE nor PSA is sensitive or specific enough to be used alone as a screening test. Therefore, the combination of a DRE and PSA is recommended if and when the evaluation of the prostate is deemed necessary.

Chemoprevention

The 5-α reductase inhibitors work by inhibiting an enzyme that converts testosterone to DHT, which is involved in prostate epithelial proliferation. Finasteride and dutasteride falsely lower the PSA in patients and this needs to be accounted for when measuring the PSA. Studies reveal that 5-α reductase inhibitors reduce the rate of prostate cancer, but may increase the cancer grade (Gleason grade 7-10) in those who develop prostate cancer. Therefore, finasteride and dutasteride use is debatable and the benefits, side effects, and risks should be discussed prior to initiating therapy. Common side effects include impotence, ejaculation disorders, decreased libido, and breast enlargement or tenderness (Table 14-1). Finasteride and dutasteride are not currently approved for this indication.

TREATMENT

The initial treatment for prostate cancer depends on the disease stage, the Gleason score, the presence of symptoms, and life expectancy of the patient. Asymptomatic patients with a low risk of recurrence, a Gleason score of 2 through 6, and a PSA of less than 10 ng/mL (10 mcg/L) may be managed by active surveillance, radiation (external beam or brachytherapy), or radical prostatectomy. Individuals with moderate disease or a Gleason score of 7 or a PSA ranging from 10 to 20 ng/mL (10-20 mcg/L) are at intermediate risk for prostate cancer recurrence. Individuals with less than a 10-year expected survival may be offered active surveillance, radical prostatectomy, or radiation therapy with or without 4 to 6 months of neoadjuvant androgen deprivation therapy (ADT) with or without brachytherapy. Those individuals with a greater than or equal to 10-year life expectancy may be offered either radical prostatectomy with or without a pelvic lymph node dissection or radiation therapy with or without 4 to 5 months of neoadjuvant ADT with or without brachytherapy. The treatment of patients at high risk of recurrence (Gleason score ranging from 8-10, or a PSA value greater than 20 ng/mL, or 20 mcg/L) should be treated with androgen ablation for 2 to 3 years combined with radiation therapy with or without brachytherapy (Table 14-2).

ADT can be used to provide palliation for patients with advanced (stage D$_2$) prostate cancer. Deprivation therapy includes either orchiectomy, an LH-RH agonist alone, or an

LH-RH agonist plus an antiandrogen (combined androgen blockade [CAB]). Patients who develop metastatic disease often have tumor progression and develop castration resistant prostate cancer. Castration resistant prostate cancer is defined as disease progression despite multiple antihormonal therapies or disease growth despite a testosterone level less than 50 ng/mL. Denosumab (RANK ligand inhibitor) or an intravenous bisphosphonate (such as zoledronic acid) is added in patients with bone metastases. Importantly, further therapy is determined by the presence of symptomatic disease or whether the metastatic progression is manifested as only a rising PSA.

Castrate resistant prostate cancer may be treated with either intravenous chemotherapy or oral agents such as enzalutamide or abiraterone. Docetaxel with prednisone, enzalutamide, or abiraterone with prednisone may be utilized first-line despite the presence of visceral or non-visceral metastases (Table 14-3). Potential side effects and on-going medical conditions should be considered prior to drug selection. If failure with primary therapy occurs, treatment should be rotated to an agent that has not been utilized. Cabazitaxel, an intravenous chemotherapy agent, may be utilized as a second-line option. Patients who are asymptomatic or minimally symptomatic may receive treatment with sipuleucel-T as first-line therapy. Radium-223, an α emitter, may be recommended in patients to target specific bone metastases or those in need of pain relief.

Pharmacologic Therapy

Luteinizing Hormone–Releasing Hormone Agonists

LH-RH agonists are a reversible method of androgen deprivation and are as effective as orchiectomy in treating prostate cancer. Table 14-2 lists available LH-RH formulations and dosing. Direct comparative trials of LH-RH agonists are lacking;

TABLE 14-3	Hormonal Agents		
Drug	**Trade Name**	**Dose**	**Adverse Effects**
Antiandrogens			
Flutamide	Eulexin	250 mg three times daily	Gynecomastia Hot flushes Gastrointestinal disturbances (diarrhea) Liver function test abnormalities Breast tenderness Methemoglobinemia
Bicalutamide	Casodex	50 mg/d	Gynecomastia Hot flushes Gastrointestinal disturbances (diarrhea) Liver function test abnormalities Breast tenderness
Nilutamide	Nilandron	300 mg/d × 1 mo, then 150 mg/d	Gynecomastia Hot flushes Gastrointestinal disturbances (nausea or constipation) Liver function test abnormalities Breast tenderness Visual disturbances (impaired dark adaptation) Alcohol intolerance Interstitial pneumonitis
Enzalutamide	Xtandi	160 mg/d	Gastrointestinal disturbances (diarrhea) Musculoskeletal disorders (back pain, arthralgias, muscle pain, weakness) Asthenia Peripheral edema Central nervous system (headache, dizziness) Seizures Liver function test abnormalities
Androgen Synthesis Inhibitor			
Abiraterone	Zytiga	1000 mg/d	Gastrointestinal disturbances (diarrhea) Edema Hypokalemia Hypophosphatemia Liver function test abnormalities Hypertriglyceridemia

therefore, an agent is selected on cost, provider preference, and dosing schedule.

Common adverse effects reported with LH-RH agonist therapy include a disease flare during the first week of therapy, hot flashes, impotence, decreased libido, and injection-site reactions. The disease flare is caused by an initial increase in the release of LH and FSH by the LH-RH agonist leading to increased testosterone production, and manifests clinically as increased bone pain or increased urinary symptoms. Initiating an antiandrogen prior to the administration of the LH-RH agonist and continuing for 7 days of overlap is utilized to minimize this initial tumor flare. Utilizing an antiandrogen with an LH-RH agonist is known as CAB and is used to maximize androgen deprivation.

ADT may decrease the bone-mineral density leading to an increased risk for skeletal fractures or osteoporosis. Most clinicians recommend that men starting long-term ADT should have a baseline bone mineral density assessment and be initiated on a calcium and vitamin D supplement. Additionally, an antiresorptive agent (zoledronic acid or denosumab) should be considered. Patients should be monitored for osteonecrosis of the jaw when on zoledronic acid and hypocalcemia while receiving denosumab.

Gonadotrophin-Releasing Hormone Antagonists

An alternative to LH-RH agonists is the gonadotrophin-releasing hormone (GnRH) antagonist degarelix (Table 14-2). Degarelix works by binding to GnRH receptors on cells in the pituitary gland, reducing the production of testosterone to castrate levels. The advantage of degarelix over LH-RH agonists is the speed at which testosterone levels are decreased. Castrate levels are achieved in 7 days or less with degarelix, compared to 28 days with leuprolide, eliminating the tumor flare and need for antiandrogens with LH-RH agonists. Additionally, degarelix does not cause tumor flare. Degarelix adverse reactions include injection sites reactions and osteoporosis (consider calcium and vitamin D supplementation). Degarelix has not been studied in combination with antiandrogens and routine use of the combination is not recommended.

Antiandrogens

Four antiandrogens are currently available flutamide, bicalutamide, nilutamide, and enzalutamide (Table 14-3). For advanced prostate cancer, flutamide and bicalutamide are indicated in combination with an LH-RH agonist, and nilutamide is indicated in combination with orchiectomy. Antiandrogen adverse effects are listed in Table 14-3. Antiandrogens reduce symptoms from the flare phenomenon associated with initiation of LH-RH agonist therapy. Enzalutamide is approved as a single agent for patients with metastatic hormone resistant prostate cancer. As with the other antiandrogens, enzalutamide does not lower androgen levels but inhibits androgen-receptor signaling by competitively inhibiting the binding of androgens without stimulation of the androgen receptor. Enzalutamide may have an advantage over the currently available antiandrogen agents because it inhibits nuclear translocation of the androgen receptor, DNA binding, and coactivator recruitment.

Secondary Therapies

Secondary or salvage therapies are utilized in patients that progress after initial therapy. For localized prostate cancer patients, radiotherapy can be used in failed radical prostatectomy. Alternatively, androgen ablation can be used in patients who progress after either radiation therapy or radical prostatectomy.

In patients treated initially with one hormonal modality, secondary hormonal manipulations may be attempted including adding an antiandrogen to an LH-RH agonist. If the patient initially received CAB with an LH-RH agonist and an antiandrogen, then androgen withdrawal is the first salvage manipulation. Objective and subjective responses have been noted following the discontinuation of flutamide, bicalutamide, or nilutamide in patients receiving these agents as part of combined androgen ablation with an LH-RH agonist. A potential explanation for response when antiandrogen therapy is discontinued may be mutations in the androgen receptor. These mutations allow antiandrogens to become agonists and activate the androgen receptor.

Adding an agent that blocks adrenal androgen synthesis at the time that androgens are withdrawn may produce a better response than androgen withdrawal alone. Androgen synthesis inhibitors (aminoglutethimide, ketoconazole, or abiraterone) can provide symptomatic relief for a short time in approximately 50% of patients with progressive disease despite previous androgen-ablation therapy. Central nervous system effects that include lethargy, ataxia, and dizziness and a self-limiting rash are the major adverse reactions of aminoglutethimide. Ketoconazole adverse reactions include gastrointestinal intolerance, transient rises in liver and renal function tests, and hypoadrenalism. Ketoconazole is combined with replacement doses of hydrocortisone to prevent symptomatic hypoadrenalism. Abiraterone is an androgen synthesis inhibitor that targets CYP17A1 resulting in a decrease in circulating levels of testosterone. Abiraterone is indicated in patients with metastatic castrate resistant prostate cancer and should be taken with prednisone 5 mg twice daily. Hypertension, hypokalemia, and edema may occur due to hypoadrenalism. Abiraterone is available as the prodrug, abiraterone acetate, and should be taken on an empty stomach as food increases bioavailability by up to 10-fold. Monitoring of liver function tests (LFT) is recommended at baseline, every 2 weeks for the first 3 months, and then monthly thereafter. Since abiraterone is an inhibitor of CYP 2D6, medication profiles should be reviewed for potential drug interactions prior to initiation of abiraterone therapy.

Chemotherapy

Intravenous chemotherapy with docetaxel and prednisone improves survival in patients with castrate-refractory prostate cancer may be utilized as a first-line therapy for these patients. Adverse events with this regimen are nausea, alopecia, and bone marrow suppression. Additional adverse effects of docetaxel include fluid retention and peripheral neuropathy. Docetaxel is metabolized in the liver; therefore, patients with hepatic impairment may not be eligible for treatment because of an increased risk for toxicity (Table 14-4).

Cabazitaxel is a taxane with demonstrated activity in docetaxel resistant cell lines and animal models of human cancer. Cabazitaxel has lower affinity for P-glycoprotein multidrug resistance transporter than docetaxel, which may explain

TABLE 14-4	Chemotherapy Agents		
Regimen	**Usual Dose**	**Adverse Effects**	**Dose Adjustments**
Docetaxel	75 mg/m^2 every 3 wk	Fluid retention Alopecia Mucositis Neuropathy	Do not administer for: AST/ALT >1.5 × upper limit of normal Alk Phos >2.5 × upper limit of normal Assure complete blood count recovery
Mitoxantrone	12 mg/m^2 every 3 wk	Myelosuppression Alopecia Cardiotoxicity Blue/green secretions	EKG prior to initiation Administered with caution in hepatic impairment Assure complete blood count recovery
Cabazitaxel	25 mg/m^2/dose every 3 wk	Myelosuppression Hypersensitivity Diarrhea	Assure complete blood count recovery Diarrhea

Abbreviations: ALT, alanine transaminase; Alk Phos, alkaline phosphatase; AST, aspartate transaminase; EKG, electrocardiogram.

Note: Agents are in combination with prednisone.

why cabazitaxel is active in the setting of docetaxel resistance. In patients previously treated with docetaxel and prednisone, treatment with cabazitaxel 25 mg/m² every 3 weeks with prednisone 10 mg daily improved progression-free survival and overall survival as compared to mitoxantrone and prednisone. Neutropenia, febrile neutropenia, neuropathy, and diarrhea are the significant toxicities. Hypersensitivity reactions may occur and premedication with an antihistamine, a corticosteroid, and an H₂ antagonist is recommended. Cabazitaxel is extensively metabolized in the liver and should be avoided in patients with hepatic dysfunction.

CASE Application

1. A 62-year-old man with a recent diagnosis of prostate cancer presents to oncologist. His oncologist tells him that his prostate cancer has a Gleason score of 3 + 3 or 6. A prostate cancer with a Gleason score of 6 is considered:

   a. Not differentiated
   b. Poorly differentiated
   c. Differentiated
   d. Moderately differentiated
   e. Well differentiated

2. HH is a 72-year-old African American man with a family history of prostate cancer who presents to his primary care physician for his annual examination. He has a past medical history of hypertension, diabetes, and heart failure. He asks about prostate cancer screening. According to the AUA, Which of the following is the most appropriate course of action? Select all that apply.

   a. Observation because he is not eligible for prostate cancer screening due to his age being >70.
   b. Patient should be screened with a DRE and a PSA level.
   c. Observation because he is not eligible for prostate cancer screening due to his family history.
   d. Patient should be screened with a DRE alone.
   e. Observation because his life expectancy is less than 10 to 15 years.

3. JJ is a 52-year-old man with a history of BPH. His most recent DRE was normal, but last PSA was 5.1 ng/mL. JJ is concerned about getting prostate cancer and wants to discuss preventative therapy. Which of the following is true pertaining to the use of 5-α reductase inhibitors for prostate cancer prevention?

   a. 5-α reductase inhibitors are approved for prostate cancer prevention.
   b. 5-α reductase inhibitors increase libido.
   c. 5-α reductase inhibitors decrease prostate cancer, but increase the Gleason score in patients who develop cancer.
   d. 5-α reductase inhibitors increase the risk of prostate cancer.
   e. 5-α reductase inhibitors can increase the PSA level.

4. Which of the following agents is considered a GnRH antagonist?

   a. Goserelin
   b. Degarelix
   c. Leuprolide
   d. Triptorelin
   e. Sipuleucel-T

5. BD is a 59-year-old man with hypertension and dyslipidemia. He reports to the ER in status epilepticus. Which medication is the most likely cause?

   a. Bicalutamide
   b. Flutamide
   c. Nilutamide
   d. Enzalutamide
   e. Abiraterone

6. What is the trade name of abiraterone?

   a. Xtandi
   b. Nilandron
   c. Avodart
   d. Casodex
   e. Zytiga

7. MN is a newly diagnosed prostate cancer patient being treated with androgen deprivation. Which of the following are appropriate counseling points for a new patient starting on an LH-RH agonist? Select all that apply.

   a. Patient may experience side effects such as a loss in libido, hot flushes, and impotence.
   b. ADT is associated with osteoporosis and therefore the patient should take a calcium/vitamin D supplement.
   c. Patient may experience worsening symptoms during the first week related to "tumor flare."
   d. Patient may experience nausea/vomiting, alopecia, and weight loss.

8. SL is a 69-year-old man who was recently diagnosed with prostate cancer and is initiated on a hormone agent for the first time for androgen deprivation. The pharmacist tells the patient he should not experience tumor flare with this new medication. Which of the following agents was this patient initiated on?

   a. Leuprolide
   b. Goserelin
   c. Triptorelin
   d. Degarelix
   e. Enzalutamide

9. CC is a 56-year-old man with metastatic castrate resistant prostate cancer. He has several other comorbid diseases including chronic heart failure (CHF), diabetes, and hypertension. Which of the following chemotherapy or systemic agents is the most appropriate for this patient? Select all that apply.

   a. Abiraterone
   b. Enzalutamide

c. Cabazitaxel

d. Docetaxel + prednisone

10. BB is a 69-year-old man with metastatic prostate cancer who is receiving chemotherapy and denosumab. Which of the following side effects may potentially occur while on denosumab?

a. Hypocalcemia

b. Osteonecrosis of the jaw

c. Loss of libido

d. Hypokalemia

e. Hypertriglyceridemia

11. Which of the following side effects is associated with docetaxel use? Select all that apply.

a. Myelosuppression

b. Gynecomastia

c. Alopecia

d. Cardiotoxicity

e. Blue/Green secretions

12. Which of the following antiandrogens is associated with interstitial pneumonitis?

a. Flutamide

b. Bicalutamide

c. Nilutamide

d. Enzalutamide

e. Abiraterone

13. Which of the following patients with prostate cancer can be managed with observation alone?

a. Patient with a Gleason score of 3 and PSA of 5 ng/mL

b. Patient with a Gleason score of 8 and PSA of 40 ng/mL

c. Patient with a Gleason score of 2 and PSA of 15 ng/mL

d. Patient with a Gleason score of 5 and PSA of 20 ng/mL

e. Patient with a Gleason score of 6 and a PSA of 100 ng/mL

14. A 61-year-old is seeing his primary care physician for an annual physical today. As part of the shared-decision making, the physician reviews the data pertaining to prostate cancer screening. Which of the following is true?

a. DRE is highly specific and highly sensitive for detecting prostate cancer and should be used alone for diagnosis.

b. PSA is highly specific and highly sensitive for detecting prostate cancer and should be used alone for diagnosis.

c. DRE and PSA are highly specific and highly sensitive for detecting prostate cancer and should be used in combination for diagnosis.

d. Neither DRE nor PSA are highly specific or highly sensitive when used alone for detecting prostate cancer. Therefore, these agents should be used in combination for diagnosis.

e. DRE is highly specific and PSA is low is sensitivity and therefore it doesn't matter if these screening methods are used separately or in combination.

15. Which of the following agents has an adherence concern due to the dosing concern?

a. Flutamide

b. Bicalutamide

c. Nilutamide

d. Enzalutamide

e. Abiraterone

16. Which of the following agents should be utilized in patients with castrate resistant prostate cancer with bone pain for assistance with pain reduction?

a. Flutamide

b. Bicalutamide

c. Docetaxel

d. Radium-223

e. Sepulture-T

17. MN is seeing his oncologist today and receives a prescription for both leuprolide and flutamide. The use of an antiandrogen and an LH-RH agonist together is called:

a. Concurrent chemoprevention

b. Concurrent chemoradiotherapy

c. CAB

d. Castrate resistant prostate cancer

e. Concurrent chemotherapy

18. Which of the following agents should only be utilized as second-line therapy for metastatic castrate resistant prostate cancer? Select all that apply.

a. Docetaxel plus prednisone

b. Abiraterone plus prednisone

c. Enzalutamide plus prednisone

d. Mitoxantrone plus prednisone

e. Cabazitaxel plus prednisone

19. Which of the following hormonal therapies is administered via depot? Select all that apply.

a. Lupron

b. Zoladex

c. Trelstar

d. Viadur

e. Firmagon

20. GS is a 58-year-old man who was diagnosed with prostate cancer several years ago. He was recently referred to oncology as his disease was deemed castrate resistant. The physician recommends docetaxel with prednisone for GS every 3 weeks. Which of the following premedication regimens would you recommend?

a. Diphenhydramine and ranitidine

b. Loperamide

c. Allopurinol

d. Calcium and magnesium

e. Mesna

TAKEAWAY POINTS »

- Prostate cancer can be graded systematically according to the histologic appearance of the malignant cell and grouped into well, moderately, or poorly differentiated grades based on the Gleason score.
- Skeletal metastases are the most common site of distant spread of prostate cancer.
- The testes and the adrenal glands are the major sources of circulating androgens.
- Hormonal regulation of androgen synthesis is mediated by a negative feedback loop involving the hypothalamus, pituitary gland, adrenal glands, and testes.
- Ureteral dysfunction, frequency, hesitancy, dribbling, and impotence are common symptoms in patients with prostate cancer.
- The combination of a DRE plus PSA determination is the preferred method for detecting prostate cancer.
- The AUA does not recommend routine screening for any man with a life expectancy less than 10 to 15 years, men under 40, men between 40 and 54 years at average risk, or men over the age of 70. Shared decision making is recommended for men age 55 to 69 years who are considering screening based on patients' values and preferences.

- 5-α reductase inhibitors can be used for the prevention of prostate cancer, although not approved for this indication.
- Prostate cancer managed by active surveillance, radiation (external beam or brachytherapy), radical prostatectomy, androgen ablation, or chemotherapy depending on the stage and grade of the disease.
- LH-RH agonists are a reversible method of androgen ablation and are as effective as orchiectomy in treating prostate cancer.
- "Tumor flare" can be treated with antiandrogens.
- Common side effects of antiandrogens include gynecomastia, hot flushes, gastrointestinal disturbances, and LFT abnormalities.
- Docetaxel and prednisone, enzalutamide, or abiraterone and prednisone may be utilized first-line in castrate resistant prostate cancer.
- Bisphosphonates or a RANK-L inhibitor may prevent skeletal related events and improve bone mineral density.
- Radium-223 may be utilized in castrate resistant prostate cancer with bone metastases to reduce bone pain.

BIBLIOGRAPHY

Chabner BA, Bertino J, Cleary J, et al. Cytotoxic agents. In: Brunton LL, Chabner BA, Knollmann BC, eds. *Goodman & Gilman's The Pharmacological Basis of Therapeutics*. 12th ed. New York, NY: McGraw-Hill; 2011:chap 61.

Chu E, Sartorelli AC. Cancer Chemotherapy. In: Katzung BG, Masters SB, Trevor AJ, eds. *Basic & Clinical Pharmacology*. 13th ed. New York, NY: McGraw-Hill; 2015:chap 54.

Norris LB, Kolesar JM. Prostate cancer. In: DiPiro JT, Talbert RL, Yee GC, Matzke GR, Wells BG, Posey L, eds. *Pharmacotherapy:*

A Pathophysiologic Approach. 10th ed. New York, NY: McGraw-Hill; 2017:chap 131.

Scher HI. Benign and malignant diseases of the prostate. In: Longo DL, Fauci AS, Kasper DL, Hauser SL, Jameson J, Loscalzo J, eds. *Harrison's Principles of Internal Medicine*. 19th ed. New York, NY: McGraw-Hill; 2015:chap 115.

The NCCN Clinical Practice Guidelines in Oncology™ Prostate Cancer (Version 1.2017)®. National Comprehensive Cancer Network. www.NCCN.org. Accessed April 28, 2017.

KEY ABBREVIATIONS

ADT = androgen deprivation therapy
ALT = alanine transaminase
Alk Phos = alkaline phosphatase
AST = aspartate transaminase
AUS = American Urologic System
BPH = benign prostatic hyperplasia
CAB = combined androgen blockade
CHF = chronic heart failure
DRE = digital rectal examination
DHT = dihydrotestosterone

EKG = electrocardiogram
FSH = follicle-stimulating hormone
GnRH = gonadotrophin-releasing hormone
LFT = liver function tests
LH = luteinizing hormone
LH-RH = luteinizing hormone–releasing hormone
PSA = prostate specific antigen
SQ = subcutaneous
TNM = tumor, node, metastases
USPSTF = United States Preventive Services Task Force

15

Leukemias

David L. DeRemer

FOUNDATION OVERVIEW

Acute Lymphoblastic Leukemia

Leukemia is the most common malignancy in pediatrics and the exact cause of acute lymphoblastic leukemia (ALL) is unknown. Less than 5% of cases have been associated with inherited genetic syndromes (Down or Bloom syndrome) or with exposure to ionizing radiation and chemotherapeutic agents. In the development of B cells and T cells, various events occur to develop a competent immune system. In ALL, mutations occur in the development of B- and T-cell progenitors leading to dysregulated proliferation and clonal expansion.

Patients present with malaise, fever, weight loss, palpitations, bruising, petechiae, bone pain, and lymphadenopathy. Many symptoms represent malignant cells replacing normal hematopoiesis. Electrolyte disturbances such as hyperkalemia, hyperphosphatemia, hyperuricemia, and hypocalcemia may occur and patients may experience tumor lysis syndrome (TLS). Physical examination findings include hepatomegaly, splenomegaly, and a mediastinal mass. Leukocytosis (WBC >30,000-50,000/μL) confers a poor prognosis, particularly in B-cell ALL. Other factors conferring a poor prognosis include age (>30), immunophenotype (B lineage worse), Philadelphia chromosome (Ph+) disease, and central nervous system (CNS) disease.

Diagnosis is determined by evaluating the complete blood count (CBC) with differential, coagulation studies, bone marrow biopsy and aspiration, and lumbar puncture. Cytochemical studies, immunophenotyping, and cytogenetics are performed on bone marrow samples. A lumbar puncture should be performed to assess CNS involvement.

TREATMENT

The primary goal of treatment is to induce and maintain a complete remission (CR). A CR can be induced in 96% to 99% of children and 78% to 93% of adults. Treatment of pediatric ALL is divided into induction, consolidation, interim maintenance, delayed intensification, and maintenance. Adult ALL is divided into induction, consolidation, and maintenance. CNS treatment is performed throughout all phases of therapy. Intrathecal therapy consists of methotrexate and cytarabine which can be given alone or in combination. Patients with T-cell ALL have an increased incidence of CNS disease and should receive systemic high-dose methotrexate to penetrate the CNS. Multiple intensive chemotherapy regimens have been shown to provide benefit in adult ALL. Specific agents used in the initial treatment of ALL are summarized in Table 15-1. Treatment of relapsed ALL typically includes aggressive chemotherapy. Single-agent treatment for relapsed ALL includes nelarabine (T-cell origin), clofarabine (B-cell origin), and blinatumomab (B-cell origin). Blinatumomab is a new monoclonal antibody that improved survival compared to standard chemotherapy in patients with B-cell origin ALL that had received multiple prior chemotherapy regimens.

Special Populations

Approximately 5% of children and 30% of adult ALL will have Ph+ disease. These patients may receive oral tyrosine kinase inhibitors (TKIs) in combination with traditional chemotherapy. For pediatric patients, there is no standard regimen, rather these patients will be enrolled in a clinical trial and must maintain strict adherence to protocol. In adults (55-65 years) dose reductions may be necessary due to toxicities of adult ALL regimens. Elderly patients rarely achieve a CR and goals of therapy include control of leukemia and maintaining acceptable quality of life.

Acute Myelogenous Leukemia

The incidence of acute myelogenous leukemia (AML) increases with age and is typically diagnosed in elderly patients and more frequently found in males. Risk factors include ionizing radiation, benzene, and cytotoxic chemotherapy. Specifically, alkylating agents and topoisomerase II inhibitors have been associated with the development of AML. AML arises from a leukemic cell which expands and acquires additional mutations. Genetic alterations lead to AML blasts which are ineffective in generating mature neutrophils, platelets, and red blood cells.

Clinical presentation is nonspecific and related to decreased production of normal hematopoietic cells. Patients often describe an infection characterized by fatigue and elevated temperature. Other symptoms include weight loss, dyspnea on exertion, bleeding and bruising, joint and bone pain, gingival hypertrophy, and headache. Unlike ALL, AML is less

TABLE 15-1 **Commonly Used Agents in Treatment of ALL**

Agent	Classification	Route of Administration	Adverse Reactions
Asparaginase (*Escherichia coli* strain)	Other	IM/IV/SQ	Allergic reactions, coagulopathy (increased prothrombin time), depression, fatigue, hyperglycemia, pancreatitis, thrombotic events
Cyclophosphamide	Alkylating agent	IV	Alopecia, hemorrhagic cystitis, impairment of fertility, myelosuppression, N/V, secondary malignancies
Cytarabine	Antimetabolite	IV/IT	Cerebellar dysfunction, conjunctivitis, diarrhea, myelosuppression, pulmonary edema, N/V
Daunorubicin	Topoisomerase II inhibitor	IV	Alopecia, cardiotoxicity, discoloration of urine, extravasation, myelosuppression, N/V, secondary malignancies
Doxorubicin	Topoisomerase II inhibitor	IV	Alopecia, cardiotoxicity, discoloration of urine, extravasation, myelosuppression, N/V, secondary malignancies
Mercaptopurine	Antimetabolite	po	Hyperbilirubinemia, increased hepatic transaminases, intrahepatic cholestasis, myelosuppression
Methotrexate	Antimetabolite	IV/IT	IV: Acute renal failure, dermatologic reactions, diarrhea, hepatotoxicity, impaired fertility, mucositis, neurotoxicity IT or high-dose MTX: Headache, motor paralysis of extremities, cranial nerve palsy, seizure
Prednisone	Corticosteroid	po	Cushing syndrome, diabetes mellitus, fluid retention, insomnia, mood swings, myopathy, osteoporosis, ulcerative esophagitis, wound healing impairment
Vincristine	Antimicrotubule	IV	Alopecia, constipation and paralytic ileus, CNS depression, extravasation, peripheral neuropathy Note: Do not give intrathecally; it may cause severe neurological toxicity and/or death

Abbreviation: N/V, nausea/vomiting.

commonly associated with CNS involvement. Metabolic and electrolyte abnormalities are common. Patients may present with hyperuricemia, hyperkalemia, and hyperphosphatemia. A CBC with differential will reveal anemia, thrombocytopenia, and leukopenia or leukocytosis (20% of patients will present with a high WBC).

The diagnostic work-up for AML includes CBC with differential, coagulation studies, examination of a peripheral blood smear, and examination of a bone marrow aspirate and biopsy. Cytochemical studies to determine leukemia lineage (myeloid or lymphoid) and immunophenotyping are also performed. Cytogenetic analysis to determine chromosomal abnormalities assists in diagnosis and prognosis. Molecular testing for the presence of mutations such as FLT-3, NPM1, C-KIT, and CEBPA is utilized for determining prognostic risk.

TREATMENT

Treatment is immediately initiated following definitive diagnosis. Treatment consists of three phases: (1) induction, (2) post-remission, and (3) refractory/relapsed disease. The goal of induction therapy is to induce a CR with a return of normal hematopoiesis. A CR is defined as achieving a platelet count more than 100,000 µL, neutrophil count more than 1000 µL, and a bone marrow specimen less than 5% blasts. Patients that achieve a CR post-induction have a better prognosis. For the past 30 years, induction therapy has consisted of the combination of cytarabine with an anthracycline (daunorubicin or idarubicin). A common regimen is "7+3" which combines cytarabine (100 mg/m^2 days 1-7) with idarubicin (12 mg/m^2

days 1-3) or daunorubicin (60-90 mg/m^2 days 1-3). Patients 60 years of age and older with significant comorbidities should not receive 7+3 due to poor outcomes. These patients may benefit from supportive care or investigational treatment.

Post-remission therapy consists of multiple cycles of high-dose cytarabine (HDAC). The optimal dose (g/m^2) and the number of cycles to be given are controversial. Patients will typically receive 6 to 18 g/m^2 of cytarabine per cycle for 3 to 4 cycles. Toxicities of HDAC include cerebellar dysfunction, pulmonary edema, pericardial effusion, and conjunctivitis. Renal function should be closely monitored following HDAC administration since renal dysfunction has correlated to cerebellar dysfunction. For patients who are unable to achieve a CR, refractory/relapsed treatments are available. Cytarabine alone or in combination with fludarabine, mitoxantrone, etoposide, or clofarabine are options. Response rates in the relapsed setting range from 10% to 50% and often have a short duration. Depending on age and cytogenetic risk factors (good, intermediate, or poor) patients may benefit from either an autologous or allogeneic stem cell transplant. The development of novel targeted therapies and immunotherapy-based options are actively being investigated.

Acute promyelocytic leukemia (APL or AML-M3) represents approximately 10% of AML cases. In general, APL has a better prognosis than other AML subtypes. Rather than receiving standard 7+3 induction therapy, APL patients should receive tretinoin (all-trans retinoic acid, or ATRA) with an anthracycline or with arsenic trioxide depending upon patient risk status. Tretinoin is given orally at 45 mg/m^2, divided into two doses after a full meal. At the initiation of tretinoin, patients need to be monitored for differentiation syndrome (DS, formerly known as retinoic acid syndrome). DS is associated with respiratory distress, pleural effusions, pulmonary infiltrates, and fever. This syndrome can be fatal; patients should immediately receive dexamethasone 10 mg IV Q12 for 3 to 5 days to improve symptoms and decrease mortality. Tretinoin may need to be held during this period, but will need to be reinstituted following symptom improvement and continued. The addition of arsenic trioxide to tretinoin has led to impressive CR rates in low/intermediate risk patients. Arsenic trioxide has been associated with QT prolongation thus periodic monitoring with a 12-lead ECG and correction of hypokalemia or hypomagnesemia is recommended.

Following induction therapy, consolidation therapy should be administered due to high rates of relapse in APL. Consolidative therapies consists of additional anthracycline cycles, tretinoin, and in some regimens arsenic trioxide. Patients may receive tretinoin daily for 15 days every 3 months ± oral 6-mercaptopurine (100 mg/m^2) and methotrexate for maintenance therapy.

SPECIAL CONSIDERATIONS

Supportive care and monitoring is essential in patients with acute leukemias. Patients with high WBC counts are particularly susceptible to TLS. Aggressive hydration and diuresis are important in the prevention and management of TLS. TLS is characterized by increased uric acid, hyperphosphatemia, hyperkalemia, hypocalcemia, increased serum creatinine, and decreased urine output. Patients should receive allopurinol to prevent the formation of uric acid. In patients who present with hyperuricemia, rasburicase should be used in select patients. Rasburicase is contraindicated with glucose-6-phosphate dehydrogenase (G6PD) deficiency.

Patients will receive platelet and red cell transfusions as clinically indicated. Also, prophylactic antimicrobial therapy is recommended in patients who may have prolonged neutropenia. The use of granulocyte colony-stimulating factors (filgrastim, sargramostim) should be considered in older patients to decrease the duration of hospitalization.

Chronic Lymphocytic Leukemia

Chronic lymphocytic leukemia (CLL) is the most common form of leukemia in the United States. The disease is typically diagnosed in the elderly with a median age of onset between 65 and 75. The etiology of CLL is elusive since no causal relationship has been found with exposure of radiation, chemicals, or viral oncogenesis. CLL is thought to arise from a polyclonal expansion of CD5+ B lymphocytes. A majority of patients will be asymptomatic upon diagnosis. Patients with symptoms will most often present with lymphadenopathies. Other symptoms include splenomegaly, hepatomegaly, fever, night sweats, and increased frequency of infections. Laboratory examinations may reveal lymphocytosis, anemia, thrombocytopenia, and hypogammaglobulinemia. The diagnostic workup includes a physical examination, laboratory studies including CBC, bone marrow biopsy and aspirate, immunophenotyping, and cytogenetics.

TREATMENT

CLL is considered incurable and the goals of treatment include palliation and increase duration of life. Standard treatment for CLL may include a period of watchful waiting until progression of disease (eg, high WBC, bulky lymph nodes, symptomatic splenomegaly). Early treatment has not resulted in survival benefit. In advanced stages (Rai stage III-IV), treatment is warranted in attempt to obtain disease remission. Both traditional cytotoxic chemotherapy and monoclonal antibodies offer effective treatment options.

Cytotoxic Chemotherapy

Purine analogs are effective agents in treating CLL. Specifically, fludarabine has been shown as monotherapy and in combination to provide benefit. As single-agent therapy, fludarabine is given once daily for 5 days intravenously. Adverse events associated with fludarabine include myelosuppression, autoimmune effects, and neurologic toxicities. Fludarabine monotherapy is associated with an increased risk of infections; in combination with other immunosuppressive or cytotoxic agents the risk escalates. Therefore, patients need to be counseled on infection prevention strategies. Due to risk of opportunistic infections patients should receive phencyclidine (PCP), antifungal, and antiviral prophylaxis. Oral alkylating agents (cyclophosphamide and chlorambucil) are also a treatment option but have been shown to be inferior to fludarabine. Fludarabine with IV cyclophosphamide has resulted in improved overall survival and CR rates when compared to fludarabine alone. An additional alkylating agent, bendamustine, which has low cross-resistance with other alkylating agents, is recommended as monotherapy for first-line therapy and in combination for relapsed disease. Bendamustine has been associated with myelosuppression, skin reactions, infections, infusion reactions, and TLS.

Monoclonal Antibodies

Rituximab is a chimeric monoclonal antibody that targets CD20 surface antigen expressed on B lymphocytes. Single agent weekly rituximab has demonstrated modest clinical benefit and is commonly used in combination regimens. Adverse events associated with rituximab include infusion-related reactions, TLS, flu-like symptoms, skin rash, and cytopenias. Hepatitis B reactivation has been reported in patients treated with rituximab in combination with chemotherapy. As a result, it is recommended that hepatitis B testing be performed prior to the initiation of rituximab.

Alemtuzumab is a humanized monoclonal antibody that targets CD52 antigen expressed on B and T lymphocytes. Severe infusion-related reactions are associated with alemtuzumab. Patients should receive acetaminophen and diphenhydramine 30 minutes prior to the initiation of infusion. Due to the infusion-related reactions associated with intravenous administration, some investigators sought to improve adverse events with subcutaneous administration. Additional adverse events include pancytopenias, fever, rigors, hypotension, and immunosuppression. Patients who receive alemtuzumab have a significant increased risk of infection. It is recommended that patients receive PCP prophylaxis and herpes viral prophylaxis for a minimum of 2 months following the completion of alemtuzumab in addition to appropriate antifungal prophylaxis. Reactivation of cytomegalovirus (CMV) has also been reported and warrants monitoring and preemptive therapy. Alemtuzumab is frequently used as second-line agent, but is recommended as first line in specific patient populations. In 2013, obinutuzumab was approved in combination with chlorambucil for untreated CLL. As with rituximab, it is recommended that patients be screened for Hepatitis B and monitored during treatment with obinutuzumab.

Combination Therapy

The combination of fludarabine, cyclophosphamide, and rituximab (FCR regimen) is recommended as first-line regimen following a study which demonstrated superiority over fludarabine and cyclophosphamide (FC) in untreated patients. Multiple rituximab based combinations have demonstrated clinical benefit. Alemtuzumab has also been combined with fludarabine or rituximab for additional treatment options. Factors taken into consideration for treatment options include comorbidities, age (≥70), and cytogenetics.

Targeted Therapy

Recently, there has been the emergence of novel oral therapies for the treatment of CLL which has changed the landscape of treatment. Ibrutinib, a novel Bruton's tyrosine kinase (BTK) inhibitor was approved by the FDA in 2014 and is now indicated as frontline therapy option in CLL. Several clinical studies have demonstrated positive efficacy even in patients with high-risk cytogenetics (17 p deletion) CLL. Ibrutinib is associated with diarrhea, fatigue, fever, and nausea. In select CLL patients receiving ibrutinib, lymphocytosis will occur but is not an indicator of disease progression.

Idelalisib is an oral phosphatidylinositol 3-kinase (PI3K) inhibitor indicated for relapsed CLL. In combination with rituximab, idelalisib (150 mg po twice daily) has significantly improved 12-month overall survival in relapsed CLL patients who were unable to tolerate other therapies. Toxicities are significant concern with idelalisib which has the following FDA Black Box Warnings—hepatotoxicity, severe diarrhea or colitis, pneumonitis, infections, and GI perforations. Both idelalisib and ibrutinib are substrates to CYP3A4 and thus require vigilance in the monitoring of drug interactions.

Venetoclax is an oral BCL-2 inhibitor approved for the treatment of CLL with 17p deletion who have received at least one prior therapy. This agent is associated with a high risk of TLS and requires prophylactic hydration and antihyperuricemics prior to the first dose. Venetoclax is initiated at a dose of 20 mg/d for 1 week prior to weekly dose escalations up to a maximum of 400 mg/d. Other Grade 3/4 adverse events include neutropenia, anemia, and thrombocytopenia. To avoid increased toxicity potential, concurrent administration of strong CYP3A4 and p-glycoprotein (P-gp) inhibitors are contraindicated.

SPECIAL CONSIDERATIONS

Appropriate supportive care for CLL patients is essential. It is recommended that patients with hypogammaglobulinemia who experience reoccurring infections particularly with encapsulated organisms receive monthly intravenous immunoglobulins (IVIG) 0.3 to 0.5 g/kg. Dosing should be titrated to maintain a serum IgG level of approximately 500 mg/dL. Patients should also be given an annual influenza vaccine and a pneumococcal vaccine every 5 years. Also, patients should receive the appropriate aforementioned antimicrobial prophylaxis secondary to drug toxicities.

Chronic Myelogenous Leukemia

Chronic myelogenous leukemia (CML) is a myeloproliferative disorder, which represents approximately 15% of all adult leukemias with a median age of diagnosis of 66 years. The disease results from a translocation of genetic material between the long arms of chromosomes 9 and 22, which is referred to as Ph+. This translocation generates in the BCR-ABL fusion gene which encodes a protein that has constitutively active tyrosine kinase activity. The activated tyrosine kinase triggers multiple downstream pathways which lead to cellular proliferation. BCR-ABL is found in approximately more than 90% of CML patients as well as 15% of patients with ALL.

Patients are often asymptomatic and are diagnosed incidentally. However, some patients will present with symptoms such as early satiety, fatigue, weight loss, night sweats, and bleeding or bruising. Upon physical examination, patients may present with splenomegaly and hepatomegaly. CML has three clinical phases: (1) chronic (CP), (2) accelerated (AP), and (3) blast (BP). Criteria commonly used to define these include the presence of blasts in peripheral blood and bone marrow, peripheral basophilia, thrombocytopenia, clonal evolution, splenomegaly, and anemia. It is recommended as a part of initial evaluation that a physical examination, CBC, platelet count, bone marrow aspirate and biopsy, and cytogenetic analysis be performed.

TREATMENT

Historically, treatment options for CML included busulfan, hydroxyurea, interferon based combinations, and allogeneic stem cell transplants. Imatinib is an oral TKI targeting BCR-ABL and approved following a phase III study demonstrating superiority over interferon-α in combination with cytarabine. Imatinib is first-line treatment for chronic phase CML and continues to demonstrate durable response rates. However, BCR-ABL kinase mutations have been identified that confer differing levels of resistance to imatinib. Second-generation TKIs (eg, dasatinib, nilotinib, bosutinib) have been developed and offer new treatment options for select patients. All three second-generation TKIs have demonstrated clinical

TABLE 15-2   Comparison of BCR-ABL Tyrosine Kinase Inhibitors

	Dose	Indication(s)	Adverse Reactions	Drug Interactions	Contraindications
Imatinib (Gleevec)	400-800 mg po every day	CML-CP, AP, BP Ph+ALL	Cardiovascular, diarrhea, fluid retention, myelosuppression, nausea, rash	Substrate and inhibitor of CYP3A4	None
Dasatinib (Sprycel)	100-140 mg po every day	CML-CP, AP, BP Ph+ ALL	Diarrhea, fluid retention, myelosuppression, pleural effusion, rash	Substrate of CYP3A4	None
Nilotinib (Tasigna)	300- 400 mg po bid	CML-CP, AP	Elevated bilirubin, and lipase, hypokalemia, hypophosphatemia, increased transaminases, myelosuppression, rash, QT prolongation	Substrate of CYP3A4, inhibits CYP3A4, 2C8, 2C9, 2D6	Hypokalemia, hypomagnesium, long QT interval
Bosutinib (Bosulif)	500 mg po every day	CML-CP, AP, BP	Diarrhea, nausea, thrombocytopenia, vomiting, abdominal pain, rash, anemia	Substrate of CYP3A4	None
Ponatinib (Iclusig)	45 mg po every day	CML-CP, AP, BP or Ph+ ALL for whom no other TKI is indicated	Hypertension, cardiac arrhythmias, pancreatitis, neuropathy, rash, abdominal pain, myelosuppression	Substrate CYP2C8 (minor), CYP2D6 (minor), CYP3A4 (minor)	None

Abbreviations: AP, accelerated phase; BP, blast phase; CP, chronic phase.

benefit in patients with resistance and/or intolerance to imatinib. Furthermore, data from the ENESTnd and DASISION studies support frontline therapy for nilotinib and dasatinib in CML-CP patients. The BELA trial demonstrated that bosutinib is effective in CML-CP patients but is associated with higher rates of gastrointestinal toxicity. Until recently, the T315I mutation conferred resistance to all available TKIs and required patients to seek allogeneic stem cell transplants or clinical trials for effective treatment. In February 2012, the FDA approved ponatinib, which appears effective in patients harboring the T315I mutation. Data from clinical trials and postmarketing adverse event reporting indicate that ponatinib is associated with cardiovascular toxicities such as myocardial infarction, blood clots, and stroke. The FDA continues to monitor the risks of benefits of ponatinib. See Table 15-2 for a comparison of these TKIs. Omacetaxine is given subcutaneously and offers a novel treatment option for patient with CML-CP or -AP with resistance and/or intolerance to two or more TKIs. Disease monitoring is essential for the evaluation of the efficacy of current therapy and detection of relapse. Goals included achieving a hematologic response (normalization of blood counts), cytogenetic response (decrease number of Ph+ cells), and molecular response (decrease number of BCR-ABL transcripts by quantitative reverse-transcriptase polymerase chain reaction [RT-PCR]).

SPECIAL CONSIDERATIONS

Treatment options for CML are expensive; the approximate annual costs are the following—imatinib ($92,000), dasatinib ($123,000), nilotinib ($115,000), bosutinib ($118,000), ponatinib ($138,000), and omacetaxine ($28,000—induction, $14,000 per maintenance course). For uninsured patients, pharmacists should encourage and assist in patient enrollment into industry sponsored patient assistance programs. Patients with insurance may incur high copays and seek financial support as well. Pharmacists should be vigilant in monitoring for patient adherence to these agents.

The decision as to which particular agent should be individualized and take into consideration patient-specific information. Patients with a history of hypertension, smoking, cardiovascular disease, chronic obstructive pulmonary disease would be better candidates for nilotinib, to avoid the possible development of pleural effusions. Monitoring is warranted in nilotinib or dasatinib patients with a previous history of congestive heart failure or left ventricular dysfunction because QTc elongation has been noted with both agents. For diabetes patients, hyperglycemia needs to be carefully monitored because it could be exacerbated with the initiation of nilotinib.

CASE Application

For questions 1 to 7 use patient DC vignette.

1. DC is a 59-year-old Caucasian man who reports to his primary care physician complaining of 2-week history of fatigue and fever. A CBC with differential reveals an elevated WBC (25,000 U/L) and profound thrombocytopenia (platelets 30,000 U/L). His peripheral blood has 20% blasts. A bone marrow biopsy was performed and DC was diagnosed with acute myeloid leukemia (AML-M4). Molecular testing revealed—FLT3 negative, NPML1 negative, C-KIT negative. Initial induction therapy should consist of the following:

   a. Mitoxantrone
   b. Cytarabine + idarubicin
   c. Cytarabine + imatinib
   d. Asparaginase

2. Physician asks you about tumor lysis syndrome (TLS) prevention and management for patient DC. Which of the following suggestions should include? Select all that apply.

   a. Initiating allopurinol
   b. Treating electrolyte disturbances

c. Aggressive hydration

d. Minimize hydration

3. TLS is characterized by the following:

a. Hypocalcemia, hypouricemia, hyperkalemia

b. Hyperphosphatemia, hyperkalemia, hyperuricemia

c. Hypercalcemia, hyperkalemia, hypomagnesium

d. Hypokalemia, hyperphosphatemia, hypouricemia

4. Following induction therapy, DC achieves a complete remission. Next month he arrives at your institution to receive high-dose cytarabine (HDAC) for consolidation therapy. You receive the following order—

Cytarabine 3000 mg/m^2 IV Q12 hours days 1, 3, and 5 Patient characteristics: Height 6'0", Weight 165 lb

Which of the following represents a correct dosing strategy for patient DC?

a. Cytarabine 5850 mg IV days 1, 3, and 5

b. Cytarabine 5850 mg IV Q12 hours days 1, 3, and 5

c. Cytarabine 5550 gm IV days 1, 3, and 5

d. Cytarabine 5550 mg IV Q12 hours days 1, 3, and 5

5. Which type of biological safety cabinet (BSC) should the cytarabine be prepared in?

a. Vertical flow, class I

b. Vertical flow, class II

c. Horizontal flow, class II

d. Horizontal flow, class I

6. What toxicities should DC be counseled on prior to receiving high-dose cytarabine?

a. Infusion-related reactions, paralytic ileus, cardiotoxicity

b. Cerebellar toxicity, peripheral neuropathy, infusion-related reactions

c. Nausea, peripheral neuropathy, ocular toxicity

d. Cerebellar toxicity, nausea, ocular toxicity

7. A newly diagnosed patient with acute promyelocytic leukemia (APL) begins treatment with tretinoin 40 mg orally twice daily. Within 48 hours of the initiation, the patient develops fever, dyspnea, and respiratory distress. Which of the following should be immediately initiated to treat apparent differentiation syndrome (DS)?

a. Dexamethasone

b. Acetaminophen

c. Diphenhydramine

d. Epinephrine

For questions 8 to 10 use patient AB vignette.

8. AB is a 60-year-old African American man newly diagnosed with acute lymphoblastic leukemia (ALL). His physician has recommended part A hyper-CVAD regimen (cyclophosphamide, vincristine, doxorubicin, and dexamethasone). Which of the following is a correct dose for doxorubicin?

Patient specifics: Height 5'8", Weight 180 lb

Notable labs: SrCr 1 mg/dL, Total bilirubin 2.5 mg/dL

Dosing recommendations: CrCl <50 mL/min: No dosage adjustment necessary; Serum bilirubin 1.2-3 mg/dL: Administer 50% of dose; Serum bilirubin 3.1-5 mg/dL: Administer 25% of dose.

Regimen

Cyclophosphamide 300 mg/m^2 IV Q12 hours days 1-3

Mesna 600 mg/m^2 CIVI days 1-3

Vincristine 2 mg IV day 4 and 11

Doxorubicin 50 mg/m^2 IV over 24 hours day 4

Dexamethasone 40 mg po days 1-4 and days 11-14

a. 50 mg doxorubicin IV over 24 hours

b. 100 mg doxorubicin IV over 24 hours

c. 75 mg doxorubicin IV over 24 hours

d. 100 mg doxorubicin IV push

9. Why is AB receiving mesna given continuously with cyclophosphamide on days 1-3?

a. Prevention of renal toxicity associated with cyclophosphamide

b. Chemotherapy induced nausea and vomiting prevention

c. Neutropenic fever prophylaxis

d. Reduce incidence of cyclophosphamide-induced hemorrhagic cystitis

10. AB is to receive CNS prophylaxis. Which of the following can be safely administered intrathecally (IT)? Select all that apply.

a. Cytarabine

b. Methotrexate

c. Vincristine

d. Vinblastine

11. You are an oncology pharmacist counseling a parent and their child undergoing treatment for pediatric ALL. Patient will be treated with a Children's Oncology Group (COG) protocol. All of the following adverse events should be discussed with them regarding asparaginase? Select all that apply.

a. Hyperglycemia

b. Risk of allergic reactions

c. Potential for bleeding

d. Alopecia

For questions 12 to 15 use patient TC vignette.

12. TC is a 62-year-old man recently diagnosed with Stage 3 CLL. TC has been recently complaining of painful lymphadenopathies as well as easy bruising. His physician has chosen to begin rituximab for 6 cycles. Which of the following adverse events should be discussed with the patient prior to first cycle infusion? Select all that apply.

a. Hepatitis B reactivation

b. Infusion-related reactions

c. Tumor lysis syndrome
d. Flu-like symptoms

13. Which of the following is true regarding the monoclonal antibody rituximab (Rituxan®)?

    a. Humanized, targets CD33+ myeloid cells
    b. Chimeric, targets CD20+ B cells
    c. Humanized, targets CD52+ lymphocytes
    d. Chimeric, targets CD33+ myeloid cells

14. Patient TC relapses following rituximab therapy and now their oncologist is contemplating an oral therapy option such as ibrutinib, idelalisib, or ventoclax. TC has been experiencing diarrhea episodes from irritable bowel syndrome. Which of the following novel oral therapies should not be recommended for patient TC?

    a. Ibrutinib
    b. Idelalisib
    c. Ventoclax
    d. None of the above

15. For CLL patients such as TC, which of the following agents should be recommended for patients who present with recurrent infections? Select all that apply.

    a. Annual influenza vaccine
    b. Monthly intravenous immunoglobulin (when serum IgG <400 mg/dL)
    c. Pneumococcal vaccine every 5 years
    d. Annual pneumococcal vaccine

For questions 16 to 19, please refer to patient DD vignette.

16. DD is a 55-year-old woman who has been in excellent health until 2 weeks ago. Since that time she has complained about fatigue, night sweats, and early satiety. She presented to her PCP where labs revealed the following—WBC 62,000 mm³, platelets 190,000 mm³, and hemoglobulin 12.3 g/dL.

    She was referred to an oncologist where a bone marrow biopsy was performed.

Cytogenetics: + translocation (9;22)

Diagnosis: chronic myelogenous leukemia (CML)

Which of the following is an approved first-line treatment for CML?

    a. Allogeneic stem cell transplant
    b. Interferon-α + cytarabine
    c. Imatinib (Gleevec)
    d. Sunitinib (Sutent)

17. It is established that DD has chronic phase (CP-CML). Which of the following BCR-ABL inhibitors are FDA labeled for the treatment of CP-CML?

    a. Imatinib only
    b. Imatinib and dasatinib only
    c. Imatinib, dasatinib, and nilotinib
    d. Imatinib, dasatinib, nilotinib, and erlotinib

18. Select the brand name for nilotinib.

    a. Tasigna
    b. Sprycel
    c. Gleevec
    d. Nexavar

19. Which of the following adverse events associated with dasatinib should be discussed with DD? Select all that apply.

    a. Pleural effusion
    b. Bruising
    c. Alopecia
    d. Fatigue

20. QTc monitoring is warranted with which BCR-ABL inhibitor?

    a. Imatinib
    b. Dasatinib
    c. Nilotinib
    d. Bosutinib

TAKEAWAY POINTS ››

- The primary goal of treatment is to induce and maintain a CR.
- Treatment of pediatric ALL is divided into the following phases: induction, consolidation, interim maintenance, delayed intensification, and maintenance. Adult ALL is divided into induction, consolidation, and maintenance.
- Multiple intensive chemotherapy regimens have been shown to provide benefit in adult ALL.
- CNS treatment is performed throughout all phases of ALL therapy. Intrathecal therapy consists of methotrexate and cytarabine, which can be given alone or in combination. Patients with T-cell ALL have an

increased incidence of CNS disease and should receive systemic high-dose methotrexate to penetrate the CNS.

- Treatment of AML is immediately initiated following definitive diagnosis. AML treatment consists of three phases: (1) induction, (2) post-remission, and (3) refractory/relapsed disease. The goal of induction therapy is to induce a CR with a return of normal hematopoiesis.
- AML induction therapy has consisted of the combination of cytarabine with an anthracycline (daunorubicin or idarubicin). A common regimen is "7+3" which combines cytarabine at (100 mg/m²

days 1-7) with idarubicin (12 mg/m² days 1-3) or daunorubicin (60-90 mg/m² days 1-3).

- Post-remission therapy consists of multiple cycles of HDAC.
- Patients will typically receive 6-18 g/m² of cytarabine per cycle in 3 to 4 cycles. Toxicities of HDAC include cerebellar dysfunction, pulmonary edema, pericardial effusion, and conjunctivitis. Renal function should be closely monitored following HDAC administration since renal dysfunction has correlated to cerebellar dysfunction.
- For AML patients who are unable to achieve a CR, refractory/relapsed treatments are available. Cytarabine alone or in combination with fludarabine, mitoxantrone, etoposide, or clofarabine are options.
- At the initiation of tretinoin, patients need to be monitored for retinoic acid syndrome (or differentiation syndrome, DS). DS is associated with respiratory distress, pleural effusions, pulmonary infiltrates, and

fever. This syndrome can be fatal; patients should immediately receive dexamethasone 10 mg IV Q 12 for 3 to 5 days to improve symptoms and decrease mortality.

- CLL is considered incurable and the goals of treatment include palliation and increase duration of life. Standard treatment for CLL may include a period of watchful waiting until progression of disease (eg, high WBC, bulky lymph nodes, symptomatic splenomegaly).
- Imatinib is considered first-line treatment for chronic phase CML and continues to demonstrate durable response rates. However, *BCR-ABL* kinase mutations have been identified that confer differing levels of resistance to imatinib. Second-generation TKIs (eg, dasatinib, nilotinib) have been developed and offer new treatment options for patients. The T315I mutation confers resistance to these TKIs and other therapies, such as ponatinib or omacetaxine, should be considered.

BIBLIOGRAPHY

Chabner BA, Barnes J, Neal J, et al. Targeted therapies: tyrosine kinase inhibitors, monoclonal antibodies, and cytokines. In: Brunton LL, Chabner BA, Knollmann BC, eds. *Goodman & Gilman's The Pharmacological Basis of Therapeutics.* 12th ed. New York, NY: McGraw-Hill; 2011:chap 62.

Chabner BA, Bertino J, Cleary J, et al. Cytotoxic agents. In: Brunton LL, Chabner BA, Knollmann BC, eds. *Goodman & Gilman's The Pharmacological Basis of Therapeutics.* 12th ed. New York, NY: McGraw-Hill; 2011:chap 61.

Kiel PJ, Fausel CA. Chronic leukemias. In: DiPiro JT, Talbert RL, Yee GC, Matzke GR, Wells BG, Posey L, eds. *Pharmacotherapy:*

A Pathophysiologic Approach. 10th ed. New York, NY: McGraw-Hill; 2017:chap 135.

Seung A. Acute leukemias. In: DiPiro JT, Talbert RL, Yee GC, Matzke GR, Wells BG, Posey L, eds. *Pharmacotherapy: A Pathophysiologic Approach.* 10th ed. New York, NY: McGraw-Hill; 2017:chap 134.

Shord SS, Medina PJ. Cancer treatment and chemotherapy. In: DiPiro JT, Talbert RL, Yee GC, Matzke GR, Wells BG, Posey L, eds. *Pharmacotherapy: A Pathophysiologic Approach.* 10th ed. New York, NY: McGraw-Hill; 2017:chap 104.

KEY ABBREVIATIONS

ALL = acute lymphoblastic leukemia
AML = acute myelogenous leukemia
APL = acute promyelocytic leukemia
ATRA = all-trans retinoic acid
BTK = Bruton's tyrosine kinase
CBC = complete blood count
CLL = chronic lymphocytic leukemia
CML = chronic myelogenous leukemia
CNS = central nervous system

CR = complete remission
DS = differentiation syndrome
G6PD = glucose-6-phosphate dehydrogenase
HDAC = high-dose cytarabine
IVIG = intravenous immunoglobulins
PI3K = phosphatidylinositol 3-kinase
TKIs = tyrosine kinase inhibitors
TLS = tumor lysis syndrome

16

Breast Cancer

Robert K. Sylvester, Kyle J. LaPorte, and Lisa Narveson

FOUNDATION OVERVIEW

Mutations of genes controlling cell proliferation and apoptosis are the primary causes of neoplastic diseases and specific gene mutations (*BRCA1, BRCA2, p53, PTEN*) have been identified in breast cancer. Women with mutations in the tumor suppressor genes *BRCA1* and *BRCA2* have a four- to five-fold increased risk for the development of breast cancer (approximate lifetime risk increases from 12% to 45%-65%). In addition, family history, prolonged exposure to estrogen (early menarche, nulliparity, late first pregnancy, late menopause), and age over 40 have been established as risk factors for breast cancer.

Clinical Presentation/Diagnosis

Prior to the development of mammography, breast cancer was diagnosed after a tissue biopsy of a painless breast mass that was palpated during self or clinical breast examination. The increased survival and improved quality of life for women whose breast cancer was diagnosed before it had spread to lymph nodes (micrometastatic disease) or to distant organs (metastatic disease) led to efforts to increase early detection of localized breast cancers. Since the widespread implementation of screening mammography guidelines in the mid-1980s, the majority of breast cancers are diagnosed after tissue biopsy of a suspicious lesion identified by mammography.

After a breast mass is identified, the diagnosis of breast cancer is made by microscopic examination of a tissue biopsy. Breast cancers are categorized by the histologic and biologic characteristics of the cells present in the biopsy specimen. They arise from lobular and ductal epithelial cells and thus are classified as adenocarcinomas. Furthermore, adenocarcinomas of the breast are classified as in situ (cancer confined to site of origin) or invasive (cancer that has spread through tissue barriers and invaded surrounding areas). The pathologic description of breast adenocarcinoma also includes the quantification of receptors present on the surface of the breast cancer cells. Specifically, the pathology report will determine the level of expression of the estrogen receptor (ER), progesterone receptor (PR), and human epidermal growth factor receptor-2 (HER-2). These biologic markers are prognostic for a patient responding to drugs that target these receptors.

Following a positive pathologic review, various imaging strategies (eg, computed tomography [CT] scan, magnetic resonance imaging [MRI], positron-emission tomography [PET] scan, bone scan) are conducted to determine the extent of cancer spread and disease stage.

Pharmacotherapy Overview

The stage of a patient's breast cancer is determined by the size of the primary lesion (T), whether regional lymph nodes contain micrometastatic cancer (N), and whether metastatic disease is present (M). Stage I breast cancer is characterized by a breast tumor less than or equal to 2 cm and regional lymph nodes that do not contain micrometastatic cancer. Stage II breast cancer exists when regional lymph nodes contain cancer or when the primary lesion is more than 5 cm, even though lymph nodes do not contain cancer. Stage III breast cancer exists when either the primary tumor extends into the chest wall or when regional lymph nodes are fixed to surrounding tissue (immobile). Stage IV disease is present when the tumor cells have invaded distant tissue (metastatic disease). Common sites of breast cancer metastases include the bone, liver, and lungs. Survival of women with invasive breast cancer correlates with the stage of disease. Five-year survival rates for women with localized breast cancer (stages I, II), locally advanced breast cancer (stage III), and metastatic breast cancer (stage IV) are 98.8%, 85.2%, and 26.3%, respectively.

The term systemic adjuvant therapy describes the administration of antineoplastic therapy to women after surgical resection of the primary cancer (lumpectomy or modified mastectomy). Systemic adjuvant therapy is administered to eradicate or suppress the growth of breast cancer cells that have spread beyond the breast at the time of surgery. Patients with breast cancers larger than 1 cm or cancer that has spread to lymph nodes at the time of surgery are at an increased risk for cancer recurrence. Administration of systemic adjuvant antineoplastic therapy results in significant improvement in disease free survival (DFS) and overall survival (OS). Genomic tests capable of detecting genes linked to an increased risk for recurrence are useful in identifying patients who may benefit from adjuvant therapy.

The term neoadjuvant therapy describes the administration of antineoplastic therapy prior to surgery. Neoadjuvant therapy has been proven to decrease tumor size,

TABLE 16-1 **Pharmacotherapeutic Classes/Indications for Management of Breast Cancer**

Antineoplastic Class	Effective Drugs	Indications			
		Stage IV (Metastatic)	Stages I-III (Adjuvant)	Stages I-III Neoadjuvant	Prevention
Alkylating agent	Cyclophosphamide (Cytoxan)	√	√	√	
Anthracycline antibiotics	Doxorubicin (Adriamycin)	√	√	√	
	Doxorubicin liposomal (Doxil)	√			
	Epirubicin (Ellence)	√	√		
Antimetabolites	5-Fluorouracil	√	√		
	Capecitabine (Xeloda)	√			
	Methotrexate	√	√		
	Gemcitabine (Gemzar)	√			
Platinum analogs	Carboplatin (Paraplatin)	√	√	√	
	Cisplatin (Platinol)	√			
Microtubule inhibitors (Taxanes)	Paclitaxel (Taxol)	√	√	√	
	Albumin-bound paclitaxel (Abraxane)	√			
	Docetaxel (Taxotere)	√	√		
Microtubule inhibitors (Nontaxane)	Eribulin (Halaven)	√			
Vinca alkaloid	Vinorelbine (Navelbine)	√			
Epothilone	Ixabepilone (Ixempra)	√			
Monoclonal antibodies	Trastuzumab (Herceptin)	√	√	√	
	Bevacizumab (Avastin)	√			
	Pertuzumab (Perjeta)[a]	√		√	
	Ado-trastuzumab emtansine (Kadcyla)	√			
Selective estrogen receptor modulators (SERMs)	Tamoxifen (Nolvadex)	√	√	√	√
	Toremifene (Fareston)	√			
	Raloxifene (Evista)				√
Aromatase inhibitors	Anastrozole (Arimidex)	√	√	√	
	Letrozole (Femara)	√	√	√	
	Exemestane (Aromasin)	√	√	√	
Estrogen receptor antagonist	Fulvestrant (Faslodex)	√			
Signal transduction inhibitor	Lapatinib (Tykerb)	√			
	Everolimus (Afinitor)	√			
	Palbociclib (Ibrance)	√			
	Ribociclib (Kisqali)	√			
	Neratinib (Nerlynx)		√		

[a]First agent to receive FDA label as neoadjuvant therapy.

making possible less extensive surgery and improved post-surgical outcomes. As with adjuvant therapy, neoadjuvant regimens have achieved significant improvements in patient DFS and OS.

Currently, 30 antineoplastic agents are labeled for the treatment of patients with metastatic disease. At least 12 agents are effective in slowing the progression of micrometastatic breast cancer (systemic adjuvant therapy), and two selective estrogen receptor modulators (SERMs) are effective in reducing the risk of women at high risk for developing breast cancer (Table 16-1). The National Comprehensive Cancer Network (NCCN) practice guidelines provide valuable evidence-based recommendations for the use of these agents in the management of breast cancer.

PREVENTION

Tamoxifen is a SERM that is Food and Drug Administration (FDA) indicated for the treatment of metastatic breast cancer and reduction in risk of invasive breast cancer. The recommended duration of tamoxifen administration to reduce the risk of invasive breast cancer is 5 years. SERMs inhibit proliferation of breast cancer by blocking the binding of estrogens to the ER. Tamoxifen is associated with increased risks of the following adverse effects: endometrial cancer, hot flashes, cataracts, vaginal discharge, and thromboembolic events (deep venous thrombosis and pulmonary emboli) in women aged 50 years and older. Women taking tamoxifen who experience changes in vision should have an ophthalmologic examination and women with an intact uterus reporting vaginal spotting should undergo a gynecologic examination.

Raloxifene is a second-generation SERM initially approved by the FDA for treating postmenopausal osteoporosis. Subsequently, raloxifene was also proven as effective as tamoxifen in reducing the risk of invasive breast cancer but associated with a lower incidence of endometrial cancer, thromboembolic events, and cataracts.

Women who are considered "high-risk" can reduce their risk of developing breast cancer by 50% by taking tamoxifen or raloxifene for 5 years. No data have been published establishing that either drug lowers the death rate from breast cancer. While raloxifene has been established as the preferred agent in postmenopausal women because of its superior side effect profile, inadequate data exist to support its use in premenopausal high-risk women. Prior thromboembolic events (deep venous thrombosis, pulmonary emboli, and stroke) are contraindications to the administration of tamoxifen and raloxifene for the prevention of breast cancer. Raloxifene is not indicated in premenopausal women.

The NCCN Breast Cancer Risk Reduction Guidelines also include the aromatase inhibitors (AIs) anastrozole and exemestane as options for postmenopausal women based on published clinical trial data. However, neither medication is FDA labeled for this indication.

TREATMENT

Pharmacotherapy for Patients at Increased Risk of Developing Recurrent Breast Cancer after Surgery (Stages I, II, and III)

At the time of lumpectomy or modified mastectomy, a pathologist determines the size of the patient's mass and performs a microscopic evaluation of regional lymph nodes removed at the time of surgery. If any lymph nodes contain breast cancer, that patient has micrometastatic disease. Women diagnosed with micrometastatic disease or a primary breast cancer more than 1 cm are at an increased risk of subsequently developing metastatic breast cancer.

Systemic adjuvant therapy describes the administration of antineoplastic therapy to women at an increased risk of developing metastatic breast cancer after surgery. Adjuvant hormonal, chemotherapy, and trastuzumab regimens have resulted in statistically significant improvements in both the duration of DFS and OS.

The majority of drugs proven effective in treating patients with metastatic disease have also been proven effective in prolonging the DFS and OS of women at risk of disease recurrence (see Table 16-1). A patient's menopausal status and biologic characteristics of the cancer (ER status, HER-2 status) are critical for selecting appropriate systemic adjuvant antineoplastic regimens.

Adjuvant Endocrine Therapy

Tamoxifen and AIs (anastrozole, letrozole, and exemestane) are effective systemic adjuvant agents for women with ER positive breast cancer. Tamoxifen has achieved improvements in the DFS and OS of both premenopausal and postmenopausal women. The recommended duration of therapy is 5 to 10 years. Adjuvant therapy with AIs is also effective in increasing the DFS and OS of postmenopausal women with ER positive breast cancers. Typically, they are administered for 5-10 years, either as initial therapy or following tamoxifen. Comparative studies have demonstrated that AIs are superior to tamoxifen in postmenopausal women and should be used preferentially. AIs should not be used in premenopausal women.

Neoadjuvant/Adjuvant Cytotoxic Chemotherapy

Many combination cytotoxic chemotherapy regimens are effective in prolonging the DFS and OS. Combinations of cyclophosphamide, doxorubicin, and a taxane administered for 4 to 6 months are examples of preferred regimens.

Neoadjuvant/Adjuvant Targeted Therapy

Combination cytotoxic chemotherapy followed by trastuzumab and pertuzumab has resulted in a significant improvement in the OS of women with early stage HER-2 positive, ER negative breast cancer. Specifically, pertuzumab has been proven effective as neoadjuvant therapy, while trastuzumab has been proven effective in both neoadjuvant and adjuvant combination regimens.

PHARMACOTHERAPY FOR PATIENTS WITH METASTATIC BREAST CANCER (STAGE IV)

Metastatic breast cancer is rarely curable in spite of the availability of drugs that target breast cancer cells. Although at least 50% of women diagnosed with metastatic disease will respond to their initial antineoplastic therapy, most will have progression of the disease within 6 to 8 months. Typically, the duration of remission achieved after subsequent second- and third-line therapies becomes progressively shorter. The median survival of women diagnosed with metastatic breast cancer is approximately 2 years. The biologic characteristics of the breast cancer cells (ER and HER-2 status) and the woman's menopausal status are essential in determining the appropriate treatment.

If a woman's breast cancer expresses ERs and there is no disease in visceral organs, endocrine therapy is the initial therapy. If the breast cancer does not express ERs, or the cancer has spread to visceral organs, cytotoxic chemotherapy is recommended as initial therapy. Trastuzumab, pertuzumab, and ado-trastuzumab emtansine are only indicated for women with breast cancers that overexpress HER-2.

Endocrine Therapy

Fifty to seventy percent of patients with primary or metastatic breast cancer have hormone receptor positive tumors. Three types of endocrine therapy are effective in treating breast cancer. Table 16-2 provides specific dosing regimens and toxicity profiles for these drugs. Sixty to seventy percent of

TABLE 16-2	Medications That Alter Estrogen Effects and Associated Side Effects		
		Dose	**Class Side Effects**
SERMs	Tamoxifen (Nolvadex)	20 mg orally daily	Hot flashes, vaginal discharge, blood coagulation, endometrial cancer
	Toremifene (Fareston)	60 mg orally daily	
Aromatase inhibitors	Anastrozole (Arimidex)	1 mg orally daily	Hot flashes
	Letrozole (Femara)	2.5 mg orally daily	Arthralgias
	Exemestane (Aromasin)	25 mg orally daily	Myalgias
Estrogen antagonist	Fulvestrant (Faslodex)	500 mg IM every 28 d	Hot flashes, injection site reactions

women with ER positive disease respond to initial endocrine treatment. The duration of response is approximately 1 year. A therapeutic trial of several months is recommended since the full therapeutic benefit may not be evident earlier. When disease progression occurs, a trial of an alternative endocrine treatment is recommended until the disease becomes refractory to hormonal treatments. Patients with ER positive disease that progresses during treatment with letrozole or anastrozole may benefit from the combined regimen of exemestane and everolimus or palbociclib and fulvestrant. Ultimately all patients develop refractory ER positive disease and become candidates for cytotoxic chemotherapy.

Selective Estrogen Receptor Modulators Tamoxifen is the SERM of choice for premenopausal women with ER positive breast cancer. The standard dosage regimen is an oral dose of 20 mg administered daily until the patient experiences disease progression. While generally well tolerated, it is imperative that pharmacists counsel women about potential adverse effects and significant drug interactions with paroxetine, fluoxetine, and sertraline. These drugs inhibit CYP2D6 activity, decreasing the conversion of tamoxifen into its active metabolite endoxifen.

Aromatase Inhibitors Anastrozole, letrozole, and exemestane are AIs effective as systemic adjuvant therapy in treating micrometastatic and metastatic breast cancer. Aromatase is an enzyme present in nonovarian tissues (eg, fat and adrenal glands) and is responsible for producing estradiol in postmenopausal women by converting androgen precursors to estradiol. These agents produce their benefit by depleting estradiol production from nonovarian tissues in postmenopausal women. The AIs are considered to be therapeutically equivalent. Commonly prescribed dosing regimens and associated side effects are detailed in Table 16-2. Typically, arthralgias and myalgias are reported by 10% to 20% of women 1 to 2 months after beginning therapy. A trial with an alternative AI is recommended if a patient develops arthralgias and/or myalgias based on reports of individual differences in tolerability.

Pure Estrogen Antagonist Fulvestrant is a pure estrogen antagonist that inhibits ER-mediated gene transcription by binding to and downregulating ERs. It is effective in the treatment for postmenopausal women with ER positive metastatic breast cancer whose disease progresses after antiestrogen therapy. Fulvestrant is administered monthly as a 500 mg intramuscular injection. Common side effects include injection site reactions and hot flashes.

Cytotoxic Chemotherapy

Cytotoxic antineoplastic drugs disrupt DNA replication. Their action is nonspecific and disrupts the replication of neoplastic and normal cells, especially normal cells with more rapid growth rates. Cytotoxic chemotherapy agents share many of the same dose-dependent toxicities. Among these are myelosuppression (neutropenia, thrombocytopenia, anemia), alopecia, mucositis, nausea, and vomiting. Neutropenia and thrombocytopenia are potentially life threatening. Consequently, it is generally recommended that patient's absolute neutrophil count is more than 1500 cells/mm^3 and platelets more than 100,000 cells/mm^3 before any additional doses are administered.

These drugs can be administered as single agents or in combination with one or two additional drugs. In patients with advanced disease, the administration of single-agent chemotherapy offers the advantage of less toxicity while providing efficacy comparable to combination regimens. The NCCN guidelines identify seven "preferred" single chemotherapy agents and multiple "preferred" chemotherapy combinations as appropriate for the treatment of metastatic breast cancer. Approximately 50% of women respond to initial chemotherapy treatment. However, progression of disease typically occurs within 8 months. Patients are switched to a chemotherapy agent from another class if the initial chemotherapy agent is not effective or when their disease progresses. Table 16-3 provides specific dosing regimens and toxicity profiles for these agents.

Alkylating Agents Numerous alkylating agents provide palliative benefit for women with metastatic breast cancer. Cyclophosphamide has proven superior to other agents in this class by achieving overall response rates (partial plus complete responses) in one-third of treated patients. Subsequently, trials of combinations of cyclophosphamide with other cytotoxic chemotherapy agents resulted in response rates up to 50%. Cyclophosphamide is metabolized to reactive electrophilic alkyl groups that bind to nucleophilic groups on nucleotide bases in DNA, thereby disrupting DNA replication.

Antimetabolites Numerous antimetabolites have been proven effective in providing palliative benefit to patients with metastatic breast cancer. Methotrexate and 5-fluorouracil have long been combined with cyclophosphamide and was the standard of care until doxorubicin combinations resulted in higher response rates.

Methotrexate impedes cell growth by inhibiting dihydrofolate reductase, the enzyme needed to reduce folates to the active form (tetrahydrofolic acid) required for purine and

TABLE 16-3 **Cytotoxic Chemotherapy Agents and Associated Side Effects**

Chemotherapy Agent	Dosage Regimen[a]	Side Effects[b]
Alkylating Agent		
Cyclophosphamide (Cytoxan)	500-600 mg/m² IV every 21 d 75-100 mg/m² po days 1-14	Nausea, vomiting, rarely hemorrhagic cystitis
Anthracycline Antibiotics		
Doxorubicin[c] (Adriamycin)	60-75 mg/m² IV every 21 d	Cardiomyopathy, tissue necrosis if extravasation occurs
Doxorubicin liposomal[c] (Doxil)	50 mg/m² IV every 28 d	Cardiomyopathy, tissue necrosis if extravasation occurs, hand-foot syndrome
Epirubicin (Ellence)[c]	60-90 mg/m² IV every 21 d	Cardiomyopathy, tissue necrosis if extravasation occurs
Antimetabolites		
5-Fluorouracil	500-600 mg/m² IV	Diarrhea
Capecitabine[d] (Xeloda)	2000-2500 mg/m² per day po divided twice daily for 14 d of 21 d cycle	Hand-foot syndrome, diarrhea
Gemcitabine (Gemzar)	800-1200 mg/m² IV per week days 1, 8, and 15 of 28 d cycle	Diarrhea
Methotrexate[c,d]	40 mg/m² IV d 1, and 8 every 28 d	Diarrhea
Antimicrotubule Agents		
Taxanes		
Paclitaxel[c] (Taxol)	175 mg/m² IV over 3 h every 3 wk or 80 mg/m² IV over 1 h weekly	Hypersensitivity/infusion reactions, diarrhea, peripheral neuropathy, myalgias, arthralgias, elevated ALT/AST
Albumin-bound paclitaxel[c] (Abraxane)	260 mg/m² over 30 min every 3 wk	Diarrhea, peripheral neuropathy, myalgias, arthralgias, elevated ALT/AST, hypersensitivity/infusion reactions
Docetaxel[c] (Taxotere)	60-100 mg/m² IV over 1 h every 21 d or 35 mg/m² IV over 0.5 h weekly	Hypersensitivity/infusion reactions, diarrhea, peripheral neuropathy, myalgias, arthralgias, elevated ALT/AST, fluid retention
Nontaxane		
Vinorelbine[c] (Navelbine)	25-30 mg/m² IV bolus weekly	Peripheral neuropathy
Eribulin (Halaven)	1.4 mg/m² d 1, and 8 of 21 d cycle	Asthenia/fatigue, peripheral neuropathy, constipation
Ixabepilone[c] (Ixempra)	40 mg/m² IV over 3 h every 21 d	Hypersensitivity/infusion reactions, diarrhea, peripheral neuropathy, myalgias, arthralgias
Platinum analogs		
Carboplatin (Paraplatin)	AUC 2 d 1, 8, and 15 every 21 d or AUC 6 d 1 every 21 d	Peripheral neuropathy, ototoxicity, renal impairment
Cisplatin	75 mg/m² d 1 of 21 d cycle	Peripheral neuropathy, ototoxicity, renal impairment

[a]Multiple single-agent and combination regimens have been proven effective. Confirmation of specific dosage schedule detailed in NCCN Breast Cancer Guidelines or protocol required to ensure patient safety.

[b]Side effects other than common shared toxicities of myelosuppression (neutropenia, thrombocytopenia, anemia), nausea, vomiting, alopecia, and stomatitis.

[c]Dosage adjustment recommended for patients with hepatic dysfunction characterized by elevated serum bilirubin, alanine or aspartate transaminase; see manufacturer's package insert for specifics.

[d]Dosage adjustment recommended for patients with renal dysfunction.

thymidylate synthesis. 5-Fluorouracil is a pyrimidine analogue that is metabolized to fluorodeoxyuridine monophosphate (FdUMP). This metabolite inhibits the enzyme thymidylate synthase which is responsible for thymidine synthesis. Capecitabine is a fluoropyrimidine analog that is administered orally and metabolized to FdUMP, the same active metabolite as 5-fluorouracil. Nonhematologic side effects of note are painful swelling and redness of the hands and feet (hand-foot syndrome), stomatitis (inflammation of mouth), and diarrhea. Patients experiencing painful hand-foot syndrome, stomatitis, or more than four to six stools daily should be instructed to stop taking capecitabine immediately.

The enzyme dihydropyrimidine dehydrogenase (DPD) is responsible for the degradation of 5-fluorouracil to inactive metabolites. Approximately 5% of the population has a DPD deficiency, a contraindication to the administration of capecitabine because of an increased risk of potentially life-threatening mucositis, diarrhea, and myelosuppression. It is also contraindicated in patients with creatinine clearances below 30 mL/min. The ability of 5-fluorouracil and capecitabine to significantly increase warfarin's anticoagulant effects is well documented. Closer monitoring of a patient's international normalized ratio (INR) is required when these drugs are given concomitantly.

Anthracycline Antibiotics Doxorubicin and epirubicin are two anthracycline antibiotics administered as single agents or in combination with other antineoplastic agents as systemic adjuvant treatment or for palliation of symptoms in patients with metastatic breast cancer. They damage DNA by inhibiting the enzyme topoisomerase II that is needed for the normal coiling/uncoiling of DNA and by binding of reactive electrophilic sites on the drugs to nucleophilic nucleotides in DNA.

Cardiomyopathy resulting in congestive heart failure is a dose-related toxicity of anthracyclines. The incidence of cardiomyopathy increases with cumulative doses of both doxorubicin and epirubicin. Therefore, cumulative doses of doxorubicin exceeding 400 mg/m^2 and epirubicin exceeding 900 mg/m^2 should be administered cautiously. These drugs are potent vesicants and can result in severe tissue necrosis at sites of extravasation. They are cleared hepatically. Specific recommendations for dose modification of doxorubicin and epirubicin based on a patient's serum bilirubin and aspartate transaminases are published in the products' FDA approved package inserts.

Microtubule Inhibitors Microtubules are structures critical to the successful completion of cell division (mitosis). Four subclasses of cytotoxic chemotherapy agents that disrupt normal microtubule function are effective in treating breast cancer. Table 16-3 provides commonly prescribed dosing regimens and associated side effects of these agents.

Taxanes Paclitaxel, albumin-bound paclitaxel, and docetaxel bind to β-tubulin, a protein needed to form microtubules. As a result, taxanes inhibit depolymerization of the microtubules, a terminal phase in cell division. Taxanes are effective agents in treating patients with locally advanced and advanced disease.

A prominent side effect of paclitaxel is the occurrence of infusion-related hypersensitivity reactions. Typically, these reactions are characterized by the onset of symptoms (eg, dyspnea, flushing, tachycardia, chest pain) within 1 hour of administration. These symptoms are attributed to mast cell degranulation caused by Cremophor EL, the surfactant used to increase the solubility of paclitaxel. Premedication with corticosteroids, an H1, and an H2 antagonist, is standard of care for any patient receiving paclitaxel.

Abraxane, a nanoparticle albumin-bound paclitaxel formulation, is a paclitaxel formulation that does not contain Cremophor EL and does not require premedication. The reported incidence of hypersensitivity reactions are 4% for nanoparticle albumin-bound paclitaxel and 12% for paclitaxel. Paclitaxel is contraindicated in patients with a documented history of a hypersensitivity reaction to Cremophor EL and/or paclitaxel.

Docetaxel is contraindicated in patients with a history of severe hypersensitivity reactions. Fluid retention occurs in nearly 25% of patients. Dexamethasone the day before, the day of, and the day after docetaxel therapy is recommended to attenuate this adverse effect.

Epothilones Ixabepilone is the prototype semisynthetic analog of epothilone B. It inhibits the depolymerization of microtubules by binding to a β-tubulin site different than the taxane binding site. Ixabepilone should be dose adjusted in patients with impaired hepatic function. Cremophor EL is used to increase ixabepilone solubility. Premedication with an H1 and an H2 antagonist an hour prior to administering ixabepilone is recommended in order to minimize hypersensitivity reactions. If a patient develops a hypersensitivity reaction, the addition of dexamethasone to the pretreatment regimen is recommended. Ixabepilone is contraindicated in patients with a history of hypersensitivity reactions to drugs formulated with Cremophor EL.

Vinca Alkaloids Vinorelbine is a semisynthetic vinca alkaloid that impedes mitosis by inhibiting the formation of functioning microtubules. It should be administered with caution to patients with elevated serum bilirubin levels. If a patient's serum bilirubin level is between 2.1 and 3 mg/dL, a 50% dosage reduction is recommended; if a patient's serum bilirubin level exceeds 3 mg/dL, a 75% dosage reduction is recommended.

Halichondrins Eribulin is a microtubule inhibitor that works similar to vinca alkaloids. Its side effects are similar to the vinca alkaloids but with a lower incidence of neuropathy.

Targeted Therapies

Monoclonal Antibodies Trastuzumab, ado-trastuzumab, pertuzumab, and bevacizumab are humanized monoclonal antibodies approved for the treatment of metastatic breast cancer. Table 16-4 provides specific dosing regimens and toxicity profiles of these agents.

Twenty to thirty percent of patients have breast cancers that overexpress the HER-2. Trastuzumab was developed to bind to the HER-2 receptor. This interaction may cause cell death by several mechanisms. Cell lysis may result from the activation of the complement cascade and/or the enhanced recognition of the antibody-tagged cells by cytotoxic T lymphocytes. Cell growth may also be impeded by the inhibition of normal intracellular signaling pathways that occurs when the binding of growth factor to growth factor receptor is blocked.

In 2013, pertuzumab became the first antineoplastic agent to receive an FDA label for neoadjuvant treatment of patients with early stage HER-2-positive breast cancer. Pertuzumab administered in combination with trastuzumab and docetaxel resulted in superior pathological complete response rates compared to competing regimens. This combination is also approved for the treatment of patients with metastatic breast cancer.

Ado-trastuzumab emtansine is a HER-2-targeted antibody-drug conjugate. The antibody is the humanized anti-HER-2, trastuzumab that has the microtubule inhibitor DM1 attached to it. After binding to HER-2, ado-trastuzumab emtansine undergoes internalization and subsequent lysosomal degradation, resulting in intracellular release of DM1 containing cytotoxic catabolites. Binding of DM1 to tubulin disrupts microtubule function leading to cell cycle arrest and apoptotic cell death. This drug is indicated, as a single agent, for the treatment of patients with HER-2-positive, metastatic breast cancer who previously received trastuzumab and a taxane therapy.

TABLE 16-4	Monoclonal Antibodies and Associated Side Effects	
Monoclonal Antibody	Dosage Regimen[a]	Side Effects
Targets HER-2		
Trastuzumab (Herceptin)	Initial dose of 4 mg/kg as a 90 min IV infusion followed by subsequent weekly doses of 2 mg/kg as 30 min IV infusions (as tolerated)	Infusion reactions, fever, chills, congestive heart failure, cough, diarrhea, headache
Pertuzumab (Perjeta)	Initial dose of 840 mg administered as a 60-min intravenous infusion, followed every 3 wk by a dose of 420 mg administered as an intravenous infusion over 30 to 60 min	Infusion reactions, fever, chills, left ventricular dysfunction, stomatitis, diarrhea, headache, dysgeusia, rash, hypersensitivity
Ado-trastuzumab emtansine (Kadcyla)	3.6 mg/kg as an intravenous infusion every 3 weeks	Nausea, fatigue, musculoskeletal pain, thrombocytopenia, increased transaminases, anemia, headache constipation, peripheral neuropathy, infusion reaction
Targets VEGF		
Bevacizumab (Avastin)	10 mg/kg every 2 wk as IV infusion: First infusion: Administer over 90 min Subsequent infusions: Administer second infusion over 60 min if first infusion is tolerated; administer all subsequent infusions over 30 min if infusion over 60 min is tolerated as IV infusion	Infusion reactions, chills, fever, hypertension, proteinuria, thromboembolic events, gastrointestinal perforation

[a]Multiple regimens have been proven effective. Confirmation of specific dosage schedule detailed in NCCN Breast Cancer Guidelines or protocol required to ensure patient safety.

Bevacizumab is a monoclonal antibody developed to bind to and inhibit vascular endothelial growth factor (VEGF). VEGF is the endogenous protein produced by cells to stimulate the growth of blood vessels in the vicinity of its release. The scientific term for this process is angiogenesis. Bevacizumab possesses antiangiogenic activity by binding to and blocking VEGF from binding to cell receptors that stimulate angiogenesis. Bevacizumab was granted accelerated approval for the treatment of metastatic breast cancer based on improvement of patient progression-free survival. That indication was withdrawn in 2011 after data ultimately documented that bevacizumab did not increase OS.

Signal Transduction Inhibitors Lapatinib is the first signal transduction inhibitor active against breast cancer cells. It is approved to be given with capecitabine as a combination treatment of metastatic breast cancer for patients with HER-2 positive disease that has progressed after therapy with an anthracycline, a taxane, and trastuzumab. It inhibits intracellular tyrosine kinase activity of epidermal growth factor receptor-1 (EGFR-1) and EGFR-2. Lapatinib should be taken at least 1 hour before or after a meal. This instruction is important because lapatinib taken within 1 hour of a meal has resulted in mean area under the curve (AUC) increases ranging from 167% to 325%. Lapatinib is extensively metabolized by CYP3A4. Consequently, significant drug interactions can occur when lapatinib is administered concurrently with strong inhibitors or inducers of CYP3A4. It is recommended that concurrent administration of lapatinib with strong CYP3A4 inhibitors (eg, azole antifungal agents, protease inhibitors) and strong CYP3A4 inducers (ie, carbamazepine, dexamethasone, phenytoin, rifampin, phenobarbital) be avoided. If concurrent administration cannot be avoided, it is imperative to cautiously titrate the dose of lapatinib based on patient tolerability.

Approved for the extended adjuvant treatment of patients with early stage HER-2-positive breast cancer following adjuvant trastuzumab-based therapy, neratinib is an irreversible tyrosine kinase inhibitor of HER-1, HER-2, HER-4, and EGFR receptors. Neratinib is given orally once daily with food for a total duration of 1 year. Dose reduction may be needed for patients who exhibit hepatic impairment prior to, or during therapy. Additionally, neratinib is extensively metabolized by CYP3A4. Consequently, significant drug interactions can occur when administered concurrently with strong inhibitors or inducers of CYP3A4. Therefore, it is recommended that concurrent administration with strong CYP3A4 inhibitors and strong CYP3A4 inducers be avoided. Common adverse reactions include diarrhea, nausea, vomiting, abdominal pain, fatigue, rash, stomatitis, and increase in liver function tests. With the most common adverse reaction leading to discontinuation being diarrhea, it is recommended that patients receive antidiarrheal prophylaxis with loperamide for the first 2 cycles.

The combination of everolimus and exemestane has been proven effective in benefiting patients with ER positive disease that progressed during treatment with letrozole or anastrozole. Everolimus is an inhibitor of mammalian target of rapamycin (mTOR), a serine-threonine kinase, downstream of the PI3K/AKT pathway. The mTOR pathway is dysregulated in several human cancers including breast cancer.

Palbociclib is approved for treatment of HR-positive, HER-2-negative metastatic breast cancer, in combination with an AI as initial endocrine therapy in postmenopausal women or in combination with fulvestrant in women with disease progression following endocrine therapy. It is an inhibitor of cyclin-dependent kinases (CDK) 4 and 6, which are downstream signaling pathways leading to cellular proliferation. Plasma concentrations of palbociclib may be increased when administered concomitantly with strong CYP3A4 inhibitors (ie, itraconazole, posaconazole, voriconazole). Plasma concentrations of palbociclib may be decreased when coadministered with strong CYP3A4 inducers (ie, phenytoin, rifampin, carbamazepine, enzalutamide).

TABLE 16-5	**Signal Transduction Inhibitors and Associated Side Effects**	
Signal Transduction Inhibitor	**Dosage Regimen**	**Side Effects**
Targets EGFR-1, EGFR-2		
Lapatinib (Tykerb)	1250 mg po once daily at least 1 h before or 1 h after a meal on days 1-21 continuously	Maculopapular rash, diarrhea, decreased left ventricular ejection fraction, rarely severe hepatotoxicity
Neratinib (Nerlynx)	240 mg po once daily with food. Antidiarrheal prophylaxis with loperamide recommended for first 2 cycles	Diarrhea, nausea, vomiting, abdominal pain, skin rash, fatigue, hepatotoxicity
Targets mTOR		
Everolimus (Afinitor)	10 mg po once daily at the same time every day. Administer either consistently with food or consistently without food	Stomatitis, infections, rash, fatigue, diarrhea, decreased appetite, hyperglycemia, dyspnea, pneumonitis, increased transaminases, leukopenia, thrombocytopenia
Targets CDK 4 and 6		
Palbociclib (Ibrance)	125 mg po once daily at the same time on days 1-21 of 28-d cycle in combination with letrozole or fulvestrant. Should be taken with food	Fatigue, nausea, anemia, stomatitis, headache, diarrhea, thrombocytopenia, constipation, alopecia, vomiting, rash, and decreased appetite
Ribociclib (Kasqali)	600 mg po once daily at the same time on days 1-21 of 28-d cycle in combination with aromatase inhibitor. May be taken with or without food	Fatigue, nausea, headache, diarrhea, leukopenia, neutropenia, constipation, alopecia, vomiting, back pain, decreased appetite, abnormal liver function tests, and QT interval prolongation

Similarly to palbociclib, ribociclib is approved for treatment of HR-positive, HER-2-negative, metastatic breast cancer, in combination with an AI as initial endocrine-based therapy in postmenopausal women. It also is an inhibitor of CDK 4 and 6. In the same manner as palbociclib, plasma concentrations of ribociclib may be increased when administered concomitantly with strong CYP3A4 inhibitors, and coadministration should be avoided if possible. Similarly, plasma concentrations of ribociclib may be decreased when coadministered with strong CYP3A4 inducers.

Table 16-5 provides the recommended dosing regimens and associated adverse events for signal transduction inhibitors approved for the treatment of breast cancer.

CASE Application

1. Select the agent that is administered via intramuscular injection for the treatment of metastatic ER positive breast cancer.

    a. Anastrozole
    b. Avastin
    c. Herceptin
    d. Faslodex

2. Which of the following conditions would be a contraindication to administration of tamoxifen for the prevention of breast cancer in a "high-risk" premenopausal patient?

    a. History of deep venous thrombosis
    b. First-degree relative with ER negative breast cancer
    c. History of diabetes mellitus
    d. History of seizures

3. A premenopausal woman with ER negative, node positive breast cancer is starting doxorubicin and cyclophosphamide adjuvant treatment. What would you recommend to determine the severity of the most common toxicity associated with this treatment regimen?

    a. An electrocardiogram
    b. A complete blood count including platelets 1 week after administration of the chemotherapy
    c. Serum bilirubin and aspartate transaminase
    d. Urinalysis

4. Select the toxicity that has been associated with the administration of both trastuzumab and bevacizumab.

    a. Myelosuppression
    b. Gastrointestinal (GI) perforation
    c. Alopecia
    d. Infusion reactions

5. Which of the following medications are recommended to be administered prior to an infusion of paclitaxel in order to prevent infusion reactions? Select all that apply.

    a. Dexamethasone
    b. Ranitidine
    c. Meperidine
    d. Diphenhydramine
    e. Acetaminophen

6. A patient taking capecitabine for metastatic breast cancer describes to you the development of tenderness on her hands and feet, making it difficult for her to be on her feet. Select the most appropriate recommendation for this patient.

    a. Her symptoms describe the onset of a known side effect of capecitabine. You recommend she call her physician and describe the onset of these symptoms before taking any more doses of capecitabine.

b. Her symptoms are classic for individuals with vitamin B6 deficiency. You recommend she schedule an appointment with her physician to discuss these symptoms.

c. Her symptoms are commonly caused by capecitabine. You reassure her that there is nothing to worry about and recommend she avoid standing as much as possible while she completes the last week of capecitabine.

d. Her symptoms are commonly caused by capecitabine. You recommend the symptoms are self-limiting and easily managed by spraying her hands and feet with benzocaine first-aid spray four times daily.

7. A patient presents her prescription for capecitabine to you. Review of her medication profile documents she is also taking 5 mg of warfarin daily for atrial fibrillation and metformin for type II diabetes mellitus. Select the appropriate assessment of potential drug interactions for this patient.

a. Capecitabine has been shown to increase metabolism of warfarin and result in subtherapeutic INRs. More frequent monitoring of this patient's INRs is recommended.

b. Capecitabine has been shown to decrease metabolism of warfarin and result in elevated INRs and bleeding. More frequent monitoring of this patient's INRs is recommended.

c. Capecitabine has been shown to decrease metabolism of metformin and result in hypoglycemia. The importance of scheduled blood glucose monitoring and possible need for holding metformin doses needs to be discussed with this patient.

d. Capecitabine has been shown to increase metabolism of metformin and result in hyperglycemia. The importance of daily blood glucose monitoring and possible need for increasing metformin doses needs to be discussed with this patient.

e. Metformin has been shown to decrease metabolism of capecitabine and result in the increased severity of capecitabine induced-myelosuppression. A 25% reduction in the dose of capecitabine is indicated.

8. A patient presents a new prescription to you for tamoxifen. Her doctor said he was prescribing it as adjuvant treatment for breast cancer following her surgery last month. You review her medication profile and document that she is also taking metoprolol, hydrochlorothiazide, and fluoxetine. Select the appropriate assessment of potential drug interactions for this patient.

a. There are no clinically significant drug interactions to alter her medication regimen.

b. You explain that a number of selective serotonin reuptake inhibitors (SSRIs) including fluoxetine decrease the effectiveness of tamoxifen by interfering with its metabolism to an active metabolite. You will call the patient's physician to consider alternative antidepressant options.

c. You explain that hydrochlorothiazide has been documented to decrease the effectiveness of tamoxifen by interfering with its metabolism to an active metabolite. You will call the patient's physician to consider alternative diuretic.

d. You explain that metoprolol has been documented to decrease the effectiveness of tamoxifen by interfering with its metabolism to an active metabolite. You will call the patient's physician to consider alternative β-blocker.

9. Select the endocrine therapy associated with an increased incidence of endometrial cancer.

a. Letrozole
b. Raloxifene
c. Toremifene
d. Fulvestrant
e. Tamoxifen

10. Which of following conditions would be a contraindication for prescribing an AI?

a. The development of arthralgias and myalgias
b. A patient with a history of thromboembolic events
c. A premenopausal patient
d. A postmenopausal patient with a history of thromboembolic events
e. There are no contraindications for the administration of AIs

11. Which of the following statements are true regarding palbociclib? Select all that apply.

a. It is a signal transduction inhibitor that inhibits CDK 4 and 6.
b. It is a signal transduction inhibitor that inhibits intracellular tyrosine kinase activity at EGFR-1 and EGFR-2.
c. It is approved for treatment of ER positive and HER-2 negative metastatic breast cancer, in combination with letrozole as initial endocrine therapy for postmenopausal women.
d. It is approved in combination with fulvestrant for metastatic disease, following progression on endocrine therapy.
e. It is approved as monotherapy for patients with metastatic disease.

12. Select the brand name for letrozole.

a. Arimidex
b. Nolvadex
c. Avastin
d. Evista
e. Femara

13. Select the taxane effective in treating advanced breast cancer that is formulated as an albumin nanoparticle product.

a. Abraxane
b. Taxol

c. Jevtana

d. Taxotere

14. A 69-year-old woman is taking anastrozole for ER positive/PR positive, HER-2 negative stage IV breast cancer. Upon returning for her third refill she tells you that she has noticed increased stiffness and joint pain in knees. She started taking ibuprofen 400 mg four times daily and at bedtime without much benefit for the past week. Your recommendation is to:

   a. Increase the ibuprofen dosage to 800 mg four times daily and at bedtime.

   b. The symptoms of joint and muscle pain are likely caused by anastrozole. You offer to call her physician to discuss switching to letrozole or exemestane.

   c. The symptoms are consistent with a hypersensitivity reaction to anastrozole. You recommend she take some diphenhydramine and go to the emergency room for evaluation.

   d. The symptoms have not been associated with anastrozole; she is likely developing rheumatoid arthritis.

15. MK is a 63-year-old woman with newly diagnosed metastatic breast cancer scheduled to receive her first dose of trastuzumab. She is 5' 6" tall and weighs 175 lb. You receive the following order: trastuzumab 440 mg IV infusion over 1.5 hours. Select the appropriate assessment to discuss with the prescriber.

   a. Trastuzumab causes significant nausea and vomiting warranting premedication with a serotonin antagonist antiemetic. It would be best to call the prescriber and suggest administration of an antiemetic.

   b. Trastuzumab can safely be administered as an IV bolus injection. It would be appropriate to call the prescriber and suggest the order be changed to be administered as an IV bolus injection.

   c. Trastuzumab has been shown effective as an adjuvant treatment but not treatment of metastatic disease. It would be appropriate to call the prescriber and clarify the indication for trastuzumab for this patient.

   d. The recommended initial dose of trastuzumab is 4 mg/kg (320 mg total for this patient). It would be appropriate to call the prescriber and clarify dosage for this patient.

   e. Trastuzumab ordered appropriately for this patient. No clarification is indicated.

16. JK is a 48-year-old woman scheduled to receive her first 175 mg/m^2 dose of paclitaxel for metastatic breast cancer. She is 5'3" tall and weighs 127 lb. Using the Mosteller formula (BSA (m^2) = $\sqrt{\text{Ht [cm]} \times \text{Wt [kg]}/3600}$) what dose of paclitaxel would you prepare?

   a. 2780 mg

   b. 278 mg

   c. 412 mg

   d. 4120 mg

17. You receive the following order for a patient with stage IV breast cancer. Albumin-bound paclitaxel 470 mg administer as an IV infusion at a rate of 10 mg/min. You verify that an appropriate dose is 260 mg/m^2 administered over 30 minutes. The patient has a BSA of 1.81 m^2. Is this dose and infusion rate ordered correctly?

   a. Yes, the order is correct.

   b. No, the order is incorrect because the dose and the infusion rate are miscalculated.

   c. No, the order is incorrect because the dose is correct, but the infusion rate should be 15 mg/min.

   d. No, the order is incorrect because the infusion rate is correct but the dose is miscalculated.

18. A 65-year-old patient brings in her tamoxifen prescription for a refill. Upon reviewing her medication profile, you discover that she began taking tamoxifen 20 mg daily in June 2000 for the prevention of breast cancer and she has been having it refilled regularly since then. What if anything should you discuss with the patient's physician?

   a. The recommended duration of tamoxifen when prescribed to decrease the risk of breast cancer is 10 years. There is no need to clarify this patient's tamoxifen regimen.

   b. The merits of increasing the dose to 40 mg daily based on results of a recent study documenting superior efficacy of a 40 mg daily dose.

   c. Switching this patient to an AI based on recent studies that have documented improvement in efficacy and tolerability with AIs.

   d. The merits of decreasing the dose to 10 mg daily based on results of a recent study documenting equal efficacy but superior tolerability of a 20 mg daily dose.

   e. The recommended duration of tamoxifen when prescribed to decrease the risk of breast cancer is 5 years.

19. This patient asks you if you could recommend a dietary supplement that has been proven effective in decreasing the risk of breast cancer.

   a. You explain that vitamin A 100 IU daily has been proven effective to decrease the risk of breast cancer.

   b. You explain that vitamin D 200 mg daily has been proven effective to decrease the risk of breast cancer.

   c. You explain that vitamin C 500 IU daily has been proven effective to decrease the risk of breast cancer.

   d. You explain that there are not any dietary supplements that have been proven effective in lowering the risk of breast cancer.

   e. You explain that vitamin E 100 IU daily has been proven effective to decrease the risk of breast cancer.

20. Which of the following organizations publishes on their website evidence-based clinical practice guidelines for cancers that affect over 90% of patients with cancer?

   a. The American Cancer Society

   b. The Eastern Cooperative Oncology Group

c. NCCN

d. The National Cancer Institute

e. The American Society of Health-System Pharmacy

21. Which of the following antineoplastic agents are likely to cause arthralgias and myalgias? Select all that apply.

a. Docetaxel, ixabepilone, letrozole, exemestane

b. Paclitaxel, ixabepilone, anastrozole

c. Anastrozole, exemestane

d. Letrozole, anastrozole, exemestane

22. Which of the following antineoplastic agents are vesicants? Select all that apply.

a. 5-Fluorouracil

b. Fulvestrant

c. Doxorubicin

d. Methotrexate

e. Epirubicin

23. Which of the following antineoplastic agents would be effective as adjuvant therapy for postmenopausal patients with breast cancer that is ER negative and does not over-express HER-2? Select all that apply.

a. Cyclophosphamide

b. Epirubicin

c. Doxorubicin

d. Letrozole

24. The goal of neoadjuvant chemotherapy is to:

a. Eradicate micrometastatic disease following localized modalities such as surgery or radiation or both.

b. Attempt to shrink large tumors and make them more amenable to subsequent surgical resection.

c. Reduce the symptoms of the cancer without affecting the underlying tumor.

d. Rapidly treat and reduce tumor volume for a cure without other treatment modalities.

TAKEAWAY POINTS »

- Thirty antineoplastic agents representing nine distinct classes of antineoplastic agents are effective in managing breast cancer.

- Multiple antineoplastic regimens are effective in neoadjuvant, adjuvant, and advanced stage patients. Confirmation of specific dosage schedule detailed in clinical practice guidelines or protocols such as NCCN Breast Cancer Guidelines is required to ensure patient safety.

- The selection of an antineoplastic regimen for a patient is individualized based on the size and anatomical location (staging) of the cancer, the patient's menopausal status, and biologic markers (ERs, HER-2) identified on the breast cancer cells.

- Cytotoxic chemotherapy is the preferred treatment regimen for women with breast cancer that is ER negative or hormone refractory.

- Myelosuppression is the most common dose-related toxicity associated with cytotoxic chemotherapy.

- Single-agent endocrine therapy with a selective ER modulator is the preferred initial treatment for premenopausal women with ER positive disease.

- Single-agent endocrine therapy with an AI is the preferred initial treatment for postmenopausal women with ER positive disease.

- The monoclonal antibodies trastuzumab, ado-trastuzumab emtansine, and pertuzumab, and the signal transduction inhibitors lapatinib and neratinib are only indicated for the treatment of women who overexpress the HER-2. Approximately 30% of women with breast cancer overexpress HER-2.

- The administration of antineoplastic agents effective in treating metastatic breast cancer is palliative, not curative.

- Clinically significant drug interactions have been documented with capecitabine, 5-fluorouracil, tamoxifen, lapatinib, neratinib, palbociclib, and ribociclib.

BIBLIOGRAPHY

Barnett CM, Michaud L. Breast cancer. In: DiPiro JT, Talbert RL, Yee GC, Matzke GR, Wells BG, Posey L, eds. *Pharmacotherapy: A Pathophysiologic Approach.* 10th ed. New York, NY: McGraw-Hill; 2017:chap 128.

Breast Cancer. NCCN Practice Guidelines in Oncology—V.2.2016. http://www.nccn.org/professionals/physician_gls/pdf/breast.pdf.

Breast Cancer Risk Reduction. NCCN Practice Guidelines in Oncology—V.1.2017. http://www.nccn.org/professionals/physician_gls/pdf/breast_risk.pdf.

Chabner BA, Bertino J, Cleary J, et al. Cytotoxic agents. In: Brunton LL, Chabner BA, Knollmann BC, eds. *Goodman & Gilman's The Pharmacological Basis of Therapeutics.* 12th ed. New York, NY: McGraw-Hill; 2011:chap 61.

Chu E, Sartorelli AC. Cancer chemotherapy. In: Katzung BG, Masters SB, Trevor AJ, eds. *Basic & Clinical Pharmacology.* 12th ed. New York, NY: McGraw-Hill; 2012:chap 54.

Higa G. Breast cancer. In: Chisholm-Burns MA, Wells BG, Schwinghammer TL, Malone PM, Kolesar JM, DiPiro JT, eds. *Pharmacotherapy Principles and Practice.* 3rd ed. New York, NY: McGraw-Hill; 2013:chap 89.

KEY ABBREVIATIONS

CT = computed tomography
DFS = disease free survival
DNA = deoxyribonucleic acid
DPD = dihydropyrimidine dehydrogenase
EFGR = epidermal growth factor receptor
ER = estrogen receptor
FDA = Food and Drug Administration
FdUMP = fluorodeoxyuridine monophosphate
GI = gastrointestinal
INR = international normalized ratio

MRI = magnetic resonance imaging
mTOR = mammalian target of rapamycin
NCCN = National Comprehensive Cancer Network
NSABP = National Surgical Adjuvant Breast Project
OS = overall survival
PET = positron-emission tomography
PR = progesterone receptor
SERM = selective estrogen receptor modulator
SSRI = selective serotonin reuptake inhibitor
VEGF = vascular endothelial growth factor

17

Solid Organ Transplantation

Jeong M. Park and Natalia M. Jasiak

FOUNDATION OVERVIEW

Rejection is a primary barrier to success of solid organ transplantation. There are three types of graft rejection that can occur after solid organ transplantation: antibody-mediated, acute cellular, and chronic rejection. Antibody-mediated rejection is mediated by donor-specific antibodies against human leukocyte antigens or other antigens and typically occurs intraoperatively or within days after receiving ABO blood type mismatched or positive crossmatch organ transplant. Avoiding mismatched transplant or desensitizing recipients with known detectable donor-specific antibodies may prevent this mode of rejection, but treating antibody-mediated rejection remains challenging. Acute cellular rejection (ACR) is the most common type of rejection and is generally reversible with appropriate diagnosis and timely treatment. It results from an orchestrated immune response that involves alloantigen presentation by antigen presenting cells (APCs) that leads to alloreactive T cells. The cytotoxic T cells infiltrate the graft and cause direct tissue damage, whereas the helper T cells produce cytokines to cause subsequent immunological and inflammatory events. Although ACR can occur anytime following transplant, the risk is highest in the first several months after transplant. Prevention and treatment of ACR is of utmost importance, as it is a significant predictor of chronic rejection. The exact etiology of chronic rejection is unknown. It is a slow process of graft fibrosis and arteriopathy, which results in graft dysfunction, usually manifested years after transplantation. While ACR can be treated pharmacologically, the only therapy for chronic rejection is retransplantation.

Signs and symptoms of rejection are nonspecific pain and tenderness over graft site, fever, and lethargy. The diagnosis of rejection is made based on histologic evidence of tissue injury from a biopsy specimen of the transplant organ. Presence of circulating donor-specific antibodies is also required for the diagnosis of antibody-mediated rejection. If left untreated, rejection leads to clinically significant organ dysfunction and graft loss.

PREVENTION OF REJECTION

Immunosuppression Regimen

Over the last 40 years, advances in immunosuppression have contributed to the improvement in patient and graft survival rates following solid organ transplantation largely by preventing ACR. The goal of immunosuppression after solid organ transplantation is to prevent graft rejection and to minimize the undue side effects such as infection, malignancy, and drug toxicity. In order to achieve this goal, a combination of immunosuppressant drugs with different mechanisms of action is employed at relatively low doses. The mainstay of current maintenance immunosuppressive regimens (the "triple drug regimen") includes a calcineurin inhibitor (tacrolimus or cyclosporine), an antiproliferative agent (mycophenolate or azathioprine), and corticosteroids (Table 17-1). The most common initial regimen consists of tacrolimus, mycophenolate mofetil, and prednisone. Typically, these agents are used in high doses in the early weeks post-transplant, with dosages tapering down as the risk of ACR decreases. In addition to the maintenance immunosuppression, antibody induction (antithymocyte globulins [ATGs], alemtuzumab, or basiliximab) can be used at the time of transplant in select patients. Antibody induction therapy has shown to reduce ACR rates compared to no induction at all. In an effort to further minimize the negative sequelae of immunosuppression, steroid- and calcineurin inhibitor-sparing regimens (including belatacept or mammalian target of rapamycin [mTOR] inhibitors) may be used in carefully selected patients.

Corticosteroids

Corticosteroids are the oldest element of the triple drug regimen and suppress both inflammation and immune activation. Their immunosuppressive effects are exerted on the entire process of immune activation, including antigen presentation by APCs, cytokine release including but not limited to interleukins (such as IL-1, IL-2, IL-6) and tumor necrosis factor α (TNF α), and subsequently lymphocyte proliferation. Typically, doses are higher during the immediate post-transplant period and then are tapered down. Side effects vary by both the dose and the duration of therapy. At high doses, patients can experience neurotoxicity ranging from headache, mood disturbance, and insomnia to psychosis. Additional adverse events include electrolyte disturbances and fluid retention, glucose intolerance, and leukocytosis. The severity of these adverse effects will diminish as the dose is reduced. Long-term use of corticosteroids can lead to Cushingoid type effects such as growth suppression, osteoporosis, loss of muscle mass,

TABLE 17-1	Commonly Used Immunosuppressive Agents in Solid Organ Transplantation									
			Dosage Forms			**Indication**				
Drug	**Brand Name**	**Generic**	**IV**	**PO**	**PO liquid**	**Induction**	**Maintenance**	**ACR**	**TDM**	**REMS**
Calcineurin Inhibitors										
Cyclosporine	Sandimmune	X	X	X	X		X		X	
Cyclosporine (modified)	Neoral Gengraf	X		X	X		X		X	
Tacrolimus	Prograf	X	X	X			X		X	
Tacrolimus (extended release)	Astagraf XL Envarsus XR			X			X		X	
Antiproliferatives										
Azathioprine	Imuran	X	X	X			X			
Mycophenolate mofetil	CellCept	X	X	X	X		X			X
Mycophenolate sodium	Myfortic	X		X			X			X
Corticosteroids										
Prednisone	Deltasone	X		X	X		X			
Methylprednisolone	Solu-Medrol	X	X	X		X	X	X		
mTOR Inhibitors										
Sirolimus	Rapamune	X		X	X		X		X	
Everolimus	Zortress			X			X		X	
Costimulation Blocker										
Belatacept	Nulojix		X				X			X
IL-2 Receptor Antagonist										
Basiliximab	Simulect		X			X				
Antithymocyte Globulins										
Rabbit ATG	Thymoglobulin		X			X		X		
Equine ATG	Atgam		X			X		X		

Abbreviations: ACR, acute cellular rejection; ATG, antithymocyte globulin; IL-2, interleukin-2; IV, intravenous; mTOR, mammalian target of rapamycin; PO, oral; REMS, risk evaluation and mitigation strategy; TDM, therapeutic drug monitoring.

fragile skin, and lipodystrophy. For side effects associated with corticosteroids, immunosuppressive regimens including steroid withdrawal or avoidance are employed in select patients with good outcomes. Steroid minimization protocols typically taper prednisone rapidly during the first week post-transplant as late steroid withdrawal has been associated with increased rejection risk.

Calcineurin Inhibitors (Tacrolimus or Cyclosporine)

The calcineurin inhibitor is the backbone of the triple drug regimen. Calcineurin, a phosphatase, dephosphorylates nuclear factor of activated T cells (NFAT), which is a required transcription factor in the production of cytokines by T cells. By inhibiting calcineurin, cyclosporine (as cyclosporine-cyclophilin complex) and tacrolimus (as tacrolimus-FKBP12 complex) suppresses synthesis of IL-2, the cytokine that is responsible for lymphocyte activation.

The introduction of cyclosporine (Sandimmune) in the early 1980s improved patient and graft survival rates dramatically. This original formulation was highly dependent on bile acids for absorption, leading to extreme inter- and intrapatient pharmacokinetic variability. The newer modified cyclosporine products (Neoral and Gengraf) improved intrapatient variability, allowing more reliable drug absorption; however, interpatient pharmacokinetic variability due to gut metabolism persisted. It is important to note that the original formulation and newer formulations are not considered equivalent, and should not be substituted for one another.

Tacrolimus (Prograf), also known as FK506, is an alternative calcineurin inhibitor that is widely used in all types of solid organ transplantation. Its use has increased steadily since the *Food and Drug Administration* (FDA) approval in the early 1990s. Several multicenter randomized controlled trials and meta-analyses comparing tacrolimus to cyclosporine demonstrated lower acute rejection rates and potentially better graft survival rates with tacrolimus; however, tacrolimus was associated with development of post-transplant diabetes mellitus.

In addition to the immediate-release twice-daily tacrolimus (Prograf), two extended-release once-daily tacrolimus formulations are available in the US market, Astagraf XL and Envarsus XR. Both formulations are FDA-approved for the prophylaxis of rejection in kidney transplant patients and showed similar efficacy and safety to Prograf. Due to significantly different pharmacokinetics, these three tacrolimus products are not interchangeable and dosing conversions among the products should be done carefully to avoid medication errors.

Both calcineurin inhibitors demonstrate pharmacokinetic variability and a narrow therapeutic index (the window between toxicity and efficacy is small), thus requiring therapeutic drug monitoring. Typically, a trough concentration before the morning dose is monitored and goals vary by type of organ transplant, time elapsed since transplant, concomitant immunosuppression, history of rejection, and complications. Further aspects of calcineurin inhibitor pharmacokinetics include poor oral bioavailability, high plasma protein binding (cyclosporine to lipoproteins and tacrolimus to albumin and α-1 glycoprotein), extensive intestinal and hepatic metabolism primarily by cytochrome P-450 3A4 and 3A5 (CYP 3A4/3A5), and substrates for multiple drug transporters including P-glycoprotein. Additionally, tacrolimus expresses significant pharmacogenetic interindividual variability and patients with the *CYP3A5*1* allele often require much higher doses to attain therapeutic trough concentrations.

As a class, calcineurin inhibitors have similar adverse effects. Common and significant adverse effects are nephrotoxicity, electrolyte disturbances (hyperkalemia and hypomagnesemia), hypertension, and neurotoxicity (usually manifesting as tremor or headache). These effects are generally dose-dependent, and can complicate diagnosis, especially in renal transplant patients for whom calcineurin inhibitor-induced nephrotoxicity can be confused with renal graft rejection. Adverse effects that are specific to cyclosporine include hyperlipidemia, hyperuricemia, hirsutism, and gingival hyperplasia. Adverse effects that are specific to tacrolimus include hyperglycemia, alopecia, and diarrhea.

Drug interactions with calcineurin inhibitors can be both pharmacokinetic and pharmacodynamic in nature. Drugs that are inducers or inhibitors of CYP 3A4/3A5 or P-glycoprotein are expected to affect cyclosporine or tacrolimus levels (Table 17-2). While some potent and rapid-acting inhibitors, such as voriconazole, require preemptive calcineurin inhibitor dosage adjustment, other less potent agents, such as fluconazole, can be concomitantly administered with close monitoring of calcineurin-inhibitor levels. Pharmacodynamic interactions include increased nephrotoxicity with concomitant nephrotoxins, such as aminoglycosides and nonsteroidal anti-inflammatory agents (NSAIDs). The calcineurin inhibitors can also block the metabolism of other agents, such as the 5-hydroxy-3-methylglutaryl-coenzyme A (HMG-CoA) reductase inhibitors (or statins), resulting in an increased risk for myopathy and rhabdomyolysis when used with cyclosporine.

TABLE 17-2	**Effects of Concomitant Drugs on Cyclosporine, Tacrolimus, Sirolimus, and Everolimus Levels**
Increase Levels	**Decrease Levels**
Calcium channel blockers	Rifampin
Diltiazem	Phenytoin
Verapamil	Carbamazepine
Nicardipine	St. John's wort (herbal)
Azole antifungals	
Ketoconazole	
Voriconazole	
Itraconazole	
Fluconazole	
Macrolide antibiotics	
Clarithromycin	
Erythromycin	
Grapefruit (food)	

Antiproliferative Agents (Azathioprine, Mycophenolate Mofetil, or Mycophenolate Sodium)

Azathioprine

Azathioprine (Imuran) is an older generation antiproliferative agent that can be used as part of a triple drug immunosuppressive regimen and has other implications such as rheumatoid arthritis. With the availability of more specific mycophenolate products, azathioprine is not commonly used in solid organ transplantation, although it has a role as an alternative to more teratogenic immunosuppressant agents if a transplant patient becomes pregnant. Azathioprine is metabolized to 6-mercaptopurine, then to the active metabolites 6-thioguanine nucleotides. 6-Thioguanine nucleotides disrupt both the salvage and de novo deoxy ribonucleic acid (DNA) and ribonucleic acid (RNA) synthesis, resulting in nonspecific cell cycle arrest at the G2-M phase. Leukopenia, anemia, and thrombocytopenia are common and often dose-dependent. Less common side effects of azathioprine include skin cancer, hepatotoxicity, pancreatitis, and alopecia. Thiopurine methyltransferase (TPMT) is involved in two major inactivation routes of 6-mercaptopurine to the inactive metabolites, methyl-6-mercaptopurine and methyl-6-mercaptopurine nucleotide. TPMT activity correlates inversely with 6-thioguanine nucleotide level and therefore hematological toxicity of azathioprine. Patients with two nonfunctional alleles of *TPMT*2, TPMT*3A, TPMT*3C, and TPMT*4* have low or absent TPMT activity. Azathioprine dosing based on TPMT genotype or phenotype should be considered to minimize risk of severe pancytopenia.

Mycophenolic Acid Derivatives

Mycophenolate mofetil (CellCept) and mycophenolate sodium (Myfortic) are converted to mycophenolic acid (MPA) in vivo. MPA inhibits inosine monophosphate dehydrogenase (IMPDH), an enzyme required for the de novo synthesis of purines. MPA derivatives, therefore, selectively inhibit lymphocyte proliferation, as these cells are unable to utilize salvage pathways of purine synthesis. MPA undergoes enterohepatic recirculation and is cleared via hepatic glucuronidation as well as renal excretion. MPA derivatives should not be administered concurrently with aluminum or magnesium containing antacids (separate by 2 hours) or binding resins such as cholestyramine due to decreased serum levels of MPA. Noticeable adverse effects of both MPA derivatives are gastrointestinal distress, such as diarrhea and bone marrow suppression leading to pancytopenia, although not to the same extent as azathioprine. Mycophenolate sodium was initially touted by the manufacturer as an enteric delayed-release MPA formulation with decreased gastrointestinal side effects. However, this advantage was not evident in the phase III clinical trials. Mycophenolate sodium 720 mg is therapeutically equivalent to mycophenolate mofetil 1000 mg.

MPA derivatives are associated with the increased risks of first trimester pregnancy loss and congenital malformations and are subject to a risk evaluation and mitigation strategy (REMS) by the FDA. Female patients of reproductive potential should be provided with information about the pregnancy risks and counseling on pregnancy planning, and must take acceptable contraception during the entire treatment with mycophenolate and for 6 weeks after they stop taking mycophenolate. Pregnancy tests are required immediately before initiation of mycophenolate, 8 to 10 days later, and at routine follow-up visits.

mTOR Inhibitors (Sirolimus or Everolimus)

Sirolimus (Rapamune) and everolimus (Zortress) inhibit lymphocyte proliferation by arresting the G1-S phase of cell cycle. Their greatest utility in clinical practice is to allow sparing of calcineurin inhibitors. mTOR inhibitors are less likely to cause nephrotoxicity than calcineurin inhibitors. However, mTOR inhibitors are known to cause proteinuria and enhance calcineurin inhibitor-associated nephrotoxicity. Therefore, reduced doses of calcineurin inhibitors are required when used in combination with mTOR inhibitors to reduce nephrotoxicity. Common side effects of mTOR inhibitors are hypercholesterolemia, hypertriglyceridemia, leukopenia, anemia, thrombocytopenia, and mouth sores. The most troubling adverse effect is impaired wound healing. Sirolimus has been associated with hepatic artery thrombosis in liver transplant patients and bronchial anastomotic dehiscence in lung transplant patients. Both sirolimus and everolimus are substrates for CYP 3A4/3A5 and P-glycoprotein with the similar drug interaction potential to calcineurin inhibitors (see Table 17-2). Therapeutic drug monitoring is recommended for all patients taking sirolimus or everolimus.

Costimulation Blocker (Belatacept)

By blocking CD86-mediated costimulation, belatacept (Nulojix) inhibits cytokine production by T cells. Belatacept is the first FDA approved intravenous maintenance immunosuppressant and offers a benefit that therapeutic drug monitoring is not required. When compared to cyclosporine-based maintenance immunosuppression, belatacept regimen had comparable patient and graft survival and superior renal function despite a higher rate of ACR in kidney transplant recipients on basiliximab induction, mycophenolate mofetil, and corticosteroids. Due to the risk of post-transplant lymphoproliferative disorder (PTLD) predominantly involving the central nervous system, belatacept is contraindicated in patients who are Epstein-Barr virus (EBV) seronegative or with unknown EBV serostatus and a REMS is required by the FDA. A clinical trial evaluating belatacept regimen in comparison to tacrolimus-based maintenance immunosuppression is currently underway.

Antibody Induction

There is an increasing trend toward the use of induction therapy with antibodies in most solid organ transplantation, except for liver transplant. Rabbit ATG is the most commonly used antibody in induction, followed by basiliximab and alemtuzumab. The use of equine ATG has decreased significantly in recent years.

Antithymocyte Globulins

ATGs are polyclonal antithymocyte antibodies derived from animals. ATGs interact with lymphocyte surface antigens, including CD2, CD3, CD4, CD8, CD16, CD25, and CD45, thereby depleting the number of circulating T cells. Rabbit ATG (thymoglobulin) has the more profound lymphopenic effect than equine ATG (Atgam). Residual immunosuppressive effects after rabbit ATG can persist for years. The superior efficacy of rabbit ATG to equine ATG and basiliximab in prevention of ACR has been demonstrated in kidney transplant. The most common adverse effect of ATGs is cytokine release syndrome. The symptoms include fever, chills, rigors, dyspnea, nausea, vomiting, diarrhea, hypotension or hypertension, malaise, rash, and headache. Slow infusion rates and pretreatment with corticosteroids, acetaminophen, and diphenhydramine can prevent severe cytokine release syndrome. Other common adverse effects are leukopenia, thrombocytopenia, and serum sickness. ATGs may also increase the risk of infections and malignancy.

Alemtuzumab

Alemtuzumab (Campath) is a recombinant monoclonal antibody against CD52 on the surface of B and T cells. By binding to CD52, it induces depletion of lymphocytes. Although alemtuzumab is FDA-approved for B-cell chronic lymphocytic leukemia, it is commonly used "off-label" as an induction agent for the prophylaxis of rejection in kidney transplant patients. Some of the reported side effects include infusion-related reactions, cytopenias (eg, anemia, neutropenia, thrombocytopenia), cancer, and infectious complications. Premedication with corticosteroid, acetaminophen, and diphenhydramine reduces risk of infusion reactions. Compared to ATGs, alemtuzumab has a higher risk for chronic allograft injury and infectious complications.

Basiliximab

Basiliximab (Simulect) is a chimeric monoclonal antibody that binds specifically to the α chain (CD25) of the IL-2 receptor and inhibits T-cell activation. Unlike ATGs and alemtuzumab, basiliximab is well tolerated without significant risk for infusion-related reactions. While induction with IL-2 receptor antagonists have shown to lower rejection rates, they have not been studied adequately for treatment of rejection.

TREATMENT OF REJECTION

ACR is one of the most common complications of solid organ transplantation. The incidence of ACR varies depending on the organ transplanted and rejection criteria employed. Another type of rejection called antibody-mediated rejection may also occur post-transplant. A biopsy of the transplanted organ will distinguish between the two rejection types. Classifying the rejection as ACR versus antibody-mediated rejection is important as treatment modalities differ based on type of rejection present.

Steroid Pulses

When treating ACR episodes, large doses of intravenous corticosteroids are given over a series of days (eg, methylprednisolone 250-1000 mg/dose). This treatment course is commonly referred to as "steroid pulses". Patients receiving steroid pulses are at risk for the earlier mentioned side effects of corticosteroids.

Antithymocyte Globulins

ATGs are typically used for more severe forms or steroid-resistant ACR. The dose of equine ATG (10-15 mg/kg) is ten times that of rabbit ATG (1.25-1.5 mg/kg) and skin testing is strongly recommended prior to equine ATG.

Treatment Option for Antibody-Mediated Rejection

Treatment for antibody-mediated rejection is not well established. Plasmapheresis in conjunction with intravenous immunoglobulin is commonly utilized in treatment of antibody-mediated rejection. Rituximab (Rituxan), Bortezomib (Velcade), and eculizumab (Soliris) have been used "off-label" as adjunct therapy for antibody-mediated rejection.

PREVENTION OF INFECTION

In addition to immunosuppressive medications, transplant recipients also receive infection prophylaxis to prevent viral, bacterial, and fungal infections. Depending on center protocol, patients may receive valganciclovir to prevent cytomegalovirus infection for 3 to 6 months. Sulfamethoxazole-trimethoprim, pentamidine inhalation, or dapsone is commonly administered to prevent *Pneumocystis jiroveci* pneumonitis. Nystatin solution, clotrimazole troches, fluconazole, or voriconazole may be used to prevent fungal infections.

Furthermore, immunization history must be assessed for each patient evaluated for transplant. As live vaccines are contraindicated post-transplant, every effort should be made to complete required series of live vaccinations such as measles, mumps, rubella (MMR) and varicella prior to transplant.

CASE Application

1. JP is a kidney transplant patient whose biopsy showed cellular rejection. Select the statement that most accurately describes mechanism of JP's rejection.

   a. An orchestrated immune response that involves allo-antigen presentation via APCs that then leads to allo-reactive T lymphocytes.

   b. A cytotoxic immune response mediated via pre-formed antibodies against antigens present on vascular endothelium.

   c. A slow process of graft fibrosis and arteriopathy, which results in graft dysfunction.

   d. A process which inhibits the entire process of immune activation, including antigen presentation by APCs, the release of cytokines such as IL-1, IL-2, IL-6, and TNF α, and subsequently lymphocyte proliferation.

2. SK is a 16-year-old boy who is waiting for kidney transplantation. He states that he has been doing research on the internet and heard that ACR is a major complication of kidney transplantation. What can a pharmacist counsel him regarding the time frame for risk of ACR after transplant?

   a. The risk is greatest during the first hours to days after transplantation

   b. The risk is greatest during the first several months after transplantation

   c. The risk increases with increased time from transplant

   d. The risk is the same regardless of time after transplant

3. SK received kidney transplantation from his brother today. Which "triple drug regimen" describes the most commonly used maintenance immunosuppression?

   a. Cyclosporine, prednisone, and basiliximab

   b. Cyclosporine, tacrolimus, and prednisone

   c. Tacrolimus, mycophenolate mofetil, and rabbit ATG

   d. Tacrolimus, mycophenolate mofetil, and prednisone

4. GH presents to your pharmacy with a prescription for clarithromycin. He says that his primary care physician prescribed this medication to treat community-acquired pneumonia. You review GH's medication profile and you see that he received a renal transplant 2 years ago and his immunosuppressive regimen includes tacrolimus, mycophenolate mofetil, and prednisone. Which of the following would be most appropriate as your next course of action?

   a. Dispense clarithromycin and counsel on avoiding grapefruit juice.

   b. Contact the prescriber about the interactions between clarithromycin and tacrolimus as clarithromycin will inhibit the metabolism of tacrolimus resulting in supratherapeutic levels and toxicity.

c. Contact the prescriber about the interactions between clarithromycin and mycophenolate mofetil as clarithromycin will inhibit the metabolism of mycophenolate mofetil resulting in supratherapeutic levels and toxicity.

d. Recommend an alternative as clarithromycin is not an appropriate therapy for community-acquired pneumonia in an immunosuppressed host.

5. AJ is a lung transplant recipient who is found to have *Aspergillus* on routine bronchoscopy. AJ's transplant physician wants to begin treatment with the antifungal voriconazole. The patient is currently taking prednisone, cyclosporine, azathioprine, clotrimazole, rabeprazole, cotrimoxazole, valganciclovir, and inhaled amphotericin. Which of the following medications will interact with voriconazole?

a. Prednisone
b. Azathioprine
c. Cyclosporine
d. Valganciclovir

6. PW is a transplant patient taking a stable dose of cyclosporine and rosuvastatin was recently added. Which counseling information should a pharmacist provide to PW? Select all that apply.

a. Avoid grapefruit and grapefruit juice.
b. Report unexplained muscle pain, muscle weakness, or dark urine.
c. Cyclosporine dose should be decreased within days after starting rosuvastatin.
d. Inform the prescriber of rosuvastatin that PW is taking cyclosporine.

The following case pertains to Questions 7 through 11.

CJ is a 24-year-old female patient who received kidney transplantation 3 months ago. She fills her prescription for tacrolimus, mycophenolate sodium, and prednisone at your pharmacy.

7. Which of the following represents two adverse effects specific to tacrolimus that CJ may experience?

a. Diarrhea and leukopenia
b. Alopecia and hyperglycemia
c. Hypertriglyceridemia and nephrotoxicity
d. Hirsutism and gingival hyperplasia

8. Which of the following represents two adverse effects specific to corticosteroids that CJ may experience?

a. Diarrhea and leukopenia
b. Alopecia and hyperglycemia
c. Water retention and osteoporosis
d. Hirsutism and nephrotoxicity

9. Which of the following should be included in patient counseling about mycophenolate sodium for CJ? Select all that apply.

a. Educate CJ regarding higher risks of miscarriage and birth defects.
b. Counsel CJ regarding pregnancy planning.
c. Ensure the use of acceptable contraception during the first 6 weeks of starting mycophenolate.
d. Perform pregnancy tests only before starting mycophenolate.

10. CJ approaches the counter at your pharmacy and would like you to suggest an over-the-counter remedy for her mild headache. What would you suggest for her headache?

a. That she should proceed immediately to a local emergency room as this might be a symptom of severe tacrolimus toxicity.
b. That she may take OTC acetaminophen, and alert the transplant physician if the headache does not resolve.
c. That she may take OTC naproxen, and alert the transplant physician if the headache does not resolve.
d. That she may take OTC ibuprofen, and alert the transplant physician if the headache dose not resolve.

11. CJ presents to the hospital with symptoms concerning for a bowel obstruction. She is receiving mycophenolate sodium 720 mg po bid. The physician wants to convert the patient from oral mycophenolate sodium to IV due to po intolerance resulting from her bowel obstruction. Which of the following would result in comparable plasma concentrations of MPA?

a. Mycophenolate sodium 720 mg IV bid
b. Mycophenolate sodium 1000 mg IV bid
c. Mycophenolate mofetil 720 mg IV bid
d. Mycophenolate mofetil 1000 mg IV bid

12. Which of the following agents would be most appropriate to prevent a gout flare in a transplant patient who is currently receiving tacrolimus, azathioprine, and prednisone?

a. Indomethacin
b. Allopurinol
c. Diclofenac
d. Probenecid

13. You are counseling HD who is being discharged today. He received a living related renal transplant 3 days ago, and his postoperative course has been uncomplicated except for mild hypertension. When reconciling his home medications, you notice that the medical team has not restarted his home diltiazem. What is the most appropriate action to control his blood pressure at this point?

a. Notify the patient's medical team and request a discharge prescription for amlodipine.
b. Notify the patient's medical team and instruct the patient to resume his home regimen of diltiazem after discharge.

c. Notify the patient's medical team and request a discharge prescription for verapamil.

d. Notify the patient's medical team and request addition of diltiazem at discharge.

14. Which of the following statement is correct about sirolimus?

a. Sirolimus is not metabolized via cytochrome P450 enzymes, thus decreasing the propensity for drug interactions.

b. Sirolimus is less nephrotoxic than calcineurin inhibitors.

c. Sirolimus is available in many different formulations, thereby facilitating ease of dosing.

d. Sirolimus does not require therapeutic drug monitoring.

15. What is the drug target for the immunosuppressive agent MPA?

a. mTOR
b. Cyclophilin
c. FKBP-12
d. IMPDH

16. Which of the following is generally considered as a narrow therapeutic ratio drug?

a. Cyclosporine
b. Prednisone
c. Mycophenolate mofetil
d. Mycophenolate sodium

17. DD is a liver transplant patient who presents with elevated liver function tests. She admits to not taking her immunosuppressive regimen for the past week as she was out of town and forgot her medications. The medical team wants to treat her for ACR. Which of the following would treat ACR most effectively?

a. Basiliximab
b. Rabbit ATG
c. Belatacept
d. Rituximab

18. Which of the following should be confirmed before administering belatacept in a kidney transplant patient? Select all that apply.

a. Positive cytomegalovirus serostatus
b. Positive EBV serostatus

c. Normal renal and liver function
d. Absence of any new or worsening neurological abnormalities

19. During interdisciplinary rounds, the medical resident states that TK has a low white blood cell (WBC) count. TK received a combined kidney pancreas transplant for juvenile onset diabetes mellitus 2 months ago and presented 2 days ago with hyperglycemia and elevated amylase and lipase. ACR of the pancreas transplant was confirmed on a subsequent biopsy. Her rejection episode is being treated with rabbit ATG. Her home immunosuppressive regimen consists of tacrolimus, mycophenolate mofetil, and prednisone. She is receiving antiviral prophylaxis with valganciclovir, antibacterial prophylaxis with trimethoprim-sulfamethoxazole, and antifungal prophylaxis with nystatin. Which of the following approach is most appropriate for this patient's new onset leukopenia?

a. Suggest the physician to hold her prednisone until her WBC count normalizes.

b. Suggest the physician to hold her mycophenolate mofetil until her WBC count normalizes.

c. Suggest the physician to hold her current therapy, but to closely monitor her WBC count.

d. Suggest the physician to hold her valganciclovir until her WBC count normalizes.

20. Which of the following medications require a REMS by FDA? Select all that apply.

a. Mycophenolate mofetil
b. Mycophenolate sodium generic products
c. Belatacept
d. Tacrolimus

21. Which of the following vaccines will need to be administered prior to transplant as they are relatively contraindicated post-transplant? Select all that apply.

a. Pneumococcal polysaccharide
b. Varicella
c. MMR
d. Meningococcal conjugate

TAKEAWAY POINTS ››

- To promote patient and graft survival, solid organ transplantation requires balance between rejection prevention and the adverse sequelae from immunosuppression, such as infection, malignancy, and drug side effects.

- There are three types of allograft rejection: antibody-mediated, acute cellular, and chronic.

- Induction with an ATG, alemtuzumab, or basiliximab reduces ACR.

- Corticosteroids and ATGs are indicated for the treatment of ACR.

- ACR is prevented by utilizing a multidrug maintenance immunosuppressive regimen, which maximizes the immunosuppressive effect of each agent while minimizing adverse effects by including drugs with different mechanisms of action and toxicities.

- The gold standard "triple drug" immunosuppressive regimen includes a calcineurin-inhibitor (eg,

- tacrolimus), an antiproliferative agent (eg, mycophenolate), and corticosteroids.
- Drug interactions with calcineurin inhibitors can be both pharmacokinetic (via CYP 3A4/3A5 and P-glycoprotein) and pharmacodynamic (via common adverse effects).
- Therapeutic drug monitoring is required for calcineurin inhibitors and mTOR inhibitors because they have variable pharmacokinetics, a narrow therapeutic index, and high potential for drug interactions.
- mTOR inhibitors can be used in place of the calcineurin inhibitor or the antiproliferative agent in a triple drug immunosuppressive regimen if a patient has intolerable adverse effects to either of these classes.
- Immunosuppressive agents are associated with various adverse effects, which require close monitoring.
- REMS is required for mycophenolate (due to the increased risks of first trimester pregnancy loss and congenital malformations), and belatacept (due to the risk of PTLD and progressive multifocal leukoencephalopathy).
- Live-vaccines are relatively contraindicated post-transplant and every effort should be made to vaccinate patients prior to transplant.
- Pharmacists can play an important role in post-transplant patient care by assessing the appropriateness of their medication therapy, monitoring signs and symptoms of rejection and other negative sequelae of immunosuppression, and educating patients on immunosuppressants and compliance.

BIBLIOGRAPHY

2015 Annual Data Report. Scientific Registry of Transplant Recipients http://srtr.transplant.hrsa.gov/annual_reports/Default.aspx. Accessed March 1, 2017.

Birdwell KA, Decker B, Barbarino JM, et al. Clinical pharmacogenetics implementation consortium (CPIC) guidelines for *CYP3A5* genotype and tacrolimus dosing. *Clin Pharmacol Ther.* 2015;98(1):19-24.

Dansinger-Isakov L, Kumar D, the AST Infectious Diseases Community of Practice. Guidelines for vaccination of solid organ transplant candidates and recipients. *Am J Transplant.* 2009;9(Suppl 4):S258-S262.

Jasiak NM, Park JM. Immunosuppression in solid-organ transplantation: essentials and practical tips. *Crit Care Nurs Q.* 2016;39(3):227-240.

Johnson HJ, Schonder KS. Solid-organ transplantation. In: Dipiro JT, Talbert RL, Yee GC, Matzke GR, Wells BG, Posey LM, eds. *Pharmacotherapy: A Pathophysiologic Approach.* 10th ed. New York, NY: McGraw-Hill; 2017:chap 89.

Lee RA, Gabardi S. Current trends in immunosuppressive therapies for renal transplant recipients. *Am J Health-Syst Pharm.* 2012;69:1961-1975.

Relling MV, Gardner EE, Sandborn WJ, et al. Clinical pharmacogenetics implementation consortium guidelines for thiopurine methyltransferase genotype and thiopurine dosing. *Clin Pharmacol Ther.* 2011;89(3):387-391.

Wagner SJ, Brennan DC. Induction therapy in renal transplant recipients. How convincing is the current evidence? *Drugs.* 2012;72:671-683.

KEY ABBREVIATIONS

ACR = acute cellular rejection
APC = antigen presenting cell
ATG = antithymocyte globulin
CYP = cytochrome P-450
DNA = deoxy ribonucleic acid
EBV = Epstein-Barr virus
FDA = Food and Drug Administration
HMG-CoA = 5-hydroxy-3-methylglutaryl-coenzyme A
IL = interleukin
IMPDH = inosine monophosphate dehydrogenase
IV = intravenous
MPA = mycophenolic acid

mTOR = mammalian target of rapamycin
NFAT = nuclear factor of activated T cells
NSAID = nonsteroidal anti-inflammatory agent
OTC = over-the-counter
PO = orally
PTLD = post-transplant lymphoproliferative disorder
REMS = risk evaluation and mitigation strategy
RNA = ribonucleic acid
TDM = therapeutic drug monitoring
TNF = tumor necrosis factor
TPMT = thiopurine methyltransferase

18

Skin and Melanoma

Betty M. Chan, Hansen Ho, and Samantha Y. Shi

FOUNDATION OVERVIEW

Melanoma is a serious form of skin cancer and is the sixth most common cancer in men and seventh most common cancer in women. The outcome and survival rate of melanoma is dependent on the stage of the disease at diagnosis (Table 18-1).

Melanoma arises from melanocytes located at the epidermal and dermal layers of the skin and the choroids of the eyes. Melanocytes help synthesize melanin, a brown pigment deeper layers of tissues from ultraviolet radiation damage (eg, sun damage). Melanoma is a result of malignant skin transformation from skin melanocytes or preexisting nevocellular nevi (moles). Although the etiology of melanoma is not fully understood, many risk factors have been identified. Risk for melanoma includes personal or family history of melanoma, presence of multiple atypical moles or dysplastic nevi, previous history of nonmelanoma skin cancer (eg, basal cell and squamous cell), and immunosuppression. Incidence of melanoma increases with intermittent intense ultraviolet sun exposure over chronic periods.

Normal nevi present as an evenly colored brown, tan, or black spot on the skin. They are round or oval in shape, and appear flat or raised. Nevi are generally less than 6 mm in diameter and stay about the same size, shape, and color. However, any nevi that change size, shape, or color are suspicious and require evaluation by a dermatologist. The ABCDE rule of melanoma is a useful tool to identify suspicious lesions. *A* is asymmetry where one-half of the mole does not match the other half; *B* is border irregularity where the edges of the mole are often irregular, blurred, ragged, or notched; *C* is color where the color of the mole is not uniform, it may appear with different shades of tan or blue-black, and sometimes mixed with colors of red, purple, and white; *D* is diameter where lesions are often more than 6 mm in diameter, although melanoma can sometimes present with lesions of less than 6 mm in diameter; *E* is evolving or changing characteristics of a lesion.

Classification of Melanoma

Depending on the location and presentation of the lesions, the classification of melanoma can be different. Superficial spreading melanoma is the most common type of melanoma. The lesions arise from a preexisting flat nevus that develops into an irregular and asymmetrical nevus. Nodular melanoma is the second most common type of melanoma. Nodular melanoma has an aggressive and rapid growth pattern. The lesions are uniform in color and are commonly located on the head, neck, and trunk. Lentigo maligna melanomas occur in older individuals and are located on the face. Compared to other melanoma subtypes, lentigo maligna does not usually metastasize due to its slow growing nature. Acral lentiginous melanoma is the most common type of melanoma in African Americans, Hispanics, and Asians. The lesions are observed on the palms of the hands, soles of the feet, or beneath the nail beds. Uveal melanoma is an ocular melanoma which arises from the pigmented epithelium of the choroids with metastases frequently occurring in the liver.

Diagnosis and Staging

Suspicious lesions should be evaluated by a dermatologist. Excisional biopsy of suspicious lesions is the only way to confirm the diagnosis of melanoma. Melanomas may be staged by using the American Joint Commission on Cancer (AJCC) TNM staging system, where T stands for tumor, N stands for nodal involvement, and M stands for metastases. In addition to TNM, sentinel lymph node biopsy is also used as a staging procedure in patients with subclinical nodal metastases at high risk of recurrence. The two most important prognostic factors influencing staging are the Breslow tumor thickness and the presence or absence of ulceration of the overlying epithelium. Sentinel lymph node biopsy should be considered in patients whose tumor thickness is more than or equal to 0.76 mm.

PREVENTION

The American Cancer Society (ACS) recommends practicing sun safety when you are outdoors by remembering to:

1. Protect your skin from sun exposure by wearing clothing. Long-sleeved shirts, long skirts, or long pants offer the most protection. Dark colored clothing offers more protection than light colored clothing. Avoid direct sun exposure between 10 AM to 4 PM when the ultraviolet radiations are the strongest.
2. Wear a hat with a minimum of at least 2- to 3-inch brim to protect sun-exposed areas such as neck, ears, eyes, forehead, nose, and scalp.

To access your complimentary online question exams, visit https://accesspharmacy.mhmedical.com/NAPLEX.aspx

TABLE 18-1	Stages of Melanoma and Mortality

- Early stage—localized disease[a]
  - Primary tumors ≤1 mm in thickness
    - 5-y survival >90%
  - Primary tumors >1 mm in thickness
    - 5-y survival rate 50%-90%
- Advanced disease
  - Disease with nodal involvement
    - 5-y survival rate 20%-70%
  - Distant metastases[b]
    - 5-y survival rate <10%

[a]Majority (82%-85%) of patients.
[b]2%-5% of patients.

3. Use sunscreen and lip balms with sun protection factor (SPF) of 15 or higher on areas where skin is exposed to the sun. Apply sunscreen 20 to 30 minutes prior to sun exposure, and reapply every 2 hours or more frequently if you sweat or swim.

4. Wear sunglasses that wrap around the eyes for additional sun protection with at least 99% ultraviolet A and B absorption.

Other recommendations include the avoidance of using tanning beds or sunlamps, a monthly self-examination of the skin to identify any suspicious markings, and annual clinical examination by a dermatologist for high-risk patients.

TREATMENT

The treatment and management of melanoma is dependent on the stage and disease involvement. Surgical excision is the primary treatment option for early stage melanoma.

Adjuvant Treatment of Melanoma

High-dose interferon-alfa 2b is Food and Drug Administration (FDA) approved for adjuvant treatment of melanoma within 56 days after surgical resection of primary melanoma in patients at high risk of recurrence, such as those with nodal involvement. The dose of interferon-alfa 2b is 20 million international units (IU)/m² intravenously five times weekly for 4 weeks, followed by 10 million IU/m² subcutaneously three times weekly for 48 weeks. Majority of patients (>80%) develop flu-like symptoms (eg, fever, chills, headache, myalgias, and arthralgias). Premedication with an antipyretic, such as acetaminophen or nonsteroidal anti-inflammatory agent (NSAID), minimizes the risk and severity of fever and chills. Other side effects associated with high-dose interferon-alfa 2b include fatigue, anorexia (can be dose limiting), and neuropsychiatric symptoms (eg, depression, confusion, and somnolence). Other effects associated with interferon include myelosuppression (eg, neutropenia and thrombocytopenia), hepatotoxicity, and thyroid disorders (both hypo- and hyperthyroidism). Duration of treatment is 1 year or until recurrence of disease or unacceptable toxicities.

Ipilimumab (Yervoy) is a monoclonal antibody that targets the cytotoxic T lymphocyte antigen-4 (CTLA-4) receptor

TABLE 18-2	Summary of Current Guideline Recommendation on Treatment Algorithm for Patients With Unresectable Metastatic Melanoma	
First-line Treatment	**Second-line or Subsequent Treatment**	
	Good PS	**Poor PS**
Nivolumab	First-line options not already used	Consider best supportive care
Pembrolizumab	Pembrolizumab	
Nivolumab/ ipilimumab	Nivolumab	
Dabrafenib/ trametinib[a]	Nivolumab/ ipilimumab	
Vemurafenib/ cobimetinib[a]	Dabrafenib/ trametinib[a]	
Clinical trial	Vemurafenib/ cobimetinib[a]	
	Ipilimumab	
	High-dose IL-2	
	Biochemotherapy	
	Cytotoxic agents	
	Clinical trial	

[a]Preferred over immunotherapy for patients with BRAF V600 activating mutation and if clinically needed for early response due to symptoms or tumor burden.

resulting in an immune response directed against melanoma. Ipilimumab is FDA approved for adjuvant treatment of resected melanoma. In the adjuvant setting, ipilimumab is dosed at 10 mg/kg intravenously every 3 weeks for 4 cycles then every 12 weeks for 3 years.

Metastatic Treatment of Melanoma

Treatment options for metastatic melanoma are determined based on patients' performance status (PS), molecular marker, whether the lesions are resectable or unresectable, and the presence or absence of distant metastases. Both single agent and combinational chemotherapeutic agents have been used; however, median duration of response remains low (<1 year). Recent research with immunotherapy and molecular targeted treatment have demonstrated improved survival (>1 year) with different and distinct toxicities compared to chemotherapy (Table 18-2).

Molecular Targeted Agents

Molecular agents (Table 18-3) primarily target mutations in the proto-oncogene BRAF and downstream redundant MEK (mitogen activated extracellular kinase) pathway. The current standard of care is now dual BRAF and MEK inhibition to prevent early BRAF resistance via redundant MEK pathway. Vemurafenib (Zelboraf) and cobimetinib (Cotellic) are oral BRAF and MEK inhibitors, respectively. FDA approved in combination for the treatment of BRAF positive metastatic or unresectable melanoma. Vemurafenib is dosed at 960 mg orally twice daily and cobimetinib is dosed at 60 mg once daily given three of every 4-week cycles. Long term follow-up demonstrated a median overall survival was 22.3 months compared to 17.3 months with vemurafenib alone. The median progression free survival was also significant at 12.3 months versus 7.2 months with vemurafenib alone. Before the approval of

TABLE 18-3   Summary of Oral Kinase Inhibitor Dosing and Administration Guidelines

Drug	Dose	Administration	Storage	Missed doses
Vemurafenib (Zelboraf)	960 mg orally bid (morning and evening 12 h apart)	Swallow whole, with whole glass of water; with or without meals, do not crush or chew	Room temperature in original container with lid closed	Missed doses can be taken up to 4 h prior to next scheduled dose
Dabrafenib (Tafinlar)	150 mg orally bid (morning and evening 12 h apart)	Swallow whole, with a whole glass of water; take 1 h before or 2 h after a meal; do not break or crush capsule	Room temperature in original container with lid closed	Missed doses can be taken up to 6 h prior to next scheduled dose
Trametinib (Mekinist)	2 mg orally once daily	Swallow whole, with whole glass of water; take 1 h before or 2 h after a meal; do not crush or chew	Room temperature in original container with lid closed	Missed doses can be taken up to 12 h of next scheduled dose
Cobimetinib (Cotellic)	60 mg once daily	Swallow whole, with or without food; do not crush tablets	Room temperature	Missed doses can be taken if within 4 h of the scheduled time, otherwise resume with the next scheduled dose

cobimetinib, single-agent vemurafenib was FDA approved demonstrating superiority compared to the former standard of care, dacarbazine. Cobimetinib and vemurafenib are cytochrome P450 3A4 substrate. Caution when administering 3A4 inducers or inhibitors with cobimetinib. Adverse effects associated with vemurafenib and cobimetinib include:

- Dermatologic toxicity includes severe photosensitivity, rash, squamous cell carcinoma, keratoacanthomas, and basal cell carcinomas. Avoid sun exposure and use broad-spectrum long wave ultraviolet A/short wave ultraviolet B (UVA/UVB) SPF more than or equal to 30 sunscreen and lip balm when outdoors. Perform dermatologic evaluations periodically while on therapy. Manage skin lesions with excision and dermatopathologic evaluation.

- Cardiac abnormalities include QTc prolongation and asymptomatic decline in left ventricular dysfunction. Consider withholding treatment if QTc is more than 500 msec. Monitor and replete electrolytes particularly potassium and magnesium. Monitor electrocardiogram (EKG) at and echocardiogram at baseline and periodically while on treatment.

- Hepatotoxicity include transaminitis, hyperbilirubinemia, and functional hepatic impairment including coagulopathy. Monitor liver function tests monthly.

- Musculoskeletal toxicity include rhabdomyolysis and arthralgia (most common noncutaneous adverse effect observed). Monitor Cr and **creatine phosphokinase** (CPK) periodically during treatment.

- Ophthalmologic reactions include uveitis, blurry vision, and photophobia. Conduct periodic ophthalmological examination and interrupt therapy until resolution of symptoms.

Dabrafenib (Tafinlar) and trametinib (Mekinist) are also oral BRAF and MEK inhibitors, respectively, indicated for metastatic or unresectable melanoma with BRAF mutation (+) disease. Dabrafenib is dosed 150 mg twice daily and trametinib is given 2 mg daily. Unlike vemurafenib and cobimetinib, there is no break during each treatment cycle. As described previously, BRAF and MEK inhibitors are most beneficial when used together. Long term follow-up demonstrated the combination of dabrafenib and trametinib provided a robust overall survival of 25.1 months compared to 18.1 months with dabrafenib alone. Median progression free survival was 11.1 months with combination therapy versus 8.8 months with dabrafenib alone. Without head-to-head trials it is difficult to determine which combination BRAF/MEK inhibitor is most beneficial. Dabrafenib is also a major substrate of cytochrome p450 3A4, caution when administering with inhibitors and inducers. Adverse effects associated with dabrafenib and trametinib include:

- Dermatologic toxicity has been observed with the combination include rash, dermatitis, acneiform rash, palmar-plantar erythrodysesthesia syndrome, and erythema, and secondary skin infections have also been reported. Dose reduction, interruption of treatment, or discontinuation of treatment may be necessary depending on severity of symptoms.

- Fever and febrile reactions accompanied by hypotension, rigors, chills, and dehydration is common. Monitor patients and interrupt treatment for severe febrile reactions (T >104°F). Administer corticosteroids for subsequent febrile events. Many consider prophylactic use of antipyretic (eg, acetaminophen and/or nonsteroidal anti-inflammatory drugs [NSAIDs]) on restart.

- Cutaneous squamous cell carcinoma and basal cell carcinoma can occur with dabrafenib or in combination with trametinib. Perform dermatologic evaluations prior to initiations and periodically while on therapy. Dose interruption and reduction is not necessary. Excision of carcinoma is preferred treatment.

- Cardiomyopathy has been observed and defined as a decrease in left ventricular ejection fraction (LVEF) with combination. Perform echocardiogram at baseline and periodically during treatment. Withhold treatment for up to 1 month for LVEF decrease of more than or equal to 10% until resolution.

- Venous thromboembolism with both deep vein thrombosis (DVT) and pulmonary embolism (PE) has been reported. Monitor for symptoms; discontinue treatment for complicated life-threatening PE. Therapy may be restarted for uncomplicated PE or DVT after 3 weeks.

- Ocular toxicities include retinopathy and retinal-vein occlusion has been reported with the combination. Urgent referrals to ophthalmology is essential for patient reporting vision loss or visual disturbance.

- Colitis and gastrointestinal perforation can occur with trametinib. Monitor closely for events.

Immunotherapy Targeted Agents

Interleukin-2 (IL-2, Proleukin) is FDA approved for treatment of metastatic melanoma. The dose of IL-2 is 600,000 IU/kg intravenously every 8 hours for a maximum of 14 doses; repeats after 9 days for a total of 28 doses per course. Treatment with IL-2 is associated with flu-like symptoms and premedication with an antipyretic may decrease symptoms. Vascular or capillary leak syndrome is a dose-limiting toxicity observed with high-dose IL-2. Vascular or capillary leak syndrome may present as weight gain, ascites, arrhythmias, hypotension, oliguria, and pleural effusions. Early intervention with dopamine 1 to 5 mcg/kg/min may be necessary to maintain renal perfusion and minimize renal toxicities. Myelosuppression (eg, neutropenia, anemia, and thrombocytopenia), reversible hepatotoxicity, neuropsychiatric symptoms (eg, somnolence, delirium, and confusion) have been observed. Continuous neurologic, cardiac, and pulmonary monitoring is recommended during therapy. Avoid concomitant use of:

- Nonsteroidal anti-inflammatory agents as they may increase the risk of capillary leak syndrome

- Antihypertensives as IL-2 potentiate the effect of antihypertensives

- Corticosteroids as they may decrease the antitumor effects of IL-2 due to corticosteroids inhibitory effect on the immune system

Ipilimumab (Yervoy) is a monoclonal antibody that targets the CTLA-4 receptor resulting in an immune response directed against melanoma. Ipilimumab is FDA approved for adjuvant treatment of resected melanoma and metastatic or unresectable melanoma. In the adjuvant setting, ipilimumab is dosed at 10 mg/kg intravenously every 3 weeks for 4 cycles then every 12 weeks for 3 years. In metastatic disease, ipilimumab is dosed at 3 mg/kg every 3 weeks for 4 cycles. As with most immunotherapy, treatment response may be delayed and a transient worsening of disease may develop before responses are observed and the disease stabilizes. Adverse effects associated with ipilimumab include:

- Immune-related enterocolitis (eg, diarrhea) was reported as the most common adverse reaction observed with ipilimumab. Median onset occurs about 6 to 7 weeks after initiation of treatment. Moderate cases of noninfectious enterocolitis (diarrhea ≤ six stools) can be treated with antidiarrheals. For severe cases of diarrhea, high-dose corticosteroids (eg, methylprednisolone 1-2 mg/kg/d) should be given intravenously until symptoms subsided,

then continue steroids taper over more than or equal to 1 month to avoid exacerbation of symptoms. Treatment should be withheld for moderate and severe enterocolitis.

- Severe peripheral motor neuropathy has been reported. Monitor for signs and symptoms of both sensory and motor neuropathy. Consider withholding treatment for moderate neuropathy. For severe neuropathy, treatment should be discontinued and high-dose corticosteroids (eg, methylprednisolone 1-2 mg/kg/d) given intravenously can be initiated if necessary.

- Endocrine disorders (eg, hypopituitarism, adrenal insufficiency, hypogonadism, and hypothyroidism) have been reported. Median onset was 11 weeks after initiation of treatment. Monitor for signs and symptoms and initiate appropriate treatment with either high-dose corticosteroids or hormone replacement therapy in symptomatic patients.

- Severe immune-mediated hepatitis has been reported. Monitor liver function test and assess symptoms of hepatotoxicity prior to treatment. Consider discontinuation of treatment for severe hepatotoxicity and initiate high-dose corticosteroids with steroid tapering over more than or equal to 1 month. Mycophenolate mofetil can be added if transaminases do not decrease within 48 hours of steroid initiation.

- Toxicity of ipilimumab is dose related and was greater at 10 mg/kg versus 3 mg/kg.

Nivolumab (Opdivo) is a fully human immunoglobulin G4 (IgG4) monoclonal antibody that selectively inhibits programmed cell death-1 (PD-1) activity by binding to the PD-1 receptor to block the ligands PD-L1 and PD-L2 from binding. The negative PD-1 receptor signaling that regulates T-cell activation and proliferation is disrupted. This releases the suppression on immune system, thus allowing propagation of antimelanoma immune response.

Nivolumab is FDA approved as monotherapy for treatment of BRAF V600 wild-type or BRAF V600 mutation (+) unresectable or metastatic melanoma, and also as combination therapy with ipilimumab for treatment of unresectable or metastatic melanoma. Nivolumab monotherapy is dosed at 240 mg intravenously every 2 weeks until disease progression or unacceptable toxicity. Nivolumab/ipilimumab combination regimen is dosed at nivolumab 1 mg/kg, followed by ipilimumab 3 mg/kg on the same day, every 3 weeks for 4 doses, then nivolumab 240 mg every 2 weeks. Nivolumab has minimal emetogenicity and does not require premedication. Corticosteroids should be avoided during treatment due to their immunosuppressive properties to reduce the antitumor effects of nivolumab, unless in the case of life-threatening hypersensitivity or anaphylactic reaction or severe immune-mediated adverse effects. Like ipilimumab, nivolumab is also associated with immune-mediated adverse reactions that are autoimmune in nature, often due to reduction in self-tolerance, proliferation of activated T-cells, and proinflammatory reactions (release of cytokines) in normal organs and tissues. Adverse effects associated with nivolumab include:

- Fatigue, rash, pruritus, cough, diarrhea, decreased appetite, constipation, and arthralgia have been reported in more than 20% of patients. Depending on the severity of the reaction, nivolumab should be discontinued.

- Moderate to severe immune-mediated pneumonitis, colitis, hepatitis, endocrinopathies, nephritis, and hypo/hyperthyroidism have been reported. Nivolumab should be discontinued and high-dose systemic steroids (eg, 1-2 mg/kg/d prednisone equivalents) should be administered and tapered gradually.

- Severe immune-mediated colitis has been reported. Monitor for signs and symptoms of colitis. Infliximab 5 mg/kg is preferred for treatment in patients who do not respond within 1 week to high-dose corticosteroid therapy. A single dose of infliximab is sufficient to resolve immune-related colitis in most patients. Treatment should be held for moderate or severe colitis, and permanently discontinued for life-threatening or for recurrent colitis.

- Immune-mediated dermatitis sometimes responds to topical corticosteroids. For patients who do not respond or who have a history of autoimmune skin disorders, consider referral to a dermatologist for management. Severe immune-mediated rash, including Stevens-Johnson syndrome (SJS) and toxic epidermal necrolysis (TEN), have been reported and some cases with fatal outcome. If SJS or TEN is confirmed, permanently discontinue nivolumab.

- Immune-mediated pneumonitis and nephritis have been reported. They tend to be more common with nivolumab compared to ipilimumab monotherapy. Monitor for signs with radiographic imaging and for symptoms of pneumonitis. Treatment should be held for moderate and permanently discontinued for severe or life-threatening pneumonitis. Monitor for elevated serum creatinine prior to and periodically during treatment. Hold treatment for moderate or severe increased serum creatinine, and permanently discontinue for life-threatening increased serum creatinine.

- Immune-mediated hepatitis has been reported. Monitor for abnormal liver tests prior to and periodically during treatment. Treatment should be held for moderate and permanently discontinued for severe or life-threatening hepatitis.

- Immune-mediated endocrinopathies may require long-term hormone replacement therapy. Monitor thyroid function prior to and periodically during treatment. Discontinuation of nivolumab is not required if symptoms can be controlled with hormone replacement therapy.

- Immune-mediated toxicities occur more frequently in nivolumab/ipilimumab combination therapy. Gastrointestinal and cutaneous adverse effects tend to manifest earlier in treatment, whereas the onset tends to be later for endocrinopathies and other rarer toxicities (eg, hepatic, renal, and respiratory).

Similar to nivolumab, pembrolizumab (Keytruda) is a highly selective anti-PD-1 humanized monoclonal antibody that inhibits PD-1 activity by binding to the PD-1 receptor on T-cells to block PD-L1 and PD-L2 from binding. Pembrolizumab is FDA approved as monotherapy for treatment of unresectable or metastatic melanoma. It is dosed at 2 mg/kg administered intravenously over 30 minutes every 3 weeks until disease progression or unacceptable toxicity. Adverse effects associated with pembrolizumab were less than ipilimumab (10% vs 20%). Adverse effects associated with pembrolizumab are very similar to nivolumab.

Single-Agents Chemotherapy

Dacarbazine (DTIC) is an alkylating agent FDA approved for treatment of metastatic melanoma. Dacarbazine is dosed at 150 to 250 mg/m² intravenous piggyback (IVPB) on days 1 to 5 every 3 to 4 weeks. Response rates with single-agent dacarbazine range from 15% to 25%, with duration of response lasting 3 to 6 months. Adverse effects associated with dacarbazine are:

- Myelosuppression (eg, leukopenia and thrombocytopenia) is a dose-limiting toxicity.

- Nausea and vomiting can be severe and dacarbazine is classified as a highly emetogenic chemotherapeutic agent.

- Antiemetic therapy with a 5-HT3 receptor antagonist and a corticosteroid given 30 to 60 minutes prior to dacarbazine is recommended.

- Flu-like symptoms (eg, fever, chills, malaise, myalgia, and arthralgia).

- Local pain and burning sensation at injection site.

- Risk of extravasation (extravasation may lead to severe tissue necrosis around injection site).

- Hepatotoxicity with hepatocellular necrosis and hepatic vein thrombosis.

Temozolomide (Temodar) is an oral alkylating agent structurally similar to dacarbazine. Temozolomide and dacarbazine have demonstrated similar response rates. The dose of temozolomide is 200 mg/m²/d orally for 5 days; repeat every 28 days up to 12 cycles. Dose-limiting myelosuppression (eg, leukopenia and thrombocytopenia) is associated with temozolomide. Temozolomide is classified as a moderately emetogenic agent. The use of antiemetics prior to drug administration is recommended to minimize the risk of nausea and vomiting. Fatigue, headache, mild elevation of hepatic transaminases, and photosensitivity has also been associated with temozolomide.

Other chemotherapy with paclitaxel (Taxol) and docetaxel (Taxotere) have been used for treatment of metastatic melanoma; however, response rates are relatively low (6%-18%). With the advent of immunotherapy and molecularly targeted BRAF and MEK inhibition, standard chemotherapy has fallen by the wayside.

Combination Chemotherapy and Biochemotherapy

Similar to single-agent chemotherapies, combination chemotherapy and biochemotherapy regimens have fallen out of favor with the advent of immunotherapy and new molecularly targeted therapies. They are utilized in attempts to improve treatment response of metastatic melanoma, but at the expense of increased toxicity and questionable overall survival benefits.

Dacarbazine has been used in combination with the Dartmouth regimen (dacarbazine 220 mg/m^2 IVPB on day 1-3, carmustine 150 mg/m^2 IVPB on day 1 of every other cycle, cisplatin 25 mg/m^2 IVPB on days 1-3, and tamoxifen 10 mg po bid with cycle repeat every 3 weeks). Evidence demonstrated equivalent response rates between the Dartmouth regimen and dacarbazine; however, side effects were higher in the combination group. Other combination regimens such as CVD (cisplatin, vinblastine, and dacarbazine) have been used for treatment of metastatic melanoma; however, there is no survival advantage with the use of CVD over single-agent dacarbazine. The most commonly used biochemotherapy regimen is the CVD regimen with IL-2 and interferon-alfa 2b. However, the addition of immunotherapy to combination chemotherapy did not improve quality of response or overall survival, but increased side effects.

Follow-up Care

Lifetime annual skin examination is recommended for all patients with melanoma regardless of melanoma stage. Frequency of follow-up surveillance should be individualized and determined based on patients' risk factors, family history, presence of dysplastic nevi, and history of nonmelanoma skin cancers. Health care professionals should educate patients to perform monthly self-examination of their skin and suspicious lesions should be evaluated by a health care professional.

CASE Application

1. AE is a 28-year-old woman in clinic today for routine annual check-up with her general practitioner. AE's older brother was recently treated for basal cell carcinoma. Which of the following are risk factor(s) associated with melanoma AE should be educated about?

   a. Presence of multiple dysplastic nevi
   b. Presence of genetic factors
   c. Individuals with fair skin type who sunburns easily
   d. Individuals who are immunosuppressed

2. Which of the following statement(s) is (are) true regarding the subtypes of melanoma? Select all that apply.

   a. Superficial spreading melanomas are the most common type of melanomas with lesions usually arising from preexisting nevus.
   b. Nodular melanomas are slow-growing lesions that develop and spread in a vertical growth phase pattern.
   c. Lentigo maligna melanomas are more commonly reported in children, with lesions less likely to metastasize.
   d. Uveal melanomas are rare lower extremity malignancies arising from pigmented epithelium of the choroids, with lesions more likely to metastasize to liver.

3. FB is a 25-year-old woman presented to dermatology clinic for her initial check-up after noticing multiple lesions and dark spot on her skin after 1 month of tanning session. Which of the following is not a part of the ABCDE rule used to identify and evaluate a suspicious lesion? Select all that apply.

   a. Asymmetry
   b. Border irregularity
   c. Color of lesions
   d. Depths of the lesions
   e. Evolving or changing characteristics of a lesion

4. TS is a 35-year-old man in dermatology clinic today for follow-up visit on a suspicious lesion that was identified last week. Which is the best method in confirming the diagnosis?

   a. Obtain a complete clinical examination, and medical history of patient and family members.
   b. Obtain complete laboratory studies with hematology, electrolytes, liver function test, and lactate dehydrogenase (LDH).
   c. Consider full-thickness excisional biopsy with 1 to 3 mm margin of normal-appearing skin.
   d. Consider ordering a chest x-ray and a computerized tomography (CT) scan for confirming diagnosis.

5. According to the ACS, what is the latest recommendation for the prevention and screening of melanoma? Select all that apply.

   a. Wear proper protective clothing to cover as much exposed skin as possible (ie, sun glasses, hat with wide brim, long sleeve clothing, etc.).
   b. Use sunscreen lotion with an SPF of at least 15 or higher.
   c. Avoid direct sun exposure between 10 AM to 4 PM when ultraviolet rays are the most intense.
   d. Avoid the use of tanning beds or sunlamps to minimize exposure to ultraviolet radiation.

6. Which of the following molecular targeted marker is relevant for the treatment of metastatic melanoma?

   a. EGFR (+) mutation
   b. Kras wild-type
   c. BRAF V600 (+) mutation
   d. VEGF (+) mutation
   e. ALK (+) mutation

7. TN is a 54-year-old man with newly diagnosed stage IV metastatic melanoma. TN has good PS with no comorbid conditions, thought to be perfect candidate for immunotherapy. Which of the following immunotherapy would be treatment of choice for TN?

   a. Interferon alfa-2b
   b. Dacarbazine
   c. Carmustine
   d. IL-2
   e. Paclitaxel

8. Which of the following oral chemotherapeutic agent has been used in the treatment of unresectable melanoma?

   a. Capecitabine
   b. Lapatinib
   c. Erlotinib
   d. Procarbazine
   e. Vemurafenib

9. KT is a 45-year-old woman with newly diagnosed stage III melanoma; KT tumor was surgically resected 3 months ago but was found to have (+) lymph node 4/10 involvement. KT is in clinic today to discuss adjuvant treatment. Which of the following is the best treatment option for KT?

   a. Ipilimumab
   b. IL-2
   c. Interferon-alpha 2b
   d. Procarbazine
   e. Trametinib

10. DS is a 35-year-old man with stage IV unresectable melanoma who is in dermatology clinic for follow-up visit and assessment for his second treatment with ipilimumab. What side effect(s) would you monitor in DS prior to treatment?

    a. Immune-mediated constipation
    b. Immune-mediated enterocolitis
    c. Capillary leak syndrome
    d. Myelosuppression
    e. Immune-mediated depression

11. CD is a 28-year-old woman who is to start immunotherapy treatment with high-dose interferon-alfa 2b. Select the side effect(s) associated with interferon. Select all that apply.

    a. Flu-like symptoms requiring premedication with antipyretic
    b. Fatigue
    c. Depression
    d. Somnolence and confusion

12. HM is a 52-year-old man with newly diagnosed BRAF V600E mutation (+) unresectable melanoma. HM has untreated CNS involvement, with poor PS. Which of the following treatment option is appropriate for HM?

    a. IL-2
    b. Temozolomide

   c. Vemurafenib
   d. Dacarbazine
   e. Ipilimumab

13. LG is a 40-year-old woman in dermatology clinic today to discuss vemurafenib treatment with her oncologist. Which of the following are side effect(s) associated with vemurafenib in the treatment of unresectable melanoma? Select all that apply.

    a. Arthralgia
    b. Cutaneous squamous cell carcinoma
    c. QTc prolongation
    d. Photosensitivity

14. Which of the follow is the only FDA-approved combination tyrosine kinase oral chemotherapy regimen approved for the treatment of unresectable or metastatic V600E or V600K mutated melanoma?

    a. Ipilimumab + Dacarbazine
    b. IL-2 + Temozolomide
    c. Interferon-alpha 2b + Temozolomide
    d. Vemurafenib + Dabrafenib
    e. Dabrafenib + Trametinib

15. PF is a 42-year-old man with newly resected stage III melanoma who is in dermatology clinic today to discuss adjuvant treatment option. Which of the following is the correct FDA-approved dosing of interferon-alfa 2b when used as single agent for adjuvant treatment of melanoma?

    a. 375 mg/m^2 IVPB on days 1 and 15 with cycle repeat every 28 days
    b. 20 million IU/m^2 IVPB five times weekly for 4 weeks, then 10 million IU/m^2 subcutaneously three times weekly for 48 weeks
    c. 250 mg/m^2 IVPB on days 1 to 5 with cycle repeat every 21 days
    d. 600,000 IU/kg IVPB every 8 hours for a maximum of 14 doses; repeat after 9 days for a total of 28 doses per course
    e. 150 mg/m^2 po daily for 5 days with cycle repeat every 28 days

16. WK is a 36-year-old man with newly diagnosed unresectable BRAF V600E (+) melanoma. He is in excellent health with no comorbid conditions. WK is being admitted to oncology unit to start treatment with IL-2. Which of the following is the correct FDA-approved dosing of IL-2 when used as single agent for treatment of unresectable melanoma?

    a. 375 mg/m^2 IVPB on days 1 and 15 with cycle repeat every 28 days
    b. 20 million IU/m^2 IVPB five times weekly for 4 weeks, then 10 million IU/m^2 subcutaneously three times weekly for 48 weeks
    c. 250 mg/m^2 IVPB on days 1 to 5 with cycle repeat every 21 days

d. 600,000 IU/kg IVPB every 8 hours for a maximum of 14 doses; repeat after 9 days for a total of 28 doses per course

e. 150 mg/m² po daily for 5 days with cycle repeat every 28 days

17. GK is a 62-year-old man who has just completed his adjuvant treatment for advanced stage III melanoma. Which of the following is (are) appropriate follow-up care recommendations for patients with melanoma? Select all that apply.

a. Annual skin examination and surveillance by a dermatologist for all patients with melanoma regardless of stage of lesions.

b. Educate patients to perform monthly self-examination of their skin and lymph nodes.

c. Educate patients about skin cancer prevention including sun protection and proper use of sunscreen with at least SPF of 15 or higher.

d. None of the above is appropriate follow-up care recommendations for patients with melanoma.

18. RC is a 47-year-old man with stage IV unresectable melanoma who is in the hospital for his treatment with high-dose IL-2. Select the side effect associated with IL-2 that can lead to hypotension and reduced organ perfusion.

a. Capillary leak syndrome

b. Myelosuppression

c. Anemia

d. Hepatotoxicity

e. Delirium

19. AC is a 35-year-old woman with newly diagnosed stage IV metastatic melanoma who presents to clinic

for treatment with Nivolumab. Which of the following is the correct FDA-approved dosing for Nivolumab monotherapy?

a. 240 mg IVPB every 2 weeks

b. 240 mg IVPB every 3 weeks

c. 200 mg IVPB every 2 weeks

d. 1 mg/kg IVPB every 2 weeks

e. 1 mg/kg IVPB every 3 weeks

20. GS is a 52-year-old man who has developed severe immune-mediated colitis after receiving 12 cycles of pembrolizumab. He was started on prednisone 2 mg/kg/d, but has not improved after 1 week of treatment. Which of the following is the most appropriate treatment option for GS now?

a. Prednisone 4 mg/kg/d

b. Infliximab 5 mg/kg IVPB

c. Tacrolimus 0.06 mg/kg po twice daily

d. Loperamide 2 mg po every 2 hours

e. Atropine 0.4 mg IV

21. DK is a 45-year-old woman with stage IV unresectable melanoma who presents to clinic today for her third cycle of Pembrolizumab. She has tolerated the previous 2 cycles of treatment very well, except for some mild nausea. Which of the following is the most appropriate supportive care to add to DK's treatment today?

a. Acetaminophen 650 mg po

b. Hydrocortisone 100 mg IV

c. Dexamethasone 10 mg IV

d. Diphenhydramine 25 mg po

e. Ondansetron 8 mg IV

TAKEAWAY POINTS »

- Melanoma is a serious form of skin cancer.
- Risk factors include personal or family history of melanoma, genetic factors, atypical dysplastic nevi, previous history of nonmelanoma skin cancer, and individuals who are immunosuppressed.
- Practice sun protective safety measures if you have to be outdoors by wearing sun protective clothing and using sunscreen with an SPF of 15 or higher.
- The ABCDE rule of melanoma identifies clinical features of any suspicious lesions.
- Biopsy is the only way to confirm the diagnosis of melanoma.
- The outcome and survival rate is dependent on stage of disease at diagnosis; outcome is best if melanoma is diagnosed at its earliest stages of disease when 5-year survival rate is more than 90%.
- The two most important prognostic factors influencing staging and outcome are the Breslow tumor thickness

and the presence or absence of ulceration of the overlying epithelium.

- Molecular marker BRAF V600 E or V600K mutation has been identified to be associated with melanoma.
- High-dose interferon-alfa 2b is FDA approved for adjuvant treatment of melanoma.
- Ipilimumab is a CTLA-4 inhibitor used in adjuvant and metastatic or unresectable melanoma in treatment with ipilimumab is associated with immune-mediated adverse events requiring continuous monitoring prior to treatment.
- Nivolumab and pembrolizumab are anti-PD-1 immunotherapy agents with FDA approval for treatment of metastatic or unresectable melanoma. Treatment with anti-PD-1 agents is associated with immune-mediated adverse events, which depending on the severity of symptoms may require withholding or permanently discontinuing treatment.

- Immune-mediated adverse events associated with immunotherapy can be managed with high-dose corticosteroids or other immunosuppressants.
- Both vemurafenib and dabrafenib are BRAF kinase inhibitor FDA approved for treatment of metastatic or unresectable melanoma with BRAF V600E or V600K mutation (+) disease.
- Trametinib and cobimetinib are MEK inhibitor with FDA approval for treatment of metastatic or unresectable melanoma with BRAF V600E or V600K mutations.
- Combination use of BRAF and MEK inhibitors obtained FDA accelerated approval for use in the treatment of metastatic or unresectable melanoma as the combination therapy allows for greater inhibition of the MAPK pathway, and improved outcome in patients with BRAF mutation (+) disease.
- Temozolomide has been used in treatment of advanced or metastatic or unresectable melanoma and has a similar response rate compared to dacarbazine.
- High-dose IL-2 has been used in treatment of metastatic melanoma in selected patients with good PS; treatment with IL-2 is associated with many severe side effects requiring continuous monitoring.
- National Comprehensive Cancer Network (NCCN) guidelines recommended follow-up care with lifetime annual skin examination for patients with melanoma regardless to stage of lesions.

BIBLIOGRAPHY

American Cancer Society. Skin cancer–melanoma 2014. www.cancer.org. Accessed January 27, 2014.

Atallah E, Flaherty L. Treatment of metastatic malignant melanoma. *Curr Treat Options Oncol.* 2005;6:185-193.

Balch CM, Soong SJ, Atkins MB, et al. An evidence-based staging system for cutaneous melanoma. *CA Cancer J Clin.* 2004;54:131-149.

Coit DG, Andtbacka R, Bichakjian CK, et al. Melanoma: clinical practice guidelines in oncology. *JNCCN.* 2009;7:250-275.

Kaufman HL, Kirkwood JM, Hodi FS, et al. The Society for Immunotherapy of Cancer consensus statement on tumour immunotherapy for the treatment of cutaneous melanoma. *Nat Rev Clin Oncol.* 2013;10:588-598.

Li Y, McClay EF. Systemic chemotherapy for the treatment of metastatic melanoma. *Semin Oncol.* 2002;29:413-426.

National Comprehensive Cancer Network. Melanoma (Version 1.2017), November 10, 2016. http://www.nccn.org. Accessed March 26, 2017.

Serrone L, Zeuli M, Sega FM, et al. Dacarbazine-based chemotherapy for metastatic melanoma: thirty-year experience overview. *J Exp Clin Cancer Res.* 2000;19:21-34.

Weber JS, Kahler KC, Hauschild A. Management of immune-related adverse events and kinetics of response with ipilimumab. *J Clin Oncol.* 2012;30(21):2691-2697.

KEY ABBREVIATIONS

AJCC = American Joint Commission on Cancer
CPK = creatine phosphokinase
CT = computerized tomography
CTLA-4 = cytotoxic T lymphocyte antigen-4
CVD = cisplatin, vinblastine, and dacarbazine
DVT = deep vein thrombosis
EKG = electrocardiogram
FDA = Food and Drug Administration
IG4 = immunoglobulin G4
IL-2 = interleukin-2
IVPB = intravenous piggyback
LVEF = left ventricular ejection fraction
MEK = mitogen activated extracellular kinase

MRI = magnetic resonance imaging
NSAID = nonsteroidal anti-inflammatory agent
PD-1 = programmed cell death-1
PE = pulmonary embolism
PET = positron emission tomography
PS = performance status
SJS = Stevens-Johnson syndrome
SPF = sun protection factor
TEN = toxic epidermal necrolysis
TNFα = tumor necrosis factor alpha
UVA = long wave ultraviolet A
UVB = short wave ultraviolet B

Colorectal Cancer

Keith A. Hecht

FOUNDATION OVERVIEW

General Overview

Colorectal cancer (CRC) involves the colon, rectum, and anal canal. Colon and rectal cancer are grouped together in epidemiological studies and share similar pathophysiology, but there are distinct approaches to treatment. Conventional therapies including surgery, radiation, and chemotherapy are used depending on the stage and type of cancer. Targeted therapies, such as monoclonal antibodies and kinases inhibitors, are of increasing importance in treating advanced CRCs.

Pathophysiology

CRCs are the result of an accumulation of genetic mutations that transforms normal epithelial cells into nonmalignant adenomas or polyps, then finally malignant adenocarcinomas. Mutations originate due to hereditary syndromes or acquired through lifestyle or environmental risk factors.

Key Definitions

Adenocarcinoma—malignant neoplasm of epithelial cells with glandular or glandlike features.

Adjuvant—in oncology, treatment added after primary therapy, usually a surgery, with the goal to reduce recurrence.

CEA—carcinoembryonic antigen, tumor marker found in the serum for CRC but is also elevated in other malignant and nonmalignant conditions such as smoking.

Chemoradiation—chemotherapy given concomitantly with radiation, usually with radiosensitizing agents like fluoropyrimidines or platinums.

Microsatellite instability—when microsatellites, repeated sequences of DNA that are usually of a set length, accumulate errors and become longer or shorter than normal.

Neoadjuvant—in oncology, treatment added before primary therapy, usually a surgery, with the goal to improve outcomes of that curative therapy.

TNM staging—method of classifying cancers by T: tumor size, N: lymph node involvement, and M: presence of distant metastases; the combination of these three factors categorizes a cancer into "stages"; the higher the stage number the more widespread the cancer and generally the worse the prognosis.

Clinical Presentation/Signs and Symptoms

The clinical presentation of CRCs can be nonspecific including gastrointestinal (GI) bleeding, abdominal pain, and change in bowel habits (constipation, abnormal stools). Patients sometimes experience significant weight loss and a partial or complete bowel obstruction. The pattern of spread to distant sites primarily involves the liver and lungs (liver more common for colon and lung for rectal cancer).

Diagnosis

The diagnosis of CRC is accomplished through colonoscopy and biopsies. A colonoscopy can visualize the entire colon and remove polyps for pathology review. If a full colonoscopy is not possible (eg, due to an obstruction), a postoperative colonoscopy is still recommended to rule out any synchronous tumors that may occur. Barium enemas with flexible sigmoidoscopy (FSIG) can diagnose tumors in the sigmoid colon but could miss any tumors in the remaining two-thirds of the colon. Sometimes a bowel obstruction or other barriers preclude a complete colonoscopy necessitating a radiographic diagnosis.

During colonoscopy, a biopsy of the suspicious mass is taken to confirm diagnosis of CRC. CRCs typically arise from glandular tissue and are thusly classified as adenocarcinomas. Additional pathologic testing should be performed to determine if the tumor has mutations in KRAS, NRAS, or BRAF. Testing to determine if the patient is positive for microsatellite instability-high (MSI-H) and mismatch repair deficiency (dMMR) should also be performed.

Colon and rectal cancers are staged clinically using radiographic, endoscopic, and intraoperative techniques prior to the definitive pathologic staging. CRC staging utilizes the TNM criteria and this provides prognostic information and aids treatment decisions. An important component of staging is the number of lymph nodes resected. Inadequate lymph node sampling can miss advanced disease and should be considered high risk for metastases and tumor recurrence. The tumor-marker CEA is used to monitor response to treatment and to detect recurrence.

Screening

Screening can prevent CRC through early detection and removal of noninvasive adenomatous polyps and can reduce

---

TABLE 19-1 | **Patient Counseling Points Prior to Guaiac-Based Stool Tests**

To Avoid False Positives	To Avoid False Negatives

• **Dietary restrictions**
  • Avoid red meat (beef, lamb, liver) and raw vegetables with peroxidase activity (turnips, broccoli, cauliflower, and radishes) for 3 d prior to testing[a]
• **Medical restrictions**
  • Avoid rectal enemas, rectal medications, and digital rectal examinations for 3 d prior to testing
  • Avoid aspirin and nonsteroidal anti-inflammatory drugs for up to 7 d prior to testing
  • Avoid testing if blood from hemorrhoids is evident in stool
  • Delay testing until 3 d after menstrual bleeding has ended
	• Avoid vitamin C in excess of 250 mg supplements and from citrus juices and fruit for 3 d prior to testing
	• Avoid testing dehydrated samples (rehydrating of samples is not recommended)

Procedure for Guaiac-Based Stool Testing
Patient uses an applicator stick to apply stool to two test cards on three separate occasions, usually from different bowel movements on consecutive days (total of six test cards or samples). After the sample dries, the card is mailed or returned to the healthcare professional.

[a]Test instructions for several products no longer contain dietary vegetable or fruit restrictions.

Reproduced with permission from DiPiro JT, Talbert RL, Yee GC, et al: *Pharmacotherapy: A Pathophysiologic Approach*, 10th ed. New York, NY: McGraw-Hill; 2017.

mortality by preventing progression to advanced disease. Screening methods include stool tests (fecal occult blood tests, stool DNA tests) and structural examinations (FSIG, colonoscopy, virtual colonoscopy [VC]). Fecal occult blood tests detect hemoglobin products in the stool through consecutive sampling of three bowel movements. Aspirin, non-steroidal anti-inflammatory drugs (NSAIDs), vitamin C, red meat, poultry, fish, and some raw vegetables can interact with versions of this test (Table 19-1). Stool tests must be repeated at regular intervals, and require follow-up with colonoscopy for abnormal results. Newly available fecal blood testing, called fecal immunochemical testing (FIT) is more sensitive than traditional testing methods and less prone to false positives. FIT testing should be considered the preferred method of screening for blood in the stool. It has been reported that the incidence of CRC may be reduced by 20% with stool testing, and mortality from CRC decreased by 15% to 33% over a period of 8 to 13 years. FSIG is an endoscopic procedure that can be performed in an outpatient visit with a standard bowel preparation, and usually without sedation. It can reduce mortality from CRC by 60% to 80% over a period of 10 years. However, its drawbacks include limited viewing of only the rectum, sigmoid, and descending colon, and the need to be followed-up by a colonoscopy if adenomas are discovered.

Colonoscopy is also an endoscopic procedure which allows for examination of the entire tract of the bowel. Colonoscopy requires more extensive bowel preparation as well as procedural sedation. Additionally, removal of adenomatous polyps can be performed during this procedure. Colonoscopy is considered the gold standard for screening procedures of CRC.

VC is an imaging technique that produces two and three dimensional images of the entire colon and rectum using computed tomography or magnetic resonance imaging. Patients undergoing VC also have to have extensive bowel preparation. VC has been shown effective at detecting polyps and cancer; however, positive results must be confirmed with colonoscopy.

Screening should start at age 50 for average-risk patients and the frequency of screening depends on the method utilized (eg, stool testing should be preformed annually, if stool testing is the screening method utilized; colonoscopy should be performed at least every 10 years, if colonoscopy is the screening method utilized). All abnormal tests should be followed-up with a colonoscopy. Persons with above average risk for CRC (history of adenomatous polyps, history of CRC, family history of CRC, inflammatory bowel disease, hereditary syndromes predisposing to CRC) should have more frequent screenings that begin at an earlier age.

Risk Factors

Obesity, higher body mass index (BMI), hyperinsulinemia, increased C-peptide levels, diabetes, and lack of fiber intake increase CRC risk. The American Gastroenterological Association recommends a total daily fiber intake of at least 30 to 35 g. Additionally, some people are predisposed to CRC from hereditary conditions such as hereditary nonpolyposis colon cancer (HNPCC, also called Lynch syndrome) or familial adenomatous polyposis (FAP). Other risk factors for CRC include inflammatory bowel disease, alcohol, and smoking.

PREVENTION

Aspirin or Nonsteroidal Anti-Inflammatory Drugs

Consistent use of aspirin and NSAIDs has been noted to reduce the incidence of colorectal adenoma. Longer-term use and higher doses are positively associated with greater risk reductions. However, the adverse effects of aspirin (GI bleeding and hemorrhagic stroke) and NSAIDs (GI bleeding and cardiovascular outcomes) are also increased with longer use and higher doses. The US Preventive Services Task Force (USPSTF) and American Cancer Society do not recommend the routine use of these agents for primary prevention of CRC due to the significant risk associated and lack of evidence of decreased mortality from CRC.

Hormone Therapy

Several landmark studies have noted that women who used hormone replacement (estrogen plus progestin) have lower incidences of CRC than those who did not. However, the USPSTF recommends against combined estrogen and progestin as prevention of any chronic conditions (including CRC) in postmenopausal women due to the associated increased risk of harm.

Other

Dietary factors may play a role in the risk of CRC, including protective effects. There have been inconsistencies in the data for supplemental fiber despite the recommendations. Vitamin D levels have been shown to be lower in patients with CRC; however, clinical trials to date have not shown benefit in vitamin D supplementation to prevent CRC. Calcium and magnesium have shown promise and the American College of Gastroenterology recommends calcium supplementation to prevent polyps.

TREATMENT

Colon Cancer

Many early stage colon cancers are resectable and the therapy of choice is surgery. Low risk, localized disease with no lymph node involvement does not usually require adjuvant systemic therapy. Adjuvant chemotherapy is a consideration for higher-risk colon cancer with no nodal or metastatic involvement, for example, high-grade tumors, tumors with microsatellite instability, or inadequate lymph node dissection. Stage III colon cancers, having lymph node involvement, have documented benefit from adjuvant chemotherapy, and therefore 6 months of chemotherapy following surgical resection is recommended. Stage II colon cancers have a less clear documented benefit with adjuvant therapy, although research is currently ongoing. Future guidelines may assist in treatment decisions for these patients. Currently, treatment decisions should be made on a case-by-case basis.

Metastatic disease, unlike most other cancers, will still be surgically resected if the spread is limited. Local therapy for the primary tumor and metastases can translate into long-term remission and survival. Neoadjuvant chemotherapy may be given to shrink unresectable disease with the goal to make the patient eligible for surgery. Metastatic disease almost always warrants the use of systemic therapy.

Chemotherapy usually consists of combination therapy including a fluoropyrimidine, like fluorouracil, or capecitabine. See Table 19-2 for a list of medications used in the treatment of CRCs. If fluorouracil is used, leucovorin is usually added to increase its efficacy, although also increasing toxicity. Historically, fluorouracil was given in bolus regimens (Mayo Clinic and Roswell Park regimens), but are now mostly given as 2-day continuous infusions due to a better safety and perhaps efficacy profile. Oxaliplatin or irinotecan may be combined with fluoropyrimidine in patients with advanced CRC. Targeted therapies are considered in patients with metastatic or relapsed disease.

Infusional fluorouracil, leucovorin, and oxaliplatin (FOLFOX) is the recommended regimen for all stage III and some high-risk stage II colon cancers. FOLFOX is also a first-line regimen for metastatic disease. Acute neurotoxicity (cold sensitivity) and cumulative neurotoxicity (peripheral neuropathies) are unique side effects with this regimen and can be dose limiting. Researchers have investigated various strategies to mitigate these effects with mixed success.

Irinotecan has also shown to increase the efficacy of fluoropyrimidine-based therapies. Bolus fluorouracil plus leucovorin when combined with irinotecan (IFL) has shown unacceptable high rates of severe adverse events including fatal diarrhea. Infusional fluorouracil (FOLFIRI) regimens are used in its place. Irinotecan regimens are considered acceptable first-line therapy for metastatic colon cancer or used as a second-line agent after failing oxaliplatin-based therapy. Irinotecan's dose limiting toxicity is diarrhea. Early diarrhea occurs due to a cholinergic syndrome and is best treated with an anticholinergic drug such as atropine. Diarrhea can also occur later due to enterohepatic recirculation of irinotecan and its main active metabolite SN-38. Late diarrhea should be treated with an aggressive loperamide regimen, dosed 4 mg at the onset of diarrhea, and 2 mg every 2 hours until diarrhea free for 12 hours. Patients with severe diarrhea may require hospital admission for rehydration and therapy with octreotide. Irinotecan also can cause significant bone marrow suppression.

Substituting orally administered capecitabine for fluorouracil may add to convenience. Most current evidence suggests capecitabine regimens have similar efficacy to fluorouracil based therapy, but with different side effects. Capecitabine has higher rates of palmar-plantar erythrodysesthesias (PPE, or hand-foot syndrome), GI toxicity, and thrombocytopenia.

Targeted agents are now standard therapy for metastatic and/or recurrent colon cancer. Bevacizumab was the first targeted agent approved for use in metastatic colon cancer and works by inhibiting angiogenesis, an important step in tumor biology. Toxicities include delayed wound healing, bleeding and thrombotic complications, hypertension, proteinuria, and bowel perforation. Epidermal growth factor receptor 1 (EGFR1) targeting agents, namely cetuximab and panitumumab, also have activity and are used as part of standard therapy in metastatic and/or recurrent disease. These agents should not be used in patients with mutation in KRAS, NRAS, or BRAF as these mutations confers resistance to the EGFR therapy. These agents are recommended for left-sided CRC only, tumors arising from the splenic flexure of the colon or later. EGFR1 agents commonly cause a unique rash described as acneiform, although not caused by bacteria. This rash is managed with moisturizers, tetracyclines for anti-inflammatory effects, topical antibiotics to prevent superinfections, and in severe cases, corticosteroids. Drying agents like benzoyl peroxide or retinoids should not be used. Cetuximab can also cause infusion reactions that can be serious and fatalities have been reported. EGFR1 antibodies can also cause electrolyte wasting, most commonly hypomagnesemia. Regular monitoring of magnesium, potassium, and calcium is recommended. Ziv-aflibercept (a soluble recombinant fusion protein) and ramucirumab (a monoclonal antibody) have similar mechanisms of action to bevacizumab. They are each indicated with FOLFIRI in patients who have failed an oxaliplatin containing regimen. Their side effect profile is similar to bevacizumab. Regorafenib is an oral kinase inhibitor that is indicated as a single agent in the third- or fourth-line setting. Notable

TABLE 19-2 **CRC Drug Summary**

Drug	Drug Class/MOA	Adverse Effects	Other Considerations
Fluorouracil (Adrucil)	Antimetabolite	Bone marrow suppression, mucositis, diarrhea	Infusional less toxic than bolus regimens, contraindicated in DPD deficiency
Capecitabine (Xeloda)	Antimetabolite	Fluorouracil toxicities, hand-foot rash	Drug accumulation with renal impairment, oral therapy, interacts with warfarin, contraindicated in DPD deficiency, take with food
Trifluridine/ Tipiracil (Lonsurf)	Antimetabolite	Bone marrow suppression, mucositis, diarrhea	Oral therapy, trifluridine is chemotherapy agent, tipiracil inhibits trifluridine metabolism, dose based on trifluridine component, take with food
Oxaliplatin (Eloxatin)	Platinum agent	Acute cold sensitivity, cumulative peripheral neuropathy, hypersensitivity reactions	Oxaliplatin-free intervals can decrease neurotoxicity
Irinotecan (Camptosar)	Topoisomerase I inhibitor	Early and late diarrhea, dehydration, severe neutropenia	Early diarrhea is cholinergically mediated, late diarrhea is secretory. Dose reduction with elevated serum bilirubin, dose reduction in UGT1A1*28 homozygous patients
Bevacizumab (Avastin)	VEGF inhibitor, humanized monoclonal antibody	Bleeding, arterial thrombotic events, impaired wound healing, gastrointestinal perforation	Treat hypertension and monitor for proteinuria. Consider holding dose with uncontrolled elevations. Wait at least 4-6 weeks after surgery to initiate therapy
Ramucirumab (Cyramza)	VEGF inhibitor, fully human monoclonal antibody	Treat hypertension and monitor for proteinuria. Consider holding dose with uncontrolled elevations. Wait at least 4-6 weeks after surgery to initiate therapy	Treat hypertension and monitor for proteinuria. Consider holding dose with uncontrolled elevations. Wait at least 4-6 weeks after surgery to initiate therapy
Ziv-Aflibercept (Zaltrap)	VEGF inhibitor, soluble recombinant fusion protein	Bleeding, arterial thrombotic events, impaired wound healing, gastrointestinal perforation	Treat hypertension and monitor for proteinuria. Consider holding dose with uncontrolled elevations. Wait at least 4-6 weeks after surgery to initiate therapy
Regorafenib (Stivarga)	VEGF inhibitor, oral kinase inhibitor	Hepatotoxicity, bleeding, hypertension, hand-foot syndrome	Monitor hepatic function before and during therapy.
Cetuximab (Erbitux)	EGFR inhibitor, chimeric monoclonal antibody	Infusion reactions, skin rash, magnesium wasting	KRAS, NRAS, BRAF gene mutations leads to tumor insensitivity to EGFR therapy, decreased efficacy in right-sided colon cancer
Panitumumab (Vectibix)	EGFR inhibitor, fully human monoclonal antibody	Infusion reactions, skin rash, magnesium wasting	KRAS, NRAS, BRAF gene mutations leads to tumor insensitivity to EGFR therapy, decreased efficacy in right-sided colon cancer
Nivolumab (Opdivo)	PD-1 inhibitor, fully human monoclonal antibody	Immune-mediated toxicities including pneumonitis, colitis, hepatitis, endocrinopathies, nephritis, encephalitis, and skin toxicity	Effective in MSI-H/dMMR tumors
Pembrolizumab (Keytruda)	PD-1 inhibitor, fully human monoclonal antibody	Immune-mediated toxicities including pneumonitis, colitis, hepatitis, endocrinopathies, nephritis, encephalitis, and skin toxicity	Effective in MSI-H/dMMR tumors

toxicities for regorafenib include potentially fatal hepatotoxicity, bleeding, hypertension, and hand-foot syndrome. Tumors that are MSI-H or dMMR positive are likely to respond to programmed cell death protein 1 (PD-1) inhibitors, nivolumab and pembrolizumab. These agents inhibit the PD-1 receptor on the T-lymphocyte, preventing the tumor from deactivating it. These agents have both shown promising efficacy in patients with heavily pretreated CRC. Their side effect profiles are similar with immune-mediated side effects being of primary concern. These include immune-mediated pneumonitis, colitis, hepatitis, endocrinopathies, nephritis, encephalitis, and skin toxicity.

Rectal Cancer

Rectal cancer is often treated with a combination of surgery, radiation therapy (RT), chemoradiation, and chemotherapy.

Many of the therapies for rectal cancer are the same or similar to colon cancer except for the emphasis on radiation or chemoradiation as a standard modality in treatment. Preoperative chemotherapy may be recommended for 2 to 3 months, and an additional 4 to 6 months of chemotherapy when adjuvant treatment is appropriate. An interesting approach in rectal cancer is the use of radiation sensitizing chemotherapy regimens along with RT, such as fluorouracil.

SPECIAL CONSIDERATIONS

Pharmacogenetic information is increasingly being used to steer treatment decisions by predicting toxicities or response when treating CRC. Irinotecan and its principle active metabolite, SN-38, are primarily eliminated through glucuronidation by UGT1A1. Homozygous mutant varieties of this gene can significantly decrease clearance of the drug, leading to serious adverse reactions. Similarly, dihydropyrimidine dehydrogenase (DPD) deficiency predicts intolerance to fluoropyrimidines and these agents are contraindicated in patients with known deficiencies. Routine testing for UGT1A1 or DPD polymorphisms is not considered standard and debate remains on the optimal patient for testing.

CASE Application

Use the following scenario to answer questions 1 through 3.

GC is a 58-year-old man with a recent diagnosis of stage IV colon cancer. His prior medical history is significant for hypertension (on lisinopril and hydrochlorothiazide [HCTZ]), deep vein thrombosis (on warfarin), and atrial fibrillation (on amiodarone). The oncologist informs the patient the plan is for him to receive neoadjuvant chemotherapy followed by surgery. The oncologist informs GC that he will receive the chemotherapy regimen XELOX (capecitabine and oxaliplatin).

XELOX:

Capecitabine 1000 mg/m^2 orally twice daily for 14 days

Oxaliplatin 130 mg/m^2 IV on day 1

Repeat cycle every 3 weeks

1. GC presents to your pharmacy with a prescription for capecitabine. Which of his home medications has a significant drug interaction with his capecitabine?

    a. Lisinopril
    b. HCTZ
    c. Warfarin
    d. Cetirizine

2. Which of the following points should the pharmacist council GC on regarding his capecitabine?

    a. Take tablets with food.
    b. If he has trouble swallowing the tablets, crush them and mix in applesauce.
    c. Avoid eating grapefruit or drinking grapefruit juice while taking capecitabine.
    d. Avoid drinking cold liquids while taking capecitabine.

3. How many 500 mg capecitabine tablets are required to fill GC's capecitabine prescription for 1 cycle of XELOX? GC's BSA is 2.0 m^2.

    a. 28 tablets
    b. 56 tablets
    c. 112 tablets
    d. 168 tablets

4. PL is a 67-year-old man with a history of diabetes and alcoholism. PL presents to the clinic for his seventh cycle of oxaliplatin. He is currently taking capecitabine at home. PL's complete blood count (CBC) with differential is within normal limits. Before preparing the oxaliplatin for infusion, which parameters would determine if he requires a dose reduction or for this dose to be held? Select all that apply.

    a. Total bilirubin
    b. Renal function estimated by creatinine clearance
    c. Assessment of neurotoxicity side effects
    d. Liver function estimated by aspartate transaminase (AST), alanine transaminase (ALT)

5. PY is a 62-year-old woman diagnosed with stage IV colon cancer with a primary tumor in the sigmoid colon that has spread to the liver. The patient has undergone surgery 2 weeks ago to remove the solitary tumor in the liver and is ready to begin drug therapy including combination chemotherapy (FOLFOX) and a monoclonal antibody. The patient tested negative for KRAS, NRAS, BRAF, MSI, and MMR. What is the most appropriate monoclonal antibody for PY to receive with FOLFOX?

    a. Bevacizumab
    b. Nivolumab
    c. Cetuximab
    d. Ramucirumab

6. Which of the following monoclonal antibodies used in the treatment of CRC is associated with causing hypomagnesemia? Select all that apply.

    a. Panitumumab
    b. Bevacizumab
    c. Cetuximab
    d. Nivolumab

7. During a routine colonoscopy, KG was diagnosed with stage I colon cancer but is otherwise healthy. He is experiencing no symptoms and has no complications from his cancer so far. His oncologist will likely recommend which therapy?

    a. Surgery
    b. Radiation
    c. Neoadjuvant chemotherapy
    d. Adjuvant chemotherapy

8. Which of the following medications is part of the CRC regimen FOLFIRI?

    a. Fludarabine
    b. Lomustine
    c. Oxaliplatin
    d. Irinotecan

9. Which of the following targeted therapies can delay wound healing and should not be used until at least 4 weeks after a surgical procedure. Select all that apply.

    a. Cetuximab
    b. Ramucirumab
    c. Bevacizumab
    d. Pembrolizumab

10. GW is a 58-year-old man with metastatic colon cancer on irinotecan plus cetuximab therapy. When he arrives to the infusion center, he is complaining of new "pimples" appearing all over his chest and face. The oncology nurse asks you to counsel him on managing this new finding. Your counseling points would include which of the following? Select all that apply.

    a. Reassure him that this side effect actually may be predictive of a positive tumor response to this regimen.
    b. Warn him to use sunscreen since direct sunlight can exacerbate his condition.
    c. Recommend him to ask his doctor about isotretinoin, give him the FDA approved med guide, and explain about the iPLEDGE program to reduce birth defects.
    d. Recommend him to ask his doctor about initiating a tetracycline such as doxycycline or minocycline.

11. Which of the following may increase a person's risk of CRC? Select all that apply.

    a. Family history of CRC
    b. Hormone replacement therapy (HRT)
    c. Obesity
    d. HNPCC

12. KY is a 74-year-old man with a diagnosis of relapsed metastatic rectal cancer. His tumor is positive for KRAS mutation. The patient has undergone extensive prior therapies including fluorouracil/leucovorin, XELOX with bevacizumab, and FOLFIRI with ramucirumab. The patient wishes to receive further therapy; however, he is not interested in having to come to the clinic to receive intravenous medications. Which of the following medications is most appropriate for KY at this time?

    a. Capecitabine
    b. Trifluridine/tipiracil
    c. Regorafenib
    d. Ziv-aflibercept

13. SL is 53-year-old woman with advanced CRC that has progressed despite multiple prior chemotherapy regimens. Pathologic review of her tumor reveals she is positive for mutation in KRAS, negative for mutation in BRAF, and positive for deficiency in mismatch repair (dMMR). Which of the following medications is most likely to benefit SL at this time? Select all that apply.

    a. Cetuximab
    b. Nivolumab
    c. Pembrolizumab
    d. Trastuzumab

14. According to national guidelines, what is the recommended age to begin screening for CRC in a person with average risk?

    a. No later than 21 years old
    b. 40 years old
    c. 45 years old
    d. 50 years old

15. Which of the following chemotherapy agents is safe to use in patients with dihydropyridine dehydrogenase (DPD) deficiency? Select all that apply.

    a. Fluorouracil
    b. Trifluridine/tipiracil
    c. Capecitabine
    d. Irinotecan

Use the following scenario to answer questions 16 through 18.

JM is a 63-year-old woman with a recent diagnosis of stage IV CRC with widespread metastatic disease. She has a prior medical history of hypertension, type 2 diabetes, peripheral neuropathy, and inflammatory bowel disease. She is scheduled to begin chemotherapy with FOLFOX and bevacizumab.

FOLFOX and Bevacizumab:

Fluorouracil 400 mg/m^2 bolus then 600 mg/m^2 continuous infusion day 1 and 2

Leucovorin 200 mg/m^2 intravenous infusion day 1 and 2

Oxaliplatin 85 mg/m^2 intravenous infusion day 1

Bevacizumab 10 mg/kg intravenous infusion day 1

Repeat every 2 weeks

16. Which of the medications JM is scheduled to receive does not have anticancer activity when used by itself?

    a. Fluorouracil
    b. Leucovorin
    c. Oxaliplatin
    d. Bevacizumab

17. Which of the conditions from JM's prior medical history may be exacerbated by her receiving bevacizumab?

    a. Hypertension
    b. Diabetes
    c. Peripheral neuropathy
    d. Inflammatory bowel disease

18. Avastin is the brand name of which medication that JM is receiving for her CRC?

    a. Fluorouracil
    b. Leucovorin
    c. Oxaliplatin
    d. Bevacizumab

19. Which of the following statements about CRC is *correct*? Select all that apply.

    a. FOLFOX with bevacizumab can be used as a first-line therapy.
    b. FOLFIRI with bevacizumab can be used as a first-line therapy.
    c. Surgery and other local therapies are almost never a valid option.
    d. Colon cancer tends to first spread to the liver.

20. JL is a 55-year-old African American man concerned about CRC screening. He inquires about screening recommendations for someone his age. Which of the following screening tests is most appropriate for JL?

a. FSIG
b. Digital rectal examination
c. CEA blood test
d. Colonoscopy

TAKEAWAY POINTS »

- Regular screening for CRC can prevent disease and progression to advanced disease. There are various methods for screening, but all abnormal results should be followed-up by a colonoscopy.
- Risk factors for CRC include hereditary predisposition, obesity, diabetes, diet, and alcohol intake.
- Regular use of aspirin and NSAIDs at high doses can reduce the incidence of CRC, but does not decrease mortality and carries significant risk. Primary prevention is not recommended.
- Despite the reduction of incidence in CRC with hormone replacement therapy, use of these drugs for primary prevention of CRC is not recommended due to significant risks.
- Early CRC is often treated with surgery. Adjuvant or neoadjuvant chemotherapy may be considered in stage II CRC and is recommended in stage III disease.

- Metastatic disease is sometimes treated with surgery or other local therapies for limited disease. All metastatic colorectal patients will receive systemic therapy with chemotherapy.
- Fluoropyrimidines are agents in most chemotherapy regimens for both colon and rectal cancers.
- Leucovorin is used with fluorouracil to enhance efficacy, with some increase in toxicity.
- Infusional fluorouracil is preferred over bolus regimens due to lessened toxicity and perhaps better efficacy.
- Oxaliplatin and irinotecan are frequently combined with fluoropyrimidines in colon cancer.
- Agents targeting biological pathways including angiogenesis, EGFR1, and PD-1 are used in CRC.
- Pharmacogenomics in CRC may personalize treatment to predict efficacy and/or toxicities.

BIBLIOGRAPHY

Borders EB, Medina PJ. Colorectal cancer. In: Chisholm-Burns MA, Schwinghammer TL, Wells BG, Malone PM, Kolesar JM, DiPiro JT, eds. *Pharmacotherapy Principles and Practice.* 4th ed. New York, NY: McGraw-Hill; 2016:chap 91.

Chabner BA, Bertino J, Cleary J, et al. Cytotoxic agents. In: Brunton LL, Chabner BA, Knollmann BC, eds. *Goodman & Gilman's The Pharmacological Basis of Therapeutics.* 12th ed. New York, NY: McGraw-Hill; 2011:chap 61.

Chu E, Sartorelli AC. Cancer chemotherapy. In: Katzung BG, Trevor AJ, eds. *Basic & Clinical Pharmacology.* 13th ed. New York, NY: McGraw-Hill; 2015:chap 54.

Holle LM, Clement JM, Davis LE. Colorectal cancer. In: DiPiro JT, Talbert RL, Yee GC, Matzke GR, Wells BG, Posey L, eds. *Pharmacotherapy: A Pathophysiologic Approach.* 10th ed. New York, NY: McGraw-Hill; 2017:chap 130.

National Comprehensive Cancer Network. Breast Cancer (Version 2.2017). https://www.nccn.org/professionals/physician_gls/pdf/colon.pdf. Accessed April 2017.

Rex DK, Boland CR, Dominitz JA, et al. Colorectal cancer screening: Recommendations for physicians and patients from the U.S. Multi-Society Task Force on Colorectal Cancer. *Am J Gastroenterol.* 2017. Published online ahead of print: http://gi.org/wp-content/uploads/2017/06/ajg2017174a.pdf. Accessed August 2017.

KEY ABBREVIATIONS

BMI = body mass index
CEA = carcinoembryonic antigen
dMMR = mismatch repair deficiency
DPD = dihydropyrimidine dehydrogenase
EGFR = epidermal growth factor receptor
FAP = familial adenomatous polyposis
FIT = fecal immunochemical testing

HNPCC = hereditary nonpolyposis colon cancer
MSI-H = microsatellite instability-high
PD-1 = programmed cell death protein 1
PPE = palmar-plantar erythrodysesthesias
PSA = prostate-specific antigen
RT = radiation therapy
USPSTF = US Preventive Services Task Force

Antimicrobial Principles

S. Scott Sutton and Christopher M. Bland

FOUNDATION OVERVIEW

Antimicrobials vary in their ability to inhibit or kill different species of bacteria. Antimicrobials that kill many different species of bacteria are called broad-spectrum antimicrobials; whereas, antimicrobials that kill fewer different species of bacteria are called narrow-spectrum antimicrobials. Empirically treating infectious diseases and monitoring therapy requires knowledge of antimicrobial properties, host factors, patient's normal flora, differentiating infection versus colonization, and understanding clinical presentation and diagnostic tests (microbiologic and nonmicrobiologic laboratory studies). Broad-spectrum antimicrobial coverage increases the likelihood of empirically targeting a causative pathogen; unfortunately, the development of secondary infections caused by selection of antimicrobial-resistant pathogens is a common complication. In addition, adverse events may complicate up to 10% of antimicrobial therapy (adverse event rate is higher for select agents).

TREATMENT

Antimicrobial Properties

Drug-specific considerations in antimicrobial therapy include spectrum of activity, pharmacokinetic (PK) and pharmacodynamic properties, adverse effects, drug interactions, and cost.

Spectrum of Activity

Patients who receive initial antimicrobial therapy that provides coverage against the causative pathogen survive at twice the rate of patients who do not receive adequate therapy initially. Because empiric antimicrobial therapy selection is critical to patient outcomes, broad-spectrum antimicrobials are often utilized because it will increase the likelihood of empirically targeting a causative pathogen. However, if all patients receive broad-spectrum antimicrobials, resistance would become an even more difficult problem. Therefore, it is important to understand the difference in antimicrobial spectrum of activity and select agent(s) that target the pathogens most likely causing the infection. Table 20-1 lists the spectrum of activity for select antimicrobials.

Collateral Damage Collateral damage is defined as the development of resistance occurring in a patient's nontargeted antimicrobial flora that may cause a secondary infection. For example, clindamycin may be utilized to treat gram-positive cocci infections. See Figure 20-1 for a list of gram-positive and gram-negative bacteria. However, clindamycin also readily selects for resistance in a nontargeted organism that may be present in the intestinal tract, *Clostridium difficile*. If several different antimicrobials possess activity against a targeted pathogen, the antimicrobial that is least likely to be associated with collateral damage is preferred.

Antimicrobial Dose

Antimicrobial dosage regimens with the same agent may be different depending upon the infection or pathogen. For example, cefepime (Maxipime), a fourth-generation cephalosporin, has various dosage regimens based on the site of infection. The usual cefepime dosage range for adults is 1 to 2 g intravenously every 8 to 12 hours. Dosage recommendations for cefepime based upon site of infection are:

- Febrile neutropenia: 2 g every 8 hours
- Intra-abdominal infections: 2 g every 12 hours
- Nosocomial pneumonia: 1 to 2 g every 8 to 12 hours
- Community-acquired pneumonia: 1 to 2 g every 12 hours
- Skin and skin structure: 2 g every 12 hours
- Urinary tract infections (UTIs): 2 g every 12 hours (severe) and 500 to 1000 mg every 12 hours (mild-moderate)

Pharmacokinetic and Pharmacodynamic Properties

Integration of PK and pharmacodynamic properties of an agent is important when choosing antimicrobial therapy to ensure efficacy and to prevent resistance.

Pharmacokinetic Properties Pharmacokinetics describes *in vivo* drug exposure in terms of absorption, distribution, metabolism, and elimination.

Bioavailability refers to the amount of antimicrobial that is absorbed orally compared to an equivalent intravenous (IV) dose. Drug factors that affect oral bioavailability include the

To access your complimentary online question exams, visit https://accesspharmacy.mhmedical.com/NAPLEX.aspx

TABLE 20-1 Drugs of Choice, First Choice, Alternative(s)

Gram-Positive Cocci

Enterococcus faecalis (generally not as resistant to antibiotics as *Enterococcus faecium*)

    Serious infection (endocarditis, meningitis, pyelonephritis with bacteremia)

    Ampicillin (or penicillin G) + (gentamicin or streptomycin)

    Vancomycin + (gentamicin or streptomycin), linezolid, daptomycin, tigecycline

    Urinary tract infection (UTI)

    Ampicillin, amoxicillin

    Fosfomycin or nitrofurantoin

E. faecium (generally more resistant to antibiotics than *E. faecalis*)

    Recommend consultation with infectious disease specialist

    Linezolid, quinupristin/dalfopristin, daptomycin, tigecycline

Staphylococcus aureus/Staphylococcus epidermidis

    Methicillin (oxacillin)-sensitive

    PRP[a]

    FGC,[b,c] trimethoprim-sulfamethoxazole, clindamycin,[d] ampicillin-sulbactam, or amoxicillin-clavulanate

    Methicillin (oxacillin)-resistant

    Vancomycin ± (gentamicin or rifampin)

    Trimethoprim-sulfamethoxazole, doxycycline[e] or clindamycin,[d] Linezolid, quinupristin-dalfopristin, daptomycin, or tigecycline

Streptococcus (groups A, B, C, G, and *Streptococcus bovis*)

    Penicillin G[f] or V[g] or ampicillin

    FGC,[b,c] erythromycin, azithromycin, clarithromycin[h]

Streptococcus pneumoniae

    Penicillin-sensitive (MIC <0.1 mcg/mL)

    Penicillin G or V or ampicillin/amoxicillin

    Erythromycin, FGC,[b,c] doxycycline, azithromycin, clarithromycin[h]

    Penicillin intermediate (MIC 0.1-1.0 mcg/mL)

    High-dose penicillin (12 million units/d for adults) or ceftriaxone[c] or cefotaxime[c]

    Levofloxacin,[i] moxifloxacin,[i] gemifloxacin,[i] telithromycin, or vancomycin

    Penicillin-resistant (MIC ≥1.0 mcg/mL)

    Recommend consultation with infectious disease specialist

    Vancomycin ± rifampin

    Per sensitivities: TGC,[c,j] telithromycin, levofloxacin,[i] moxifloxacin,[i] or gemifloxacin[i]

Streptococcus, viridans group

    Penicillin G ± gentamicin[k]

    TGC,[c,j] erythromycin, azithromycin, clarithromycin,[h] or vancomycin ± gentamicin

Gram-Negative Cocci

Moraxella (Branhamella) catarrhalis

    Amoxicillin-clavulanate, ampicillin-sulbactam

    Trimethoprim-sulfamethoxazole, erythromycin, azithromycin, clarithromycin,[h] doxycycline,[e] SGC,[c,j] TGC,[c,j] or TGC po[c,m]

Neisseria gonorrhoeae (also give concomitant treatment for *Chlamydia trachomatis*)

    Disseminated gonococcal infection

    Ceftriaxone[c] or cefotaxime[c]

    Oral follow-up: Cefpodoxime,[c] ciprofloxacin,[i] or levofloxacin[i]

    Uncomplicated infection

    Ceftriaxone[c] or cefotaxime,[c] or cefpodoxime[c]

    Ciprofloxacin[i] or levofloxacin[i]

    Neisseria meningitides

    Penicillin G

    TGC[c,j]

Gram-Positive Bacilli

Clostridium perfringens

    Penicillin G ± clindamycin

    Metronidazole, clindamycin, doxycycline,[e] cefazolin,[c] imipenem,[n] meropenem,[n] or ertapenem[n]

Clostridium difficile

    Oral metronidazole

    Oral vancomycin

    Oral fidaxomicin

    Oral vancomycin + IV metronidazole (severe complicated)

Gram-Negative Bacilli

Acinetobacter spp.

    Imipenem or meropenem ± aminoglycoside[o] (amikacin usually most effective)

    Ciprofloxacin,[i] ampicillin-sulbactam, colistin, or tigecycline

Bacteroides fragilis (and other Bacteroides species)

    Metronidazole

    BLIC,[p] clindamycin, cephamycins,[c,q] or carbapenem[n]

Enterobacter spp.

    Imipenem, meropenem, ertapenem, or cefepime ± aminoglycoside[p]

    Ciprofloxacin,[i] levofloxacin,[i] piperacillin-tazobactam, ticarcillin-clavulanate, or tigecycline

Escherichia coli

    Meningitis

    TGC[c,j] or meropenem

    Systemic infection

    TGC[c,j]

    Ampicillin-sulbactam, FGC,[b,c] BL/BLI,[p] fluoroquinolone,[i,n,r] imipenem,[n] meropenem[n]

    Urinary tract infection

    Most oral agents: check sensitivities

    Amoxicillin, amoxicillin-clavulanate, doxycyline,[e] or cephalexin[c]

    Aminoglycoside,[p] FGC[b,c] nitrofurantoin, fluoroquinolone[i,n,r]

Gardnerella vaginalis

    Metronidazole

    Clindamycin

Haemophilus influenzae

    Meningitis

    Cefotaxime[c] or ceftriaxone[c]

    Meropenem[n] or chloramphenicol[s]

    Other infections

    BLIC,[p] or if β-lactamase-negative, ampicillin or amoxicillin

    Trimethoprim-sulfamethoxazole, cefuroxime,[c] azithromycin, clarithromycin,[h] or fluoroquinolone[i,n,r]

Klebsiella pneumoniae

    TGC[e,k] (if UTI only: aminoglycoside[p])

    Cefuroxime,[e] fluoroquinolone,[b,r] BLIC,[q] imipenem,[o] meropenem,[o] or ertapenem

Legionella spp.

    Erythromycin ± rifampin or fluoroquinolone[i,r]

    Trimethoprim-sulfamethoxazole, clarithromycin,[h] azithromycin, or doxycycline[e]

Pasteurella multocida

    Penicillin G, ampicillin, amoxicillin

    Doxycycline,[e] BLIC,[p] trimethoprim-sulfamethoxazole, or ceftriaxone[c,j]

Proteus mirabilis

    Ampicillin

    Trimethoprim-sulfamethoxazole, most antibiotics except PRP[a]

(Continued)

TABLE 20-1   Drugs of Choice, First Choice, Alternative(s) (Continued)

Proteus (indole-positive) (including *Providencia rettgeri, Morganella morganii, and Proteus vulgaris*)
TGC^{c,h} or fluoroquinolone^{f,r}
BLIC,^{p} aztreonam,^{t} imipenem,^{n} or TGC po^{c,m}

Providencia stuartii
TGC^{c,j} or fluoroquinolone^{i,r}
Trimethoprim-sulfamethoxazole, aztreonam,^{t} imipenem,^{n} meropenem,^{n} or ertapenem

Pseudomonas aeruginosa
Cefepime,^{c} fluoroquinolones, ceftazidime,^{c} piperacillin-tazobactam, or ticarcillin-clavulanate plus aminoglycoside^o
Ciprofloxacin,^{i} levofloxacin,^{i} aztreonam,^{t} imipenem,^{n} meropenem,^{n} or colistin
UTI only: aminoglycoside^o
Ciprofloxacin,^{i} levofloxacin^i

Salmonella typhi
Ciprofloxacin,^{i} levofloxacin,^{i} ceftriaxone,^{c} or cefotaxime^c
Trimethoprim-sulfamethoxazole

Serratia marcescens
Piperacillin-tazobactam, ticarcillin-clavulanate, or TGC^{c,j} ± gentamicin
Trimethoprim-sulfamethoxazole, ciprofloxacin,^{i} levofloxacin,^{i} aztreonam,^{t} imipenem,^{n} meropenem,^{n} or ertapenem

Stenotrophomonas (Xanthomonas) maltophilia
Trimethoprim-sulfamethoxazole
Generally very resistant to all antimicrobials; check sensitivities to fluoroquinolones, ceftazidime,^{e} ticarcillin-clavulanate, doxycycline,^{e} and minocycline^e

Miscellaneous Microorganisms

Chlamydia pneumoniae
Doxycycline^e
Erythromycin, azithromycin, clarithromycin,^{h} telithromycin, or fluoroquinolone^{f,r}

C. trachomatis
Doxycycline^e or azithromycin
Levofloxacin^i or ofloxacin^i

Mycoplasma pneumoniae
Erythromycin, azithromycin, clarithromycin^h
Doxycycline^e or fluoroquinolone^{f,r}

Spirochetes

Treponema pallidum
  Neurosyphilis (must be desensitized if allergic)
  Penicillin G
  Ceftriaxone^c
  Primary or secondary
  Benzathine penicillin G
  Doxycycline^e or ceftriaxone^c

Borrelia burgdorferi (choice depends on stage of disease)
  Ceftriaxone^c or cefuroxime axetil,^{c} doxycycline,^{e} amoxicillin
  High-dose penicillin, cefotaxime,^{c} or azithromycin

Abbreviations: BLIC, β-lactamase inhibitor combination; BL/BLI, β-lactamase/β-lactamase inhibitor; FGC, first-generation cephalosporin; MIC, minimal inhibitory concentration; po, orally; PRP, penicillinase-resistant penicillin; SGC, second-generation cephalosporin; TGC, third-generation cephalosporin.

^{a}Penicillinase-resistant penicillin: nafcillin or oxacillin.

^{b}First-generation cephalosporins—IV: cefazolin; po: cephalexin, cephradine, or cefadroxil.

^{c}Some penicillin-allergic patients may react to cephalosporins.

^{d}Not reliably bactericidal; should not be used for endocarditis.

^{e}Not for use in pregnant patients or children younger than 8 years old.

^{f}Either aqueous penicillin G or benzathine penicillin G (pharyngitis only).

^{g}Only for soft tissue infections or upper respiratory infections (pharyngitis, otitis media).

^{h}Do not use in pregnant patients.

^{i}Not for use in pregnant patients or children younger than 18 years old.

^{j}Third-generation cephalosporins—IV: cefotaxime, ceftriaxone.

^{k}Gentamicin should be added if tolerance or moderately susceptible (MIC >0.1 g/mL) organisms are encountered; streptomycin is used but can be more toxic.

^{l}Second-generation cephalosporins—IV: cefuroxime; po: cefaclor, cefditoren, cefprozil, cefuroxime axetil, and loracarbef.

^{m}Third-generation cephalosporins—po: cefdinir, cefixime, cefetamet, cefpodoxime proxetil, and ceftibuten.

^{n}Reserve for serious infection.

^{o}Aminoglycosides: gentamicin, tobramycin, and amikacin; use per sensitivities.

^{p}Beta-lactam/β-lactamase inhibitor combination—IV: ampicillin-sulbactam, piperacillin-tazobactam, ticarcillin-clavulanate; po: amoxicillin-clavulanate.

^{q}Cefoxitin.

^{r}IV/po: ciprofloxacin, levofloxacin, and moxifloxacin.

^{s}Reserve for serious infection when less toxic drugs are not effective.

^{t}Generally reserved for patients with hypersensitivity reactions to penicillin.

Adapted with permission from DiPiro JT, Talbert RL, Yee GC, et al: *Pharmacotherapy: A Pathophysiologic Approach*, 7th ed. New York, NY: McGraw-Hill; 2008.

salt formulation, dosage form, and stability of agent in gastrointestinal tract. Patients manifesting systemic signs of infection such as hypotension or hypoperfusion should receive IV antimicrobials. Patients with a functioning gastrointestinal tract and without hemodynamic instability may receive oral antimicrobials, especially if the agent has good bioavailability. Examples of anti-infectives with good bioavailability include fluoroquinolones, fluconazole, and linezolid. Antimicrobials with poor bioavailability should be administered intravenously for systemic infections (eg, vancomycin—IV vancomycin is utilized for systemic infections; oral vancomycin is utilized to treat *C. difficile* gastrointestinal infections).

Tissue penetration (distribution) relevance varies with the site of infection. The central nervous system (CNS) is one body site where antimicrobial penetration is defined and correlations with clinical outcomes are established. Anti-infectives that do not reach significant concentrations in the cerebrospinal fluid (CSF) should either be avoided or instilled directly. Caution must be utilized when selecting an antimicrobial on the basis of tissue or fluid penetration. Body fluids where drug concentrations are clinically relevant include the CSF, urine, synovial fluid, and peritoneal fluid. Apart from these areas, more attention should be paid to clinical efficacy, antimicrobial spectrum, adverse effects, and cost than to comparative data on penetration.

Oral or parenteral administration of anti-infectives depends on the severity of illness and location of the infection. In sequestered infections, higher concentrations may be required to reach the infected source (meningitis, osteomyelitis, endocarditis, pneumonia) and may require parenteral anti-infectives. Patients treated for upper respiratory tract infections (pharyngitis, bronchitis, sinusitis, and otitis media),

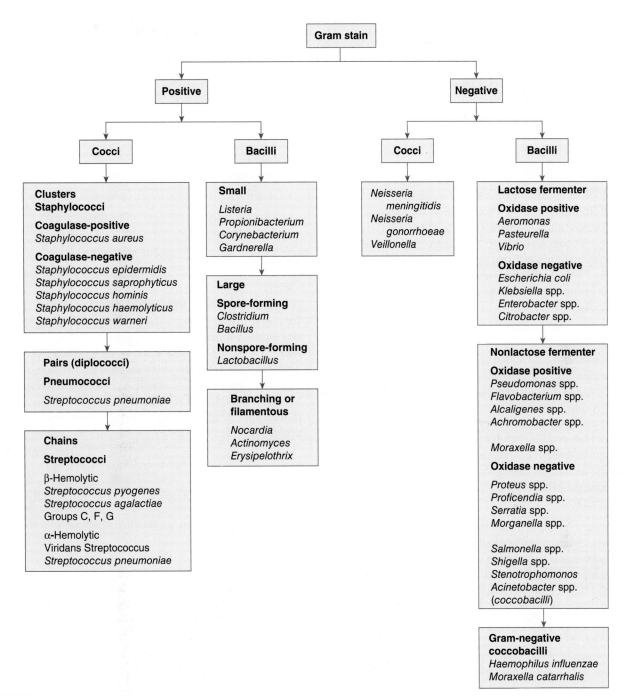

FIGURE 20-1 Bacterial pathogen classification—gram stain and morphologic characteristics. Reproduced with permission from DiPiro JT, Talbert RL, Yee GC, et al: *Pharmacotherapy: A Pathophysiologic Approach,* 7th ed. New York, NY: McGraw-Hill; 2008.

skin and soft tissue infections, uncomplicated UTIs, and selected sexually transmitted diseases can receive oral therapy.

Pharmacodynamic Properties Pharmacodynamics (PD) describes the relationship between drug exposure and pharmacologic effect of antibacterial activity or human toxicology. Antimicrobials are categorized based upon their concentration related effects of bacteria. Concentration-dependent PD activity occurs where higher drug concentrations are associated with greater rates and extents of bacterial killing. Concentration-dependent activity is maximized when peak antimicrobial concentrations are high. In contrast, time-dependent activity refers to a minimal increase in the rate or extent of bacterial killing with an increase in dose. Time-dependent activity is maximized when antimicrobials are dosed to maintain blood and/or tissue concentrations above the minimal inhibitory concentration (MIC) in a time-dependent manner. Fluoroquinolones, aminoglycosides, and metronidazole are examples of antimicrobials that exhibit concentration-dependent activity. β-Lactams and glycopeptides exhibit time-dependent activity.

PD properties have been optimized to develop new dosing strategies for antimicrobials. Examples include extended dosing *interval* aminoglycosides and extended *infusion* β-lactam therapy.

- Aminoglycoside antimicrobials (gentamicin, tobramycin, and amikacin) display concentration-dependent activity and may be dosed by *traditional* or *extended interval* methods. *Traditional* dosing in patients with normal renal function is often 1.5 to 2 mg/kg IV every 8 hours. *Traditional* dosing is monitored by obtaining peaks and troughs after a patient has reached steady state. *Extended interval* dosing is 7 mg/kg IV every 24, 36, or 48 hours. A 7 mg/kg dose is administered and an aminoglycoside level between 6 and 14 hours after administration is obtained and plotted on the Hartford nomogram to determine the dosing interval. The administration of 7 mg/kg of a medication that has a 2 to 3 hour half-life is a clinical example of utilizing PD properties of aminoglycosides (concentration-dependent activity).

- β-Lactam antimicrobials are often administered intravenously as 30 minute infusions. Examples include piperacillin/tazobactam (Zosyn) 4.5 g IV over 30 minutes every 6 hours and imipenem/cilastatin (Imipenem) 500 mg IV over 60 minutes every 6 hours. In efforts to optimize the time-dependent activity of β-lactams, *extending the infusion interval* is being clinically utilized (piperacillin/tazobactam 3.375 g IV every 8 hours administered as a 4-hour infusion). *Extending the infusion interval* allows for the concentration to remain above the MIC for longer periods of time (time-dependent activity).

Antimicrobials are also classified as bactericidal or bacteriostatic. Bactericidal antibiotics kill at least 99.9% of a bacterial population, whereas bacteriostatic antibiotics inhibit further replication of bacteria. Clinically, bactericidal antibiotics may be necessary to achieve success in infections such as endocarditis or meningitis.

Adverse effects

Antimicrobials with a low propensity of causing adverse events or drug interactions should be selected if possible, particularly for patients with risk factors for a particular complication. Risk factors include coadministration of other drugs that are associated with a similar type of adverse event. For example, coadministration of the known nephrotoxin gentamicin with vancomycin increases the risk for nephrotoxicity compared with administration of either drug alone. Other drug interactions may predispose the patient to dose-related toxicity through inhibition of drug metabolism. For example, erythromycin has the potential to prolong cardiac QT intervals in a dose-dependent manner, potentially increasing the risk of sudden cardiac death. Patients prescribed with medications that inhibit the metabolism of erythromycin exhibited a fivefold increase in cardiac death versus controls. See Table 20-2 for a list of selected drug interactions with anti-infectives. Examples of selected adverse effects from anti-infectives include:

- Antibiotic associated CNS toxicities (usually when not dose-adjusted for renal function—penicillins, cephalosporins, quinolones, and imipenem)
- Hematologic toxicities (neutropenia) manifested by prolonged use of nafcillin
- Piperacillin and platelet dysfunction
- Cefotetan and hypoprothrombinemia
- Chloramphenicol and bone marrow suppression
- Trimethoprim and megaloblastic anemia
- Aminoglycosides and nephrotoxicity/ototoxicity
- Photosensitivity and quinolones, tetracyclines, trimethoprim
- *Clostridium difficile* and all antibiotics

Cost

A final consideration with antimicrobial properties in selecting therapy relates to cost. The total cost of antimicrobial therapy includes more than just the acquisition cost of the agent. Many ancillary costs and factors affect the cost of therapy. These include factors such as storage, preparation, distribution, and administration, as well as costs incurred from monitoring for adverse effects and factors such as therapeutic drug monitoring, length of hospitalization, readmissions, and all directly provided health-care goods and services.

Host Factors

Host factors should be considered when evaluating a patient for antimicrobial therapy. Important host factors are: drug allergies, age, pregnancy, genetic/metabolic abnormalities, and organ dysfunction.

Allergy

Allergy to an antimicrobial agent generally precludes its use. Assessment of allergy histories must be performed because patients confuse adverse drug effects (gastrointestinal disturbance) with true allergic reactions. Penicillin and penicillin-related compounds are the most commonly cited antimicrobial allergies. Recommendations for administration of cephalosporin antibiotics in penicillin allergic patients depend on the type of reaction. Patients with a history of immediate or accelerated reactions (eg, anaphylaxis) to penicillin should in nearly all cases avoid cephalosporins. Patients with a delayed hypersensitivity reaction (rash) to penicillin may be given cephalosporins under supervision.

Age

Age is an important factor in determining causative pathogens for certain infections and PK/physiologic factors for certain antibiotics. Causative pathogens in bacterial meningitis differ based upon age. For example, *Listeria monocytogenes* is a possible cause of meningitis in neonates and patients greater than 55 years of age. PK factors affected by age may alter concentrations of the agent. For example, hepatic functions are not well developed in neonates and the use of chloramphenicol

TABLE 20-2 **Antimicrobial Adverse Drug Reactions**

Antimicrobial Class	Adverse Drug Reaction	Monitoring Parameters	Comments
Penicillins	Hypersensitivity reactions and rash, drug fever, diarrhea, emesis, abdominal pain, hepatitis, interstitial nephritis, leukopenia, thrombocytopenia, Coomb's positive-hemolytic anemia, C. difficile colitis, electrolyte abnormalities, seizures	Monitor for hypersensitivity reactions (eg, bronchospasm, anaphylaxis, angioneurotic edema, immediate urticaria). During prolonged therapy and/or high-dose regimens, periodically monitor renal function, hepatic function, and CBC	Most serious reaction is immediate IgE-mediated anaphylaxis. Incidence is 0.05%, but 5%-10% can be fatal
Cephalosporins	Hypersensitivity reactions and rash, drug fever, diarrhea, interstitial nephritis, Coomb's positive-hemolytic anemia, leukopenia, thrombocytopenia, coagulopathy, hepatitis, C. difficile colitis	Monitor for hypersensitivity reactions (eg, bronchospasm, anaphylaxis, angioneurotic edema, immediate urticaria) and rash, renal function, hepatic function, and CBC	Patients with a history of IgE-mediated allergic reactions to penicillins should not receive a cephalosporin
Carbapenems	Hypersensitivity reactions and rash, headache, nausea, diarrhea, seizures, drug fever, eosinophilia, thrombocytopenia, hepatitis, C. difficile colitis	Monitor for hypersensitivity reactions (eg, bronchospasm, anaphylaxis, angioneurotic edema, immediate urticaria) and rash, renal function, hepatic function, and CBC	Skin test cross-sensitivity with penicillin reported to be up to 50%, but clinically significant cross-sensitivity reactions in penicillin-allergic patients reported to be as low as 1%. Highest incidence of seizures with use of imipenem–cilastatin. More frequent in patients who are elderly, have history of seizure disorders and renal dysfunction
Monobactams	Rash, diarrhea, nausea, hepatitis, thrombocytopenia, C. difficile colitis	Monitor renal and hepatic function	May be used in patients with allergy to penicillins/cephalosporins
Aminoglycosides	Tubular necrosis and renal failure, vestibular and cochlear toxicity, neuromuscular blockade, vertigo, anemia, hypersensitivity	Monitor renal function, serum drug concentrations, serum calcium, magnesium, sodium. Monitor for nausea, vomiting, nystagmus, and vertigo	Nephrotoxicity can be reversible. More frequent in patients with the following risk factors: elderly, history of renal dysfunction, concomitant administration of nephrotoxic drug (ie, cyclosporine, amphotericin B, radiocontrast, vancomycin), and duration of therapy. Ototoxicities can be irreversible
Glycopeptides	Red man syndrome, phlebitis, renal dysfunction, neutropenia, leukopenia, eosinophilia, thrombocytopenia, drug fever	Monitor renal function, CBC, and serum drug concentrations	Red man syndrome is associated with rapid infusion and nonspecific histamine release. May be prevented by prolonging infusions to over at least 60 minutes and pretreatment with antihistamines
Lipopeptides (daptomycin)	Hepatotoxicity, CPK elevation with or without myopathy, diarrhea, eosinophilic pneumonia, C. difficile colitis	Monitor LFTs, development of muscle pain/weakness, or neuropathy. Obtain serum CPK levels at baseline and weekly (or more frequently in patients with prior or concomitant statin, renal dysfunction, or patients with elevations in CPK)	CPK elevation is dose-dependent. Obtain baseline and weekly CPK levels. Discontinue daptomycin if CPK exceeds 10 times normal level or if patient develops myopathy and CPK >1,000 international units/L (>16.7 μkat/L). Consider stopping statin therapy during treatment with daptomycin
Oxazolidinones	Myelosuppression (thrombocytopenia, leukopenia, and anemia), peripheral neuropathy, optic neuropathy, blindness, lactic acidosis, diarrhea, nausea, serotonin syndrome, interstitial nephritis	Monitor for signs and symptoms of serotonin syndrome particularly in patients with prior or concomitant serotonergic agents, CBC with differential. For prolonged therapy, perform visual function tests, monitor visual acuity and visual field defect	Myelosuppression is reversible and associated with treatment duration >2 wk. Caution with use of other serotonergic agents due to potential additive interaction
Tetracyclines	GI upset, nausea, vomiting, diarrhea, hepatotoxicity, esophageal ulcerations, photosensitivity, azotemia, visual disturbances, vertigo, hyperpigmentation, deposition on teeth, hemolytic anemia, pseudotumor cerebri, pancreatitis, C. difficile colitis	Monitor CBC with differential, LFTs, and renal function	Doxycycline preferred in patients with renal dysfunction. Vestibular symptoms more frequent in women than in men. Avoid use during pregnancy and in children

(Continued)

TABLE 20-2   Antimicrobial Adverse Drug Reactions (Continued)

Antimicrobial Class	Adverse Drug Reaction	Monitoring Parameters	Comments
Chloramphenicol	Myelosuppression, aplastic anemia, "gray baby syndrome," optic neuritis, peripheral neuropathy, digital paresthesias, GI upset, *C. difficile* colitis, hypersensitivity	Obtain baseline CBC with differential and every 2 d during therapy. Monitor SDC (particularly in children and in patients with hepatic or renal insufficiency), liver and renal function	Bone marrow suppression associated with doses >4 g/d. Serum levels >50 mcg/mL (mg/L; 155 μmol/L) are associated with increased risk for "gray baby syndrome"
Rifamycins	Discoloration of urine, tears, contact lens, sweat, hepatotoxicity, GI upset, flu-like syndrome, hypersensitivity, thrombocytopenia, leukopenia, drug fever, interstitial nephritis, thrombocytopenia	Monitor LFTs, bilirubin, renal function, CBC at baseline; continue to monitor every 2-4 wk in patients with hepatic impairment or receiving concomitant hepatotoxic drugs	Increased potential for hepatitis with concomitant hepatotoxic drugs (ie, TB drugs)
Macrolides/azalides	GI intolerance, diarrhea, prolonged QTc, cholestatic hepatitis, reversible ototoxicity, torsade de pointes, rash, hypothermia, exacerbation of myasthenia gravis	Monitor LFTs and ECG in high-risk patients	
Clindamycin	Diarrhea, *C. difficile* colitis, nausea, vomiting, generalized rash, hypersensitivity	For prolonged therapy, monitor liver and renal function	
Fluoroquinolones	GI intolerance, headache, malaise, insomnia, dizziness, photosensitivity, QTc prolongation, tendon rupture, peripheral neuropathy, crystalluria, seizure, interstitial nephritis, Stevens-Johnson syndrome, allergic pneumonitis, *C. difficile* colitis	Monitor renal function, encephalopathic changes (eg, confusion, hallucinations, and tremor)	Tendon rupture more frequently seen in the elderly and kidney, heart, and lung transplant recipients, and with concurrent use of corticosteroids
Polymyxins	Nephrotoxicity, neurotoxicity (paresthesia, vertigo, ataxia, blurred vision, slurred speech), neuromuscular blockade, bronchospasm (administered via inhalation)	Obtain baseline renal function tests regularly during therapy. Monitor for signs of neuromuscular blockade (eg, respiratory depression, apnea, muscle weakness)	Nephrotoxicity is dose-dependent
Sulfonamides and trimethoprim	GI intolerance, rash, hyperkalemia, bone marrow suppression (anemia with folate deficiency, thrombocytopenia, and leukopenia), serum sickness, hepatitis, photosensitivity, crystalluria with azotemia, urolithiasis, methemoglobinemia, Stevens-Johnson syndrome, toxic epidermal necrolysis, aseptic meningitis, pancreatitis, interstitial nephritis, Sweet syndrome, neurologic toxicity	Monitor for hypersensitivity reactions and rash, CBC, renal and hepatic function, serum potassium, serum glucose	HIV-infected patients are at increased risk for developing hypersensitivity drug reactions. Methemoglobinemia due to severe G6PD deficiency
Metronidazole	GI intolerance, headache, metallic taste, dark urine, peripheral neuropathy, disulfiram reactions with alcohol, insomnia, stomatitis, aseptic meningitis, dysarthria	Monitor hepatic function, mental/neurologic status	Peripheral neuropathy is reversible and associated with prolonged treatment

Abbreviations: CBC, complete blood count; CPK, creatine phosphokinase; LFT, liver function test; SDC, serum drug concentrations; TB, tuberculosis.
Reproduced with permission from DiPiro JT, Talbert RL, Yee GC, et al: *Pharmacotherapy: A Pathophysiologic Approach,* 10th ed. New York, NY: McGraw-Hill; 2017.

may lead to shock and cardiovascular collapse (gray baby syndrome). This is caused by the inability of the newborn's liver to metabolize and detoxify the drug. Neonates may also develop kernicterus when administered sulfonamides. Physiologic changes in persons older than 65 years of age may impact anti-infective properties. A decrease in the number of nephrons resulting in decreased renal function is a common physiologic change in elderly patients. The decrease in renal function may increase the incidence of side effects of renally eliminated anti-infectives.

Pregnancy

Antimicrobial agents must be used with caution in pregnant and nursing women. Some agents are known or likely to be teratogenic (eg, metronidazole), and others pose potential threats to the fetus or infant (eg, quinolones, tetracyclines, and sulfonamides). PK variables also are altered during pregnancy. Both the clearance and volume of distribution are increased during pregnancy. As a result, increased dosages and/or more frequent administration of certain drugs may be required to achieve adequate concentrations.

Metabolic Abnormalities

Inherited or acquired metabolic abnormalities influence infectious diseases therapy. Patients with peripheral vascular disease may not absorb drugs given by intramuscular injection. Other examples include:

- Patients who are phenotypically slow acetylators of isoniazid are at greater risk for peripheral neuropathy.
- Patients with glucose-6-phosphate dehydrogenase (G6PD) deficiency can develop hemolysis when exposed to sulfonamides and dapsone.

Organ Dysfunction

Patients with diminished renal or hepatic function (or both) will accumulate certain drugs unless the dosage is adjusted. Recommendations for dosing antibiotics in patients with liver dysfunction are not as formalized as guidelines for patients with renal dysfunction. Antibiotics that should be adjusted in severe liver disease include clindamycin, erythromycin, metronidazole, and rifampin.

Normal Flora

Normal flora represents bacteria colonized in areas of the human body. Infections arise from normal flora (also called endogenous flora). Knowing what organisms reside where can help guide empirical antimicrobial therapy (Figure 20-2).

Infections acquired from an external source are referred to as exogenous infections. These infections occur as a result of human-to-human transmission, contact with exogenous bacterial populations in the environment, and animal contact. Resistant pathogens such as methicillin-resistant *Staphylococcus aureus* (MRSA) and vancomycin-resistant *Enterococcus* species (VRE) may colonize hospitalized patients. Patients colonized with MRSA, VRE, or other multidrug resistant organisms often require different empiric therapy and should

be placed in isolation to minimize transmission to other patients.

Patients with a history of recent antimicrobial use may have altered normal flora. If a patient develops a new infection while on therapy, fails therapy, or has received antimicrobials recently, it is prudent to utilize a different class of antimicrobials because of bacterial resistance. Previous hospitalization or home health care utilization are risk factors for the acquisition of exogenous pathogens.

Colonization Versus Infection

It is important to differentiate infection from colonization because antimicrobial therapy targeting bacterial colonization is inappropriate and may lead to the development of resistant bacteria. Infection refers to the presence of bacteria that are causing disease. Colonization refers to the presence of bacteria that are not causing disease.

Clinical Presentation

Findings on physical examination, along with the clinical presentation, can help to provide the anatomic location of the infection. Once the anatomic site is identified, the most probable pathogens associated with disease can be determined based upon likely endogenous or exogenous flora.

Fever often accompanies infection and is defined as a rise in body temperature above the normal 98.6°F (37°C). Oral and axillary temperatures may underestimate core temperature by at least 1°F, whereas rectal temperatures best approximate core temperatures. Fever is a host response to bacterial toxins. Fever may also be caused by other infections (eg, fungal or viral), medications (eg, penicillins, cephalosporins, salicylates, phenytoin), trauma, or other medical conditions (autoimmune disease, malignancy, hyperthyroidism). Patients with infections may also present with hypothermia (eg, patients with overwhelming infection, sepsis). Elderly patients may be afebrile, as well as patients with localized infection (eg, uncomplicated UTIs). For some patients, fever may be the only indication of infection. For example, neutropenic patients may not have the ability to mount normal immune responses to infection and the only finding may be fever.

Diagnosis

Microbiologic studies that allow for direct examination of a specimen may aid in the diagnosis and give an indication of the infecting organism. A gram stain can give rapid information that can be applied immediately to patient care. A gram stain is performed to identify if bacteria are present and to determine morphologic characteristics of bacteria (such as gram-positive or negative, or shape—cocci, bacilli). Figure 20-1 identifies bacterial pathogens as classified by gram stain and morphologic characteristics. The presence of white blood cells (WBCs) on a gram stain indicates inflammation and suggests that the identified bacteria are pathogenic. The gram stain may be useful in judging a sputum specimen's adequacy. For example, the presence of epithelial cells on sputum gram stain suggests that the specimen is either poorly collected or

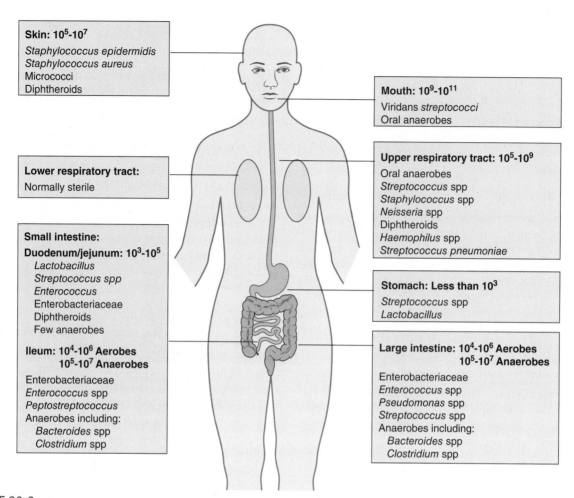

Skin: 10^5-10^7

Staphylococcus epidermidis
Staphylococcus aureus
Micrococci
Diphtheroids

Mouth: 10^9-10^{11}

Viridans *streptococci*
Oral anaerobes

Lower respiratory tract:

Normally sterile

Upper respiratory tract: 10^5-10^9

Oral anaerobes
Streptococcus spp
Staphylococcus spp
Neisseria spp
Diphtheroids
Haemophilus spp
Streptococcus pneumoniae

Small intestine:
Duodenum/jejunum: 10^3-10^5

Lactobacillus
Streptococcus spp
Enterococcus
Enterobacteriaceae
Diphtheroids
Few anaerobes

Ileum: 10^4-10^6 **Aerobes**
      10^5-10^7 **Anaerobes**

Enterobacteriaceae
Enterococcus spp
Peptostreptococcus
Anaerobes including:
  Bacteroides spp
  Clostridium spp

Stomach: Less than 10^3

Streptococcus spp
Lactobacillus

Large intestine: 10^4-10^6 **Aerobes**
          10^5-10^7 **Anaerobes**

Enterobacteriaceae
Enterococcus spp
Pseudomonas spp
Streptococcus spp
Anaerobes including:
  Bacteroides spp
  Clostridium spp

FIGURE 20-2   Normal flora and concentrations of bacteria (organisms per millimeter).   Reproduced with permission from Chisholm-Burns MA, Schwinghammer TL, Wells BG, et al: *Pharmacotherapy Principles & Practice,* 2nd ed. New York, NY: McGraw-Hill; 2010.

contaminated. A poor specimen can give misleading information with regard to the underlying pathogen and is a waste of laboratory personnel time and patient cost.

Culture and susceptibility testing provides additional information for clinicians to guide therapy. Specimens are placed on culture media that provide the proper growth conditions. Once the bacteria grow on culture media, they can be identified through a variety of biochemical tests. Once a pathogen is identified, susceptibility tests can be performed to various antimicrobial agents. The minimum inhibitory concentration (MIC) is a standard susceptibility test. The MIC is the lowest concentration of antimicrobial that inhibits visible bacterial growth. Breakpoint and MIC values determine if the organism is susceptible (S), intermediate (I), or resistant (R) to an antimicrobial. The breakpoint represents the concentration that leads to clinical cure of the infection when given FDA-approved dosages of the antibiotic. If the MIC is below the breakpoint, the organism is considered to be susceptible to that agent. If the MIC is above the breakpoint, the organism is said to be resistant. Bacterial cultures should be obtained prior to initiating antimicrobial therapy. The decision to culture depends on the sensitivity and specificity of the physical findings, diagnostic examination findings, and

whether or not the pathogens are predictable. For example, culture and susceptibility testing usually is not warranted in a young, otherwise healthy woman who presents with signs and symptoms consistent with a UTI because the primary pathogen, *Escherichia coli*, is readily predictable. Cultures need to be interpreted with caution. Poor specimen collection technique can result in misleading information and inappropriate use of antimicrobials.

Common nonmicrobiologic laboratory tests include the WBC count and differential, erythrocyte sedimentation rate (ESR), and determination of the C-reactive protein level (CRP). In most cases, the WBC count is elevated in response to infection, but it may be normal in localized infections or decreased in overwhelming infection. In response to infection, neutrophils leave the bloodstream and enter the tissue to fight against the offending pathogens (ie, leukocytosis). The ESR and CRP are nonspecific markers of inflammation. They increase as a result of the acute-phase reactant response, which is a response to inflammatory stimuli such as infection or tissue injury. These tests may be used as markers of infectious disease response because they are elevated when the disease is active and usually fall in response to treatment. These tests should not be used to diagnose infection because they may be elevated in noninfectious conditions (autoimmune disorders).

There has been a recent explosion of Food and Drug Administration (FDA)-approved rapid diagnostic testing methodologies for infectious diseases. In the current era of managed care and antimicrobial stewardship programs, the need for rapid diagnostic tests (RDTs) is critical. A major focus of RDT is on pathogens associated with increased morbidity and mortality, which include influenza virus, MRSA, VRE, *C. difficile*, extended-spectrum β-lactamase (ESBL)-producing *Klebsiella* spp., and *Mycobacterium tuberculosis*. The benefit of rapid diagnostic technology is to quickly identify and/or rule out infectious pathogens, streamline antimicrobial therapy, and improve infection control measures such as isolation. Utilization of rapid diagnostic testing significantly reduces the time required to identifying the infecting pathogen, thus improving clinician's ability to more rapidly diagnose and treat infections. Pathogen RDT also prompts de-escalation of antibiotic therapy and if the test is negative, discontinuation of therapy, which decreases the potential for antimicrobial resistance. The process of RDT often requires the evaluation of a clinical specimen such as blood (ie, serum or plasma), stool, or bodily fluids (ie, as saliva, urine). These specimens are processed in a qualitative or quantitative manner, to provide a result that is available within 15 minutes to a few hours (depending on the technology). This is in contrast to traditional culture methodologies discussed above which may take 4 to 6 days (ie, for *Staphylococcus* in the blood) or up to 6 weeks (ie, mycobacterium). The most current RDT involves genomic testing methodologies, which include immunologic, molecular technologies, and mass spectrometry.

SPECIAL CONSIDERATIONS

Patients must be monitored for a therapeutic response. Culture and susceptibility reports must be reviewed (if obtained) and the therapy changed accordingly. Use of agents with the narrowest spectrum of activity against the identified pathogen is recommended. Patient monitoring should include many of the same parameters to diagnose the infection. The WBC count and temperature should start to normalize. Physical complaints from the patient should diminish (cough, sputum production, shortness of breath). Determinations of serum levels of antimicrobials can be useful in ensuring outcome, preventing adverse events, or both. Anti-infectives that require serum concentration monitoring are the aminoglycosides, flucytosine, and chloramphenicol (vancomycin is often monitored as well). Changes in the volume of distribution can have a significant impact on the efficacy, safety, or both. A low volume of distribution (eg, dehydrated patient) results in higher drug concentrations, whereas a larger than expected volume of distribution (eg, edema) results in lower concentrations.

As patients improve clinically, the route of administration of the antimicrobial should be re-evaluated for patients receiving parenteral agents. Streamlining therapy from parenteral to oral should be considered in patients who display clinical improvement, lack of fever for 8 to 24 hours, decreased WBC, and have a functioning gastrointestinal tract. Drugs that exhibit excellent oral bioavailability when compared with IV formulations include the fluoroquinolones, clindamycin, doxycycline, metronidazole, linezolid, and trimethoprim-sulfamethoxazole.

CASE Application

1. Select the antimicrobial that may cause collateral damage by selecting for a nontargeted organism (ie, *Clostridium difficile*) leading to a colitis infection. Select all that apply.

    a. Clindamycin
    b. Levofloxacin
    c. Ciprofloxacin
    d. Ceftriaxone

2. Select the correct dose of cefepime (Maxipime) for a patient with normal renal function and empirically treated for an infection (at this time the site or source of infection have not been identified). Select all that apply.

    a. 1 g IV every 12 hours
    b. 2 g IV every 12 hours
    c. 2 g IV every 8 hours
    d. 4.5 g every 6 hours

3. Select the antimicrobial PK property that impacts the dose and/or interval. Select all that apply.

    a. Bioavailability
    b. Volume of distribution
    c. Metabolism
    d. Elimination

4. Select the factor that may affect the bioavailability of an oral anti-infective.

    a. A medication that is a substrate of the CYP-450 system
    b. Dosage formulation of the anti-infective
    c. A patient that has peripheral vascular disease
    d. A patient that has renal dysfunction

5. Select the factor that would usually necessitate a patient to be given IV anti-infectives.

    a. Fever of 101.9°F
    b. Severe cough
    c. G6PD deficiency
    d. Blood pressure of 91/52 mm Hg with signs of hypoperfusion (baseline blood pressure for patient is 129/86 mm Hg)

6. Select the oral anti-infective(s) that displays good bioavailability. Select all that apply.

    a. Fluconazole
    b. Linezolid
    c. Levofloxacin
    d. Vancomycin

7. Select the infection that requires excellent tissue penetration (distribution). Select all that apply.

    a. Meningitis
    b. Acute cystitis
    c. Bronchitis
    d. Cellulitis

8. Select the anti-infective that exhibits the pharmacodynamic property of concentration dependent activity.

    a. Ceftriaxone
    b. Amoxicillin
    c. Ciprofloxacin
    d. Meropenem

9. Select the anti-infective that exhibits the pharmacodynamic property of time-dependent activity.

    a. Levofloxacin
    b. Doripenem
    c. Amikacin
    d. Metronidazole

10. A patient with a health care-associated pneumonia infection is found to have a multidrug resistant organism (this was found by the culture and susceptibility and the pathogen *P. aeruginosa* exhibits high MIC to all antibiotics). Since the pathogen exhibits high-level resistance, modifications to the dose or interval will be required to achieve successful outcomes. Currently, the patient is receiving the β-lactam piperacillin/tazobactam 4.5 g intravenously every 6 hours infused over 30 minutes. Select the factor that may be done to piperacillin/tazobactam that could optimize the pharmacodynamic property.

    a. Increase the infusion time
    b. Increase the dose
    c. Add combination therapy with another β-lactam
    d. Decrease the dose to 3.375 g

11. CNS side effects (seizures and mental status changes) are associated with β-lactam and quinolone anti-infectives. A risk factor for development of the CNS reactions is:

    a. Duration of therapy
    b. Infusion interval
    c. Bioavailability
    d. Renal dysfunction

12. Select the anti-infective that is associated with the adverse effects of nephrotoxicity and ototoxicity.

    a. Amoxicillin/clavulanate
    b. Cefpodoxime
    c. Moxifloxacin
    d. Gentamicin

13. Select the anti-infective(s) that is associated with the adverse reaction of AAD (*C. difficile*). Select all that apply.

    a. Augmentin
    b. Levaquin
    c. Cleocin
    d. Vancocin

14. JG is a patient with an immediate allergic reaction to ticarcillin/clavulanate (Timentin). Select the antimicrobial that JG may take in relation to his allergy.

    a. Piperacillin/tazobactam
    b. Amoxicillin/clavulanate
    c. Cephalexin
    d. Aztreonam

15. Select the host factor(s) that may impact antimicrobial therapy. Select all that apply.

    a. Age
    b. Pregnancy
    c. Metabolic abnormalities
    d. Organ dysfunction

16. Select the risk factor(s) for the acquisition of exogenous pathogens. Select all that apply.

    a. Nursing home admission
    b. Pregnancy
    c. Recent antimicrobial use
    d. Hospital admission for 7 days

17. Select the potential cause of a fever. Select all that apply.

    a. Infection
    b. Piperacillin
    c. Trauma
    d. Cancer

18. Select the information that is revealed by a gram stain.

    a. MIC
    b. Genre and species of the bacteria
    c. Morphologic characteristics of the bacteria
    d. Antibiotic susceptibility

19. Select the pathogen(s) that is classified as an atypical organism.

    a. *Escherichia coli*
    b. *Klebsiella pneumoniae*
    c. *Mycoplasma pneumoniae*
    d. *Streptococcus pneumoniae*

20. Select the pathogen that represents an exogenous bacteria flora (ie, acquired from the hospital). Characteristics of this pathogen are nonlactose fermenting gram-negative bacilli.

    a. *Neisseria meningitidis*
    b. *Enterobacter cloacae*
    c. *Streptococcus pneumoniae*
    d. *Pseudomonas aeruginosa*

21. Select the penicillin antimicrobial that is broad spectrum and has coverage against nonlactose negative (oxidase-positive) gram-negative bacilli.

    a. Amoxicillin
    b. Nafcillin
    c. Cefepime

d. Doripenem

e. Piperacillin/tazobactam

22. Select the pathogen(s) that is part of the normal (endogenous) flora of the large intestine. Select all that apply.

a. *Escherichia coli*

b. Viridans streptococci

c. *Neisseria meningitidis*

d. *Enterococcus* species

23. Select the best answer that represents part of the normal (endogenous) flora of the lower respiratory tract.

a. Enterobacteriaceae

b. *Streptococcus pneumoniae*

c. *Enterococcus* species

d. Normally sterile

24. Select the drug interaction(s) with aminoglycosides. Select all that apply.

a. Amphotericin B

b. Vancomycin

c. Furosemide

d. Cisplatin

25. RL is a patient with a past medical history of iron deficiency anemia. He is being treated with ferrous sulfate. Select the antimicrobial(s) that would have a decreased bioavailability when combined with ferrous sulfate. Select all that apply.

a. Moxifloxacin

b. Tetracycline

c. Azithromycin

d. Doxycycline

TAKEAWAY POINTS »

- Antimicrobials that kill many different species of bacteria are called broad-spectrum, whereas antimicrobials that kill only a few different species of bacteria are called narrow-spectrum antimicrobials.

- Empirically treating infectious diseases and monitoring therapy requires knowledge of anti-infective properties, host factors, patient's normal flora, differentiating infection versus colonization, and understanding clinical presentation and diagnostic tests (microbiologic and nonmicrobiologic laboratory studies).

- It is important to understand the difference in antimicrobial spectrum of activity and select agent(s) that target the pathogens most likely causing the infection.

- Antimicrobial dosage regimens with the same agent may be different depending upon the infection or pathogen.

- Integration of PK and PD properties of an agent is important when choosing antimicrobial therapy to ensure efficacy and to prevent resistance.

- Pharmacokinetics refers to a mathematical method of describing in vivo drug exposure in terms of absorption, distribution, metabolism, and elimination.

- PD describes the relationship between drug exposure and pharmacologic effect of antibacterial activity or human toxicology.

- Concentration-dependent PD activity occurs where higher drug concentrations are associated with greater rate and extent of bacterial killing. Fluoroquinolones, aminoglycosides, and metronidazole are examples of antimicrobials that exhibit concentration-dependent activity.

- Time-dependent activity is maximized when these antimicrobials are dosed to maintain blood and/or tissue concentrations above the MIC in a time-dependent manner. β-Lactams and glycopeptides exhibit time-dependent activity.

- Antimicrobials with a low propensity of causing adverse events or drug interactions should be selected if possible, particularly for patients with risk factors for a particular complication.

- Host factors should be considered when evaluating a patient for antimicrobial therapy. Important host factors are: drug allergies, age, pregnancy, genetic/metabolic abnormalities, and organ dysfunction.

- Patients with a history of immediate or accelerated reactions (eg, anaphylaxis) to penicillin should not be given cephalosporin antibiotics. Patients with a delayed hypersensitivity reaction (rash) to penicillin may be given cephalosporin under close supervision.

- Normal flora are bacteria that are colonized in areas of the human body. Infections arise from normal flora (also called endogenous flora).

- A gram stain is performed to identify if bacteria are present and to determine morphologic characteristics of bacteria (such as gram-positive or negative, or shape—cocci, bacilli).

- Once a pathogen is identified, susceptibility tests can be performed to various antimicrobial agents. The MIC is a standard susceptibility test. The MIC is the lowest concentration of antimicrobial that inhibits visible bacterial growth. Breakpoint and MIC values determine if the organism is susceptible (S), intermediate (I), or resistant (R) to an antimicrobial.

BIBLIOGRAPHY

Gumbo T. General principles of antimicrobial therapy. In: Brunton LL, Chabner BA, Knollmann BC, eds. *Goodman & Gilman's The Pharmacological Basis of Therapeutics.* 12th ed. New York, NY: McGraw-Hill; 2011:chap 48.

Lampiris HW, Maddix DS. Clinical use of antimicrobial agents. In: Katzung BG, Masters SB, Trevor AJ, eds. *Basic & Clinical Pharmacology.* 12th ed. New York, NY: McGraw-Hill; 2012:chap 51.

Lee GC, Burgess DS. Antimicrobial regimen selection. In: DiPiro JT, Talbert RL, Yee GC, Matzke GR, Wells BG, Posey L, eds. *Pharmacotherapy: A Pathophysiologic Approach.* 10th ed. New York, NY: McGraw-Hill; 2017.

McAdam AJ, Onderdonk AB. Laboratory diagnosis of infectious diseases. In: Longo DL, Fauci AS, Kasper DL, Hauser SL, Jameson J, Loscalzo J, eds. *Harrison's Principles of Internal Medicine.* 18th ed. New York, NY: McGraw-Hill; 2012:chap e22.

Rybak MJ, Aeschlimann JR, LaPlante KL. Laboratory tests to direct antimicrobial pharmacotherapy. In: DiPiro JT, Talbert RL, Yee GC, Matzke GR, Wells BG, Posey L, eds. *Pharmacotherapy: A Pathophysiologic Approach.* 10th ed. New York, NY: McGraw-Hill; 2017.

KEY ABBREVIATIONS

AAD = antibiotic-associated diarrhea
AUC = area under the curve
CRP = C-reactive protein
ESBL = extended-spectrum β-lactamase
ESR = erythrocyte sedimentation rate
FDA = Food and Drug Administration
G6PD = glucose-6-phosphate dehydrogenase
GFR = glomerular filtration rate
IV = intravenous

MDRD = modification of diet in renal disease
MIC = minimal inhibitory concentration
MRSA = methicillin-resistant *Staphylococcus aureus*
PD = pharmacodynamics
RDT = rapid diagnostic test
UTI = urinary tract infection
VRE = vancomycin-resistant *Enterococcus* species
WBC = white blood cell

21 Lower Respiratory Tract Infections

Christopher M. Bland and S. Scott Sutton

FOUNDATION OVERVIEW

A lower respiratory tract infection (LRTI) is an infection below the level of the larynx and includes bronchitis, bronchiolitis, and pneumonia. LRTIs result from viral or bacterial invasion of lung parenchyma. Viral infections are diagnosed by the recognition of characteristic constellation of clinical signs and symptoms and treatment consists of supportive care measures (except for influenza, antivirals may be given). Bacterial LRTIs (in particular bacterial pneumonia) requires expedient, effective, and specific antimicrobial therapy. An appropriate treatment regimen for the patient with an LRTI can be established with the aid of a thorough medical history, physical examination, chest radiograph, knowledge of common bacterial pathogens, and results of properly collected cultures. This chapter will focus on pneumonia; see the special considerations section for information on bronchitis and bronchiolitis.

Pneumonia

Pneumonia is inflammation of the lung with consolidation and is classified by the setting in which it develops (eg, community-acquired or hospital-acquired). The etiology of bacterial pneumonia varies in accordance with the type of pneumonia. Table 21-1 lists common bacterial pathogens associated with the various classifications of pneumonia. Viruses are a common cause of community-acquired pneumonia (CAP) in adults (often co-infecting with bacteria) and in children (65%). Viral pneumonia in children is frequently caused by respiratory syncytial, influenza or parainfluenza virus.

Pathophysiology

Microorganisms gain access to the lower respiratory tract by three routes:

1. Aspiration of oropharyngeal secretions. Aspiration of small volumes of saliva (microaspiration) is the major mechanism by which pulmonary pathogens gain access to the normally sterile lungs.
2. Inhalation of aerosolized particles.
3. Metastatic spread to the lungs via the bloodstream from an extrapulmonary site of infection.

When pulmonary defense mechanisms are functioning optimally, aspirated microorganisms are cleared before infection is established. Local host defenses of the upper and lower respiratory tracts and anatomy of the airway are important in preventing pneumonia. Upper respiratory tract defenses include: mucociliary apparatus of the nasopharynx, nasal hair, normal bacterial flora, IgA antibodies, and complement. Lower respiratory tract defenses include: cough, mucociliary apparatus of the trachea and bronchi, antibodies (IgA, IgM, and IgG), complement, and alveolar macrophages. If microorganisms are not contained/eliminated by host defenses, the pathogen(s) may descend to the alveolar sacs of the lung and infection may ensue.

Hospitalized patients become colonized with bacteria that exist in the hospital setting. These bacteria are repeatedly exposed to antibiotics when they infect other patients and often evolve resistance to antibiotics. Patients who develop pneumonia during a hospital stay are therefore at risk for infection with highly resistant pathogens (Table 21-2).

A major aspiration of the oropharyngeal or gastric contents may lead to pneumonitis and ultimately to aspiration pneumonia. Dysphagia caused by neurologic impairment, seizures, or alcoholism is a common risk factor for the development of aspiration pneumonia. Other factors that may lead or predispose to aspiration pneumonia are: (1) oropharyngeal colonization altered by oral/dental disease; (2) poor oral hygiene; (3) tube feedings; or (4) medications.

Once breakdown of the local host defenses occurs and organisms invade the lung tissue, an inflammatory response is generated either by the exotoxins produced by the organism or by the immune response to the presence of organisms. This inflammatory response can remain localized in the lung (and potentially cause tissue damage) or become systemic.

Clinical Presentation

Patients with pneumonia present with respiratory and nonrespiratory symptoms. With increasing age, some respiratory and nonrespiratory symptoms decrease in frequency due to an attenuated immune response. Patients who are intubated may not be able to demonstrate many of these signs and symptoms, making diagnosis difficult.

Symptoms of pneumonia include:

1. Respiratory: Cough (productive or nonproductive), shortness of breath, difficulty breathing

TABLE 21-1   Etiology and Treatment of Pneumonia in Adults

Clinical Setting	Usual Pathogens	Empirical Therapy
Outpatient/Community Acquired		
Previously healthy	*S. pneumoniae, M. pneumoniae, H. influenzae, C. pneumoniae, M. catarrhalis*	Macrolide/azalide,[a] or tetracycline[b]
Comorbidities (eg, diabetes, heart/lung/liver/renal disease, and/or alcoholism)	Viral MDR *S. pneumoniae*	Oseltamivir or zanamivir if <48° from onset of symptoms Fluoroquinolone[c] or β-lactam[d] + macrolide[a]
Elderly Regions with >25% rate of macrolide-resistant *S. pneumoniae*	*S. pneumoniae,* gram-negative bacilli	Fluoroquinolone[c] or β-lactam + macrolide[a]/doxycycline
Inpatient/Community Acquired		
Non-ICU	*S. pneumoniae, H. influenzae, M. pneumoniae, C. pneumoniae, Legionella* sp.	Fluoroquinolone[c] or β-lactam[d] + macrolide[a]/doxycycline
ICU	*S. pneumoniae, S. aureus, Legionella* sp., gram-negative bacilli, *H. influenzae*	β-Lactam + macrolide[a]/fluoroquinolone[c]
	If *P. aeruginosa* suspected	Piperacillin/tazobactam or meropenem or cefepime + fluoroquinolone[c]/AMG/azithromycin; or β-lactam + AMG + azithromycin/respiratory fluoroquinolone[c]
	If MRSA suspected	Above + vancomycin or linezolid
	Viral	Oseltamivir or zanamivir ± antibiotics for 2° infection
Hospital Acquired or Ventilator Associated		
No risk factors for MDR pathogens (single-agent *Pseudomonal* coverage)	*S. pneumoniae, H. influenzae,* MSSA enteric gram-negative bacilli	Piperacillin/tazobactam, cefepime, levofloxacin, imipenem or meropenem
Risk factors for MDR pathogen (dual-agent *Pseudomonal* coverage) or septic shock	*P. aeruginosa, K. pneumoniae* (ESBL), *Acinetobacter* sp.	Antipseudomonal cephalosporin[e] or antipseudomonal carbapenem or Antipseudomonal β-lactam/β-lactamase inhibitor + antipseudomonal fluoroquinolone[c] or AMG[g]
	If MRSA or *Legionella* sp. suspected	Above + vancomycin or linezolid
Aspiration	*S. aereus,* enteric gram-negative bacilli Anaerobes	Penicillin or clindamycin or piperacillin/tazobactam + AMG[g] Clindamycin, β-lactam/β-lactamase inhibitor, or carbapenem
Atypical Pneumonia[h]		
Legionella pneumophila		Fluoroquinolone,[c] doxycycline, or azithromycin
Mycoplasma pneumoniae		Fluoroquinolone,[c] doxycycline, or azithromycin
Chlamydophila pneumoniae		Fluoroquinolone,[c] doxycycline, or azithromycin
SARS		Fluoroquinolone[c] or macrolides[a]
Avian influenza		Oseltamivir
H1N1 influenza		Oseltamivir

Abbreviations: MRSA, methicillin-resistant *Staphylococcus aureus*; AMG, aminoglycoside; SARS, severe acute respiratory syndrome; ESBL, extended-spectrum β-lactamases; MDR, multidrug resistant; MSSA, methicillin-sensitive *Staphylococcus aureus*.

[a]Macrolide/azalide: erythromycin, clarithromycin, and azithromycin.

[b]Tetracycline: doxycycline.

[c]Fluoroquinolone: levofloxacin and moxifloxacin.

[d]β-lactam: high-dose amoxicillin, amoxicillin/clavulanate, ceftriaxone (inpatient only), cefpodoxime, or cefuroxime.

[e]Antipseudomonal cephalosporin: cefepime and ceftazidime.

[f]Antipseudomonal carbapenem: imipenem and meropenem.

[g]Aminoglycoside: amikacin, gentamicin, and tobramycin.

[h]For tuberculosis, see Chapter 30.

Data from Mandell L, Wunderink R, Anzeuto A, et al. Infectious Diseases Society of America/American Thoracic Society consensus guidelines on the management of community-acquired pneumonia in adults. Clin Infect Dis 2007;44(Suppl 2):S27–S72; Kalil AC, Metersky ML, Klompas M, et al. Management of adults with hospital-acquire and ventilator-associated pneumonia: 2016 Clinical practice guidelines by the Infections Diseases Society of America and the American Thoracic Society. Clin Infect Dis. Advanced Access published July 14, 2016; Marrie TJ, Costain N, La Scola B, et al. The role of atypical pathogens in community-acquired pneumonia. Semin Respir Crit Care Med 2012;33:244–256.

2. Nonrespiratory: Fever, fatigue, sweats, headache, myalgias, mental status changes

Signs of pneumonia include:

1. Fever: Temperature may increase or decrease from baseline, but most often is elevated.
2. Respiratory rate is increased. Cyanosis, increased respiratory rate, and use of accessory muscles of respiration are suggestive of severe respiratory compromise.

3. Breath sounds may be diminished.
4. Confusion, lethargy, and disorientation are common in elderly patients.

Diagnosis

Key parameters for the diagnosis of pneumonia include clinical presentation, diagnostic tests, laboratory tests, and microbiology tests. Key diagnostic tests for pneumonia include: chest x-ray, oxygen saturation, and arterial blood gases. In addition

TABLE 21-2 Pneumonia Classifications and Risk Factors

Type of Pneumonia	Definition	Risk Factors
Community acquired pneumonia (CAP)	Pneumonia developing in patients with no contact to a medical facility	- Age > 65 y - Diabetes mellitus - Asplenia - Chronic cardiovascular, pulmonary, renal, or liver disease - Smoking and /or alcohol abuse
Hospital-acquired pneumonia (HAP)	Pneumonia developing > 48 h after hospital admission	- COPD, ARDS, or coma - Administration of antacids, H2 antagonists, or proton pump inhibitors - Supine position - Witnessed aspiration - Enteral nutrition, nasogastric tube - Reintubation, tracheostomy, or patient transport - Head trauma, ICP monitoring - Age > 60 y - MDR risk (eg, MRSA, Pseudomonas) if intravenous antibiotic use within 90 d
Ventilator-associated pneumonia (VAP)	Pneumonia developing > 48 h after intubation and mechanical ventilation	- Same as hospital acquired - MDR risk with septic shock, ARDS, acute renal replacement therapy, or ≥5 d of hospitalization, intravenous antibiotic use within 90 d

Abbreviations: ARDS, acute respiratory distress syndrome; CAP, community-acquired pneumonia; COPD, chronic obstructive pulmonary disease; HAP, hospital-acquired pneumonia; ICP, intracranial pressure; MDR, multidrug resistant; MRSA, methicillin-resistant *Staphylococcus aureus*; VAP, ventilator-associated pneumonia; VAP, ventilator-associated pneumonia.

to a constellation of suggestive clinical features, a demonstrable infiltrate on imaging is required for the diagnosis of pneumonia. The chest x-ray would reveal single or multiple infiltrates in a patient with pneumonia. Oxygen saturation and arterial blood gases are obtained to evaluate gas exchange in select patients. Laboratory tests obtained to aid in the diagnosis or treatment of patients with pneumonia include: the white blood cell (WBC) count with differential and basic metabolic panel (BMP). Microbiologic tests that may be utilized in patients with pneumonia include:

1. *Gram stain of respiratory secretions:* A sputum Gram stain should demonstrate the presence of WBCs and few squamous epithelial cells. It will also reveal if the bacteria are gram-positive or gram-negative and the morphology (eg, cocci or bacilli). For patients with severe pneumonia, bronchoscopy may be performed to obtain tracheal secretions. Tracheal secretions are better specimens compared to sputum samples because they lack oral contamination. However, a sample of either that does not reveal bacteria does not rule out pneumonia.
2. *Culture and susceptibility (C&S) tests:* C&S tests (sputum and/or blood cultures) may reveal the genus and species of the bacteria and the degree of susceptibility of the bacteria to antimicrobials (susceptible/intermediate/resistant). Positive cultures could indicate colonization; should be correlated with clinical symptoms consistent with pneumonia. Negative culture results do not rule out infection. C&S reports are not routinely ordered for outpatient pneumonia cases.
3. Serology (IgM and IgG) is useful in determining the presence of difficult-to-culture atypical pathogens such as *Mycoplasma* and *Chlamydia*.
4. Urinary direct fluorescence antigen is used to diagnose *Legionella pneumophila*, which is also difficult to

culture. Urinary antigen can be used to diagnose *Streptococcus pneumoniae* as well.

PREVENTION

Prevention of pneumonia is possible though the use of vaccines and infection control/prevention measures. Vaccines directed against strains of *Streptococcus pneumoniae* are administered to children and select adult populations. Influenza vaccine is also effective in preventing pneumonia and should be offered to persons at hospital discharge or during outpatient treatment during the fall and winter. Respiratory hygiene measures, including the use of hand hygiene and masks or tissues for patients with cough, should be used in outpatient settings and emergency departments as a means to reduce the spread of respiratory infections caused by viruses. However, since pneumonia is not principally spread via respiratory droplets, isolation is not generally required. There are also recommendations for preventing pneumonia in the hospital (infection control measures, patients should be kept in semirecumbent position, and enteral nutrition is preferred over parenteral).

TREATMENT

The goal of antimicrobial treatment is to eliminate the patient's symptoms, minimize or prevent complications, and prevent mortality. The treatment of bacterial pneumonia involves the empirical use of antimicrobial(s) that is or are effective against probable pathogens. Antimicrobials exhibiting activity against the suspected pathogens without having activity against nontargeted pathogens is preferred. Table 21-2 lists the common bacterial pathogens associated with the different classifications of pneumonia. Numerous antimicrobials are available, and many are effective in the treatment of bacterial pneumonia.

Superiority of one antibiotic over another when both demonstrate similar in vitro activity and tissue distribution characteristics is difficult to define and has rarely been shown.

The response and outcome of patients with pneumonia depend on the antimicrobial agent involved and the patient status at presentation. Poor prognostic factors include age greater than 65 years; coexisting disease such as diabetes, renal failure, heart failure, or chronic obstructive pulmonary disease (COPD); multiple lobes involved; bacteremia; alcoholism; and neutropenia. Most patients with pneumonia improve clinically (decreased temperature and systemic symptoms) 24 to 72 hours after the initiation of effective antibiotic therapy. Chest radiograph resolution lags, however, taking up to 3 weeks in healthy young adults and 12 weeks in elderly patients and those with complicated infections. Community-acquired and hospital-acquired pneumonia treatment regimens are based upon patient characteristics, severity of illness, and risk factors (see Tables 21-1 and 21-2). Outpatient aspiration pneumonia may be treated with amoxicillin/clavulanate or clindamycin. Once the microbial etiology of the pneumonia has been identified and susceptibilities are known, antimicrobial therapy should be directed at the specific pathogen(s) isolated. Table 21-3 lists key characteristics for antimicrobials recommended for treatment of pneumonia.

SPECIAL CONSIDERATIONS

Duration of Treatment

The duration of therapy for pneumonia should be kept as short as possible and depends on several factors: type of pneumonia, inpatient or outpatient status, patient comorbidities, bacteremia/sepsis, and the antibiotic chosen. Many patients with CAP can be treated with 5 days of antibiotic therapy. Patients with CAP and aspiration pneumonia should be treated for 5 to 10 days. Patients should be afebrile for 48 to 72 hours and should have clinically improved before treatment is discontinued. A longer duration of therapy may be needed if initial therapy was not active against the identified pathogen. Patients with hospital-acquired pneumonia should be treated for 8 to 15 days, depending on severity of the disease, response to therapy, and the organisms isolated. Positive culture results should be used to choose definitive therapy that is targeted to the pathogen isolated.

Hospital-Acquired Pneumonia

When feasible, a lower respiratory tract culture should be collected from all patients before antibiotic therapy for health care-associated pneumonia, but the initiation of therapy should not be delayed by the need to collect cultures. Negative lower respiratory tract cultures for 72 hours can be used to stop antibiotic therapy. Early, appropriate, broad-spectrum antimicrobial therapy should be prescribed with adequate doses to optimize therapy.

Antibiotic Resistance Issues

Resistance to commonly used antibiotics for pneumonia presents a major consideration in choosing empirical therapy.

Resistance patterns vary by geography. Therefore, antibiotic recommendations must be modified on the basis of local susceptibility patterns.

Drug-Resistant *Streptococcus pneumoniae*

The most problematic resistant pathogen in the community setting is *S. pneumoniae*. The definition of resistance to penicillin in *S. pneumoniae* changed after it was noticed that the breakpoint overcalled resistance and that isolates labeled as penicillin-resistant were successfully treated with penicillin. Resistance to macrolides in most settings remains high (30%-40%) and patients who are at risk for resistant-*S. pneumoniae* or who have more severe disease should not receive monotherapy with a macrolide for this reason. High doses of amoxicillin (1g q8h) and amoxicillin/clavulanate XR (2g q12h) are recommended for the possibility of drug-resistant *S. pneumoniae*.

Methicillin-Resistant *Staphylococcus aureus* (MRSA)

Methicillin-resistant *Staphylococcus aureus* (MRSA) is a common cause of hospital-acquired pneumonia in some centers. The predominant strain of community-associated MRSA (CA-MRSA) rarely causes CAP, but it can cause a form of necrotizing pneumonia that is very severe and rapidly fatal. If this is suspected, an agent with activity against MRSA such as linezolid or vancomycin +/− clindamycin for potential exotoxin production should be given empirically in addition to other antibiotics.

Resistant Gram-Negative Rods

Among the more problematic pathogens in late-onset hospital-acquired and health care-associated pneumonia are highly resistant gram-negative rods such as *Pseudomonas aeruginosa*, *Acinetobacter baumannii*, and *Klebsiella pneumoniae*. Empiric double-coverage with two anti-gram-negative agents is recommended to ensure that at least one active antibiotic is given when infection is first suspected.

Pediatric Bacterial Pneumonia

Pediatric pneumonia is caused by the same bacterial pathogens that cause adult CAP. Fluoroquinolones and tetracyclines should not be used in children. High-dose amoxicillin, amoxicillin-clavulanate, intramuscular ceftriaxone, azithromycin, and clarithromycin are potential agents for use in children (Table 21-4).

Bronchitis/Bronchiolitis

Acute bronchitis and bronchiolitis are inflammatory conditions of the large and small elements of the tracheobronchial tree and do not involve the alveoli. Acute bronchitis is most commonly a self-limiting viral illness. Treatment is symptomatic and supportive. Bronchiolitis is an acute viral infection of the lower respiratory tract that affects children. Respiratory syncytial virus (RSV) is the most common cause. Treatment of bronchiolitis is symptomatic and supportive.

TABLE 21-3 Antimicrobials Recommended for Treatment of Pneumonia

Antibiotic	Indication(s)[a]	Route of Administration (RA); Formulation (F); Dose (D)[b]	Mechanism of Action	Side Effects (SE) and Contraindications (CI)	Excretion (E); Drug Interactions (DI); General Information (GI)
Clarithromycin (Biaxin)	CAP	RA: Oral F: Suspension, tablets, extended release tablets D: 250-500 mg every 12 h; 1000 mg every 24 h (XL)	Inhibits protein synthesis	SE: Headache, rash, abnormal taste, gastrointestinal, C. diff CI: Hypersensitivity to macrolide	E: H & R DI: P450 substrate: 3A4 (major); P450 inhibitor: 3A4 (strong), 1A2 (weak) GI: Pregnancy category C
Azithromycin (Zithromax; ZPak)	CAP	RA: Oral, IV F: Injection, suspension, tablet D: 250-500 mg every 24 h	Inhibits protein synthesis	SE: Headache, rash, gastrointestinal, C. diff CI: Hypersensitivity to macrolide	E: H; use with caution in patients with preexisting liver disease DI: P450 substrate: 3A4 (minor), P450 inhibitor: 3A4 (weak) GI: Pregnancy category B
Doxycycline (Vibramycin and others)	CAP	RA: Oral, IV F: Capsule, tablet, suspension, syrup, injection D: 100 mg every 12 h	Inhibits protein synthesis	SE: Rash (photosensitivity), GI pill esophagitis, C. diff, BMS (rare), hepatotoxicity (rare), autoimmune disease reported CI: Hypersensitivity to doxycycline/tetracyclines, children ≤ 8 y of age	E: R and feces DI: P450 inhibitor 3A4 (moderate), levels decreased by cations GI: Pregnancy category D; avoid in children ≤8 years of age
Amoxicillin (Amoxil)	CAP	RA: Oral F: Capsule, tablet, suspension D: 500 mg every 8 h or 875 every 12 h (1000 mg every 8 h for DRSP)	Inhibits bacterial cell wall synthesis	SE: Rash, GI, C. diff, BMS (rare), allergic reaction (immediate—anaphylaxis or delayed—rash) CI: Hypersensitivity to amoxicillin or penicillin compounds	E: R (dose reductions required for renal dysfunction) GI: Pregnancy category B; high percentage of patients with infectious mononucleosis develop rash on amoxicillin.
Ampicillin (Principen and others)	CAP	RA: Oral, IV F: Capsule, suspension, injection D: 2 g IV every 6 h	Inhibits bacterial cell wall synthesis	SE: Rash, GI, C. diff, BMS (rare), allergic reaction (immediate—anaphylaxis or delayed—rash) CI: Hypersensitivity to amoxicillin or penicillin compounds	E: R (dose reductions required for renal dysfunction) GI: Pregnancy category B; high percentage of patients with infectious mononucleosis develop rash on ampicillin
Amoxicillin/ Clavulanate (Augmentin)	CAP; aspiration	RA: Oral F: Suspension, tablet, XR tablet D: 500 mg every 8 h, 875 mg every 12 h, 2000 mg every 12 h	Inhibits bacterial cell wall synthesis; addition of clavulanate extends coverage of amoxicillin to include β-lactamase producing bacteria[c]	SE: Rash, GI, C. diff, BMS (rare), allergic reaction (immediate—anaphylaxis or delayed—rash) CI: Hypersensitivity to amoxicillin or penicillin compounds	E: R (dose reductions required for renal dysfunction) GI: Pregnancy category B; high percentage of patients with infectious mononucleosis develop rash on amoxicillin/clavulanate
Ampicillin/ Sulbactam (Unasyn)	CAP	RA: IV F: Injection D: 1.5-3 g every 6 h	Inhibits bacterial cell wall synthesis; addition of sulbactam extends coverage of ampicillin to include β-lactamase-producing bacteria[c]	SE: Rash, GI, C. diff, BMS (rare), allergic reaction (immediate—anaphylaxis or delayed—rash) CI: Hypersensitivity to ampicillin or penicillin compounds	E: R (dose reductions required for renal dysfunction) GI: Pregnancy category B; high percentage of patients with infectious mononucleosis develop rash on ampicillin/sulbactam

(Continued)

TABLE 21-3   Antimicrobials Recommended for Treatment of Pneumonia (Continued)

Antibiotic	Indication(s)[a]	Route of Administration (RA); Formulation (F); Dose (D)[b]	Mechanism of Action	Side Effects (SE) and Contraindications (CI)	Excretion (E); Drug Interactions (DI); General Information (GI)
Piperacillin/ Tazobactam (Zosyn)	HAP, VAP	RA: IV F: Injection D: 3.375-4.5 g every 4-6 h	Inhibits bacterial cell wall synthesis; addition of tazobactam extends coverage of piperacillin to include β-lactamase-producing bacteria[c]	SE: Rash, GI, *C. diff*, BMS (rare), allergic reaction (immediate—anaphylaxis or delayed—rash) CI: Hypersensitivity to piperacillin or penicillin compounds	E: R (dose reductions required for renal dysfunction) GI: Pregnancy category B; high percentage of patients with infectious mononucleosis develop rash on piperacillin; bleeding disorders have been observed, particularly in patients with renal dysfunction, discontinue if thrombocytopenia or bleeding occurs; 4.5 g injection contains 11.17 mEq of sodium, 3.375 g contains 8.38 mEq of sodium
Cefpodoxime (Vantin)	CAP	RA: Oral F: Suspension, tablet D: 200 mg every 12 h	Inhibits bacterial cell wall synthesis	SE: Rash, GI, *C. diff*, BMS (rare), allergic reaction (immediate—anaphylaxis or delayed—rash) CI: Hypersensitivity to cefpodoxime or cephalosporin compounds; if allergic to penicillin: delayed reaction (rash) 3%-5% chance of cross reactions, immediate reaction (anaphylaxis) do not use	E: R (dose reductions required for renal dysfunction); GI: Pregnancy category B
Cefuroxime (Ceftin and others)	CAP	RA: Oral, IV F: Tablet, suspension, injection D: 500 mg every 12 h (po), 750 mg every 8 h (IV)	Inhibits bacterial cell wall synthesis	SE: Rash, GI, *C. diff*, BMS (rare), allergic reaction (immediate—anaphylaxis or delayed—rash) CI: Hypersensitivity to cefuroxime or cephalosporin compounds; if allergic to penicillin: delayed reaction (rash) 3%-5% chance of cross reactions, immediate reaction (anaphylaxis) do not use	E: R (dose reductions required for renal dysfunction) GI: Pregnancy category B; cefuroxime axetil film coated tablets and oral suspension are not bioequivalent and are not substitutable on a mg/mg basis
Ceftriaxone (Rocephin)	CAP	RA: IV F: Injection D: 1-2 g daily	Inhibits bacterial cell wall synthesis	SE: Rash, GI, *C. diff*, BMS (rare), allergic reaction (immediate—anaphylaxis or delayed—rash) CI: Hypersensitivity to ceftriaxone or cephalosporin compounds; if allergic to penicillin: delayed reaction (rash) 3%-5% chance of cross reactions, immediate reaction (anaphylaxis) do not use	E: R (dose reductions *not* required for renal dysfunction), feces GI: Pregnancy category B; do not use in hyperbilirubinemic neonates and concomitant use with calcium containing solutions/products in neonates is contraindicated
Cefotaxime (Claforan)	CAP	RA: IV F: Injection D: 1-2 g every 8 h	Inhibits bacterial cell wall synthesis	SE: Rash, GI, *C. diff*, BMS (rare), allergic reaction (immediate—anaphylaxis or delayed—rash) CI: Hypersensitivity to cefotaxime or cephalosporin compounds; if allergic to penicillin: delayed reaction (rash) 3%-5% chance of cross reactions, immediate reaction (anaphylaxis) do not use	E: R (dose reductions required for renal dysfunction) GI: Pregnancy category B
Cefepime (Maxipime)	HAP, VAP	RA: Injection F: IV D: 1-2 g every 8-12 h	Inhibits bacterial cell wall synthesis	SE: Rash, GI, *C. diff*, BMS (rare), allergic reaction (immediate—anaphylaxis or delayed—rash); neurotoxicity (including seizures) CI: Hypersensitivity to cefepime or cephalosporin compounds; if allergic to penicillin: delayed reaction (rash) 3%-5% chance of cross reactions, immediate reaction (anaphylaxis) do not use	E: R (dose reductions required for renal dysfunction) GI: Pregnancy category B; may be used for CAP, however since cefepime has activity against *Pseudomonas aeruginosa*, it should be reserved for HCAP, use ceftriaxone or cefotaxime for CAP

Drug	Indication	Route/Form/Dose	Mechanism	Side Effects/Contraindications	Elimination/Other
Ertapenem (Invanz)	CAP	RA: Injection F: IV D: 1 g daily	Inhibits bacterial cell wall synthesis	SE: Headache, Rash, GI, *C. diff* BMS (rare), allergic reaction (immediate—anaphylaxis or delayed—rash); neurotoxicity (including seizures) CI: Hypersensitivity to ertapenem or carbapenem compounds; if allergic to penicillin, <1% chance of cross-reactivity	E: R, feces (dose reduction, required for renal dysfunction) GI: Pregnancy category B
Imipenem/ Cilastatin (Primaxin)	HAP, VAP	RA: Injection F: IV D: 500-1000 mg every 6 h	Inhibits bacterial cell wall synthesis	SE: Headache, seizure, rash, GI, *C. diff*, BMS (rare), allergic reaction (immediate—anaphylaxis or delayed—rash) CI: Hypersensitivity to imipenem or carbapenem compounds; if allergic to penicillin: <1% chance of cross-reactivity	E: R (dose reduction required for renal dysfunction) GI: Pregnancy category C; has been associated with seizures—use with caution in patients with history of seizures, (highest risk among carbapenems)
Meropenem (Merrem)	HAP, VAP	RA: Injection F: IV D: 1-2 g every 8 h	Inhibits bacterial cell wall synthesis	SE: Headache, rash, GI, *C. diff*, BMS (rare), allergic reaction (immediate—anaphylaxis or delayed—rash); neurotoxicity (including seizures) CI: Hypersensitivity to meropenem or carbapenem compounds; if allergic to penicillin: <1% chance of cross-reactivity	E: R (dose reduction required for renal dysfunction) GI: Pregnancy category B
Doripenem (Doribax)	HAP,VAP	RA: Injection F: IV D: 500 mg every 8 h	Inhibits bacterial cell wall synthesis	SE: Headache, rash, GI, *C. diff*, BMS (rare), allergic reaction (immediate—anaphylaxis or delayed—rash); neurotoxicity (including seizures) CI: Hypersensitivity to doripenem or carbapenem compounds; <1% chance of allergic to penicillin: cross-reactivity	E: R (dose reduction required for renal dysfunction) GI: Pregnancy category B; administration is over 1 h (most antimicrobials are administered over 30 min, except for highly resistant bacteria; HCAP use is unlabeled/investigational at time of writing
Levofloxacin (Levaquin)	CAP; HAP, VAP	RA: Oral, injection F: Solution, tablet, IV D: 500-750 mg daily	Inhibits DNA gyrase; inhibits relaxation of supercoiled DNA and promotes breakage of DNA strands	SE: Headache, confusion, mental status changes, GI, *C. diff*, BMS (rare), allergic reaction (immediate or delayed), glucose (hypo or hyperglycemia), Photosensitivity CI: Hypersensitivity to levofloxacin or other quinolones	E: R (dose reduction required for renal dysfunction) DI: QTc prolonging agents, cations, rare cases of torsade de pointes reported (use caution in patients with known prolongation of QT interval, bradycardia, hypokalemia, hypomagnesemia, or receiving Class 1a or Class III antiarrhythmics) GI: Pregnancy category C; black box warning: reports of tendon inflammation and rupture (Achilles tendon); fluoroquinolones have been associated with the development of serious (sometimes fatal) hypoglycemia

(Continued)

TABLE 21-3 Antimicrobials Recommended for Treatment of Pneumonia (*Continued*)

Antibiotic	Indication(s)[a]	Route of Administration (RA); Formulation (F); Dose (D)[b]	Mechanism of Action	Side Effects (SE) and Contraindications (CI)	Excretion (E); Drug Interactions (DI); General Information (GI)
Ciprofloxacin (Cipro)	HAP/VAP	RA: Oral, injection F: Suspension, tablet, IV D: Oral: 500-750 mg every 12 h, IV: 400 mg every 8-12 h	Inhibits DNA gyrase; inhibits relaxation of supercoiled DNA and promotes breakage of DNA strands	SE: Headache, confusion, mental status changes, GI, C. *diff*, BMS (rare), allergic reaction (immediate or delayed), glucose (hypo- or hyperglycemia), photosensitivity CI: Hypersensitivity to ciprofoxacin or other quinolones	E: R, feces (dose reduction required for renal dysfunction) DI: Inhibits CYP-450 1A2 (strong) and 3A4 (weak), QTc prolonging agents, cations, theophylline, rare cases of torsade de pointes reported (use caution in patients with known prolongation of QT interval, bradycardia, hypokalemia, hypomagnesemia, or receiving Class 1a or Class III antiarrhythmics) GI: Pregnancy category C; black box warning: reports of tendon inflammation and rupture (Achilles tendon); fluoroquinolones have been associated with the development of serious (sometimes fatal) hypoglycemia
Moxifloxacin (Avelox)	CAP	RA: Oral, injection F: Tablet, IV	Inhibits DNA gyrase; inhibits relaxation of supercoiled DNA and promotes breakage of DNA strands	SE: Headache, confusion, mental status changes, GI, C. *diff*, BMS (rare), allergic reaction (immediate or delayed), glucose (hypo- or hyperglycemia), photosensitivity CI: Hypersensitivity to moxifoxacin or other quinolones	E: R (20%), H, feces DI: QTc prolonging agents, cations, rare cases of torsade de pointes reported (use caution in patients with known prolongation of QT interval, bradycardia, hypokalemia, hypomagnesemia, or receiving Class 1a or Class III antiarrhythmics) GI: Pregnancy category C; black box warning: reports of tendon inflammation and rupture (Achilles tendon); fluoroquinolones have been associated with the development of serious (sometimes fatal) hypoglycemia
Gemifloxacin (Factive)	CAP	RA: Oral F: Tablet	Inhibits DNA gyrase; inhibits relaxation of supercoiled DNA and promotes breakage of DNA strands	SE: Headache, confusion, mental status changes, GI, C. *diff*, BMS (rare), allergic reaction (immediate or delayed), glucose (hypo or hyperglycemia), Photosensitivity CI: Hypersensitivity to gemifloxacin or other quinolones	E: R (dose reduction required for renal dysfunction) DI: QTc prolonging agents, cations, rare cases of torsade de pointes reported (use caution in patients with known prolongation of QT interval, bradycardia, hypokalemia, hypomagnesemia, or receiving Class 1a or Class III antiarrhythmics) GI: Pregnancy category C; black box warning: reports of tendon inflammation and rupture (Achilles tendon); fluoroquinolones have been associated with the development of serious (sometimes fatal) hypoglycemia

		Inhibits protein synthesis by binding to 30s and 50s ribosomal subunit	RA: Injection F: IV D: 1-2.5 mg/kg every 8-12 h (conventional) to produce peak of 8-10 mg/L and trough ≤2 mg/L, 4-7 mg/kg every 24, 36, 48 h (extended interval); check random level between 6-14 h to determine dosing interval based on nomogram	SE: Neurotoxicity (vertigo, ataxia), ototoxicity, nephrotoxicity, rash, BMS (rare), GI, C. diff CI: Hypersensitivity to gentamicin, tobramycin or other aminoglycosides	E: R (dose modifications required for renal dysfunction) GI: Pregnancy category D; risk factors for nephrotoxicity: preexisting renal impairment, concomitant nephrotoxic drug, advanced age, dehydration; may cause neuromuscular blockade and respiratory paralysis; dosage individualization is critical because of low therapeutic index, initial and periodic plasma drug levels should be determined, particularly in critically ill patients or in disease states known to significantly alter aminoglycoside pharmacokinetics (cystic fibrosis, burns, or major surgery)
Gentamicin (Garamycin) and Tobramycin (Tobrex)	HAP/VAP				
Amikacin (Amikin)	HAP/VAP	Inhibits protein synthesis by binding to 30s and 50s ribosomal subunit	RA: Injection F: IV D: 5-7.5 mg/kg every 8 h (conventional), 15-20 mg/kg every 24, 36, 48 h (extended interval) and dose based on levels drawn in dosing interval to be adjusted by nomogram	SE: Neurotoxicity (vertigo, ataxia), ototoxicity, nephrotoxicity, rash, BMS (rare), GI, C. diff CI: Hypersensitivity to amikacin or other aminoglycosides	E: R (dose modifications required for renal dysfunction) GI: Pregnancy category D: risk factors for nephrotoxicity: preexisting renal impairment, concomitant nephrotoxic drug, advanced age, dehydration; may cause neuromuscular blockade and respiratory paralysis; dosage individualization is critical because of low therapeutic index, initial and periodic plasma drug levels should be determined, particularly in critically ill patients or in disease states known to significantly alter aminoglycoside pharmacokinetics (cystic fibrosis, burns, or major surgery)
Vancomycin (Vancocin)	HAP/VAP	Inhibits bacterial cell wall synthesis	RA: Oral, injection F: Capsule (treatment of C. diff only), IV D: IV: 15-20 mg/kg every 8-12 h to produce trough of 15-20 mg/L or AUC/MIC ratio ≥ 400	SE: Red-man syndrome (rash), BMS (rare, except with high dose), ototoxicity, nephrotoxicity, increase nephrotoxic potential when combined with aminoglycoside, thrombocytopenia, leukopenia CI: Hypersensitivity to vancomycin	E: R (dose modifications required for renal dysfunction) GI: Pregnancy category C, pharmacokinetics may be altered during pregnancy; dosing in dialysis patients is variable, poorly dialyzable by conventional hemodialysis, increased removal with high flux membranes and continuous renal replacement; Red-man syndrome is not an allergic reaction but is associated with too rapid infusion of the drug

(Continued)

TABLE 21-3   Antimicrobials Recommended for Treatment of Pneumonia (Continued)

Antibiotic	Indication(s)[a]	Route of Administration (RA); Formulation (F); Dose (D)[b]	Mechanism of Action	Side Effects (SE) and Contraindications (CI)	Excretion (E); Drug Interactions (DI); General Information (GI)
Linezolid (Zyvox)	HAP/VAP	RA: Oral, injection F: Suspension, tablet, IV D: 600 mg every 12 h	Inhibits bacterial protein synthesis by binding to 23s ribosomal RNA of the 50s subunit	SE: Headache, GI, C. diff, rash, BMS. BMS (including anemia, leukopenia, pancytopenia, and thrombocytopenia may be more common in patients receiving for > 2 wk CI: Hypersensitivity to linezolid, concurrent use if within 2 wk of monoamine oxidase inhibitors, patients with uncontrolled hypertension, taking sympathomimetics, vasopressive agents, or dopaminergic agents unless closely monitored for increase in blood pressure, patients taking antidepressants with serotonin mechanism, meperidine unless closely monitored for serotonin syndrome	E: R (30% parent drug, 50% inactive metabolites), feces DI: Sympathomimetics, antidepressants with serotonin activity, meperidine, tyramine containing foods (hypertensive crisis) GI: Pregnancy category C; monitoring: weekly complete blood count, particularly in patients at increased risk of bleeding, preexisting myelosuppression, on concomitant medications that cause BMS, those requiring more than 2 wk of therapy
Clindamycin (Cleocin)	Aspiration	RA: Oral, injection F: Capsule, solution, IV D: Oral: 300-450 mg every 6-8 h, IV: 600-900 mg every 8 h	Reversibly binds to 50s ribosomal subunit preventing peptide bond formation thus inhibiting bacterial protein synthesis	SE: Rash, GI pill esophagitis, C. diff, BMS (rare) CI: Hypersensitivity to clindamycin	E: R (10%), H, feces GI: Pregnancy category B; can cause severe and possibly fatal colitis (C. diff infection)

Abbreviations: AUC, area under the curve; BMS, bone marrow suppression; CAP, community-acquired pneumonia; C. diff, Clostridium difficile; DRSP, drug-resistant Streptococcus pneumonia; GI, gastrointestinal; H, hepatic; MIC, minimum inhibitory concentration; R, renal; P450, CYP-450 system.

[a]Indication lists the type of pneumonia for which the antimicrobial is most commonly used and recommended by treatment guidelines. The antimicrobials listed have other indications besides pneumonia.

[b]Adult dose.

[c]Bacteria (eg, Staphylococcus, Enterics: Klebsiella pneumonia, Escherichia coli, Enterobacter species, Proteus species, Serratia marcescens, and gram-negative anaerobes (Bacteroides fragilis).

TABLE 21-4	Etiology and Treatment of Pneumonia in Pediatric Patients	
Clinical Setting	**Usual Pathogen(s)**	**Empirical Therapy**
Outpatient/Community Acquired		
<1 mo	Group B *Streptococcus, H. influenzae* (nontypable), *E. coli, S. aureus, Listeria monocytogenes*, RSV, adenovirus	Preferred therapy: Ampicillin plus gentamicin; Alternative: Cephalosporin,[a] carbapenem[b] Ribavirin for RSV[c]
1-3 mo	*C. pneumoniae*, possibly *Ureaplasma*, CMV, *Pneumocystis carinii* (afebrile pneumonia syndrome) *S. pneumoniae, S. aureus*	Macrolide/azalide,[d] trimethoprim–sulfamethoxazole Semisynthetic penicillin[e] or cephalosporin[f]
Preschool-aged children	Viral (rhinovirus, RSV, influenza A and B, *H. parainfluenzae*, adenovirus, human metapneumovirus, coronavirus)	Antimicrobial therapy not routinely required
Previously healthy, fully immunized infants and preschool children with suspected mild–moderate bacterial CAP	*S. pneumoniae* *M. pneumoniae*, other atypical organisms	Amoxicillin, cephalosporin[a,f] Macrolide/azalide
Previously healthy, fully immunized school-aged children and adolescents with mild–moderate CAP	*S. pneumoniae* *M. pneumoniae*, other atypical	Amoxicillin, cephalosporin,[a,f] Macrolide/azalide or tetracycline
Moderate–severe CAP during influenza virus outbreak	Influenza A and B, other viruses	Oseltamivir or zanamivir
Inpatient/Community Acquired		
Fully immunized infants and school-aged children	*S. pneumoniae* CA-MRSA *M. pneumoniae, C. pneumoniae*	Ampicillin, penicillin G, cephalosporin[a] β-Lactam + vancomycin/clindamycin for those at risk of MRSA β-Lactam + macrolide/doxycycline
Not fully immunized infants and children; regions with invasive penicillin-resistant pneumococcal strains; patients with life-threatening infections	*S. pneumoniae*, PCN resistant MRSA *M. pneumoniae*, other atypical pathogens	Cephalosporin[a] Add vancomycin/clindamycin for those at risk of MRSA Macrolide/azalide[d] + β-lactam/doxycycline

Abbreviations: CMV, cytomegalovirus; RSV, respiratory syncytial virus; CAP, community-acquired pneumonia; MRSA, methicillin-resistant *Staphylococcus aureus*.
[a]Third-generation cephalosporin: ceftriaxone and cefotaxime (preferred in infants <1 month). Note that cephalosporins are not active against *Listeria monocytogenes*.
[b]Carbapenem: imipenem–cilastatin and meropenem.
[c]See text for details regarding possible ribavirin treatment for RSV infection.
[d]Macrolide/azalide: erythromycin and clarithromycin/azithromycin.
[e]Semisynthetic penicillin: nafcillin and oxacillin.
[f]Second-generation cephalosporin: cefuroxime and cefprozil.
Data from Bradley JS, Byington Cl, Shah SS, et al. The management of community-acquired pneumonia in infants and children older than 3 months of age: Clinical practice guidelines by the Pediatric Infectious Diseases Society and the Infectious Diseases Society of America. Clin Infect Dis 2011;53:e25–e76.

CASE Application

1. Select the infection(s) that is/are an LRTI. Select all that apply.

   a. Pneumonia
   b. Sinusitis
   c. Bronchitis
   d. Otitis

2. AS is a 54-year-old man with fever, cough, and shortness of breath. He has been diagnosed with an LRTI. Select bacterial pathogen(s) that is a common cause of LRTI. Select all that apply.

   a. *Haemophilus influenzae*
   b. *Moraxella catarrhalis*
   c. Influenza
   d. *Streptococcus pneumoniae*

3. QW is a patient admitted to a rehabilitation hospital to improve strength after cardiac surgery. He does not want to develop an infection (especially pneumonia) because it hurts when he coughs. He questions how he can prevent the development of pneumonia. Which of the following may prevent pneumonia? Select all that apply.

   a. Infection control/prevention measures
   b. *Streptococcus pneumoniae* vaccine
   c. Influenza vaccine
   d. Levofloxacin

4. A pharmacy student is on his pediatric acute care clerkship and is charged with developing a list of antibiotics that may be used to treat pediatric pneumonia. Select anti-infectives that may be used to treat pediatric CAP. Select all that apply.

   a. Levofloxacin
   b. Doxycycline

c. Ceftriaxone

d. Azithromycin

5. AQ is a 44-year-old female patient with a past medical history of hypertension (HTN) and dyslipidemia. Medications include lisinopril and simvastatin. AQ has developed pneumonia and would like to take an oral agent that will not interact with her medications. Which of the following antibiotics used in the treatment of CAP is a strong inhibitor of the CYP-450 3A4 hepatic enzyme and would have a drug interaction with her medications?

a. Azithromycin

b. Clarithromycin

c. Amoxicillin

d. Cefpodoxime

6. KC is a 33-year-old pregnant female with a bacterial LRTI. Select the antimicrobial that is preferred in LRTIs in pregnant patients. Select all that apply.

a. Clarithromycin

b. Azithromycin

c. Doxycycline

d. Cefuroxime

7. Which of the following antibiotics has the same oral and IV dose?

a. Doxycycline

b. Amoxicillin/clavulanate

c. Piperacillin/tazobactam

d. Ceftriaxone

e. Ciprofloxacin

8. Select the antimicrobial(s) that is associated with the adverse effect of photosensitivity. Select all that apply.

a. Doxycycline

b. Ciprofloxacin

c. Cefepime

d. Sulfamethoxazole/trimethoprim

9. Select the antimicrobials that are associated with a *C. difficile* infection. Select all that apply.

a. Ciprofloxacin

b. Clindamycin

c. Cefotaxime

d. Cephalexin

10. ZT is a patient with an LRTI. She has a past medical history for HTN and reflux. Medications include amlodipine and pantoprazole. She has an allergy to Unasyn (delayed/rash). Select the antimicrobial(s) that a patient with a delayed allergic hypersensitivity reaction to Unasyn may receive. Select all that apply.

a. Ceftriaxone

b. Moxifloxacin

c. Piperacillin/tazobactam

d. Oral vancomycin

11. Select the penicillin antimicrobial that is combined with a β-lactamase inhibitor. Select all that apply.

a. Zosyn

b. Unasyn

c. Augmentin

d. Primaxin

12. Select the β-lactam antimicrobial that requires dose or interval modifications in patients with significant renal dysfunction. Select all that apply.

a. Amoxicillin

b. Azithromycin

c. Ceftriaxone

d. Moxifloxacin

e. Cefepime

13. Select the side effect(s) associated with fluoroquinolone antimicrobials. Select all that apply.

a. Hypoglycemia

b. *Clostridium difficile* infection

c. Confusion in the elderly

d. QTc prolongation

Use the patient case scenario to answer questions 14 and 15.

KP is a 78-year-old man who was admitted to the hospital 6 days ago for a COPD exacerbation. Today KP is complaining of shortness of breath and cough. A chest X-ray reveals a left lower lobe infiltrate. His vitals today are: Tmax 100.9, blood pressure (BP) 132/80, heart rate (HR) 97, respiratory rate (RR) 20.

Labs

143	102	19	Glucose 140 WBC 15 H/H 12.7/39 Plt 220K
4.2	30	1.0	

KP is diagnosed with pneumonia.

14. What type of pneumonia does KP have?

a. CAP

b. Influenza pneumonia

c. Aspiration pneumonia

d. Hospital-acquired pneumonia

15. Based on the above patient case, what MDR pathogen may be causing his pneumonia? Select all that apply.

a. *Pseudomonas aeruginosa*

b. *Klebsiella pneumoniae*

c. *Acinetobacter* species

d. Methicillin-resistant *Staphylococcus aureus*

Use the patient case scenario to answer questions 16 and 17.

AL is a 67-year-old WM in the emergency room with a 3-day history of subjective fever, productive cough, chills, and increasing shortness of breath, to the point where he now has difficulty walking up the stairs in his home.

History of previous illness (HPI): 2 weeks ago AL was diagnosed with bronchitis and a Z-Pak was prescribed by his primary care physician. He states that he "hasn't felt completely better since."

Past medical history (PMH):

Diabetes mellitus (DM), type II

Hx of venous thromboembolism (VTE) (*deep vein thrombosis* [DVT] 5 years ago)

HTN

Past cerebrovascular accident (CVA)

Allergies: Unknown

Meds (home):

Metformin XL 1 g po daily

Glipizide 5 mg po daily

Lisinopril 10 mg po daily

Warfarin 5 mg po MWF

Warfarin 7.5 mg po TThSS

ASA 81 mg 1 po daily

Physical examination:

Ht 5'9", Wt 170 lb, T=101°F, BP 110/72, HR 100, RR 21, Pulse Ox 95% Room Air

Gen: WDWN WM in obvious distress

Cardiac: RRR, no murmurs, rubs or gallops

Lungs: Decreased bilateral breath sounds

Ext: normal

Labs:

$$\frac{143 \mid 102 \mid 19}{4.2 \mid 30 \mid 1.0} \quad \text{Glucose 180} \quad \text{WBC 14.2} \quad \text{H/H 13/38} \quad \text{Plt 180 K}$$

Sputum and blood cultures are sent, and a chest radiograph shows a right lower lobe (RLL) infiltrate, suggestive of pneumonia. AL is admitted to the internal medicine service.

16. What pathogen is the likely cause of the pneumonia this patient is presenting with?

    a. *Streptococcus pneumoniae*
    b. *Mycoplasma pneumoniae*
    c. MRSA
    d. *Acinetobacter baumannii*

17. What empiric antibiotic regimen would you start on AL?

    a. Azithromycin + ceftriaxone
    b. Clarithromycin + ceftriaxone
    c. Azithromycin + ceftriaxone + vancomycin
    d. Vancomycin + piperacillin/tazobactam

Use the patient case scenario to answer questions 18 through 22.

ZX is a 29-year-old man with no significant past medical history who was in a serious motor vehicle collision 3 weeks ago, and has been in the ICU sedated and on a ventilator since.

Recently he has been spiking fevers up to 103.2°F, producing purulent sputum, and he has a WBC that has been trending upward. A chest x-ray is performed and shows an RLL infiltrate. The team diagnoses him with pneumonia, collects a deep sputum sample and blood cultures, and wishes to begin therapy.

Chem 7 = normal   CBC = elevated WBC and bands
Tmax = 103.2°F

18. Based on the above case which bacterial organisms should be covered? Select all that apply.

    a. *Streptococcus pneumoniae*
    b. *Pseudomonas aeruginosa*
    c. MRSA
    d. *Klebsiella pneumoniae*

19. ZX is allergic to penicillin (type I/anaphylaxis). Based on this, what antibiotic regimen would be most appropriate for him?

    a. Cefepime + tobramycin + vancomycin
    b. Azithromycin + ceftriaxone
    c. Levofloxacin + gentamicin + vancomycin
    d. Gentamicin + vancomycin

20. ZX is placed on a regimen of linezolid, tobramycin, and ciprofloxacin. What are potential adverse effects associated with the drugs in this regimen? Select all that apply.

    a. Ototoxicity
    b. Nephrotoxicity
    c. QTc prolongation
    d. Thrombocytopenia

21. A sputum Gram stain shows few epithelial cells, many WBCs, and moderate gram-negative rods. Two days later, the following data are known:

    Sputum: *K. pneumoniae*

    Susceptible to: ampicillin/sulbactam, piperacillin/tazobactam, imipenem, cefepime, levofloxacin, gentamicin, tobramycin, amikacin

    Resistant to: ampicillin, piperacillin

    Blood cultures (2/2): No growth

    Chem 7 normal CBC normal Tmax = 37.8°C

    Based on the susceptibility report, what should his therapy be now?

    a. Continue current therapy
    b. Stop current therapy, start Levaquin
    c. Stop current therapy, start Rocephin
    d. Stop current therapy, start Unasyn

22. How many days in total should ZX receive antibiotics?

    a. 3 days
    b. 5 days
    c. 7 days
    d. 14 to 21 days

TAKEAWAY POINTS ›››

- The main classifications of pneumonia are: community-acquired and hospital-acquired.
- The etiology of bacterial pneumonia varies in accordance with the type of pneumonia.
- Therapy choices for pneumonia are dictated by the setting in which the disease occurred.
- Key parameters for the diagnosis of pneumonia include the clinical presentation, diagnostic tests, laboratory tests, and microbiology tests.

- Prevention of some cases of pneumonia is possible through the use of vaccines and infection control/prevention measures.
- Treatment of bacterial pneumonia involves the empirical use of antimicrobial(s) that is/are effective against probable pathogens. Antimicrobials exhibiting activity against the suspected pathogens without having activity against nontargeted pathogens are preferred.

BIBLIOGRAPHY

Attridge RT. Pneumonia. In: Attridge RL, Miller ML, Moote R, Ryan L, eds. *Internal Medicine: A Guide to Clinical Therapeutics.* New York, NY: McGraw-Hill; 2013:chap 26.

Blackford MG, Glover ML, Reed MD. Lower respiratory tract infections. In: DiPiro JT, Talbert RL, Yee GC, Matzke GR, Wells BG, Posey L, eds. *Pharmacotherapy: A Pathophysiologic Approach.* 10th ed. New York, NY: McGraw-Hill; 2017.

Bradley JS, Byington CL, Shah SS, et al. The management of community-acquired pneumonia in infants and children older than 3 months of age: Clinical Practice Guidelines by the Pediatric Infectious Diseases Society and the Infectious Diseases Society of America. *Clin Infect Dis.* 2011;53(7):e25-e76.

Kalil AC, Metersky ML, Klompas M, et al. Management of adults with hospital-acquire and ventilator-associated pneumonia: 2016 Clinical practice guidelines by the Infections Diseases Society of America and the American Thoracic Society. *Clin Infect Dis.* 2016;63(5):e61-e111.

Mandell LA, Wunderink RG, Anzueto A, et al. Infectious Diseases Society of America/American Thoracic Society Consensus Guidelines on the Management of Community-Acquired Pneumonia in Adults. *Clin Infect Dis.* 2007;44(suppl 2):S27–S72.

KEY ABBREVIATIONS

BMP = basic metabolic panel
BP = blood pressure
C&S = culture and susceptibility
CA-MRSA = community-associated MRSA
CAP = community-acquired pneumonia
COPD = chronic obstructive pulmonary disease
CVA = cerebrovascular accident
DM = diabetes mellitus
DVT = deep vein thrombosis
ESBL = extended-spectrum β-lactamase
FDA = Food and Drug Administration
GNR = gram-negative rod

HMG-CoA = hydroxymethylglutaryl-coenzyme A
HR = heart rate
HTN = hypertension
ICU = intensive care unit
LRTI = lower respiratory tract infection
MDR = multidrug resistant
MRSA = methicillin-resistant *Staphylococcus aureus*
PMH = past medical history
RR = respiratory rate
RSV = respiratory syncytial virus
VTE = venous thromboembolism
WBC = white blood cell

22

Upper Respiratory Tract Infections

S. Scott Sutton and Christopher M. Bland

FOUNDATION OVERVIEW

Upper respiratory tract infections (URTIs) include otitis media (OM), sinusitis, pharyngitis, laryngitis, rhinitis, and epiglottitis. Most URTIs have a viral etiology and resolve spontaneously; therefore, antibiotics are not appropriate for the majority of URTIs. Nevertheless, URTIs are responsible for the majority of antimicrobials prescribed in ambulatory practice. This practice is concerning as the use and overuse of antimicrobials contribute to the development of microbial resistance. Guidelines have been developed to reduce inappropriate antimicrobial use for viral URTIs. This chapter will focus on acute otitis media (AOM), sinusitis, and pharyngitis because they are more frequently associated with bacterial infection and circumstantially necessitate appropriate antimicrobial therapy to minimize complications.

Otitis Media

OM is an inflammation of the middle ear and represents the most common reason for prescribing antimicrobials to children. OM occurs after a viral infection of the nasopharynx and is subclassified as AOM or otitis media with effusion (OME). AOM is a symptomatic middle ear infection that occurs rapidly with inflammation and effusion. OME is the presence of fluid in the middle ear without symptoms of an acute illness. It is important to differentiate between AOM and OME because antimicrobials are only useful for AOM. OM is common in children, but occurs in all age groups. Bacteria frequently are isolated from middle ear fluid in AOM, but viruses play a predominant role. *Streptococcus pneumoniae, Haemophilus influenzae,* and *Moraxella catarrhalis* are the three most common bacterial pathogens causing AOM. Viruses are isolated from middle ear fluid with or without concomitant bacteria in over half of AOM cases. Examples of AOM viruses are respiratory syncytial virus (RSV), influenza virus, rhinovirus, and adenovirus. Lack of improvement with antimicrobial therapy is often a sign of viral infection with subsequent inflammation rather than antimicrobial resistance.

Viral infection of the nasopharynx impairs Eustachian tube function and causes mucosal inflammation; this then impairs mucociliary clearance, which promotes bacterial proliferation and infection. Children are predisposed to AOM because their Eustachian tubes are shorter and more horizontal compared to adults; this makes them less functional for drainage and protection of the middle ear from bacterial entry. Increased incidence of AOM is observed with bottle-feeding, pacifier use, day care attendance, and exposure to cigarette smoke.

AOM presents as an acute onset of symptoms such as fever, otalgia (earache), irritability, and tugging on the ear. Accompanying otoscopic examination demonstrates a gray, bulging, nonmobile tympanic membrane. Since AOM often follows a viral URTI, the child may experience symptoms of rhinorrhea, nasal congestion, and cough. Resolution of AOM symptoms usually occurs over 1 week. Pain and fever tend to resolve after 2 to 3 days, with most children becoming asymptomatic by day 7. The diagnosis of AOM and OME are easily confused; therefore, careful attention to history, signs and symptoms, as well as results from pneumatic otoscopy are important. Diagnosis of AOM requires either moderate to severe bulging of the tympanic membrane, new onset of otorrhea not due to acute otitis externa, or a mild bulging of the tympanic membrane with new onset of ear pain within the preceding 48 hours. Complications of AOM are infrequent but include mastoiditis, bacteremia, meningitis, and auditory sequelae with potential for speech and language impairment.

PREVENTION

There are several preventative measures that may reduce the occurrence of URTIs, including proper hand hygiene and practices of infection control. Moreover, there are vaccinations that target bacterial and viral pathogens involved in URTIs. Specifically, there are vaccines available targeting *H. influenzae, S. pneumoniae,* and influenza virus. Additional information regarding immunization practices can be found on the United States Centers for Disease Control and Prevention website (www.cdc.gov).

TREATMENT

AOM treatment goals are to alleviate ear pain and fever, eradicate infection, prevent complications, and minimize unnecessary antimicrobial use. Treatment of AOM depends on patient's age, illness severity, viral and/or bacterial etiology, and certainty of diagnosis. Children 24 months of age or greater should be prescribed antimicrobials if they have severe signs or symptoms such as high fever (≥39°C/102°F), moderate to severe otalgia, or otalgia lasting at least 48 hours. Children younger than 2 years of age have higher clinical and bacteriologic failure rates when not treated initially with antimicrobials as compared to older children, and are often treated.

Nonpharmacologic Treatment

Watchful waiting approaches are being used to attenuate microbial resistance, limit unwarranted health care expenditures, and avoid unnecessary adverse events caused by antimicrobials. Watchful waiting involves monitoring for 48 to 72 hours after diagnosing AOM to see if spontaneous resolution will occur. Observation or delayed antimicrobial therapy should only be considered in healthy children, without recurrent disease, when proper follow-up and good communication exist among the clinician(s), patient, and caregiver(s). Surgical treatment includes tympanostomy tubes for patients with recurrent disease or chronic OME with impaired hearing or speech. Adenoidectomy may be necessary for children with tympanostomy tubes and chronic nasal obstruction.

Pharmacologic Treatment

Amoxicillin is the drug of choice for AOM for patients without concurrent purulent conjunctivitis who have not received amoxicillin in the previous 30 days. Aminopenicillins like amoxicillin are an excellent treatment option for AOM due to their proven effectiveness when used in sufficient doses, their excellent safety profile, low cost, palatable suspension, multiple dosage formulations, and narrow spectrum of activity. High-dose amoxicillin/clavulanate is preferred for cases of treatment failure, otitis-conjunctivitis syndrome, severe illness, recent exposure to amoxicillin, or when coverage of β-lactamase producing organisms is otherwise desired. Patients with penicillin allergies require alternative treatment with cephalosporins (delayed penicillin allergic reaction only) or clindamycin (only for *S. pneumoniae*). Treatment with respiratory fluoroquinolones is unconventional and should be reserved for patients with severe penicillin allergies and prescribers should consider consulting with pediatric medical subspecialists, such as an otolaryngologist or an infectious disease expert, before using a fluoroquinolone. Due to increasing resistance with *S. pneumoniae*, trimethoprim-sulfamethoxazole and macrolides are no longer recommended. Table 22-1 lists properties of antibiotics utilized for the treatment of AOM.

Pain is a central feature of AOM and may be alleviated by acetaminophen or ibuprofen. The use of aspirin is contraindicated in children with fever due to the risk of Reye syndrome. Topical anesthetic drops such as benzocaine provide relief within 30 minutes and may be preferred over systemic analgesics when fever is absent. However, topical benzocaine is not recommended for use in children less than

TABLE 22-1	Select Antibiotics for the Treatment of AOM		
Antibiotic	**Usual Dose and Schedule[a]**	**Common Adverse Effects[b]**	**Comments**
Amoxicillin (Amoxil)	C: 80-90 mg/kg/d in 2-3 divided doses A: 875 mg twice daily	Gastrointestinal, rash, allergic reactions	Drug of choice of AOM; experts recommend high dose (80-90 mg/kg) over conventional dose (40-45 mg/kg); high dose is utilized for PRSP
Amoxicillin/ clavulanate (Augmentin)	C: 90 mg/kg/d (with 6.4 mg/kg/d of clavulanate) in 2 divided doses A: 875 mg twice daily	Gastrointestinal, rash, allergic reactions	More diarrhea than amoxicillin because of clavulanate (goal ratio of amoxicillin to clavulanate of 14:1 to lessen this side effect)
Cefdinir (Omnicef)	C: 14mg/kg/d in 1-2 divided doses A: 600 mg daily in 1-2 divided doses	Gastrointestinal, rash, allergic reactions	
Cefuroxime axetil (Ceftin)	C: 30 mg/kg/d in 2 divided doses (max 1 g/d with suspension) A: 250-500 mg twice daily	Gastrointestinal, rash, allergic reactions	Suspension gritty and bitter tasting and not interchangeable with tablets (less bioavailable)
Cefpodoxime proxetil (Vantin)	C: 10 mg/kg/d in 2 divided doses A: 200 mg twice daily	Gastrointestinal, rash, allergic reactions	Suspension is bitter tasting
Ceftriaxone (Rocephin)	C: 50 mg/kg IM or IV once daily	Gastrointestinal, rash, allergic reactions	3-d regimen preferred for PRSP; avoid in children under 2 mo
Clindamycin (Cleocin)	C: 30-40 mg/kg/d in 3 divided doses A: 300-450 mg 3-4 times per day	Gastrointestinal	Oral liquid has poor taste; only utilized for *S. pneumoniae*

Abbreviations: A, adults; AOM, acute otitis media; C, children; IM, intramuscular; IV, intravenous; PRSP, penicillin-resistant *Streptococcus pneumoniae*.
[a]All doses are oral unless otherwise specified.
[b]Side effects listed are the common side effects. There are numerous other side effects of these antibiotics used for URTIs. For example, all of the antimicrobials listed may cause *Clostridium difficile* colitis, with clindamycin having the highest incidence. Bone marrow suppression (neutropenia, thrombocytopenia) is a rare side effect of antibiotics. Please see other infectious diseases chapters in this book for more inclusive side effects.

2 years of age due to a heightened risk of methemoglobinemia. Other medications such as decongestants, antihistamines, and corticosteroids have no role in the management of AOM.

SPECIAL CONSIDERATIONS

Bacterial Resistance

Bacterial resistance has significantly affected treatment guidelines for AOM. Penicillin-resistant *S. pneumoniae* (PRSP) encompasses intermediate and high-level resistance. The mechanism of resistance for *S. pneumoniae* is through altered penicillin-binding proteins (PBP3) which cannot be overcome via the addition of a β-lactamase inhibitor. PRSP is also commonly resistant to other antibiotic classes (sulfonamides, macrolides, clindamycin).

Conversely, β-lactamase (penicillinase) production is the mechanism of bacterial resistance for *H. influenzae* and *M. catarrhalis* and can be overcome with the addition of clavulanate to amoxicillin (Augmentin). Although infections caused by these organisms are more likely to resolve without treatment compared to *S. pneumoniae*, they must be considered in cases of treatment failure.

Sinusitis

Sinusitis is an inflammation and/or infection of the paranasal sinus mucosa. The term rhinosinusitis is also used to describe sinusitis because the nasal mucosa is often involved. Even though the majority of sinus infections are viral, antimicrobials are frequently prescribed. Therefore, it is important to differentiate between viral and bacterial sinusitis to aid in optimizing treatment. Viral sinusitis and bacterial sinusitis are difficult to differentiate because their clinical presentations are similar. Viral infections tend to resolve in 7 to 10 days. Persistence of symptoms beyond this time or worsening of symptoms likely indicates a bacterial infection. Acute bacterial sinusitis lasts less than 30 days with complete resolution of symptoms, whereas chronic sinusitis is an episode of inflammation lasting more than 3 months with persistence of respiratory symptoms.

Chronic sinusitis may be recognized by:

- Nonspecific symptoms that are similar to acute sinusitis
- Rhinorrhea, which is associated with acute exacerbations of chronic sinusitis
- Chronic unproductive cough, laryngitis, and headache may occur
- Chronic/recurrent infections typically occur three to four times a year
- Symptoms are unresponsive to steam/vapor and decongestants

Bacterial sinusitis is often over-diagnosed and thus antimicrobials are overprescribed. Compared to the gold standard sinus aspiration, no single clinical finding can accurately diagnose bacterial sinusitis. Clinical presentations that predict a diagnosis of bacterial sinusitis include any one of the following three:

1. Nonspecific upper respiratory signs and symptoms that persist consistently, without any evidence of clinical improvement for 10 or more days
2. Severe onset illustrated by a high fever (≥39°C/102°F) and purulent nasal discharge or facial pain lasting 3 to 4 consecutive days at the beginning of illness
3. Worsening signs and/or symptoms after initial improvement from a typical, viral URTI that lasted 5 to 6 days characterized by a new onset of fever, headache, or increased nasal discharge

Sinusitis is caused by mucosal inflammation and local damage to mucociliary mechanisms usually as a result of viral infection or allergy. Increased mucus production and reduced clearance of secretions can lead to blockage of sinus ostia. Bacterial pathogens that cause sinusitis are similar to those that cause AOM. *Streptococcus pneumoniae*, *H. influenzae*, and *M. catarrhalis* are responsible for approximately 40%, 35%, and 15% of cases respectively, with a growing prevalence of *Staphylococcus aureus* (10%) within the adult patient. However, routine empiric therapy with antistaphylococcal agents for suspected acute bacterial rhinosinusitis is not currently recommended.

TREATMENT

The goals of therapy are to reduce the signs and symptoms of sinusitis, limit antimicrobial exposure to those that would benefit from treatment, eradicate the bacteria when a bacterial infection is present, and minimize the duration of illness. Initial management of sinusitis focuses on symptom relief for patients with mild disease lasting less than 10 days. Routine antibiotic use is not recommended for all patients because viral sinusitis is self-limiting and bacterial infection often resolves spontaneously. Antimicrobial therapy should be reserved for persistent, worsening, or severe cases. When indicated, empiric antimicrobial treatment should target likely pathogens since cultures are rarely obtained.

Nonpharmacologic Treatment

Ancillary treatments such as humidifiers, vaporizers, and saline nasal sprays are used to moisturize the nasal canal and inhibit crusting of secretions, along with promoting ciliary function. While these nonpharmacologic treatments are often used, there is limited evidence to support their effectiveness alone or as adjunctive therapy.

Pharmacologic Treatment

Supportive medications that target symptoms of viral URTIs are used in patients with sinusitis. There is a lack of evidence supporting their use in sinusitis, but they may provide temporary relief in certain patients. Examples of supportive medications include:

- Analgesics can be used to treat fever and pain from sinus pressure.

TABLE 22-2   Antibiotics for the Treatment of Acute Bacterial Sinusitis

Antibiotic	Adult Dose[a]	Pediatric Dose[a,b]	Comments
Amoxicillin/Clavulanate (Augmentin)	500 mg/125 mg 3 times daily or 875 mg/125 mg twice daily 2 g XR twice daily for PRSP	90 mg/kg/d in 2 divided doses or 180 mg/kg/d in 2 divided doses for PRSP	Broad coverage particularly with high doses
Ampicillin/Sulbactam (Unasyn)	6-12 g IV daily in 4 divided doses	200-400 mg/kg/d in 4 divided doses	
Cefixime (Suprax)	400 mg daily	8 mg/kg/d in 2 divided doses	
Cefpodoxime proxetil (Vantin)	200 mg twice daily	10 mg/kg/d in 2 divided doses	
Ceftriaxone (Rocephin)	1-2 g IV or IM daily in 1-2 divided doses	50 mg/kg IV or IM in 2 divided doses	The recommended duration of therapy is 5-7 d for adults and 10-14 d for children
Doxycycline (Vibramycin)	200 mg daily in 1-2 divided doses	Avoid in children under 8 y of age	Can cause photosensitivity, many drug interactions
Levofloxacin (Levaquin)	500 mg daily	20 mg/kg/d in 1-2 doses	Can cause photosensitivity, many drug interactions
Moxifloxacin (Avelox)	400 mg daily	Avoid	Can cause photosensitivity, many drug interactions
Clindamycin (Cleocin)	150-450 mg 3-4 times daily	30-40 mg/kg/d in 3 divided doses	Not active against *H. influenza* or *M. catarrhalis*

Abbreviations: IM, intramuscular; IV, intravenous; PRSP, penicillin-resistant *Streptococcus pneumoniae*.
[a]All doses are oral unless otherwise specified.
[b]Maximum dose not to exceed adult dose.

- Intranasal saline irrigation with either isotonic or hypertonic saline is recommended.

- Intranasal corticosteroids are reserved for patients with allergic rhinitis.

- Oral and intranasal decongestants are not recommended as adjunctive treatment as they have not been proven as clinically effective and, therefore, the potential risk outweighs the potential benefit. Topical treatment may also further induce inflammation in the nasal cavity.

- Antihistamines should be avoided because they thicken mucus and impair its clearance. Risks of drowsiness, xerostomia, and other potential adverse effects outweigh any potential benefit.

Amoxicillin/clavulanate is a first-line antimicrobial for acute bacterial sinusitis. Amoxicillin is no longer recommended *empirically* due to the increasing prevalence of β-lactamase producing respiratory pathogens (*H. influenzae* and *M. catarrhalis*). The advantages of amoxicillin/clavulanate include proven efficacy and safety, targeted spectrum of activity, good tolerability, and low cost.

Patients with a non-type I penicillin allergy may receive treatment with an oral cephalosporin such as cefixime or cefpodoxime, in combination with clindamycin. Otherwise, in patients with a confirmed history of an IgE-mediated reaction to penicillin (eg, hives or anaphylaxis), doxycycline (avoid in children ≤8 years of age) or a respiratory fluoroquinolone may be used as an alternative. Macrolides (clarithromycin and azithromycin) are not recommended for empiric therapy due to high rates of resistance among *S. pneumoniae*. Similarly, trimethoprim-sulfamethoxazole is not recommended for empiric therapy due to high rates of resistance among both *S. pneumoniae* and *H. influenzae*. Use of fluoroquinolones should be restricted to patients with drug resistant *S. pneumoniae* or patients with a type I penicillin allergy. Table 22-2 lists antibiotics recommended for the treatment of acute bacterial sinusitis.

SPECIAL CONSIDERATIONS

High-dosed amoxicillin/clavulanate is recommended to overcome potential bacterial resistance when PRSP is a concern given any of the following scenarios:

- Geographic regions with high endemic rates [≥10%] of invasive PRSP

- Less than 2 years of age or greater than 65 years of age

- Immunocompromised host

- Severe infection

- Daycare exposure

- Recent hospitalization within the past 5 days

- Receipt of antibiotics in the past 30 days

Clindamycin may also be utilized for PRSP; however, it is important to note that this drug is not active against *H. influenzae* or *M. catarrhalis*.

Broader spectrum antimicrobial coverage may also be required in patients that fail (worsening symptoms after 2-3 days of treatment or lack of improvement after 3-5 days) conventional treatment with amoxicillin/clavulanate for sinusitis. Improved coverage of *H. influenzae* and *M. catarrhalis* with either high-dose amoxicillin/clavulanate, levofloxacin, or a β-lactamase stable cephalosporin that covers *S. pneumoniae*. (cefixime, cefpodoxime) in combination with clindamycin are potential alternative options.

Pharyngitis

Pharyngitis is an acute throat infection that can be of viral or bacterial etiology. Pharyngitis is generally self-limiting without serious sequelae; however, antibiotics are often prescribed due to the inability to easily distinguish viral and bacterial pathogens and the fear of untreated streptococcal illness. While viruses are the most common cause of pharyngitis, group A β-hemolytic *Streptococcus* (GAS) is the primary bacterial cause and is the focus of this section. GAS is also called *Streptococcus pyogenes* or strep throat. GAS is also referred to as the flesh-eating bacteria in skin and soft-tissue infections.

Pharyngeal colonization with GAS occurs in children and is a risk factor for developing streptococcal pharyngitis after a break in mucosal integrity. Symptoms of streptococcal pharyngitis are usually self-limited and resolve within a few days of onset, even without treatment. Historically, untreated or mistreated streptococcal pharyngitis caused acute rheumatic fever, potential heart valve damage, and complications such as peritonsillar abscesses.

Children between 5 and 15 years of age have the highest incidence of streptococcal pharyngitis. Parents and adults with significant pediatric contact are also at increased risk. The signs and symptoms of streptococcal pharyngitis are:

- Sudden onset of sore throat with severe pain on swallowing
- Fever
- Headache, abdominal pain, nausea, vomiting
- Pharyngeal and tonsillar erythema with possible patchy exudates
- Tender, enlarged anterior cervical lymph nodes
- Swollen, red uvula
- Soft palate petechiae
- Scarlatiniform rash

The diagnosis of streptococcal pharyngitis consists of a throat swab and the identification of GAS via rapid antigen detection test and/or culture. Clinical features alone do not reliably differentiate GAS from viral pharyngitis. Therefore, diagnostic testing for GAS should be routinely performed when streptococcal pharyngitis is suspected prior to treatment with antimicrobials. Likewise, testing is not recommended in children or adults when overt viral features are present such as rhinorrhea, cough, oral ulcers, and/or hoarseness. Children and adolescents with a negative rapid antigen detection test should have an additional throat culture performed. If the rapid antigen test is positive, no additional cultures are needed. For adults, a negative rapid antigen detection test alone is sufficient due to the low incidence of GAS pharyngitis and the low risk of developing secondary complications such as rheumatic fever in this patient population. Testing is also not routinely recommended in children under 3 years of age because streptococcal pharyngitis is rare in this patient population.

TREATMENT

The goals of therapy for streptococcal pharyngitis are to eradicate infection in order to prevent complications, shorten the disease course, and reduce the spread of infection to close contacts. Sequelae that can be prevented by antimicrobials are peritonsillar abscess, cervical lymphadenitis, and rheumatic fever. Antimicrobial therapy is not effective at preventing poststreptococcal glomerulonephritis.

Antimicrobial therapy should only be used in cases of laboratory confirmed streptococcal pharyngitis associated with clinical symptoms in order to avoid overtreatment. Penicillin or amoxicillin are the antibiotic of choice because of their narrow spectrum of activity, low cost, and documented safety and efficacy. Non-type I penicillin-allergic individuals should be treated with a first-generation cephalosporin such as cephalexin, which will also result in bacteriological and clinical cure. For individuals with anaphylactic sensitivity to penicillins, other alternative agents include clindamycin, clarithromycin, or azithromycin. Table 22-3 lists selected antibiotics used for the treatment of streptococcal pharyngitis.

TABLE 22-3	Antibiotics for the Treatment of Streptococcal Pharyngitis			
Antibiotic	**Adult Dose[a]**	**Pediatric Dose[a,b]**	**Duration**	**Comments**
Penicillin V (PEN VK)	250 mg 4 times daily or 500 mg twice daily	250 mg 2-3 times daily	10 d	Drug of choice
Penicillin G benzathine (Bicillin LA)	1.2 million units (if 27 kg or greater)	600,000 units (if under 27 kg)	1 IM dose	Drug of choice; useful for nonadherence or emesis; painful injection
Amoxicillin (Amoxil)	1000 mg in 1-2 doses	50 mg/kg/d in 1-2 doses	10 d	Drug of choice; preferred over penicillin for young children (more palatable)
Cephalexin (Keflex)	500 mg twice daily	40 mg/kg/d in 2 doses	10 d	Consider in the penicillin allergic (if allergy is delayed reaction)
Azithromycin (Zithromax)	500 mg once daily	12 mg/kg once daily	5 d	Increasing resistance; consider if severe penicillin allergy
Clindamycin (Cleocin)	300 mg 3 times daily	21 mg/kg/d in 3 doses	10 d	Increasing resistance; consider if severe penicillin allergy; useful for recurrent infections (typical dose for chronic carriers is 20-30 mg/kg/d in 3 doses)

[a]All doses are oral unless otherwise specified.
[b]Maximum dose not to exceed adult dose.

CASE Application

1. Select the upper respiratory tract condition that is defined as the presence of fluid in the middle ear without symptoms of acute illness.

   a. OME
   b. Sinusitis
   c. Pharyngitis
   d. Laryngitis
   e. Rhinitis

2. JH is a 4-year-old patient that is brought to his pediatrician with a 36-hour history of rhinorrhea, nasal congestion, cough, and mild otalgia. He does not have any concurrent purulent conjunctivitis. His current temperature is 38°C (100.4°F). He has no known drug allergies and no known past medical conditions. He has not received amoxicillin in the previous 30 days. He is 36 lb. Which of the following would be the most appropriate option for JH?

   a. Acetaminophen 10 mg/kg po qid prn
   b. Amoxicillin 30 mg/kg po tid
   c. Pseudoephedrine HCl 15 mg po qid
   d. Diphenhydramine 6.25 mg po qid
   e. Levofloxacin 10 mg/kg po bid

Questions 3 and 4 pertain to the following case:

JM is a 6-year-old patient that presents to his pediatrician with a 5 days history of otalgia and otorrhea. Upon otoscopic review, his pediatrician notices moderate bulging of his tympanic membrane. His temperature is 38.5°C (101.3°F). He has a history of penicillin allergy, and his reaction was itchy legs. He does not have concurrent purulent conjunctivitis and he has not received amoxicillin in the previous 30 days. He is 44 lb.

3. Which of the following would be the most appropriate treatment option for JM?

   a. Amoxicillin 600 mg po tid
   b. Amoxicillin 1375 mg po tid
   c. Cefdinir 300 mg po bid
   d. Cefdinir 140 mg po bid
   e. Levofloxacin 600 mg po bid

4. Which of the following pathogens might be the cause of JM's AOM. Select all that apply.

   a. *Streptococcus pneumoniae*
   b. *Moraxella catarrhalis*
   c. *Haemophilus influenzae*
   d. Influenza virus
   e. Adenovirus

5. When considering treatment failure and mechanisms of bacterial resistance, which of the following might be present in any one of the three most common bacterial pathogens for AOM? Select all that apply.

   a. Reduction in antimicrobial drug accumulation due to the upregulation of bacterial efflux pumps
   b. Inability of the antimicrobial to bind to the targeted bacteria due to bacterial alterations of their PBPs
   c. Enzymatic inactivation of the antimicrobial via bacterial production of β-lactamase
   d. Reduction in antimicrobial drug accumulation due to decreased bacterial membrane permeability
   e. Enzymatic inactivation of the antimicrobial via bacterial production of penicillinase

Questions 6 through 8 pertain to the following case:

JS is a 16-year-old patient with purulent nasal discharge, headache, cough and congestion, bad breath, and anosmia (loss of smell) for the past 2 days. He has a temperature of 38.3°C (100.9°F). He has no known drug allergies. He has no known past medical history; however, he did receive 5 days of an unknown antibiotic to treat a skin and soft tissue infection about 20 days ago. He is 140 lb.

6. Which of the following treatment options should be recommended?

   a. Acetaminophen 325 mg po q4h prn
   b. Amoxicillin 875 po tid
   c. Pseudoephedrine HCl 60 mg po qid
   d. Amoxicillin/clavulanate 875 mg po bid
   e. Amoxicillin/clavulanate 2 g XR po bid

7. After providing JS with an appropriate treatment option, 4 to 5 days after his initial presentation, he started to feel much better. On day 5, he even decided to go outside and ride his scooter with his friends. However, the next morning he woke up with chills, nausea, headache, and increased nasal discharge. He had a temperature of 38.3°C (100.9°F). Which of the following is the most appropriate recommendation?

   a. Acetaminophen 325 mg po q4h prn
   b. Amoxicillin 875 mg po tid
   c. Levofloxacin 500 mg po daily
   d. Amoxicillin/clavulanate 875 mg po bid
   e. Amoxicillin/clavulanate 2 g XR po bid

8. Which of the following are common side effects that JS could experience while taking this recommended treatment? Select all that apply.

   a. Hepatotoxicity
   b. Diarrhea
   c. Prolonged QT interval
   d. Tendon rupture
   e. Candidiasis

Questions 9 through 11 pertain to the following case:

TM is a 17-year-old patient who initially presented to the ED with a fever of ≥40°C/104°F, severe headache, purulent nasal discharge, and facial pain for the last four consecutive days. He is 143 lb, has no known drug allergies, and no significant past medical history. He was originally worked up for meningitis and received the following medications:

1. Vancomycin 30 mg/kg IV over 2 hours (placed in 500 mL of normal saline [NS])
2. Ceftriaxone 2 g IV over 30 minutes (placed in 50 mL of D5W [5% dextrose in water])
3. Dexamethasone 10 mg IV over 5 minutes (10 mg/1 mL)

Unfortunately, after his lumbar puncture TM got increasingly nauseous which prompted an intern to give an additional:

4. Piperacillin/tazobactam 4.5 g IV over 4 hours (placed in 100 mL of D5W)

Fortunately, after his lumbar puncture returned grossly negative and consulting with an otolaryngologist, TM was diagnosed with severe acute sinusitis and was ultimately given:

5. Ampicillin/sulbactam 3 g IV over 30 minutes Q 6 hours (placed in 100 mL of NS)

9. Calculate each IV dose in "mg/min" that TM received and then order the medications from highest to lowest "mg/min" given.

Unordered Options	Ordered Response
Vancomycin 30 mg/kg IV over 2 h	
Ceftriaxone 2 g IV over 30 min	
Dexamethasone 10 mg IV over 5 min	
Piperacillin/tazobactam 4.5 g IV over 4 h	
Ampicillin/sulbactam 3 g IV over 30 min	

10. Which of the following vaccines may have prevented TMs sinusitis? Select all that may apply.
    a. Comvax
    b. Prevnar 13
    c. Fluzone
    d. Ipol
    e. Twinrix

11. Calculate each drip rate in "mL/min" that TM received and then order the medications from fastest to slowest drip rate.

Unordered Options	Ordered Response
Vancomycin 30 mg/kg IV over 2 h	
Ceftriaxone 2 g IV over 30 min	
Dexamethasone 10 mg IV over 5 min	
Piperacillin/tazobactam 4.5 g IV over 4 h	
Ampicillin/sulbactam 3 g IV over 30 min	

Questions 12 and 13 pertain to the following case:

ES is a 12-year-old patient who was brought to her pediatrician with complaints of sore throat, odynophagia, and vomiting for 24 hours. She has a temperature of 38.5°C (101.3°F).

Upon physical examination, she is noted to have enlarged cervical lymph nodes and red uvula.

12. In an ideal situation, which of the following would occur first?
    a. Give penicillin 250 mg po tid
    b. Give saline nasal spray each nostril qid
    c. Obtain a rapid antigen detection test or throat culture
    d. Give a diphenhydramine 25 mg po qid
    e. Give Comvax

13. Given that ES has bacterial pharyngitis, what are the goals of therapy? Select all that apply.
    a. Eradicate infection
    b. Prevent infectious complications
    c. Shorten the disease course
    d. Reduce infectivity and spread to others
    e. Reduce sore throat and odynophagia

14. Historically, which of the following rare sequelae might be prevented with full treatment of "strep throat"? Select all that apply.
    a. Peritonsillar abscess
    b. Cervical lymphadenitis
    c. Rheumatic fever
    d. Poststreptococcal glomerulonephritis
    e. Appendicitis

Questions 15 and 16 pertain to the following case:

MM is a 15-year-old patient that was recently diagnosed with acute bacterial sinusitis. She has a complicated past medical history including venous thromboembolism (left leg) 2/2 severe systemic lupus erythematosus/antiphospholipid antibody syndrome, lupus nephritis, seizures, and depression. At age 13, she has had an anaphylactic reaction to amoxicillin resulting in an intensive care unit (ICU) admission, requiring intubation and mechanical ventilation; she has no other known drug allergies. She is 115 lb. Her current medications include:

1. Prednisone 15 mg po daily
2. Ibuprofen 400 mg po tid
3. Warfarin 5 mg po daily
4. Sertraline 50 mg po daily
5. Flintstones + iron multivitamin po daily

15. A concerned otolaryngologist would like to treat MM's sinusitis with levofloxacin 500 mg po daily to avoid any potential risk of anaphylaxis. Which of the following medications could potentially interact with levofloxacin 500 mg po daily? Select all that apply.
    a. Prednisone
    b. Ibuprofen
    c. Warfarin
    d. Sertraline
    e. Flintstones + iron

16. While receiving levofloxacin, which of the following might MM be at risk for given her past medical history and current medication history? Select all that apply.

    a. Tendinitis
    b. Bleeding/bruising
    c. Clotting
    d. QTc prolongation
    e. Seizures

17. Select the parenteral cephalosporin that is often administered intramuscularly for AOM.

    a. Clarithromycin
    b. Amoxicillin/clavulanate
    c. Trimethoprim-sulfamethoxazole
    d. Clindamycin
    e. Ceftriaxone

18. Correctly assign the following antimicrobials that can be used (either alone or in combination) for the treatment of sinusitis with their assigned mechanisms of actions: cefixime, clavulanate, clindamycin, doxycycline, levofloxacin

Unordered Options	Ordered Response
Inhibits protein synthesis by primarily binding to the 30S ribosomal subunit	
Inhibits DNA-gyrase, promoting the breakage of DNA strands	
Binds and inhibits β-lactamase production	
Inhibits protein synthesis by reversibly binding to the 50S ribosomal subunit	
Inhibits bacterial cell wall synthesis by binding to penicillin-binding proteins	

19. Correctly rank the following antimicrobials based on their respective half-lives in order from shortest to longest. (Hint, consider appropriate dosing intervals and available dosage formulations.)

Unordered Options	Ordered Response
Amoxicillin/clavulanate	
Cefixime	
Clindamycin	
Doxycycline	
Levofloxacin	

20. DV is a 26-year-old patient with chronic/recurrent sinus infections. Which of the following are most likely to occur? Select all that apply.

    a. Sinus infections three to four times yearly
    b. Excellent symptomatic response to steam/vapor
    c. Symptomatic cure with nasal decongestions
    d. Chronic unproductive cough
    e. Frequent headaches

TAKEAWAY POINTS »

- URTIs include OM, sinusitis, pharyngitis, laryngitis, rhinitis, and epiglottitis.
- Most URTIs have a viral etiology and tend to resolve spontaneously; therefore, antibiotics would not be appropriate for the majority of URTIs.
- OM is an inflammation of the middle ear and represents the most common reason for prescribing antimicrobials to children.
- AOM is a symptomatic middle ear infection that occurs rapidly with effusion. OME is the presence of fluid in the middle ear without symptoms of acute illness. It is important to differentiate between AOM and OME because antibiotics are only useful for AOM.
- Amoxicillin is the drug of choice because of its proven effectiveness in AOM when used in sufficient doses, as well as its excellent safety profile, low cost, good-tasting suspension, and narrow spectrum of activity.
- Bacterial resistance has significantly affected treatment guidelines for AOM (altered binding site of *S. pneumoniae* and β-lactamase production of *H. influenzae* and *M. catarrhalis*).
- Sinusitis is an inflammation and/or infection of the paranasal sinus mucosa.

- Initial management of sinusitis focuses on symptom relief for patients with mild disease lasting less than 10 days. Routine antimicrobial use is not recommended for all patients because viral sinusitis is self-limiting and bacterial infection often resolves spontaneously. Antimicrobial therapy should be reserved for persistent, worsening, or severe cases.
- Amoxicillin/clavulanate is a first-line antibiotic for acute bacterial sinusitis.
- Broader spectrum antimicrobial coverage may be required in patients that fail conventional treatment for sinusitis with amoxicillin/clavulanate, or in patients who have received antibiotic therapy in the previous 4 to 6 weeks. Improved coverage of *H. influenzae* and *M. catarrhalis* with either high-dose amoxicillin/clavulanate, levofloxacin, or a β-lactamase stable cephalosporin that covers *S. pneumoniae*.
- Pharyngitis is an acute throat infection caused by viruses or bacteria.
- Antimicrobials should only be used in cases of laboratory confirmed streptococcal pharyngitis associated with clinical symptoms in order to avoid overtreatment.

- Penicillin is the antibiotic of choice because of its narrow spectrum of activity, documented safety and efficacy, and low cost.
- Patients with penicillin allergies require alternative antibiotics for treatment of URTIs

and examples include cephalosporins (delayed penicillin-allergic reaction only), doxycycline, and fluoroquinolones.

BIBLIOGRAPHY

Chow AW, Benninger MS, Brook I, et al. IDSA clinical practice guideline for acute bacterial rhinosinusitis in children and adults. *Clin Infect Dis.* 2012;54:72-112.

Frei C, Frei B. Upper respiratory tract infections. In: DiPiro JT, Talbert RL, Yee GC, Matzke GR, Wells BG, Posey L, eds. *Pharmacotherapy: A Pathophysiologic Approach.* 10th ed. New York, NY: McGraw-Hill; 2017.

Inamdar S, Best BM. Otitis media and sinusitis. In: Linn WD, Wofford MR, O'Keefe M, Posey L, eds.

Pharmacotherapy in Primary Care. New York, NY: McGraw-Hill; 2009:chap 38.

Lieberthal AS, Carroll AE, Chonmaitree T, et al. The diagnosis and management of acute otitis media. *Pediatrics.* 2013;131(3):964-999.

Shulman ST, Bisno AL, Clegg HW, et al. Practice guidelines for the diagnosis and management of group A streptococcal pharyngitis: 2012 update by the Infectious Diseases Society of America. *Clin Infect Dis.* 2012;55:86-102.

KEY ABBREVIATIONS

AOM = acute otitis media
GAS = group A β-hemolytic *Streptococcus*
ICU = *intensive care unit*
OM = otitis media
OME = otitis media with effusion

PBP3 = penicillin-binding proteins
PRSP = penicillin-resistant *S. pneumoniae*
RSV = respiratory syncytial virus
URTI = upper respiratory tract infection

23

Urinary Tract Infections

S. Scott Sutton and Christopher M. Bland

FOUNDATION OVERVIEW

A urinary tract infection (UTI) is the presence of urinary microorganisms that cannot be accounted for by contamination. UTIs occur in all individuals, but age, sex, pregnancy, diabetes, urinary catheter, and vaginal intercourse increase the risk of development. UTIs are divided into cystitis (lower tract and bladder) and pyelonephritis (upper tract and kidneys). Cystitis symptoms include dysuria, increased frequency, urgency, and occasionally suprapubic tenderness. Pyelonephritis is characterized as cystitis symptoms plus fever, flank pain, nausea, and/or vomiting. Elderly patients frequently do not experience specific urinary symptoms, but may present with altered mental status, change in eating habits, or gastrointestinal symptoms. In addition, patients with indwelling catheters or neurologic disorders commonly will not have lower tract symptoms. Instead, they may present with flank pain and fever.

Uncomplicated UTIs are infections occurring in women of childbearing age with structurally and neurologically normal urinary tracts. Complicated UTIs occur in patients with functional or structural abnormalities. In general, UTIs in men, pregnant women, children, and patients in health care–associated settings are considered complicated.

Symptoms are unreliable for the diagnosis of bacterial UTIs. A UTI diagnosis requires a patient with a positive urinalysis and urine culture. A urinalysis will identify pyuria, which is defined as more than or equal to 10 leukocytes/mm^3 of urine. Pyuria is nonspecific, and patients with pyuria may not have an infection (note the urine in the bladder is normally sterile). Patients with a UTI usually have more than or equal to 10^5 bacteria/mL identified by culture. Leukocyte esterase found in the urine is an additional sign of UTI. Any organism colonizing the urinary tract can cause a UTI, but most are caused by bacteria. The majority of uncomplicated UTIs are caused by gram-negative bacteria, with *Escherichia coli* being isolated in 70% to 95% of cultures. The most common gram-positive bacteria isolated are *Staphylococcus saprophyticus* and enterococci (Table 23-1).

Asymptomatic bacteriuria is the isolation of bacteria in an appropriately collected urine specimen obtained from a person without symptoms. The diagnosis of asymptomatic bacteriuria should be based on results of a urine culture. Pyuria accompanying asymptomatic bacteriuria is not an indication for therapy. Pregnant women should be screened for bacteriuria by urine culture at least once during early pregnancy (12-16 weeks gestation) or at their first prenatal visit. All positive urine cultures, including asymptomatic bacteriuria, should be treated in pregnant women. Screening for and treatment of asymptomatic bacteriuria before transurethral resection of the prostate is recommended.

PREVENTION

Recurrent UTI is defined as at least three UTIs in 12 months, without evidence of structural abnormalities. This is the primary category of patients that are candidates for antimicrobial prophylaxis. Prophylaxis should be considered in all renal transplant patients to prevent infection of the graft. Systemic antimicrobial prophylaxis should not be routinely used in patients with Foley catheters because of concern about selection of antimicrobial resistance. The following regimens may be considered for prophylaxis of recurrent UTIs in *select* patients:

- Nitrofurantoin 50 mg orally once daily.
- One-half trimethoprim-sulfamethoxazole (TMP-SMX) single-strength (SS) tablet (Trimethoprim 40 mg-sulfamethoxazole 200 mg) orally once daily.

TREATMENT

There are four responses of bacteriuria to antimicrobial therapy: cure, persistence, relapse, and reinfection. Bacteriologic cure is defined as negative urine cultures while on therapy and during the follow-up period (usually 1-2 weeks). Bacteriologic persistence is defined as persistence of bacteriuria after 48 hours of therapy. Sites of persistence within the urinary tract are the renal parenchyma, calculi, and the prostate. Bacteriologic relapse is defined as recurrence of bacteriuria 1 to 2 weeks post therapy by the same infecting bacteria. Relapse is often associated with renal infection, structural abnormalities, or chronic bacterial prostatitis. Reinfection occurs after the initial sterilization of the urine and is defined as the development of bacteriuria during therapy or at any time thereafter. Reinfection can be due to the same organism, different serotype of the same organism, or a different organism.

There are many antimicrobials effective for the treatment of UTIs. There is no evidence to support superiority

TABLE 23-1	Bacterial Causes of UTIs	
	Uncomplicated (%)	Complicated (%)
Gram-Negative		
Escherichia coli	70-95	21-54
Proteus mirabilis	1-2	1-10
Klebsiella spp	1-2	2-17
Citrobacter spp	<1	5
Enterobacter spp	<1	2-10
Pseudomonas aeruginosa	<1	2-19
Other	<1	6-20
Gram-Positive		
Staphylococcus saprophyticus	5-10	1-4
Enterococci	1-2	1-23
Group B streptococci	<1	1-4
Staphylococcus aureus	<1	1-2
Other	<1	2

of bactericidal medications over bacteriostatic medications for the treatment of UTIs. Nonpharmacological treatment options include hydration, urine acidification, and urinary analgesics. There is no evidence that hydration improves the results of antimicrobial therapy, and continuous hydration is inconvenient. Urinary acidification is difficult to achieve and urinary analgesics (phenazopyridine) have little place in the routine treatment of symptomatic infections.

Three days of therapy with TMP-SMX or fluoroquinolones is effective treatment for uncomplicated lower UTIs in women. TMP-SMX is the recommended first-line therapy. Trimethoprim alone can be used in patients allergic to sulfa drugs; however, it is possible to have allergic reactions to trimethoprim. Due to increasing resistance to TMP-SMX among *E. coli* isolates, ciprofloxacin may be considered pending resistance rates in local area. It is important to know your local sensitivity patterns when making treatment recommendations. Nitrofurantoin is an antibiotic used specifically for uncomplicated UTIs in 5-day treatment courses. It is *not* indicated for the treatment of pyelonephritis or perinephric abscesses, and it is contraindicated in patients with a creatinine clearance less than 30 mL/min. Ciprofloxacin and levofloxacin are the two fluoroquinolones indicated for UTIs. Moxifloxacin is metabolized in the liver via glucuronide and sulfate conjugation, and it is not indicated for the treatment of UTIs.

Tables 23-2 to 23-4 summarizes treatment of UTIs. Short-course therapy (eg, 3 days) is not appropriate for women with a history of UTIs caused by antibiotic-resistant bacteria, 7 days of symptoms, complicated UTIs, or male UTIs. These patients should receive 7 to 14 days of therapy. Pyelonephritis should be treated for 7 to 14 days with most agents. Severely ill patients with pyelonephritis may need to be hospitalized and require IV antimicrobial therapy. Appropriate IV antimicrobial therapy includes aminoglycosides, piperacillin-tazobactam, ceftriaxone, or a parenteral fluoroquinolone.

Special Populations

UTIs in men are considered complicated. Urine cultures should always be obtained in men because the causative organism is not as predictable as in women. Initial therapy should be for 10 to 14 days. Short-course therapy (3 days) has not been adequately studied in men and is not recommended.

The most important factors influencing the prevalence of UTIs in children are age and gender. In newborns, the rate for premature infants (2.9%) exceeds that for full-term infants (0.7%), and boys are five to eight times more likely than girls to be infected. Male predominance persists for the first 3 months of life, after which the prevalence among girls exceeds that in boys. Young children with a UTI often do not present with specific urinary tract symptoms (dysuria, urgency, or urinary frequency) and a urine culture is necessary to diagnose a UTI in a young child. Oral treatment options for UTIs in children include a TMP-SMX or a cephalosporin. Fluoroquinolones are not recommended for use in children less than or equal to 18 years of age due to an increased risk of musculoskeletal disorders. Initial therapy should be for 7 to 14 days.

The goal of UTI treatment during pregnancy is to maintain sterile urine throughout gestation. Complications associated with UTIs during pregnancy include premature delivery, low birth weight, and stillbirth. Sulfonamides, amoxicillin, amoxicillin/clavulanic acid, cephalexin, and nitrofurantoin are effective in 70% to 80% of patients. Initial therapy should be for 7 days, and a follow-up urine culture 1 to 2 weeks post therapy and then monthly until birth is recommended. Caution with sulfonamides is warranted near term due to a potential increased risk of kernicterus. During pregnancy, tetracyclines should be avoided due to teratogenic effects, and fluoroquinolones should be avoided due to the risk of arthropathies and the potential to inhibit cartilage and bone development in the newborn. Nitrofurantoin is contraindicated in pregnant patients at term (38-42 weeks gestation) and during labor and delivery due to the risk of hemolytic anemia via immature erythrocyte enzyme systems (glutathione instability). Nitrofurantoin has been detected in breast milk, and it is recommended that mothers nursing infants under 1 month of age should avoid using nitrofurantoin.

Eighty percent of hospital-acquired UTIs are attributable to an indwelling Foley catheter. Patients with an indwelling catheter acquire UTIs at a rate of 5% per day. Bacteriuria in patients with an indwelling catheter is usually asymptomatic. When asymptomatic bacteriuria occurs in short-term catheterized patients (<30 days), the use of systemic antimicrobials should be withheld and the catheter should be removed immediately. If the patient becomes symptomatic, the catheter should be removed prior to the initiation of therapy. In patients with chronic indwelling catheters (≥30 days), asymptomatic bacteriuria is universal in patients. Antimicrobial therapy will not prevent bacteriuria or symptomatic infection, but will facilitate antimicrobial resistance. Symptomatic patients must have their catheter removed, be recatheterized,

TABLE 23-2   Commonly Used Antimicrobial Agents in the Treatment of UTIs

Drug	Adverse Drug Reactions	Monitoring Parameters	Comments
Oral Therapy			
Trimethoprim–sulfamethoxazole	Rash, Stevens–Johnson Syndrome, renal failure, photosensitivity, hematologic (neutropenia, anemia, etc.)	Serum creatinine, BUN, electrolytes, signs of rash, and CBC	This combination is highly effective against most aerobic enteric bacteria except *P. aeruginosa*. High urinary tract tissue concentrations and urine concentrations are achieved, which may be important in complicated infection treatment. Also effective as prophylaxis for recurrent infections
Nitrofurantoin	GI intolerance, neuropathies, and pulmonary reactions	Baseline serum creatinine and BUN	This agent is effective as both a therapeutic and a prophylactic agent in patients with recurrent UTIs. Main advantage is the lack of resistance even after long courses of therapy
Fosfomycin trometamol	Diarrhea, headache, and angioedema	No routine tests recommended	Single-dose therapy for uncomplicated infections, low levels of resistance, use with caution in patients with hepatic dysfunction
Fluoroquinolones			
Ciprofloxacin Levofloxacin	Hypersensitivity, photosensitivity, GI symptoms, dizziness, confusion, and tendonitis (black box warning)	CBC, baseline serum creatinine, and BUN	The fluoroquinolones have a greater spectrum of activity, including *P. aeruginosa*. These agents are effective for pyelonephritis and prostatitis. Avoid in pregnancy and children. Moxifloxacin should not be used owing to inadequate urinary concentrations
Penicillins			
Amoxicillin–clavulanate	Hypersensitivity (rash, anaphylaxis), diarrhea, superinfections, and seizures	CBC, signs of rash, or hypersensitivity	Due to increasing *E. coli* resistance, amoxicillin–clavulanate is the preferred penicillin for uncomplicated cystitis
Cephalosporins			
Cefaclor Cefpodoxime-proxetil	Hypersensitivity (rash, anaphylaxis), diarrhea, superinfections, and seizures	CBC, signs of rash, or hypersensitivity	There are no major advantages of these agents over other agents in the treatment of UTIs, and they are more expensive. These agents are not active against enterococci
Parenteral Therapy			
Aminoglycosides			
Gentamicin Tobramycin Amikacin	Ototoxicity, nephrotoxicity	Serum creatinine and BUN, serum drug concentrations, and individual pharmacokinetic monitoring	These agents are renally excreted and achieve good concentrations in the urine. Amikacin generally is reserved for multidrug-resistant bacteria
Penicillins			
Ampicillin–sulbactam Piperacillin–tazobactam	Hypersensitivity (rash, anaphylaxis), diarrhea, superinfections, and seizures	CBC, signs of rash, or hypersensitivity	These agents generally are equally effective for susceptible bacteria. The extended-spectrum penicillins are more active against *P. aeruginosa* and enterococci and often are preferred over cephalosporins. They are very useful in renally impaired patients or when an aminoglycoside is to be avoided
Cephalosporins			
Ceftriaxone Ceftazidime Cefepime	Hypersensitivity (rash, anaphylaxis), diarrhea, superinfections, and seizures	CBC, signs of rash, or hypersensitivity	Second- and third-generation cephalosporins have a broad spectrum of activity against gram-negative bacteria, but are not active against enterococci and have limited activity against *P. aeruginosa*. Ceftazidime and cefepime are active against *P. aeruginosa*. They are useful for nosocomial infections and urosepsis due to susceptible pathogens
Carbapenems/monobactams			
Imipenem–cilastatin Meropenem Doripenem Ertapenem Aztreonam	Hypersensitivity (rash, anaphylaxis), diarrhea, superinfections, and seizures	CBC, signs of rash, or hypersensitivity	Carbapenems have a broad spectrum of activity, including gram-positive, gram-negative, and anaerobic bacteria. Imipenem, meropenem, and doripenem are active against *P. aeruginosa* and enterococci, but ertapenem is not. Aztreonam is a monobactam that is only active against gram-negative bacteria, including some strains of *P. aeruginosa*. Generally useful for nosocomial infections when aminoglycosides are to be avoided and in penicillin-sensitive patients
Fluoroquinolones			
Ciprofloxacin Levofloxacin	Hypersensitivity, photosensitivity, GI symptoms, dizziness, confusion, and tendonitis (black box warning)	CBC, baseline serum creatinine, and BUN	These agents have broad-spectrum activity against both gram-negative and gram-positive bacteria. They provide urine and high-tissue concentrations and are actively secreted in reduced renal function

Abbreviations: BUN, blood urea nitrogen; CBC, complete blood count; GI, gastrointestinal; UTIs, urinary tract infections.
Reproduced with permission from DiPiro JT, Talbert RL, Yee GC, et al: *Pharmacotherapy: A Pathophysiologic Approach,* 10th ed. New York, NY: McGraw-Hill; 2017.

TABLE 23-3 Evidence-Based Empirical Treatment of UTIs and Prostatitis

Diagnosis	Pathogens	Treatment Recommendation	Comments
Acute uncomplicated cystitis	*Escherichia coli, Staphylococcus saprophyticus*	1. Nitrofurantoin × 5 d (A,I)[a] 2. Trimethoprim–sulfamethoxazole × 3 d (A,I)[a] 3. Fosfomycin trometamol × 1 dose (A,I)[a] 4. Fluoroquinolone × 3 d (A,I)[a] 5. β-Lactams × 3-7 d (B,I)[a] 6. Pivmecillinam × 3-7 d (A,I)	Short-course therapy more effective than single dose Reserve fluoroquinolones as alternatives to development of resistance (A-III)[a] β-Lactams as a group are not as effective in acute cystitis then trimethoprim–sulfamethoxazole or the fluoroquinolones, do not use amoxicillin or ampicillin[a] Pivmecillinam not available in United States
Pregnancy	As above	1. Amoxicillin–clavulanate × 7 d 2. Cephalosporin × 7 d 3. Trimethoprim–sulfamethoxazole × 7 d	Avoid trimethoprim–sulfamethoxazole during the third trimester
Acute pyelonephritis			
Uncomplicated	*E. coli*	1. Quinolone × 5-7 d (A,I)[a] 2. Trimethoprim–sulfamethoxazole (if susceptible) × 14 d (A,I)[a]	Can be managed as outpatient
	Gram-positive bacteria	1. Amoxicillin or amoxicillin–clavulanic acid × 14 d	
Complicated	*E. coli* *P. mirabilis* *K. pneumoniae* *P. aeruginosa* *Enterococcus faecalis*	1. Quinolone × 14 d 2. Extended-spectrum penicillin plus aminoglycoside	Severity of illness will determine duration of IV therapy; culture results should direct therapy Oral therapy may complete 14 d of therapy
Prostatitis	*E. coli* *K. pneumoniae* *Proteus* spp. *P. aeruginosa*	1. Trimethoprim–sulfamethoxazole × 4-6 wk 2. Quinolone × 4-6 wk	Acute prostatitis may require IV therapy initially Chronic prostatitis may require longer treatment periods or surgery

Abbreviation: UTI, urinary tract infection.

[a]Strength of recommendations: A, good evidence for; B, moderate evidence for; C, poor evidence for and against; D, moderate against; E, good evidence against. Quality of evidence: I, at least one proper randomized, controlled study; II, one well-designed clinical trial; III, evidence from opinions, clinical experience, and expert committees.

Reproduced with permission from DiPiro JT, Talbert RL, Yee GC, et al: *Pharmacotherapy: A Pathophysiologic Approach,* 10th ed. New York, NY: McGraw-Hill; 2017.

and then treated to prevent the development of pyelonephritis or bacteremia.

Prostatitis

Bacterial prostatitis is an inflammation of the prostate gland and surrounding tissue as a result of infection. It is classified as either acute or chronic. By definition, pathogenic bacteria and significant inflammatory cells must be present in prostatic secretions and urine to make the diagnosis of bacterial prostatitis. The acute form is characterized by a sudden onset of fever, tenderness, and urinary and constitutional symptoms. Chronic prostatitis presents with non-prostate related symptoms including urinating difficulty, low back pain, perineal pressure, or a combination of these. The chronic form represents a recurring infection with the same organism that results from incomplete eradication of bacteria from the prostate gland. Gram-negative enteric organisms (eg, *E. coli*) are the most frequent pathogens in acute bacterial prostatitis. The goals in the management of bacterial prostatitis are the same as those for UTIs. Acute bacterial prostatitis responds to antimicrobial therapy that is directed at the most commonly isolated organisms. Prostatic penetration of antimicrobials occurs because the acute inflammatory reaction alters the cellular membrane

barrier between the bloodstream and the prostate. Most patients can be managed with oral antimicrobial agents such as TMP-SMX and the fluoroquinolones (eg, ciprofloxacin, levofloxacin). Other effective agents include cephalosporins and β-lactam–β-lactamase combinations, but their use is second-line. The total course of antibiotic therapy should be 4 weeks in order to reduce the risk of development of chronic prostatitis, although in some cases 2 weeks may be sufficient. Therapy may be prolonged with chronic prostatitis (6-12 weeks). Long-term suppressive therapy also may be initiated for recurrent infections, such as three times weekly ciprofloxacin, TMP-SMX regular-strength tablet daily, or nitrofurantoin 100 mg daily. The choice of antibiotics in chronic bacterial prostatitis should include agents that are capable of reaching therapeutic concentrations in the prostatic fluid and which possess the spectrum of activity to be effective. Agents that achieve therapeutic prostatic concentrations include trimethoprim and the fluoroquinolones. Sulfamethoxazole penetrates poorly and probably contributes very little to trimethoprim activity when used in combination. Therapy should be continued for 4 to 6 weeks initially. Longer treatment periods may be necessary in some cases. If therapy fails with these regimens, chronic suppressive therapy may be used or surgery considered.

TABLE 23-4   Overview of Outpatient Antimicrobial Therapy for Lower Tract Infections in Adults

Indications	Antibiotic	Dose	Interval	Duration
Lower tract infections				
Uncomplicated	Trimethoprim–sulfamethoxazole	1 DS tablet	Twice a day	3 d
	Nitrofurantoin monohydrate	100 mg	Twice a day	5 d
	Nitrofurantoin macrocrystals	50 mg	Four times a day	5 d
	Fosfomycin trometamol	3 g	Single dose	1 d
	Ciprofloxacin	250 mg	Twice a day	3 d
	Levofloxacin	250 mg	Once a day	3 d
	Amoxicillin–clavulanate	500 mg	Every 8 h	5-7 d
	Pivmecillinam	400 mg	Twice a day	3 d
Complicated	Trimethoprim–sulfamethoxazole	1 DS tablet	Twice a day	7-10 d
	Ciprofloxacin	250-500 mg	Twice a day	7-10 d
	Levofloxacin	250 mg	Once a day	10 d
		750 mg	Once a day	5 d
	Amoxicillin–clavulanate	500 mg	Every 8 h	7-10 d
Recurrent infections	Nitrofurantoin	50 mg	Once a day	6 mo
	Trimethoprim–sulfamethoxazole	1/2 SS tablet	Once a day	6 mo
Acute pyelonephritis	Trimethoprim–sulfamethoxazole	1 DS tablet	Twice a day	14 d
	Ciprofloxacin	500 mg	Twice a day	14 d
		1000 mg ER	Once a day	7 d
	Levofloxacin	250 mg	Once a day	10 d
		750 mg	Once a day	5 d
	Amoxicillin–clavulanate	500 mg	Every 8 h	14 d

Abbreviations: DS, double strength; SS, single strength.
Dosing intervals for normal renal function.
Reproduced with permission from DiPiro JT, Talbert RL, Yee GC, et al: *Pharmacotherapy: A Pathophysiologic Approach,* 10th ed. New York, NY: McGraw-Hill; 2017.

POSTEXPOSURE PROPHYLAXIS

In some women, reinfection is associated with sexual intercourse. Voiding immediately after intercourse may help prevent reinfection. A single dose of TMP-SMX single strength or nitrofurantoin 50 to 100 mg can be given prophylactically post-intercourse.

CASE Application

Questions 1 through 3 are related to the same case.

1. GB is a 28-year-old woman with a chief complaint of dysuria. Symptoms started 3 days ago. The physician orders a urinalysis and a urine culture. What is the most likely bacterial cause of the UTI?

   a. *Acinetobacter baumannii (A. baumannii)*
   b. *Escherichia coli (E. coli)*
   c. *Pseudomonas aeruginosa (P. aeruginosa)*
   d. *Staphylococcus saprophyticus (S. saprophyticus)*

2. What is appropriate empiric therapy for GB? Patient has normal renal function and no medication allergies. Medications include metoprolol and omeprazole.

   a. Cefdinir
   b. Linezolid
   c. Amoxicillin
   d. TMP-SMX

3. What is the appropriate duration of therapy for GB?

   a. 1 day
   b. 3 days
   c. 7 days
   d. 14 days

4. Who should be screened for asymptomatic bacteriuria?

   a. College students
   b. Men
   c. Patients with indwelling catheters
   d. Pregnant women

5. Which of the following patient groups are considered to have complicated UTIs? Select all that apply.

   a. Children
   b. Men
   c. Pregnant women
   d. Catheter-associated

Questions 6 through 10 are related to the same case.

6. NK is a 62-year-old man presenting to urgent care today with dysuria, increased urinating frequency, and flank pain. His past medical history includes hyperlipidemia and migraines. He is allergic to penicillin and sulfa drugs. The patient has a high fever and severe nausea and vomiting (N&V). What is the probable diagnosis?

   a. Benign prostatic hyperplasia (BPH)
   b. Cystitis

c. Prostate cancer

d. Pyelonephritis

7. What is the most appropriate therapy for NK?

a. Amoxicillin 500 mg po tid

b. Ciprofloxacin 500 mg po bid

c. Ciprofloxacin 400 mg IV twice daily

d. TMP-SMX 1 double strength (DS) tablet po bid

8. What is the most appropriate duration of therapy for NK?

a. 7 days

b. 3 days

c. 14 days

d. 1 day

9. NK completes prescribed therapy and feels better. Two weeks later, he returns to the emergency department (ED) with general malaise, a temperature of 101.7°F, pelvic pain, dysuria, and increased urination. The basic metabolic panel was within the references ranges for each laboratory. Additionally, the complete blood count laboratory values were also within the reference rages. The prostate specific antigen was 12 ng/mL (reference less than 4.0 ng/mL), the erythrocyte sedimentation rate was 10 mm/h (reference range less than 15 mm/h) and the C-reactive protein was 11 mg/dL (reference range less than 3.0 mg/dL). What is the probable diagnosis?

a. Acute bacterial prostatitis

b. Benign prostatic hyperplasia

c. Cystitis

d. Epididymitis

10. NK is admitted to the hospital. Blood and urine cultures are collected. He is started on ceftriaxone 1 g IV daily. On day 3, blood cultures are negative, and the urine culture is positive for *E. coli*. The isolate is resistant to amoxicillin. On day 4, NK is ready for discharge. What is the most appropriate outpatient therapy for NK?

a. Ciprofloxacin 500 mg po bid for 3 days

b. Ciprofloxacin 500 mg po bid for 14 days

c. Ciprofloxacin 500 mg po bid for 28 days

d. Nitrofurantoin 100 mg po bid for 28 days

11. What is the most common gram-positive cause of a UTI?

a. *Streptococcus aureus*

b. *Staphylococcus epidermidis*

c. *Staphylococcus saprophyticus*

d. *Streptococcus pneumoniae*

12. Which antibiotic is most appropriate for prophylaxis of recurrent UTIs?

a. Amoxicillin/clavulanic acid

b. Levofloxacin

c. Moxifloxacin

d. Nitrofurantoin

13. Select the correct statement regarding nitrofurantoin.

a. Does not have a renal dosing recommendations/requirements

b. Appropriate throughout pregnancy

c. Is not indicated for the treatment of pyelonephritis

d. Is an antifungal

Questions 14 through 16 are related to the same case.

14. LA is 30-year-old pregnant woman. She is 16 weeks pregnant and reports dysuria at her appointment today. Urinalysis and urine culture are conducted, and she is started on TMP-SMX 1 DS tablet po bid. What is the appropriate duration of therapy?

a. 3 days

b. 7 days

c. 14 days

d. 28 days

15. Three days later, the clinic calls LA to tell her the culture results are back and she needs to change therapy. The culture was positive for *E. coli*, and it is resistant to TMP-SMX only. What would be the new appropriate therapy for LA?

a. Amoxicillin 500 mg po tid for 3 days

b. Ciprofloxacin 500 mg po bid for 7 days

c. Nitrofurantoin 100 mg po bid for 7 days

d. TMP-SMX 2 DS tablets po bid for 7 days

16. Does LA need a follow-up culture? If so, when?

a. No follow-up culture is needed

b. Yes, in 2 days

c. Yes, a day after the therapy is complete

d. Yes, 7 to 14 days after the therapy is complete

17. Which antibiotic is appropriate for UTI treatment in pregnant women who are not near-term? Select all that apply.

a. Amoxicillin/clavulanic acid

b. Doxycycline

c. Nitrofurantoin

d. TMP-SMX

18. Patients with chronic indwelling catheters usually have asymptomatic bacteriuria. What should be done if the patient becomes symptomatic? Select all that apply.

a. Remove the catheter; insert new sterile catheter before treatment

b. Remove the catheter; insert new sterile catheter after treatment

c. Start antibiotic therapy

d. Leave the same catheter in place

19. What is the brand name for TMP-SMX? Select all that apply.

a. Bactrim

b. Macrobid

c. Septra

d. Trimprex

20. Short-course therapy (3 days) is appropriate for which patient group.

    a. Women with a history of UTIs caused by antibiotic-resistant bacteria
    b. Men
    c. Women with >7 days of symptoms
    d. Women with uncomplicated cystitis

21. TC is a 19-year-old woman diagnosed with acute cystitis. She is allergic to sulfa drugs. What is an appropriate empiric regimen for her? Select all that apply.

    a. Ciprofloxacin 250 mg po bid for 3 days
    b. Trimethoprim 100 mg po bid for 3 days
    c. Sulfamethoxazole/trimethoprim 1 DS tablet twice daily for 3 days
    d. Moxifloxacin 400 mg daily for 3 days

22. YI is a 26-year-old patient being treated with TMP-SMX for a UTI. The current dose is 1 DS tablet twice daily. What gram-negative organisms would TMP-SMX treat that are potentially causes of a complicated UTI? Select all that apply.

    a. *Staphylococcus saprophyticus*
    b. *Escherichia coli*
    c. *Klebsiella pneumoniae*
    d. *Pseudomonas aeruginosa*
    e. *Proteus mirabilis*

23. Place the following antibiotics in order of dosing frequency. Start with the antibiotic that should be dosed most frequently in a patient with an estimated glomerular filtration of 100 mL/min (calculated by the Cockcroft-Gault equation).

Unordered Response	Ordered Response
Macrodantin 50 mg	
Levaquin 500 mg	
Septra 160/800 mg	

24. Select the antibiotic that is available as a 3-gram single dose for management of adult acute uncomplicated cystitis?

    a. Nitrofurantoin
    b. Ciprofloxacin
    c. Amoxicillin/clavulanate
    d. Fosfomycin

TAKEAWAY POINTS ››

- UTIs are divided into cystitis (lower tract and bladder) and pyelonephritis (upper tract and kidneys).
- Cystitis symptoms include dysuria, increased frequency, urgency, and occasionally suprapubic tenderness. Pyelonephritis is characterized as cystitis symptoms plus fever, flank pain, nausea, and vomiting.
- Uncomplicated UTIs occur in structurally and neurologically normal urinary tracts, and complicated UTIs occur in a urinary tract with functional or structural abnormalities.
- UTIs in men, pregnant women, children, and hospitalized patients are considered complicated.
- The most common cause of UTIs is gram-negative bacteria, with *E. coli* being isolated in 70% to 95% of cultures.
- Nitrofurantoin and TMP-SMX are recommended for prophylaxis of recurrent UTIs in *select* patients.
- Short-course (3 days) therapy at standard doses is effective treatment for uncomplicated lower UTIs in women, but is not recommended in women with more than 7 days of symptoms or a history of UTIs caused by antibiotic-resistant bacteria. Short-course therapy is not recommended in men.
- TMP-SMX is the recommended first-line therapy for complicated and uncomplicated UTIs, and trimethoprim alone can be used in patients allergic to sulfa drugs.
- Due to increasing resistance to TMP-SMX among *E. coli* isolates, fluoroquinolones (such as ciprofloxacin or levofloxacin) may be considered as first-line therapy.
- Nitrofurantoin is an antibiotic used specifically for uncomplicated UTIs. It is not indicated for the treatment of pyelonephritis or perinephric abscesses and contraindicated in patients with a creatinine clearance less than 30 mL/min.
- Pregnant women should be screened for bacteriuria by urine culture at least once during early pregnancy (12-16 weeks gestation) or at their first prenatal visit. All positive urine cultures, including asymptomatic bacteriuria, should be treated in pregnant women.
- Symptomatic patients with a catheter-associated UTI must have their catheter removed, be recatheterized, and then treated to prevent the development of pyelonephritis or bacteremia.

BIBLIOGRAPHY

Coyle EA, Prince RA. Urinary tract infections and prostatitis. In: DiPiro JT, Talbert RL, Yee GC, Matzke GR, Wells BG, Posey L, eds. *Pharmacotherapy: A Pathophysiologic Approach.* 10th ed. New York, NY: McGraw-Hill.

Gumbo T. General principles of antimicrobial therapy. In: Brunton LL, Chabner BA, Knollmann BC, eds. *Goodman & Gilman's The Pharmacological Basis of Therapeutics.* 12th ed. New York, NY: McGraw-Hill; 2011:chap 48.

Gupta K, Hooton TM, Naber KG, et al. International clinical practice guidelines for the treatment of acute uncomplicated cystitis and pyelonephritis in women: A 2010 update by the Infectious Diseases Society of America and the European Society for Microbiology and Infectious Diseases. *Clin Infect Dis.* 2011;52(5):e103–e120.

Lampiris HW, Maddix DS. Clinical use of antimicrobial agents. In: Katzung BG, Masters SB, Trevor AJ, eds. *Basic & Clinical Pharmacology.* 12th ed. New York, NY: McGraw-Hill; 2012:chap 51.

Petri WA, Jr. Sulfonamides, trimethoprim-sulfamethoxazole, quinolones, and agents for urinary tract infections. In: Brunton LL, Chabner BA, Knollmann BC, eds. *Goodman & Gilman's The Pharmacological Basis of Therapeutics.* 12th ed. New York, NY: McGraw-Hill; 2011:chap 52.

KEY ABBREVIATIONS

BPH = Benign prostatic hyperplasia
CRP = C-reactive protein
DS = double strength
ED = emergency department
IDSA = Infectious Disease Society of America
MIC = minimum inhibitory concentrations

MRSA = methicillin-resistant *S. aureus*
PSA = prostate specific antigen
TMP-SMX = trimethoprim-sulfamethoxazole
UTI = urinary tract infection
VRE = vancomycin-resistant enterococci

24 Skin and Soft Tissue Infections

Jennifer Le and Quang Dam

FOUNDATION OVERVIEW

Skin and soft tissue infections (SSTIs), also called skin and skin structure infections, are among the most common infections encountered in clinical practice. While most cases present as mild infections, severity of SSTIs can range extensively, from minor and superficial infections that are self-limiting, to severe and deep-seated infections that may be life threatening.

The skin serves as a primary defense mechanism against infections by acting as a barrier between the hosts and their environment. The skin consists of three layers: the epidermis, dermis, and subcutaneous fat. SSTIs may involve any or all layers of the skin, as well as the fascia and muscle underneath it. In rare instances, SSTIs may spread from the initial site of infection and cause severe complications such as sepsis, bacteremia, osteomyelitis, endocarditis, and glomerulonephritis.

The intact skin is generally impervious to infectious pathogens; however, disruption of this normal host defense (eg, excessive moisture, decreased skin perfusion, or physical damage) predisposes the skin to infections. Most SSTIs originate from a mechanical disruption of the skin, such as a puncture or abrasion, but can also commence as a complication of an underlying disease, such as diabetes mellitus.

Two categories of SSTIs exist: primary and secondary. In primary infections, healthy skin is infected, typically by a single microorganism. Secondary infections occur in pre-existing damaged skin and are often polymicrobial. Table 24-1 lists the common etiologic pathogens responsible for specific types of SSTIs. Gram-positive organisms present on skin, particularly *Staphylococcus aureus* (including community-associated methicillin-resistant *S. aureus* [caMRSA]) and *Streptococcus pyogenes* (also known as group A streptococci [GAS] or β-hemolytic streptococci) cause the majority of SSTIs. In the following sections, different types of SSTIs and their treatment strategies will be presented.

SPECIFIC INFECTIONS AND TREATMENTS

Folliculitis, Furuncles, and Carbuncles

Folliculitis is a superficial inflammatory infection involving hair follicles. Furuncles and carbuncles occur when the infection spreads to the subcutaneous tissue around the follicle. Furuncles describe lesions that occur in individual hair follicles. Carbuncles are larger than furuncles and form when furuncles adjacent to each other coalesce into one large lesion. *Staphylococcus aureus* is the most common cause of these infections. Other organisms, such as *Pseudomonas aeruginosa* and *Candida*, may also cause them.

The treatment of folliculitis and small furuncles is mainly nonpharmacologic with warm, moist compresses to facilitate drainage of pus. Topical antimicrobials, such as mupirocin, may be utilized for more severe infections. Large furuncles and carbuncles may require incision and drainage. Pharmacologic treatment may be employed if the patient exhibits systemic symptoms such as fever, or have an associated cellulitis. Treatment with systemic antibiotics active against *S. aureus* (eg, dicloxacillin, cephalexin) should be employed. When caMRSA is suspected, trimethoprim-sulfamethoxazole (TMP-SMX), clindamycin, doxycycline, or minocycline may be substituted as empiric treatment until cultures return.

Impetigo

Impetigo is a superficial skin infection that most frequently occurs in children and individuals with poor hygiene during hot and humid weather months, which facilitates microbial colonization and overgrowth. The microorganisms invade through breaks in the skin (eg, minor abrasions or insect bites) and cause blisters that rupture and form a golden-yellow crust over the lesions. Impetigo may present as bullous, non-bullous, or a deeper ulcerative form called ecthyma. The most common causes of impetigo are GAS and *S. aureus*. The treatment of impetigo consists of soaking the lesions with soap and water, using skin emollients to dry areas, and systemic antimicrobials. For mild cases of impetigo, topical antibiotics may be used. For more severe cases, systemic antimicrobials active against GAS and *S. aureus* (eg, cephalexin or dicloxacillin) are preferred.

Lymphangitis

Lymphangitis is an inflammation of the lymphatic channels that occurs when a local skin infection spreads into the lymphatics. Lymphangitis is characterized by erythematous streaks that extend from the original infection site to

TABLE 24-1 | **Bacterial Classification of Skin and Soft Tissue Infections**

Primary Infections	Pathogen
Folliculitis, furuncles, carbuncles	S. aureus (including caMRSA), Pseudomonas aeruginosa, Candida species
Impetigo	S. aureus, group A streptococci
Lymphangitis	Group A streptococci, occasionally S. aureus
Erysipelas	Group A streptococci
Cellulitis	Group A streptococci, S. aureus (including caMRSA), occasionally other gram-positive, gram-negative, or anaerobic pathogens
Necrotizing fasciitis	
Type I	Anaerobes (eg, Bacteroides spp., Peptostreptococcus spp.), streptococci, Enterobacteriaceae
Type II	Group A streptococci, caMRSA
Osteomyelitis	
Hematogenous	S. aureus
Contiguous	S. aureus, streptococci, Enterobacteriaceae, anaerobes
Vascular insufficiency	S. aureus, streptococci, Enterobacteriaceae, anaerobes
Secondary Infections	
Diabetic foot infections	S. aureus, streptococci, Enterobacteriaceae, anaerobes, P. aeruginosa
Pressure sores	S. aureus, streptococci, Enterobacteriaceae, anaerobes, P. aeruginosa
Bite wounds	
Animal (dog, cat)	Pasteurella multocida, S. aureus, streptococci, Bacteroides species, oral anaerobes
Human	Eikenella corrodens, S. aureus, streptococci, Corynebacterium species, Bacteroides species, Peptostreptococcus, oral anaerobes
Burn wounds	P. aeruginosa, Enterobacteriaceae, Acinetobacter species, S. aureus, streptococci

Abbreviations: caMRSA, community-associated methicillin-resistant S. aureus.

the lymph nodes. Lymphangitis is typically caused by GAS. Uncontrolled infection can progress rapidly to cause serious complications; therefore, the goal of therapy is to promptly eradicate the infecting organism to prevent further damage. Parenteral treatment with penicillin should be started within 48 to 72 hours. With clinical improvement, the patient can be switched to oral penicillin to complete a 7- to 10-day course. Clindamycin is an alternative for patients allergic to penicillin.

Erysipelas

Erysipelas is an infection that is limited to the most superficial layer of the skin (ie, epidermis) and the cutaneous lymphatics. In contrast to cellulitis, erysipelas presents as an intensely red and burning lesion with clearly demarcated, raised margins. The most common etiologic pathogen is GAS. Mild to moderate cases of erysipelas are treated with oral penicillin or

intramuscular penicillin for 7 to 10 days. Patients with severe infections usually require treatment with intravenous penicillin. Clindamycin and macrolides are alternatives for patients who are penicillin allergic.

Cellulitis

Cellulitis is an acute, infectious process that initially affects the epidermis and dermis, and potentially spread to the superficial fascia. Cellulitis represents a serious type of SSTI because of the propensity of the infection to spread through the lymphatic tissue and bloodstream, if left untreated. GAS and S. aureus are the most frequent etiologic pathogens; however, many other pathogens have been implicated. Cellulitis is described as painful and tender with rapidly spreading signs of redness, edema, and warmth. Unlike erysipelas, the cellulitis lesion has poorly defined margins and is not raised. While it is often hard to distinguish the etiologic pathogen on presentation alone, cellulitis associated with abscesses and/or those purulent in nature may be indicative of infection caused by S. aureus rather than streptococci.

The goals of therapy for cellulitis are prompt and successful eradication of the infection, and prevention of progression to complications, such as osteomyelitis or septic arthritis. Nonpharmacological treatments of cellulitis consist of elevating and immobilizing the limb to decrease swelling, placement of sterile saline dressings on open lesions, surgical debridement for severe infection, and drainage of abscesses (if present). Pharmacologic treatment of cellulitis should provide coverage against the most common pathogens. In areas where MRSA is highly prevalent, or if there is a high suspicion of MRSA infection, empiric treatment against MRSA should be initiated. If MRSA infection is not suspected, β-lactams active against penicillinase-producing strains of S. aureus (ie, methicillin-sensitive S. aureus [MSSA]) and GAS are sufficient in most cases. Table 24-2 provides empiric treatment strategies for cellulitis. The duration of therapy ranges from 7 to 10 days. For complicated cellulitis, initiate intravenous and then convert to oral therapy once the patient is stable and skin symptoms begin to resolve.

Necrotizing Fasciitis

Necrotizing fasciitis (NF) is a rare, rapidly progressive, and life-threatening infection of the subcutaneous tissue and fascia. Although the incidence of NF is higher in patients with chronic underlying diseases (eg, diabetes, alcoholism, and peripheral vascular disease), healthy individuals can become infected as well. NF commences after an initial trauma, which may vary from a minor abrasion to a deep penetrating wound. Bacteria introduced into the fascia replicate and release toxins that facilitate their spread along the fascial planes. There are two types of NF: types I and II. Type I is polymicrobial and develops after surgery or deep penetrating wounds in the bowel, decubitus ulcer, or injection site of an intravenous drug user. Type II is monomicrobial, caused by GAS, and usually occurs after minor trauma from an abrasion or insect bite.

TABLE 24-2 **Empiric Antimicrobial Therapy for Cellulitis**

Probable Pathogen	Mild Infection (Oral)[a]	Moderate-Severe Infection (IV)[a]
MSSA, GAS[b]	Dicloxacillin 500 mg every 6 h *or* cephalexin 500 mg every 6 h	Nafcillin/oxacillin 1-2 g every 4-6 h *or* cefazolin 1-2 g every 8 h
caMRSA	TMP-SMX DS 1-2 tablets every 12 h *or* doxycycline 100 mg every 12 h *or* minocycline 100 mg every 12 h *or* clindamycin 300-450 mg every 6 h	Vancomycin 15-20 mg/kg every 12 h[c] *or* linezolid 600 mg every 12 h *or* daptomycin 4 mg/kg daily *or* ceftaroline 600 mg every 12 h
Streptococci (documented)[b]	Penicillin VK 500 mg every 6 h *or* procaine penicillin G 600,000 units IM every 8-12 h	Aqueous penicillin G 1-2 million units every 4-6 h
Polymicrobial infection (*S. aureus*, streptococci, gram-negatives, anaerobes)	Amoxicillin/clavulanic acid 500 mg every 8 h or 875 mg every 12 h[d] *or* ciprofloxacin 500-750 mg every 12 h + clindamycin 300-600 mg every 6-8 h *or* levofloxacin 500-750 mg daily[e] *or* moxifloxacin 400 mg daily **If caMRSA suspected, ADD:** TMP-SMX DS 1-2 tablets every 12 h *or* doxycycline 100 mg every 12 h *or* minocycline 100 mg every 12 h *or* clindamycin 300-450 mg every 6 h	Ampicillin-sulbactam 1.5-3 g every 6 h *or* ceftriaxone 1 g daily[e] *or* ertapenem 1 g daily *or* moxifloxacin 400 mg every day **If *Pseudomonas* suspected CHOOSE:** Piperacillin-tazobactam 3.375-4.5 g every 4-6 h *or* cefepime 2 g every 8-12 h[e] *or* imipenem-cilastatin 500 mg every 6 h *or* meropenem 1 g every 8 h *or* doripenem 500 mg every 8 h *or* levofloxacin 500-750 mg daily **If MRSA suspected, ADD:** Vancomycin 15 mg/kg every 12 h[c] *or* linezolid 600 mg every 12 h *or* daptomycin 4 mg/kg daily *or* ceftaroline 600 mg every 12 h

Abbreviations: caMRSA, community acquired methicillin-resistant *S. aureus*; DS, double strength; GAS, group A streptococci; MRSA, methicillin-resistant *S. aureus*; MSSA, methicillin-sensitive *S. aureus*; TMP-SMX, trimethoprim-sulfamethoxazole.

[a]Adult dose with normal renal function.

[b]For patients who have severe penicillin allergies, use clindamycin for mild infections and vancomycin for moderate to severe infections. Other antibiotics may also be options.

[c]Vancomycin dose should be individualized to patient's parameters and goals.

[d]Narrow gram-negative pathogen coverage.

[e]If anaerobes suspected, add clindamycin or metronidazole.

Notably, caMRSA is an increasing cause of type II NF and it should be empirically covered.

The goals of therapy for NF include eradication of infection, and reduction in morbidity and mortality. Prompt surgical intervention is essential to effectively treat NF. Delay in surgical intervention increases mortality. Empiric antimicrobial therapy should also be initiated immediately for suspected NF. The most common regimens include a parenteral β-lactam/β-lactamase inhibitor or a carbapenem, in combination with clindamycin and a parenteral MRSA-active antibiotic such as vancomycin, linezolid, or daptomycin. As a protein synthesis inhibitor, clindamycin is empirically added to decrease bacterial toxin production in order to minimize further tissue damage that occurs with NF. Moreover, clindamycin enhances antibacterial activity, which may be important for infections with a high bacterial inoculum like NF. Once the causative organisms are identified, antimicrobial treatment should be streamlined to target those organisms. Since optimal treatment duration has not been well defined, antibiotic therapy should be continued until substantial clinical improvement is observed, with clinical stability for at least 48 to 72 hours and no additional planned surgical intervention. Adjunct treatments include hyperbaric oxygen and intravenous immunoglobulin.

Diabetic Foot Infections

Infections from chronic foot ulcers are among the most common, severe, and costly complications of diabetes mellitus.

The pathogenesis of diabetic foot infections (DFIs) stems from three factors that result from poorly controlled diabetes: neuropathy, angiopathy, and immunopathy. While aerobic gram-positive bacteria, such as *S. aureus* and streptococci (both group A and non-GAS), are predominant pathogens in acutely infected ulcers, chronically infected ulcers are polymicrobial involving other pathogens. These organisms include Enterobacteriaceae, *P. aeruginosa*, and anaerobes. Spread of infection, osteomyelitis, and amputation are all complications that can result from DFIs. The goals of therapy are resolution of infection, avoidance of complications, and prevention of future infections. In the treatment of DFIs, nonpharmacologic therapy, such as debridement, plays a crucial role.

Comprehensive foot care programs have shown to have significant role in reducing the rate of DFIs. Periodic foot examinations with monofilament testing and patient education on proper foot care, optimal glycemic control, and smoking cessation are key preventive strategies. Multiple antibiotic options exist for the treatment of DFIs. Table 24-3 provides examples of antimicrobials of DFIs. Depending on the severity of the infection, the treatment duration can vary greatly, from 7 to 28 days or longer.

Infected Pressure Sores

Pressure sores, also known as decubitus ulcers or bedsores, are chronic wounds that result from continuous pressure on the tissue overlying a bony prominence. This pressure impedes

TABLE 24-3	Empiric Pharmacologic Treatment of Diabetic Foot Infection	
IDSA Infection Severity (PEDIS grade)	**General Approach to Therapy**	**Examples of Empiric Regimens[a]**
Uninfected (1)	None. Avoid treating uninfected diabetic foot ulcers.	Not applicable.
Mild (2)	Usually treat as an outpatient with oral, narrow-spectrum antibiotics with activity against *S. aureus* and streptococcal species. **Include coverage for MRSA (caMRSA or haMRSA) according to patient history and resistance patterns in the area.**	**If MRSA not *or* suspected, CHOOSE:** cephalexin 500 mg every 6 h *or* dicloxacillin 500 mg every 6 h *or* amoxicillin-clavulanic acid 875 mg every 12 h **If MRSA suspected, CHOOSE:** TMP-SMX DS 1-2 tablets every 12 h *or* doxycycline 100 mg every 12 h *or* minocycline 100 mg every 12 h *or* clindamycin 300-600 mg every 6-8 h *or* linezolid 600 mg oral every 12 h
Moderate to severe (3-4)	While some moderate infections may be treated as an outpatient basis, many are treated initially as an inpatient with parenteral antibiotics then transitioned to oral. Severe infections often require parenteral therapy for full duration of therapy. Generally select antibiotics with activity against gram-positive, gram-negative, and anaerobic bacteria. **Include coverage for MRSA according to patient history and resistance patterns in the area.**	Ampicillin-sulbactam 3 g every 6 h[b] *or* ertapenem 1 g daily[b] *or* ceftriaxone 2 g daily + clindamycin 600-900 mg every 6-8 h or metronidazole 500 mg every 8 h[b] *or* piperacillin-tazobactam 3.375-4.5 g every 6 h *or* imipenem-cilastatin 500 mg every 6 h *or* meropenem 1 g every 8 h *or* doripenem 500 mg every 8 h *or* ciprofloxacin 400 mg IV every 8-12 h or levofloxacin 750 mg daily + clindamycin 600-900 mg every 8 h or metronidazole 500 mg every 8 h *or* tigecycline 100 mg load, then 50 mg every 12 h[b,c] *or* moxifloxacin 400 mg daily[b] **If MRSA suspected, ADD:** vancomycin 15-20 mg/kg q12h[d] *or* linezolid 600 mg every 12 h *or* daptomycin 4 mg/kg daily *or* ceftaroline 600 mg every 12 h

Abbreviations: caMRSA, community acquired methicillin-resistant *S. aureus*; DS, double strength; haMRSA, health care-associated methicillin-resistant *S. aureus*; MRSA, methicillin-resistant *S. aureus*; TMP-SMX, trimethoprim-sulfamethoxazole.

[a]Adult dose with normal renal function.

[b]This regimen does not cover *P. aeruginosa*.

[c]Tigecycline covers MRSA but should be reserved for last-line therapy.

[d]Vancomycin dose should be individualized to patient's parameters and goals.

blood flow to the dermis and subcutaneous fat, resulting in tissue damage and necrosis. Pressure sores are heavily colonized and in some cases, the colonizing bacteria invade tissue and cause infection. Pressure sore infections generally are polymicrobial. The goals of therapy for infected pressure sores include resolution of infection, promotion of wound healing, and establishment of effective infection control. Prevention is the most effective way to manage pressure sores. Key prevention strategies include monitoring of high-risk patients, reducing skin exposure to pressure and moisture, and promoting good nutritional status. Systemic antimicrobials are indicated for pressure sores associated with spreading cellulitis, osteomyelitis, or bacteremia. Because the infections are polymicrobial, empiric therapy should be broad spectrum and total duration of therapy should be 10 to 14 days. Mild superficial infections may be treated with wound care and topical antimicrobial agents. Table 24-4 lists empiric therapy for pressure sores.

Infected Bite Wounds

Animal bites are common causes of trauma to the skin and underlying tissue. Dogs are the most common causes of animal bites; however, cat and human bites have higher risk of infections and complications. Thorough irrigation and debridement of the bitten tissue should be performed as soon as possible. Most wounds do not require antibiotic therapy in absence of infection. However, in some cases, such as cat and human bites, deep puncture wounds, bites to the hand or other critical anatomy, and bites requiring surgical repair require prophylactic therapy. The normal mouth flora of the biting animal, and the victim's skin flora to a lesser extent, are the etiologic pathogens of bite wound infections. Amoxicillin/clavulanic acid or ampicillin-sulbactam are considered the drugs of choice for dog, cat, and human bites. Second- and third-generation cephalosporins, fluoroquinolones, TMP-SMX, or doxycycline in combination with clindamycin or metronidazole are some alternatives for patients who are intolerant to penicillins (depending on the severity of intolerance).

SPECIAL CONSIDERATIONS

Antimicrobial Properties and Antimicrobial Resistance

The armamentarium of antibiotics that may be utilized to treat SSTIs is considerable. The properties of a drug may influence the preference for one agent over the other. Key properties include side effect profile, drug interactions, formulation, and

TABLE 24-4	Empiric Therapy for Infected Pressure Sores
Formulation	Antibiotic[a]
Topical	Silver sulfadiazine 1% cream *or* combination antibiotic ointments
Oral[b]	Amoxicillin/clavulanic acid 500 mg every 8 h or 875 mg every 12 h *or* ciprofloxacin 500-750 mg every 12 h *or* levofloxacin 500-750 mg daily + clindamycin 300-450 mg every 6 h *or* metronidazole 500 mg every 8 h[c] *or* moxifloxacin 400 mg daily **If MRSA suspected, CHOOSE:** TMP-SMX DS 1-2 tablets every 12 h *or* doxycycline 100 mg every 12 h *or* minocycline 100 mg every 12 h *or* clindamycin 300-600 mg every 6-8 h *or* linezolid 600 mg oral every 12 h
Parenteral[b]	Cefoxitin 1-2 g every 8 h *or* piperacillin-tazobactam 3.375-4.5 g every 6 h[c] *or* imipenem-cilastatin 500 mg every 6 h[c]; meropenem 1 g every 8 h[c] *or* doripenem 500 mg every 8 h[c] *or* ciprofloxacin 400 mg IV every 8-12 h or levofloxacin 500-750 mg daily + clindamycin 600-900 mg every 8 h or metronidazole 500 mg every 8 h[c] *or* moxifloxacin 400 mg daily **If MRSA suspected, ADD:** vancomycin 15-20 mg/kg q12h[d] *or* linezolid 600 mg every 12 h *or* daptomycin 4 mg/kg daily *or* ceftaroline 600 mg every 12 h[d]

[a]Include coverage for caMRSA or haMRSA according to patient history and resistance patterns in the area.
[b]Adult dose with normal renal function.
[c]Regimens with activity against *P. aeruginosa*
[d]The use of two β-lactam antibiotics has not been well studied and thus not recommended.

pregnancy category. Table 24-5 describes the properties of antibiotics that can be used to treat SSTIs.

Antimicrobial resistance is another important consideration in selecting an antibiotic treatment for an SSTI. SSTIs caused by caMRSA has rapidly increased in the past two decades. Therefore, local high prevalence of caMRSA may prompt the use of a MRSA-active antibiotic for empiric treatment. Resistance to specific antibiotics may influence the decision in choosing one agent over another as well. For example, clindamycin should be avoided in regions with local resistance rates exceeding 10% to 15%, or infections caused by *S. aureus* isolates with positive double disk diffusion tests (D-tests), which denote rapid development of inducible resistance to clindamycin from the *erm* gene.

Cellulitis in Injection Drug Users and Immune Compromised Patients

Injection drug users are at increased risk for a number of infectious complications, including cellulitis and abscess formation at site of injection. SSTIs in injection drug users may be polymicrobial, encompassing a wide variety of organisms like the normal oral flora, *S. aureus* (including MRSA), GAS, and anaerobes.

Comparable to injection drug users, immunocompromised patients are at increased risk for polymicrobial cellulitis. In this population, antibiotics with broad spectrum of activity may be warranted for severe cellulitis that is accompanied by systemic symptoms. Table 24-2 provides empiric antibiotic options for cellulitis.

Osteomyelitis

Osteomyelitis, an infection of the bone, can be a severe complication of SSTIs. Gram-positive bacteria, particularly *S. aureus* and streptococci, are predominant pathogens identified in osteomyelitis. Osteomyelitis can be divided into three

categories: hematogenous, contiguous, and secondary to vascular insufficiency. Hematogenous osteomyelitis often occurs in children and affects the long bones. Contiguous osteomyelitis, affecting mostly adults, arises from infections of adjacent tissues or organs, and is most commonly encountered after surgery. Osteomyelitis secondary to vascular insufficiency occurs mostly in older adults or those with diabetes. It affects the lower limbs and can be difficult to treat due to decreased blood flow to the area. Deep culture and surgical intervention (if possible) should be performed prior to treatment with systemic antibiotics. Empiric therapy should target causative pathogen(s), depending on the type of osteomyelitis and patient-specific risk factors. Table 24-6 lists common empiric treatment options for osteomyelitis. The total duration of therapy, which is typically 4 to 6 weeks, should be based on the clinical presentation, type of surgical intervention performed, and clinical imaging.

PREVENTION

Prevention of SSTIs is primarily nonpharmacological. In general, patients should maintain good personal hygiene which includes showering daily, frequent hand washing, using clean dressings, avoiding the sharing of personal hygiene products, washing linens and clothing in hot water, and frequent cleaning of shared areas. In addition, modifying underlying risk factors (such as diabetes) should be optimized.

Pharmacologic measures for prevention of SSTIs are controversial because of inconsistent evidence for effectiveness and concern for increasing resistance. However, some patients may benefit from pharmacologic interventions. For example, patients who suffer from recurrent MRSA SSTIs, despite optimizing nonpharmacologic therapy, may be decolonized using intranasal mupirocin with or without chlorhexidine baths.

Antimicrobial	Formulations	Mechanism of Action	Side Effects	Contraindications (CI); Warnings (W)	Drug Interactions (DI); General Information (GI); Monitoring (M)
First-Generation Cephalosporins					
Cephalexin (Keflex); Cefazolin (Ancef)	Cephalexin: capsule, tablet, suspension; Cefazolin: parenteral	Inhibits bacterial cell wall synthesis by binding to one or more PBPs which inhibits the final transpeptidation step of peptidoglycan synthesis in bacterial cell wall synthesis	CNS (confusion, dizziness), rash, GI, CDI; BMS (rare)	CI: IgE-mediated hypersensitivity to cephalosporins or penicillin derivatives W: Modify dosage in renal dysfunction, use with caution in patients with a delayed penicillin allergy (rash) and avoid in immediate allergic (anaphylaxis/ IgE-mediated) penicillin reaction, may be associated with increased INR, especially in nutritionally malnourished patients, prolonged treatment, hepatic or renal disease, use with caution in patients with a history of seizure disorder (high levels, especially in the presence of renal dysfunction, may increase risk of seizures)	DI: Food—peak cephalexin levels are decreased with food, but total absorption is not affected GI: Pregnancy category B, renal elimination M: With prolonged therapy, monitor renal hepatic function periodically, CBC with differential for cytopenias or signs of allergic reaction
Second-Generation Cephalosporins					
Cefuroxime (Ceftin, Zinacef); Cefoxitin (Mefoxin)	Cefuroxime axetil: tablet, suspension; Cefuroxime sodium: parenteral; Cefoxitin: parenteral	Inhibits bacterial cell wall synthesis by binding to one or more PBPs which inhibits the final transpeptidation step of peptidoglycan synthesis in bacterial cell wall synthesis	CNS (confusion, dizziness), rash, GI, CDI; BMS (rare)	CI: IgE-mediated hypersensitivity to cephalosporins or penicillin derivatives W: Modify dosage in renal dysfunction, use with caution in patients with a delayed penicillin allergy (rash) and avoid in immediate allergic (anaphylaxis/ IgE-mediated) penicillin reaction, may be associated with increased INR, especially in nutritionally malnourished patients, prolonged treatment, hepatic or renal disease	GI: Pregnancy category B, renal elimination, cefuroxime axetil film-coated tablets and oral suspension are not bioequivalent and are not substitutable on a mg/mg basis M: With prolonged therapy, monitor renal hepatic function periodically, CBC with differential for cytopenias or signs of allergic reaction
Third-Generation Cephalosporins					
Cefpodoxime (Vantin); Cefdinir (Omnicef); Ceftriaxone (Rocephin); Cefotaxime (Claforan)	Cefpodoxime: tablet, suspension; Cefdinir: capsule, suspension; Ceftriaxone: parenteral; Cefotaxime: parenteral	Inhibits bacterial cell wall synthesis by binding to one or more PBPs which inhibits the final transpeptidation step of peptidoglycan synthesis in bacterial cell wall synthesis	CNS (confusion, dizziness), rash, GI, CDI; BMS (rare) Ceftriaxone—biliary toxicities/ obstructions	CI: IgE-mediated hypersensitivity to cephalosporins or penicillin derivatives W: Modify dosage in renal dysfunction (cefpodoxime/ cefotaxime), use with caution in patients with a delayed penicillin allergy (rash) and avoid in immediate allergic (anaphylaxis/IgE-mediated) penicillin reaction, do not use ceftriaxone in hyperbilirubinemia neonates—particularly those who are premature since ceftriaxone can displace bilirubin from albumin sites, ceftriaxone may complex with calcium causing precipitation—fatal lung and kidney damage has been observed in premature and term neonates	DI: Ceftriaxone—avoid concomitant use with calcium salts (IV) and lactated ringers injection GI: Pregnancy category B, renal elimination (ceftriaxone is 33%-67% eliminated via kidney and does not require dose reduction in renal dysfunction) M: With prolonged therapy, monitor renal hepatic function periodically, CBC with differential for cytopenias or signs of allergic reaction

(Continued)

TABLE 24-5   Properties of Antimicrobials Used in the Treatment of Skin and Soft Tissue Infections (*Continued*)

Antimicrobial	Formulations	Mechanism of Action	Side Effects	Contraindications (CI); Warnings (W)	Drug Interactions (DI); General Information (GI); Monitoring (M)
Fourth-Generation Cephalosporins					
Cefepime (Maxipime)	Parenteral	Inhibits bacterial cell wall synthesis by binding to one or more PBPs which inhibits the final transpeptidation step of peptidoglycan synthesis in bacterial cell wall synthesis	CDI, rash, CNS (encephalopathy, myoclonus, seizures), BMS (rare)	CI: IgE-mediated hypersensitivity to cephalosporins or penicillin derivatives W: Modify dosage in renal dysfunction—increased risk of encephalopathy, myoclonus, and seizures; use with caution in patients with a delayed penicillin allergy (rash) and avoid in immediate allergic (anaphylaxis/IgE-mediated) penicillin reaction, may be associated with increased INR, especially in nutritionally malnourished patients, prolonged treatment, hepatic or renal disease	GI: Pregnancy category B, renal elimination M: With prolonged therapy, monitor renal hepatic function periodically, CBC with differential for cytopenias or signs of allergic reaction
Fifth-Generation Cephalosporin					
Ceftaroline (Teflaro)	Parenteral	Inhibits bacterial cell wall synthesis by binding to one or more PBPs (binding to PBP2a grants anti-MRSA activity) which inhibits the final transpeptidation step of peptidoglycan synthesis in bacterial cell wall synthesis	CDI, rash, hypokalemia, elevated LFTs, CNS (seizures), BMS (rare), hepatitis (rare)	CI: IgE-mediated hypersensitivity to cephalosporins or penicillin derivatives W: Modify dosage in renal dysfunction—increased risk of encephalopathy, myoclonus, and seizures; use with caution in patients with a delayed penicillin allergy (rash) and avoid in immediate allergic (anaphylaxis/IgE-mediated) penicillin reaction, may be associated with increased INR, especially in nutritionally malnourished patients, prolonged treatment, hepatic or renal disease	GI: Pregnancy category B, renal elimination M: With prolonged therapy, monitor renal hepatic function periodically, CBC with differential for cytopenias or signs of allergic reaction
Penicillin Antimicrobials					
Penicillin (Pen VK, Bicillin CR or Bicillin LA, and Aqueous penicillin G)	Parenteral, oral (tablet, solution)	Inhibits bacterial cell wall synthesis by binding to one or more PBPs which inhibits the final transpeptidation step of peptidoglycan synthesis in bacterial cell wall synthesis	CNS (confusion, dizziness), rash, GI, CDI; BMS (rare)	CI: Hypersensitivity to penicillin W: Use with caution in patients with renal dysfunction (modify dose) or history of seizures, serious and occasionally severe or fatal hypersensitivity reactions have been reported in patients on penicillin therapy, especially with a history of β-lactam allergies, or previous IgE-mediated reactions (anaphylaxis, urticaria); Bicillin CR (procaine) and Bicillin LA (benzathine) are not interchangeable	GI: Pregnancy category B, renal elimination M: With prolonged therapy, monitor renal function periodically, CBC with differential for neutropenias or signs of allergic reaction
Penicillinase-Stable Penicillins					
Dicloxacillin (Dycill, others); Nafcillin (Unipen); Oxacillin (Bactocill)	Dicloxacillin: capsule; Nafcillin: parenteral; Oxacillin: parenteral	Inhibits bacterial cell wall synthesis by binding to one or more PBPs which inhibits the final transpeptidation step of peptidoglycan synthesis in bacterial cell wall synthesis	CNS (confusion, dizziness), rash, GI, CDI; BMS (rare), renal—acute interstitial nephritis (AIN), hepatotoxicity (oxacillin)	CI: Hypersensitivity to penicillins W: Serious and occasionally severe or fatal hypersensitivity reactions have been reported in patients on penicillin therapy, especially with a history of β-lactam allergies, history of sensitivity to multiple allergens, or previous IgE-mediated reactions (anaphylaxis, urticaria)	DI: Nafcillin—CYP-450 3A4 inducer GI: Dicloxacillin—Poor oral absorption, pregnancy category B nafcillin/oxacillin—Primarily eliminated via the liver; biliary and feces; minimal renal elimination (no renal adjustments required) M: With prolonged therapy, monitor renal function periodically (interstitial nephritis), LFT, CBC with differential for neutropenia or signs of allergic reaction

Aminopenicillins

Drug	Mechanism of Action	Adverse Effects	Contraindications/Warnings	Notes
Amoxicillin (Amoxil, Trimox); Ampicillin (Principen)	Inhibits bacterial cell wall synthesis by binding to one or more PBPs which inhibits the final transpeptidation step of peptidoglycan synthesis in bacterial cell wall synthesis	CNS—rare (confusion, dizziness), rash, GI (high incidence), CDI or superinfections, BMS (rare)	CI: Hypersensitivity to penicillins W: Serious and occasionally severe or fatal hypersensitivity reactions have been reported in patients on penicillin therapy, especially with a history of β-lactam allergies, history of sensitivity to multiple allergens, or previous IgE-mediated reactions (anaphylaxis, urticaria), high percentage of infectious mononucleosis patients have developed rash while taking ampicillin-class antibiotics	GI: Diarrhea, pregnancy category B, renal elimination M: With prolonged therapy, monitor renal function periodically, CBC with differential for neutropenias or signs of allergic reaction

β-Lactam/β-Lactamase Inhibitor Combinations

Drug	Mechanism of Action	Adverse Effects	Contraindications/Warnings	Notes
Amoxicillin/clavulanate (Augmentin); Ampicillin-sulbactam (Unasyn); Piperacillin-tazobactam (Zosyn)	Clavulanic acid, sulbactam, and tazobactam binds and inhibits β-lactamases that inactivate amoxicillin, ampicillin, or piperacillin resulting in an expanded spectrum of activity. Amoxicillin, ampicillin, and piperacillin inhibits bacterial cell wall synthesis by binding to one or more of the PBPs	CNS (confusion, dizziness), rash, GI, CDI; BMS (rare)	CI: Hypersensitivity to penicillins W: Use with caution in patients with renal dysfunction (modify dose) or history of seizures, serious and occasionally severe or fatal hypersensitivity reactions have been reported in patients on penicillin therapy, especially with a history of β-lactam allergies, history of sensitivity to multiple allergens, or previous IgE-mediated reactions (anaphylaxis, urticaria), high percentage of infectious mononucleosis patients have developed rash while taking ampicillin-class antibiotics; due to differing content of clavulanate—not all formulations are interchangeable CI for piperacillin only: Bleeding disorders have been observed, particularly in patients with renal dysfunction, discontinue if thrombocytopenia or bleeding occurs due to high sodium load and to adverse effects of high serum concentrations, dosage modifications are required in renal dysfunction	GI: Pregnancy category B, renal elimination M: With prolonged therapy, monitor renal and hematologic function periodically, signs of allergic reaction; piperacillin-tazobactam has 11.17 mEq of sodium in 4.5 g and 8.38 mEq in 3.375 g

Carbapenems

Drug	Mechanism of Action	Adverse Effects	Contraindications/Warnings	Notes
Imipenem-cilastatin (Primaxin); Meropenem (Merrem); Doripenem (Doribax); Ertapenem (Invanz)	Inhibits bacterial cell wall synthesis by binding to PBPs, which inhibits the final transpeptidation step of peptidoglycan synthesis. Cilastatin prevents renal metabolism of imipenem by inhibition of dehydropeptidase along the brush border of the renal tubules	CNS (confusion, dizziness), rash, GI, CDI; BMS (rare)	CI: Hypersensitivity to carbapenems W: Dosage reduction required in renal dysfunction has been associated with CNS adverse effects (confusion and seizures), use caution in patients with a history of seizures or hypersensitivity to β-lactams	GI: Pregnancy category C (imipenem) B (others), renal elimination; ertapenem does not cover *Pseudomonas* species M: With prolonged therapy, monitor renal and hematologic function periodically, signs of allergic reaction

(Continued)

TABLE 24-5 Properties of Antimicrobials Used in the Treatment of Skin and Soft Tissue Infections *(Continued)*

Antimicrobial	Formulations	Mechanism of Action	Side Effects	Contraindications (CI); Warnings (W)	Drug Interactions (DI); General Information (GI); Monitoring (M)
Fluoroquinolones					
Ciprofloxacin (Cipro); Levofloxacin (Levaquin); Moxifloxacin (Avelox)	Ciprofloxacin: parenteral, suspension, tablet; Levofloxacin: parenteral, suspension, tablet; Moxifloxacin: parenteral, tablet	Inhibits DNA gyrase—inhibits relaxation of supercoiled DNA and promotes breakage of double-stranded DNA	Headache, confusion, mental status changes, GI, CDI, BMS (rare), allergic reaction (immediate or delayed), hypoglycemia (early) or hyperglycemia (delayed), photosensitivity, peripheral neuropathy	CI: Hypersensitivity to quinolones W: Reports of tendon inflammation and/or rupture (black box warning), CNS stimulation may occur (tremor, restlessness, confusion, and rarely hallucination or seizures); use with caution in patients with CNS disorders; quinolones prolong QTc interval—avoid use in patients with a history of QTc prolongation, uncorrected hypokalemia, hypomagnesemia, or concurrent administration of medications known to prolong QT interval (Class 1a and Class III antiarrhythmics, erythromycin, antipsychotics, tricyclic antidepressants); adverse effects are increased in pediatric patients and should not be considered first-line agents in children (exception is anthrax treatment); dose reduction required in renal dysfunction, may exacerbate myasthenia gravis symptoms, peripheral neuropathy	DI: Divalent/trivalent cations, ciprofloxacin—inhibits CYP-450 1A2 (strong) and 3A4 (weak) GI: pregnancy category C, renal elimination M: With prolonged therapy, monitor renal and hematologic function periodically, signs of allergic reaction, drug interactions, neuropathy, EKG
MRSA Antimicrobials					
Clindamycin (Cleocin)	Capsule, solution, parenteral	Reversibly binds to 50s ribosomal subunits preventing peptide bond formation thus inhibiting bacterial protein synthesis	Rash, GI, CDI, BMS (rare), pill esophagitis (rare)	CI: Hypersensitivity to clindamycin W: Dosage adjustment necessary for severe hepatic dysfunction, can cause fatal colitis (C. difficile) (black box warning)	GI: Pregnancy category B, hepatic metabolism, with prolonged therapy monitor renal and hematologic function periodically, observe for changes in bowel frequency
Doxycycline (Vibramycin, others); Minocycline (Minocin, Dynacin)	Doxycycline: capsule, parenteral, suspension, syrup, tablet Minocycline: capsule, tablet, parenteral	Inhibits protein synthesis by binding with the 30s and 50s ribosomal subunit	Rash (photosensitivity), GI, CDI, BMS (rare), hepatotoxicity (rare), autoimmune disease reported, pill esophagitis (rare)	CI: Hypersensitivity to doxycycline or tetracycline, children ≤8 y (except in treatment of anthrax) W: Photosensitivity reaction may occur—avoid prolonged exposure to sunlight or tanning equipment, antianabolic effects may increase BUN, hepatotoxicity has been reported; Minocycline: CNS effects (lightheadedness, vertigo) may occur Outdated tetracycline can cause Fanconi syndrome (renal compromise)	DI: Divalent/trivalent cations, doxycycline—inhibits CYP-450 3A4 (moderate) GI: Pregnancy category D M: Complete blood count, renal, liver function tests periodically with prolonged therapy
Trimethoprim-sulfamethoxazole (Septra, Bactrim)	Parenteral, tablet, suspension	Sulfamethoxazole interferes with bacterial folic acid synthesis and growth via inhibition of dihydrofolic acid formation from para-aminobenzoic acid; trimethoprim inhibits dihydrofolic acid reduction to tetrahydrofolate resulting in inhibition of enzymes of the folic acid pathway	GI, CDI, rash, photosensitivity, hyperkalemia, BMS, hepatitis, renal failure, allergic reaction	CI: Hypersensitivity to any sulfa drug, trimethoprim, megaloblastic anemia due to folate deficiency W: Use with caution in patients with G6PD deficiency, impaired renal or hepatic function or potential folate deficiency (malnourished, chronic anticonvulsant therapy, or elderly), adjust dose in renal impairment, fatalities associated with severe reactions including Stevens-Johnson syndrome, toxic epidermal necrolysis, agranulocytosis, and aplastic anemia—discontinue use at first sign of rash or serious adverse reaction	DI: Sulfamethoxazole—substrate CYP 2C9 (major), 3A4 (minor), inhibits 2C9 (moderate) Trimethoprim—substrate 2C9 (major), 3A4 (major), inhibits 2C8 (moderate), 2C9 (moderate) GI: Pregnancy category C/D, may falsely increase SCr levels due to competitive inhibition for active tubular secretion; no activity against GAS M: Complete blood count, potassium, serum creatinine, signs/symptoms of allergic reaction

Drug	Route/Formulation	Mechanism	Adverse Effects	CI/W	Other
Daptomycin (Cubicin)	Parenteral	Binds to components of the cell membrane and causes rapid depolarization, inhibiting intracellular synthesis of DNA, RNA, and protein	GI, CDI, anemia, BMS, headache, rash, CPK elevation—muscle pain	CI: Hypersensitivity to daptomycin. W: Associated with myopathy, discontinue in patients with signs and symptoms of myopathy in conjunction with increase in CPK >5 times upper limit of normal or in asymptomatic patients with CPK >10 times upper limit of normal, not indicated for treatment of pneumonia, use caution in renal dysfunction (dosage adjustment required)	GI: Pregnancy category B. M: CPK at least weekly (more frequent if on a statin), muscle weakness/pain
Tigecycline (Tygacil)	Parenteral	Binds to 30s ribosomal subunit, inhibiting protein synthesis	GI, CDI, headache, dizziness, rash, BMS, increased LFTs	CI: Hypersensitivity to tigecycline. W: Due to structural similarity with tetracyclines, use caution in patients allergic to tetracyclines, other tetracyclines' effects are possible as well—photosensitivity, antianabolic effects, discoloration of teeth; increased all-cause mortality versus comparators (black box warning)	GI: Pregnancy category D, systemic clearance reduced in hepatic impairment—adjust dose in severe hepatic impairment (Child-Pugh C), no dosing adjustment required in renal dysfunction
Linezolid (Zyvox)	Parenteral, tablet, suspension	Inhibits bacterial protein synthesis by binding to 23s ribosomal RNA of the 50s subunit	Headache, GI, CDI, rash, BMS. BMS (including anemia, leukopenia, pancytopenia, and thrombocytopenia) may be more common in patients receiving therapy for >2 wk	CI: Hypersensitivity to linezolid, concurrent use if within 2 wk of monoamine oxidase inhibitors, patients with uncontrolled hypertension, taking sympathomimetics, vasopressive agents, or dopaminergic agents unless closely monitored for increase in blood pressure, patients taking antidepressants with serotonin mechanism, meperidine unless closely monitored for serotonin syndrome. W: Lactic acidosis has been reported with use (rare), myelosuppression has been reported and is more common with >2 wk of therapy but can occur earlier, peripheral and optic neuropathy has been reported, especially with >28 d of therapy. Any neuropathic symptoms require immediate evaluation	DI: Sympathomimetics, antidepressants with serotonin activity, meperidine, tyramine-containing foods (hypertensive crisis). GI: Pregnancy category C. M: Weekly CBC, particularly in patients at increased risk of bleeding, preexisting myelosuppression, on concomitant medications that cause BMS, those requiring more than 2 wk of therapy
Vancomycin (Vancocin)	Parenteral, capsule (capsule is not absorbed and used for treatment of CDI)	Inhibits bacterial cell wall synthesis by blocking glycopeptide polymerization through binding of D-alanyl-D-alanine portion of cell wall precursor	Red-man syndrome (rash), BMS (rare, except with high dose), ototoxicity, nephrotoxicity, increase nephrotoxic potential when combined with aminoglycoside	CI: Hypersensitivity to vancomycin. W: May cause nephrotoxicity, usual risk factors are pre-existing renal dysfunction, concurrent nephrotoxic agent, advanced age, and dehydration; ototoxicity is proportional to the amount of drug given and duration of treatment—tinnitus or vertigo may be indications of vestibular injury and impending bilateral irreversible damage	GI: Pregnancy category C, reduce dose in renal dysfunction, administer vancomycin by intravenous infusion over at least 60 min, if maculopapular rash appears on the face, neck, trunk, and/or upper extremities (Redman syndrome), slow infusion rate to over 1.5-2 h +/- antihistamines. M: Renal function, complete blood count, serum vancomycin concentrations, audiogram

Abbreviations: BMS, bone marrow suppression; BUN, blood urine nitrogen; CBC, complete blood count; CDI, *Clostridium difficile* infection; CNS, central nervous system; CPK, creatine phosphokinase; DNA, deoxynucleic acid; EKG, electrocardiogram; GAS, group A streptococci; GI, gastrointestinal; INR, international normalized ratio; LFT, liver function test; mEq, milliequivalent; PBP, penicillin-binding protein; RNA, ribonucleic acid; SCr, serum creatinine.

TABLE 24-6 **Empirical Therapy for Osteomyelitis**

Type of Osteomyelitis	Probable Pathogen	Potential Empirical Regimens[a]
Hematogenous	S. aureus (MSSA or MRSA)	**MRSA not suspected:** Nafcillin/oxacillin 2 g IV every 4 h *or* Cefazolin 2 g IV every 8 h **Penicillin allergic:** Clindamycin 600-900 mg IV every 6-8 h *or* Vancomycin 15-20 mg/kg IV every 12 h[b] **MRSA suspected:** Vancomycin 15-20 mg/kg IV every 12 h[b] *or* linezolid 600 mg every 12 h *or* daptomycin 4 mg/kg *or* ceftaroline 600 mg every 12 h
Contiguous or vascular insufficiency	S. aureus (MSSA or MRSA), streptococci, Enterobacteriaceae, anaerobes	General approach: start parenteral, broad-spectrum antibiotics with activity against gram-positive, gram-negative, and anaerobic bacteria that are likely to cause infections of the adjacent skin or organ. Include coverage for MRSA according to patient history and resistance patterns in the area. Ampicillin-sulbactam 3 g every 6 h[c] *or* ertapenem 1 g daily[c] *or* ceftriaxone 2 g daily + clindamycin 600-900 mg every 6-8 h *or* metronidazole 500 mg every 8 h[c] *or* piperacillin-tazobactam 3.375-4.5 g every 6 h *or* imipenem-cilastatin 500 mg every 6 h *or* meropenem 1 g every 8 h *or* doripenem 500 mg every 8 h *or* ciprofloxacin 400 mg every 8-12 h or levofloxacin 750 mg daily + clindamycin 600-900 mg every 6-8 h or metronidazole 500 mg every 8 h *or* tigecycline 100 mg load, then 50 mg every 12 h[c,d] *or* moxifloxacin 400 mg daily[c] **If MRSA suspected:** ADD vancomycin 15-20 mg/kg q12h[b] *or* linezolid 600 mg every 12 h *or* daptomycin 4 mg/kg *or* ceftaroline 600 mg every 12 h

Abbreviations: MRSA, methicillin-resistant *S. aureus*; MSSA, methicillin-sensitive *S. aureus*; IV, intravenous.

[a]Adult dose with normal renal function.

[b]Vancomycin dose should be individualized to patient's parameters and goals.

[c]This regimen does not cover *P. aeruginosa*.

[d]Tigecycline covers MRSA but should be reserved for last-line therapy.

CASE Application

1. Which organism(s) is(are) the most common cause of SSTIs? Select all that apply.

   a. *Streptococcus pyogenes*
   b. *Staphylococcus aureus*
   c. *Pasteurella multicida*
   d. *Enterobacter cloacae*

2. TR is a 29-year-old pregnant patient with a diagnosis of cellulitis. TR has no drug allergies and is not on any other medications. Select the most appropriate antibiotic that may be used to treat TR's infection.

   a. Cefazolin
   b. Doxycycline
   c. Imipenem-cilastatin
   d. Levofloxacin

The following patient case pertains to questions 3 through 5.

AB, a 30-year-old man who does not have any significant previous medical history nor drug allergies, was admitted to the hospital with an abscess and associated cellulitis. After appropriate drainage of the abscess, AB was initiated on intravenous vancomycin therapy. The culture from the incision and drainage grew caMRSA. AB's clinical status improved with 2 days of vancomycin therapy and thus will be discharged home with an oral antibiotic to finish his therapy.

3. Which of the following antibiotic(s) is(are) appropriate step-down options for AB? Select all that apply.

   a. Cephalexin
   b. Minocycline
   c. Tigecycline
   d. Trimethoprim-sulfamethoxazole

4. Doxycycline is chosen as the step-down therapy for AB's cellulitis. What pertinent counseling point(s) should be provided to AB regarding this medication? Select all that apply.

   a. Doxycycline may cause your teeth to turn brown.
   b. Avoid direct sunlight for prolonged periods and wear sunscreen.
   c. Doxycycline may turn your urine and tears into an orange-red color.
   d. Avoid taking this medication with antacids.

5. During discharge counseling, AB expresses concern that he may spread his infection to others. What are some measures he can take to minimize this risk? Select all that apply.

   a. Wash linens with cold water.
   b. Keep wound covered with a clean and dry dressing until it has healed.
   c. Avoid sharing personal hygiene products with others.
   d. As the infection is being treated with antibiotics, there are no precautions needed.

6. RD is an 18-year-old woman who presents to a clinic with cellulitis. The local antibiogram reveals that <1% of *S. aureus* that were isolated last year were methicillin resistant. The treating physician would like to prescribe an oral antibiotic regimen that covers both *S. aureus* and GAS. Which of the following regimens is the most appropriate for monotherapy?

   a. Amoxicillin
   b. Cephalexin
   c. Ciprofloxacin
   d. Trimethoprim-sulfamethoxazole

7. What is the brand name of linezolid?

   a. Teflaro
   b. Tygacil
   c. Zosyn
   d. Zyvox

8. OT is a 45-year-old man with diabetes who was diagnosed with a mild foot infection. Since he has a history of chronic renal insufficiency, the provider would like to use an antibiotic that does not have to be adjusted for renal dysfunction. To treat his diabetic foot infection, select the antibiotic(s) that does(do) not require adjustment for renal dysfunction.

   a. Cefazolin
   b. Linezolid
   c. Nafcillin
   d. Vancomycin

9. Select the antibiotic that may cause an adverse reaction during or soon after infusion characterized by itching, warmth, flushing, and rash (among other symptoms), especially if infused at a rate faster than recommended.

   a. Ampicillin
   b. Cefazolin
   c. Daptomycin
   d. Vancomycin

The following patient case pertains to questions 10 and 11.

BC is a 40-year-old woman, who has hypertension and drug allergies to penicillins (angioedema, hives) and sulfa drugs (rash), presents to urgent care with a dry and intensely red lesion about 5 cm by 5 cm in size, with well-demarcated and raised borders on her right lower extremity. She describes having pain and burning sensation.

10. What is the most likely type of SSTI that BC is experiencing?

   a. Cellulitis
   b. Folliculitis
   c. Impetigo
   d. Erysipelas

11. What is the most appropriate oral antibiotic for BC's SSTI?

   a. Amoxicillin
   b. Cefuroxime
   c. Clindamycin
   d. Vancomycin

12. Among the following, select the β-lactam(s) that have activity against penicillinase-producing *Staphylococcus aureus*. Select all that apply.

   a. Ampicillin
   b. Cefazolin
   c. Dicloxacillin
   d. Doxycycline

13. GT is a 60-year-old man who was initiated on vancomycin and piperacillin-tazobactam for a rapidly progressing cellulitis in the emergency department. Upon arrival to the critical care unit, GT was determined to have necrotizing fasciitis. What, if anything, should be adjusted to the patient's antibiotic regimen?

   a. Add clindamycin.
   b. Change piperacillin-tazobactam to cefepime.
   c. Discontinue piperacillin-tazobactam.
   d. The current regimen is optimal, with no changes necessary.

14. What is the generic name of Omnicef?

   a. Cefdinir
   b. Cefpodoxime
   c. Cefuroxime
   d. Cephalexin

The following patient case pertains to questions 15 and 16.

15. HW is a 7-year-old girl who was bitten on the forearm by a dog. While the wound was superficial, it now shows signs of infection. The wound was thoroughly irrigated and cleaned. The patient does not have any allergies. What are the most common organisms that may cause the infection? Select all that apply.

   a. *Pasteurella multocida*
   b. *Escherichia coli*
   c. *Eikenella corrodens*
   d. Streptococci

16. What is the most appropriate antibiotic monotherapy for HW's dog bite wound infection?

   a. Augmentin
   b. Avelox
   c. Cleocin
   d. Doxycycline

The following patient case pertains to questions 17 and 18.

17. PT is a 58-year-old woman with diabetes who will be started on Zosyn and an MRSA-active antibiotic for her diabetic foot infection with osteomyelitis. The patient's other medications include simvastatin, metoprolol, fenofibrate, escitalopram, and metformin. The team is concerned with potential drug interactions and wants to avoid medications that interact with the patient's chronic

medications. Which of the following medications is the most appropriate for MRSA coverage?

a. Daptomycin
b. Linezolid
c. Moxifloxacin
d. Vancomycin

18. Which of the following is a reasonable duration of antimicrobial therapy for PT's infection?

a. 1 week
b. 2 weeks
c. 3 weeks
d. 6 weeks

19. ZD is a 50-year-old man (83.3 kg) who was admitted into the hospital for cellulitis and was empirically initiated on vancomycin 15 mg/kg every 12 hours. Because of an adverse reaction he suffered when he previously received vancomycin, the medical team would like to infuse vancomycin at a rate of 500 mg/h. The pharmacy policy for final concentration of reconstituted vancomycin is at 5 mg/mL. What is the correct rate of infusion (mL/h) for his vancomycin and how long will it take to infuse each dose?

a. 50 mL/h for 5 hours
b. 100 mL/h for 2.5 hours
c. 125 mL/h for 2 hours
d. 200 mL/h for 2.5 hours

20. TY is a 29-year-old woman with a mild penicillin allergy who is being treated with an intravenous antibiotic in the hospital for a severe lymphangitis. The patient is not receiving any other medications. One week into therapy, TY's creatine phosphokinase (CPK) elevated to six times above the normal level and she complains of muscle aches. Which antimicrobial agent is TY most likely receiving and contributing to this lab abnormality and symptom?

a. Cefuroxime
b. Daptomycin
c. Linezolid
d. Vancomycin

21. DM is a 51-year-old man with uncontrolled diabetes, 20-year 1 pack/d smoking history who just finished treatment for his first episode of a mild diabetic foot infection. He is interested in learning preventive strategies to reduce his chances of another infection. Which counseling point is appropriate for DM? Select all that apply.

a. Obtain periodic foot exams.
b. Work toward improving his control of diabetes.
c. Work toward smoking cessation.
d. Walk in open-toed shoes or barefoot as much as possible to keep feet dry.

TAKEAWAY POINTS ››

- SSTIs can range in severity from mild to severe, and may involve any or all layers of the skin, as well as the underlying fascia and muscle. They may also spread and lead to severe complications, such as sepsis, bacteremia, glomerulonephritis, endocarditis, or osteomyelitis.
- *Staphylococcus aureus* and *Streptococcus pyogenes* (also known as GAS and β-hemolytic streptococci) account for the majority of SSTIs. Depending on the type of SSTI, empiric antibiotic therapy (if necessary) should target these pathogens.
- Folliculitis, furuncles, and carbuncles are caused by *S. aureus* and treated with nonpharmacologic therapy, such as moist heat and incision and drainage. For severe infections, antibiotics active against *S. aureus* are also utilized.
- Impetigo is a superficial skin infection caused by β-hemolytic *Streptococcus* and *S. aureus* and treated with first-generation cephalosporins or penicillinase-stable penicillins. Topical mupirocin may be used alone when there are minimal lesions.
- Lymphangitis is an inflammation of the lymphatic channel that ensues when a local skin infection is not contained, most often caused by GAS and treated with penicillin.
- Erysipelas is an infection of the superficial layer of the skin and cutaneous lymphatics. Erysipelas is treated with penicillin.

- Cellulitis is an acute, infectious process that represents a serious type of SSTI most commonly caused by *S. aureus* and GAS. Empiric pharmacologic treatment should be directed against these organisms and possibly other organisms depending on patient-specific risk factors and severity of infection.
- NF is an uncommon, rapidly progressive, life-threatening infection of the subcutaneous tissue and fascia. Prompt surgical intervention and appropriate antibiotic therapy are essential to successfully treat NF. A high-dose, β-lactam/β-lactamase inhibitor or carbapenem may be used in combination with clindamycin to treat NF. Vancomycin, daptomycin, ceftaroline, or linezolid should be included until MRSA is excluded.
- DFIs are among the most common, severe, and costly complications of diabetes mellitus. They are usually polymicrobial and caused by pathogens like Enterobacteriaceae, MRSA, and *P. aeruginosa*.
- Osteomyelitis is most often caused by *S. aureus*, but the patient's age, predisposing factors, type (eg, hematogenous), and location of the infection may change the primary causative pathogen, which includes polymicrobial infection.
- Several different antibiotics may be utilized in the treatment of SSTIs. Properties of an antibiotic influence

the preference for one agent over the other. Key characteristics, such as the side effect profile, drug interactions, formulation, and pregnancy category, may influence the selection of an antibiotic.

- caMRSA is rapidly increasing in prevalence as a cause of SSTIs (including cellulitis). Local prevalence and susceptibility should be considered when selecting empiric treatment.

- Optimizing personal hygiene and modifiable risk factors (such as control of diabetes) are key strategies in preventing SSTIs.

BIBLIOGRAPHY

Fish DN. Skin and soft-tissue infections. In: DiPiro JT, Talbert RL, Yee GC, Matzke GR, Wells BG, Posey L, eds. *Pharmacotherapy: A Pathophysiologic Approach.* 10th ed. New York, NY: McGraw-Hill; 2017.

Lipsky BA, Berendt AR, Cornia PB, et al. 2012 Infectious Diseases Society of America clinical practice guideline for the diagnosis and treatment of diabetic foot infections. *Clin Infect Dis.* 2012;54(12):e132-e173.

Liu C, Bayer A, Cosgrove SE, et al. Clinical practice guidelines by the infectious diseases society of America for the treatment of methicillin-resistant Staphylococcus aureus infections in adults and children. *Clin Infect Dis.* 2011;52(3):e18-e55.

Stevens DL, Bisno AL, Chambers HF, et al. Practice guidelines for the diagnosis and management of skin and soft tissue infections. *Clin Infect Dis.* 2005;41:1373-1406.

Stevens DL, Bisno AL, Chambers HF, et al. Practice guidelines for the diagnosis and management of skin and soft-tissue infections: 2014 update by the Infectious Diseases Society of America. *Clin Infect Dis.* 2014;59:e10-e52.

KEY ABBREVIATIONS

caMRSA = community-associated methicillin-resistant *Staphylococcus aureus*
CPK = creatine phosphokinase
DFI = diabetic foot infection
GAS = group A streptococcus
haMRSA = health care-associated methicillin-resistant *Staphylococcus aureus*

MRSA = methicillin-resistant *Staphylococcus aureus*
MSSA = methicillin-sensitive *Staphylococcus aureus*
NF = necrotizing fasciitis
PBP = penicillin-binding protein
SSTI = skin and soft tissue infection
TMP-SMX = trimethoprim-sulfamethoxazole

25 Central Nervous System Infections

Julie Ann Justo and Daniel B. Chastain

FOUNDATION OVERVIEW

Central nervous system (CNS) infections are often differentiated by the cause and type of infection (meningitis or encephalitis). Meningitis is a CNS infection characterized by inflammation of the meninges, or the layers of tissue that surround the brain and spinal cord. In contrast, encephalitis is an infection and inflammation of the brain. Aseptic meningitis occurs secondary to pathogens or other causes that do not grow in the microbiology laboratory when cultured (eg, viruses, atypical bacteria, fungi, drug causes). Meningitis (aseptic more than bacterial) is the most common type of CNS infection, followed by viral encephalitis.

Bacterial Meningitis

Pathogens associated with bacterial meningitis vary based upon the age of the patient. In neonates and infants less than 3 months of age, the most common isolated bacteria is *Streptococcus agalactiae* (also known as group B *Streptococcus*), followed by *Escherichia coli*, *Streptococcus pneumoniae*, and *Listeria monocytogenes*. Specifically, early onset meningitis (first week of life) is associated with pathogens found in the maternal genital tract (eg, *S. agalactiae, E. coli, L. monocytogenes*). Meningitis occurring from 1 to 4 weeks of age is associated with maternal and community-associated pathogens (eg, *S. pneumoniae*) or with nosocomial pathogens (eg, *Staphylococcus aureus, Enterobacter* species) in hospitalized infants. From 2 to 3 months of age, the likelihood of pathogens from the maternal genital tract decrease and the community-associated pathogens become prevalent. In children over 3 months old and adults, the most common causes of bacterial meningitis are *S. pneumoniae* and *Neisseria meningitidis*. Common bacterial causes of meningitis in patients older than 50 years include *S. pneumoniae, N. meningitidis,* and *L. monocytogenes.*

In order to cause meningitis, a bacteria must be able to avoid the patient's normal barriers to infection and cause systemic infection. Next, the bacteria are able to cross the blood–brain barrier, multiply, stimulate inflammation in the subarachnoid and ventricular space, and cause damage. In the neonate, the blood–brain barrier is not well developed and allows bacteria to cross more readily than in an older patient. *Neisseria meningitidis* and *S. pneumoniae* are common causes of bacterial meningitis in older infants and adults because they are surrounded by a polysaccharide capsule that assists in avoiding the usual immune system response to bacterial invasion. Additionally, when patients are immunosuppressed (by disease, drugs, or functional/anatomical asplenia) or have interrupted barriers, such as broken skin (eg, cochlear implants, recent trauma), bacteria are more likely to be able to cause disease.

Aseptic Meningitis and Viral Encephalitis

Viral meningitis is the most frequent infectious cause of aseptic meningitis and is common in infants less than 1 year old. The most common cause of viral meningitis in children are enteroviruses. Two common types of enteroviruses are coxsackie and echoviruses. Additionally, nonviral infectious causes of aseptic meningitis include mycobacterial and spirochetal (eg, *Borrelia burgdorferi*).

Viral encephalitis is the least frequent of the CNS infections and the majority of cases have an unknown etiology. The most frequent virus identified is herpes simplex virus (HSV). Other viral causes include: enteroviruses, other herpes viruses (eg, varicella, cytomegalovirus, Epstein-Barr virus, and human herpes virus 6), adenoviruses, arboviruses (eg, West Nile virus, St. Louis encephalitis virus, Eastern equine encephalitis virus, and Western equine encephalitis virus), measles, mumps, and rubella viruses, influenza viruses, bunyaviruses, reoviruses, arenaviruses, and rabies viruses.

Pathogens that cause aseptic meningitis and viral encephalitis enter the body as they would usually cause infection (eg, orally for enterovirus, tick bite for *B. burgdorferi*). The pathogen, however, moves from the usual site of infection via the blood to the CNS where it leads to encephalitis or meningitis. Herpes viruses are unusual as they can travel to the CNS by either the blood or travel along the neuron. Additionally, herpes viruses are also unique as they can cause meningitis/encephalitis during initial disease or by reactivation of disease. A summary of the typical infectious causes of meningitis and encephalitis by age are shown in Table 25-1.

Clinical Presentation

The clinical presentation of a CNS infection is dependent upon age. Neonates and young infants with meningitis or encephalitis may have nonspecific symptoms such as poor feeding,

---

To access your complimentary online question exams, visit https://accesspharmacy.mhmedical.com/NAPLEX.aspx

TABLE 25-1 Common Infectious Causes of Meningitis and Encephalitis by Age

Neonates

Bacteria: *S. agalactiae*, aerobic gram-negative bacilli[a], *L. monocytogenes*

Viral: HSV, CMV, enterovirus, adenovirus, rubella virus

Other: *T. gondii, T. pallidum*

Young Infants

Bacteria: *S. pneumoniae, N. meningitidis, H. influenzae, S. agalactiae, E. coli*

Viral: enteroviruses, HSV, EBV, adenovirus

Older Infants, Children, and Adults

Bacterial: *S. pneumoniae, N. meningitidis*

Viral: enteroviruses, adenovirus, HSV, WNV, EEEV, influenza virus, La Crosse virus

Other: *B. burgdorferi*

Adults >50 y

Bacterial: *S. pneumoniae, N. meningitidis*, aerobic gram-negative bacilli[a], *L. monocytogenes*

Viral: enteroviruses, HSV, WNV, EEEV, St. Louis encephalitis virus

Other: *B. burgdorferi*

Abbreviations: CMV, cytomegalovirus; EBV, Epstein-Barr virus; HSV, herpes simplex virus; EEEV, Eastern equine encephalitis virus; WNV, West Nile virus.
[a]Such as *E. coli* or *Klebsiella* spp.

fever, or irritability. Older children and adults with meningitis usually present with the classic signs of meningitis including a temperature more than 101.3°F, headache, neck stiffness, and altered consciousness. Other symptoms including seizures are less common. Older children and adults are more likely to also have positive Kernig or Brudzinski signs. Similar to meningitis, patients with infectious encephalitis usually have fever, headache, altered consciousness, and seizures, but they also have specific focal neurologic signs.

Diagnosis

Meningitis is diagnosed based on symptoms plus laboratory data from the cerebrospinal fluid (CSF) (Table 25-2). These laboratory data assist in the differentiation between viral and bacterial meningitis. Generally, in bacterial meningitis the CSF is cloudy, CSF white blood cell (WBC) count elevated (often >1000 cells/mm³) with a predominance of neutrophils,

TABLE 25-2 Typical CSF Laboratory Values for Bacterial and Viral Meningitis

	WBC/mm³	Neutrophils (%)	CSF Glucose	CSF Protein
Bacterial	1000-10,000	80-90[a]	<40 mg/dL	>100 mg/dL
Viral	100-1000	<40[a]	Normal	<100 mg/dL[b]

[a]Although it may be lower in partially treated bacterial meningitis or higher in early enteroviral meningitis.
[b]Or appropriate for age, as infants <6 months old may have higher normal CSF protein.

the CSF glucose concentration is decreased (<40 mg/dL) with a CSF:serum glucose ratio of less than or equal to 0.4, while the CSF protein is elevated (>100 mg/dL). In viral meningitis, the CSF WBC is also increased (although not usually as high) with a monocytic or lymphocytic predominance. Additionally, the CSF glucose and protein concentrations are less likely to be abnormal. It is important to note that these are the usual findings, as 10% patients with enteroviral meningitis have a predominance of neutrophils while some patients with bacterial meningitis may not, especially if they have received prior antibiotic therapy.

The Gram stain and culture from the CSF is another tool used to assist in differentiating the type of meningitis. The Gram stain is more likely to be positive in patients with high concentrations of bacteria in the CSF. When the Gram stain is positive, many practitioners find it helpful in focusing antibiotic therapy. In most patients with bacterial meningitis, an organism will be grown from the CSF culture. There are two significant limitations of the CSF culture. First, the results are not quickly available, so empiric antibiotic therapy must be determined prior to culture results. Secondly, patients that received prior antibiotic treatment are less likely to grow bacteria. Additionally, as enteroviruses are the most likely cause of viral meningitis, enteroviral polymerase chain reaction (PCR) and/or culture is useful to assist in solidifying a diagnosis of viral meningitis.

It is much more difficult to identify a causative pathogen in infectious encephalitis. Since many etiologies of encephalitis exist, initial testing is often based on patient history and common pathogens. Tests often include bacterial and fungal cultures of the CSF fluid, and PCR of common viruses (including HSV and enterovirus). Additional cultures (blood, respiratory, stool), serologic testing, or other tests are also often performed.

PREVENTION

The focus for prevention of neonatal meningitis has been to decrease exposure to pathogens in the birth canal. Specifically, rates of early group B streptococcal meningitis have decreased significantly by identifying and treating mothers colonized with the bacteria with either intravenous (IV) penicillin or ampicillin during the delivery period.

Vaccination against common bacteria is the primary means of prevention of some CNS diseases including meningitis in older infants and adults. Specifically, the vaccines against encapsulated bacteria (*Haemophilus influenzae* type b, *N. meningitidis, S. pneumoniae*) decrease the likelihood of bacterial meningitis. The *H. influenzae* type b (Hib) vaccine has had such efficacy in reducing systemic infections due to this pathogen that it is no longer a common cause of bacterial meningitis in developed countries. The meningococcal vaccines and pneumococcal vaccines also provide protection against the strains covered by the vaccines. Vaccine specifics are provided in Table 25-3. Vaccine recommendations are updated annually and available at www.cdc.gov/vaccines. Currently, the minimum approved age for both the meningococcal and the pneumococcal conjugate vaccines is 6 weeks.

TABLE 25-3	Comparison of Pneumococcal and Meningococcal Vaccines				
	Pneumococcal Vaccines		**Meningococcal Vaccines**		
Abbreviated name	PCV13	PPSV23	Hib-MenCY	MCV4	MPSV4
Type of inactive vaccine	Conjugated	Polysaccharide	Conjugated	Conjugated	Polysaccharide
Strains included	13	23	2 (plus Hib)	4	4
Indication(s)	Routine pediatric vaccination; Vaccination for patients in other age groups at risk for pneumococcal disease[a]	Routine for patients ≥65 y; Vaccination for patients ≥2 y at risk for pneumococcal disease[a]	Patients at risk for meningococcal disease[b]	Routine adolescent vaccination; Vaccination for patients in other age groups at risk for meningococcal disease[b]	Patients at risk for meningococcal disease[b] (preferred for vaccine-naïve patients ≥56 y)
Age group	≥6 wk	≥2 y	6 wk-18 mo	9 mo-55 y	≥2 y (preferred ≥56 y)
Route of administration	Intramuscular	Intramuscular	Intramuscular	Intramuscular	Subcutaneous
Adverse effects	Injection site reactions, fever	Injection site reactions (Note: fever and muscle pain are uncommon)	Injection site reactions, fever, irritability, drowsiness, decreased appetite	Injection site reactions, fever, headache, malaise, reports of Guillain-Barré	Injection site reactions, fever, headache, malaise
Contraindications	Severe allergic reaction (eg, anaphylaxis) to prior dose of vaccine or to a vaccine component.				
Precautions	Moderate to severe illness. For MCV4 vaccine products, a history of Guillain-Barré Syndrome (GBS) is listed as a precaution in FDA labeling; yet, current guideline recommendations state the benefits of vaccination may outweigh the risk of recurrent GBS, if vaccination is otherwise indicated.				

[a]At-risk patients defined by age group and often include those who have a chronic disease (eg, cardiovascular, respiratory, diabetes mellitus, alcoholism, cirrhosis, CSF leak, or cochlear implants), are immunocompromised (eg, medication-induced, asplenia), reside in nursing homes or long-term care facilities, or smoke cigarettes.

[b]At-risk patients defined by age group and often include those with persistent complement deficiencies, anatomic or functional asplenia (eg, sickle cell disease), college freshmen living in dorms, military recruits, microbiologists that work with *N. meningitidis*, those present during outbreak caused by a vaccine serogroup, and those traveling to the African meningitis belt or to the Hajj (Hib-MenCY is insufficient for travelers).

Additionally, other routine vaccinations including measles, mumps, rubella (MMR), and varicella are thought to have decreased encephalitis infections due to these organisms. All of these vaccines are subcutaneous, live-virus vaccines included in the routine immunization schedules for children older than 1 year. Adverse reactions to the live vaccines are most likely to occur between days 5 and 12. Injection site reaction, fever, and rash are common, occurring in 5% to 33% of patients. Transient arthralgias and arthritis have been reported in one-fourth of postpubertal females. Rare adverse effects include thrombocytopenia (MMR), anaphylaxis, and CNS dysfunction. Cases of disseminated disease in immunocompromised patients receiving the vaccines have been reported. Since both vaccines contain live viruses, neither should be given to patients with most immunodeficiencies (some HIV patients can receive the vaccines and patients with isolated humoral immunodeficiency may be able to receive varicella vaccine), immunosuppressing conditions (including radiation and medications), those who are pregnant, and in those with moderate to severe illness. Additionally, vaccines should be avoided in patients with a prior allergic reaction to the vaccine or its components. Both the MMR vaccine and the varicella vaccine contain neomycin and gelatin, so both should be avoided in patients allergic to either component. It is also important to note that although there has been much media attention surrounding vaccines and autism, scientific groups have independently investigated the data and have not found any link between any vaccine and autism.

TREATMENT

Guidelines for bacterial meningitis and encephalitis provide empiric antibiotic recommendations for bacterial meningitis based upon age. The IV route of administration is recommended for treatment of patients with bacterial meningitis.

In neonates, empiric therapy includes ampicillin plus either an aminoglycoside (eg, gentamicin) or cefotaxime. The ampicillin is necessary to cover for *L. monocytogenes*. Patients between 1 month old and 50 years old should receive vancomycin plus either cefotaxime or ceftriaxone. Adult patients over the age of 50 years should receive ampicillin in addition to the vancomycin and cefotaxime or ceftriaxone. Again the ampicillin is to provide additional coverage against the *L. monocytogenes*. Further, monotherapy with IV ceftriaxone is recommended in patients with aseptic meningitis with a suspicion of Lyme meningitis (as long as there is no concern for HSV).

It is important to note that the recommendation of adding vancomycin to the antibiotic regimen when *S. pneumoniae* is a likely pathogen is due to the possibility of multidrug-resistant *S. pneumoniae* (resistant to the third generation cephalosporins). Although most pneumococcal isolates are susceptible to the third-generation cephalosporins, increases in nonsusceptibility for some serotypes (19A) have been reported. Therefore, vancomycin should be added to any empiric meningitis antibiotic regimen where *S. pneumoniae* is a likely pathogen. Finally, once the pathogen is identified and susceptibilities are determined therapy should be appropriately narrowed.

The use of dexamethasone in bacterial meningitis has been debated. In theory, the dexamethasone decreases the inflammation, which is thought to be the cause for many of the meningitis sequelae. However, some clinicians are concerned with using dexamethasone because when inflammation is decreased the penetration of medications into the CNS is also diminished. In children, dexamethasone has only demonstrated benefit against *H. influenzae* meningitis. Since this pathogen is no longer a common cause of meningitis in children, no consensus exists regarding the routine use of dexamethasone in children. Initially shown in one randomized controlled trial, and reinforced by two meta-analyses, adjunctive dexamethasone has decreased mortality and improved outcomes in adults with pneumococcal meningitis. If adjunctive dexamethasone is used, it should be administered before or with the first dose of antibiotics.

Guidelines suggest that IV acyclovir be started on patients with suspected encephalitis, pending appropriate tests. This recommendation stems from the lower rates of mortality observed in patients that received acyclovir therapy early in the course of their disease (<4 days vs ≥4 days). The guidelines also suggest that addition of doxycycline be considered if age, location, and season are appropriate for tick-borne diseases.

The medications utilized for CNS infections are well tolerated. Allergic reactions are possible, but appear more often with the β-lactams (ampicillin, penicillin, ceftriaxone, and cefotaxime). Since most antibiotics can alter the bacterial flora of the gut, it is important to remember that this could result in drug interactions with warfarin and contraceptives. Gentamicin is associated with nephrotoxicity and ototoxicity which is common when administered for long durations or with other toxic medications. Vancomycin is also associated with nephrotoxicity in high troughs and/or with other concurrent nephrotoxic medications. Patients receiving vancomycin should have trough concentrations monitored, with goals of 15 to 20 mcg/mL for CNS infections and as such should be monitored for signs of nephrotoxicity (serum creatinine, urine output). Acyclovir can cause nephrotoxicity by precipitating in the renal tubules and is more common with the doses used in treating encephalitis. The nephrotoxicity can be minimized by hydration and slow infusion. Doxycycline causes upset stomach and phototoxicity. Patients taking aluminum, calcium, magnesium, or iron containing products should take them 2 hours before or after doxycycline because they can decrease the concentrations of the antibiotic. With a short course of dexamethasone, the likelihood of adverse effects is reduced; however, patients should be monitored for gastrointestinal bleeding and hyperglycemia.

Special Considerations

Although ceftriaxone has similar antibacterial coverage to cefotaxime, it is not recommended in neonates because of the potential to displace bilirubin, possibly leading to kernicterus. Ceftriaxone administered at high doses with IV calcium solutions is associated with causing lethal precipitates in neonates and young infants. Therefore, IV ceftriaxone should not be administered to any neonate nor should it be used in any infant within 48 hours of any calcium containing IV product. Additionally, patients of any age with trauma to the brain, CNS surgery, or immunocompromised state are at risk for meningitis as a result of additional pathogens (*Pseudomonas aeruginosa*) and will require broad-spectrum initial therapy.

If a neonate is determined to have HSV infection, even of just the skin, they should be treated empirically for encephalitis as disseminated infection is common and can have devastating consequences if it is not appropriately managed.

POSTEXPOSURE PROPHYLAXIS

Antibiotic prophylaxis for *N. meningitidis* is recommended for close contacts (those who live in the same household, seated next to a patient on prolonged airplane travel, children in day care with a patient, and those exposed to oral secretions of a patient). Intramuscular ceftriaxone, oral rifampin, or oral ciprofloxacin can be used. Additionally, vaccination with any meningococcal vaccine is recommended for control of community outbreaks of *N. meningitidis* types A, C, Y, or W135.

Haemophilus influenzae is a rare cause of meningitis in developed countries due to routine vaccination. Since *H. influenzae* invasive disease was common in young children (that are now immune) or immunocompromised individuals, chemoprophylaxis of contacts is limited to a small group of patients. Specifically, chemoprophylaxis with rifampin should be provided to individuals exposed, if they have incompletely immunized young children or immunocompromised close contacts. Additionally, if more than one day care attendee has Hib invasive disease (such as meningitis) everyone that attends or works in the day care should receive oral rifampin. No prophylaxis is recommended for pneumococcal or viral meningitis. Unimmunized persons exposed to measles, mumps, or varicella who do not have contraindications of receiving the vaccine should receive it as soon as possible. Additionally, IV immune globulin or hyperimmune globulins (VariZig for varicella) can be used for immunocompromised patients exposed to these viruses.

Special Considerations

When choosing an agent for meningococcal prophylaxis, a few considerations should be made. Intramuscular ceftriaxone is painful and should not be used in patients less than 1 month of age. Rifampin is a microsomal enzyme inducer, can color body secretions, and requires compounding if a suspension is required. Finally, although the fluoroquinolones have been used extensively in children, they are still not recommended to be used as first-line agents.

CASE Application

1. A 13-day-old former 35-week gestational age baby presents to the emergency room with a temperature of 102°F. The mother reports that the baby has been feeding less, is constipated, and is very irritable. Which of the following

is a common symptom of meningitis in a neonate? Select all that apply.

a. Temperature of 102°F
b. Decreased feeding
c. Constipation
d. Irritable appearance

2. The emergency physician is unable to obtain CSF after multiple attempts. Based on clinical findings, the team believes that the 13-day-old former 35-week gestational age baby may have meningitis. What is the best empiric therapy to begin in this baby before sending her to a pediatric hospital?

a. Ampicillin and gentamicin
b. Ceftriaxone and gentamicin
c. Vancomycin and cefotaxime
d. Ampicillin and ceftriaxone

3. When the 13-day-old former 35-week gestational age baby is examined at the pediatric hospital, she is also noted to have some lesions. The team has just sent cultures of the lesions as well as HSV PCR of the CSF. Which of the following is an appropriate pharmacologic approach in this patient?

a. Wait for the cultures and PCR results to come back, then modify therapy if needed.
b. Change antibiotic therapy to ceftriaxone and vancomycin.
c. Add IV acyclovir to the current antibiotic regimen.
d. Add oral voriconazole therapy to the current antibiotic regimen.

4. If a neonate is begun on acyclovir for HSV-associated encephalitis, which of the following should be routinely monitored? Select all that apply.

a. Serum creatinine
b. WBC count
c. Urine output
d. International normalized ratio (INR)

5. What is the brand name for ceftriaxone?

a. Ceftin
b. Keflex
c. Maxipime
d. Rocephin

6. Which of the following patients are recommended to receive a vaccine against *Streptococcus pneumoniae*? Select all that apply.

a. Healthy infants
b. A 40 year old with chronic obstructive pulmonary disease (COPD)
c. A healthy 55 year old
d. A 35-year-old asplenic patient

7. A 66-year-old woman with coronary artery disease, peripheral artery disease, diabetes, and hypertension is transferred from a nursing home to the hospital secondary to fever and altered mental status. A lumbar puncture was performed and CSF was sent for fluid analysis and culture. Which of the following findings are consistent with bacterial meningitis in this patient? Select all that apply.

a. CSF WBC 5000 cells/mm³
b. CSF WBC with 70% lymphocytes
c. CSF glucose of 23 mg/dL
d. CSF protein of 250 mg/dL

8. The physician decides to start the patient on vancomycin, ampicillin, and ceftriaxone, but the patient has a history of difficult IV access. Which of the following is an appropriate plan for treatment of this patient's bacterial meningitis?

a. Attempt immediate IV line placement and administer antibiotics IV for the duration of therapy.
b. Administer antibiotics orally for the duration of therapy.
c. Administer antibiotics intramuscularly for the duration of therapy.
d. Immediately insert an external ventricular drain into the brain and administer antibiotics intraventricularly for the duration of therapy.

9. Nephrotoxicity is one of the common side effects for which of the following IV antimicrobial agents? Select all that apply.

a. Acyclovir
b. Ceftriaxone
c. Gentamicin
d. Vancomycin

10. A 12-year-old boy presents to his pediatrician for a routine follow-up visit. The patient denies having any complaints. Physical examination, vital signs, and laboratory values are all within normal limits. Which of the following vaccinations should the patient receive today as part of routine care for a healthy adolescent?

a. MCV4
b. MPSV4
c. PCV13
d. PPSV23

11. A 22-year-old man (94 kg) with no significant past medical history presents to your hospital with fever, severe headache, photophobia, and neck pain. The physician does a lumbar puncture and sends the CSF collections to the laboratory. Based upon clinical diagnosis, the patient is suspected to have bacterial meningitis. Which of the following are likely pathogens associated with bacterial meningitis in this patient?

a. *Streptococcus pneumoniae* and *Haemophilus influenzae*
b. *Neisseria meningitidis* and *Listeria monocytogenes*

c. *L. monocytogenes* and *Streptococcus agalactiae* (group B)

d. *S. pneumoniae* and *N. meningitidis*

12. What is an appropriate empiric antibiotic therapy for this 22-year-old patient with suspected bacterial meningitis?

    a. Ceftriaxone

    b. Ceftriaxone and ampicillin

    c. Cefotaxime and vancomycin

    d. Ampicillin and gentamicin

13. The physician orders vancomycin 1500 mg IV Q12h for this 22-year-old man (among other antimicrobials). In order to minimize the risk of infusion-related reactions, for example, Red Man Syndrome, the drug will be administered at a concentration of 5 mg/mL and rate of 10 mg/min. What is the resulting infusion rate and duration for each vancomycin dose?

    a. 120 mL/h over 150 minutes

    b. 300 mL/h over 90 minutes

    c. 120 mL/h over 90 minutes

    d. 300 mL/h over 150 minutes

14. The 22-year-old male patient received antibiotics prior to CSF collection. CSF, blood, sputum, and urine specimens were sent for Gram stain and culture. Which of the following is correct regarding diagnosis of bacterial meningitis?

    a. The likelihood of a bacteria being identified from CSF Gram stain and/or culture is unchanged, despite the patient receiving antibiotics prior to CSF collection.

    b. CSF Gram stain and culture are not reliable for diagnosis of bacterial meningitis.

    c. There is no role for blood cultures in the diagnosis of bacterial meningitis.

    d. A bacteria will be identified in majority of CSF cultures in bacterial meningitis cases.

15. The CSF culture is growing *N. meningitidis*. Close contacts of this patient needing chemoprophylaxis for meningococcal disease are identified. Which of the following are therapeutic options for chemoprophylaxis? Select all that apply.

    a. Ceftriaxone

    b. Vancomycin

    c. Ciprofloxacin

    d. Rifampin

16. A 4-year-old girl with no significant past medical history is admitted for suspected bacterial meningitis and started on empiric therapy with ceftriaxone and vancomycin. What is the purpose of adding vancomycin to this empiric regimen for bacterial meningitis?

    a. To provide coverage against resistant *L. monocytogenes*

    b. To provide coverage against resistant *N. meningitidis*

    c. To provide coverage against resistant *S. pneumoniae*

    d. Vancomycin is not needed in a 4 year old with bacterial meningitis because *S. aureus* is unlikely

17. The 4-year-old patient is diagnosed with bacterial meningitis secondary to *N. meningitidis*. This case is identified as being part of an outbreak in the patient's day care center. Which meningococcal vaccine is recommended for use in control of an outbreak caused by a vaccine-preventable serogroup of *N. meningitidis* (ie, A, C, Y, and W135)? Select all that apply.

    a. Hib-MenCY

    b. MCV4

    c. MPSV4

    d. MCV4, followed by administration of MPSV4

18. In which of the following groups has dexamethasone demonstrated a mortality benefit?

    a. A 2 week old with *S. agalactiae* (group B) meningitis

    b. A 17 year old with *N. meningitidis* meningitis

    c. A 35 year old with *S. pneumoniae* meningitis

    d. It has not demonstrated clear benefit for any type of bacterial meningitis

19. A 70-year-old man presents with fever, nausea, vomiting, severe headache, and extreme photophobia. CSF results: WBC 2500 cells/mm^3, 87% neutrophils, glucose 37 mg/dL, and protein 240 mg/dL. What type of CNS infection is considered based upon the information provided?

    a. Bacterial meningitis

    b. Aseptic meningitis

    c. Viral encephalitis

    d. HSV Encephalitis

20. Which of the following is consistent with the recommended antibacterial therapy for a 70-year-old patient with bacterial meningitis?

    a. Vancomycin and ceftriaxone

    b. Vancomycin, ceftriaxone, and ampicillin

    c. Ampicillin and ceftriaxone

    d. Ceftriaxone

21. The 70-year-old patient also has a significant past medical history of hypertension, diabetes, and stroke. What is the *optimal* order of events for delivery of care for this patient (assuming no delays in any of these procedures)?

Unordered Response	Ordered Response
Dexamethasone	
Lumbar puncture for CSF culture	
Restart chronic home medications	
Antibiotic therapy	

TAKEAWAY POINTS »

- Bacterial meningitis is a serious infection that causes significant morbidity and mortality.
- Preventative measures against meningitis include preventative perinatal care and appropriate routine vaccinations.
- Pneumococcal conjugate vaccine should be given to all infants beginning between 6 and 8 weeks of age.
- Pneumococcal polysaccharide 23 valent vaccine should be given to any patient over 2 years old that (1) has a chronic disease, including adult asthma; (2) is immunocompromised; (3) resides in a nursing home; or (4) is an adult smoker.
- Prompt empiric IV antibiotic therapy is necessary when bacterial meningitis is suspected.
- Empiric antibiotic therapy should be chosen based upon common age-related pathogens.
- Ampicillin with either gentamicin or cefotaxime is recommended to cover the group B *Streptococcus*, *E. coli*, and *L. monocytogenes* that are likely in neonates.
- Vancomycin and either ceftriaxone or cefotaxime are recommended for empiric therapy against

S. pneumoniae and *N. meningitidis* in older infants, children, and adults.
- In addition to the common bacteria that cause meningitis in adults, *L. monocytogenes* is possible in older adults and, therefore, ampicillin should be added to empiric antibiotic therapy in patients older than 50 years.
- Controversy exists regarding whether dexamethasone should be used in pediatric bacterial meningitis since *H. influenzae* is now uncommon.
- Dexamethasone has shown to improve mortality and other clinical outcomes in adult patients with pneumococcal meningitis.
- If dexamethasone is used, it should be given before or with the first dose of antibiotics.
- Viral meningitis is commonly caused by enterovirus and is usually self-limiting.
- When herpes simplex is considered as a possible cause of a CNS infection, IV acyclovir should be started.
- Chemoprophylaxis with rifampin, ceftriaxone, or ciprofloxacin is recommended for certain *N. meningitidis* contacts.

BIBLIOGRAPHY

Centers for Disease Control and Prevention. Prevention of Pneumococcal Disease Among Infants and Children—Use of 13-Valent Pneumococcal Conjugate Vaccine and 23-Valent Pneumococcal Polysaccharide Vaccine: Recommendations of the Advisory Committee on Immunization Practices (ACIP). *MMWR Weekly.* 2010;59:1-24.

Centers for Disease Control and Prevention. Use of 13-Valent Pneumococcal Conjugate Vaccine and 23-Valent Pneumococcal Polysaccharide Vaccine for Adults with Immunocompromising Conditions: Recommendations of the Advisory Committee on Immunization Practices (ACIP). *MMWR Weekly.* 2012;61(40):816-819.

Centers for Disease Control and Prevention. Advisory Committee on Immunization Practices (ACIP) Recommended Immunization Schedules for Persons Aged 0 Through 18 Years and Adults Aged 19 Years and Older - United States, 2013. *MMWR Weekly.* 2013;62:1-21.

Centers for Disease Control and Prevention. Prevention and Control of Meningococcal Disease: Recommendations on the Advisory Committee on Immunization Practices (ACIP). *MMWR Weekly.* 2013;62(2):1-32.

Centers for Disease Control and Prevention. Infant Meningococcal Vaccination: Advisory Committee on Immunization Practices

(ACIP) Recommendations and Rationale. *MMWR Weekly.* 2013;62(3):52-54.

Centers for Disease Control and Prevention. Use of 13-Valent Pneumococcal Conjugate Vaccine and 23-Valent Pneumococcal Polysaccharide Vaccine Among Children Aged 6-18 Years with Immunocompromising Conditions: Recommendations of the Advisory Committee on Immunization Practices (ACIP). *MMWR Weekly.* 2013;62(25):521-524.

Elshaboury RH, Ahiskali AS, Holt JS, Rotschafer JC. Central nervous system infections. In: DiPiro JT, Talbert RL, Yee GC, Matzke GR, Wells BG, Posey L, eds. *Pharmacotherapy: A Pathophysiologic Approach.* 10th ed. New York, NY: McGraw-Hill; 2017.

Sucher AJ. Meningitis. In: Attridge RL, Miller ML, Moote R, Ryan L, eds. *Internal Medicine: A Guide to Clinical Therapeutics.* New York, NY: McGraw-Hill; 2013:chap 30.

Tunkel AR, Glaser CA, Bloch KC, et al. The management of encephalitis: clinical practice guidelines by The Infectious Diseases Society of America. *Clin Infect Dis.* 2008;47:303-327.

Tunkel AR, Hartman BJ, Kaplan SL, et al. Practice guidelines for the management of bacterial meningitis. *Clin Infect Dis.* 2004;39:1267-1284.

KEY ABBREVIATIONS

CNS = central nervous system	HSV = herpes simplex virus
COPD = chronic obstructive pulmonary disease	INR = international normalized ratio
CSF = cerebrospinal fluid	MMR = measles, mumps, rubella
Hib = *H. influenzae* type b	PCR = polymerase chain reaction

26

Sepsis Syndromes

S. Scott Sutton, Christopher M. Bland, April M. Quidley, Brianne L. Dunn, and Trisha N. Branan

FOUNDATION OVERVIEW

Sepsis is a continuum of physiologic stages characterized by infection, systemic inflammation, and hypoperfusion leading to tissue injury and organ failure (Table 26-1 for definitions to utilize for sepsis syndromes). Risk factors for sepsis include extremes of age, cancer, immunodeficiency, chronic organ failure, genetic factors (male and non-white ethnic origin in North America), patients with bacteremia, and genetic polymorphisms associated with immune regulation. Pulmonary, gastrointestinal, genitourinary, and bloodstream infections account for the majority of sepsis cases.

The development of sepsis is complex and multifactorial. The key factor in the development of sepsis is inflammation. Infection or injury is controlled through pro- and anti-inflammatory mediators. Systemic responses ensue when there is an overwhelming pro-inflammatory response.

The clinical presentation of sepsis varies and the development of clinical manifestations may differ from patient to patient (see Table 26-1). Recently international consensus definitions have been updated for sepsis and septic shock. The Sequential (Sepsis-Related) Organ Failure Assessment (SOFA) score now defines those patients with sepsis-related organ dysfunction identified with a score more than or equal to 2. This score is calculated from various organ system functional assessments including respiratory function, coagulation, hepatic function, cardiovascular function, central nervous system function, and renal function. A rapid, bedside screening tool to identify patients at risk for sepsis-related organ dysfunction is known as the qSOFA or "quick" SOFA score and is considered positive in the presence of any 2 of the 3 following criteria: respiratory rate more than or equal to 22, altered mentation, or systolic blood pressure less than or equal to 100 mm Hg. The cumulative burden of sepsis complications is the leading factor in mortality. The most common complications are disseminated intravascular coagulation (DIC), acute respiratory distress syndrome (ARDS), acute kidney injury (AKI), and hemodynamic compromise.

Gram-positive and gram-negative bacteria are major causes of sepsis, but fungal species and viruses can also cause sepsis. Microbiologic cultures should be obtained before anti-infective therapy is initiated; however, antibiotic therapy should not be delayed until the return of gram stain or culture data. Cultures take 6 to 48 hours for results to be returned and often reveal no growth of bacterial organisms but negative cultures do not rule out infection. Rapid identification of bacteria or fungi from blood cultures can be performed on positive blood cultures with results available within 1 to 3 hours of initial growth depending on the rapid diagnostic platform used.

TREATMENT

The goal of sepsis treatment is to decrease morbidity and mortality. Treatment is aimed at early fluid resuscitation; reduction or elimination of organ failure; treatment and elimination of the source of infection; avoidance of adverse treatment reactions; and provision of cost-effective therapy. The speed and appropriateness of therapy influences the outcome (similar to acute myocardial infarction and cerebrovascular accidents). Pertinent issues in the management of septic patients are: (1) early resuscitation during the first 3 hours after recognition; (2) early administration of broad-spectrum anti-infective therapy; (3) hydrocortisone for septic shock patients refractory to resuscitation and vasopressors; (4) glycemic control using continuous insulin infusion to maintain a glucose level less than 180 mg/dL; (5) adjunctive therapies such as nutrition, deep vein thrombosis (DVT) prophylaxis, stress ulcer prophylaxis (SUP), and sedation for mechanically ventilated patients (Figure 26-1).

Early Fluid Resuscitation

Early intervention with fluid resuscitation decreases mortality in septic patients. Crystalloid (such as 0.9% sodium chloride or Lactated Ringer's solutions) or colloid fluids (5% albumin) can be used for resuscitation. Crystalloid solutions are preferred due to equivalence with decreased cost, reserving albumin for patients requiring substantial amounts of fluid. Upon recognition, septic patients should receive at least 30 mL/kg of IV crystalloid fluid within the first 3 hours. Hydroxyethyl starch solutions are no longer recommended due to the risk of renal failure and bleeding. Crystalloid solutions require more volume thus increasing risk of edema; therefore, utilize caution in patients at risk for fluid overload (eg, heart failure and ARDS). To avoid volume overload, a fluid challenge of 500 to 1000 mL of crystalloid solution should be administered to hypovolemic patients after the initial resuscitative period.

TABLE 26-1	Definitions Related to Sepsis
Condition	**Definition**
Bacteremia (fungemia)	Presence of viable bacteria (fungi) within the bloodstream
Infection	Inflammatory response to invasion of normally sterile host tissue by the microorganisms
Sepsis	Life-threatening organ dysfunction caused by a dysregulated host response noted by ≥2 point increase in Sequential Organ Failure Assessment (SOFA) score
Septic shock	Septic patients who display underlying cardiovascular, cellular, and/or metabolic derangements requiring volume resuscitation, have a serum lactate >2 mmol/L, and require vasopressor support to maintain a mean arterial pressure ≥65 mm Hg
Multiple-organ system failure	Presence of altered organ function requiring intervention to maintain homeostasis

Additional fluids should be given based on response including increased blood pressure and urine output. Aggressive infusion rates of resuscitation fluids and blood may be needed in patients with severe hypoperfusion.

When volume resuscitation fails to provide adequate arterial pressure and organ perfusion, vasopressors and/or inotropic agents should be initiated. Vasopressors and inotropes are effective in treating life-threatening hypotension and improving cardiac index, but complications such as tachycardia and myocardial ischemia require slow titration to restore mean arterial pressure (MAP) to minimize tachycardia and avoid impairing stroke volume. These agents may also cause peripheral vasoconstriction and ischemia leading to impaired gut motility, hypotension, or organ and tissue necrosis. Intravascular volume status should be continually reassessed to ensure optimal vasopressor response and minimize adverse effects. Norepinephrine is the recommended initial vasopressor in patients with septic shock refractory to fluid resuscitation. Dopamine or epinephrine are alternative vasopressors that may be added to patients refractory to norepinephrine therapy but are not first-line therapies due to increased potential for arrhythmias compared to norepinephrine. Vasopressin at a dose of 0.03 units/minute should be avoided in sepsis as monotherapy. Low-dose vasopressin is not recommended as the single initial vasopressor for treatment of sepsis-induced hypotension. Phenylephrine is not recommended in the treatment of septic shock except in circumstances where (a) norepinephrine is associated with serious arrhythmias, (b) cardiac output is known to be high and blood pressure persistently low, or (c) as salvage therapy when combined inotrope/vasopressor drugs and low-dose vasopressin have failed to achieve MAP target. In patients with myocardial dysfunction, inotropic therapy with dobutamine is recommended.

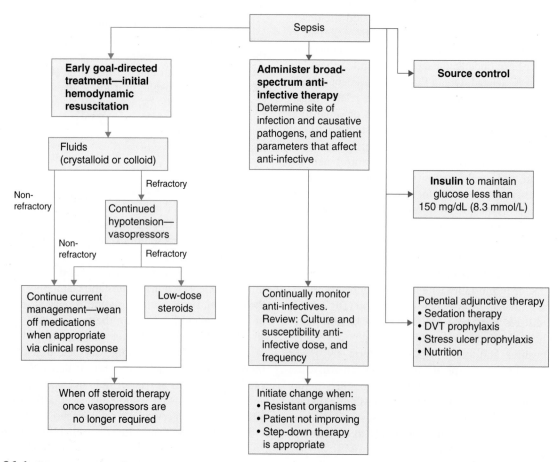

FIGURE 26-1   Therapeutic approach to sepsis.   Reproduced with permission from Chisholm-Burns MA, Wells BG, Schwinghammer TL, et al: *Pharmacotherapy Principles and Practice*, 3rd ed. New York, NY: McGraw-Hill; 2013.

TABLE 26-2	Empirical Intravenous Antimicrobial Regimens in Septic Shock	
Infection (Site or Type)	**Community-Acquired**	**Hospital-Acquired**
Urinary tract	Third-generation cephalosporin (ceftriaxone) *or* fluoroquinolone (levofloxacin or ciprofloxacin)	Antipseudomonal penicillin *or* antipseudomonal cephalosporin *or* antipseudomonal carbapenem *plus* aminoglycoside
Community-acquired pneumonia	Third-generation cephalosporin *plus* a macrolide *or* doxycycline *or* levofloxacin/moxifloxacin	
Ventilator-associated pneumonia or Nosocomial pneumonia		Antipseudomonal penicillin *or* antipseudomonal cephalosporin *or* antipseudomonal carbapenem *plus* aminoglycoside *or* antipseudomonal fluoroquinolone *plus* vancomycin *or* linezolid
Intra-abdominal	Cefoxitin *or* ciprofloxacin/levofloxacin *plus* metronidazole	Piperacillin-tazobactam *or* imipenem or meropenem *or* cefepime *plus* metronidazole *or* ciprofloxacin/levofloxacin *plus* metronidazole
Skin and soft-tissue	Nafcillin or cefazolin or vancomycin (for MRSA)	Vancomycin or daptomycin
Unknown source of infection	Local antibiogram along with risk factors for resistant pathogens should determine empiric regimen	Antipseudomonal penicillin or antipseudomonal cephalosporin or antipseudomonal carbapenem *plus* aminoglycoside *plus* vancomycin

Abbreviation: MDR, multidrug resistant.

Early Administration of Broad-Spectrum Anti-Infective Therapy

Appropriate empiric anti-infective therapy decreases mortality compared to inappropriate empiric therapy. Administration of broad-spectrum anti-infectives for initial therapy should occur within the first hour of recognition of sepsis. Cultures should be obtained prior to initiating antimicrobial therapy, if they can be obtained without delaying therapy (obtained in <45 minutes). Rapid identification of blood cultures within 1 to 3 hours of a positive culture is available in some hospitals but susceptibility testing still takes up to 72 hours. Anti-infective clinical trials in sepsis and septic shock patients are scarce and have not demonstrated differences among agents. Empiric therapy includes combination regimens to ensure coverage of causative organisms, but monotherapy is equivalent to combination therapy once a causative pathogen has been identified. Table 26-2 and Figure 26-1 provide guidelines for selecting appropriate empiric coverage. Factors that determine selection are site of infection, causative pathogens, community- or nosocomial-acquired infection, immune status of patient, patient history, cost and antibiogram data for the institution. Clinicians should be cognizant of bacterial resistance in community and health care setting.

Average duration of anti-infective therapy for septic patients is 7 to 10 days. However, durations vary depending on the site of infection and response to therapy (eg, *Staphylococcus aureus* bacteremia often requires 2 weeks minimum of parenteral therapy). In addition to antimicrobial therapy, an anatomical site for infection should be identified. If feasible and indicated, this source should be contained (eg, removal of infected devices, tissue debridement, abscess drainage).

Pharmacokinetics of antimicrobials may be altered because of increased volume of distribution due to initial resuscitation or change in renal function (augmented renal clearance or acute kidney injury). Reevaluation of the initial regimen daily should occur to optimize activity, prevent development of resistance, reduce toxicity, and decrease costs.

Initiation of step-down therapy based on microbiologic cultures is critical to prevent resistance, reduce toxicity and decrease overall costs.

Hydrocortisone for Septic Shock Patients Refractory to Resuscitation and Vasopressors

Septic patients with shock refractory to resuscitation and vasopressors can be considered for administration of corticosteroid administration with IV hydrocortisone 200 mg per day (generally divided as 50 mg every 6 hours but may be given as a continuous infusion). Patients should be weaned from steroid therapy when vasopressors are no longer required. Previously, the adrenocorticotropic hormone (ACTH) stimulation test was recommended to identify candidates for hydrocortisone therapy. Its use in sepsis is no longer recommended.

Glycemic Control

Following initial stabilization of sepsis/septic shock patients, maintain blood glucose levels between 140 and 180 mg/dL. Septic patients with two consecutive blood glucose levels more than 180 mg/dL should receive intravenous insulin with frequent blood glucose monitoring (every 1-2 hours until glucose values and insulin infusion rates are stable, then every 4 hours).

Adjunctive Therapy

Adjunctive therapy for patients with sepsis consists of enteral nutrition, DVT prophylaxis, SUP, and analgesia/sedation in mechanically ventilated patients. Oral or enteral (if necessary) nutrition is recommended in septic patients to meet the increased energy and protein requirements. Early administration of parenteral nutrition alone or parenteral nutrition in combination with enteral feedings is not recommended.

DVT prophylaxis is recommended for septic patients. Low-dose unfractionated heparin or low-molecular-weight heparin (such as enoxaparin or dalteparin) may be utilized along with mechanical prophylaxis. Patients with contraindications to chemical prophylaxis should receive mechanical prophylaxis using graduated compression stockings or intermittent compression devices.

Patients with sepsis and septic shock have risk factors placing them at high risk for stress ulcers, including coagulopathy, mechanical ventilation, hypotension, and in some patients, corticosteroid therapy. Histamine-receptor antagonists (such as ranitidine) or proton pump inhibitors (such as omeprazole) are recommended when SUP is indicated. The benefit of prophylaxis must be weighed against the potential effect of an increased gastric pH leading to the development of ventilator-associated pneumonia or *Clostridium difficile* infection.

Critically ill patients often require analgesia/sedation when complex ventilator settings are used, when patients are difficult to ventilate, or for acute agitation and delirium. Patients with progressive hypoxia leading to ARDS frequently require uncomfortable modes of mechanical ventilation. Adoption of a sedation protocol that uses the smallest amount of sedation required to maintain patient comfort and safety should be utilized. The sedation protocol should include daily interruption or lightening of a sedative infusion until the patient is awake.

SPECIAL POPULATIONS

Pediatric definitions of sepsis syndromes are similar to adult definitions but depend on age-specific heart rate, respiratory rate, and white blood cell cutoff values. Key points relative to pediatric sepsis that differ from adult sepsis include:

1. Clindamycin and antitoxin therapy for toxic shock syndromes with refractory hypotension. Children are prone to toxic shock because of lack of circulating antibodies to toxins. Children with sepsis should be treated with clindamycin to reduce toxin production. Role of IVIG is unclear, but may be considered.
2. No firm recommendations are available on the use of DVT prophylaxis or SUP.

CASE Application

1. Select the definition that describes a patient with septic shock.

    a. GH has the presence of bacteria within the blood.
    b. HH has a systemic inflammatory response to a clinical insult.
    c. JA has an infection associated with organ dysfunction.
    d. KS has an infection with persistent hypotension despite fluid resuscitation.

2. ZB is a patient with sepsis in the intensive care unit. ZB is currently receiving piperacillin/tazobactam, tobramycin, and vancomycin to treat his infection. The source of his infection is currently unknown. What type of organism(s) may cause septic shock? Select all that apply.

    a. Gram-positive bacteria
    b. Gram-negative bacteria
    c. Fungal species
    d. Viruses

3. Which of the following components make up the qSOFA score? Select all that apply.

    a. Respiratory rate ≥22
    b. Altered mentation
    c. Systolic blood pressure ≤100 mm Hg
    d. Diastolic blood pressure ≤60 mm Hg
    e. Heart rate ≥100 beats per minute

4. Which of the following may reduce or prevent morbidity and mortality associated with sepsis? Select all that apply.

    a. Preventing organ failures
    b. Early fluid resuscitation
    c. Acquisition of microbiologic cultures
    d. Administration of narrow spectrum anti-infectives

5. XJ is a 33-year-old woman (weight 70 kg) who presents with sepsis (hypotension and decreased urine output). Past medical history is significant for diabetes, hypertension, hypothyroidism, and gastroesophageal reflux. Medications include metformin, lisinopril, levothyroxine, and omeprazole. Select the appropriate initial regimen for fluid resuscitation in XJ.

    a. 5% dextrose 500 mL
    b. 5% albumin 1000 mL
    c. 0.9% sodium chloride 2000 mL
    d. 0.45% sodium chloride 2000 mL

6. AA is a patient with hypotension secondary to sepsis. Past medical history is significant for heart failure with active fluid overload, hypertension, diabetes, previous myocardial infarction, and dyslipidemia. Medications include lisinopril, spironolactone, glipizide, metoprolol succinate, atorvastatin, and a baby aspirin. Labs were within normal limits except for a SCr of 1.9 mg/dL, glucose 180 mg/dL, and potassium of 5.6 mEq/L. Select the appropriate colloid therapy for fluid resuscitation in this patient.

    a. 5% albumin 500 mL
    b. 5% dextrose 500 mL
    c. 0.45% sodium chloride with 5% dextrose 500 mL
    d. 0.45% sodium chloride 500 mL

7. KT is a 65-year-old man with a history of end-stage renal disease on hemodialysis admitted with sepsis likely secondary to an infected dialysis catheter. KT was diagnosed 30 minutes ago and has not yet received intervention. Which of the following represents the best order of events to manage KT?

    a. Vasopressors, fluids, microbiologic cultures, antimicrobial therapy

b. Vasopressors, antimicrobial therapy, microbiologic cultures, fluids

c. Fluids, microbiologic cultures, antimicrobial therapy, insulin for glucose >180 mg/dL

d. Fluids, antimicrobial therapy, microbiologic cultures, insulin for glucose >180 mg/dL

8. TP is a 63-year-old male patient with a past medical history of hypertension, diabetes, chronic obstructive pulmonary disease, and dyslipidemia. Medications include amlodipine, metformin, tiotropium, albuterol as needed, and pravastatin. TP is diagnosed with sepsis. Pertinent labs include a pH of 7.25, white blood cell count of 13,500 cells/mm³, glucose of 170 mg/dL, serum creatinine of 2.3 mg/dL, and blood pressure of 85/43 mm Hg. What therapy should be administered within 1 hour of the recognition of sepsis?

a. Broad-spectrum antimicrobial therapy

b. Corticosteroids

c. Sodium bicarbonate

d. Vasopressor therapy

9. SL is a 32-year-old man with sepsis secondary to an intra-abdominal abscess. He has no significant past medical history and currently has been fluid resuscitated with an MAP of 70 mm Hg. What is the best treatment plan for SL?

a. Cefoxitin 2 g IV every 6 hours and transfer to the intensive care unit

b. Cefoxitin 2 g IV every 6 hours and surgical drainage of the abscess

c. Amoxicillin/clavulanic acid 875 mg/125 mg po every 12 hours and transfer to the intensive care unit

d. Amoxicillin/clavulanic acid 875 mg/125 mg po every 12 hours and surgical drainage of the abscess

10. XC is a 41-year-old patient admitted to the intensive care unit for septic shock. Appropriate therapy was initiated within the desired times. The critical care attending asks the pharmacy student during rounds how long antimicrobial therapy should be continued for XC. Select the duration of antimicrobial therapy in most patients with septic shock.

a. 1 to 3 days

b. 3 to 5 days

c. 7 to 10 days

d. 24 to 28 days

11. UC is a patient in the medical intensive care unit with a diagnosis of septic shock. During rounds the pulmonary critical care attending questions the pharmacy student about the utilization of corticosteroids. Which corticosteroid should be used to treat patients with septic

shock refractory to aggressive fluid resuscitation and vasopressor therapy?

a. Prednisone

b. Hydrocortisone

c. Methylprednisolone

d. Dexamethasone

12. What is the brand name for hydrocortisone?

a. Deltasone

b. Sterapred

c. Solu-Medrol

d. Solu-Cortef

The Following Case Pertains to Questions 13 and 14.

13. LA is a patient in the medical intensive care unit with sepsis. Past medical history includes hypertension, myocardial infarction 3 years ago, dyslipidemia, and gastroesophageal reflux. Medications include lisinopril, metoprolol, atorvastatin, aspirin and omeprazole. Labs include: white blood cell count of 12,000 cells/mm³, serum creatinine 1.8 mg/dL, and blood glucose 190 mg/dL. What is the goal blood glucose for patients with sepsis?

a. 80 to 110 mg/dL

b. ≤120 mg/dL

c. ≤150 mg/dL

d. 140 to 180 mg/dL

14. Select the most appropriate regimen for glycemic control in LA. Select all that apply.

a. Metformin 1000 mg po bid

b. Sitagliptin 100 mg po daily

c. Insulin glargine 50 units qhs

d. Regular insulin infusion

15. VB is admitted to the medical intensive care unit with sepsis and acute respiratory failure requiring mechanical ventilation. She is currently receiving crystalloid resuscitation, doripenem and amikacin. The critical care attending requests pharmacy to handle the nutrition recommendations for VB as it has been nearly a week prior to admission that VB has had any nutritional intake. Which of the following nutrition regimens is (are) most appropriate in a patient with sepsis secondary to pneumonia with a functioning GI tract?

a. Continuous tube feeding via a nasoduodenal tube

b. Parenteral nutrition via a central IV catheter

c. Parenteral nutrition via a peripheral IV catheter

d. Intravenous glucose

16. Which of the following is a risk factor for stress-induced gastrointestinal bleeding? Select all that apply.

a. Mechanical ventilation ≥48 hours

b. Coagulopathy

c. Warfarin therapy (Therapeutic INR)

d. Hypertension

17. RE is a patient with sepsis from an *Escherichia coli* urinary tract infection. RE is receiving ertapenem for management of the infection. Select the medication that may be used for RE for stress-ulcer prophylaxis. RE does not have any risk factors for the development of a stress ulcer. Select all that apply.

a. Proton pump inhibitor

b. H$_2$ blocker

c. Sucralfate

d. Prophylaxis is not recommended

18. QP is a 68-year-old man diagnosed with sepsis. Past medical history includes heart failure (ejection fraction 25%), diabetes, and dyslipidemia. Patient was initially hospitalized for a heart failure exacerbation (20 lb of fluid overload). Select the initial fluid resuscitation for QP.

a. Dextrose

b. Albumin

c. Hydroxyethyl starch

d. 0.45% normal saline

19. CX is an adult patient in septic shock. Crystalloid fluid resuscitation at 40 mL/kg did not improve hemodynamics. Further assessment of CX's clinical variables indicate that he is not fluid responsive. Select the agent to increase CX's blood pressure.

a. Normal saline

b. Norepinephrine

c. Dopamine

d. Phenylephrine

20. ER is a patient in septic shock currently receiving vasopressor therapy and broad spectrum anti-infective therapy. ER has continued signs of hypoperfusion (although he has achieved adequate intravascular volume and MAP). ER is currently receiving a low dose of norepinephrine. What inotropic agent should be utilized to manage his continued hypoperfusion?

a. Vasopressin

b. Dopamine

c. Dobutamine

d. Phenylephrine

21. KJ is an 87-kg man receiving a norepinephrine infusion (4 mg/250 mL) at 2 mcg/kg/min for management of his septic shock. At what rate (mL/h) should the infusion be administered?

a. 652.5 mL/h

b. 652,500 mL/h

c. 7.5 mL/h

d. 10.9 mL/h

22. JZ is a 48-year-old man admitted to the hospital with sepsis. He receives initial therapy with fluid resuscitation and antibiotic therapy but remains hypotensive. The physician decides to initiate therapy with a norepinephrine continuous infusion and phones the pharmacy for dosing recommendations. What reference(s) would be appropriate to find information on appropriate dosing? Select all that apply.

a. *Drug Information Handbook*

b. *Micromedex*

c. *PubMed*

d. *Drug Facts and Comparisons*

e. *Lexi-Comp*

23. BD is a 44-year-old man with severe alcoholism who is intubated due to hypoxia from community-acquired pneumonia complicated by sepsis. Which of the following sedation regimens if given via continuous infusion may induce a metabolic acidosis?

a. Ativan

b. Precedex

c. Valium

d. Versed

24. Which of the following is the generic name of Precedex?

a. Dexamethasone

b. Dexmedetomidine

c. Dextroamphetamine

d. Dextromethorphan

25. LL is an 80-year-old woman who was admitted to the ICU with presumed sepsis due to a urinary tract infection. Upon review of the medical record, you note that the patient has several allergies including heparin (history of heparin-induced thrombocytopenia 1 month ago) and also penicillin (anaphylaxis). Which of the following is recommended in LL to prevent the occurrence of venous thromboembolism?

a. Unfractionated heparin 5000 units SQ every 8 hours

b. Enoxaparin 40 mg SQ every 24 hours

c. Rivaroxaban 20 mg po daily with food

d. Mechanical prophylaxis only (eg, graduated compression stockings or intermittent compression devices)

26. Which of the following best describes the hemodynamic properties of norepinephrine?

a. Minimal α- and β-adrenergic agonist effects

b. Potent α-adrenergic activity with less potent β-adrenergic agonist properties

c. Potent β-adrenergic agonist effects and minimal α-adrenergic effects

d. Potent α- and β-adrenergic agonist properties

TAKEAWAY POINTS »

- Sepsis is a continuum of physiologic stages characterized by infection, systemic inflammation, and hypoperfusion leading to tissue injury and organ failure.
- The majority of sepsis cases occur as a result of bacterial infection.
- Early resuscitation with IV fluids is essential to improving morbidity and mortality in sepsis.
- Either crystalloids (0.9% sodium chloride, Lactated Ringer's) or colloids (5% albumin) can be used as fluids for resuscitation, although crystalloids are preferred first-line due to lower cost.
- Broad-spectrum, empiric antimicrobial therapy should be administered within 1 hour of the recognition of sepsis. If the source of sepsis is known, initial therapy may be narrowed.

- Once pathogen(s) have been identified, antimicrobial therapy can be tailored to specific organisms. Therapy should typically be continued for 7 to 10 days.
- Patients with shock and hypotension refractory to fluid resuscitation and vasopressors may be considered for corticosteroid therapy with intravenous hydrocortisone 200 mg per day.
- The optimal target for blood glucose in sepsis patients is between 140 and 180 mg/dL.
- Adult patients with sepsis should often receive adjunctive therapies such as enteral nutrition, deep vein thrombosis prophylaxis, and stress ulcer prophylaxis.

BIBLIOGRAPHY

Attridge RL. Sepsis and septic shock. In: Attridge RL, Miller ML, Moote R, Ryan L, eds. *Internal Medicine: A Guide to Clinical Therapeutics.* New York, NY: McGraw-Hill; 2013:chap 36.

Branan TN, Bland CM, Sutton SS. Sepsis and septic shock. In: Chisholm-Burns MA, Schwinghammer TL, Wells BG, Malone PM, Kolesar JM, DiPiro JT, eds. *Pharmacotherapy Principles and Practice.* 4th ed. New York, NY: McGraw-Hill; 2016:chap 82.

Ely EW, Goyette RE. Sepsis with acute organ dysfunction. In: Hall JB, Schmidt GA, Wood LD, eds. *Principles of Critical Care.* 3rd ed. New York, NY: McGraw-Hill; 2005:chap 46.

Kalil AC, Metersky ML, Klompas M, et al. Management of Adults with Hospital-acquired and Ventilator-associated Pneumonia:

2016 Clinical Practice Guidelines by the Infectious Diseases Society of America and the American Thoracic Society. *Clin Infect Dis.* 2016;63:e61-111.

Kang-Birken SL. Sepsis and septic shock. In: DiPiro JT, Talbert RL, Yee GC, Matzke GR, Wells BG, Posey LM, eds. *Pharmacotherapy: A Pathophysiologic Approach.* 10th ed. New York, NY: McGraw-Hill; 2017:chap 119.

Rhodes A, Evans LE, Alhazzani W, et al. Surviving Sepsis Campaign: International guidelines for Management of Sepsis and Septic Shock: 2016. *Intensive Care Med.* 2017;43:304-377.

Singer M, Deutschman C, Seymour C, et al. The third international consensus definitions for sepsis and septic shock (Sepsis-3). *JAMA.* 2016;315:801-810.

KEY ABBREVIATIONS

ACTH = adrenocorticotropic hormone
AKI = acute kidney injury
ARDS = acute respiratory distress syndrome
DIC = disseminated intravascular coagulation
DVT = deep vein thrombosis

MAP = mean arterial pressure
qSOFA = quick sequential organ failure assessment
SOFA = sequential organ failure assessment
SUP = stress ulcer prophylaxis

27 Human Immunodeficiency Virus

P. Brandon Bookstaver

FOUNDATION OVERVIEW

The human immunodeficiency virus (HIV or HIV-1) is a **retrovirus** that causes the acquired immunodeficiency syndrome (AIDS), a condition in which progressive failure of the immune system leads to life-threatening opportunistic infections. A second retrovirus, HIV-2, also is recognized to cause AIDS, although it is less virulent, transmissible, and prevalent than HIV-1. Modern antiretroviral regimens have decreased the morbidity and mortality of HIV; however, HIV infection cannot be cured due to the integration of the HIV genome into host cells, creating a latent reservoir. An AIDS diagnosis is made when the presence of HIV is laboratory-confirmed and the cluster of differentiation 4 (CD4 cell) count drops below 200 cells/mm³ (200×10^6/L) for those older than or equal to 6 years of age or after the development of an opportunistic infection.

Infection with HIV occurs through three primary modes: sexual, parenteral, and perinatal. **Sexual intercourse**, primarily anal and vaginal intercourse, is the most common method for transmission. The probability of HIV transmission depends upon the type of sexual exposure and the highest risk is from receptive anorectal intercourse. Transmission risk is lower for receptive vaginal intercourse, and insertive sex acts have lower risk than receptive acts. Condom use reduces risk of transmission by approximately 80%. The viral load in the index partner is an additional risk factor for transmission. For example, transmission is higher when the index partner has early or late HIV compared with asymptomatic HIV, as these disease stages are associated with higher viral loads. Individuals with genital ulcers or sexually transmitted diseases (STDs) are at greater risk for contracting HIV. **Parenteral transmission** of HIV broadly encompasses infections due to infected blood exposure from needle sticks, intravenous (IV) injection with used needles, receipt of blood products, and organ transplants. Use of contaminated needles has been the main cause of parenteral transmissions. Blood and tissue products in the healthcare system are now rigorously screened for HIV and the risk for receiving tainted blood or blood products is very low. Healthcare workers have a small but definite occupational risk of contracting HIV through accidental exposure. Most cases of occupationally acquired HIV have been the result of a percutaneous needle stick injury. **Perinatal infection,** or vertical transmission, is the most common cause of pediatric HIV

infection. Most infections occur during or near to the time of birth, although a fraction can occur in utero. Casual contact with patients with HIV is not a risk factor for transmission.

The life cycle of HIV is illustrated in Figure 27-1. HIV has an outer glycoprotein (gp160) on its surface and is composed of two subunits (gp120 and gp41). The glycoprotein has affinity for CD4 receptors and the gp120 subunit is responsible for CD4 binding after exposure. Once initial binding occurs, the association of HIV with the cell is enhanced by additional binding to chemokine coreceptors. The two major chemokine receptors are chemokine receptor 5 (CCR5) and chemokine receptor 4 (CXCR4). HIV may contain a mixture of viruses that target one or the other of these coreceptors, and some viral strains may be dual-tropic (ie, can use both coreceptors). The HIV strain that preferentially uses CCR5, R5 viruses, is macrophage-tropic and typically implicated in most cases of sexually transmitted HIV. The HIV strain that targets CXCR4, designated X4 virus, is T-cell–tropic and often is predominant in the later stage of disease. CD4 and coreceptor attachment of HIV to the cell promotes membrane fusion, which is mediated by gp41, and finally internalization of the viral genetic material and enzymes necessary for replication. After internalization, the viral protein shell surrounding the nucleic acid (capsid) is uncoated in preparation for replication. The genetic material of HIV is single-stranded RNA and the virus must transcribe RNA into DNA (transcription normally occurs from DNA to RNA; HIV works backward, hence the name *retrovirus*). The enzyme reverse transcriptase completes the RNA to DNA step by synthesizing a complementary strand of DNA using the viral RNA as a template. The consistency of HIV reverse transcriptase is poor, and many mistakes are made during the process. These errors in the final DNA product contribute to the rapid mutation of the virus, which enables the virus to evade the immune response, promotes drug resistance during partially suppressive therapy, and complicates vaccine development. Following reverse transcription, the final double-stranded DNA virus migrates into the nucleus and is integrated into the host cell chromosome by integrase. The integration of HIV into the host chromosome establishes a persistent, latent infection in long-lived cells of the immune system (eg, memory T lymphocytes). The virus is effectively hidden in these cells; therefore, continuous suppressive therapy is ideal because the virus reemerges from this reservoir

To access your complimentary online question exams, visit https://accesspharmacy.mhmedical.com/NAPLEX.aspx

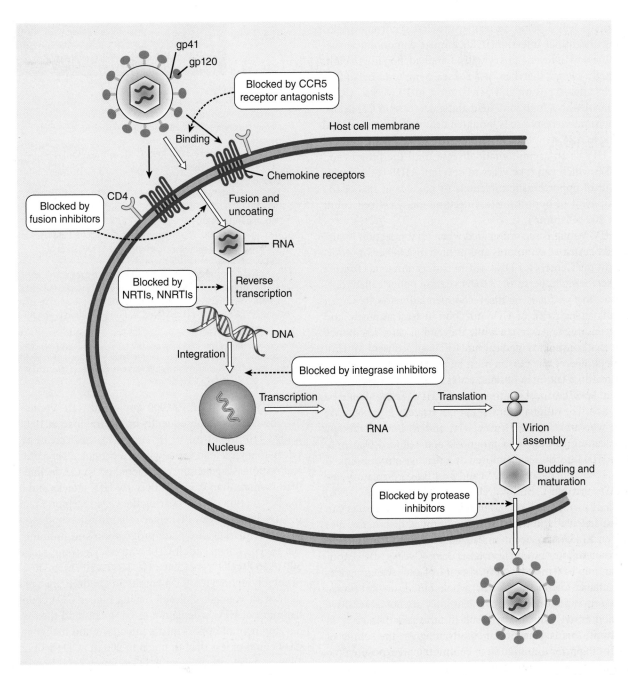

FIGURE 27-1 Life cycle of HIV. Binding of viral glycoproteins to host cell CD4 and chemokine receptors leads to fusion of the viral and host cell membranes via gp41 and entry of the virion into the cell. After uncoating, reverse transcription copies the single-stranded HIV RNA genome into double-stranded DNA, which is integrated into the host cell genome. Gene transcription by host cell enzymes produces messenger RNA, which is translated into proteins that assemble into immature noninfectious virions that bud from the host cell membrane. Maturation into fully infectious virions is through proteolytic cleavage. NNRTIs, nonnucleoside reverse transcriptase inhibitors; NRTIs, nucleoside/nucleotide reverse transcriptase inhibitors. Reproduced with permission from Katzung BG, Trevor AJ: *Basic & Clinical Pharmacology*, 13th ed. New York, NY: McGraw-Hill; 2015.

if therapy is suspended. After integration into the nucleus of a CD4 cell, the transcription of DNA occurs (eg, replication) causing nuclear release of viral genomic RNA and mRNA. Translation of the RNA and mRNA into viral proteins occurs and are assembled by viral protease and packaged into a budding virion. Protease is responsible for cleaving a precursor polypeptide (gag-pol) into functional proteins that are necessary to produce mature, infectious virus. Once mature, the virus will infect other susceptible cells causing immune system destruction with approximately 10 billion new viruses produced each day.

Clinical Presentation/Diagnosis

Acute symptoms of HIV infection are nonspecific, making the diagnosis difficult. Although symptoms are nonspecific, the presence of aseptic meningitis, oral or genital ulcers, rash, and leukopenia should raise suspicion of acute HIV infection in the setting of a potential exposure. Approximately 40% to 90%

of patients will develop an acute retroviral syndrome (ARS) during the initial infection. ARS mimics a mononucleosis-like illness with fevers, pharyngitis, lymphadenopathy, weight loss, night sweats, diarrhea, and nausea. Symptoms occur 2 to 6 weeks after exposure and persist for 2 to 10 weeks. ARS is associated with a high viral load and a decrease in CD4 cells, but an immune response is mounted decreasing the viral load leading to ARS symptom resolution. Therefore, after the initial ARS, HIV is an asymptomatic disease until the progression to AIDS which can take years to develop. AIDS is the development of opportunistic infections or patients at risk of the development of opportunistic infections (ie, CD4 cell count below 200 cells/mm³).

HIV testing is recommended when HIV infection is suspected because of symptoms and/or high-risk behavior. Additionally, the Centers for Disease Control recommends routine HIV screening in persons 13 to 64 years, a policy called "opt-out" testing. A focus of the recommendations is to screen persons at high risk of HIV infection at least annually and to screen pregnant women while they are in care. The policy states that consent for medical care will imply consent for HIV testing; however, the person must be informed of the test and can opt out of taking it. Because states may have different HIV consent laws, the local requirements for HIV testing should be consulted. The rationale for the opt-out strategy is to diagnose those who unknowingly carry HIV and to initiate therapy early leading to improved prognosis and reduced transmissions. HIV infection is diagnosed by a reactive enzyme-linked immunosorbent assay (ELISA) and positive confirmatory test (eg, Western blot). ELISA tests are highly sensitive (<99%) and highly specific (>99%), but rare false-positive results can occur particularly in those with autoimmune disorders. False negative ELISA tests occur and are attributed to new infection because antibody production takes 3 to 4 weeks after exposure and up to 6 months. Several point-of-care screening kits are available for serum, plasma, whole blood, or oral fluids. While oral fluid tests are convenient, they are not as sensitive as blood assays, which may result in false negatives early in infections; this is a particular disadvantage in the setting of HIV testing prior to initiating or continuing preexposure prophylaxis (PrEP). Once diagnosed with HIV, a patient should receive counseling, a complete medical history, and a baseline physical and laboratory evaluation (Table 27-1).

Once HIV is diagnosed and a baseline evaluation is complete, HIV progression is routinely monitored by viral load and CD4 cell count. Viral load is a major prognostic factor for disease progression, CD4 count decline, and death. It is also the predominant way to assess the effectiveness of treatment. The viral load test quantifies the degree of viremia by measuring the number of copies of viral RNA (HIV RNA) in the plasma. The viral load is reported as the number of viral RNA copies per milliliter of plasma and a viral load laboratory assay has a lower limit of quantitation. Unfortunately, results can vary between different viral load assays; therefore, it is recommended that the same assay method be used consistently for each patient. Reductions in viral load often are reported in base 10 logarithm. For example, if a patient presents initially

TABLE 27-1	CDC Recommendations for Baseline Laboratory Evaluation of Newly Diagnosed HIV Patient

- CD4 T-cell count
- Plasma HIV RNA (viral load)
- Complete blood count
- Complete chemistry profile including transaminase levels
- Urinalysis
- Syphilis screening test (eg, RPR, VDRL, or Treponema EIA)
- TST or IGRA unless history of:
  prior disease or positive tests
  Anti-*Toxoplasma gondii* IgG
- Hepatitis A, B, and C serologies
- Pap smear (women)
- Fasting blood glucose and serum lipids at risk for cardiovascular disease and for baseline evaluation prior to initiation of combination antiretroviral therapy
- Genotypic resistance testing in patients with pretreatment HIV RNA >1000 copies/mL, regardless if therapy will be immediately initiated
  - Patients with HIV RNA levels of 500-1000 copies/mL, resistance testing also can be considered, but amplification is not always successful

Abbreviations: EIA, enzyme immunoassay; HIV, human immunodeficiency virus; IgG, immunoglobulin G; IGRA, interferon-γ release assay; RNA, Ribonucleic acid; RPR, rapid plasma regain; TST, tuberculin skin test; VDRL, venereal disease research laboratory

with a viral load of 100,000 copies/mL (10^5 copies/mL or 10^8 copies/L) and subsequently has a viral load of 10,000 copies/mL (10^4 copies/mL or 10^7 copies/L), the decrease is 1 $\log_{10}$. Given that viral load varies within a patient, a perceptible clinical response is generally considered when the decline in viral load is more than 0.5 $\log_{10}$. Because HIV attacks and leads to the destruction of cells bearing the CD4 receptor, the number of CD4 lymphocytes (T-helper cells) in the blood is a critical surrogate marker of disease progression and immune system status. The normal adult CD4 lymphocyte count ranges from 500 to 1600 cells/mm³ (500×10^6-1600×10^6/L), or 40% to 70% of total lymphocytes. CD4 counts in children are age dependent, with younger children having higher CD4 counts. The hallmark of HIV is depletion of CD4 cells and the associated development of opportunistic infections and malignancies. A CD4 count of less than or equal to 200 µL, CD4% of less than 14%, or development of an AIDS defining condition indicates an AIDS classification. AIDS defining conditions include but are not limited to: *Pneumocystis jiroveci* pneumonia, *Mycobacterium avium* complex, esophageal candidiasis, Toxoplasmosis, and Kaposi's sarcoma. An AIDS diagnosis is forever, regardless of restoration of immune status or increase in CD4 cell count.

PREVENTION

Currently there are no effective strategies that will cure HIV infection; therefore, prevention of virus acquisition is key. Prevention strategies differ based on the mode of transmission. Sexual transmission predominately occurs by receptive anal or vaginal intercourse; however, transmission can occur through any sexual contact including oral. Abstinence is the only 100% effective way to prevent sexual transmission of HIV;

however, barrier methods (male and female condoms), reducing or eliminating high-risk behaviors (anal intercourse), and decreasing the number of sexual partners can reduce the risk of transmission. Coinfection with other STDs can increase the risk of transmission, so treating other STDs can reduce transmission rates. Any persons engaging in any high-risk behavior or having multiple sexual partners should be routinely screened for HIV and other STDs.

Parenteral transmission includes IV drug injection with used needles, shared drug paraphernalia, needle stick exposure in the healthcare setting, and receipt of contaminated blood products or organs. Prevention of parenteral transmission includes stopping IV drug abuse, obtaining clean needles and not reusing any paraphernalia, and using personal protective equipment (PPE) in the healthcare setting when obtaining blood or injecting medication in a patient. The risk of HIV transmission secondary to receipt of blood products or organs has been dramatically reduced due to rigorous screening mechanisms.

Perinatal transmission can be dramatically reduced by screening all pregnant mothers for HIV during the pregnancy and providing antiretroviral therapy (ART) to those infected. Mothers with HIV should not breastfeed because HIV can be transmitted through breast milk.

Pre-exposure Prophylaxis

PrEP is a method of prevention allowing HIV-negative individuals to take antiretrovirals to prevent acquisition. Tenofovir (TVF) plus emtricitabine (Truvada®) is FDA-approved PrEP therapy. High-risk individuals in serodiscordant heterosexual relationships and injection drug users may benefit from therapy. Patients considering PrEP should have a documented negative HIV screening test and should not be provided more than 90 days of therapy without a repeat negative test. Continuous adherence to therapy on a daily basis is associated with a reduction in HIV transmission.

TREATMENT

Potent combination ART (also termed highly active antiretroviral therapy, HAART; combination antiretroviral therapy, cART) has revolutionized treatment for patients diagnosed with HIV/AIDS. Treatment goals include a decrease in morbidity and mortality, improvement in quality of life, restoration and preservation of immune function, and prevention of further transmission. The most effective way to achieve these goals is maximal and durable suppression of HIV replication by having the viral load less than the lower limit of quantitation (ie, undetectable; usually less than 50 copies/mL [less than 50×10^3/L]). While undetectable HIV RNA almost always corresponds with a rise in CD4 lymphocytes, some patients respond virologically or immunologically without the other. There are six antiretroviral classes approved for therapy and include: nucleoside/tide reverse transcriptase inhibitors (NRTIs), nonnucleoside reverse transcriptase inhibitors (NNRTIs), protease inhibitors (PIs), fusion inhibitors, integrase strand transfer

TABLE 27-2	Combination HIV Medications

Single Tablet Regimens (STRs)
Abacavir, dolutegravir, lamivudine (Triumeq)
Efavirenz, emtricitabine, tenofovir (TDF) (Atripla)
Elvitegravir, cobicistat, emtricitabine, tenofovir (TAF) (Genvoya)
Elvitegravir, cobicistat, emtricitabine, tenofovir (TDF) (Stribild)
Emtricitabine, rilpivarine, tenofovir (TAF) (Odefsey)
Emtricitabine, rilpivirine, tenofovir (TDF) (Complera)

Multiple Tablet Regimens (MTRs)
Abacavir, lamivudine (Epzicom)
Abacavir, lamivudine, zidovudine (Trizivir)
Atazanavir, cobicistat (Evotaz)
Darunavir, cobicistat (Prezcobix)
Emtricitabine, tenofovir (tenofovir alafenamide [TAF]) (Descovy)
Emtricitabine, tenofovir (tenofovir disoproxil fumarate [TDF]) (Truvada)
Lamivudine, zidovudine (Combivir)
Lopinavir, ritonavir (Kaletra)

inhibitors (INSTI), and CCR5-receptor antagonists. However, there are four classes of ARTs that are primarily utilized: NRTIs, NNRTIs, INSTIs, and PIs. Additionally, single tablet regimens (STRs) were developed in 2006 and now are the predominant type of ART formulation utilized. STRs are a single pill consisting of multiple different HIV medications. STRs are one pill per day and have improved patient adherence and associated with improved clinical outcomes compared to multiple tablet regimens (MTRs). It is very important to know the different types of combination formulation products available for HIV (Table 27-2).

The initial step of viral entry into the CD4 cell is inhibited by fusion inhibitors (bind to portion of gp-41 on the viral surface) and CCR5-receptor antagonists (bind to CCR5 protein on CD4 cell to prevent virion binding). NRTIs *indirectly* target reverse transcriptase causing termination of DNA chain elongation acting as false nucleoside/tide analogues. NNRTIs directly act on reverse transcriptase, binding to and inhibiting enzymatic activity, preventing viral conversion from RNA to DNA. Viral DNA integration into CD4 DNA is inhibited by INSTI targeting the enzyme by the same name, integrase. The final step prior to viral budding from the CD4 cell is a viral packaging step, which is inhibited by the PIs. The Department of Health and Human Services (DHHS) Guidelines recommend (preferred or alternative) a backbone of therapy with two NRTIs (TVF plus emtricitabine or Truvada® is preferred) plus either the NNRTI, efavirenz (Sustiva®), an INSTI, or a PI boosted with ritonavir (Norvir®) for treatment of naïve patients. Fusion inhibitors and the CCR5-receptor antagonists are recommended in treatment experienced patients. Tables 27-3 to 27-10 summarize treatment initiation recommendations and key antiretroviral characteristics.

ART should be individualized based on patient factors including pre-existing comorbid conditions, potential drug-drug interactions, socioeconomic status, and antiretroviral adverse effects. Drug-drug interactions are an important consideration facilitating treatment and dosing modifications (Tables 27-5 to 27-10). Antiretrovirals have clinically relevant drug interactions because of cytochrome P450 3A4 inhibition and induction (PIs, NNRTIs, select INSTIs, and maraviroc).

TABLE 27-3	Recommendations on When to Initiate Antiretroviral Therapy[a]
Condition and/or Laboratory Data	**Treatment Decision (DHHS Guidelines)**
CD4 <500 cells/mm³	Treat
CD4 >500 cells/mm³	Treat
AIDS-defining illness	Treat
HIV-associated nephropathy	Treat
Coinfected with HBV	Treat
Pregnancy	Treat

Abbreviations: AIDS, acquired immunodeficiency syndrome; DHHS, Department of Health and Human Services; HBV, hepatitis B virus; HIV, human immunodeficiency virus.

*Strongly consider in HIV RNA >100,000 c/mL; CD4 decrease 100 cells/mm³ in 12 months; excessive sexually transmitted infections

[a]Please refer to DHHS guidelines (https://aidsinfo.nih.gov/) for up-to-date recommendations on when to initiate treatment as this may (and often does) change based upon new information.

Some interactions are beneficial and used purposely (eg, ritonavir and cobicistat as pharmacokinetic enhancers); others may be harmful, leading to dangerously elevated or inadequate drug concentrations. Potential drug-drug and/or drug-food interactions should be taken into consideration when selecting an antiretroviral regimen. A thorough review of concomitant medications can help in designing a regimen that minimizes undesirable interactions. In addition, the potential for drug interactions should be assessed when a new antiretroviral is added to an existing antiretroviral combination, as well as when any drug (including over-the-counter agents) is added to a patient's medication regimen. Most drug interactions are mediated through inhibition or induction of hepatic drug metabolism. The PIs (except nelfinavir), the NNRTIs etravirine, and rilpivirine, the CCR5 antagonist maraviroc, and the INSTI elvitegravir are metabolized by CYP3A. In general: (1) efavirenz, etravirine, and nevirapine are inducers of CYP3A; (2) ritonavir is a potent mechanism-based inhibitor of CYP3A-mediated metabolism and is now used exclusively at lower doses as a pharmacokinetic enhancer of other PIs; and (3) cobicistat, which is an analog of ritonavir without antiretroviral activity, is also a potent mechanism-based inhibitor of CYP3A activity and is used also as a pharmacokinetic enhancer. Some antiretroviral drugs require acidic environments for optimal absorption leading to interactions with antacids, particularly proton-pump inhibitors (eg, atazanavir, rilpivirine). However, some antiretroviral agents chelate polyvalent cations in antacids, reducing absorption following concomitant dosing (eg, raltegravir, dolutegravir, elvitegravir); dosing can be separated for these cases. This summary of drug interactions is not complete. Clinicians who treat HIV must stay up to date with antiretroviral drug interaction data. Websites are available that catalog and update HIV drug-interaction information (http://www.hiv-druginteractions.org/), and the DHSS guidelines for antiretroviral use provide, and regularly update, excellent summaries of known clinically relevant drug interactions.

Adverse events are common with ARTs and should be well recognized to allow for appropriate patient counseling.

TABLE 27-4	Recommended, Alternative, and Other Antiretroviral Regimen Options for Treatment-Naïve Patients

Selection of a regimen should be individualized based on virologic efficacy, potential adverse effects, pill burden, dosing frequency, drug-drug interaction potential, comorbid conditions, cost, and resistance test results. Some regimens listed in this table may not be appropriate for patients with renal impairment. See the product prescribing information for recommendations on ARV dose modification in the setting of renal impairment. Drug classes and regimens within each class are arranged first by evidence rating and when ratings are equal, in alphabetical order.

Recommended Regimen Options
Recommended regimens are those with demonstrated durable virologic efficacy, favorable tolerability and toxicity profiles, and ease of use

INSTI plus two-NRTI Regimen:
- DTG/ABC/3TC[a] **(AI)**—if HLA-B*5701 negative
- DTG plus either TDF/FTC[a] **(AI)** or TAF/FTC[b] **(AII)**
- EVG/c/TAF/FTC **(AI)** or EVG/c/TDF/FTC **(AI)**
- RAL plus either TDF/FTC[a] **(AI)** or TAF/FTC[b] **(AII)**

Boosted PI plus two NRTIs:
DRV/r plus either TDF/FTC[a] **(AI)** or TAF/FTC[b] **(AII)**

Alternative Regimen Options
Alternative regimens are effective and tolerable, but have potential disadvantages when compared with the recommended regimens, have limitations for use in certain patient populations, or have less supporting data from randomized clinical trials. **However, an alternative regimen may be the preferred regimen for some patients.**

NNRTI plus two NRTIs:
- EFV/TDF/FTC[a] **(BI)**
- EFV plus TAF/FTC[b] **(BII)**
- RPV/TDF/FTC[a] **(BI)** or RPV/TAF/FTC[b] **(BII)**—if HIV RNA <100,000 copies/mL and CD4 >200 cells/mm³

Boosted PI plus two NRTIs:
- (ATV/c or ATV/r) plus either TDF/FTC[a] **(BI)** or TAF/FTC[b] **(BII)**
- DRV/c **(BIII)** or DRV/r **(BII)** plus ABC/3TC[a]—if HLA-B*5701 negative
- DRV/c plus either TDF/FTC[a] **(BII)** or TAF/FTC[b] **(BII)**

[a] 3TC may be substituted for FTC, or vice versa, if a non-fixed dose NRTI combination is desired.

[b] The evidence supporting this regimen is based on relative bioavailability data coupled with data from randomized, controlled switch trials demonstrating the safety and efficacy of TAF-containing regimens.

Note: The following are available as coformulated products: ABC/3TC, ATV/c, DRV/c, DTG/ABC/3TC, EFV/TDF/FTC, EVG/cTAF/FTC, EVG/c/TDF/FTC, LPV/r, RPV/TAF/FTC, RPV/TDF/FTC, TAF/FTC, and TDF/FTC.

Abbreviations: 3TC, lamivudine; ABC, abacavir; ATV/c, atazanavir/cobicistat; ATV/r, atazanavir/ritonavir; CD4, CD4 T lymphocyte; DRV/c, darunavir/cobicistat; DRV/r, darunavir/ritonavir; DTG, dolutegravir; EFV, efavirenz; EVG, elvitegravir; FTC, emtricitabine; INSTI, integrase strand transfer inhibitor; LPV/r, lopinavir/ritonavir; NNRTI, non-nucleoside reverse transcriptase inhibitor; NRTI, nucleoside reverse transcriptase inhibitor; RAL, raltegravir; RPV, rilpivirine; TAF, tenofovir alafenamide; TDF, tenofovir disoproxil fumarate.

Common ART-associated effects are listed in Tables 27-5 to 27-9. Adherence to therapy is the cornerstone for successful outcomes in suppressing the HIV virus and helping to prevent opportunistic infections. Therefore, patient desire and willingness to engage in treatment and maintain adherence must be evaluated and confirmed prior to initiating treatment. Resistance testing is recommended prior to initiating ART. The goal of ART is to have three active agents in the regimen (not including the pharmacokinetic enhancers ritonavir or cobicistat). Three active agents are associated with increased viral

TABLE 27-5	Advantages and Disadvantages of Antiretroviral Components Recommended as Initial Antiretroviral Therapy		

Note: All drugs within an ARV class are listed in alphabetical order.

ARV Class	ARV Agent(s)	Advantage(s)	Disadvantage(s)
Dual–NRTI	ABC/3TC	▪ Coformulated with DTG	▪ May cause life-threatening hypersensitivity reaction in patients positive for the HLA-B*5701 allele. As a result, HLA-B*5701 testing is required before use. ▪ In the ACTG 5202 study, patients with baseline HIV RNA ≥100,000 copies/mL showed inferior virologic responses when ABC/3TC was given with EFV or ATV/r as opposed to TDF/FTC. This difference was not seen when ABC/3TC was used in combination with DTG. ▪ ABC use has been associated with cardiovascular disease and cardiac events in some, but not all, observational studies.
	TAF/FTC	▪ Coformulated with EVG/c or RPV ▪ Active against HBV ▪ Smaller decline in renal function, less proteinuria, and smaller reductions in BMD than after initiation of TDF/FTC ▪ Safe in patients with eGFR ≤30 mL/min	▪ Fasting lipid levels, including LDL and HDL cholesterol and triglycerides, increased more in the TAF group than in the TDF group. Total cholesterol to HDL ratio was unchanged.
	TDF/FTC	▪ Coformulated with EFV, EVG/c, and RPV as STRs ▪ Active against HBV; recommended dual-NRTI for HIV/HBV coinfected patients ▪ Better virologic responses than with ABC/3TC in patients with baseline viral load ≥100,000 copies/mL when combined with ATV/r or EFV ▪ Associated with more favorable lipid effects than ABC or TAF	▪ Renal toxicity, including proximal tubulopathy and acute or chronic renal insufficiency ▪ Osteomalacia has been reported as a consequence of proximal tubulopathy ▪ Decreases BMD more than other NRTI combinations
INSTI	DTG	▪ Once-daily dosing ▪ Higher barrier to resistance than EVG or RAL ▪ Coformulated with ABC and 3TC ▪ No food requirement ▪ No CYP3A4 interactions	▪ Oral absorption of DTG can be reduced by simultaneous administration with products containing polyvalent cations (eg, Al, Ca, or Mg-containing antacids or supplements, or multivitamin tablets with minerals). ▪ Inhibits renal tubular secretion of Cr and can increase serum Cr without affecting glomerular function ▪ UGT substrate; potential for drug interactions ▪ Depression and suicidal ideation (rare, usually in patients with pre-existing psychiatric conditions)
	EVG/c	▪ Coformulated with TDF/FTC or TAF/FTC ▪ Once-daily dosing ▪ Compared with ATV/r, causes smaller increases in total and LDL cholesterol	▪ EVG/c/TDF/FTC is only recommended for patients with baseline CrCl ≥70 mL/min; this regimen should be discontinued if CrCl decreases to <50 mL/min. ▪ COBI is a potent CYP3A4 inhibitor, which can result in significant interactions with CYP3A substrates. ▪ Oral absorption of EVG can be reduced by simultaneous administration with products containing polyvalent cations (eg, Al, Ca, or Mg-containing antacids or supplements, or multivitamin tablets with minerals). ▪ COBI inhibits active tubular secretion of Cr and can increase serum Cr, without affecting renal glomerular function. ▪ May have lower genetic barrier to resistance than boosted PI- or DTG-based regimens ▪ Food requirement ▪ Depression and suicidal ideation (rare; usually in patients with preexisting psychiatric conditions)
	RAL	▪ Compared to other INSTIs, has longest postmarketing experience ▪ No food requirement ▪ No CYP3A4 interactions	▪ Twice-daily dosing ▪ May have lower genetic barrier to resistance than boosted PI- or DTG-based regimens ▪ Increases in creatine kinase, myopathy, and rhabdomyolysis have been reported. ▪ Rare cases of severe hypersensitivity reactions (including SJS and TEN) have been reported. ▪ Oral absorption of RAL can be reduced by simultaneous administration with products containing polyvalent cations (eg, Al, Ca, or Mg-containing antacids or supplements, or multivitamin tablets with minerals). ▪ UGT substrate; potential for drug interactions ▪ Depression and suicidal ideation (rare; usually in patients with preexisting psychiatric conditions)

(Continued)

TABLE 27-5 Advantages and Disadvantages of Antiretroviral Components Recommended as Initial Antiretroviral Therapy (*Continued*)

Note: All drugs within an ARV class are listed in alphabetical order.

ARV Class	ARV Agent(s)	Advantage(s)	Disadvantage(s)
INSTI, contd.	EFV	<ul><li>Once-daily dosing</li><li>Coformulated with TDF/FTC</li><li>Long-term clinical experience</li><li>EFV-based regimens (except for EFV plus ABC/3TC) have well documented efficacy in patients with high HIV RNA.</li></ul>	<ul><li>Transmitted resistance more common than with PIs and INSTIs</li><li>Short- and long-term neuropsychiatric (CNS) side effects, including depression and, in some studies, suicidality</li><li>Teratogenic in nonhuman primates; avoid use in women who are trying to conceive or who are sexually active and not using contraception</li><li>Dyslipidemia</li><li>Greater risk of resistance at the time of treatment failure than with PIs</li><li>Skin rash</li><li>Potential for CYP450 drug interactions</li><li>Should be taken on an empty stomach (food increases drug absorption and CNS toxicities)</li></ul>
NNRTIs	RPV	<ul><li>Once-daily dosing</li><li>Coformulated with TDF/FTC and TAF/FTC</li><li>RPV/TDF/FTC and RPV/TAF/FTC have smaller pill size than other coformulated ARV drugs</li><li>Compared with EFV:<ul><li>Fewer discontinuations for CNS adverse effects</li><li>Fewer lipid effects</li><li>Fewer rashes</li></ul></li></ul>	<ul><li>Not recommended in patients with pre-ART HIV RNA >100,000 copies/mL or CD4 count <200 cells/mm^3 because of higher rate of virologic failure in these patients</li><li>Transmitted resistance more common than with PIs and INSTIs</li><li>More NNRTI-, TDF-, and 3TC-associated mutations at virologic failure than with regimen containing EFV and two NRTIs</li><li>Potential for CYP450 drug interactions</li><li>Meal requirement (>390 kcal)</li><li>Requires acid for adequate absorption<ul><li>Contraindicated with PPIs</li><li>Use with H2 antagonists or antacids with caution</li></ul></li><li>Use caution when coadministering with a drug known to increase the risk of Torsades de Pointes</li><li>Depression and suicidality</li></ul>
PIs	ATV/c or ATV/r	<ul><li>Once-daily dosing</li><li>Higher genetic barrier to resistance than NNRTIs, EVG, and RAL</li><li>PI resistance at the time of treatment failure uncommon with PK-enhanced PIs</li><li>ATV/c and ATV/r have similar virologic activity and toxicity profiles</li></ul>	<ul><li>Commonly causes indirect hyperbilirubinemia, which may manifest as scleral icterus or jaundice</li><li>Food requirement</li><li>Absorption depends on food and low gastric pH</li><li>Nephrolithiasis, cholelithiasis, nephrotoxicity</li><li>GI adverse effects</li><li>CYP3A4 inhibitors and substrates: potential for drug interactions</li></ul>
	ATV/c (Specific considerations)	<ul><li>Coformulated tablet</li></ul>	<ul><li>COBI inhibits active tubular secretion of Cr and can increase serum Cr, without affecting renal glomerular function.</li><li>Coadministration with TDF is not recommended in patients with CrCl <70 mL/min</li><li>Less long-term clinical experience than for ATV/r</li><li>COBI is a potent CYP3A4 inhibitor, which can result in significant interactions with CYP3A substrates.</li></ul>
	DRV/c or DRV/r	<ul><li>Once-daily dosing</li><li>Higher genetic barrier to resistance than NNRTIs, EVG, and RAL</li><li>PI resistance at the time of treatment failure uncommon with PK-enhanced PIs</li></ul>	<ul><li>Skin rash</li><li>Food requirement</li><li>GI adverse effects</li><li>CYP3A4 inhibitors and substrates: potential for drug interactions</li></ul>
	DRV/c-specific considerations	<ul><li>Coformulated tablet</li></ul>	<ul><li>Less long-term clinical experience than for DRV/r</li><li>COBI inhibits active tubular secretion of Cr and can increase serum Cr, without affecting renal glomerular function.</li><li>Coadministration with TDF is not recommended in patients with CrCl <70 mL/min</li><li>Approval primarily based on PK data comparable to that for DRV/r rather than on trials comparing the efficacy of DRV/c and DRV/r</li><li>COBI is a potent CYP3A4 inhibitor, which can result in significant interactions with CYP3A substrates.</li></ul>
	LPV/r	<ul><li>Only RTV-coformulated PI</li><li>No food requirement</li><li>Once or twice daily dosing</li></ul>	<ul><li>Requires 200 mg per day of RTV</li><li>Possible higher risk of MI associated with cumulative use of LPV/r</li><li>PR and QT interval prolongation have been reported. Use with caution in patients at risk of cardiac conduction abnormalities or in patients receiving other drugs with similar effect</li><li>Possible nephrotoxicity</li><li>CYP3A4 inhibitors and substrates: potential for drug interactions</li></ul>

Abbreviations: 3TC, lamivudine; ABC, abacavir; AI, aluminum; ART, antiretroviral therapy; ARV, antiretroviral; ATV, atazanavir; ATV/c, atazanavir/cobicistat; ATV/r, atazanavir/ritonavir; BMD, bone mineral density; Ca, calcium; CaCO$_3$, calcium carbonate; CD4, CD4 T lymphocyte; CNS, central nervous system; c or COBI, cobicistat; Cr, creatinine; CrCl, creatinine clearance; CYP, cytochrome P450; DRV darunavir; DRV/c, darunavir/cobicistat: DRV/r, darunavir/ritonavir; DTG, dolutegravir; EFV, efavirenz; EVG, elvitegravir; EVG/c, elvitegravir/cobicistat; FTC, emtricitabine; GI, gastrointestinal; HBV, hepatitis B virus; HDL, high-density lipoprotein; HSR, hypersensitivity reaction; INSTI, integrase strand transfer inhibitor; LDL, low-density lipoprotein; LPV/r, lopinavir/ritonavir; Mg, magnesium; MI, myocardial infarction; NNRTI, non-nucleoside reverse transcriptase inhibitor; NRTI, nucleoside reverse transcriptase inhibitor; PI, protease inhibitor; PPI, proton pump inhibitor; RAL, raltegravir; RPV, rilpivirine; RTV, ritonavir; SJS, Stevens-Johnson syndrome; STRs, single-tablet regimens; TAF, tenofovir alafenamide; TDF, tenofovir disoproxil fumarate; TEN, toxic epidermal necrosis.

TABLE 27-6   Characteristics of Nucleoside Reverse Transcriptase Inhibitors

Generic Name (Abbreviation) *Trade Name*	Formulations	Dosing Recommendations	Elimination	Serum/ Intracellular Half-Lives	Adverse Event
Abacavir (ABC) *Ziagen* Note: Generic available in tablet formulation **Also available as a component of fixed-dose combinations (by trade name and abbreviation):** *Triazivir* (ABC/ZDV/3TC) **Note:** Generic available *Epzicom* (ABC/3TC) *Triumeq* (ABC/3TC/DTG)	**Ziagen:** ■ 300 mg tablet ■ 20 mg/mL oral solution **Trizivir:** ■ (ABC 300 mg plus ZDV 300 mg plus 3TC 150 mg) tablet **Epzicom:** ■ (ABC 600 mg plus 3TC 300 mg) tablet **Triumeq:** ■ (ABC 600 mg plus 3TC 300 mg plus DTG 50 mg) tablet	**Ziagen:** ■ 300 mg bid, *or* ■ 600 mg once daily ■ Take without regard to meals **Trizivir:** ■ 1 tablet bid **Epzicom:** ■ 1 tablet once daily **Triumeq:** ■ 1 tablet once daily	Metabolized by alcohol dehydrogenase and glucuronyl transferase Renal excretion of metabolites: 82% Dosage adjustment for ABC is recommended in patients with hepatic insufficiency	1.5 h/12–26 h	■ HSRs: Patients who test positive for HLA-B*5701 are at highest risk. HLA screening should be done before initiation of ABC. ■ For patients with history of HSR, re-challenge is not recommended. ■ Symptoms of HSR may include fever, rash, nausea, vomiting, diarrhea, abdominal pain, malaise, fatigue, or respiratory symptoms such as sore throat, cough, or shortness of breath. ■ Some cohort studies suggest increased risk of MI with recent or current use of ABC, but this risk is not substantiated in other studies.
Didanosine (ddI) *Videx* *Videx EC* **Note:** Generic available; dose same as Videx or Videx EC	**Videx EC:** ■ 125, 200, 250, and 400 mg capsules **Videx:** ■ 10 mg/mL oral solution	**Body Weight ≥60 kg:** ■ 400 mg once daily *With TDF:* ■ 250 mg once daily **Body Weight <60 kg:** ■ 250 mg once daily *With TDF:* ■ 200 mg once daily Take 1/2 h before or 2 h after a meal. **Note:** Preferred dosing with oral solution is bid (total daily dose divided into 2 doses).	Renal excretion: 50% Dosage adjustment in patients with renal insufficiency is recommended	1.5 h/>20 h	■ Pancreatitis ■ Peripheral neuropathy ■ Retinal changes, optic neuritis ■ Lactic acidosis with hepatic steatosis with or without pancreatitis (rare but potentially life–threatening toxicity) ■ Nausea, vomiting ■ Potential association with noncirrhotic portal hypertension; in some cases, patients presented with esophageal varices ■ One cohort study suggested increased risk of MI with recent or current use of ddI, but this risk is not substantiated in other studies. ■ Insulin resistance/diabetes mellitus

(Continued)

TABLE 27-6 Characteristics of Nucleoside Reverse Transcriptase Inhibitors (*Continued*)

Generic Name (Abbreviation) *Trade Name*	Formulations	Dosing Recommendations	Elimination	Serum/ Intracellular Half-Lives	Adverse Event
Emtricitabine (FTC) *Emtriva* Also available as a component of fixed-dose combinations (by trade name and abbreviation):	**Emtriva:** ▪ 200 mg hard gelatin capsule ▪ 10 mg/mL oral solution	**Emtriva:** *Capsule:* ▪ 200 mg once daily *Oral Solution:* ▪ 240 mg (24 mL) once daily Take without regard to meals.	Renal excretion: 86% Dosage adjustment in patients with renal insufficiency is recommended	10 h/>20 h	▪ Minimal toxicity ▪ Hyperpigmentation/skin discoloration ▪ Severe acute exacerbation of hepatitis may occur in HBV-coinfected patients who discontinue FTC.
Atripla (FTC/EFV/TDF)	**Atripla:** ▪ (FTC 200 mg plus EFV 600 mg plus TDF 300 mg) tablet	**Atripla:** ▪ 1 tablet at or before bedtime ▪ Take on an empty stomach to reduce side effects.			
Complera (FTC/RPV/TDF)	**Complera:** ▪ (FTC 200 mg plus RPV 25 mg plus TDF 300 mg) tablet	**Complera:** ▪ 1 tablet once daily with a meal			
Descovy (FTC/TAF)	**Descovy:** ▪ (FTC 200 mg plus TAF 25 mg) tablet	**Descovy:** ▪ 1 tablet once daily			
Genvoya (FTC/EVG/c/TAF)	**Genvoya:** ▪ (FTC 200 mg plus EVG 150 mg plus COBI 150 mg plus TAF 10 mg) tablet	**Genvoya:** ▪ 1 tablet once daily with food			
Odefsey (FTC/RPV/TAF)	**Odefsey:** ▪ (FTC 200 mg plus RPV 25 mg plus TAF 25 mg) tablet	**Odefsey:** ▪ 1 tablet once daily with a meal			
Stribild (FTC/EVG/c/TDF)	**Stribild:** ▪ (FTC 200 mg plus EVG 150 mg plus COBI 150 mg plus TDF 300 mg) tablet	**Stribild:** ▪ 1 tablet once daily with food			
Truvada (FTC/TDF)	**Truvada:** ▪ (FTC 200 mg plus TDF 300 mg) tablet	**Truvada:** ▪ 1 tablet once daily			
Lamivudine (3TC) *Epivir* **Note:** Generic available Also available as a component of fixed-dose combinations (by trade name and abbreviation):	**Epivir:** ▪ 150 and 300 mg tablets ▪ 10 mg/mL oral solution	**Epivir:** ▪ 150 mg bid, or ▪ 300 mg once daily ▪ Take without regard to meals.	Renal excretion: 70% Dosage adjustment in patients with renal insufficiency is recommended	5-7 h/18-22 h	▪ Minimal toxicity ▪ Severe acute exacerbation of hepatitis may occur in HBV-coinfected patients who discontinue 3TC.
Combivir (3TC/ZDV) **Note:** Generic available	**Combivir:** ▪ (3TC 150 mg plus ZDV 300 mg) tablet	**Combivir:** ▪ 1 tablet bid			
Epzicom (3TC/ABC)	**Epzicom:** ▪ (3TC 300 mg plus ABC 600 mg) tablet	**Epzicom:** ▪ 1 tablet once daily			
Trizivir (3TC/ZDV/ABC) **Note:** Generic available	**Trizivir:** ▪ (3TC 150 mg plus ZDV 300 mg plus ABC 300 mg) tablet	**Trizivir:** ▪ 1 tablet bid			
Triumeq (3TC/ABC/DTG)	**Triumeq:** ▪ (3TC 300 mg plus ABC 600 mg plus DTG 50 mg) tablet	**Triumeq:** ▪ 1 tablet once daily			

Drug	Preparations	Dosing	Pharmacokinetics	Adverse Effects
Stavudine (d4T) *Zerit* **Note:** Generic available	**Zerit:** • 15, 20, 30, and 40 mg capsules • 1 mg/mL oral solution	**Body Weight ≥60 kg:** • 40 mg bid **Body Weight <60 kg:** • 30 mg bid Take without regard to meals. **Note:** WHO recommends 30 mg bid dosing regardless of body weight.	Renal excretion: 50% Dosage adjustment in patients with renal insufficiency is recommended. 1 h/7.5 h	• Peripheral neuropathy • Lipoatrophy • Pancreatitis • Lactic acidosis/severe hepatomegaly with hepatic steatosis (rare but potentially life-threatening toxicity) • Hyperlipidemia • Insulin resistance/diabetes mellitus • Rapidly progressive ascending neuromuscular weakness (rare)
Tenofovir Alafenamide (TAF) Only available as a component of fixed-dose combinations (by trade name and abbreviation). *Descovy (TAF/FTC)*	See fixed-dose combinations below. **Descovy:** • (FTC 200 mg plus TAF 25 mg) tablet	See fixed-dose combinations below. **Descovy:** • 1 tablet once daily	Metabolized by cathepsin A; P-glycoprotein substrate Not recommended in patients with CrCl < 30 mL/min 0.5 h/150-130 h	• Renal insufficiency, Fanconi syndrome, proximal renal tubulopathy, less likely than from TDF • Osteomalacia, decrease in bone mineral density, lesser effect than from TDF • Severe acute exacerbation of hepatitis may occur in HBV-coinfected patients who discontinue TAF • Diarrhea, nausea, headache
Genvoya (TAF/EVG/c/FTC)	• (TAF 10 mg plus EVG 150 mg plus COBI 150 mg plus FTC 200 mg) tablet	**Genvoya:** • 1 tablet once daily with food		
Odefsey (TAF/RPV/FTC)	• (TAF 25 mg plus RPV 25 mg plus FTC 200 mg) tablet	**Odefsey:** • 1 tablet once daily with a meal		
Tenofovir Disoproxil Fumarate (TDF) *Viread* Also available as a component of fixed-dose combinations (by trade name and abbreviation):	**Viread:** • 150, 200, 250, and 300 mg tablets • 40 mg/g oral powder	**Viread:** • 300 mg once daily, or • 7.5 level scoops once daily (dosing scoop dispensed with each prescription; 1 level scoop contains 1 g of oral powder). • Take without regard to meals. Mix oral powder with 2-4 ounces of a soft food that does not require chewing (eg, applesauce, yogurt). **Do not mix oral powder with liquid.**	Renal excretion is primary route of elimination. Dosage adjustment in patients with renal insufficiency is recommended 17 h/>60 h	• Renal insufficiency, Fanconi syndrome, proximal renal tubulopathy • Osteomalacia, decrease in bone mineral density • Severe acute exacerbation hepatitis may occur in HBV-coinfected patients who discontinue TDF. • Asthenia, headache, diarrhea, nausea, vomiting, and flatulence
Atripla (TDF/EFV/FTC)	**Atripla:** • (TDF 300 mg plus EFV 600 mg plus FTC 200 mg) tablet	**Atripla:** • 1 tablet at or before bedtime • Take on an empty stomach to reduce side effects.		
Complera (TDF/RPV/FTC)	**Complera:** • (TDF 300 mg plus RPV 25 mg plus FTC 200 mg) tablet	**Complera:** • 1 tablet once daily • Take with a meal.		
Stribild (TDF/EVG/c/FTC)	**Stribild:** • (TDF 300 mg plus EVG 150 mg plus COBI 150 mg plus FTC 200 mg) tablet	**Stribild:** • 1 tablet once daily • Take with food.		
Truvada (TDF/FTC)	**Truvada:** • (TDF 300 mg plus FTC 200 mg) tablet	**Truvada:** • 1 tablet once daily • Take without regard to meals.		

(Continued)

TABLE 27-6 **Characteristics of Nucleoside Reverse Transcriptase Inhibitors** (*Continued*)

Generic Name (Abbreviation) *Trade Name*	Formulations	Dosing Recommendations	Elimination	Serum/ Intracellular Half-Lives	Adverse Event
Zidovudine (ZDV) *Retrovir* **Note:** Generic available **Also available as a component of fixed-dose combinations (by trade name and abbreviation):** *Combivir* (ZDV/3TC) **Note:** Generic available *Trizivir* (ZDV /3TC/ ABC) **Note:** Generic available	**Retrovir:** ▪ 100 mg capsule ▪ 300 mg tablet (only available as generic) ▪ 10 mg/mL intravenous solution ▪ 10 mg/mL oral solution **Combivir:** ▪ (ZDV 300 mg plus 3TC 150 mg) tablet **Trizivir:** ▪ (ZDV 300 mg plus 3TC 150 mg plus ABC 300 mg) tablet	**Retrovir:** ▪ 300 mg bid, or ▪ 200 mg tid ▪ Take without regard to meals. **Combivir:** ▪ 1 tablet bid ▪ Take without regard to meals. **Trizivir:** ▪ 1 tablet bid ▪ Take without regard to meals.	Metabolized to GAZT Renal excretion of GAZT Dosage adjustment in patients with renal insufficiency is recommended	1.1 h/7 h	▪ Bone marrow suppression: macrocytic anemia or neutropenia ▪ Nausea, vomiting, headache, insomnia, asthenia ▪ Nail pigmentation ▪ Lactic acidosis/severe hepatomegaly with hepatic steatosis (rare but potentially life-threatening toxicity) ▪ Hyperlipidemia ▪ Insulin resistance/diabetes mellitus ▪ Lipoatrophy ▪ Myopathy

Abbreviations: 3TC, lamivudine; ABC, abacavir; bid, twice daily; c, COBI, cobicistat; CrCl, creatinine clearance; d4T, stavudine; ddI, didanosine; DTG, dolutegravir; EC, enteric coated; EFV, efavirenz; EVG, elvitegravir; FTC, emtricitabine; GAZT, azidothymidine glucuronide; HBV, hepatitis B virus; HLA, human leukocyte antigen; HSR, hypersensitivity reaction; MI, myocardial infarction; RPV, rilpivirine; TAF, tenofovir alafenamide; TDF, tenofovir disoproxil fumarate; tid, three times a day; WHO, World Health Organization; ZDV, zidovudine.

TABLE 27-7 Characteristics of Non-Nucleoside Reverse Transcriptase Inhibitors

Generic Name (Abbreviation) Trade Name	Formulations	Dosing Recommendations	Elimination Metabolic Pathway	Serum Half-Life	Adverse Events
Efavirenz (EFV) *Sustiva* Also available as a component of fixed-dose combination (by trade name and abbreviation): *Atripla* (EFV/TDF/FTC)	**Sustiva:** ▪ 50 and 200 mg capsules ▪ 600 mg tablet **Atripla:** ▪ (EFV 600 mg plus TDF 300 mg plus FTC 200 mg) tablet	**Sustiva:** ▪ 600 mg once daily, at or before bedtime ▪ Take on an empty stomach to reduce side effects. **Atripla:** ▪ 1 tablet once daily, at or before bedtime	Metabolized by CYPs 2B6 (primary), 3A4, and 2A6 CYP3A4 mixed inducer/inhibitor (more an inducer than an inhibitor) CYP2C9 and 2C19 inhibitor; 2B6 inducer	40-55 h	▪ Rash[a] ▪ Neuropsychiatric symptoms[b] ▪ Increased transaminase levels ▪ Hyperlipidemia ▪ False-positive results with some cannabinoid and benzodiazepine screening assays reported. ▪ Teratogenic in nonhuman primates and potentially teratogenic during the first trimester of pregnancy in humans
Etravirine (ETR) *intelence*	▪ 25, 100, and 200 mg tablets	▪ 200 mg bid ▪ Take following a meal.	CYP3A4, 2C9, and 2C19 substrate 3A4 inducer; 2C9 and 2C19 inhibitor	41 h	▪ Rash, including Stevens-Johnson syndrome[a] ▪ HSRs, characterized by rash, constitutional findings, and sometimes organ dysfunction (including hepatic failure) have been reported. ▪ Nausea
Nevirapine (NVP) *Viramune or Viramine XR* Generic available for 200 mg tablets and oral suspension	▪ 200 mg tablet ▪ 400 mg XR tablet ▪ 50 mg/5 mL oral suspension	▪ 200 mg once daily for 14 d (lead-in period); thereafter, 200 mg bid, or 400 mg (Viramune XR tablet) once daily ▪ Take without regard to meals. ▪ Repeat lead-in period if therapy is discontinued for >7 d. ▪ In patients who develop mild-to-moderate rash without constitutional symptoms, continue lead-in period until rash resolves but not longer than 28 d total.	CYP450 substrate, inducer of 3A4 and 2B6; 80% excreted in urine (glucuronidated metabolites, <5% unchanged); 10% in feces	25-30 h	▪ Rash, including Stevens-Johnson syndrome[a] ▪ Symptomatic hepatitis, including fatal hepatic necrosis, has been reported: ▪ Rash reported In approximately 50% of cases. ▪ Occurs at significantly higher frequency in ARV-naive female patients with pre-NVP CD4 counts >250 cells/mm³ and in ARV-naive male patients with pre-NVP CD4 counts >400 cells/mm³. NVP should not be initiated in these patients unless the benefit clearly outweighs the risk.
Rilpivirine (RPV) *Edurant* Also available as a component of fixed-dose combinations (by trade name and abbreviation): *Complera* (RPV/TDF/FTC) *Odefsey* (RPV/TAF/FTC)	**Edurant:** ▪ 25 mg tablet **Complera:** ▪ (RPV 25 mg plus TDF 300 mg plus FTC 200 mg) tablet **Odefsey:** ▪ (RPV 25 mg plus TAF 25 mg plus FTC 200 mg) tablet	**Edurant:** ▪ 25 mg once daily ▪ Take with a meal. **Complera:** ▪ 1 tablet once daily ▪ Take with a meal. **Odefsey:** ▪ 1 tablet once daily ▪ Take with a meal.	CYP3A4 substrate	50 h	▪ Rash[a] ▪ Depression, insomnia, headache ▪ Hepatotoxicity

Abbreviations: ARV, antiretroviral; bid, twice daily; CD4, CD4 T lymphocyte; CYP, cytochrome P; DLV, delavirdine; EFV, efavirenz; ETR, etravirine; FDA, Food and Drug Administration; FTC, emtricitabine; HSR, hypersensitivity reaction; NNRTI, nonnucleoside reverse transcriptase inhibitor; NVP, nevirapine; RPV, rilpivirine; TAF, tenofovir alafenamide; TDF, tenofovir disoproxil fumarate; XR, extended release.

[a]Rare cases of Stevens-Johnson syndrome have been reported with most NNRTIs; the highest incidence of rash was seen with NVP.

[b]Adverse events can include dizziness, somnolence, insomnia, abnormal dreams, depression, suicidality (suicide, suicide attempt or ideation), confusion, abnormal thinking, impaired concentration, amnesia, agitation, depersonalization, hallucinations, and euphoria. Approximately 50% of patients receiving EFV may experience any of these symptoms. Symptoms usually subside spontaneously after 2 to 4 weeks but may necessitate discontinuation of EFV in a small percentage of patients.

TABLE 27-8 Characteristics of Protease Inhibitors

Generic Name (Abbreviation) / Trade Name	Formulations	Dosing Recommendations	Elimination/ Metabolic Pathway	Serum Half-Life	Storage	Adverse Events
Atazanavir (ATV) / *Reyataz* / Also available as a component of fixed-dose combination (by trade name and abbreviation): / *Evotaz* (ATV/c)	**Reyataz:** • 100, 150, 200, and 300 mg capsules • 50 mg single packet oral powder / **Evotaz:** • (ATV 300 mg plus COBI 150 mg) tablet	**In ARV-Naive Patients:** • (ATV 300 mg plus RTV 100 mg) once daily; or • ATV 400 mg once daily **With TDF or in ARV-Experienced Patients:** • (ATV 300 mg plus RTV 100 mg) once daily **With EFV in ARV-Naive Patients:** • (ATV 400 mg plus RTV 100 mg) once daily Take with food. For recommendations on dosing with H2 antagonists and PPIs, refer to Table 19a. **Evotaz:** • 1 tablet once daily • Take with food. **With TDF:** • **Not recommended** for patients with baseline CrCl <70 mL/min.	CYP3A4 inhibitor and substrate; weak CYP2C8 inhibitor; UGT1A1 inhibitor Dosage adjustment in patients with hepatic insufficiency is recommended ATV: as above COBI: substrate of CYP3A, CYP2D6 (minor); CYP3A inhibitor	7 h	Room temperature (up to 25° C or 77° F)	▪ Indirect hyperbilirubinemia ▪ PR interval prolongation: First-degree symptomatic AV block reported. Use with caution in patients with underlying conduction defects or on concomitant medications that can cause PR prolongation. ▪ Hyperglycemia ▪ Fat maldistribution ▪ Cholelithiasis ▪ Nephrolithiasis ▪ Renal insufficiency ▪ Serum transaminase elevations ▪ Hyperlipidemia (especially with RTV boosting) ▪ Skin rash ▪ Increase in serum creatinine (with COBI)
Darunavir (DRV) / *Prezista* / Also available as a component of fixed-dose combination (by trade name and abbreviation): / *Prezcobix* (DRV/c)	• 75, 150, 600, and 800 mg tablets • 100 mg/mL oral suspension / **Prezcobix:** • (DRV 800 mg plus COBI 150 mg) tablet	**In ARV-Naive Patients or ARV-Experienced Patients with No DRV Mutations:** • (DRV 800 mg plus RTV 100 mg) once daily **In ARV-Experienced Patients with One or More DRV Resistance Mutations:** • (DRV 600 mg plus RTV 100 mg) bid Unboosted DRV **is not recommended.** Take with food. **Prezcobix:** • 1 tablet once daily • Take with food. **Not recommended** for patients with one or more DRV resistance-associated mutations. **With TDF:** • **Not recommended** for patients with baseline CrCl <70 mL/min.	CYP3A4 inhibitor and substrate CYP2C9 inducer DRV: As above COBI: substrate of CYP3A, CYP2D6 (minor); CYP3A inhibitor	15 h (when combined with RTV)	Room temperature (up to 25° C or 77° F)	▪ Skin rash (10%): DRV has a sulfonamide moiety; Stevens-Johnson syndrome, toxic epidermal necrolysis, acute generalized exanthematous pustulosis, and erythema multiforme have been reported. ▪ Hepatotoxicity ▪ Diarrhea, nausea ▪ Headache ▪ Hyperlipidemia ▪ Serum transaminase elevation ▪ Hyperglycemia ▪ Fat maldistribution ▪ Increase in serum creatinine (with COBI)

Drug	Formulations		Half-life	Metabolism	Dosing	Storage	Adverse Effects
Fosamprenavir (FPV) *Lexiva* (a prodrug of APV)	▪ 700 mg tablet ▪ 50 mg/mL oral suspension		7.7 h (APV)	APV is a CYP3A4 substrate, inhibitor, and inducer. Dosage adjustment in patients with hepatic insufficiency is recommended	**In ARV-Naive Patients:** ▪ FPV 1400 mg bid, or ▪ (FPV 1400 mg plus RTV 100–200 mg) once daily, or ▪ (FPV 700 mg plus RTV 100 mg) bid **In PI-Experienced Patients (Once-Daily Dosing Not Recommended):** ▪ (FPV 700 mg plus RTV 100 mg) bid **With EFV:** ▪ (FPV 700 mg plus RTV 100 mg) bid, or ▪ (FPV 1400 mg plus RTV 300 mg) once daily *Tablet:* ▪ Without RTV tablet: Take without regard to meals. ▪ With RTV tablet: Take with meals. *Oral Suspension:* ▪ Take without food.	Room temperature (up to 25° C or 77° F)	▪ Skin rash (12%-19%): FPV has a sulfonamide moiety. ▪ Diarrhea, nausea, vomiting ▪ Headache ▪ Hyperlipidemia ▪ Serum transaminase elevation ▪ Hyperglycemia ▪ Fat maldistribution ▪ Possible increased bleeding episodes in patients with hemophilia ▪ Nephrolithiasis
Indinavir (IDV) *Crixivan*	▪ 100, 200, and 400 mg capsules		1.5-2 h	CYP3A4 inhibitor and substrate Dosage adjustment in patients with hepatic insufficiency is recommended	▪ 800 mg every 8 h ▪ Take 1 h before or 2 h after meals; may take with skim milk or a low-fat meal. **With RTV:** ▪ (IDV 800 mg plus RTV 100-200 mg) bid ▪ Take without regard to meals.	Room temperature (15°-30° C or 59°-86° F) Protect from moisture.	▪ Nephrolithiasis ▪ GI intolerance, nausea ▪ Hepatitis ▪ Indirect hyperbilirubinemia ▪ Hyperlipidemia ▪ Headache, asthenia, blurred vision, dizziness, rash, metallic taste, thrombocytopenia, alopecia, and hemolytic anemia ▪ Hyperglycemia ▪ Fat maldistribution ▪ Possible increased bleeding episodes in patients with hemophilia
Lopinavir/ Ritonavir (LPV/r) *Kaletra*	**Tablets:** ▪ (LPV 200 mg plus RTV 50 mg), or ▪ (LPV 100 mg plus RTV 25 mg) Oral solution: ▪ Each 5 mL contains (LPV 400 mg plus RTV 100 mg). ▪ Oral solution contains 42% alcohol.		5-6 h	CYP3A4 inhibitor and substrate	▪ (LPV 400 mg plus RTV 100 mg) bid, *or* ▪ (LPV 800 mg plus RTV 200 mg) once daily Once-daily dosing is not recommended for patients with ≥3 LPV-associated mutations, pregnant women, or patients receiving EFV, NVP, FPV, NFV, carbamazepine, phenytoin, or phenobarbital. **With EFV or NVP (PI-Naive or PI-Experienced Patients):** ▪ LPV/r 500 mg/125 mg tablets bid (use a combination of 2 LPV/r 200 mg/50 mg tablets plus 1 LPV/r 100 mg/25 mg tablet to make a total dose of LPV/r 500 mg/125 mg), *or* ▪ LPV/r 520 mg/130 mg oral solution bid *Tablet:* ▪ Take without regard to meals. *Oral Solution:* ▪ Take with food.	Oral tablet is stable at room temperature. Oral solution is stable at 2°-8° C (36°-46° F) until date on label and is stable for up to 2 mo when stored at room temperature (up to 25° C or 77° F).	▪ GI intolerance, nausea, vomiting, diarrhea ▪ Pancreatitis ▪ Asthenia ▪ Hyperlipidemia (especially hypertriglyceridemia) ▪ Serum transaminase elevation ▪ Hyperglycemia ▪ Insulin resistance/diabetes mellitus ▪ Fat maldistribution ▪ Possible increased bleeding episodes in patients with hemophilia ▪ PR interval prolongation ▪ QT interval prolongation and torsades de pointes have been reported; however, causality could not be established.

(Continued)

TABLE 27-8 Characteristics of Protease Inhibitors (*Continued*)

Generic Name (Abbreviation) *Trade Name*	Formulations	Dosing Recommendations	Elimination/ Metabolic Pathway	Serum Half-Life	Storage	Adverse Events
Nelfinavir (NFV) *Viracept*	▪ 250 and 625 mg tablets ▪ 50 mg/g oral powder	▪ 1250 mg bid, *or* ▪ 750 mg tid Dissolve tablets in a small amount of water, mix admixture well, and consume immediately. Take with food.	CYP2C19 and 3A4 substrate-metabolized to active M8 metabolite; CYP3A4 inhibitor	3.5-5 h	Room temperature (15°-30° C or 59°-86° F)	▪ Diarrhea ▪ Hyperlipidemia ▪ Hyperglycemia ▪ Fat maldistribution ▪ Possible increased bleeding episodes in patients with hemophilia ▪ Serum transaminase elevation
Ritonavir (RTV) *Norvir* Also available as a component of fixed-dose combination (see Lopinavir/ Ritonavir)	▪ 100 mg tablet ▪ 100 mg soft gel capsule ▪ 80 mg/mL oral solution Oral solution contains 43% alcohol.	As Pharmacokinetic Booster (or Enhancer) for Other PIs: ▪ 100-400 mg per day in 1 or 2 divided doses (refer to other PIs for specific dosing recommendations). *Tablet:* ▪ Take with food. *Capsule and Oral Solution:* ▪ To improve tolerability, take with food if possible.	CYP3A4 >2D6 substrate; potent 3A4, 2D6 inhibitor; Inducer of CYPs 1A2, 2c8, 2C9, and 2C19 and UGT1A1	3-5 h	Tablets do not require refrigeration. Refrigerate capsules. Capsules can be left at room temperature (up to 25° C or 77° F) for up to 30 d. **Oral solution should not be refrigerated.**	▪ GI intolerance, nausea, vomiting, diarrhea ▪ Paresthesia (circumoral and extremities) ▪ Hyperlipidemia (especially hypertriglyceridemia) ▪ Hepatitis ▪ Asthenia ▪ Taste perversion ▪ Hyperglycemia ▪ Fat maldistribution ▪ Possible increased bleeding episodes in patients with hemophilia
Saquinavir (SQV) *invirase*	▪ 500 mg tablet ▪ 200 mg capsule	▪ (SQV 1000 mg plus RTV 100 mg) bid ▪ Unboosted SQV is **not recommended.** ▪ Take with meals or within 2 h after a meal.	CYP3A4 substrate	1-2 h	Room temperature (15°-30° C or 59°-86° F)	▪ GI intolerance, nausea, and diarrhea ▪ Headache ▪ Serum transaminase elevation ▪ Hyperlipidemia ▪ Hyperglycemia ▪ Fat maldistribution ▪ Possible increased bleeding episodes in patients with hemophilia ▪ PR interval prolongation ▪ QT interval prolongation, torsades de pointes have been reported. Patients with pre- SQV QT interval >450 msec should not receive SQV.

| Tipranavir (TPV) Aptivus | • 250 mg capsule
• 100 mg/mL oral solution | • (TPV 500 mg plus RTV 200 mg) bid
Unboosted TPV **is not recommended.**
With RTV Tablets:
• Take with meals.
With RTV Capsules or Solution:
• Take without regard to meals. | CYP P450 3A4 inducer and substrate
CYP2D6 inhibitor; CYP3A4, 1A2, and 2C19 inducer
Net effect when combined with RTV (CYP3A4, 2D6 inhibitor) | 6 h after single dose of TPV/r | Refrigerate capsules.
Capsules can be stored at room temperature (25° C or 77° F) for up to 60 d.
Oral solution should not be refrigerated or frozen and should be used within 60 d after bottle is opened. | • Hepatotoxicity: Clinical hepatitis (including hepatic decompensation and hepatitis- associated fatalities) has been reported; monitor patients closely, especially those with underlying liver diseases.
• Skin rash (3%–21%): TPV has a sulfonamide moiety; use with caution in patients with known sulfonamide allergy.
• Rare cases of fatal and nonfatal intracranial hemorrhages have been reported. Risks include brain lesion, head trauma, recent neurosurgery, coagulopathy, hypertension, alcoholism, and the use of anti-coagulant or anti-platelet agents (including vitamin E).
• Hyperlipidemia
• Hyperglycemia
• Fat maldistribution
• Possible increased bleeding episodes in patients with hemophilia |

Abbreviations: APV, amprenavir; ARV, antiretroviral; ATV, atazanavir; ATV/c, atazanavir/cobicistat; AV, atrioventricular; bid, twice daily; COBI, cobicistat; CYP, cytochrome P; DRV, darunavir; DRV/c, darunavir/cobicistat; EFV, efavirenz; FPV, fosamprenavir; GI, gastrointestinal; IDV, indinavir; LPV, lopinavir; LPV/r, lopinavir/ritonavir; msec, millisecond; NFV, nelfinavir; NVP, nevirapine; PI, protease inhibitor; PK, pharmacokinetic; PPI, proton pump inhibitor; RTV, ritonavir; SQV, saquinavir; TDF, tenofovir disoproxil fumarate; tid, three times a day; TPV, tipranavir.

TABLE 27-9   Characteristics of Integrase Inhibitors

Generic Name (Abbreviation) *Trade Name*	Formulations	Dosing Recommendations	Elimination/ Metabolic Pathways	Serum Half-Life	Adverse Events
Dolutegravir (DTG) *Tivicay* Also available as a component of fixed-dose combination (by trade name and abbreviation):	▪ 50 mg tablet	ARV-Naive or ARV-Experienced, INSTI-Naive Patients: ▪ 50 mg once daily ARV-Naive or ARV-Experienced. INSTI-Naive Patients when Coadministered with EFV, FPV/r, TPV/r, or Rifampin: ▪ 50 mg bid INSTI-Experienced Patients with Certain INSTI Mutations (See Product Label) or with Clinically Suspected INSTI Resistance: ▪ 50 mg bid Take without regard to meals.	UGT1A1 mediated glucuronidation Minor contribution from CYP3A4	~14 h	▪ HSRs, including rash, constitutional symptoms, and organ dysfunction (including liver injury) have been reported (for Triumeq). ▪ Insomnia ▪ Headache ▪ Depression and suicidal ideation (rare; usually in patients with pre-existing psychiatric conditions)
Triumeq (DTG/ ABC/3TC)	**Triumeq:** ▪ (DTG 50 mg plus ABC 600 mg plus 3TC 300 mg) tablet	**Triumeq:** ▪ Take 1 tablet daily without regard to meals.			
Elvitegravir (EVG) *Vitekta* Also available as a component of fixed-dose combinations (by trade name and abbreviation):	▪ 85 and 150 mg tablets	With Once Daily ATV/r or bid LPV/r: ▪ 85 mg once daily with food With bid DRV/r, FPV/r, orTPV/r: ▪ 150 mg once daily with food Unboosted EVG **is not recommended.**	CYP3A, UGT1A1/3 substrate	~9 h	▪ Nausea ▪ Diarrhea ▪ Depression and suicidal ideation (rare, usually in patients with pre-existing psychiatric conditions)
Genvoya (EVG/c/FTC/ TAF)	**Genvoya:** ▪ (EVG 150 mg plus COBI 150 mg plus FTC 200 mg plus TAF 10 mg) tablet	**Genvoya:** ▪ 1 tablet once daily with food **Not recommended** for patients with CrCl <30 mL/min. **Not recommended for use with other ARV drugs.**	EVG: As above COBI: CYP3A, CYP2D6 (minor); CYP3A inhibitor	~13 h	
Stribild (EVG/c/FTC/ TDF)	**Stribild:** ▪ (EVG 150 mg plus COBI 150 mg plus FTC 200 mg plus TDF 300 mg) tablet	**Stribild:** ▪ 1 tablet once daily with food **Not recommended** for patients with baseline CrCl <70 mL/min. **Not recommended for use with other ARV drugs.**		~13 h	
Raltegravir (RAL) *Isentress*	▪ 400 mg tablet ▪ 25 and 100 mg chewable tablets ▪ 100 mg single packet for oral suspension	▪ 400 mg bid With Rifampin: ▪ 800 mg bid Take without regard to meals.	UGT1A1-mediated glucuronidation	~9 h	▪ Rash, including Stevens-Johnson syndrome, HSR, and toxic epidermal necrolysis ▪ Nausea ▪ Headache ▪ Diarrhea ▪ Pyrexia ▪ CPK elevation, muscle weakness, and rhabdomyolysis ▪ Insomnia ▪ Depression and suicidal ideation (rare; usually in patients with preexisting psychiatric conditions)

TABLE 27-9 Characteristics of Integrase Inhibitors (*Continued*)

Generic Name (Abbreviation) Trade Name	Formulations	Dosing Recommendations	Elimination/ Metabolic Pathways	Serum Half-Life	Adverse Events
Maraviroc (MVC) *Selzentry*	■ 150 and 300 mg tablets	■ **150 mg bid** when given with drugs that are strong CYP3A inhibitors (with or without CYP3A inducers) including PIs (except TPV/r) ■ **300 mg bid** when given with NRTIs, T20, TPV/r, NVP, RAL, and other drugs that are not strong CYP3A inhibitors or inducers ■ **600 mg bid** when given with drugs that are CYP3A inducers, including EFV, ETR, etc. (without a CYP3A inhibitor) ■ Take without regard to meals.	14-18 h	CYP3A4 substrate	■ Abdominal pain ■ Cough ■ Dizziness ■ Musculoskeletal symptoms ■ Pyrexia ■ Rash ■ Upper respiratory tract infections ■ Hepatotoxicity, which may be preceded by severe rash or other signs of systemic allergic reactions ■ Orthostatic hypotension, especially in patients with severe renal insufficiency

Abbreviations: 3TC, lamivudine; ABC, abacavir; ARV, antiretroviral; ATV/r, atazanavir/ritonavir; bid, twice daily; c, COBI, cobicistat; CPK, creatine phosphokinase; CrCl, creatinine clearance; CYP, cytochrome P; DRV/r, darunavir/ritonavir; DTG, dolutegravir; EFV, efavirenz; ETR, etravirine; FPV/r, fosamprenavir/ritonavir; FTC, emtricitabine; HBV, hepatitis B virus; HSR, hypersensitivity reaction; INSTI, integrase strand transfer inhibitor; LPV/r, lopinavir/ritonavir; MVC, maraviroc; NRTI, nucleoside reverse transcriptase inhibitor; NVP, nevirapine; PI, protease inhibitor; RAL, raltegravir; T20, enfuvirtide; TAF, tenofovir alafenamide; TPV/r, tipranavir/ritonavir; UGT, uridine diphosphate gluconyltransferase.

suppression and CD4+ cell count. Therefore, naïve and treatment experienced patients should have therapy guided by a genotype or phenotype resistance profile.

SPECIAL POPULATIONS

Pediatrics and Newborns

Most children born with HIV are asymptomatic. On physical examination, children often present with nonspecific signs, such as lymphadenopathy, hepatomegaly, splenomegaly, failure to thrive, weight loss or unexplained low birth weight (in prenatally exposed infants), and fever of unknown origin.

Laboratory findings include anemia, hypergammaglobulinemia (primarily immunoglobulin [Ig]A and IgM), altered mononuclear cell function, and altered T-cell subset ratios. All children more than 1 year of age with AIDS or symptomatic disease should be initiated on therapy. Additionally, children 1 to 5 years of age with a CD4% less than 25% and children more than 5 years with a CD4 count less than 350 cells/mm^3 should also be initiated on ART. Those with mild or asymptomatic disease and a high viral load (HIV RNA >100,000 c/mL) should be initiated on therapy. Treatment principles are similar to that of adults, with a backbone of two NRTIs plus either a boosted PI or NNRTI. Typically, zidovudine is recommended as one of the two NRTIs in the backbone because it is

TABLE 27-10 Characteristics of Fusion Inhibitor (Last updated January 29, 2008; last reviewed April 8, 2015)

Generic Name (Abbreviation) Trade Name	Formulation	Dosing Recommendation	Serum Half-Life	Elimination	Storage	Adverse Events[a]
Enfuvirtide (T20) *Fuzeon*	■ Injectable; supplied as lyophilized powder ■ Each vial contains 108 mg of T20; reconstitute with 1.1 mL of sterile water for injection for delivery of approximately 90 mg/1 mL.	■ 90 mg (1 mL) subcutaneously bid	3.8 h	Expected to undergo catabolism to its constituent amino acids, with subsequent recycling of the amino acids in the body pool	Store at room temperature (up to 25° C or 77° F). Reconstituted solution should be refrigerated at 2°-8° C (36°-46° F) and used within 24 h	■ Local injection site reactions (eg, pain, erythema, induration, nodules and cysts, pruritus, ecchymosis) in almost 100% of patients ■ Increased incidence of bacterial pneumonia ■ HSR (<1% of patients): Symptoms may include rash, fever, nausea, vomiting, chills, rigors, hypotension, or elevated serum transaminases. Rechallenge is not recommended.

Abbreviations: bid, twice daily; HSR, hypersensitivity reaction; T20, enfuvirtide.
[a] Also see Table 14.

highly researched in pediatrics. Peripartum use of zidovudine is recommended to reduce vertical transmission during delivery from HIV-infected mothers. Nevirapine therapy should also be considered in addition to zidovudine in high-risk newborns to further reduce the risk of transmission.

Renal and Hepatic Insufficiency

Pre-existing renal and hepatic insufficiency should be considered when selecting ART. TVF may cause nephrotoxicity and should be used with caution in renal disease patients. Cobicistat is a pharmacokinetic enhancer (boosting agent without HIV activity) and is associated with increased serum creatinine (SCr) due to altered tubular secretion. This effects the *estimated* glomerular filtration, but not the *actual* glomerular filtration. Dosing of NRTIs except abacavir (ABC) should be modified in patients with moderate to severe renal dysfunction. Combination products containing NRTIs with other antiretrovirals should not be used in patients with renal dysfunction due to differences in renal dosing adjustment of each individual agent. All PIs, specifically when boosted with ritonavir, should be used with caution in hepatic dysfunction. Nevirapine is associated with severe hepatic dysfunction, especially in women with CD4+ counts more than 250 cells/mm^3 and men more than 400 cells/mm^3. Other ARVs, including ABC and additional NNRTIs, have been associated with elevated hepatic enzymes. Dosing recommendations are available in Table 27-4 and the DHHS guidelines.

Pregnancy

Pregnant women should be tested in the first and third trimester (if initially negative). ART is recommended in pregnant women regardless of CD4+ cell count. Teratogenic effects should be considered when selecting ART. Efavirenz should be avoided in pregnancy, especially during the first trimester, because of its potential teratogenicity. The risk of neural tube defects is restricted to the first 5 to 6 weeks of pregnancy, a time when pregnancy is rarely recognized. Adherence is critical to reduce the risk of transmission to the newborn. Vaginal delivery is recommended, as opposed to Caesarean section, in mothers with undetectable viral loads.

Postexposure Prophylaxis

Postexposure prophylaxis (PEP) is categorized as either occupational PEP or nonoccupational PEP. Three or more active drugs should be used for all exposures, regardless of severity. Treatment should be started within 72 hours of exposure, but delayed treatment may still provide a benefit, particularly in high-risk exposure settings, and should be continued for 4 weeks. PEP consists of the NRTI backbone TVF plus emtricitabine plus twice daily raltegravir. Once daily raltegravir, dolutegravir, or PI-based regimens are alternatives. Nevirapine should be avoided due to high risk of hepatotoxicity. Regimens can be modified if resistance patterns of the potentially transmitted virus are known. Follow-up HIV-1 antibody testing is recommended for at least 4 to 6 months after the exposure.

Tenofovir (Tenofovir Disoproxil Fumarate and Tenofovir Alafenamide)

Tenofovir disoproxil fumarate (TDF), the first approved oral prodrug of TFV, has been used in combination ART for the treatment of HIV-1 infection since 2001. Despite being overall well tolerated, TDF can cause clinically significant renal toxic effects and a decline in bone mineral density (BMD). After oral administration, TDF is metabolized to TFV which, in turn, is phosphorylated intracellularly to the active moiety TFV diphosphate (TFV-DP). Tenofovir alafenamide (TAF), a novel oral prodrug of TFV, is metabolized to TFV intracellularly, rather than in the plasma, which results in substantially higher intracellular concentrations of the active metabolite TFV-DP and lower plasma levels of TFV compared with TDF. As a result, the dose of TAF is less than one-tenth of the dose of TDF, which is believed to reduce the risk of renal and bone toxicity. Treatment guideline recommendations currently recommend TDF or TAF for treatment as one of the NRTI backbones (Table 27-4). Importantly, TAF is not currently recommended for PrEP due to substantially lower TDF concentrations in cervicovaginal fluid. An understanding of the different types of TFV and respective formulations is critical (Table 27-2).

CASE Application

1. YP is a patient recently diagnosed with HIV. The patient presents to your pharmacy to fill a prescription for Triumeq. During the counseling session, YP ask the pharmacist, when is a person living with HIV classified as having AIDS? Select all that apply.

   a. Diagnosis of *Pneumocystis jiroveci* pneumonia
   b. CD4 count of 350 μL
   c. HIV viral load of >100,000 copies/mL
   d. CD4 count of 150 μL
   e. CD4% of 10%

2. LF is a 31-year-old male patient recently diagnosed with HIV. He presents to the HIV clinic for the first time and is eager to start treatment, what is your most appropriate course of action? Select all that apply.

   a. Begin therapy with TFV, emtricitabine, and efavirenz
   b. Counsel the patient regarding HIV, transmission, prevention of transmission to others, answer his questions, and schedule another follow-up visit
   c. Obtain baseline viral load and CD4
   d. Begin therapy with emtricitabine, lamivudine, darunavir/ritonavir
   e. Obtain genotype

3. Select the signs and symptoms of primary HIV infection (acute infection) in an adult patient. Select all that apply.

   a. Mononucleosis-like illness (fever, sore-throat, fatigue, weight loss)
   b. GI-upset (nausea, vomiting, diarrhea)
   c. Lymphadenopathy
   d. Night sweats

4. Which of the following statements about HIV prevention is TRUE?

   a. Condoms are 100% effective in preventing HIV transmission.
   b. All pregnant women should be screened for HIV.
   c. Only pregnant women who engage in high-risk behaviors should be screened for HIV.
   d. IV drug abusers can reuse/share syringe hubs as long as a new needle is used.

5. A patient presents to the hospital with a 2-week history of a mono-like illness. Basic metabolic and complete blood count tests are within normal limits and an ELISA test is negative (nonreactive). The patient reports being sexually active with multiple partners. Which of the following counseling points should be discussed with the patient? Select all that apply.

   a. Inform her she most likely had viral sinusitis.
   b. Inform her that she does not have HIV.
   c. Inform her that she will need to complete a follow-up ELISA in 1 month to evaluate for HIV.
   d. Provide counseling on HIV and STD prevention.

6. In a patient receiving zidovudine therapy, which of the following could you expect to be elevated on laboratory evaluation?

   a. Blood urea nitrogen (BUN)
   b. Mean corpuscular volume (MCV)
   c. SCr
   d. Potassium

7. A treatment experienced patient receiving atazanavir therapy should avoid the addition of which of the following medications?

   a. Omeprazole
   b. Metronidazole
   c. Pravastatin
   d. Metoprolol

8. Which of the following treatment regimens would be considered appropriate in a treatment naîve patient?

   a. Maraviroc + Efavirenz + Nevirapine
   b. Raltegravir + ABC + Indinavir + Ritonavir
   c. TFV + Zidovudine + ABC
   d. Lamviudine + Zidovudine + Lopinavir + Ritonavir

9. In a patient with a history of acute or chronic pancreatitis, which of the following medications should be avoided?

   a. Didanosine
   b. Darunavir
   c. TFV
   d. Enfuvirtide

10. Which of the following properties are true regarding efavirenz? Select all that apply.

    a. Should be taken with a high fat meal
    b. Is a common cause of vivid dreams and hallucinations
    c. Is the NNRTI of choice in pregnancy
    d. Lacks significant drug interactions
    e. Teratogenic in nonhuman primates and potentially teratogenic in first trimester of pregnancy

11. Which of the following antiretrovirals is/are available in a parenteral form? Select all that apply.

    a. Zidovudine
    b. Etravirine
    c. Dolutegravir
    d. Rilpivirine
    e. Enfuvirtide

12. Which of the following patients would be at highest risk for developing hepatotoxicity secondary to nevirapine therapy?

    a. 31-year-old woman with a CD4+ = 91 cells/mm^3
    b. 21-year-old man with CD4+ = 270 cells/mm^3
    c. 50-year-old man with CD4+ = 260 cells/mm^3
    d. 25-year-old woman with CD4+ = 265 cells/mm^3

13. Which of the following combinations of antiretrovirals should be avoided because of contraindications?

    a. Rilpivirine and TFV
    b. Efavirenz and nevirapine
    c. Lamivudine and zidovudine
    d. Fosamprenavir and ritonavir

14. Which of the following regarding Truvada® PrEP is true?

    a. Should only be given to HIV-positive patients.
    b. Should be administered under direct medical supervision in an emergency situation.
    c. Should be taken daily in high-risk patients to prevent acquisition of HIV.
    d. A negative HIV screening test is required monthly prior to prescribing.

15. Dosing of *maraviroc* should be increased to 600 mg twice daily when combined with which of the following medications?

    a. Ketoconazole
    b. Clarithromycin
    c. Rifampin
    d. Warfarin

16. Which of the following is true regarding PEP?

    a. PEP should be administered within 1 week of HIV exposure.
    b. A two-drug regimen of TFV plus zidovudine is preferred for PEP.
    c. A three-drug regimen of TFV, emtricitabine, and raltegravir is preferred for PEP.
    d. Nevirapine should be included in PEP regimen when possible.

17. Which of the following is true regarding Stribild® therapy?

    a. This medication should be taken on an empty stomach at bedtime.
    b. This medication will commonly increase SCr value.

c. This medication should only be used in patients with an eGFR <60 mL/min.

d. This medication will commonly increase indirect bilirubin.

18. Which of the following laboratory tests should be evaluated on a patient prior to starting ABC therapy?

a. MCV
b. Hemoglobin
c. SCr
d. HLA-B*5701

19. Which of the following medications has hepatitis B virus (HBV) activity and if stopped in a patient with HBV, may cause a hepatitis flare? Select all that apply.

a. Emtricitabine
b. Nevirapine
c. Lamivudine
d. TFV
e. ABC

20. Which of the following HIV medications is associated with increased bilirubin?

a. Acyclovir
b. Atazanavir
c. ABC
d. TFV

21. Based upon the development of central nervous system side effects, which of the following NNRTIs would you expect to have the highest concentration distributed into the CNS? Select all that apply.

a. Viramune
b. Sustiva
c. Atripla
d. Stribild

22. Place the following NNRTIs in order based upon initial starting dose. Start with the lowest mg NNRTI.

Unordered Response	Ordered Response
Nevirapine	
Efavirenz	
Rilpivirine	
Etravirine	

23. Which of the following medication regimen(s) contain efavirenz?

a. Triumeq
b. Atripla
c. Genvoya
d. Complera
e. Odefsey

24. Which of the following medication(s) contain TFV? Select all that apply.

a. Stribild
b. Triumeq
c. Genvoya
d. Prezcobix
e. Descovy

25. Which of the following medication(s) contact TFV alafenamide (taf)? Select all that apply.

a. Evotaz
b. Kaletra
c. Truvada
d. Odefsey
e. Genvoya

26. Which of the following antiretrovirals are STRs?

a. Epzicom
b. Sustiva
c. Triumeq
d. Complera
e. Atripla

27. A patient presents to your pharmacy with severe muscle weakness. The patient has a past medical history of hypertension and HIV. Medications include lisinopril, TFV alafenamide, emtricitabine, and raltegravir. The patient was referred to you to evaluate the medications and see if the symptom is associated with one of his medications. Which of the following medications may be causing the patients symptom of muscle weakness?

a. Emtricitabine
b. TFV alafenamide
c. Simvastatin
d. Raltegravir
e. Daptomycin

TAKEAWAY POINTS »

- HIV is an RNA retrovirus with three primary modes of transmission (sexual, parenteral, and perinatal).
- Viral load and CD4 cell counts are the laboratory surrogate markers used to monitor HIV progression.
- Symptoms of acute HIV (ARS) mimic a mononucleosis illness with fevers, pharyngitis, lymphadenopathy, weight loss, night sweats, diarrhea, and nausea.

- Abstinence is the only 100% effective way to prevent sexual transmission of HIV.
- Barrier methods, reducing or eliminating high-risk behaviors like anal intercourse and decreasing the number of sexual partners can reduce the risk of sexual transmission.

- Perinatal transmission can be reduced if HIV-positive mothers take ART and do not breastfeed.
- Combination ART has decreased the incidence of opportunistic infections, increased life expectancy and quality of life.
- The backbone of therapy in treatment naïve patients should consist of two NRTI plus either an NNRTI, an INSTI, or boosted PI.
- At least three active agents (excluding ritonavir or cobicistat) should be the goal of every regimen.
- Ritonavir is given at a low-dose in combination with other PIs as a boosting or pharmacokinetic enhancer due to potent CYP3A4 inhibition.

- Cobicistat is a boosting agent similar to ritonavir.
- The PIs and many of the NNRTIs are substrates and/or inducers/inhibitors of the CYP 3A system and associated with significant drug interactions.
- Acid suppressing agents and food can have significant alterations to several antiretrovirals and careful attention is required with coadministration.
- Treatment should be initiated in pregnancy and efavirenz and nevirapine should be avoided in pregnancy.
- TAF has a similar tolerability, safety, and effectiveness to TDF and probably less adverse events related to renal and bone density outcomes in the treatment of HIV.

BIBLIOGRAPHY

Anderson PL, Kakuda TN, Fletcher CV. Human immunodeficiency virus infection. In: DiPiro JT, Talbert RL, Yee GC, Matzke GR, Wells BG, Posey L, eds. *Pharmacotherapy: A Pathophysiologic Approach.* 10th ed. New York, NY: McGraw-Hill.

Fauci AS, Lane H. Human immunodeficiency virus disease: AIDS and related disorders. In: Longo DL, Fauci AS, Kasper DL, Hauser SL, Jameson J, Loscalzo J, eds. *Harrison's Principles of Internal Medicine.* 18th ed. New York, NY: McGraw-Hill; 2012:chap 189.

Flexner C. Antiretroviral agents and treatment of HIV infection. In: Brunton LL, Chabner BA, Knollmann BC, eds. *Goodman & Gilman's The Pharmacological Basis of Therapeutics.* 12th ed. New York, NY: McGraw-Hill; 2011:chap 59.

Panel on Antiretroviral Guidelines for Adults and Adolescents. Guidelines for the use of antiretroviral agents in HIV-1-infected adults and adolescents. Department of Health and Human Services. Available at http://aidsinfo.nih.gov/ContentFiles/AdultandAdolescentGL.pdf.

Safrin S. Antiviral agents. In: Katzung BG, Masters SB, Trevor AJ, eds. *Basic & Clinical Pharmacology.* 12th ed. New York, NY: McGraw-Hill; 2012:chap 49.

KEY ABBREVIATIONS

ABC HSR = abacavir hypersensitivity reaction
AIDS = acquired immunodeficiency syndrome
ARS = acute retroviral syndrome
BMD = bone mineral density
BUN = blood urea nitrogen
cART = combination antiretroviral therapy
CCR5 = chemokine receptor 5
CD4 = cluster of differentiation 4
CXCR4 = chemokine receptor 4
eGFR = estimated glomerular filtration
ELISA = enzyme-linked immunosorbent assay
FDA = Food and Drug Administration
gp = glycoprotein
HBV = hepatitis B virus
HIV = human immunodeficiency virus

HSR = hypersensitivity reaction
INSTI = integrase strand transfer inhibitors
IV = intravenous
MHC = major histocompatibility complex
MTRs = multiple tablet regimen
NNRTIs = non-nucleoside reverse transcriptase inhibitors
NRTIs = nucleoside/tide reverse transcriptase inhibitors
PI = protease inhibitors
PPE = personal protective equipment
PrEP = preexposure prophylaxis
SCr = seum creatinine
STD = sexually transmitted disease
STRs = single tablet regimens
TAF = Tenofovir alafenamide
TDF = Tenofovir disoproxil fumarate

FOUNDATION OVERVIEW

People with healthy immune systems can be exposed to certain viruses, bacteria, or parasites and have minimal reactions to them; however, people living with human immunodeficiency virus (HIV) can face serious health threats from *opportunistic infections* (OIs). These infections are called opportunistic because they take advantage of a weakened immune system. Opportunistic pathogens are traditionally encountered at CD_4 levels below certain thresholds (Figure 28-1). Besides contributing to morbidity and mortality, OIs accelerate the progression of HIV disease. For this reason, guidelines emphasize concurrent antiretroviral therapy (ART) with prophylaxis, treatment, and secondary prophylaxis of OIs.

MUCOCUTANEOUS CANDIDIASIS

Mucocutaneous candidiasis is a fungal infection caused by *Candida* species (most commonly *Candida albicans*). Candidiasis presents as thrush (a creamy, white plaque-like lesion on the tongue or buccal surface). The most common location for thrush is the oropharynx and esophagus. Esophageal candidiasis may present as retrosternal pain or dysphagia. The diagnosis of thrush is a clinical diagnosis based on the appearance of plaques. A culture may be needed to identify the *Candida* species. The lesions are painless and can be scraped off with a tongue depressor.

Prophylaxis

Primary prophylaxis is not routinely recommended for Candidiasis. Routinely administering prophylaxis would increase the likelihood of drug interactions with ART and may promote drug-resistant species. Secondary prophylaxis is recommended for patients with severe recurrences (fluconazole 100-200 mg/d).

Treatment

Topical treatment may be used for the *initial* episode of oropharyngeal candidiasis. Topical agents primarily include clotrimazole troches or nystatin suspension. Systemic treatment options include oral fluconazole for 7 to 14 days. Itraconazole and posaconazole are alternatives for oropharyngeal candidiasis. Systemic therapy is recommended for esophageal candidiasis (fluconazole 200-400 mg/d for 14-21 days). Treatment failure may occur in patients with previous azole exposure. Alternative treatment options include itraconazole, voriconazole, caspofungin, micafungin, anidulafungin, and amphotericin B (Table 28-1).

PNEUMOCYSTIS JIROVECII

Pneumocystis jirovecii (PJP) is an opportunistic fungal pathogen that is an important cause of pneumonia in the immunocompromised host. Patients with PJP develop dyspnea, fever, and a nonproductive cough. Patients infected with HIV are usually ill for several weeks and may have subtle manifestations. A high index of suspicion and a thorough history are key factors in early detection. Physical findings include tachypnea, tachycardia, and cyanosis, but lung auscultation reveals few abnormalities. Due to the nonspecific nature of the clinical picture, the diagnosis is based on specific identification of the organism. A definitive diagnosis is chiefly made by histopathologic staining. The classic findings on chest radiography consist of bilateral diffuse infiltrates beginning in the perihilar regions.

Prophylaxis

Prophylaxis is indicated for HIV-infected patients with CD_4 counts of less than 200 cells/mm³ (Reference range: 500-1500 cells/mm³), a history of oropharyngeal candidiasis, and for patients who have recovered from PJP. Prophylaxis may be discontinued in HIV-infected patients once CD_4 counts have risen to more than 200 cells/mm³ and remained at that level for 3 months or more. Trimethoprim/sulfamethoxazole (TMP/SMX) is the drug of choice for primary and secondary prophylaxis. Protection against toxoplasmosis and some bacterial infections is also provided by TMP/SMX. Alternative regimens are available for individuals intolerant of TMP/SMX (Table 28-2).

Treatment

The drug of choice for PJP is TMP/SMX. Therapy is continued for 14 days in non–HIV-infected patients and for 21 days in patients infected with HIV. Non–HIV-infected patients are usually tolerant of TMP-SMX; however, more than half of

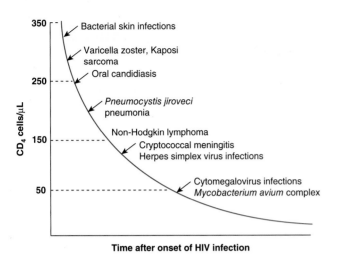

FIGURE 28-1 History of opportunistic infections associated with human immunodeficiency virus. Reproduced with permission from DiPiro JT, Talbert RL, Yee GC, et al: *Pharmacotherapy: A Pathophysiologic Approach,* 9th ed. New York, NY: McGraw-Hill; 2014.

HIV-infected patients experience serious adverse reactions. Alternative treatment options are listed in Table 28-3.

CRYPTOCOCCAL MENINGITIS

Cryptococcal meningitis (CM) is a central nervous system (CNS) infection caused by the fungus *Cryptococcus neoformans.* Transmission occurs via inhalation of infected particles in the environment. The mortality observed with CM at 10 weeks is high (10%-25%) despite optimal treatment. India ink preparations and lumbar punctures aid in the diagnosis of CM (findings: low glucose, normal to high protein, detectable white blood cell count, normal red blood cell count, positive for yeast).

Prophylaxis

Routine primary prophylaxis is not recommended because the incidence of cryptococcal infections is low. Secondary prophylaxis is recommended and patients commonly receive oral

TABLE 28-1	Drug Treatment for Oropharyngeal Candidiasis			
Drug and Availability	**Dose**	**Adverse Effects**	**Drug/Drug Interactions**	**Clinical Notes**
Clotrimazole troches po: 10 mg troche	10 mg po 5 × daily			Poor taste Compliance with multiple daily dosing
Nystatin suspension po: 100,000 units/mL (5, 60, 480 mL)	4-6 mL qid	GI distress		Swish and retain in mouth before swallowing
Fluconazole (Diflucan®) po: 50, 100, 150, 200 mg tabs IV: 200, 400 mg	Oropharyegal: 100-200 mg qd Esophageal: 200-400 mg qd	↑ LFTs, GI distress, rash, alopecia	Amiodarone, benzodiazepines, phenytoin, warfarin, rifampin	Inhibits many CYP isoenzymes (2C9, 2C19, 3A4); CI with cisapride, *ergot* derivatives, quinidine Monitor LFTs for all azoles
Itraconazole (Sporanox®) po: 100 mg cap, 10 mg/mL soln. IV: 10 mg/mL	200 mg po qd	Hepatotoxicity, GI distress, rash, edema	Benzodiazepines, *calcium* channel blockers, digoxin, ritonavir, warfarin, sulfonylureas	Strong 3A4 inhibitor; CI with cisapride, *ergot* derivatives, quinidine
Posaconazole (Noxafil®) po: 40 mg/mL susp	100 mg bid × 1 d, then 100 mg qd × 13 d	GI distress, hepatotoxicity, QTc prolongation, rash	Rifampin, *calcium* channel blockers, statins, cimetidine	Take with food CI with cisapride, *ergot* derivatives, quinidine
Voriconazole (Vfend®) po: 50, 200 mg tabs, 200 mg/5 mL susp IV: 200 mg	200 mg po/IV bid	Hallucinations, visual changes, rash, hepatotoxicity, photophobia	Efavirenz, rifampin, barbiturates, carbamazepine, warfarin, calcium channel blockers	Inhibits many CYP isoenzymes (2C9, 2C19, 3A4); CI with cisapride, *ergot* derivatives, quinidine & pregnancy Food ↓ absorption
Caspofungin (Cancidas®) IV: 50, 70 mg	50 mg IV qd	Fever, chills, ↑ LFTs	Tacrolimus, cyclosporine	May ↓ dose to 35 mg for moderate hepatic impairment (Child-Pugh score 7–9)
Micafungin (Mycamine®) IV: 50, 100 mg	150 mg IV qd	Fever, ↓ K/Mg, neutropenia, thrombocytopenia	Nifedipine	Monitor LFTs, BUN, SCr
Anidulafungin (Eraxis®) IV: 50 mg	100 mg IV × 1, then 50 mg IV qd	Transaminitis, electrolyte disturbances, diarrhea	None	Monitor LFTs
Amphotericin B deoxycholate (Amphocin®, Fungizone®) IV: 50 mg	0.6 mg/kg IV qd	Renal failure, infusion reactions (including anaphylaxis), anemia, electrolyte wasting	Additive with other nephrotoxins	Premedicate with APAP, diphenhydramine, or hydrocortisone Monitor BUN, SCr, CBC throughout therapy

Reproduced with permission from Attridge RL, Miller ML, Moote R, et al: *Internal Medicine: A Guide to Clinical Therapeutics.* New York, NY: McGraw-Hill; 2013.

TABLE 28-2 Prophylaxis for *Pneumocystis Jirovecii* Pneumonia

Drug(s), Dose, Route	Comments
First Choice	
TMP-SMX, 1 DS tablet or 1 SS tablet qd po[a]	TMP-SMX can be safely reintroduced for treatment of some patients who have had mild to moderate side effects.
Other Agents	
Dapsone, 50 mg bid or 100 mg qd po	—
Dapsone, 50 mg qd po; plus pyrimethamine, 50 mg weekly po; plus leucovorin, 25 mg weekly po	Leucovorin prevents bone marrow toxicity from pyrimethamine.
Dapsone, 200 mg weekly po; plus pyrimethamine, 75 mg weekly po; plus leucovorin, 25 mg weekly po	Leucovorin prevents bone marrow toxicity from pyrimethamine.
Pentamidine, 300 mg monthly via Respirgard II nebulizer	Adverse reactions include cough and bronchospasm.
Atovaquone, 1500 mg qd po	—
TMP-SMX, 1 DS tablet 3 times weekly po	TMP-SMX can be safely reintroduced for treatment of some patients who have had mild to moderate side effects.

Abbreviations: DS, double-strength; SS, single-strength; TMP-SMX, trimethoprim-sulfamethoxazole.

Reproduced with permission from Longo DL, Fauci AS, Kasper DL, et al: *Harrison's Principles of Internal Medicine,* 18 ed. New York, NY: McGraw-Hill; 2012.

TABLE 28-3 Treatment of *Pneumocystis Jirovecii* Pneumonia

Drug Name and Availability	Dose	Adverse Effects	Contraindications	Drug/Drug Interactions	Clinical Notes
SMX/TMP (Bactrim, Septra) 80 mg/16 mg/mL IV 200 mg/40 mg/5 mL po susp; 400 mg/80 mg, 800 mg/160 mg (DS) tabs MOA: interferes with folic acid synthesis and growth	15 mg/kg (trimethoprim component) po or IV divided Q8h *Renal adjustment:* CrCl <30: use 50% of recommended dose CrCl <15: not recommended	Fever, rash, SJS, leucopenia, thrombocytopenia, hyperkalemia, crystalluria, hepatotoxicity	Megaloblastic anemia due to folate deficiency, porphyria, marked hepatic damage	Warfarin, amiodarone, fluoxetine, phenytoin, ACE inhibitors, *potassium* sparing diuretics	Monitor CBC, chemistry, renal function Inhibits CYP 2C9
Dapsone (**Aczone**) 25, 100 mg tabs MOA: interference with folic acid synthesis and growth	100 mg po daily	Rash, G6PD anemia, methemaglobinemia, hepatotoxicity, peripheral neuropathy, acute tubular necrosis	G6PD deficiency	Azole antifungals, macrolides, *calcium* channel blockers, carbamazepine, phenytoin, rifamycins	Monitor CBC, renal function, LFTs Assess for G6PD deficiency Substrate of multiple CYP isoenzymes
Pentamidine (Nebu-Pent, Pentam-300) 300 mg powder for injection; 300 mg powder for nebulization	3-4 mg/kg IV daily *Renal adjustment:* CrCl <50: 4 mg/kg Q24-36h CrCl <10: 4 mg/kg Q48h	Arrhythmias, rash, SJS, nephrotoxicity, hyper-/hypoglycemia, pancreatitis, bone marrow suppression, hepatotoxicity	None	QTc prolonging agents, azole antifungals, phenytoin, carbamazepine, rifampin	Monitor CBC, chemistry, pancreatic enzymes, and EKG Major 2C19 substrate
Clindamycin (Cleocin) 300, 600, 900 mg premixed IV; 150 mg/mL IV soln; 150, 300 mg caps MOA: binds 50S ribosomal subunit and inhibits protein synthesis	600 mg IV Q8h or 300-450 mg po Q6h	Fever, rash, diarrhea (including *Clostridium difficile-* associated diarrhea), hepatotoxicity	Previous pseudomembranous colitis, regional enteritis, ulcerative colitis	None	Monitor LFTs, assess GI adverse effects
Primaquine 26.3 mg (15 mg base) tabs MOA: not clearly understood; may interfere with DNA synthesis	30 mg base po qd	N/V, hemolytic anemia, visual accommodation changes	G6PD deficiency, concomitant use of bone marrow-suppressive agents	Ciprofloxacin, theophylline, carbamazepine, phenytoin, mirtazapine	Monitor CBC Major 3A4 substrate; inhibits 1A2 Assess for G6PD deficiency
Atovaquone (Mepron) 750 mg/5 mL po susp MOA: inhibition of pyrimidine synthesis	750 mg po bid	HA, nausea, diarrhea, rash, transaminase elevations	None	Rifamycins	Monitor LFTs

Reproduced with permission from Attridge RL, Miller ML, Moote R, et al: *Internal Medicine: A Guide to Clinical Therapeutics.* New York, NY: McGraw-Hill; 2013.

TABLE 28-4	Drug Treatment for Cryptococcal Meningitis				
Drug	**Dose**	**Adverse Effects**	**Contraindications**	**Drug/Drug Interactions**	**Clinical Notes**
Fluconazole (Diflucan)	Suppressive: 400 mg po qd Maintenance: 200 mg po qd	See Table 28-1			
Amphotericin B-deoxycholate (Amphocin, Fungizone)	0.7 mg/kg daily	See Table 28-1			
Liposomal amphotericin B (Ambisome) IV: 50 mg	3-6 mg/kg IV daily × 14 d	See Table 28-1 Delayed nephrotoxicity compared with conventional amphotericin B			
Fluocytosine (Ancobon) po: 250, 500 mg tab	25 mg/kg po q6h × 14 d *Renal adjustment:* CrCl 20-40: 37.5 mg/kg bid CrCl 10-20: 37.5 mg/kg daily CrCl <10: 37.5 mg/kg q36-48h	Bone marrow suppression, rash, nephrotoxicity	Do not use as monotherapy—rapid resistance occurs	↑ Toxicity with other myelosuppressive agents	Monitor CBC, renal and hepatic function
Itraconazole (Sporanox)	po: 200 mg bid	Less effective than fluconazole			

Reproduced with permission from Attridge RL, Miller ML, Moote R, et al: *Internal Medicine: A Guide to Clinical Therapeutics*. New York, NY: McGraw-Hill; 2013.

fluconazole 200 mg daily. The duration of prophylaxis is not clearly defined. Discontinuation may be considered if immune reconstitution with ART occurs.

Treatment

Nonpharmacologic treatment includes daily lumbar puncture for opening pressures more than 25 cm H_2O. The lumbar puncture aims to relieve the increased intracranial pressure. Pharmacologic treatment includes an induction, suppressive, and maintenance phase (Table 28-4).

- Induction: intravenous amphotericin B daily × 14 days ± oral flucytosine.
- Suppressive: oral fluconazole × 8 weeks; alternative: itraconazole.
- Maintenance: oral fluconazole indefinitely.
- Echinocandins are not largely ineffective for treatment of CM.

TOXOPLASMA GONDII

Toxoplasmosis is a CNS infection caused by the parasite *Toxoplasma gondii*. In persons with intact immune systems, acute toxoplasmosis is customarily asymptomatic and self-limiting. Patients with acquired immunodeficiency syndrome (AIDS) and those receiving immunosuppressive therapy are at greatest risk for developing acute toxoplasmosis. In most of these cases, encephalitis develops when the CD_4 counts fall below 100 cells/mm^3 and may be rapidly fatal if untreated. Signs and symptoms of acute toxoplasmosis in immunocompromised patients involve the CNS and include altered mental status, fever, seizures, headaches, and focal neurologic findings (motor deficits, cranial nerve palsies, movement disorders, visual-field loss). The diagnosis of acute toxoplasmosis is made predominantly by culture, serologic testing, and polymerase chain reaction. A clinical diagnosis of Toxoplasma encephalitis in AIDS

patients is guided by presentation, history of exposure, and radiologic evaluation. *Toxoplasma gondii* routinely is transmitted via ingestion of undercooked meats and poor hand hygiene after handling cat feces (feline primary carrier). The majority of HIV patients will have anti-toxoplasma IgG antibodies and all patients should be tested for antibodies. Most cases of active infection are reactivation of latent disease.

Prophylaxis

All HIV-infected persons, including those who lack IgG antibody to *Toxoplasma*, should be counseled regarding sources of *Toxoplasma* infection. The chances of primary infection with *Toxoplasma* can be reduced by not eating undercooked meat. Specifically, lamb, beef, and pork should be cooked to an internal temperature of 165°F to 170°F. Hands should be washed thoroughly with soap and water after work in the garden and fruits and vegetables should be washed. If the patient owns a cat, the litter box should be cleaned or changed daily, preferably by an HIV-negative, nonpregnant person. Alternatively, patients should wash their hands thoroughly with soap and water after changing the litter box. Primary prophylaxis is recommended for patients with a CD_4 count less than 100 cells/mm^3 (TMP/SMX) and may be discontinued when CD_4 greater than 200 cells/mm^3 for more than 3 months (Table 28-5). Secondary prophylaxis is

TABLE 28-5	Primary Prophylaxis for *Toxoplasma* Encephalitis
Preferred Therapy	**Alternative Therapy**
TMP- SMX 1 DS po qd	TMP-SMX 1 DS po tiw
TMP-SMX 1 SS po qd	Dapsone 50 mg po bid or 100 mg po qd
	Dapsone 50 mg po daily + pyrimethamine 50 mg + leucovorin 25 mg po weekly
	Atovaquone 1500 mg po daily with food

Abbreviations: DS, double strength; po, per oral; qd, four times a day; SS, single strength; tiw, three times a week; TMP-SMX, trimethoprim/sulfamethoxazole.

TABLE 28-6	Drug Treatment of Toxoplasmosis				
Drug	**Dose**	**Adverse Effects**	**Contraindications**	**Drug/Drug Interactions**	**Clinical Notes**
Pyrimethamine (Daraprim) 25 mg tab	50-75 mg po qd	Hematologic toxicity, GI upset, rash, SJS, arrhythmias (at high doses)	Megaloblastic anemia	↑ hematological toxicity with zidovudine, SMX-TMP	Inhibits 2D6, 2C9 Monitor CBC, platelets MOA: inhibits parasitic dihydrofolate reductase, decreases folic acid synthesis
Leucovorin 5, 10, 15, 25 mg tabs; 10 mg/mL IV soln	10-20 mg po qd	Rash, thrombocytosis, nausea/vomiting	Pernicious anemia, B_{12}–deficient anemia	↓ efficacy of SMX-TMP for PCP treatment	Not an anti-infective agent Used to prevent hematological toxicity caused by pyrimethamine
Sulfadiazine 500 mg tabs	1000-1500 mg po qd	Aplastic anemia, rash (SJS & toxic epidermal necrolysis), neutropenia, thrombocytopenia	Sulfa allergy, porphyria, pregnancy (at term)	SSRIs, dapsone, phenytoin, warfarin	MOA: competitively inhibits PABA; inhibits folic acid synthesis Inhibits 2C9
Atovaquone (Mepron)	1500 mg po bid	see Table 28-3			
Clindamycin (Cleocin)	600 mg IV Q6h	see Table 28-3			
SMX/TMP (Bactrim)	15 mg/kg (trimethoprim component) po/IV, divided Q8h	see Table 28-3			
Azithromycin (Zithromax) 250, 500, 600 mg tabs; 100, 200 mg/5mL susp; 500 mg IV	1200 mg po qd	GI distress, rash, vaginitis	None	Tacrolimus, phenytoin, carbamazepine, cyclosporine, bromocriptine, benzodiazepines	Weakly inhibits 3A4 Monitor QTc interval

Reproduced with permission from Attridge RL, Miller ML, Moote R, et al: *Internal Medicine: A Guide to Clinical Therapeutics.* New York, NY: McGraw-Hill; 2013.

recommended indefinitely unless immune reconstitution with ART occurs (CD_4 >200 cells/mm³ for 6 months).

Treatment

Preferred therapy for toxoplasmosis is pyrimethamine, leucovorin, and sulfadiazine for at least 6 weeks (Table 28-6). Alternative treatment regimens include: (1) Pyrimethamine + leucovorin plus clindamycin or azithromycin or atovaquone; or (2) TMP/SMZ, atovaquone, and sulfadiazine.

MYCOBACTERIUM AVIUM COMPLEX

Mycobacterium avium complex (MAC) is a slow-growing aerobic bacilli transmitted via inhalation or ingestion of organisms. Presenting as a pulmonary infection and disseminated disease (liver, spleen, bone marrow), MAC is likely to be isolated in patients with HIV and CD_4 counts less than 50 cells/mm³. Signs and symptoms of infection include fever, weight loss, abdominal pain, night sweats, fatigue, diarrhea, increased liver function tests, anemia, hepatosplenomegaly, and leukopenia.

Prophylaxis

Primary prophylaxis for MAC is recommended for patients with a CD_4 counts less than 50 cells/mm³. Prophylaxis options include azithromycin, clarithromycin, or rifabutin (Table 28-7). Prophylaxis may be discontinued when the CD_4 count is greater than 100 cells/mm³ for 3 months or more. Secondary prophylaxis is indefinitely unless the patient has immune reconstitution. Secondary prophylaxis may be discontinued if a patient has completed 12 months of treatment and the CD_4 greater than 100 cells/mm³ for 6 months or more (restart prophylaxis if CD_4 count drops <50).

TABLE 28-7	Primary Prophylaxis for *Mycobacterium avium* Complex
Preferred Therapy	**Alternative Therapy**
Azithromycin 1200 mg po qw	Rifabutin 300 mg po qd[a,b]
Clarithromycin 500 mg po bid	
Azithromycin 600 mg po biw	

Abbreviations: biw, twice a week; qw, once a week.
[a]Active TB should be ruled out before initiation.
[b]Dosage adjustment may be necessary based on drug interactions.

TABLE 28-8	Drug Treatment for *Mycobacterium avium* Complex				
Drug	**Dose**	**Adverse Effects**	**Contraindications**	**Drug/Drug Interactions**	**Clinical Notes**
Clarithromycin (Biaxin®) 125 mg/5 mL, 250 mg/5 mL susp; 250, 500 mg tab	500 mg po bid CrCL <30: 50% of normal dose OR double dosing interval	GI distress, bitter taste, rash, hearing loss	Use with *ergot* derivatives, cisapride	*Calcium* channel blockers, benzodiazepines, statins, azoles, SSRIs, QTc prolonging agents	Inhibits 3A4 Monitor QTc interval Max 1g/d MOA: bind 50s ribosomal subunit, inhibit protein synthesis
Azithromycin (Zithromax®) 250, 500, 600 mg tabs; 100 mg/5 mL, 200 mg/5 mL susp; 500 mg IV	500-600 mg po daily	GI distress, rash, vaginitis	None	Tacrolimus, phenytoin, carbamazepine, cyclosporine, bromocriptine, benzodiazepines	Weakly inhibits 3A4 Monitor QTc interval
Ethambutol (Myambutol®) 100, 400 mg tabs	15 mg/kg po daily CrCL 10-50: Q24-36h CrCl <10: Q48h	GI distress, optic neuritis at high doses	Optic neuritis, use in patients whose vision cannot be assessed	Decreased absorption with aluminum hydroxide	Consider ophthalmic examination prior to therapy initiation D/C if vision changes occur MOA: Interferes with RNA synthesis
Rifabutin (Mycobutin®) 150 mg caps	300 mg po daily CrCl <30: 50% of normal dose	GI distress, hepatitis, neutropenia, arthralgias, uveitis at high doses	WBC <100 K Platelets <50 K	Efavirenz, amprenavir, indinavir	Major 3A4 substrate & inhibitor Monitor LFTs MOA: inhibit DNA dependent RNA polymerase, halt transcription of RNA
Rifampin (Rifadin®) 150, 300 mg tabs and caps; 600 mg IV	600 mg po daily	GI distress, hepatitis, neutropenia	Concurrent use with amprenavir, saquinavir/ ritonavir	Clopidogrel, isoniazid, protease inhibitors, amiodarone, warfarin, SSRIs, hormonal contraceptives, benzodiazepines, corticosteroids, statins	Induces 1A2, 2C9/19, 3A4 Monitor CBC, LFTs
Amikacin (Amikin®) 50 mg/mL, 250 mg/mL IV	15 mg/kg IV 3×/wk (Use IBW)	Vestibular and auditory abnormalities, renal toxicity	None	Additive effects with other nephrotoxins	Monitor BUN, SCr, hearing changes Therapeutic monitoring MOA: bind to 30s ribosomal subunit, inhibit protein synthesis
Streptomycin 1 g powder	15 mg/kg IM 3×/wk Max dose: 1 g				

Reproduced with permission from Attridge RL, Miller ML, Moote R, et al: *Internal Medicine: A Guide to Clinical Therapeutics.* New York, NY: McGraw-Hill; 2013.

Treatment

Treatment recommendations include at least two active agents to decrease the chances of resistance. Preferred therapy includes clarithromycin, ethambutol, ± rifabutin for 12 months (Table 28-8). Alternative therapy includes azithromycin and select aminoglycosides.

CASE Application

1. Pyrimethamine has been shown to cause bone marrow suppression. Which agent can be given in conjunction with pyrimethamine to lessen the suppressive effects?

    a. Vitamin B_{12}
    b. Levofloxacin
    c. Dapsone
    d. Leucovorin

2. Treatment for PCP during pregnancy has been associated with hemolytic anemia in G6PD deficient states. Select the medication that may be implicated in this condition. Select all that apply.

    a. Azithromycin
    b. Primaquine
    c. Dapsone
    d. Atovaquone

3. What is the brand name for moxifloxacin?

    a. Avelox
    b. Septra

c. Mepron
d. Aczone

4. JK is a patient at a local clinic with a recent diagnosis of AIDS. His past medical history includes hypertension, dyslipidemia, and depression. Medications include losartan, atorvastatin, and escitalopram. Labs include: CD_4 count of 120 cells/mm^3, serum and potassium 4.8 mEq/L (increased from 3.5 mEq/L). Which agent is recommended as a preferred therapy for PCP prophylaxis?

a. Clindamycin
b. TMP-SMX
c. Amikacin
d. Levofloxacin

5. RA is a nonpregnant female with a past medical history of AIDS (diagnosed 5 years ago). Due to denial of her status, she refused treatment. RA presents to the clinic today with a CD_4 count of 80 cells/mm^3. Which of the following primary prophylaxis medications should be recommended for RA? Select all that apply.

a. MAC
b. TE
c. PCP
d. No prophylaxis is recommended for RA

6. LZ is a 52-year-old patient admitted to the hospital with complications of AIDS. The nurse informs the pharmacy resident that he is being treated for a PJP infection. She is unclear of the duration of therapy and asks the pharmacy resident for clarification. Select the approximate duration of antimicrobial therapy in most patients with PJP infection.

a. 7 days
b. 10 days
c. 14 days
d. 21 days

7. The diagnostic criterion for which of the following opportunistic infections is seropositive for immunoglobulin G (IgG)?

a. Candidiasis
b. Toxoplasmosis
c. MAC
d. PJP

8. Which of the agents listed below is available in an aerosolized preparation used in the primary prophylaxis of PJP?

a. Dapsone
b. Leucovorin
c. Trimethoprim
d. Pentamidine

9. Which of the agents listed below are utilized for primary prophylaxis in both PJP and toxoplasmosis? Select all that apply.

a. Atovaquone
b. Dapsone
c. Leucovorin
d. Pentamidine

10. Which of the agents listed below can be given once weekly in primary prophylaxis for MAC?

a. Azithromycin
b. Aztreonam
c. Clindamycin
d. Cefazolin

11. What is the generic name for Biaxin?

a. Clindamycin
b. Sulfamethoxazole-Trimethoprim
c. Clarithromycin
d. Vancomycin

12. IT is a male patient with a past medical history of HIV. CD_4 count is 115 cells/mm^3 and HIV RNA is currently undetectable (3 months ago he was started on tenofovir (TDF)/emtricitabine/rilpivirine). He presents to the clinic today with pain upon swallowing and white patches in his mouth. He is diagnosed with oropharyngeal candidiasis (first episode). Which of the following medications may be used for an initial episode of oropharyngeal candidiasis and is available as a troche?

a. Fluconazole
b. Clotrimazole
c. Itraconazole
d. Posaconazole
e. Voriconazole

13. GY is an HIV patient with a past medical history of HIV (CD4 150). Medications include tenofovir (TDF)/emtricitabine and lopinavir/ritonavir, TMP/SMZ (PJP prophylaxis), Amiodarone (history of atrial fibrillation), and clarithromycin (started 3 days for a respiratory tract infection—day 3 of 10 day treatment course). He presents to the clinic with complaints of thrush. This is his third case of thrush this year. Which of the following medications may be utilized for the management of GY's esophageal candidiasis and would have a potential drug interaction with his medications? Select all that apply.

a. Fluconazole
b. Clotrimazole
c. Itraconazole
d. Voriconazole

14. Select the brand name for amphotericin B products. Select all that apply.

a. Amphocin
b. Fungizone
c. Ambisome
d. Ancobon

15. RT is a patient with HIV on the following medications: simvastatin, pantoprazole, TMP/SMZ, and as needed ibuprofen. Because his CD_4 count has decreased, he is to be placed on MAC primary prophylaxis. Which of the following medications may be utilized for MAC prophylaxis in RT?

    a. Azithromycin
    b. Clarithromycin
    c. Clindamycin
    d. Clotrimazole

16. Which of the following medications is available in a powder for nebulization formulation?

    a. Dapsone
    b. Pentamidine
    c. Clindamycin
    d. Primaquine

17. What is the brand name of posaconazole?

    a. Diflucan
    b. Vfend
    c. Sporanox
    d. Noxafil

18. Place the following echinocandins in order based upon day 1 initial dose for esophageal candidiasis. Start with the lowest mg dose.

Unordered Response	Ordered Response
Micafungin	
Anidulafungin	
Caspofungin	

19. Which of the following azole antifungal medication is associated with hallucinations? Select all that apply.

    a. Voriconazole
    b. Metronidazole
    c. Clotrimazole
    d. Fluconazole

20. Which of the following medications is associated with optic neuritis?

    a. Clarithromycin
    b. Itraconazole
    c. Ethambutol
    d. Amphotericin

TAKEAWAY POINTS »

- Prophylactic and treatment efforts of OIs are guided by patients' CD_4 counts.
- Mucocutaneous candidiasis is a fungal infection caused by *Candida* species (most commonly *Candida albicans*).
- Primary prophylaxis is not routinely recommended for Candidiasis. Secondary prophylaxis is recommended for patients with severe recurrences (fluconazole 100-200 mg/d).
- Topical treatment may be used for the initial episode of oropharyngeal candidiasis.
- *Pneumocystis* is an opportunistic fungal pulmonary pathogen that is an important cause of pneumonia in the immunocompromised host.
- Pneumocystis prophylaxis is indicated for HIV-infected patients with CD_4 counts of less than 200 cells/mm³ or a history of oropharyngeal candidiasis and for both HIV-infected and non–HIV-infected patients who have recovered from PJP.
- CM is a CNS infection caused by the fungus *Cryptococcus neoformans*.
- Pharmacologic treatment of CM includes an induction, suppressive, and maintenance phase.
- Toxoplasmosis is a CNS infection caused by the parasite *Toxoplasma gondii*.
- All HIV-infected persons, including those who lack IgG antibody to *Toxoplasma*, should be counseled regarding sources of *Toxoplasma* infection.
- Toxoplasma primary prophylaxis is recommended for patients with a CD_4 counts less than 100 cells/mm³ (TMP/SMX) and may be discontinued when CD_4 greater than 200 cells/mm³ for more than 3 months.
- The preferred therapy for toxoplasma infection is pyrimethamine, leucovorin, and sulfadiazine for at least 6 weeks.
- MAC is a slow-growing aerobic bacilli transmitted via inhalation or ingestion of organisms. MAC presents as a pulmonary infection.
- Primary prophylaxis for MAC is recommended for patients with a CD_4 count less than 50 cells/mm³.
- Treatment recommendations for MAC include at least two active agents to lower the possibility of resistance.

BIBLIOGRAPHY

Anderson PL, Kakuda TN, Fletcher CV. Human immunodeficiency virus infection. In: DiPiro JT, Talbert RL, Yee GC, Matzke GR, Wells BG, Posey L, eds. *Pharmacotherapy: A Pathophysiologic Approach.* 10th ed. New York, NY: McGraw-Hill; 2017.

Brooks GF, Carroll KC, Butel JS, Morse SA, Mietzner TA. AIDS and lentiviruses. In: Brooks GF, Carroll KC, Butel JS, Morse SA, Mietzner TA, eds. *Jawetz, Melnick, & Adelberg's Medical Microbiology.* 26th ed. New York, NY: McGraw-Hill; 2013:chap 44.

Hand E, Dzintars K. HIV infection and AIDS. In: Attridge RL, Miller ML, Moote R, Ryan L, eds. *Internal Medicine: A Guide to Clinical Therapeutics.* New York, NY: McGraw-Hill; 2013:chap 35.

Panel on Opportunistic Infections in HIV-Infected Adults and Adolescents. Guidelines for the prevention and treatment of opportunistic infections in HIV-infected adults and adolescents: recommendations from the Centers for Disease Control and Prevention, the National Institutes of Health, and the HIV Medicine Association of the Infectious Diseases Society of America. Available at http://aidsinfo.nih.gov/contentfiles/lvguidelines/adult_oi.pdf. Accessed April 18, 2018.

KEY ABBREVIATIONS

AIDS = acquired immunodeficiency syndrome
ART = antiretroviral therapy
CM = cryptococcal meningitis
CNS = central nervous system
HIV = human immunodeficiency virus

MAC = *Mycobacterium avium* complex
OIs = opportunistic infections
PJP = *Pneumocystis jirovecii*
TMP/SMX = trimethoprim/sulfamethoxazole

29

Invasive Fungal Infections

Douglas Slain

FOUNDATION OVERVIEW

Invasive fungal infections are associated with significant morbidity and mortality, occurring most frequently in immunocompromised patients. Advances in medical technology, including organ and bone marrow transplantation, cytotoxic chemotherapy, the widespread use of indwelling intravenous (IV) catheters, and the increased use of broad-spectrum antibiotics have contributed to the increase of fungal infections.

Fungi are eukaryotic organisms that exist in two basic forms, yeasts and molds. Figure 29-1 displays how pathogenic fungi can be grouped based on their morphological characteristics. Yeasts are unicellular in nature whereas molds are filamentous. Some fungal organisms exist in both forms and are referred to as dimorphic fungi. Dimorphic fungi exist as molds in the environment and convert to parasitic yeast in the human body. Common dimorphic fungi that cause invasive infection are *Blastomyces dermatitidis*, *Histoplasma capsulatum*, and *Coccidioides immitis*. Exposure to these organisms occurs in certain regions of the country and as such is termed endemic fungi.

The most common invasive fungal infections are caused by yeasts (*Candida* species). Examples of *Candida* species include *C. albicans, C. glabrata, C. parapsilosis, C. tropicalis,* and *C. krusei. Candida* are normal inhabitants of mucocutaneous surfaces of the human body and frequently colonize the female genital tract, gastrointestinal (GI) tract, and skin. These organisms cause infections if they overwhelm host defenses and invade sterile areas. A classic example is seen with a proliferation in the number of *Candida* in the GI tract after treatment with broad-spectrum antibiotics. Common invasive infections include bloodstream infections (candidemia) and/or invasive candidiasis (eg, peritonitis and hepatosplenic). Risk factors for invasive candidiasis include neutropenia, diabetes, immunodeficiency diseases, high-dose corticosteroids, immunosuppressants, antineoplastic agents, total parenteral nutrition, antimicrobials, surgery, and burns.

Cryptococcus neoformans is an encapsulated yeast found in soil or bird excrement that causes invasive infections less frequently than *Candida. Cryptococcus neoformans* most often causes meningitis in immunocompromised patients.

Molds cause fewer infections than yeasts because they affect patients with severely suppressed immune systems.

The most common molds that cause clinical infections are the *Aspergillus* species. *Aspergillus* is a ubiquitous mold that grows well on a variety of substrates, including soil, water, decaying vegetation, and organic debris. Common species of *Aspergillosis* infections are: (1) *A. fumigatus,* (2) *A. flavus,* and (3) *A. niger.* The term aspergillosis may be broadly defined as a spectrum of diseases attributed to allergy, colonization, or tissue invasion. Invasive infections with *Aspergillus* are associated with a high mortality.

Diagnosis

Invasive fungal infections are suspected in at-risk patients that show signs of infection despite broad-spectrum antibiotic therapy. This is especially true in immunocompromised patients. *Candida* and *Cryptococcus* may be isolated in a culture of body fluid (blood or cerebral spinal fluid [CSF]). Generally, fungi take longer to grow in specimen cultures than bacteria. India ink is a stain that helps to identify the capsule of *C. neoformans.*

Diagnosis of molds and the endemic fungi may involve identifying organisms in blood or tissue. Serologic antibody testing or antigen detection may also be used in the diagnosis. Two examples are the *Histoplasma capsulatum* antigen assay and the galactomannan antigen assay which is used in the diagnosis of aspergillosis. Computed tomography (CT) is a radiologic test that is often used to provide a better diagnostic yield than conventional x-rays. Classic findings in pulmonary aspergillosis are the halo and/or crescent signs.

Prevention

Prophylactic use of antifungal agents is employed for preventing fungal infections in bone marrow transplant (BMT) or hematopoietic stem cell transplantation (HSCT), high-risk leukemia, and liver and lung transplant patients. The primary preventative agents have been oral or IV azoles (fluconazole or posaconazole). Another preventative use of antifungals is the practice of secondary prophylaxis (suppression) of cryptococcal disease in human immunodeficiency virus (HIV) patients. After a patient is treated for cryptococcal disease, they receive oral fluconazole 200 mg daily until their CD4 cell count is more than 100 cells/mm^3 for 6 months (sometimes longer).

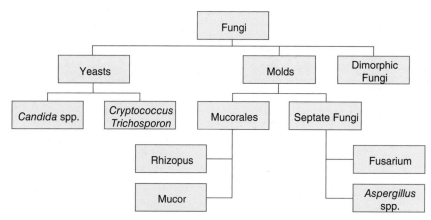

FIGURE 29-1 Morphologically, pathogenic fungi can be grouped as either filamentous molds or unicellular yeasts. Molds grow as multicellular branching, thread-like filaments (hyphae) that are either septate (divided by transverse walls) or coenocytic (multinucleate without cross walls). Reproduced with permission from DiPiro JT, Talbert RL, Yee GC, et al: *Pharmacotherapy: A Pathophysiologic Approach,* 9th ed. New York, NY: McGraw-Hill; 2014.

Treatment

The approach to antifungal therapy for invasive fungal infections is determined by the type of fungal infection (yeast vs mold), severity of clinical presentation, patient's underlying immunosuppression, susceptibility data, potential toxicities, and drug interactions. Antifungals are associated with significant drug interactions and toxicities, especially with prolonged treatment courses. A majority of patients are treated empirically for invasive candidiasis before conclusive evidence of infection is available to direct therapy. Empiric therapy for

invasive candidiasis should be considered in patients with persistent, unexplained fever and host deficits that predispose patients to candidemia (eg, broad-spectrum antibiotics, presence of central venous catheter, patients with severe organ dysfunction, dialysis, neutropenia). Response to antifungal therapy for patients with invasive candidiasis is more rapid than for endemic fungal infections. Resolution of fever and sterilization of cultures are indications of response to fungal therapy. Key characteristics of antifungal medications are listed in Table 29-1.

TABLE 29-1	**Characteristics of Antifungal Agents**			
Drug/Drug Class	**Mechanism of Action**	**Clinical Applications**	**Pharmacokinetics and Interactions**	**Toxicities**
Amphotericin B	Binds to ergosterol in fungal cell membranes, forming "leaky pores"	Candidemia and infections caused by *Aspergillus, Blastomyces, Cryptococcus, Histoplasma, Mucor,* etc.	Multiple forms, IV for systemic infections (liposomal forms less nephrotoxic) Topical for ocular/bladder infections	Nephrotoxicity is dose limiting, additive with other nephrotoxic drugs; infusion reactions (chills, fever, muscle spasms, hypotension)
Azoles Ketoconazole Fluconazole Itraconazole Posaconazole Voriconazole Isavuconazole	Inhibit fungal P450-dependent enzymes blocking ergosterol synthesis Resistance can occur with long-term use	Aspergillosis (voriconazole) Blastomycosis (itraconazole, fluconazole) Mucormycosis (posaconazole and isavuconazole) Alternative drugs in candidemia and infections caused by *Aspergillus, Blastomyces, Cryptococcus,* and *Histoplasma*	Various topical and oral forms for dermatophytoses Oral, parenteral forms for mycoses (fluconazole, itraconazole [oral only], posaconazole, voriconazole, isavuconazole) Most azoles undergo hepatic metabolism Fluconazole eliminated in urine unchanged	Ketoconazole rarely used in systemic fungal infections owing to its inhibition of hepatic and adrenal P450s Other azoles are less toxic, but may cause gastrointestinal (GI) upsets and rash Voriconazole causes visual disturbances and is class D for pregnancy risk
Echinocandins Caspofungin Micafungin Anidulafungin	Inhibit β-glucan synthase decreasing fungal cell wall synthesis	Treatment of candidemia Caspofungin is also used as "salvage" therapy in aspergillosis	IV forms Micafungin increases levels of nifedipine and cyclosporine	GI distress, flushing from histamine release
Flucytosine	Inhibits DNA and RNA polymerases	Synergistic with amphotericin B in candidemia and cryptococal infections	Oral; enters cerebrospinal fluid Renal elimination	Bone marrow suppression
Terbinafine	Inhibits epoxidation of squalene	Mucocutaneous fungal infections Accumulates in keratin	Oral Long duration of action (weeks)	GI upset

Reproduced with permission from Trevor AJ, Katzung BG, Kruidering-Hall MM, et al: *Katzung & Trevor's Pharmacology: Examination & Board Review,* 10th ed. New York, NY: McGraw-Hill; 2013.

Amphotericin B

Amphotericin B is a polyene antifungal that binds to fungal cell membrane ergosterol and promotes enhanced permeability leading to fungal cell death. Amphotericin B is regarded as the gold standard systemic antifungal because of its fungicidal activity and broad spectrum of antifungal activity (molds and yeasts). Amphotericin B is administered intravenously and available as an injection (eg, 50 mg powder for reconstitution). The conventional formulation of amphotericin B is the deoxycholate (deoxycholate) formulation. This formulation must be prepared in dextrose 5% to facilitate the proper micellular dispersion. Lipid-based formulations are also available and include liposomal (Ambisome) and lipid-complex (Abelcet) formulations. All formulations of amphotericin B are nephrotoxic and can be associated with infusion-related toxicities (fever, chills, and rigors). Premedication with acetaminophen and diphenhydramine may help lessen infusion-related toxicities. Administration of normal saline boluses (500-1000 mL) before (and sometimes after) amphotericin B infusions may help ameliorate the nephrotoxicity. The lipid-based agents appear less nephrotoxic than the conventional formulation of amphotericin B. Unfortunately liposomal products are considerably more expensive than conventional amphotericin B. The liposomal formulation (AmBisome) has a lower rate of infusion-related reactions than other amphotericin B formulations. Despite the improved safety profile, lipid-based amphotericin B formulations have not improved survival rates. Lipid-based formulations are dosed at 3 to 5 mg/kg versus the 0.5 to 1.5 mg/kg dose of conventional amphotericin B. Amphotericin B is the treatment of choice for pregnant patients with fungal infections, because the other classes of antifungal agents have risk of teratogenicity (categories C and D). Anaphylaxis has been reported with amphotericin B products; therefore, the drug should be administered under close clinical observation. Other key drug parameters for amphotericin B products include:

- Try to avoid use with other nephrotoxic medications;
- Drug-induced renal toxicity improves with interrupting therapy, switching to a lipid-based formulation (if on deoxycholate formulation), decreasing dosage, or increasing dosing interval;
- Electrolyte wasting is associated with amphotericin products (hypokalemia, hypomagnesemia).

Flucytosine

Flucytosine (5-flucytosine, 5-FC, Ancobon) is a pyrimidine analog that penetrates fungal cells and is converted to 5-fluorouracil (5-FU) which interferes with fungal RNA and protein synthesis. Flucytosine is used as adjunctive treatment of systemic fungal infections (eg, susceptible strains of *Candida* or *Cryptococcus*). 5-FC is not used as monotherapy because resistance rapidly develops. The drug is available as an oral capsule and has good absorption and distribution (penetrates well into the CSF). 5-FC is associated with bone marrow suppression (black box warning) leading to blood dyscrasias (neutropenia, thrombocytopenia, and anemia). GI adverse effects are also common. Flucytosine is dosed 50 to 100 mg/kg in divided doses every 6 hours in patients with a creatinine clearance (CrCl) greater than 40 mL/min. Use caution in patients with renal dysfunction and adjust dose as required.

Azole Antifungals

Azole antifungals interfere with the fungal enzyme 14α-demethylase thereby decreasing ergosterol synthesis and inhibiting cell membrane formation. Azoles are well tolerated, but are associated with cytochrome P-450 drug interactions and occasionally hepatotoxicity. Most of the drug interactions are due to enzyme inhibition of CYP 3A4 metabolism. Itraconazole and voriconazole are also substrates of some of the P-450 isoenzymes and can have their metabolism affected by other drugs (Table 29-2).

TABLE 29-2	Drug Interactions, Administration, and Dietary Recommendations for Azole Antifungals	
Azole Antifungal	**Drug Interactions (CYP 450)**	**Oral Administration**
Fluconazole (Diflucan)	I: 1A2 (weak); 2C9 (strong); 2C19 (strong); 3A4 (moderate)	Take with or without regard to meals
Itraconazole (Sporanox)	S: 3A4 (major)	Capsule: Absorption enhanced by food and possibly gastric acidity. Cola drinks have been shown to increase the absorption of the capsules in patients with achlorhydria or those taking H₂ receptor antagonists
	I: 3A4 (strong)	Solution: Take on an empty stomach
		Capsules and oral solutions are not interchangeable; doses greater than 200 mg are given in two divided doses
Voriconazole (Vfend)	S: 2C9 (major); 2C19 (major); 3A4 (minor) I: 2C9 (weak); 2C19 (weak); 3A4 (moderate)	Oral: Should be taken 1 h before or 1 h after a meal
		Dietary: Tablets contain lactose—avoid in lactose intolerance; suspension contains sucrose—use caution in sucrose/fructose malabsorption
Posaconazole (Noxafil)	I: 3A4 (strong)	Administer with food; food and/or nutritional supplement increases absorption; fasting states do not provide sufficient absorption to ensure adequate plasma concentration.
Isavuconazole (Cresemba)	S: 3A4, I: 3A4 (weak-moderate); 2B6 (weak)	Oral capsules can be taken with or without food

Abbreviations: I, inhibitor of CYP isoenzyme; S, substrate of CYP isoenzyme.

Fluconazole (Diflucan) is the most commonly used triazole antifungal and is used for candidiasis, cryptococcal meningitis, and antifungal prophylaxis in allogenic BMTs. Fluconazole is well tolerated, available in oral (tablet and suspension) and IV formulations, and has a lower rate of drug interactions compared to other triazoles. Fluconazole penetrates into the CSF (thus used for meningitis) and is eliminated renally (dosage adjustments are required for renal dysfunction). Fluconazole is effective against *Cryptococcus* and most *Candida* species (*C. albicans*, *C. parapsilosis*, and *C. tropicalis*), but is inactive against molds and *C. krusei*. Fluconazole's susceptibility to *C. glabrata* is usually defined as "susceptible-dose-dependent" (S-DD), meaning that larger dose may be needed to achieve cure in serious infections. The daily dose for fluconazole is the same for oral and IV administration and depends upon the type of fungal infection (400-800 mg daily for candidemia, 150 mg for vaginal candidiasis; 400 mg for cryptococcosis [step-down therapy from amphotericin B + flucytosine]).

Despite having activity against *Candida* species and some molds including *Aspergillus*, itraconazole (Sporanox) is not used much because of its lack of predictable pharmacokinetics (eg, bioavailability). The capsule formulation of itraconazole displays wide interpatient oral absorption. The bioavailability of the capsule formulation may be enhanced by administering itraconazole with soda, meals, or nutritional supplements and by avoiding concomitant acid-suppressing agents (eg, proton pump inhibitors, H_2 antagonists, antacids). A newer oral solution provides more predictable absorption. Due to differences in bioavailability, oral capsules and oral solution cannot be used interchangeably. Itraconazole can display negative inotropic effects and should be used with caution in patients with left ventricular dysfunction or a history of heart failure (black box warning). The daily dose of itraconazole depends upon the type of fungal infection (eg, 200-400 mg daily for aspergillosis; 200 mg daily for endemic fungal infections; 100-200 mg daily for esophageal candidiasis). Trough serum concentrations may be performed to assure therapeutic levels, especially in the face of oral therapy. Itraconazole has largely been relegated to treating the endemic fungi infections.

Voriconazole (VFEND) is an analog of fluconazole that has a broader spectrum of activity against *Candida* species. In addition, the drug has activity against *Aspergillus* and has become a drug of first choice for invasive aspergillosis. Voriconazole is subject to a large number of drug interactions and has been associated with reversible visual disturbances. Voriconazole drug interactions are dose dependent, as they exhibit unpredictable nonlinear pharmacokinetics; thus, drug interactions are more difficult to predict and manage. Studies indicate that CYP 2C19 is significantly involved in the metabolism of voriconazole. This enzyme exhibits genetic polymorphism; about 3% to 5% of Caucasians and 12% to 23% of Asians are expected to be poor metabolizers of voriconazole. Voriconazole is available in both oral and cyclodextrin IV formulations. There are concerns about the IV cyclodextrin carrier accumulating in and exacerbating renal failure. Visual changes, including blurred vision, changes in visual acuity,

color perception, and photophobia, are commonly associated with treatment. Patients should be warned to avoid tasks which depend on vision, including operating machinery or driving. Changes are reversible on discontinuation following brief exposure (less than 28 days). The daily dose of voriconazole depends upon the type of fungal infection (aspergillosis: 6 mg/kg IV every 12 hours on day 1 followed by 4 mg/kg IV every 12 hours; esophageal candidiasis: 200 mg po every 12 hours). Patients with mild-moderate hepatic dysfunction (Child Pugh class A and B) should receive a normal loading dose followed by 2 mg/kg every 12 hours. Voriconazole should only be used in severe hepatic dysfunction when the benefits outweigh the risks. In patients with CrCl less than 50 mL/min, accumulation of the IV vehicle cyclodextrin occurs. After the initial IV loading dose, oral voriconazole should be administered to these patients, unless an assessment of the benefit-risk ratio to the patient justifies the use of IV voriconazole.

Posaconazole (Noxafil) is approved for prophylaxis of *Candida* and *Aspergillus* infections in high-risk neutropenic patients and in the treatment of oropharyngeal candidiasis. Posaconazole oral suspension has a variable absorption. The absorption can be enhanced by administering with meals or nutritional supplements and by avoiding concomitant acid-suppressing agents. The dose of posaconazole depends upon the type of fungal infection. Posaconazole solution is dosed 200 mg tid for prophylaxis (*Aspergillus* and *Candida*) and 400 mg twice daily for treatment of *Candida* infections. Delayed-release tablets and an IV formulation are available. These formulations provide better drug exposure and are dosed 300 mg once daily (after a twice daily loading dose on day 1). The IV formulation has a cyclodextrin carrier, so it should not be used if CrCL is less than 50 mL/min. Posaconazole can prolong QTc interval.

Recently, the new triazole, isavuconazole (Cresemba) was approved. This agent is administered as the prodrug isavuconazonium sulfate, and is available as an oral capsule formulation and as an IV formulation. Isavuconazole is similar to voriconazole, but has less pharmacokinetic variability and does not require cyclodextrin in the IV formulation. This agent can also be used to treat some Mucorales mold species.

Echinocandins

There are three echinocandin antifungals: caspofungin (Cancidas), micafungin (Mycamine), and anidulafungin (Eraxis). Echinocandins inhibit the fungal enzyme (1, 3) β-D-glucan synthase; which inhibits the formation (1, 3) β-D-glucan fibrils, which are essential components for outer cell walls of some fungi. These agents are effective against most *Candida* species and *Aspergillus* species. Echinocandins are well tolerated with minimal drug interaction potential. Echinocandins are available as parenteral formulations and do not require dosage adjustments in patients with renal insufficiency. The dose of caspofungin is 70 mg daily on day 1, followed by 50 mg daily. Patients with a Child-Pugh score of 7 to 9 should be given a maintenance dose of 35 mg/d, instead of 50 mg/d. The dose of micafungin is 50 to 150 mg daily depending upon the indication and the dose of anidulafungin is 50 to 200 mg daily depending upon the indication.

Special Considerations

There are studies with all of the antifungal agents in children; amphotericin B, fluconazole, and echinocandins are recommended in neonatal candidiasis. Amphotericin B carries a pregnancy category B, whereas most azoles, echinocandins and flucytosine all carry category C status. Voriconazole is category D. Clinicians must weigh the potential benefit/risks of therapy in pregnant patients when using azoles, echinocandins and flucytosine.

CASE Application

1. TI is a 44-year-old patient with an aspergillosis infection. She is to receive treatment with amphotericin B. Which one of the following adjunctive measures is used to lessen the occurrence of nephrotoxicity associated with amphotericin B?

   a. Test dose of amphotericin B
   b. Diphenhydramine premedication
   c. Normal saline boluses
   d. Furosemide

2. PT is a 33-year-old HIV patient. He has a high viral load and low CD4. He has been nonadherent with medication and provider appointments. PT is admitted to the medical center for a change in mental status. He is undergoing a complete work-up to identify the cause. An India Ink stain is reported as positive. Which one of the following organisms is likely to manifest a positive India ink stain on a CSF sample?

   a. *Candida albicans*
   b. *Candida glabrata*
   c. *Aspergillosis fumigatus*
   d. *Candida neoformans*

3. When preparing an IV formulation of amphotericin B deoxycholate, the lyophilized amphotericin B powder must first be reconstituted with sterile water. What type of IV fluid must the reconstituted amphotericin B be placed in for IV administration?

   a. 0.9% sodium chloride
   b. 5% dextrose in water
   c. Lactated Ringer's solution
   d. Any of the above solutions

4. Which of the following agents is recommended as therapy for invasive aspergillosis? Select all that apply.

   a. Amphotericin B
   b. Fluconazole
   c. Voriconazole
   d. Liposomal amphotericin B
   e. Terbinafine

5. IT is receiving initial therapy for *Cryptococcus*. His provider has been monitoring for toxicity and identified that IT has a low granulocyte count (previously within normal limits). Which of the following antifungal agents is associated with bone marrow suppression?

   a. Fluconazole
   b. Amphotericin B
   c. Voriconazole
   d. Flucytosine

6. Lipid-based or liposomal amphotericin B formulations have what advantage over conventional amphotericin B (deoxycholate)?

   a. Less expensive than conventional amphotericin B
   b. Decreased mortality
   c. Decreased rates of nephrotoxicity
   d. More efficacious than conventional amphotericin B

7. Which antifungal preparation carries a relative contraindication against use in patients with severe renal insufficiency (due to risk of renal complications from a carrier molecule)?

   a. IV posaconazole
   b. IV voriconazole
   c. Oral itraconazole
   d. IV caspofungin
   e. Oral voriconazole

8. A patient with a histoplasmosis infection is to be discharged from the hospital and started on oral itraconazole capsules. Which one of the following statements would you tell the patient about his medication to maximize the oral absorption?

   a. Take with food and avoid concomitant use of antacids
   b. Take on an empty stomach
   c. Food will not affect the oral absorption
   d. Do not take this with cola

9. A patient is to receive home infusion therapy with amphotericin B. What laboratory values should be monitored? Select all that apply.

   a. Serum creatinine
   b. Serum potassium
   c. Serum magnesium
   d. Serum creatine phosphokinase (CPK)

10. Which of the following antifungal agents has been shown to cause visual acuity side effects? Select all that apply.

    a. Amphotericin B
    b. Flucytosine
    c. Fluconazole
    d. Voriconazole
    e. Caspofungin

11. A 54-year-old man with leukemia developed neutropenia 10 days ago after a chemotherapy course. His absolute neutrophil count (ANC) is 200, and he has been febrile for 7 days despite empiric bacterial therapy

with imipenem and vancomycin. He was ordered amphotericin B 5 days ago. His CrCl has diminished to <30 mL/min. Which one of the following antifungal agents would be an option for a febrile neutropenic patient with renal insufficiency? The provider would like a broad-spectrum antifungal that covers yeasts and molds and an agent that does not affect the kidneys as much as conventional amphotericin B.

a. Liposomal amphotericin B
b. Fluconazole
c. Posaconazole
d. Ketoconazole

12. A 58-year-old febrile woman in the surgical intensive care unit has one out of two blood culture bottles growing yeast and is hemodynamically stable. A urine sample collected 2 days ago is growing *C. glabrata*. What is the best empiric decision for this patient?

a. Start fluconazole 400-800 mg daily
b. Wait for a susceptibility report and then start with a sensitive antifungal agent
c. The one out of two blood bottles and the urine culture do not require therapy
d. Initiate caspofungin 70 mg × 1 dose, then 50 mg daily

13. Genetic variability in cytochrome P-450 CYP 2C19 has been linked to significant interpatient pharmacokinetic differences for which antifungal agent?

a. Fluconazole
b. Voriconazole
c. Micafungin
d. Flucytosine

14. A 55-year-old man is to be treated for invasive aspergillosis. He weighs 100 kg. What amphotericin B formulation dose(s) would be appropriate for this patient? Select all that apply.

a. Amphotericin B deoxycholate 80 mg
b. Amphotericin B deoxycholate 400 mg
c. Liposomal Amphotericin B 400 mg
d. Liposomal Amphotericin B 80 mg
e. Liposomal Amphotericin 800 mg

15. The fungal cell wall component (1, 3) β-D-glucan is not a key structure in *C. neoformans* and therefore explains the poor activity of what class of antifungal agents for *Cryptococcus*?

a. Triazoles
b. Amphotericin B
c. Echinocandins
d. 5-Flucytosine

16. What drug interaction would be exhibited by adding fluconazole to a person's medication regimen that includes warfarin (stabilized at an INR of 2.5)?

a. Fluconazole and warfarin concentrations would both be reduced
b. An increase in INR would be expected
c. Warfarin cytochrome P-450 metabolism would be induced
d. An interaction would not be expected

17. BK is a 40-year-old HIV-positive patient. He develops CSF culture-positive cryptococcal meningitis. He has no hepatic or renal insufficiency and his complete blood count is within normal limits. Select the preferred antifungal regimen for a patient with cryptococcal meningitis.

a. Amphotericin B deoxycholate + flucytosine
b. Amphotericin B deoxycholate
c. Liposomal amphotericin B
d. Fluconazole

18. Which antifungal agent is only available as a parenteral formulation? Select all that apply.

a. Amphotericin B lipid-complex
b. Voriconazole
c. Posaconazole
d. Fluconazole

19. Which antifungal agent has the greatest 24-hour urinary excretion percentage?

a. Amphotericin B deoxycholate
b. Fluconazole
c. Voriconazole
d. Caspofungin

20. At the end of initial treatment (amphotericin and flucytosine) for cryptococcal meningitis (CSF-sterilized) in an HIV-positive patient, what is generally recommended in terms of cryptococcal infection? Select all that apply.

a. Once weekly doses of azithromycin
b. Four weeks of fluconazole oral therapy
c. Indefinite low-dose suppressive fluconazole therapy
d. No further antifungal therapy is needed
e. Once weekly doses of fluconazole for 4 weeks

21. What is the generic name for Cresemba?

a. Itraconazole
b. Isavuconazole
c. Posaconazole
d. Ketoconazole

TAKEAWAY POINTS »

- Invasive fungal infections are associated with high morbidity and mortality in immunocompromised patients.
- Amphotericin B deoxycholate has been the gold standard antifungal agent due to broad-spectrum and fungicidal killing.
- Amphotericin B deoxycholate is associated with significant infusion-related reactions and nephrotoxicity.
- Lipid-based (liposomal) formulations of amphotericin B have a lower rate of nephrotoxicity. Liposomal amphotericin B (Ambisome) has less infusion-related reactions than amphotericin B deoxycholate.
- Lipid-based formulations are given in a higher mg/kg dosage than amphotericin B deoxycholate.
- Flucytosine is adjunctive therapy used in combination with amphotericin B to treat cryptococcal meningitis. Once patients are stable, step-down therapy to an oral azole may be utilized.
- Flucytosine can cause blood dyscrasias.

- All azole antifungal agents are subject to cytochrome P-450 drug interactions. Fluconazole has less interaction potential than voriconazole or itraconazole.
- Voriconazole and posaconazole have been associated with QTc prolongation.
- Fluconazole has excellent activity against *C. albicans* but may be less effective against *C. glabrata* and other *Candida* species.
- Oral itraconazole is not well absorbed and benefits from coadministration with food or acidic beverages. Acid-suppressing agents (proton pump inhibitors and H$_2$-antagonists) may decrease absorption of this azole.
- Voriconazole and amphotericin B are the drugs of first choice for invasive aspergillosis.
- IV voriconazole and IV posaconazole are formulated with a cyclodextrin-carrier molecule that may accumulate in renal insufficiency.
- Echinocandins are well tolerated and have excellent activity against most *Candida* species.

BIBLIOGRAPHY

Bennett JE. Antifungal agents. In: Brunton LL, Chabner BA, Knollmann BC, eds. *Goodman & Gilman's The Pharmacological Basis of Therapeutics.* 12th ed. New York, NY: McGraw-Hill; 2011:chap 57.

Carver PL. Invasive fungal infections. In: DiPiro JT, Talbert RL, Yee GC, Matzke GR, Wells BG, Posey L, eds. *Pharmacotherapy: A Pathophysiologic Approach.* 10th ed. New York, NY: McGraw-Hill; 2017:chap 121.

Pappas PG, Kauffman CA, Andes D, et al. Clinical Practice Guideline for the Management of Candidiasis: 2016 Update by the Infectious Diseases Society of America. *Clin Infect Dis.* 2016;62(4):e1-50.

Sheppard D, Lampiris HW. Antifungal agents. In: Katzung BG, Trevor AJ, eds. *Basic & Clinical Pharmacology.* 13th ed. New York, NY: McGraw-Hill; 2015:chap 48.

Trevor AJ, Katzung BG, Kruidering-Hall MM, Masters SB. Antifungal agents. In: Trevor AJ, Katzung BG, Kruidering-Hall MM, Masters SB, eds. *Katzung & Trevor's Pharmacology: Examination & Board Review.* 10th ed. New York, NY: McGraw-Hill; 2013:chap 48.

KEY ABBREVIATIONS

5-FC = 5-flucytosine
ANC = absolute neutrophil count
BMT = bone marrow transplant
CPK = creatine phosphokinase
CrCl = creatinine clearance
CSF = cerebral spinal fluid
CT = computed tomography

GI = gastrointestinal
HIV = human immunodeficiency virus
HSCT = hematopoietic stem cell transplantation
IV = intravenous
MAC = *Mycobacterium* avium-intracellulare complex
S-DD = susceptible-dose-dependent

CHAPTER 30

Tuberculosis

Kristen Cook

FOUNDATION OVERVIEW

Tuberculosis (TB) is an infection caused by the acid-fast bacillus (AFB) *Mycobacterium tuberculosis*. Transmission of TB is person to person through inhalation of droplet nuclei in the air. The majority of patients infected with *M. tuberculosis* develop latent tuberculosis infection and do not develop active, symptomatic, disease. Approximately 10% of patients develop active disease if not treated with isoniazid. Risk of active disease is highest in the first 2 years after infection.

Tuberculosis primarily affects the lungs. The clinical presentation of pulmonary TB includes: productive cough, fever, weight loss, night sweats, and hemoptysis. Extrapulmonary TB develops in genitourinary, skeletal, central nervous system, and the pericardial system. Disseminated TB occurs in several parts of the body.

Targeted tuberculin skin testing is used to identify patients with TB. The Mantoux test injects a tuberculin purified protein derivative (PPD) intradermally on the inner portion of the forearm. The induration at the injection site is evaluated in 48 to 72 hours. The size of the induration and the patient's risk determine whether the test is read as positive (Table 30-1). Patients who have previously received the bacillus Calmette-Guerin vaccine in another country can have a positive skin test due to the vaccine. This vaccination is not recommended for most of the US population. The QuantiFERON TB-Gold test measures the level of interferon gamma released in a blood sample in response to PPD. This test provides a rapid diagnosis confirmation compared to skin testing. The Centers for Disease Control has said it can be used in place of skin testing in individuals greater than 5 years of age. Sputum cultures, chest radiographs, and drug susceptibilities are obtained at first suspicion of active disease.

TREATMENT

The goals of TB treatment include: controlling the spread of TB, reducing the development of drug resistance, and preventing relapse to active disease. A four-drug regimen comprised of isoniazid, pyrazinamide, rifampin, and ethambutol is initiated in suspected active TB infection. Combination therapy prevents selecting out drug-resistant organisms. Typical treatment for active disease includes an initial 2-month phase of four drugs and a continuation phase of 4 months (18 weeks)

with two drugs. The continuation phase is extended to 7 months in the following patient groups: cavitary pulmonary TB with positive-sputum culture at the end of 2-month initial phase, if the initial phase did not include pyrazinamide, and those taking isoniazid-rifapentine once-weekly regimens who have positive-sputum cultures at the end of initial phase. Directly observed therapy (DOT) is recommended in patients receiving regimens of five times per week or less. Ethambutol can be discontinued after drug susceptibility reveals the TB is susceptible to isoniazid and rifampin. Baseline laboratory values before initiating treatment include: liver function tests, creatinine, bilirubin, and platelets. Routine monitoring of these parameters is not needed unless they are abnormal initially or clinical situation warrants rechecking. For example, if any symptoms of liver toxicity are found at follow-up visits, this situation would warrant rechecking of baseline labs. Treatment in children includes isoniazid, rifampin, and pyrazinamide. First-line drug treatment regimens are listed in Table 30-2 and key characteristics in Table 30-3.

Latent TB infection treatment should not be initiated until active disease has been ruled out. Latent TB infection recommendation is isoniazid monotherapy for 9 months unless contraindicated. A once weekly regimen is approved for treatment of latent infection (isoniazid and rifapentine). This regimen can be used as a preferred regimen as well, with the exception of a few patient populations (Table 30-4). Daily or twice-weekly isoniazid for 9 months is the preferred regimen for children. Patients taking isoniazid for treatment of latent disease who drink alcohol regularly, are HIV positive, pregnant, post partum less than 3 months, or who have liver disease should have baseline liver enzymes evaluated.

Outcome Evaluation

Effectiveness of TB therapy is determined by AFB smears and cultures. Acid-fast bacteria retain their staining color after being washed with acid-alcohol washes. Sputum cultures should be sent for AFB staining and microscopic examination every 1 to 2 weeks until two consecutive smears are negative. This provides evidence of a response to treatment. If sputum cultures continue to be positive after 2 months, drug susceptibility testing should be repeated, and serum concentration of the drugs should be checked. Table 30-5 lists monitoring for TB medications.

TABLE 30-1	Criteria for Tuberculin Positivity by Risk Group	
Reaction 5 mm of Induration	**Reaction ≥10 mm of Induration**	**Reaction ≥15 mm of Induration**
HIV-positive persons	Recent immigrants (ie, within the last 5 years) from high-prevalence countries	Persons with no risk factors for TB
Recent contacts of TB case patients	Injection-drug users	
Fibrotic changes on chest radiograph consistent with prior TB	Residents and employees[a] of the following high-risk congregate settings: prisons and jails, nursing homes and other long-term care facilities for the elderly, hospitals and other health care facilities, residential facilities for patients with AIDS, homeless shelters	
Patients with organ transplants and other immunosuppressed patients (receiving the equivalent of ≥15 mg/d of prednisone for 1 month or more)[b]	Mycobacteriology laboratory personnel Persons with the following clinical conditions that place them at high risk: silicosis, diabetes mellitus, chronic renal failure, some hematologic disorders (eg, leukemias and lymphomas), other specific malignancies (eg, carcinoma of the head or neck and lung), weight loss of ≥10% of ideal body weight, gastrectomy, jejunoileal bypass Children younger than 4 years or infants, children, and adolescents exposed to adults at high risk	

Abbreviations: AIDS, acquired immunodeficiency syndrome; HIV, human immunodeficiency virus; TB, tuberculosis.

[a]For persons who are otherwise at low risk and who are tested at the start of employment, a reaction of ≥15 mm induration is considered positive.

[b]Risk of TB for patients treated with corticosteroids increases with higher dose and longer duration.

Data from Screening for tuberculosis and tuberculosis infection in high-risk populations. Recommendations of the Advisory Council for the Elimination of Tuberculosis, *MMWR Recomm Rep.* 1995 Sep 8;44(RR-11):19-34.

Patient nonadherence is a serious problem with TB therapy. The most effective way to achieve adherence is with directly observed therapy. DOT also provides opportunities to observe the patient for toxicity, thus improving overall care.

Hepatotoxicity

Hepatotoxicity should be suspected in patients whose transaminases exceed five times the upper limit of normal or whose bilirubin is significantly elevated and in patients with symptoms such as nausea, vomiting, and jaundice. At this point, the offending agent(s) should be discontinued.

Specific Agents

Isoniazid

Isoniazid is a first-line agent against latent TB and also one of the first-line drugs in combination therapy for active TB. Isoniazid (INH) inhibits production of mycolic acids, which

form a large part of the mycobacterial cell wall. Metabolism of isoniazid occurs by acetylation and may be affected by genetic differences in slow and fast acetylators. Currently there are no recommendations in testing for genetic differences that affect treatment. Dosing is 300 mg daily or 900 mg for the once, twice, and three times weekly regimens in adults. Caution should be used with this agent in patients with liver disease. Pyridoxine (vitamin B6) 25 to 50 mg daily is recommended to be taken with isoniazid to help prevent drug-induced peripheral neuropathy. Adverse effects of isoniazid include: rash, neuropathy, gastrointestinal upset, and hepatotoxicity. Isoniazid-induced hepatitis is rare, but rates are increased in the elderly, pregnant women, postpartum women, alcohol abusers, patients with underlying liver disease, and when used in combination with rifampin. Isoniazid should be discontinued immediately and not used again with confirmation of INH-induced hepatitis. Table 30-6 lists drug interactions with isoniazid.

TABLE 30-2	First-Line Regimens for Active Pulmonary Tuberculosis				
Drugs	**Frequency**	**Time**	**Drugs**	**Frequency**	**Interval**
Isoniazid, Rifampin, Pyrazinamide, Ethambutol	7 d/wk or 5 d/wk	8 wk	Isoniazid, Rifampin	7 d/wk or 5 d/wk or twice weekly[a]	18 wk
Isoniazid, Rifampin, Pyrazinamide, Ethambutol	5-7 d/wk for 2 wk then twice weekly	8 wk	Isoniazid, Rifampin	Twice weekly[b]	18 wk
Isoniazid, Rifampin, Pyrazinamide, Ethambutol	3 d/wk	8 wk	Isoniazid, Rifampin	3 d/wk	18 wk
Isoniazid, Rifampin, Ethambutol	7 d/wk or 5 d/wk	8 wk	Isoniazid, Rifampin	7 d/wk or 5 d/wk or twice weekly	18 wk

[a]Should not be used in HIV-positive patients.

[b]Twice weekly rifampin in the continuation phase of treatment is not recommended for HIV-positive patients with CD4 counts <100 cells/m3.

Reproduced with permission from American Thoracic Society; CDC; Infectious Diseases Society of America: Treatment of tuberculosis, MMWR Recomm Rep 2003 Jun 20;52(RR-11):1-77.

TABLE 30-3   Characteristics of Tuberculosis Medications

Subclass	Mechanism of Action	Effects	Clinical Applications	Pharmacokinetics, Toxicities, Interactions
Isoniazid	Inhibits synthesis of mycolic acids, an essential component of mycobacterial cell walls	Bactericidal activity against susceptible strains of *M. tuberculosis*	First-line agent for tuberculosis • treatment of latent infection • less active against other *mycobacteria*	Oral, IV • hepatic clearance (half-life 1 h) • reduces levels of phenytoin • *Toxicity*: Hepatotoxic, peripheral neuropathy (give pyridoxine to prevent)
Rifamycins Rifampin	Inhibits DNA-dependent RNA polymerase, thereby blocking production of RNA	Bactericidal activity against susceptible bacteria and mycobacteria • resistance rapidly emerges when used as a single drug in the treatment of active infection	First-line agent for tuberculosis • atypical mycobacterial infections • eradication of meningococcal colonization, staphylococcal infections	Oral, IV • hepatic clearance (half-life 3.5 h) • potent cytochrome P450 inducer • turns body fluids orange color • *Toxicity*: Rash, nephritis, thrombocytopenia, cholestasis, flu-like syndrome with intermittent dosing
Rifabutin: Oral; similar to rifampin *but less cytochrome P450 induction and fewer drug interactions* *Rifapentine*: Oral; long-acting analog of rifampin *that may be given once weekly in the continuation phase of tuberculosis treatment*				
Pyrazinamide	Not fully understood • pyrazinamide is converted to the active pyrazinoic acid under acidic conditions in macrophage lysosomes	Bacteriostatic activity against susceptible strains of *M. tuberculosis* • may be bactericidal against actively dividing organisms	"Sterilizing" agent used during first 2 months of therapy • allows total duration of therapy to be shortened to 6 months	Oral • hepatic clearance (half-life 9 h), but metabolites are renally cleared so use doses 3 × weekly if creatinine clearance <30 mL/min • *Toxicity*: Hepatotoxic, hyperuricemia
Ethambutol	Inhibits mycobacterial arabinosyl transferases, which are involved in the polymerization reaction of arabinoglycan, an essential component of the mycobacterial cell wall	Bacteriostatic activity against susceptible mycobacteria	Given in four-drug initial combination therapy for tuberculosis until drug sensitivities are known • also used for atypical mycobacterial infections	Oral • mixed clearance (half-life 4 h) • dose must be reduced in renal failure • *Toxicity*: Retrobulbar neuritis
Streptomycin	Prevents bacterial protein synthesis by binding to the S12 ribosomal subunit	Bactericidal activity against susceptible mycobacteria	Used in tuberculosis when an injectable drug is needed or desirable and in treatment of drug-resistant strains	IM, IV • renal clearance (half-life 2.5 h) • administered daily initially, then 2 × week • *Toxicity*: Nephrotoxic, ototoxic

Reproduced with permission from Katzung BG, Masters SB, Trevor AJ: *Basic & Clinical Pharmacology*, 12th ed. New York, NY: McGraw-Hill; 2012.

TABLE 30-4   Treatment Regimens for Latent Tuberculosis

Drug	Length of Treatment	Adult Dose
Isoniazid[a]	9 mo	300 mg daily
Isoniazid	9 mo	900 mg twice weekly
Isoniazid[b]	6 mo	300 mg daily
Isoniazid[b]	6 mo	900 mg twice weekly
Rifampin	4 mo	600 mg daily
Isoniazid + Rifapentine[c]	3 mo	INH 900 mg weekly + Rifapentine 10.0-14.0 kg: 300 mg 14.1-25.0 kg: 450 mg 25.1-32.0 kg: 600 mg 32.1-49.9 kg: 750 mg ≥50.0 kg: 900 mg

[a]Preferred regimen for children 2-11 years of age.

[b]Not recommended in HIV-positive patients.

[c]Not recommended for those younger than 2 years of age or those with HIV on antiretrovirals or those who are pregnant. Must be directly observed therapy.

Data from Centers for Disease Control and Prevention. Targeted tuberculin testing and treatment of latent tuberculosis infection, *MMWR Recomm Rep.* 2000 Jun 9;49(RR-6):1-51 and Recommendations for use of an isoniazid-rifapentine regimen with direct observation to treat latent mycobacterium tuberculosis infection, *MMWR Morb Mortal Wkly Rep* 2011 Dec 9;60(48):1650-1653.

Rifamycins

Rifampin is a first-line agent against active TB (used in combination). Rifampin inhibits DNA-dependent RNA polymerase in bacterial cells. Dosing is 600 mg once daily and twice or three times weekly regimens in adults. Rifabutin and rifapentine are other rifamycins which can be used in place of rifampin. Rifampin, rifabutin, and rifapentine significantly induces the cytochrome P-450 and increases metabolism of several drugs including: oral anticoagulants, anticonvulsants, antiretrovirals, cyclosporine, and oral contraceptives. Rifabutin is the least potent enzyme inducer. The alternative rifamycins can also be used with intolerance to rifampin. Adverse reactions to rifamycins include: pruritus, rash, gastrointestinal upset, flu-like syndrome, and rarely hepatotoxicity. Rifamycins give urine, sweat, and tears a harmless reddish-orange color.

Pyrazinamide

Pyrazinamide (PZA) is a first-line agent for active TB (used in combination). PZA exerts its effects against dormant organisms inside macrophages. Dosing is 20 to 25 mg/kg/d in adults rounded to the nearest 500 mg tablets. PZA is contraindicated

TABLE 30-5	Drug Monitoring	
Drug	**Adverse Effects**	**Monitoring**
Isoniazid	Asymptomatic elevation of aminotransferases, clinical hepatitis, fatal hepatitis, peripheral neurotoxicity, CNS effects, lupus-like syndrome, hypersensitivity, monoamine poisoning, diarrhea	LFT monthly in patients who have preexisting liver disease or who develop abnormal liver function that does not require discontinuation of drug; dosage adjustments may be necessary in patients receiving anticonvulsants or warfarin
Rifampin	Cutaneous reactions, GI reactions (nausea, anorexia, abdominal pain), flu-like syndrome, hepatotoxicity, severe immunologic reactions, orange discoloration of bodily fluids (sputum, urine, sweat, tears), drug interactions due to induction of hepatic microsomal enzymes	Liver enzymes and interacting drugs as needed (eg, warfarin)
Rifabutin	Hematologic toxicity, uveitis, GI symptoms, polyarthralgias, hepatotoxicity, pseudojaundice (skin discoloration with normal bilirubin), rash, flu-like syndrome, orange discoloration of bodily fluids (sputum, urine, sweat, tears)	Drug interactions are less problematic than rifampin
Rifapentine	Similar to those associated with rifampin	Drug interactions are being investigated and are likely similar to rifampin
Pyrazinamide	Hepatotoxicity, GI symptoms (nausea, vomiting), nongouty polyarthralgia, asymptomatic hyperuricemia, acute gouty arthritis, transient morbilliform rash, dermatitis	Serum uric acid can serve as a surrogate marker for adherence; LFTs in patients with underlying liver disease
Ethambutol	Retrobulbar neuritis, peripheral neuritis, cutaneous reactions	Baseline visual acuity testing and testing of color discrimination; monthly testing of visual acuity and color discrimination in patients taking >15-20 mg/kg, having renal insufficiency, or receiving the drug for >2 months
Streptomycin	Ototoxicity, neurotoxicity, nephrotoxicity	Baseline audiogram, vestibular testing, Romberg testing, and SCr Monthly assessments of renal function and auditory or vestibular symptoms
Amikacin/kanamycin	Ototoxicity, nephrotoxicity	Baseline audiogram, vestibular testing, Romberg testing, and SCr; monthly assessments of renal function and auditory or vestibular symptoms
Capreomycin	Nephrotoxicity, ototoxicity	Baseline audiogram, vestibular testing, Romberg testing, and SCr Monthly assessments of renal function and auditory or vestibular symptoms Baseline and monthly serum K^+ and Mg^{2+}
p-Aminosalicylic acid	Hepatotoxicity, GI distress, malabsorption syndrome, hypothyroidism, coagulopathy	Baseline LFTs and TSH TSH every 3 months
Moxifloxacin	GI disturbance, neurologic effects, cutaneous reactions	No specific monitoring recommended

Abbreviations: CNS, central nervous system; GI, gastrointestinal; LFT, liver function test; SCr, serum creatinine; TSH, thyroid-stimulating hormone.

Adapted with permission from American Thoracic Society, Centers for Disease Control and Prevention, Infectious Diseases Society of America. Treatment of tuberculosis. *MMWR Recomm Rep* 2003;June 20;52(RR-11):1-77.

TABLE 30-6	Isoniazid-Drug Interactions via Inhibition and Induction of CYPs	
Co-Administered Drug	**CYP Isoform**	**Adverse Effects**
Acetaminophen	CYP2E1 inhibition-induction	Hepatotoxicity
Carbamazepine	CYP3A inhibition	Neurological toxicity
Diazepam	CYP3A and CYP2C19 inhibition	Sedation and respiratory depression
Ethosuximide	CYP3A inhibition	Psychotic behavior
Isoflurane and enflurane	CYP2E1 induction	Decreased effectiveness
Phenytoin	CYP2C19 inhibition	Neurological toxicity
Theophylline	CYP3A inhibition	Seizures, palpitation, nausea
Vincristine	CYP3A inhibition	Limb weakness and tingling
Warfarin	CYP2C9 inhibition	Possibility of increased bleeding (single case reported)

Reproduced with permission from Brunton LL, Chabner BA, Knollmann BC: *Goodman & Gilman's The Pharmacological Basis of Therapeutics,* 12th ed. New York, NY: McGraw-Hill; 2011.

in patients with severe liver disease and acute gout attacks. Caution should be taken in those with a history of gout. Adverse reactions include: hepatotoxicity, gastrointestinal upset, and hyperuricemia. Baseline liver function tests should be performed in patients with preexisting liver disease and if used with rifampin.

Ethambutol

Ethambutol is a first-line treatment of active tuberculosis (used in combination). Ethambutol targets mycobacterial arabinosyl transferase to inhibit cell wall production. Ethambutol is added to the TB regimen to prevent rifampin resistance. Dosing in adults is 15 to 20 mg/kg/d rounded to the nearest dose using whole tablets (100 mg, 400 mg). Dose adjustments are required for renal dysfunction. Ethambutol is contraindicated in patients with optic neuritis as well as with those who would have difficulty determining visual acuity (children). Ethambutol causes a retrobulbar neuritis, which presents as decreased visual acuity or red–green color blindness. Patients should have baseline visual acuity and color blindness assessed as well as continued monitoring for this adverse effect.

Special Populations

Immunocompromised

HIV patients should receive TB testing. Patients with HIV and other immunocompromised diseases may be managed with chemotherapeutic agents similar to those utilized in immunocompetent individuals. However, the treatment duration is extended to 9 months. Highly intermittent regimens (twice or once weekly) are not recommended for HIV-positive TB patients.

HIV-positive patients can have a paradoxical reaction when antiretroviral therapy is initiated in TB-positive patients (a self-limited inflammatory response). Treatment is with a nonsteroidal anti-inflammatory or corticosteroid. HIV treatment is still recommended to be initiated during TB treatment within the first 2 weeks if CD4 counts are less than 50 cells/µL and 8 to 12 weeks for those with a CD4 count greater than or equal to 50 cells/µL. The exception to this is patient who have tubercular meningitis.

Drug interactions with rifamycins are important in HIV patients. Interactions among rifamycins, HIV-protease inhibitors, and non-nucleoside reverse transcriptase inhibitors are common and require dose and frequency modifications. Rifabutin provides an alternative rifamycin, but careful attention is required for drug adjustments.

Pregnant/Breast-feeding

Drug therapy is warranted in pregnant women with active TB. Treatment in pregnant patients with latent TB is controversial. Patients with latent TB who are HIV positive or recently infected with latent TB should be considered for treatment. All pregnant and postpartum women should have baseline liver function tests before therapy initiation. The first-line drug regimen in pregnancy consists of isoniazid, rifampin, and ethambutol. Pyrazinamide is not recommended. Known teratogens that should not be used include several second-line drugs: streptomycin, kanamycin, amikacin, and capreomycin. Patients taking TB therapy can breast-feed.

Multidrug Resistant TB

There are no standardized treatment regimens for multidrug resistant (MDR) TB. MDR-TB treatment is based on the previous drug therapy, exposure history, geographic resistance patterns, and drug-susceptibility data. An important treatment principle in MDR-TB is to never change one drug at a time. Two or more new drugs should be added to a regimen to lessen the likelihood of resistance development.

Treatment of MDR-TB consists of second-line antituberculosis drugs including cycloserine, ethionamide, streptomycin, amikacin/kanamycin, capreomycin, p-aminosalicylic acid (PAS), and select fluoroquinolones.

Bedaquiline was approved in December 2012 for use in MDR-TB when other agents are unavailable or ineffective. Bedaquiline inhibits mycobacterial ATP synthase. Bedaquiline is a major substrate of CYP 3A4 and drug interactions must be taken into account (including QTc prolongation). There was an increased risk of death in trials with bedaquiline and it should only be used when other medications are not options.

CASE Application

1. JK is a 32-year-old HIV-negative patient presenting to your clinic. He receives a Mantoux skin test that returns positive 2 days later. He was born in the United States and works as a prison guard. He injects heroin on a regular basis. His chest x-ray comes back normal, he has no symptoms of tuberculosis, and his smear culture is negative. What type of drug therapy would be appropriate for this patient?

   a. Isoniazid 300 mg daily × 9 months
   b. Rifampin 100 mg daily × 4 months
   c. No drug therapy needed
   d. Isoniazid 300 mg and rifampin 600 mg × 6 months
   e. Isoniazid, rifampin, ethambutol, and pyrazinamide

2. BCG vaccine should be routinely given to which patient in the United States?

   a. A 10-year-old child
   b. A 2-month-old infant
   c. A 65-year-old man
   d. A 6-month-old infant
   e. BCG vaccine is not routinely recommended in the United States

3. RL is a 37-year-old man who presents to your pharmacy with a prescription for rifampin. His other medications include: acetaminophen 1000 mg four times daily, phenytoin 100 mg twice daily, warfarin 3 mg daily, and omeprazole 20 mg once daily. Which of the following is important to counsel RL on his new medication? Select all that apply.

a. This medication can cause your body secretions to be an orange-red color.
b. You should limit your acetaminophen use as much as possible during therapy with this medication.
c. This medication can cause you to need a decrease in your warfarin dose.
d. This medication may cause gastrointestinal upset.
e. This medication can cause your phenytoin concentrations to go down.

4. RS is a 25-year-old Hispanic woman who is recently diagnosed with active tuberculosis. Her physician asks what drug regimen you would recommend to treat her disease. She does not have any contraindications to any of the tuberculosis medications. You do not have susceptibility testing back yet.

a. INH, RIF, PZA × 8 weeks, then INH, RIF ×18 weeks
b. INH × 9 months
c. INH, RIF × 9 months
d. INH, RIF, EMB, FQ × 8 weeks, then INH, RIF × 18 weeks
e. INH, RIF, EMB, PZA × 8 weeks, then INH, RIF × 18 weeks

5. Which of the following is true regarding acid-fast bacteria?

a. They cause the majority of bacterial infectious diseases in the United States.
b. *Mycobacterium tuberculosis* is the only type of acid-fast bacteria.
c. Cultures of acid-fast bacteria grow faster than other bacteria.
d. They retain their stained color even with acid-alcohol washes.

6. Select the primary method for transmission of tuberculosis.

a. Inhalation
b. Exposure to blood and/or bodily fluids
c. Exposure to dead birds
d. Hospitalization

7. What time period is the risk highest for conversion to active disease in those patients with latent tuberculosis infection?

a. 10 years after exposure
b. 8 years after exposure
c. 6 years after exposure
d. 4 years after exposure
e. 2 years after exposure

8. Which of the following is a sign/symptom of pulmonary tuberculosis? Select all that apply.

a. Weight loss
b. Productive cough
c. Headache
d. Fever
e. Night sweats

9. How long after a Mantoux skin test for TB infection is placed should it be read?

a. 12 hours
b. 24 hours
c. 48 hours
d. 96 hours
e. 120 hours

10. Which patient group should get drug-susceptibility testing?

a. All latent tuberculosis patients
b. Latent tuberculosis patients over age 35
c. All active tuberculosis disease patients
d. Active tuberculosis patients over age 35
e. Foreign-born cases of latent and active tuberculosis

11. TF is a 10-year-old girl recently diagnosed with active tuberculosis. Her other medications include: methylphenidate 10 mg twice daily. She is HIV negative. Which medication should not be included in her regimen for active TB?

a. Isoniazid
b. Rifampin
c. Pyrazinamide
d. Ethambutol

12. The addition of which of the following drugs necessitates follow-up liver function tests in a patient being treated for latent TB infection treated with isoniazid?

a. Naproxen
b. Multivitamin
c. Sertraline
d. Acetaminophen
e. Lisinopril

13. What is the preferred regimen for treating latent tuberculosis infection in adults?

a. Isoniazid 300 mg daily × 6 months
b. Isoniazid 300 mg daily × 9 months
c. Rifampin 600 mg daily × 6 months
d. Rifampin 600 mg daily × 9 months

14. RS is a 45-year-old woman who was placed on isoniazid for latent tuberculosis. Medications include: metformin 1000 mg twice daily, glipizide 10 mg twice daily, lisinopril 20 mg daily, and atorvastatin 40 mg daily. She presents to your pharmacy to purchase some vitamin B6 (pyridoxine) as recommended by her doctor. Which adverse effect of isoniazid does pyridoxine reduce?

a. Hepatotoxicity
b. Peripheral neuropathy
c. Gastrointestinal upset
d. Rash

15. Which rifamycin is the least potent in terms of CYP450 induction?

    a. Rifampin
    b. Rifabutin
    c. Rifapentine
    d. Rocephin

16. ZK is a 56-year-old woman who has been on treatment for active TB for the past month. Her regimen includes: isoniazid, rifampin, ethambutol, and pyrazinamide. She reports to her doctor for routine monitoring. She reports no adverse effects. Which of the following tests should be done?

    a. Creatinine
    b. Foot examination
    c. Snellen visual chart examination
    d. Complete blood count
    e. Triglycerides

17. Which of the following is a contraindication to pyrazinamide therapy? Select all that apply.

    a. Acute gout attacks
    b. Chronic obstructive pulmonary disease
    c. Rheumatoid arthritis
    d. Asthma

18. Place the following patient groups in order of lowest reaction to highest reaction size (that defines a positive PPD reaction).

Unordered Response	Ordered Response
No risk factor	
HIV	
Injection drug user	

19. Place the following latent TB treatments in order based upon duration of therapy. Start with the shortest duration.

Unordered Response	Ordered Response
Rifampin	
Isoniazid + Rifapentine	
Isoniazid	

20. Which of the following medications would be expected to interact with INH? Select all that apply.

    a. Carbamazepine
    b. Warfarin
    c. Phenytoin
    d. Theophylline

TAKEAWAY POINTS »

- TB is caused by *M. tuberculosis*, an acid-fast bacilli and is a public health concern worldwide.
- Tuberculosis is transmitted by inhalation and not all people who are exposed develop active tuberculosis.
- The majority of patients exposed with competent immune systems develop latent TB infection. Latent TB infection is not contagious.
- Latent TB infection should be treated with INH to prevent people from converting to active disease later on in life. The risk for active disease is greatest 2 years after exposure.
- Mantoux skin tests are used to identify patients who have TB infection. The skin tests need to be read within 48 to 72 hours of placement. The Quantiferon-TB test can now be used in select clinical situations for testing.
- Common symptoms of active pulmonary TB include productive cough, night sweats, fever, fatigue, weight loss, and hemoptysis. Pulmonary TB is the most common type of active tuberculosis disease.
- The following diagnostic test should be done when active TB is suspected: chest x-ray, culture, and drug susceptibility.

- Drug treatment for active tuberculosis typically includes isoniazid, rifampin, ethambutol, and pyrazinamide for the first 2 months, and isoniazid and rifampin for an extra 4-month continuation phase.
- HIV-positive patients typically have this continuation phase last for 7 months.
- Directly observed therapy is recommended for any regimen in which meds are given five times per week or less.
- Isoniazid hepatotoxicity is rare but increased in the following circumstances: rifampin use, increasing age, pregnant women, postpartum women, alcohol abusers, and underlying liver disease.
- Pyridoxine is given with isoniazid to help prevent peripheral neuropathy caused by isoniazid.
- Rifamycins induce cytochrome P450 significantly and can decrease the concentration of several medications. Rifabutin is often the preferred rifamycin in patients on antiretroviral regimens.
- Pregnant women with active TB disease should receive treatment at time of diagnosis. Pyrazinamide is not included in TB treatment regimens of pregnant patients.

BIBLIOGRAPHY

Deck DH, Winston LG. Antimycobacterial drugs. In: Katzung BG, Masters SB, Trevor AJ, eds. *Basic & Clinical Pharmacology*, 12th ed. New York, NY: McGraw-Hill; 2012:chap 47.

Gumbo T. Chemotherapy of tuberculosis, mycobacterium avium complex disease, and leprosy. In: Brunton LL, Chabner BA, Knollmann BC, eds. *Goodman & Gilman's The Pharmacological Basis of Therapeutics*, 12th ed. New York, NY: McGraw-Hill; 2011:chap 56.

Lewinsohn DM, Leonard MK, LoBue PA, et al. Official American Thoracic Society/Infectious Diseases Society of America/Centers for Disease Control and Prevention Clinical Practice Guidelines: Diagnosis of Tuberculosis in Adults and Children. *Clin Infect Dis.* 2017;64(2):e1-e33.

Namdar R, Lauzardo M, Peloquin CA. Tuberculosis. In: DiPiro JT, Talbert RL, Yee GC, Matzke GR, Wells BG, Posey L, eds. *Pharmacotherapy: A Pathophysiologic Approach*, 10th ed. New York, NY: McGraw-Hill; 2017.

Trevor AJ, Katzung BG, Kruidering-Hall MM, Masters SB. Antimycobacterial drugs. In: Trevor AJ, Katzung BG, Kruidering-Hall MM, Masters SB, eds. *Katzung & Trevor's Pharmacology: Examination & Board Review*, 10th ed. New York, NY: McGraw-Hill; 2013:chap 47.

KEY ABBREVIATIONS

AFB = acid-fast bacillus
DOT = directly observed therapy
MDR = multidrug resistant

PAS = p-aminosalicylic acid
PPD = purified protein derivative
TB = tuberculosis

31

Sexually Transmitted Diseases

Hana Rac

FOUNDATION OVERVIEW

Sexually transmitted diseases (STDs) describe a range of infections acquired through sexual contact and have a major impact on public health and the utilization of health care resources. STDs are associated with symptomatic disease, infertility, and deleterious effects on pregnancy and childbirth, among other complications. Four STDs will be reviewed in this chapter: chlamydia, gonorrhea, genital herpes, and syphilis.

Chlamydia

Chlamydial genital infection is caused by *Chlamydia trachomatis*, an obligate intracellular pathogen and the most common bacterium responsible for STDs. Infection is transmissible through vaginal, anal, or oral sex. Chlamydia can manifest as cervicitis in women and urethritis in men; however, asymptomatic infection is common, occurring in up to 70% of women and 50% of men. In symptomatic disease, women present with mucopurulent vaginal discharge, postcoital bleeding, and urethral infection. Symptoms in men include dysuria and urethral discharge. Without appropriate and timely treatment, complications such as pelvic inflammatory disease (PID), ectopic pregnancy, premature delivery, and infertility can result.

Testing methods for diagnosis of chlamydia include cell culture, antigen-based tests, molecular methods such as nucleic acid hybridization (deoxyribonucleic acid [DNA] probing), and nucleic acid amplification tests (NAATs). NAATs are recommended for diagnosing chlamydial genital infection due to high sensitivity and specificity.

Gonorrhea

Gonorrhea is caused by *Neisseria gonorrhoeae*, a gram-negative diplococcus, and is transmissible through contact with genitals, mouth, or anus. After contact is made, the organism attaches to mucosal epithelium causing a strong neutrophil response with pus production. Gonococcal infection causes cervicitis in women and urethritis in men. In men, symptoms include dysuria and urethral discharge which becomes purulent within days. Because of the early presentation and discomfort associated with symptoms in men, treatment is sought early enough to prevent complications. Women

are asymptomatic or have minor symptoms. Symptoms occur within 10 days in those who develop them and include vaginal discharge, dysuria, and vaginal bleeding (sometimes postcoital). Asymptomatic infection in women can lead to PID, ectopic pregnancy, tubal scarring, and infertility. In both men and women, gonorrhea can cause increased susceptibility to and transmission of human immunodeficiency virus (HIV) infection.

In symptomatic men, a urethral specimen Gram stain showing neutrophils and gram-negative diplococci can be considered diagnostic, but a negative Gram stain is not sufficient to rule out infection in asymptomatic men. Other diagnostic tests for gonococcal urethritis and cervicitis include culture, nucleic acid hybridization, and NAATs. NAATs offer the widest range of specimen types for diagnosis. Nonculture diagnostic tests cannot provide antibiotic susceptibility results, which may be necessary in cases of infection that persists after treatment.

Genital Herpes

Genital herpes is a chronic, lifelong viral infection due to double-stranded DNA viruses of the *Herpesviridae* family. Two types of virus cause clinical disease: herpes simplex virus-1 (HSV-1) and herpes simplex virus-2 (HSV-2). While most genital herpes is due to HSV-2, cases of genital herpes due to HSV-1 are increasing. The type of herpes virus (HSV-1 vs HSV-2) does not impact treatment recommendations. Genital herpes is transmissible through sexual contact, including oral sex. Most transmissions originate from individuals not aware that they are infected. The HSV viruses enter the body through mucosa or abraded skin and replicate at the entry site. Subsequent skin cell damage causes epithelial detachment and blister formation. The viruses then penetrate the dermis and enter peripheral sensory nerves, where they lie dormant between outbreaks (recurrences).

During the first episode of genital herpes, clusters of papular and vesicular lesions on the external genitalia are accompanied by pain, itching, and burning. Involvement may also include perianal, buttock, and thigh areas. Within 2 to 3 weeks, lesions typically transform into ulcers before healing. In most patients, recurrences are within 1 year of the first episode and are associated with fewer lesions and milder pain. The rate of recurrence generally decreases over time.

The diagnosis of genital herpes can be made through virologic and/or serologic tests. Virologic tests detect the presence of the virus using specimens from genital lesions, while serologic tests detect antibodies to HSV viruses. Additionally, some serologic tests can distinguish between HSV-1 and HSV-2 viruses.

Syphilis

Syphilis is caused by *Treponema pallidum*, a spiral-shaped bacterium. Syphilis is transmissible through vaginal and anal intercourse, oral sex, and kissing at or near infectious lesions. The disease can also be transmitted in utero. After contact, *T. pallidum* enters the host through compromised skin or intact mucosa. After acquisition of *T. pallidum*, untreated syphilitic disease passes through a series of four stages: primary syphilis, secondary syphilis, latent syphilis, and tertiary syphilis. Neurosyphilis can occur at any stage of the disease. The characteristic lesion of primary syphilis is the chancre (ulcer). The chancre is painless and appears at the site of *T. pallidum* entrance into the body approximately 3 weeks after transmission. Regional lymphadenopathy may also develop 7 to 10 days after the chancre appears. In secondary syphilis, a diffuse rash, classically affecting the palms and soles, appears approximately 8 weeks after transmission. Other systemic symptoms may also be present. Latent syphilis refers to patients with a positive serologic diagnosis for syphilis, but no clinical symptoms. This stage occurs after secondary syphilis symptoms have subsided and there are two possible outcomes: progression to tertiary syphilis or clinical cure. Tertiary syphilis encompasses the long-term complications of syphilitic disease such as granulomatous disease (also called gummatous syphilis) and cardiovascular syphilis. Tertiary syphilis is uncommon due to antibiotic treatment and is not transmissible. Central nervous system (CNS) involvement can present at any stage of syphilis. Early neurosyphilis occurs within the first few years of infection and usually coexists with primary or secondary syphilis. The meninges and cerebrospinal fluid (CSF) are primarily affected. Early neurosyphilis can present with symptomatic meningitis or be asymptomatic. Late neurosyphilis occurs years to decades after the initial infection and represents a tertiary manifestation of syphilis. Symptoms include general paresis, dementia, and sensory ataxia with incontinence and pain.

Treponema pallidum cannot be cultured, so indirect diagnostic techniques must be used. Syphilis can be diagnosed based on microscopic examination of a lesion exudate or tissue. Serologic testing, including treponemal and nontreponemal tests, provides a presumptive diagnosis and is the standard method of detecting primary, secondary, latent, and tertiary syphilis in the United States. Nontreponemal tests, such as the venereal disease research laboratory (VDRL) and rapid plasma reagin (RPR) are used for initial syphilis screening. Nontreponemal tests should be confirmed by treponemal-specific tests (such as the *T. pallidum* particle agglutination or fluorescent treponemal antibody absorption test) due to the rate of false-positive results. Since there is no single diagnostic test for neurosyphilis, a combination of clinical manifestations, CSF evaluation, and serologic tests are typically used. Detection of an elevated leukocyte count with lymphocyte predominance and increased protein upon CSF evaluation is suggestive of syphilis. The VDRL-CSF is the standard serologic test (CSF specimen) for neurosyphilis.

PREVENTION

STDs are highly transmissible and can lead to serious complications; therefore, effective preventative strategies are essential. Goals of prevention include the avoidance of disease transmission to partners and children as well as prevention of long-term disease complications. There are no available vaccines for chlamydia, gonorrhea, genital herpes, or syphilis. The most reliable methods to prevent transmission of these STDs are abstinence, monogamy with an uninfected partner, and barrier contraception (condoms). Condom use and STD/HIV counseling have been shown to be effective in reducing the acquisition and transmission of STDs. Diaphragms cannot be relied upon, and hormonal contraception, hysterectomy, and surgical sterilization are not effective preventative measures. Of great concern is the prevention of perinatal transmission. Chlamydia, gonorrhea, genital herpes, and syphilis can be passed by mothers to children during childbirth (vertical transmission). Syphilis can also be passed to the unborn fetus in utero. Specific strategies to prevent perinatal STD transmission are discussed in the treatment section of this chapter.

TREATMENT

STD treatment is indicated at time of diagnosis and/or symptom presentation. STD patients should also be screened for HIV infection. Goals of therapy include: (1) symptom resolution, (2) prevention of disease transmission, and (3) prevention of long-term disease complications. Additionally, gonorrhea, chlamydia, and syphilis, have a treatment goal of disease eradication. Genital herpes cannot be eradicated; therefore, the goals of therapy include viral suppression and decreased frequency and severity of recurrences. Antimicrobial therapies for individual STDs will be reviewed in this section; however, specific dose and regimen information is presented in Table 31-1.

Treatment Agents for Chlamydia

Azithromycin and doxycycline are the drugs of choice for the treatment of chlamydia. Erythromycin, ofloxacin, and levofloxacin are alternatives. Because azithromycin is administered in a single dose, it may have advantages over doxycycline in patients with compliance difficulties. Erythromycin may be less effective than the azithromycin and doxycycline due to frequency of gastrointestinal side effects. Because patients infected with *N. gonorrhea* are commonly coinfected with *C. trachomatis*, presumptive therapy for chlamydia should be considered when treating patients with gonorrhea.

Azithromycin and Erythromycin

Azithromycin and erythromycin are macrolide antibiotics that inhibit protein synthesis. They exert their mechanism

TABLE 31-1   Adult Treatment Regimens for Select Sexually Transmitted Diseases (STDs)

Infection	Recommended Regimen(s)	Alternative Regimen(s)
Chlamydia	▪ Azithromycin 1 g po × 1 dose ▪ Doxycycline 100 mg po bid × 7 d[a]	▪ Erythromycin base 500 mg po qid × 7 d ▪ EES 800 mg po qid × 7 d ▪ Ofloxacin 300 mg po bid × 7 d[a] ▪ Levofloxacin 500 mg po once daily × 7 d[a]
Gonorrhea[b,c]	▪ Ceftriaxone 250 mg IM × 1 dose *plus* azithromycin 1 g po x 1 dose	▪ Cefixime 400 mg po × 1 dose *plus* azithromycin 1 g po × 1 dose or doxycycline 100 mg po bid × 7d[a]
Genital herpes[d]	First episode: ▪ Acyclovir 400 mg po tid × 7-10 d ▪ Acyclovir 200 mg po five times daily × 7-10 d ▪ Famciclovir 250 mg po tid × 7-10 d ▪ Valacyclovir 1 g po bid × 7-10 d	n/a
	Recurrence: ▪ Acyclovir 400 mg po tid × 5 d ▪ Acyclovir 800 mg po bid × 5 d ▪ Acyclovir 800 mg po tid × 2 d ▪ Famciclovir 125 mg po bid × 5 d ▪ Famciclovir 1000 mg po bid × 1 d ▪ Famciclovir 500 mg po once, followed by 250 mg po bid × 2 d ▪ Valacyclovir 500 mg po bid × 3 d ▪ Valacyclovir 1 g po once daily × 5 d	n/a
	Suppressive therapy: ▪ Acyclovir 400 mg po bid ▪ Famciclovir 250 mg po bid ▪ Valacyclovir 500 mg po once daily ▪ Valacyclovir 1 g po once daily	n/a
Syphilis	Primary and secondary syphilis: ▪ Benzathine penicillin G, 2.4 MU IM × 1 dose Early latent syphilis (<1 y duration): ▪ Benzathine penicillin G, 2.4 MU IM × 1 dose Late latent syphilis (>1 y duration) or unknown duration: ▪ Benzathine penicillin G, 2.4 MU IM once weekly × 3 wk (7.2 MU total) Tertiary syphilis (not including neurosyphilis): ▪ Benzathine penicillin G, 2.4 MU IM once weekly × 3 wk (7.2 MU total) Neurosyphilis: ▪ Aqueous crystalline penicillin G, 18-24 MU IV daily (3-4 MU IV every 4 h or by CI) × 10-14 d	Primary and secondary syphilis—PCN-allergy[e]: ▪ Doxycycline 100 mg po bid × 14 d[a] ▪ Tetracycline 500 mg po qid × 14 d[a] ▪ Ceftriaxone 1-2 g IV/IM once daily × 10-14 d Early latent syphilis—PCN allergy: ▪ Same as primary and secondary syphilis Late latent syphilis (or unknown duration)—PCN allergy: ▪ Doxycycline 100 mg po bid × 28 d[a] ▪ Tetracycline 500 mg po qid × 28 d[a] Tertiary syphilis (not including neurosyphilis)—PCN allergy: ▪ Same as late latent syphilis Neurosyphilis: ▪ Procaine penicillin 2.4 MU IM once daily × 10-14 d + probenecid 500 mg po qid × 10-14 d PCN allergy[e]: ▪ Ceftriaxone 2 g IV/IM once daily × 10-14 d

Abbreviations: bid, twice daily; CI, continuous infusion; EES, erythromycin ethylsuccinate; IM, intramuscularly; IV, intravenously; MU, million units; PCN, penicillin; po, orally; qid, four times daily; tid, three times daily; wk, weeks.

[a]Fluoroquinolones and tetracyclines are generally not recommended for use during pregnancy.
[b]Regimens are for uncomplicated gonococcal infections of the cervix, urethra, and rectum only.
[c]Fluoroquinolones are no longer recommended for the treatment of gonorrhea in the United States due to increasing rates of fluoroquinolone-resistant *N. gonorrhoeae.*
[d]The use of topical antiviral agents (eg, acyclovir ointment) is discouraged, as it offers minimal clinical benefit. Treatment with oral agents can be extended if healing is incomplete at the end of recommended therapy.
[e]The possibility of cross-allergenicity between ceftriaxone and penicillin exists and desensitization may be necessary.

intracellularly by binding to the 23S component of the 50S ribosomal subunit, thereby inhibiting RNA-dependent protein synthesis. Their effects can be bacteriostatic or bactericidal. Gastrointestinal side effects include nausea, vomiting, and diarrhea (more commonly encountered with erythromycin). Prolongation of the QTc interval also may occur with macrolides including azithromycin and has been associated with sudden cardiac death in select studies. Erythromycin is metabolized by and is an inhibitor of the cytochrome P450 3A4 (CYP 3A4) enzyme system, and drug interactions are possible. Azithromycin is associated with fewer drug interactions because it is metabolized by CYP 3A4 to a lesser extent.

Azithromycin's long half-life allows less frequent dosing than erythromycin.

Doxycycline and Tetracycline

Doxycycline and tetracycline are tetracycline antibiotics that reversibly bind to the 30S bacterial ribosomal subunit, ultimately inhibiting bacterial protein synthesis. This intracellular mechanism of action results in bacteriostatic effects. Dose-related gastrointestinal side effects can occur (least common with doxycycline). The calcium-binding effects of tetracyclines cause permanent darkening of teeth in children and effects on developing bone. For this reason, tetracyclines are contraindicated in pregnancy (formerly pregnancy category D) and in children under the age of eight. Photosensitivity can also occur with the tetracyclines, but can be decreased by using skin protective measures. Tetracyclines bind multivalent cations (eg, calcium, aluminum, magnesium, iron) causing interactions with foods and vitamins that decrease antibiotic absorption. Patients should be instructed to separate cation-containing products from tetracycline antibiotics. Patients should also be instructed to take tetracycline antibiotics with an adequate amount of fluid and remain upright to reduce the risk of esophageal irritation and ulceration.

Ofloxacin and Levofloxacin

Ofloxacin and levofloxacin are fluoroquinolone antibiotics that exhibit bactericidal action due to their effects on bacterial DNA. Fluoroquinolones bind and stabilize DNA complexes with topoisomerase II and topoisomerase IV enzymes, causing DNA strand breakage and subsequent cell death. Gastrointestinal side effects and CNS effects (dizziness and headache) have been associated with their use. Prolongation of the QTc interval can also occur. Caution should be used when administering fluoroquinolones with other QTc interval-prolonging drugs or electrolyte disorders (hypokalemia and hypomagnesemia). Fluoroquinolones bind multivalent cations (eg, calcium, aluminum, magnesium, iron) leading to decreased antibiotic absorption. Patients should be instructed to separate cation-containing products from fluoroquinolone antibiotics. Fluoroquinolones have the potential to cause dysglycemia (hypo- or hyperglycemia), and this adverse effect has been most commonly reported in patients with underlying diabetes mellitus. Arthropathy and tendon injury may be experienced in specific populations. Arthropathy is most common in patients under 30 years old and presents as joint pain, swelling, and stiffness of the knees. Tendon injury generally occurs in older persons and is associated with additional risk factors. Clinical manifestations include severe and sudden pain, most often affecting the Achilles tendon. Fluoroquinolones have not adequately been studied in pregnancy (formerly pregnancy category C), and their use is generally discouraged. Fluoroquinolones should not be used as first-line antimicrobial agents in children younger than 18 years of age. Although emerging data suggest that these agents can possibly be safely administered to children, extreme caution is advised. Use of fluoroquinolones in children should be limited to life threatening or difficult to treat infections where the benefits of therapy outweigh the risks.

Treatment Agents for Gonorrhea

Therapy for gonococcal urethritis and cervicitis is complicated by the ability of N. gonorrhoeae to develop resistance to antimicrobials. The Centers for Disease Control and Prevention (CDC) no longer recommend the use of fluoroquinolones due to resistant N. gonorrhoeae. Presumptive therapy for chlamydia should be considered when treating gonorrhea since coinfection with C. trachomatis in patients with N. gonorrhoeae is common.

Cephalosporins

Cephalosporins represent the primary antibiotic recommended for the treatment of gonorrhea; however, the recommendation is only for parenteral cephalosporins. Along with penicillins, carbapenems, and monobactams, cephalosporins are members of the β-lactam antibiotic group. β-Lactams bind and inactivate a family of enzymes, called penicillin-binding proteins, which are required for bacterial cell wall synthesis. This action causes cell death and is bactericidal. Cephalosporins are well tolerated; however, there is potential for cross-allergenicity in patients with penicillin allergy. This is most common with first- and second-generation cephalosporins. While penicillin allergy (hypersensitivity) is reported in up to 10% of the general population, the frequency of a life-threatening reaction (anaphylaxis) is much less (0.01%-0.05%).

Treatment Agents for Genital Herpes

The antiviral agents recommended for the management of genital herpes are acyclovir, valacyclovir, and famciclovir. These drugs inhibit viral DNA replication by competitively inhibiting viral DNA polymerase. Subsequent incorporation of the drug into the growing viral DNA chain causes chain termination. Famciclovir has a lower affinity for viral DNA polymerase than acyclovir, but has a longer intracellular half-life. Valacyclovir is a prodrug of acyclovir that has increased oral bioavailability. Acyclovir, valacyclovir, and famciclovir are well tolerated. Neurologic toxicity has been reported with acyclovir and valacyclovir administration due to drug accumulation in renal failure. Adequate hydration should be maintained during oral and intravenous therapy.

Antiviral therapy does not eradicate latent herpes viral infection, but aids in disease management. Therapy is divided into three approaches: treatment for the initial episode, intermittent therapy for recurrence, and daily suppressive therapy. All treatment approaches provide symptom improvement during genital herpes episodes. Daily suppressive therapy also reduces the frequency and severity of recurrences and decreases HSV viral shedding, thereby reducing the risk of disease transmission. Daily suppressive therapy is associated with an improved quality of life in patients who have frequent recurrences. Use of topical antiviral therapy (eg, acyclovir ointment) is discouraged due to limited clinical benefit.

Treatment Agents for Syphilis

Parenteral penicillin is the drug of choice for syphilis. Tetracyclines and cephalosporins (reviewed earlier) are alternative therapies. Penicillins are β-lactam antimicrobials with the same mechanism of action as cephalosporins.

Parenteral Penicillin Preparations

Three parenteral penicillin preparations are used for the treatment of syphilis: aqueous crystalline penicillin G, procaine penicillin, and benzathine penicillin G. Aqueous crystalline penicillin G is used in the treatment of neurosyphilis and is administered intravenously. Its short half-life necessitates administration every 4 hours or by continuous infusion. Procaine penicillin, with the addition of oral probenecid, is an alternative for the treatment of neurosyphilis and is administered intramuscularly. The addition of procaine delays intramuscular drug absorption, allowing for less frequent administration, as infrequently as once daily. Benzathine penicillin G is used in the treatment of primary, secondary, latent, and tertiary syphilis. It is administered intramuscularly. Penicillin is released slowly after intramuscular administration of the benzathine preparation, providing sustained concentrations and allowing for single-dose therapy or once weekly dosing. Other parenteral penicillin preparations exist, and health care professionals should be aware of their differences in order to avoid mix-ups and inappropriate therapy. The inadvertent administration of a procaine-benzathine penicillin mix (Bicillin C-R) instead of benzathine penicillin (Bicillin L-A) to patients with syphilis has been reported. Bicillin C-R contains only half the dose of benzathine penicillin recommended for the treatment of syphilis and is inappropriate therapy for this indication. Penicillins are well tolerated, as are other β-lactam antibiotics. Neither procaine nor benzathine penicillin should be administered intravenously due to the potential for cardiorespiratory arrest and death. As mentioned previously, up to 10% of the population reports a penicillin allergy, but life-threatening reactions are much less common. Penicillin desensitization may be considered in select patients with a confirmed or suspected penicillin allergy who require penicillin therapy.

Jarisch-Herxheimer Reaction

An acute febrile reaction may occur within hours of initiation of therapy for syphilis. This reaction occurs because of the release of cytokines from dying *T. pallidum* organisms. The reaction is common in patients with early syphilis. Symptoms such as myalgia, headache, and tachycardia may accompany the fever. The reaction usually subsides within a 24-hour period. Analgesics and antipyretics may provide symptomatic improvement, but have not been shown to be effective for prevention. Complications of the Jarisch-Herxheimer reaction include induction of early labor and fetal distress in pregnant women.

Special Populations

Pregnancy

The treatment of STDs in pregnancy can decrease pregnancy complications and prevent disease transmission to the child.

Of note, pregnancy categories are being replaced with more specific language to better help providers make decisions on whether medications would be appropriate for use in pregnant patients.

Chlamydia Treating pregnant women for chlamydial infection usually prevents transmission to infants during birth. Doxycycline and fluoroquinolones should generally be avoided during pregnancy, and azithromycin or amoxicillin (500 mg po tid × 7 days) are recommended. Both azithromycin and amoxicillin were formerly classified in pregnancy category B.

Gonorrhea Spontaneous abortion, preterm labor, and postpartum infection are associated with untreated *N. gonorrhoeae* infection. The disease is also transmissible to the newborn, commonly manifesting as a scalp abscess, ophthalmic infection, or disseminated gonococcal disease. Ceftriaxone plus azithromycin is recommended first line for treatment of gonococcal infection during pregnancy. Both ceftriaxone and azithromycin were formerly classified in pregnancy category B.

Genital Herpes Herpes transmission from an infected mother can cause symptomatic disease in the neonate. The risk of transmission is highest in mothers who have the initial outbreak at the time of delivery. Although a lower risk, transmission also occurs in mothers who have a disease recurrence at the time of delivery. The risk in a mother with recurrent disease but no visible lesions is thought to be low. Use of antiviral therapy late in pregnancy decreases herpes recurrences near term as well as transmission to the neonate. Acyclovir, famciclovir, and valacyclovir were formerly classified in pregnancy category B.

Syphilis In addition to transmission during delivery, syphilis can be transmitted in utero during pregnancy. Exposure to syphilis before birth can lead to preterm labor, fetal death, and neonatal infection. Penicillin regimens, appropriate for the stage of disease, are recommended for the treatment of syphilis in pregnant women. No proven alternatives to penicillin exist for the treatment of syphilis during pregnancy. It is recommended that pregnant patients with a penicillin allergy undergo desensitization and subsequent treatment with penicillin.

Children

Children, including neonates and infants, who are diagnosed with congenital or acquired STDs should be treated according to guideline recommendations. In children who acquire STDs after the neonatal period, and for which a nonsexual explanation does not exist, the possibility of sexual abuse and/or assault should be considered.

Adolescents

In general, pharmacologic treatment for STDs in adolescent patients is the same as in adults. As with adults, appropriate education and counseling on STD risk reduction are important components of the treatment plan.

HIV Infection

Because severe or prolonged herpes episodes may occur in immunocompromised patients, doses for patients with HIV infection are typically higher and/or treatment durations longer than in patients who are HIV-negative. Treatment guidelines should be consulted for specific recommendations. Patients infected with HIV and diagnosed with chlamydia, gonorrhea, or syphilis should be treated in the same manner as patients who are HIV negative.

POSTEXPOSURE PROPHYLAXIS

Postexposure prophylaxis is not recommended for chlamydia, gonorrhea, genital herpes, or syphilis infections. However, patients diagnosed with these STDs are encouraged to inform their sexual partner(s) of the diagnosis so that they may seek treatment. In some cases, evaluation and treatment of sexual partners may be facilitated by health care providers or public health authorities.

SPECIAL CONSIDERATIONS

Although not specifically reviewed in this chapter, practitioners should also be familiar with treatment and prevention recommendations for genital human papillomavirus (HPV). Most HPV infections are asymptomatic and self-resolving; however, persistent infection can lead to cervical cancer in women as well as anogenital cancer in men and women. Topical therapies are available for symptomatic infections (ie, genital and anal warts). Additionally, a quadrivalent HPV vaccine (Gardasil) and a 9-valent HPV vaccine (Gardasil 9) are approved for the prevention of HPV-related cancer in females ages 9 to 26 and in males ages 9 to 21.

CASE Application

1. AS is a 27-year-old patient with a new diagnosis of a chlamydia infection. The patient is concerned about the infection, the treatment, and complications from the infection. Complications of chlamydia genital infection include which of the following?

   a. Granulomatous and cardiovascular diseases
   b. Vesicular lesions on the external genitalia
   c. Pelvic inflammatory disease and infertility
   d. General paresis, dementia, and sensory ataxia

2. TD is 27-year-old man who presents to a local STD clinic with complaints of painful urination and urethral discharge over the past 4 days. He is sexually active, reporting one partner within the past 30 days. He has no known drug allergies. A diagnosis of chlamydia is made. Select the most appropriate therapy for TD.

   a. Doxycycline
   b. Azithromycin + cefixime
   c. Ceftizoxime
   d. Acyclovir + ofloxacin

3. Which of the following is a contraindication to doxycycline therapy? Select all that apply.

   a. Age less than 8 years
   b. Concomitant use of QTc interval-prolonging drugs
   c. Diabetes mellitus
   d. Documented penicillin allergy

4. JM is a 23-year-old woman who is 28 weeks pregnant. She presents to her primary care physician (PCP) with symptoms of dysuria and unusual vaginal discharge. A diagnosis of chlamydia is made. JM has no medication allergies. Select appropriate therapy for JM.

   a. Doxycycline
   b. Amoxicillin
   c. Cefixime
   d. Levofloxacin

5. Which of the following represents an adverse effect associated with fluoroquinolone use? Select all that apply.

   a. Permanent tooth darkening
   b. Esophageal ulceration
   c. Dysglycemia
   d. Jarisch-Herxheimer reaction

6. Which of the following is true regarding gonococcal urethritis and/or cervicitis?

   a. Gonorrhea infections are treated with oral vancomycin.
   b. Men are typically asymptomatic or have minor symptoms.
   c. Increased transmission of HIV infection is associated with gonococcal infection.
   d. Antibiotic susceptibility data can be obtained using nonculture diagnostic tests for gonorrhea.

7. IT is a patient that reports to her primary care provider for evaluation of a vaginal discharge, dysuria, and vaginal bleeding. The provider orders several labs and cultures. A Gram stain reveals gram-negative diplococci. The presence of gram-negative diplococci on Gram stain is suggestive of which organism?

   a. *Treponema pallidum*
   b. *Chlamydia trachomatis*
   c. Herpes simplex virus-2
   d. *Neisseria gonorrhoeae*

8. AF is a 19-year-old college student who is considering becoming sexually active. During her annual Pap smear, she asks her gynecologist for information on STD and pregnancy prevention. Which of the following statements is true regarding STD prevention? Select all that apply.

   a. Vaccines are currently available for chlamydia, gonorrhea, and syphilis.
   b. Diaphragm use is a reliable method of STD prevention.

c. Hormonal contraception is effective in preventing pregnancy and STDs.

d. Condom use reduces the acquisition and transmission of STDs.

9. Select the mechanism of action for cephalosporin antibiotics.

a. Bind to the 30S bacterial ribosomal subunit, ultimately inhibiting bacterial protein synthesis

b. Bind and inactivate a family of enzymes required for bacterial cell wall synthesis, causing cell death

c. Bind and stabilize DNA complexes with topoisomerase II and topoisomerase IV enzymes, causing DNA-strand breakage and cell death

d. Bind to the 23S component of the 50S ribosomal subunit, inhibiting RNA-dependent protein synthesis

10. SA is a 33-year-old man with no known drug allergies who presents to the local STD clinic with complaints of extreme pain on urination and urethral discharge for 2 days. A diagnosis of gonococcal urethritis is made. Select the most appropriate therapy for SA.

a. Ceftriaxone + azithromycin

b. Benzathine penicillin

c. Azithromycin

d. Levofloxacin + azithromycin

11. TE is a 33-year-old patient with genital herpes. Which of the following describes a current goal of therapy for genital herpes infection? Select all that apply.

a. Disease eradication

b. Viral suppression

c. Transmission prevention

d. Decrease recurrence frequency

12. Which of the following is true regarding genital herpes infection?

a. Genital herpes is an acute, self-limiting disease.

b. Genital lesions are typically vesicular in nature and accompanied by pain, itching, and burning.

c. The rate of recurrence increases over time in most patients.

d. Transmission risk in a mother with recurrent disease but no visible lesions is high.

13. EV is a 29-year-old pregnant patient with a past medical history of genital HSV herpes. Which of the following is true regarding genital herpes infection and pregnancy?

a. The risk of herpes transmission is lowest in mothers who have the initial outbreak at the time of delivery.

b. Acyclovir, famciclovir, and valacyclovir are classified in pregnancy category D.

c. Use of antiviral therapy late in pregnancy decreases herpes transmission to the neonate.

d. Herpes disease in the neonate commonly manifests as a scalp abscess or ophthalmic infection.

14. HF is a 29-year-old woman who was diagnosed with genital herpes 6 years ago. She reports approximately one to two recurrences each year since diagnosis. Recently she has experienced an increase in outbreaks, having three in a 6-month period. The decision is made to start HF on daily suppressive therapy. Select the most appropriate therapy for HF.

a. Valacyclovir po

b. Erythromycin ointment

c. Tetracycline po

d. Acyclovir ointment

15. Which of the following is true regarding the stages of syphilis infection?

a. The characteristic lesion of primary syphilis is a diffuse rash, usually affecting the palms and soles.

b. Manifestations of latent syphilis include regional lymphadenopathy and meningitis.

c. Tertiary syphilis is highly transmissible.

d. Neurosyphilis can present at any stage of syphilis.

16. Which of the following is true regarding the diagnosis of syphilis?

a. The diagnosis of syphilis is made through direct techniques such as culture.

b. Serologic testing is the standard method of detecting primary, secondary, latent, and tertiary syphilis in the United States.

c. The VDRL-CSF is the standard serologic test for secondary syphilis.

d. Nontreponemal serologic testing alone is sufficient for a definitive diagnosis of syphilis.

17. Select the brand name for benzathine penicillin.

a. Bicillin C-R

b. Wycillin

c. Bicillin L-A

d. Pen-VK

18. TP is a 26-year-old woman who is 31 weeks pregnant. She visits her obstetrician-gynecologist because of a sore throat, generalized weakness, and a rash on her palms and soles for the past week. Testing is performed and a diagnosis of secondary syphilis is made. The treating physician requests pharmacist consultation because the patient is allergic to penicillin. Select the most appropriate therapy for TP.

a. Doxycycline

b. Cefoxitin + probenecid

c. Levofloxacin

d. Desensitization + benzathine penicillin G

19. The Jarisch-Herxheimer reaction is an acute febrile reaction associated with therapy for which STD?

a. Genital herpes

b. Gonorrhea

c. Chlamydia

d. Syphilis

20. Which of the following is true regarding the treatment of STDs in special populations?

   a. The treatment of STDs in pregnancy can decrease pregnancy complications and prevent disease transmission to the child.

   b. Children diagnosed with congenital or acquired STDs should not be treated until they reach 2 years of age due to antimicrobial toxicities.

   c. In general, adolescent patients require lower doses of recommended antimicrobials for the treatment of STDs.

   d. Management of genital herpes in patients with HIV infection is the same as the management in patient who are HIV negative.

TAKEAWAY POINTS »

- STDs are acquired through sexual contact and associated with symptomatic disease, infertility, and deleterious effects on pregnancy and childbirth.

- Effective STD preventative measures include abstinence, monogamy with an uninfected partner, and barrier methods (condoms).

- Chlamydia and gonorrhea are the first and second most common bacterial STDs and typically present as cervicitis in women and urethritis in men. However, asymptomatic infection is common.

- Recommended agents for the treatment of chlamydia are azithromycin and doxycycline. Erythromycin, ofloxacin, and levofloxacin are alternatives.

- Cephalosporins are the recommended agents for the treatment of gonorrhea. Fluoroquinolones are no longer recommended due to the emergence of resistance.

- Because people infected with *N. gonorrhoeae* are frequently coinfected with *C. trachomatis,* treatment for chlamydia is recommended when gonorrhea is diagnosed.

- Genital herpes is a chronic, lifelong viral infection characterized by an initial episode followed by periodic recurrences. The typical disease manifestation includes clusters of painful papular and vesicular lesions on the external genitalia.

- Genital herpes cannot be cured, but antiviral therapy decreases the frequency and severity of recurrences as well as the risk of disease transmission.

- Four stages are associated with syphilitic disease: primary syphilis, secondary syphilis, latent syphilis, and tertiary syphilis. Neurosyphilis can occur at any stage of the disease. Distinct clinical manifestations are associated with each stage of disease as well as neurosyphilis.

- Penicillin is the drug of choice for syphilis treatment. Different preparations and regimens are recommended depending on the stage of disease.

- Patients with penicillin allergy who require penicillin therapy (eg, for syphilis in pregnancy) should be desensitized and subsequently treated with penicillin.

- Treatment of STDs during pregnancy can decrease complications and prevent disease transmission to the child.

- Tetracyclines and fluoroquinolones should be avoided in pregnancy.

BIBLIOGRAPHY

Centers for Disease Control and Prevention. Sexually transmitted diseases treatment guidelines, 2015. MMWR Recomm Rep. 2015;64(3):1-137.

Gaydos CA, Quinn TC. Chlamydial infections. In: Longo DL, Fauci AS, Kasper DL, Hauser SL, Jameson J, Loscalzo J, eds. *Harrison's Principles of Internal Medicine.* 18th ed. New York, NY: McGraw-Hill; 2012:chap 176.

Knodel LC, Duhon B, Argamany J. Sexually transmitted diseases. In: DiPiro JT, Talbert RL, Yee GC, Matzke GR, Wells BG, Posey L, eds. *Pharmacotherapy: A Pathophysiologic Approach.* 10th ed. New York, NY: McGraw-Hill; 2017.

MacDougall C, Chambers H. Protein synthesis inhibitors and miscellaneous antibacterial agents. In: Brunton LL, Chabner BA, Knollmann BC, eds. *Goodman & Gilman's The Pharmacological Basis of Therapeutics.* 12th ed. New York, NY: McGraw-Hill; 2011:chap 55.

Safrin S. Antiviral agents. In: Katzung BG, Masters SB, Trevor AJ, eds. *Basic & Clinical Pharmacology.* 12th ed. New York, NY: McGraw-Hill; 2012:chap 49.

KEY ABBREVIATIONS

CDC = Centers for Disease Control and Prevention
CNS = central nervous system
CSF = cerebrospinal fluid
CYP 3A4 = cytochrome P450 3A4
DNA = deoxyribonucleic acid
HIV = human immunodeficiency virus

HPV = human papillomavirus
HSV = herpes simplex virus
NAAT = nucleic acid amplification test
PCP = primary care physician
PID = pelvic inflammatory disease
STD = sexually transmitted disease

32 Influenza

Hana Rac, P. Brandon Bookstaver, and S. Scott Sutton

FOUNDATION OVERVIEW

Influenza is a viral infection that attacks your respiratory system (nose, throat, and lungs) causing significant morbidity and mortality, particularly among children and elderly. Influenza occurs at any time during the year, but the highest rates occur between December and March. Influenza A and B are the two types of influenza viruses and influenza A is further categorized into subtypes based upon two surface antigens (hemagglutinin and neuraminidase). Immunity to influenza occurs from antibody development directed at the surface antigens.

Influenza transmission is person-to-person via inhalation of respiratory droplets with an average incubation period of 2 days (range 1 and 4). Classic signs and symptoms of influenza include rapid onset of fever, myalgia, headache, malaise, nonproductive cough, sore throat, and rhinitis. Nausea, vomiting, and otitis media are commonly reported in children. Signs and symptoms resolve in 3 to 7 days; however, cough and malaise may persist for more than 2 weeks. Influenza increases the risk for pneumonia (including methicillin resistant *Staphylococcus aureus* pneumonia). The gold standard for the diagnosis of influenza is viral culture, but the clinical utility of the culture is limited because of the length of time to receive results. Tests such as the rapid antigen and point-of-care (POC) tests, direct fluorescence antibody (DFA) test, and the reverse transcriptase polymerase chain reaction (RT-PCR) assay may be used for rapid detection of the influenza virus.

PREVENTION

Annual vaccination is the most effective method to prevent influenza; unfortunately, the annual rate of vaccination is 30% to 40%. Vaccination should be administered to any person who wishes to reduce the likelihood of becoming ill with influenza or transmitting influenza to others. While it is important for all to receive influenza vaccination, emphasis should be placed upon vaccinating groups at higher risk of influenza infection and influenza-related complications (Table 32-1). The inactivated and live-attenuated formulations are the commercially available vaccines. The inactivated vaccines are trivalent or quadrivalent while the live-attenuated vaccine is quadrivalent. Most trivalent vaccines are grown in hens eggs and contain equivalent strains (influenza A H1N1, influenza A H3N2, and influenza B). The quadrivalent vaccines are grown in an identical manner and contain strains of influenza A H1N1, influenza A H3N2, and two influenza B strains. See Table 32-2 for a comparison of influenza vaccines. Tables 32-2 to 32-5 present key information regarding the influenza vaccines and Figure 32-1 discusses dosing for children aged 6 months through 8 years.

Optimally, vaccination should occur before onset of influenza activity in the community. Health care providers should offer vaccination by the end of October, if possible. Children aged 6 months through 8 years who require 2 doses (see Figure 32-1) should receive their first dose as soon as possible after vaccine becomes available, to allow the second dose (which must be administered ≥4 weeks later) to be received by the end of October.

Trivalent and Quadrivalent Inactivated Influenza Vaccine

The trivalent (IIV$_3$) and quadrivalent (IIV$_4$) inactivated influenza vaccines are approved for use in people 6 months of age and older. The cell culture-based trivalent vaccine (ccIIV$_3$) is approved for people 18 years of age and older while the recombinant hemagglutinin trivalent influenza vaccine (RIV) is approved for people 18 to 49 years of age. Both the ccIIV$_3$ and RVI are manufactured using technologies that reduce or completely avoid the use of eggs, respectively. Most trivalent and quadrivalent inactivated vaccines are administered intramuscularly and made with killed influenza viruses. They cannot cause signs and symptoms of influenza or influenza-like illness. The most frequent adverse effect associated with IIV (IIV$_3$, IIV$_4$, ccIIV$_3$) and RIV is injection site soreness that may last up to 48 hours. They may also cause fever and malaise in those who have not previously been exposed to the viral antigens in the vaccine.

Live-Attenuated Influenza Vaccine

Live-attenuated influenza vaccine (LAIV), or the nasal spray vaccine, is *not* recommended for use during the 2017-2018 season because of concerns about its effectiveness. For subsequent influenza seasons, please refer to the Centers for Disease Control and Prevention (CDC) recommendations.

TABLE 32-1 Target Groups for Vaccination

Persons at High Risk of Complications From Influenza
- All children age 6-59 mo
- Adults aged more than 50 y of age
- Residents of any age of nursing homes or other long-term care institutions
- Women who are or will be pregnant during the influenza season
- American Indians/Alaska Natives
- Persons with:
  - Asthma or other chronic pulmonary diseases, such as cystic fibrosis in children or chronic obstructive pulmonary disease in adults
  - Hemodynamically significant cardiac disease
  - Immunosuppressive disorders or who are receiving immunosuppressive therapy
  - HIV
  - Sickle cell anemia and other hemoglobinopathies
  - Diseases that require long-term aspirin therapy, such as rheumatoid arthritis or Kawasaki disease (especially persons age 6-18 y who may be at risk of Reye syndrome after influenza virus infection)
  - Chronic renal and/or liver dysfunction
  - Cancer
  - Chronic metabolic disease, such as diabetes mellitus
  - Neuromuscular disorders, seizure disorders, or cognitive dysfunction that may compromise handling of respiratory secretions
  - Morbid obesity (BMI greater than or equal to 40)

Persons who Live With or Care for Persons at Higher Risk
- Health care personnel
- Household contacts (including children) and caregivers of children aged ≤59 mo and adults aged greater than or equal to 50 y
- Household contacts (including children) and caregivers of persons with medical conditions that put them at higher risk for severe complications from influenza

LAIV is a live, weakened virus approved for intranasal administration in healthy, nonpregnant persons between 2 and 49 years of age. It is available in a quadrivalent formulation. Advantages of LAIV include ease of administration and the potential induction of broad mucosal and systemic immune response. Adverse events associated with LAIV administration include runny nose, congestion, sore throat, and headache. LAIV should not be given to those who are immunocompromised (eg, HIV infection) or those with close contact to immunocompromised persons who require a restricted environment.

Contraindications

IIV and LAIV should not be administered to a person with hypersensitivity to eggs. RIV can be used in people 18 to 49 years of age with hypersensitivity to eggs. Allergic type reactions (hives, systemic anaphylaxis) rarely occur after influenza vaccination; however, when allergic reactions occur it is likely a result of residual egg protein in the vaccine. Table 32-3 lists contraindications for LAIV, IIV, and RIV.

Guillain-Barre syndrome (GBS) has been linked to influenza vaccination; however, there is insufficient evidence to establish causality. Vaccination (IIV, LAIV, or RIV) should be avoided in persons who experienced GBS within 6 weeks of receiving a previous influenza vaccine and are not at high risk for influenza complications.

TABLE 32-2 Comparison of Influenza Vaccines

Factor	LAIV	IIV/RIV
Route of administration	Intranasal spray	Intramuscular injection (one IIV product is given via intradermal route)
Type of vaccine	Live-attenuated virus	Killed virus
Number of included virus strains	Four (two influenza A, two influenza B)	Three or four (two influenza A, one or two influenza B)
Vaccine virus strains updated	Annually	Annually
Frequency of administration	Annually	Annually
Approved age	Persons aged 2-49 y (healthy, nonpregnant)	IIV: Persons ≥6 mo of age ccIIV$_3$: Persons ≥18 y RIV: Persons 18-49 y
Interval between 2 doses recommended for children aged ≥6 mo-8 y who are receiving influenza vaccine for the first time	4 wk	4 wk[a]
Can be administered to children with asthma or children aged 2-4 y with wheezing during the preceding year	No	Yes[a]
Can be administered to family members or close contacts of immunosuppressed persons not requiring a protected environment	Yes	Yes[a]
Can be administered to family members or close contacts of immunosuppressed persons requiring a protected environment (eg, hematopoietic stem cell transplant recipient)	No	Yes[a]
Can be simultaneously administered with other vaccines	Yes[b]	Yes[b]
If not simultaneously administered, can be administered within 4 wk of another live vaccine	Prudent to space 4 wk apart	Yes
If not simultaneously administered, can be administered within 4 wk of an inactivated vaccine	Yes	Yes

[a]ccIIV$_3$ and RIV should not be used in children
[b]LAIV coadministration has been evaluated systematically only among children aged 12 to 15 months who received measles, mumps, and rubella vaccine or varicella vaccine. IIV coadministration has been evaluated systematically only among adults who received pneumococcal polysaccharide or zoster vaccine. Live-attenuated influenza vaccine (LAIV), or the nasal spray vaccine, is *not* recommended for use during the 2017-2018 season because of concerns about its effectiveness. For subsequent influenza seasons, please refer to the CDC recommendations.

TABLE 32-3   Persons Who Should Not Receive Influenza Vaccine

IIV (including IIV₃, IIV₄, and ccIIV₃)

- Persons known to have anaphylactic hypersensitivity to eggs.
- Persons with moderate to severe acute febrile illness usually should not be vaccinated until their symptoms have abated. Minor illnesses with or without fever do not contraindicate use of influenza vaccine.
- Persons who experienced Guillain-Barre syndrome within 6 wk following a previous dose of IIV is considered to be a precaution for use of IIV.

RIV

- Persons with moderate to severe acute febrile illness usually should not be vaccinated until their symptoms have abated. Minor illnesses with or without fever do not contraindicate use of influenza vaccine.
- Persons who experienced Guillain-Barre syndrome within 6 wk following a previous dose of RIV is considered to be a precaution for use of RIV.

LAIV

- Live-attenuated influenza vaccine (LAIV), or the nasal spray vaccine, is **not** recommended for use during the 2017-2018 season because of concerns about its effectiveness. For subsequent influenza seasons, please refer to the CDC recommendations.
- Persons with a history of hypersensitivity to any components of LAIV or to eggs.
- Persons less than 2 y of age or more than 49 y of age.
- Persons with any of the underlying medical conditions that serve as an indication for routine influenza vaccination:
  - Asthma
  - Reactive airway disease
  - Chronic disorders of pulmonary system
  - Chronic disorders of cardiovascular system (except hypertension)
  - Metabolic diseases (eg, diabetes)
  - Liver/renal dysfunction
  - Hemoglobinopathies
  - Known or suspected immunodeficiency
- Children aged 2-4 y whose parents or caregivers report that a health care provider has told them during the preceding 12 mo that their child had wheezing or asthma, or whose medical record indicates a wheezing episode has occurred in the preceding 12 mo.
- Children or adolescents receiving aspirin or other salicylates.
- Persons with a history of Guillain-Barre syndrome after influenza vaccination.
- Pregnant women.

TABLE 32-4   Influenza Vaccines–United States, 2007-18 Influenza Season[a]

Trade Name	Manufacturer	Presentation	Age Indication	Mercury (From Thimerosal, mcg/0.5 mL)	Latex	Route
Inactivated influenza vaccines, quadrivalent (IIV4s), standard-dose[b]						
Afluria Quadrivalent	Seqirus	0.5 mL prefilled syringe	≥5 y	NR	No	IM[c]
		5.0 mL multidose vial	≥5 y (by needle/syringe) 18 through 64 y (by jet injector)	24.5	No	IM
Fluarix Quadrivalent	GlaxoSmithKline	0.5 mL prefilled syringe	≥6 mo	NR	No	IM
FluLaval Quadrivalent	ID Biomedical Corp. of Quebec (distributed by GlaxoSmithKline)	0.5 mL prefilled syringe	≥6 mo	NR	No	IM
		5.0 mL multidose vial	≥6 mo	<25	No	IM
Fluzone Quadrivalent	Sanofi Pasteur	0.25 mL prefilled syringe	6 through 35 mo	NR	No	IM
		0.5 mL prefilled syringe	≥3 y	NR	No	IM
		0.5 mL single-dose vial	≥3 y	NR	No	IM
		5.0 mL multidose vial	≥6 mo	25	No	IM
Inactivated influenza vaccine, quadrivalent (ccIIV4), standard-dose,[b] cell culture-based						
Flucelvax Quadrivalent	Seqirus	0.5 mL prefilled syringe	≥4 y	NR	No	IM
		5.0 mL multidose vial	≥4 y	25	No	IM
Inactivated influenza vaccine, quadrivalent (IIV4), standard-dose, intradermal[d]						
Fluzone Intradermal Quadrivalent	Sanofi Pasteur	0.1 mL single-dose prefilled microinjection system	18 through 64 y	NR	No	ID[e]
Inactivated influenza vaccines, trivalent (IIV3s), standard-dose[b]						
Afluria	Seqirus	0.5 mL prefilled syringe	≥5 y	NR	No	IM
		5.0 mL multidose vial	≥5 y (by needle/syringe) 18 through 64 y (by jet injector)	24.5	No	IM

TABLE 32-4	Influenza Vaccines–United States, 2007-18 Influenza Season[a] (*Continued*)					
Trade Name	Manufacturer	Presentation	Age Indication	Mercury (From Thimerosal, mcg/0.5 mL)	Latex	Route
Fluvirin	Seqirus	0.5 mL prefilled syringe	≥4 y	≤1	Yes[f]	IM
		5.0 mL multidose vial	≥4 y	25	No	IM
Adjuvanted inactivated influenza vaccine, trivalent (aIIV3),[b] standard-dose						
Fluad	Seqirus	0.5 mL prefilled syringe	≥65 y	NR	Yes[f]	IM
Inactivated influenza vaccine, trivalent (IIV3), high-dose[g]						
Fluzone high-dose	Sanofi Pasteur	0.5 mL prefilled syringe	≥65 y	NR	No	IM
Recombinant influenza vaccine, quadrivalent (RIV4)[h]						
Flublok Quadrivalent	Protein Sciences	0.5 mL prefilled syringe	≥18 y	NR	No	IM
Recombinant influenza vaccine, trivalent (RIV3)[h]						
Flublok	Protein Sciences	0.5 mL single-dose vial	≥18 y	NR	No	IM
Live-attenuated influenza vaccine, quadrivalent (LAIV4)[i] (not recommended for use during the 2017-18 season)						
FluMist Quadrivalent	MedImmune	0.2 mL single-dose prefilled intranasal sprayer	2 through 49 y	NR	No	NAS

Abbreviations: ACIP = Advisory Committee on Immunization Practices; ID = intradermal; IM = intramuscular; NAS = intranasal; NR = not relevant (does not contain thimerosal).

[a]Immunization providers should check Food and Drug Administration–approved prescribing information for 2017-18 influenza vaccines for the most complete and updated information, including (but not limited to) indications, contraindications, warnings, and precautions. Package inserts for U.S.-licensed vaccines are available at https://www.fda.gov/BiologicsBloodVaccines/Vaccines/ApprovedProducts/ucm093833.htm. Availability of specific products and presentations might change and differ from what is described in this table and in the text of this report.

[b]Standard dose intramuscular IIVs contain 15 mcg of each vaccine HA antigen (45 mcg total for trivalents and 60 mcg total for quadrivalents) per 0.5 mL dose.

[c]For adults and older children, the recommended site for intramuscular influenza vaccination is the deltoid muscle. The preferred site for infants and young children is the anterolateral aspect of the thigh. Specific guidance regarding site and needle length for intramuscular administration is available in the ACIP General Best Practice Guidelines for Immunization, available at https://www.cdc.gov/vaccines/hcp/acip-recs/general-recs/index.html.

[d]Quadrivalent inactivated influenza vaccine, intradermal: a 0.1-mL dose contains 9 mcg of each vaccine HA antigen (36 mcg total).

[e]The preferred injection site is over the deltoid muscle. Fluzone Intradermal Quadrivalent is administered per manufacturer's instructions using the delivery system included with the vaccine.

[f]Syringe tip cap might contain natural rubber latex.

[g]High-dose IIV3 contains 60 mcg of each vaccine antigen (180 mcg total) per 0.5 mL dose.

[h]RIV contains 45 mcg of each vaccine HA antigen (135 mcg total for trivalent 180 mcg total for quadrivalent) per 0.5 mL dose.

[i]ACIP recommends that FluMist Quadrivalent (LAIV4) not be used during the 2017-18 season.

Special Populations

Pregnant women, regardless of trimester, should receive annual influenza vaccination with IIV or RIV but not with LAIV. IIV or RIV is also safe for breast-feeding mothers. Immunocompromised hosts should receive annual vaccination with IIV or RIV but not LAIV. Children 6 months of age and greater should receive annual influenza vaccination. Children greater than 6 months of age may receive IIV and children greater than 24 months of age may receive LAIV. Multidose vials and a few of the single-dose preparations of IIV contain trace to small amounts of the preservative thimerosal. No scientifically persuasive evidence is linked between thimerosal and autism. Children 6 months through 8 years of age who are receiving the influenza vaccine for the first time require 2 doses of vaccine administered greater than or equal to 4 weeks apart. Due to demonstrated lower titers against influenza virus strains included in seasonal influenza vaccines in adults 65 years of age or greater, high-dose IIV may be an acceptable option for these persons even though it is not explicitly recommended by the CDC.

TREATMENT

The four goals of therapy for influenza are: control symptoms, prevent complications, decrease work and/or school absenteeism, and prevent the spread of infection. Treatment options for influenza consist of neuraminidase inhibitors and the adamantanes. Antiviral drugs shorten the duration of illness (1 day), provide symptom control, and are most effective if started within 48 hours of the onset of illness. Adjunctive agents may be used concomitantly with the antiviral drugs and include acetaminophen for fever or antihistamines for rhinitis.

Adamantanes

Amantadine and rimantadine are adamantanes that have activity against influenza A only. Rapid emergence of resistance is a problem with these agents because cross-resistance is conferred by a single-point mutation. Ninety-two percent of the circulating influenza A viruses are resistant to the adamantanes, which is why these agents are not currently

TABLE 32-5	Contraindications and Precutions to the Use of Influenza Vaccines–United States, 2017-18 Influenza Season[a]	
Vaccine Type	**Contraindications**	**Precautions**
IIV	History of severe allergic reaction to any component of the vaccine[b] or after previous dose of any influenza vaccine	Moderate-to-severe acute illness with or without fever History of Guillain-Barré syndrome within 6 wk of receipt of influenza vaccine
RIV	History of severe allergic reaction to any component of the vaccine	Moderate-to-severe acute illness with or without fever History of Guillain-Barré syndrome within 6 wk of receipt of influenza vaccine
LAIV for the 2017-18 season, ACIP recommends that LAIV not be used. Content is provided for information. For subsequent influenza seasons, please refer to the CDC recommendations.	History of severe allergic reaction to any component of the vaccine[b] or after a previous dose of any influenza vaccine Concomitant aspirin or salicylate-containing therapy in children and adolescents Children aged 2 through 4 y who have received a diagnosis of asthma or whose parents or caregivers report that a health care provider has told them during the preceding 12 mo that their child had wheezing or asthma or whose medical record indicates a wheezing episode has occurred during the preceding 12 mo Children and adults who are immunocompromised due to any cause (including immunosuppression caused by medications or by HIV infection) Close contacts and caregivers of severely immunosuppressed persons who require a protected environment Pregnancy Receipt of influenza antiviral medication within the previous 48 hours	Moderate-to-severe acute illness with or without fever History of Guillain-Barré syndrome within 6 wk of receipt of influenza vaccine Asthma in persons aged ≥5 y Other underlying medical conditions that might predispose to complications after wild-type influenza infection (eg, chronic pulmonary, cardiovascular [except isolated hypertension], renal, hepatic, neurologic, hematologic, or metabolic disorders [including diabetes mellitus])

Abbreviations: ACIP, Advisory Committee on Immunization Practices; IIV, inactivated influenza vaccine; LAIV, live-attenuated influenza vaccine; RIV, recombinant influenza vaccine.

[a]Immunization providers should check Food and Drug Administration–approved prescribing information for 2017-18 influenza vaccines for the most complete and updated information, including (but not limited to) indications, contraindications, and precautions. Package inserts for US-licensed vaccines are available at https://www.fda.gov/BiologicsBloodVaccines/Vaccines/ApprovedProducts/ucm093833.htm.

[b]History of severe allergic reaction (eg, anaphylaxis) to egg is a labeled contraindication to the use of IIV and LAIV. However, ACIP recommends that any licensed, recommended, and appropriate IIV or RIV may be administered to persons with egg allergy of any severity.

BOX Abbreviation conventions for influenza vaccines used in this report
- Inactivated influenza vaccines are abbreviated IIV. For the 2017-18 season, IIVs as a class will include:
    - egg-based, unadjuvanted, and adjuvanted trivalent influenza vaccines (IIV3s); and
    - egg-based or cell culture-based unadjuvanted quadrivalent influenza vaccines (IIV4s).
- RIV refers to recombinant hemagglutinin influenza vaccine, available in trivalent (RIV3) and quadrivalent (RIV4) formulations for the 2017-18 season.
- LAIV refers to live-attenuated influenza vaccine, available as a quadrivalent formulation (LAIV4) since the 2013-14 season.
- IIV, RIV, and LAIV denote vaccine categories; numeric suffix specifies the number of hemagglutinin (HA) antigens in the vaccine.
- When necessary to refer specifically to cell culture-based vaccine, the prefix "cc" is used (eg, ccIIV4).
- When necessary to refer specifically to adjuvanted vaccine, the prefix "a" is used (eg, aIIV3).
- When necessary to refer specifically to standard-dose or high-dose vaccines, the prefixes "SO-" or "HD-" are used (eg, SD-IIV3 and HD-IIV3).

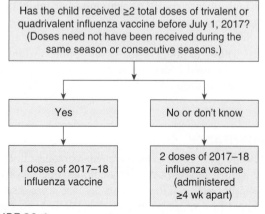

FIGURE 32-1 Influenza vaccine dosing algorithm for children aged 6 months through 8 years. Reproduced with permission from Grohskopf LA, Sokolow LZ, Broder KR, et al: Prevention and Control of Seasonal Influenza with Vaccines: Recommendations of the Advisory Committee on Immunization Practices—United States, 2017–18 Influenza Season, *MMWR Recomm Rep* 2017 Aug 25;66(2):1-20.

recommended as monotherapy for treatment of influenza in the United States. Central nervous system toxicity is the primary adverse reaction to adamantanes. Rimantadine causes fewer central nervous system side effects than amantadine.

Neuraminidase Inhibitors

Oseltamivir and zanamivir are neuraminidase inhibitors that have activity against influenza A and B viruses. Without neuraminidase, release of the virus from infected cells is impaired; therefore, viral replication is decreased. Oseltamivir is approved for treatment in those more than 1 year of age, while zanamivir is approved for treatment in those older than 7 years of age. The recommended dosages vary by agent and age, but dosing frequency of these agents is twice daily and the duration of treatment is 5 days. Between 2007-2009, seasonal influenza A (H1N1) virus strains tested from the United States and other countries were resistant to oseltamivir. As of

December 2010, no evidence existed of ongoing transmission of these strains worldwide.

Adverse effects of neuraminidase inhibitors are typically mild, although serious side effects have been described. Zanamivir can cause bronchospasm and a decline in respiratory function in patients with asthma and other chronic respiratory disorders. Oseltamivir can also cause nausea and vomiting but these side effects have not generally resulted in discontinuation of therapy. The manufacturer of oseltamivir notified health care professionals and the Food and Drug Administration (FDA) of postmarketing reports of self-injury and delirium in patients (primarily children) receiving the drug for treatment of influenza. Most of these reports came from Japan, where the drug is used more commonly than in the United States. However, a subsequent study has not demonstrated a causal association between neuraminidase inhibitors and abnormal behavior.

Special Populations

Inadequate data exist regarding the use of adamantanes or the neuraminidase inhibitors in immunocompromised patients. No clinical studies have been conducted evaluating the safety and efficacy of adamantanes or the neuraminidase inhibitors during pregnancy. All of the agents are pregnancy category C. Both the adamantanes and the neuraminidase inhibitors are excreted in breast milk and should be avoided by mothers who are breast-feeding their infants.

POSTEXPOSURE PROPHYLAXIS

The two classes of antiviral drugs for influenza prophylaxis are the adamantanes and the neuraminidase inhibitors (because of high-level resistance, the adamantanes are not recommended as monotherapy). The recommended dosages of the neuraminidase inhibitors for prophylaxis vary by agent and age, but dosing frequency is once daily in this instance. Antiviral drugs used for prophylaxis should be considered adjuncts and not a replacement for annual vaccination with IIV, RIV, or LAIV.

SPECIAL CONSIDERATIONS

Influenza antiviral drugs should not be administered for 2 weeks after administration of LAIV because the antiviral drugs inhibit influenza virus replication and LAIV should not be administered until 48 hours after influenza antiviral therapy has been stopped. No contraindication exists for concomitant use of IIV or RIV and influenza antiviral drugs.

Novel Influenza Strains

Antigenic shift, the acquirement of new hemagglutinin and/or neuraminidase via genetic reassortment by influenza virus, results in the emergence of novel influenza viruses and always carries the potential to cause a pandemic (eg, 2009 H1N1). However, the new novel virus must be able to replicate in humans, spread person-to-person, and affect a susceptible population. Influenza information may change frequently because of resistance or new information. Please refer to www.cdc.gov/flu for the most up-to-date recommendations for novel strains and seasonal influenza.

Everyday Prevention

There are everyday actions that can help prevent the spread of germs that cause respiratory illnesses like influenza. Take these everyday steps to protect your health:

- Cover your nose and mouth with a tissue when you cough or sneeze. Throw the tissue in the trash after you use it.
- Wash your hands often with soap and water. If soap and water are not available, use an alcohol-based hand rub.
- Avoid touching your eyes, nose, or mouth. Germs spread this way.
- Try to avoid close contact with sick people.
- If you are sick with flu-like illness, CDC recommends that you stay home for at least 24 hours after your fever is gone except to get medical care or for other necessities. (Your fever should be gone without the use of a fever-reducing medicine.) Keep away from others as much as possible to keep from making others sick.

CASE Application

1. Select the statement that accurately describes a patient with influenza.

   a. MP has a bacterial illness caused by *Haemophilus influenzae.*
   b. BA has a viral illness caused by respiratory syncytial virus (RSV).
   c. JJ has a viral illness caused by rhinovirus.
   d. FJ has a viral illness caused by influenza A and B.

2. ZC is a 35-year-old woman. She does not have a significant past medical history and is currently taking a multivitamin and calcium supplementation. She has a 3-year-old child. Based upon the information provided, provide influenza vaccination recommendations.

   a. ZC is 35 years old and influenza only affects the elderly and young children. Vaccination not recommended.
   b. ZC does not have comorbidities that place her at risk for influenza complications. Vaccination not recommended.
   c. ZC has a child that is at risk for influenza complications. Vaccination recommended for ZC.
   d. ZC has a child that is at risk for influenza complications. Vaccination recommended for ZC and her 3-year-old child.

The following case should be used for questions 3 and 4:
A 33-year-old woman who runs a daycare for children 6 months of age to 5 years of age calls your pharmacy for information pertaining to the transmission of influenza.

3. What primary method of transmission for seasonal influenza should she be most concerned with?

   a. Inhalation
   b. Exposure to blood
   c. Exposure to dead birds
   d. Exposure to body fluids

4. What other information should be provided to this caller to help reduce the transmission of seasonal influenza? Select all that apply.

   a. Influenza vaccination is strongly encouraged given the caller's place of work.
   b. Cover your nose and mouth with a tissue when you cough or sneeze.
   c. Wash your hands often with soap and water.
   d. Stay at home when worker or child has a fever.

5. DB is a 40-year-old man with a history of hypertension. DB has not been feeling well for the past 2 days and decides to go to his doctor. Based on his symptoms, DB's doctor diagnoses him with influenza. What could be some of DB's symptoms that led to his diagnosis? Select all that apply.

   a. Rapid onset of fever
   b. Myalgia
   c. Headache
   d. Nonproductive cough

6. BC is a 28-month-old child with no significant past medical history. BC has not had a wheezing episode in the last 12 months. Select the best statement as it relates to influenza vaccination.

   a. BC should be vaccinated with IIV.
   b. BC should be vaccinated with LAIV.
   c. BC should be vaccinated with RIV or ccIIV$_3$.
   d. BC should be administered oseltamivir for prophylaxis.

7. Select the agent that is administered via intramuscular injection for influenza prevention or postexposure prophylaxis.

   a. IIV
   b. LAIV
   c. Zanamivir
   d. Amantadine

8. XW is a 28-year-old pregnant patient. She is currently receiving amoxicillin for a urinary tract infection caused by *Escherichia coli*. She comes to your pharmacy wanting an influenza vaccination. She hates shots and prefers not to receive any injection. During last year's influenza season, she received treatment with oseltamivir. What is the appropriate agent for influenza vaccination for XW? Select all that apply.

   a. LAIV
   b. IIV

c. RIV
d. Oseltamivir

9. Which of the following condition(s) would be a contraindication for receiving LAIV? Select all that apply.

   a. Diabetes mellitus
   b. Development of GBS within 6 weeks of receiving previous influenza vaccine
   c. Egg allergy
   d. Recently received amantadine (within 48 hours)

10. Which of the following condition(s) would be a contraindication for receiving IIV?

    a. Diabetes mellitus
    b. Egg allergy
    c. Recently received amantadine (within 48 hours)
    d. Concerned about development of autism from thimerosal in IIV

11. Adamantanes have activity against which influenza types?

    a. Influenza A
    b. Influenza B
    c. Influenza C
    d. *Haemophilus influenzae*

12. Select the brand name for zanamivir.

    a. Relenza
    b. Tamiflu
    c. Symmetrel
    d. Fluzone

13. Select the anti-influenza agent that is formulated as a Rotadisk inhaler.

    a. Rimantadine
    b. Amantadine
    c. Oseltamivir
    d. Zanamivir

14. YQ is a 59-year-old man with a past medical history significant for COPD, diabetes mellitus, hypertension, and hyperlipidemia. YQ wanted to receive influenza vaccination, but the United States has a short supply of IIV and RIV. YQ's physician recommended postexposure prophylaxis if he is exposed to influenza. If YQ is exposed to influenza, which agent should be used as postexposure prophylaxis?

    a. Amantadine
    b. Rimantadine
    c. Oseltamivir
    d. Zanamivir

15. A 24-year-old woman with a history of asthma presents to your pharmacy to ask a question about influenza prevention and symptom resolution. She was diagnosed

with influenza B. She still has cough and malaise. What should you discuss with the patient? Select all that apply.

a. Influenza symptoms will disappear within 48 hours. If you are still having symptoms, see your provider.
b. Influenza symptoms typically last 3 to 7 days. Cough and malaise may last up to 2 weeks. If your symptoms have increased/worsened, you may need to see your provider.
c. As long as a patient does not have a fever, there is no need to worry. Cough and malaise symptoms will go away.
d. Influenza vaccination on an annual basis is strongly encouraged given the patient's history of asthma.

16. SW is a 32-year-old woman who is in her third trimester of pregnancy. Her doctor suggested that she be vaccinated with the seasonal influenza vaccine since she is at a higher risk of having influenza and influenza-related complications due to pregnancy. She comes to your pharmacy for the vaccination and inquires about side effects. Select the most common adverse reaction of IIV.

a. Injection site soreness
b. Birth defects
c. GBS
d. Autism

17. Which of the following patient(s) should receive influenza vaccination? Select all that apply.

a. CH who is 8-year-old boy with a history of cystic fibrosis
b. GS who is a healthy 10-month-old baby girl
c. KL who is a 48-year-old man with diabetes
d. RC who is a healthy 65-year-old woman

18. LWS is a 28-year-old man returning home from a military tour of duty from overseas. LWS is an OEF (operation enduring freedom) veteran. He received IIV 7 days ago. Today he presents with symptoms of influenza. Select the reason LWS could develop influenza symptoms, even if he received the appropriate vaccine.

a. IIV is a dead virus and can cause influenza.
b. LWS was not a candidate for influenza vaccination; therefore, he should not have received IIV.
c. LWS does not have influenza. He has the common cold.
d. Influenza vaccines are not 100% effective.

19. Select the surface antigens that categorize influenza A. Select all that apply.

a. Hemagglutinin
b. Thimerosal
c. Neuraminidase
d. GBS

20. TK is a 59-year-old HIV-positive patient. He does not want to develop influenza and would like to be vaccinated since he is immunocompromised. He has a severe egg allergy (wheezing). Select the appropriate vaccination for TK.

a. LAIV
b. RIV
c. IIV
d. Immunocompromised patients should not be vaccinated

21. You are working in an outpatient clinic and a 27-year-old man comes in with a 2-day history of myalgia, headache, malaise, nonproductive cough, sore throat, and rhinitis. He also has a fever that started this morning. The doctor at the clinic diagnoses him with influenza after a positive rapid antigen test and wants to prescribe oseltamivir therapy for 5 days to the patient. The doctor asks you for a dose. What reference(s) would you consult to find this information?

a. PubMed
b. *Drug Information Handbook*
c. Index Medicus
d. *Martindale: The Complete Drug Reference*

TAKEAWAY POINTS ❱❱

- Influenza is a viral illness associated with a high morbidity/mortality.
- The primary route of influenza transmission is person-to-person via inhalation of respiratory droplets.
- Classic signs and symptoms include abrupt onset of fever, muscle pain, headache, malaise, nonproductive cough, sore throat, and rhinitis.
- Annual influenza vaccination is the primary mechanism for prevention.
- IIV, RIV, and LAIV are the three commercially available vaccines for prevention of influenza.
- Most IIV can be administered to persons greater than 6 months of age.
- IIV should not be administered to patients with egg allergy, patients who experience GBS within 6 weeks of receiving influenza vaccine, and persons with moderate to severe febrile illness.
- RIV can be used in people 18 to 49 years of age with hypersensitivity to eggs.
- LAIV can be administered to healthy persons between 2 and 49 years of age.

- LAIV should not be administered to patients with an egg allergy, patients less than 2 years of age, patients more than 49 years of age, persons with chronic obstructive pulmonary disease (COPD), asthma, diabetes, cardiovascular, or renal disease, children with a wheezing and/or asthma episode in the preceding 12 months, children or adolescents receiving aspirin or other salicylates, persons with a history of GBS after influenza vaccination, or pregnant women.

- Antiviral drugs (adamantanes and neuraminidase inhibitors) for prophylaxis should be considered adjuncts to vaccine and are not replacements for annual vaccination.
- Neuraminidase inhibitors are the agents of choice for treatment of influenza. They are most effective if started within 48 hours of the onset of illness.

BIBLIOGRAPHY

Acosta EP, Flexner C. Antiviral agents (Nonretroviral). In: Brunton LL, Chabner BA, Knollmann BC, eds. *Goodman & Gilman's The Pharmacological Basis of Therapeutics.* 12th ed. New York, NY: McGraw-Hill; 2011:chap 49.

Dolin R. Influenza. In: Fauci AS, Jameson JL, Longo DL, Hauser SL, eds. *Harrison's Principles of Internal Medicine.* 18th ed. New York, NY: McGraw-Hill; 2012:chap 187.

Fiore AE, Fry A, Shay D, et al. Antiviral agents for the treatment and chemoprophylaxis of influenza—recommendations of the Advisory Committee on Immunization Practices (ACIP)—United States, 2013-2014. *MMWR Recomm Rep.* 2013;60:1-24.

Grohskopf LA, Sokolow LZ, Broder KR, et al. Prevention and control of seasonal influenza with vaccines. Recommendations of the Advisory Committee on Immunization Practices (ACIP)—United States, 2017-2018. *MMWR Recomm Rep.* 2017;66:1-20.

Njoku JC, Hermsen ED. Influenza. In: DiPiro JT, Talbert RL, Yee GC, Matzke GR, Wells BG, Posey LM, eds. *Pharmacotherapy: A Pathophysiologic Approach.* 9th ed. New York, NY: McGraw-Hill; 2014:chap 87.

Safrin S. Antiviral agents. In: Katzung BG, Masters SB, Trevor AJ, eds. *Basic & Clinical Pharmacology.* 12th ed. New York, NY: McGraw-Hill; 2012:chap 49.

KEY ABBREVIATIONS

DFA = direct fluorescence antibody
FDA = Food and Drug Administration
GBS = Guillain-Barre syndrome
HIV = human immunodeficiency virus

LAIV = live-attenuated influenza vaccine
POC = point-of-care
RSV = respiratory syncytial virus
RT-PCR = reverse transcriptase polymerase chain reaction

Renal and Nutritional Disorders

Estimating Renal Function

Christopher M. Bland, Caitlin Jenkins, and S. Scott Sutton

FOUNDATION OVERVIEW

Estimating renal function is important for patients taking renally eliminated medications in order to maximize effectiveness while limiting toxicity. The glomerular filtration rate (GFR) is an effective indicator of renal function and normal values are approximately 130 mL/min/1.73 m² for men and 120 mL/min/1.73 m² for women. The gold standard for approximating GFR is the inulin clearance method. Inulin is filtered by the glomerulus and is not secreted or reabsorbed, making it an ideal agent for approximating GFR. The inulin clearance method is rarely done because it is costly, invasive, and requires technical expertise. Additional markers used to estimate GFR include iothalamate, iohexol, and ethylenediaminetetraacetic acid. Like inulin, these markers are expensive and have limited availability, making them impractical in the clinical setting. Numerous methods have been developed to estimate GFR and examples include the Cockcroft-Gault and the Modification of Diet in Renal Disease (MDRD) equations.

Serum Creatinine

Creatinine is an endogenous substance that is eliminated primarily by glomerular filtration and serves an important role in estimating renal function. Creatinine is not as precise as inulin because it undergoes some tubular secretion. The range of serum creatinine (SCr) is approximately 0.6 to 1.2 mg/dL in normal, healthy adults. SCr is affected by age, gender, race, diet, muscle mass, and certain drugs; therefore, SCr is not used alone in predicting GFR. High doses of trimethoprim, for example, may increase SCr values due to competition for active tubular secretion into the urine; however, renal function is unchanged. Muscle mass is an important consideration when analyzing SCr values. Creatinine is a by-product of creatine metabolism and is influenced by the amount of muscle mass in a patient. Patients with low muscle mass would be expected to have lower SCr values. Low muscle mass can occur in elderly, cachectic (eg, acquired immunodeficiency patients), or individuals with limited muscle use (eg, spinal cord injury). Therefore, low muscle mass patients may have SCr values in the normal range but actually have renal insufficiency.

Urinary Clearance of Creatinine

GFR can be estimated via the combination of a timed urine collection and blood sampling of creatinine. The most common time interval utilized is a 24-hour urine collection. This practice has decreased due to the difficulty with accurate collection.

Creatinine Clearance and Glomerular Filtration Rate Prediction Equations

Equations estimating GFR based on SCr, age, weight, and race are more accurate than SCr alone. The Cockcroft-Gault method calculates a creatinine clearance (CrCl) and is a widely used equation to estimate GFR.

$$CrCl\,(mL/min) = \frac{[(140 - age) \times ideal\,body\,weight\,(kg)][0.85\,(for\,women)]}{(72 \times SCr)}$$

If a patient's actual body weight is below the ideal body weight (IBW), then the actual body weight should be used when calculating CrCl. The Cockcroft-Gault equation may be used for determining drug dosing in obese patients; however, it becomes less accurate with increasing weight. It is important to understand the manufacturer's recommendation for an individual medication as actual body weight has been used by some when giving dosage recommendations based on the Cockcroft-Gault equation. An example of this are the direct-acting oral anticoagulants. Therefore, an overestimation of renal function could occur resulting in toxicity in obese patients especially morbidly obese patients as many of these patients are not well represented in the clinical studies that gained that particular medication FDA approval.

Ideal body weight (IBW) (men) = 50 kg + (2.3 kg × height in inches over 5 ft)
Ideal body weight (women) = 45.5 kg + (2.3 kg × height in inches over 5 ft)

Cockcroft and Gault published this equation in 1976, using data primarily from approximately 250 healthy men. The equation has subsequently been validated in other patient populations. In clinical practice, it is customary to round the SCr up to 1.0 mg/dL in patients with actual values less than 1.0 mg/dL (eg, patients with low muscle mass or age >65), although some believe this underestimates renal function.

The MDRD equation is another calculation utilized to estimate GFR; however, this is used primarily to stage kidney disease. Some manufacturers are beginning to use MDRD to base their dosage adjustment recommendations for newer antimicrobials (eg, delafloxacin) but these are rare at the current time.

$$\text{GFR (mL/min/1.73m}^2) = 186 \times (\text{Scr})^{-1.154} \times (\text{age})^{-0.203} \times 0.742$$
(if patient is female) × 1.210 (if patient is African American)

The MDRD was originally validated in patients with chronic kidney disease, but was subsequently validated in a large group of patients. The MDRD factors race into the equation accounting for increased muscle mass (and therefore SCr) in African American patients.

When dosing medications based on renal function, either Cockcroft-Gault or MDRD are appropriate; however, most pharmacokinetic studies used the Cockcroft-Gault method. Also most manufacturers of pharmacotherapeutic agents provide renal dosage adjustments utilizing the Cockcroft-Gault equation.

SPECIAL CONSIDERATIONS

Children

The Cockcroft-Gault and MDRD equations are not validated in children and therefore should be used with caution when estimating renal function in pediatrics. The most common equation used to estimate renal function in children is the Schwartz equation.

$$\text{Schwartz GFR (mL/min/1.73m}^2) = [\text{length (in cm)} \times k]/\text{Scr},$$
where k = 0.45 (age <1 year), 0.55 (age 1–13 years),
0.7 (adolescent male), or 0.55 (adolescent female).

The Schwartz equation is convenient and provides a relatively good estimate of GFR in the pediatric population. Height (length) is used in the Schwartz equation as it has been shown to be proportional to muscle mass.

Unstable Renal Function

Using traditional methods for estimating GFR can be problematic in patients with rapidly changing renal function. SCr levels do not correlate well with GFR because there can be a lag in the rise and fall of SCr during acute kidney injury. Equations such as Cockcroft-Gault and MDRD overestimate GFR during periods of renal function decline and underestimate GFR during periods of recovery. If a SCr doubles within 24 hours, the GFR is likely close to zero. Numerous equations have been developed in an attempt to accurately estimate renal function in this patient population. The most commonly accepted is the Jelliffe equation. Clinical judgment must be used to adjust medication dosages in patients with rapidly changing renal function as even the Jelliffe equation has limited supporting data. For example, critically ill patients receiving volume resuscitation may recover renal function rapidly and are at risk for underdosing of antibiotics in sepsis. The effect of unstable renal function on drug clearance and the potential ramifications of overdosing or underdosing the

patient must be considered before making a decision regarding renal dose-adjustment.

CASE Application

Questions 1 through 3 apply to the following case.

BG is a 50-year-old African American woman who is 63 in tall and weighs 130 lb. Her current SCr is 1.6 mg/dL.

1. What is BG's IBW?

   a. 125 lb
   b. 115 lb
   c. 135 lb
   d. 165 lb

2. What is BG's CrCl as estimated by the Cockcroft-Gault equation?

   a. 41 mL/min
   b. 35 mL/min
   c. 50 mL/min
   d. 58 mL/min

3. What is BG's GFR as estimated by the MDRD equation?

   a. 25 mL/min
   b. 35 mL/min
   c. 45 mL/min
   d. 55 mL/min

Questions 4 through 6 apply to the following case.

GS is a 79-year-old African American man who is 71 in tall and weighs 190 lb. His current SCr is 1.2 mg/dL.

4. What is GS's IBW?

   a. 145 lb
   b. 156 lb
   c. 166 lb
   d. 254 lb

5. What is GS's CrCl as estimated by the Cockcroft-Gault equation?

   a. 69 mL/min
   b. 45 mL/min
   c. 81 mL/min
   d. 53 mL/min

6. What is GS's GFR as estimated by the MDRD equation?

   a. 45 mL/min
   b. 55 mL/min
   c. 65 mL/min
   d. 75 mL/min

7. JK is a 4-year-old girl who is 42 in tall and weighs 50 lb. Her current SCr is 0.6 mg/dL. What is JK's estimated GFR based on the Schwartz equation?

   a. ~30 mL/min
   b. ~60 mL/min

   c. ~80 mL/min

   d. ~100 mL/min

8. LO is a 6-month-old infant who is 25 in long and weighs 15 lb. His current SCr is 0.4 mg/dL. What is LO's estimated GFR based on the Schwartz equation?

   a. 60 mL/min

   b. 70 mL/min

   c. 80 mL/min

   d. 90 mL/min

9. Which of the following factors independent from GFR affect SCr? Select all that apply.

   a. Age

   b. Diet

   c. Gender

   d. Race

10. Which of the following patients would be most likely to have a baseline SCr of <0.8 mg/dL?

   a. A 25-year-old man in very good health

   b. A 36-year-old man adhering to the Atkins diet

   c. A 92-year-old woman who is wheelchair bound

   d. A bodybuilder taking creatine supplements

11. Which of the following is considered the gold standard for measurement of GFR?

   a. Cockcroft-Gault equation

   b. MDRD equation

   c. 24-Hour urine creatinine

   d. Inulin clearance

12. Which of the following factors are important to consider when dosing a medication based on renal function? Select all that apply.

   a. The extent to which the drug is renally eliminated

   b. SCr

   c. The manufacturer-recommended dosing guidelines for the agent

   d. Aspartate aminotransferase (AST)

13. GU is a 50-year-old man who is admitted with SCr of 1.1 mg/dL. Twenty-four hours later, his SCr is 2.2 mg/dL. GU is on several medications that need to be dose-adjusted for renal function. What is the most appropriate course of action?

   a. Calculate GU's GFR using the MDRD equation and dose adjust based on the result.

   b. Calculate GU's CrCl using the Cockcroft-Gault equation and dose-adjust based on the result.

   c. Discontinue all of GU's medications until his renal function improves.

   d. Assess each of GU's medications and use clinical judgment to determine the best course of action, balancing the risk of treatment failure with drug toxicity.

14. LN is an 88-year-old man who weighs 70 kg and is 71 in tall. His current SCr is 0.6 mg/dL. What is his CrCl as estimated by the Cockcroft-Gault equation?

   a. 101 mL/min

   b. 51 mL/min

   c. 92 mL/min

   d. 46 mL/min

15. FW is a 33-year-old woman with a SCr of 1.3 mg/dL. She is 64 in tall and weighs 118 lb. She has no past medical history. Which of the following methods is the most appropriate way to estimate her renal function? Select all that apply.

   a. Schwartz equation

   b. MDRD equation

   c. Cockcroft-Gault equation

   d. Jelliffe equation

Questions 16 through 18 apply to the following case.

DA is a 32-year-old African American woman who is 67 in tall and weighs 88 lb. Her current SCr is 0.8 mg/dL.

16. What is DA's IBW?

   a. 135 lb

   b. 125 lb

   c. 145 lb

   d. 85 lb

17. What is DA's CrCl as estimated by the Cockcroft-Gault equation?

   a. 98 mL/min

   b. 115 mL/min

   c. 64 mL/min

   d. 75 mL/min

18. What is DA's GFR as estimated by the MDRD equation?

   a. 54 mL/min

   b. 66 mL/min

   c. 75 mL/min

   d. 88 mL/min

19. Select the normal SCr for an adult patient.

   a. 0.3 mg/dL

   b. 0.7 mg/dL

   c. 1.7 mg/dL

   d. 2.0 mg/dL

20. Select the weight that should be used to calculate the CrCl via the Cockcroft-Gault method.

   a. IBW

   b. Actual body weight

   c. Adjusted body weight

   d. No weight should be used

TAKEAWAY POINTS ››

- The GFR is the best indicator of renal function; however, since it cannot be readily measured, surrogate markers must be used to estimate GFR.
- Inulin clearance is the gold standard for estimating GFR since it is filtered by the glomerulus. Inulin clearance is rarely measured in clinical practice due to cost and need for technical expertise.
- SCr is affected by several factors including age, gender, race, diet, muscle mass, and certain drugs.
- The most practical way to estimate renal function is to use GFR and CrCl estimation equations.

- The MDRD and Cockcroft-Gault equations provide a reasonable estimate of GFR in most patients with stable renal function.
- Both the Cockcroft-Gault and the MDRD equations are *estimates* of renal function.
- In children with stable renal function, the Schwartz equation can be used to estimate GFR.
- In patients with unstable renal function, the standard equations used to estimate GFR become very inaccurate and clinical judgment must be used to assess renal function.

BIBLIOGRAPHY

Cockcroft DW, Gault MH. Prediction of creatinine clearance from serum creatinine. *Nephron.* 1976;16:31-41.

Jelliffe RW. Estimation of creatinine clearance in patients with unstable renal function, without a urine specimen. *Am J Nephrol.* 2002;22(4):320-324.

Jones CA, McQuillan GM, Kusek JW, et al. Serum creatinine levels in the US population: Third National Health and Nutrition Examination Survey. *Am J Kidney Dis.* 1998;32:992-999.

Lemann J, Bidani AK, Bain RP, Lewis EJ, Rohde RD. Use of the serum creatinine to estimate glomerular filtration rate in health and early diabetic nephropathy. *Am J Kidney Dis.* 1990;16:236-243.

Levey AS, Bosch JP, Lewis JB, Greene T, Rogers N, Roth D. A more accurate method to estimate glomerular filtration rate from serum creatinine: a new prediction equation. *Ann Intern Med.* 1999;130:461-470.

National Kidney Foundation. K/DOQI Clinical practice guidelines for chronic kidney disease: evaluation, classification, and stratification. *Am J Kidney Dis.* 2002;39(suppl 1):S1-S266.

Schwartz GJ, Brion LP, Spitzer A. The use of plasma creatinine concentration for estimating glomerular filtration rate in infants, children, and adolescents. *Pediatr Clin North Am.* 1987;34:571-590.

KEY ABBREVIATIONS

AST = aspartate aminotransferase
CrCl = creatinine clearance
GFR = glomerular filtration rate

IBW = ideal body weight
MDRD = modification of diet in renal disease
SCr = serum creatinine

34

Acute Kidney Injury

Trisha N. Branan and W. Anthony Hawkins

FOUNDATION OVERVIEW

Acute kidney injury (AKI) occurs when there is a sudden and significant decrease in kidney function. An increase in the serum creatinine (SCr) concentration is the result of accumulation due to a decrease in the glomerular filtration rate (GFR). The diagnosis of AKI is based on the change in SCr from baseline and/or changes in urinary output (UOP). AKI can occur because the kidneys are vulnerable to certain types of injury. First, they are dependent upon the heart and vasculature to deliver sufficient blood supply to drive glomerular filtration. Second, they are exposed to numerous endogenous and exogenous substances, which are eliminated from the body via the urine.

A classification system has been developed to describe the severity of AKI utilizing SCr, estimated GFR, and UOP. AKI is classified into one of five strata via the acronym RIFLE: *r*isk, *i*njury, *f*ailure, *l*oss, and *e*nd-stage renal disease. The first three categories rate the severity of kidney injury, while the last two categories refer to the time sensitive clinical outcomes. Both AKI defined by the RIFLE criteria and increasing severity of AKI have been associated with increased mortality rates.

PATHOPHYSIOLOGY AND CLASSIFICATION OF ACUTE KIDNEY INJURY

AKI is classified into three types based on location and type of injury: prerenal, intrinsic, and postrenal. Many medications can cause or worsen various types of AKI (Table 34-1).

Prerenal Acute Kidney Injury

Prerenal implies damage or defect occurring before the kidney and is the most commonly encountered type of AKI. A decrease in blood flow/pressure to the kidneys results in a decrease in intraglomerular pressure as well as a decrease in UOP and GFR. Prerenal AKI can occur with total body fluid overload. However, the important factor is the effective arterial blood volume (EABV), not the total body fluid volume. Patients with heart failure, renal artery stenosis, nephrotic-range proteinuria, or advanced liver disease may have an increase in total body water with decreased EABV. This is secondary to decreased cardiac output and/or the fluid shift from the intravascular to extravascular compartment. Although such patients appear fluid overloaded (presenting with edema, rales, ascites, etc.), the decrease in EABV results in decreased perfusion to the kidney and may result in prerenal AKI.

Functional prerenal AKI describes a subtype of prerenal AKI. The mechanism is hypoperfusion and intraglomerular hypotension; however, the pathophysiology occurs at the microscopic level of the glomerulus. Intraglomerular pressure is dependent on the pressure of the blood flow entering Bowman's capsule (via the afferent arteriole) and the pressure of the blood flow leaving Bowman's capsule (via the efferent arteriole). The tone of the afferent arteriole is maintained by vasodilatory prostaglandins such as PGE_2 and prostacyclin (PGI_2). Agents such as nonsteroidal anti-inflammatory drugs (NSAIDs) that inhibit prostaglandin synthesis may cause vasoconstriction of the afferent arteriole and therefore decrease the pressure in Bowman's capsule. Other agents that can cause vasoconstriction of the afferent arteriole include cyclosporine and tacrolimus, though these act by a slightly different mechanism. The tone in the efferent arteriole is maintained by the vasoconstrictive properties of angiotensin II. Agents that decrease the production of angiotensin II or antagonize its effects (angiotensin-converting enzyme inhibitors [ACE-I], angiotensin II receptor antagonists [ARB]) may cause the efferent arteriole to vasodilate. The vasodilation causes decreased pressure in Bowman's capsule (Figure 34-1). Signs and symptoms will be consistent with prerenal AKI, as the decreased perfusion to the glomeruli causes activation of the renin-angiotensin-aldosterone axis with subsequent increases in sodium and water reabsorption.

Intrinsic Acute Kidney Injury

Intrinsic AKI is direct damage to one or more areas of the kidney, including the glomerulus, the tubules, or the interstitium. Examples include glomerulonephritis (GN), acute tubular necrosis (ATN), and acute interstitial nephritis (AIN).

Glomerulonephritis

GN occurs from an immune-mediated process or another precipitating event, such as an acute infection that causes inflammation and direct damage to the glomerulus. Deposits of immune complexes may accumulate and damage the

TABLE 34-1 | **Medications Associated With Acute Kidney Injury**

Pre-renal	Acute Glomerulonephritis	Acute Tubular Necrosis	Acute Interstitial Nephritis
ACE-Is	Gold compounds	Aminoglycosides	Ciprofloxacin
ARBs	Lithium	Amphotericin B	Levofloxacin
Calcineurin inhibitors		Cisplatin	Agents that contain a sulfonamide moiety
NSAIDs		Carboplatin	PCNs
Diuretics		Bisphosphates (IV)	Cephalosporins
		Tenofovir	NSAIDs
		Pentamidine	Proton pump inhibitors
		Sucrose (IV immunoglobulin)	
		Radiocontrast media[a]	
		Vancomycin	
		Polymyxins (IV)	

Abbreviations: ACE-I, angiotensin-converting enzyme inhibitor; ARB, angiotensin receptor blocker; NSAIDs, nonsteroidal anti-inflammatory drugs; IV, intravenous; PCN, penicillins.
[a]Diagnostic agent.

glomerulus causing filtering defects. Large molecules such as proteins and blood cells pass through the glomerulus into the proximal tubule and may be visualized on microscopic urinalysis (UA).

Acute Tubular Necrosis

ATN signifies death of tubular epithelial cells and is the most common form of intrinsic AKI. Cellular debris (muddy brown casts) is specific to ATN and is important to the diagnosis. There are two mechanisms that destroy tubular epithelial cells: 1) prolonged ischemia; 2) direct toxic effects of a substance.

Prolonged ischemia is an extreme form of prerenal AKI that is commonly seen postcardiac arrest. ATN may develop as a consequence of a prerenal AKI that could not be reversed in a timely manner. Aminoglycosides, cisplatin, and radiocontrast media may cause tubular cell apoptosis by a direct toxic effect.

Acute Interstitial Nephritis

AIN is a hypersensitivity reaction manifesting predominantly in the kidneys. AIN is caused by medications or infections. Antimicrobial agents, especially penicillins, are commonly associated with drug allergy and AIN. Because the

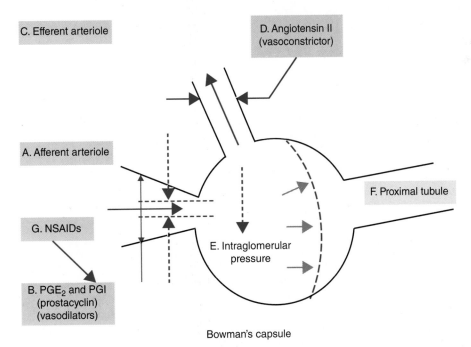

FIGURE 34-1 Physiology and regulation of intraglomerular pressure. Intraglomerular pressure (E), and therefore glomerular filtration rate, depend on the pressure in Bowman capsule. (A) Blood enters the glomerulus via the afferent arteriole. (B) Vasodilatory prostaglandins (PGE$_2$ and prostacyclin) maintain appropriate vascular tone of the afferent arteriole. Substances that cannot pass through the glomerulus into the proximal tubule (F) are returned to systemic circulation via the efferent arteriole (C). Angiotensin II (D) acts to vasoconstrict the efferent arteriole to maintain pressure in Bowman capsule. The effect of angiotensin-converting enzyme inhibitors or angiotensin receptor blockers is seen on regulation of intraglomerular pressure. By inhibiting angiotensin II, these agents cause vasodilation of the efferent arteriole and a subsequent decrease in intraglomerular pressure. The effect of nonsteroidal anti-inflammatory agents (G) occurs in the regulation of intraglomerular pressure. By inhibiting the synthesis of vasodilatory prostaglandins (PGE$_2$ and prostacyclin) these agents cause vasoconstriction of the afferent arteriole and a subsequent decrease in the intraglomerular pressure.

hypersensitivity reaction causes an inflammatory response in the interstitium of the kidney, it is imperative that the causative agent be identified and discontinued as soon as possible.

Postrenal Acute Kidney Injury

Postrenal AKI occurs when an obstruction occurs in the urinary tract below the kidneys that affects the normal flow of urine. There are a variety of substances and situations that cause obstruction of urine flow. The formation of calculi (kidney stones), precipitation of crystals, benign or malignant masses, misplaced indwelling catheters, or hypertrophic prostatic disease can partially or completely block urine flow. The impedance of urine excretion will result in backflow of urine into the kidney. This reverse pressure can damage the kidneys and cause AKI or chronic kidney disease (CKD) if left untreated. As with prerenal AKI, postrenal AKI may resolve completely or cause significant long-term kidney damage depending on the duration of the insult and timeliness of reversal and supportive care.

Urine Output

Anuria is defined as the production of less than 50 mL of urine per day and is associated with complications of hyperkalemia, hypertension, and acid–base disorders. Oliguria is defined as the production of 50 to 400 mL of urine per day.

DIAGNOSIS

The process of differentiating between AKI types involves evaluation of the past medical history, medication history, physical examination, laboratory values, and diagnostic tests (Table 34-2). AKI may be asymptomatic, especially if

TABLE 34-2	Examples of Signs and Symptoms Indicative of Each Type of AKI				
	Prerenal	**GN**	**ATN**	**AIN**	**Postrenal**
Chief complaint/ history of present illness	Dehydration, blood loss, infection, hypotension	Vasculitis/ inflammation, (ie, arthralgias, myalgias)	Infection, hospitalization, procedure with IV contrast, muscular damage	Infection, new medications	Difficulty in urinating, decreased force of stream or intermittent stream
Medical history	Heart failure, renal artery stenosis, severe liver disease	Systemic immune disorder			Genitourinary or GI masses, lithotripsy
Surgical history	Recent surgery—blood loss, hypotension		Procedure with IV contrast		Recent urinary catheter, TURP
Allergies				PCN, sulfa	
Medications	Diuretics, ACE-Is, ARBs, cyclosporine, tacrolimus, NSAIDs	Gold/Lithium	Radiocontrast media, aminoglycosides cisplatin, amphotericin	PCNs, cephalosporins, proton pump inhibitors	α reductase inhibitors, α_1 antagonists, TCAs
Vitals	Low BP, tachycardia			+/- Increased temperature	
Review of systems	Decreased urination, syncopal episode, thirst, blood loss	Unusual arthralgias, myalgias, viral illness			Decreased urination, decreased force of stream, pain on urination
Physical examination	Dehydration/ decreased EABV		Prolonged prerenal state	Possible rash/urticaria	Enlarged prostate, palpable abdominal masses, indwelling bladder catheter
Laboratory values	BUN:SCr >15 (AST/ ALT abnormalities in hepatic dysfunction)	WBC serum markers of immune activation		Increased WBC, eosinophilia	Elevated PSA, elevated urate concentration
Urinalysis	No sediment, SpGr >1.013 >350 mOsm/Kg	Active sediment + protein	Active sediment, muddy brown casts SpGr <1.013 <250 mOsm/kg	Active sediment, +WBC, +/-eosinophils	Active sediment, variable crystalluria
Urine electrolytes	Na <20 mEq/L FENa <1%		Na >20 mEq/L FENa >1-2%		
Urine output	Scant urine		Anuria, oliguria, or polyuria		Anuria or decreased force of stream or painful urination
Tests	Echo: decreased EF				KUB: hydronephrosis

Abbreviations: ALT, alanine aminotransferase; AST, aspartate aminotransferase; BP, blood pressure; BUN, blood urea nitrogen; EABV, effective arteriole blood volume; Echo, echocardiogram; EF, ejection fraction; FENa, fractional excretion of sodium; GI, gastrointestinal; KUB, X-ray of kidney ureters and bladder; Na, sodium; PCN, penicillins; PSA, prostate-specific antigen; SpGr, specific gravity; TCA, tricyclic antidepressant; TURP, transurethral resection of prostate; WBC, white blood cells.

the patient presents early or if the symptoms are masked by other medical conditions. Generally, the first noticeable sign of AKI is a decrease in UOP, which may occur before subsequent increases in blood urea nitrogen (BUN) and SCr. The BUN and SCr concentrations are dependent on the steady state homeostasis of muscle synthesis and breakdown. There are certain circumstances that may cause an increase in the BUN and SCr, confounding the interpretation and clinical correlation. Diseases or drug therapy that may cause muscle breakdown can elevate BUN and SCr concentrations. The use of corticosteroids, diets high in protein, upper gastrointestinal bleeding, and rhabdomyolysis can cause elevated concentrations without altering kidney function. Likewise, BUN and SCr concentrations may be decreased in situations of malnutrition or muscle wasting. Additionally, there are medications that can interfere with the laboratory assay used to quantify the SCr concentration, such as cefazolin, cephalexin, and ascorbic acid.

In addition to assessing and quantifying renal function, BUN and SCr can be useful in differentiating between prerenal and other causes of AKI. Although both parameters may be elevated in any type of AKI, the ratio of BUN to SCr is increased (generally >15:1) in prerenal AKI. In response to hypoxia or poor perfusion, the kidney will compensate by increasing the amount of water that is reabsorbed in the proximal tubule. An increased amount of urea (not creatinine) will be absorbed with the water due to passive diffusion resulting in the disproportionate rise of BUN compared to SCr.

Analysis of Urine

Obtaining and analyzing a urine sample is important in classifying the type of AKI. An analysis comprises three basic components: macroscopic, microscopic, and chemical. Findings from a UA may be nonspecific especially in the case of postrenal obstructive AKI. The UA may be useful in differentiating between prerenal and intrinsic damage, specifically ATN (Table 34-3). In addition to the UA, urine electrolyte (sodium, chloride, potassium) analysis should be performed.

TABLE 34-3	Comparison of Laboratory Results Between Prerenal and Acute Tubular Necrosis Types of AKI	
Laboratory Test	**Prerenal AKI**	**ATN**
Color of urine	Dark, concentrated	Pale, clear
Volume of urine	Scant	Varies (anuria to polyuria)
Urine sediment	Bland (no cells/casts)	Active (cells, casts)
Urine sodium	<20 mEq/L	>40 mEq/L
FENa[a]	<1%	>2%
Urine:serum osmolality	>1.5	<1.5
BUN:SCr	>15-20:1	<15:1
		"Muddy brown casts"[b]

[a]May be falsely high if receiving diuretic therapy. Measurement of urine urea indicated if on diuretic therapy.

[b]Casts of tubular epithelial cells sloughed off and excreted in urine.

Evaluating the urine sodium concentration and calculating the fractional excretion of sodium (FENa) is helpful in differentiating between a prerenal AKI and ATN. In a prerenal state, the kidneys excrete very little sodium as a compensatory mechanism to increase water reabsorption and restore EABV. The FENa is calculated as an accurate means of determining the kidneys' ability to reabsorb sodium, as it takes into account the decrease in urinary sodium excretion due to a decrease in creatinine excretion. Notably, drugs that enhance sodium excretion, namely diuretics, may decrease the clinical utility of the FENa calculation. Under normal conditions, the kidneys excrete approximately 1% to 2% of the total sodium intake (normal FENa value). In a prerenal AKI, the FENa should be lower than 1% as the kidneys should reabsorb more sodium to absorb more water. In contrast, a FENa of greater than 1% occurs in ATN as the tubules are not able to reabsorb the sodium as efficiently. The expected urine findings in prerenal injury would be oliguria/anuria, decreased urinary sodium concentration and low FENa, a high specific gravity, and high urine osmolality (uOsmol). In contrast, the damaged tubules are unable to reabsorb sodium and water in ATN and therefore the urinary sodium concentration and FENa will generally be higher than normal and both the specific gravity and osmolality will be lower than normal.

A urine sample of a patient with prerenal AKI should not contain cells, casts, or other particulate matter. The presence of these substances in the urine may be used to rule out a prerenal AKI and may be consistent with another type of AKI. Unfortunately, the presence of white blood cells, red blood cells, protein, and casts (with the exception of muddy brown casts) occur in many other types of AKI. Urine eosinophils may be caused by a hypersensitivity reaction, supporting the diagnosis of possible AIN. However, lack of urine eosinophils does not rule out AIN. Serum urate concentrations may be helpful if postrenal obstruction from uric acid crystallization is suspected. Other crystals or calculi may be indicative of oversaturation and/or precipitation of particular compounds.

Two diagnostic tests that are helpful to detect a postrenal obstructive AKI are a renal ultrasound or an x-ray of the kidneys, ureters, and bladder (often referred to as a "KUB"). These tests measure the size of the kidneys and can detect the presence of abdominal masses, free air, and fluid collections. Fluid around the kidneys is called hydronephrosis and often signifies reverse flow of urine due to a postrenal obstructive AKI.

A kidney biopsy may be used to determine the type of AKI. This procedure is invasive and is contraindicated in many patients, such as those with uncontrolled hypertension, bleeding diatheses, or those with a solitary kidney. Because this procedure has risks, it is reserved for situations in which the diagnosis is indeterminate by less invasive means.

PREVENTION

The best treatment of AKI is *prevention*. Strategies to protect high-risk patients should include the judicious use (or complete avoidance) of known nephrotoxins and maintenance of optimal fluid status. For example, fluid hydration, sodium

TABLE 34-4	Strategies to Prevent Contrast-Induced Nephropathy
Minimize volume of contrast utilized	
Use agents that are iso-osmolar or have low osmolarity	
Discontinue/avoid the use of nephrotoxins or agents that can alter kidney perfusion	
▪ Diuretics, ACE-I, ARB, NSAIDs, vancomycin, aminoglycosides	
Hydration: fluid hydration with isotonic crystalloid preferred	
▪ 1 mL/kg/h up to 150 mL/h	
▪ Begin 3-6 h pre-procedure and continue for at least 8 h postexposure	
Other potentially beneficial therapies:	
▪ N-acetylcysteine: 600-1200 mg po every 12 h. First dose preprocedure	
▪ Sodium bicarbonate 150 mEq/L in either sterile water or dextrose 5% water IV infusion 3 mL/kg × 1 h before procedure then 1 mL/kg/h for 6 h after procedure	

Abbreviations: ACE-I, angiotensin-converting enzyme inhibitor; ARB, angiotensin receptor blocker; IV, intravenous; NSAIDs, nonsteroidal anti-inflammatory drugs; po, oral.

bicarbonate, and avoidance of hyperosmolar contrast may reduce the risk of contrast-induced nephropathy, with hydration being the best preventative therapy (Table 34-4).

TREATMENT

For all cases of AKI, the first treatment should be supportive care consisting of proper fluid and electrolyte management, acid–base balance, and protection of the kidneys from further insult. Identifying the cause of AKI and stopping/minimizing the damage is imperative in preserving renal function.

Prerenal Acute Kidney Injury

Improving perfusion to the kidneys and optimizing intraglomerular pressure is imperative to mitigating kidney damage. If allowed to persist, hypoxia and ischemia may cause ATN. Efforts to improve perfusion and glomerular pressure may include optimizing cardiac output, volume repletion, and discontinuation/monitoring of agents that can negatively affect EABV or intraglomerular pressure (diuretics, ACE-I, ARBs, calcineurin inhibitors, NSAIDs). Efforts to restore EABV and optimize renal perfusion include the administration of isotonic crystalloid fluids, blood products, inotropes, or the use of vasopressors to maintain systemic blood pressure. Judicious use of albumin in conjunction with diuretics may be beneficial in cases of total body fluid overload with a decrease in EABV such as liver failure or nephrotic syndrome.

Glomerulonephritis

There are many causes and types of GN. As the damage in the glomerulus causes inflammation, corticosteroids or other immunosuppressive agents may be helpful in certain situations. The exact agent/regimen should be determined depending on the specific type of GN.

Acute Interstitial Nephritis

Discontinuation of the offending agent is the first and most important step. As AIN is the result of an inflammatory process, there is some evidence that corticosteroids may be used early in the process to limit damage to the kidney. This treatment is not standard of care, and underlying disease states (such as infection, diabetes) should be considered.

Acute Tubular Necrosis

Once ATN has developed, there is little that can be done to promote or hasten recovery other than supportive care and protecting the kidneys from additional insults. Please refer to the supportive care section below.

Postrenal Acute Kidney Injury

As with prerenal AKI, the most important treatment for postrenal AKI is to identify and reverse/discontinue the cause. Depending on the etiology, there may be specific treatments or pharmacologic agents that can be employed. For example, if the obstruction is caused by prostatic hypertrophy, agents such as tamsulosin may be beneficial. If the obstruction is caused by a neoplasm pressing on the ureter, placement of a ureteral stent or surgical resection might be necessary. If the obstruction is caused in part by the anticholinergic effects of a tricyclic antidepressant used for neuropathic pain, an alternative agent to treat neuropathic pain should be given.

Fluid and Electrolytes

Utilization of diuretics allows for pharmacologic control of fluid and electrolytes (and perhaps drug elimination) and may avoid the need for renal replacement therapy. The patient's total fluid volume as well as an estimation of EABV must be considered before diuretics are instituted. Fluid management may be particularly difficult in heart failure, cirrhosis, and nephrotic syndrome because these disease states make estimation of EABV difficult in the setting of excess total body water. Diuretics should be used with caution in these situations to avoid intravascular depletion acutely. Fluid is slow to redistribute from the tissue back into the vasculature due to capillary leak, third-spacing, and loss of intravascular oncotic pressure. This could lead to hypotension and a new renal insult. Fluid overload may occur rapidly as kidney function declines. The intravenous (IV) fluids administered for volume expansion and hemodynamic support can rapidly accumulate. Additionally, many patients with AKI are critically ill and may require the administration of numerous IV medications that add significantly to the total daily fluid intake. Provided that the patient is not hyponatremic, a sodium restriction of 2 to 3 g/d may be applied. Diuretics should be used judiciously to remove excess fluid, with careful consideration of EABV. Most patients with AKI are prone to hyperkalemia. For this reason, diuretics that antagonize aldosterone (spironolactone, eplerenone), and those that inhibit potassium excretion (triamterene) are often avoided. Thiazide-type diuretics have been shown to be less effective as monotherapy in patients with decreased kidney function. They are, however, often used in combination with a loop diuretic to provide synergistic natriuresis and diuresis. By blocking sodium reabsorption in the loop of Henle (blocking the Na-K-Cl transporter), there is a greater delivery of sodium to the distal tubule. By blocking sodium reabsorption in the distal tubule first, the excretion of sodium and water is greater than what could have been achieved by loop or thiazide alone. If this strategy is utilized, it is important to administer the thiazide-type prior to the loop diuretic.

Any of the loop diuretics can be utilized in AKI. Although there may be a perception that one agent is more effective than another, they all have similar efficacy when given in equipotent doses. There are differences in oral bioavailability, and care should be taken when converting patients from IV to oral preparations. Generally, ethacrynic acid has been reserved for patients with a severe allergy to sulfa moieties. In patients with oliguria/anuria, higher doses may be required as the flow of water and sodium reaching the tubules is decreased. Initial bolus, IV doses are used and then titrated based on response. While higher doses are often needed to achieve the desired effect, ototoxicity is a dose-dependent adverse reaction and the risk to benefit ratio should be considered. In an effort to limit toxicity and enhance receptor blockade, continuous infusions of loop diuretics can be utilized.

Electrolyte Abnormalities

Depending on the type of AKI and the UOP, electrolyte homeostasis may be affected. Generally, electrolytes such as potassium, sodium, magnesium, and phosphorus will accumulate in prerenal AKI (generally low UOP). In cases of intrinsic or postrenal AKI, the effect on electrolytes may vary depending on the UOP as well as the exact location of the damage. ATN may cause significant losses of potassium, magnesium, and even phosphorus, as the tubules are unable to reabsorb the substances appropriately.

Hyperkalemia

The accumulation of potassium in AKI is common and potentially life threatening. Once hyperkalemia develops (or is suspected) an electrocardiogram should be completed immediately to evaluate cardiac effects. Peaked T waves or widened QRS complexes connote a potential life-threatening situation and emergent treatment of hyperkalemia should be initiated.

The first agent that should be given is 1 g of IV calcium (either chloride or gluconate) over 2 to 5 minutes. Calcium antagonizes the cardiac membrane effects of hyperkalemia and stabilizes the heart. The next steps involve shifting potassium from the extracellular to intracellular compartment. While this can be achieved by a variety of means, the most common approach is to first administer 10 units of regular human insulin with 25 g of dextrose 50% IV push over 2 to 5 minutes. Insulin acts to stimulate Na^+/K^+-ATPase receptors to exchange more potassium into the cell and more sodium outside the cell. Although β_2-agonists have the same action, the excitatory effects on the β_2-receptors in the heart may be deleterious. Sodium bicarbonate can also be utilized to cause an intracellular shift of potassium. This agent is generally reserved for patients with an underlying acidosis or in situations when the patient has been hypoxic and presumably in an anaerobic metabolic state. Doses of 50 mEq of sodium bicarbonate can be given by IV injection over 2 to 5 minutes in life-threatening scenarios. While these interventions acutely antagonize the effect of potassium on the myocardium (calcium) or force extracellular potassium into cells, the only way to remove potassium from the body is through the urine, feces, or renal replacement therapy (dialysis). Removal methods have a slower time of onset for potassium correction and should be used in conjunction with the acute management measures discussed above in patients with symptomatic hyperkalemia. If the patient has residual UOP, loop diuretics (and hydration if appropriate) can be utilized to enhance potassium excretion. Sodium polystyrene sulfonate in sorbitol can be given orally or as a retention enema to bind potassium in the gastrointestinal tract to be excreted in the feces. This agent is an exchange resin, binding potassium ions in exchange for sodium ions. For this reason it should be used with caution in patients with heart failure or cirrhosis as it may enhance fluid overload. Renal replacement therapy (RRT) is generally a last line treatment option unless the patient already has vascular or peritoneal access.

Renal Replacement Therapy

RRT, the general term used to refer to any renal dialytic/hemofiltration therapy, is reserved for specific indications. The acronym "AEIOU" is used to remember these indications: *a*cid/base abnormalities, *e*lectrolyte imbalances, *i*ntoxications, fluid *o*verload, and *u*remia (Table 34-5). Any RRT can be used as supportive therapy depending on the hemodynamic stability of the patient, the resources available, and other patient factors. Hemodialysis provides solute and water clearance. However, patients must be hemodynamically stable to withstand the rapid fluid shifts caused by this modality. Continuous renal replacement therapies (CRRT) provide excellent clearance as they run continuously, utilizing slower blood flow and fluid rates and add additional solute removal due to increased convective clearance. These therapies are reserved for patients who are hemodynamically unstable and in an intensive care setting with individualized nursing care. Less commonly, peritoneal dialysis can be used during AKI, provided there are no contraindications (recent abdominal surgery, intra-abdominal infections, ascites).

INDIVIDUALIZING DRUG DOSAGE IN ACUTE KIDNEY INJURY

Pharmacokinetic parameters may be altered due to kidney dysfunction or the use of RRT. Absorption and bioavailability from enteral sources may be diminished secondary to edema and decreased motility in the gastrointestinal tract. Volume of distribution may fluctuate due to edema or fluid removal. While urinary excretion may be altered, other organs may be more active to compensate. One strategy to avoid dosage

TABLE 34-5	"AEIOU"—Indications for Renal Replacement Therapy
A	*Acid–base abnormalities*
	Metabolic acidosis is the most common disorder seen and can predispose patients to cardiac arrhythmias.
E	*Electrolyte abnormalities*
	Hyperkalemia is the most common abnormality seen as the kidneys are responsible for ~95% of the total body elimination. Hyperkalemia can be life threatening, leading to fatal arrhythmias.
I	*Intoxication or ingestion*
	Whether toxic concentrations are intentional, accidental, or simply a consequence of decreased elimination, renal replacement therapy may be employed to remove water soluble or renally excreted compounds that have a low molecular weight. Volume of distribution and protein binding may not preclude clearance with dialysis under toxic conditions.
O	*Overload—fluid overload*
	Pulmonary edema is a life-threatening complication of disease (heart failure) or volume resuscitation that can occur quickly.
U	*Uremia*
	Uremia is a clinical syndrome that occurs due to the accumulation of all of the substances that the body cannot eliminate in severe kidney insufficiency. While all of the toxic substances have not been identified, metabolic wastes, drugs, and other substances may cause symptoms such as intractable nausea/vomiting, pruritus, pericarditis, asterixis, encephalopathy, and seizures. Patients are also at increased bleeding risk due to platelet inhibition.

adjustment is to identify alternative agents that do not require dose adjustment for kidney dysfunction. All medications should be reviewed and evaluated for the potential to cause toxicity, if accumulation occurs due to AKI.

The SCr concentration is of limited use to assess renal function. Although a quick calculation can be used as a basis for determining kidney function, clinical factors and professional judgment should be used in conjunction with common formulas to quantify renal function. The trend in SCr concentrations and UOP should be utilized to assess renal function.

The SCr concentration should not be used to determine kidney function during RRT. The fluctuations in this value reflect the creatinine clearance (CrCl) achieved by the RRT as well as the patient's own clearance. Determining appropriate drug doses during RRT is confounded by numerous factors, including mode of RRT, flow rate, and filter size. Primary literature may provide information regarding dosing regimens successfully employed during RRT. Review articles that compile dosing recommendations for frequently prescribed agents (such as antibiotics) may be especially helpful.

While there are a number of formulas that can be utilized to predict drug dosing during RRT, accurate assessment is difficult. Clinical factors and professional judgment are important in making final recommendations. Factors that can alter drug clearance include the flow rates of blood, dialysate and other solutions, the amount of ultrafiltration (fluid removal),

residual urine output, length of dialysis, and the specific dialyzer pore size. Many times RRT may be interrupted due to clotting within the system or if the patient becomes hemodynamically unstable. When a drug is deemed necessary (no alternative appropriate), a thorough risk versus benefit analysis should be conducted. The risk of subtherapeutic concentrations versus dose-related toxicity must be weighed. Reference texts often recommend initial doses based on a CrCl of 10 to 50 mL/min. Once the drug is initiated, therapeutic drug monitoring of serum concentrations may be useful if available. The clinician must rely on careful monitoring for subjective signs and symptoms as well as objective measures to assess the safety and efficacy of the regimen.

PROGNOSES AND OUTCOMES

The mortality rate of AKI is highly dependent upon the etiology, severity, and duration of the damage as well as the existing comorbidities of the patient. Prerenal AKI is generally reversible, and most patients regain independent kidney function.

CASE Application

1. AH is a 72-year-old woman who presents to the emergency room complaining of severe nausea and vomiting for 3 days. On admission, her SCr is 2.5 mg/dL (her baseline is 1.1 mg/dL). She has not been able to eat or drink for 3 days and has lost 2.5 kg. Her medications on admission include: hydrochlorothiazide 25 mg po every day, lisinopril 10 mg po every day. Which of the following statements is *true* regarding AH at this time? Select all that apply.

   a. Nausea and vomiting may have caused a decrease in her EABV leading to prerenal AKI.
   b. AH should not receive radiocontrast media unless absolutely necessary until her kidneys recover.
   c. Hydrochlorothiazide may have caused vasoconstriction of the afferent arteriole leading to prerenal AKI.
   d. Lisinopril should be discontinued until AH's kidney function returns near her baseline.
   e. AH's weight loss suggests fluid volume depletion.

2. Which of the following findings is consistent with the diagnosis of prerenal AKI?

   a. Specific gravity 1.029, FENa 0.85%, uOsmol 550 mOsm/kg
   b. Specific gravity 1.013, FENa 1.75%, uOsmol 350 mOsm/L
   c. Specific gravity 1.009, FENa 2.04%, uOsmol 213 mOsm/L
   d. UA: 1+ protein, 10 to 15 RBC, 10 to 15 WBC

3. A patient in the intensive care unit develops AKI. You review the medications the patient has been taking to

evaluate for drug-induced AKI. Which of the following agents would be *most likely* to cause AIN?

a. Labetalol
b. Diltiazem
c. Nafcillin
d. Propofol

4. Which of the following statements is *true* regarding the use of diuretics in patients with oliguric AKI?

a. Diuretics increase urine output and reverse kidney damage.
b. Diuretics can be used in very high doses with little concern for toxicity.
c. Thiazides and potassium-sparing diuretics are the preferred agents in AKI.
d. Diuretics may improve urine output and help manage fluid and electrolyte abnormalities.

5. Which of the following agents can cause constriction of the *afferent* arteriole? Select all that apply.

a. Ibuprofen
b. Tacrolimus
c. Captopril
d. Rocephin
e. Cyclosporine

6. Which of the following combinations would be effective to enhance urine production in a patient who has oliguric AKI secondary to ATN?

a. Furosemide and ethacrynic acid
b. Triamterene and hydrochlorothiazide
c. Bumetanide and spironolactone
d. Furosemide and metolazone

7. A patient with ATN with anuria has a serum potassium concentration of 6.8 mEq/L with associated electrocardiogram changes of peaked T waves. Which intervention should be initiated first?

a. Regular insulin 10 units and 25 g of dextrose 50% IV push over 2 to 5 minutes
b. Sodium bicarbonate 8.4% 50 mEq IV push over 2 to 5 minutes
c. Calcium gluconate 1 g IV push over 2 to 5 minutes
d. Sodium polystyrene sulfonate 15 g po

8. Which of the following regimens would be the most appropriate prophylaxis option for contrast-induced nephropathy in a high-risk patient?

a. Acetadote 150 mg/kg IV for 6 hours preprocedure
b. Sodium chloride 0.9% IV infusion 6 hours before and 8 hours after
c. Theophylline 200 mg po every 12 hours, two doses before, two doses after
d. Dopamine 0.5 mcg/kg/min IV infusion 6 hours before and 6 hours after

9. Which of the following circumstances can lead to ATN? Select all that apply.

a. Administration of a direct nephrotoxin
b. Prolonged hypotension
c. Prolonged prerenal AKI
d. Metronidazole
e. Colistin

10. Which of the following statements is *true* regarding drug dosing in AKI?

a. All patients should be dosed for a CrCl <10 mL/min.
b. Pharmacokinetic parameters do not usually change so dose adjustment is not needed.
c. Although elimination may be decreased, the volume of distribution should remain unchanged in AKI.
d. The estimation of kidney function should include urine output.

11. Which of the following UA findings would be *indicative* of acute GN?

a. Protein
b. Muddy brown casts
c. pH 8.0
d. Eosinophils

12. Which of the following statements appropriately defines urine volume?

a. Anuria is defined as <50 mL of urine per day.
b. Oliguria is defined as <50 mL of urine per day.
c. Polyuria is defined as <50 mL of urine per day.
d. Anuria is defined as no urea in the urine.

13. Place the acronym "AEIOU" in the correct order as it relates to the indications for RRT.

a. A, *a*cid–base imbalance; E, *E*KG changes; I, *i*nflammation; O, *o*btundation; U, *u*remia
b. A, *a*cute distress; e, *e*lectrolyte disturbance; I, *i*nflammation; O, *o*vert proteinuria; U, *u*remia
c. A, *a*cid–base imbalance; E, *e*lectrolyte disturbance; I, *i*ngestion/intoxication; O, *f*luid overload; U, *u*remia
d. A, *a*cid–base imbalance; E, *E*KG abnormality; I, *i*ngestion/intoxication; O, *o*liguria; U, *u*remia

14. CB is a 24-year-old man brought to the hospital by his roommate. He states that he has been having diarrhea and vomiting for 3 days. He reports a 3 kg weight loss and cannot keep down anything, even water. In the emergency department (ED) his BP is 96/46 mm Hg, HR 120 beats/min, temp is 102.6°F, weight is 65 kg. On examination, his mucous membranes are dry and he has no peripheral edema. He does not recall the last time that he urinated but thinks it may have been yesterday. Which of the following findings would you expect from his serum and urine laboratory analysis?

a. SpGr 1.035, 0 protein, dark yellow urine, no casts, FENa <1%

b. SpGr 1.035, 0 protein, hazy-red urine, granular casts, FENa >2%

c. SpGr 1.016, 2+ protein, light-yellow urine, many WBC and RBCs

d. SpGr 1.005, 0 protein, hazy-red urine, granular casts, FENa >1%

15. Which of the following statements best describes the BUN to SCr ratio?

a. In situations of dehydration, the BUN:SCr ratio will be <10:1.

b. In situations of dehydration, the BUN:SCr ratio will be >15:1.

c. In situations of volume overload, the BUN:SCr ratio will be <10:1.

d. In situations of volume overload, the BUN:SCr ratio will be >15:1.

16. MT is a 38-year-old man brought to the ED after being found at the bottom of the stairs to his apartment. Apparently, while he was intoxicated, MT fell down the stairs, and remained unresponsive for approximately 6 to 12 hours. In the ED, he was diagnosed with rhabdomyolysis. Which of the following statements best describes rhabdomyolysis?

a. Rhabdomyolysis may cause AIN.

b. Rhabdomyolysis may cause ATN.

c. Rhabdomyolysis may cause eosinophilia and eosinophiluria.

d. MT should undergo RRT for his rhabdomyolysis.

17. Hyperkalemia may result from AKI and can lead to which one of the following life-threatening complications?

a. Seizures

b. Arrhythmias

c. Hypertension

d. Acidosis

18. TB is a 62-year-old woman with a history of CKD and heart failure. Her baseline SCr is 1.8 mg/dL with a corresponding CrCl of approximately 50 mL/min. Today she is brought by ambulance to the emergency room with dyspnea at rest (currently has an oxygen saturation of 100% on 2 L room air of oxygen) and lower extremity edema all the way up to her thighs. Laboratory analysis shows a SCr of 3.6 mg/dL and she does not recall urinating at all in the past 24 hours. Which of the following best describes TB's kidney injury?

a. Her CrCl is essentially zero as she is not making urine.

b. Her CrCl is approximately 25 mL/min.

c. Her CrCl is still approximately 50 mL/min.

d. Acute hemodialysis is indicated.

19. CG is a 58-year-old woman with a history of stage 4 ovarian cancer. She has metastases in her colon, abdominal cavity, liver, and bone. Recently, she has undergone chemotherapy and radiation as palliative treatment. Today she is admitted due to 1-week history of fatigue, malaise, nausea, vomiting, and she notes that she has not urinated for days. Upon examination, the doctor notes that her bladder is palpable and distended. Which of the following tests would be best to confirm a postrenal obstruction in this patient? Select all that apply.

a. MRI with contrast media

b. CT abdomen with contrast media

c. KUB

d. Renal ultrasound

e. MRI of the bladder without contrast

20. Which of the following agents may be used to treat AIN?

a. Prednisone

b. Furosemide

c. Lisinopril

d. Ibuprofen

TAKEAWAY POINTS »

- The best treatment for AKI is prevention.
- AKI can result in permanent kidney damage and CKD.
- The first step in treating AKI is to identify the cause and stop/reverse it.
- Unnecessary exposure to nephrotoxins should be avoided during AKI.
- Supportive care includes management of fluid and electrolyte abnormalities, acid–base balance, blood pressure support/control, avoidance of potential nephrotoxins/further insults, and proper drug dosing.
- Diuretic therapy may be used to enhance fluid and electrolyte excretion.
- Targeted pharmacotherapy may be considered for AIN and GN.
- Drug dosing should be individualized for each patient and close monitoring is necessary.

BIBLIOGRAPHY

Bagshaw SM, George C, Dinu I, Bellomo R. A multi-centre evaluation of the RIFLE criteria for early acute kidney injury in critically ill patients. *Nephrol Dial Transplant.* 2008;23:1203-1210.

Bellomo R, Kellum J, Ronco C. Acute kidney injury. *Lancet.* 2012;380:756-766.

Bentley M, Corwin H, Dasta J. Drug-induced acute kidney injury in the critically ill adult: Recognition and prevention strategies. *Crit Care Med.* 2010;38(6):S169-174.

Coca SG, Singanamala S, Parikh CR. Chronic kidney disease after acute kidney injury: A systematic review and meta-analysis. *Kidney Int.* 2012;81:442-448.

Hoste EA, Clermont G, Kersten A, et al. RIFLE criteria for acute kidney injury are associated with hospital mortality in critically ill patients: A cohort analysis. *Crit Care.* 2006;10:R73.

Kellum J, Lameire N. Diagnosis, evaluation, and management of acute kidney injury: a KDIGO summary (Part 1). *Crit Care.* 2013;17:204.

Kidney Disease: Improving Global Outcomes (KDIGO) Acute Kidney Injury Workgroup. KDIGO clinical practice guideline for acute kidney injury. *Kidney Int Suppl.* 2012;2:1-138.

Mehta RL, Kellum JA, Shah SV, et al. Acute Kidney Injury Network: Report of an initiative to improve outcomes in acute kidney injury. *Crit Care.* 2007;11:R31.

Ricci Z, Ronco C. Year in review 2007: Critical Care—Nephrology. *Crit Care.* 2008;12:230.

Siew ED, Matheny ME, Ikizler TA, et al. Commonly used surrogates for baseline renal function affect the classification and prognosis of acute kidney injury. *Kidney Int.* 2010;77:536-542.

Zavada J, Hoste E, Cartin-Ceba R, et al. A comparison of three methods to estimate baseline creatinine for RIFLE classification. *Nephrol Dial Transplant.* 2010;25:3911-3918.

KEY ABBREVIATIONS

ACE-I = angiotensin converting enzyme-inhibitor
ARB = angiotensin receptor blockers
AIN = acute interstitial nephritis
AKI = acute kidney injury
ATN = acute tubular necrosis
BUN = blood urea nitrogen
CKD = chronic kidney disease
CRRT = continuous renal replacement therapy

EABV = effective arterial blood volume
FENa = fractional excretion of sodium
GFR = glomerular filtration rate
GN = glomerulonephritis
NSAIDs = nonsteroidal anti-inflammatory drugs
RRT = renal replacement therapy
SCr = serum creatinine
UOP = urinary output

35

Chronic Kidney Disease/End-Stage Renal Disease

Melinda (Mindy) J. Burnworth and Ted Walton

FOUNDATION OVERVIEW

Chronic kidney disease (CKD) is a progressive disease staged on the patient's glomerular filtration rate (GFR) and presence of albuminuria. The National Kidney Foundation's Kidney Disease Outcomes Quality Initiative (KDOQI) and the global nonprofit foundation, Kidney Disease: Improving Global Outcomes (KDIGO), define CKD as: (1) pathological abnormalities or markers of kidney damage such as proteinuria present for more than or equal to 3 months with or without a decreased GFR, or (2) a GFR less than 60 mL/min/1.73 m^2 for more than or equal to 3 months. Staging of CKD identifies patients at higher risk of worsening clinical manifestations and disease complications. Stages are determined by GFR and albuminuria categories. See Table 35-1 for CKD staged by GFR. Albuminuria is categorized by urine albumin-to-creatinine ratio (ACR) as mg/g or urinary albumin excretion rate (AER) as mg/24 hour. A1 is less than 30 ACR or AER (normal to mildly increased protein). A2 is 30 to 300 ACR or AER (moderately increased). A3 is greater than 300 ACR or AER (including nephrotic syndrome) (severely increased). Kidney failure is defined as: (1) a GFR less than 15 mL/min/1.73 m^2, or (2) a need for kidney replacement therapy (KRT) such as continuous renal replacement therapy (CRRT), intermittent hemodialysis (IHD), peritoneal dialysis (PD), or kidney transplantation to maintain renal homeostasis and avoid complications. End-stage renal disease (ESRD) is an administrative term that determines reimbursement conditions for health care by the Medicare ESRD Program. ESRD includes patients treated by dialysis or transplantation, irrespective of the level of GFR.

Diabetes and hypertension (HTN) are the most common causes of CKD that lead to kidney failure. Diabetic nephropathy is thought to be caused by vascular changes from chronic hyperglycemia. Renal afferent arteriole vasodilation is hypothesized to result from hyperglycemia and high insulin-like growth factor-1 (IGF-1) concentrations resulting in glomerular hyperfiltration. Alterations in hemodynamics, solute transport, and growth factors eventually cause proteinuria and an inflammatory process which results in activation of the renin-angiotensin-aldosterone system (RAAS), fibrosis, and loss of renal function. HTN is both a cause and a complication of CKD. HTN is a risk factor for progression of kidney disease by accelerating proteinuria and activation

of the RAAS. Uncontrolled HTN in the patient with renal disease can lead to cardiovascular (CV) complications such as heart attacks and strokes. Other causes include various kidney pathologies such as polycystic kidney disease, glomerulonephritis, and renal arterial stenosis. Medications such as nonsteroidal anti-inflammatory drugs (NSAIDS), lithium, calcineurin inhibitors, and herbal or over-the-counter medicines containing aristolechic acid can also cause long-term kidney damage.

The diagnosis of CKD can vary depending upon the underlying etiologic disease state and the stage at which the patient presents. In general, patient workup should include laboratory studies such as a basic chemistry panel, calculation of GFR, measurement of proteinuria/albuminuria, and radiologic studies.

The clinical manifestations of CKD worsen as renal function declines and can include nausea/vomiting, anorexia, fatigue, insomnia, decreased urination, swelling of legs/feet, itching, shortness of breath, and muscle cramping. Kidney failure may cause significant fluid overload and severe uremia. Uremia is a clinical syndrome associated with fluid, electrolyte, and hormone imbalances and metabolic abnormalities that occur in patients with advanced kidney failure due to the inadequate clearance of toxic metabolites. Furthermore, additional complications of impaired renal function include anemia, mineral and bone disorders, CV complications, and vitamin irregularities.

PREVENTION

Although CKD is generally progressive and irreversible, there are steps to slow progression to kidney failure. There are several strategies for slowing progression which include improving blood pressure control and improving glucose control for patients with diabetes. Delaying the progression to kidney failure and dialysis has been shown to improve quality of life and decrease mortality in patients with CKD.

Controlling blood pressure is the most effective intervention to slow the progression of CKD. When tolerated, angiotensin-converting enzyme (ACE) inhibitors or angiotensin II receptor blockers (ARBs) are considered first-line therapy for blood pressure control and to reduce albuminuria. In addition to treating HTN, these drugs have shown

TABLE 35-1 Glomerular Filtration Rate Categories Based on KDIGO Classification

GFR Category[a]	GFR (mL/min/1.73 m²)	Terms
1	>90	Normal or high
2	60-89	Mildly decreased
3a	45-59	Mildly to moderately decreased
3b	30-44	Moderately to severely decreased
4	15-29	Severely decreased
5	<15	Kidney failure

Abbreviations: CKD, chronic kidney disease; GFR, glomerular filtration rate; KDIGO, Kidney Disease: Improving Global Outcomes.

[a]To meet criteria for CKD, there must be a significant reduction in GFR (categories 3a-5) or there must also be evidence of kidney damage (categories 1 and 2) for 3 months or greater.

Data from Kidney Disease: Improving Global Outcomes (KDIGO) CKD Work Group. KDIGO 2012 Clinical Practice Guideline for the Evaluation and Management of Chronic Kidney Disease. Kidney Int Suppl 2013;3:1-150.

benefit in albuminuric kidney disease in patients without HTN. See Table 35-2 for a comparison of ACE inhibitors and ARBs as first-line antihypertensive agents in CKD. Optimal glucose control for patients with diabetes prior to the development of kidney disease may delay or prevent its occurrence. However, once kidney disease is present, it is unclear if tight glucose control may be more beneficial than less control in the progression of kidney disease. See Table 35-3 for selected treatment goals for HTN and diabetes mellitus (DM) in the setting of CKD.

TREATMENT

The purpose of nonpharmacologic and pharmacologic treatment is identical, namely, to slow progression of CKD and to prevent/treat complications of reduced renal function. Clinical practice guidelines provided by KDOQI and KDIGO are designed to assist clinician decision making in patients with renal disease. However, the needs of individual patients, available resources, and limitations unique to an institution or type of practice may appropriately lead to variations in management.

Nonpharmacologic Treatment

The main nonpharmacologic interventions include diet therapy and lifestyle modifications. Patients with CKD should be referred to a clinical nutritionist for counseling and optimal diet choices.

The National Kidney Disease Education Program (NKDEP) recommends that dietary sodium be limited to 2300 mg/d to help control blood pressure. Salt substitutes are usually rich in potassium and should generally be avoided with lower GFR values or if the patient is taking medications that retain potassium such as ACE inhibitors or ARBs. Potassium free salt substitutes are available and patient counseling is helpful in choosing the correct product.

Reduction of protein intake may reduce albuminuria and slow progression of CKD. KDIGO recommends an adequate protein intake of 0.8 g/kg/d in all patients with CKD who have a GFR less than 30 mL/min/1.73 m².

As CKD progresses, the kidney's ability to regulate phosphorus (Phos) and calcium (Ca) levels may lead to bone

TABLE 35-2 ACE inhibitors and ARBs as First-Line Antihypertensive Agents in CKD

Class	Drug (Brand Name)	Usual Dose Range (mg/d)	Daily Frequency	Comments
ACE inhibitors	Benazepril (Lotensin)	10-40	1 or 2	May cause hyperkalemia in patients with CKD or in those receiving a potassium-sparing diuretic, aldosterone antagonist, ARB, or direct renin inhibitor; can cause acute kidney failure in patients with severe bilateral renal artery stenosis or severe stenosis in artery to solitary kidney; do not use in pregnancy or in patients with a history of angioedema; cough is a bothersome side effect; starting dose should be reduced 50% in patients who are on a thiazide, are volume depleted, or are very elderly due to risks of hypotension.
	Captopril (Capoten)	12.5-150	2 or 3	
	Enalapril (Vasotec)	5-40	1 or 2	
	Fosinopril (Monopril)	10-40	1	
	Lisinopril (Prinivil, Zestril)	10-40	1	
	Moexipril (Univasc)	7.5-30	1 or 2	
	Perindopril (Aceon)	4-16	1	
	Quinapril (Accupril)	10-80	1 or 2	
	Ramipril (Altace)	2.5-10	1 or 2	
	Trandolapril (Mavik)	1-4	1	
ARB	Azilsartan (Edarbi)	40-80	1	May cause hyperkalemia in patients with CKD or in those receiving a potassium-sparing diuretic, aldosterone antagonist, ACE inhibitor, or direct renin inhibitor; can cause acute kidney failure in patients with severe bilateral renal artery stenosis or severe stenosis in artery to solitary kidney; do not cause a dry cough like an ACE inhibitor may; do not use in pregnancy; starting dose should be reduced 50% in patients who are on a thiazide, are volume depleted, or are very elderly due to risks of hypotension.
	Candesartan (Atacand)	8-32	1 or 2	
	Eprosartan (Teveten)	600-800	1 or 2	
	Irbesartan (Avapro)	150-300	1	
	Losartan (Cozaar)	50-100	1 or 2	
	Olmesartan (Benicar)	20-40	1	
	Telmisartan (Micardis)	20-80	1	
	Valsartan (Diovan)	80-320	1	

Abbreviations: ACE, angiotensin-converting enzyme; ARB, angiotensin II receptor blocker; CKD, chronic kidney disease.
Adapted with permission from DiPiro JT, Talbert RL, Yee GC, et al: *Pharmacotherapy: A Pathophysiologic Approach*, 10th ed. New York, NY: McGraw-Hill; 2017.

TABLE 35-3	Selected BP and Glucose Goals in CKD
Recommendation Area	**Specific Recommendation**
Glycemic goals	HbA$_{1c}$ goal for nonpregnant adults in general is <7%.
	HbA$_{1c}$ goal should be individualized, with <6.5% if achieved without significant hypoglycemia or adverse effects in younger, long-life expectancy, and no CVD patients.
	Less stringent HbA$_{1c}$ goal (<8%) may be appropriate in patients with a history of severe hypoglycemia, limited life expectancy, advanced micro/macrovascular complications or comorbidities, or in difficult to reach goal patients despite adequate therapy.
Blood pressure	Systolic blood pressure should be treated to <140 mm Hg.
	Diastolic blood pressure should be treated to <90 mm Hg.
	Lower systolic blood pressure <130 mm Hg and/or diastolic blood pressure <80 mm Hg goals may be appropriate for some, such as younger patients or patients with diabetes and urine albumin excretion >30 mg/24 h, if attained without undue treatment burden.

Abbreviations: BP, blood pressure; CKD, chronic kidney disease; HbA$_{1c}$, hemoglobin A1C.
Data from DiPiro JT, Talbert RL, Yee GC, et al: *Pharmacotherapy: A Pathophysiologic Approach*, 10th ed. New York, NY: McGraw-Hill; 2017.

disease and calcification of vascular and soft tissues. If serum Phos levels become elevated, avoiding food with Phos food additives may be an appropriate first step before progressing to pharmacologic therapy, renal replacement therapy, or parathyroidectomy. Limiting potassium intake may be necessary as hyperkalemia may contribute to cardiac abnormalities such as arrhythmias.

Smoking cessation is an important intervention as cigarette smoking is associated with abnormal albuminuria and progression of CKD. Smoking also increases the risk for heart attacks and strokes in this population.

Patients should be encouraged to participate in physical activity, both aerobic and strength training, at a goal of 20 to 30 minutes every day. Physical activity may help prevent CV disease, improve glucose control in patients with diabetes, and maintain muscle mass.

Ultimately, patients with advanced CKD/kidney failure will require KRT such as CRRT, IHD, or PD. These modalities are most effective to maintain renal homeostasis and avoid complications when used in combination with diet therapy and lifestyle modifications. IHD is the most common modality performed three times per week for about 4 hours per session in a dialysis center. The dialysis machine and dialyzer filter remove uremic waste products and extra fluid from the blood. While KRT is beneficial at removing toxins, clinicians must be mindful that these therapies may also remove therapeutic medications.

Specifically, IHD may alter the pharmacokinetics (absorption, distribution, metabolism, elimination) of medications. For example, IHD can result in a decreased volume of distribution (Vd) for medications resulting from fluid removal. In addition, certain drugs such as phenytoin have a larger Vd in patients who have elevated blood urea nitrogen levels. After IHD, the Vd of phenytoin can shrink and result in higher nonprotein bound drug levels than expected. IHD can also change drug elimination by resulting in the rapid removal of small molecule drugs. Pharmacists should be aware of the type of IHD (high flux or low flux) being used. High-flux dialysis uses dialysis filters that have more permeable membranes that allow for additional solute (and medication) removal. Pharmacists may suggest appropriate timing of medication administration (typically after IHD on dialysis days) or medication prescribing alterations (lower daily dose or supplemental dosing after IHD, increased administration interval such as every other day, or a combination of change in dosing and interval) to facilitate adequate drug concentrations while minimizing toxicities. In addition, avoidance of some medications may be recommended in the setting of CKD/kidney failure based on accumulation of active drug or metabolites. Pharmacists will individualize medications based on drug parameters (eg, side effects and pharmacokinetics) and patient-specific parameters (eg, trends in renal function and clinical condition).

As a last resort, kidney transplantation may be necessary and requires an interdisciplinary health care approach.

Pharmacologic Treatment

The mainstay of pharmacologic interventions aim to prevent and/or treat complications of impaired renal function such as anemia, mineral and bone disorders, CV complications, and vitamin irregularities. Several medications have shown benefit depending upon the complication.

Anemia of Chronic Kidney Disease

As an individual's stage of CKD progresses and approximates a GFR less than 60 mL/min/1.73 m^2, anemia develops. Anemia of CKD occurs in approximately 90% of patients receiving dialytic therapy. Symptoms of anemia include fatigue, weakness, angina, and shortness of breath. Anemia in patients with CKD is usually the result of decreased production of erythropoietin in the kidneys but can be multifactorial including blood loss, iron deficiency, folate and B12 deficiency, and aluminum toxicity. Patients with CKD who develop anemia should be evaluated for other causes of anemia prior to the initiation of erythropoiesis-stimulating agents (ESAs). Data have shown that over 50% of patients with hematocrit values less than 25 g/dL have iron deficiency. Hemoglobin (Hgb) formation is dependent on both effective erythropoiesis and adequate iron stores. Therefore, the initiation of ESAs and iron replacement therapies are effective in treating anemia of CKD.

Erythropoiesis Stimulating Agents

Treatment of anemia in patients with CKD requires effective use of exogenous ESAs, guided by appropriate monitoring of

TABLE 35-4	Erythropoiesis-Stimulating Agents in Chronic Kidney Disease			
Drug Name	**Brand Name(s)**	**Starting Dose**	**Route of Administration**	**Half-Life (Hours)**
Epoetin alfa	Epogen, Procrit	Adults: 50-100 units/kg three times per wk Pediatrics: 50 units/kg three times per wk	IV or SubQ	8.5 (IV) 24 (SubQ)

Darbepoetin alfa	Aranesp	Adults:
		 ND-CKD: 0.45 mcg/kg once every 4 wk
		 CKD 5HD or CKD 5PD: 0.45 mcg/kg once per wk or
		   0.75 mcg/kg every 2 wk
		 Pediatrics:
		 0.45 mcg/kg once weekly; may give 0.75 mcg/kg once
		   every 2 wk in ND-CKD patients
			IV or SubQ	25 (IV)
				 48 (SubQ)

Methoxy PEG-epoetin beta	Mircera	All adult CKD patients: 0.6 mcg/kg every 2 wk; once Hgb stabilizes, double the dose and administer monthly (eg, if administering 0.6 mcg/kg every 2 wk, give 1.2 mcg/kg every mo)	IV or SubQ	134 (IV) 139 (SubQ)

Abbreviations: CKD, chronic kidney disease; HD, hemodialysis; Hgb, hemoglobin; IV, intravenous; mcg, microgram; mo, month; ND-CKD, nondialysis CKD patients; PD, peritoneal dialysis; PEG, Polyethylene glycol; SubQ, subcutaneous; wk, week.

Adapted with permission from DiPiro JT, Talbert RL, Yee GC, et al: *Pharmacotherapy: A Pathophysiologic Approach*, 10th ed. New York, NY: McGraw-Hill; 2017.

blood indices including Hgb. ESAs induce erythropoiesis by stimulating the division and differentiation of committed erythroid progenitor cells and the release of reticulocytes from bone marrow into the bloodstream.

Various ESAs therapy including recombinant human erythropoietin (rHuEPO) (ie, epoetin alfa or Procrit®, Epogen®), novel erythropoiesis-stimulating protein (NESP) (ie, darbepoetin alfa or Aranesp®), and methoxy polyethylene glycol-epoetin beta (Mircera®) are used for the management of patients with anemia secondary to renal disease. It is important to note that, in patients with CKD, ESAs carry a blackbox warning for increased mortality, serious CV events, thromboembolic events, and stroke when administered ESAs to target an Hgb level of greater than 11 g/dL. Common side effects with ESAs include elevated blood pressure, nausea/vomiting, diarrhea, headache, muscle pain, swelling, or rash. While there is a consensus among various sources for individualized doses of ESAs to ensure safety and efficacy, there does not seem to be a general agreement on the target Hgb values (ranges from 9 to 11.5 g/dL).

Guidelines recommend monthly monitoring of Hgb with ESAs, minimum interval of 2 weeks between dosage adjustments, no more than a 1 to 2 g/dL increase in Hgb monthly, decreasing dosage (instead of holding) when reduction in Hgb is needed as well as replacing missed doses as soon as possible and consideration for intravenous (IV) administration of ESAs for patients receiving dialytic therapy. Table 35-4 provides an overview of ESAs.

Iron Replacement Therapies

Patients with CKD commonly are iron deficient (functional and/or absolute) due to multiple factors including blood loss and administration of ESAs. Treatment of anemia in patients with CKD/ESRD requires effective use of iron agents, guided by appropriate testing of iron status. Efficacy of iron therapy appears not to be limited to patients with evidence of iron deficiency. Thus, the goals of iron therapy are to avoid storage iron depletion, prevent iron-deficient erythropoiesis, and achieve and maintain target Hgb levels.

Due to the limitations of oral iron therapy (variable elemental iron content, poor absorption, gastrointestinal (GI) side effects, drug-drug interactions, and unintended toxicities), guidelines recommend regular use of small doses of parenteral iron to prevent iron deficiency and promote better erythropoiesis with ESAs especially in patients receiving dialytic therapy. Oral iron therapy may be effective in patients with the beginning stages of CKD. Assessment of iron status is evaluated through periodic laboratory parameter monitoring such as serum ferritin (goal ≥500 ng/mL) and percent transferrin saturation (TSAT) more than or equal to 30%.

Common side effects associated with parenteral iron products include hypotension, peripheral edema, headache, nausea, and muscle cramps. Although rare (<1%), anaphylactic/anaphylactoid reactions including serious or life-threatening responses have been reported. Cardiopulmonary resuscitation equipment and personnel should be available during initial administration until tolerance has been demonstrated. Tables 35-5 and 35-6 provide an overview of IV and oral iron products, respectively.

Mineral and Bone Disorders

Patients with CKD have reduced plasma levels of vitamin D resulting in reduced intestinal absorption of Ca and also decreased Phos elimination. This combined with reduced elimination of Phos by the kidney leads to hyperphosphatemia and hypocalcemia. These abnormalities negatively affect parathyroid hormone (PTH) production and the body tries to compensate by altering Ca and Phos concentrations in the kidney and bone. As bones are the major source for Ca in the body, elevated PTH will increase osteoclasts to break down bone to release Ca into the serum. This results in secondary hyperparathyroidism, which is a subset of the syndrome more commonly referred to as mineral and bone disorders

TABLE 35-5   Overview of Intravenous Iron Products

Iron Compounds	Brand Name(s)	Half-Life (Hours)	Molecular Weight (Daltons)	FDA-Approved Indications	FDA-Approved Dosing[a]	Dose Ranges (mg)[b]
Ferric carboxymaltose	Injectafer	7-12	150,000	Adult patients with intolerance to oral iron or who have had an unsatisfactory response to oral iron and in adult patients with CKD not on dialysis	Give two doses separated by at least 7 d of 750 mg per dose (if body weight is ≥50 kg) or 15 mg/kg per dose (if body weight is <50 kg) not to exceed 1500 mg per course. Give either IV push (100 mg per min) or diluted in not more than 250 mL of 0.9% NaCl as an infusion over at least 15 min	750
Ferumoxytol	Feraheme	15	750,000	Adult patients with iron-deficiency anemia associated with chronic kidney disease	510 mg (17 mL) as a single dose, followed by a second 510 mg dose 3-8 d after the initial dose. Dilute in 50-200 mL of 0.9% NaCl or 5% dextrose and administer as an IV infusion over 15 min	510
Iron dextran	INFeD Dexferrum	40-60	96,000 265,000	Patients with iron deficiency in whom oral iron is unsatisfactory or impossible	100 mg over 2 min (25-mg test dose required) Note: Equation provided by manufacturer to calculate dose based on desired Hgb	25-1000
Iron sucrose	Venofer	6	43,000	Adult and pediatric CKD 5HD patients aged 2 y and older	Adult: 100 mg over 2-5 min or 100 mg in maximum of 100 mL of 0.9% NaCl over 15 min per consecutive HD session Pediatric: 0.5 mg/kg not to exceed 100 mg per dose over 5 min or diluted in 25 mL of 0.9% NaCl administered over 5-60 min (give dose every 2 wk for 12 wk)	25-1000
Iron sucrose				Adult and pediatric ND-CKD patients aged 2 y and older	Adult: 200 mg over 2-5 min on five different occasions within 14-day period. There is limited experience with administration of 500 mg diluted in a maximum of 250 mL of 0.9% NaCl over 3.5-4 h on day 1 and day 14 Pediatric: see pediatric dosing for CKD 5HD (give dose every 4 wk for 12 wk)	
Iron sucrose				Adult and pediatric CKD 5PD patients aged 2 y and older	Adult: Give three divided doses within 28 d as 2 infusions of 300 mg over 1.5 h 14 d apart followed by one 400 mg infusion over 2.5 h 14 d later. Dilute in a maximum of 250 mL of 0.9% NaCl Pediatric: see pediatric dosing for CKD 5HD (give dose every 4 wk for 12 wk)	
Sodium ferric gluconate	Ferrlecit Intravenous Sodium Ferric Gluconate Complex in Sucrose Intravenous	1	350,000	Adult and pediatric CKD 5HD patients aged 6 y and older receiving ESA therapy	Adult: 125 mg over 10 min or 125 mg in 100 mL of 0.9% NaCl over 60 min Pediatric: 1.5 mg/kg in 25 mL of 0.9% NaCl over 60 min; maximum dose 125 mg per dose	62.5-1000

Abbreviations: CKD, chronic kidney disease; d, days; ESA, erythropoiesis stimulating agent; FDA, Food and Drug Administration; HD, hemodialysis; Hgb, hemoglobin; IV, intravenous; KDIGO, Kidney Disease: Improving Global Outcomes; ND-CKD, nondialysis CKD patients; PD, peritoneal dialysis; wk, weeks

[a]Monitor for 30 minutes following an infusion; KDIGO guidelines recommend monitoring for 60 minutes (1B recommendation for iron dextran, 2C recommendation for nondextran products).

[b]With the exception of ferric carboxymaltose and ferumoxytol, small doses (eg, 25-150 mg/wk) are generally used for maintenance regimens. Larger doses (eg, 1 g) should be administered in divided doses.

Adapted with permission from DiPiro JT, Talbert RL, Yee GC, et al: *Pharmacotherapy: A Pathophysiologic Approach*, 10th ed. New York, NY: McGraw-Hill; 2017.

TABLE 35-6 | Overview of Oral Iron Products

Iron Salt	Percent Elemental Iron	Elemental Iron Provided/ Common Formulations
Ferrous sulfate	20	60-65 mg/324-325 mg tablet 60 mg/5 mL syrup 44 mg/5 mL elixir 15 mg/1 mL solution
Ferrous sulfate (exsiccated)	30	65 mg/200 mg tablet 50 mg/160 mg tablet
Ferrous gluconate	12	38 mg/325 mg tablet 28-29 mg/240-246 mg tablet
Ferrous fumarate	33	66 mg/200 mg tablet 106 mg/324-325 mg tablet

Abbreviations: mg, milligram; mL, milliliter.
Adapted with permission from DiPiro JT, Talbert RL, Yee GC, et al: *Pharmacotherapy: A Pathophysiologic Approach*, 10th ed. New York, NY: McGraw-Hill; 2017.

in patients with chronic kidney disease (CKD–MBD). CKD–MBD refers to the clinical syndrome encompassing mineral, bone, and vascular calcification abnormalities that develop as complications of CKD. Clinical symptoms manifest as itchy skin, bone pain/fractures, neuropathies, and heart problems.

Pharmacologic therapy aimed at regulating PTH levels include phosphate binders (calcium carbonate, calcium acetate; non-Ca binders such as sevelamer, lanthanum carbonate, aluminum hydroxide; iron-based binders such as ferric citrate, sucroferric oxyhydroxide), vitamin D analogs (calcitriol, paricalcitol, doxercalciferol), and calcimimetic agents (cinacalcet). An alternative to calcitriol and its analogs is "nutritional" vitamin D supplementation (ergocalciferol, cholecalciferol); however, limited evidence support this therapy.

Each class of agents has unique dosing and administration, variable side effects, and targeted mechanism of actions. For example, phosphate binders and cinacalcet are best administered with or immediately after food, whereas calcitriol may be administered without regard to food. See Tables 35-7 and 35-8 for a complete review of phosphate binders and vitamin D agents. Cinacalcet hydrochloride (Sensipar) is the only calcimimetic agent approved for treatment of secondary hyperparathyroidism in patients with CKD on dialysis. The typical starting dose is 30 mg by mouth daily with titration every 2 to 4 weeks to a maximum dose of 180 mg once daily until the desired PTH values are achieved and to maintain goal serum Ca. Cinacalcet increases the sensitivity of the parathyroid gland to extracellular Ca, subsequently reducing PTH secretion and decreasing serum Ca. The most frequent adverse events associated with cinacalcet are nausea/vomiting and hypocalcemia (do not initiate if the serum Ca is less than 8.4 mg/dL). Cinacalcet is known to interact with other medications utilizing the cytochrome P450 CYP3A4 pathway.

In general, regardless of which regulatory agent is used, careful serum monitoring of Ca, albumin, Phos, and PTH are essential for safe and effective medication management. Guidelines recommend that therapeutic decisions be based on trends rather than on a single laboratory value, taking into account all available CKD–MBD assessments. In patients with CKD stages 3 to 5, the goal PTH is "greater than two times and less than nine times the upper limit of normal" or 150 to 700 pg/mL, Ca goals (total, ionized, or corrected for albumin levels) "normal" or 8.4 to 10.2 mg/dL, and Phos should be "lowered toward the normal range" or 2.5 to 5.5 mg/dL.

Cardiovascular Mortality

Data shows that in patients with CKD, mortality secondary to CV disease is 10 to 30 times greater in dialysis patients than the general population. In addition to renal disease contributing to mineral imbalances that affect the heart and blood vessels, this patient population typically has other comorbidities (HTN) that increase CV risk. Although CV risk is elevated, some data suggest possible negative consequences of using agents known to lower cardiac risk, such as aspirin. If the clinician initiates aspirin therapy, consider low dose of 81 mg by mouth daily to minimize bleeding risk while providing heart protection.

Vitamin Considerations

Deficiency and/or altered metabolism of vitamins in CKD/ESRD is caused by various factors (uremic toxins, dietary restrictions, illness, losses during KRT, and drug interactions). The amount of vitamins to avoid and/or supplement should be individualized for the patient with renal disease.

Avoid vitamins A and E The fat soluble vitamins, A and E, have been found to be elevated in patients with CKD/ESRD and should not be supplemented. Elevated vitamin A and E levels can lead to toxicity and harm.

Supplement Vitamin C, B Complex, and Folic Acid Patients with CKD have greater requirements for some water-soluble vitamins such as B1 (thiamine), B2 (riboflavin), B6 (pyridoxine), B12 (cyanocobalamin), folic acid, niacin, pantothenic acid, biotin, and vitamin C. Deficiencies of these vitamins often result from poor nutritional intake or removal by HD. There are several specialized once daily orally available renal vitamins which provide the needed supplements for the CKD/ESRD population.

SPECIAL CONSIDERATIONS

Other Pharmacologic Therapies

Kidney failure interferes with the body's immune system. Therefore, CKD/ESRD patients are more prone to certain infectious diseases secondary to impaired immunity and more at risk for others due to exposure during dialysis sessions. It is important that patients with renal disease receive a yearly influenza vaccine, are current on pneumococcal and hepatitis B immunizations, and are screened appropriately for hepatitis C and human immunodeficiency virus infection/acquired immune deficiency syndrome (HIV/AIDS).

TABLE 35-7	Phosphate-Binding Agents for Treatment of Hyperphosphatemia in Patients with Chronic Kidney Disease					
Category	Drug	Brand Name(s)	Compound Content	Starting Doses	Dose Titration[a]	Comments[b]
Calcium-based binders	Calcium acetate (25% elemental calcium)	PhosLo	25% elemental calcium (169 mg elemental calcium per 667 mg capsule)	1334 mg three times a day with meals	Increase or decrease by 667 mg per meal (169 mg elemental calcium)	Comparable efficacy to calcium carbonate with lower dose of elemental calcium Approximately 45 mg phosphorus bound per 1 g calcium acetate Evaluate for drug interactions with calcium Avoid in patients with hypercalcemia
		Phoslyra	169 mg elemental calcium per 5 mL of 667 mg calcium acetate solution			Same as PhosLo
	Calcium carbonate[c]	Tums, Os-Cal, Caltrate	40% elemental calcium	0.5-1 g (elemental calcium) three times a day with meals	Increase or decrease by 500 mg per meal (200 mg elemental calcium)	Dissolution characteristics and phosphate binding may vary from product to product Approximately 39 mg phosphorus bound per 1 g calcium carbonate Evaluate for drug interactions with calcium Avoid in patients with hypercalcemia
Iron-based binders	Ferric citrate	Auryxia	210 mg tablets (= 1 g ferric citrate)	420 mg ferric iron three times daily with meals	Increase or decrease dose by one or two tablets per meal	May increase serum iron, ferritin, and TSat May cause discolored (dark) stools Evaluate for drug interactions with iron
	Sucroferric oxyhydroxide	Velphoro	500 mg chewable tablets	500 mg three times daily with meals	Increase or decrease by 500 mg/d	May cause discolored (dark) stools Evaluate for drug interactions with iron
Resin binders	Sevelamer carbonate	Renvela	800 mg tablet 0.8 and 2.4 g powder for oral suspension	800-1600 mg three times a day with meals (once-daily dosing also effective)	Increase or decrease by 800 mg per meal	Also lowers low-density lipoprotein cholesterol Consider in patients at risk for extraskeletal calcification Risk of metabolic acidosis with sevelamer hydrochloride (less risk with carbonate formulation) May interact with ciprofloxacin and mycophenolate mofetil
	Sevelamer hydrochloride	Renagel	400 and 800 mg tablets	800-1600 mg three times a day with meals	Increase or decrease by 800 mg per meal	Same as sevelamer carbonate
Other elemental binders	Lanthanum carbonate	Fosrenol	500, 750, and 1000 mg chewable tablets 750 and 1000 mg oral powder	1500 mg daily in divided doses with meals	Increase or decrease by 750 mg/d	Potential for accumulation of lanthanum due to GI absorption (long-term consequences unknown) Evaluate for drug interactions (eg, cationic antacids, quinolone antibiotics) Higher rate of nausea/vomiting
	Aluminum hydroxide	AlternaGel	Content varies (range 100-600 mg/unit)	300-600 mg three times a day with meals	Not for long-term use	Not a first-line agent; risk of aluminum toxicity; do not use concurrently with citrate-containing products Reserve for short-term use (4 wk) in patients with hyperphosphatemia not responding to other binders Evaluate for drug interactions

Abbreviations: d, day; g, gram; mg, milligram; mL, milliliter; TSat, transferrin saturation; wk, weeks.

[a]Based on phosphorus levels, titrate every 2-3 wk until phosphorus goal reached.

[b]GI side effects are possible with all agents (eg, nausea, vomiting, abdominal pain, diarrhea, or constipation).

[c]Multiple preparations available that are not listed.

Adapted with permission from DiPiro JT, Talbert RL, Yee GC, et al: *Pharmacotherapy: A Pathophysiologic Approach*, 10th ed. New York, NY: McGraw-Hill; 2017.

TABLE 35-8	Vitamin D Agents					

Generic Name	Brand Name	Form of Vitamin D	Dosage Forms	Initial Dose[a]	Dosage Range	Frequency of Dosing
Nutritional Vitamin D						
Ergocalciferol	Drisdol	D_2	po	Varies based on 25(OH) D levels	400-50,000 international units	Daily (doses of 400-2000 international units) Weekly or monthly for higher doses (50,000 international units)
Cholecalciferol[b]	Generic	D_3	po	Varies based on 25(OH) D levels	400-50,000 international units	Daily (doses of 400-2000 international units) Weekly or monthly for higher doses (50,000 international units)

Vitamin D and Analogs						
Generic Name	Brand Name	Form of Vitamin D	Dosage Forms	Initial Dose[a,c]	Dosage Range	Dose Titration[d]
Calcitriol	Rocaltrol	D_3	po	0.25 mcg daily	0.25-5 mcg	Increase by 0.25 mcg/d at 4-8 wk intervals
	Calcijex		IV	1-2 mcg three times per wk	0.5-5 mcg	Increase by 0.5-1 mcg at 2-4 wk intervals
Doxercalciferol[e]	Hectorol	D_2	po	ND-CKD: 1 mcg daily ESRD: 10 mcg three times per wk	5-20 mcg	Increase by 0.5 mcg at 2-wk intervals for daily dosing or by 2.5 mcg at 8-wk intervals for three times per wk dosing
			IV	ESRD: 4 mcg three times per wk	2-8 mcg	Increase by 1-2 mcg at 8-wk intervals
Paricalcitol	Zemplar	D_2	po	ND-CKD: 1 mcg daily or 2 mcg three times per wk if PTH ≤500 pg/mL; 2 mcg daily or 4 mcg three times per wk if PTH >500 pg/mL	1-4 mcg	Increase by 1 mcg (for daily dosing) or 2 mcg (for three times per wk dosing) at 2-4 wk intervals
			IV	ESRD: 0.04-1 mcg three times per wk	2.5-15 mcg	Increase by 2-4 mcg at 2-4 wk intervals

Abbreviations: ESRD, end-stage renal disease; IV, intravenous; mcg, microgram; ND-CKD, nondialysis chronic kidney disease; po, oral; PTH, parathyroid hormone; wk, week

[a]Dose ratios are as follows: 1:1 for IV paricalcitol to oral doxercalciferol, 1.5:1 for IV paricalcitol to IV doxercalciferol, and 1:1 for IV to oral calcitriol.

[b]Multiple preparations are available that are not listed.

[c]Daily orally dosing most common for nonhemodialysis CKD patients, IV dosing three times per week more often used in the hemodialysis population.

[d]Based on PTH, calcium, and phosphorus levels. Decreases in dose are necessary if PTH is oversuppressed and/or if calcium and phosphorus are elevated.

[e]Prodrug that requires activation by the liver.

Adapted with permission from DiPiro JT, Talbert RL, Yee GC, et al: *Pharmacotherapy: A Pathophysiologic Approach*, 10th ed. New York, NY: McGraw-Hill; 2017.

All patients who are currently or potentially could receive hemodialysis should receive hepatitis B vaccine due to possible exposure to blood. Studies have shown that patients with ESRD have a decreased immune response to the vaccine so it is recommended that CKD patients receive the vaccine course as early as possible. Once the patient is receiving dialysis or becomes uremic, the patient should receive the vaccine at twice the standard dose (40 mcg doses in a four-dose schedule). Patients may require periodic serologic testing to ensure an adequate response to the vaccine.

Patients with CKD/kidney failure are also at a higher risk of developing pneumococcal disease and should receive both the pneumococcal 13-valent (PCV13) and 23-valent (PCV23) vaccines with the PCV23 given at least 8 weeks after PCV13 regardless of age. PCV23 doses should be continued at a minimum 5-year interval.

PHARMACIST'S ROLE IN CHRONIC KIDNEY DISEASE/END-STAGE RENAL DISEASE

Pharmacists have a major role in the management of patients with CKD/ESRD including patient education to enhance adherence, review of patient medication regimens to reduce polypharmacy when possible, adjustment of medication dosing or frequency as necessary based on impaired renal function, and review of long-term health maintenance goals such as immunization screening. With the complexity of medication regimens in this population, the pharmacist is able to evaluate drug dosing based on pharmacokinetic principles to ensure appropriate drug dosing based on renal function and indication. The pharmacist can tailor regimens individually or provide system-wide influence through management of renal dosing protocols in the institution's electronic medical record. In patients with CKD, the pharmacist can help manage pharmacologic and nonpharmacologic interventions to delay the progression of disease and can help manage long-term complications such as anemia, mineral and bone disease, CV complications, and malnutrition.

CASE Application

The following case should be used for questions 1 through 6 below.

A 79-year-old African American woman with HTN and diabetes presents to her primary care physician for a routine visit. Her spot urine albumin:urine creatinine ratio is 200 mg/g and GFR is estimated at 50 to 55 mL/min/1.73 m². The patient reports that she does not drink alcohol. She is a smoker but is willing to quit. She participates in an aerobics and strength training class for 30 minutes every day and enjoys a low-sodium diet. Pt denies medication allergies. Medications include lisinopril, metformin, aspirin, and nicotine replacement therapy.

1. Which of the following are risk factors for development of CKD as related to this patient? Select all that apply.

   a. HTN
   b. DM
   c. Smoking
   d. Diet and exercise

2. Based on this patient's ACR, she would be classified as having what category of albuminuria?

   a. A1 (normal to mildly increased)
   b. A2 (moderately increased)
   c. A3 (severely increased)
   d. Classification cannot be determined

3. Based on this patient's GFR, she would be categorized as having what stage of CKD?

   a. Stage 1
   b. Stage 2
   c. Stage 3a
   d. Stage 3b
   e. Stage 4

4. Due to a change in formulary medications, the patient will have to be switched to an alternative antihypertensive. Which of the following agents is classified as first-line therapy for patients with HTN in the setting of CKD and will inhibit the RAAS to slow the progression of proteinuria? Select ALL that apply.

   a. Benazepril
   b. Mavik
   c. Losartan
   d. Amlodipine
   e. Toprol XL

5. In general, common patient counseling pearls that should be shared regarding the use of an ACE inhibitor include which of the following? Select all that apply.

   a. ACE inhibitors are safe to use during pregnancy.
   b. Monitoring of potassium levels is necessary while taking an ACE inhibitor.
   c. A common side effect associated with ACE inhibitor use includes dry cough.
   d. Per the KDIGO guidelines, the ideal blood pressure in patients with diabetes, HTN, and CKD is less than 140/90 mm Hg (with a lower goal of less than 130/80 mm Hg, if the patient has proteinuria).

6. Which of the following medications may provide CV protection by inhibiting platelet aggregation in the setting of CKD?

   a. Lisinopril
   b. Metformin
   c. Aspirin
   d. Amlodipine

The following case should be used for questions 7 through 17 below.

A 44-year-old man with comorbid diabetes, HTN, and peripheral neuropathy was recently diagnosed with ESRD requiring hemodialysis on Monday-Wednesday-Friday. You receive a pharmacy consult for medication therapy management for this complicated patient. The patient states that he does not like taking medications with meals and experienced two episodes of hypoglycemia in the last month. He denies medication or food allergies and does not recall his recent immunizations.

Height 5'11" Weight 90 kg
Vitals: BP 160/89 (baseline BP prior to hemodialysis 145/80); heart rate, 72; respiratory rate, 18; temperature, 98.6
Pertinent labs:

Hgb	Hematocrit	T_{sat}	Serum ferritin	Retic count	Albumin	Phos	Ca²⁺	iPTH	HbA1c
9.2	30	18	69	1.01	2.9	7.5	7.8	420	10.5

Current Medications
EC aspirin 81 mg po daily
Insulin glargine 30 units subcutaneous (SubQ) QHS
Regular insulin 10 units SubQ QAC
Metoprolol tartrate 25 mg po bid
Losartan 50 mg po daily
Iron dextran 100 mg IV QHD to be initiated today (was receiving oral ferrous sulfate)
Epoetin alfa 4000 units IV QHD
Amitriptyline 50 mg po QHS
Calcium carbonate 500 mg po tid

7. Which of the following would be the most appropriate vitamin supplement to recommend for this patient?

   a. Prenatal vitamin 1 tab po daily
   b. Vitamin A 4000 units po daily
   c. Multivitamin with iron 1 tab po daily
   d. Vitamin B complex-folic acid-vitamin C 1 tab po daily

8. Assuming the patient does not have any contraindications, which of the following preventive health measures does the patient qualify for? Select all that apply.

    a. Influenzae vaccine
    b. PCV13
    c. PCV23
    d. Hepatitis B series (standard dose)
    e. Hepatitis B series (twice the standard dose)

9. The patient expresses frustration with taking medications around mealtimes. Which medication is most effective when taken with meals and may require motivational interviewing to change the patient's mindset?

    a. EC aspirin
    b. Calcium carbonate
    c. Iron dextran
    d. Epoetin alfa

10. The nephrologist is considering starting cinacalcet for this patient to help regulate PTH and treat mineral and bone disorders common in patients with chronic kidney disease (CKD–MBD). Select the best recommendation to the provider in regards to initiation of cinacalcet.

    a. It is safe to start cinacalcet but it is best to administer with food.
    b. The starting dose of cinacalcet is 180 mg by mouth daily with aggressive titration to goal PTH and serum Ca levels.
    c. Cinacalcet is typically well-tolerated with low incidence of GI irritation and minimal drug-drug interactions.
    d. It is unsafe to start cinacalcet as the patient has hypocalcemia that may be worsened by this calcimimetic.

11. Of the following brand name medications that may be used for the treatment of hyperphosphatemia in patients with CKD, which contain a non-Ca based or iron-based binder? Select all that apply.

    a. Auryxia
    b. Tums
    c. Renvela
    d. Fosrenol
    e. AlternaGel

12. This patient is receiving pharmacotherapy for the treatment of mineral and bone disorders that are common in patients with chronic kidney disease (CKD–MBD). Starting with reduced renal function, identify the sequence of pathophysiological events that can result in this complication.

    a. Increased PTH production resulting in increased bone breakdown
    b. Elevations of Phos concentrations in the blood as the result of reduced renal function
    c. Reduction in intestinal absorption of Ca and reduced serum Ca levels
    d. Reduction in plasma levels of vitamin D due to decreased activation by the kidney

13. This patient is receiving pharmacotherapy to manage anemia of CKD. In patients with anemia where endogenous stores of erythropoietin are adequate, the body is able to compensate for hypoxic states. Identify the correct sequence of this normal compensatory mechanism.

    a. Erythropoietin acts on E-progenitor cells in the bone marrow to produce new red blood cells
    b. Kidney decreases erythropoietin production
    c. Kidney senses increased tissue oxygenation
    d. Kidney senses hypoxia and increases endogenous erythropoietin production

14. The patient is receiving IV epoetin alfa (Procrit) with each hemodialysis session for anemia of CKD. Identify the correct statement regarding the use of ESAs for the treatment of anemia of CKD. Select all that apply.

    a. ESAs have a boxed warning that highlights increased risk of CV events (death, heart attacks, stroke, venous thromboembolism, thrombosis of vascular access).
    b. Prior to ESAs initiation and during treatment with ESAs, evaluation of and maintenance of iron stores is necessary.
    c. Common side effects with ESAs include elevated blood pressure, nausea/vomiting, diarrhea, headache, muscle pain, swelling, or rash.
    d. In general, a target Hgb value of less than 11.5 g/dL when on ESAs allows for individualized patient dosing and monitoring for safety and efficacy.

15. This patient was previously receiving oral ferrous sulfate with initiation of IV iron dextran at the current visit. Which of the following statements is accurate regarding common patient counseling tips for patients with CKD receiving oral iron replacement products? Select all that apply.

    a. Oral ferrous sulfate contains approximately 65 mg elemental iron per 325 mg tablet.
    b. Oral iron replacement products may cause constipation, darkening of stools, nausea/vomiting, and stomach cramps.
    c. Absorption of ferrous gluconate is best when given with a concomitant proton pump inhibitor like lansoprazole.
    d. It is important to keep oral iron replacement products out of children's reach and in child-resistant containers as severe toxicity may occur if inadvertently ingested.

16. This patient will be initiated on IV iron dextran today. Which of the following IV iron products require monitoring of the patient for 30 to 60 minutes following an infusion to ensure tolerance? Select all that apply.

    a. INFed
    b. Venofer
    c. Sodium ferric gluconate
    d. Ferric carboxymaltose

17. In this patient with ESRD (hemodialysis) and insulin-requiring diabetes, HTN, and peripheral neuropathy,

select the most appropriate hemoglobin A1c (HbA1c) goal (in percentage)?

a. Less than 6
b. Less than 6.5
c. Less than 7
d. Less than 8

18. Which of the following medications are best to avoid in patients with Stage 4 or Stage 5 CKD? Select ALL that apply.

a. Ibuprofen
b. Phenazopyridine
c. Glucophage
d. Doxycycline
e. Macrobid

19. In the setting of CKD, some medications require careful assessment. By ordering the answers, select which adverse event is appropriately matched with each medication and its metabolite.

Medication	Metabolite	Adverse Drug Event
Allopurinol	Oxypurinol	
Glipizide	Norglipizide	
Meperidine	Normeperidine	

a. Hypoglycemia
b. Kidney stone
c. Seizure

The following case should be used for question 20 below.

20. A 67-year-old man with community acquired pneumonia and CKD due to diabetic nephropathy is admitted to the hospital for failure of standard outpatient treatment with oral levofloxacin. The patient will be initiated on piperacillin/tazobactam (Zosyn).

Patient specific information: NKDA, Height 5'11", Weight 80 kg

Renal function trends:

Baseline serum creatinine (SCr) = 1.5; Yesterday SCr = 2.0; Today SCr = 2.3

Baseline urine output (UOP) 2000 mL/24 h; Yesterday UOP 1000 mL/24 h; Today UOP 300 mL/24 h

As the hospital pharmacist assigned the renal dosing queue, which of the following parameters may be considered when making a renal dose adjustment recommendation? Select all that apply.

a. Piperacillin/tazobactam-induced adverse effects if drug accumulates in renal insufficiency
b. Renal function trends as determined by SCr and UOP (improving or declining)
c. Clinical status of the patient (mild infection or severe infection)
d. Availability of alternative drug that does not require renal dose adjustment

TAKEAWAY POINTS »

- CKD is a progressive disease staged on the patient's GFR and albuminuria with complications of anemia and mineral and bone disorders starting at a GFR less than 60 mL/min/1.73 m².

- Kidney failure is defined as: (1) a GFR less than 15 mL/min/1.73 m², or (2) a need for KRT. ESRD is used for reimbursement and includes patients treated by dialysis or transplantation, irrespective of the level of GFR.

- DM and HTN are the most common causes of CKD. Appropriate blood pressure control and achievement of glycemic goals are ideal.

- ACE inhibitors or ARBs are the most effective treatment for reducing the progression of CKD by providing blood pressure control and reduction in proteinuria especially in patients with diabetes.

- Anemia of CKD is common and typically responds to exogenous ESA therapy (goal Hgb 9-11.5 g/dL) when concomitant iron therapy is used to maintain adequate iron stores (TSAT, ferritin).

- Mineral and bone disorders related to CKD may be treated with monotherapy or combination therapy of phosphate binders, vitamin D analogues, and/or calcimimetics dosed to maintain near normal Ca, Phos, and PTH levels.

- Patients with CKD/ESRD are at increased risk of CV disease and may benefit from low-dose aspirin therapy to provide CV protection.

- Fat soluble vitamins (A, E) should be avoided in patients with renal disease. Supplementation of water-soluble vitamins (B complex, folic acid, vitamin C) may be necessary in patients requiring KRT.

- Patients with CKD/ESRD should be screened appropriately for administration of influenza, pneumococcal, and hepatitis B immunizations as well as risk stratification for other infectious diseases such as hepatitis C and HIV/AIDS.

- In addition to pharmacotherapy, dietary and lifestyle modifications may slow the progression of and complications related to CKD/ESRD.

- Pharmacists play an integral role in the acute and chronic management of patients with CKD/ESRD by providing medication therapy management.

BIBLIOGRAPHY

Centers for Disease Control and Prevention (CDC). Use of 13-valent pneumococcal conjugate vaccine and 23-valent pneumococcal polysaccharide vaccine for adults with immunocompromising conditions: Recommendations of the Advisory Committee on Immunization Practices (ACIP). *MMWR*. 2012;61:816-819.

Clase CM, Ki V, Holden RM. Water-soluble vitamins in people with low glomerular filtration rate or on dialysis: a review. *Semin Dial*. 2013;26:546-567.

Foley RN, Parfrey PS, Sarnak MJ. Clinical epidemiology of cardiovascular disease in chronic renal disease. *AJKD*. 1998;32:S112-S119.

Hudson JQ, Wazny LD. Chronic kidney disease. In: DiPiro JT, Talbert RL, Yee GC, Matzke GR, Wells BG, Posey L, eds. *Pharmacotherapy: A Pathophysiologic Approach*. 10th ed. New York, NY: McGraw-Hill; 2017:chap 44.

KDIGO 2017 Clinical Practice Guideline Update for the Diagnosis, Evaluation, Prevention and Treatment of Chronic Kidney Disease–Mineral and Bone Disorder (CKD–MBD). *Kidney Int Suppl*. 2017;7:1-59.

Kidney Disease: Improving Global Outcomes (KDIGO) Anemia Work Group. KDIGO Clinical Practice Guidelines for Anemia in Chronic Kidney Disease. *Kidney Int*. 2012;2:279-335.

Kidney Disease: Improving Global Outcomes (KDIGO) Chronic Kidney Disease Work Group. KDIGO 2012 Clinical Practice Guideline for the Evaluation and Management of Chronic Kidney Disease. *Kidney Int Suppl*. 2013;3:1-150.

National Kidney Foundation: Kidney Disease Outcomes Quality Initiative (NKF-KDOQI). Clinical Practice Guidelines for Bone Metabolism and Disease in Chronic Kidney Disease. Guideline 8B. Vitamin D Therapy in Patients on Dialysis (CKD Stage 5). *AJKD*. 2003;42:S1-S201.

National Kidney Foundation: Kidney Disease Outcomes Quality Initiative (NKF-KDOQI). KDOQI US Commentary on the 2012 KDIGO Clinical Practice Guideline for Anemia in CKD. *AJKD*. 2013;62:849-859.

National Kidney Foundation: Kidney Diseases Outcomes Quality Initiative, Clinical Practice Guidelines and Clinical Practice Recommendations for Anemia in Chronic Kidney Disease: 2007 Update of Hemoglobin Target. *AJKD*. 2007;50:471-530.

KEY ABBREVIATIONS

ACE = angiotensin-converting enzyme
ACR = albumin-to-creatinine ratio
AER = albumin excretion rate
ARBs = angiotensin II receptor blockers
CKD = chronic kidney disease
CKD–MBD = mineral and bone disorders in patients with chronic kidney disease
CRRT = continuous renal replacement therapy
CV = cardiovascular
ESA = erythropoiesis-stimulating agent
ESRD = end-stage renal disease
GFR = glomerular filtration rate
HbA1c = hemoglobin A1c
HIV/AIDS = human immunodeficiency virus infection/ acquired immune deficiency syndrome
IGF-1 = insulin-like growth factor-1

IHD = intermittent hemodialysis
IV = intravenous
KDIGO = Kidney Disease: Improving Global Outcomes
KDOQI = Kidney Disease Outcomes Quality Initiative
KRT = kidney replacement therapy
NESP = novel erythropoiesis-stimulating protein
NKDEP = National Kidney Disease Education Program
NSAIDs = nonsteroidal anti-inflammatory drugs
PCV13 = pneumococcal 13-valent vaccine
PCV23 = pneumococcal 23-valent vaccine
PD = peritoneal dialysis
rHuEPO = recombinant Human Erythropoietin
TSAT = transferrin saturation
UOP = urine output
Vd = volume of distribution

36

Acid–Base Disorders

Kurt A. Wargo

FOUNDATION OVERVIEW

This chapter reviews the mechanisms responsible for the maintenance of acid–base balance and the laboratory analyses that aid clinicians in their assessment of these disorders. The complexity of acid–base concepts may be intimidating, but having a basic understanding will allow you to optimize the care of critically ill patients.

When discussing any complicated process, it is best to start from a reference point. For acid–base disturbances, that reference point is the bicarbonate–carbon dioxide buffer system, shown in Equation 36-1.

$$CO_2 + H_2O \leftrightarrow H_2CO_3 \leftrightarrow H^+ + HCO_3^- \qquad \text{(Equation 36-1)}$$

The buffering equation holds the foundation for all acid–base physiology within the human body. The processes that occur in the body drive this equation either to the left or the right in order to maintain a neutral pH. Think in terms of the left side of the equation occurring in the lungs and the right side occurring in the kidneys. Anytime the body loses hydrogen ions, the equation shifts to the right. That is to say, the lungs retain more CO_2 in order to convert it into carbonic acid, which is then converted to hydrogen ions and bicarbonate, thereby replacing the lost hydrogen ions. Likewise, anytime an extra hydrogen ion is gained, the equation shifts to the left and the respiratory center is activated to increase ventilation in an effort to get rid of excess acid (CO_2). However, an important point needs to be made; CO_2 and HCO_3^- are excreted independent of one another. If excess CO_2 exists, it cannot be excreted in the kidneys; rather it must be exhaled by the lungs. Similarly, if there is an increase in H^+, the body cannot convert it to CO_2 for excretion in the lungs; it must be excreted by the kidneys.

From this equation all acid–base disturbances can be explained. Metabolic acidosis results from either an excess in H^+ or a deficiency in HCO_3^-. On the other hand, metabolic alkalosis results from an excess in HCO_3^- or a deficiency in H^+. Respiratory acidosis results from an excess in arterial carbon dioxide (P_aCO_2), whereas respiratory alkalosis results from a deficiency in P_aCO_2. The determination of all acid–base disturbances can be done through evaluation of electrolyte panels, arterial blood gases (ABG), and patient assessment.

Two final concepts that need to be discussed are the compensatory response that occurs in response to the primary acid–base disorder, as well as mixed acid–base disorders. Primary metabolic disorders can be seen as disturbances in the serum bicarbonate level, with compensation occurring via the respiratory route and reflected in the P_aCO_2. Likewise, all respiratory disturbances will be reflected in the P_aCO_2 level, with compensation occurring metabolically as reflected in the serum bicarbonate level. Sometimes it may be unclear which disturbance is the primary problem by simply evaluating the laboratory values; thus it is crucial to assess the patient in order to get a good history of their present illness to determine which acid–base disorder may be primary. Unfortunately, some acid–base disorders are not as clear as others and may actually be mixed disorders. This chapter will provide a stepwise approach to assessing ABGs and will provide actual case examples in order to familiarize you with the concepts of acid–base disorders. At the completion, you will have the tools necessary to assess *any* ABG that may be encountered in clinical practice.

STEPWISE APPROACH TO ASSESSING ACID–BASE DISORDERS

In order to interpret acid–base disorders, a basic understanding of general concepts is necessary. Many hospital laboratories report ranges in normal laboratory values, such as pH 7.35 to 7.45 and P_aCO_2 35 to 45 mm Hg. What is important to understand is that under normal physiologic conditions, the human body attempts to maintain homeostasis by keeping the pH and P_aCO_2 as close as possible to 7.40 and 40 mm Hg, respectively. Therefore, any variation from those values should be considered abnormal for the purposes of blood gas evaluation. Serum bicarbonate levels, on the other hand, may vary from 22 to 28 mEq/L on a daily basis, based upon a number of metabolic variables. In general terms, it is best to always keep in mind that *acidemia* is defined as the existence of a pH <7.40, whereas an *alkalemia* is defined as having a pH >7.40. Acidosis is the process leading to acidemia while alkalosis describes the process leading to alkalemia. For purposes of this chapter, the terms will be used interchangeably.

When presented with an ABG, your task is to determine the primary acid–base disturbance and whether compensation has occurred. *Compensation* is a process that the body undergoes in an effort to maintain homeostasis (pH = 7.40). For any

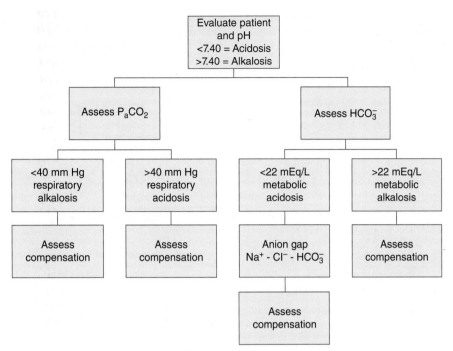

FIGURE 36-1 Stepwise approach to assessing acid-base disturbances.

respiratory abnormality, the body will compensate metabolically with changes in serum HCO_3^- through renal regulation. This compensation may take 3 to 5 days to completely occur. On the other hand, for any metabolic disorder, the body compensates through pulmonary regulation of P_aCO_2. This compensation occurs more rapidly than metabolic compensation, taking minutes to begin, with full compensation seen in hours.

Determining the primary acid–base disturbance and whether or not compensation has occurred is not an easy task; however, if a stepwise approach is utilized, outlined in Figure 36-1, both simple and complex acid–base disorders can be determined. First, and most important, is the assessment of the patient in order to determine what may be physiologically occurring at that moment in time. At the same time, assessment of the pH points one in the direction of a primary acidosis (pH <7.40) or alkalosis (pH >7.40). Second, assessment of P_aCO_2 and HCO_3^- will allow you to determine the primary disturbance and whether compensation has occurred. Third, if a metabolic acidosis is present, you must calculate an anion gap in an effort to further differentiate the cause of the disturbance and better determine treatment options. Finally, check to see if the patient is compensating for the primary disorder.

Example: A patient with community-acquired pneumonia presents with a pH of 7.46, P_aCO_2 of 32 mm Hg, and serum HCO_3^- of 26 mEq/L. Upon assessment of the patient (step 1), it is determined that the patient has a pulmonary process occurring (pneumonia). In addition, through assessment of the pH, it is evident that this patient has an alkalosis, as the pH is >7.40. In the second step, assessment of both the P_aCO_2 and HCO_3^- must be done in order to determine which is causing the acid–base abnormality. In this case, the P_aCO_2 is lower than normal and the HCO_3^- is normal, indicating the major driving force for the pH increase is respiratory alkalosis. It does not appear that the patient is compensating for

the primary respiratory problem as the bicarbonate is normal. This is likely due to a lack of time for compensation to occur. Treatment of the patient's underlying pneumonia with antimicrobials (if bacterial in origin) should resolve this acid–base disturbance.

There are five acid–base disturbances that can occur in the human body listed in Table 36-1: (1) metabolic acidosis, (2) metabolic alkalosis, (3) respiratory acidosis, (4) respiratory alkalosis, and (5) mixed acid–base disturbances. If the stepwise approach to assessing ABGs is used, all of these disturbances can be determined.

Metabolic Acidosis

Case 1

A 58-year-old woman presented with a 4-day history of lethargy, anorexia, abdominal pain, and nausea. Her medical history was positive for type 2 diabetes and osteoarthritis for which she was taking metformin 500 mg twice daily and celecoxib respectively (unknown dose). Her laboratory values on admission were the following: Electrolytes: sodium 140 mEq/L (136-145 mEq/L); potassium 4.4 mEq/L (3.5-5 mEq/L); chloride 100 mEq/L (98-106 mEq/L); bicarbonate 5 mEq/L (22-28 mEq/L); blood urea nitrogen 77 mg/dL (10-20 mg/dL); creatinine 9 mg/dL (0.5-1.2 mg/dL); glucose 112 mg/dL (70-110 mg/dL); lactic acid 178 mg/dL (5-20 mg/dL). Arterial blood gas: pH 6.8; P_aCO_2 20 mm Hg; P_aO_2 77 mm Hg.

Metabolic acidosis can be defined either by an increased amount of unmeasured anions (increased anion gap metabolic acidosis) or by a normal anion gap. In the case of an increased anion gap, several variables lead to an increase in unmeasured anions. A useful way to remember the potential causes is through the use of the mnemonic "KILU", where "K" signifies *ketoacidosis* (caused by diabetes, starvation, and chronic

TABLE 36-1 **Etiologies of Various Acid–Base Disorders**

Metabolic Acidosis		Metabolic Alkalosis	Respiratory Acidosis	Respiratory Alkalosis
Normal Anion Gap	**Increased Anion Gap**			
Drugs	Ketoacidosis	Drugs	Drugs	Drugs
▪ Acetazolamide	▪ Alcoholism	▪ Corticosteroids	▪ Aminoglycosides	▪ Catecholamines
▪ Amphotericin B	▪ Starvation	▪ Diuretics	▪ Anesthetics	▪ Methylphenidate
▪ Cholestyramine	▪ Diabetic	Volume contraction	▪ Beta-blockers	▪ Nicotine
▪ Lithium	Ingestions	Vomiting or NG suction[b]	▪ Sedatives	▪ Salicylates (early toxicity)
▪ Topiramate	▪ Methanol	Alkali administration	▪ Opioids	CNS diseases[d]
▪ Zonisamide	▪ Ethylene glycol	Hypokalemia	NMBAs[c]	Anxiety/panic disorders
Diarrhea	▪ Salicylates (late toxicity)	Hyperaldosteronism	Neuromuscular diseases	Pneumonia
Renal tubular acidosis	Lactic acidosis		CNS diseases[d]	Pulmonary embolism
Lead poisoning	▪ Metformin		Pneumonia	Tissue hypoxia/severe anemia
Saline infusions	▪ Lorazepam (Intravenous)		Restrictive airway diseases	Thyrotoxicosis
Adrenal insufficiency	▪ Isoniazid		▪ COPD	
	▪ NRTIs[a]		▪ Obesity	
	Uremia		▪ Ascites	
			Hypothyroidism	

[a]Nucleoside reverse transcriptase inhibitors, especially didanosine.
[b]Nasogastric.
[c]Neuromuscular blocking agents.
[d]Central nervous system.

alcoholism), "I" signifies *ingestions* (typically from salicylates, ethylene glycol, and methanol), "L" signifies *lactic acidosis*, and "U" signifies *uremia*. Some refer to the mnemonic "MUD-PILES" (methanol, uremia, DKA, paraldehyde, INH/Iron, lactic acid, ethylene glycol/ethanol, salicylates) for elevated anion gap metabolic acidosis. When faced with a serum electrolyte panel that reveals a lower than normal serum HCO_3^-, indicating a metabolic acidosis, an anion gap must be calculated by calculating the difference in serum concentrations of the major cation, sodium (Na^+), and anions, chloride (Cl^-) and bicarbonate (HCO_3^-), see Equation 36-2.

$$\text{Anion gap} = ([Na^+] - [Cl^-] - [HCO_3^-]) \quad \text{(Equation 36-2)}$$

Under normal circumstances, the anion gap should be 8 to 16 mEq/L; however, negatively charged proteins, specifically albumin, can have a significant impact on the anion gap, such that a 1 g/dL drop in albumin will lower the anion gap by 2.5 mEq/L. If the albumin of a patient is known, the *normal* anion gap can be calculated by multiplying the serum albumin by 3. This proves to be crucial when calculating the *delta gap*, which is the difference between the observed and the expected anion gap, Equation 36-3. The delta gap is used, whenever an increased anion gap is observed, in order to determine what the bicarbonate level would be, in the absence of unmeasured anions. That is, the result of the delta gap is added back to the measured bicarbonate, resulting in the *revealed bicarbonate*, the serum bicarbonate without an anion gap, Equation 36-3. This is especially useful in determining if treatment with sodium bicarbonate should be given to correct the acidosis.

$$\text{Delta gap} = \text{Observed anion gap} - \text{Expected anion gap}$$
$$\text{(Equation 36-3)}$$
$$\text{Revealed } HCO_3^- = \text{Delta gap} + \text{Serum } HCO_3^-$$

From Equation 36-2, the following can be calculated:

Anion gap = 140 mEq/L – 100 mEq/L – 5 mEq/L
Anion gap = 35 mEq/L

Now, utilizing Equation 36-3, the following can be calculated:

Expected anion gap = 12 mEq/L (no albumin is provided)
Delta gap = 35 mEq/L – 12 mEq/L
Delta gap = 23 mEq/L
Revealed HCO_3^- = 23 mEq/L + 5 mEq/L
Revealed HCO_3^- = 28 mEq/L

Based upon this case example, the increased anion gap observed (35 mEq/L) is secondary to unmeasured anions, in this case lactic acid, secondary to metformin in the setting of acute kidney injury. When the delta gap equation is used, an HCO_3^- of 28 is revealed, indicating that if all the lactic acid were removed, the patient's HCO_3^- would be on the high-end of normal. Therefore, if the pH were >6.9, it may be inappropriate to administer sodium bicarbonate; however, due to the severity of the acidosis, the administration would be justified. To complete this case example, it is necessary to assess the P_aCO_2 to determine respiratory compensation. In this case it is lower than 40 mm Hg; therefore, the patient has been appropriately compensated for the metabolic acidosis with a respiratory alkalosis.

Metformin is an extremely rare cause of lactic acidosis. Particular care should be taken when using it in patients where renal blood flow has been altered, such as in acute kidney injury, sepsis, iodinated contrast studies, and acutely decompensated heart failure. More commonly, isoniazid and nucleoside reverse transcriptase inhibitors, such as didanosine and stavudine, can cause lactic acidosis. Another type of lactic acidosis, D-lactic acidosis (the "D" isomer of lactic acid), can rarely be encountered in practice as well. This type of lactic acidosis is caused by intravenous (IV) infusions of products containing the excipient propylene glycol, such as IV lorazepam and IV diazepam, and typically occurs after high doses of continuous infusions. Typical presentation is an increased osmolar gap, increased anion gap, and renal failure. Although propylene glycol can cause either a lactic acidosis or D-lactic acidosis, the D-isomer is not detected in the routine assay, and thus lactic acidosis may or may not be identified. In these patients, it is recommended to check a lactic acid level or determine the osmolar gap, which if elevated, would indicate the presence of D-lactic acid.

Case 2

A 42-year-old man with HIV is admitted to the hospital with headache and fever. He is diagnosed with cryptococcal meningitis and initiated on amphotericin B and flucytosine. One week later, the patient is found to be confused and the following laboratory values were drawn: Electrolytes: sodium 152 mEq/L; potassium 3.4 mEq/L; chloride 120 mEq/L; bicarbonate 20 mEq/L; blood urea nitrogen 32 mg/dL; creatinine 1.4 mg/dL; glucose 112 mg/dL. Arterial blood gas: pH 7.30; P_aCO_2 36; P_aO_2 85.

Normal anion gap metabolic acidosis is a result of either bicarbonate loss or inadequate buffering. The most common cause of bicarbonate loss is excessive diarrhea, but can also be seen in proximal (type 2) renal tubular acidosis (RTA). Because stool has a basic pH, large volume diarrhea can result in a loss of HCO_3^-, resulting in a normal anion gap acidosis. In type 2 RTA, there is a disruption in the proximal tubular reabsorption of HCO_3^-, resulting in lower serum HCO_3^- levels. Medications such as carbonic anhydrase inhibitors and ifosfamide are common iatrogenic causes of type 2 RTA. A common mnemonic for normal gap metabolic acidosis is USED CAR: *u*reteral diversion, *s*aline infusion, *e*xogenous acid, *d*iarrhea, *c*arbonic anhydrase inhibitors, *a*drenal insufficiency, and *r*enal tubular acidosis.

Inadequate buffering in a normal anion gap acidosis is a result of decreased distal H^+ secretion by luminal H^+-ATPase pumps in the collecting duct of the kidneys, defined as distal RTA (type 1). This decreased secretion of H^+ results in the inability to establish normally acidic urine and therefore a urine pH that is typically above 5.3. Another mechanism of type 1 RTA is secondary to increased permeability of the luminal membrane, resulting in back diffusion of secreted H^+ and distal secretion of K^+. Amphotericin B is an agent which inserts into cell membranes and creates pores, ultimately decreasing the membrane's permeability. The net result is H^+ retention and K^+ excretion resulting in normal anion gap acidosis and hypokalemia.

In Case 2, the first step in the approach to evaluating ABGs leads the reader to determine the patient has a metabolic

process occurring with cryptococcal meningitis, and no reason to suspect a respiratory problem. In addition to evaluating the patient, evaluation of the pH reveals an acidosis is present. When assessing the metabolic component of the ABG, it is discovered the patient has a lower than normal HCO_3^-, indicating a metabolic acidosis is present. Evaluation of the respiratory component of the ABG shows that the P_aCO_2 is lower than normal, indicating a respiratory alkalosis may be present due to compensation. Therefore, we determine that the patient has a metabolic acidosis with respiratory compensation. The next step, according to our approach, is to calculate an anion gap because of the presence of a metabolic acidosis. When this is calculated, it is determined that a normal anion gap is present (12 mEq/L). Therefore, it is evident that the acid–base disturbance present is a normal gap metabolic acidosis with appropriate respiratory compensation. The most likely cause in this case is RTA secondary to amphotericin B, and so alternative therapy may be warranted.

Metabolic Alkalosis

Case 3

A 65-year-old man is admitted to the hospital for abdominal pain and diarrhea. He has a history of chronic constipation for which he takes lactulose. Three weeks prior to admission, an exploratory laparotomy revealed no obstruction. He then developed pneumonia and received 5 days of moxifloxacin. Five days prior to admission he developed large-volume, watery diarrhea, without nausea or vomiting. He had the following laboratory values upon admission: Electrolytes: sodium 143 mEq/L; potassium 3.3 mEq/L; chloride 102 mEq/L; bicarbonate 33 mEq/L; urea nitrogen 19 mg/dL; creatinine 1 mg/dL; glucose 109 mg/dL. Arterial blood gas: pH 7.44; P_aCO_2 42 mm Hg; P_aO_2 53 mm Hg. *Clostridium difficile* toxin: negative via polymerase chain reaction (PCR) test.

Metabolic alkalosis is characterized by a pH >7.40 and HCO_3^- >28 mEq/L. Causes of metabolic alkalosis can be divided into gastrointestinal loss of H^+, renal loss of H^+, intracellular shift of H^+, or retention of HCO_3^-. Gastrointestinal loss of H^+ usually is a result of vomiting, nasogastric (NG) suctioning, or antacid use. Renal H^+ loss is associated with a number of conditions including diseases of mineralocorticoid excess, such as primary hyperaldosteronism or Cushing disease. In these conditions, the presence of hypokalemia exists, which acts as a stimulus for H^+ secretion and HCO_3^- reabsorption. Diuretics also promote renal H^+ loss through distal secretion. This condition, referred to as "contraction alkalosis," occurs secondary to increased production of aldosterone and reabsorption of Na^+ and HCO_3^- in the proximal tubule, in response to hypovolemia. Additionally, diuretics can cause hypokalemia that may result in the previously mentioned H^+ secretion and HCO_3^- reabsorption. In addition to diuretic use, vomiting can also lead to a condition of contraction alkalosis where Na^+, Cl^-, and H_2O are lost without HCO_3^-. Finally, retention of bicarbonate, due to excessive administration of sodium bicarbonate, can also result in metabolic alkalosis.

Because the most common causes of metabolic alkalosis include vomiting, NG suction, and diuretics, the usual treatment involves administration of IV fluids containing NaCl. However, in some cases, patients may be resistant to administration of IV NaCl, usually due to edematous states or hypokalemia. In those patients, withholding conventional diuretics and possibly administering a carbonic anhydrase inhibitor, acetazolamide, is recommended.

In the case above, the stepwise approach indicates the patient currently has a metabolic process occurring (large volume diarrhea), as well as a pH that shows alkalosis. The second step of the approach demonstrates that the P_aCO_2 is slightly higher than normal, representing a potential respiratory acidosis, with an HCO_3^- that is higher than normal, demonstrating a metabolic alkalosis. Because the pH is elevated, this leads us to the conclusion that the patient has metabolic alkalosis with respiratory compensation. It is puzzling, however, that this patient has had large amounts of diarrhea and has an alkalosis, a state in which one would normally expect to see metabolic acidosis (through loss of bicarbonate in the stool). Nevertheless, upon closer examination, the etiology becomes clear. The metabolic alkalosis that was present in this patient was most likely a result of hypokalemia combined with lactulose therapy. Lactulose creates an acidic stool, thereby converting ammonia (NH_3) into ammonium (NH_4^+) for excretion. Therefore, the patient was losing H^+ through diarrhea, in a way that was analogous to vomiting or NG suctioning. The patient was given IV fluids, lactulose therapy was discontinued, and the metabolic alkalosis resolved.

Respiratory Acidosis

Case 4

An 89-year-old man with a history of heart failure and chronic kidney disease (baseline creatinine 1.6 mg/dL) was being treated in the hospital for a left femoral neck fracture. While in the hospital, he developed a urinary tract infection with *Pseudomonas aeruginosa*, and began to experience decreased mental status, a temperature of 103°F (39°C), and a white blood cell count (WBC) of 41,000 cells/mm³. At that time he was on room air and his ABG demonstrated the following: pH 7.43, P_aCO_2 19 mm Hg, P_aO_2 57 mm Hg. Therapy with gentamicin was begun and the patient's WBC began to drop and his mental status began to improve. Days later he began to experience acute kidney injury secondary to gentamicin as evidenced by a serum creatinine of 4.5 mg/dL and a gentamicin trough of 6 mg/dL; therefore, gentamicin was discontinued. His mental status began to deteriorate and he began to go into respiratory failure. The ABG revealed pH 7.19, P_aCO_2 57 mm Hg, and P_aO_2 59 mm Hg. After 3 days of mechanical ventilation, the patient improved and was extubated.

Respiratory acidosis is characterized by a pH <7.40 with an elevated P_aCO_2 with multiple potential etiologies. Acutely, respiratory acidosis is most commonly associated with severe asthma exacerbations (after diaphragm fatigue), pneumonia, pulmonary edema, and suppression of the respiratory center secondary to medications such as opioids, benzodiazepines,

paralytics, and neuromuscular blockers. Chronic respiratory acidosis is most commonly associated with chronic obstructive pulmonary disease (COPD) and extreme obesity. Because the renal compensation may take days, through secretion of H^+, acute respiratory acidosis must be treated by removal of the offending agent, or treating the underlying cause. Supplemental oxygenation may be required in severe cases.

In the case presented, the stepwise approach demonstrates the patient has a pulmonary process occurring (respiratory failure), as well as a pH that is acidemic after his respiratory failure. Evaluation of the P_aCO_2 from the time of respiratory failure indicates a respiratory acidosis. Although the HCO_3^- is not available for assessment, one would not expect to see much of a change from normal, as metabolic compensation would take several days to occur. Through assessment of the patient we know a pulmonary process is occurring; therefore, the patient has a primary respiratory acidosis, with no evidence of metabolic compensation. The acute respiratory failure was secondary to a rare adverse effect of gentamicin therapy, neuromuscular blockade. After gentamicin was discontinued and mechanical ventilation was employed, the patient improved. While it is rare, aminoglycosides have been associated with neuromuscular blockade, an adverse effect of which all clinicians should be cognizant, although more commonly seen with gentamicin and neomycin than with tobramycin and amikacin. This is most commonly seen when combined with neuromuscular blocking agents such as cisatracurium.

Respiratory Alkalosis/Mixed Acid–Base Disorders

Case 5

A 58-year-old schizophrenic man was brought to the hospital because of strange behavior. He was completely disoriented and provided no history. The following laboratory values were collected: Electrolytes: sodium 139 mEq/L; potassium 4.7 mEq/L; chloride 90 mEq/L; bicarbonate 14 mEq/L; urea nitrogen 18 mg/dL; creatinine 1 mg/dL; glucose 100 mg/dL. Arterial blood gas: pH 7.49; P_aCO_2 15 mm Hg; P_aO_2 169 (2 L nasal O_2).

Respiratory alkalosis is characterized by a pH >7.40 and hyperventilation resulting in a lower than normal P_aCO_2. This is commonly seen during states of hypoxia, such as in pneumonia, pulmonary thromboembolism, heart failure, and severe anemia. Other causes include psychogenic hyperventilation, pregnancy, hepatic failure, salicylate overdose, fever, infections, cerebrovascular events, and drugs such as catecholamines, methylphenidate, nicotine, and progesterone. Treatment of respiratory alkalosis should be solely aimed at correcting the underlying cause.

The case provided above is complicated, in the sense that it is a mixed acid–base disorder. If the stepwise approach is used, we see the patient's pH is elevated, indicating alkalosis. Unfortunately, it is difficult to assess the patient due to his current mental status; therefore, we must rely exclusively upon laboratory values. The P_aCO_2 is markedly decreased, indicating a respiratory alkalosis. Furthermore, the HCO_3^- is also markedly decreased indicating metabolic acidosis. After recognizing a metabolic acidosis, the next step is calculation of the anion gap, which in this case is 35 mEq/L which is elevated. At first glance it is difficult to ascertain which came first, though one might simply state the patient has a metabolic acidosis with respiratory compensation. However, upon further laboratory analysis, it was noted that his salicylate level was extremely elevated. The classic presentation of salicylate overdose involves respiratory alkalosis followed by an increased anion gap metabolic acidosis. A family member then brought in an empty bottle of *Alka-Seltzer* that was found near the patient's bedside, which contains aspirin. Thus, the patient experienced respiratory alkalosis and an increased anion gap acidosis secondary to aspirin overdose.

CONCLUSION

Acid–base pathophysiology can be complicated and overwhelming to both the novice and the experienced clinician alike. Recalling the five major disorders that can occur and utilizing this stepwise approach proposed in this chapter will help clinicians at any level of training assess and develop treatment options for any acid–base disturbance encountered in practice.

CASE Application

Questions 1 and 2 pertain to the following case.

A 35-year-old woman is in the intensive care unit, intubated after a recent abdominal surgery. While in the operating room, she received more than 8 L of fluid and blood products, but has been aggressively diuresed since that time. In the past 3 days she has generated 6 L of urine output, her BUN and Cr have *increased* to 35 mg/dL and 1.4 mg/dL, respectively (baseline of 10 mg/dL and 0.7 mg/dL), and her blood pressure has decreased to 100/60 mm Hg. This morning, her ABG shows the following: pH 7.50, P_aCO_2 48 mm Hg, and HCO_3 37 mEq/L.

1. Which of the primary acid–base disturbances is present in this patient?

   a. Metabolic acidosis
   b. Metabolic alkalosis
   c. Respiratory acidosis
   d. Respiratory alkalosis

2. Has the patient appropriately compensated for the primary disorder?

   a. Yes, the P_aCO_2 is elevated, indicating appropriate compensation.
   b. Yes, the HCO_3 is elevated, indicating appropriate compensation.
   c. No, the HCO_3 is low, indicating the patient has not yet been compensated.
   d. No, the P_aCO_2 is low, indicating the patient has not yet been compensated.

3. Which of the following acid–base disturbances would *most likely* be exhibited in a person with GOLD 3 (severe) chronic obstructive pulmonary disease (COPD)? Select all that apply.

   a. Respiratory alkalosis
   b. Respiratory acidosis
   c. Respiratory acidosis compensation
   d. Metabolic alkalosis compensation
   e. Metabolic acidosis compensation

4. Which of the following acid–base disturbances would you expect to see in the early stages of an acute asthma exacerbation?

   a. Respiratory acidosis
   b. Respiratory alkalosis
   c. Metabolic acidosis
   d. Metabolic alkalosis

5. A patient presents to the emergency department unconscious, after ingesting a bottle of temazepam. What acid–base disturbance would you expect to see?

   a. Increased anion gap metabolic acidosis
   b. Respiratory alkalosis
   c. Normal gap metabolic acidosis
   d. Respiratory acidosis

Questions 6 to 8 pertain to the following case.

A 62-year-old woman has been hospitalized in the ICU for several weeks. She has had a complicated hospital course with sepsis secondary to pneumonia, requiring prolonged courses of antibiotics. Over the past few days, she began spiking fevers and is having a lot of diarrhea. Her stool was positive for *C. difficile* by polymerase chain reaction. Laboratory values include:

Na^+ 140 mEq/L, Cl^- 110 mEq/L, HCO_3^- 17 mEq/L, albumin 4.1 g/dL, pH 7.32, and P_aCO_2 33 mm Hg.

6. Place the following answers in the correct order to assess the acid–base disorder:

   a. Calculate the anion gap
   b. Assess the patient
   c. Assess P_aCO_2 and HCO_3^-
   d. Assess the pH to determine if acidotic or alkalotic

7. What is the *most likely primary* acid–base disturbance?

   a. Increased anion gap metabolic acidosis
   b. Normal anion gap metabolic acidosis
   c. Metabolic alkalosis
   d. Respiratory acidosis

8. Has the patient appropriately compensated for the primary disorder?

   a. No, the P_aCO_2 is elevated, indicating the patient has not yet been compensated.
   b. Yes, the HCO_3 is elevated, indicating appropriate compensation.

c. No, the HCO_3 is low, indicating the patient has not yet been compensated.

d. Yes, the P_aCO_2 is low, indicating appropriate compensation.

Questions 9 and 10 pertain to the following case.

A 17-year-old girl with no known medical history is brought to the emergency department (ED) in a difficult-to-arouse state. Her parents report she was been complaining of a vague abdominal pain earlier in the morning, and then began vomiting and urinating frequently in the hours before admission. Urine and blood were positive for ketones. The following laboratory values were taken: Na^+ 145 mEq/L, K^+ 4.7 mEq/L, Cl^- 105 mEq/L, HCO_3^- 8 mEq/L, glucose 625 mg/dL, pH 7.22, and P_aCO_2 22 mm Hg.

9. What is the *most likely primary* acid–base disturbance?

 a. Increased anion gap metabolic acidosis
 b. Normal anion gap metabolic acidosis
 c. Metabolic alkalosis
 d. Respiratory alkalosis

10. Has the patient appropriately compensated for the primary disorder?

 a. Yes, the P_aCO_2 is elevated, indicating appropriate compensation.
 b. Yes, the HCO_3 is elevated, indicating appropriate compensation.
 c. Yes, the P_aCO_2 is low, indicating appropriate compensation.
 d. Yes, the HCO_3 is low, indicating appropriate compensation.

Questions 11 and 12 pertain to the following case.

A 22-year-old man with no medical history is admitted after being "found down" at a party after drinking a lot of alcohol over a 20-minute time period. Upon arrival to the emergency department, he was neurologically unresponsive and had the following laboratory values: pH 7.15, P_aO_2 55, P_aCO_2 60 mm Hg, HCO_3^- 25 mEq/L, Na^+ 132 mEq/L, Cl^- 95 mEq/L, and albumin 4.2 g/dL. Urine drug screen is positive for benzodiazepines.

11. What is the *primary* acid–base disturbance?

 a. Increased anion gap metabolic acidosis
 b. Normal anion gap metabolic acidosis
 c. Metabolic alkalosis
 d. Respiratory acidosis

12. Has the patient appropriately compensated for the primary acid–base disorder?

 a. Yes, the P_aCO_2 is elevated, indicating appropriate compensation.

b. Yes, the P_aCO_2 is low, indicating appropriate compensation.

c. Yes, the HCO_3 is elevated, indicating appropriate compensation.

d. Unsure, it is too soon after the acute respiratory event to assess metabolic compensation at this time.

Questions 13 and 14 pertain to the following case.

A 45-year-old woman with previous peptic ulcer disease was admitted with persistent vomiting. She looked dehydrated, with dry mucus membranes and skin tenting. Her blood results were Na^+ 142 mEq/L, K^+ 2.6 mEq/L, Cl^- 88 mEq/L, pH 7.52, P_aCO_2 51 mm Hg, and HCO_3^- 42 mEq/L.

13. What is the primary acid–base disorder?

 a. Increased anion gap metabolic acidosis
 b. Normal anion gap metabolic acidosis
 c. Metabolic alkalosis
 d. Respiratory acidosis

14. Has the patient appropriately compensated for the primary acid–base disorder?

 a. Yes, the P_aCO_2 is elevated, indicating appropriate compensation.
 b. Yes, the P_aCO_2 is low, indicating appropriate compensation.
 c. Yes, the HCO_3^- is elevated, indicating appropriate compensation.
 d. Yes, the HCO_3^- is low, indicating appropriate compensation.

Questions 15 and 16 pertain to the following case.

A 55-year-old man was admitted to the hospital with a 3-day history of persistent vomiting. The following laboratory values are taken: pH 7.40, P_aCO_2 40 mm Hg, HCO_3 24 mEq/L, Na 149 mEq/L, Cl 100 mEq/L, BUN 110 mg/dL, and Cr 8.7 mg/dL.

15. What would you *expect* the pH, P_aCO_2, and HCO_3 to be in a patient who has persistent vomiting ($\uparrow$, $\downarrow$, or N)?

 a. pH $\uparrow$; P_aCO_2 $\downarrow$; HCO_3 $\uparrow$
 b. pH $\downarrow$; P_aCO_2 $\downarrow$; HCO_3 $\downarrow$
 c. pH $\uparrow$; P_aCO_2 N; HCO_3 $\uparrow$
 d. pH $\downarrow$; P_aCO_2 N; HCO_3 $\downarrow$

16. What acid–base disturbance would you expect in this patient who has acute-on-chronic kidney failure?

 a. Increased anion gap metabolic acidosis
 b. Normal anion gap metabolic acidosis
 c. Metabolic alkalosis
 d. Respiratory acidosis

17. A 55-year-old woman with a history of severe chronic obstructive pulmonary disease is admitted after several

days of worsening shortness of breath. Recently, she was discharged from the hospital with a similar episode and was doing fine until 3 days before admission when she developed a productive cough, requiring an increase in her home O_2, and more frequent albuterol/ipratropium use. What would you *expect* the pH, P_aCO_2, and HCO_3 to be in this patient ($\uparrow$, $\downarrow$, N)?

a. pH $\uparrow$; P_aCO_2 $\downarrow$; HCO_3 $\uparrow$
b. pH $\downarrow$; P_aCO_2 $\uparrow$; HCO_3 $\uparrow$
c. pH $\uparrow$; P_aCO_2 N; HCO_3 $\uparrow$
d. pH $\downarrow$; P_aCO_2 N; HCO_3 $\downarrow$

18. What acid–base disturbance might you see in a person from New Orleans, LA (1 ft. below sea level) who just flew to Denver, CO and is hiking up Pike's Peak (over 14,000 ft. above sea level)?

a. Increased anion gap metabolic acidosis
b. Normal anion gap metabolic acidosis
c. Metabolic alkalosis
d. Respiratory alkalosis

19. Which of the following antifungals may cause a normal anion gap metabolic acidosis?

a. Flucytosine
b. Amphotericin B
c. Caspofungin
d. Voriconazole

20. Which of the following analgesics is associated with a respiratory alkalosis especially with toxic doses?

a. Acetaminophen
b. Aspirin
c. Hydrocodone
d. Fentanyl

21. Excessive use of bumetanide may lead to what acid–base disorder?

a. Metabolic acidosis
b. Metabolic alkalosis
c. Respiratory acidosis
d. Respiratory alkalosis

TAKEAWAY POINTS ➤➤

- Acid–base disorders are primarily due to either metabolic or respiratory processes as manifested by disorders in HCO_3^- or P_aCO_2; however, a combination of the two may also result in an acid–base disorder.

- Acidemia is defined by a pH <7.40, whereas alkalemia is defined by a pH >7.40. Acidosis and alkalosis refers to the process causing the acidemia and alkalemia respectively.

- Respiratory acidosis occurs when the P_aCO_2 >40 mm Hg, while respiratory alkalosis occurs when the P_aCO_2 <40 mm Hg.

- Metabolic acidosis occurs when the HCO_3^- <22 mEq/L, whereas metabolic alkalosis occurs when it is >28 mEq/L.

- Metabolic acidosis is further characterized by the anion gap ($[Na^+]$ – $[Cl^-]$ – $[HCO_3^-]$).

- Increased anion gap metabolic acidosis is caused by "KILU," while normal anion gap acidosis is caused by "USED CAR."

- A stepwise approach should be employed when assessing acid–base disturbances:
  1. Evaluate the patient. Do they have a pulmonary process occurring at that particular point in time, or a metabolic one?
  2. Evaluate pH. Is the patient acidemic or alkalemic?
  3. Evaluate P_aCO_2. Is it less than or greater than 40 mm Hg? Assess possible causes.
  4. Evaluate HCO_3^-.
     a. Is it <22 mEq/L? If so, check the anion gap. If the gap is elevated, check the delta gap, and add the result to the HCO_3^-, to reveal the true level (if all the anions were removed).
     b. Is it >28 mEq/L? Assess causes of metabolic alkalosis.
  5. Evaluate compensation.

BIBLIOGRAPHY

Devlin JW, Matzke GR. Acid–base disorders. In: DiPiro JT, Talbert RL, Yee GC, Matzke GR, Wells BG, Posey L, eds. *Pharmacotherapy: A Pathophysiologic Approach.* 10th ed. New York, NY: McGraw-Hill; 2017:chap 52.

McConville JF, Solway J. Disorders of ventilation. In: Longo DL, Fauci AS, Kasper DL, Hauser SL, Jameson J, Loscalzo J, eds. *Harrison's Principles of Internal Medicine.* 18th ed. New York, NY: McGraw-Hill; 2012:chap 264.

Rose BD, Post TW. *Clinical Physiology of Acid-Base and Electrolyte Disorders.* 5th ed. New York, NY: McGraw-Hill; 2001.

Wargo KA, Centor RM. ABCs of ABGs: a guide to interpreting acid-base disorders. *Hosp Pharm.* 2008;43:808-815.

KEY ABBREVIATIONS

ABG = arterial blood gases
COPD = chronic obstructive pulmonary disease
IV = intravenous
NG = nasogastric

PCR = polymerase chain reaction
RTA = renal tubular acidosis
WBC = white blood cell

37

Enteral Nutrition

Rickey A. Evans

FOUNDATION OVERVIEW

Enteral nutrition (EN) refers to the act of taking nutrients into the body through the gastrointestinal (GI) tract. When a patient cannot ingest the necessary nutrients by eating food, either because of illness, injury, surgery, dysphagia, or changes in absorption, EN can be used to fill the void. In medical terms, we typically think of EN as supplying specialized nutrition support via tube feedings. Parenteral nutrition (PN) provides nutrition intravenously, entirely bypassing the GI tract. In general, if the GI system is functional, it is preferable to use EN rather than parenteral feedings.

EN is used in various clinical situations. It may be used to provide nutrition acutely when a patient cannot ingest or absorb adequate nutrition from oral intake or to provide nutrition during periods of extended illness. In general, if an otherwise well-nourished patient cannot take food by mouth for 7 to 14 days, EN should be considered. EN may be the only means of energy intake, or may be used as a supplement to food when oral intake alone is insufficient. Enteral feedings are preferred to parenteral feedings (provision of nutrients through the venous system) for several reasons. Enteral feedings make use of a functional or partially functional gut, reducing the risk of gut atrophy. EN also reduces the risk of infection by removing the need for venous access, and it is also less costly than PN. Additionally, EN is associated with significantly less metabolic complications, particularly glucose intolerance and increased requirements for insulin given it is more physiologic compared to PN in terms of nutrient utilization.

TREATMENT

The decision to initiate EN therapy must be based on determination of risk:benefit ratio. The potential benefit for the patient must outweigh the risks of tube placement as well as risk of complications. There are a variety of factors that must be considered when initiating EN in any patient. These issues are discussed below.

Route of Administration

Several considerations dictate the route of administration. The level of GI dysfunction and disease state determines where nutrients should enter the GI tract. Feeding should be initiated at the highest level of functional gut, consistent with the patient's disease. This will maximize the nutrient absorption as well as maintain the gut function at the highest level possible. Patients with gastroparesis or other motility disorders may benefit from tube placement in the jejunum or duodenum as opposed to the stomach. Another consideration is anticipated length of treatment; short-term therapy is typically achieved through use of a nasogastric, orogastric, nasojejunal, or orojejunal tube, but longer therapy usually requires percutaneous placement of a gastrostomy or jejunostomy tube (Table 37-1). Feeding tubes that are intended for short-term therapy are typically placed manually at the bedside as opposed to surgical or endoscopic placement of gastrostomy or jejunostomy tubes that are intended for provision of long-term EN.

The type of enteral feed as well as the route of feeding is determined by the level at which the normal process has broken down. For instance, in a patient whose jaw is wired shut, the mouth is the portion of the GI tract that needs to be bypassed, so a nasogastric tube would be appropriate, whereas a patient with gastric cancer may require feeding at the level of the duodenum, bypassing the stomach completely.

The tubes used for EN are classified by their external diameter, which is measured in French units (Fr); 1 French unit equals 0.33 mm. The inner lumen size is dependent upon the material used; the smallest practical size is used for patient comfort. While small-bore tubes are more likely to become clogged, they are preferred for oral or nasal feedings. Larger nasogastric or orogastric tubes are typically reserved for suctioning or decompression. While these tubes clog significantly less than small-bore tubes, they are associated with more discomfort for the patient.

Administration Methods

For critically ill patients, continuous feeds are usually the preferred method of administration. Most patients tolerate continuous feeds better than intermittent or bolus regimens, but continuous feeding regimens are restrictive. They require that the patient remain attached to the feeding source, which in the case of ambulatory patients is extremely limiting. Continuous feeds may also need to be interrupted for medication administration. Recommendations for the initiation and advancement of continuous tube feeds are variable as it is highly dependent on how well the patient tolerates the regimen. The general

TABLE 37-1 | **Enteral Feeding Routes**

Tube	Type/Insertion Technique	Clinical Uses	Potential Complications
Nasogastric	Placed into the stomach through the nose Position verified by injecting air and auscultation or by x-ray	Short-term (up to 4 wk) or longer periods with intermittent insertion; bolus feeding simpler, but continuous drip with pump better tolerated	Aspiration; ulceration of nasal and esophageal tissues, leading to stricture; sinusitis
Nasoduodenal	Placed into the duodenum through the nose, usually endoscopically	Short-term clinical situations where gastric emptying is impaired Requires continuous drip with pump Decreased aspiration risk compared to gastric insertion	Spontaneous pulling back into stomach (position verified by aspirating content, pH >6); sinusitis Diarrhea common, fiber-containing formulas may help
Nasojejunal	Placed into the jejunum through the nose, usually endoscopically	Short-term clinical situations where gastric emptying is impaired Requires continuous drip with pump	Spontaneous pulling back into stomach Diarrhea common, fiber-containing formulas may help; sinusitis
Gastrostomy	Percutaneous endoscopic gastrostomy (PEG) Endoscopic placement directly into the stomach	Long-term clinical situations, swallowing disorders, or impaired small-bowel absorption requiring continuous drip	Aspiration; irritation around tube exit site; peritoneal leak; balloon migration and obstruction of pylorus
Jejunostomy	Percutaneous endoscopic jejunostomy (PEJ) Endoscopic placement directly into the jejunum	Long-term clinical situations where gastric emptying is impaired Requires continuous drip with pump; direct endoscopic placement (PEJ) is the most comfortable for patient	Clogging or displacement of tube; jejunal fistula if large-bore tube used; diarrhea from dumping; irritation of surgical anchoring suture
Combined gastrojejunostomy	Double-lumen line, one lumen in stomach for gastric suction, the other in the jejunum to provide nutrition	Used for patients with impaired gastric emptying and at high risk for aspiration or patients with acute pancreatitis or proximal leaks	Clogging, especially of small bore jejunal tube

Note: All small tubes are at risk for clogging, especially if used for crushed medications. In long-term enteral patients, gastrostomy and jejunostomy tubes can be exchanged for a low-profile "button" (access port) once the tract is established.

Adapted with permission from Fauci AS, Braunwald E, Kasper DL, et al: *Harrison's Principles of Internal Medicine*, 17th ed. New York, NY: McGraw-Hill Professional; 2008.

recommendation is to start at 20 to 50 mL/h and advance by 10 to 25 mL/h every 4 to 8 hours until the desired goal is achieved.

Other mechanisms of tube feed administration include cyclic, intermittent, and bolus administration. Cyclic EN may be beneficial in patients who may not eat well throughout the day due to inability to consume enough calories to meet increased needs during illness or simply lack of appetite. As a result, cyclic feeds can be administered by pump only at night as a supplement to the calories that the patient is able to consume throughout the day. Intermittent feedings provide more flexibility as they are scheduled for specific times and durations. Bolus feeds mimic meals as a relatively large amount of formula is provided over a short amount of time. Initially, bolus feeds are not tolerated as well as other methods, but many patients who are on long-term EN come to accept them as their diet is advanced.

Contraindications

EN is contraindicated in patients with a mechanical bowel obstruction, bowel ischemia, active peritonitis, necrotizing enterocolitis, and uncorrectable coagulopathy. Although not absolute contraindications, intractable nausea and vomiting, severe diarrhea, gastrointestinal bleeding, and hemodynamic instability may result in challenges to providing optimal EN to a patient.

REGIMEN SELECTION

The choice of nutritional products must be made on an individual basis, taking into account not only nutritional requirements (Table 37-2), but individual patient preferences as well.

Fluid Requirements

Daily fluid requirements vary by age and body weight (Table 37-3). Individual requirements can diverge from these estimations dramatically in acutely ill patients, as the formulas do not account for fluid losses from sources such as diarrhea, vomiting, nasogastric suction, or wound drainage. These basic calculations also cannot account for fluid retention in diseases such as heart, renal, or hepatic failure.

TABLE 37-2	**Enteral Formula Components**				
Formula	**Carbohydrate**	**Protein**	**Fat**	**Indication**	**Comments**
Standard polymeric	Corn syrup solids	Casein	Corn oil	Patients with functional GI tract	Isotonic 1-2 kcal/mL
	Hydrolyzed corn starch	Whey	Soybean oil		
	Sucrose	Soy protein	Canola oil		
	Fructose	Egg white	MCT		
Elemental or peptide based	Hydrolyzed corn starch Maltodextrin fructose	Hydrolyzed casein Hydrolyzed whey	Corn oil Soybean oil	Patients who cannot digest intact proteins	
		Hydrolyzed soy protein	Canola oil		
		Hydrolyzed lactalbumin	MCT		
		Crystalline amino acids			
High protein				Patients who require ≥1. 5 g/kg protein daily	
Modular formulas				Those who need supplementation of specific nutrient (protein, fat, or carbohydrate) to supplement other EN formula	

Assessment of the fluid needs of each patient must be made on an individual basis, and all sources of fluid intake (oral intake, tube feeding, intravenous infusion) must be taken into account.

Energy Requirements

Adult energy requirements in well-nourished adults on bed rest average 30 to 35 kcal/kg. Critical illness, trauma (burns especially), catabolic states such as some cancers, and preexisting malnutrition can increase energy requirements, while those with chronic illnesses or wasting with a loss of lean body tissue may have significantly lower energy requirements.

Enteral formulas are available commercially with a caloric density of 0.5 to 2.0 kcal/mL, while most standard formulas are around 1 kcal/mL. The availability of various caloric densities is useful for those with fluid restrictions, or those unable to tolerate more concentrated feedings.

Proteins and Amino Acids

In patients who require nutritional support, at least 1 g protein per kilogram body weight per day is recommended. This level of protein repletion can minimize protein loss and muscle wasting. Up to 1.5 g/kg may be recommended in malnourished patients or those in catabolic states, reserving 1 g/kg or less for those with renal or hepatic failure.

Protein in enteral nutritional formulas is provided in several different forms. Standard enteral formulas (also known as polymeric formulas) are appropriate for those who do not have any difficulty with digestion, because they contain intact proteins. These proteins are most often derived from milk, meat, egg, or soybeans sources. For those unable to digest intact proteins, the proteins may be hydrolyzed to peptides or specific amino acids. Smaller molecular forms of protein provide higher osmolar loads. Many products contain combinations of protein forms.

Essential amino acids are those that must be provided by the diet and cannot be synthesized in the body. Conditionally, essential amino acids are those that can become depleted. Essentially the body's production of these amino acids cannot keep up with the demand. Therefore, in times of high demand, conditionally essential amino acids must be supplemented by the diet.

Glutamine and arginine may become conditionally essential amino acids in times of physiological stress such as trauma or infection, and are often present in EN formulas used for critical illness even though clinical trials have not shown consistent benefit.

Carbohydrates

Carbohydrates provide the majority of calories in EN; usually 40% to 60%. These calories are provided as monosaccharides and polysaccharides depending on the formulation. Polysaccharides are preferred in patients who have the ability to digest them; monosaccharides are more osmotically active than polysaccharides, increasing the osmolality of the formulation.

Care must be taken in those with insulin resistance or diabetes to minimize glucose excursions, which expose the patient to hyper- or hypoglycemia and may complicate the course of recovery.

Most enteral formulas are lactose free. This is important because of the high prevalence of lactase deficiency in the population. There is also decreased lactase production during critical illness, which decreases the tolerability of lactose-containing products.

TABLE 37-3	**Daily Maintenance Fluid Requirements**	
Age	**Weight**	**Calculation**
Neonates	1-10 kg	100 mL/kg body weight
Child	10-20 kg	1000 mL + 50 mL/kg >10 kg
Adult	>20 kg	1500 mL + 20 mL/kg >20 kg

Lipids

Most EN products derive 30% to 40% of their calories from fat, although specialty products with different levels are available. Lipid content is usually derived from corn, soybean, or canola oil. Medium-chain triglycerides (MCT) are available in elemental formulas and are easier to digest than lipids in standard formulas given they are more water soluble when compared to long-chain triglycerides; they may be especially beneficial for those with hepatic failure.

Fiber

Fiber requirements for EN patients are driven by several factors. EN products containing fiber may be beneficial for those who experience GI intolerance to EN such as diarrhea or constipation. Fiber supplementation may also help to maintain GI function in those on long-term EN, but may be inappropriate for patients at risk for GI obstruction.

Disease-Specific Considerations

Patients with chronic renal disease, particularly those with nephrotic syndrome, are at risk of protein malnutrition. Malnutrition risk must be balanced with the possible benefit of protein restriction (potential decrease in disease progression) depending on disease stage. This is done by providing enteral feeds with low protein and high amino acid content. Formulas for dialysis patients have higher protein content (closer to usual protein diet) to replace protein lost during dialysis. All renal preparations are calorically dense to decrease fluid load and have low electrolyte content.

Hepatic disease causes irregularities in protein metabolism and synthesis which can not only lead to protein malnutrition, but also to hepatic encephalopathy from accumulation of nitrogenous waste, particularly from aromatic amino acids (AAA). Hepatic patients tend to have low levels of branched chain amino acids (BCAA) and high levels of aromatic AAA. Formulations high in BCAA and low in AAA are available; the results of randomized clinical trials using these products are mixed.

Trauma patients are in a state of catabolism with high caloric needs; the products for these patients are calorically dense and provide high levels of nitrogen to prevent protein malnutrition.

Malnutrition in pulmonary disease is common, and many advanced COPD patients are in a hypermetabolic state. Carbohydrate metabolism produces more CO_2 than fat or protein metabolism. Pulmonary formulations provide a lower percent of calories from carbohydrate and higher percent from fat (approximately 50%) when compared to a standard nutritional product to help ease this strain on the respiratory system.

DRUG ADMINISTRATION

As pharmacists, some of the most common questions that arise regarding EN surround the medications that can and cannot be administered via feeding tubes.

When drugs are administered orally, they are delivered directly to the stomach. Once in the stomach, medications must contend with a relatively low pH environment. Many drugs have been designed with this in mind; bypassing the stomach may delay or decrease drug dissolution.

When administering drugs via feeding tube, special attention must be paid to timing of drugs versus timing of feedings, especially in those receiving continuous feedings. In those on continuous feeding regimens, feeding should be held at least 15 minute prior to and after drug administration. A few drugs require administration on an empty stomach. In those cases feeding needs to be stopped 1 to 2 hours before and after drug administration.

The size of the feeding tube also needs to be taken into account. While very narrow tubes may be more comfortable for the patient, they are more likely to clog with drug administration. Flushing with 30 mL of water (10-15 mL for children) before and after drug administration can minimize clogging. When administering drugs that are provided in tablet form, special attention needs to be paid to whether or not the tablet is crushable. Numerous lists of "do not crush" drugs have been published, and the package insert for the specific drug will also provide this information. Tablets that can be crushed must be ground to a fine powder and mixed with 15 to 30 mL of water (or other solvent, check package insert) for tube administration. It is imperative to verify "crushability" of each specific medication. Crushing delayed-release medications will result in a bolus effect of the medication. Some capsules can be opened, and the intact beads administered via the feeding tubes, but with small-bore tubes, the granules may clog the tube. Intuitively, liquid medication would be more appropriate for tube administration than other forms, but this is not always the case, as some liquid medications may cause GI intolerance (especially those containing sorbitol); primarily when administered to the small intestine rather than the stomach. In addition, liquid medications are likely to have physical incompatibilities with the EN product itself, becoming insoluble in the GI tract or clogging the feeding tube; diluting the liquid prior to administration may avoid this complication.

One of the most well-known drug–tube feed interactions is oral phenytoin (Table 37-4). When oral phenytoin is administered in the presence of EN products, drug absorption may be decreased by up to 75%. When oral phenytoin is administered to patients receiving EN, consistent timing between feeds and drug administration must be maintained. Vigilant patient monitoring is also required to minimize toxicity and maintain therapeutic phenytoin concentrations. Administering phenytoin via the intravenous route may be required in some circumstances in order to guarantee therapeutic concentrations.

Another drug that requires vigilant monitoring in those receiving EN is warfarin. Many EN products have above the adequate intake level (90-120 mcg/d) of vitamin K; most products contain approximately 200 mcg/1000 kcal. Warfarin resistance is commonly reported in those using EN.

Aside from some of the more obvious interactions, drugs administered via tube feedings often cause diarrhea, especially liquid medications that contain sorbitol and those with high osmolality.

TABLE 37-4	Medications with Special Considerations for Enteral Feeding Tube Administration	
Drug	**Interaction**	**Comments**
Phenytoin	■ Reduced bioavailability in the presence of tube feedings ■ Possible phenytoin binding to *calcium* caseinates or protein hydrolysates in enteral feeding	■ To minimize interaction, holding tube feedings 1-2 hours before and after phenytoin has been suggested; this has no proven benefit ■ Adjust tube-feeding rate to account for time held for phenytoin administration ■ Monitor phenytoin serum concentration and clinical response closely ■ Consider switching to IV phenytoin if unable to reach therapeutic serum concentration
■ Fluoroquinolones ■ Tetracyclines	Potential for reduced bioavailability because of complexation of drug with divalent and trivalent cations found in enteral feeding	■ Consider holding tube feeding 1 hour before and after administration ■ Avoid jejunal administration of ciprofloxacin ■ Monitor clinical response
Warfarin	Decreased absorption of warfarin because of enteral feeding; therapeutic effect antagonized by vitamin K in enteral formulations	■ Adjust warfarin dose based on INR ■ Anticipate need to increase warfarin dose when enteral feedings are started and decrease dose when enteral feedings are stopped ■ Consider holding tube feeding 1 hour before and after administration
■ Omeprazole ■ Lansoprazole	Administration via feeding tube complicated by acid-labile medication within delayed-release, base-labile granules	■ Granules become sticky when moistened with water and may occlude small-bore tubes ■ Granules should be mixed with acidic liquid when given via a gastric feeding tube ■ An oral liquid suspension can be extemporaneously prepared for administration via a feeding tube

Abbreviation: INR, International Normalized Ratio.
Reproduced with permission from DiPiro JT, Talbert RL, Yee GC, et al: *Pharmacotherapy: A Pathophysiologic Approach*, 9th ed. New York:, NY McGraw-Hill; 2014.

COMPLICATIONS

Many complications of EN are a direct result of mechanical problems related to the feeding process itself while others are GI or metabolic complications that may be related to the specific formula being used or patient's disease state.

Gastrointestinal

Motility disorders are frequent adverse effects of EN and include both constipation and diarrhea. Diarrhea from malabsorption, medications, or bacterial overgrowth is common. Less commonly, diarrhea may be caused by administration of a hypertonic formula. It can often be managed by the use of continuous administration versus intermittent feedings or by using a formula that contains fiber. Likewise, constipation may be caused by drugs, or it may be precipitated by low volume status, obstruction, or low fiber intake.

Nausea and vomiting, also commonly seen in EN, is believed to be a result of high gastric residual (high volume of formula left in the stomach). In acute situations, gastric residuals are monitored every 4 to 6 hours, or prior to the next scheduled feeding time. High gastric residual is also considered a culprit in aspiration.

Aspiration

Aspiration is a frequent complication of tube feeding. The risks for aspiration increase with delayed gastric emptying (and subsequent high gastric residual), impaired lower esophageal sphincter tone, inhibition of cough reflex, decreased consciousness, and mechanical ventilation. All patients should be evaluated for risk of aspiration.

The most serious complication of aspiration and of EN itself is aspiration pneumonia. This is a chemical pneumonitis initially, as gastric pH is not conducive to bacterial growth. The ubiquitous use of proton pump inhibitors and H_2 blockers may contribute to bacterial involvement early in the infection process. Most cases of aspiration result in pneumonitis not pneumonia; therefore, antibiotic therapy is only rarely indicated.

Risks of aspiration can be minimized by elevating the head of the bed to 30° to 45° during feeding and for at least 30 to 60 minutes after feeding. The use of continuous feeding versus intermittent or bolus feeds and regular assessment for correct tube placement can also decrease the risk of aspiration as can duodenal tube placement.

Metabolic

Metabolic complications seen with EN include hyperglycemia along with fluid and electrolyte imbalances. These complications are more common in the critically ill patient than patients managed long-term on EN.

Mechanical

By far the most common mechanical complication seen in EN is clogging of the feeding tube. This may be due to incorrect medication administration such as insufficient flushing of the tube or crushing/mixing of tablets. Malfunctioning feeding tubes and physical irritation from the tube itself may complicate therapy. Management for unclogging tubes includes sterile water, pancreatic enzymes, and sodium bicarbonate solutions.

CASE Application

1. Which of the following statements is <u>NOT</u> true regarding enteral nutrition?

   a. Enteral nutrition should be used only if parenteral nutrition is contraindicated in the patient.
   b. Enteral nutrition is associated with less glucose intolerance compared to parenteral nutrition.
   c. Enteral nutrition is associated with lower rates of infection compared to parenteral nutrition.
   d. Enteral nutrition can be used even if the patient is eating by mouth.

2. While administering medications via nasogastric tubes:

   a. The medication must be compatible with basic fluids.
   b. Tablets must be fully crushed and mixed with 15 to 30 mL of water.
   c. The tube must be flushed with 250 mL of water before and after medication administration.
   d. Capsule beads should be crushed and mixed with 15 to 30 mL of water.

3. JK is a 28 yo admitted with seizures secondary to alcohol withdrawal. The medical team starts JK on oral phenytoin regimen of 100 mg three times daily and also initiates the patient on continuous tube feedings since his oral food intake is inadequate at this time to provide optimal nutrition. All of the following counseling points are appropriate to give the medical team <u>EXCEPT</u>:

   a. The patient's phenytoin should always be converted to IV when on continuous tube feedings.
   b. Tube feedings should be held 1-2 hours before and after the patient's phenytoin dose.
   c. It is important that the nurse adjust the patient's tube feeding rate to adjust for the time held for phenytoin administration.
   d. Tube feedings lead to reduced bioavailability of phenytoin.

4. When administering drugs via enteral feeding tube:

   a. Liquid medications are always preferable to solid dosage forms.
   b. As long as tablets are crushed very finely they will retain their pharmacokinetic properties.
   c. All drugs that a patient receives should be given simultaneously to minimize feeding interruptions.
   d. Liquid medications may interact with nutritional formula.

5. Which of the following statements is correct?

   a. Modular formulas contain a balanced mixture of carbohydrates and lipids.
   b. Calorically dense formulas provide nutrition targeted to a specific disease state.
   c. Elemental formulas contain intact proteins and polysaccharides.
   d. Standard formulas contain intact proteins.

6. Aspiration risks during enteral nutrition feedings are increased by which of the following?

   a. Feeding in an elevated or upright position
   b. High gastric residual prior to feeding
   c. Continuous feeding regimens
   d. High-protein modular feeding

7. Which of the following statements is true regarding aspiration pneumonia?

   a. Is usually viral
   b. Is usually preceded by a bacterial infection
   c. Is a chemical pneumonitis initially
   d. Is decreased by H_2 antagonists

8. Which of the following factors is most important for initial selection of an enteral formulation?

   a. Formula osmolality
   b. Cost of formulation
   c. Location of tube
   d. Nutritional needs

9. Enteral nutrition may be contraindicated or cautioned against use in which of the following situations?

   a. Gastrointestinal bleeding
   b. Gastric cancer
   c. Short bowel syndrome
   d. Colostomy

10. MJ is a hospitalized man who weighs 78 kg and has a BMI of 24 kg/m². What is his calculated daily fluid requirement?

    a. 2160 mL
    b. 2660 mL
    c. 3160 mL
    d. 3660 mL

11. Which of the following daily calorie counts would be most appropriate for MJ (from Question 10)?

    a. 1500 kcal
    b. 2000 kcal
    c. 2500 kcal
    d. 3000 kcal

12. Which of the following is a common complication of enteral nutrition therapy?

    a. Weight loss
    b. Diarrhea
    c. Weight gain
    d. Hypoglycemia

13. Fluid retention associated with enteral nutrition is a problem that is commonly encountered in which of the following disease states?

    a. Heart failure
    b. Respiratory distress

  c. Hyperthyroidism
  d. Diabetic ketoacidosis

14. ED is a 62-year-old woman with type 2 diabetes and end-stage renal disease who requires enteral nutrition. She was recently placed on hemodialysis therapy 3 times/wk. Please select the most appropriate nutrition combination.

  a. Low protein, high carbohydrate
  b. Low protein, low carbohydrate
  c. Moderate protein, low carbohydrate
  d. High protein, high carbohydrate

15. Patients with hepatic encephalopathy may benefit from nutritional formulations containing:

  a. High branched chain amino acids (BCAA), low aromatic amino acids (AAA)
  b. Low branched chain amino acids, high aromatic amino acids
  c. High protein, low amino acids
  d. Protein and amino acid content does not affect hepatic encephalopathy

16. TR is a 72-year-old man with diabetes and COPD. He is currently hospitalized and on a ventilator for community-acquired pneumonia. Which of the following regimens would be most appropriate dietary therapy?

  a. 50% carbohydrate, 30% fat, 20% protein
  b. 65% carbohydrate, 30% fat, 35% protein
  c. 35% carbohydrate, 25% fat, 40% protein
  d. 35% carbohydrate, 50% fat, 15% protein

17. TR (from Question 16) has been in your facility on the ventilator for 4 days and the resident asks how the risk of aspiration can be decreased. Which of the following methods is an appropriate intervention for this patient?

  a. Elevating head of the bed during and after feedings
  b. Initiating intermittent bolus feedings rather than continuous feedings
  c. Placing gastric tube and stopping proton-pump inhibitor use
  d. Placing gastric tube instead of duodenal tube

18. Which of the following statements applies to fiber in enteral formulations?

  a. Decreases tolerability in most patients
  b. May increase diarrhea
  c. May increase constipation
  d. May contribute to GI obstruction

19. Which of the following tubes are correctly matched to their preferred use or tube type?

  a. Nasogastric tube, long-term use
  b. Orogastric tube, small bore
  c. Percutaneous gastric tube, short-term use
  d. Nasojejunal tube, large bore

20. Which of the following patient groups have increased metabolic needs? Select all that apply.

  a. Type 1 diabetics
  b. Trauma patients
  c. Burn patients
  d. Critically ill patients

TAKEAWAY POINTS »

- EN is preferred to PN in those with a functional gut.
- EN should be provided at the highest gut level consistent with the patient's disease state.
- Transnasal tube insertion is appropriate for short-term EN.
- Nausea, vomiting, diarrhea, and constipation are common adverse effects of EN feeding.
- Aspiration pneumonia is the most devastating complication encountered with EN.

- Risk for aspiration is increased with decreased mental status, prolonged supine position, and bolus feeding regimens.
- Standard enteral formulas provide proteins in their intact form that must be hydrolyzed in the gut.
- Fluid content of EN feeds must be individualized based on the disease state and patient-specific parameters.

BIBLIOGRAPHY

ASPEN Board of Directors and the Clinical Guidelines Task Force. Guidelines for the use of parenteral and enteral nutrition in adult and pediatric patients. *J Parenter Enteral Nutr.* 2002;26(suppl):1SA-138SA.

Bankhead R, Boullata J, Brantley S, et al. Clinical guidelines for the use of parenteral and enteral nutrition in adult and pediatric patients. *J Parenter Enteral Nutr.* 2009;33:122-167.

Bistrian BR, Driscoll DF. Enteral and parenteral nutrition therapy. In: Longo DL, Fauci AS, Kasper DL, Hauser SL, Jameson J, Loscalzo J., eds. *Harrison's Principles of*

Internal Medicine. 18th ed. New York, NY: McGraw-Hill; 2012:chap 76.

Kumpf VJ, Chessman KH. Enteral nutrition. In: DiPiro JT, Talbert RL, Yee GC, Matzke GR, Wells BG, Posey L., eds. *Pharmacotherapy: A Pathophysiologic Approach.* 10th ed. New York, NY: McGraw-Hill; 2017.

Walroth TA, Ryan L, Miller ML. Enteral and parenteral nutrition. In: Attridge RL, Miller ML, Moote R, Ryan L., eds. *Internal Medicine: A Guide to Clinical Therapeutics.* New York, NY: McGraw-Hill; 2013:chap 19.

KEY ABBREVIATIONS

AAA = aromatic amino acids
BCAA = branched chain amino acids
EN = enteral nutrition

GI = gastrointestinal
MCT = medium-chain triglycerides

38 Parenteral Nutrition

Sarah J. Miller

FOUNDATION OVERVIEW

Parenteral nutrition (PN) involves delivery of nutrients by the intravenous (IV) route. The term total parenteral nutrition (TPN) implies that all of the patient's nutritional needs are being met by this route even though the term is often used when the patient is receiving both oral feedings or tube feedings (enteral nutrition or EN) and IV feedings simultaneously.

PN may be delivered by either the central (CPN) or peripheral (PPN) route. When delivered centrally, the feeding catheter is typically placed into the subclavian vein with the tip of the catheter near the opening of the right atrium. For PPN, the catheter is placed into a peripheral vein; because hypertonic solutions of PN can cause phlebitis when administered peripherally, the osmolarity of PPN solutions in adults is generally limited to about 900 mOsm/L. The osmolarity of dextrose/amino acid containing PPN can be estimated by adding 100 mOsm/L for each 1% final concentration of amino acid and 50 mOsm/L for each 1% final concentration of dextrose. Peripherally inserted central catheters (PICC lines) are often utilized for PN administration. PICC lines provide central venous access through which hypertonic PN formula may be administered.

PN is preferred over EN *only* when EN cannot be used safely. PN is indicated in situations when EN is not possible or feasible. When to start PN in these situations is patient and situation specific and is controversial. North American guidelines discourage use of PN in a well-nourished patient and in those not at high nutritional risk during the first 7 days of an intensive care unit (ICU) admission in which EN cannot be established. For ICU patients who were malnourished prior to admission or whose illness puts them at high nutritional risk, the guidelines recommend initiation of PN as soon as possible if EN is not feasible. Typically, if resumption of EN is anticipated within 5 to 7 days, PN should not be initiated as it is unlikely to improve outcomes, is expensive, and is associated with potentially significant adverse events. See Table 38-1 for a list of more common situations in which PN is indicated. CPN may be used long term; patients with short bowel syndrome may receive home PN for decades. On the other hand, PPN is usually a short-term therapy lasting no more than 7 to 10 days.

COMPONENTS AND DESIGNING A REGIMEN

PN solutions contain macrosubstrates and microsubstrates. Macrosubstrates consist of a carbohydrate source, lipid emulsion, and amino acid solution. Microsubstrates include electrolytes, vitamins, and trace elements.

Fluid

Fluid requirements of PN patients can vary widely. Some fluid-restricted patients may receive as little as 1000 or 1250 mL of PN per day. Typical PN volumes for patients without fluid restrictions are 1500 to 3000 mL/d. In the hospital, PN is most commonly infused continuously over 24 hours. In the home setting, PN may be cycled over a shorter period of time (eg, 12-16 hours), often at night, to allow the patient more freedom in mobility.

Carbohydrate

The carbohydrate source of most PN solutions is dextrose. IV dextrose provides 3.4 kcal/g. Stock solutions of 10%, 20%, 30%, 50%, and 70% dextrose are commonly used in compounding. Dextrose and amino acid cannot come premixed from the manufacturer because of stability issues with heat sterilization. On the other hand, glycerin and amino acid can be mixed by the manufacturer and heat sterilized; the trade name of such a product is ProcalAmine.

Lipid

IV lipid emulsions (Intralipid, Liposyn III, Smoflipid) contain fat, glycerin, and phospholipid. When calculating calories from IV lipid emulsions, the following caloric densities are used: 10% emulsion—1.1 kcal/mL; 20% emulsion—2 kcal/mL; and 30% emulsion—2.9 kcal/mL.

Amino Acids

Standard amino acid solutions (Aminosyn, Aminosyn II, Travasol, FreAmine III, Clinisol, Novamine) contain essential and nonessential amino acids and are supplied by the manufacturer in concentrations ranging from 3.5% to 15%. Some of these products contain standard concentrations of electrolytes already added, whereas others do not. Specialized amino acid

TABLE 38-1	Indications for Parenteral Nutrition in Adults

- Bowel obstruction
  - Physical or mechanical (eg, tumor compressing intestinal lumen)
  - Functional (eg, ileus, colonic pseudo-obstruction)
- Major small bowel resection (eg, short-bowel syndrome)
  - Adult patients with <100 cm of small bowel distal to the ligament of Treitz without a colon
  - Adult patients with <50 cm of small bowel if the colon is intact
- Diffuse peritonitis
- Intestinal fistulas if EN cannot be provided above or below the fistula
- Pancreatitis—if patients have failed EN beyond the ligament of Treitz or cannot receive EN (eg, because of intestinal obstruction)
- Severe intractable vomiting
- Severe intractable diarrhea
- Preoperative nutrition support in patients with moderate to severe malnutrition who cannot tolerate EN and in whom surgery can be delayed safely for at least 7 days
- In critically ill patients without malnutrition who cannot receive oral or EN in the first 7 days of ICU admission, PN should only be initiated after the first 7 days of admission and if oral or EN is still not feasible

Abbreviations: EN, enteral nutrition; ICU, intensive care unit; PN, parenteral nutrition.
Reproduced with permission from Chisholm-Burns MA, Schwinghammer TL, Wells BG, et al: *Pharmacotherapy Principles and Practice*, 4th ed. New York, NY: McGraw-Hill; 2016.

formulations designed for pediatrics (TrophAmine, Aminosyn-PF, Premasol) are widely utilized. Specialized amino acid formulations designed for adults with renal failure, hepatic failure, and stress are expensive and are rarely clinically useful. Hepatic formulations contain higher amounts of branched chain amino acids and lower amounts of aromatic amino acids compared to standard formulas. Stress formulas contain higher amounts of branched chain amino acids with amounts of aromatic amino acids similar to those found in standard solutions. Renal formulas contain mainly essential amino acids. Amino acid solutions provide 4 kcal/g.

Macrosubstrate Provision Recommendations

Guidelines call for provision of energy via PN for nonobese adults between 20 and 35 total kcal per kg body weight per day (kcal/kg/d). Guidelines for calorie provision in the obese patient are shown in Table 38-2. Calories should be divided between dextrose and lipid (as well as protein) such that dextrose does not exceed 7 g/kg/d and lipid does not exceed 2.5 g/kg/d. Lipid kilocalories typically make up about 15% to 30% of nonprotein kilocalories; North American guidelines discourage IV soybean lipid (eg, Intralipid, Liposyn III) administration during the first 7 days of an ICU admission. The recent approval in the United States of Smoflipid, which contains soybean oil, medium chain triglycerides, olive oil, and fish oil, gives a potentially less proinflammatory lipid option for use in the early days of an ICU admission. Note that propofol, a medication used in the ICU for sedation, is compounded in a 10% soybean lipid emulsion; these lipid kilocalories (1.1 kcal/mL) should be taken into account when calculating total kilocalories in a patient's regimen. Likewise, many medications are

TABLE 38-2	Guidelines for Calorie and Protein Provision in Obese Critically Ill Patients: Hypocaloric, High Protein Feedings[a]	
	Calorie Recommendation per Day	**Protein Recommendation per Day**
	11-14 kcal/kg/d actual body weight if body mass index is 30-50 kg/m²	2 g/kg/d ideal body weight for body mass index 30-40 kg/m²
	22-25 kcal/kg/d ideal body weight if body mass index is >50 kg/m²	Up to 2.5 g/kg/d ideal body weight if body mass index >40 kg/m²

[a]Recommendations are for patients without severe renal or hepatic dysfunction.

compounded in dextrose 5% which may provide significant calories.

Amino acids are generally supplied in PN solutions at amounts up to about 2 g/kg/d. Guidelines for ICU patients with body mass index (BMI) less than 30 kg/m² call for 1.2 to 2 g/kg actual body weight per day or perhaps higher in burn and trauma patients. Protein guidelines for obese patients are given in Table 38-2. Patients receiving hemodialysis or continuous renal replacement therapy may require up to 2.5 g protein per kg body weight per day to account for protein losses through the dialysis process itself. Nitrogen balance studies can be useful in determining protein requirements. In these studies, "nitrogen out" (urinary urea nitrogen in grams) is augmented by a factor of 4 g (to account for nonurinary urea nitrogen.) This sum is then subtracted from "nitrogen in" (number of grams of amino acid infused divided by 6.25) to arrive at the nitrogen balance.

Electrolytes, Vitamins, and Trace Elements

The electrolytes, vitamins, and trace elements commonly included in PN solutions are listed in Table 38-3. Addition of thiamine, folic acid, and pyridoxine are the most critical vitamins in the short-term PN situation. Note that vitamin K added to PN solution can counteract the effect of the anticoagulant warfarin.

Other Additives

Medications commonly added to PN formulations are listed in Table 38-4.

ORDERING, COMPOUNDING, LABELING, AND ADMINISTRATION

Hospitals administering PN solutions should utilize an order form. Compounding of PN solutions may occur by a manual system (eg, not using a pump and utilizing volumes of macrosubstrates supplied by the manufacturers) or by using an automated compounder by which volumes of the various macrosubstrates and microsubstrates can be more tightly controlled. A commercially available, two-chambered, premixed system (Clinimix, Clinimix E) comprised of various concentrations of dextrose and amino acids separated by a septum is also commonly

TABLE 38-3	Electrolytes, Vitamins, and Trace Elements Commonly Included in PN Solutions

Electrolytes

Sodium (from sodium chloride, sodium acetate, sodium phosphate)

Potassium (from potassium chloride, potassium acetate, potassium phosphate)

Magnesium (from magnesium sulfate, magnesium chloride)

Calcium (from calcium gluconate, calcium chloride)

Phosphorus (from potassium phosphate, sodium phosphate)

Chloride (from potassium chloride, sodium chloride, calcium chloride, magnesium chloride)

Acetate (from sodium acetate, potassium acetate)

Vitamins

Vitamin A

Vitamin D

Vitamin E

Vitamin K

Thiamine

Riboflavin

Niacin

Pyridoxine

Cyanocobalamin (Vitamin B_{12})

Folic acid

Pantothenic acid

Biotin

Ascorbic acid (Vitamin C)

Trace elements

Zinc

Copper[a]

Chromium

Manganese[a]

Selenium

[a]Copper and manganese are commonly omitted with cholestasis, that is, if serum total bilirubin exceeds about 5 mg/dL.

TABLE 38-4	Medications Most Commonly Added to PN

Regular insulin

Histamine$_2$-receptor antagonists

Heparin[a]

Hydrocortisone[a]

Iron dextran[b]

[a]Sometimes added to PPN to help prevent thrombophlebitis.
[b]Can be added to dextrose/amino acid solutions but is incompatible with TNA.

utilized. A three-chambered system (Kabiven, Perikabiven) which includes lipid is also available. Simple breakage of the septa allows the components to mix together. Lipid can be added to the two-chambered dextrose/amino acid mixture or infused separately. Clinimix E, Kabiven, and Perikabiven are manufactured with standard amounts of electrolytes already included in the solutions. Some health care institutions outsource PN compounding to entities outside the institution. Sterility in compounding PN is important because these solutions may support microbial growth and may hang for up to 24 hours.

PN solutions may be compounded as a combination of dextrose, amino acids, lipid, and additives in a single container. These are referred to as three-in-one emulsions or total nutrient admixtures (TNA). A TNA will be most stable if it meets the following final concentration criteria: amino acids more than or equal to 4%, dextrose more than or equal to 10%, and lipid more than or equal to 2%. Another method

for administration mixes dextrose and amino acids together; the lipid emulsion is then piggybacked onto a primary IV line. Whereas TNA or dextrose plus amino acid solutions can hang for 24 hours, lipid emulsion alone generally should only hang for 12 hours due to the higher potential of microbial growth in the isotonic environment of lipid emulsion which has a pH near the physiologic range.

Addition of electrolytes, particularly calcium and phosphate, to PN solutions must be done with care. Calcium and phosphate can form a precipitate if added in large quantities. Factors increasing calcium/phosphate solubility include decreased temperature, decreased pH, and increased amino acid concentration of the solution. When compounding PN, it is typically recommended to add phosphate first, and then to add calcium near the end of the compounding sequence when the volume of the PN is maximized. Also, calcium gluconate leads to a better solubility profile in PN compared to calcium chloride.

TNAs present other stability concerns. Destabilization of the negative charge on the surface of lipid emulsion globules in the admixture can lead to creaming or cracking of the emulsion. A creamed emulsion can be made homogeneous again by gently inverting the bag containing the emulsion several times; such an emulsion may be safely administered to a patient. On the other hand, gentle inversion of a cracked emulsion does not result in the emulsion returning to its initial state and cannot be safely administered to a patient.

Dextrose/amino acid solutions should be administered through a 0.22-µm filter; such filters remove particulates as well as microorganisms introduced into the solution during the compounding process. TNAs cannot be administered through 0.22-µm filters because lipid globules within these admixtures are larger than 0.22 µm. Thus, TNA should be administered through 1.2 µm filters which remove particulates but not smaller microbes.

PN labels should reflect daily amounts of components. This should decrease errors, particularly when transferring a patient from one health care setting to another (eg, hospital to home or vice versa). Listing concentrations and amounts per liter of components may lead to more errors due to misinterpretation.

COMPLICATIONS AND MONITORING

Metabolic

PN can be associated with various metabolic complications. Hyperglycemia is common; blood sugar is typically monitored several times daily at initiation of PN. Frequency of blood sugar monitoring can be decreased when stability is demonstrated. Goal blood glucose range is 140 to 180 mg/dL in patients receiving PN. Regular insulin is frequently added to PN solutions, and subcutaneous sliding scale insulin is also frequently administered. Use of long-acting insulin, such as insulin glargine, may be useful in selected patients on PN, although this use is problematic if the PN is unexpectedly discontinued, held or if patients have renal dysfunction which impairs insulin elimination. Separate insulin drips utilizing regular insulin are frequently utilized in ICU patients receiving PN. Hypoglycemia can occur when PN is abruptly discontinued. Although this is not commonly a problem, some institutions cut the rate of PN in half for an hour or so before discontinuing. Home PN patients often run their solution at lower rates for the first and last hours of their daily infusion cycle.

Abnormalities of electrolytes are frequently seen in PN patients. Hypophosphatemia, hypokalemia, and hypomagnesemia may require increases in the amounts of these electrolytes added to the PN, additional bolus dosages, or both. These electrolyte abnormalities, especially hypophosphatemia, can be associated with the so-called refeeding syndrome in chronically malnourished patients. These electrolytes should be monitored at least twice a week upon initiation of PN; frequency of monitoring can be cut back when levels have demonstrated stability. Hyperphosphatemia, hyperkalemia, and hypermagnesemia occur primarily during renal insufficiency and require decreasing these electrolytes in the PN solution. Mild hyponatremia is common in PN patients. Addition of more sodium to the PN is not always appropriate; the patient could already be fluid-overloaded and thus the decreased serum sodium is due to dilution. Acid–base imbalances are not typically secondary to PN therapy itself. Acetate in PN solutions is converted to bicarbonate in the liver. Decreasing the acetate to chloride ratio in the PN may help correct metabolic alkalosis, whereas increasing this ratio may be helpful in metabolic acidosis.

Hypertriglyceridemia, defined as a serum triglyceride concentration above 400 to 500 mg/dL, may occur in patients receiving IV lipid. Hypertriglyceridemia of this magnitude should be avoided, if possible, to prevent an increased risk of pancreatitis. With hypertriglyceridemia in this range, generally the amount of lipid emulsion infused is decreased. Triglycerides should be measured prior to initiation of lipid emulsion, after a day of administration, and approximately weekly thereafter in hospitalized patients. Caution is warranted if lipid emulsion is completely withheld in patients receiving PN for more than a couple of weeks; essential fatty acid deficiency could develop if there is no intake of fat.

Liver function abnormalities have been associated with PN therapy. Two general patterns have been described. The first pattern, characterized by elevation of aspartate and alanine aminotransferase, typically occurs within a few days of initiation of PN and is associated with hepatic steatosis, or fat accumulation in the liver. This pattern is seen in patients being overfed especially with dextrose. The second pattern is cholestasis characterized by an increase in alkaline phosphatase and total bilirubin. This pattern tends to develop after two or

more weeks of PN in adult patients. Liver function tests should be monitored weekly in hospitalized patients receiving PN.

Mechanical

Mechanical complications of PN include problems with insertion of the central venous catheter such as pneumothorax (punctured lung). Catheter occlusion or thrombosis may also occur. Occlusion may be treated by infusion of a thrombolytic agent or hydrochloric acid, depending on the nature of the occlusion.

Infectious

Catheter-related infections are common in patients receiving PN and are the most common cause of hospitalization in patients receiving home PN. Such infections present with symptoms such as fever, chills, and rigors. Because placement of a permanent central venous catheter is expensive and invasive, attempts to salvage infected catheters are frequently made in long-term home PN patients where IV access sites may also be limited. Administration of IV antibiotics and/or placement of a small amount of antibiotic as an antibiotic lock of the catheter may be utilized. Most catheter-related infections are secondary to gram-positive bacteria, although gram-negative bacteria or fungi may also be culprits. Typically, fungal infection requires catheter removal and replacement.

CASE Application

1. LC is a 48-year-old man who underwent small bowel resection for a volvulus (gut twisting) that caused bowel necrosis. He is receiving PN and has required a nasogastric tube for suction. He develops metabolic alkalosis. Which of the following is the most appropriate adjustment to LC's PN solution?

   a. Add sodium bicarbonate
   b. Decrease acetate and increase chloride
   c. Increase acetate and decrease chloride
   d. Increase sodium and potassium

2. Which of the following statements is true regarding macrosubstrates found in PN solutions? Select all that apply.

   a. Dextrose and amino acids can be mixed together by the manufacturer, heat sterilized, and then shipped to hospitals.
   b. Glycerin and amino acids can be mixed together by the manufacturer, heat sterilized, and then shipped to hospitals.
   c. Clinimix is a two compartment PN solution containing dextrose and amino acid that is available in the United States.
   d. Kabiven is a three compartment PN solution containing dextrose, amino acid, and lipid that is available in the United States.
   e. Glycerin and dextrose can be mixed together by the manufacturer, heat sterilized, and then shipped to hospitals.

3. A patient is receiving ProcalAmine postoperatively at 100 mL/h. ProcalAmine contains 3% final concentration of glycerin (4.3 kcal/g) and 3% final concentration of amino acid. How many total calories and how much protein are provided per day by this solution?

   a. 598 kcal and 72 g amino acid
   b. 533 kcal and 72 g amino acid
   c. 720 kcal and 60 g amino acid
   d. 747 kcal and 60 g amino acid

4. A 51-year-old patient has hepatic encephalopathy that is refractory to standard medical therapy including lactulose. He is intolerant of enteral feedings and is being considered for PN. When compared to a standard amino acid formulation, which of the following amino acid profiles best describes a specialty formulation designed for patients such as this?

   a. Higher in branched chain amino acids, same level of aromatic amino acids
   b. Higher in branched chain amino acids, lower in aromatic amino acids
   c. Higher in essential amino acids, lower in nonessential amino acids
   d. Fortified with dipeptides containing glutamine

5. MF is a 68-year-old woman with cancer cachexia. She has lost 10% of her body weight since her diagnosis with colon cancer about 6 months ago. Her cancer treatments are causing severe nausea and vomiting. The physician wants to start PN. The dietitian expresses concern regarding refeeding syndrome. Which electrolyte abnormalities are characteristic of this syndrome? Select all that apply.

   a. Hypomagnesemia
   b. Hypercalcemia
   c. Hypokalemia
   d. Hypophosphatemia
   e. Hypernatremia

6. A national shortage of IV multivitamin products leads a hospital to ration this product in patients receiving PN. Which vitamins would be most crucial to supplement as individual entities to a hospitalized patient receiving PN for a few weeks in the setting of an IV multivitamin shortage? Select all that apply.

   a. Pantothenic acid
   b. Biotin
   c. Folic acid
   d. Thiamine
   e. Phytonadione

7. Which of the following increases the solubility of calcium and phosphate in a PN solution? Select all that apply.

   a. Increased temperature
   b. Decreased pH

   c. Use of calcium gluconate instead of calcium chloride
   d. Increased amino acid concentration in the PN
   e. Decreased acidity

8. A hospital is transitioning from use of dextrose/amino acid solutions plus piggybacked lipid for PN to a system utilizing TNA. The former practice was to use 0.22 μm filters for dextrose/amino acid solutions and to use 1.2 μm filters for piggybacked lipid emulsion. Which one of the following best describes proper use of final filters with the new TNA system?

   a. A switch from use of 0.22 μm filters to use of 1.2 μm filters is appropriate.
   b. A switch from use of 0.22 μm filters to use of 5 μm filters is appropriate.
   c. No switch in filtration practices is necessary; use of 0.22 μm filters may continue.
   d. Switching from the current 0.22 μm filters to no filters is most appropriate.

9. PS is a 28-year-old man receiving PN because of intolerance to enteral feeding following multiple trauma. He is receiving 150 g of protein each day. A 24-hour urine collection for urea nitrogen (UUN) yields a value of 20 g. What is the estimated nitrogen balance in grams per day for this patient?

   a. +4
   b. 0
   c. −30
   d. −120

10. TL is a 41-year-old mechanically ventilated woman receiving propofol for sedation. The drug is provided as 10 mg/mL propofol and is being delivered at 100 mg/h. Propofol is commercially provided in a 10% lipid emulsion vehicle. How many calories per day is TL receiving via the propofol infusion?

   a. 22
   b. 43
   c. 216
   d. 264

11. Which of the following statements is true regarding TNA?

   a. A cracked TNA may be safely administered to a patient, but a creamed TNA is unsafe for administration.
   b. A creamed TNA may be safely administered to a patient, but a cracked TNA is unsafe for administration.
   c. Neither a creamed nor a cracked TNA may be safely administered to a patient.
   d. Both creamed and cracked TNA may be safely administered to a patient.

12. A 19-year-old patient is involved in a serious motor vehicle accident. He is admitted to the ICU and is

initiated on tube feeding. However, on day 8 of hospitalization, he remains in the ICU and is not tolerating tube feeding. A TNA is ordered. Which of the following additives to the TNA would be expected to remain stable for at least 24 hours and also not adversely affect stability of the TNA? Select all that apply.

a. Famotidine
b. Regular insulin
c. Iron dextran
d. Manganese
e. Glargine insulin

13. AM is to receive cycled PN over 16 h/d at home. The PN is to be infused at half the goal rate for the first and last hours of the 16-hour cycle. If the final concentration of amino acid in the solution is 5%, what goal rate of PN (in mL/h) will supply about 80 g of protein per day?

a. 62
b. 77
c. 92
d. 107

14. A 71-year-old woman is in the intensive care receiving PN following surgical repair of a fistula. Which of the following most closely reflects the current recommendation for the optimal goal blood glucose range for this critically ill PN patient?

a. 80 to 110 mg/dL
b. 90 to 130 mg/dL
c. 140 to 180 mg/dL
d. 180 to 240 mg/dL

15. LF is a 56-year-old man who is receiving PN following a bowel resection for mesenteric ischemia. He is receiving a dextrose/amino acid solution with final concentrations of 15% dextrose and 5% amino acid. This solution is being administered at 75 mL/h continuously over 24 hours. He is also receiving 200 mL of 20% lipid each day. Renal function is normal. LF weighs 60 kg, which is near his ideal body weight of 62 kg. Which of the following best describes the amount of kcal, protein, and dextrose that LF is receiving?

a. Calories are excessive, but the amounts of protein and dextrose are within recommended ranges.
b. The amounts of dextrose and protein are lower than recommended ranges as is the amount of calories.
c. Protein is below the recommended range, but calories and dextrose are adequate.
d. The number of calories, as well as the amounts of protein and dextrose, are within recommended ranges.

16. Which of the following vitamins commonly included in PN solutions could interfere with warfarin anticoagulation?

a. Vitamin A
b. Vitamin K

c. Riboflavin
d. Vitamin B_6

17. Which of the following trace elements are commonly included in PN solutions? Select all that apply.

a. Iron
b. Zinc
c. Manganese
d. Copper
e. Chloride

18. YN is a 38-year-old man with short bowel syndrome who receives home PN. What is the most common PN-related reason that patients on home PN require hospitalization?

a. Metabolic bone disease
b. Catheter-related sepsis
c. Trace element deficiency
d. Hyperglycemia

19. HS is a 61-year-old critically ill, morbidly obese woman (BMI 42 kg/m²) with severe acute pancreatitis in whom EN has failed. On day 7 of hospitalization, PN is initiated. HS weighs 150 kg; ideal body weight is 82 kg. The PN regimen consists of 1800 kcal/d and 180 g protein per day. The patient's renal and liver functions are not severely compromised. What is the most appropriate assessment of this PN regimen?

a. Appropriate calories and protein
b. Appropriate calories; too much protein
c. Appropriate protein; too many calories
d. Too little protein; too many calories

20. Order the following components of a typical PN solution from highest to lowest volume contribution.

Unordered Options	Ordered Response
Electrolytes	
Amino acids	
Vitamins	
Water	

21. A TNA is compounded using 1000 mL of dextrose 10%, 1000 mL of amino acid 8.5%, and 250 mL of 20% lipid emulsion. Which one of the following is true regarding stability of this TNA?

a. Should be stable.
b. Could be unstable because of low concentrations of dextrose and amino acids.
c. Could be unstable because of low concentrations of amino acids and fat.
d. Could be unstable because of high concentrations of dextrose and fat.

22. A peripheral PN solution has final concentrations of 4.25% amino acid and 5% dextrose; no fat is included in this

admixture. What is the approximate osmolarity of this solution (without electrolytes and other additives), and is that osmolarity appropriate for peripheral administration?

a. 675; appropriate
b. 675; inappropriate
c. 1025; appropriate
d. 1025; inappropriate

23. UN is a 34-year-old man admitted to the ICU following a motor vehicle accident in which he suffers major trauma. He was well nourished prior to the accident, and although his injuries are significant, it is anticipated that he is not at high nutritional risk. Enteral feedings (tube feedings) are started on day 2 of admission, but on day 4 they are discontinued due to intolerance. What is the best approach at this time?

a. Start PN with dextrose, amino acids, and soybean oil fat emulsion as soon as possible.
b. Start PN with dextrose and amino acids as soon as possible; hold soybean oil fat emulsion for now.
c. Keep trying to reinitiate enteral feedings and wait on starting PN until about day 8 of admission if the tube feedings are still not successful.
d. Because the patient was previously well nourished, hold both PN and enteral feedings until about day 14 of the hospitalization.

TAKEAWAY POINTS »

- PN is a potentially lifesaving modality of feeding for the patient with severe gastrointestinal compromise precluding adequate oral or enteral feeding.

- EN is preferred over PN if EN can be administered safely, mainly due to a lesser chance of infectious complications with EN and possibly less stimulation of proinflammatory conditions.

- PN may be delivered through either a central or peripheral venous access. Peripheral delivery is limited by the osmolarity of solution that can be administered by this route.

- In patients for whom PN is appropriate, timing of PN is controversial. In general, patients who are previously malnourished should be started on PN sooner than those who are not previously malnourished.

- Caloric contribution of the major macrosubstrates used in PN is as follows: dextrose 3.4 kcal/g, lipid emulsion 20% 2 kcal/mL, and amino acid 4 kcal/g.

- Calories are generally provided via PN at 20 to 35 kcal/kg/d. For the obese patient, recommendations call for less than 14 kcal/kg actual body weight.

- Dextrose is generally limited to less than 7 g/kg/d. Lipid is generally limited to less than 2.5 g/kg/d.

- Amino acids are generally administered at 1.2 to 2 g/kg/d based on actual body weight. Higher amounts (2-2.5 g/kg ideal body weight per day) are appropriate for obese patients. Patients receiving renal replacement therapy also require higher amounts of amino acid.

- Standard amino acid formulations are appropriate for most patients; specialized amino acid formulations (eg, hepatic, renal, stress formulas) are more expensive and rarely indicated.

- TNAs are inherently less stable than dextrose/amino acid solutions. A TNA that has creamed may be administered to a patient after redispersion, whereas a cracked TNA should never be administered to a patient.

BIBLIOGRAPHY

Ayers P, Adams S, Boullata J, et al. A.S.P.E.N. parenteral nutrition safety consensus recommendations. *JPEN J Parenter Enteral Nutr.* 2014;38:296-333.

Boullata JI, Gilbert K, Sacks G, et al. A.S.P.E.N. clinical guidelines: parenteral nutrition ordering, order review, compounding, labeling, and dispensing. *JPEN J Parenter Enteral Nutr.* 2014;38:334-377.

Choban P, Dickerson R, Malone A, et al. A.S.P.E.N. clinical guidelines: nutrition support of hospitalized adult patients with obesity. *JPEN J Parenter Enteral Nutr.* 2013;37:714-744.

Critical Care Nutrition. Clinical practice guidelines. Available at: http://www.criticalcarenutrition.com/index.php?option=com_content&task=view&id=17&Itemid=100. Accessed on February 8, 2017.

Institute for Safe Medication Practices. IV fat emulsion needs a filter. *Acute Care ISMP Medication Safety Alert.* 2016;21(1):3-4.

McClave SA, Taylor BE, Martindale RG, et al. Guidelines for the provision and assessment of nutrition support therapy in the adult critically ill patient: Society of Critical Care Medicine (SCCM) and American Society for Parenteral and Enteral Nutrition (A.S.P.E.N.). *JPEN J Parenter Enteral Nutr.* 2016;40:159-211.

McMahon MM, Nystrom E, Braunschweig C, et al. A.S.P.E.N. clinical guidelines: nutrition support of adult patients with hyperglycemia. *JPEN J Parenter Enteral Nutr.* 2013;37:23-36.

O'Grady NP, Alexander M, Burns LA, et al. 2011 Guidelines for the prevention of intravenous catheter-related infections. Available at: http://www.cdc.gov/hicpac/pdf/guidelines/bsi-guidelines-2011.pdf. Accessed on February 8, 2017.

Trissel LA. Calcium chloride and calcium gluconate. *Handbook on Injectable Drugs.* 18th ed. Bethesda, MD: American Society of Health-Systems Pharmacists; 2014:184-197.

KEY ABBREVIATIONS

ASPEN = American Society for Parenteral and Enteral Nutrition
BMI = body mass index
CPN = central parenteral nutrition
EN = enteral nutrition
ICU = intensive care unit
IV = intravenous
NICE-SUGAR = Normoglycemia in Intensive Care
 Evaluation—Survival Using Glucose Algorithm Regulation

PICC = peripherally inserted central catheter
PN = parenteral nutrition
PPN = peripheral parenteral nutrition
TNA = total nutrient admixture
TPN = total parenteral nutrition
UUN = urinary urea nitrogen

Electrolyte Disorders

Kendrea Jones

FOUNDATION OVERVIEW

Electrolytes are involved in numerous metabolic and homeostatic processes throughout the body. Abnormalities are associated with excessive or reduced intake, altered absorption and excretion, or changes in hormonal and neurological homeostasis. Signs and symptoms of electrolyte disorders range from asymptomatic to life threatening, depending on the speed of onset and degree of electrolyte loss or excess. The goals of therapy for electrolyte disorders are to prevent the development and/or treat life-threatening complications, identify and treat the underlying cause of the disturbance, correct concomitant abnormal electrolyte findings, and attain a normal electrolyte concentration while preventing overcorrection. The rapidity of development, severity of symptoms present, concomitant medical conditions, medications, dietary factors, and consideration for patient compliance should all be considered when selecting a treatment strategy. This chapter provides a review of the pathophysiology, clinical manifestations, and treatment of the most common electrolyte disorders. Listed in Table 39-1 are the normal serum concentrations of the common electrolytes.

SODIUM DISORDERS

General Overview

Sodium is the major extracellular cation and is responsible for the majority of the extracellular fluid (ECF) osmolality. Under normal conditions, the serum sodium concentration is maintained between 135 and 145 mEq/L. Disorders of sodium balance are the most common electrolyte disturbances encountered in clinical practice and occur in both inpatient and ambulatory patients. Hyponatremia can be classified by the patient's serum osmolality and volume status (Figure 39-1). Pseudohyponatremia may be caused by hyperparaproteinemia, and hyperlipidemia (mainly hypertriglyceridemia). Hypernatremia always causes hypertonicity, and can be classified by the patient's volume status (Figure 39-2). Common causes of sodium disorders are listed in Table 39-2.

Pathophysiology

Maintenance of ECF tonicity and sodium concentration is controlled by homeostatic mechanisms that regulate the intake and excretion of free water. Antidiuretic hormone (ADH), also known as arginine vasopressin, plays a major role in determining serum sodium concentration by regulating the renal handling of water. ADH and the thirst mechanism are efficient at maintaining a normal serum osmolality despite large variations in sodium and water intake. While a loss or excess of total body sodium may occur, sodium disorders are primarily caused by abnormalities of water balance. Patients with marked hyperglycemia often exhibit hyponatremia. The most often cited correction factor is a decrease in sodium of 1.6 meq/L for every 100 mg/dL increase in glucose concentration.

When brain cells are threatened with swelling from hyponatremia or shrinkage from hypernatremia, adaptive measures are taken to maintain normal cell volume. In sodium disorders, intracellular electrolytes and organic osmolyte concentrations are altered to reduce osmotic fluid shifts between the extracellular and intracellular space. This adaptive process normalizes cell volume and is responsible for the relatively mild symptoms seen in chronic sodium disorders. It is also responsible for life-threatening complications that arise from correcting serum sodium too quickly in chronic sodium disorders.

Signs and Symptoms

Clinical manifestations of sodium disorders are related to central nervous system (CNS) dysfunction. Cases can range from asymptomatic to life threatening. Symptoms are more apparent when the change in serum sodium is large or develops rapidly. Symptoms associated with sodium disorders are listed in Table 39-3.

TREATMENT OF HYPONATREMIA

Serum sodium should be corrected at a rate that improves symptoms but does not place the patient at risk for osmotic demyelination. In patients with chronic hyponatremia (>48 hours), neurologic complications can be avoided by limiting the correction rate to 10 to 12 mEq/L in 24 hours or 18 mEq/L in 48 hours. A correction rate of 2 to 4 mEq/L within 2 to 4 hours may be beneficial in patients with severe symptoms such as seizures. Available intravenous (IV) solutions are listed in Table 39-4.

TABLE 39-1	**Electrolyte Serum Concentrations**
Electrolytes	**Normal Values**
Sodium (Na)	135-145 mEq/L
Potassium (K)	3.5-5.0 mEq/L
Magnesium (Mg)	1.4-1.8 mEq/L
Calcium (Ca)	8.5-10.5 mg/dL
Phosphate (PO_4)	2.6-4.5 mg/dL

Hypovolemic Hypotonic Hyponatremia

The cornerstone of therapy for hypovolemic hyponatremia is isotonic (0.9%) saline infusion. Additionally, specific therapies for underlying causes should be initiated. Due to a high rate of recurrence, thiazide diuretics should be permanently discontinued. Gastrointestinal (GI) losses can be treated with antiemetics and antidiarrheals as appropriate.

Isovolemic Hypotonic Hyponatremia

Fluid restriction is generally considered the cornerstone of therapy for mild or moderate cases of isovolemic hyponatremia. Patients with syndrome of inappropriate diuretic hormone (SIADH) should have fluid restricted to 1 L/d to ensure a negative fluid balance of 500 mL daily. Dietary intake should be relatively high unless otherwise contraindicated, to augment free water excretion. Medications associated with SIADH should be discontinued. Pharmacologic therapy is reserved for patients not responding to fluid restriction. Demeclocycline

is the preferred agent. It interferes with the action of ADH in the collecting duct and increases water excretion. Demeclocycline should be given orally in doses of 600 to 1200 mg/d in divided doses. Because of its delayed onset, doses should not be increased for 3 to 4 days. Adverse effects include reversible azotemia and nephrotoxicity, especially in patients with renal insufficiency. Lithium has a similar renal effect, but is less efficacious than demeclocycline and is poorly tolerated. Vasopressin receptor antagonists represent an additional treatment option for isovolemic hyponatremia. Agents available in the United States include IV conivaptan and oral tolvaptan. All vasopressin receptor antagonists are contraindicated in stage 4 or 5 chronic kidney disease (CKD). Acute symptomatic SIADH should be treated with hypertonic (3%) saline. IV furosemide 20 to 40 mg can be added to treat or prevent volume overload.

Hypervolemic Hypotonic Hyponatremia

The cornerstone of therapy for hyponatremia associated with edema is dietary sodium restriction, water restriction, and diuretic therapy. Vasopressin receptor blockers represent an additional option for the treatment of hypervolemic hyponatremia.

TREATMENT OF HYPERNATREMIA

Treatment should correct serum sodium at a rate sufficient to alleviate symptoms and not place the patient at risk for cerebral edema. In patients with chronic hypernatremia,

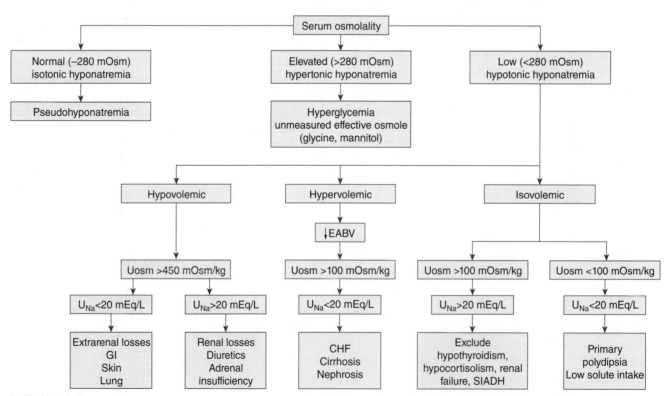

FIGURE 39-1   Diagnosis of hyponatremia.   Reproduced with permission from DiPiro JT, Talbert RL, Yee GC, et al: *Pharmacotherapy: A Pathophysiologic Approach*, 10th ed. New York, NY: McGraw-Hill; 2017.

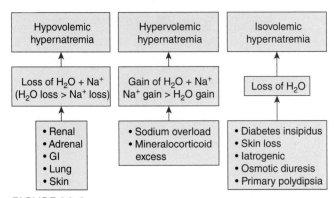

FIGURE 39-2 Diagnosis of hypernatremia. Reproduced with permission from DiPiro JT, Talbert RL, Yee GC, et al: *Pharmacotherapy: A Pathophysiologic Approach*, 7th ed. New York, NY: McGraw-Hill; 2008.

neurologic complications can be avoided by not exceeding a correction rate of 0.5 mEq/L/h. Sodium correction should be limited to 10 mEq/L/d. A faster correction rate of 1 mEq/L/h may be beneficial in patients with acute hypernatremia.

Hypovolemic Hypernatremia

Patients with hemodynamic instability should first receive normal saline until volume status is restored and vital signs are stable. Subsequently, the patient should be switched to hypotonic fluids to correct serum sodium. Oral or enteral replacement with hypotonic fluids is the preferred route. IV is appropriate when oral replacement is not possible. Patients receiving concentrated enteral feedings due to volume restrictions often result in hypovolemic hypernatremia.

Isovolemic Hypernatremia

Access to free water or replacement with IV hypotonic fluids is the cornerstone of therapy for isovolemic hypernatremia. Patients with central diabetes insipidus require exogenous ADH. Desmopressin is the drug of choice and is typically initiated at a dose of 10 mcg intranasally in the evening. Most adults require a dose of 10 mcg twice daily. Desmopressin is also available in injectable and oral forms. Injectable desmopressin is given at a dose of 2 to 4 mcg daily in two divided doses. The dose of oral desmopressin ranges from 0.1 to 1.2 mg daily in divided doses, with a common starting dose of 0.05 mg twice daily. Since unsuppressed ADH activity can cause water intoxication from excess water retention, patients should be monitored for signs and symptoms of hyponatremia and hypervolemia. Thiazide diuretics and sodium restriction are used in nephrogenic diabetes insipidus to cause modest volume depletion. This results in proximal tubule sodium and water reabsorption and diminishes water delivery to the collecting tubules. The overall effect is a reduction in water excretion. Medications used to treat diabetes insipidus are listed in Table 39-5.

Hypervolemic Hypernatremia

Treatment consists of 5% dextrose infusion with loop diuretics added to promote renal sodium excretion. Since this disorder is commonly iatrogenic and develops within a few hours, rapid correction of serum sodium is safe and appropriate.

POTASSIUM DISORDERS

General Overview

Potassium is the most plentiful intracellular cation in the body. Total body stores of potassium are estimated at 3,000 to 4,000 mEq with approximately 2% being distributed in the extracellular compartment. Potassium homeostasis is maintained through intra- and extracellular shifting, predominantly regulated by the sodium-potassium-adenosine triphosphatase (Na^+-K-ATPase) pump; therefore, serum potassium concentrations do not accurately reflect total body content. Potassium is responsible for many cellular functions, including protein synthesis, cellular metabolism, and conduction of the electrical action potential. The normal range for serum potassium concentration is 3.5 to 5.0 mEq/L.

Pathophysiology

Maintenance of the normal range for potassium is affected by diet, acid–base balance, aldosterone, insulin, catecholamines, tonicity of body fluids, and GI and renal excretion. The recommended daily intake of potassium is 50 mEq/d. The primary route of potassium elimination is the kidney, though small amounts are excreted via the GI tract. Hypokalemia is the finding of a serum potassium concentration less than 3.5 mEq/L and can be classified as mild (serum potassium 3-3.5 mEq/L), moderate (2.5-3 mEq/L), or severe (<2.5 mEq/L). It is caused by a total body deficit of potassium when there is insufficient intake of potassium in the diet or excessive loss through the renal or GI tracts. Hypokalemia caused by the intracellular shift of serum potassium is known as *false hypokalemia* because there is no true deficit in total body content. Hypokalemia is commonly iatrogenic with the most common causes being loop and thiazide diuretics. Hypokalemia may also increase the risk of digoxin toxicity. Increased GI loss of potassium is also a common cause. Hypomagnesemia contributes to the development of hypokalemia by increasing renal potassium wasting and decreasing the intracellular uptake of potassium. If both disorders are present, hypomagnesemia should be addressed first to facilitate correction of the potassium deficiency.

Hyperkalemia is defined as a serum potassium concentration more than 5.5 mEq/L and can be classified as mild (5.5-6 mEq/L), moderate (6.1-6.9 mEq/L), or severe (>7 mEq/L). It is caused by excessive potassium intake in comparison to potassium elimination or when the compartmental distribution of potassium is disrupted. Elevated serum potassium resulting from cellular shifts is known as *false hyperkalemia* since there is no true excess in total body potassium, such as that present in some diabetic ketoacidosis patients upon presentation. Hyperkalemia is commonly associated with acute or chronic kidney disease, especially if patients are noncompliant with dietary restrictions. Potassium disorders are commonly induced by drugs as well as iatrogenic

TABLE 39-2   **Causes and Contributing Factors for Electrolyte Disorders**

Electrolyte	Decreased	Increased
Sodium	*Hypovolemic hypotonic hyponatremia* Excessive sweating GI losses Renal losses *Isovolemic hypotonic hyponatremia* SIADH secondary to malignancy, pulmonary disease, CNS disorders, iatrogenic sources *Hypervolemic hypotonic hyponatremia* Cirrhosis Congestive heart failure	*Hypovolemic hypernatremia* Dermal losses Vomiting NG suction Lactulose Osmotic diuresis—hyperglycemia, mannitol Loop diuretics Concentrated enteral feedings *Isovolemic hypernatremia* Insensible water loss Diabetes insipidus *Hypervolemic hypernatremia* Hypertonic saline
Potassium	Poor dietary intake β-Agonists Loop and thiazide diuretics Sorbitol Theophylline intoxication Caffeine intoxication Insulin overdose Mineralocorticoids Amphotericin B Cisplatin Aminoglycosides	Dietary noncompliance Spironolactone Amiloride Triamterene Angiotensin-converting enzyme inhibitors Angiotensin receptor antagonists Trimethoprim Heparin Renal insufficiency Metabolic acidosis (can be falsely high in diabetic ketoacidosis (DKA) as patients often have low total body stores) β-blockers
Magnesium	Alcoholism Protein malnutrition Malabsorptive disease Vomiting Laxative abuse Diarrhea Bartter syndrome Amphotericin B Aminoglycosides Loop and thiazide diuretics Hyperthyroidism Hypercalcemia Proton pump inhibitors	Renal insufficiency Treatment of eclampsia Severe preeclampsia Cathartics Lithium therapy Hypothyroidism Milk-alkali syndrome Addison disease DKA
Calcium	Decreased parathyroid activity Vitamin D deficiency Hyperphosphatemia Hypoalbuminemia Hypomagnesemia Loop diuretics Glucocorticoids Calcitonin Phenobarbital Phenytoin Proton pump inhibitors	Malignancy Increased parathyroid activity Thiazide diuretics Lithium Excessive calcium intake Paget disease Increased thyroid activity Adrenal insufficiency Sarcoidosis
Phosphate	Renal tubular dysfunction Increased parathyroid activity Refeeding syndrome Insulin and dextrose treatment for hyperkalemia Alcoholism Malnutrition Phosphate binders Decreased vitamin D intake	Chronic kidney disease Tumor lysis syndrome Rhabdomyolysis Septic shock Excessive phosphate administration Increased vitamin D intake

TABLE 39-3	Signs and Symptoms of Electrolyte Disorders	
Electrolyte	Low	High
Sodium	Disorientation Headache Lethargy Malaise Nausea Restlessness Coma Respiratory arrest Seizures	Anorexia Weakness Nausea Restlessness Vomiting Altered mental status Coma Irritability Lethargy
Potassium	Muscle cramps Weakness Malaise Myalgias Impaired muscle function ECG changes Arrhythmias	Palpitations ECG changes Arrhythmias Asystole
Magnesium	Tetany Muscular fasciculation Convulsions Trousseau and/or Chvostek sign Palpitations ECG changes Arrhythmias Hypertension	Hypotension Flushing ECG changes Complete heart block Asystole Sedation Coma Hypotonia/hyporeflexia Paralysis Respiratory failure
Calcium	Paresthesia Muscle cramps Tetany Laryngeal spasm Depression Confusion Memory loss Brittle nails Hair loss Eczema Seizures Myocardial infarction Arrhythmias Hypotension	Nausea Vomiting Abdominal pain Dyspepsia Anorexia Acute pancreatitis Lethargy Obtundation Ataxia Coma ECG changes Arrhythmias Hypertension Polyuria/polydipsia Nephrolithiasis Renal dysfunction
Phosphate	Arrhythmias Respiratory failure Myalgias Confusion Hallucinations Weakness Platelet/WBC dysfunction Hemolysis	Calcium-phosphate precipitation

administration of potassium supplements. Causes of potassium disorders are listed in Table 39-2.

Signs and Symptoms

Patients with potassium disorders are often asymptomatic; however, alterations in serum potassium concentration can affect neuromuscular, cardiac, and smooth muscle tissue. Signs and symptoms of potassium disorders are listed in Table 39-3.

TREATMENT

Hypokalemia

The treatment options for hypokalemia consist of increased dietary intake of potassium-rich foods, oral potassium supplements, and IV potassium. A general rule for replacement is that there is a total body potassium deficit of 100 to 400 mEq for every 1 mEq/L decrease in the serum potassium concentration below the normal range. For every 10 meq of potassium supplemented, the average increase in potassium concentration is 0.1 meq/L. This does not apply in patients with severe hypokalemia as these patients often require much more supplementation. However, a patient's renal function, acid–base status, concomitant medications, or disease processes must all be considered before recommending an estimated dose for replacement. For patients with concomitant hypomagnesemia, the magnesium deficit should be corrected to prevent refractory hypokalemia.

Dietary Potassium

Dietary supplementation is recommended for patients with low-normal serum potassium concentrations and may be considered for those with serum potassium concentrations of 3 to 3.5 mEq/L.

Oral Potassium Replacement

Oral potassium supplements are preferred whenever possible, especially for asymptomatic patients. It should be given to patients with potassium concentrations of 3 to 3.5 mEq/L who have underlying risk for cardiac arrhythmias. Patients with serum potassium concentrations below 3 mEq/L should receive supplementation to target a goal of 4 to 4.5 mEq/L. Of the three salt forms available, chloride is used more frequently because it is effective for common causes of hypokalemia. Phosphate should be reserved for patients with concomitant hypophosphatemia, and bicarbonate is advantageous for patients with concurrent metabolic acidosis. In stable patients receiving preventative supplementation, serum potassium and magnesium concentrations and renal function parameters should be obtained every 1 to 2 months. Hospitalized patients being treated for mild hypokalemia should be monitored every 2 to 3 days. When more aggressive replacement is warranted, the potassium concentration should be obtained 1 to 2 hours following the administration of an immediate-release oral dose to allow time for absorption and distribution. Oral potassium replacement may result in nausea, vomiting, and GI erosions.

Intravenous Potassium Replacement

IV potassium can be used in patients with severe deficiency, those exhibiting severe symptoms such as electrocardiogram (ECG) changes, or patients unable to tolerate oral supplements.

TABLE 39-4 | **Intravenous Replacement Solutions**

Solution	Dextrose (g/100 mL)	Na⁺ (mEq/L)	Cl⁻ (mEq/L)	Tonicity	Distribution		Free Water/L
					% ECF	% ICF	
D5W	5	0	0	Hypotonic	40	60	1000 mL
0.45% Sodium chloride	0	77	77	Hypotonic	73	37	500 mL
0.9% Sodium chloride	0	154	154	Isotonic	100	0	0 mL
3% Sodium chloride[a]	0	513	513	Hypertonic	100	0	−2331 mL

[a]This solution will result in osmotic removal of water from the intracellular space.

Abbreviations: Cl⁻, chloride; D5W, 5% dextrose in water; ECF, extracellular fluid; ICF, intracellular fluid; Na⁺, sodium.

Reproduced with permission from DiPiro JT, Talbert RL, Yee GC, et al: *Pharmacotherapy: A Pathophysiologic Approach*, 7th ed. New York, NY: McGraw-Hill; 2008.

IV therapy is more likely to cause hyperkalemia and may cause damage to the veins and infusion site pain. Typically, 10 to 20 mEq of potassium is diluted in at least 100 mL of 0.9% sodium chloride and administered through a peripheral vein over 1 hour. Patients should be monitored for burning pain and phlebitis at the injection site. Larger amounts can be diluted in larger total volumes and infused at a rate not exceeding 40 mEq/h for severe hypokalemia. For IV infusion rates exceeding 10 mEq/h, ECG monitoring is recommended. These infusions should employ a central venous line due to the risk of pain and peripheral venous sclerosis. After each 30 to 40 mEq infusion, the serum potassium concentration should be reevaluated to guide further dosing needs. Following completion of the infusion, at least 30 minutes should elapse before drawing the serum level to allow time for potassium distribution. Observing recommendations regarding the amount, site (peripheral or central), and rate of potassium infusion is instrumental in preventing untoward effects of potassium replacement.

Alternative Therapies

Potassium-sparing diuretics such as spironolactone, triamterene, and amiloride are alternatives to chronic exogenous potassium. They may be particularly useful when patients are concomitantly receiving potassium-depleting medications.

TABLE 39-5 | **Central and Nephrogenic Diabetes Insipidus Treatment**

Drug	Indication	Dose
Desmopressin acetate	Central and nephrogenic	5-20 mcg intranasally every 12-24 h
Chlorpropamide	Central	125-250 mg po daily
Carbamazepine	Central	100-300 mg po bid
Clofibrate	Central	500 mg po qid
Hydrochlorothiazide	Central and nephrogenic	25 mg po every 12-24 h
Amiloride	Lithium-related nephrogenic	5-10 mg po daily
Indomethacin	Central and nephrogenic	50 mg po every 8-12 h

Reproduced with permission from DiPiro JT, Talbert RL, Yee GC, et al: *Pharmacotherapy: A Pathophysiologic Approach*, 7th ed. New York, NY: McGraw-Hill; 2008.

Hyperkalemia

Along with addressing underlying causes, the treatment options for hyperkalemia consist of dietary restriction, pharmacotherapy, and hemodialysis. Asymptomatic patients with mild hyperkalemia may be managed with dietary education and careful monitoring of potassium concentration. A loop diuretic may be added to increase urinary potassium elimination. For patients unable to tolerate loop diuretics, a cation-exchange resin like sodium polystyrene sulfonate (SPS) may be administered orally or rectally. In patients with severe hyperkalemia or acute ECG changes, IV calcium is administered for stabilization of the cardiac membrane and hemodynamics. Calcium gluconate is preferred over calcium chloride due to an increased risk of tissue necrosis with the chloride salt if extravasation occurs. Concomitantly, an additional therapy should be instituted to shift potassium intracellularly and attain a serum potassium concentration less than 5.5 mEq/L. Sodium bicarbonate, insulin with dextrose, and albuterol are available options. Comorbid disease processes may influence the choice of therapy. Sodium bicarbonate is advantageous for patients with concomitant metabolic acidosis; however, the effects on potassium-lowering are significantly delayed in patients with advanced renal insufficiency. Additionally, renal patients are at increased risk of sodium and volume overload. Insulin and dextrose administration does not adversely impact volume status, but blood glucose levels must be monitored carefully. β-Agonists have a dual mechanism for lowering potassium by stimulating the Na⁺-K⁺-ATPase pump and stimulating increased secretion of pancreatic insulin, but the effects can be unpredictable secondary to variable bioavailability of inhaled agents. Finally, excess potassium is removed from the body with diuretics, a resin binder, or hemodialysis. Dosing information and utility of available therapies for potassium disorders is described in Tables 39-6 and 39-7.

Adverse effects associated with treatment of hyperkalemia include hypo- or hyperglycemia from administration of insulin and dextrose, SPS-induced diarrhea, cardiac excitability from albuterol, volume depletion or electrolyte abnormalities following diuretic therapy, and hypercalcemia from IV calcium. Additionally, skin necrosis may occur if calcium extravasates.

During emergent treatment, the serum potassium concentration should be evaluated hourly, and ECG monitored continuously until the serum concentration is less than 5 mEq/L

TABLE 39-6	Available Treatment Modalities for Hypokalemia
Source	**Utility**
Dietary	
Dried fruits—figs, dates, prunes, raisins	Food sources are often insufficient for replacement and may cause increased weight
Nuts	
Vegetables—lima beans, spinach, potatoes	
Fruits—bananas, cantaloupe, oranges	
Meats—beef, pork, lamb	
Potassium chloride salt substitutes	
Oral Replacement	
Controlled-release tablets	Microencapsulated formulations cause fewer GI erosions than wax-matrix tablets Wax-matrix tablet may appear in stool (empty of medication)
Elixir	Elixir is inexpensive and works quickly but poor taste often results in poor compliance
Effervescent tablets	
Chloride, phosphate, bicarbonate salts	Chloride salts are most effective for most causes of hypokalemia; bicarbonate is useful for hypokalemia with concomitant metabolic acidosis
Intravenous Replacement	
Chloride, phosphate, bicarbonate salts	Most useful in severe deficiency; requires continuous monitoring at rates >10 mEq/h; concentrations >10 mEq/100 mL should be administered via a central line to avoid pain and vein necrosis
Potassium-Sparing Diuretics	
Spironolactone, triamterene, amiloride	Used as alternatives to exogenous supplementation; may be especially useful when administered concomitantly with potassium-depleting medications

and ECG changes have resolved. Patients who receive SPS and are asymptomatic should have serum potassium concentrations obtained within 4 hours to guide the need for readministration.

MAGNESIUM

General Overview

Magnesium is the second most abundant intracellular cation and is mainly distributed in bone and muscle. The normal range for the serum magnesium concentration is 1.4 to 1.8 mEq/L, or 1.7 to 2.3 mg/dL. Magnesium is responsible for many physiologic functions including protein synthesis, function of the cell membrane and mitochondria, and secretion of parathyroid hormone (PTH). Magnesium abnormalities are common because allocation of magnesium between extracellular and intracellular compartments is not hormonally regulated. It is estimated that up to 65% of intensive care unit patients have hypomagnesemia. Compared with hypomagnesemia, hypermagnesemia is rare. Serum magnesium concentrations outside the normal range can result in significant alterations in neuromuscular and cardiovascular activity.

TABLE 39-7	Available Treatment Modalities for Hyperkalemia				
Therapy	**Dose**	**Route**	**Onset/Duration**	**Monitoring**	**Physiologic Effect**
Albuterol	10-20 mg	Inhalation	30 min/1-2 h	Palpitations/heart rate	Increases intracellular K^+ uptake
Calcium	1 g	IV	1-2 min/10-30 min	Serum calcium, ECG	Increases cardiac membrane potential
Furosemide	20-40 mg	IV	5-15 min/4-6 h	Urine output, serum chemistry	Increases renal K^+ elimination
Insulin	5-10 U	IV	30 min/2-6 h	Hourly blood glucose	Increases intracellular K^+ uptake
Dextrose	25 g	IV	30 min/2-6 h	Hourly blood glucose	Increases intracellular K^+ uptake following insulin release
Sodium bicarbonate	50-100 mEq	IV	30 min/2-6 h	Volume status, pH, serum chemistry	Increases intracellular K^+ concentration
Sodium polystyrene sulfonate	15-60 g	po or PR	1 h/ –	Stool output	Increases K^+ elimination by exchanging Na^+ for K^+
Hemodialysis	4 h	–	Immediate	Volume status, serum chemistry	Increases K^+ elimination

These changes can have life-threatening consequences including cardiac arrhythmias and paralysis.

Pathophysiology

Like other electrolytes, magnesium homeostasis is dependent upon the balance of intake versus output with approximately 30% to 40% of dietary magnesium absorbed in the small bowel. Renal reabsorption of magnesium occurs predominantly in the loop of Henle, with only about 20% of filtered magnesium reabsorbed in the proximal tubule. Like potassium, magnesium is principally located intracellularly; therefore, the serum concentration may not accurately reflect the total body content. The recommended daily intake of magnesium is approximately 310 mg/d for women and 400 mg/d for men.

Hypomagnesemia is usually associated with decreased absorption secondary to small bowel disease or increased renal elimination as occurs with diuretic therapy. Hypermagnesemia occurs when magnesium intake is greater than relative elimination by the kidney. Causes of magnesium disorders are listed in Table 39-2.

Signs and Symptoms

Signs and symptoms of magnesium disorders involve the neuromuscular and cardiovascular systems and are listed in Table 39-3. Hypomagnesemia (serum magnesium concentration <1.4 mEq/L) is commonly asymptomatic. Concomitant electrolyte abnormalities, such as hypokalemia and hypocalcemia, are often associated with hypomagnesemia and complicate the discrimination of symptoms specific to hypomagnesemia. Hypermagnesemia (serum magnesium concentration >2 mEq/L) is an uncommon finding, and symptoms often do not present until the serum magnesium concentration exceeds 4 mEq/L. Pregnant women receiving continuous magnesium infusions for eclampsia or preeclampsia have to be monitored hourly with serum levels as well as signs/symptoms (eg, deep tendon reflexes) to prevent magnesium toxicity.

TREATMENT

Hypomagnesemia

The treatment of hypomagnesemia can be accomplished by supplementation via oral, intramuscular (IM), or IV routes. The selection of a route of delivery is dependent on the severity of deficiency and associated signs and symptoms. Because approximately half of the dose administered is eliminated in the urine, magnesium replacement should occur over several days. A description of magnesium replacement strategies is described in Table 39-8. Ongoing supplementation may be necessary if the patient is unable to ingest maintenance requirements of magnesium or has ongoing losses. Empiric dosing should be reduced by half for patients with renal insufficiency.

Oral Magnesium Replacement

Oral magnesium supplementation can be given to patients with magnesium concentrations more than 1 mEq/L who are asymptomatic. Available products include magnesium-containing antacids or laxatives as well as magnesium oxide. Diarrhea is the most common side effect of oral replacement and more likely with large doses. Usual oral dosing is 400 to 800 mg three to four times daily. In hospitalized patients, serum magnesium concentrations should be evaluated at least daily until released from the hospital.

Intramuscular Magnesium Replacement

Because IM administration is painful, it should be limited to patients with limited IV access who warrant more aggressive replacement than can be accomplished with oral supplementation.

Intravenous Magnesium Replacement

Patients with severe magnesium deficiency (<1 mEq/L) or signs and symptoms of hypomagnesemia should receive IV repletion until signs and symptoms resolve. IV administration is associated with rate-related flushing and sweating. Bolus administration should be avoided if possible, and IV solutions should be diluted to 20% before infusion to prevent sclerosis of the vein. Serum magnesium concentrations should be monitored hourly until symptoms resolve and the serum concentration is at least 1.5 mEq/L. For the next 24 hours, serum magnesium concentration should be obtained every 6 to 12 hours, and then daily, once the concentration has returned to normal.

Hypermagnesemia

The treatment of hypermagnesemia is typically addressed in three ways: reduction of intake, enhanced elimination, and

TABLE 39-8	Magnesium Replacement		
Serum Magnesium Concentration		<1 mEq/L	>1 mEq/L and <1.5 mEq/L
Symptoms	Life-threatening (seizures, arrhythmias)	Asymptomatic	Asymptomatic
Day 1	2 g magnesium sulfate[a] followed by 1 mEq/kg IV over 24 h	1 mEq/kg/d continuously or IM every 4 h × 5 doses	1 mEq/kg/d continuous IV or divided IM doses, or milk of magnesia 5 mL qid, or magnesium-based antacid 15 mL tid, or magnesium oxide tablets 400 mg up to four times daily as tolerated
Days 2-5	0.5 mEq/kg/d in maintenance fluids	0.5 mEq/kg/d as continuous IV or divided IM doses	May increase magnesium oxide tablets to 800 mg qid as tolerated; monitor need for continued supplementation

[a]Initial replacement given over 5 to 60 minutes. For torsades de pointes with cardiac arrest, shorten to 5 to 20 minutes IV push. For seizures, give over 10 minutes.

antagonism of the adverse effects of elevated magnesium concentrations. Patient-specific therapy is dependent upon associated signs and symptoms of hypermagnesemia. Education regarding magnesium-rich foods, beverages, and over-the-counter products is essential to prevent recurrent episodes of hypermagnesemia. Available therapies for acute treatment include IV calcium and forced diuresis using saline and loop diuretics. Dialysis patients may require emergency hemodialysis using a magnesium-free dialysate. Adverse effects of hypermagnesemia treatment are similar to those of hyperkalemia.

Intravenous Calcium

IV calcium can be employed to antagonize the neuromuscular and cardiac signs and symptoms of hypermagnesemia. Because the effect is transient, doses may need to be repeated as frequently as hourly until the signs and symptoms resolve and the magnesium concentration returns to normal. The typical dose is 100 to 200 mg of elemental calcium. If life-threatening adverse effects of elevated serum magnesium are present, additional care measures such as ventilatory and hemodynamic support may be required. Continuous ECG and hourly serum magnesium concentrations should be monitored until symptoms resolve and the serum magnesium concentration is less than 4 mg/dL.

Forced Diuresis

Diuresis to enhance magnesium elimination can be employed in patients without kidney dysfunction. This is usually accomplished via administration of saline accompanied by an IV loop diuretic such as furosemide, similar to hyperkalemia treatment. Patients with chronic renal insufficiency may require continued administration of diuretic therapy to maintain normal electrolyte concentrations. Urine output and signs and symptoms of volume overload should be monitored closely.

CALCIUM DISORDERS

Pathophysiology

Calcium is involved in numerous processes including propagation of neuromuscular activity, regulation of the blood coagulation cascade, bone and tooth metabolism, and endocrine and exocrine functions. Under normal conditions, the total serum calcium concentration is 8.5 to 10.5 mg/dL. Only 0.5% of calcium stores may be found in the ECF, while 99% of calcium stores are found in skeletal bone. ECF calcium is transported in three different forms: bound to plasma proteins, mostly albumin (45%); ionized or free state (40%); and bound to small anions including phosphates, citrates, and bicarbonates (6%). The unbound or ionized calcium is the physiologically active form and regulated through complex interactions between PTH, vitamin D, and serum phosphate levels.

Any disease state or factor that alters albumin concentrations or its affinity to bind to calcium may change the concentration of serum calcium in the ionized form. The total calcium concentration may not accurately reflect the

metabolically active or free concentration. Despite decreased levels of albumin, ionized calcium concentration may actually remain normal. The serum total calcium concentration decreases approximately 0.8 mg/dL for every 1 g/dL fall in serum albumin below 4 g/dL. Thus, in patients with hypoalbuminemia, total serum calcium concentration should be corrected using the following equation:

$$\text{Corrected calcium} = [(4 - \text{albumin}) \times 0.8 \text{ mg/dL}] + \text{measured calcium}$$

If a laboratory can reliably measure an ionized calcium concentration (reference range 1.12–1.3 mmol/L), many clinicians prefer this measure in patients with hypoalbuminemia and acid–base disturbances. Ionized calcium concentrations are often available with blood gas measurements.

Hormonal Regulation of Calcium and Phosphate

The three major hormones that regulate serum calcium and phosphate concentrations are PTH, vitamin D, and calcitonin (Table 39-9). PTH is released from the parathyroid gland in response to a reduction in serum-ionized calcium. Upon release, it acts on the kidneys to stimulate reabsorption of calcium in the distal tubule and increases intestinal absorption of calcium by increasing renal production of

TABLE 39-9	Hormonal Regulation of Calcium and Phosphate	
Hormone	**Effects on Calcium**	**Effects on Phosphate**
PTH	▪ Promotes absorption of calcium by intestine ▪ Mobilizes Ca²⁺ salts from the bones by activating osteoclasts ▪ Increases Ca²⁺ reabsorption in the distal tubules ▪ Stimulates the release of vitamin D *Net effect*: ↑ Serum calcium levels	▪ Decrease PO₄ reabsorption in the proximal tubule *Net effect*: ↓ Serum phosphate levels
Vitamin D	▪ Increases intestinal absorption of calcium ▪ Facilitates reabsorption of calcium in the proximal tubules ▪ Activates osteoclasts to mobilize calcium from bone *Net effect*: ↑ Serum calcium levels	▪ Increases intestinal absorption of phosphate ▪ Facilitates reabsorption of phosphate in the proximal tubules *Net effect*: ↑ Serum phosphate levels
Calcitonin	▪ Inhibits osteoclasts and stimulates osteoblasts ▪ Increases renal excretion of Ca²⁺ *Net effect*: ↓ Serum calcium levels	

1-25-dihydroxycholecalciferol (1,25-DHCC or calcitriol), the active form of vitamin D. In addition, it stimulates osteoclast and osteoblast activity to increase calcium mobilization from skeletal bone. PTH acts in the kidneys to increase phosphate excretion by blocking renal reabsorption.

Vitamin D refers to a group of closely related sterols that are hormones, not vitamins. Vitamin D_2 and vitamin D_3 can be ingested in the diet or formed as a result of ultraviolet radiation of the skin, converting 7-dehydrocholesterol (D_2) to cholecalciferol (D_3). Cholecalciferol must be converted to calcitriol via hepatic and renal hydroxylation. Active vitamin D increases calcium and phosphate levels by increasing intestinal absorption and renal reabsorption. Additionally, vitamin D regulates the synthesis and release of PTH. Calcitonin is released in response to increased ionized calcium concentrations. It inhibits osteoclast activity and decreases calcium levels. An alteration in any of these hormones may result in calcium and phosphate abnormalities.

Causes of Calcium Disorders

The most common causes of hypocalcemia are due to hypoparathyroidism and vitamin D deficiency seen in rickets, GI disorders, and CKD. The most common causes of hypercalcemia are malignancy and primary hyperparathyroidism. Malignancy-associated hypercalcemia may be caused by tumor invasion of bone leading to osteolysis and calcium release from the bone, tumor production of PTH-like substances, or substances that increase osteoclast development and activity. Primary hyperparathyroidism is characterized by inappropriate release of PTH from the parathyroid gland resulting in increased calcium levels. Additionally, these patients may experience increased production of calcitriol. Other causes of calcium disorders are listed in Table 39-2.

Signs and Symptoms

Patients with acute hypocalcemia exhibit symptoms associated with the neuromuscular system. Chronic hypocalcemia is associated with CNS and dermatological disturbances. Chvostek and Trousseau signs may be observed on physical examination. Chvostek sign is the unilateral twitch of the facial muscles when the facial nerve is slightly tapped. Trousseau sign is a carpal spasm that occurs when a blood pressure cuff is compressed on the upper arm. Patients with hypercalcemia, especially those with a serum calcium level more than 14 mg/dL, may present with GI symptoms, including acute pancreatitis. In addition to GI symptoms, hypercalcemia may be associated with neuromuscular, cardiovascular, or renal manifestations. Common symptoms of calcium disorders are listed in Table 39-3. Renal insufficiency is associated with an increased calcium-phosphate product (usually >55 mg/dL) which may lead to soft-tissue calcification and deposits in the coronary arteries, myocardial fibers, and aortic valves. Increased serum calcium levels may inhibit antidiuretic hormone's effects on the collecting ducts, leading to polyuria and polydipsia. Chronic hypercalcemia may cause renal tubular dysfunction.

TREATMENT

Hypocalcemia

In patients with hypocalcemia and low albumin levels, an ionized calcium should be obtained and treatment based on the ionized calcium level. Acute symptomatic hypocalcemia requires IV administration of calcium until signs and symptoms resolve. Administration of 100 to 300 mg of elemental calcium over 10 minutes will usually alleviate symptoms. IV calcium is available in two salt forms: calcium gluconate (1 g Ca gluconate = 90 mg elemental calcium) and calcium chloride (1 g of Ca chloride = 270 mg elemental calcium). Calcium gluconate administration is preferred over calcium chloride because it is associated with less risk of tissue necrosis. Calcium chloride is often stored in crash carts for administration in code situations. Rapid administration of calcium may result in cardiac dysfunction. Additionally, IV calcium should not be administered with bicarbonate or phosphate containing solutions due to the risk of precipitation. Bolus doses of calcium only last about 2 hours, and ionized calcium and magnesium levels should be monitored closely after IV administration.

Patients with chronic or asymptomatic hypocalcemia due to hypoparathyroidism or vitamin D deficiency may be managed with oral calcium salts or vitamin D replacement. Calcium replacement may begin with 1 to 3 g/d of elemental calcium and progress to a maintenance dose of 2 to 8 g/d in divided doses. Numerous oral calcium-containing products are available, with calcium carbonate containing more elemental calcium and being the least expensive. A complete list of oral calcium supplements are listed in Table 39-10. Calcium carbonate requires an acidic environment for absorption. Adverse effects of calcium salts include GI upset, constipation, and hypercalcemia.

Vitamin D supplementation should be reserved for patients with vitamin D deficiency. Several different products are available including: ergocalciferol, calcitriol, paricalcitol, and doxercalciferol. Usual oral dosage ranges from 0.5 to 3 mcg daily, with adjustments made every 4 weeks. In patients with reduced hepatic metabolism, calcitriol is preferred.

Hypercalcemia

Hypercalcemia treatment involves definitive treatment of primary hyperparathyroidism or malignancy. In patients with

TABLE 39-10 **Calcium Salt Formulations**

Calcium Salt	Calcium Content per Gram	
	mg	mEq
Acetate	250	12.7
Carbonate	400	20
Chloride	270	13.5
Citrate	211	10.6
Glubionate	64	3.2
Gluconate	90	4.5
Lactate	130	6.5
Phosphate tribasic	390	19.3

TABLE 39-11	Treatment of Hypercalcemia			
Drug	**Starting Dose**	**Initial Response**	**Contraindications**	**Adverse Effects**
NS ± electrolytes	200-300 mL/h	24-48 h	Renal insufficiency; chronic heart failure	Electrolyte abnormalities; fluid overload
Loop diuretics	40-80 mg IV every 1-4 h	NA		Electrolyte abnormalities
Calcitonin	4 U/kg every 12 h SQ/IM 10-12 U/h IV	1-2 h		Facial flushing, N/V, allergic reaction
Pamidronate	30-90 mg IV over 2-24 h	2 d	Renal insufficiency	Fever
Etidronate	7.5 mg/kg IV over 2 h	2 d	Renal insufficiency	Fever
Zoledronate	4-8 mg IV over 15 min	1-2 d	Renal insufficiency	Fever, fatigue, skeletal pain
Gallium nitrate	200 mg/m² daily IV for 5 days as continuous infusion	Variable	Severe renal insufficiency	Nephrotoxicity; hypophosphatemia; N/V/D; metallic taste
Mithramycin	25 mcg/kg IV over 4-6 h	12 h	Decreased liver function; renal insufficiency, thrombocytopenia	Nausea/vomiting; stomatitis; thrombocytopenia; nephrotoxicity; hepatotoxicity
Glucocorticoids	40-60 mg po prednisone equivalents	Variable	Serious infections	Hyperglycemia, osteoporosis; infection
Denosumab	120 mg SQ every 4 weeks; with additional 120 mg on day 8 and 15	Within 10 days	Caution in renal insufficiency	Osteonecrosis of the jaw; hypocalcemia

Abbreviations: D, diarrhea; IV, intravenous; IM, intramuscular; N, nausea; NS, normal saline; po, per oral; SQ, subcutaneous; V, vomiting
Reproduced with permission from DiPiro JT, Talbert RL, Yee GC, et al: *Pharmacotherapy: A Pathophysiologic Approach*, 7th ed. New York, NY: McGraw-Hill; 2008.

drug-induced hypercalcemia, the offending agent should be discontinued. The initial treatment for hypercalcemia in patients without severe renal dysfunction is volume expansion with saline-containing fluids and loop diuretics to enhance urinary excretion of calcium. Loop diuretics block calcium reabsorption in the ascending limb of the loop of Henle. Calcitonin is an alternative treatment that increases renal excretion of calcium by inhibiting bone resorption. It has a rapid onset of action but an unpredictable effect on serum calcium levels. Calcitonin may be administered intramuscularly, subcutaneously, intranasally, or intravenously. IV calcitonin is associated with an infusion-related syndrome and is therefore not preferred.

Bisphosphonates are first-line treatment in prevention and treatment of malignancy-induced hypercalcemia. They lower calcium levels by inhibiting bone resorption and the formation of osteoclasts. The onset of action of bisphosphonates may be delayed, so saline hydration with loop diuretics or calcitonin may be necessary if a rapid decline in calcium levels is warranted. IV therapy is associated with fever, and serum creatinine monitoring is recommended for all bisphosphonate therapy. Bisphosphonates are contraindicated in patients with a creatinine clearance less than 30 mL/min. Osteonecrosis of the jaw is a severe complication of bisphosphonate therapy, most commonly seen in patients with multiple myeloma.

Denosumab is an additional agent approved for hypercalcemia of malignancy. It is a monoclonal antibody that has shown success in hypercalcemia patients that did not respond to bisphosphonate therapy. Like the bisphosphonates, it has been associated with osteonecrosis of the jaw and need for careful monitoring of calcium levels specifically in patients with renal impairment.

Gallium nitrate reduces serum calcium levels by inhibiting bone resorption. Due to its adverse effects, it is reserved for patients with hypercalcemia of malignancy that is unresponsive to hydration and other therapies. Mithramycin (plicamycin) is an antibiotic that inhibits osteoclast activity. It is recommended for short-term use due to adverse effects including renal and hepatotoxicity and platelet dysfunction. Glucocorticoids may be effective in treatment of hypercalcemia associated with malignancy, sarcoidosis, and syndromes of increased vitamin A and D. Glucocorticoids increase bone resorption, decrease osteoblast proliferation, and reduce estrogen and testosterone levels. Glucocorticoid therapy is not preferred due to its slow onset of action in lowering calcium levels and numerous adverse effects. Potassium and magnesium serum levels should be monitored closely in all patients receiving treatment for hypercalcemia.

A list of the most commonly used agents for the management of hypercalcemia may be found in Table 39-11.

PHOSPHATE DISORDERS

Many of the factors that regulate serum calcium levels also influence serum phosphate levels (see Table 39-9). Phosphate is a major intracellular anion, and normal serum concentrations are 2.6 to 4.5 mg/dL. Phosphate is involved in numerous functions including regulation of enzymatic reactions and metabolism of protein, fats, and carbohydrates. It is a major component of phospholipid membranes of all cells and 2,3 diphosphoglycerate, which regulates the oxygen-carrying capacity of hemoglobin. In addition, it is required for the formation of high-energy bonds in adenosine triphosphate (ATP) production. The majority of dietary phosphate is absorbed in the small intestine, and absorption may be increased by 1,25-DHCC. In the kidneys, the elimination of phosphate is dependent on both glomerular filtration and reabsorption in the proximal tubule.

Causes of Hypo- and Hyperphosphatemia

Phosphate disorders are commonly caused by disorders of excretion, altered intake, and cellular shifting. Common disorders associated with hypo- and hyperphosphatemia are listed in Table 39-2.

Signs and Symptoms

Symptoms of hypophosphatemia may present as the serum phosphate level falls below 2 mg/dL. Most of the symptoms are due to decreased formation of ATP and depletion of 2,3-diphosphoglycerate, which increases the affinity of oxygen for hemoglobin, leading to tissue hypoxia. Symptoms of hypophosphatemia are listed in Table 39-3. The most common clinical manifestation of hyperphosphatemia is hypocalcemia due to the formation of a calcium-phosphate precipitate, which may lead to tetany. Patients with a serum calcium and phosphate product that exceeds 55 mg/dL are at increased risk for precipitate formation and soft tissue calcification. Patients receiving parenteral nutrition therapy should have a calcium/phosphate solubility calculation performed before compounding to limit precipitation of the product.

TREATMENT

Hypophosphatemia

Administration of phosphate is key to preventing hypophosphatemia in hospitalized patients at risk, including patients with a history of alcoholism or receiving parenteral nutrition.

Asymptomatic, mild hypophosphatemia may be treated with oral phosphate supplementation. Oral phosphate supplements are associated with diarrhea and unpredictable absorption. Severe, symptomatic hypophosphatemia should be treated with IV phosphate administration, which are available as a potassium or sodium salt. One mmol of IV potassium phosphate contains 1.47 mEq of potassium, and 1 mmol of sodium phosphate contains 1.33 mEq of sodium. Potassium phosphate is reserved for patients with concomitant hypokalemia. Usually, 15 to 45 mmols of phosphorus is infused over 4 to 6 hours to reduce infusion-related adverse effects and formation of a calcium-phosphate precipitate. The available therapies for hypophosphatemia are listed in Table 39-12.

Hyperphosphatemia

Elevated serum phosphate is common in CKD. Dietary restriction of phosphate intake is key to preventing and treating hyperphosphatemia. If tetany is present, IV calcium is required to increase serum calcium levels. The mainstay of pharmacological treatment of hyperphosphatemia is phosphate binders administered with each meal and snack to bind dietary phosphate (Table 39-13). Oral calcium supplements are considered first-line therapy for long-term treatment. Calcium carbonate and calcium acetate are two commonly used agents and are adjusted based on phosphate levels. Recently, concerns have risen that calcium-based salts may be associated with increased risk of vascular calcification and hypercalcemia. Aluminum-containing antacids also bind phosphate in the intestines and may be more beneficial for acute management of hyperphosphatemia. Long-term use should be avoided because of the risk of aluminum intoxication. Sevelamer is a

TABLE 39-12	Pharmacological Treatment of Hypophosphatemia		
Product	**PO_4^- (mmol)**	**Na^+ (mEq)**	**K^+ (mEq)**
Oral Therapy			
Neutra-Phos cap/packet	8	7.1	7.1
Neutra-Phos-K	8	0	14.2
K-Phos Original tab	3.6	0	3.7
K-Phos MF tab	4	2.9	1.1
K-Phos Neutral tab	8	13	1.1
K-Phos No. 2 tab	8	5.8	2.3
Phospho-Soda	16	32	0
Uro-KP-Neutral tab	8	10.8	1.3
Intravenous Therapy			
Sodium phosphate	3 mmol/mL	4 mEq/mL	
Potassium phosphate	3 mmol/mL		4.4 mEq/mL

Note: 250 mg elemental phosphorus = ~ 8 mmol phosphate.

TABLE 39-13	Oral Phosphate Binders	
Phosphate Binder	**Advantages**	**Disadvantages**
Aluminum salts	High efficacy	Aluminum toxicity
Calcium carbonate	Aluminum free Inexpensive	pH influences efficacy Hypercalcemia Constipation Drug interactions
Calcium acetate	Aluminum free Absorption less Dependent on pH Reduced calcium content than carbonate Lower cost than newer agents	Hypercalcemia Constipation Drug interactions
Sevelamer	Calcium and aluminum free Increased efficacy over calcium products	Expensive Bind fat-soluble vitamins pH influences efficacy Drug interactions
Lanthanum carbonate	Calcium and aluminum free Chewable Increased efficacy Lower pill burden	Expensive Drug interactions

noncalcium, nonaluminum-containing phosphate binder. It is more costly than calcium products, but efficacious in patients with persistent hyperphosphatemia secondary to CKD. After approximately 5 days, it will decrease dietary absorption of phosphate, with peak effects seen in 2 weeks.

Lanthanum carbonate is another noncalcium, nonaluminum-containing phosphate binder that dissociates in the upper GI tract to lanthanum ions (La^{3+}) which bind to dietary phosphate. This results in insoluble lanthanum-phosphate complexes and a net decrease in serum phosphate.

Antacids and lanthanum may bind to some drugs in the GI tract and decrease their absorption. Therefore, patients should be counseled not to take interacting medications within 2 hours of antacids or lanthanum.

MONITORING

In general, patients receiving treatment for electrolyte disorders should be monitored aggressively when these agents are initiated and during titration. Once a stable dose is achieved, patients with normal renal function should have serum concentrations evaluated at least monthly. Patients with renal insufficiency should be evaluated more frequently.

PREVENTION

Prevention of electrolyte disorders involves proper dietary intake, careful monitoring of patients receiving medications which contribute to alterations in serum concentrations, and aggressive monitoring and treatment of disease processes which alter electrolyte homeostasis.

SPECIAL POPULATIONS

Aside from patients with concomitant disease processes or electrolyte disorders which influence the choice of salt for replacement or guide the selection of therapy for lowering serum concentrations, there are no recommendations of note for special populations.

CASE Application

1. A 72-year-old man is admitted for a low serum sodium level at a routine check-up. The patient states he feels fine. Past medical history includes chronic obstructive pulmonary disease, depression, gout, and hypertension. Current medications are albuterol, allopurinol, lisinopril, and sertraline. Physical examination is unremarkable. Pertinent laboratory values include a serum sodium of 123 mEq/L, urine sodium of 90 mEq/L, and a urine osmolarity of 585 mOsm/L. The patient is diagnosed with SIADH. Which of the following represents appropriate treatment to correct this patient's sodium abnormality?

    a. 3% Saline infusion
    b. Demeclocycline

    c. Stopping the offending agent and fluid restriction
    d. Normal saline infusion

2. Choose the statement that best describes SIADH based on the underlying disorder and common cause.

    a. Hypervolemic hypotonic hypernatremia and hydrochlorothiazide
    b. Hypervolemic hypotonic hypernatremia and cirrhosis
    c. Euvolemic hypotonic hyponatremia and lithium
    d. Euvolemic hypotonic hyponatremia and sertraline

3. A 68-year-old woman is brought to the hospital because of progressive drowsiness and syncope. She complains of diarrhea for the past 3 days. She is lethargic but has no focal neurologic deficits. Past medical history is significant for lung cancer, depression, hypertension, gastroesophageal reflux disease (GERD), and osteoarthritis. Medications include acetaminophen, hydrochlorothiazide, fluoxetine, ranitidine, and magnesium oxide. Physical examination reveals a blood pressure of 96/56 mm Hg, pulse of 110 beats/min, dry mucous membranes, and reduced skin turgor. Laboratory value is significant for serum sodium of 125 mEq/L. The most appropriate treatment to correct this patient's sodium abnormality includes which of the following?

    a. 3% Saline infusion
    b. Demeclocycline
    c. Fluid restriction of <1000 mL/d
    d. Normal saline infusion

4. A 54-year-old man is admitted to the hospital from the outpatient clinic with abdominal swelling, weight gain, and abnormal laboratory values. Medical history is significant for cirrhosis and hepatitis C. Medications include furosemide and propranolol. His physical examination is significant for distended abdomen with shifting dullness. Significant laboratory values include serum sodium of 124 mEq/L, INR of 1.9, and albumin of 2.1. The most appropriate treatment to correct this patient's sodium abnormality includes:

    a. 3% Saline with IV furosemide
    b. Fluid restriction
    c. Normal saline infusion
    d. Sodium restriction and diuretics

5. An 82-year-old man was brought to the emergency department by his daughter for worsening confusion and diarrhea. The daughter reports he has had poor oral intake over the last week. Medical history is significant for hypertension, ischemic stroke, reflux, and chronic constipation. Medications include aspirin, lactulose, lisinopril, omeprazole, and simvastatin. His physical examination is significant for orthostatic hypotension, tachycardia, and dry mucous membranes. Significant laboratory values include serum sodium of 162 mEq/L, blood urea nitrogen (BUN) of 66, and serum creatinine

of 2.5. Appropriate initial treatment for this patient would include:

a. 0.45% Saline infusion
b. 5% Dextrose infusion
c. Desmopressin
d. Normal saline infusion

6. A 39-year-old man presents to the emergency department with abnormal laboratory values from a local psychiatric hospital. He is 4 days post neurosurgical repair of intraventricular hemorrhage secondary to bilateral self-enucleation. He is currently constrained to the hospital bed and hallucinating. Medical history includes hypertension and schizophrenia. Medications include haloperidol, fluphenazine, and benztropine. Physical examination is normal. Pertinent laboratory values include sodium of 158 mEq/L and a urine osmolarity of 76 mOsm/kg. Urine output was 6500 mL over the last 24 hours. The patient is admitted for the treatment of central diabetes insipidus. The most appropriate treatment to correct this patient's sodium abnormality includes:

a. Desmopressin
b. Free water orally
c. Hydrochlorothiazide
d. Normal saline infusion

7. What is the drug of choice for lithium-induced diabetes insipidus when lithium must be continued?

a. Amiloride
b. Desmopressin
c. Hydrochlorothiazide
d. Indomethacin

8. Which of the following are potential side effect(s) of potassium replacement (all dosage forms)? Select all that apply.

a. Irritation of the vein
b. Constipation
c. Nausea/vomiting
d. Cardiac arrhythmias
e. Dyspepsia

9. A 66-year-old man is seen for annual follow-up. He has a history of hypertension, type 2 diabetes, coronary artery disease, and heart failure (EF 30%). Current medications include spironolactone 25 mg daily, lisinopril 20 mg daily, metoprolol succinate XL 100 mg once daily, furosemide 40 mg daily, simvastatin 40 mg daily, metformin 500 mg twice daily, and aspirin 81 mg daily. Laboratory values reveal Na 141, K 6, BUN 11, serum creatinine (SCr) 1.1, Phos 3.5, and Mg 2.2. Patient has no complaints at this time. What is the most likely cause of this patient's potassium disorder?

a. Spironolactone
b. Metoprolol
c. Albuterol
d. Furosemide

10. Which hyperkalemia treatment results in the permanent removal of potassium from the body?

a. Insulin and dextrose
b. Calcium gluconate
c. Kayexalate
d. Nebulized albuterol

11. Which statement best describes a mechanism of potassium homeostasis? Select all that apply.

a. Insulin increases the intracellular uptake of potassium.
b. Aldosterone increases potassium excretion.
c. Calcitonin increases the tubular reabsorption of potassium.
d. Increasing the plasma pH decreases the uptake of potassium into the cells.
e. β-Receptor stimulation increases movement of potassium extracellularly.

12. A 48-year-old man presents to the ambulatory clinic with complaints of palpitations over the past few days. Current medications are ramipril 10 mg daily, aspirin 325 mg daily, and omeprazole 20 mg daily. Vitals are blood pressure 152/90 mm Hg, pulse 90, temp 98.6°F, and respiratory rate 14 breaths/min. Laboratory values reveal Na 141, K 5.9, Cl 101, HCO_3 25, BUN 12, SCr 1.1, and glucose 115. ECG showed peaked T waves. Which is the most appropriate initial management for this patient's potassium disorder?

a. PO SPS
b. Calcium chloride
c. Sodium bicarbonate
d. Albuterol

13. Which of the following is an expected symptom of significant (>10 meq/L) hypermagnesemia? Select all that apply.

a. Hypotension
b. Flushing
c. Coma
d. ECG changes
e. Diarrhea

14. Which commonly causes hypomagnesemia? Select all that apply.

a. Amphotericin B
b. Amiloride
c. Lithium
d. Ethacrynic acid
e. Amoxicillin

15. Loop diuretics are commonly associated with which of the following effects? Select all that apply.

a. Hypokalemia
b. Hypocalcemia
c. Hypermagnesemia

d. Hypomagnesemia

e. Hyperkalemia

16. Which statement accurately describes hormonal regulation of calcium and phosphate homeostasis?

    a. Vitamin D reduces calcium and phosphate serum levels.
    b. Calcitonin decreases serum calcium levels.
    c. PTH decreases calcium levels and increases phosphate levels.
    d. Vitamin D causes renal wasting of potassium, calcium, and magnesium.

17. A 55-year-old woman with a past medical history of multiple myeloma is admitted to the hospital with nausea, abdominal pain, and severe constipation. Current laboratory values are Na 140, K 4.2, Cl 103, CO_2 24, BUN 13, SCr 0.9, Glu 123, Mg 2.2, Ca 11.5, Phos 4, and albumin 1.3. She is currently receiving normal saline and furosemide 20 mg IV q4h with adequate urine output. Select the best treatment to prevent recurrence of her calcium disorder.

    a. Intranasal calcitonin
    b. IV potassium phosphate
    c. Sevelamer
    d. IV pamidronate 90 mg

18. Which adverse effect may be associated with pamidronate therapy?

    a. Constipation
    b. Tachycardia
    c. Osteonecrosis of the jaw
    d. Increased blood sugar

19. A patient with hyperparathyroidism is admitted to the medical intensive care unit with pneumonia and respiratory distress requiring mechanical ventilation. Current laboratory values are Na 144, K 3.4, Cl 105, CO_2 24, BUN 16, SCr 0.9, Glu 130, Mg 1.9, Ca 9, Phos 0.8, and albumin 4. Select the best medication to manage this patient's phosphate disorder.

    a. IV sodium phosphate
    b. IV potassium phosphate
    c. IV calcium chloride
    d. PO Neutra-Phos

20. A 70-year-old man on hemodialysis with Stage 5 CKD presents to the nephrology clinic for routine follow-up. Past medical history includes end-stage renal disease (ESRD), hypertension, and type II diabetes. Current medications include amlodipine 10 mg daily, lisinopril 20 mg daily, glipizide 10 mg daily, and aspirin 325 mg daily. Current laboratory values are BUN 60, SCr 4.5, Ca 9, Phos 8, and albumin 2. Which is the best initial management of this patient's phosphate disorder?

    a. Calcium acetate
    b. Sevelamer

c. Discontinuation of lisinopril

d. Calcium carbonate

21. Which of the following represents an appropriate counseling point for patients prescribed a phosphate binder?

    a. Take with meals to reduce phosphate absorption
    b. Take with meals to increase phosphate absorption
    c. Take with meals to reduce GI side effects
    d. Take between meals to reduce food–drug interactions

22. Which electrolyte abnormalities commonly occur in patients with CKD? Select all that apply.

    a. Hyperkalemia
    b. Hyperphosphatemia
    c. Hypomagnesemia
    d. Hypercalcemia
    e. Hypernatremia

23. Which drug/disease state is matched with the correct drug-induced electrolyte disorder?

    a. Lisinopril and hyperkalemia
    b. Fluoxetine and hypernatremia
    c. Alcoholism and hypermagnesemia
    d. Diabetes insipidus and hyponatremia

24. Place the following electrolytes in order based upon their normal serum concentration. Start with the lowest concentration.

Unordered Response	Ordered Response
Sodium	
Potassium	
Magnesium	

25. Place the following NaCl solution in order based upon the chloride concentration. Start with the lowest.

Unordered Response	Ordered Response
0.9% NaCl	
3% NaCl	
0.45% NaCl	

26. Place the following calcium products in order based upon their Meq calcium concentration. Start with the lowest.

Unordered Response	Ordered Response
Acetate 250 mg	
Gluconate 90 mg	
Carbonate 400 mg	

TAKEAWAY POINTS »

- To avoid possibly fatal neurologic consequences, chronic sodium disorders should be corrected slowly in patients without life-threatening symptoms.
- Medications are a common cause of hyponatremia. Thiazide diuretics cause hypovolemic hyponatremia. Antidepressants, chemotherapy, and anticonvulsants may be the cause of SIADH.
- Normal saline is used to restore volume and correct serum sodium in hypovolemic hyponatremia.
- Hypertonic saline is reserved for hyponatremic patients with life-threatening symptoms.
- Fluid restriction is the mainstay of therapy for patients with isovolemic hyponatremia.
- Patients with hypovolemic and isovolemic hypernatremia require free water to correct serum sodium. Patients with central diabetes insipidus require exogenous ADH.
- Thiazides and NSAIDs are useful for the treatment of nephrogenic diabetes insipidus.
- Amiloride is useful in lithium-induced nephrogenic diabetes insipidus.

- IV potassium replacement at a rate of more than 10 mEq/h requires ECG monitoring.
- It is necessary to correct concomitant hypomagnesemia in order to successfully treat hypokalemia.
- Hyperkalemia and hypermagnesemia commonly occur in patients with renal disease.
- Hypokalemia is commonly induced by drugs.
- Hypomagnesemia is typically caused by excessive GI or renal elimination.
- Serum calcium and phosphate levels are regulated by PTH, vitamin D, and calcitonin.
- Classic signs and symptoms of calcium and phosphate disorders involve neurological, neuromuscular, renal, cardiac, and dermatological manifestations.
- Hypercalcemia is most commonly managed with volume expansion, diuretics, and bisphosphonates.
- Hyperphosphatemia commonly occurs in patients with renal disease and may be treated with phosphate binders.

BIBLIOGRAPHY

Brophy DF. Disorders of potassium and magnesium homeostasis. In: DiPiro JT, Talbert RL, Yee GC, Matzke GR, Wells BG, Posey L, eds. *Pharmacotherapy: A Pathophysiologic Approach*. 9th ed. New York, NY: McGraw-Hill; 2014:chap 36.

Chessman KH, Matzke GR. Disorders of sodium and water homeostasis. In: DiPiro JT, Talbert RL, Yee GC, Matzke GR, Wells BG, Posey L, eds. *Pharmacotherapy: A Pathophysiologic Approach*. 9th ed. New York, NY: McGraw-Hill; 2014:chap 34.

Cohn JN, Kowey PR, Whelton PKK, Prisant LM. New guidelines for potassium replacement in clinical practice: a contemporary review by the National Council on Potassium in Clinical Practice. *Arch Intern Med*. 2000;160:2429-2436.

Lau A, Chan LN. Electrolytes, other minerals, and trace elements. In: Lee M, ed. *Basic Skills in Interpreting Laboratory Data*. 4th ed. Bethesda, MD: American Society of Health-System Pharmacists; 2009;119.

Pai AB. Disorders of calcium and phosphorus homeostasis. In: DiPiro JT, Talbert RL, Yee GC, Matzke GR, Wells BG, Posey L, eds. *Pharmacotherapy: A Pathophysiologic Approach*. 9th ed. New York, NY: McGraw-Hill; 2014:chap 35.

Verbalis JG, Goldsmith SR, Greenberg A, Schrier RW, Sterns RH. Hyponatremia treatment guidelines 2007: expert panel recommendations. *Am J Med*. 2007;120:S1-S21.

KEY ABBREVIATIONS

ACE-I = angiotensin-converting enzyme inhibitor
ADH = antidiuretic hormone
ATP = adenosine triphosphate
BUN = blood urea nitrogen
cAMP = cyclic adenosine monophosphate
CNS = central nervous system
1,25-DHCC = 1-25-dihydroxycholecalciferol
ECF = extracellular fluid

ECG = electrocardiogram
ESRD = end-stage renal disease
Glu = glucose
ICF = intracellular fluid
PTH = parathyroid hormone
SCr = serum creatinine
SIADH = syndrome of inappropriate diuretic hormone
SPS = sodium polystyrene sulfonate

Gastrointestinal Disorders

40 Liver Cirrhosis and Complications

Julie Sease and David Eagerton

FOUNDATION OVERVIEW

Cirrhosis (or end-stage liver disease) is an advanced state of liver fibrosis. Fibrosis, the replacement of injured tissue by scar tissue, is accompanied by a distortion of the hepatic vasculature leading to shunting of hepatic blood supply. The shunting compromises exchange between hepatic sinusoids and hepatocytes altering the functions of the liver. The complications of cirrhosis include impaired hepatocyte function, portal hypertension, esophageal varices, ascites, spontaneous bacterial peritonitis, hepatic encephalopathy, thrombocytopenia, coagulopathies, hepatocellular carcinoma, hepatorenal syndrome, and hepatopulmonary syndrome. Cirrhosis may be asymptomatic or encompass a variety of symptoms. Symptoms of cirrhosis include jaundice, spider angiomas splenomegaly, ascites, palmar erythema, gynecomastia, hypogonadism, anorexia, fatigue, weight loss, muscle wasting, and type 2 diabetes.

Alcoholism and hepatitis C are the most common causes of cirrhosis. Examples of medications that cause liver injury are listed in Table 40-1. Drug-induced liver disease resembles acute hepatitis, cholestatic liver disease, or mixed hepatitis/cholestasis. Additionally, drug-induced liver disease may also resemble cirrhosis and fibrosis (eg, methotrexate).

Acute and chronic liver injuries increase serum concentrations of aspartate aminotransferase (AST) and alanine aminotransferase (ALT). Abnormal AST and ALT liver enzymes *may* signal liver damage. ALT elevation is more specific for liver damage because AST is present in heart, skeletal muscle, kidneys, brain, and red blood cells. AST and ALT elevations greater than 10 times the normal limit are associated with acute hepatic injury (eg, toxic liver injury or acute viral hepatitis). Cirrhosis and chronic hepatitis also increase AST and ALT, but to a lower degree than acute injury. AST and ALT levels may be within the normal range in patients with cirrhosis or chronic liver disease. Elevations in alkaline phosphatase (ALP) and gamma-glutamyl transpeptidase (GGT) may accompany cholestatic liver disease (eg, drug-induced cholestatis, cholangitis). ALP and GGT are present in other tissues; therefore, they lack specificity for liver disease. Though also nonspecific for liver disease, decreased serum albumin, increased conjugated bilirubin, and increased prothrombin time are potential findings in end-stage liver disease.

QUANTIFICATION OF LIVER DYSFUNCTION AND DRUG DOSE ADJUSTMENT

The Child-Pugh classification system quantifies cirrhosis by evaluation of laboratory parameters and clinical manifestations (Table 40-2). Drug dosing recommendations and adjustments for hepatically metabolized medications are based upon the Child-Pugh score. However, the model for end-stage liver disease (MELD) scoring system is the classification used by the United Network for Organ Sharing in the allocation of livers for transplantation and determines mortality risk.

Cirrhosis alters several physiologic parameters associated with medications including changes in blood flow through the liver, decreased hepatic intrinsic clearance, and decreased albumin leading to decreased protein binding. The fibrosis of cirrhosis can cause abnormal blood flow through the liver causing blood carrying drug not to be able to interact with hepatocytes where drug metabolism takes place. Hepatic intrinsic clearance is reduced because of decreased phase I metabolism (eg, oxidation) and decreased phase II conjugation reactions (eg, glucuronidation). Complicating matters further, alterations in drug metabolism are inconsistent with oxidative CYP-450 mediated reactions being affected to a greater degree than glucuronidation reactions. Also, bound versus unbound drug concentrations are altered by decreased albumin production which occurs in cirrhosis. Less albumin results in reduced protein binding and increased free drug concentrations. Patients with cirrhosis may also exhibit pharmacodynamic changes. Examples of pharmacodynamic changes include: a decreased therapeutic effect to β-blockers and diuretics; increased sensitivity to opioid analgesics, anxiolytics, and sedatives; and increased kidney side effects from non-steroidal anti-inflammatory drugs.

Select medications contain dosage adjustment recommendations based on the Child-Pugh score. Guidelines for dosage adjustment in patients with hepatic dysfunction are summarized in Table 40-3. Additionally, the manufacturer's prescribing information should be reviewed for recommendations in patients with hepatic dysfunction. Patients that develop hepatorenal syndrome may need medication dosing

TABLE 40-1	**Medications Associated with Liver Damage (list not all inclusive)**

Acetaminophen
Amiodarone
Azathioprine
Darunavir
Didanosine
Estrogens
HMG-CoA reductase inhibitors (eg, [statins])
Isoniazid
Ketoconazole
Nevirapine
Nicotinic acid
Phenytoin
Retinol
Rifampin
Stavudine
Tipranavir
Valproic acid

adjustment based upon decreased hepatic *and* renal dysfunction. Unfortunately, hepatorenal syndrome complicates drug dosing because serum creatinine measurements are often inaccurate in patients with severe liver disease.

TREATMENT OF CIRRHOSIS COMPLICATIONS

Portal Hypertension and Esophageal Varices

Fibrotic changes within the hepatic sinusoids during cirrhosis increases the pressure gradient between portal and central venous pressures. The pressure gradient results in gastrointestinal and esophageal varices. Varices occur because the body attempts to find outlets to relieve the pressure of portal hypertension. Additional outlets include retroperitoneal vessels, hemorrhoidal venous plexus, recanalized umbilical vein, and intrahepatic shunts. The management of varices involves three strategies: (1) primary prophylaxis (prevention of the first bleeding episode); (2) treatment of acute variceal hemorrhage; and (3) secondary prophylaxis (prevention of rebleeding). Recommendations for the management of portal hypertension and variceal bleeding are listed in Table 40-4.

Primary Prophylaxis

Primary prophylaxis utilizes nonselective β-adrenergic blocking agents (eg, propranolol, nadolol, or carvedilol). Nonselective β-blockers reduce portal pressure by diminishing portal venous inflow via two mechanisms: (1) decreasing cardiac output through β_1-adrenergic blockade and (2) decreasing splanchnic blood flow through β_2-adrenergic blockade. Patients with contraindications (eg, asthma, peripheral vascular disease) or intolerance to therapy with nonselective β-adrenergic blockers may be managed with endoscopic variceal ligation (EVL).

Treatment

Vasoactive drug therapy may be considered in the management of variceal bleeding to stop or slow bleeding. Octreotide is the vasoactive drug used to manage acute variceal bleeding and is dosed intravenously. Octreotide is a splanchnic vasoconstrictor thereby decreasing portal blood flow and pressure. Octreotide monitoring should include blood glucose (hypo- or hyperglycemia) and cardiac conduction abnormalities. Patients with cirrhosis with active bleeding are at high risk for bacterial infections. Prophylactic antibiotic therapy should be prescribed for all patients with cirrhosis and acute variceal bleeding. A short course (7 days) of oral norfloxacin, intravenous ciprofloxacin, or intravenous ceftriaxone is recommended.

Secondary Prophylaxis

The use of EVL plus pharmacologic therapy to prevent rebleeding is the recommended therapeutic approach. Pharmacologic therapy should be initiated with an oral nonselective β-blocker (eg, propranolol, nadolol, or carvedilol). Patients receiving nonselective β-blockers should be monitored for heart failure, bronchospasm, and glucose intolerance. EVL should be conducted every 1 to 2 weeks until variceal obliteration, followed by surveillance endoscopy in 1 to 3 months and then surveillance endoscopy every 6 to 12 months. Those who cannot tolerate or fail EVL plus oral nonselective β-blocker are considered for surgical shunting to prevent rebleeding.

TABLE 40-2	**Criteria and Scoring[a] for the Child-Pugh Grading of Chronic Liver Disease**		
Score	1	2	3
Total bilirubin (mg/dL)	<2	2-3	>3
Albumin (g/dL)	>3.5	2.8-3.5	<2.8
Ascites	None	Mild/Moderate (diuretic-sensitive)	Severe (diuretic-refractory)
Encephalopathy (grade[b])	None	1 and 2 (or precipitant-induced)	3 and 4 (or chronic)
Prothrombin time (seconds prolonged)	<4	4-6	>6

[a]Grade A, <7 points; Grade B, 7-9 points; Grade C, 10-15 points.
[b]Encephalopathy Grade 0: Minimal, may go unnoticed; Encephalopathy Grade 1: Mild, short attention span, mood changes; Encephalopathy Grade 2: Moderate, forgetting, decreased energy, inappropriate behavior; Encephalopathy Grade 3: Severe, Confusion, drowsiness, anxiety, strange behavior; Encephalopathy Grade 4: Coma.
Data from https://www.hepatitis.va.gov/pdf/Child-Pugh-score.pdf; http://he123.liverfoundation.org/diagnosis/what-are-the-stages-of-he/.

TABLE 40-3 | **Drug Dosage Adjustment Guidelines for Hepatic Dysfunction**

1	The oral bioavailability of high hepatic extraction ratio drugs can be greatly increased; therefore, dosage should be reduced accordingly.
2	Pharmacokinetic evaluation of low hepatic extraction and highly plasma protein bound drugs should be based on unbound concentrations and dosage adjustment may be necessary even though total blood/plasma concentrations are within the normal range.
3	Dosage adjustment of low hepatic extraction ratio/low plasma protein bound drugs should be aimed at maintaining normal total (bound plus unbound) plasma concentrations.
4	Elimination of drugs partly excreted unchanged by the kidneys will be impaired in patients with hepatorenal syndrome. Creatinine clearance significantly overestimates glomerular filtration rate in these patients. Cystatin C based formulas perform better to estimate renal function in cirrhotic patients.
5	Volume of distribution of hydrophilic drugs may be increased in patients with cirrhosis and edema or ascites. Loading doses of these drugs may need to be increased if a rapid effect of the drug is required. Renal function should also be taken into consideration.
6	Extreme caution is recommended when using drugs with a narrow therapeutic index.

Ascites and Spontaneous Bacterial Peritonitis

Ascites is the development of fluid retention in the setting of cirrhosis. Physical examination findings of ascites include a full, bulging abdomen, and shifting flank dullness. Diagnostic paracentesis is utilized to evaluate ascitic fluid (eg, infection). Treatment of ascites includes alcohol avoidance, sodium restriction, and oral diuretic therapy or therapeutic paracentesis. The combination of spironolactone and furosemide (ratio of 100 mg:40 mg) is recommended by practice guidelines.

Electrolytes (eg, potassium, sodium, and magnesium) should be monitored in patients on diuretic therapy.

Spontaneous bacterial peritonitis (SBP) is an infection of ascitic fluid and is diagnosed by a positive ascitic fluid bacterial culture and an elevated ascitic fluid absolute polymorphonuclear count. SBP is caused by *Escherichia coli, Klebsiella pneumonia*, and Pneumococci and empiric antibiotic therapy (eg, cefotaxime, ceftriaxone, and ofloxacin) should target these pathogens. Long-term antibiotic therapy for the *prevention* of SBP should be considered in patients at high risk.

TABLE 40-4 | **Therapeutic Recommendations for Variceal Bleeding in Portal Hypertension**

Recommendation	Notes
Prevention of variceal bleeding in patients with varices Propranolol 20 mg po bid Or Nadolol 40 mg po daily Or Carvedilol 3.125 mg po bid	Titrate nonselective β-blocker to maximal tolerated dose or heart rate of 55-60 beats/min. Nadolol is renally eliminated and dosing adjustments are required in patients with renal dysfunction. Carvedilol has hepatic dose adjustments cited in its packaging. Endoscopic variceal ligation may be used instead of drug therapy in the case of medium/large varices and high risk of bleeding.
Treatment of variceal bleeding Antibiotic prophylaxis[a] Norfloxacin 400 mg po bid (or ciprofloxacin dose is 400 mg IV bid route not available) Or Ceftriaxone 1 g IV daily Vasoactive drugs: Octreotide IV bolus of 50 mcg and followed by a continuous infusion of 50 mcg/h × 3-5 d *Plus* Endoscopic variceal ligation	
Secondary prophylaxis of variceal bleeding Propranolol 20 mg po bid or nadolol 40 mg po daily or carvedilol 3.125 mg po bid *Plus* Endoscopic variceal ligation	Titrate nonselective β-blocker to maximal tolerated dose or heart rate of 55-60 beats/min. Nadolol is renally eliminated and dosing adjustments are required in patients with renal dysfunction. Carvedilol has hepatic dose adjustments cited in its packaging.

[a]Consider ceftriaxone in areas with high fluoroquinolone resistance rates.

TABLE 40-5	Therapeutic Recommendations for Ascites and Spontaneous Bacterial Peritonitis
Recommendation	**Notes**
Ascites	
Initial therapeutic paracentesis should be performed in patients with tense ascites. Sodium restriction of 2000 mg/d should be instituted as well as oral diuretic therapy. Diuretic-sensitive patients should be treated with sodium restriction and diuretics rather than serial paracentesis.	Diuretic therapy: Spironolactone 100 mg po daily with or without furosemide 40 mg po daily. Therapy can be titrated every 3-5 days (maintaining the 100 mg: 40 mg ratio) to reach adequate natriuresis and weight loss. Maximal doses are spironolactone 400 mg po daily and furosemide 160 mg po daily.
Refractory Ascites	
Serial therapeutic paracentesis may be performed. Post-paracentesis albumin infusion of 6-8 g/L of fluid removed can be considered if large volumes of fluid (eg, >5 L) are removed during paracentesis.	
Treatment of Spontaneous Bacterial Peritonitis	
If ascitic fluid PMN counts are greater than 250 cells/mm^3, empiric antibiotic therapy should be instituted. If ascitic fluid PMN counts are <250 cells/mm^3, but signs or symptoms of infection exist, empiric antibiotic therapy should be initiated while awaiting culture results. If (1) ascitic fluid PMN counts are >250 cells/mm^3, (2) clinical suspicion of spontaneous bacterial peritonitis is present, and (3) the patient has a serum creatinine >1 mg/dL, blood urea nitrogen of >30 mg/dL or total bilirubin >4 mg/dL, 1.5 g/kg albumin should be infused within 6 h of detection and 1 g/kg albumin infusion should also be given on day 3.	Community acquired: cefotaxime 2 g IV every 8 h (or comparable third generation cephalosporin such as ceftriaxone) recommended. Ofloxacin 400 mg po twice daily may be substituted for cefotaxime in patients without prior exposure to quinolones, vomiting, shock, grade 2 or higher encephalopathy, or serum creatinine >3 mg/dL. Nosocomial setting and/or in presence of recent β-lactam antibiotic exposure: empiric choice should be based on local susceptibility testing of patients with cirrhosis.
Prophylaxis Against Spontaneous Bacterial Peritonitis	
Long-term prophylaxis with norfloxacin 400 mg po daily (or daily oral trimethoprim/sulfamethoxazole) may be considered in any patient with history of spontaneous bacterial peritonitis. Long-term prophylaxis may also be justified in patients without history of peritonitis who have ascitic total protein less than 1.5 g/dL and at least one of the following present: (1) serum creatinine ≥1.2 mg/dL, (2) blood urea nitrogen greater than or equal to 25 mg/dL, (3) serum sodium ≤130 mg/dL, or (4) Child-Pugh score ≥9 with serum bilirubin ≥3 mg/dL.	

Abbreviation: PMN, polymorphonuclear.

High-risk patients include those with prior SBP or those with low-protein ascites (<1.5 g/dL) plus at least one of the following: (1) serum creatinine greater than or equal to 1.2 mg/dL, (2) blood urea nitrogen greater than or equal to 25 mg/dL, (3) serum sodium less than or equal to 130 mEq/L, or (4) Child-Pugh score of greater than or equal to 9 with bilirubin greater than or equal to 3 mg/dL. Oral norfloxacin or trimethoprim/sulfamethoxazole daily may be utilized for long-term SBP prevention. Albumin infusion may be considered in refractory ascites cases following large volume paracentesis and in select patients with SBP. Drug therapy recommendations for the management of ascites and SBP are listed in Table 40-5.

Hepatic Encephalopathy

Hepatic encephalopathy (HE) is a disturbance in central nervous system function because of hepatic dysfunction. The primary treatment for episodic and persistent HE is reducing ammonia blood concentrations. Ammonia levels are decreased by dietary restriction of protein and drug therapy is aimed at inhibiting ammonia production or enhancing removal. As a first-line agent, lactulose administration (oral or rectal enema) lowers ammonia blood levels by: (1) creation of a laxative effect which reduces ammonia absorption, (2) leaching of ammonia into the colon and increasing bacterial uptake of ammonia in the gut, and (3) reducing ammonia production by interfering with the uptake of glutamine in the intestinal wall. Patients on lactulose therapy should have their electrolytes (eg, sodium, potassium, and magnesium) monitored periodically. Inhibiting urease-producing bacteria by using neomycin, metronidazole, or rifaximin can also decrease production of ammonia. Despite poor absorption, chronic use of neomycin can lead to ototoxicity and nephrotoxicity. Therefore, neomycin is not first-line therapy for HE. Metronidazole may produce a favorable clinical response in HE. However, neurotoxicity caused by impaired hepatic clearance of the drug may be problematic. Orally administered rifaximin is effective for HE and has a favorable side effect profile as compared to neomycin and metronidazole and is therefore considered second-line therapy. Rifaximin is recommended in combination with lactulose in patients with recurrent HE following a second recurrence.

TABLE 40-6 | **Therapeutic Recommendations for Hepatic Encephalopathy**

Recommendations	Notes
Nutritional Management	
Patients with HE should receive the maximally tolerated amount of protein (goal 1.2-1.5 g/kg/d)	Patients with zinc deficiency (eg, <0.66 mcg/mL) should receive supplementation (eg, 220 mg po bid).
Reduction of Nitrogenous Load from the Gut	
Lactulose	Lactulose dosing:
	45 mL (30 g) po followed by hourly dosing until evacuation occurs. Then dosing adjusted to achieve 2-3 soft bowel movements per day (typically 15-45 mL [10-30 g] every 8-12 h). May also be provided via 1 h retention enema (200 g in 300 mL).
Antibiotics	
Neomycin	Neomycin dosing:
	1 g po every 6 h for up to 6 days for acute HE.
	1-2 g po once daily for persistent HE.
	Patients should be monitored for renal function periodically and annually for ototoxicity.
Metronidazole	Metronidazole dosing: 250 mg po bid
Rifaximin	Rifaximin dosing: 550 mg po bid (in conjunction with lactulose)

Abbreviation: HE, hepatic encephalopathy.

Oral zinc supplementation is recommended for long-term management in patients with cirrhosis who are zinc deficient (eg, <50 mcg/dL). Therapeutic recommendations for the management of HE are listed in Table 40-6.

CASE Application

Utilize the following case to answer the next three questions.

DT is a 42-year-old man with a 20-year history of alcohol abuse who presents with altered mental status, anorexia, mild weight loss over the past 3 months, recent abdominal swelling, and general malaise. Current medications include rosuvastatin, niacin, acetaminophen, and diazepam. Upon examination he was found to have palmar erythema and splenomegaly and his labs were significant for mildly elevated AST, ALT, bilirubin, and blood glucose. He is diagnosed with hepatic cirrhosis.

1. Which of the following is the most likely cause of DT's cirrhosis?
   a. Rosuvastatin
   b. Ethanol
   c. Acetaminophen
   d. Niacin

2. An arterial ammonia level is drawn for DT with the following results:
   125 mcg/dL (Normal: 15-60 mcg/dL)
   This laboratory abnormality is most closely associated with which of the symptoms reported by DT?
   a. Abdominal swelling
   b. Altered mental status
   c. Jaundice
   d. Palmar erythema

3. A consultation with DT should include recommendations to prevent the exacerbation or progression of his cirrhosis and complications. Select the counseling points that should be discussed by the pharmacist. Select **ALL** that apply.
   a. Limit alcohol intake
   b. Limit protein intake
   c. Limit total caloric intake
   d. Limit sodium intake
   e. Limit fluid intake

4. Your patient is a 52-year-old woman who presents with the following liver function test results:
   AST: 200 U/L (Normal: 8-20 U/L)
   ALT: 520 U/L (Normal: 5-40 U/L)
   Your patient's liver function test results are most likely associated with which of the following?
   a. Acute acetaminophen toxicity
   b. Cirrhosis
   c. Chronic hepatitis C infection
   d. Nonalcoholic fatty liver disease

Utilize the following case to answer the next four questions.

KD is a 65-year-old man who has been diagnosed with cirrhosis for the past 2 years. KD presents with mild ascites, esophageal and gastric varices with no bleeding, and no apparent encephalopathy. Pertinent laboratory values are: total bilirubin 2.5 mg/dL (normal: 0.3-1.2 mg/dL), albumin 2.9 g/dL (normal: 3.2-4.6 g/dL), prothrombin time 19.5 seconds (normal:12.5-15.2 seconds).

5. KD is currently having difficulty with overactive bladder and his physician is considering starting him on darifenacin. Based on the patient's Child-Pugh score and the

following information from darifenacin's dosing information, what dose will you recommend for KD.

No Liver Disease	Mild Hepatic Insufficiency	Moderate Hepatic Insufficiency	Severe Hepatic Insufficiency
15 mg daily	15 mg daily	7.5 mg daily	No clinical experience

a. KD has grade A cirrhosis and should be started on 15 mg daily.
b. KD has grade B cirrhosis and should be started on 7.5 mg daily.
c. KD has grade C cirrhosis and should be started on 7.5 mg daily.
d. KD has grade A cirrhosis and should not be given darifenacin.

6. Which of the following drugs would be expected to have a decreased therapeutic effect in KD due to pharmacodynamic changes associated with chronic liver disease?

a. Hydromorphone
b. Propranolol
c. Alprazolam
d. Zolpidem

7. Which of the following statements is true for KD regarding volume of distribution and half-life of drugs highly protein bound to albumin in the blood?

a. Albumin is increased in chronic liver disease leading to increased protein binding, increased volume of distribution, and potentially decreased half-life.
b. Albumin is decreased in chronic liver disease leading to decreased protein binding, increased volume of distribution, and potentially increased half-life.
c. Albumin is decreased in chronic liver disease leading to decreased protein binding, decreased volume of distribution, and potentially decreased half-life.
d. No changes in albumin concentrations, volume of distribution, or half-life normally occur in chronic liver disease.

8. Which of the following is true about the oral bioavailability of high hepatic ratio drugs in KD if portal-systemic shunting has occurred?

a. Oral bioavailability will be unchanged and no initial dosage adjustment should be considered.
b. Oral bioavailability will be decreased and initial dosage should be increased.
c. Oral bioavailability will be increased but no dosage adjustment need be considered.
d. Oral bioavailability will be increased and initial dosage should be decreased.

9. Hepatic drug elimination is dependent upon which of the following?

a. Blood flow, drug binding in blood, and hepatic extraction ratio

b. Blood flow, drug binding in blood, and bioavailability
c. Drug binding in blood, bioavailability, and hepatic extraction ratio
d. Blood flow, drug binding in blood, hepatic intrinsic clearance

10. Patients who have cirrhosis and edema may have an increased volume of distribution for hydrophilic drugs. In this situation, what adjustments should be made to the loading doses if a rapid drug effect is required?

a. Loading doses should be eliminated in these patients
b. Loading doses should be increased
c. Loading doses should be decreased
d. Hydrophilic drugs are contraindicated in patients with cirrhosis

11. Dosage adjustment of low hepatic extraction ratio/low plasma protein bound drugs should be aimed at maintaining which of the following?

a. Normal unbound plasma concentrations
b. Normal bound plasma concentrations
c. Normal total (bound plus unbound) plasma concentrations
d. No dosage adjustments need be considered

12. Which of the following statements is true?

a. In liver disease, phase II conjugation metabolism is affected to a greater extent than phase I oxidative reactions.
b. In liver disease, phase I oxidative metabolism is affected to a greater extent than phase II conjugation reactions.
c. Chronic liver disease is associated with uniform reductions in metabolism via the different cytochrome P450 pathways.
d. Serum creatinine is an accurate reflection of renal function in chronic liver disease.

13. Your patient has just been diagnosed with cirrhosis and undergoes an endoscopy. Several large esophageal varices are noted and his hepatologist decides that he should be started on drug therapy to prevent variceal bleeding. Which of the following describes appropriate therapy for primary prevention of variceal bleeding in this patient?

a. No primary prevention therapy needed; only patients who have experienced an episode of variceal bleeding in the past should receive prophylaxis therapy.
b. Norfloxacin 400 mg po bid.
c. Sucralfate 1 g po four times daily.
d. Propranolol 20 mg po bid.

14. The physician decides to treat your patient's ascites with oral diuretic therapy and starts him on 100 mg spironolactone and 40 mg furosemide every day. After 5 days the patient is re-evaluated and the physician decides to increase the spironolactone to 150 mg/d and a further adjustment to 200 mg/d occurs after an additional

3 days. What is the appropriate dose of oral furosemide that should be given with this dose of spironolactone?

a. Furosemide 100 mg/d
b. Furosemide 40 mg/d
c. Furosemide 60 mg/d
d. Furosemide 80 mg/d

15. A 65-year-old man with a 20-year history of heavy alcohol use, cirrhosis, and portal hypertension presents for emergent care after experiencing hematemesis and is diagnosed with acute esophageal variceal bleeding. Which of the following is appropriate therapy for this patient at this time?

a. Nadolol 40 mg po daily plus norfloxacin 400 mg po bid
b. Octreotide 50 mcg IV bolus, then 50 mcg/h infusion plus norfloxacin 400 mg po bid
c. Octreotide 50 mcg IV bolus, then 50 mcg/h infusion plus pantoprazole 40 mg IV daily
d. Octreotide 50 mcg IV bolus then 50 mcg/h infusion plus propranolol 20 mg po bid

16. Octreotide is ordered to be infused at a rate of 50 mcg/h and the pharmacy prepares 1 mg of Octreotide in 1 L of normal saline. What amount of the preparation will need to be infused per hour in order to attain the prescribed rate?

a. 10 mL/h
b. 25 mL/h
c. 50 mL/h
d. 250 mL/h

Use the following questions to answer the next three questions.

AB is a 65-year-old woman with a history of cirrhosis who was just admitted with severe ascites and undergoes paracentesis. AB's polymorphonuclear count is found to be 300 cells/mm^3 and she is diagnosed with spontaneous bacterial peritonitis.

17. Which of the following antibiotics is available in IV formulation and is appropriate empiric therapy for AB's spontaneous bacterial peritonitis?

a. Vancomycin
b. Cephalexin
c. Tigecycline
d. Cefotaxime

18. Which of the following resources would be appropriate to use to determine compatibility for an IV solution for AB's antibiotic? Select **ALL** that apply.

a. King Guide
b. Red Book
c. Orange Book
d. Trissel's
e. Sanford Guide

19. The treatment for AB is effective and she recovers from her spontaneous bacterial peritonitis but develops symptoms of hepatic encephalopathy. Place the following drug options for hepatic encephalopathy in proper order from first line, to second line, to third line.

a. Neomycin, lactulose, rifaximin
b. Lactulose, rifaximin, neomycin
c. Rifaximin, lactulose, neomycin
d. Lactulose, neomycin, rifaximin

20. Your patient presents with a prescription for Flagyl® which his physician has chosen in the management of his hepatic encephalopathy. The script indicates substitution permitted. Which of the following generic agents would be an appropriate substitution for Flagyl®?

a. Neomycin
b. Rifaximin
c. Metronidazole
d. Cefotaxime

21. PA is a 42-year-old woman who is at risk for developing cirrhosis. Identify the correct sequence of events that can result in the development of cirrhosis.

a. Shunting of hepatic blood supply
b. Distortion of hepatic vasculature
c. Hepatic cell injury
d. Replacement of injured tissue by scar tissue

22. Which of the following decreases splanchnic blood flow through mechanisms other than β-adrenergic antagonism?

a. Inderal®
b. Corgard®
c. Sandostatin®
d. Xifaxan®

23. Which of the following medications is useful in the prevention of esophageal variceal bleeding? Select **ALL** that apply.

a. Sandostatin®
b. Pravastatin
c. Corgard®
d. Calan®
e. Carvedilol

24. KR is a 45-year-old man who has been diagnosed with chronic hepatitis C. Which of the following would indicate that KR is developing or has developed cirrhosis? Select **ALL** that apply.

a. Gynecomastia
b. Hypogonadism
c. Aplastic anemia
d. Type 2 diabetes
e. Thrombocytopenia

TAKEAWAY POINTS »

- The primary causes of cirrhosis include alcohol abuse and hepatitis C infection.
- Acute toxicities or acute damage to the liver causes increases in aminotransferase levels. Chronic disease, such as cirrhosis, is likely to cause moderate increases in the aminotransferases or they may remain normal.
- The Child-Pugh classification and MELD scoring systems can be used to stage the severity of liver disease in a patient with cirrhosis.
- Dosing recommendations for drugs metabolized by the liver are based on Child-Pugh classification.
- Complications of cirrhosis include portal hypertension, esophageal varices/variceal bleeding, ascites, spontaneous bacterial peritonitis, encephalopathy, hepatorenal syndrome, hepatopulmonary syndrome, hepatocellular carcinoma, thrombocytopenia, and coagulopathies.
- Octreotide is used in acute variceal hemorrhage to control bleeding.

- Nonselective β-adrenergic blocking agents (eg, propranolol, nadolol, or carvedilol) are utilized to prevent variceal bleeding, both in those who have never had variceal bleeding and in those who have suffered variceal bleeding in the past.
- Sodium restriction and oral diuretic therapy are used to control ascites in patients with cirrhosis.
- Spontaneous bacterial peritonitis is most often caused by *Escherichia coli, Klebsiella pneumonia,* and Pneumococci and empiric antibiotic therapy (eg, cefotaxime, ceftriaxone, ofloxacin) is used which targets these pathogens.
- Lactulose is first-line therapy for hepatic encephalopathy.
- Rifaximin therapy is second-line therapy, in combination with lactulose, for those patients who suffer a second occurrence of hepatic encephalopathy.

KEY ABBREVIATIONS

ALP = alkaline phosphatase
ALT = alanine aminotransferase
AST = aspartate aminotransferase
EVL = endoscopic variceal ligation

GGT = gamma-glutamyl transpeptidase
HE = hepatic encephalopathy
MELD = model for end-stage liver disease
SBP = spontaneous bacterial peritonitis

41

Inflammatory Bowel Disease

Sheila M. Wilhelm and Sean McConachie

FOUNDATION OVERVIEW

Inflammatory bowel disease (IBD) is a chronic relapsing and remitting inflammatory condition of the gastrointestinal (GI) tract and consists of ulcerative colitis (UC) and Crohn disease (CD). The incidence of UC in the United States is estimated to be 8 to 12 cases per 100,000 population per year, while CD is reported as approximately 5 cases per 100,000 population per year. While the underlying pathophysiology of IBD involves an abnormal immune inflammatory response directed against the intestinal tract, the true cause of IBD has not been identified. Genetic and environmental factors have been implicated as contributors to the development of IBD. IBD has been observed to occur more commonly in patients who report a positive family history of IBD. Another leading theory is that the inflammatory response is induced by the local bacterial flora that inhabit the human GI tract. Ultimately, the inflammatory response results in injury to the GI tract that may vary in location, depth, severity, and duration.

While both UC and CD involve inflammation of the GI tract, there are some key differences between the two. UC is localized to the colon and is characterized by diffuse continuous mucosal inflammation with the absence of granulomatous changes. The rectal area is involved in 95% of patients with UC. In contrast, CD may affect any area of the GI tract, but most frequently involves the ileum or colon. The inflammation in CD is often discontinuous in nature, resulting in "skip lesions," and often penetrates much deeper into the intestinal wall compared to UC. Inflammation confined to the intestinal wall is referred to as luminal CD, and may progress to fibrostenotic disease with development of strictures and luminal obstruction. Likewise, severe inflammation resulting in fistula formation occurs in 20% to 40% of patients with CD, while patients with UC do not develop fistulae.

Due to the location and inflammatory nature of the disease, most patients with UC will present with bloody diarrhea, urgency, and tenesmus as their main symptoms. Patients with CD may exhibit similar symptoms, but most commonly present with diarrhea, abdominal pain, weight loss, fever, perianal lesions, and signs of malnutrition. In addition to GI tract involvement, patients with IBD may also develop inflammation in various other organ systems, referred to as extraintestinal symptoms. Examples include arthritis, erythema nodosum, pyoderma gangrenosum, uveitis, episcleritis, and primary sclerosing cholangitis, among others.

The diagnosis of IBD is based collectively on presenting signs and symptoms, along with radiographic and endoscopic findings. Endoscopy is particularly helpful in characterizing the extent and location of the disease, as well as ruling out other potential causes of intestinal inflammation. Disease location also directly impacts selection of drug therapy. Patients with UC can be classified as having "extensive" disease if inflammation extends proximal to the splenic flexure. The term "distal" or "left-sided" disease is used if inflammation is distal to the splenic flexure. Lastly, ulcerative proctitis denotes inflammation localized to the rectum, while proctosigmoiditis involves both the rectum and sigmoid colon. While these terms are used for denoting the subtype of UC based on extent and location of inflammation, the extent and location of CD is also determined via endoscopy in a similar manner.

Disease severity of UC is classified based on various parameters, such as the number and characteristics of stools per day, presence of systemic signs of inflammation, such as fever or elevated erythrocyte sedimentation rate, among others. The designations used for UC are mild, moderate, moderate severe, and fulminant. While a validated scoring system, the CD Activity Index, may be used to classify CD severity, a similar designation to UC also exists and includes classifications of mild-moderate, moderate-severe, and severe/fulminant disease.

TREATMENT

Once disease extent, location, and severity have been determined, pharmacologic therapies may be instituted to address the underlying inflammation. Drug therapy does not provide a cure for IBD, so the major goals of treatment are to suppress acute inflammation, improve patient symptoms and quality of life, avoid or minimize toxicities, and prevent complications of the disease. Drug therapies should aim to induce disease remission, and then maintain long-term remission if possible. Extraintestinal manifestations of IBD also need to be managed in conjunction with the GI aspects of the disease. In some instances, patients who are refractory to medical therapy or develop severe complications may require surgical intervention.

An important aspect of drug therapy for IBD is that the choice of therapy depends on the disease subtype, as well as the severity and location of the disease. More severe or extensive forms of IBD may require administration of systemic medications, either in oral or parenteral forms. Alternatively, disease that is mild or moderate in nature and is located in areas distal to the splenic flexure may be treated with rectal dosage forms, also referred to as "topical" therapies. Suppositories can be used to treat up to 20 cm of the rectal area and are preferred for patients with proctitis. Enemas may reach inflammation that extends to the splenic flexure and thus may be used for patients with left-sided disease. Oral formulations of some drugs used in the management of IBD are designed to release in specific areas of the small or large intestine and should be chosen based on the target area of inflammation. Systemic and topical therapies may be combined for maximal effectiveness. As many drug therapies for IBD may have serious adverse effects or complicated dosing regimens, counseling to promote patient adherence is key to optimizing outcomes.

Aminosalicylates

The aminosalicylate drug class consists of the prototypical agent sulfasalazine and other agents formulated to deliver mesalamine, also known as 5-aminosalicylate or 5-ASA, the active component of sulfasalazine, to various locations within the GI tract (Table 41-1). Sulfasalazine consists of mesalamine bound to sulfapyridine via a diazo bond. When administered orally, bacteria located in the colon cleave the diazo bond and release mesalamine which acts locally in the colon. The sulfapyridine component is systemically absorbed. Patients with allergies to sulfonamides should avoid sulfasalazine, as the sulfapyridine component may lead to hypersensitivity reactions. Adverse effects from sulfasalazine are mainly related to the sulfapyridine component and may be dose related or idiosyncratic. Common adverse effects are nausea, diarrhea, headache, and abdominal pain.

Newer formulations of mesalamine lack the sulfapyridine component and deliver the drug to the GI tract through various delayed release mechanisms. All of these formulations are safe to use in patients with allergies to sulfonamides. Some products use inert carrier molecules in place of sulfapyridine, such as balsalazide (Colazal), while others, such as olsalazine (Dipentum), use two molecules of mesalamine linked via a diazo bond to deliver the drug to the colon. Other formulations use pH-dependent coated tablets (Asacol, Delzicol) or microgranules (Pentasa). The newest formulations of mesalamine use pH-dependent multimatrix tablets (Lialda) or granules with a polymer matrix (Apriso) to allow for once daily dosing and improved patient adherence. Lastly, mesalamine is also available as a suppository or an enema, which are preferred formulations for patients with distal disease. The nonsulfa-containing aminosalicylates are better tolerated than sulfasalazine and thus are used more often.

The choice of an aminosalicylate is based on the type of disease, as well as the location and severity. The formulation of drug chosen should release or deliver mesalamine to the site of inflammation. The aminosalicylates can be used in UC

TABLE 41-1 Aminosalicylate Products Used in the Treatment of IBD

Brand Name(s)	Formulation	Site of Action
Topical Mesalamine Therapies		
Rowasa	Enema	Rectum, distal colon
Canasa	Suppository	Rectum
Oral Products		
Sulfasalazine Azulfidine Azulfidine En-tabs Mesalamine	Immediate release or enteric-coated tablets	Colon
Asacol HD Delzicol	Tablet coated with Eudragit-S (delayed-release acrylic resin)	Terminal ileum and colon
Pentasa	Encapsulated ethylcellulose microgranules (capsule)	Small bowel and colon
Dipentum	Dimer of mesalamine (capsule)	Colon
Colazal	Mesalamine bound to inert carrier molecule (capsule)	Colon
Lialda	Once daily tablet with pH-dependent coating and MMX, mutimatrix core	Terminal ileum and colon
Apriso	Once daily pH-dependent tablet with mesalamine granules in a Intellicor polymer matrix	Colon

for both induction and maintenance of remission in patients with both distal and extensive mild to moderate disease. The aminosalicylates can also be used in mild to moderate CD, but appear to be less efficacious than in UC. Patients should be instructed to take the appropriate number of tablets or capsules and not to crush or break them. Likewise, proper instruction on use of suppositories and enemas will ensure maximal effectiveness.

Corticosteroids

Corticosteroids have potent anti-inflammatory effects and have specific roles in the management of IBD. Corticosteroids are mainly used to rapidly suppress inflammation in patients with moderate to severe symptoms or in those patients unresponsive to aminosalicylates. There are many different formulations of corticosteroids available including oral, parenteral, and topical agents. In general, short courses (7-10 days) of oral prednisone at doses of 40 to 60 mg daily are used for moderate to severe UC and CD. Parenteral hydrocortisone or methylprednisolone can be used for hospitalized patients with severe disease. Budesonide (Entocort EC), a corticosteroid with limited systemic bioavailability, is formulated to release in the terminal ileum and ascending colon and can be considered a first-line agent in the management of mild-moderate CD in place of an aminosalicylate, especially in CD affecting the ileum and ascending colon. Uceris is a multimatrix formulation of budesonide which distributes throughout the colon and is used in the management of mild to moderate active UC. Topical hydrocortisone products, available as enemas or suppositories, can be used for patients with distal disease who do not initially respond to aminosalicylates. Corticosteroids are generally ineffective for treatment of fistulae associated with CD.

Despite their ability to rapidly suppress inflammation, corticosteroids are ineffective as long-term treatments and have no role in the maintenance of remission of IBD. The potential for serious adverse effects precludes the long-term use of these agents. Patients who become corticosteroid dependent may develop hypertension, osteoporosis, glucose intolerance, and psychiatric disturbances, among others. Thus, efforts should be made to limit corticosteroid exposure and to utilize other agents that may have steroid-sparing effects should patients become dependent on steroids for controlling their disease.

Immunomodulators

Immunomodulators, such as azathioprine, 6-mercaptopurine (6-MP), and methotrexate, have potent immunosuppressive effects and are used as maintenance therapy in IBD, particularly for patients who are resistant to or dependent on corticosteroids (Table 41-2).

Azathioprine is the pro-drug of 6-MP, and requires hepatic activation to 6-MP following absorption. 6-MP is then taken up into the cell and further metabolized by various enzymes, including xanthine oxidase and thiopurine methyltransferase (TPMT). Genetic polymorphisms in the TPMT enzyme may predispose patients to toxicity from azathioprine and 6-MP, so patients should have TPMT activity or genotype evaluated prior to initiating therapy.

Oral azathioprine 2 to 3 mg/kg/d or 6-MP 1 to 1.5 mg/kg/d are recommended as maintenance therapy, following steroid-induced remission, in patients with moderate to severe IBD or

in those who have failed corticosteroids or aminosalicylates. Recent data have shown that azathioprine in combination with infliximab is better than either drug alone in biologic or immunomodulator naïve patients with CD. It is now recommended that azathioprine should be initiated concomitantly with a tumor necrosis factor-alfa (TNF-α) antagonist or in patients already on TNF-α antagonists who require additional therapy for their CD. Both azathioprine and 6-MP have delayed effects and often take more than 3 to 4 months to work. Toxicities associated with azathioprine and 6-MP include bone marrow suppression, hepatitis, pancreatitis, rash, fever, arthralgia, lymphoma, and diarrhea. Patients should have complete blood cell counts and liver transaminases monitored regularly during treatment.

Methotrexate is a folate antagonist that is used mostly in CD as a maintenance therapy. Like azathioprine and 6-MP, methotrexate has a slow onset of action and thus is not used as an induction therapy in patients with active disease. Methotrexate has steroid sparing effects in patients with steroid dependence and can be also used in patients who are steroid refractory. Weekly intramuscular or subcutaneous doses of 15 to 25 mg are recommended for patients with CD. Potential toxicities associated with methotrexate therapy include nausea, abdominal pain, diarrhea, bone marrow suppression, pneumonitis, and hepatotoxicity. Complete blood cell counts, liver transaminases, and chest radiography should be assessed at baseline and periodically during methotrexate therapy. Methotrexate is teratogenic and should be avoided in women of child-bearing age. If therapy is deemed necessary, then reliable forms of contraception should be used.

Cyclosporine is an immunosuppressant medication that may be used in patients with severe or fulminant UC who have not responded to 3 to 5 days of intravenous steroids. Intravenous cyclosporine at doses of 2 to 4 mg/kg/d has been shown to reduce the need for acute colectomy in patients who did not respond to intravenous steroids. The success rate of cyclosporine in reducing the need for urgent surgical intervention is increased with the concomitant use of azathioprine or 6-MP but is decreased in the face of systemic symptoms including persistent fevers, elevated CRP, and hypoalbuminemia. Cyclosporine is associated with significant adverse effects including hypertension, seizures, hyperkalemia, nephrotoxicity, and increased susceptibility to infections and should be reserved as a last line resort to avoiding surgical intervention in refractory severe or fulminant disease.

TABLE 41-2	**Immunomodulator and Biologic Therapies Used in the Treatment of IBD**	
Drug	**Brand Name(s)**	**Formulation**
Immunomodulator Therapies		
Azathioprine	Imuran, Azasan	Tablet
6-Mercaptopurine	Purinethol	Tablet
Methotrexate	Trexall	Tablet, injection (IM, SC)
Cyclosporine	Sandimmune, Neoral, Gengraf	Injection (IV), capsule
Biologic Therapies		
Infliximab	Remicade	Injection (IV)
Adalimumab	Humira	Injection (SC)
Certolizumab	Cimzia	Injection (SC)
Golimumab	Simponi	Injection (SC)
Natalizumab	Tysabri	Injection (IV)
Vedolizumab	Entyvio	Injection (IV)
Ustekinumab	Stelara	Injection (IV, SC)

Abbreviations: IM, intramuscular; IV, intravenous; SC, subcutaneous.

Biologic Therapies

Several biologic agents have now been approved for both the treatment of acute, active IBD and maintenance of remission (Table 41-2). The most widely used biologic agents are designed to antagonize the effects of TNF-α and include infliximab, adalimumab, certolizumab, and golimumab. These agents are typically indicated for patients with moderate to severe disease as an alternative to corticosteroids, for patients who are steroid dependent, or those that have failed other therapies. The TNF-α antagonists are the drugs of choice for patients with fistulizing CD. All of the TNF-α antagonists require parenteral administration and are very costly compared to the available oral therapies; however, the advent of biosimilar medications may lower the cost of these agents and improve access to many patients due to price reductions from market competition.

Infliximab is a chimeric antibody that is given intravenously and is indicated in both moderate to severe UC and CD, with specific indications in pediatric and fistulizing CD. Doses of 5 mg/kg intravenously given at 0, 2, and 6 weeks, followed by 5 mg/kg every 8 weeks are typically used. Due to its chimeric structure, antibodies to infliximab may develop over time, which may lead to subsequent loss of efficacy. Adalimumab is a fully humanized antibody to TNF-α that is also approved for moderate to severe CD and UC. Adalimumab is given subcutaneously at dose of 160 mg on day 1, then 80 mg on day 15 of therapy, followed by 40 mg subcutaneously every other week starting on day 29 of therapy. Since it is a humanized molecule, it may be used in patients who develop loss of efficacy to infliximab due to antibody development or as a first-line biologic agent. Certolizumab is a pegylated, humanized, antigen-binding fragment with complementary determining regions derived from a murine source that is used in moderate to severe CD. Certolizumab is given subcutaneously at a dose of 400 mg initially, and then at 2 and 4 weeks followed by 400 mg subcutaneously every 4 weeks if an initial response is achieved. Patients with initial C-reactive protein concentrations more than 10 mg/dL tend to respond better to certolizumab compared to those with concentrations less than 10 mg/dL. Golimumab is a humanized antibody to TNF-α approved for use in moderate to severe UC. Golimumab is administered subcutaneously at a dose of 200 mg initially, 100 mg at 2 weeks, then 100 mg every 4 weeks. As mentioned above, TNF-α antagonists are more effective in combination with azathioprine, although this combination may increase the risk of cancer and opportunistic infections.

Biosimilar medications are medications deemed by the FDA to be "highly similar" to a reference product in terms of both nonclinical (structure and function) and clinical (pharmacokinetics, immunogenicity, safety, and efficacy) parameters. There are currently two FDA-approved biosimilar TNF-α antagonists in the United States: Inflectra—a biosimilar product to infliximab and Amjevita—a biosimilar product to adalimumab. These biosimilar products were not studied in IBD disease states prior to market approval; however, early studies in IBD indicate that they are effective in both CD and UC, and patients have been safely converted from the reference product to the biosimilar product with good results. These medications have the potential to decrease the price of immunologic therapies and increase access to these medications for a large number of patients.

All of the TNF-α antagonists, and their biosimilar counterparts, carry a risk of serious potential adverse effects, particularly predisposition to infections. Prior to initiating therapy with a TNF-α antagonist, patients should be evaluated for latent tuberculosis and hepatitis B. Patients being evaluated for possible TNF-α therapy should not have a current serious infection or sepsis. Heart failure may be precipitated or worsened, so use should be avoided in patients with advanced heart failure. Infliximab may cause infusion-related reactions, such as urticaria, erythema, dizziness, and nausea, which can be managed by slowing the infusion or premedicating with acetaminophen and diphenhydramine. Delayed infusion reactions may also occur, ranging from 3 to 14 days after the injection, and may consist of myalgia, fever, rash, urticaria, and pruritus. Due to their administration as subcutaneous injections, adalimumab, certolizumab, and golimumab carry a lower risk of injection-related adverse effects. Other less common adverse effects of TNF-α antagonists include a lupus-like syndrome, lymphoma, and nerve demyelination.

In addition to the TNF-α antagonists, the integrin inhibitors, natalizumab and vedolizumab, are also approved for use in IBD. Natalizumab is a humanized monoclonal antibody that prevents leukocyte α-4 mediated adhesion, preventing transmigration across endothelial cells. It is approved for the induction and maintenance of remission of moderate to severely active CD in patients who have failed other therapies, including TNF-α antagonists. It is administered intravenously at a dose of 300 mg initially, and then 300 mg intravenously every 4 weeks. Patients who do not respond to natalizumab within 12 weeks of treatment have little chance of experiencing efficacy and should have therapy discontinued. Natalizumab also carries a risk of progressive multifocal leukoencephalopathy and is only available by registering through the manufacturer's prescribing program. Patients should be monitored for any signs of neurologic abnormality while receiving natalizumab. Infusion-related reactions and hepatotoxicity have also been reported.

Vedolizumab also prevents leukocyte adhesion to integrins via the α4 subunit, but is more specific to integrin α4β7, which is localized to the gut. This specificity allows for more targeted therapy and also reduces the risk of progressive multifocal leukoencephalopathy as α4β7 is not expressed at the blood-brain barrier. At this point, there have been no reported cases of vedolizumab-induced PML, which has led to the recommendation to use vedolizumab over natalizumab in patients requiring anti-integrin therapy for either UC or CD. Vedolizumab is administered as a single 300 mg IV infusion at weeks 0, 2, and 6 and then every 8 weeks thereafter. If therapeutic response is not achieved by week 14, treatment should be stopped. Adverse effects are usually mild and include headache, nasopharyngitis, arthralgia, and fatigue. Vedolizumab should not be coadministered with TNF-α antagonists due to the potential for additive immunosuppression.

The anti-interleukin monoclonal antibody, ustekinumab, is indicated in the treatment of moderately to severely active CD in patients who have failed previous immunomodulator and corticosteroid therapies. Ustekinumab is a humanized antibody targeted at the p40 shared subunit of IL-12 and IL-23, two molecules involved in the differentiation and maturation of T-cells. Both interleukins have been linked to the pathogenesis of CD and IL-12 is overexpressed by intestinal lamina propria cells in CD patients. Ustekinumab is administered as an initial weight-based intravenous infusion followed by a 90-mg subcutaneous dose at week 8 and every 8 weeks thereafter. Ustekinumab carries a risk of adverse effects similar to the TNF-α inhibitors including a risk for serious infections, infusion reactions, and the need to rule-out tuberculosis prior to initiation of therapy.

Antibiotics

Given that bacteria may play a role in the pathogenesis of IBD, antibiotics have been observed to be effective IBD treatment. Metronidazole and ciprofloxacin are the two most-studied antimicrobial agents used, and are recommended in patients with UC who develop pouchitis following ileal pouch-anal anastomosis. In patients with CD, metronidazole alone or in combination with ciprofloxacin has the most favorable effects as short-term adjunctive therapy in patients with colonic, perianal, or fistulizing disease. Common adverse effects of metronidazole include nausea, diarrhea, and metallic taste. Long-term use is associated with the development of peripheral neuropathy and should be avoided if possible. Ciprofloxacin may be associated with diarrhea, particularly overgrowth of *Clostridium difficile*, and may also rarely precipitate tendon rupture.

Special Considerations

Patients with active IBD may be at risk for development of acute colonic dilation, also known as toxic megacolon, particularly if medications are used that decrease intestinal motility. Patients with active disease should have drugs such as loperamide, narcotics, and anticholinergic agents discontinued. Patients who receive prolonged courses of corticosteroids may require calcium and vitamin D supplementation for prevention of bone loss and possible use of a bisphosphonate as preventative therapy. Patients who smoke have a higher risk of steroid dependence, so efforts should be made to institute smoking cessation techniques or therapies, particularly in patients with CD. Nicotine replacement therapy, typically with a patch, is a viable adjunctive treatment option in UC, and appears to be most efficacious in ex-smokers. Patients who require long-term immunosuppressive therapies are at increased risk for infection and must remain vigilant about the need for vaccination or prophylactic therapy prior to travel. All immunosuppressed patients should receive annual inactivated influenza vaccine as well as both variants of the pneumococcal vaccine, PCV 13 and PPSV 23, 1 year apart and patients who will require live vaccines, such as varicella zoster, should ideally be vaccinated prior to the initiation of immunosuppressive therapy. Lastly, patients who undergo multiple surgeries for IBD may require long-term parenteral or enteral nutrition, particularly if they develop short bowel syndrome.

CASE Application

1. A 67-year-old man, RJ, presents with complaints of 2 months of 2 to 3 loose bloody stools per day without accompanying fever or weight loss. His gastroenterologist performs a colonoscopy to determine the extent and severity of his suspected IBD. RJ is found to have UC, which is confined to the rectum. Select all of the characteristics that are features of UC but not of CD.

   a. Disease distribution limited to the colon
   b. Inflammation interspersed with healthy tissue
   c. Inflammation affecting only the mucosal layer
   d. Inflammation penetrating below the mucosal layer

2. Which drug formulation of mesalamine is most effective as initial therapy for RJ's UC confined to the rectum?

   a. Suppository
   b. Enema
   c. Tablet
   d. Intravenous injection

3. Three years later, RJ's UC has advanced to moderately severe disease. After a course of steroids, his gastroenterologist wants to start him on azathioprine. Which enzyme should be tested to determine RJ's ability to metabolize azathioprine?

   a. Rasburicase
   b. Dihydrofolate reductase
   c. Thiopurine methyltransferase
   d. Hyaluronidase

4. A 33-year-old African American woman is newly diagnosed with moderate extensive UC. She reports a drug allergy to sulfonamide-containing medications, which manifests as a rash. Which product would be most appropriate as initial therapy for this patient?

   a. Canasa
   b. Colazal
   c. Entocort
   d. Azulfidine

5. Which of the following products is available only as an intravenous solution for injection?

   a. Flagyl
   b. Purinethol
   c. Colazal
   d. Remicade

6. A 56-year-old man, QC, has a history of CD and is maintained in remission with daily oral mesalamine 800 mg daily and oral prednisone 30 mg daily. He is interested in trying weekly subcutaneous injections of methotrexate with a goal of discontinuing his prednisone therapy. Which monitoring parameters should be assessed prior to intiating and periodically during methotrexate therapy? (Please choose all that apply)

   a. Liver transaminases
   b. Chest radiography
   c. Complete blood count
   d. Serum potassium

7. Eight months later, JJ presents to the gastroenterologist's office again. He complains that his symptoms are not controlled on methotrexate therapy. His physician is considering initiating JJ on infliximab. Which of the following conditions is considered a contraindication to receiving a TNF-α antagonist?

   a. Asthma
   b. Migraine headache
   c. Previous myocardial infarction
   d. Sepsis

8. A 49-year-old woman has been receiving maximal doses of Delzicol for treatment of UC, but continues to have daily moderate symptoms including urgency, abdominal pain, and rectal bleeding. Which therapy would be best for treatment of her symptoms at this time?

   a. Trexall
   b. Remicade
   c. Entocort EC
   d. Apriso

9. A 38-year-old female patient with CD is prescribed Humira for treatment of severe symptoms. Which counseling point is best to provide to this patient prior to starting this therapy?

   a. Correct number of tablets to take on a daily basis
   b. The next dose should be given in 8 weeks
   c. Proper injection technique
   d. Monitor for development of diarrhea

10. A 53-year-old man with CD for 25 years is experiencing draining, non-healing fistulas. He is interested in beginning therapy with infliximab. Which of the following are important to discuss with this patient prior to starting infliximab therapy? (Please choose all that apply)

    a. Rule out tuberculosis prior to infliximab therapy
    b. Infliximab may be self-administered subcutaneously
    c. Premedication with acetaminophen and diphenhydramine prevents infusion reactions
    d. Administration of a test dose is required before the initial injection

11. A 27-year-old man presents with an 8-week history of new-onset cramping abdominal pain together with 2 to 3 bloody stools per day. He is diagnosed with left-sided UC. Which one of the following is the most appropriate initial therapy?

    a. Sulfasalazine orally 1 g 4 times per day
    b. Mesalamine enema rectally 4 g every night
    c. Hydrocortisone enema rectally 100 mg every night
    d. 6-Mercaptopurine (6-MP) orally 75 mg/d

12. A 38-year-old male patient is newly diagnosed with mild to moderate CD confined to the ileum and ascending colon. What is the best recommendation for this patient?

    a. Mesalamine enema 1 g PR at bedtime
    b. Prednisone 40 mg daily orally

    c. Certolizumab pegol 400 mg subcutaneously
    d. Budesonide 9 mg daily orally

13. Order the following formulations of mesalamine from least to most area of exposure within the GI tract:

Unordered Options	Ordered Response
Asacol	
Rowasa	
Pentasa	
Canasa	

14. A 42-year-old patient presents to his community pharmacy with a prescription for Entocort. What is the generic drug name for Entocort EC?

    a. Methylprednisolone
    b. Prednisone
    c. Hydrocortisone
    d. Budesonide

15. A patient receiving Tysabri for CD develops mental status changes after 24 weeks of therapy. This may indicate development of which adverse effect of Tysabri?

    a. Progressive multifocal leukoencephalopathy
    b. Central pontine myelinolysis
    c. Cerebrovascular accident
    d. Multi-infarct dementia

16. A 41-year-old woman with UC affecting most of her colon (pancolitis) has been taking balsalazide 6.75 g/d for 2 years and prednisone 40 mg/d for 1 year. When the dose of prednisone is reduced to less than 40 mg, the patient develops fever, abdominal pain, and five or six bloody bowel movements a day. Which modification to this patient's drug regimen is the most appropriate at this time?

    a. Initiate therapy with methotrexate 25 mg intramuscularly once weekly.
    b. Initiate infliximab 5 mg/kg intravenous infusion.
    c. Change balsalazide to sulfasalazine orally 6 g/d.
    d. Add mesalamine suppository 1000 mg rectally once daily.

17. A 34-year-old woman presents to the emergency department with a 2-day history of cramping abdominal pain, fever, fatigue, and 10 to 12 bloody stools a day. She has had CD for 5 years; typically, she is maintained on mesalamine (Pentasa) 250 mg 4 capsules two times/day. On admission, her vital signs include temperature 101°F, heart rate 110 beats/min, respiratory rate 18 breaths/min, and blood pressure 118/68 mm Hg. Which therapeutic choice is best?

    a. Administer cyclosporine 4 mg/h by continuous infusion.
    b. Increase the dose of mesalamine (Pentasa) to 4 g/d.

c. Obtain a surgery consult for immediate colectomy.

d. Administer hydrocortisone 100 mg intravenously every 8 hours.

18. A 58-year-old male patient is receiving long-term therapy with metronidazole for the prevention of pouchitis following ileal pouch-anal anastomosis. This patient should be monitored for the development of which adverse effect?

a. Anemia

b. Peripheral neuropathy

c. Hepatitis

d. Pulmonary fibrosis

19. A 56-year-old woman with a history of UC presents to the emergency department with 1 day of abdominal pain, which she rates as 10 out of 10. The pain worsens when she eats and improves slightly when she lies down. She denies alcohol, tobacco, and illicit drug use. Her laboratory findings include a serum lipase level of 3,794 U/L (normal 0-160 U/L). She states that she started taking a new medication to control her UC but cannot recall the name of it. Which drug is most likely causing this adverse effect?

a. Methotrexate

b. Adalimumab

c. Azathioprine

d. Natalizumab

20. A 26-year-old woman has been able to maintain remission of her UC for the past year with the use of oral mesalamine, oral azathioprine, and intravenous infliximab therapy. This patient is not up to date with her vaccines. Which of the following vaccines are recommended for this patient? (Please choose all that apply.)

a. Injectable influenza vaccine

b. Human papilloma virus (HPV)

c. Measles, mumps, rubella (MMR)

d. Tetanus, diphtheria, pertussis (Tdap)

21. A 38-year-old man with moderate to severe CD has been experiencing numerous relapses on his current medication regimen. He is taking azathioprine and infliximab for maintenance therapy. What changes would be best to make to his maintenance regimen?

a. Stop infliximab and initiate intravenous cyclosporine

b. Stop infliximab and azathioprine and initiate dexamethasone

c. Stop infliximab and azathioprine and initiate vedolizumab

d. Continue azathioprine and infliximab and begin natalizumab

22. A 58-year-old woman, AK, with a history of severe UC presents to the emergency department with profuse, bloody diarrhea. She is hypotensive and tachycardic on admission, and is initiated on intravenous fluids. The decision is made to start the patient on glucocorticoid therapy. Rank the following steroids in order of glucocorticoid potency from least potent (1) to most potent (4).

Unordered Options	Ordered Response
Prednisone	
Dexamethasone	
Hydrocortisone	
Methylprednisolone	

23. AK is initiated on intravenous methylprednisolone for her UC exacerbation; however, she continues to decompensate and the surgery team is considering colectomy. Which medication can you recommend to potentially eliminate the need for surgical intervention?

a. Intraveous natalizumab

b. Oral methotrexate

c. Intraveous cyclosporine

d. Intraveous infliximab

TAKEAWAY POINTS »

- IBD consists of both UC and CD and is considered an inflammatory disorder with no known definitive cause.
- Differences exist between UC and CD in regards to disease location, depth and pattern of inflammation, and presenting signs and symptoms.
- Patients may also manifest extraintestinal symptoms of IBD, such as arthritis.
- Choice of drug therapy for active IBD should be based on the subtype of IBD, the disease location and severity, and considerations of potential contraindications to therapy.

- Aminosalicylates are generally first-line agents for UC and CD and should be chosen based on the formulation that will deliver the active component, mesalamine, to the site of inflammation.
- Topical mesalamine products are preferred for patients with distal disease.
- Corticosteroids are used for short term in the setting of active IBD and should not be used as maintenance therapy.
- Immunomodulators, such as azathioprine and methotrexate, are used for long-term maintenance

therapy, particularly for patients who are steroid dependent.

- Biologic agents that antagonize TNF-α can be used as first-line therapies for moderate to severe IBD and are the drugs of choice for fistulizing CD.
- TNF-α antagonist use predisposes patients to the development of serious infections.

- Other biologic agents targeting integrin and IL-12 and IL-23 are available for use in patients who fail to respond to TNF-α antagonist therapy.
- Antibiotics are considered adjunctive therapies in patients with fistulizing or perianal CD.

BIBLIOGRAPHY

Farraye FA, Melmed GY, Lichtenstein GR. ACG Clinical Guideline: preventive care in inflammatory bowel disease. *Am J Gastroenterol.* 2017. doi: 10.1038/ajg.2016.53.

Greenley RN, Junz JH, Walter J, Hommel KA. Practical strategies for enhancing adherence to treatment regimen in inflammatory bowel disease. *Inflamm Bowel Dis.* 2013;19:1534-1545. doi: 10.1097/MIB.0b013e3182813482.

Hemstreet BA. Inflammatory bowel disease. In: DiPiro JT, Talbert RL, Yee GC, Matzke GR, Wells BG, Posey L, eds. *Pharmacotherapy: A Pathophysiologic Approach.* 10th ed. New York, NY: McGraw-Hill; 2017:chap 34. http://accesspharmacy.mhmedical.com/content.aspx?bookid=1861&sectionid=146059124. Accessed January 28, 2017.

Kornbluth A, Sachar DB. Ulcerative colitis practice guidelines in adults: American College of Gastroenterology, Practice Parameters Committee. *Am J Gastroenterol.* 2010;105:501-523.

Lichtenstein GR, Hanauer SB, Sandborn WJ; The Practice Parameters Committee of the American College of Gastroenterology. Management of Crohn's disease in adults. *Am J Gastroenterol.* 2009;104:465-483.

Nielsen OH, Ainsworth MA. Tumor necrosis factor inhibitors for inflammatory bowel disease. *N Engl J Med.* 2013;369:754-762. doi: 10.1056/NEJMct1209614.

Pham C, Efros C, Berardi RR. Cyclosporine for severe ulcerative colitis. *Ann Pharmacother.* 2006;40:96-101.

Podolsky DK. Inflammatory bowel disease. *N Engl J Med.* 2002;347:417-429.

Regueiro M, Loftus EV, Steinhart AH, Cohen RD. Clinical guidelines for the medical management of left-sided ulcerative colitis and ulcerative proctitis: summary statement. *Inflamm Bowel Dis.* 2006;12:972-978.

Shahidi N, Bressler B, Panaccione R. The role of vedolizumab in patients with moderate-to-severe Crohn's disease and ulcerative colitis. *Ther Adv Gastroenterol.* 2016;9:330-338.

Simon EG, Ghosh S, Iacucci M, et al. Ustekinumab for the treatment of Crohn's disease: can it find its niche? *Ther Adv Gastroenterol.* 2016;9:26-36.

Terdiman JP, Gruss CB, Heidelbaugh JJ, et al. American Gastroenterological Association Institute Guideline of the use of thiopurines, methtrexate, and anti-TNA-a biologic drugs for the induction and maintenance of remission in inflammatory Crohn's disease. *Gastroenterology.* 2013;145:1459-1463.

KEY ABBREVIATIONS

5-ASA = 5-aminosalicylate
6-MP = 6-mercaptopurine
CD = Crohn disease
GI = gastrointestinal

IBD = inflammatory bowel disease
TNF-α = tumor necrosis factor-alfa
TPMT = thiopurine methyltransferase
UC = ulcerative colitis

Nausea and Vomiting

Kelly K. Nystrom

FOUNDATION OVERVIEW

Nausea and vomiting is caused by numerous factors, with two of the most common factors being chemotherapy and surgery. Nausea and vomiting can lead to serious medical complications such as dehydration, electrolyte imbalances, and esophageal tears. It is easier to prevent nausea and vomiting than to treat it once it has started. Although significant progress has been made in the management of nausea and vomiting, these side effects are some of the most worrisome and undesirable effects reported by patients receiving chemotherapy or a surgical procedure.

The etiology of nausea and vomiting is complex. The chemoreceptor trigger zone (CTZ), located outside of the blood-brain barrier, is activated by chemotherapy and other irritants. The CTZ is triggered by various neurotransmitters including dopamine, serotonin, histamine, and neurokinin-1 (substance P), which then stimulates the vomiting center (Figure 42-1). In addition to the CTZ, the gastrointestinal (GI) tract releases serotonin in response to stimulants such as chemotherapy and anesthesia, which can activate the vomiting center, also causing nausea and vomiting. Current antiemetic medications block the neurotransmitter receptors with the intent to mitigate nausea and vomiting.

There are several risk factors that increase the possibility of experiencing chemotherapy-induced nausea and vomiting (CINV) and postoperative nausea and vomiting (PONV). Things that increase the risk of both despite adequate antiemetic treatment are female gender, age less than 50, a history of motion sickness or nausea with pregnancy, and a history CINV or PONV. In terms of CINV, the emetic potential of the chemotherapy agent or agents is the most important factor. Agents are classified into high, moderate, low, or minimal risk for causing CINV (Table 42-1). Dose of the agent can also affect risk (the higher the dose, the higher the risk of CINV). Bolus infusions also tend to have higher risk of CINV than extended infusions. For PONV, certain anesthesia agents, how the anesthesia is delivered and non-smokers tend to have a higher incidence of PONV.

CHEMOTHERAPY-INDUCED NAUSEA AND VOMITING

There are several types of CINV: acute, delayed, anticipatory, breakthrough, and refractory. Acute CINV is defined as nausea and vomiting that occurs within the first 24 hours following the administration of chemotherapy. Delayed CINV develops greater than 24 hours after chemotherapy is administered and can be seen up to 7 days following chemotherapy. Chemotherapeutic agents that commonly cause delayed CINV include cisplatin, carboplatin, cyclophosphamide, and doxorubicin or epirubicin in combination with cyclophosphamide. Anticipatory CINV occurs after a negative experience with chemotherapy, and thus can only occur if chemotherapy has been previously received. The incidence of this type of nausea or vomiting ranges from 10% to 45%. Breakthrough CINV occurs when patients have at least one episode of nausea and/or vomiting that may require antiemetic treatment despite preventative antiemetic premedication. Refractory CINV occurs when premedications and breakthrough therapy fail to prevent or control CINV.

Antiemetics

Serotonin (5-HT3) Receptor Antagonists

Serotonin is a common neurotransmitter involved in CINV. The serotonin (5-HT3) receptor antagonists block serotonin in the GI tract and the CTZ to prevent CINV. The 5-HT3 receptor antagonists (Table 42-2) are effective in the prevention of acute CINV, but have a limited role in delayed CINV (with the exception of palonosetron). Palonosetron is superior to other 5-HT3 receptor antagonists in the prevention of *delayed CINV* because of a longer half-life and higher receptor affinity. It is the only one in the class FDA-approved for the prevention of both acute and delayed CINV in patients receiving moderately emetic chemotherapy (MEC) in addition to the prevention of acute CINV in patients receiving highly emetic chemotherapy (HEC). When a substance P neurokinin-1 (NK-1) receptor antagonist is not used with MEC, there is lack of consensus whether palonosetron is the preferred 5HT-3 receptor antagonist. It is a reasonable option when an NK-1 receptor inhibitor is not used, but until more studies are completed, any of the 5-HT3 receptor antagonists may be used.

Choice of agent should be based on availability and cost. The oral route is as effective as the intravenous route. Therefore, the oral route is preferred for prevention of CINV because of ease of administration and decreased cost. Another option available is a long-acting granisetron available as an injection or topical granisetron patch that lasts up to 7 days. The patch should be applied 24 to 48 hours prior to chemotherapy

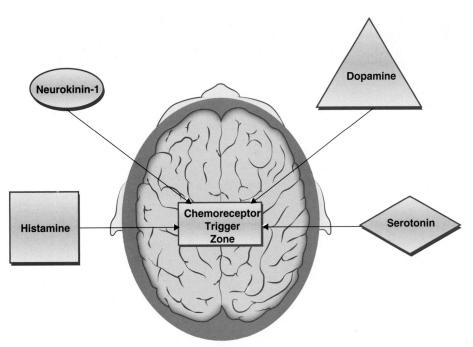

FIGURE 42-1 Chemoreceptor trigger zone and activating neurotransmitters with the vomiting center.

TABLE 42-1	Emetic Risk of Commonly Administered Chemotherapy Agents		
Emetic Risk	Incidence Without Antiemetics	Intravenous Agent	Oral Agent
High	>90%	Cisplatin	
High	>90%	Cyclophosphamide (>1500 mg/m²)	
High	>90%	Cyclophosphamide and epirubicin or doxorubicin combination	
High	>90%	Dacarbazine	
Moderate	30%-90%	Alemtuzumab	Bosutinib
Moderate	30%-90%	Bendamustine	Ceritinib
Moderate	30%-90%	Carboplatin	Crizotinib
Moderate	30%-90%	Cytarabine (>200 mg/m²)	Imatinib
Moderate	30%-90%	Doxorubicin (<60 mg/m²)	
Moderate	30%-90%	Irinotecan	
Moderate	30%-90%	Oxaliplatin	
Low	10%-30%	Belinostat	Afatinib
Low	10%-30%	Cabazitaxel	Capecitabine
Low	10%-30%	Carfilzomib	Everolimus
Low	10%-30%	Docetaxel	Ibrutinib
Low	10%-30%	Etoposide	Lenalidomide
Low	10%-30%	Fluorouracil	Nilotinib
Low	10%-30%	Paclitaxel	Pazopanib
Minimal	<10%	Bevacizumab	Erlotinib
Minimal	<10%	Bortezomib	Gefitinib
Minimal	<10%	Ipilimumab	Pomalidomide
Minimal	<10%	Pembrolizumab	Sorafenib
Minimal	<10%	Rituximab	Vemurafenib
Minimal	<10 %	Pertuzumab	
Minimal	<10%	Trastuzumab	

TABLE 42-2	Antiemetics Used for Prevention of Chemotherapy-Induced Nausea and Vomiting			
Antiemetic	**Trade Name**	**Dose**	**Route**	**Frequency**
5-HT3 Receptor Antagonists				
Ondansetron	Zofran	8-16 mg	IV	30-60 min before chemotherapy
		0.15 mg/kg	IV	Maximum IV dose of 16 mg
		16-24 mg	po	
Granisetron	Kytril	2 mg	po	30-60 min before chemotherapy
		1 mg bid	po	
	Sustol	1 mg	IV	Do not repeat within 7 d
		10 mg	SQ	
	Sancuso	Delivers 3.1 mg/24 h	Topical	24-48 h before chemotherapy
				Can be used for up to 7 d
Dolasetron	Anzemet	100 mg	po	30-60 min before chemotherapy
Palonosetron	Aloxi	0.25 mg	IV	30 min before chemotherapy
Neurokinin-1 Receptor Antagonists				
Aprepitant	Emend	125 mg	po	30-60 min before chemotherapy
		80 mg	po	On days 2 and 3
Fosaprepitant dimeglumine	Emend	150 mg	IV	30 min before chemotherapy (with no additional aprepitant)
Rolapitant	Varubi	180 mg	po	60-120 min before chemotherapy
Combination 5-HT3 Receptor Antagonist/Neurokinin-1 Receptor Antagonist				
Netupitant-Palonosetron	Akynzeo	300 mg-0.5 mg	po	60 min before chemotherapy
Corticosteroid				
Dexamethasone	Decadron	12-20 mg	IV/po	30-60 min before chemotherapy
		12 mg	IV/po	30-60 min before chemotherapy with all NK-1 receptor antagonists except rolapitant

Abbreviations: IV, intravenous; po, oral; SQ, subcutaneous.

and can remain on the skin for up to 7 days; the injection should be given shortly prior to chemotherapy. Common toxicities for the 5-HT3 receptor antagonists include headache, constipation, and mild dizziness. An infrequent, but more serious, toxicity is the ability of the 5-HT3 receptor antagonists to cause QT prolongation. The FDA recommended that the 32 mg IV dose of ondansetron no longer be used because of QT prolongation and has recommended a maximum of 16 mg per dose. QT prolongation in cancer patients has been reported infrequently for those patients receiving palonosetron, so this may be a safer alternative for patients who already have a prolonged QT interval, those with cardiac disease or those who are taking other medications that increase the risk of QT prolongation

Neurokinin-1 Receptor Antagonists

The NK-1 receptor antagonists are approved to prevent CINV with HEC and certain MEC regimens (in conjunction with a 5-HT3 receptor antagonist and dexamethasone). Substance P exerts its effect on the NK-1 receptors causing nausea and vomiting, thus the NK-1 receptor antagonists exert their effect by blocking substance P and preventing nausea and vomiting (Figure 42-1). Aprepitant and fosaprepitant dimeglumine (intravenous prodrug of aprepitant) were the first NK-1 receptor antagonists approved (Table 42-2). All agents are approved as a one-time dose given before chemotherapy

except aprepitant (Tables 42-2 and 42-3). Common side effects include headache, anorexia, abdominal pain, hiccups, and mild transaminase elevations. Aprepitant and fosaprepitant are substrates of CYP3A4, moderate inhibitors of CYP3A4, and inducers of CYP2C9. Therefore, drug interactions include oral contraceptives, warfarin, dexamethasone, and other 3A4 and 2C9 medications. This is why the dexamethasone dose should be decreased by 50% when given with any NK-1 receptor antagonist except rolapitant.

Rolapitant is a newer oral NK-1 receptor antagonist and is approved on day 1 of chemotherapy only (Tables 42-2 and 42-3). Rolapitant is metabolized by CYP3A4, but unlike aprepitant and fosaprepitant, it does not inhibit or induce CYP3A4, so the dose of dexamethasone does not need to be adjusted. It is an inducer of CYP2C9, so there are still drug interactions possible with drugs like digoxin and warfarin. Side effects are similar to other NK-1 receptor antagonists.

Combination 5-HT3 Receptor Antagonist/ Neurokinin-1 Receptor Antagonist

Netupitant and palonosetron, also referred to as NEPA, is the only combination product on the market (Tables 42-2 and 42-3). It is approved for HEC and MEC regimens in combination with dexamethasone. Like aprepitant and fosaprepitant, it is a moderate inhibitor of CYP3A4 so a reduced dose of dexamethasone should be used. Side effects are similar to

TABLE 42-3 Dexamethasone Dosing with NK-1 Receptor Antagonists for Prevention of Acute and Delayed Nausea and Vomiting

NK-1 Receptor Antagonist	Dexamethasone Dosing
Aprepitant 125 mg po on day 1, then aprepitant 80 mg po daily on days 2 and 3	12 mg day 1 then 8 mg daily days 2 to 4
Fosaprepitant 150 mg IV on day 1	12 mg day 1; 8 mg daily day 2, then 8 mg bid days 3-4
Netupitant 300 mg/palonosetron (NEPA) 0.5 mg po on day 1	12 mg day 1 then 8 mg daily days 2 to 4
Rolapitant 180 mg po on day 1	20 mg day 1 then 8 mg bid days 2 to 4

those seen with the 5-HT3 and NK-1 receptor antagonists, with constipation and headache being the most commonly reported adverse effects.

Corticosteroids

Corticosteroids are used as monotherapy for the prevention of CINV with low-risk emetic agents. Dexamethasone is the most commonly used corticosteroid and is often used in conjunction with 5-HT3 receptor antagonists with or without aprepitant for the prevention of acute and delayed CINV with HEC or MEC. Oral and IV routes are considered equivalent. Since the use of corticosteroids for CINV is short-term, the common toxicities are limited to GI discomfort, insomnia, fluid retention, increased appetite, acne, and increased blood sugars.

Dopamine Receptor Antagonists

Dopamine is a neurotransmitter affecting the CTZ resulting in CINV (Figure 42-1). Dopamine receptor antagonists include the phenothiazines (prochlorperazine, promethazine), the butyrophenones (droperidol, haloperidol), and metoclopramide (see Table 42-4). These agents are used for breakthrough nausea and vomiting. Toxicities include sedation and extrapyramidal side effects. A black box warning has been added to the package insert for metoclopramide warning of tardive dyskinesia with high doses or long-term use (>3 months). These dyskinesias may continue after the metoclopramide is discontinued.

Miscellaneous

Cannabinoids produce their antiemetic activities through effects on the central nervous system and GI tract, including activity at the cannabinoid receptor (CB1) (Table 42-4). The cannabinoid, dronabinol, is a Schedule III controlled substance that is helpful for patients with refractory nausea and vomiting (Table 42-4). Nabilone is also an option in this class, but it is classified as a Schedule II controlled substance, which may make it harder to use. Side effects include sedation, dysphoria, dizziness, and dry mouth; elderly patients may be more sensitive to these side effects. These agents may also increase appetite, which may be beneficial in patients with refractory nausea and vomiting resulting in weight loss.

Olanzapine is an atypical antipsychotic that has shown efficacy in the management of CINV by blocking dopamine, serotonin and histamine receptors. It can be used both before chemotherapy and as an option for breakthrough or refractory

TABLE 42-4 Select Antiemetics Used for Breakthrough Chemotherapy-Induced Nausea and Vomiting

Drug	Trade Name	Dose	Route	Frequency	Special Notes
Dopamine Antagonists					
Droperidol	Inapsine	0.625-1.25 mg	IV	Every 4-6 h prn	Black box warning for risk of QT prolongation
Haloperidol	Haldol	1-5 mg	IV/IM/po	Every 4-6 h prn	
Metoclopramide	Reglan	10-20 mg	IV/po	Every 4-6 h prn	Black box warning for permanent EPSE
Prochlorperazine	Compazine	5-10 mg / 25 mg	IV/IM/po / PR	Every 4-6 h prn / Every 12 h prn	
Promethazine	Phenergan	12.5-25 mg	IV/deep IM/po/PR	Every 4-6 h prn	Concentrated solution may cause tissue damage if extravasated; dilute in 10 mL normal saline before administration
Benzodiazepines					
Lorazepam	Ativan	0.5-2 mg	IV/IM/po/SL	Every 4-6 h prn	Works well for anticipatory CINV
Miscellaneous					
Dronabinol	Marinol	5-10 mg	po	Every 3-6 h prn	Works well to increase appetite; use with caution in elderly as may see increased side effects; schedule III medication
Nabilone	Cesamet	1-2 mg	po	bid prn	Same issues as dronabinol; schedule II medication
Olanzapine	Zyprexa	2.5-5 mg	po	bid prn	May be used for acute and refractory, although it is not FDA-approved for this indication
Scopolamine	Transderm Scop	1.5 mg	Transdermal	q72hrs	Effect is seen within 4 h

Abbreviations: CINV, chemotherapy-induced nausea and vomiting; EPSE, extrapyramidal side effects; IM, intramuscular; IV, intravenous; po, oral.

CINV (Tables 42-3 and 42-4). The manufacturer recommends avoiding use of olanzapine concurrently with metoclopramide or haloperidol to avoid excessive dopamine blockade. The most common side effects are drowsiness, sleep disturbances, and akathisia.

Scopolamine transdermal patch is a nice option for refractory CINV because of the route of administration (Table 42-4). The antiemetic effect will be seen within 4 hours of application and may last up to 72 hours. Because of its anticholinergic effects, dry mouth is the most common adverse effect. Patients may also see urinary retention, constipation, and drowsiness with this medication.

Prevention of Acute Chemotherapy-Induced Nausea and Vomiting

Guidelines exist from several organizations on the treatment and prevention of CINV. Commonly used guidelines are the Multinational Association of Supportive Care in Cancer (MASCC)/European Society of Medical Oncology (ESMO) guidelines. The American Society of Clinical Oncology (ASCO) guidelines and the National Comprehensive Cancer Network (NCCN) guidelines are also commonly used. NCCN guidelines can be found at their website (www.nccn.org). For HEC regimens or for patients with additional risk factors receiving MEC regimens, the recommendation is to give a 5-HT3 receptor antagonist, dexamethasone and an NK-1 receptor antagonist prior to the chemotherapy (Table 42-3). Certain MEC agents such as carboplatin, doxorubicin and cyclophosphamide can cause delayed nausea and vomiting, and these patients may be appropriate to receive an NK-1 receptor antagonist as well. An agent for breakthrough nausea and vomiting, with a different mechanism of action than the drug(s) prescribed for prophylaxis of acute CINV, should be prescribed for use on an as needed basis (Table 42-4).

For MEC, a 5-HT3 receptor antagonist with dexamethasone should be used (Table 42-3). There is lack of consensus whether palonosetron is the preferred 5HT-3 receptor antagonist, but it is a reasonable option when an NK-1 receptor antagonist is not used. Until more studies are completed though, any of the 5-HT3 receptor antagonists may be used. An agent for breakthrough nausea and vomiting, with a different mechanism of action than the drug(s) prescribed for prophylaxis of CINV, should be prescribed for use on an as needed basis.

For low-emetic risk agents, the recommendation is a single-agent antiemetic, such as dexamethasone or a dopamine receptor antagonist. The medication should be administered 30 to 60 minutes prior to chemotherapy. An agent for breakthrough nausea and vomiting, with a different mechanism of action than the drug prescribed for prophylaxis of CINV, should be prescribed for use on an as needed basis. For minimal risk agents, scheduled antiemetics should be avoided, and antiemetics should only be used on an as needed basis.

The prevention of acute CINV for multi-day chemotherapy regimens is similar to the recommendations above. Thus, selected antiemetics should be given every day prior to chemotherapy. For a 3-day regimen, the current recommendation is to give a 5-HT3 receptor antagonist and dexamethasone with or without aprepitant on each day of chemotherapy unless palonosetron or a long-acting granisetron is used, and then the 5-HT3 receptor antagonist would not be repeated on days 2 and 3. If an NK-1 receptor antagonist other than aprepitant is used, then administration is needed on day 1 only as well. Dexamethasone should be continued for 2 to 3 days after the completion of chemotherapy.

Even with adequate prevention for CINV, patients may experience breakthrough CINV within the first 24 hours after chemotherapy. There are agents available for treatment of breakthrough CINV and a variety of factors should be considered when choosing an agent (Table 42-4). When choosing an agent, it is important to remember to use an agent with a different mechanism of action than was prescribed for prevention of acute CINV. In order to get the breakthrough CINV controlled, it may be helpful to schedule the breakthrough antiemetic around the clock until the breakthrough CINV subsides.

Prevention of Delayed Chemotherapy-Induced Nausea and Vomiting

For HEC and for MEC regimens that can cause delayed CINV, if aprepitant 125 mg orally was given on day 1 of chemotherapy, then aprepitant 80 mg orally daily should be continued on days 2 and 3. No further aprepitant is needed if a different NK-1 receptor antagonist was given on day 1. Dexamethasone should also be continued for 2 to 3 days after chemotherapy to prevent delayed CINV and the dose depends on the NK-1 receptor antagonist used (Tables 42-2 and 42-3).

For MEC, when an NK-1 receptor antagonist is used, there is lack of consensus whether palonosetron is the preferred 5HT-3 receptor antagonist. It is a reasonable option when an NK-1 receptor antagonist is not used, but until more studies are completed, any of the 5-HT3 receptor antagonists may be used. Dexamethasone should also be continued for 2 to 3 days after chemotherapy to prevent delayed CINV and the dose depends on which NK-1 receptor antagonist is used (Table 42-3). If an NK-1 receptor antagonist is not used, then dexamethasone 8 mg po bid should be used for 2 to 3 days after chemotherapy. Antiemetic therapy for the prevention of delayed CINV is not well established for multi-day regimens. For a 3-day regimen, the current recommendation is to give a 5-HT3 receptor antagonist and dexamethasone with or without aprepitant on each day of chemotherapy unless palonosetron or long-acting granisetron is used, and then the 5-HT3 receptor antagonist would not be repeated on days 2 and 3. If an NK-1 receptor antagonist other than aprepitant is used, then administration is needed on day 1 only. Dexamethasone should be continued for 2 to 3 days after the completion of chemotherapy.

Treatment of Delayed Chemotherapy-Induced Nausea and Vomiting

Treatment includes the same breakthrough medications used in the treatment of acute CINV, keeping in mind that it is much harder to treat delayed CINV than acute CINV (Table 42-4).

Anticipatory Nausea and Vomiting

Anticipatory nausea is more common than anticipatory vomiting, but both are conditioned responses, so they occur only after a poor experience with chemotherapy. Benzodiazepines can help control this type of nausea and vomiting. Lorazepam is the most commonly used benzodiazepine for this purpose, and is usually given in combination with other antiemetics for prevention of anticipatory CINV (Table 42-4). Common side effects include sedation, dizziness, and amnesia.

POSTOPERATIVE NAUSEA AND VOMITING

PONV can occur following surgery and anesthesia. The most recent consensus guidelines for the management of PONV were published in 2014. Patients at increased risk of PONV include female sex, nonsmokers, history of PONV or motion sickness, and postoperative opioid use. Patients with one risk factor have a risk of PONV of 20%, and each additional risk factor increases the risk of PONV by 20%. Risk is further stratified into low (0-1 risk factors), medium (2 risk factors) or high (≥3 risk factors). Additional risk factors for PONV include the type of anesthetic used (volatile anesthetics and nitrous oxide), the duration of surgery (the longer the surgery, the higher the risk), patient age (<50 years old) and the type of surgery (cholecystectomy, laparoscopic, gynecological).

Prevention of Postoperative Nausea and Vomiting

Strategies used to decrease the risk of PONV include avoiding select anesthetics, minimizing intraoperative and postoperative opioids, use of regional anesthetics, use of propofol for induction and maintenance of anesthesia and adequate hydration. Patients with low risk of PONV will not benefit from prophylaxis and should not receive this treatment unless they are at risk of medical adverse effects from vomiting including patients with wired jaws and increased intracranial pressure. Patients with moderate to high risk of PONV should receive prophylactic antiemetic therapy (Table 42-5). For patients with moderate risk, prophylaxis with one or two agents is recommended; for patients with high risk, combination prophylaxis with two or more agents from different classes is recommended. Gabapentin and midazolam have been shown to be effective in the prevention of PONV, and are an option if adverse effects or allergies limit the use of standard antiemetics.

Treatment of Postoperative Nausea and Vomiting

When a 5-HT3 receptor antagonist is used for prophylaxis and PONV is experienced within 6 hours of initial administration, then a drug with a different mechanism of action should be used and the 5-HT3 receptor antagonist dose should not be

TABLE 42-5	Antiemetics Used for Prevention of Postoperative Nausea and Vomiting			
Antiemetic	**Trade Name**	**Dose**	**Route**	**Frequency**
5-HT3 Receptor Antagonists				
Granisetron	Kytril	0.35-3 mg	IV	End of surgery
Ondansetron	Zofran	4 mg	IV	End of surgery
		8 mg	ODT	End of surgery
Palonosetron	Aloxi	0.075 mg	IV	At induction
Corticosteroid				
Dexamethasone	Decadron	4-5 mg	IV	At induction
Neurokinin-1 Receptor Antagonist				
Aprepitant	Emend	40 mg	po	Within 3 h of induction
Dopamine Antagonists				
Droperidol*	Inapsine	0.625-1.25 mg	IV	End of surgery
Haloperidol*	Haldol	0.5-2 mg	IV/IM	Not specified
Metoclopramide	Reglan	10 mg	IV/IM	End of surgery
Promethazine	Phenergan	6.25-12.5 mg	IV	At induction
Antihistamines				
Hydroxyzine	Vistaril	25-50 mg	IM	After induction
Miscellaneous				
Scopolamine transdermal patch	Trans Scop	1.5 mg patch	Topical	Applied prior evening or 2-4 h before surgery

Abbreviations: IV, intravenous; ODT, oral disintegrating tablet; po, oral.

*QT prolongation warnings.

repeated. In this situation, if a patient is still in post-anesthesia care, propofol 20 mg as needed, may be used for PONV.

Propofol may also be needed if initial triple antiemetic therapy fails. When PONV occurs more than 6 hours after the initial treatment was given, any of these drugs can be used again for treatment of PONV.

CASE Application

Questions 1 to 6 pertain to the following case.

MR is a 42-year-old woman diagnosed with stage 2 breast cancer. Past medical history is significant for heavy alcohol use. She is single and has no children. She presents to clinic today to begin treatment with doxorubicin and cyclophosphamide.

1. Which of the following are risk factors MR has for developing nausea and vomiting? Select all that apply.
   a. Heavy alcohol use
   b. Female gender
   c. Age
   d. No children

2. Select which antiemetic combination will give MR optimal prevention of acute and delayed CINV?
   a. Aprepitant, prochlorperazine, and dexamethasone
   b. Fosaprepitant, dolasetron, and prochlorperazine
   c. Netupitant/palonosetron and haloperidol
   d. Rolapitant, palonosetron, and dexamethasone

3. You note that MR is appropriately treated for acute CINV, but not delayed CINV. Her day 1 regimen includes ondansetron, dexamethasone, and fosaprepitant 150 mg IV prior to chemotherapy. What is the best regimen to prevent delayed CINV for MR?
   a. Dexamethasone 8 mg po daily on days 2 through 4
   b. Dexamethasone 8 mg po daily on day 2 and 8 mg bid on days 3 and 4
   c. Ondansetron 8 mg po bid and dexamethasone 8 mg po daily on day 2 and 8 mg bid on days 3 and 4
   d. No treatment is needed as MR is not at risk for delayed nausea and vomiting

4. MR tolerated cycle 2 well, but had significant nausea and vomiting with cycle 3 requiring hospitalization. When MR arrives to the clinic for cycle 4, she immediately feels nauseous. This is an example of what kind of CINV?
   a. Acute
   b. Anticipatory
   c. Breakthrough
   d. Delayed

5. What is the best treatment for the type of CINV that MR is experiencing?
   a. Dexamethasone
   b. Dronabinol
   c. Lorazepam
   d. Palonosetron

6. MR is ready to go home from the clinic and would like a prescription for something in case she gets sick at home. What would be the most appropriate antiemetic for MR?
   a. Aprepitant
   b. Droperidol
   c. Ondansetron
   d. Prochlorperazine

7. Which of the following statements is correct concerning delayed CINV?
   a. Is easier to prevent than acute nausea and vomiting
   b. Occurs ≥24 hours following drug administration
   c. Occurs more commonly with etoposide and docetaxel
   d. No 5-HT3 receptor antagonist has been shown to be more effective in the prevention of delayed CINV

8. Which neurotransmitter(s) are involved in CINV? Select all that apply.
   a. Dopamine
   b. Neurokinin-1
   c. Norepinephrine
   d. Serotonin

Questions 9 and 10 pertain to the following case.

9. MB is a 42-year-old woman undergoing a laparoscopic cholecystectomy. She has a history of PONV and motion sickness and denies alcohol or tobacco use. Which drug(s) should be administered at induction or at the end of surgery for the prevention of PONV? Select all that apply.
   a. Dexamethasone
   b. Ondansetron
   c. Aprepitant
   d. Scopolamine

10. You receive a call from the physician who cannot remember the correct dose of aprepitant for the prevention of PONV and when it should be administered. What is your response?
    a. 40 mg orally within 3 hours of induction
    b. 80 mg orally within 3 hours of induction
    c. 40 mg IV at the end of surgery
    d. 150 mg IV at the end of surgery

11. RL is a 72-year-old man being treated for non-small cell lung cancer. He is scheduled to receive carboplatin and etoposide today. You receive the following antiemetic orders: ondansetron 32 mg IV and dexamethasone 12 mg IV 30 minutes before chemotherapy. What is your assessment of the regimen for prophylaxis of acute CINV? Select all that apply.
    a. Aprepitant 125 mg IV prior to chemotherapy should be added to the regimen.

b. Ondansetron should be decreased to 16 mg po prior to chemotherapy.

c. Rolapitant 180 mg po should be added to the regimen prior to chemotherapy and the dexamethasone dose should be increased to 20 mg po prior to chemotherapy.

d. Ondansetron must be changed to palonosetron and the dexamethasone dose should be increased to 20 mg.

12. Which statement concerning 5-HT3 receptor antagonist therapy for CINV is correct?

a. Dolasetron has similar efficacy to ondansetron when used at equipotent doses.

b. Granisetron is the only 5-HT3 receptor antagonist approved for prevention of delayed CINV with HEC.

c. Palonosetron is superior to prochlorperazine for the treatment of breakthrough CINV.

d. The IV route of administration of ondansetron is superior to oral administration.

Questions 13 and 14 pertain to the following case.

RN is a 64-year-old man who will be coming to clinic to receive a 3-day chemotherapy regimen that includes cisplatin on all 3 days. He has no history of alcohol use and is otherwise healthy.

13. The oncologist contacts you and asks for your antiemetic regimen recommendations to prevent acute and delayed CINV for RN. Which regimen(s) is/are appropriate? Select all that apply.

a. Dolasetron 100 mg po prior to chemotherapy each day and fosaprepitant 150 mg IV on day 1 before chemotherapy. Dexamethasone 12 mg po given daily prior to chemotherapy each day and then continued on days 4 through 6 alone after chemotherapy.

b. Granisetron transdermal patch applied 24 hours before chemotherapy, dexamethasone 12 mg po and aprepitant 125 mg po on day 1 before chemotherapy, then aprepitant 80 mg po daily on days 2 and 3 and dexamethasone 8 mg po daily on days 2 through 6.

c. Ondansetron 32 mg IV and dexamethasone 20 mg IV daily before chemotherapy. Aprepitant 125 mg po on day 1 and 80 mg po on days 2 and 3.

d. Palonosetron 0.25 mg IV, dexamethasone 12 mg IV and fosaprepitant 150 mg IV on day 1 before chemotherapy, then dexamethasone 8 mg po daily on day 2 and dexamethasone 8 mg po bid on days 3 through 6.

14. RN is sent home with prescriptions for lorazepam and prochlorperazine. He calls 3 days later to say that the lorazepam and prochlorperazine are not working. The nurse tells RN to take the prochlorperazine q6h scheduled and calls in a prescription for ondansetron as needed. He calls back the next day to say he is not getting

any relief. What agent is commonly used for refractory nausea and vomiting?

a. Droperidol

b. Olanzapine

c. Palonosetron

d. Promethazine

15. Which antiemetic(s) should be avoided in patients with the potential for a prolonged QT-interval? Select all that apply.

a. Aprepitant 150 mg IV

b. Palonosetron 0.25 mg IV

c. Droperidol 1.25 mg IV

d. Ondansetron 24 mg IV

16. VP is a 47-year-old woman and is admitted for abdominal pain. She denies alcohol or tobacco use but does have issues with motion sickness. CT scan shows an inflamed gall bladder, and the patient is scheduled for a cholecystectomy. With the information you have, what is VP's risk of developing PONV?

a. Low

b. Moderate

c. High

d. Very high

Questions 17 and 18 pertain to the following case.

JS is a 64-year-old woman who presents to the clinic for cycle 1 of single-agent gemcitabine for pancreatic cancer. She has no history of nausea and vomiting with pregnancy or motion and no heavy alcohol use.

17. Categorize this patient's risk for CINV based on the chemotherapy agent to be given.

a. Minimal risk

b. Low risk

c. Moderate Risk

d. High risk

18. Based on the emetic risk classification of gemcitabine, what medication(s) should JS receive for prevention of acute nausea and vomiting?

a. Ondansetron, aprepitant, and dexamethasone

b. Dexamethasone

c. Lorazepam

d. Olanzapine

19. Which antiemetic should be diluted when given intravenously to minimize extravasation potential?

a. Droperidol

b. Fosaprepitant

c. Palonosetron

d. Promethazine

20. A 34-year-old woman is admitted for a total abdominal hysterectomy and bilateral oophorectomy. The nurse calls and tells you she is asked to write antiemetic orders

for ondansetron to prevent PONV but she can't remember the dose. What do you tell her?

a. Ondansetron 16 mg IV given at the beginning of surgery
b. Ondansetron 32 mg IV given in postoperative recovery
c. Ondansetron 8 mg IV given 2 hours before surgery
d. Ondansetron 4 mg IV given at the end of surgery

21. Rank the 5-HT3 receptor antagonists in order of mg dose. Start with the lowest mg.

Unordered Response	Ordered Response
Rolapitant	
Netupitant (as part of NEPA)	
Fosaprepitant	
Aprepitant	

TAKEAWAY POINTS »

- Nausea and vomiting is a common side effect experienced by patients receiving chemotherapy or a surgical procedure.
- Neurotransmitters are involved in the pathogenesis of nausea and vomiting and include dopamine, serotonin, histamine, and neurokinin-1.
- Risk factors for CINV include chemotherapy agent, rate of infusion, dose of drug, younger patients, female patients, and those with a history of motion sickness or nausea with pregnancy.
- Acute and delayed CINV are easier to prevent than to treat. Antiemetic drug therapy should be directed toward the prevention of acute and delayed CINV.
- Serotonin (5-HT3) receptor antagonists and dexamethasone should be used in the prevention, not treatment, of CINV.

- Neurokinin-1 (NK-1) receptor antagonists are useful in the prevention (not treatment) of acute and delayed nausea and vomiting and the use of one is a reasonable option in HEC or MEC regimens that are known to cause delayed CINV.
- Dopamine antagonists such as promethazine are used in the treatment of breakthrough nausea and vomiting.
- When treating breakthrough CINV, a drug with a different mechanism of action than prescribed previously should be used.
- Benzodiazepines such as lorazepam are useful in the prevention of anticipatory CINV.
- Risk factors for developing PONV include type of anesthetic used, duration of surgery, type of surgery, female patients, nonsmokers, and history of PONV.

BIBLIOGRAPHY

Clinical Pharmacology [Internet]. Tampa (FL): Elsevier. c2017- [cited Feb 27, 2017]. Available from: http://www.clinicalpharmacology.com

Gan TJ, Diemunsch P, Habib AS, et al: Consensus Guidelines for the Management of Postoperative Nausea and Vomiting. *Anesth Analg.* 2014;118:85-113.

Grunberg SM, Slusher B, Rugo HS. Emerging treatments in chemotherapy-induced nausea and vomiting. *Clin Adv Hematol Oncol.* 2013;11(2 Suppl 1):1-19.

Hesketh PJ, Bohlke K, Lyman GH, et al. Antiemetics: American Society of Clinical Oncology Focused Guideline Update. *J Clin Oncol.* 2016;34:381-386.

Hylton Gravatt LA, Donohoe KL, DiPiro CV. In: DiPiro JT, Talbert RL, Yee GC, Matzke GR, Wells BG, Posey LM, eds. *Nausea and*

Vomiting in Pharmacotherapy: A Pathophysiologic Approach. 10th ed. New York, NY: McGraw-Hill; 2017.

Jordan K, Jahn F, Aapro M. Recent developments in the prevention of chemotherapy-induced nausea and vomiting (CINV): a comprehensive review. *Ann Oncol.* 2015 Jun;26(6):1081-90.

Roila F, Molassiotis A, Herrstedt J, et al. 2016 MASCC and ESMO guideline update for the prevention of chemotherapy- and radiotherapy-induced nausea and vomiting and of nausea and vomiting in advanced cancer patients. *Ann Oncol.* 2016;27(suppl 5):v119-v133.

Shaikh SI, Nagarekha D, Hegade G, Marutheesh M. Postoperative nausea and vomiting: a simple yet complex problem. *Anesth Essays Res.* 2016;10(3):388-396.

KEY ABBREVIATIONS

CINV = chemotherapy-induced nausea and vomiting
CTZ = chemoreceptor trigger zone
GI = gastrointestinal

HEC = highly emetic chemotherapy
MEC = moderately emetic chemotherapy
PONV = postoperative nausea and vomiting

43

Upper Gastrointestinal Disorders

Bryan L. Love

FOUNDATION OVERVIEW: PEPTIC ULCER DISEASE

Peptic ulcers are lesions in the stomach or duodenum that extend deeper into the gastrointestinal (GI) tract than other acid related disorders. These lesions develop in response to damage by gastric acid and pepsin. *Gastric* ulcers occur primarily on the lesser curvature, but may occur anywhere in the stomach. In contrast, *duodenal* ulcers occur in the first part of the duodenum. *Peptic ulcer disease* (PUD) is divided into three forms: (1) *Helicobacter pylori* (*H. pylori)* induced; (2) nonsteroidal anti-inflammatory drug (NSAID) induced; and (3) stress related mucosal damage (SRMD). A comparison of characteristics of peptic ulcer are summarized in Table 43-1.

Helicobacter pylori *Helicobacter pylori* is a spiral-shaped, pH-sensitive, gram-negative, urease producing bacteria that resides between the mucus layer and the gastric epithelium. The exact mechanism of gastric injury is unknown, but theories include: the production of enzymes/cytotoxins, increased gastric acid production, and alterations in the host immune response. *Helicobacter pylori* infection is recognized as a risk factor for gastric cancer.

Nonsteroidal Anti-inflammatory Drugs Damage from NSAIDs occurs by two mechanisms: (1) direct irritation of the gastric epithelium; and (2) systemic inhibition of prostaglandin cyclooxygenase-1 (COX-1) and cyclooxygenase-2 (COX-2) synthesis. Up to 25% of *chronic* NSAID users will develop ulcer disease. NSAIDs are associated with gastric ulcers.

Stress Related Mucosal Damage Stress ulcers are superficial lesions in the mucosal layer of the stomach. The most common cause of GI bleeding in the intensive care unit is stress ulcers.

Signs and Symptoms

The clinical presentation of PUD includes nonlocalized epigastric pain, heartburn, belching, bloating, nausea, and anorexia. Duodenal ulcer pain may be worse with an empty stomach (at night or between meals). Gastric ulcer pain occurs at any time and may be worsened with eating. Both types of ulcers can occur in the absence of symptoms, especially gastric ulcers in the elderly. Patients can present with varied symptoms; therefore, no symptom can differentiate between *H. pylori*, NSAID, or SRMD ulcers.

GI bleeding, perforation, and obstruction can occur with *H. pylori* or NSAID-induced ulcer disease. Evidence of bleeding may appear as vomiting blood (hematemesis) or black-colored stools (melena). Perforation may begin as a sharp sudden pain, but then the pain spreads to the abdomen area. Obstruction tends to occur over time and may present with bloating, nausea, and vomiting.

Diagnosis

Upper GI radiography and upper endoscopy can be used to diagnose PUD. Patients with active ulcer disease and gastric mucosa associated lymphoid tissue (MALT) lymphoma should be tested for *H. pylori*. Diagnostic tests for presence of *H. pylori* can be endoscopic (rapid urease test, histology, and culture) or nonendoscopic (serologic testing, urea breath test, stool antigen assay). Endoscopic tests are expensive, uncomfortable, and invasive.

PREVENTION

Prevention of NSAID-induced ulcers includes using an NSAID with low GI toxicity at the lowest effective dose. Partially selective and nonacetylated products may be associated with lower GI toxicity (Table 43-2).

The selection of an agent to use with an NSAID for prevention of GI toxicity depends on GI and cardiovascular (CV) risk factors. Risk factors that can cause NSAID GI complications include prior history of GI event (ulcer, hemorrhage), age more than 60, high-dose NSAID, and concurrent use of antiplatelet agents, anticoagulants, corticosteroids, or selective serotonin reuptake inhibitors. Table 43-3 provides recommendations for preventive strategies stratifying patients according to GI and CV risk profile. To minimize the risk of CV events in patients treated with celecoxib, the total daily dose should not exceed 400 mg per day. Patients with low risk of NSAID-induced ulcers and low CV risk do not require protective measures.

Compared to traditional NSAIDs, selective COX-2 inhibitors have a lower incidence of duodenal and gastric ulcers. However, the gastroprotective effect of COX-2 inhibitors

To access your complimentary online question exams, visit https://accesspharmacy.mhmedical.com/NAPLEX.aspx

TABLE 43-1	Comparison of Common Forms of Peptic Ulcer		
Characteristic	***H. pylori* Induced**	**NSAID Induced**	**SRMD**
Condition	Chronic	Chronic	Acute
Site of damage	Duodenum > stomach	Stomach > duodenum	Stomach > duodenum
Intragastric pH	More dependent	Less dependent	Less dependent
Symptoms	Usually epigastric pain	Often asymptomatic	Asymptomatic
Ulcer depth	Superficial	Deep	Most superficial
GI bleeding	Less severe, single vessel	More severe, single vessel	More severe, superficial mucosal capillaries

Abbreviations: GI, gastrointestinal; NSAID, nonsteroidal anti-inflammatory drug; SRMD, stress-related mucosal damage.
Reproduced with permission from DiPiro JT, Talbert RL, Yee GC, et al: *Pharmacotherapy: A Pathophysiologic Approach*, 10th ed. New York, NY: McGraw-Hill; 2017.

is lost in patients taking low-dose aspirin. The Food and Drug Administration (FDA) requires all NSAIDs, including COX-2 inhibitors, to include a boxed warning highlighting the increased risk of CV events. Results from the PRECISION (Prospective Randomized Evaluation of Celecoxib Integrated Safety Versus Ibuprofen or Naproxen) study, comparing GI and CV risk among over 24,000 patients randomized to celecoxib, ibuprofen, or naproxen, found that celecoxib was noninferior with regard to CV safety. The risk of GI events was significantly lower with celecoxib than with naproxen (p = 0.01). This remains controversial, but recent guidelines recommend naproxen combined with misoprostol or proton pump inhibitor (PPI) for patients on low-dose aspirin therapy and at low or moderate risk of GI toxicity from an NSAID.

Ibuprofen reduces the antiplatelet effect of low-dose aspirin. The American Heart Association recommends patients to take aspirin 30 minutes before the ibuprofen or at least 8 hours after to avoid the interaction and maintain the cardioprotective effects of aspirin. The FDA has concluded that all NSAIDs, including COX-2 inhibitors, are contraindicated for pain management in patients immediately after coronary artery bypass grafting (CABG) surgery due to the increased risk of myocardial infarction (MI) and stroke.

Misoprostol

Misoprostol is a prostaglandin E1 analog indicated to prevent NSAID-induced gastric ulcers by enhancing gastric mucous production and mucosal secretion of bicarbonate. Side effects of misoprostol include nausea, abdominal cramping, headache, and flatulence. Diarrhea occurs in 10% to 30% of patients taking misoprostol; taking misoprostol with food can minimize this side effect. Misoprostol is category X in pregnancy and should be avoided in women of childbearing age unless the patient is at high risk of complications from gastric ulcers. Patients should receive both written and oral warnings of the dangers of misoprostol and should be capable of complying

TABLE 43-2	Comparison of Gastrointestinal and Cardiovascular Risk for NSAIDs		
Drug/Class	**COX-2 Selectivity (in vitro)**	**Gastrointestinal Risk**	**Cardiovascular Risk**
Acetylated Salicylates			
Aspirin	Low	Moderate	Low
Nonacetylated Salicylates			
Salsalate (Disalcid)	Unavailable	Low	Data not available
Diflunisal (Dolobid)	Moderate	Moderate	Data not available
Non-COX-2 Selective NSAIDs			
Flurbiprofen (Ansaid)	Low	High	Data not available
Ibuprofen (Motrin)	Moderate	Low	Moderate to high
Indomethacin (Indocin)	Low	Moderate to high	Moderate
Ketoprofen (Orudis)	Low	Moderate	Data not available
Ketorolac (Toradol)	Low	High	Data not available
Nabumetone (Relafen)	Moderate	Low	Data not available
Naproxen (Naprosyn)	Low	Moderate	Low to moderate
Oxaprozin (Daypro)	Low	High	Data not available
Piroxicam (Feldene)	Moderate	High	Low
Sulindac (Clinoril)	Moderate	Moderate	Data not available
COX-2 Selective NSAIDs			
Celecoxib (Celebrex)	High	Low	Moderate to High
Diclofenac (Voltaren)	High	Moderate	High
Etodolac (Lodine)	High	Low	Moderate
Meloxicam (Mobic)	High	Low	Moderate

Abbreviations: COX-2, cyclooxygenase-2; NSAID, nonsteroidal anti-inflammatory drug.

TABLE 43-3	Prevention of Peptic Ulcer Disease in Patients Receiving Chronic NSAID Therapy	
	Low Gastrointestinal Risk[a]	High Gastrointestinal Risk[b,c]
Low cardiovascular risk	Nonselective NSAIDs	Nonselective NSAIDs plus PPI; celecoxib plus PPI[d]
High cardiovascular risk[e]	Naproxen; add PPI if patient is taking aspirin	No NSAIDs; naproxen plus PPI; low-dose celecoxib plus aspirin plus PPI may be an alternative option[f]

Abbreviations: NSAID, nonsteroidal anti-inflammatory drug; PPI, proton pump inhibitor.

[a]No risk factors.

[b]Presence of risk factors (patients 60 years or older, history of peptic ulcers, receiving concomitant antiplatelet agents, anticoagulants, corticosteroids, or selective serotonin reuptake inhibitors).

[c]In patients with prior history of ulcers, adopt test-and-treat strategy to exclude *H. pylori* infection.

[d]Consider when patients have complicated ulcer history or presence of multiple risk factors.

[e]Use risk calculator (eg, Framingham or ASCVD risk calculators) to estimate cardiovascular risk on the basis of several variables. Patients with a history of cardiovascular events or diabetes are considered high cardiovascular risk.

[f]NSAIDs with increasing selectivity for COX-2 (ie, celecoxib) have been associated with increased cardiovascular risk, and this risk appears to be increased in patients with established cardiovascular disease. In patients with cardiovascular disease or risk factors, recommendations for pain management (in the order listed) include: acetaminophen, aspirin, tramadol, opioids (short-term), nonacetylated salicylates (eg, diflunisal), NSAIDs with low COX-2 selectivity (eg, naproxen), NSAIDs with some COX-2 selectivity (eg, nabumetone), and COX-2 selective agents (ie, celecoxib).

Reproduced with permission from Lanas A, Chan FKL: *Peptic ulcer disease,* Lancet 2017 Aug 5;390(10094):613-624

with effective contraceptive measures. A negative serum pregnancy test within 2 weeks prior to starting therapy is required and female patients should start misoprostol on the second or third day of their next normal menstrual cycle. Arthrotec is a combination product containing diclofenac and misoprostol.

Stress Ulcers

Two independent risk factors for SRMD include patients with respiratory failure (mechanical ventilation for longer than 48 hours) or coagulopathy defined as a platelet count less than 50,000 mm³, an international normalized ratio of more than 1.5, or a partial thromboplastin time of more than two times normal. Patients with these risk factors should receive prophylaxis for stress ulcers. Other risk factors include severe burns (>35% of body surface area), multiple trauma, sepsis, surgery, or organ failure. It is not cost effective to use prophylaxis for all patients; therefore, prophylaxis should be reserved for those patients at high risk of SRMD. Adverse effects, drug interactions, and frequent dosing make antacids and sucralfate less favorable compared to H2-receptor antagonists (H2RAs) and PPIs for the prevention of SRMB. Clinical trials demonstrate that H2RAs significantly reduce the risk of GI bleeding in critically ill patients. However, tolerance can develop within 42 hours and pH control can deteriorate with the use of H2RAs. PPIs provide more consistent acid suppression and unlike H2RAs tolerance does not develop. Both H2RAs and PPIs may be given by mouth, nasogastric tube, or intravenously.

TREATMENT

The goals of PUD treatment include relief of symptoms, ulcer healing, prevention of ulcer recurrence, and reduction of complications.

NSAID-Induced Ulcers

In regards to therapy, two issues that most often need to be addressed are prevention of NSAID-induced ulcers and treatment of the ulcers once they occur. When the NSAID is stopped, most uncomplicated ulcers will heal. If the NSAID must be continued, as in the case of arthritis, a PPI is the agent of choice. Treatment for *H. pylori* is recommended for patients on NSAIDs, if they test positive for the organism.

Sucralfate

Sucralfate is indicated for the management of duodenal ulcers, but is also used in the treatment of gastric ulcers, gastroesophageal reflux disease (GERD), and esophagitis. Adding sucralfate to NSAID therapy is not effective in preventing gastric or duodenal ulcers. Sucralfate does not effect acid secretion, but forms a physical barrier over ulcerated tissue. The most common side effect with sucralfate is constipation. Other side effects include dry mouth, nausea, rash, and metallic taste. Elderly patients who have difficulty in swallowing the large tablets may tolerate the suspension. Sucralfate may reduce the absorption of other drugs (digoxin, fluoroquinolones, ketoconazole, levothyroxine, phenytoin, quinidine, tetracycline, theophylline, and warfarin) and should be administered 2 hours after the interacting medication(s). In order to prevent a delay in onset and reduced efficacy, sucralfate should be dosed 30 minutes after a PPI. Sucralfate use should be limited in patients with chronic renal failure or receiving dialysis due to risk of aluminum accumulation and toxicity.

H2-Receptor Antagonists

H2RAs reversibly inhibit H2 receptors on the parietal cell, which results in a decrease of basal and food stimulated acid secretion. After 30 days of therapy, some patients develop a tolerance to H2RAs. H2RAs are not very effective for healing or preventing gastric ulcers, but do prevent duodenal ulcers. The overall incidence of side effects is less than 3% but can include confusion, headache, dizziness, fatigue, somnolence, and either diarrhea or constipation. Adverse effects are more likely in elderly patients and those with reduced renal function. Cimetidine has numerous drug interactions (eg, warfarin, phenytoin, theophylline, and lidocaine) due to the inhibition of several CYP450 isoenzymes. Famotidine, ranitidine, and nizatidine are excreted renally and require dose reduction or extension of the dosing interval in renal insufficiency.

Proton Pump Inhibitors

PPIs irreversibly inhibit the final step in gastric acid secretion. These agents inhibit greater than 90% of gastric acid secreted in 24 hours. PPIs are effective for healing duodenal and gastric ulcers. Additionally, they have a protective effect against NSAID-related mucosal injury. All PPIs provide similar ulcer healing rates and relief of symptoms. Compared to H2RAs, PPIs relieve symptoms and heal more quickly, and most are available as generics. Patients should take PPIs 30 to 60 minutes before eating. Elimination of PPIs is predominantly hepatic and dosage adjustment is recommended in severe liver disease. Dosage adjustment for hepatic impairment varies between PPIs and is not always correlated to a Child-Pugh score. Pantoprazole requires no dosage adjustment for hepatic impairment, but esomeprazole, omeprazole, and dexlansoprazole recommends a maximum dose of 20 to 30 mg per day. Omeprazole and esomeprazole decrease the elimination of phenytoin, diazepam, and warfarin by inhibiting the CYP2C19. Currently, there is conflicting data from retrospective studies suggesting that PPIs decrease the effectiveness of clopidogrel, increasing the risk of MI or death. The only prospective, randomized clinical trial to evaluate this interaction did not demonstrate an increased risk of MI or death, but there were fewer GI events in the clopidogrel group receiving omeprazole cotherapy. Clopidogrel is a prodrug requiring hepatic conversion by the CYP2C19 to its active metabolite. One theory suggests some PPIs inhibit the CYP2C19, which would decrease the antiplatelet effect of clopidogrel. In general, PPIs are well tolerated and the side effects are similar to H2RAs, which include headache, nausea, dizziness, somnolence, diarrhea, constipation, and nutrient malabsorption (ie, calcium, magnesium, vitamin B_{12}).

Helicobacter pylori-Induced Ulcers

Selection of first-line treatment for confirmed *H. pylori* should incorporate prior antibiotic exposure, particularly exposure to macrolides, and history of allergy. Due to increasing resistance, clarithromycin-based triple therapy (PPI, clarithromycin, and amoxicillin or metronidazole) for 14 days is no longer recommended in areas where clarithromycin resistance exceeds 15%, which is thought to include most of the United States. Instead, bismuth quadruple therapy (PPI or H2RA, bismuth, metronidazole, and tetracycline) for 10 to 14 days is recommended as a first-line option. Concomitant therapy (PPI, amoxicillin, clarithromycin, and metronidazole) for 10 to 14 days is a recommended regimen. Sequential therapy (PPI and amoxicillin for 5 days, then PPI, clarithromycin, and metronidazole for 5 days) is a recommended first-line alternative regimen. Hybrid therapy (PPI and amoxicillin for 7 days, then PPI, amoxicillin, clarithromycin, and metronidazole for 7 days) is also an option. Levofloxacin triple therapy (PPI, levofloxacin, and amoxicillin for 10-14 days) and levofloxacin sequential therapy (PPI and amoxicillin for 5-7 days, followed by PPI, amoxicillin, metronidazole, and levofloxacin for 5-7 days) are recommended first-line options.

In general, longer treatment durations (ie, 10-14 days) are preferred for all treatment regimens, since eradication rates are lower with shorter durations and the initial regimen offers the best opportunity for *H. pylori* eradication. For true penicillin allergic patients, there are two therapeutic options: (1) Bismuth quadruple therapy or (2) substitution of metronidazole

for amoxicillin in clarithromycin-based triple therapy. Confirmation of eradication should occur at least 4 weeks following completion of antibiotics and after withholding PPI for 1 to 2 weeks. If initial treatment is unsuccessful, then the second course of therapy (salvage therapy) should avoid antibiotics that were previously used. See Table 43-4 for initial treatment regimens to eradicate *H. pylori*.

In general, the most common adverse effects associated with antibiotics for infection are GI in nature (eg, nausea, dysgeusia, dyspepsia/abdominal pain, diarrhea). Clarithromycin may also cause a prolonged QTc interval and a metallic taste. Metronidazole can cause metallic taste, dyspepsia, peripheral neuropathy, and a disulfiram-like reaction with alcohol consumption. Bismuth may darken the tongue and stool.

SPECIAL CONSIDERATIONS

The incidence of *H. pylori* infection, PUD, and gastric malignancy is uncommon in children in the United States. Even though the same agents used to treat *H. pylori* in adults appears to be effective in children, there are no standard guidelines. Gastric ulcers generally do not develop before age 40 and the incidence of duodenal ulcers increases with age up to 60 years of age. H2RAs and PPIs are pregnancy category B or C and both are excreted in breast milk.

FOUNDATION OVERVIEW: GASTROESOPHAGEAL REFLUX DISEASE

GERD is a disorder caused by abnormal reflux of gastric contents into the esophagus and often results from a defect in lower esophageal sphincter (LES) function. Additionally, abnormal defense mechanisms may promote the development of gastroesophageal reflux and include anatomic factors (hiatal hernia), reduced esophageal clearance, delayed gastric emptying, inadequate mucus secretion, and decreased salivary buffering. The classic symptom of GERD is heartburn described as substernal warmth or burning starting in the epigastric area radiating to the neck. Warning signs and symptoms of complicated GERD include dysphagia, early satiety, GI bleeding, iron deficiency anemia, odynophagia, vomiting, or weight loss. There is no standard method for diagnosing GERD; rather diagnosis is made based upon symptoms. Endoscopy, manometry, and other diagnostic testing should be reserved for patients with complicated GERD or those refractory to initial therapy.

Excessive reflux of acid and pepsin resulting in mucosal damage and inflammation is termed reflux esophagitis. Less commonly, reflux can even lead to erosion of squamous epithelium lining the esophagus or erosive esophagitis. Long-term complications of reflux include development of strictures, Barrett esophagus, and esophageal adenocarcinoma. Additionally, chronic reflux may cause extraesophageal syndromes such as chronic cough, laryngitis, asthma, and erosion of dental enamel.

TABLE 43-4	Recommended First-Line Drug Regimens to Eradicate *H. pylori*				
Regimen	Duration	Drug #1	Drug #2	Drug #3	Drug #4
Proton Pump Inhibitor–Based Triple Therapy[a]	14 d	PPI once or twice daily[b]	Clarithromycin 500 mg twice daily	Amoxicillin 1 g twice daily *or* metronidazole 500 mg twice daily	
Bismuth Quadruple Therapy[a]	10-14 d	PPI or H$_2$RA once or twice daily[b,c]	Bismuth subsalicylate[d] 525 mg four times daily	Metronidazole 250-500 mg four times daily	Tetracycline 500 mg four times daily
Nonbismuth Quadruple or "Concomitant" Therapy[e]	10-14 d	PPI once or twice daily on days 1-10[b]	Clarithromycin 250-500 mg twice daily on days 1-10	Amoxicillin 1 g twice daily on days 1-10	Metronidazole 250-500 mg twice daily on days 1-10
Sequential Therapy[e]	10 d	PPI once or twice daily on days 1-10[b]	Amoxicillin 1 g twice daily on days 1-5	Metronidazole 250-500 mg twice daily on days 6-10	Clarithromycin 250-500 mg twice daily on days 6-10
Hybrid Therapy[e]	14 d	PPI once or twice daily on days 1-14[b]	Amoxicillin 1 g twice daily on days 1-14	Metronidazole 250-500 mg twice daily on days 7-14	Clarithromycin 250-500 mg twice daily on days 7-14
Levofloxacin triple	10-14 d	PPI twice daily	Levofloxacin 500 mg qd	Amoxicillin 1 g twice daily	
Levofloxacin Sequential	10 d	PPI twice daily on days 1-10	Amoxicillin 1 g twice daily on days 1-5	Levofloxacin 500 mg once daily on days 6-10	Metronidazole 500 mg twice daily on days 6-10
LOAD	7-10 d	Levofloxacin 250 mg once daily	Omeprazole (or other PPI) at high dose once daily	Nitazoxanide (Alinia) 500 mg twice daily	Doxycycline 100 mg once daily

Abbreviations: H2RA, H2-receptor antagonist; PPI, proton pump inhibitor.

[a]May be used when clarithromycin resistance is known to be less than 15%. Prior antibiotic exposure, particularly macrolides, should be determined prior to regimen selection. Treatment duration of 10 to 14 days is recommended. The antisecretory drug may be continued beyond antimicrobial treatment for patients with a history of a complicated ulcer, for example, bleeding, or in heavy smokers.

[b]Standard PPI peptic ulcer healing dosages given once or twice daily.

[c]Standard H2RA peptic ulcer healing dosages may be used in place of a PPI.

[d]Bismuth subcitrate potassium (biskalcitrate) 140 mg, as the bismuth salt, is contained in a prepackaged capsule (Pylera), along with metronidazole 125 mg and tetracycline 125 mg; three capsules are taken with each meal and at bedtime; a standard PPI dosage is added to the regimen and taken twice daily. All medications are taken for 10 days.

[e]Requires validation as first-line therapy in the United States.

PREVENTION

Lifestyle modifications are recommended for GERD. These measures include weight loss in individuals who are overweight or have had recent weight gain, head of bed elevation, and avoidance of meals 2 to 3 hours before bed in patients with nocturnal GERD (Table 43-5). Other lifestyle recommendations may be effective for individual patients. For example, patients who experience GERD following ingestion of alcohol or caffeinated beverages will benefit from avoidance of these triggers. However, empiric elimination of known foods (eg, acidic and/or spicy foods) that can trigger reflux is no longer recommended.

TREATMENT

The goals of GERD treatment include relieving symptoms, reducing the frequency of symptoms, promoting healing of mucosal injury, and preventing complications. Reducing gastric acidity decreases reflux symptoms and allows esophagitis to heal. An empiric trial of PPI therapy for 8 weeks is indicated for patients with typical symptoms and the absence of atypical symptoms suggesting complications. Traditional PPI formulations should be administered 30 to 60 minutes prior to a meal for optimal acid suppression. Once daily dosing is appropriate for most patients, but pharmacotherapy can be tailored for individual patients (eg, twice daily PPI) for patients with partial response or have breakthrough symptoms later in the day (eg, night-time symptoms, sleep disturbance). Nonresponders to PPI should be referred for further evaluation. GERD is considered a chronic disease and maintenance acid suppression may be required in patients with complications (eg, erosive esophagitis, Barrett esophagus) or patients with symptom recurrence after initial PPI treatment course. Maintenance therapy with acid suppression maintains relief of symptoms and prevents the recurrence of esophagitis. H2RAs may be used for maintenance only in patients without erosive disease. See Table 43-6 for a list of medications commonly utilized in GERD.

Antacids

Over-the-counter (OTC) antacid and antacid-alginic acid preparations are effective for GERD. Antacids are beneficial for immediate symptomatic relief and may be used in conjunction with other acid-suppression regimens; however, they are not recommended as treatment for erosive esophagitis. GI adverse effects are commonly encountered (diarrhea or constipation) and vary depending on the product used. Electrolyte disturbances and drug interactions are important considerations when selecting a product.

TABLE 43-5	Therapeutic Lifestyle Changes Recommended for the Treatment of Gastroesophageal Reflux Disease	
Dietary and Medication Aggravating Factors		**Lifestyle Changes**
Directly irritating foods:	Directly irritating medications:	General:
Citrus fruits	Bisphosphonates	Smoking cessation
Carbonated beverages	Aspirin/NSAIDs	Weight reduction if overweight
Onions	Iron	Reduction of alcohol consumption
Spicy foods	Potassium	Avoid aggravating factors
Tomatoes	Medications which lower esophageal sphincter tone:	Nighttime symptoms:
Foods which lower esophageal sphincter tone:	Anticholinergics	Avoid eating within 3 h before bedtime
Caffeinated beverages	Estrogen/progesterone	Elevate head of bed
Chocolate	Nicotine	Postprandial symptoms:
Fried or fatty foods	Nitrates	Eat smaller and more frequent meals
Mint	Tetracyclines	Avoid lying down after meals
	Theophylline	

Sucralfate

Sucralfate (Carafate) is a prescription product which acts by creating a barrier to acid penetration in the esophagus. Clinical studies of sucralfate have demonstrated little or no efficacy in patients with GERD; thus, it is not routinely recommended. Anecdotally, sucralfate suspension may be used for symptomatic relief for a short duration in patients with endoscopically confirmed erosive esophagitis.

H2-Receptor Antagonists

Cimetidine (Tagamet), famotidine (Pepcid), nizatidine (Axid), and ranitidine (Zantac) are approved OTC products for heartburn. Higher doses taken more frequently are often needed for mild to moderate GERD. Esophageal healing rates and heartburn symptoms are improved with H2RAs when compared with placebo; however, they are less effective than PPIs. Esophageal healing rates are approximately 50% with standard doses of H2RAs and are, therefore, not recommended when erosions are present. Available H2RAs have similar efficacy and are interchangeable, although cimetidine is often avoided due to an increased risk of drug interactions (inhibition of cytochrome P-450 enzymes) and gynecomastia.

Proton Pump Inhibitors

PPIs inhibit H^+/K^+-adenosine triphosphatase in gastric parietal cells thereby blocking gastric acid secretion. PPIs are superior to H2RAs in treating patients with moderate to severe GERD symptoms, including patients with erosive esophagitis. Approximately, 80% of patients achieve symptomatic relief and endoscopic healing following 8 weeks of prescription-strength therapy. Although the incidence is similar to placebo, the most common adverse effects of PPIs are abdominal pain, constipation, diarrhea, and headache. In general, long-term use of PPIs is considered safe; however, there are potential and confirmed risks associated with continuous use. In theory, potent acid suppression with PPIs poses additional risks with long-term use including malabsorption, excessive gastrin secretion (hypergastrinemia) leading to gastric carcinomas, and hypochlorhydria resulting in bacterial overgrowth. More recently, large studies have revealed a 40% increase in hip fractures in patients over 50 years of age thought to be related to calcium malabsorption. Additionally, PPIs increase the risk of infectious gastroenteritis by 50% and double the risk of *Clostridium difficile* colitis.

Miscellaneous Therapy

Diminished esophageal sphincter tone, esophageal clearance, and delayed gastric emptying may also contribute to GERD. Metoclopramide, bethanechol, and baclofen have been used to improve these factors; however, central nervous system side effects (drowsiness, confusion, and dystonia) limit their usefulness. Side effects occur in a dose-dependent manner and are common in elderly or renal insufficiency patients. Although these agents may provide symptomatic improvement in GERD, they are last-line therapy and should be used in conjunction with acid suppressive therapy.

Surgery

Surgery is an alternative option for GERD patients with chronic symptoms, particularly, patients who initially respond to PPIs, but prefer not to take PPIs long-term. Surgical treatments possess risks not associated with medical therapy, including need for repeat surgery, increased flatulence, inability to belch, severe dysphagia, and changes in bowel habits (diarrhea, bloating, abdominal pain, or constipation).

SPECIAL CONSIDERATIONS

GERD occurs in 18% of pediatric patients. Dietary adjustments and postural changes during and after feedings are usually effective first-line management strategies. Additionally, smaller and more frequent feedings may also be beneficial. A similar approach to medical management is useful in pediatric patients, although combined use of a promotility agent and an acid suppressant provides quicker relief of symptoms. H2RAs and PPIs are considered safe and are used in pediatric and neonatal patients, although most PPIs are only indicated for patients over 1 year of age. Available H2RAs and PPIs are classified as either pregnancy category B or C and are considered safe in pregnant patients if indicated. Both classes of agents are passed into breast milk.

TABLE 43-6 | **Medications Commonly Utilized in Upper GI Disorders**

Drug	Brand Name	Initial Dose (oral)	Usual Range	Special Population Dose	Other
Proton Pump Inhibitors					
Omeprazole, sodium bicarbonate	Prilosec, Zegerid	40 mg daily	20-40 mg/d	Consider adjustment for hepatic disease	Pregnancy Category C
Lansoprazole	Prevacid, various	30 mg daily	15-30 mg/d	Consider adjustment for hepatic disease	Pregnancy Category B
Rabeprazole	Aciphex	20 mg daily	20-40 mg/d	Use with caution in severe hepatic disease	Pregnancy Category B
Pantoprazole	Protonix, various	40 mg daily	40-80 mg/d	Consider adjustment for severe hepatic disease	Pregnancy Category B
Esomeprazole	Nexium	40 mg daily	20-40 mg/d	Limit dose to 20 mg/d in severe hepatic disease	Pregnancy Category B
Dexlansoprazole	Dexilant	30-60 mg daily	30-60 mg/d	Consider dose limit of 30 mg/d in moderate hepatic impairment, dose not established in severe hepatic disease	Pregnancy Category B
H2-Receptor Antagonists					
Cimetidine	Tagamet, various	300 mg four times daily, 400 mg twice daily, or 800 mg at bedtime	800-1600 mg/d in divided doses	Adjust dose for renal and severe hepatic impairment	Pregnancy Category B
Famotidine	Pepcid, various	20 mg twice daily, or 40 mg at bedtime	20-40 mg/d	Adjust dose for renal impairment	Pregnancy Category B
Nizatidine	Axid, various	150 mg twice daily, or 300 mg at bedtime	150-300 mg/d	Adjust dose for renal impairment	Pregnancy Category B
Ranitidine	Zantac, various	150 mg twice daily, or 300 mg at bedtime	150-300 mg/d	Adjust dose for renal impairment	Pregnancy Category B
Mucosal Protectants					
Sucralfate	Carafate, various	1 g four times daily, or 2 g twice daily	2-4 g/d		Aluminum may accumulate in renal failure, Pregnancy Category B
Misoprostol	Cytotec	100-200 mcg four times daily	400-800 mcg/d		Pregnancy Category X

Adapted with permission from DiPiro JT, Talbert RL, Yee GC, et al: *Pharmacotherapy: A Pathophysiologic Approach*, 10th ed. New York, NY: McGraw-Hill; 2017.

CASE Application

1. Patients with NSAID-induced ulcers are more likely to have which of the following? Select all that apply.
   a. Superficial ulcer depth
   b. A duodenal ulcer
   c. Stress related mucosal bleeding
   d. Damage to the gastric mucosa
   e. More severe GI bleeding involving a single vessel

2. You are asked for pharmacotherapy recommendations for a 59-year-old man with a documented NSAID-induced ulcer who is *H. pylori* negative. He needs to continue taking an NSAID for severe osteoarthritis. Which is the preferred medication for treating an NSAID-induced ulcer?
   a. Lansoprazole
   b. Misoprostol
   c. Ranitidine
   d. Sucralfate

3. A 43-year-old woman with epigastric pain was just diagnosed with a duodenal ulcer. A urea breath test confirmed *H. pylori*. The patient denies any allergies to medications, and recently completed a course of azithromycin for community-acquired pneumonia. In addition to PPI, which of the following is/are recommended as primary initial therapy for *H. pylori*? Select all that apply.
   a. Amoxicillin + levofloxacin for 14 days
   b. Metronidazole + clarithromycin for 7 days
   c. Amoxicillin + clarithromycin for 14 days
   d. Metronidazole + bismuth + tetracycline for 14 days
   e. Levofloxacin + nitazoxanide + doxycycline for 10 days

4. Which of the following is a nonendoscopic test used to diagnose active *H. pylori* PUD?
   a. Urea breath test
   b. Mucosal biopsy
   c. Culture
   d. Antibody detection

5. A patient calls the pharmacy to complain about her tongue turning black after starting a new regimen for PUD. Which medication is causing the side effect?

   a. Amoxicillin
   b. Metronidazole
   c. Bismuth subsalicylate
   d. Clarithromycin

6. A patient was treated initially with PPI, amoxicillin, and clarithromycin for 10 days but failed to eradicate *H. pylori*. Which regimen(s) would you recommended for salvage therapy? Select all that apply.

   a. PPI + amoxicillin for 10 days
   b. PPI + tetracycline + metronidazole + bismuth for 14 days
   c. PPI + metronidazole + clarithromycin for 14 days
   d. PPI + nitazoxanide + levofloxacin + doxycycline for 10 days
   e. PPI + amoxicillin + clarithromycin for 14 days

7. What is the recommended duration of treatment for *H. pylori* if clarithromycin-based triple therapy is initially used?

   a. 5 days
   b. 7 days
   c. 10 days
   d. 14 days

8. A 62-year-old woman with rheumatoid arthritis and atrial fibrillation (AF) requires chronic NSAID therapy. She controls her arthritis pain with high-dose nabumetone and takes warfarin for AF. Patient is considered as low CV risk. Which medication regimen(s) is/are recommended for prevention of NSAID ulcer complications? Select all that apply.

   a. Change to celecoxib plus PPI
   b. Add PPI to current NSAID
   c. Change to celecoxib
   d. No change is needed
   e. Change to indomethacin

9. A patient heard on television that indomethacin can cause ulcers. She calls the pharmacy to find out if there is a better alternative to treat her arthritis. She prefers an NSAID with a similar treatment effect but a lower risk of GI toxicity. The patient is aged 55 and does not have any other significant medical problems. What recommendation would be most appropriate?

   a. Sulindac
   b. Etodolac
   c. Piroxicam
   d. Naproxen

10. A 55-year-old woman with prior PUD, hyperlipidemia, MI (2 years ago), and hypertension (HTN) requires chronic NSAID therapy for hip pain. Medications include atorvastatin 20 mg once daily, acetylsalicylic acid (ASA) 81 mg once daily, and metoprolol 100 mg bid.

What would you recommended for treatment of her hip pain +/- ulcer prevention?

   a. Celecoxib 100 mg daily
   b. Naproxen
   c. Celecoxib 100 mg daily plus omeprazole 20 mg daily
   d. Naproxen plus ranitidine

11. Which of the following describes the clinical presentation of duodenal ulcers?

   a. Pain may be accompanied by coughing up blood.
   b. Pain is worse at night or between meals.
   c. Pain is worse with food.
   d. Pain is caused by damage from NSAIDs.

12. Which of the following requires a negative pregnancy test prior to starting therapy?

   a. Celecoxib
   b. Misoprostol
   c. PPIs
   d. Amoxicillin

13. A patient is admitted to the intensive care unit after a car accident. The patient has been on mechanical ventilation for 72 hours and has a head injury. Which of the following is recommended for this patient for stress ulcer prophylaxis?

   a. Ranitidine by mouth
   b. Intravenous pantoprazole
   c. Sucralfate by nasogastric tube
   d. Patient does not require stress ulcer prophylaxis

14. Which of the following factors may worsen symptoms in GERD patients? Select all that apply.

   a. Alcohol consumption
   b. Caffeine consumption
   c. Obesity or recent weight gain
   d. Smoking
   e. Furosemide

15. A 45-year-old obese woman with HTN and diabetes presents with complaints of "severe" heartburn after meals and occasionally at night. She admits to smoking and occasional alcohol consumption. She consumes four to five caffeinated beverages daily. Medications include: hydrochlorothiazide (HCTZ) 12.5 mg daily and metformin 850 mg twice daily. Which of the following represents the best initial treatment option with the highest probability of symptom control?

   a. Ranitidine
   b. Metoclopramide
   c. Lansoprazole
   d. Sucralfate

16. A 65-year-old woman with osteoporosis, GERD, and HTN is taking alendronate 70 mg weekly, calcium carbonate 600 mg + vitamin D 400 units twice daily, omeprazole 20 mg daily, and enalapril 10 mg twice daily.

Which of the following are possible consequences of this regimen? Select all that apply.

a. Alendronate may worsen GERD symptoms.
b. Enalapril may worsen GERD symptoms.
c. Omeprazole may reduce calcium absorption.
d. Omeprazole may decrease alendronate metabolism.
e. Omeprazole may decrease absorption of vitamin D.

17. Which of the following is a typical sign or symptom of patients with GERD?

a. Iron deficiency anemia
b. Dysphagia
c. Regurgitation
d. Weight loss

18. Which of the following acts by competitively inhibiting histamine at the H2 receptor of gastric parietal cells? Select all that apply.

a. Omeprazole
b. Rabeprazole
c. Cimetidine
d. Ranitidine
e. Misoprostol

19. A 50-year-old woman presented to her physician approximately 8 weeks ago with complaints of heartburn, regurgitation, and dysphagia which resulted in an endoscopy. At that time, her physician diagnosed GERD with erosive esophagitis and prescribed 2 months of lansoprazole 30 mg daily. Today at her follow-up visit, she reports improvement in her symptoms. What would you recommend as an initial trial of maintenance therapy for NJ?

a. Famotidine 20 mg twice daily
b. Lansoprazole 30 mg daily

c. No further therapy required
d. Sucralfate 1 g twice daily

20. Select the brand name for pantoprazole.

a. Axid
b. Aciphex
c. Prevacid
d. Protonix

21. Which of the following would be appropriate health information to discuss with a patient presenting to your pharmacy with GERD symptoms? Select all that apply.

a. Eating smaller meals more often
b. Elevating the head of the bed 6 inches if nighttime symptoms are present
c. Weight reduction for patients who are overweight
d. Smoking cessation for those who smoke
e. Avoid eating within 6 hours before bedtime

22. Select the counseling points for a patient receiving omeprazole 40 mg daily.

a. Take in the evening 30 minutes prior to going to bed.
b. The capsule may be chewed or crushed.
c. Administer with food.
d. Delayed release capsule may be opened and added to 1 tablespoon of applesauce.

23. Order the following NSAIDs in order of risk of GI toxicity. Place in order starting with the lowest to highest risk: Salsalate, Piroxicam, Aspirin.

a. Salsalate < Piroxicam < Aspirin
b. Salsalate < Asprin < Piroxicam
c. Aspirin < Piroxicam < Salsalate
d. Piroxicam < Aspirin < Salsalate

TAKEAWAY POINTS »

- PUD is divided into three forms: *H. pylori* induced, NSAID induced, and SRMD.
- Symptoms cannot differentiate between *H. pylori* and NSAID-induced ulcer.
- Misoprostol is a prostaglandin analog indicated to prevent NSAID-induced gastric ulcers.
- Misoprostol is pregnancy category X.
- Respiratory failure (mechanical ventilation for longer than 48 hours) or coagulopathy are risk factors for SRMD.
- Treatment options for prophylaxis of SRMD are H2RAs and PPIs.
- For the treatment of NSAID-induced ulcer disease, if the NSAID must be continued, a PPI is the agent of choice.
- Sucralfate is indicated for the management of duodenal ulcers, but constipation and frequent dosing limit the use of this agent.
- H2RAs are not very effective for healing or preventing gastric ulcers, but do prevent duodenal ulcers.

- All PPIs provide similar ulcer healing rates and relief of symptoms for gastric and duodenal ulcers.
- Compared to H2RAs, PPIs relieve symptoms and heal more quickly.
- Although controversial, PPIs may decrease the effectiveness of clopidogrel.
- Primary treatment for *H. pylori* should be triple therapy for 14 days or quadruple therapy for 10 to 14 days.
- Lifestyle modifications may be beneficial in patients with GERD, although additional pharmacologic therapy is required for symptom control in most patients.
- Acid suppression with PPI is the foundation of GERD treatment, and either a step-up or step-down approach to therapy may be used for the 8-week empirical trial.
- Although less effective overall when compared to PPIs, H2RAs in divided doses may be beneficial in mild to moderate GERD without erosive disease.

- PPIs typically provide the greatest symptomatic relief and have the highest healing rates in patients with reflux esophagitis.
- Antacids and OTC acid suppressants are options for patient-directed therapy for heartburn.
- Promotility agents (metoclopramide) may be useful in selected patients when used as an adjunct to acid suppression.

- A PPI is the drug of choice for maintenance therapy in patients with moderate to severe GERD. The lowest effective dose of acid suppressive therapy should be used.

BIBLIOGRAPGY

AGA Institute Medical Position Panel. American Gastroenterological Association Medical Position Statement on the management of gastroesophageal reflux disease. *Gastroenterology.* 2008;135:1383-1391.

Chey WD, Leontiadis GI, Howden CW, Moss SF. ACG Clinical Guideline: Treatment of Helicobacter pylori Infection. *Am J Gastroenterol.* 2017;112:212-238.

DeVault KR, Castell DO. Updated guidelines for the diagnosis and treatment of gastroesophageal reflux disease. *Am J Gastroenterol.* 2005;100:190-200.

Dunleavy AA, Mack D. Peptic ulcer disease. In: Linn WD, Wofford MR, O'Keefe M, Posey L, eds. *Pharmacotherapy in Primary Care.* New York, NY: McGraw-Hill; 2009:chap 11.

Lanas A, Chan FLK. Peptic ulcer disease. *Lancet.* 2017;390:613-624.

Love BL, Mohorn PL. Peptic ulcer disease and related disorders. In: DiPiro JT, Talbert RL, Yee GC, Matzke GR, Wells BG, Posey L, eds. *Pharmacotherapy: A Pathophysiologic Approach.* 10th ed. New York, NY: McGraw-Hill; 2014:chap 33.

Wallace JL, Sharkey KA. Pharmacotherapy of gastric acidity, peptic ulcers, and gastroesophageal reflux disease. In: Brunton LL, Chabner BA, Knollmann BC, eds. *Goodman & Gilman's The Pharmacological Basis of Therapeutics.* 12th ed. New York, NY: McGraw-Hill; 2011:chap 45.

KEY ABBREVIATIONS

ACE = angiotensin-converting enzyme
AF = atrial fibrillation
ASA = acetylsalicylic acid
CABG = coronary artery bypass grafting
COX = cyclooxygenase
FDA = Food and Drug Administration
GERD = gastroesophageal reflux disease
GI = gastrointestinal

HCTZ = hydrochlorothiazide
HTN = hypertension
LES = lower esophageal sphincter
MALT = mucosa associated lymphoid tissue
NSAID = nonsteroidal anti-inflammatory drug
OTC = over-the-counter
PUD = peptic ulcer disease
SRMD = stress related mucosal damage

44

Viral Hepatitis

Bryan L. Love

FOUNDATION OVERVIEW

Hepatitis is the inflammation and damage of hepatocytes in the liver caused by hepatitis A, B, C, D, E viruses, alcohol, and medications. Viral hepatitis occurs at any age and is the most common cause of liver disease. The prevalence and incidence may be underreported because patients are often asymptomatic. Acute hepatitis is associated with all five types of viral hepatitis and rarely exceeds 6 months in duration. Chronic viral hepatitis is associated with hepatitis B, C, and D and may lead to the development of ascites, jaundice, hepatic encephalopathy, esophageal varices, cirrhosis, and hepatocellular carcinoma. This chapter focuses on the most common viral forms of hepatitis (hepatitis A, B, and C).

Hepatitis A

Hepatitis A virus (HAV) is an acute viral infection spread via the fecal-oral route. In the United States, HAV has declined considerably since the development of the hepatitis A vaccine, but HAV remains prevalent in underdeveloped countries. HAV is an RNA virus that impacts areas with inadequate sanitation and persons with poor hygienic practices. Other risk factors include IV drug use, exposure to infected individuals, and homosexual activity in men.

Hepatitis B

Hepatitis B virus (HBV) causes an acute and chronic viral infection. In the United States, acute HBV is transmitted through exposure to blood and bodily secretions, sexual activity, IV drug use, and occupational exposure. Despite having an effective vaccine against HBV, more than 300,000 newly diagnosed infections emerge annually. Approximately 10% to 15% of patients develop chronic HBV disease; therefore, 85% to 90% of acute HBV infections resolve without complications.

Hepatitis C

Hepatitis C virus (HCV) infection is the most common blood-borne infection in the United States. There are six geographically specific genotypes of HCV; however, only genotypes 1 to 4 are commonly encountered in the United States. For example, genotype 1 represents 75% of infections within the United States, whereas genotype 4 is common in the Middle East. HCV genotype is used to determine the duration of therapy and the likelihood of therapeutic response. The most common modes of transmission of HCV are IV drug use and blood transfusion prior to 1992 before blood banks began screening for HCV. Other HCV risk factors include tattoos, body piercings, and shared drug paraphernalia. HCV is rarely transmitted through sexual intercourse in heterosexual monogamous relationships. Approximately 10% to 15% of patients with acute HCV resolve without any further sequelae; therefore, 85% to 90% of HCV cases develop into chronic disease.

Clinical Presentation and Diagnosis

Signs and symptoms vary among patients and range from asymptomatic to liver failure. Asymptomatic patients may only present with mildly elevated liver enzymes. Common acute symptoms include fatigue, jaundice, nausea and vomiting, weight loss, fever, right upper quadrant pain, and splenomegaly. An overview of HAV, HBC, and HCV can be found in Table 44-1.

Diagnosing viral hepatitis is difficult because patients may be asymptomatic. Symptoms cannot identify the type of hepatitis; therefore, laboratory serology must be obtained. Viral hepatitis is diagnosed by the presence of antibodies, antigens, and measured virus. Elevated liver enzymes (eg, AST and ALT) are not specific to viral hepatitis but of hepatocellular injury. In the presence of persistently elevated liver enzymes, lack of antibody production, and continued presence of viral particles in the blood, chronic HBV or HCV can be diagnosed. A liver biopsy is useful for assessing the grade and stage of liver disease in chronic HBV or HCV. The grade reflects the degree of liver inflammation, and the stage reflects extent of fibrosis or presence of cirrhosis.

PREVENTION

Prevention of HAV, HBV, and HCV includes avoiding risk factors for transmission and immunization of children and at-risk adults against HAV and HBV (there is no vaccine for HCV). Screening is recommended for individuals with risk factors for acquiring viral hepatitis. Pregnant females should be screened for HBV to prevent perinatal HBV transmission. Patients acquiring HBV or HCV should be screened for other

TABLE 44-1   **Overview of Hepatitis A, B, and C**

	Hepatitis A	Hepatitis B	Hepatitis C
Route of transmission	Oral-fecal	Blood, bodily secretions	Blood
Risk factors	Geographic areas with poor sanitation, poor hygienic practices, IV drug use, homosexual activity in men	IV drug use, sexual activity, occupational exposure to infected blood or bodily secretions, uterine exposure to infected female	IV drug use, blood transfusion prior to 1992, intranasal drug users who share paraphernalia, tattoos or body piercings if performed without proper infection control practices
Signs and symptoms of acute infection	Elevated liver enzymes, fatigue, jaundice, nausea, vomiting, weight loss, fever, right upper quadrant pain, splenomegaly; may be asymptomatic		
Chronic form (% incidence)	No	Yes (10%); 90% (if acute HBV was perinatally acquired)	Yes (80%-85%)
Screening	Not necessary unless assessing need for vaccine	Patients with above risk factors, pregnant females, patients with HCV or HIV	Recommended for patients who have ever used IV drugs, are on hemodialysis, had a blood transfusion prior to 1992, received blood clotting factors prior to 1987, unexplained elevated liver enzymes, organ transplant, children born to HCV infected mothers, have occupational exposure to HCV infected blood or a needle stick, persons born between 1945-1965
Prevention for at-risk children and adults	**Havrix** *Adult:* 1440 ELISA units (1 mL) IM with a booster dose of 1440 ELISA units to be given 6-12 mo following primary immunization *Pediatric:* 720 ELISA units (0.5 mL) IM with a booster dose of 720 ELISA units to be given 6-12 mo following primary immunization **Vaqta** *Adult:* 50 units (1 mL) IM with a booster dose of 50 units (1 mL) to be given 6-18 mo after primary immunization *Pediatric:* 25 units (0.5 mL) IM with a booster dose of 25 units (0.5 mL) to be given 6-18 mo after primary immunization **Twinrix** (combination HAV and HBV vaccine) *Adult:* 1 mL IM given on a 0-, 1-, and 6-mo schedule	**Engerix-B** **Recombivax HBA** *Adult (>19):* 1 mL IM at 0, 1, and 6 mo *Pediatric (0-19 y):* 0.5 mL IM at 0, 1, and 6 mo	None available
Diagnosis	IgM anti-HAV, elevated liver enzyme (nonspecific)	HBsAg, HBcAg, HbeAg, HBV DNA, elevated liver enzymes (nonspecific)	HCV RNA, anti-HCV, elevated liver enzymes (nonspecific)

Abbreviation: DNA, deoxyribonucleic acid; HAV, hepatitis A virus; HBV, hepatitis B virus; HCV, hepatitis C virus; IM, intramuscular; IV, intravenous drug; RNA, ribonucleic acid.

forms of viral hepatitis because coinfection is common and harder to treat.

Hepatitis A Prevention

Good personal hygiene and proper disposal of sanitary waste are required to prevent fecal-oral transmission of HAV. This includes frequent hand washing with soap and water after using the bathroom and prior to eating meals. Drinking bottled water in areas where HAV is most endemic will also minimize the risk of becoming infected with HAV. Individuals

at high risk of acquiring HAV should receive either serum immune globulin (IG) or HAV vaccine.

Immune Globulin

IG contains antibodies from pooled human plasma that provides passive immunization against various infectious diseases, including HAV. IG is available in intravenous (IVIG) or intramuscular (IGIM) formulations, but only IGIM is used for prevention of HAV. IGIM is effective in providing pre- and postexposure prophylaxis against HAV, but it does not confer lifelong immunity. Adverse effects of IGIM are rare; however, there have been reports of anaphylaxis in individuals who have immunoglobulin A deficiency. IgA deficient patients should not receive IGIM.

HAV Vaccine

HAV vaccine (Havrix; Vaqta) is an inactivated virus administered intramuscularly for adults and children older than 1 year of age. HAV vaccine is recommended for children, persons traveling to countries with endemic HAV, men who have sex with men, chronic liver disease patients, intravenous drug users, patients who receive clotting factors, and people with occupational exposure to primates or HAV. For pretravel vaccination, the HAV vaccine should be administered at least 2 weeks prior to expected exposure.

Hepatitis B Prevention

Hepatitis B vaccine (Engerix-B; Recombivax HB) is an inactivated virus administered intramuscularly in multiple doses. Hepatitis B vaccine is indicated for children and adults with occupational exposure to HBV, household and sexual contact of HBV carriers, men who have sex with men, people with multiple heterosexual partners, partners of patients with a newly acquired sexually transmitted disease, patients diagnosed with HIV, intravenous drug users, children born after 1991, infants born to mothers with HBV, patients on hemodialysis, patients with chronic liver disease, and people arriving to the United States from endemic HBV areas. Twinrix is a preparation for adults that contains immunizations for HAV and HBV in one vaccine. The preparation contains a trace amount of neomycin and should be used with caution in patients who are allergic to neomycin.

Vaccine Adverse Reactions

Adverse reactions to the HAV and HBV vaccines include soreness, warmth, and erythema at the injection site, drowsiness, headache, and fever. Rare cases (<1%) of Guillain-Barré syndrome have been reported. The only contraindication to HAV and HBV vaccines includes hypersensitivity to HAV or HBV and yeast (HBV and Twinrix vaccines).

HAV and HBV vaccines are pregnancy category C. Pregnancy is not a contraindication for the HAV and HBV vaccines and none of the products contain the preservative thimerosal.

TREATMENT

The treatment goals of viral hepatitis vary by the infecting virus. HAV treatment is supportive or preventative in nature. Management of chronic forms of hepatitis consists of viral suppression (HBV), and virus eradication (HCV) to prevent long-term complications (eg, cirrhosis and hepatocellular carcinoma). Surrogate endpoints indicating treatment response include normalization of serum liver function tests (eg, ALT), reduced viral load, and histologic improvement. Treatment initiation for HBC and HCV is based upon viral load, liver histology from biopsy, and liver function tests. Tables 44-2 and 44-3 summarize treatment regimens for HBV and HCV.

TABLE 44-2	**Drug Therapy for Chronic HBV**
	Hepatitis B
Treatment	Pegylated-interferon α-2a (Pegasys) or one of the following: lamivudine (Epivir), adefovir (Hepsera), entecavir (Baraclude), telbivudine (Tyzeka), tenofovir (Viread)
Duration	Pegylated-interferon α-2a (Pegasys): 48 wk, NRTIs: 6-12 mo after HBeAg seroconversion if HBeAg positive patient or until loss of HBsAg if HBeAg negative patient
Efficacy	Varies per agent and the presence of HBeAg

Chronic Hepatitis B

Patients with chronic HBV have either e-antigen positive or negative disease. E-antigen negative disease is more difficult to treat and requires longer treatment duration. Chronic HBV can be treated with peg-interferon α-2a (Pegasys) or a nucleoside/nucleotide reverse transcriptase inhibitor (NRTI). Peg-interferon α-2a and the NRTIs are similar in efficacy for e-antigen positive and negative HBV; however, seroconversion of the e-antigen occurs more often at 1 year for peginterferon α-2a and 2 years for NRTIs. Viral resistance does not develop to peg-interferon α-2a, but is associated with NRTIs. Lamivudine was the first NRTI used to treat chronic HBV, but it is plagued with a high incidence of viral resistance and cross-resistance. Adefovir is structurally similar to tenofovir, but is less potent than tenofovir in suppressing HBV levels. Telbivudine offers another option in select patients, but viral resistance was reported in 25% of patients after 2 years of treatment. When treatment with NRTIs is indicated, tenofovir and entecavir are preferred agents due to decreased chance of resistance, favorable side effect profile, and once daily dosing. Tenofovir may be used preferentially in patients previously exposed to lamivudine due to potential cross-resistance with entecavir. If entecavir is used in patients in whom lamivudine resistance is suspected, the higher dose of entecavir 1 mg/d should be used. Studies involving combination therapy with NRTIs have not shown improved results compared to monotherapy; therefore, combination therapy is not warranted in most patients.

The most common interferon adverse effects are flu-like symptoms (fever, headache, nausea, musculoskeletal pain, myalgia, and weakness), thrombocytopenia, neutropenia, depression, alopecia, fatigue, anxiety, and insomnia. Severe adverse effects include hepatic decompensation, bone marrow suppression, gastrointestinal hemorrhage or ischemic colitis, hemorrhagic or ischemic stroke, pulmonary disease including respiratory failure, and severe psychiatric side effects (depression, suicidal ideation, and suicide attempt). There are black box warnings for caution in patients with neuropsychiatric disorders, autoimmune disease, persistent severe infections, and ischemic disorders. Contraindications to interferon therapy include hypersensitivity to the drug, autoimmune hepatitis, and decompensated cirrhosis.

The NRTIs, including lamivudine (Epivir), adefovir (Hepsera), entecavir (Baraclude), telbivudine (Tyzeka), and

TABLE 44-3	AASLD/IDSA Recommended Treatment Regimens for Treatment-Naïve Patients with Hepatitis C (in Alphabetical Order)	
HCV Genotype	**No Cirrhosis**	**Compensated Cirrhosis**
1a	Elbasvir/grazoprevir for 12 wk[a] Glecaprevir/pibrentasvir for 8 wk Ledipasvir/sofosbuvir for 12 wk Ledipasvir/sofosbuvir for 8 wk[b] Sofosbuvir/velpatasvir for 12 wk	Elbasvir/grazoprevir for 12 wk[a] Glecaprevir/pibrentasvir for 12 wk Ledipasvir/sofosbuvir for 12 wk Sofosbuvir/velpatasvir for 12 wk
1b	Elbasvir/grazoprevir for 12 wk Glecaprevir/pibrentasvir for 8 wk Ledipasvir/sofosbuvir for 12 wk Ledipasvir/sofosbuvir for 8 wk[b] Sofosbuvir/velpatasvir for 12 wk	Elbasvir/grazoprevir for 12 wk Glecaprevir/pibrentasvir for 12 wk Ledipasvir/sofosbuvir for 12 wk Sofosbuvir/velpatasvir for 12 wk
2	Glecaprevir/pibrentasvir for 8 wk Sofosbuvir/velpatasvir for 12 wk	Glecaprevir/pibrentasvir for 12 wk Sofosbuvir/velpatasvir for 12 wk
3	Glecaprevir/pibrentasvir for 8 wk Sofosbuvir/velpatasvir for 12 wk	Glecaprevir/pibrentasvir for 12 wk Sofosbuvir/velpatasvir for 12 wk

Abbreviations: HCV, hepatitis C virus; wk, weeks

[a]Negative baseline viral resistance testing to elbasvir is required for all genotype 1a patients.

[b]Duration can be shortened to 8 weeks for patients who are non-black, HIV-negative, and have HCV RNA level < 6 million IU/mL.

Data from AASLD/IDSA/IAS-USA. Recommendations for testing, managing, and treating hepatitis C. Available at: http://www.hcvguidelines.org. Accessed Sept. 15, 2015.

tenofovir (Viread), inhibit HBV polymerase. Administered orally, they are well tolerated with few adverse effects. Headache and gastrointestinal problems are the most commonly reported side effects. Rare, but serious side effects include lactic acidosis, hepatomegaly with steatosis, and HBV exacerbation upon discontinuation of the NRTI (black box warning). Adefovir and tenofovir can cause nephrotoxicity; therefore serum creatinine should be monitored closely. Telbivudine may cause peripheral neuropathy and increased creatine kinase.

Chronic Hepatitis C

The primary goal of therapy is to eradicate HCV infection. Virologic cure, or sustained virologic response (SVR), is defined as a nondetectable HCV RNA at least 12 weeks after completing HCV therapy. The treatment of chronic HCV was revolutionized with the approval of direct-acting antivirals (DAAs). Previously, HCV treatment included the injection of peg-interferon and was associated with a substantial side-effect profile. The current standard of care for all chronic HCV infections, regardless of genotype, is an all-oral regimen. Tables 44-3 and 44-4 list therapeutic regimens for HCV patients. The need for concomitant ribavirin use varies. Patients who are treatment-experienced, in whom prior peg-IFN and ribavirin therapy failed, and who have cirrhosis may require either a longer treatment duration or the addition of ribavirin. Ribavirin is a weak antiviral drug indicated for treatment of HCV when used in combination. Ribavirin requires dosage modifications in renal dysfunction with CrCl less than 50 mL/min. Other contraindications include pregnancy, male partners of pregnant females, autoimmune hepatitis, decompensated cirrhosis, and sickle cell anemia. Adverse effects to ribavirin include rash, dry skin, nausea, anorexia, decreased weight, alopecia, and dose-related hemolytic anemia. There are black box warnings for hemolytic anemia, pregnancy, and warnings against ribavirin monotherapy.

The treatment of hepatitis C has significantly changed over the last several years and continues to change very rapidly. Please refer to the hepatitis C treatment guidelines for the most recent additions—www.hcvguidelines.org.

SPECIAL CONSIDERATIONS

Pregnant females with chronic HBV should be treated with an NRTI during the third trimester to prevent perinatal transmission. Approximately 90% of children whose mothers were not treated with antiviral therapy during the third trimester will develop HBV within 6 months of birth. Most of the safety data in pregnancy has been collected with lamivudine and tenofovir.

Peg-interferon is pregnancy category C, but severe birth defects have occurred in fetuses exposed to ribavirin (pregnancy category X) either directly from the pregnant female or indirectly from the male sexual partner. All men and women of childbearing age should use two forms of contraception during ribavirin therapy and for 6 months following discontinuation of ribavirin. A Ribavirin Registry is required by the FDA to collect and evaluate in utero exposure to ribavirin during gestation and up to 6 months preconception. Both health care providers and patients can provide information to this important registry.

HBV or HCV coinfection with HIV is common and presents a treatment challenge secondary to drug interactions and side effects from complex drug regimens. In HBV/HIV coinfection, NRTI monotherapy should be avoided because HIV may develop resistance to the NRTIs used to treat HBV (exception—telbivudine). Therefore, unless telbivudine is used, combination NRTI therapy with HBV activity is warranted. Tenofovir/emtricitabine is often used in HBV/HIV coinfected patients due to dual activity against both viruses; however, this combination requires the addition of at least one additional agent (eg, HIV NNRTI or Protease inhibitor) for optimal HIV suppression. Continued long-term therapy with

				Comparison of Recommended Hepatitis C Virus Direct Acting Antivirals[a]	

TABLE 44-4   **Comparison of Recommended Hepatitis C Virus Direct Acting Antivirals**[a]

Trade Name	Generic Name & Adult Dose	Drug Class	Use in Cirrhosis	Use in Renal Insufficiency	Adverse Effects[b]
Zepatier	Elbasvir 50 mg Grazoprevir 100 mg	NS5A inhibitor Protease inhibitor	Not recommended in CTP Class B or C	No dosage adjustment needed	Fatigue, headache, nausea
Mavyret	Glecaprevir 300 mg Pibrentasvir 120 mg	Protease inhibitor NS5A inhibitor	Not recommended in CTP Class B or C	No dosage adjustment needed	Fatigue, headache
Harvoni	Ledipasvir 90 mg Sofosbuvir 400 mg	NS5A inhibitor NS5B inhibitor	No dosage adjustment needed	Not recommended if eGFr < 30 mL/min/1.73 m^2	Fatigue, headache, nausea, diarrhea, insomnia
Epclusa	Sofosbuvir 400 mg Velpatasvir 100 mg	NS5B inhibitor NS5A inhibitor	No dosage adjustment needed	Not recommended if eGFr < 30 mL/min/1.73 m^2	Headache, fatigue, nausea, insomnia
Vosevi	Sofosbuvir 400 mg Velpatasvir 100 mg Voxilaprevir 100 mg	NS5B inhibitor NS5A inhibitor Protease inhibitor	Not recommended in CTP Class B or C	Not recommended if eGFr < 30 mL/min/1.73 m^2	Headache, fatigue, nausea, insomnia

Abbreviations: CTP, Child-Turcotte-Pugh; eGFR, estimated glomerular filtration rate; NS, nonstructural protein.
[a]All recommended regimens listed are co-formulated tablets taken once daily.
[b]Listed in order of frequency reported in clinical trials. Frequency of adverse effects increases with increased duration.
Reproduced with permission from DiPiro JT, Talbert RL, Yee GC, et al: *Pharmacotherapy: A Pathophysiologic Approach*, 10th ed. New York, NY: McGraw-Hill; 2017.

the NRTIs is common because the HBV poorly responds to treatment in the HBV/HIV coinfected patient population.

HCV treatment in HCV/HIV coinfected patients should not begin until the patient's HIV is well controlled on medications. If the HIV regimen contains didanosine, either an alternative HIV medication should be chosen or ribavirin should be excluded from the HCV treatment regimen due to additive and profound anemia. The only peg-interferon treatment indicated for HCV/HIV coinfection is peg-interferon α-2a (Pegasys). Limited studies with DAAs suggest that HCV/HIV coinfected patients have a similar cure rate when compared to HCV monoinfected patients.

HBV/HCV coinfection leads to more severe liver disease and an increased risk of hepatocellular carcinoma. There are no treatment guidelines for treating HBV/HCV coinfected patients, treatment should be individualized to the patient.

POSTEXPOSURE PROPHYLAXIS

Postexposure prophylaxis for HAV and HBV includes vaccination and IG within 14 days of exposure to the virus. IG (GamaSTAN) and hepatitis B IG (HepaGam B; HyperHEP B S/D; Nabi-HB) provide protection by imparting passive immunity for patients exposed to HBV and HAV, respectively.

Adverse reactions to intramuscular IG and HBIG include pain and swelling at the injection site, headache, muscle pain, nausea, and vomiting. Because IGs are prepared from human plasma, a risk exists for acquiring HIV or viral hepatitis. The only contraindications to IG and HBIG are hypersensitivity to the products. IG and HBIG are pregnancy category C.

CASE Application

1. Select the most common mode of transmission for the hepatitis A virus (HAV).

   a. Blood
   b. Fecal-oral route
   c. Perinatal exposure
   d. Semen

2. Which of the following forms of viral hepatitis can be cured with drug therapy?

   a. Chronic hepatitis A
   b. Chronic hepatitis B
   c. Chronic hepatitis C
   d. Viral hepatitis can never be cured

3. Which of the following represent a rare side effect associated with Twinrix (hepatitis A/B vaccine)?

   a. Stevens-Johnson syndrome
   b. Neuroleptic syndrome
   c. Guillain-Barré syndrome
   d. Red-man syndrome

4. Which of the following best represents the pregnancy category when ribavirin is added to a HCV regimen?

   a. B
   b. C
   c. D
   d. X

5. A 58-year-old man diagnosed with chronic hepatitis C (HCV) genotype 1a is to begin therapy with ledipasvir/sofosbuvir + ribavirin. Which of the following counseling topics is appropriate? Select all that apply.

   a. He should use two forms of birth control.
   b. His HCV treatment will last 48 weeks.
   c. He likely developed HCV from a contaminated food source.
   d. He should not share razors or toothbrushes with anyone.

6. LO is a 28-year-old woman who found out her boyfriend has chronic hepatitis B (HBV). They are sexually active

and plan to marry in 6 months. Which of the following is the best course of action? Select all that apply.

a. Administer HBIG
b. Begin the HBV vaccine series
c. Initiate lamivudine
d. Offer HBV screening

7. Which of the following signs and symptoms may LO experience if she develops HBV? Select all that apply.

a. Jaundice
b. Nausea
c. Elevated liver enzymes
d. She may experience no physical symptoms

8. MO is a 19-year-old Asian man diagnosed with chronic HBV acquired from perinatal exposure. He will begin therapy with entecavir today. Entecavir will likely

a. Be combined with ribavirin
b. Eradicate the HBV virus
c. Develop resistance
d. Cause minimal side effects

9. Rank the following HCV treatment regimens based on their likelihood of clinical cure (SVR) from lowest to highest cure rate. (ALL options must be used.)

Unordered Options	Ordered Response
Interferon α monotherapy	
Peg-interferon α-2b, ribavirin, and telaprevir	
Peg-interferon α-2b and ribavirin	
Sofosbuvir/velpatasvir	

10. Immune globulin (GamaSTAN) is indicated for postexposure prophylaxis for which of the following?

a. Autoimmune hepatitis
b. Hepatitis A virus
c. Hepatitis B virus
d. Hepatitis C virus

11. Which of the following drugs has the highest incidence of hemolytic anemia?

a. Ribavirin
b. Peg-interferon α-2a
c. Lamivudine
d. Tenofovir

12. DP is a 42-year-old woman who has developed chronic HBV from longstanding intravenous drug use. Her physician asks you to recommend an NRTI that has both high potency and low viral resistance. Rank the following HBV treatment regimens from best to worse choice. (ALL options must be used.)

Unordered Options	Ordered Response
Telbivudine	
Lamivudine	
Entecavir	
Adefovir	

13. A 54-year-old man with HCV genotype 2 infection, treatment-naive and no cirrhosis presents for treatment initiation. Which of the following would be the best treatment option?

a. Peg-interferon and ribavirin for 24 weeks
b. Peg-interferon and ribavirin for 48 weeks
c. Glecaprevir/pibretansvir for 8 weeks
d. Sofosbuvir and ribavirin for 24 weeks

14. RM is a man who has just learned he is coinfected with HIV/HCV. When should RM's chronic HCV be treated?

a. Immediately.
b. As soon as his HIV is well controlled with medication.
c. Never. His HCV is not treatable.
d. After he develops decompensated cirrhosis.

15. DA has been diagnosed with chronic HCV genotype 1. His past medical and social histories include a history of IV drug abuse, alcoholism, a wife (married 30 years) with chronic HCV, and a blood transfusion in 2002. During your patient counseling session, DA asks you how he most likely acquired HCV. You correctly tell him.

a. Blood transfusion in 2002
b. Sexually transmitted from his wife
c. Intravenous drug abuse
d. Alcoholism

16. BR is a 47-year-old woman coinfected with HBV and HIV. The physician wants to prescribe a nucleoside reverse transcriptase inhibitor (NRTI) monotherapy to treat BR's chronic HBV. Which of the following NRTIs should you recommend?

a. Lamivudine
b. Entecavir
c. Telbivudine
d. Tenofovir

17. Which of the following drugs has been given a black box warning by the FDA for the risk of severe depression and suicidal risk?

a. Ribavirin
b. Peg-interferons
c. Nucleoside reverse transcriptase inhibitors
d. Hepatitis B immune globulin (HBIG)

18. Which of the following products should not be given concomitantly with live vaccines?

a. Engerix-B
b. Recombivax HB
c. Twinrix
d. GamaSTAN

19. MM, a 21-year-old woman, has been exposed to hepatitis C. Which of the following is the most appropriate course of action?

    a. Do nothing unless MM acquires hepatitis C.
    b. Administer immune globulin.
    c. Begin peg-interferon and ribavirin.
    d. Begin lamivudine.

20. TO is a 42-year-old patient prescribed lamivudine for HBV. Which of the following products contain lamivudine and may be used for HBV in TO?

    a. Viread
    b. Combivir
    c. Epivir
    d. Emtriva

TAKEAWAY POINTS »

- HAV, HBV, and HCV are the most common forms of viral hepatitis.
- HAV is an acute disease; while HBV and HCV can cause acute and chronic diseases.
- Viral hepatitis is spread via the following route(s): HAV (fecal-oral route), HBV (blood and bodily secretions), and HCV (blood).
- Acute and chronic viral hepatitis patients are often asymptomatic with elevated liver enzymes being the first indicator of disease.
- Prevention vaccines are available for HAV and HBV, but there is no vaccine for HCV.
- The duration of chronic HBV treatment is 1 year for peg-interferon α-2a, but is usually greater than 1 year for monotherapy with nucleoside/nucelotide reverse transcriptase inhibitors (NRTIs).
- The NRTIs drugs have few side effects, but viral resistance and cross-resistance are common.
- Pregnant females with HBV should be treated with NRTIs in the third trimester to reduce the transmission of HBV to the fetus.
- NRTI monotherapy should be avoided in patients with HIV/HBV coinfection because HIV can develop resistance to all of the NRTIs used to treat HBV with the exception of telbivudine. Therefore, unless telbivudine is used, combination NRTI therapy is warranted.
- Current treatment for chronic HCV treatment should include triple-therapy with daily oral ribavirin, weekly subcutaneous peg-interferon, and either sofosbuvir or simeprevir for 12 to 48 weeks in genotype 1 or 4. For genotype 2 infected HCV patients, treatment should consist of sofosbuvir and ribavirin for 12 weeks. In genotype 3 infected patients should receive sofosbuvir and ribavirin extended to 24 weeks.
- Interferon products are associated with serious adverse effects including hepatic decompensation, bone marrow suppression, gastrointestinal hemorrhage or ischemic colitis, hemorrhagic or ischemic stroke, pulmonary disease including respiratory failure, and severe psychiatric side effects (depression, suicidal ideation, and suicide attempt).
- Ribavirin is pregnancy category X. Pregnant women should forgo treatment for chronic HCV until after delivery. All men and women of childbearing age should use two forms of contraception during therapy and for 6 months following discontinuation of ribavirin. A Ribavirin Registry is required by the FDA to collect and evaluate in utero exposure to ribavirin during gestation and up to 6 months preconception.
- Patients coinfected with HIV/HCV should not be treated for chronic HCV unless HIV is well controlled with medication.
- Postexposure prophylaxis for HAV and HBV involves the provision of passive immunity with an IG and the HAV and HBV vaccines. There is no postexposure prophylaxis for HCV.

BIBLIOGRAPHY

Acosta EP, Flexner C. Antiviral agents (nonretroviral). In: Brunton LL, Chabner BA, Knollmann BC, eds. *Goodman & Gilman's The Pharmacological Basis of Therapeutics*. 12th ed. New York, NY: McGraw-Hill; 2011:chap 58.

Deming P. Viral hepatitis. In: DiPiro JT, Talbert RL, Yee GC, Matzke GR, Wells BG, Posey L, eds. *Pharmacotherapy: A Pathophysiologic Approach*. 10th ed. New York, NY: McGraw-Hill; 2017.

Dienstag JL. Acute viral hepatitis. In: Longo DL, Fauci AS, Kasper DL, Hauser SL, Jameson J, Loscalzo J, eds. *Harrison's Principles of Internal Medicine*. 18th ed. New York, NY: McGraw-Hill; 2012:chap 304.

Safrin S. Antiviral agents. In: Katzung BG, Masters SB, Trevor AJ, eds. *Basic & Clinical Pharmacology*. 12th ed. New York, NY: McGraw-Hill; 2012:chap 49.

KEY ABBREVIATIONS

DAAs = direct-acting antivirals
HAV = hepatitis A virus
HBV = hepatitis B virus
HCV = hepatitis C virus
IG = immune globulin

IGIM = intramuscular immune globulin
IVIG = intravenous immune globulin
NRTI = nucleoside/nucleotide reverse transcriptase inhibitor
SVR = sustained virologic response

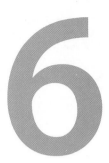

PART

6

Respiratory Disorders

45 Chronic Obstructive Pulmonary Disease

Miranda R. Andrus and Nathan A. Pinner

FOUNDATION OVERVIEW

Chronic obstructive pulmonary disease (COPD) is a preventable chronic disease of the airways characterized by gradual, progressive loss of lung function. COPD patients have airflow limitation that is not fully reversible. The airflow limitation is associated with an abnormal inflammatory response of the lung to noxious particles or gases. Emphysema and chronic bronchitis are often present in COPD, but patients must also have abnormal spirometry to be formally diagnosed with COPD. Emphysema is an abnormal permanent enlargement of the airspaces distal to the terminal bronchioles, accompanied by destruction of their walls and without fibrosis. Chronic bronchitis is inflammation of the bronchioles with mucus hypersecretion and chronic productive cough. Because most patients exhibit some features of emphysema and chronic bronchitis, the appropriate emphasis of COPD pathophysiology is on small airway disease and parenchymal damage that contributes to chronic airflow limitation.

The most common risk factor for COPD is cigarette smoking; however, not all smokers develop COPD. Inhalation exposure risk factors include occupational dusts and chemicals (chemical agents and fumes), indoor air pollution (wood, animal dung, crop residues, and coal burned in open fires), and outdoor air pollution. A rare genetic disorder called alpha 1 antitrypsin (AAT) deficiency is also a risk factor for COPD. AAT deficiency causes patients to develop COPD at an early age (20-50 years). Patients presenting with COPD at an early age or a strong family history should be screened for this disorder. Another potential risk factor is impaired lung growth during gestation, birth, and childhood. Oxidative stress, or a depletion of antioxidants in the lungs plays a role in the development of COPD and can initiate lung inflammation and injury. Respiratory infections (viral and bacterial) may contribute to the pathogenesis of COPD and are considered a risk factor.

COPD is caused by amplification of the normal inflammatory response to chronic irritants such as cigarette smoke. Inflammatory mediators increased in COPD patients include neutrophils, macrophages, and lymphocytes. Oxidative stress generated by oxidants released by cigarette smoke and other inhaled substances and a reduction in endogenous antioxidants also contribute to lung inflammation. An imbalance between the proteases that break down connective tissue in the lung and the antiproteases that protect against this is also seen in COPD. These characteristics lead to airflow limitation and air trapping, resulting in hyperinflation of the lungs. This reduces the capacity of the lungs to fill during inspiration, resulting in dyspnea, particularly during exertion. Gas exchange abnormalities also result, with hypoxemia and hypercapnia common in COPD. Finally, mucus hypersecretion and chronic productive cough are often present due to chronic irritation of the airway.

Symptoms characteristic of COPD are dyspnea, chronic cough, and sputum production. Dyspnea is usually present every day, worsened by exertion, and progressively worsens over time. Patients describe an increased effort to breathe or gasping. Patients with symptoms of COPD and exposure to risk factors should be tested with spirometry to confirm a diagnosis. The Global Initiative for Chronic Obstructive Lung Disease (GOLD) guidelines define COPD as a post-bronchodilator forced expiratory volume in 1 second (FEV_1) to forced vital capacity (FVC) ratio of less than 0.7 in the presence of characteristics symptoms of COPD. The GOLD guidelines also classify the severity of airflow limitation by reduction in post-bronchodilator FEV_1 (Table 45-1).

COPD is a progressive disease, and even with the best treatment, will worsen over time. Treatment is directed at managing symptoms or preventing exacerbations. The most common complication of COPD is acute exacerbations of symptoms. A COPD exacerbation is defined as an acute change from baseline in cough and/or sputum production that is beyond day-to-day variations. Exacerbations affect the prognosis of COPD, lead to poor long-term outcomes, and increase mortality. Pulmonary hypertension may develop due to hypoxic vasoconstriction of the pulmonary arteries and lead to cor pulmonale. Additionally, systemic features may develop and include skeletal muscle wasting, osteoporosis, depression, cardiovascular disease, and lung cancer.

TREATMENT

The GOLD guidelines recommend treatment groups based on risk of exacerbations (determined by history of exacerbations) and symptoms (Table 45-2). Patients are considered high risk if they experienced greater than or equal to 2 exacerbations, or 1 exacerbation requiring hospitalization, in the preceding

TABLE 45-1	GOLD Stages of Airflow Limitation	
Grade*	Description	FEV$_1$
1	Mild	≥80% predicted
2	Moderate	<80% and ≥50% predicted
3	Severe	<50% and ≥30% predicted
4	Very severe	<30% predicted

*All patients have FEV$_1$/FVC <0.70.

TABLE 45-3	Goals of Treatment for COPD
Relieve symptoms	
Improve exercise tolerance	
Improve health status	
Prevent disease progression	
Prevent and treat exacerbations	
Reduce mortality	

year. Symptoms are assessed by a variety of symptom scores, with the most common being the Modified Medical Research Council (mMRC) questionnaire. A score of greater than or equal to 2 is considered a high level of symptoms (scale 0-4, with 0 indicating breathlessness with strenuous exercise and 4 being too breathless to leave the house). The treatment goal of COPD is effective management and prevention of exacerbations. The goals of management are listed in Table 45-3.

Nonpharmacologic Treatment

Smoking cessation is the most effective treatment for reducing the progression of COPD. Tobacco dependence is a chronic condition that warrants intensive and repeated treatment with counseling and pharmacotherapy until abstinence is achieved.

Pulmonary rehabilitation improves exercise capacity, health-related quality of life, and survival. Additionally, pulmonary rehabilitation reduces hospitalizations, anxiety, and depression and should be considered for patients with COPD. A comprehensive pulmonary rehabilitation program includes exercise training, nutrition counseling, and education.

Oxygen therapy is often necessary for COPD patients with resting hypoxemia (oxygen saturation <88% on room air). Oxygen therapy for patients with chronic respiratory failure has been shown to increase survival. All patients with COPD should receive the influenza vaccine annually and the pneumococcal vaccine (PPSV 23).

Pharmacologic Treatment

COPD medications are effective for reducing or relieving symptoms, improving exercise tolerance, reducing the number and severity of exacerbations, and improving the quality of life. No medication slows the rate of decline in lung function or reduces mortality.

TABLE 45-2	GOLD Patient Groups Based on Risk and Symptoms	
	Risk Assessment	
Group	Exacerbations/year	Symptoms
A	0-1	Low
B	0-1	High
C	≥2*	Low
D	≥2*	High

*1 exacerbation if requires hospitalization.

Bronchodilators

Bronchodilators are the mainstay of treatment for symptomatic COPD. They reduce symptoms, improve exercise tolerance, and improve quality of life. Bronchodilator medications include β$_2$-agonists, anticholinergics, and theophylline. The inhaled route is the preferred route for β$_2$-agonists and anticholinergics; however, attention must be paid to proper inhaler technique. Clinicians should advise, counsel, and observe patient technique with the devices frequently and consistently. Combining different bronchodilator therapies may improve efficacy and is preferred over increasing the dose of a single agent (due to increased risk of adverse drug reactions and flat dose-response curves). Bronchodilators work by reducing the tone of airway smooth muscle (relaxation), thus minimizing airflow limitation. The initial therapy for COPD patients with intermittent symptoms and low risk of exacerbations (Group A patients) is short-acting bronchodilators as needed. Among these agents, the choices are a short-acting β$_2$-agonist or a short-acting anticholinergic. These agents have a rapid onset of action, relieve symptoms, and improve lung function. For Group B patients (still at low risk of exacerbations, but with greater symptoms), monotherapy with a long-acting bronchodilator is recommended. Finally, for patients at high risk of exacerbations (Group C-D), the preferred initial therapy is a long-acting anticholinergic or the combination of an inhaled corticosteroid and long-acting β$_2$-agonist.

β$_2$-Agonists β$_2$-Agonists cause airway smooth muscle relaxation by stimulating adenylyl cyclase to increase the formation of cyclic adenosine monophosphate (cAMP). cAMP is responsible for mediating relaxation of bronchial smooth muscle, leading to bronchodilation. β$_2$-Agonists are available in inhalation, oral, and parenteral dosage forms; the inhalation route is preferred because of fewer adverse reactions. β$_2$-Agonists are available in short-acting and long-acting formulations. Short-acting β$_2$-agonists are used for acute symptom relief and maintenance therapy. Short-acting β$_2$-agonists require frequent dosing (albuterol 2 puffs every 6 hours when prescribed on a scheduled basis) and often lose effectiveness when used regularly for more than 3 months (tachyphylaxis). Long-acting β$_2$-agonists last 12 to 24 hours, allowing for once or twice daily dosing and have not been shown to lose effectiveness with regular use. Long-acting β$_2$-agonists are more effective and convenient than short-acting β$_2$-agonists for maintenance therapy, but more expensive. If a patient has a prescription for a long-acting β$_2$-agonist, patients should also have a short-acting β$_2$-agonists available for as-needed use (rescue). Short-acting

TABLE 45-4 β₂-Agonists for COPD

Generic Name	Brand Name	Formulations	Indication	Special Considerations
Short-Acting β₂-Agonists				
Albuterol	Proventil; Ventolin	Aerosol for inhalation, nebulization, oral	Rescue and maintenance for COPD	Tachyphylaxis; requires frequent dosing for maintenance therapy. Adverse reactions: tachycardia, heart palpitations, tremor; use with caution in patients with cardiovascular disease, diabetes, hyperthyroidism, or hypokalemia.
Levalbuterol	Xopenex	Aerosol for inhalation, nebulization	Rescue and maintenance for COPD	Tachyphylaxis; requires frequent dosing for maintenance therapy. Adverse reactions (less than albuterol): tachycardia, heart palpitations, tremor; use with caution in patients with cardiovascular disease, diabetes, hyperthyroidism, or hypokalemia.
Long-Acting β₂-Agonists				
Formoterol	Foradil	Powder for inhalation	Maintenance for COPD	Should not be used as rescue inhaler. β₂ (short- and long-acting) may increase risk of arrhythmias, decrease serum potassium, prolong QTc interval, or increase serum glucose. Use with caution in patients with cardiovascular disease, diabetes, hyperthyroidism, or hypokalemia. β-Agonists may cause elevation in blood pressure, heart rate, and result in CNS stimulation/excitation.
Salmeterol	Serevent	Powder for inhalation	Maintenance for COPD	Same as formoterol
Arformoterol	Brovana	Nebulization	Maintenance for COPD	Same as formoterol
Indacaterol	Arcapta	Powder for inhalation	Maintenance for COPD	Same as formoterol
Vilanterol	Breo	Powder for inhalation	Maintenance for COPD	Same as formoterol
Olodaterol	Striverdi	Inhalation spray	Maintenance for COPD	Same as formoterol

β₂-agonists (albuterol and levalbuterol) are preferred for therapy. Adverse effects of β₂-agonists are dose-related and include palpitations, tachycardia, and tremor. Sleep disturbances may also occur and appear to be worse with higher doses of inhaled long-acting β₂-agonists. Increasing doses beyond those clinically recommended is without benefit and could be associated with increased adverse effects. Table 45-4 compares the β₂-agonists commonly used in the treatment of COPD.

Anticholinergics The anticholinergics produce bronchodilation by competitively blocking muscarinic receptors in bronchial smooth muscle. This activity blocks acetylcholine, with the net effect of a reduction in cyclic guanosine monophosphate. Cyclic guanosine monophosphate normally causes bronchial smooth muscle constriction. They may also decrease mucus secretion, although this effect is variable. Inhaled anticholinergics are well-tolerated with the most common adverse effect being dry mouth. Occasional metallic taste has also been reported with ipratropium. Anticholinergic adverse effects that occur less commonly with inhaled dosage forms include constipation, tachycardia, blurred vision, urinary retention, and precipitation of narrow-angle glaucoma symptoms. Table 45-5 compares the inhaled anticholinergics.

Methylxanthines Methylxanthines, including theophylline and aminophylline, have been available for the treatment of

TABLE 45-5 Inhaled Anticholinergics for COPD

Generic Name	Brand Name	Formulation	Duration	Indication for COPD	Special Considerations
Ipratropium	Atrovent	Aerosol for inhalation, nebulization	Short	Maintenance therapy for COPD	Paradoxical bronchospasm may occur; not indicated for initial treatment of acute episodes of bronchospasm; use with caution in patients with myasthenia gravis, narrow-angle glaucoma, and benign prostatic hyperplasia
Tiotropium	Spiriva	Powder for inhalation	Long	Maintenance therapy for COPD	Same as ipratropium
Aclidinium	Tudorza	Powder for inhalation	Long	Maintenance therapy for COPD	Same as ipratropium
Umeclidinium	Incruse	Powder for inhalation	Long	Maintenance therapy for COPD	Same as ipratropium

COPD for decades and at one time were considered first-line agents. Currently the role of methylxanthines is limited to a patient not responding to β_2-agonists, anticholinergics, or corticosteroids. Methylxanthines are nonspecific phosphodiesterase inhibitors that increase intracellular cAMP within airway smooth muscle resulting in bronchodilation. Theophylline has a modest bronchodilator effect and its use is limited due to a narrow therapeutic index and multiple-drug interactions. Theophylline's bronchodilator effects are dependent upon achieving adequate serum concentrations and therapeutic drug monitoring is needed to optimize therapy because of wide interpatient variability. If theophylline is used, serum concentrations in the range of 5 to 15 mg/L (28-83 μmol/L) provide adequate clinical response with a greater margin of safety than the traditionally recommended range of 10 to 20 mg/L (55-110 μmol/L). The most common adverse effects include heartburn, restlessness, insomnia, irritability, tachycardia, and tremor. Dose-related adverse effects include nausea and vomiting, seizures, and arrhythmias. Tobacco smoke contains a chemical that induces the cytochrome P-450 isoenzymes 1A1, 1A2, and 2E1. Theophylline is metabolized by 1A2 and 2E1, and therefore, smoking leads to increased clearance of theophylline.

Anti-Inflammatory Drugs

Corticosteroids Symptomatic patients with severe COPD (FEV_1 <50% predicted) and frequent exacerbations should be considered for treatment with inhaled corticosteroids. Regular treatment with *inhaled* corticosteroids decreases the number of exacerbations per year and improves health status; however, corticosteroid therapy does not slow the long-term decline in pulmonary function, and is associated with higher rates of pneumonia. The anti-inflammatory mechanisms of corticosteroids include: (1) reduction in capillary permeability to decrease mucus, (2) inhibition of release of proteolytic enzymes from leukocytes, and (3) inhibition of prostaglandins. Appropriate situations to consider corticosteroids in COPD include short-term systemic use for acute exacerbations and inhalation therapy for chronic management. Long-term systemic corticosteroid use should be avoided due to an unfavorable risk/benefit ratio. The steroid myopathy that can result from long-term use of oral corticosteroids weakens muscles, further decreasing the respiratory drive in patients with advanced disease. Other long-term adverse effects of systemic corticosteroid therapy include osteoporosis, thinning of the skin, development of cataracts, and adrenal suppression. Inhaled corticosteroids have an improved risk-to-benefit ratio compared to systemic corticosteroid therapy. Upon discontinuation of inhaled corticosteroids, some patients experience deterioration in lung function and an increase in dyspnea and mild exacerbations; it is reasonable to reinstitute the medication in these patients. The most common adverse effects from inhaled corticosteroid therapy include oropharyngeal candidiasis and hoarse voice. These can be minimized by rinsing the mouth after use and by using a spacer device with metered-dose inhalers (MDI). Table 45-6 lists the inhaled corticosteroids and Table 45-7 lists formulations and doses for commonly used COPD medications.

TABLE 45-6	Inhaled Corticosteroids[a,b] for COPD	
Generic Name	**Brand Name**	**Formulations**
Beclomethasone	Beconase AQ	Aerosol for inhalation
Budesonide	Pulmicort	Powder for inhalation
Ciclesonide	Alvesco	Aerosol for inhalation
Flunisolide	AeroBid	Aerosol for inhalation
Fluticasone	Flovent	Aerosol for inhalation; powder for inhalation
Mometasone	Asmanex	Powder for inhalation
Triamcinolone	Azmacort	Aerosol for inhalation

[a]Special considerations: Rinse mouth and throat after use to prevent *Candida* infection. Not for use for the relief of acute bronchospasm (oral systemic corticosteroids may be utilized for COPD exacerbations). Monitoring parameters—growth (adolescents and children[b]), signs and symptoms of adrenal suppression.
[b]Orally inhaled and intranasal corticosteroids may cause a reduction in growth velocity in pediatric patients. COPD patients are often 50 years of age or greater and therefore growth reduction would not be an issue; however, these inhalers may be utilized in younger patients diagnosed with asthma.

Phosphodiesterase-4 Inhibitors Roflumilast is currently the only phosphodiesterase-4 (PDE4) inhibitor approved for the treatment of COPD. It should only be considered in patients with severe COPD, chronic cough and sputum production, and a history of exacerbations. Inhibition of PDE4 leads to increased levels of cAMP and a reduction in inflammation, but does not cause bronchodilation. Use of roflumilast is associated with reductions in exacerbations, without improvements in quality of life scores or mortality. It is administered as a 500 mcg tablet once daily. Common adverse effects reported with roflumilast are gastrointestinal (diarrhea and nausea), weight loss, and psychiatric (insomnia, anxiety). Roflumilast is metabolized by CYP 3A4 and 1A2 and use with strong inducers of cytochrome P450 enzymes (rifampin, carbamazepine) should be avoided. The current role in therapy of roflumilast is not defined and is reserved for patients not responding to the preferred therapies.

SPECIAL CONSIDERATIONS

Other Pharmacologic Therapies

Augmentation therapy is recommended for individuals with AAT deficiency and moderate airflow obstruction (FEV_1 35%-60% predicted). Augmentation therapy consists of weekly transfusions of pooled human AAT with the goal of maintaining adequate plasma levels of the enzyme. Augmentation therapy is not recommended for individuals with AAT deficiency who does not demonstrate lung disease.

Leukotriene modifiers (zafirlukast and montelukast) have not been adequately evaluated in COPD patients and are not recommended for routine use. Nedocromil, a mast cell stabilizer, has not been adequately tested in COPD patients and is not included in the GOLD recommendations. *N*-acetylcysteine has antioxidant and mucolytic activity, which makes it a promising agent for COPD treatment, but current evidence have produced conflicting results. Routine use of *N*-acetylcysteine cannot be recommended at this time. Prophylactic antibiotics

TABLE 45-7 — Formulations and Doses for Commonly Used COPD Medications

Generic/Brand Name	Formulation	Onset	Usual Dose
Short-Acting β_2-Agonists			
Albuterol	Nebulization	5-15 min	2.5 mg every 6-8 h (max: 30 mg/d)
	Inhalation	5-15 min	MDI (90 mcg/inhalation) 1-2 puffs every 4-6 h (max: 1080 mcg/d)
	Oral	7-30 min	2-4 mg tid to qid; extended release: 4-8 mg every 12 h (max: 32 mg/d)
Levalbuterol (Xopenex)	Nebulization	10-20 min	0.63-1.25 mg tid, 6-8 h apart (max: 3.75 mg/d)
	Inhalation	5-10 min	MDI (45 mcg/inhalation) 1-2 puffs every 4-6 h (max: 540 mcg/d)
Long-Acting β_2-Agonists			
Salmeterol (Serevent)	Inhalation	10 min-2 h	Powder (50 mcg/inhalation) 1 puff every 12 h (max: 100 mcg/d)
Formoterol (Foradil)	Inhalation	1-3 min	Powder (12 mcg/inhalation) 1 puff every 12 h (max: 24 mcg/d)
Short-Acting Anticholinergics			
Ipratropium (Atrovent)	Nebulization	15 min	500 mcg every 6-8 h
	Inhalation	15 min	MDI (17 mcg/inhalation) 2 puffs every 6-8 h (max: 12 puffs/d)
Long-Acting Anticholinergics			
Tiotropium (Spiriva)	Inhalation	30 min	Powder (18 mcg/inhalation) 1 puff daily (max: 18 mcg/d)
Aclidinium (Tudorza)	Inhalation	10 min	Powder (400 mcg/inhalation) 1 puff every 12 h (max: 800 mcg/d)
Inhaled Corticosteroids			
Beclomethasone (Qvar)	Inhalation	1-7 d	MDI (40, 80 mcg/inhalation) 40-160 mcg bid (max: 640 mcg/d)
Budesonide (Pulmicort)	Inhalation	1-7 d	Powder (200 mcg/inhalation) 1-2 puffs bid
Fluticasone (Flovent)	Inhalation	1-7 d	MDI (44, 110, 220 mcg/inhalation) 88-440 mcg bid (max: 1760 mcg/d)
Mometasone (Asmanex)	Inhalation	1-7 d	MDI (110, 220 mcg/inhalation) 220-440 mcg daily
Combination Products			
Ipratropium/Albuterol (Combivent)	Inhalation (aerosol)	See individual agents	MDI (18/90 mcg/inhalation) 2 puffs qid (max 12 puffs/d)
	Inhalation (solution)		MDI (20/100 mcg/inhalation) 1 puff qid (max 6 puffs/d)
	Nebulization		0.5/2.5 mg qid
Formoterol/Budesonide (Symbicort)	Inhalation		MDI (4.5/160 mcg/inhalation) 2 puffs bid
Formoterol/Mometasone (Dulera)	Inhalation		MDI (5/100, 5/200 mcg/inhalation) 2 puffs bid
Salmeterol/Fluticasone (Advair)	Inhalation		Powder (50/100, 50/250, 50/500 mcg/inhalation) 1 puff bid MDI (21/45, 21/115, 21/230 mcg/inhalation) 2 puffs bid
Fluticasone/Vilanterol (Breo)	Inhalation		Ellipta (100/25 mcg /inhalation) 2 puffs bid
Vilanterol/Umeclidinium (Anoro)	Inhalation		Ellipta (25/62.5 mcg inhalation) 1 puff once daily
Olodaterol/tiotropium (Stiolto)	Inhalation		Respimat (2.5/2.5 mcg) 2 puffs once daily
Indacaterol/glycopyrrolate (Utibron)	Inhalation		Neohaler (27.5/15.6 mcg) 1 puff bid
Methylxanthines			
Theophylline	Oral	0.2-2 h	400-600 mcg/d divided every 6-24 h based upon the formulation. Doses vary widely and should be based upon pharmacokinetic considerations and plasma theophylline concentrations. Aminophylline is the most widely used salt of theophylline. Aminophylline is usually administered by slow IV injection. The bronchodilation effects of theophylline are proportional to the log of the theophylline concentration. This means that as the theophylline concentration increases, there will be a less than proportional increase in bronchodilation. Patients should always be maintained at the lowest possible theophylline-plasma concentration that produces a satisfactory response. There are numerous factors or disease states that impact theophylline clearance (smoking, cirrhosis, heart failure, drug interactions). The formulation Theo-24 has been associated with dose-dumping when combined with a high-fat meal, other formulations have not been associated with dose dumping.
Phosphodiesterase-4 Inhibitors			
Roflumilast (Daliresp)	Oral	Not defined	500 mcg daily

may reduce the frequency of COPD exacerbations, but due to the risks associated with the long-term use of antibiotics, and minimal benefit, they should only be used for treating infectious exacerbations. Antitussives are contraindicated in COPD because cough has an important protective role.

Pharmacologic Therapy of COPD Exacerbations

An exacerbation is a sustained worsening of the patient's symptoms from his or her usual stable state that is beyond normal day-to-day variations. Commonly reported symptoms are worsening of dyspnea, increased sputum production, and change in sputum color. The most common causes of an exacerbation are respiratory infection and air pollution. Treatment depends upon the symptoms and severity of the exacerbation. Mild exacerbations can often be treated at home with an increase in bronchodilator therapy with or without oral corticosteroids. Antibiotics are indicated only if there are clinical signs of airway infection (eg, increased volume and change in color of sputum and/or fever). Moderate to severe exacerbations require management in the emergency department or hospital. Management should consist of controlled oxygen therapy, bronchodilators, oral or IV corticosteroids, antibiotics if indicated, and consideration of mechanical ventilation.

Outcome Evaluation

COPD patients should be monitored for improvement or worsening of symptoms (dyspnea, cough, sputum production, and fatigue). Changes in the FEV_1 should not be the main outcome that is monitored. FEV_1 changes are weakly related to symptoms, exacerbations, and health related quality of life.

CASE Application

1. A patient presents with symptoms of shortness of breath, nonproductive cough, and the following spirometry results: prebronchodilator FEV_1: 69% predicted; postbronchodilator FEV_1: 70% predicted; FEV_1/FVC ratio: 0.64. How would you interpret these findings?

    a. This patient has COPD with reversible airway obstruction.
    b. This patient has COPD with irreversible airway obstruction.
    c. This patient has asthma with reversible airway obstruction.
    d. This patient does not have asthma since the airway obstruction is irreversible.
    e. This patient does not have COPD or asthma.

2. AB is a 41-year-old white male with COPD confirmed by spirometry. His physician would like to test him for alpha 1 antitrypsin (AAT) deficiency. Which of the following characterizes this disease? Select ALL that apply.

    a. Onset at an early age (<50 years)
    b. Disease caused by environmental factors
    c. Disease caused by genetic factors

    d. Prominent in African American populations
    e. Disease caused by oxidative stress

3. AF is a 59-year-old African American male who currently smokes and has recently been diagnosed with COPD. He currently is classified by the Global Initiative for Chronic Obstructive Lung Disease (GOLD) guidelines as patient group A. Which of the following would be recommended as the first-line treatment for AF?

    a. Short-acting bronchodilator
    b. Long-acting anticholinergic
    c. Long-acting β-agonist
    d. Inhaled corticosteroid
    e. Oral theophylline

4. BD is a 59-year-old man with COPD, hypertension, and dyslipidemia. He reports to your pharmacy complaining of developing a tremor since starting one of his medications. Which medication is the most likely cause?

    a. Ipratropium
    b. Tiotropium
    c. Fluticasone
    d. Prednisone
    e. Albuterol

5. ZH is a 59-year-old with COPD who was recently prescribed a fluticasone inhaler for COPD. He is concerned about the side effects of inhaled corticosteroids and you conduct inhaler counseling for him. Which of the following is the most likely side effect to be caused by inhaled corticosteroids?

    a. Oral candidiasis
    b. Glucose intolerance
    c. Tachycardia
    d. Immunosuppression
    e. Weight gain

6. Which of the following are advantages of using a spacer device with a metered-dose inhaler? Select all that apply.

    a. Decreased oropharyngeal deposition
    b. Enhanced lung delivery
    c. Less hand-lung coordination needed
    d. Reduced side effects from inhaled corticosteroids

7. SS is a 68-year-old woman who smokes and has recently been diagnosed with COPD. In addition to a short-acting bronchodilator, what would you recommend for her treatment? Select all that apply.

    a. Smoking cessation
    b. Influenza vaccine yearly
    c. Pneumococcal vaccine
    d. Oxygen therapy

8. The clinical presentation of COPD can include which of the following? Select all that apply.

    a. Dyspnea
    b. Chronic cough

c. Sputum production

d. Exposure to risk factors

9. CP is a 65-year-old man with COPD, classified by the GOLD guidelines as patient group C. He is currently using albuterol inhaler PRN, salmeterol inhaler twice a day, and tiotropium inhaler once a day. His COPD is still uncontrolled with frequent symptoms and a recent exacerbation. What recommendations would you make to his medication regimen?

a. Add theophylline once daily.

b. Change salmeterol inhaler to fluticasone/salmeterol combination inhaler scheduled twice a day.

c. Add an oral corticosteroid once daily.

d. Change tiotropium inhaler to ipratropium inhaler scheduled four times a day.

e. Do not make any changes.

10. PL is a 75-year-old man who has been experiencing increased dyspnea for the last month. He was diagnosed with COPD 3 years ago and has been taking albuterol metered-dose inhaler on an as needed (prn) basis. He has not had any exacerbations within the last year, and he has an mMRC score of 2. Which of the following is the best choice for changing his medication regimen?

a. Add scheduled inhaled tiotropium and continue prn albuterol.

b. Add scheduled inhaled fluticasone and continue prn albuterol.

c. Add prn inhaled salmeterol and continue prn albuterol.

d. Add scheduled oral theophylline and continue prn albuterol.

e. No changes are necessary at this time.

11. Select the COPD medications that can be used concurrently in a maintenance regimen for a patient classified by the GOLD guidelines as patient group C.

a. Levalbuterol and albuterol

b. Albuterol and formoterol

c. Formoterol and salmeterol

d. Fluticasone and mometasone

e. Theophylline and aminophylline

12. Select the disease state or factor that can affect the clearance of theophylline. Select all that apply.

a. Smoking history

b. Hepatic cirrhosis

c. Drug interactions (cytochrome P-450 inhibitors especially 1A2, 2E1, 3A4)

d. Occasional alcohol use

13. Select the formulation of the corticosteroid that should be utilized in maintenance therapy for COPD.

a. IV/injection (methylprednisolone)

b. Oral (prednisone)

c. Inhalation (fluticasone)

d. Nasal (fluticasone)

14. BD is a 59-year-old Caucasian man with advanced COPD who has been hospitalized with an acute exacerbation. He has been receiving IV aminophylline. His current aminophylline level is 22 mcg/mL. What adverse events would be possible at this level? Select all that apply.

a. Hypotension

b. Arrhythmias

c. Nausea and vomiting

d. Seizures

15. PW is a 49-year-old Caucasian female recently diagnosed with COPD. Her physician plans to start her on a short-acting bronchodilator. Which of the following would be appropriate for the treatment of COPD? Select all that apply.

a. Albuterol inhalation (metered-dose inhaler—90 mcg/puff) as needed "rescue" (prn)

b. Levalbuterol inhalation (metered-dose inhaler—90 mcg/puff) as needed "rescue" (prn)

c. Albuterol oral 4 mg tid

d. Ipratropium inhalation (metered-dose inhaler—17 mcg/puff) as needed "rescue" (prn)

16. AZ is a 67-year-old white male who is receiving 32 mg/h of aminophylline in the hospital. He is ready to be changed to oral theophylline. What would the daily dose of theophylline be that would equal 32 mg/h of aminophylline? Aminophylline's salt factor is 0.8.

a. 614 mg

b. 768 mg

c. 300 mg

d. 900 mg

17. Select the generic name of Symbicort.

a. Fluticasone + salmeterol

b. Albuterol + ipratropium

c. Budesonide + formoterol

d. Mometasone + formoterol

18. KT is a patient that presents to your clinic on Theo-24 (a sustained release/once a day theophylline product). She has experienced the dose-dumping effect when the agent is taken with a high-fat meal. She would like to be changed to another sustained release theophylline product that does not have the dose-dumping effect. Which of the following oral products can be used in replace of Theo-24? Select all that apply.

a. Theo-Dur twice daily

b. Slo-Bid twice daily

c. Uniphyl once daily

d. Aminophylline drip

19. Select the COPD medication that is a phosphodiesterase inhibitor.

    a. Albuterol
    b. Salmeterol
    c. Ipratropium
    d. Fluticasone
    e. Roflumilast

20. AB is a 60-year-old woman recently discharged from the hospital following an exacerbation of her COPD. She was prescribed Advair, Spiriva, and Daliresp. She also has albuterol for prn use. She complains of nausea and weight loss when she is picking up her refills and wants to know if one of these medications could be responsible. Which of the medications is most likely to cause these effects?

    a. Advair (fluticasone/salmeterol)
    b. Daliresp (roflumilast)
    c. Spiriva (tiotropium)
    d. Proair (albuterol)

TAKEAWAY POINTS »

- COPD is a preventable chronic disease of the airways that is characterized by gradual, progressive loss of lung function. It is characterized by airflow limitation that is not fully reversible.

- COPD is a progressive disease and will worsen over time. The most common complication of COPD is exacerbation of symptoms. A COPD exacerbation is defined as an acute change from baseline in cough and/or sputum production that is beyond day-to-day variations.

- Smoking cessation is the most effective treatment for reducing the progression of COPD.

- COPD patients should receive the influenza vaccine annually and the pneumococcal polysaccharide vaccination.

- Bronchodilators are the mainstay of treatment for symptomatic COPD. They reduce symptoms and improve exercise tolerance and quality of life. Bronchodilator medications utilized for COPD include β_2-agonists and anticholinergics.

- In symptomatic patients with severe COPD (FEV_1 <50% predicted) and frequent exacerbations, regular treatment with *inhaled* corticosteroids decreases the number of exacerbations per year and improves health status; however, corticosteroid therapy does not slow the long-term decline in pulmonary function, and leads to higher rates of pneumonia.

- COPD patients should be monitored for improvement or worsening of symptoms (dyspnea, cough, sputum production, and fatigue).

BIBLIOGRAPHY

Advisory committee on immunization practices (ACIP) recommended immunization schedule for adults aged 19 years and older – United States, 2013. *MMWR Surveill Summ.* 2013;62 S9-19.

Barnes PJ. Pulmonary pharmacology. In: Brunton LL, Chabner BA, Knollmann BC, eds. *Goodman & Gilman's The Pharmacological Basis of Therapeutics*, 12th ed. New York, NY: McGraw-Hill; 2011:chap 36.

Bourdet SV, Williams DM. Chronic obstructive pulmonary disease. In: DiPiro JT, Talbert RL, Yee GC, Matzke GR, Wells BG, Posey L, eds. *Pharmacotherapy: A Pathophysiologic Approach*, 10th ed. New York, NY: McGraw-Hill; 2017.

From the Global Strategy for the Diagnosis, Management, and Prevention of COPD, Global Initiative for Chronic Obstructive Lung Disease. (GOLD) 2017. Available at: http://www.goldcopd. Accessed August 29, 2017.

Trevor AJ, Katzung BG, Kruidering-Hall MM, Masters SB. Drugs used in asthma & chronic obstructive pulmonary disease. In: Trevor AJ, Katzung BG, Kruidering-Hall MM, Masters SB, eds. *Katzung & Trevor's Pharmacology: Examination & Board Review*, 10th ed. New York, NY: McGraw-Hill; 2013:chap 20.

KEY ABBREVIATIONS

AAT = alpha 1 antitrypsin
cAMP = cyclic adenosine monophosphate
COPD = chronic obstructive pulmonary disease

FVC = forced vital capacity
GOLD = Global Initiative for Chronic Obstructive Lung Disease
MDI = metered-dose inhalers

46 Asthma

Wendy Brown

FOUNDATION OVERVIEW

The characteristics of asthma are airway inflammation and bronchial hyper-responsiveness which cause variable degree of airflow obstruction. In the asthmatic response, a genetically predisposed or atopic individual is exposed to a specific reactive stimuli or trigger. Common asthma triggers include mold, pollen, animal dander, and dust mites. Minutes after repeated exposure, the immediate asthmatic response occurs causing bronchoconstriction which resolves spontaneously or easily by β_2-agonist use. Within 4 to 12 hours after the immediate asthmatic response, the late asthmatic response, caused by influx of inflammatory cells primarily eosinophils, Th2 lymphocytes, mast cells, macrophages, and mediators such as leukotrienes, histamine, and prostaglandin infiltrate the airway. The reaction is often severe and prolonged and is referred to as an asthma exacerbation. This chronic inflammation is postulated to cause hypertrophy and hyperplasia of the bronchial smooth muscle and mucus glands which may lead to permanent, irreversible obstruction termed airway remodeling. The combination of airway obstruction and inflammation leads to the common symptoms of asthma which are cough (especially one that wakes the patient at night), wheezing, chest tightness, and dyspnea. In the pediatric population, males are twice as likely to be diagnosed with asthma, however, this ratio equals between males and females in adulthood.

Diagnosis is based on a thorough history with special focus on symptoms and genetic predisposition. Spirometry is the initial test used to diagnose asthma. This is a diagnostic test where a person exhales forcefully into a machine to determine if airflow obstruction is present. To determine if obstruction is present, the ratio of the forced expiratory volume in 1 second (FEV_1) over forced vital capacity (FVC) is reviewed (Table 46-1). To determine reversibility, as in asthma, a short-acting β-agonist (SABA) (albuterol) is given and the postbronchodilator FEV_1 is evaluated. If the FEV_1 improves greater or equal to 12% and 200 mL when compared to prebronchodilator value, the person is diagnosed with asthma. Once diagnosis is made, further age-specific evaluation based on impairment and risk is determined in order to classify severity and control of asthma (Tables 46-1 and 46-2). A person is assigned to the highest step based on the most severe sign or symptom and once control has been maintained for at least 3 months, therapy is stepped down.

TREATMENT

Asthma medications are classified into two categories (quick relief and long-term control). Independent of severity, persons with asthma should have a quick relief medication readily available. The class of medication most commonly used as quick relievers is short-acting β_2-selective adrenergic agonists (Table 46-3). They stimulate the β_2-receptor on bronchial smooth muscle to cause relaxation. All are equally effective, have an onset of action within 5 minutes, a peak at 30 to 60 minutes, and duration of 4 to 6 hours. Common side effects associated with short-acting β_2-agonists include tremor, anxiety, and tachycardia. Small dose dependent decreases in serum potassium and magnesium have been observed. Overuse of short-acting β_2-agonists is defined as need for medication use for symptoms of asthma more than 2 days per week or more than twice in a month for nighttime awakenings.

Long-term controller medication should be evaluated for patients who overuse short-acting β_2-agonists. Inhaled corticosteroids (ICSs) are the most effective drug class in helping patients achieve well-controlled asthma. Through their broad effects on gene transcription, they suppress but do not cure, multiple mediators of airway inflammation. All are equally effective at controlling bronchial inflammation and decreasing airway hyperresponsiveness; however, they are not equivalent on a microgram per microgram or puff per puff basis (Table 46-4). In order to achieve maximum benefit, they must be used on a daily basis and education must be provided that it will take at least 2 weeks to 1 month for full effect. Common side effects of low to medium dose-ICSs are thrush and dysphonia. To minimize and prevent these side effects, persons with asthma should be encouraged to rinse and spit with water after inhaler use. If an ICS is delivered via a meter-dose inhaler (MDI), use of a spacer or holding chamber will decrease oral deposition of medication thus decreasing common side effects. At high doses over prolonged periods, patient's risk of developing adrenal suppression, osteoporosis, skin thinning, and cataract formation increases. To maintain a low to medium steroid dose, additional long-term medications such as long-acting β_2-agonists (LABA), leukotriene modifiers, theophylline, and/or biologic agents are added based on patient's asthma severity. LABA have a duration of action of approximately 12 hours. Due to the Salmeterol Multicenter Asthma Research Trial (SMART) trial and subsequent black box warning in regard

To access your complimentary online question exams, visit https://accesspharmacy.mhmedical.com/NAPLEX.aspx

TABLE 46-1 Asthma Severity Classification

	Age	Intermittent[a]—Step 1	Mild Persistent[a]—Step 2	Moderate Persistent[a]—Step 3	Severe Persistent[a]—Steps 4-6
FEV_1/FVC Normal 8-19 y = 85% 20-39 y = 80% 40-59 y = 75% 60-80 y = 70%	0-4 y	≤2 d/wk symptoms 0 (zero) HS awakenings ≤2 d/wk SABA use No limit on normal activity Exacerbation 0-1 × y	>2d/wk symptoms 1-2 × mo HS awakenings >2 d/wk SABA use; not qd SABA Minor limit on normal activity Exacerbation ≥2 × 6 mo; >4 wheezing episodes 1 y lasting >1 d	Daily symptoms 3-4 × mo HS awakenings Daily SABA use Some limit on normal activity Exacerbation ≥2 × 6 mo; >4 wheezing episodes 1 y lasting >1 d	Symptoms throughout the day >1 ×/wk HS awakenings Several times qd SABA use Extremely limits normal activity Exacerbation ≥2 × 6 mo; >4 wheezing episodes 1 y lasting >1 d
	5-11 y	Symptoms, HS awakenings SABA use, activity, and exacerbation same 12+ FEV_1 >80%, Normal FEV_1/FVC	Symptoms, HS awakenings SABA use, activity, and exacerbation same 12+ FEV_1 = 80%, FEV_1/FVC >80%	Symptoms, HS awakenings SABA use, activity, and exacerbation same 12+ FEV_1 60%-80%, FEV_1/FVC 75%-80%	Symptoms, HS awakenings SABA use, activity, and exacerbation same 12+ FEV_1 <60%, FEV_1/FVC <75%
	12+ y	≤2 d/wk symptoms ≤2 × mo HS awakenings ≤2 d/wk SABA No limit on normal activity FEV_1 ≥80%, Normal FEV_1/FVC Exacerbation 0-1 × y	>2d/wk symptoms 3-4 × mo HS awakenings >2 d/wk; not qd; not >1 ×/d SABA Minor limit on normal activity FEV_1 ≥80%, Normal FEV_1/FVC Exacerbation ≥2 × y	Daily symptoms >1 ×/wk not every HS awakenings Daily SABA Some limit on normal activity FEV_1 >60% and <80%, FEV_1/FVC decreased ≤5% Exacerbation ≥2 × y	Symptoms throughout the day 7 ×/wk HS awakenings Several times qd SABA use Extremely limits normal activity FEV_1 <60%, FEV_1/FVC decreased >5% Exacerbation ≥2 × y
Treatment[b]					
	0-4 y	SABA prn	Low ICS Alternatives: Cromolyn Neb/ Montelukast	Medium ICS	Step 4: Medium ICS + LABA or montelukast Step 5: High ICS + LABA or montelukast Step 6: High ICS + LABA or montelukast + po steroid
	5-11 y	SABA prn	Low ICS Alternatives: Cromolyn/LTRA/ Theophylline	Low ICS + LABA, LTRA, or theophylline or medium ICS	Step 4: Medium ICS + LABA[c] Step 5: High ICS + LABA[c] Step 6: High ICS + LABA+ po steroid[c]
	12+ y	SABA prn	Low ICS Alternatives: Cromolyn/LTRA/ Theophylline	Low ICS + LABA or Medium ICS Alternative: Low ICS + LTRA/ Theophylline or zileuton	Step 4: Medium ICS + LABA[d] Step 5: High ICS + LABA consider omalizumab Step 6: High ICS + LABA + po steroid consider omalizumab

Abbreviation: FEV_1, forced expiratory volume in 1 second; FVC, forced vital capacity HS, at bedtime; ICS, inhaled corticosteroid; LABA, long-acting β_2-agonist; LTRA, leukotriene receptor antagonist; SABA, short-acting β-agonist.

[a]Require a SABA prn regardless of need for controller therapy.

[b]Patient is reassessed in 2-6 wk for effectiveness of therapy. When patient is controlled for 3 mo, therapy is step down.

[c]Alternatives: ICS + LTRA or theophylline.

[d]Alternatives: ICS + LTRA, theophylline, or zileuton.

Reproduced with permission from Expert Panel Report 3-Diagnosis and Management of Asthma. NIH Publication Number 09-6147.

to increased risk of death, these medications should never be used alone for control of asthma. Especially in children and adolescents, a single inhaler which contains a LABA and inhaled steroid is recommended. Subsequently, there are five formulations available: Fluticasone propionate/salmeterol (Advair or AirDuo RespiClick), Fluticasone Furoate/vilanterol (Breo Ellipta), budesonide/formoterol (Symbicort), and Mometasone/formoterol (Dulera).

Leukotriene modifiers are divided into two categories to target inflammation. Two antagonize the leukotriene receptor where as the original drug, Zileuton, within this class acts as a 5-lipoxygenase inhibitor (Table 46-3). Common side effect include gastrointestinal symptoms. Patients are to be monitored for behavior and mood changes and the medication discontinued if this occurs. Zafirlukast absorption is affected by food and zileuton may elevate liver enzymes.

TABLE 46-2 Asthma Control Classification

Age	Well-Controlled	Not Well-Controlled	Very Poorly Controlled
0-4 y	≤2 d/wk symptoms ≤1 ×/mo HS awakenings ≤2 d/wk SABA No limit on normal activity 0-1 × y Exacerbation requires po steroids	>2 d/wk symptoms >1 ×/mo HS awakenings >2 d/wk SABA Some limit on normal activity 2-3/y exacerbation requires po steroids	Daily symptoms >1 × wk HS awakenings Several times per day SABA Extreme limit on normal activity >3/y exacerbation requires po steroids
5-11 y	≤2 d/wk not more than once qd symptoms ≤1 ×/mo HS awakenings ≤2 d/wk SABA No limit on normal activity 0-1 × y exacerbation requires po steroids FEV_1 or PEF >80%, FEV_1/FVC >80%	>2 d/wk or multiple times qd ≤2 d/wk symptoms ≥2 ×/mo HS awakenings >2 d/wk SABA Some limit on normal activity ≥2 × y exacerbation requires po steroids FEV_1 or PEF 60%-80%, FEV_1/FVC 75%-80%	Throughout the day ≥2 ×/wk HS awakenings Several times per day SABA Extreme limit on normal activity ≥2 × y exacerbation requires po steroids FEV_1 or PEF <60%, FEV_1/FVC <75%
12+y	≤2 d/wk symptoms ≤2 × mo HS awakenings ≤2 d/wk SABA No limit on normal activity FEV_1 or PEF ≥80% ATAQ = 0, ACQ ≤0.75, ACT ≥20 Exacerbation 0-1 × y	>2d/wk symptoms 1-3 ×/wk HS awakenings >2 d/wk SABA Some limit on normal activity FEV_1 or PEF 60%-80% ATAQ = 1-2, ACQ ≥ 1.5, ACT = 16-19 Exacerbation ≥2 × y	Throughout the day ≥4 ×/wk HS awakenings Several times per day SABA Extreme limit on normal activity FEV_1 or PEF >60% ATAQ = 3-4, ACQ=N/A, ACT ≤15 Exacerbation ≥2 × y
Treatment[a]			
	Continue current treatment Follow up 1-6 mo Step down when controlled for 3 mo	Step up one step Follow up 2-6 wk if no improvement consider alternative dx or adjusting therapy for SE consider alternative tx	Burst po corticosteroid Step up 1-2 steps Follow up 2 wk if no improvement consider alternative dx or adjusting therapy for SE consider alternative tx

Abbreviations: ACT, asthma control test; ACQ, asthma control questionnaire; ATAQ, asthma therapy assessment questionnaire; dx, diagnosis; FEV_1, forced expiratory volume in one second; FVC, forced vital capacity; ICS, inhaled corticosteroid; HS, at bedtime; LABA long-acting β-Agonist; LTRA, leukotriene receptor antagonist; SABA, short-acting β-agonist; SE, side effects; tx, treatment.

[a]Before step up on therapy review medication adherence, inhaler technique, environmental control.

Reproduced with permission from Expert Panel Report 3-Diagnosis and Management of Asthma. NIH Publication Number 09-6147.

TABLE 46-3 Asthma Medications

Mechanism of Action	Drugs	Dosage Form
Short-acting ß₂-selective adrenergic agonists	Albuterol (ProAir®, ProAir RespiClick, Proventil®, Ventolin®) Levalbuterol (Xopenex®)	MDI, DPI, Nebule MDI, Nebule
Long-acting ß₂-selective adrenergic agonists	Salmeterol (Serevent®) and Formoterol (Foradil®)	DPI
Inhaled corticosteroids	Beclomethasone (QVAR®) Budesonide (Pulmicort®) Ciclesonide (Alvesco®) Flunisolide (Aerospan®) Fluticasone Propionate (Flovent®) Fluticasone Furoate (Arnuity®, Ellipta®) Mometasone (Asmanex®)	MDI DPI, Nebule MDI MDI MDI, DPI DPI DPI
Leukotriene receptor antagonists	Montelukast (Singulair®) Zafirlukast (Accolate ®)	Granules, Chewable tables, tablet Tablet
5-Lipoxygenase inhibitor	Zileuton (Zyflo CR®)	Tablet
Methylxanthine	Theophylline (Theo-Dur, Theo-24, Uniphyl)	Tablet
Anticholinergic	Tiotropium (Spiriva*)	Respimat® Inhaler
Biologics	Omalizumab (Xolair®) Mepolizumab (Nucala®) Reslizumab (Cinqair®)	SC injection SC injection IV infusion

TABLE 46-4 Corticosteroid Dosing

Medication	Low			Medium			High		
	0-4 y	5-11 y	≥12 y	0-4 y	5-11 y	≥12 y	0-4 y	5-11 y	≥12 y
Beclomethasone HFA-Pro-drug 40 or 80 mcg/puff MDI (bid dosing)	NA	80-160 mcg	80-240 mcg	NA	>160-320 mcg	>240-480 mcg	NA	>320 mcg	>480 mcg
Budesonide-PG Cat. B 0.25, 0.5 mg, or 1 mg/2 mL Neb (Suspension qd-bid dosing with jet nebulizer only)	0.25-0.5 mg	0.5 mg	NA	>0.5-1 mg	1.0 mg	NA	>1.0 mg	2.0 mg	NA
90 or 180 mcg/inhalation DPI (bid dosing)	NA	180-360 mcg	180-540 mcg	NA	>360-720 mcg	>540-1080 mcg	NA	>720 mg	>1080 mg
Ciclesonide HFA-Pro-drug 80 or 160 mcg/puff MDI (bid dosing)	NA	80-160 mcg	160-320 mcg	NA	>160-320 mcg	>320-640 mcg	NA	>320 mcg	>640 mcg
Flunisolide HFA 80 mcg MDI (bid dosing)	NA	160 mcg	320 mcg	NA	320-480 mcg	>320-640 mcg	NA	>480 mcg	>640 mcg
Fluticasone Propionate 44, 110, 220 mcg/puff (HFA) MDI (bid dosing)	88-176 mcg	88-176 mcg	88-264 mcg	>176-352 mcg	>176-352 mcg	>264-440 mcg	>352 mcg	>352 mcg	>440 mcg
50, 100, 150 mcg/inhalation DPI (bid dosing)	NA	100-200 mcg	100-300 mcg	NA	>200-400 mcg	>300-500 mcg	NA	>400 mcg	>500 mcg
55, 113, 232 mcg/actuation (bid dosing)									
Fluticasone furoate 100, 200 mcg per actuation (Once a day dosing)									
Mometasone 110 or 220 mcg/inhalation DPI (qd-bid dosing)	NA	110 mcg	110-220 mcg	NA	220-440 mcg	220-440 mcg	NA	>440 mcg	>440 mcg

Abbreviations: bid, twice a day; DPI, dry powder inhaler; qd, four times daily; MDI, meter-dose inhaler; Neb, nebule.
Reproduced with permission from Asthma Care Quick Reference Diagnosis and Managing Asthma. NIH Publication No. 12-5075.

Theophylline is an adjunct option due to long-acting bronchial dilatory properties; however, it is not used often due to a narrow therapeutic range, dose-related side effects, and drug-drug interactions (CYP450). For patients who are not well-controlled despite high-dose inhaler corticosteroids, have an elevated IgE, and meet weight criteria, omalizumab (Xolair) may be prescribed. Omalizumab is a monoclonal antibody that attaches to free circulating IgE to prevent it from binding to mast cells, thus inhibiting part of the inflammatory response. It is given as a subcutaneous injection every 2 to 4 weeks. Common side effect are injection site reactions. The clinically significant side effect that prompted a black box warning was related to anaphylaxis that may occur at any time during treatment. In patients with elevated eosinophils, interleukin-5 (IL-5) receptor antagonists mepolizumab and reslizumab may be added to ICS therapy every 4 weeks. Common side effect of Mepolizumab are headache, injection site reactions, back pain, weakness and for reslizumab oropharyngeal pain. Both IL-5 receptor antagonists may cause anaphylaxis.

In patients 18 year and older whose severe persistent asthma is not well controlled with ICSs and long-acting β-agonists, the Alair Bronchial Thermoplasty System offers a medical device treatment which uses radiofrequency energy directed into the airways via a bronchoscopy directed catheter.

Assessment of proper inhalation technique is important for maximal deposition of medication into the respiratory tract. With meter-dose inhaler formulations, a slow deep inhalation with the aid of a spacer or holding chamber is preferred. Dry powder formulations, such as the Diskus, Ellipta, Twisthaler, Flexhaler, RespiClick, Aerolizer, require a more forceful and deep inhalation. Prior to any adjustment of medication inhaler technique, adherence to medications via asthma action plan and environmental triggers should be evaluated.

For acute exacerbation of asthma, a 7- to 10-day course of oral corticosteroid may be required for quick relief of significant lung inflammation.

SPECIAL POPULATIONS

Polymorphism of the β₂-adrenoceptor (ADRB2)

Persons with asthma who express Arg/Arg or Arg/Gly combination at codon 16 demonstrate less response to β-agonist therapy but may benefit from trial of tiotropium as an adjunct therapy to symptomatic patients on high-dose ICS/LABA combinations.

β-Blocker Use

In patients with asthma who have experienced a myocardial infarction and require a β-blocker, cardioselective β-blockers may be used. They have more affinity for the β_1 receptor versus β_2; thus at therapeutic doses their β_2-blocking effect is negligible.

Pregnancy

In pregnancy, asthma may get better, stay the same, or get worse. When a person is well controlled on current therapy, continue therapy. The majority of asthma medications are category C and maintaining oxygenation is of greatest benefit to prevent preterm labor, low birth weight, and increased risk for caesarian section deliveries. When initiating ICS therapy, budesonide (Pulmicort) has shown to be safe to use in pregnancy and has a category B designation.

Children

In children with persistent asthma, a low to medium dosage of ICS as a controller therapy provides maximal benefit with minimal systemic effects. Identifying the lowest effective dose of ICS is important in light of the recent long-term study data, 12.5 years, reported from the Childhood Asthma Management Program. The findings demonstrated that although children given ICSs continued to grow, the 1.2 cm (0.47 inch) initial reduction in growth was not regained. This was most common as the ICS dose increased and when ICS therapy was initiated in children before puberty. As with any treatment, the risks and benefits must be weighed. ICSs are the best controller medication for treating persistent asthma and have been shown to decrease mortality.

Exercise-Induced Bronchospasm

Exercise-induced asthma is diagnosed when there is a drop in FEV_1 by 15% after completion of physical activity. For prevention of bronchospasm, encourage a 10-minute warm up and cool down. One of the following medications may be given: short-acting β_2-agonist (albuterol, pirbuterol, or levalbuterol) at least 10 minutes before exercise (duration 2-3 hours or 1-2 hours, respectively), LABA at least a half an hour before exercise (last 10-12 hours), or leukotriene receptor antagonist (LTRA) montelukast more than or equal to 2 hours before exercise.

Comorbid Conditions

In persons with asthma symptoms despite appropriate management, comorbid conditions such as gastroesophageal reflux disease (GERD), obstructive sleep apnea, allergic rhinitis, aspirin exacerbated respiratory disease (AERD), and obesity should be evaluated.

IMMUNIZATIONS

All persons with asthma should receive an annual influenza vaccination. Pneumococcal polysaccharide vaccine (PPSV) is to be administered to all adults with asthma and a booster given after age 65.

CASE Application

1. Select the statement(s) that most accurately characterizes asthma. Select all that apply.

   a. Airway inflammation
   b. Esophageal hyperresponsiveness

c. Adrenal inflammation

d. Bronchial hyperresponsiveness

2. Select the mechanism(s) for development of asthma. Select all that apply.

a. Ectopy

b. Activation of natural killer cells

c. Atopy

d. Exposure to environmental triggers

The following text pertains to questions 3 and 4.

JB is started on fluticasone 220 mcg MDI 2 puffs bid, albuterol MDI 2 puff q4-6 hour prn cough, montelukast 10 mg 1 tablet at bedtime and lortadine 10 mg daily. Patient returns 1 month later with dysphonia and was recently treated for thrush.

3. Which medication is most likely to cause the patients current side effects?

a. Fluticasone

b. Loratadine

c. Montelukast

d. Albuterol

4. What intervention(s) can the pharmacist recommend to manage or prevent JB current side effects? Select all that apply.

a. Rinse and spit with water after use

b. Inhale medication quickly

c. Use a spacer or holding chamber

d. Rinse inhaler sleeve after use

5. AJ is a 5 year old who has been experiencing daytime rhinorrhea, nighttime cough that woke him two times this past week, enuresis two times in the past months, and has a history of reflux. Which symptom is most likely to warrant a work up for asthma?

a. Rhinorrhea

b. Cough

c. Reflux

d. Enuresis

6. What is the preferred treatment for an 18-year-old man with off and on chest tightness that occurred 4 days this past week with no nocturnal awakening, $FEV_1/FVC = 83\%$, and $FEV_1 = 75\%$? Select all that apply.

a. Scheduled low-dose ICS

b. Scheduled medium-dose ICS

c. Schedule low-dose ICS and LABA

d. Short-acting β-agonist as needed

7. You are providing follow-up education for a 3-year-old child with asthma who in the last month is scheduling their AccuNeb 1.25 mg tid for symptoms. Parents indicate that he wakes up at least once a night due to cough. What is/are the best treatment option(s) given the patients current asthma control? Select all that apply.

a. Continue current treatment

b. Step up one step

c. Step down one step

d. Oral steroid burst

8. CM is started on fluticasone/salmeterol DPI 100/50 mcg 1 puff bid. She returns for a follow-up visit with minimal improvement of symptoms and an FEV1 of 70% indicating not well-controlled asthma. After assessing environmental control and medication adherence, what additional factor should be addressed prior to stepping up her asthma therapy?

a. Inhaler technique assessment for slow deep inhale

b. Albuterol use in the last month

c. Adherence to morning and evening peak flows

d. Inhaler technique assessment for forceful deep inhale

9. Which medication(s) are available as an MDI and nebulization? Select all that apply.

a. Albuterol

b. Fluticasone

c. Levalbuterol

d. Budesonide

10. Select the brand name for levalbuterol.

a. Serevent

b. Flovent

c. Xolair

d. Xopenex

11. Rank the following corticosteroids as low, medium, or high potency for a 10 year old.

Unordered Options	Ordered Response
Beclomethasone MDI 80 mcg 2 puff bid	
Budesonide DPI 180 mcg 1 puff bid	
Fluticasone MDI 110 mcg 2 puffs bid	
Mometasone 220 mcg 1 puff daily	

12. A 16-year-old African American patient is admitted to the hospital for an asthma exacerbation. The patient was prescribed the following medications: albuterol MDI 2 puffs prn wheezing, mometasone DPI 1 inhalation daily, fexofenadine 180 mg 1 tablet daily, and formoterol DPI 1 capsule bid. Which has demonstrated an increased risk of death when administered as monotherapy for daily control of asthma?

a. Albuterol

b. Mometasone

c. Fexofenadine

d. Formoterol

13. Despite adherence to combination high-dose ICS/LABA therapy, a patient remains symptomatic. What is a potential cause for this patient's lack of control?

a. Polymorphism of the β-receptor (Arg/Arg or Arg/Gly combination)

b. Over production of IgG as a result of immunotherapy

c. Downregulation of muscarinic receptors (M3) on bronchial smooth muscle

d. Inability of IgE to bind to Fc receptor on mast cells

14. Using the diagram below, identify where omalizumab exerts its mechanism of action.

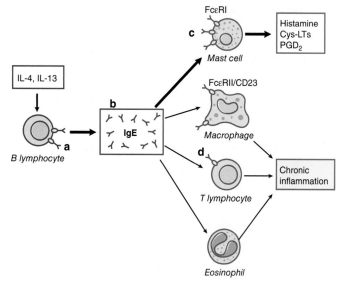

Reproduced with permission from Brunton LL, Hilal-Dandan R, Knollmann BC: *Goodman & Gilman's: The Pharmacological Basis of Therapeutics*, 13th ed. New York, NY: McGraw-Hill; 2018.

15. What is the preferred treatment option for a 46-year-old man with the diagnosis of asthma? Current complaints are wheezing in morning that gets better as day progresses. One episode of cough in last month and has required three courses of oral steroids within the last year .Current FEV_1 = 55%.

   a. Medium-dose ICS
   b. Low-dose ICS and LABA
   c. Medium-dose ICS and LABA
   d. Theophylline

16. Select the brand name for ciclesonide.

   a. Ventolin
   b. Asmanex
   c. Pulmicort
   d. Alvesco

17. What is the follow-up treatment recommendation for a 16-year-old girl currently on QVAR 80 mcg 2 puffs bid who is experiencing no limitation on activity and has not used her SABA in over 3 months?

   a. Step up therapy
   b. Step down therapy
   c. Continue current treatment
   d. Discontinue SABA

18. Which vaccination(s) are specifically recommended for a 23-year-old person with asthma? Select all that apply.

   a. MMR
   b. Influenza
   c. Herpes Zoster
   d. PPSV

19. You are counseling the parents of a 2-year-old child who will be released from the hospital with a new prescription for a medium-dose ICS. What side effect should you educate the parents about?

   a. Reduced glucose production leading to hypoglycemia
   b. Permanente growth suppression
   c. Intermitted expiratory wheezing
   d. Reduced growth over the first few years but not progressive

20. You are counseling a 25-year-old woman with asthma who is well controlled with Advair 250/50 mcg 1 puff bid and albuterol 2 puffs every 4 to 6 hours prn. She presents a prescription for prenatal vitamin from her initial obstetric appointment. What is the safest medication to recommend for *control* of her asthma?

   a. Albuterol 2 puffs qid
   b. Advair 250/50 1 puff bid
   c. Alvesco 160 mcg 1 puff daily
   d. Pulmicort 90 mg 1 puff bid

TAKEAWAY POINTS ❯❯

- The major characteristics of asthma are airway inflammation and bronchial hyperresponsiveness which cause variable degrees of airflow obstruction.
- Uncontrolled inflammation causes hypertrophy and hyperplasia of the bronchial smooth muscle and mucus glands which in susceptible individuals leads to permanent, irreversible obstruction termed airway remodeling.
- The definitive diagnosis of asthma is made through the use of spirometry when the postbronchodilator FEV_1 improves greater or equal to 12% and 200 mL when compared to the prebronchodilator value.

- All persons with asthma should have a quick relief medication (albuterol) readily available.
- ICSs are the preferred treatment for controlling inflammation in persons with persistent asthma. In children, they have been shown to decrease mortality; however, a transient reduction in growth may occur in the first few years of use which is not regained in adulthood.
- Monotherapy with LABAs is absolutely contraindicated in treatment of asthma due to increased risk of asthma-related death (black box warning). Long-acting β_2-agonists should only be used as adjuvant therapy, in a

single inhaler (combination product), in patients not adequately controlled on ICSs.

- Patients with asthma who have had a myocardial infarction and require β-blocker use may use cardioselective β-blockers without adversely affecting their asthma control.

BIBLIOGRAPHY

Barnes PJ. Asthma. In: Longo DL, Fauci AS, Kasper DL, Hauser SL, Jameson J, Loscalzo J, eds. *Harrison's Principles of Internal Medicine.* 18th ed. New York, NY: McGraw-Hill; 2012:chap 254.

Barnes PJ. Pulmonary pharmacology. In: Brunton LL, Chabner BA, Knollmann BC, eds. *Goodman & Gilman's The Pharmacological Basis of Therapeutics.* 12th ed. New York, NY: McGraw-Hill; 2011:chap 36.

Boushey HA. Drugs used in asthma. In: Katzung BG, Masters SB, Trevor AJ, eds. *Basic & Clinical Pharmacology.* 12th ed. New York, NY: McGraw-Hill; 2012:chap 20.

Expert Panel Report 3 (EPR-3): Guidelines for the Diagnosis and Management of Asthma-Summary Report 2007. National Asthma Education and Prevention Program. *J Allergy Clin Immunol.* Nov 2007;120(5 suppl):S94-S138.

Sorkness CA, Blake KV. Asthma. In: DiPiro JT, Talbert RL, Yee GC, Matzke GR, Wells BG, Posey L, eds. *Pharmacotherapy: A Pathophysiologic Approach.* 10th ed. New York, NY: McGraw-Hill; 2017.

KEY ABBREVIATIONS

AERD = aspirin exacerbated respiratory disease
CAMP = Childhood Asthma Management Program
DPI = dry powder inhaler
FEV_1 = forced expiratory volume in 1 second
FVC = forced vital capacity
GERD = gastroesophageal reflux disease
ICS = inhaled corticosteroid

IL = interleukin
LABA = long-acting β_2-agonist
LTRA = leukotriene receptor antagonist
MDI = meter-dose inhaler
PPSV = pneumococcal polysaccharide vaccine
SABA = short-acting β-agonist
SMART = Salmeterol Multicenter Asthma Research Trial

47

Cystic Fibrosis

Lisa Lubsch

FOUNDATION OVERVIEW

Cystic fibrosis (CF) is a life-threatening genetic disease of the epithelial cells in the body, especially those lining the intestinal tract and airways of the lungs. Normally, epithelial cells transport chloride through the cystic fibrosis transmembrane regulator (CFTR) with sodium and water following the ion flux. CF is the loss of the function of the CFTR with defective movement of Cl and water in the body. Thus, the composition of fluid secreted by the pancreas, hepatobiliary tree, reproductive tract, sweat glands, and the airways is thick and leads to obstruction with malfunction. This malfunction eventually leads to widespread organ system disease (Table 47-1).

Clinical presentation of CF patients is divided into early disease and disease later in life. Early disease is milder and later disease is advanced and severe. Early obstruction in the gastrointestinal system manifests as abdominal distention, pain, vomiting, and change in stool output. Early maldigestion, due to lipase deficiency, produces stools with high-fat content known as steatorrhea. Symptoms of steatorrhea are stools with foul odor, bulkiness, greasiness, and more frequent in number. Late maldigestion leads to varying degrees of malnutrition. Late pancreatic disease leads to insulin inefficiency known as cystic fibrosis-related diabetes (CFRD). Late disease in the biliary tract leads to obstruction and liver failure (Table 47-2).

Pulmonary disease is also divided into early and late disease. Early obstruction in the pulmonary system leads to coughing, sputum production, wheezing, retractions, tachypnea, dyspnea, and cyanosis. Early pulmonary infection begins with a slow cycling pattern with well-being alternating with pulmonary deterioration known as exacerbations. Initial acute pulmonary exacerbations (APE) are primarily caused by *Staphylococcus aureus*, and subsequent infection is caused by *Pseudomonas aeruginosa* and MRSA. Late pulmonary disease leads to increasing oxygen requirements, digital clubbing, increased anterior-posterior chest diameter, and flattened diaphragm. The destruction of lung tissue due to the chronic infection and inflammation leads to permanent decrease in lung function (see Table 47-2). Symptoms of chronic sinusitis may include nasal obstruction, pain, and anosmia.

The diagnosis of CF is based on elevated sweat chloride concentrations. Two samples of sweat are collected with the use of pilocarpine iontophoresis with a positive test having chloride concentrations of 60 mEq/L or more. The presence of respiratory obstruction, exocrine pancreatic dysfunction, and a positive family history provide additional support for the diagnosis of CF. CFTR mutation analysis may be required for patients with an inconclusive sweat test.

PREVENTION

Prevention of CF is based on family genetic counseling and understanding autosomal recessive inheritance. Ninety-five percent of males with CF are sterile due to obstruction of the epididymis, vas deferens, and seminal vesicles. Females with CF have reduced fertility due to abnormal cervical mucous. CF carriers who marry can produce a CF child and the incidence of the carrier state is 5% in the white population. CFTR mutation analysis can detect heterozygotes (carriers) who have no signs or symptoms of CF. For a couple where each parent is a carrier, a child has a 1:4 chance of having the disease, 1:2 chance of being a carrier, and a 1:4 chance of being normal (neither the disease nor carrier state).

TREATMENT

Treatment outcomes for CF are divided into short- and long-term outcomes. The short-term goals for the intestinal disease are normal bowel habits, weight gain, and normal vitamin levels. The long-term goal for the intestinal disease is optimal nutrition. The short-term goals for the pulmonary treatment are to reduce the airway infection, inflammation, and obstruction. The goal of an acute exacerbation is to return pulmonary function to the preexacerbation status. The long-term goal of pulmonary treatment is to arrest the persistent decline in forced vital capacity (FVC), forced expiratory volume at 1 second (FEV_1), and increase in residual volume (RV).

Gastrointestinal Disease

CFTR Modulator Therapy

CFTR therapy is indicated based on a patients mutations to improve lung function and reduce APE. Some just need a potentiator to improve the function of defective CFTR and some also need a corrector to assist delivery of CFTR to the airway apical epithelium. There are currently three modulators available approved for different CFTR mutations—Ivacaftor (Kalydeco), Ivacaftor/Lumacaftor (Orkambi), and Ivacaftor/Tezacaftor (Symdeko).

TABLE 47-1 Organ System Effects of Cystic Fibrosis

Organ Obstruction	Malfunction	Clinical Effect
Pancreatic duct	Duct obstruction	Enzyme deficiency, maldigestion
Biliary duct	Duct obstruction	Cirrhosis, portal hypertension, esophageal varices
Intestines	Viscous secretions	Distal intestinal obstructive syndrome (DIOS)
Pulmonary	Viscous secretions	Obstruction, infection
Sweat glands	Fail to reabsorb Na ("salty taste of skin")	Hyponatremia
Reproductive	♂ Obstruction epididymis, vas deferens, seminal vesicles	Aspermia
	♀ Obstruction cervix	Decreased fertility
Bone, joint	Unknown	Arthritis, osteopenia

TABLE 47-2 Early Versus Late Disease in CF Patients

Organ Malfunction	Early Disease	Late Disease
Gastrointestinal		
Obstruction	Distention, abdominal pain, nausea, and vomiting	DIOS, liver failure, CFRD
Maldigestion	Steatorrhea, malnutrition	Severe malnutrition
Pulmonary		
Obstruction	Mucus plug	Cor pulmonale
Infection	Acute exacerbations	Permanent ↓PFTs

Abbreviations: CF, cystic fibrosis; CFRD, cystic fibrosis related diabetes; COPD, chronic obstructive pulmonary disease; DIOS, distal intestinal obstruction syndrome; PFT, pulmonary function test.

Pancreatic Enzyme Replacement Therapy

Gastrointestinal treatment is accomplished with pancreatic enzyme replacement therapy. The preferred products are the microencapsulated pancreatic enzymes (Table 47-3). The enteric-coated spheres inside these capsules are protected from destruction by gastric acid; therefore, can be given in lower doses compared to noncoated products. These products are dosed based on the lipase component at an initial dose of 1000 lipase units/kg/meal; one-half of the amount is administered with snacks. For patients unable to swallow capsules, the contents may be opened and sprinkled over applesauce, jelly, or non-alkaline soft food. Side effects of sore mouth diaper rash are associated with high doses of the enzyme products. Proximal colonic stricture is associated with doses in excess of 24,000 units/kg/d. Histamine H2-receptor antagonists and proton pump inhibitors have been used to improve PERT efficacy in patients who are hypersecretors of acid. Constant acid in the GI tract prevents the enteric coating from dissolving.

TABLE 47-3 Pancreatic Enzyme Replacement Therapy

Product	Notes	Lipase (USP units)	Protease (USP units)	Amylase (USP units)
Creon	Porcine derived, delayed release, enteric-coated microspheres	3000	9500	15,000
		6000	19,000	30,000
		12,000	38,000	60,000
		24,000	76,000	120,000
		36,000	114,000	180,000
Pancrelipase	Porcine derived, delayed release, enteric-coated beads	5000	17,000	27,000
Pancreaze	Porcine derived, delayed release, enteric-coated microtablets	4200	14,200	24,000
		10,500	35,500	61,500
		16,800	56,800	98,400
		21,000	54,700	83,900
Pertzye	Porcine derived, delayed release, bicarbonate buffered, enteric coated microspheres	8000	28,750	30,250
		16,000	57,500	60,500
Ultresa	Porcine derived, delayed release, enteric-coated minitablets	13,800	27,600	27,600
		20,700	41,400	41,400
		23,000	46,000	46,000
Zenpep	Porcine derived, delayed release, enteric-coated beads	3000	10,000	16,000
		5000	17,000	27,000
		10,000	32,000	42,000
		15,000	51,000	82,000
		20,000	63,000	84,000
		25,000	79,000	105,000

Vitamin, Mineral, and Electrolyte Replacement Therapy

Fat soluble vitamins are required for patients who are pancreatic insufficient. These deficiencies become clinically evident as neurologic dysfunction (vitamin E); demineralization of the bone (vitamin D); bleeding problems (vitamin K); and dermatitis, vision difficulties (vitamin A). Vitamin K, at a dose of 5 mg twice weekly, should be given to patients with a prolonged international ratio (INR). Fat-soluble vitamins are administered in water-miscible products, such as AquADEK, Choiceful, Deka, MVW Complete, are better absorbed in the CF patient. Vitamin D3 (cholecalciferol) is more effective for increasing serum 25(OH)D and the preferred form over D2 (ergocalciferol). Sodium is given to neonates and infants by adding table salt to feeds each day.

Choleretic Therapy

The older CF patient can benefit from ursodeoxycholic acid (UDCA), a bile acid with choleretic properties. This medication has been shown to produce morphologic and functional improvement in patients with liver disease. Doses range from 15 to 20 mg/kg/d in combination with taurine supplementation. This agent is recommended to be given prophylactically to prevent end-stage liver failure.

Pulmonary Disease

Pulmonary treatment is focused on three areas: anti-obstruction, anti-inflammation, and anti-infective therapy.

Anti-Obstructive Therapy

The main treatment for removal of mucous from the airways is percussion and postural drainage. Vibrations loosen mucous (eg, percussion) and placing the head lower than the body (eg, postural drainage) facilitates removal of the mucous and secretions. The most common form of airway clearance is high-frequency chest wall oscillation (ie, vest). Nebulized mucolytics, such as sterile hypertonic sodium chloride or N-acetylcysteine (Mucomyst), can increase the results of the percussion; and short-acting beta2-agonists (SABA) can increase the results of postural drainage. Two nebulized products have been studied for long-term chronic use to prevent the accumulation of mucous in the lungs of CF patients. The first is recombinant dornase alfa to be given by inhalation (2.5 mg once) to reduce the viscosity of pulmonary secretions. This medication has been shown to improve lung function and decrease APE. The second nebulized product for chronic use is hypertonic saline in a 7% sterile solution.

Anti-Inflammatory Therapy

Anti-inflammatory treatments for CF patients can be accomplished with oral corticosteroids, azithromycin, and ibuprofen. Oral corticosteroids have shown improvements in PFTs but detrimental effects on linear growth and glucose metabolism Azithromycin is recommended for patients ≥6 years and is given three times weekly. Inhaled corticosteroids have not been studied sufficiently in this population. High-dose ibuprofen slowed the rate of decline in FEV1pp in 6 to 12 years of age but serum concentration monitoring is needed which is complicated and costly for most centers.

Antibiotic Therapy

Antibiotic therapy for APE of CF results in clinical improvement without eradicating all bacteria from the sputum (eg, suppressive therapy). The primary bacteria in the lungs of the CF patient is *P. aeruginosa*, which secretes an extracellular matrix (biofilm) that protects it from local host defenses and most antibiotics. Also, the bacteria is colonizing the airway surface, rather than penetrating the tissue as a pathogen and this is another way the bacteria is protected from host defenses and antibiotics (ie, endobronchial infection). Antibiotic therapy is aimed at *P. aeruginosa* and *S. aureus* and is accomplished with an aminoglycoside *plus* an extended-spectrum penicillin. Double antibiotic therapy is recommended to take advantage of synergy with the antibiotic combination and to prevent the emergence of resistance. Since most of the *S. aureus* encountered are β-lactamase producers, the use of an extended-spectrum penicillin plus a β-lactamase inhibitor combination (eg, piperacillin/tazobactam) should be considered. Double-drug therapy has shown superiority over treatment with single drugs and decreases the development of resistance. Unlike other lower respiratory tract infections, CF sputum cultures correlate well with lower tract organisms and should guide therapy. Older CF patients will usually have resistant organisms such as MRSA (ie, methicillin-resistant *S. aureus*), *B. cepacia*, and *S. maltophilia*. These organisms are generally resistant to antibiotics and treatment should be guided by the culture and sensitivity report. Older antibiotics with unique mechanisms of action (eg, colistin, polymyxin B) may exhibit susceptibility in patients with resistant gram-negative organisms. Patients should wear a respirator mask when with other CF patients as they have been shown to pass these organisms to other CF patients.

Oral antibiotics are prescribed in symptomatic outpatients with susceptible organisms. This prophylactic practice is discouraged because the beneficial effect does not outweigh the risk of the development of resistant organisms. Ciprofloxacin and levofloxacin are useful in all ages for treatment of *P. aeruginosa*. The earlier concern about joint or cartilage toxicity in children has not resulted in clinical trials.

Once-daily dosing of aminoglycosides is recommended in this population to achieve higher pulmonary concentrations of antibiotic. More studies are needed to determine the efficacy and safety of this method of administration.

The inhaled route of antibiotic delivery for eradication and management of chronic infection is recommended in the CF population. Topical delivery via inhalation ensures delivery of the drug in high concentrations to the site of infection while avoiding systemic toxicity. A 28-day course of inhaled tobramycin or aztreonam is provided upon initial positive respiratory culture for *P. aeruginosa* in an attempt to eradicate the organism. Once a patient has consistently grown *P. aeruginosa* (ie, ≥50% (2/4) of cultures in a year), cycled therapy is recommended. Patients are instructed to give inhaled tobramycin or aztreonam for 28-days on, followed by 28-days off, and repeat. Tobramycin is available in two formulations, a solution for nebulization and a dry powder inhaler. Benefits to chronic infection management with inhaled antibiotics are improved lung function, decrease symptoms, and decrease APE. Aerosolized vancomycin is currently under investigation for chronic MRSA.

SPECIAL CONSIDERATIONS

CF patients have volume of distribution of many antibiotics including aminoglycosides and some β-lactams. Increased volume of distribution means higher doses in most patients. β-lactams may be best administered over prolonged or continuous infusions. A CF dosing chart such as Table 47-4 should be consulted for dosing in this population and subsequent

TABLE 47-4	**Antibiotic Doses Cystic Fibrosis**					
Antibiotic	**Dose**	**Standard Interval**	**Usual Max Dose**	**Continuous Infusion**	**Extended Infusion**	**Comments**
Amikacin: Pseudomonas	35 mg/kg	24 hours				Obtain 2 hour and 4 hour level after 2nd dose. Target peak for Pseudomonas 80-120 mcg/mL and for Mycobacteria 20-30 mcg/mL, trough undetectable. Adjust frequency in renal impairment
Amikacin: Mycobacterium Children	30 mg/kg	24 hours	1500 mg			
Amikacin: Mycobacterium Adolescents	15 mg/kg	24 hours	1500 mg			
Amikacin **Inhalation**	500 mg	bid				
Aztreonam	50-75 mg/kg	6 hours	3000 mg		*	Renal adjust Clcr <30 mL/min
Aztreonam **Inhalation**	75 mg	tid				Must be used with Altera Nebulizer
Cefazolin	37.5 mg/kg	6 hours	2000 mg		*	Renal adjust Clcr <70 mL/min
Cefepime	50 mg/kg	6 hours	2000 mg		*	
Ceftazidime	75 mg/kg	6 hours	3000 mg	100-200 mg/kg/day	Over 3 hours	Obtain # hour level with CI. Target ## mg/mL. Renal adjust Clcr <50 mL/min
Ciprofloxacin **IV**	10 mg/kg	8 hours	400 mg			Renal adjust Clcr <30 mL/min
Ciprofloxacin **PO**	20 mg/kg	bid	1000 mg			
Colistimethate **Inhalation**	150 mg	bid				
Colistimethate **IV**	5 mg/kg/day divided	8 hours	100 mg			Requires a titration while monitoring UA, RFP, and neuro examination
Sulfamethoxazole/ Trimethoprim (SMX/TMP) **IV or PO**	5 mg/kg	6 hours	240 mg			Dose based on TMP. Renal adjust Clcr <30 mL/min
Doxycycline **IV or PO**	2 mg/kg	12 hours	100 mg			>8 years old
Levofloxacin **IV or PO** 6 months – 10 years	10 mg/kg	12 hours	500 mg			Renal adjust Clcr <30 mL/min
Levofloxacin **IV or PO** ≥10 years	15 mg/kg	24 hours	750 mg			
Linezolid **IV or PO** <12 years	10 mg/kg	8 hours	600 mg			CBC weekly, MAOI-caution
Linezolid **IV or PO** ≥12 years	10 mg/kg	12 hours				
Meropenem	40 mg/kg	8 hours	2000 mg		Over 3 hours	Renal adjust Clcr <50 mL/min
Oxacillin	50 mg/kg	6 hours	2000 mg		*	
Piperacillin/tazobactam	50-100 mg/kg	4 hours	4000 mg		*	Renal adjust Clcr <50 mL/min
Tobramycin **Inhalation**	300 mg	bid				May use home inhalation powder
Tobramycin*	12 mg/kg	24 hours				Obtain 2 hour and 8 hour levels after 2st dose. Target AUC 70-100 mg/L x h, peak 20-40 mcg/mL, trough undetectable.
Vancomycin* <3 months	15 mg/kg	8-24 hours			*	Obtatin trough level before 4th dose on q8h and 5th dose on q6h. Target AUC/MIC ≥400, trough of 10-20 mcg/mL. Adjust frequency in renal impairment.
Vancomycin* 3 months – 13 years	15 mg/kg	6 hours	1500 mg		*	
Vancomycin* ≥14 years	15 mg/kg	8 hours	2000 mg		*	

Use individualized regimen from preceding year.

pharmacokinetic calculations performed to further individualize the dose.

CASE Application

1. JN is a 2-year-old (8 kg) with repeat visits to her physician for pneumonia. There is a positive family history for CF. What test should be ordered in this patient to diagnose CF?

   a. Chest x-ray
   b. Sputum culture
   c. Sweat test
   d. DNA test

2. JN is diagnosed with CF and treatment for her pneumonia needs to be initiated. Which test should be ordered to guide the antibiotic selection?

   a. Sputum culture and sensitivity
   b. Chest x-ray
   c. Chest MRI
   d. Chest CAT scan

Questions 3 and 4 pertain to the same patient case.

3. TY is an 18-year-old patient with repeat visits for pneumonia. The patient has a past medical history for CF. Which organism would you empirically treat/target for in this patient with CF?

   a. *Burkholderia cepacia*
   b. *Pseudomonas aeruginosa*
   c. *Stenotrophomonas maltophilia*
   d. *Haemophilus influenza*

4. Which combination of antibiotics would be appropriate to treat TY's pneumonia?

   a. Tobramycin and amoxicillin
   b. Tobramycin and ceftriaxone
   c. Tobraymcin and piperacillin/tazobactam
   d. Ciprofloxacin

5. CF patients are unique in respect to volume of distribution and clearance. What is expected to be needed for antibiotic doses of CF patients?

   a. CF patients may require a larger dose.
   b. CF patient may require a smaller dose.
   c. CF patients have a smaller volume of distribution.
   d. CF patients have a slower rate of clearance.

6. What general statement can you make regarding the initial dose of antibiotics in CF patients? Select all that apply.

   a. Higher antibiotic doses are needed in CF patients.
   b. The same doses are needed in CF patients as other patients with pneumonia.
   c. Doses vary with each patient and should be individualized.
   d. Lower antibiotic doses are needed in CF patients.

7. Give two reasons why double IV antibiotic therapy should be used to treat an acute pulmonary exacerbation caused by Pseudomonas aeruginosa.

   a. Antibiotic synergy and decreased bacterial resistance
   b. Antibiotic synergy and increased bacterial resistance
   c. Minimize side effects of the antibiotics because of using lower doses
   d. Narrower antibacterial coverage and antibiotic synergy

8. What other therapy should be initiated along with antibiotics for an acute pulmonary exacerbation?

   a. Airway clearance (high-frequency chest wall oscillation)
   b. Pancreatic enzyme replacement therapy
   c. Vitamin replacement therapy
   d. Insulin replacement therapy

9. VC is a 3-year-old (36 months) patient with cystic fibrosis. VC is ready to be discharged from the Children's Hospital. She needs to be started on pancreatic enzyme replacement therapy. She eats three meals each day and has three snacks. How would you instruct VC's mother to administer her pancreatic enzyme replacement therapy?

   a. Administer the capsule whole with water.
   b. Administer the capsule whole with juice.
   c. Open the capsule and sprinkle over soft, non-alkaline food. Do not chew the beads.
   d. Open the capsule and sprinkle over soft, alkaline food. Do not chew the beads.

10. How would you instruct VC's mother to monitor the effectiveness of her child's pancreatic enzyme replacement therapy?

    a. $\downarrow$ Steatorrhea, $\uparrow$ weight
    b. $\downarrow$ Steatorrhea, $\downarrow$ weight
    c. $\uparrow$ Steatorrhea, $\uparrow$ weight
    d. $\uparrow$ Steatorrhea, $\downarrow$ weight

11. What side effects would you instruct VC's mother to monitor with the pancreatic enzyme replacement therapy? Select all that apply.

    a. Soar mouth
    b. Sunburn
    c. Diaper rash
    d. Decreased appetite

12. PR is a child with cystic fibrosis. The doctors would like to administer a medicine shown to decrease the frequency of pulmonary exacerbations. What would you recommend?

    a. Inhaled tobramycin
    b. Inhaled albuterol
    c. Inhaled DNAse
    d. Inhaled hypertonic saline

13. If a mother has a child with CF, what is the likelihood of development of CF in other children she may have. Neither she nor her husband has been diagnosed with CF.

    a. 25%
    b. 50%
    c. 75%
    d. 100%

14. Which vitamins should be supplemented in patients with CF? Select all that apply.

    a. Vitamin B
    b. Vitamin C
    c. Vitamin D
    d. Vitamin K

15. Which anti-inflammatory therapy is recommended and safe for patients with CF?

    a. Azithromycin
    b. High-dose ibuprofen
    c. Inhaled corticosteroids
    d. Oral corticosteroids

TAKEAWAY POINTS ››

- Cystic fibrosis is a disorder of chloride transport in all body epithelial cells. The majority of problems occur in the gastrointestinal and pulmonary systems.
- The pathology of CF results in the abnormal movement of sodium (Na) and water in the body. This results in thick secretions that obstruct systems, block exocrine gland ducts, and constantly produce infections with inflammation.
- Thick secretions in the gastrointestinal system lead to obstruction in the tract, the pancreatic duct, and the biliary duct. This leads to deficiency in digestive enzymes with malabsorption of food which leads to malnutrition.
- Treatment of the gastrointestinal system involves replacement of pancreatic enzymes and vitamins.
- Thick secretions in the pulmonary system lead to obstruction in the lungs, bacterial colonization, and chronic inflammation.
- Treatment of the pulmonary system is aimed at reducing the infection and the inflammation.
- Treatment of the pulmonary infection involves IV antibiotic therapy for CF exacerbations and prophylactic antibiotics to reduce the progression of the disease. Antibiotic therapy is aimed at *P. aeruginosa* that is the most common pathogen in the CF lung.
- Treatment of the pulmonary inflammation is aimed at decreasing the lung destruction that occurs over time.
- The overall goal of CF therapy is to slow the progression of the disease, prevent malnutrition, and help the patient to have as normal a lifestyle as possible.

BIBLIOGRAPHY

Borowitz D, Robinson KA, Rosenfeld M, Davis SD, Sabadosa KA, Spear SL, Michel SH, Parad RB, White TB, Farrell PM, Marshall BC, Accurso FJ; Cystic Fibrosis Foundation evidence-based guidelines for management of infants with cystic fibrosis. *J Pediatr* 2009; 155(6)Suppl:S73-S93.

Farrell PM, Rosenstein BJ, White TB, et al. Guidelines for the diagnosis of cystic fibrosis in newborns through older adults: Cystic Fibrosis Foundation Consensus Report. *J Pediatr.* 2008;153(2):S4-S14.

Flume PA, Mogayzel PJ, Robinson KA, Goss CH, Rosenblatt RL, Kuhn RJ, Marshall BC, Clinical Practice Guidelines for Pulmonary Therapies Committee. Cystic fibrosis pulmonary guidelines: treatment of pulmonary exacerbations. *Am J Respir Crit Care Med* 2009;180:802-808.

Lahiri T, Hempstead SE, Brady C, et al. Clinical Practice Guidelines From the Cystic Fibrosis Foundation for Preschoolers With Cystic Fibrosis. *Pediatrics.* 2016;137(4):e20151784.

Mogayzel PJ, Naureckas ET, Robinson KA, Brady C, Guill M, Lahiri T, Lubsch L, Matsui J, Oermann CM, Ratjen F, Rosenfeld M, Simon RH, Hazle L, Sabadosa K, Marshall BC. Cystic fibrosis foundation pulmonary guideline: pharmacologic approaches to prevention and eradication of initial pseudomonas aeruginosa infection. *Ann Am Thorac Soc* 2104;11(10):1640-1650.

Mogayzel PJ, Naureckas ET, Robinson KA, Mueller G, Hadjiliadis D, Hoag JB, Lubsch L, Hazle L, Sabadosa K, Marshall B, Pulmonary Clinical Practice Guidelines Committee. Cystic fibrosis pulmonary guidelines: chronic medications for maintenance of lung health. *Am J Respir Crit Care Med* 2013;187(7):680-689.

Ren CL, Morgan RL, Oermann C, et al. Use of Cystic Fibrosis Transmembrane Conductance Regulator Modulator Therapy in Patients with Cystic Fibrosis. *Ann Am Thorac Soc* 2018; 15(3):271-280

Stallings VA, Stark LJ, Robinson KA, Feranchak AP, Quinton H, Clinical practice guidelines on growth and nutrition subcommittee, ad hoc working group; Evidence-based practice recommendations for nutrition-related management of children and adults with cystic fibrosis and pancreatic insufficiency: Results of a systematic review. *J Am Diet Assoc* 2008;108:832-839.

KEY ABBREVIATIONS

CF = cystic fibrosis
CFRD = cystic fibrosis-related diabetes
CFTR = cystic fibrosis transmembrane regulator
FEV_1 = forced expiratory volume at 1 second

FVC = forced vital capacity
INR = international ratio
PFTs = pulmonary function tests
RV = residual volume

Bone and Joint Disorders

48 Gout

Michelle M. Bottenberg

FOUNDATIONAL OVERVIEW

Gout is characterized by acute and recurrent arthritis mediated by the formation of monosodium uric acid (MSU) crystals within the joints and surrounding tissues. This results in pain, erythema, and inflammation. Elevated serum uric acid (SUA) concentrations are a result of a defect in purine metabolism, a decrease in uric acid excretion, increased nucleic acid turnover, or increased purine production. Uric acid is a metabolic by-product of purine compounds derived from dietary sources or the breakdown of DNA within the body's cells. Uric acid is excreted by the kidneys and can accumulate if production exceeds excretion. A majority of patients with gout accumulate excessive uric acid due to underexcretion of the compound. Regardless of the cause, excessive intake of high purine foods contributes to hyperuricemia and gout exacerbations (Table 48-1).

SUA monitoring is an important assessment for gout. SUA concentrations are higher with increasing age, blood pressure, body weight, and alcohol intake. Gout flares can occur in individuals with normal SUA levels and elevated SUA concentrations do not always lead to the development of gout.

Clinical Presentation

Gout is a self-limiting monoarthritis disease involving a lower extremity joint (Table 48-2). Additionally, 90% of patients experience podagra (acute attacks in the great toe). Symptoms develop rapidly and include excruciating pain, erythema, warmth, and swelling near the affected joint. Although acute attacks often occur spontaneously, they can be precipitated by stress, infection, surgery, or ingestion of alcohol or medications. Exacerbations initially occur infrequently; however, gout is a chronic disease with recurrent flare-ups which increase in frequency over time. If untreated, an acute gouty attack may last 1 to 2 weeks, followed by an asymptomatic period.

In addition to traditional gout symptoms, patients may experience other complications including:

- Tophi—urate crystal deposits that can damage surrounding soft tissue and cause significant pain and joint destruction.
- Uric acid stones in the kidney (uric acid nephrolithiasis).

Diagnosis

Hyperuricemia is defined as a SUA level of more than 7 mg/dL in men or more than 6 mg/dL in women. Asymptomatic hyperuricemia is common and rarely requires medical treatment. Therefore, clinical features of gout must be considered when evaluating elevated SUA concentrations. The presence of MSU crystals on synovial fluid analysis is the gold standard for diagnosis. However, clinicians frequently diagnose gout based on physical examination, patient and family history, and current medications. Radiographs of affected joints may reveal damage consistent with gout but should not be used alone for diagnosis.

TREATMENT—ACUTE GOUT EPISODES

Goals of therapy include alleviating symptoms and preventing recurrent attacks and complications. Early, appropriate therapy is associated with decreased pain, disability, and duration of the gout attack. Pharmacologic options for acute episodes of gout include nonsteroidal anti-inflammatory drugs (NSAIDs), colchicine, and corticosteroids (Table 48-3). First-line treatment includes oral colchicine or NSAIDs to relieve pain and inflammation. Additionally, the affected joints should be rested and treated with cold packs (application of heat should be avoided).

Nonsteroidal Anti-inflammatory Drugs

Although indomethacin (Indocin) is classically described as the drug of choice in gout, any short-acting NSAID at equipotent, anti-inflammatory doses is efficacious. NSAIDs exert anti-inflammatory, analgesic, and antipyretic effects by inhibiting prostaglandin synthesis. Adverse effects include gastropathy, fluid retention, and renal dysfunction. Proton pump inhibitors or cyclooxygenase-2 (COX-2) selective inhibitors may have a role in limiting gastrointestinal (GI) toxicity, although cost and potential cardiovascular risk of COX-2 inhibitors must be considered. Caution should be used in patients with renal or hepatic dysfunction, ulcers, heart failure, or bleeding risk. Monitoring parameters include signs and symptoms of bleeding, serum creatinine, blood pressure, and electrolytes.

To access your complimentary online question exams, visit https://accesspharmacy.mhmedical.com/NAPLEX.aspx

TABLE 48-1 Dietary Components Which May Affect Serum Uric Acid (SUA) Levels

Increased SUA

- Red and organ meat (liver, kidney), seafood (shellfish, anchovies), beer, and spirits
- Sugar-sweetened soft drinks and fructose

Decreased SUA

- Vitamin C
- Coffee

TABLE 48-2 Clinical Signs and Symptoms of Gout

Signs

- Affected joint(s) are swollen, erythematous, and warm
- Mild fever
- Tophi may be present in chronic, severe disease (usually on ears, hands, wrists, elbows, or knees)

Symptoms

- Severe pain, swelling, and warmth in the affected joint(s)
- Attack is usually monoarticular; most common sites are metatarsophalangeal and knee joints
- Elderly patients may exhibit atypical presentation, such as insidious onset of symptoms and polyarticular joint involvement, often involving the hand or wrist joints

Colchicine

Oral colchicine is effective for acute gout attacks, but has a narrow therapeutic index, poor tolerability, and slow onset of action. Oral colchicine is reserved for patients at risk for NSAID-induced gastropathy or who have failed NSAID therapy. Colchicine exerts anti-inflammatory effects by reducing phagocytosis and lactic acid production in joints thereby reducing deposition of urate crystals. It is most effective when given in the first 24 to 48 hours of the attack. Colchicine causes significant GI intolerance (eg, nausea, vomiting, diarrhea, and abdominal pain), myopathy, and bone marrow suppression. The risk of toxicity is greater in patients with arrhythmias, and renal or hepatic impairment. Additionally, colchicine interacts with multiple drugs, including cyclosporine and hydroxymethylglutaryl-CoA (HMG-CoA) reductase inhibitors.

Corticosteroids

Corticosteroids are recommended as an alternative treatment option for patients who are unable to take NSAIDs or colchicine (such as those with renal insufficiency or a history

TABLE 48-3 Pharmacologic Options for Patients With Acute Gout

Drug Class	Examples	Typical Dose	Comments
NSAIDs	Indomethacin (Indocin)	50 mg po tid, then taper and discontinue once response is achieved	Any NSAID at anti-inflammatory dosing is effective Caution in patients with renal or hepatic insufficiency
	Naproxen (Naprosyn)	750 mg po initially, then 250 mg po tid until attack has subsided	Caution in patients with a history of GI bleeding or ulcers
	Sulindac (Clinoril)	200 mg bid × 7 d	
Colchicine	Colcrys	1.2 mg at first sign of flare, then 0.6 mg every hour; maximum 1.8 mg po over a 1-h period	Best used if within 24 h of the attack Avoid intravenous use; intravenous formulation no longer manufactured Most common adverse effects—nausea, vomiting, diarrhea Rare but serious adverse effects: myelosuppression, neuromyopathy Caution in patients with renal or hepatic insufficiency Potential drug interactions with erythromycin, simvastatin, and cyclosporine can increase risk of colchicine-induced toxic effects
Corticosteroids	Prednisone	40-60 mg po daily × 3 d, then decrease by 10 mg every 3 d until discontinuation	Useful for patients in whom NSAIDs and colchicine are contraindicated or in polyarticular flares
	Triamcinolone acetonide (Kenalog)	60 mg IM × 1 dose	Caution in patients subject to hyperglycemia Intra-articular therapy may be treatment of choice if only one or two accessible joints are involved
	Methylprednisolone (Depo-Medrol)	10-40 mg × 1 dose by intra-articular injection	

of GI bleeding). Corticosteroids are administered orally or via intra-articular injection. Prior to intra-articular injections, the joint fluid obtained by arthrocentesis should be examined to rule out infection. Systemic administration is recommended for patients with severe oligoarticular or polyarticular attacks and for sites not available to aspiration (eg, the midfoot). Patients taking systemic corticosteroids should be monitored for hyperglycemia, central nervous system stimulation, fluid retention, weight gain, and increased risk of infection. Although corticotropin (adrenocorticotropic hormone, ACTH) has been used for acute gouty flares, it is not a preferred agent.

PREVENTION—CHRONIC MANAGEMENT OF GOUT

The primary goal of urate-lowering therapy is to prevent urate crystal formation and deposition and to enhance dissolution of crystals. Prevention of gouty flares includes nonpharmacologic and pharmacologic management. Patients should decrease dietary intake of purine-rich foods, maintain a healthy weight, and avoid medications that increase SUA concentrations (Table 48-4).

Several pharmacologic agents are approved for the prevention of future gout attacks (Table 48-5). Urate-lowering therapy is recommended for (1) patients who experience more than or equal to two attacks per year, (2) who have tophi, or (3) radiographic evidence of joint damage. The target SUA level should be less than or equal to 6 and patients typically require 3 to 12 months of continued therapy.

TABLE 48-4	Medications That Increase Serum Uric Acid Concentrations
Thiazide diuretics	
Levodopa	
Niacin	
Low-dose aspirin	
Cytotoxic agents	
Cyclosporine	
Ethambutol	
Pyrazinamide	

Xanthine Oxidase Inhibitors

Allopurinol (Zyloprim) is a purine analogue inhibitor that blocks the conversion of xanthine to uric acid. It is effective in overproducers and underexcretors of uric acid. The dose of allopurinol is adjusted for the SUA level and renal function. Additionally, allopurinol should not be started during an acute gout attack as it can worsen arthritis. Side effects include GI intolerance and skin rash.

Febuxostat (Uloric) is a nonpurine analogue inhibitor approved for the management of chronic hyperuricemia in symptomatic gout patients. Febuxostat is metabolized by the liver; therefore, dosage adjustments are *not* required for renal insufficiency. Side effects include increased liver enzymes, nausea, and rash.

Colchicine

Colchicine (Colcrys) is approved for prophylaxis of gout, although clinical evidence is limited. When used for

TABLE 48-5	Pharmacologic Options for Urate-Lowering Therapy in Patients With Chronic Gout	
Generic Name (Trade Name)	**Typical Dose**	**Comments**
Allopurinol (Zyloprim)	100-300 mg po daily	Adjust dose for renal insufficiency
		May precipitate acute gout attack
		Adjust dose based on SUA levels
		Can cause rare life-threatening hypersensitivity reaction
		Can be used to treat both urate overproduction and renal urate underexcretion
Febuxostat (Uloric)	40-80 mg po daily	Avoid in patients with severe hepatic impairment
Probenecid (Benemid)	250-500 mg po bid	Adjust dose based on SUA levels
		May precipitate acute gout attack
		Modifies renal excretion of other drugs; monitor for drug interactions
		Maintain adequate hydration
Colchicine (Colcrys)	CrCl = 50 mL/min: 0.6 mg po bid;	Avoid IV use; IV formulation no longer manufactured
	CrCl 35-49 mL/min: 0.6 mg po daily;	Most common adverse effects—nausea, vomiting, diarrhoea
	CrCl 10-34 mL/min: 0.6 mg po every 2-3 d;	Rare but serious adverse effects: myelosuppression, neuromyopathy
	CrCl <10 mL/min: avoid use	Caution in patients with renal or hepatic insufficiency
		Potential drug interactions with erythromycin, simvastatin, and cyclosporine can increase risk of colchicine-induced toxic effects

prophylaxis, the maximum daily dose is 1.2 mg, with lower doses recommended for patients with renal insufficiency. Refer to the acute treatment and special considerations sections for specific information regarding side effects and monitoring.

Uricosuric Agents

Probenecid (Benemid) is the preferred uricosuric agent for patients with refractory hyperuricemia or intolerance to xanthine oxidase inhibitors. Probenecid is indicated for *underexcretors* of uric acid as it blocks reuptake at the proximal tubule in the kidney. It is not recommended in patients with a history of kidney stones or reduced renal function (estimated creatinine clearance less than 50 mL/min). As with xanthine oxidase inhibitors, probenecid should not be initiated during an acute gout attack.

Miscellaneous Agents

Lesinurad (Zurampic) is an FDA-approved selective uric acid reabsorption inhibitor (SURI). Lesinurad is approved as combination therapy with a xanthine oxidase inhibitor (including allopurinol and febuxostat) for treatment of hyperuricemia associated with gout in patients who have not achieved target SUA levels with xanthine oxidase inhibitor monotherapy. It works by inhibiting urate transporter 1 (URAT1), a transporter found in the proximal renal tubule. Inhibition of URAT1 results in uric acid excretion. The addition of lesinurad to daily allopurinol therapy demonstrated efficacy in reducing SUA in patients with gout and an inadequate response to allopurinol therapy. Adverse effects noted with lesinurad therapy included serum creatinine elevation, elevated lipase, increased creatinine kinase, and urticaria. Lesinurad carries a black box warning which highlights the increased risk of acute renal failure when used in the absence of xanthine oxidase inhibitor therapy.

Pegloticase (Krystexxa) is a pegylated recombinant uricase that works to reduce SUA by converting uric acid to allantoin, a water-soluble and easily excreted substance. Biweekly pegloticase therapy demonstrated efficacy in reducing SUA and resolving tophi in patients with severe gout and hyperuricemia who failed or had a contraindication to allopurinol therapy. Pegloticase infusion-related allergic reactions, may occur and patients must be treated with antihistamines and corticosteroids before therapy.

Lipid-lowering agents, in particular fenofibrate, can also be prescribed for patients with gout. Although dyslipidemia is common in gout patients, the fibrates are believed to exert their effects as an ancillary benefit by increasing the clearance of hypoxanthine and xanthine, leading to a sustained reduction in serum urate concentrations. Losartan, an angiotensin II receptor antagonist, has also demonstrated benefit in reducing serum urate concentrations independent of angiotensin receptor antagonism. Losartan inhibits renal tubular reabsorption of uric acid and increases urinary excretion, and this effect seems to be a unique property of losartan that is not shared with other angiotensin II receptor antagonists. In addition, it alkalinizes the urine, which helps reduce the risk for stone formation. Treatment guidelines support the use of fenofibrate or losartan in combination with a xanthine oxidase inhibitor in patients with refractory disease.

SPECIAL CONSIDERATIONS

Renal and Hepatic Impairment

Selecting therapy for patients with gout can be challenging in renal and hepatic impairment. NSAIDs should be avoided in patients with renal or hepatic impairment. SUA concentrations should be monitored with allopurinol and probenecid. Both of these medications require renal dosage adjustment, while colchicine should be avoided in severe renal dysfunction (creatinine clearance [CrCl] <10 mL/min). In addition, probenecid is not effective in patients with reduced kidney function (CrCl <50 mL/min). Therefore, patients with renal dysfunction are candidates for corticosteroids or febuxostat. Although febuxostat is metabolized in the liver, no dosage adjustment is needed for mild or moderate hepatic impairment (Child-Pugh Class A or B). Caution should be used in severe hepatic impairment, as no studies have been conducted in these patients.

History of Gastrointestinal Bleeding/Ulcers

NSAIDs should be avoided in patients with an increased bleeding risk or history of GI bleeding. Corticosteroids may provide a safer treatment option for these populations, although GI adverse events are still possible. Patients receiving anticoagulation therapy are at risk for bleeding; therefore, NSAIDs should be used with extreme caution.

Drug Interactions

Concurrent use of select medications may alter the elimination of colchicine resulting in an increased risk for adverse effects (Table 48-6). Allopurinol can increase concentrations of warfarin, theophylline, azathioprine, and 6-mercaptopurine. Major drug interactions of febuxostat include azathioprine, 6-mercaptopurine, and theophylline, all of which are xanthine oxidase substrates. Since coadministration can increase concentrations of these agents and potentially result in toxicity, febuxostat is contraindicated with these medications.

Since the uricosuric effect of probenecid is diminished by low-dose aspirin, this treatment combination may not be appropriate for patients taking aspirin for primary or secondary cardiovascular protection. Additionally, probenecid inhibits renal tubular secretion of penicillins, cephalosporins, rifampin, and methotrexate, thereby increasing plasma concentrations and possibly leading to increased incidence of adverse effects.

TABLE 48-6   **Colchicine Dosing Adjustments and Drug Interactions**

	Treatment of Acute Gout Flares	Prophylaxis of Gout Flares
Renal Impairment[a]		
Mild/moderate (creatinine clearance = 30-80 mL/min [0.5-1.33 mL/s])	Dose adjustment not required	Dose adjustment not required
Severe (creatinine clearance <30 mL/min [<0.5 mL/s])	Dose adjustment not required; treatment course should be repeated no more than once every 2 wk	0.3 mg daily (starting dose)
Dialysis	Single 0.6 mg dose; treatment course should not be repeated more than once every 2 wk	0.3 mg twice weekly (starting dose)
Hepatic Impairment[b]		
Mild/moderate	Dose adjustment not required	Dose adjustment not required
Severe	Dose adjustment not required; treatment course should be repeated no more than once every 2 wk	Dose reduction should be considered
Colchicine Drug Interactions		
Strong CYP3A4 inhibitors ▪ Atazanavir ▪ Clarithromycin ▪ Darunavir/ritonavir ▪ Indinavir ▪ Itraconazole ▪ Ketoconazole ▪ Lopinavir/ritonavir ▪ Nefazodone ▪ Nelfinavir ▪ Ritonavir ▪ Saquinavir ▪ Telithromycin ▪ Tipranavir/ritonavir	Single 0.6 mg dose followed by 0.3 mg 1 h later; dose to be repeated no earlier than 3 d	0.3 mg once every other day to 0.3 mg once daily
Moderate CYP3A4 inhibitors ▪ Amprenavir ▪ Aprepitant ▪ Diltiazem ▪ Erythromycin ▪ Fluconazole ▪ Fosamprenavir ▪ Grapefruit juice and related citrus products ▪ Verapamil	Single 1.2 mg dose; dose to be repeated no earlier than 3 d	0.3 mg-0.6 mg daily (0.6 mg dose may be given as 0.3 mg twice daily)
P-glycoprotein inhibitors ▪ Cyclosporine Ranolazine	Single 0.6 mg dose; dose to be repeated no earlier than 3 d	0.3 mg once every other day to 0.3 mg once daily

[a]Treatment of gout flares with colchicine is not recommended in patients with renal impairment who are receiving colchicine for prophylaxis.
[b]Treatment of gout flares with colchicine is not recommended in patients with hepatic impairment who are receiving colchicine for prophylaxis.
Reproduced with permission from DiPiro JT, Talbert RL, Yee GC, et al: *Pharmacotherapy: A Pathophysiologic Approach*, 10th ed: New York, NY: McGraw-Hill; 2017.

CASE Application

1. Which of the following is the generic name for Colcrys?

   a. Probenecid
   b. Colchicine
   c. Sulindac
   d. Febuxostat

2. JJ is a patient who is receiving medication therapy management services from your pharmacy. Since he has a past medical history of gout, which of the following foods should you counsel him to avoid eating as it contains a high purine content?

   a. Liver
   b. Apple
   c. Popcorn
   d. Potatoes

3. Which of the following is consistent with the typical clinical presentation of gout? Select all that apply.

   a. Commonly affects the great toe
   b. Bilateral joint involvement
   c. Rapid onset of symptoms
   d. Self-limiting pain and erythema

4. A 76-year-old woman with a 10-year history of gout presents to the clinic with painful MSU crystal deposits in her hand. Which of the following terms most accurately describes this complication of gout?

   a. Atheromas
   b. Podagra

c. Tophi

d. Uric acid nephrolithiasis

5. A 60-year-old man presents to the pharmacy with a past medical history of hypertension and gout. After reviewing his medication profile, which of the following medications is most likely to cause elevated SUA levels?

a. Hydrochlorothiazide

b. Lisinopril

c. Metoprolol

d. Indomethacin

6. Which of the following is the brand name for allopurinol?

a. Uloric

b. Zyloprim

c. Zebeta

d. Benemid

7. Which of the following is a *true* statement regarding allopurinol drug interactions?

a. Use of allopurinol increases warfarin levels and increases theophylline levels.

b. Use of allopurinol increases warfarin levels and decreases theophylline levels.

c. Use of allopurinol decreases warfarin levels and decreases theophylline levels.

d. Use of allopurinol decreases warfarin levels and increases theophylline levels.

8. A resident physician approaches you about a patient admitted for an acute gout flare. He wants to start the patient on corticosteroid therapy. Which of the following would be important to communicate to the resident regarding monitoring parameters?

a. Recommend to monitor serum creatinine for renal dysfunction.

b. Recommend to monitor blood glucose levels.

c. Recommend to monitor for diarrhea.

d. Recommend to monitor for presence of skin rash.

9. A 63-year-old man presents to your clinic complaining of excruciating pain in his left big toe. After being diagnosed with an acute gout flare, his physician wants to start him on therapy. His medical history is positive for hypertension, hyperlipidemia, peptic ulcer disease, and glaucoma. Which of the following is appropriate therapy for this patient?

a. Ibuprofen

b. Indomethacin

c. Allopurinol

d. Prednisone

10. In a patient with a CrCl of less than 10 mL/min, which acute gout medication is most appropriate?

a. Prednisone

b. Ibuprofen

c. Nabumetone

d. Colchicine

11. A patient is picking up a new prescription for colchicine. Which of the following are the appropriate counseling points to discuss with the patient?

a. The patient should be counseled on GI side effects of nausea, vomiting, diarrhea, and abdominal pain.

b. The patient should be counseled on possibility of a rash.

c. The patient should be counseled on signs and symptoms of bleeding.

d. The patient should be counseled on close monitoring of blood glucose levels.

12. Which of the following statements accurately describes NSAIDs mechanism of action in the treatment of gout?

a. NSAIDs work by reducing phagocytosis and lactic acid production in joints, thereby reducing deposition of urate crystals.

b. NSAIDs work by blocking the conversion of xanthine to uric acid.

c. NSAIDs work by exerting anti-inflammatory, analgesic, and antipyretic effects by inhibiting the synthesis of prostaglandin.

d. NSAIDs work by inhibiting proximal renal tubule reabsorption of uric acid to decrease serum levels.

13. Which of the following statements is *true* regarding febuxostat?

a. Febuxostat is a good choice for patients with liver failure.

b. Febuxostat is the drug of choice for acute gout.

c. Febuxostat is an option for patients with renal insufficiency.

d. Febuxostat has no drug interactions.

14. You are on the internal medicine rounding service and taking care of a patient who has developed an acute gouty flare. The resident physician on your team would like to start the patient on indomethacin. Which of the following is a *true* statement regarding the use of NSAIDs in the treatment of gout and as such, you would communicate the information to the resident physician?

a. Indomethacin is the NSAID of choice for treating gout.

b. Short-acting NSAIDs at equipotent, anti-inflammatory doses are the drugs of choice for acute gout in the absence of contraindications.

c. Intravenous administration of NSAID is the preferred route of administration for the treatment of gout.

d. NSAIDs are second-line treatment behind colchicine for the treatment of gout.

15. A 68-year-old man presents to the clinic with a history of three acute episodes of gout in the past year. He is classified as an overproducer of uric acid. He has severe

liver impairment but no renal insufficiency. Which of the following medications is appropriate for chronic prophylaxis of gout?

a. Allopurinol
b. Febuxostat
c. Probenecid
d. Sulfinpyrazone

16. What is the mechanism of action by which probenecid produces its effect?

a. Inhibition of xanthine oxidase
b. Blocks excretion of uric acid
c. Blocks reuptake of uric acid at the proximal tubule
d. Inhibits prostaglandin synthesis

Questions 17 and 18 relate to the following text.

A 75-year-old man is started on allopurinol for gout prevention. His baseline SUA level is 11.6 mg/dL. He is overweight (body mass index [BMI] 30 mg/m²) and drinks 1 to 2 cans of beer a day.

17. Which of the following statements describes allopurinol and its role in gout prevention?

a. Allopurinol is most effective when initiated within 24 to 48 hours of an acute attack.
b. The usual starting dose is 300 mg po daily.

c. Treatment with allopurinol should be continued for 3 to 12 months.
d. Serious side effects include myopathy and bone marrow suppression.

18. Which of the following measures may be recommended in a patient with gout? Select all that apply.

a. Weight loss
b. Reduction of alcohol consumption
c. Application of cold packs
d. Application of heat

19. Select the target SUA level when treating gout.

a. ≤6 mg/dL
b. ≤7 mg/dL
c. ≤8 mg/dL
d. ≤9 mg/dL

20. Place the following gout medication in order based upon their mg dose. Start with the lowest dose.

Unordered Response	Ordered Response
Methylprednisolone	
Colchicine	
Naproxen	
Indomethacin	

TAKEAWAY POINTS »

- Gout is an acute and recurrent monoarthritis caused by formation of MSU crystals in the joints and surrounding tissues.
- Hyperuricemia is defined as SUA concentrations more than 7 mg/dL in men or more than 6 mg/dL in women.
- Individuals with hyperuricemia do not always develop gout, while gouty attacks can occur with normal SUA concentrations.
- Definitive diagnosis of gout requires the observation of MSU crystals on needle aspirate, although many clinicians make the diagnosis based on clinical presentation.

- Signs and symptoms of hyperuricemia include pain, erythema, warmth, and swelling near the affected joint.
- Potential complications of gout include tophi, which can cause joint damage and uric acid nephrolithiasis.
- Treatment of gout involves a combination of nonpharmacologic and pharmacologic approaches.
- Drugs of choice for acute gouty arthritis include NSAIDs and colchicine, which help to relieve pain and inflammation.
- Urate lowering therapy can be used for the chronic gout management to prevent flare-ups.

BIBLIOGRAPHY

Fravel MA, Ernst ME. Gout and hyperuricemia. In: DiPiro JT, Talbert RL, Yee GC, Matzke GR, Wells BG, Posey L, eds. *Pharmacotherapy: A Pathophysiologic Approach.* 10th ed. New York, NY: McGraw-Hill; 2017.

Grosser T, Smyth E, FitzGerald GA. Anti-inflammatory, antipyretic, and analgesic agents; pharmacotherapy of gout. In: Brunton LL, Chabner BA, Knollmann BC, eds. *Goodman & Gilman's The Pharmacological Basis of Therapeutics.* 12th ed. New York, NY: McGraw-Hill; 2011:chap 34.

Khanna D, Fitzgerald JD, Khanna PP, et al. 2012 American College of Rheumatology guidelines for management of gout. Part 1: systemic nonpharmacologic and pharmacologic therapeutic approaches to hyperuricemia. *Arthritis Care Res (Hoboken).* 2012;64:1431-1446.

Khanna D, Khanna PP, Fitzgerald JD, et al. 2012 American College of Rheumatology guidelines for management of gout. Part 2: therapy and anti-inflammatory prophylaxis of acute gouty arthritis. *Arthritis Care Res (Hoboken).* 2012;64:1447-1461.

Schumacher H, Chen LX. Gout and other crystal-associated arthropathies. In: Longo DL, Fauci AS, Kasper DL, Hauser SL, Jameson J, Loscalzo J, eds. *Harrison's Principles of Internal Medicine.* 18th ed. New York, NY: McGraw-Hill; 2012: chap 333.

Wall GC. Gout and hyperuricemia. In: Chisholm-Burns MA, Wells BG, Schwinghammer TL, Malone PM, Kolesar JM, DiPiro JT, eds. *Pharmacotherapy Principles and Practice.* 3rd ed. New York, NY: McGraw-Hill; 2013:chap 59.

KEY ABBREVIATIONS

ACTH = adrenocorticotropic hormone
BMI = body mass index
COX-2 = cyclooxygenase-2
CrCl = creatinine clearance
HMG-CoA = hydroxymethylglutaryl-CoA

MSU = monosodium uric acid
NSAID = nonsteroidal anti-inflammatory drug
SURI = selective uric acid reabsorption inhibitor
UART1 = urate transporter 1

49

Osteoporosis

Jennifer N. Clements

FOUNDATION OVERVIEW

Osteoporosis is a reduction in bone mineral density (BMD), loss of bone strength, and deterioration of the skeletal micro-architecture resulting in fragile bones. Due to a decrease in bone strength and loss of bone quality, there is an increased risk of fractures, particularly of the hip, spine, and wrist. Women have a higher risk of an osteoporotic fracture per year, compared to men; however, men have a higher mortality associated with an osteoporotic fracture. There are two types of bone in the human skeleton—cortical and trabecular. Cortical bone, or compact bone, is a dense, strong bone and forms the outer shell found in long and flat bones. Cortical bone accounts for bone strength and is 80% of the weight for the human skeleton. Trabecular bone, also known as cancellous bone, is porous (ie, sponge-like). This type of bone is soft, weak, and flexible and, therefore, susceptible to fracture. Trabecular bone is on interior surfaces of long bones, vertebrae, and distal forearms.

Bone remodeling is controlled by osteoblasts and osteoclasts. Osteoblasts are responsible for the formation and mineralization (with calcium and phosphorous) of bone. Osteoclasts break down bone to form cavities within the tissue (ie, resorption). As bone formation exceeds resorption, the overall increase in bone mass can be achieved as 90% of bone mass can be attained by the age of 18 or 20 years, with peak bone mass achieved by the age of 25 to 35 years. In a young adult, bone remodeling is stable as new bone is generated to remove and replace damaged bone. As a person ages, there will be an imbalance in the remodeling process—driven by osteoclasts and its resorptive properties. For example, a female could lose 3% to 5% of bone mass each year during the first 5 to 7 years of menopause. Another mechanism for the development of osteoporosis involves receptor activator of nuclear factor-kappa B (RANK) ligand. RANK-L is secreted by osteoblasts and will bind to the RANK receptor on osteoclasts, therefore, inducing bone resorption by promoting the differentiation, formation, and survival of osteoclasts.

Osteoporosis is classified as primary and secondary. The classification includes:

- Primary: No known cause, but found most often in postmenopausal women and aging men.

  - Type I: Postmenopausal osteoporosis due to differentiation, formation, and prolonged survival of osteoclasts.
  - Type II: Age-related osteoporosis due to reduction in osteoblasts and changes in other contributing factors (ie, hormones, calcium, vitamin D), as well as decreased testosterone in men.
- Secondary: Known cause from medication or condition.

  - Medications: Anticoagulants, anticonvulsants, aromatase inhibitors, barbiturates, chemotherapeutic agents, depot medroxyprogesterone, glucocorticoids, gonadotropin-releasing agonists, lithium, proton pump inhibitors, and thiazolidinediones (Table 49-1).

    - Glucocorticoid-induced osteoporosis is the most common type of secondary osteoporosis. It occurs due to apoptosis of osteoblasts and osteocytes, as well as an increase in RANK-L.
  - Conditions: Endocrine (Cushing disease), gastrointestinal (GI) (inflammatory bowel disease), and rheumatologic (rheumatoid arthritis).

A patient with osteoporosis is asymptomatic, but will experience pain and immobility with fractures. Pain is localized and described as sharp, nagging, or dull. Fractures occur from bending, lifting, or falling and may lead to long-term complications (eg, depression, chronic pain, fear, nursing home placement). Height and stature (spinal kyphosis [hump-backed] or spinal lordosis [bent backward]) should be assessed at clinical visits. Baseline laboratory tests can include complete blood count (CBC), basic metabolic panel (BMP), thyroid stimulating hormone level, 25-hydroxy vitamin D level, serum creatinine, calcium, phosphorus, and alkaline phosphatase. It is important to evaluate a patient's risk factors for osteoporosis (Table 49-2). Patients should also be evaluated and assessed for the risk of falls.

The diagnosis of osteoporosis is based on a low-trauma fracture or central hip and/or spine dual energy x-ray absorptiometry (DXA) scan using World Health Organization T-score thresholds. Normal bone density or mass is defined as a T-score above −1. Osteopenia (low bone mass) is a T-score between −1 and −2.5, and osteoporosis is a T-score at or below −2.5. These definitions are based on data from postmenopausal women, but can be applied to perimenopausal women,

To access your complimentary online question exams, visit https://accesspharmacy.mhmedical.com/NAPLEX.aspx

TABLE 49-1	Medications Associated With Bone Loss and Fracture Risk
Medications	**Comments**
Anticonvulsant therapy (phenytoin, carbamazepine, phenobarbital, valproic acid)	↓ BMD and ↑ fracture risk; increased vitamin D metabolism leading to low 25(OH) vitamin D concentrations
Aromatase inhibitors (eg, letrozole, anastrozole)	↓ BMD and ↑ fracture risk; reduced estrogen concentrations
Furosemide	↑ Fracture risk; increased calcium renal elimination
Glucocorticoids (chronic oral therapy)	↓ BMD and ↑ fracture risk; dose and duration dependent; see Special Populations section
Gonadotropin-releasing hormone agonists or analogs (eg, leuprolide, goserelin)	↓ BMD and ↑ fracture risk; decreased sex hormone production
Heparin (unfractionated) or low-molecular-weight heparin	↓ BMD and ↑ fracture risk (unfractionated >>> low molecular weight) with long-term use (eg, >6 mo); decreased osteoblast function and increased osteoclast function
HIV medications Nucleoside reverse transcriptase inhibitors (ART) (zidovudine, didanosine, lamivudine) PIs (nelfinavir, indinavir, saquinavir, ritonavir, lopinavir)	↓ BMD (ART > PI), no fracture data; increased osteoclast activity and decreased osteoblast activity
Medroxyprogesterone acetate depot administration	↓ BMD, no fracture data; possible BMD recovery with discontinuation; central DXA monitoring of BMD recommended with ≥2 y of use; decreased estrogen concentrations
Proton pump inhibitor therapy (long-term therapy)	↑ Vertebral and hip fracture risk; possible calcium malabsorption secondary to acid suppression for carbonate salts
Selective serotonin reuptake inhibitors	↑ Hip fracture risk; decreased osteoblast activity
Thiazolidinediones (pioglitazone, rosiglitazone)	↓ BMD and ↑ fracture risk; risk may be greater in women than men; decreased osteoblast function
Thyroid hormone: excessive supplementation	↓ BMD and ↑ fracture risk (> in men); risk increases with TSH concentration <0.1 mIU/L; possible increase in bone resorption
Vitamin A: excessive intake (≥1.5 mg retinol form)	↓ BMD and ↑ fracture risk; decreased osteoblast activity and increased osteoclast activity

Abbreviations: ART, antiretroviral therapy; BMD, bone mineral density; DXA, dual-energy x-ray absorptiometry; HIV, human immunodeficiency virus; PIs, protease inhibitors; TSH, thyroid stimulating hormone.

Reproduced with permission from DiPiro JT, Talbert RL, Yee GC, et al: *Pharmacotherapy: A Pathophysiologic Approach*, 10th ed: New York, NY: McGraw-Hill; 2017.

men age 50 years and older, and adults from different races and ethnicities. The diagnosis of osteoporosis in children, premenopausal women, and men younger than 50 years of age should be based on a Z-score at or below −2.0 in combination with other risk factors or fracture, as Z-scores are matched to average age and sex references. An online risk assessment (FRAX score) has been provided by the World Health Organization. This assessment tool accounts for 12 risk factors, including BMD, to calculate and determine a 10-year risk of hip fracture and major osteoporotic fracture. The FRAX algorithm is useful for untreated patients. Drug therapy should be considered if the FRAX score is more than or equal to 3% for a hip or more than or equal to 20% for any major osteoporotic fracture. If therapy is initiated, patients should have a repeated BMD every 2 years.

PREVENTION

Goals will vary based on the age group. General goals for older individuals and postmenopausal women include maximizing bone mass as an adult, preserving bone mass, preventing accelerated or further bone loss, preventing falls and fractures, reducing mortality, and improving quality of life. Patients should be counseled on risk reduction through modification or elimination of risk factors for osteoporosis and falls. Nonpharmacologic interventions should be encouraged among patients with osteopenia or osteoporosis and include smoking cessation, reduction/avoidance of alcohol, limitation of caffeine, and weight-bearing exercises. These interventions can be suggested to any young adult to maximize and preserve bone mass.

Calcium is an essential mineral for achieving and maintaining bone mass, as it can decrease bone turnover. Calcium may come from dietary sources (ie, dairy products) or supplements. While dietary sources are preferred, supplements can be encouraged if an individual has inadequate intake. Approximately 1200 mg of elemental calcium is recommended on a daily basis for any adult over the age of 51 years (Table 49-3). It is important to read product labels to prevent exceeding daily calcium intake of 2500 mg per day, which could cause hypercalcemia or kidney stones. Calcium carbonate contains the most elemental calcium (40%) and has a variety of formulations (tablet, chewable, liquid). A common regimen is 500 mg (one tablet) taken with meals to increase calcium absorption.

TABLE 49-2	Risk Factors for Osteoporosis

Low bone mineral density[a]

Female sex[a]

Advanced age[a]

Race/ethnicity[a]

History of a previous fragility fracture as an adult[a] (especially clinical vertebral fracture or hip fracture)

Osteoporotic fracture in a first-degree relative (especially parental hip fracture[a])

Low body weight or body mass index[a]

Premature menopause (<45 y old)

Secondary osteoporosis[b] (especially rheumatoid arthritis[a])

Past or present systemic oral glucocorticoid therapy[a,c]

Cigarette smoking[a,c]

Alcohol intake of three or more drinks/day[a,c]

Low calcium intake

Low physical activity or immobilization

Vitamin D insufficiency

Recent falls

Cognitive impairment

Impaired vision

[a]Factors included in World Health Organization fracture risk assessment tool (FRAX).
[b]Secondary causes included in the FRAX tool are diabetes type 1, osteogenesis imperfecta as an adult, long-standing untreated hyperthyroidism, hypogonadism, premature menopause (<45 years old), chronic malnutrition, malabsorption, and chronic liver disease.
[c]Risk is larger with greater exposure.
Reproduced with permission from DiPiro JT, Talbert RL, Yee GC, et al: *Pharmacotherapy: A Pathophysiologic Approach*, 10th ed: New York, NY: McGraw-Hill; 2017.

If a patient is taking a proton pump inhibitor or acid suppressant, then calcium carbonate may not be appropriate as it requires acid dependent disintegration and dissolution for better absorption. In this situation, an alternative supplement is calcium citrate, which contains 21% elemental calcium. Calcium citrate is available in tablet and chewable formulation, but should be dosed as 950 or 1040 mg taken with or without meals. Certain medications can interact with calcium; for example, calcium can decrease the bioavailability of certain antibiotics (eg, fluoroquinolones, tetracyclines) and levothyroxine. Constipation, bloating, and flatulence are common adverse effects of calcium supplements.

Vitamin D is important in the prevention and treatment of osteoporosis. As an example, calcium absorption could be decreased by 10% to 15% if a patient has low vitamin D levels. Overall, vitamin D has a role in calcium absorption, bone health, balance, and fall risk. There are several dietary sources of vitamin D, such as fortified milk, orange juice, or cereals. However, it is difficult for a patient to have adequate vitamin D intake; therefore, supplements are generally recommended as 800 to 1000 International Units (IU) for any individual over the age of 51 years (Table 49-3). Supplements are available as single-agents, in combination with calcium or within a standard multivitamin. Over-the-counter products are available as cholecalciferol (vitamin D_3); ergocalciferol (vitamin D_2) is reserved for vitamin D insufficiency or deficiency as a prescription product. Insufficiency or deficiency can be determined by the measurement of a serum 25-hydroxy vitamin D level; the desired level is more than or equal to 30 ng/mL. A minimum of 15 minutes of sunlight exposure can increase vitamin D production, but aging and sunscreens decrease or block endogenous vitamin D production.

Antiresorptive agents are indicated for the prevention of osteoporosis. Bisphosphonates decrease the activity and

TABLE 49-3	Recommended Dietary Allowances and Upper Limits of Calcium and Vitamin D				
Group and Ages	Elemental Calcium (mg)	Calcium Upper Limit (mg)	Vitamin D (units)[a]	Vitamin D Upper Limit (units)
Infants				
Birth to 6 mo	200	1000	400	1000
6-12 mo	260	1500	400	1500
Children				
1-3 y	700	2500	600	2500
4-8 y	1000	2500	600	3000
9-18 y	1300	3000	600	4000
Adults				
19-50 y	1000	2500	600[b]	4000
51-70 y (men)	1000	2000	600[b]	4000
51-70 y (women)	1200	2000	600[b]	4000
>70 y	1200	2000	800[b]	4000

[a]Other guidelines recommend intake to achieve a 25(OH) vitamin D concentration of ≥30 ng/mL (75 nmol/L), which is higher than the Institute of Medicine goal of ≥20 ng/mL (50 nmol/L).
[b]2013 National Osteoporosis Foundation Guidelines state many adults will need more than 800 to 1000 units daily.
Reproduced with permission from DiPiro JT, Talbert RL, Yee GC, et al: *Pharmacotherapy: A Pathophysiologic Approach*, 10th ed: New York, NY: McGraw-Hill; 2017.

survival of osteoclasts to reduce bone resorption. Alendronate, ibandronate, risedronate, and zoledronic acid are indicated and approved for the prevention of postmenopausal osteoporosis (Tables 49-4 and 49-5). Alendronate is given on a daily or weekly basis (5 mg or 35 mg, respectively). Ibandronate is prescribed as an oral formulation (either 2.5 mg daily or 150 mg monthly basis). Ibandronate is available as an intravenous formulation, given as 3 mg every 3 months. Risedronate can be prescribed as 5 mg daily, 35 mg weekly, or 150 mg monthly as an oral formulation for the prevention of osteoporosis. Zoledronic acid is an intravenous formulation prescribed as 5 mg every 2 years for the prevention of osteoporosis. Certain hormonal antiresorptive agents inhibit the formation and recruitment of osteoclasts. Raloxifene is a selective estrogen receptor modulator (SERM); it has agonist properties on bone and lipids, along with antagonist properties in the breast and uterus. This agent can be used as a second-line option for the prevention of osteoporosis by reducing the risk of vertebral fractures. Raloxifene is an alternative agent, if bisphosphonates are ineffective or intolerable, but it is not as effective as bisphosphonates. For postmenopausal women, hormone replacement therapy with estrogen helps prevention of vertebral and hip fractures. Risks and benefits of raloxifene and estrogen replacement therapy should be determined as both have long-term cardiovascular and thromboembolic risk. All patients with osteopenia should be encouraged to obtain adequate calcium and vitamin D supplementation.

TREATMENT

Bisphosphonates are first-line therapy for the treatment of osteoporosis among postmenopausal women and men, as well as treatment of glucocorticoid-induced osteoporosis. Bisphosphonates are incorporated into the bone and have a long half-life of years. The antiresorptive class decreases the activity and survival of osteoclasts, and therefore, increases and stabilizes bone mass. All oral and intravenous bisphosphonates vary in efficacy, but as a class, bisphosphonates can prevent vertebral, nonvertebral, and hip fractures. Common adverse effects with oral bisphosphonates include perforation, ulceration, and bleeding in the GI tract. A patient should be encouraged to take bisphosphonates on an empty stomach, prior to breakfast with at least 8 ounces of plain water. Depending on the product, the patient should remain upright for 30 to 60 minutes. Delayed-released risedronate can be taken 30 minutes after breakfast. Intravenous formulations of bisphosphonates are available for those patients who are not able to tolerate oral bisphosphonates (eg, GI adverse effects) and not willing to follow the specific instructions for administration. Intravenous ibandronate and zoledronic acid can cause injection site reactions and acute phase reactions, such as fever or flu-like adverse effects. As a class, bisphosphonates should not be used in patients with hypocalcemia or renal insufficiency (creatinine clearance [CrCl] less than 30-35 mL/min). In addition, this class of antiresorptive agents has been associated with rare adverse effects, such as osteonecrosis of the jaw and atypical fractures.

Denosumab is an alternative agent, especially among patients who cannot tolerate or has a contraindication to bisphosphonates (eg, renal insufficiency). This agent has a unique antiresorptive activity as it mimics osteoprotegerin in preventing the maturation and activity of osteoclasts. It has been shown to be effective in preventing vertebral and hip fractures. This agent should be administered as a subcutaneous injection by a health care professional every 6 months. Denosumab can be injected into the thigh, subcutaneous portion of the arm, or the abdominal wall. The product can be kept in the refrigerator for up to 3 years or room temperature for 30 days in the original container prior to administration. This antiresorptive agent can cause back, extremity, and/or musculoskeletal pain, and cutaneous reactions. It has been associated with the rare adverse effect of osteonecrosis of the jaw. Denosumab does not require any dose adjustments for patients with renal insufficiency, but frequent monitoring of calcium levels may be warranted due to risk of hypocalcemia.

Raloxifene is an alternative agent for the prevention and treatment of osteoporosis. It decreases vertebral fractures as it has estrogen-agonist properties on bone and lipids. Additionally, raloxifene decreases total cholesterol and low-density lipoprotein levels. However, it is an antagonist in the breast and uterus. Raloxifene can reduce the risk of vertebral fractures, but is not as effective as bisphosphonates. It can be useful in reducing a patient's risk of invasive breast cancer, but can increase the risk of thrombotic events and hot flashes, the most common adverse effect. Raloxifene is contraindicated among patients with active or previous venous thromboembolism. Additionally, it should not be used among patients with coronary artery disease, cardiovascular disease, or atrial fibrillation due to the increased risk of fatal stroke. There are no dosage restrictions for raloxifene among patients with renal insufficiency.

Calcitonin is a synthetic hormone indicated for the treatment of osteoporosis. Calcitonin prevents vertebral fracture through inhibition of osteoclasts, but it can also relieve back pain associated with acute or subacute vertebral fractures. It is approved for the treatment of postmenopausal osteoporosis, specifically for women who are 5 years post menopause. Calcitonin is available as an intranasal agent and should be stored in the refrigerator. Prior to use, the bottle should be at room temperature, assembled and primed. The dose should be sprayed straight up into the nostril, as 200 units (one spray) in nostril daily. A patient should be encouraged to write the date of opening/using as the bottle is good for 35 days. Calcitonin is available in a nasal formulation and injectable formulation, but rarely used or prescribed as an injectable. As a nasal formulation, rhinitis, mucosal ulceration, and headache are common adverse effects.

Teriparatide is the only anabolic medication and is reserved for patients with severe osteoporosis (T-score below -3) and history of fractures. It can also be used among patients with multiple risk factors of osteoporosis or if the individual has failed other antiresorptive agents. Teriparatide can also be used in men with osteoporosis and for glucocorticoid-induced osteoporosis. This agent stimulates the number and

TABLE 49-4 Dosing of Medications Used in the Prevention and Treatment of Osteoporosis

Drug	Brand Name/Formulation	Dose	Comments
Antiresorptive Medications—Nutritional Supplements			
Calcium	Various	▪ *Supplement dose* is the difference between adequate daily intake, which varies by age (200-1300 mg/d) and dietary intake. ▪ Might need divided doses.	Available in different salts including carbonate and citrate and different formulations including chewable, liquid. Give calcium carbonate with meals to improve absorption.
▪ Vitamin D ▪ D₃ (cholecalciferol)	▪ Over the counter ▪ Tablets 400, 1000, and 2000 U ▪ Capsules 400, 1000, 2000, 5000, 10,000, and 50,000 U ▪ Drops 400, 1000, and 2000 U/mL ▪ Solution 400 and 5000 U/mL ▪ Spray 1000 and 5000 U/spray	▪ *Adequate daily intake:* IOM: 400-800 U/d, varies by age, to achieve adequate intake; NOF: 800-1000 U orally daily. If low 25(OH) vitamin D concentrations, malabsorption or multiple anticonvulsants might require higher doses (>2000 U daily).	
D₂ (ergocalciferol)	▪ Prescription ▪ Capsule 50,000 U ▪ Solution 8000 U/mL	▪ *Vitamin D deficiency:* 50,000 U orally once to twice weekly for 8-12 wk; repeat as needed until therapeutic concentrations.	
Antiresorptive Prescription Medications			
Bisphosphonates			
Alendronate	▪ Fosamax ▪ Binosto (effervescent tablet)	▪ *Treatment:* 10 mg orally daily or 70 mg orally weekly. ▪ *Prevention:* 5 mg orally daily or 35 mg orally weekly.	▪ 70-mg dose is available as a tablet, effervescent tablet, or combination tablet with 2800 or 5600 U of vitamin D₃. ▪ Administered first thing in the morning on an empty stomach with 6-8 oz (177-237 mL) of plain water. Do not eat and remain upright for at least 30 minutes following administration. ▪ Do not coadminister with any other medication or supplements, including calcium and vitamin D. ▪ Avoid if CrCl <35 mL/min (0.58 mL/s).
Ibandronate	Boniva	▪ *Treatment:* 150 mg orally monthly, 3 mg IV quarterly. ▪ *Prevention:* 150 mg orally monthly.	▪ Administration instructions same as for alendronate, except must delay eating and remain upright for at least 60 minutes. ▪ Avoid if CrCl <35 mL/min (0.58 mL/s).

Drug	Brand Name	Dose	Notes
Risedronate	■ Actonel ■ Atelvia (delayed release)	*Treatment and Prevention:* 5 mg orally daily, 35 mg orally weekly, 150 mg orally monthly.	■ Only 35-mg dose also available as a delayed-release product. ■ Administration instructions same as for alendronate, except delayed-release product is taken immediately following breakfast. ■ Avoid if CrCl <30 mL/min (0.5 mL/s).
Zoledronic acid	Reclast	*Treatment:* 5-mg IV infusion yearly. *Prevention:* 5-mg IV infusion every 2 y.	■ May premedicate with acetaminophen or NSAIDs to decrease infusion reaction. ■ Contraindicated if CrCl <35 mL/min (0.58 mL/s). ■ Also marketed under the brand name Zometa with different dosing for prevention of skeletal-related events from bone metastases from solid tumors.
RANK ligand inhibitor			
Denosumab	Prolia	*Treatment:* 60 mg subcutaneously every 6 mo.	■ Administered by a health care practitioner. ■ Correct hypocalcemia before administration. ■ Also marketed under the brand name Xgeva with different dosing for prevention of skeletal-related events from bone metastases from solid tumors.
Estrogen agonist antagonist			
Raloxifene	Evista	60 mg daily.	
Bazedoxifene	Viviant	20 mg daily.	
Bazedoxifene with conjugated equine estrogens	Aprela	20 or 40 mg plus 0.45 or 0.625 mg conjugated equine estrogens daily.	
Calcitonin			
Calcitonin (salmon)	■ Miacalcin ■ Fortical	■ 200 U (1 spray) intranasally daily, alternating nares every other day. ■ 100 U subcutaneously daily.	■ Refrigerate until opened for daily use, then room temperature. ■ Prime with first use.
Formation Medication			
Recombinant human PTH (1-34 U)			
Teriparatide	Forteo	20 mcg subcutaneously daily for up to 2 y.	

Abbreviations: CrCl, creatinine clearance; IOM, Institute of Medicine; NOF, National Osteoporosis Foundation; NSAID, nonsteroidal anti-inflammatory drug; PTH, parathyroid hormone; RANK, receptor activator of nuclear factor κB.

Reproduced with permission from DiPiro JT, Talbert RL, Yee GC, et al: *Pharmacotherapy: A Pathophysiologic Approach,* 10th ed: New York, NY: McGraw-Hill; 2017.

TABLE 49-5   Monitoring of Medications Used in the Prevention and Treatment of Osteoporosis

Drug	Adverse Drug Reaction	Monitoring Parameter	Comments
Antiresorptive Medications—Nutritional Supplements			
Calcium	• Constipation, gas, upset stomach • *Rare*: kidney stones	Dietary calcium intake, constipation	Education about a bowel healthy lifestyle (eg, adequate water, fiber, and exercise).
Vitamin D	Hypercalcemia (weakness, headache, somnolence, nausea, cardiac rhythm disturbance), hypercalciuria	Serum 25(OH) vitamin D concentration	Concentrations should be at least 20-30 ng/mL (50-75 nmol/L) and below 50-100 ng/mL (125-250 nmol/L).
Antiresorptive Prescription Medications			
Bisphosphonates			
Bisphosphonates	• Transient musculoskeletal pain, nausea, dyspepsia (oral), transient flu-like illness (injectable) • *Rare*: GI perforation, ulceration, and/or bleeding (oral); osteonecrosis of the jaw; atypical femoral shaft fracture; severe musculoskeletal pain; atrial fibrillation	Bone density, fractures, serum calcium for injectable products	• Pregnancy category C for alendronate, risedronate, and ibandronate. • Pregnancy category D for zoledronic acid. • Adherence is suboptimal, thus should be frequently assessed.
RANK ligand inhibitor			
Denosumab	• Flatulence, eczema, cellulitis, and infection • *Rare*: osteonecrosis of the jaw	Serum calcium, bone density, fractures	• Pregnancy category X. • REMS: Medication guide and monitoring plan due to risks of serious infections, dermatologic adverse reactions, and suppression of bone turnover.
Estrogen agonist antagonist			
Raloxifene	Hot flushes, leg pain, spasms, or cramps, peripheral edema, venous thromboembolism (warm swollen leg, chest pain, shortness of breath, coughing up blood, change in vision)	Bone density, fractures, hot flushes, leg cramps, blood clots	• Pregnancy category X. • Warning for fatal stroke; rare events predominantly seen in women at high risk for stroke.
Bazedoxifene	Similar to raloxifene	Bone density, fractures, hot flushes, blood clots	Pregnancy category TBD.
Bazedoxifene with conjugated equine estrogens	Similar to raloxifene and estrogens, plus abdominal pain, yeast infections	Bone density, fractures, hot flushes, blood clots	Pregnancy category TBD.
Calcitonin			
Calcitonin (salmon)	• Nasal: rhinitis, epistaxis • Injection: nausea, flushing, local inflammation	Bone density, fractures	Pregnancy category C. Under FDA investigation for slight increase in cancer.
Formation Medication			
Recombinant human PTH (1-34 U)			
Teriparatide	Orthostasis with first few injections, pain at injection site, nausea, headache, dizziness, leg cramps, rare increase in uric acid, slightly increased calcium	Bone density, fractures, trough serum calcium concentration 1 mo after therapy initiation	• Pregnancy category C. • If serum calcium is high (>10.6 mg/mL [>2.65 mmol/L]), calcium intake should be decreased. • Warning about osteosarcoma in rats and therefore contraindicated in patients at high risk for this adverse event. • REMS: Medication guide and communication plan due to the increased risk of osteosarcoma and to inform health care providers of the 2-y maximum lifetime treatment.

Abbreviations: FDA, Food and Drug Administration; GI, gastrointestinal; PTH, parathyroid hormone; REMS, risk evaluation and mitigation strategies; TBD, to be determined.
Reproduced with permission from DiPiro JT, Talbert RL, Yee GC, et al: *Pharmacotherapy: A Pathophysiologic Approach*, 10th ed: New York, NY: McGraw-Hill; 2017

function of osteoblasts, preventing vertebral and hip fractures. As a recombinant parathyroid hormone analog, teriparatide increases calcium absorption in the GI tract and reabsorption of calcium in the kidneys. This anabolic medication cannot be used among patients with Paget disease, metabolism bone disease, hypercalcemia, or those with elevated alkaline phosphatase levels. Teriparatide is available as a prefilled device with 28 doses; the device should be kept in the refrigerator. A patient can self-administer the dose into the thigh or abdominal wall. A patient should be encouraged to sit down for the first few doses in order to determine response, as it can cause orthostatic hypotension. Other adverse effects include nausea, headache, dizziness, and injection site discomfort.

SPECIAL CONSIDERATIONS

Women younger than age of 65 should be screened for risk factors of osteoporosis. All perimenopausal women should be counseled on nonpharmacologic interventions to preserve bone mass. There are no specific guidelines for the treatment of osteoporosis in this patient population. If a perimenopausal woman has multiple risk factors and has a T-score below −2.5, then a FRAX score can be calculated to determine if treatment should be initiated. Bisphosphonates would be preferred agents. Raloxifene could be used, but a pregnancy test should be completed for a woman of childbearing age as this agent is contraindicated among pregnant women.

Glucocorticoids increase bone resorption and decrease calcium absorption from the GI tract promoting excretion of calcium and reduction of osteoblasts. Patient taking a glucocorticoid (eg, prednisone, methylprednisolone) for longer than 3 months should be encouraged to incorporate nonpharmacologic recommendations. Alendronate and risedronate can be prescribed for a patient taking prednisone 5 mg or more for 3 months or longer. Zoledronic acid and teriparatide may also be considered as alternatives to the oral bisphosphonates.

CASE Application

1. SD is a 55-year-old woman with no significant past medical history. However, she currently smokes one pack a day and drinks alcohol socially (2 beers every other week). She attends a health fair and learns her T-score is −1.5. Which statement represents the best course of action for the patient?

    a. SD has osteopenia and should be started on alendronate 70 mg po every week.
    b. SD should be advised to quit smoking and to have her BMD checked again in 6 months.
    c. SD should be started on teriparatide 20 mcg SQ daily to rebuild her bone mass to normal levels.
    d. SD should be started on calcium 1200 mg po daily and vitamin D 800 IU po daily.

2. JR is a 58-year-old white man who presents to the emergency department with a hip fracture after rolling out of his bed in his home. He is 5' 8" and weighs 133 lb. His medical history includes rheumatoid arthritis, currently treated with prednisone 10 mg daily (× 2 years), methotrexate 15 mg weekly (× 2 years) and folic acid 1 mg daily (× 2 years). Which statement represents the best course of action for the patient?

    a. JR should have a BMD checked immediately to determine if he has osteoporosis.
    b. JR is a candidate for zoledronic acid 5 mg intravenously (IV) with repeat dosing every other year.
    c. JR is a candidate for raloxifene 60 mg po daily.
    d. JR is a candidate for teriparatide 20 mcg SQ daily.

3. Select the antiresorptive agent that can be administered monthly for osteoporosis treatment. Select all that apply.

    a. Risedronate
    b. Raloxifene
    c. Zoledronic acid
    d. Alendronate
    e. Ibandronate

4. RS is a 67-year-old Asian woman with a T-score −2.7. She is 5' 6" and 127 lb. She has a past medical history of deep vein thrombosis (DVT), 6 months ago. Her medical history includes hypertension, osteoarthritis, and diabetes. She currently takes furosemide, celecoxib, lisinopril, metformin, and aspirin. Which statement represents the best course of action for the patient?

    a. RS is a candidate for calcitonin 200 units intranasally daily.
    b. RS is a candidate for estrogen 0.625 mg po daily
    c. RS is a candidate for ibandronate 3 mg IV every 3 months.
    d. RS is a candidate for raloxifene 60 mg po daily.

5. Identify the contraindication for a bisphosphonate in the prevention and/or treatment of osteoporosis. Select all that apply.

    a. CrCl <30 mL/min
    b. Peanut allergy
    c. History of stroke
    d. History of Paget disease
    e. Hypocalcemia

6. Identify the correct statement regarding teriparatide for the treatment of osteoporosis.

    a. It may be associated with hypocalcemia.
    b. It is contraindicated in a patient with Paget disease.
    c. It is available as a monthly intramuscular injection.
    d. It should only be used for a maximum of 3 years.

7. A patient visits the pharmacy counter regarding bisphosphonates. Which statement would be correct when educating the patient about this class of medications?

    a. Ibandronate oral should be taken with food to minimize GI side effects.

b. Risedronate should be taken sitting down to minimize the risk of dizziness.

c. A patient receiving zoledronic acid should avoid drinking high-mineral water.

d. A patient taking alendronate should also routinely be taking calcium and vitamin D.

8. KG is a 59-year-old postmenopausal woman who had her BMD checked (T-score = −2.3). Her past medical history is unremarkable and she only takes a multivitamin with additional calcium and vitamin D. Her family history is remarkable for a mother who had osteoporosis and died of breast cancer. Which statement indicates the most appropriate management for the patient? Select all that apply.

a. KG has osteopenia but is taking appropriate calcium and vitamin D.

b. KG may be a good candidate for risedronate 5 mg po daily.

c. KG may be a good candidate for alendronate 70 mg po weekly.

d. KG may be a good candidate for raloxifene 60 mg po daily.

e. KG may be a good candidate for calcitonin 200 units intranasally daily.

9. MF is a 63-year-old postmenopausal woman having a T-score of −2.9 (−2.8, 1 year ago) despite being on an oral bisphosphonate, calcium, and vitamin D. Which counseling point would be the most appropriate statement to the patient?

a. Explain to her that at her age and being postmenopausal, such a small change in BMD is not surprising.

b. Suggest she talk to her doctor about taking a different bisphosphonate.

c. Recommend to her physician that raloxifene should be added to the current regimen.

d. Counsel the patient to see how she is taking her medications and review her refill records to see if she is filling the bisphosphonate as expected.

10. SM is a 65-year-old postmenopausal woman with a T-score of −3.0. Her past medical history is notable for osteoarthritis. She currently takes naproxen, as well as calcium 1200 mg po and vitamin D 1000 IU po daily. Which statement is correct regarding potential recommendations options for the patient? Select all that apply.

a. SM is on the appropriate doses of calcium and vitamin D according to WHO guidelines.

b. SM is a candidate for risedronate 150 mg po every month, despite the fact she is on naproxen.

c. SM should have her vitamin D level checked, despite the high dose of vitamin D she is currently taking.

d. SM is a candidate for zoledronic acid 5 mg IV once a year, but normal renal function should be observed prior to receiving each dose.

e. She should take a multivitamin to receive 2000 IU of vitamin D per day.

11. QW is a 43-year-old female patient with a past medical history of absence epilepsy, rheumatoid arthritis, reflux, depression, and hypertension. Medications include valproic acid, prednisone (7.5 mg daily for past year), omeprazole, sertraline, and furosemide. She presents to emergency care because of a broken bone. Which medication is the patient receiving that can increase her risk of osteoporosis and osteoporotic-related fracture? Select all that apply.

a. Valproic acid
b. Prednisone
c. Omeprazole
d. Sertraline
e. Furosemide

12. Identify the correct dosing regimen of vitamin D supplementation for a patient with vitamin D deficiency.

a. 400 IU
b. 800 IU
c. 50,000 IU one time per week
d. 50,000 IU one to two times per week

13. Identify the medication that affects osteoblast activity.

a. Teriparatide
b. Calcitonin
c. Risedronate
d. Raloxifene

14. AP is a 45-year-old patient presenting to your pharmacy to pick up a prescription for Atelvia. Identify the appropriate educational point to discuss with the patient. Select all that apply.

a. Administer first thing in the morning on an empty stomach.

b. Take immediately following breakfast.

c. Remain upright for at least 30 minutes following administration.

d. Remain upright for at least 60 minutes following administration.

e. Take with a full glass of mineral water (8 ounces).

15. A patient is taking calcium carbonate 1250 mg with breakfast and dinner due to inadequate intake from dietary sources. Calculate the daily amount of elemental calcium based on this supplement.

16. Place the following bisphosphonates in order based upon their lowest treatment milligrams dose that it available. Start with the lowest dose.

Unordered Response	Ordered Response
Alendronate	
Risedronate	
Ibandronate	

17. Identify the antiresorptive agent that would be contraindicated in a pregnant patient.

a. Ibandronate
b. Raloxifene

c. Alendronate

d. Risedronate

18. AS is a 54-year-old female patient at risk for osteoporosis and would like assistance with calcium and vitamin D supplements. Identify the correct educational point to discuss with the patient. Select all that apply.

    a. Maintain adequate hydration.
    b. Maintain adequate fiber intake.
    c. Maintain adequate exercise.
    d. Take 1000 mg of elemental calcium.
    e. Take 400 IU of vitamin D.

19. An infusion of zoledronic acid (5 mg/100 mL) will be infused over 30 minutes. How many milliliters will be administered per minute?

20. Identify the medication that can affect osteoblast activity and function.

    a. Calcitonin
    b. Teriparatide
    c. Risedronate
    d. Raloxifene

21. Identify a common adverse event associated with Prolia.

    a. Dermatitis
    b. Orthostasis
    c. Hot flashes
    d. Acute phase reactions

22. A patient is taking calcium citrate 950 mg at breakfast and dinner due to inadequate intake from dietary sources. Calculate the amount of elemental calcium in each dose. Round to the nearest whole number.

23. Identify the agents that have been associated with osteonecrosis of the jaw. Select all that apply.

    a. Teriparatide
    b. Raloxifene
    c. Alendronate
    d. Zoledronic acid
    e. Denosumab

24. RS is a 65-year-old man with a FRAX risk score of 13.5% for a major osteoporotic fracture and 1.5% for a hip fracture. Which statement would best represent a plan for this patient?

    a. Educate on a bone healthy lifestyle.
    b. Initiate an antiresorptive agent.
    c. Start an anabolic agent.
    d. Consider an antiresorptive and anabolic agent.

25. Which regimen would be the best option for a postmenopausal female (10 years since her last menses) who is at risk of vertebral fractures and has a CrCl of 25 mL/min?

    a. Calcitonin
    b. Ibandronate
    c. Teriparatide
    d. Medroxyprogesterone

26. Which medication is contraindicated in a patient with hypercalcemia?

    a. Calcitonin
    b. Alendronate
    c. Raloxifene
    d. Teriparatide

TAKEAWAY POINTS »

- Osteoporosis is a preventable, treatable, asymptomatic disease affecting the skeletal system.
- Bone formation is driven by osteoblasts, whereas bone resorption is led by osteoclasts. Osteoporosis results from bone resorption exceeding bone formation.
- Osteoporosis is based on T-score; a score below −2.5 indicates osteoporosis, which increases the risk of fractures.
- The FRAX assessment tool can evaluate a patient's risk for hip and major osteoporotic fractures to further determine if a patient is a candidate for drug therapy.

- All patients with osteopenia or osteoporosis should be encouraged to obtain adequate calcium and vitamin D intake as dietary sources or supplements.
- Patients should be counseled on nonpharmacologic interventions to preserve and prevent further bone loss from risk factors, including medications.
- Antiresorptive agents target osteoclastic function. The agents include bisphosphonates, estrogen replacement therapy, SERM (ie, raloxifene), and calcitonin.
- Teriparatide is the only one anabolic agent, which targets and increases function and activity of osteoblasts.

BIBLIOGRAPHY

Body JJ, Bergmann P, Boonen S, et al. Non-pharmacological management of osteoporosis: A consensus of the Belgian Bone Club. *Osteoporos Int.* 2011;22: 2769-2288.

Levin ER, Hammes SR. Estrogens and progestins. In: Brunton LL, Chabner BA, Knollmann BC, eds. *Goodman & Gilman's The Pharmacological Basis of Therapeutics.* 12th ed. New York, NY: McGraw-Hill; 2011:chap 40.

Lindsay R, Cosman F. Osteoporosis. In: Longo DL, Fauci AS, Kasper DL, Hauser SL, Jameson J, Loscalzo J, eds. *Harrison's Principles of Internal Medicine.* 18th ed. New York, NY: McGraw-Hill; 2012:chap 354.

Lundquist LM, Chapman LG. Osteoporosis. In: Ellis AW, Sherman JJ, eds. *Community and Clinical Pharmacy Services: A Step-by-Step Approach.* New York, NY: McGraw-Hill; 2013:chap 13.

Morello CM, Singh RF, Deftos LJ. Osteoporosis. In: Linn WD, Wofford MR, O'Keefe M, Posey L, eds. *Pharmacotherapy in Primary Care.* New York, NY: McGraw-Hill; 2009:chap 33.

O'Connell M, Borchert JS. Osteoporosis and osteomalacia. In: DiPiro JT, Talbert RL, Yee GC, Matzke GR, Wells BG, Posey L, eds. *Pharmacotherapy: A Pathophysiologic Approach.* 10th ed. New York, NY: McGraw-Hill; 2017.

Rosen CJ, Gallagher JC. The 2011 IOM report on vitamin D and calcium requirements for North America: Clinical implications for providers treating patients with low bone mineral density. *J Clin Densitom.* 2011;14:79-84.

The North American Menopause Society. Management of osteoporosis in postmenopausal women; 2010 position statement of the North American Menopause Society. *Menopause.* 2010;17:25-54.

United States Preventive Services Task Force. Summaries for patients: Screening for osteoporosis: Recommendations from the U.S. Preventive Services task force. *Ann Intern Med.* 2011;154(5):356-364.

Watts NB, Adler RA, Bilezikian JP, et al. Osteoporosis in men: An Endocrine Society clinical practice guideline. *J Clin Endocrinol Metab.* 2012;97:1802-1822.

Weaver CM, Gordon CM, Janz KF, et al. The National Osteoporosis Foundation's position statement on peak bone mass development and lifestyle factors: a systematic review and implementation recommendations. *Osteoporos Int.* 2016 Apr;27(4):1281-1286.

KEY ABBREVIATIONS

BMD = bone mineral density	IU = International Unit
BMP = basic metabolic panel	IV = intravenously
CBC = complete blood count	NOF = National Osteoporosis Foundation
CrCl = creatinine clearance	NSAID = nonsteroidal anti-inflammatory drug
DVT = deep vein thrombosis	RANK = receptor activator of nuclear factor-kappa B
DXA = dual energy x-ray absorptiometry	WHO = World Health Organization
FDA = Food and Drug Administration	

50 Rheumatoid Arthritis

Alison M. Reta, Rory O'Callaghan, Steven W. Chen, and Caitlin Mardis

FOUNDATION OVERVIEW

Rheumatoid arthritis (RA) is the presence of chronic inflammation and symmetric erosive synovitis leading to joint deterioration and deformity. The onset is usually at a young age (15-45 years) and occurs more frequently in women than in men. RA is an autoimmune disease involving T-lymphocytes, B-lymphocytes, macrophages, and cytokines, but the exact etiology is unknown. T-lymphocytes produce proinflammatory cytokines and cytotoxic substances that lead to the erosion of bone and cartilage. Activated B-lymphocytes produce plasma cells which form antibodies that attack joint tissues. Macrophages release prostaglandins and cytotoxins to cause further injury and inflammation.

Early in the disease course, patients develop vague, generalized symptoms such as fatigue, malaise, diffuse musculoskeletal pain, and morning stiffness in joints that lasts for longer than 30 minutes. In the majority of cases, symptoms develop insidiously over weeks to months. The small joints of the hands, wrists, and feet are most likely to be involved and may appear swollen and feel warm to the touch. At later stages, joints of the fingers may become deformed because of the erosive effect of the disease on bones, tendons, and ligaments. RA patients occasionally have extra-articular involvement associated with their disease such as vasculitis, Sjögren's syndrome, rheumatoid nodules, and pulmonary or cardiac complications.

There are no specific laboratory tests that establish a diagnosis of RA, but several tests suggest the diagnosis. About 60% to 70% of RA patients test positive for rheumatoid factor (RF), and 25% of patients test positive for antinuclear antibody (ANA). Erythrocyte sedimentation rates and C-reactive protein (CRP) levels may also be elevated, although these are nonspecific markers of inflammation. A complete blood count (CBC) may reveal anemia of chronic disease or thrombocytopenia.

According to the American College of Rheumatology, a diagnosis of RA is made when patients meet four of the following seven criteria for at least 6 weeks: morning stiffness (lasting >1 hour), swelling in three or more joint areas, swelling in the hand or wrist joints, symmetrical arthritis, rheumatoid nodules, positive RF, and radiological changes such as joint erosions or decalcifications.

RA varies in activity and severity among individuals and within the same patient. For this reason, it is important to assess disease duration, activity level, and prognostic factors for each patient. Disease duration is classified as early if less than 6 months, intermediate if 6 to 24 months, and long if for more than 24 months. Validated instruments (eg, RA Disease Activity Score, Simplified Disease Activity Index) are available to provide objective and consistent measures of disease activity. These instruments generate a disease activity score used to classify disease activity as low, moderate, or high, and this score is utilized for treatment decisions. Poor prognostic factors include active disease with high tender and swollen joint counts, increased RF level, extra-articular involvement, radiographic erosions, increased anti-cyclic citrullinated peptide antibodies, and functional limitation as assessed by the Health Assessment Questionnaire disability index.

TREATMENT

The five goals of therapy for RA are to minimize symptoms, alleviate pain, maintain joint function and range of motion, prevent disease progression, and create a drug treatment plan that maximizes medication efficacy, safety, and tolerance. RA treatment guidelines recommend the initiation of disease-modifying antirheumatic drugs (DMARDs) soon after RA diagnosis, but corticosteroids, NSAIDs, other analgesic medications may be used as concurrent initial therapy while waiting for the therapeutic onset of DMARDs. Biologic DMARDs are reserved for patients with moderate to high disease activity who have failed nonbiologic (sometimes referred to as traditional) DMARD therapy. Refer to Tables 50-1 to 50-3 for dosing and monitoring recommendations for medications used in the management of RA.

Nonpharmacologic Therapy

In addition to medication therapy, all RA patients and their family members should receive education about the disease, self-management training, and emotional support. Local application of heat or cold therapy, and rest of acutely inflamed joints is advisable. Both heat and cold therapy reduce pain, and patients need to try different combinations for best results. Patients should avoid physical stressors that worsen their condition, eat a healthy diet, and perform regular exercise (as tolerated) to maintain muscle strength and joint range-of-motion. Physical therapy or occupational therapy may be beneficial. Surgical repair of joints or tendons is considered a last resort for severe RA that cannot be managed by drug therapy.

TABLE 50-1 Nonbiologic DMARD Dosing Information

Generic Name	Trade Name	Dosage Range	Administration Schedule	Routes of Administration
Methotrexate	Rheumatrex, Trexall, Otrexup, Rasuvo	Initial: 7.5 mg Maximum: 20 mg	Once weekly	po, IM, SQ, IV
Leflunomide	Arava	Dose (load): 100 mg/d × 3 d Maintenance: 20 mg/d[a]	Once daily	po
Hydroxychloroquine	Plaquenil	Initial: 400-600 mg × 4-12 wk Maintenance: 200-400 mg	Once daily	po
Sulfasalazine	Azulfidine	Initial: 0.5-1 g Maintenance: 2-3 g Maximum: 3 g/d	2-3 divided doses/d	po
Gold sodium thiomalate	Myochrysine	25-50 mg	Every 2-4 wk	IM
Auranofin	Ridaura	3-6 mg Maximum: 9 mg/d	1-3 doses/d	po
D-Penicillamine	Cuprimine	Initial: 125-250 mg/d[b] Maintenance: 500-1500 mg	1-3 doses/d	po
Cyclophosphamide[c]	Cytoxan	1-2 mg/kg	Once daily	po, IV[d]
Azathioprine	Imuran	Initial: 1 mg/kg Maintenance: 1-2.5 mg/kg[e]	1-2 doses/d	po, IV
Cyclosporine[c]	Neoral	2.5-5 mg/kg	Twice daily	po, IV[d]
Minocycline[c]	Minocin	100-200 mg	Twice daily	po
Tofacitinib	Xeljanz Xeljanz XR	5 mg (IR) 11 mg (XR)	Twice daily (IR) Once daily (XR)	po

Abbreviations: IM, intramuscular; IV, intravenous; po, oral; SQ, subcutaneous.
[a]May decrease to 10 mg/d if unable to tolerate 20 mg daily.
[b]Increase dose at 1 to 3 month intervals by 125 or 250 mg/d, as patient response and tolerance indicate; if no improvement and no serious toxicity after 2 to 3 months, increases of 250 mg/d at 2 to 3 month intervals may be continued until remission or toxicity.
[c]Not FDA approved for rheumatoid arthritis.
[d]Though an IV formulation is available, dosing within the table reflects po dosing.
[e]May titrate from initial dose by 0.5 mg/kg/d after 6 to 8 weeks and every 4 weeks thereafter, maximum dose is 2.5 mg/kg/d. May decrease maintenance dose by lowering dose to 0.5 mg/kg/d every 4 weeks until lowest effective dose is reached.

TABLE 50-2 Biologic DMARD Dosing Information

Generic	Brand	Dosage Range	Administration Schedule	Routes of Administration
Anti-TNF-α Agents				
Infliximab	Remicade	3 mg/kg[a]	Wk 0, 2, and 6, and then every 8 wk	IV
Etanercept	Enbrel	50 mg once weekly or 25 mg twice weekly (off label)	1-2 doses/wk	SQ
Adalimumab	Humira	40 mg	Every 14 d[b]	SQ
Certolizumab	Cimzia	Initial: 400 mg SQ ×1 on wk 0, 2, and 4 Subsequent: 200 mg every other week or 400 mg every 4 wk	Wk 0, 2, and 4, then every 2 or 4 wk	SQ
Golimumab	Simponi	50 mg 2 mg/kg	Every 4 wk Week 0, 4, then every 8 wk	SQ IV
Other Biologic Agents				
Abatacept	Orencia	125 mg Weight based: <60 kg = 500 mg 60-100 kg = 750 mg >100 kg = 1000 mg	Weekly Wk 0, 2, and 4, and then every 4 wk	SQ IV
Rituximab	Rituxan	1000 mg IV infusion: Initial: 50 mg/h, may increase every 30 min to max 400 mg/h Subsequent: 100 mg/h, may increase every 30 min to max 400 mg/h	Repeat in 14 d; subsequent courses may be administered every 24 weeks or based on clinical evaluation (no sooner than every 16 weeks)[c]	IV
Anakinra	Kineret	100 mg	Once daily	SQ
Tocilizumab	Actemra	4 mg/kg IV infusion over 60 min Weight based: <100 kg = 162 mg >100 kg = 162 mg	Every 4 wk Every other week or weekly based on clinical response Weekly	IV SQ

Abbreviations: IV, intravenous; SQ, subcutaneous.
[a]For incomplete response: may increase dose to 10 mg/kg or decrease dosing interval to every 4 weeks.
[b]Patients not taking methotrexate concomitantly may increase dose to 40 mg every week.
[c]Labeling allows for subsequent courses based on approval trials; however, most post-marketing safety data is based on limiting the course to two doses. Premedicate with corticosteroid, acetaminophen, and an antihistamine prior to each dose.

TABLE 50-3 **Adverse Reactions and Monitoring of Rheumatoid Arthritis Medications**

Drug	Adverse Drug Reaction	Initial Monitoring	Maintenance Monitoring	Symptoms to Inquire About[a]
Non-DMARD Therapies				
NSAIDs and salicylates	GI ulceration and bleeding, renal damage	SCr and BUN, CBC q 2-4 wk p starting therapy × 1-2 mo Salicylates: serum salicylate levels if therapeutic dose and no response	Same as initial plus stool guaiac q 6-12 mo	Blood in stool, black stool, dyspepsia, nausea/vomiting, weakness, dizziness, abdominal pain, edema, weight gain, SOB
Corticosteroids	Hypertension, hyperglycemia, osteoporosis[b]	Glucose, blood pressure q 3-6 mo	Same as initial	Blood pressure if available, polyuria, polydipsia, edema, SOB, visual changes, weight gain, headaches, broken bones or bone pain
Nonbiologic DMARDs				
Methotrexate	Myelosuppression, hepatic fibrosis, cirrhosis, pulmonary infiltrates or fibrosis, stomatitis, rash	Baseline: AST, ALT, alk phos, alb, t. bili, hep B and C studies, CBC w/plt, SCr	CBC w/plt, AST, alb q 1-2 mo	Symptoms of myelosuppression, SOB, nausea/vomiting, lymph node swelling, coughing, mouth sores, diarrhea, jaundice
Leflunomide	Hepatitis, GI distress, alopecia	Baseline: ALT, CBC with platelets	CBC with platelets and ALT monthly initially and then every 6-8 wk	Nausea/vomiting, gastritis, diarrhea, hair loss, jaundice
Hydroxychloroquine	Macular damage, rash, diarrhea	Baseline: color fundus photography and automated central perimetric analysis	Ophthalmoscopy q 9-12 mo and Amsler grid at home q 2 wk	Visual changes including a decrease in night or peripheral vision, rash, diarrhea
Sulfasalazine	Myelosuppression, rash	Baseline: CBC w/plt, then q wk × 1 mo	Same as initial—q 1-2 mo	Symptoms of myelosuppression, photosensitivity, rash, nausea/vomiting
Tofacitinib	Infection, malignancy, GI perforations, upper respiratory tract infections, headache, diarrhea, nasopharyngitis	Tuberculin skin test, hepatitis C screening, neutrophil count, lymphocytes, Hgb, AST/ALT	Neutrophils, Hgb, FLP at 4-8 wk after treatment start, then lymphocytes, neutrophils, and Hgb q 3 mo	Symptoms of infection or myelosuppression, SOB, blood in stool, black stool, dyspepsia
Gold (intramuscular or oral)	Myelosuppression, proteinuria, rash, stomatitis	Baseline & until stable: UA, CBC w/plt preinjection	Same as initial—every other dose	Symptoms of myelosuppression, edema, rash, oral ulcers, diarrhea
Penicillamine	Myelosuppression, proteinuria, stomatitis, rash, dysgeusia	Baseline: UA, CBC w/plt, then q wk × 1 mo	Same as initial—q 1-2 mo, but q 2 wk if dose change	Symptoms of myelosuppression, edema, rash, diarrhea, altered taste perception, oral ulcers
Cyclophosphamide	Alopecia, infertility, GI distress, hemorrhagic cystitis, myelosuppression, nephrotoxicity, cardiotoxicity	UA, CBC w/plt q wk × 1 mo	Same as initial—q 2-4 wk	Nausea/vomiting, gastritis, diarrhea, hair loss, urination difficulties, chest pain, rash, respiratory difficulties
Cyclosporine	Hepatotoxicity, nephrotoxicity, hypertension, headache, malignancy, infections, GI distress	SCr, blood pressure q mo	Same as initial	Nausea/vomiting, diarrhea, symptoms of infection, symptoms of elevated blood pressure
Biologic DMARDs				
Etanercept, adalimumab, certolizumab, golimumab,	Local injection-site reactions, infection	Tuberculin skin test, hepatitis C screening	None	Symptoms of infection
Infliximab, rituximab, abatacept	Immune reactions, infection	Tuberculin skin test, hepatitis C screening	None	Postinfusion reactions, symptoms of infection
Anakinra	Local injection-site reactions, infection	Neutrophil count	Neutrophil count q 1 mo for 3 mo then quarterly up to 1 year	Symptoms of infection
Tocilizumab	Local injection-site reactions, infection	AST/ALT, CBC w/plt, lipids	AST/ALT, CBC w/plt, lipids q 4-8 wk	Symptoms of infection

Abbreviations: alb, albumin; alk phos, alkaline phosphatase; ALT, alanine aminotransferase; AST, aspartate aminotransferase; BUN, blood urea nitrogen; CBC, complete blood count; FLP, fasting lipid panel; GI, gastrointestinal; hep, hepatitis; Hgb, hemoglobin; p, after; plt, platelet; q, every; SCr, serum creatinine; t. bili, total bilirubin; UA, urinalysis; NSAIDs, nonsteroidal anti-inflammatory drugs; SOB, shortness of breath.

[a]Altered immune function increases risk of infection; this should be considered particularly in those patients taking azathioprine, methotrexate, and corticosteroids or other drugs as a symptom of myelosuppression.

[b]Osteoporosis is unlikely to manifest itself early in treatment, but all patients should be taking appropriate steps to prevent bone loss.

Reproduced with permission from DiPiro JT, Talbert RL, Yee GC, et al: *Pharmacotherapy: A Pathophysiologic Approach*, 10th ed: New York, NY: McGraw-Hill; 2017.

Non-DMARD Therapy

Non-DMARD therapies used in the treatment of RA do not alter the course of the disease. Therefore, these drugs must be used concomitantly with DMARDs or only temporarily during initiation of DMARD therapy. Aspirin, nonsteroidal anti-inflammatory drugs (NSAIDs), and selective COX-2 inhibitors reduce inflammation and pain by inhibiting prostaglandin synthesis. Higher doses of these agents are necessary to reduce inflammation as opposed to reducing pain, and anti-inflammatory properties require weeks of continuous therapy to manifest.

Oral corticosteroid agents such as prednisone also provide relief from inflammation and have demonstrated disease-modifying properties in RA. However, because of undesirable long-term adverse effects such as osteoporosis and adrenal suppression, corticosteroids are prescribed temporarily for acute RA flares or short term during bridge therapy as a patient awaits the onset of DMARD therapy. On occasion, long-term corticosteroid therapy at low doses may be required for patients who are refractory to NSAID or DMARD therapy but should be avoided if possible.

Patients must take NSAIDs or corticosteroids with food to minimize the risk of gastric muscosal damage. For patients requiring long-term NSAID use, concurrent proton pump inhibitor or misoprostol therapy should be considered to reduce the risk of NSAID-induced peptic ulcer disease. All NSAIDs, including COX-2 inhibitors, can cause nephropathy.

DMARD Therapy

Disease-modifying antirheumatic drugs reduce or prevent joint damage and preserve joint function and integrity. DMARD therapy should be initiated early in the course of RA, typically within 3 months of diagnosis. DMARDs generally have a slow onset of effect (1-6 months) and, as a result, bridge therapy with an NSAID or corticosteroid is often recommended until DMARD benefit is demonstrated. Patients have variable responses to different DMARDs, so trials of several DMARDs may be necessary.

It is recommended that DMARD therapy be continuously evaluated for efficacy and intensified as needed every 3 months to achieve low disease activity or remission. Disease activity should be reassessed within 3 months of DMARD initiation. For patients with moderate or high disease activity which has not improved on DMARD monotherapy in 3 months, another nonbiologic DMARD can be added, an anti-TNF biologic can be added or substituted, or a non-TNF biologic (abatacept, rituximab, or tocilizumab) can be added or substituted. If a lack or loss of benefit is noted after 3 months of anti-TNF therapy alone, it is recommended to add a traditional DMARD agent or transition to a non-TNF biologic. Patients experiencing serious adverse events from anti-TNF biologic DMARD may be switched to a non-TNF biologic DMARD, while patients experiencing non-serious adverse effects can be changed to an alternate anti-TNF agent or a non-TNF biologic. Nonbiologic DMARDs may be given alone or together with other nonbiologic or biologic DMARDs.

Nonbiologic DMARDs

Methotrexate Methotrexate is the gold standard, preferred DMARD and appears to exert anti-inflammatory effects through immunosuppression. Methotrexate is dosed on a weekly basis (which can be convenient but also challenging for adherence). Common side effects include nausea, vomiting, diarrhea, alopecia, and general malaise. Elevation of liver transaminases (alanine transaminase and aspartate transaminase), renal toxicity, and thrombocytopenia or bone marrow suppression may occur. Methotrexate should not be used in patients with transaminases more than twice the upper limit of normal, poor renal function (ClCr <40 mL/min), a white blood cell count less than 3000/mm³, or a platelet count of less than 50×10^9/L. In addition, methotrexate should not be initiated or resumed in patients with active tuberculosis, bacterial infection, herpes zoster, life-threatening fungal infection, or in patients who are pregnant (pregnancy category X). Liver transaminases, serum creatinine (SCr), and a CBC should be measured at baseline, every 2 to 4 weeks after initiation of therapy for 3 months, and then periodically (approximately every 3-6 months) thereafter. Routine liver biopsies for RA patients receiving methotrexate are no longer recommended. Liver biopsy is not cost-effective when liver transaminases are normal; however, persistently elevated liver transaminases are an indication for liver biopsy.

Methotrexate is a folic acid antagonist; therefore, its use may lead to folic acid deficiency. The use of folic acid supplementation (1 mg daily) may reduce the incidence of side effects from methotrexate, including gastrointestinal disturbances and elevations in liver enzymes, without impacting MTX efficacy.

Leflunomide Leflunomide decreases lymphocyte proliferation by inhibiting pyrimidine synthesis. Common side effects include diarrhea, rash, alopecia, headache, weight loss, and elevated liver transaminases. Leflunomide should not be used in patients with transaminase levels greater than twice the upper limit of normal, active tuberculosis, bacterial, herpes zoster, or life-threatening fungal infection, or in patients who have a white blood cell count less than 3000/mm³ or a platelet count less than 50×10^9/L. It is pregnancy category X and is teratogenic in both female and male patients; women and men should avoid leflunomide if attempting conception. Following discontinuation, up to 2 years may be required for leflunomide to clear fully from the body due to its long half-life. If a female patient intends to become pregnant, she should discontinue leflunomide at least 3 months prior to conception and must undergo a drug elimination procedure with cholestyramine. Similar to methotrexate, key laboratory tests (liver transaminases, SCr, CBC) should be measured at baseline, every 2 to 4 weeks for the first 3 months of therapy, and every 3-6 months thereafter.

Hydroxychloroquine Hydroxychloroquine may be appropriate for patients with a less active, milder form of RA. It is an antimalarial agent that has anti-inflammatory and immunomodulatory effects. Its specific mechanism of action in

RA disease processes is unknown. Following a loading dose, hydroxychloroquine is dosed daily and is well-tolerated (although some patients may experience gastrointestinal upset, diarrhea, abdominal cramping, rash, or headache). Hydroxychloroquine is not associated with hepatic or renal toxicities or bone marrow suppression. Patients receiving hydroxychloroquine should have an ophthalmological examination within 1 year of treatment initiation due to the risk of macular damage and retinal toxicity. High-risk patients should have the ophthalmological examination repeated every 6 to 12 months, while low-risk patients may repeat the examination every 5 years.

Sulfasalazine The exact mechanism of sulfasalazine for the treatment of RA is not known. Side effects include nausea, vomiting, anorexia, bone marrow suppression, rash, photosensitivity, and elevated liver transaminases. Sulfasalazine should not be used in patients with transaminases more than twice the upper limit of normal or in patients with established sulfa allergies.

Tofacitinib Tofacitinib inhibits the production of inflammatory cytokines through the inhibition of the enzyme janus kinase (JAK). It is indicated for the treatment of adults with moderate to severe RA who have experienced an inadequate response or an intolerance to methotrexate. It is administered orally at a recommended dosage of 5 mg twice daily or 11 mg once daily (XR formulation). Tofacitinib may be used alone or in combination with other nonbiologic DMARDs, but it is not recommended for use in combination with biologic DMARDs or potent immunosuppressant agents. Like the biologic DMARDs, it carries a black box warning for severe infection, lymphoma, and other malignancies. It should also be used with caution in patients who are at high risk for GI perforation.

Other agents Many other DMARD agents are available for use (some lacking Federal Drug Administration approval) but are not commonly utilized in clinical practice because of limited efficacy and/or high risk of major toxicity. These include gold compounds, penicillamine, cyclophosphamide, azathioprine, cyclosporine, and minocycline.

Biologic DMARDs

Biologic DMARDs are effective in reducing disease activity and improving function and quality of life in RA patients for whom nonbiological treatment is unsuccessful. Biologic agents are commonly separated into two groups: (1) those that attack tumor necrosis factor alpha (TNF-α) and (2) those that target other immune mediators. Biologic agents should not be used in combination with one another because of the risk of major adverse effects, particularly infections. It is recommended that patients initiating biologic DMARD therapy receive baseline liver transaminase, SCr, and CBC laboratory tests. They should also be screened for tuberculosis and have a negative tuberculin-purified protein derivative skin test before starting therapy with a biologic agent. Patients on any biologic DMARD agent should continually be monitored for signs of infection, since these drugs decrease immune response. Biologic agents should not be initiated or resumed in any patient

with active infections including bacterial, tuberculosis, herpes zoster, life-threatening fungal, or acute Hepatitis B or C. Prescribers should exercise caution when using these medications in patients with severe active upper respiratory tract infections or open skin wounds. Anti-TNF-α agents are contraindicated in patients with New York Heart Association Class III or IV heart failure. Lymphoma and other malignancies have also been reported in children and adolescents treated with anti-TNF-α agents.

Anti-TNF-α Agents

Infliximab Infliximab is an IgG anti-TNF-α human-murine chimeric antibody that binds to TNF, preventing it from binding to its receptor target. It is given as an intravenous infusion and should be taken concurrently with oral methotrexate to reduce the risk of human antichimeric antibody formation. Side effects include increased risk of infection, headache, and rash. Patients may be pretreated with acetaminophen and diphenhydramine to prevent an infusion-related reaction.

Etanercept Etanercept competitively binds to TNF, preventing it from binding to the surfaces of inflammatory cells. It is given as a weekly or biweekly subcutaneous injection. Etanercept is not associated with dose-related toxicities but can increase the risk of infection. No routine laboratory monitoring is recommended for etanercept.

Adalimumab Adalimumab is a recombinant human monoclonal antibody that binds to TNF-α receptor sites and inhibits the binding of endogenous TNF-α to those targets. Adalimumab is generally administered every other week, but some patients not receiving concurrent methotrexate may benefit from weekly dosing. Side effects include headache, rash, and injection site reactions as well as increased risk of infection.

Certolizumab pegol Certolizumab is a recombinant, humanized antibody specific for human TNF-α. It consists of a recombinant Fab fragment of a humanized anti-TNF-α monoclonal antibody which is attached to a polyethylene glycol (PEG) moiety. It is administered subcutaneously every other week and dosing may be extended to every 4 weeks after the first three doses. Certolizumab may be used as monotherapy or in combination with nonbiological DMARDs. The most common adverse reactions are upper respiratory infections, rash, and urinary tract infections.

Golimumab Golimumab is an IgG monoclonal antibody specific for human TNF-α. Golimumab is given as a 50 mg subcutaneous injection every 4 weeks. It is available as a pen for self-injection. An IV product is also available which requires weight-based dosing. The most common adverse reactions include upper respiratory infections, nasopharyngitis, and injection site reactions.

Other Biologic DMARDs

Abatacept Abatacept is an immunoglobulin protein agent that inhibits T-lymphocyte activation through blockade of its stimulation by antigen-presenting cells. It is given by IV infusion with dosages based on weight or as a weekly subcutaneous injection. Patients refractory to nonbiologic DMARDs and anti-TNF biologic agents have been successfully treated with abatacept. Common side effects include nausea, headache, and infusion-related reactions. Because of risk of major infections (even greater than anti-TNF biologic agents), abatacept is reserved for patients with at least moderate RA disease activity and poor prognostic manifestations who have experienced an inadequate response to methotrexate in combination with DMARDs or to sequential use of other nonbiologic DMARDs.

Rituximab Rituximab is a monoclonal antibody that targets the CD20 antigen on B-lymphocytes. It is given as two IV infusions 2 weeks apart. The most common side effect is infusion-related reactions. Similar to abatacept, patients refractory to nonbiologic DMARDs and anti-TNF biologic agents have been successfully treated with rituximab. Because of the risk of serious adverse effects including several black box warnings (eg, fatal infusion reactions, tumor lysis syndrome, severe mucocutaneous reactions, progressive multifocal leukoencephalopathy), rituximab is reserved for patients with high RA disease activity and poor prognostic manifestations who have experienced an inadequate response to methotrexate in combination with DMARDs or sequential use of other nonbiologic DMARDs.

Anakinra Anakinra is a recombinant human interleukin-1 (IL-1) receptor antagonist available as a daily, subcutaneous injection. Anakinra is generally less effective than anti-TNF agents; therefore, it is not included in the American College of Rheumatology recommendations and is not considered a first-line biologic agent.

Tocilizumab Tocilizumab is a humanized monoclonal antibody that selectively and competitively antagonizes interleukin-6 (IL-6) receptors. It is administered through IV infusion at 4-week intervals or subcutaneously at weekly or biweekly intervals either in combination with DMARDs including methotrexate or as monotherapy. Tocilizumab is generally well tolerated, although infusion reactions, upper respiratory tract infections, and headaches may occur. Serious adverse events such as infection occur at rates similar to those experienced with other biologic agents. Regular monitoring of liver transaminases, cholesterol levels, and CBC should be performed.

SPECIAL CONSIDERATIONS

RA patients should receive an influenza vaccine prior to starting DMARD therapy and should be revaccinated annually as long as treatment continues. They should also receive the pneumococcal vaccine if starting methotrexate, leflunomide, sulfasalazine, or any biologic DMARD. If risk factors for Hepatitis B are present, patients on a biologic DMARD should receive the vaccine series. Because of their lowered threshold for infection, patients on biologic agents should not receive live vaccines and should avoid their scheduled doses for the week before and after undergoing surgical procedures. Patients should also be screened for tuberculosis infection prior to starting therapy with a biologic agent.

CASE Application

1. Patient GS, a 50-year-old Causasian female, presents to her primary care physician with a chief complaint of generalized fatigue and malaise over the past few months. She also describes having stiffness in her fingers each morning upon waking lasting at least 1 to 2 hours and notes that her fingers and toes (right and left) sometimes appear to be swollen. The physician orders tests including a basic metabolic panel, CBC, rheumatoid factor and X-rays of the hands and feet. Which of GS' complaints could lead the physician to a diagnosis of rheumatoid arthritis? Select all that apply.

    a. Complaints of morning stiffness
    b. Swelling in fingers
    c. Duration of symptoms
    d. Swelling in toes

2. PT is a 38-year-old patient with a past medical history of rheumatoid arthritis. He is changing therapy at today's visit to an alternative agent. He had a sulfa allergic reaction 2 years ago. Which of the following DMARDs is contraindicated in a patient with a history of a sulfa allergy?

    a. Neoral
    b. Arava
    c. Rheumatrex
    d. Azulfidine
    e. Cytoxan

3. JJ was diagnosed with RA with moderate disease activity and has been exhibiting symptoms for about 2 months. Which of the following medications are appropriate to consider in the initial medication regimen for JJ?

    a. Ibuprofen
    b. Prednisone
    c. Methotrexate
    d. Etanercept

4. Which of the following nonpharmacologic therapies may be recommended to JJ? Select all that apply.

    a. Heat or cold therapy
    b. Physical therapy
    c. Weight reduction
    d. Cold therapy

5. Which of the following is the correct mechanism of action for etanercept (Enbrel)?

    a. Monoclonal antibody which targets the CD20 antigen on B-lymphocytes
    b. TNF-α inhibitor
    c. Immunoglobulin protein which inhibits T-lymphocytes
    d. Dihydrofolate reductase inhibitor

6. Which of the following is a reason that DMARDs are preferred over non-DMARD for RA management?

   a. DMARD agents cause fewer adverse reactions than non-DMARDs.
   b. Non-DMARD agents are less cost-effective than DMARDs.
   c. DMARD agents may reduce or prevent joint damage and preserve joint function.
   d. Non-DMARD agents require close laboratory monitoring.

7. Which brand/generic is correctly matched?

   a. Adalimumab/Enbrel
   b. Etanercept/Orencia
   c. Abatacept/Humira
   d. Infliximab/Remicade

8. Which of the following agents is dosed weekly?

   a. Methotrexate
   b. Leflunomide
   c. Hydroxychloroquine
   d. Sulfasalazine

9. A physician prescribes Arava 100 mg as a loading dose for her patient who is newly diagnosed with RA. A correct maintenance dose for this medication would be:

   a. Methotrexate 20 mg daily
   b. Methotrexate 20 mg weekly
   c. Leflunomide 20 mg daily
   d. Leflunomide 20 mg weekly

10. Which of the following monitoring parameters should be followed for patients receiving hydroxychloroquine?

    a. Tuberculin skin test at baseline due to the risk of serious infections.
    b. Hepatic function should be assessed at baseline, 6 months, and 12 months due to risk of hepatic toxicity.
    c. Renal function should be monitored every 6 months due to risk of renal impairment.
    d. Ophthalmological examination within 1 year of starting therapy due to the risk of retinal toxicity.

11. Which of the following are adverse reactions common to all biological DMARD agents? Select all that apply.

    a. Bone marrow suppression
    b. Heart failure exacerbation
    c. Increased susceptibility to infection
    d. Teratogenicity

12. Which of the following medications is an anti-TNF biologic DMARD?

    a. Tofacitinib
    b. Tocilizumab
    c. Rituximab
    d. Golimumab

13. Which of the following conditions would be a contraindication for receiving methotrexate?

    a. Slight renal impairment (CrCL = 50 mL/min)
    b. Mild thrombocytopenia (platelets = 100×10^9/L)
    c. Pregnancy
    d. Latent tuberculosis infection

14. Why is folic acid 1 mg po daily often recommended along with methotrexate therapy?

    a. Folic acid can prevent renal toxicity caused by methotrexate.
    b. Folic acid can prevent gastrointestinal toxicity caused by methotrexate.
    c. Most people with rheumatoid arthritis have folic acid deficiencies.
    d. Folic acid will enhance the efficacy of methotrexate.

15. A physician would like to add an anti-TNF agent which can be administered subcutaneously for a patient who has failed to respond adequately to methotrexate monotherapy after 3 months. Which of the following medications meets both of these criteria?

    a. Abatacept
    b. Cytoxan
    c. Cimzia
    d. Remicade
    e. Rituxan

16. Select the brand name for hydroxychloroquine.

    a. Arava
    b. Cytoxan
    c. Humira
    d. Plaquenil
    e. Rituxan

17. Which of the following is true about DMARD therapy?

    a. DMARDs reduce or prevent joint damage in RA.
    b. Onset of action is usually 1 to 2 weeks.
    c. Reserved for use in severe long-term RA.
    d. If a patient fails one DMARD, they will likely fail all DMARDs.

18. AA is a 34-year-old woman who regularly picks up her Arava and Ortho Tri-Cyclen refills at your pharmacy. Today she arrives to pick up her Arava and states she will no longer need her Ortho Tri-Cyclen as she and her husband have decided to start trying to have a baby. Which of the following would be an appropriate response to this information?

    a. Continue Arava at a lower dose when she becomes pregnant, as rheumatoid arthritis typically improves during pregnancy.
    b. Change Arava to methotrexate during pregnancy.
    c. Discontinue Arava 2 to 3 weeks prior to trying to get pregnant.
    d. Undergo drug-elimination with cholestyramine prior to trying to get pregnant.

19. Which of the following is true about rituximab? Select all that apply.

    a. It is available for administration intravenously.
    b. Premedication with corticosteroid, APAP, and antihistamine should be done prior to each dose.
    c. Dosing may be repeated every 7 days.
    d. It is available for administration subcutaneously.

20. DR is a 65-year-old female patient with RA which is being treated with methotrexate and Cimzia. It is November, and her doctor would like to know if DR can receive the flu vaccine. What would you recommend?

    a. DR should receive the Fluzone intramuscular vaccine.
    b. DR should receive the Flumist intranasal vaccine.
    c. DR should receive prophylactic oseltamivir.
    d. DR should not receive any vaccines while taking Cimzia for RA.

TAKEAWAY POINTS »

- RA is a chronic autoimmune disorder characterized by the presence of persistent inflammation and symmetric erosive synovitis that may eventually lead to joint deterioration and deformity.

- There are no specific laboratory tests available to establish a diagnosis of RA, but patients may test positive for RF or ANA. Erythrocyte sedimentation rates and CRP levels may also be elevated.

- Diagnosis of RA is made when patients meet four of the following seven criteria: morning stiffness that lasts more than 1 hour, swelling in three or more joint areas, swelling in the hand or wrist joints, symmetrical arthritis, rheumatoid nodules, positive RF, and radiological changes (joint erosions or decalcifications).

- RA patients should receive self-management education and training, including use of local heat or cold therapy, joint rest, proper exercise to maintain joint range of motion and muscle strength, healthy eating, and physical and occupational therapy as needed.

- Treatment guidelines recommend the initiation of DMARDs soon after RA diagnosis, but other options such as NSAIDs and corticosteroids may be used in the beginning of treatment while awaiting the therapeutic onset of DMARD agents or during flares of RA symptoms.

- A variety of DMARDs (nonbiologic and biologic) are available for RA. These agents have reduced or prevented joint damage and preserved joint function and integrity. The nonbiologic DMARDs methotrexate or leflunomide are recommended as first-line monotherapy agents for all levels of disease activity.

- Biological DMARDs are used typically after a patient has experienced treatment failure with nonbiologics, particularly methotrexate. However, triple nonbiologic DMARD therapy (methotrexate, sulfasalazine, hydroxychloroquine) may be utilized.

- Combinations of biological DMARDs are not recommended because of increased risk of serious adverse events (eg, infection) and/or lack of additive benefit.

- Abatacept and rituximab have demonstrated efficacy in RA patients refractory to nonbiologic DMARDs and anti-TNF biologic agents.

BIBLIOGRAPHY

Grosser T, Smyth E, FitzGerald GA. Anti-inflammatory, antipyretic, and analgesic agents; pharmacotherapy of gout. In: Brunton LL, Chabner BA, Knollmann BC, eds. *Goodman & Gilman's The Pharmacological Basis of Therapeutics*. 12th ed. New York, NY: McGraw-Hill; 2011:chap 34.

Schuna AA. Rheumatoid arthritis. In: Linn WD, Wofford MR, O'Keefe M, Posey L, eds. *Pharmacotherapy in Primary Care*. New York, NY: McGraw-Hill; 2009:chap 34.

Shah A, St. Clair E. Rheumatoid arthritis. In: Longo DL, Fauci AS, Kasper DL, Hauser SL, Jameson J, Loscalzo J, eds. *Harrison's Principles of Internal Medicine*. 18th ed. New York, NY: McGraw-Hill; 2012:chap 321.

Singh JA, Saag KG, Bridges SL, et al. 2015 American College of Rheumatology Guideline for the Treatment of Rheumatoid Arthritis. *Arthritis Rheumatol*. 2016 Jan;68(1):1-26.

Wahl K, Schuna AA. Rheumatoid arthritis. In: DiPiro JT, Talbert RL, Yee GC, Matzke GR, Wells BG, Posey L, eds. *Pharmacotherapy: A Pathophysiologic Approach*. 10th ed. New York, NY: McGraw-Hill; 2017.

KEY ABBREVIATIONS

ANA = antinuclear antibody
CBC = complete blood count
CRP = C-reactive protein
DMARDs = disease-modifying antirheumatic drugs
JAK = janus kinase

NSAIDs = nonsteroidal anti-inflammatory drugs
PEG = polyethylene glycol
RA = rheumatoid arthritis
RF = rheumatoid factor

51

Osteoarthritis

Anne Misher

FOUNDATION OVERVIEW

Osteoarthritis (OA) is a joint disease arising from different pathophysiological causes with manifestations of joint damage, mechanical stress, and loss of articular cartilage. A normal joint is composed of subchondral bone covered by a thin layer of articular cartilage. The interarticular space separates the adjoining subchondral bone and is cushioned with synovial fluid. Articular cartilage allows frictionless movement and uniform load distribution. Muscles, ligaments, and tendons surround the joint providing strength, maintaining stability, and absorbing load. However, there are several physiologic changes that lead to a weakened joint, instability with loss of dexterity, development of pain, and decreased mobility. Weight-bearing joints such as the knee and hip are mainly affected in OA; however, joints of the hand, foot, lumbar, and cervical spine may also be involved.

Patients with OA present with joint pain and tenderness, limited mobility, instability, and crepitus with joint movement. Symptoms may progress from absence of pain, to joint pain upon movement relieved by rest, to pain with rest. Advanced disease will manifest with joint space narrowing, formation of new bone at joint margins (osteophytosis), and subchondral sclerosis on radiographs. Risk factors associated with OA include advanced age, female gender, genetics, obesity, history of joint trauma, repetitive movement, excess mechanical stress, misalignment, and quadriceps weakness. Diagnosis of OA is based on patient history, physical examination, radiographic evidence, and laboratory testing. The American College of Rheumatology criteria for classification of OA of the knee and hip share common elements including: age more than 50 years, joint-specific pain, and joint stiffness. Diagnosis of knee or hip OA also includes bone tenderness and enlargement with radiographic evidence of osteophytes. Pain with internal rotation of the hip joint validates OA diagnosis. Hard tissue enlargement, swollen joints, and deformity in addition to hand pain with aching or stiffness, are criteria used to diagnose OA of the hand.

PREVENTION

Addressing risk factors such as obesity with weight loss, potential joint injury with joint protection, and muscle weakness with exercise are strategies for prevention of OA. Increased body mass is associated with muscle weakness, altered gait, decreased function, and fall risk and weight loss reduces the probability of developing OA. Joint injury predisposes patients for OA later in life. Current treatment of injury in those without OA may include surgery, joint rehabilitation, and muscle strengthening. Regular physical activity and muscle strengthening through resistance exercise in those without OA may be a preventative strategy. Because muscles provide movement, absorb load, and stabilize the joint, strengthening can improve muscle function.

TREATMENT

Treatment goals for OA include disease state awareness, relieving pain and stiffness, improving musculoskeletal movement and function, protecting affected joints, and maintaining and improving quality of life. These goals are accomplished by lifestyle changes, orthotics, physical and occupational rehabilitation, and pharmacologic therapy. Regular contact should be established with the patient through office visits or telephone contact to discuss pain status, compliance with pharmacologic and nonpharmacologic treatment, adverse effects of medications, and barriers to any therapy (Figures 51-1 and 51-2).

Nonpharmacologic

Obesity is a preventable risk factor of OA. Obese patients should lose weight (at least 10% of body weight) to reduce strain on joints. A fitness program focusing on improving muscle strength, mobility, and coordination should be developed for every patient. Exercise including cardiovascular (CV) and/or resistance land-based and aquatic is recommended. Physical and/or occupational therapy should be used to maintain or regain range of motion and strengthen muscles. Patients should wear appropriate footwear that supports and cushions the joints. Heat can be applied topically or through hydrotherapy during noninflammatory situations, such as immediately prior to exercise. Assistive devices such as canes, crutches, joint supports, and insoles can be used to protect joints from overuse. Surgery can be considered in patients who do not experience pain relief with medical therapy or have functional disability.

To access your complimentary online question exams, visit https://accesspharmacy.mhmedical.com/NAPLEX.aspx

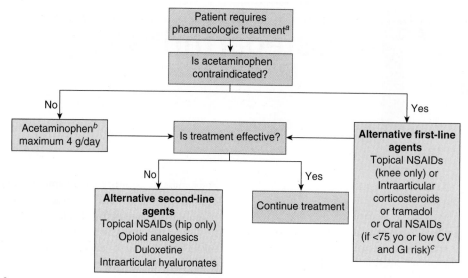

FIGURE 51-1 Treatment recommendations for knee and hip osteoarthritis. *Abbreviations:* CV, cardiovascular; GI, gastrointestinal; NSAIDs, nonsteroidal anti-inflammatory drugs. Reproduced with permission from DiPiro JT, Talbert RL, Yee GC, et al: *Pharmacotherapy: A Pathophysiologic Approach*, 10th ed: New York, NY: McGraw-Hill; 2017.

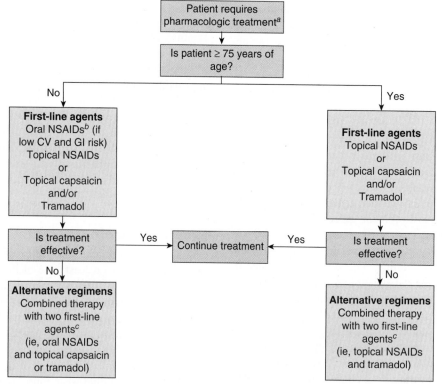

FIGURE 51-2 Treatment recommendations for hand osteoarthritis. *Abbreviations:* CV, cardiovascular; GI, gastrointestinal; NSAIDs, nonsteroidal anti-inflammatory drugs. Reproduced with permission from DiPiro JT, Talbert RL, Yee GC, et al: *Pharmacotherapy: A Pathophysiologic Approach*, 10th ed: New York, NY: McGraw-Hill; 2017

Pharmacologic

A stepwise approach should be used in order to determine the most effective patient-specific therapy. Tables 51-1 and 51-2 list key information for medications used in the management of OA.

Analgesics

Relief of pain and inflammation is a primary objective of pharmacologic treatment. First-line therapy for OA (hip and knee OA) is acetaminophen. Acetaminophen blocks the action of central cyclooxygenase preventing prostaglandin (agents that

TABLE 51-1 Drug Dosing Table

Drug	Brand Name	Starting Dose	Usual Range	Special Population Dose	Other
Oral Analgesics					
Acetaminophen	Tylenol	325-500 mg three times a day	325-650 mg every 4-6 hour or 1 g three to four times a day	Chronic alcohol intake, hepatic disease	Contained in many combination analgesics
Tramadol Tramadol ER	Ultram Ultram ER	25 mg in the morning 100 mg daily	Titrate dose in 25 mg increments to reach a maintenance dose of 50-100 mg three times a day Titrate to 200-300 mg daily	Creatinine clearance <30 mL/min (<0.5 mL/s)—maximum dose is 200 mg daily Do not use if creatinine clearance <30 mL/min (<0.5 mL/s)	May need to taper dose upon discontinuation to prevent withdrawal symptoms
Hydrocodone/ acetaminophen	Lortab, Vicodin	5 mg/325 mg three times daily	2.5-10 mg/325-650 mg three to five times daily	Titrate dose slowly in older patients	Maximum dose limited by total daily dose of acetaminophen
Oxycodone/ acetaminophen	Percocet	5 mg/325 mg three times daily	2.5-10 mg/325-650 mg three to five times daily	Titrate dose slowly in older patients	Maximum dose limited by total daily dose of acetaminophen
Topical Analgesics					
Capsaicin 0.025% or 0.075%	Capzasin-HP		Apply to affected joint three to four times per day		—
Diclofenac 1% gel	Voltaren		Apply 2 or 4 g per site as prescribed, four times daily		
Diclofenac 1.3% patch	Flector		Apply one patch twice daily to the site to be treated, as directed. Apply 40 drops to the affected knee, applying and rubbing in 10 drops		
Diclofenac 1.5% solution	Pennsaid		Apply 40 drops to the affected knee, applying and rubbing in 10 drops at a time. Repeat for a total of four times daily		
Diclofenac 2% solution	Pennsaid		Apply 40 mg (2 pump actuations) twice daily		
Intra-articular Corticosteroids					
Triamcinolone	Kenalog	5-15 mg per joint	10-40 mg per large joint (knee, hip, shoulder)	If multiple joints injected, maximum total dose is usually 80 mg	Often administered concomitantly with a local anesthetic
Methylprednisolone acetate	Depo-Medrol	10-20 mg per joint	20-80 mg per large joint (knee, hip, shoulder)	10-40 mg for medium joints (elbows, wrists)	
Nonsteroidal Anti-inflammatory Drugs (NSAIDs)					
Aspirin, plain, buffered, or enteric-coated	Bayer, Ecotrin, Bufferin	325 mg three times a day	325-650 mg four times a day		Doses of 3600 mg/d are needed for anti-inflammatory activity
Celecoxib	Celebrex	100 mg daily	100 mg twice daily or 200 mg daily		
Diclofenac XR Diclofenac IR	Voltaren-XR Cataflam	100 mg daily 50 mg twice a day	100-200 mg daily 50-75 mg twice a day		
Diflunisal	Dolobid	250 mg twice a day	500-750 mg twice a day		
Etodolac	Lodine	300 mg twice a day	400-500 mg twice a day		
Fenoprofen	Nalfon	400 mg three times a day	400-600 mg three to four times a day		

(Continued)

TABLE 51-1 | **Drug Dosing Table** (*Continued*)

Drug	Brand Name	Starting Dose	Usual Range	Special Population Dose	Other
Flurbiprofen	Ansaid	100 mg twice a day	200-300 mg/d in two to four divided doses		
Ibuprofen	Motrin, Advil	200 mg three times a day	1200-3200 mg/d in three to four divided doses		Available OTC and Rx
Indomethacin Indomethacin SR	Indocin Indocin SR	25 mg twice a day 75 mg SR once daily	Titrate dose by 25-50 mg/d until pain controlled or maximum dose of 50 mg three times a day Can titrate to 75 mg SR twice daily if needed		
Ketoprofen	Orudis	50 mg three times a day	50-75 mg three to four times a day		
Meclofenamate	Meclomen	50 mg three times a day	50-100 mg three to four times a day		
Mefenamic acid	Ponstel	250 mg three times a day	250 mg four times a day		FDA approval for 1 week of therapy
Meloxicam	Mobic	7.5 mg daily	15 mg daily		
Nabumetone	Relafen	500 mg daily	500-1000 mg one to two times a day		
Naproxen	Naprosyn	250 mg twice a day	500 mg twice a day		Available OTC and Rx
Naproxen sodium Naproxen sodium controlled-release tablets	Anaprox, Aleve Naprelan	220 mg twice a day	220-550 mg twice a day 375-750 mg twice a day		
Oxaprozin	Daypro	600 mg daily	600-1200 mg daily		
Piroxicam	Feldene	10 mg daily	20 mg daily		
Salsalate	Disalcid	500 mg twice a day	500-1000 mg two to three times a day		

Reproduced with permission from DiPiro JT, Talbert RL, Yee GC, et al: *Pharmacotherapy: A Pathophysiologic Approach*, 10th ed: New York, NY: McGraw-Hill; 2017.

enhance pain sensations) synthesis. Though effective for pain relief, acetaminophen does not target inflammation. Acetaminophen affects the hepatic, renal, and hematologic systems. Monitoring of bilirubin, alkaline phosphatase, serum creatinine, bruising, and signs and symptoms of bleeding should occur for all patients receiving chronic acetaminophen doses. Education on avoidance of alcohol and acetaminophen contents in combination products should be provided to patients.

If an acetaminophen trial of 1 to 2 weeks is ineffective, a low-dose nonselective nonsteroidal anti-inflammatory drug (NSAID) or nonacetylated salicylate may be used. NSAIDs may supersede acetaminophen as first-line treatment if inflammation is severe. Nonselective NSAIDs inhibit cyclooxygenase enzymes (COX-1 and COX-2), which block prostaglandin synthesis. Common adverse drug reactions are gastrointestinal (GI) effects, including nausea, diarrhea, cramping, and dyspepsia. Serious reactions include perforation, ulceration, obstruction, and GI bleeding. Nonselective NSAIDs can also cause renal insufficiency. NSAID monitoring include serum creatinine, blood urea nitrogen, serum potassium, blood pressure, edema, weight gain, and colored or bloody urine or stool. If pain persists on a low-dose nonselective NSAID, then a full-dose

nonselective NSAID or COX-2 inhibitor (selective NSAID) should be prescribed. Sulfonamide allergy is a contraindication to COX-2 inhibitor use. Topical rather than oral NSAIDs should be used in patients more than or equal to 75 years of age.

Tramadol is a centrally acting analgesic that inhibits the reuptake of serotonin and norepinephrine. Tramadol is used for patients with contraindications to NSAIDs or have failed previous drug trials. Adverse effects include nausea, dizziness, headache, vomiting, constipation, and somnolence. Tramadol decreases the seizure threshold necessitating appropriate precautions and monitoring. Tramadol should be avoided in patients taking other medications which increase serotonin concentrations. Opiates are reserved as a last-line therapy in OA (hip and knee OA). Opiates bind to opiate receptors in the central nervous system (CNS) causing an altered perception and response to pain. Common adverse effects associated with opioid use are constipation, nausea, somnolence, and dizziness. Topical analgesic creams, capsaicin (hand OA), and methylsalicylate are options for patients who do not wish to take systemic treatment or as adjunctive (as needed) therapy to oral medications. Topical agents deplete and prevent the reaccumulation of the CNS neurons of substance P, a mediator

TABLE 51-2	Drug Monitoring Table		
Drug	**Adverse Drug Reactions**	**Monitoring Parameters**	**Comments**
Oral Analgesics			
Acetaminophen	Hepatotoxicity	Total daily dose limits	Use caution with multiple acetaminophen-containing products—total 4 g limit
Tramadol	Nausea, vomiting, somnolence	No routine laboratory tests recommended	Drug–drug interaction with other serotonergic medications
Opioids	Sedation, constipation, nausea, dry mouth, hormonal changes	No routine laboratory tests recommended	Risks of addiction, dependence, and drug diversion
NSAIDs	Dyspepsia, cardiovascular events, GI bleeding, renal impairment	BUN/creatinine, hemoglobin/hematocrit, blood pressure	Risks higher in those older than 75 year of age
Topical Analgesics			
Capsaicin	Skin irritation and burning	Inspection of areas of application	Wash hands thoroughly after application
NSAIDs	Skin itching, rash, irritation, dyspepsia, cardiovascular events, GI bleeding, renal impairment	Inspection of areas of application As needed: blood urea nitrogen/creatinine, hemoglobin/hematocrit, blood pressure	Wash hands thoroughly after application. Avoid oral NSAID or aspirin other than cardioprotective dose. Ensure patient applying gel, solution, or patch correctly
Injectable Drugs			
Intra-articular corticosteroids	Hypertension, hyperglycemia	Glucose, blood pressure	Hypothalamic–pituitary–adrenal axis suppression if used too frequently
Intra-articular hyaluronates	Local joint swelling, stiffness, pain	No routine laboratory tests recommended	Less effective than intraarticular corticosteroids; expensive

Reproduced with permission from DiPiro JT, Talbert RL, Yee GC, et al: *Pharmacotherapy: A Pathophysiologic Approach*, 10th ed: New York, NY: McGraw-Hill; 2017.

of pain. Limited adverse effects exist with topical treatment, including burning, stinging, and erythema.

Corticosteroids

Intra-articular corticosteroids are an option (hip and knee OA) for patients experiencing an exacerbation or are not candidates for NSAIDs. A local anesthetic is often coadminstered with the corticosteroid as well as arthrocentesis (joint aspiration) prior to the injection. Improvement in pain occurs 2 to 3 days following injection and lasts between 4 and 8 weeks. Adverse effects with intra-articular administration include facial flushing, skin depigmentation, increased glucose, adrenal insufficiency, hypercorticism, sodium and fluid retention, and joint infections. Injections are limited to four times per year for one joint due to possible systemic effects and lack of response upon continued dosing.

Duloxetine

Duloxetine is an alternative for patients who have not had adequate response to alternative therapies and are unable or not willing to undergo surgery. Duloxetine is a dual-reuptake inhibitor of serotonin and norepinephrine that has its effect through blocking of these central pain transmitters. Adverse effects include nausea, dry mouth, constipation, anorexia, fatigue, and somnolence. Duloxetine should be avoided in patients taking other medications which increase serotonin concentrations.

Hyaluronic Acid

Hyaluronic acid (HA) treatment is an alternative (hip and knee OA) for patients unable to tolerate or did not response to other agents. It is a component of synovial fluid; therefore, exogenous drug stimulates HA synthesis by synoviocytes in arthritic joints. It has a slower onset of action than corticosteroids.

Glucosamine and Chondroitin

Glucosamine and chondroitin are not recommended; however, they are dietary supplements sometimes used in combination or as adjunct therapy. Glucosamine maintains elasticity, strength, and resiliency in joint cartilage and may also be anti-inflammatory. It should be avoided in patients with shellfish allergy and those taking medications that increase risk of bleeding and is contraindicated in active bleeding. Side effects are mild; GI discomfort and upset stomach are most common. Chondroitin is a compound in connective tissue and cartilage that absorbs water, increasing cartilage thickness. Chondroitin should be used with caution in patients with hemostatic problems or a history of bleeding with the most common adverse effect being nausea. It should also be avoided in those taking medications that increase bleeding risk. Numerous studies compared these agents to traditional therapies. Some studies show improvement in pain and stiffness; however, most do not show a statistically significant difference from traditional treatment.

SPECIAL CONSIDERATIONS

Celecoxib (COX-2 inhibitor) and other NSAIDs have a black box warning for GI and CV risks. Patients at high risk for GI bleeding (concomitant aspirin and NSAID therapy, prior history of GI bleeds) with low CV risk should use either a COX-2 inhibitor plus/minus a proton pump inhibitor (PPI) or an NSAID plus a PPI. Misoprostol is a gastroprotective agent that prevents NSAID GI ulceration. However, it is a prostaglandin analog and is contraindicated in pregnancy and women of child bearing potential (unless a woman is capable of complying with effective contraception measures). Patients at high risk for GI bleeding with high CV risk should avoid an NSAID, if possible; naproxen plus a PPI should be utilized if NSAID use is unavoidable.

NSAID use should be considered carefully in patients with hypertension (HTN), congestive heart failure, or renal insufficiency as NSAIDs promote sodium and water retention. Patients with these known co-morbidities or over the age of 65 should be carefully monitored and advised to hold their NSAIDs when unable to eat or drink.

CASE Application

1. EM is a 63-year-old obese man with a history of increasing pain in his left knee. He presently cares for his 85-year-old mother who has had bilateral knee replacements secondary to OA. During his college years, he played on the intramural football team and suffered several knee injuries. During his career as a radio announcer for sports, he maintained a sedentary lifestyle and does not presently exercise. Which of the following are risk factors for the development of OA in EM? Select all that apply.

   a. Age
   b. Genetics
   c. Joint injury
   d. Obesity

2. Which of the following is a sign or symptom of a patient with clinical presentation of OA?

   a. Joint stiffness with rest
   b. Normal range of motion with joint
   c. Joint stability
   d. Joint stiffness with movement
   e. Frictionless joint movement

3. Which of the following are preventative measures for OA? Select all that apply.

   a. Resistance exercise
   b. Maintaining a healthy weight
   c. Surgery
   d. Joint rehabilitation

4. SL is a 62-year-old obese man with a history of degenerative joint disease in his left knee. Past medical history (PMH) is significant for dyslipidemia treated with gemfibrozil and diabetes with NPH 10 units bid and glipizide 10 mg bid. Blood sugar readings are not at goal with HgA1c of 8.5%. Current blood pressure is 130/80 mm Hg. He receives his second injection of 40 mg of Kenalog in his left knee today. Which side effect could cause a drug–disease state interaction in this patient?

   a. Skin depigmentation
   b. Adrenal insufficiency
   c. Joint infection
   d. Hyperglycemia

5. What is the primary objective of pharmacologic therapy for OA?

   a. Improve mobility
   b. Weight loss
   c. Pain relief
   d. Improve muscle and joint strength

6. RT is a construction worker that presents to your clinic for knee pain. He is diagnosed with OA. He is currently obese and cannot take time off from work because of providing for his family. Additionally, he has a family history of OA. He would like to try nonpharmacologic therapy before starting a medication. Which of the following is (are) preventable risk factor(s) for developing OA in this patient? Select all that apply.

   a. Genetics
   b. Joint trauma history
   c. Repetitive movement
   d. Obesity

7. Select the first-line pharmacologic agent for treating OA.

   a. Acetaminophen
   b. Intra-articular corticosteroids
   c. Tramadol
   d. Ibuprofen

8. Which of the following help to reduce NSAID-induced GI toxicity? Select all that apply.

   a. Nonacetylated salicylates
   b. COX-2 inhibitors
   c. Addition of misoprostol
   d. Addition of PPI

9. Which of the following are goals of OA management? Select all that apply.

   a. Teaching patient about the disease state
   b. Curing OA
   c. Providing pain relief
   d. Improving musculoskeletal movement
   e. Maintaining ability to perform activities of daily living

10. Place the following OA management options in the *correct* order in which treatment options for acute pain should be initiated?

Unordered Response	Ordered Response
COX-2 Inhibitor	
Nonselective NSAID	
Acetaminophen	
Joint replacement	
Tramadol/opioid analgesic	

11. AZ is a 72-year-old woman with a history of atrial fibrillation treated with warfarin. Her height is 5' 2",

weight is 198 lb, blood pressure is 116/76 mm Hg, and SCr is 1.1. AZ is now complaining of pain and stiffness in her left knee. X-ray shows joint space narrowing and osteophytes at the joint. Which treatment should be initiated at this point? Select all that apply.

a. Weight reduction
b. Tylenol
c. Celebrex
d. Tramadol

12. BY is a 65-year-old man with confirmed OA. He has been pain free on his current regimen of acetaminophen 650 mg every 6 hours for 2 years. PMH is significant for GI bleed 4 years ago and HTN. He now presents to your clinic with pain in his left hip. BY's medication regimen also consists of lisinopril 40 mg daily and hydrochlorothiazide 25 mg daily. What recommendation will you present to the physician?

a. Increase acetaminophen to 1000 mg every 4 hours, reinforce fitness program.
b. Add pantoprazole 40 mg daily to his regimen, reinforce fitness program.
c. Stop acetaminophen, begin ibuprofen 400 mg tid, reinforce fitness program.
d. Stop acetaminophen, begin Anaprox 250 mg bid, Protonix 40 mg daily, reinforce fitness program.
e. Add celecoxib 200 mg daily, reinforce fitness program.

13. CK is a 58-year-old woman who presents to your pharmacotherapy clinic today with an international normalized ratio (INR) of 4.2 (she was previously stable for 6 months). She has a PMH of diabetes, atrial fibrillation, and HTN. The list of medications that she gives you from her pharmacy are as follows: metformin 1000 mg and glipizide 10 mg bid; warfarin 5 mg on Monday, Wednesday, and Friday and 2.5 mg on Sunday, Tuesday, Thursday, and Saturday; amlodipine 10 mg daily; potassium chloride 10 mEq daily; and hydrochlorothiazide 25 mg daily. CK has not had a warfarin dosage change in over 1 year. She tells you her right knee has been bothering her much more frequently than usual. Which of the following is the most likely reason for her INR fluctuation?

a. CK took 5 mg warfarin tablets every day in the past week.
b. After questioning CK about over-the-counter (OTC) use, she tells you she has been using Capsaicin-HP on her knee for the past week.
c. After questioning CK about OTC use, she tells you she has been taking acetaminophen 650 mg every 6 hours to relieve her from knee pain for the past week.
d. CK is not telling you about a herbal product she has begun taking.

14. DP is a 55-year-old man who has HTN and a positive family history of early CV disease. His medications include aspirin 81 mg daily and metoprolol 25 mg bid. DP's OA is no longer controlled with acetaminophen

650 mg every 6 hours. The physician wants to begin DP on a regimen including an NSAID. Which treatment do you recommend?

a. Naproxen 250 mg bid
b. Naproxen 500 mg tid
c. Celebrex 200 mg daily
d. Celebrex 800 mg daily

15. The physician does not take your advice for DP in Question 14. She prescribes ibuprofen 800 mg three times per day. Which of the following do you need to counsel DP concerning?

a. Do not take this medication, it might cause you harm.
b. Take ibuprofen at least 30 minutes after aspirin or aspirin. 8 hours after ibuprofen. Monitor your BP more often.
c. Stop taking your aspirin. Do not take ibuprofen on an empty stomach.
d. Stop taking your aspirin. Monitor your BP more often.

16. A 44-year-old woman with a history of GI bleed presents to your community pharmacy. She tells you her pregnancy test from last night was positive. She presents refill bottles for her prescription of ibuprofen 400 mg every 8 hours and Cytotec 200 mcg bid and asks if these are okay for her to keep taking. You respond:

a. Stop taking Cytotec. It is ok to continue ibuprofen.
b. Stop taking ibuprofen. It is ok to continue Cytotec.
c. Continue taking both medications. Call your physician as soon as you can.
d. Continue taking both medications. Your pregnancy test may not be accurate.
e. Stop taking both prescriptions. Let us call your physician together now to discuss your situation.

17. Which of the following medications is contraindicated in patients with documented sulfa allergy?

a. Ultram
b. Toradol
c. Celebrex
d. Aspirin
e. HA

18. AM is a 52-year-old woman whose medications include acetaminophen 500 mg four times per day, gabapentin 300 mg three times per day, gemfibrozil 600 mg twice daily, and fluoxetine 20 mg daily. At the direction of her physician, AM added ibuprofen 800 mg twice daily and capsaicin cream 0.025% three times per day as needed to her regimen. While putting on her contacts this morning, she experienced an immediate burning pain in her eyes. She immediately takes out her contacts, flushes her eyes, and calls you, her pharmacist. Which of the following is most likely causing her eye pain?

a. Capsaicin cream
b. Acetaminophen

c. Drug interaction between acetaminophen and gemfibrozil

d. Drug interaction between acetaminophen and gabapentin

19. KT is a 73-year-old woman with OA of the hand. Her medication list includes: salsalate 500 mg twice daily, Lantus 10 U at bedtime, hydrochlorothiazide 25 mg daily, and ibuprofen 400 mg as needed that was recently increased to 800 mg twice daily as needed because of pain. What recommendation(s) do you give to the physician during rounds? Select all that apply.

a. KT should not be on more than one NSAID at a time.

b. Ibuprofen should not be given as needed for OA.

c. Ibuprofen should be dosed three to four times daily.

d. Salsalate has a longer platelet effect than ibuprofen.

20. GM is an 81-year-old woman with history of bilateral knee OA for 25 years. She has contraindications to surgery and has received one injection of HA (Synvisc One). She calls your clinic 2 days after the intra-articular injection and states that she has not felt any pain relief. You explain:

a. She will not experience pain relief at this point.

b. She may need concomitant administration of intra-articular glucocorticoid.

c. She should take glucosamine and chondroitin in addition to the use of HA.

d. She should stop NSAID therapy while Hyalgan is administered.

21. A 59-year-old man with history of 2 months of joint pain in his knees with movement decides to treat with glucosamine chondroitin. He reports an allergy to shellfish. He asks for your recommendation. Which of the following counseling points do you discuss with the patient? Select all that apply.

a. No significant benefit is seen with use of glucosamine chondroitin as monotherapy.

b. Glucosamine chondroitin could be considered as an adjunct to other forms of therapy.

c. Glucosamine chondroitin is contraindicated in those with shellfish allergies.

d. GI symptoms of gas, bloating, and cramps may occur with use of glucosamine chondroitin.

TAKEAWAY POINTS ❯❯

- OA is a joint disease arising from different pathophysiological causes with manifestations of joint damage, mechanical stress, and loss of articular cartilage.
- Risk factors include advanced age, female gender, genetics, obesity, history of joint trauma, repetitive movement, excessive mechanical stress, malalignment, and quadriceps weakness.
- Signs and symptoms of OA are specific joint pain and tenderness, stiffness and pain with inactivity, swollen joints, and limited range of motion.
- Diagnosis of OA is made on patient history, physical examination, radiographic evidence, and laboratory monitoring.
- Preventative strategies for OA include weight loss, joint protection, muscle strengthening with exercise, and rehabilitation.
- OA treatment goals are disease state awareness, pain relief, musculoskeletal movement, function improvement, and maintain and improve quality of life.
- Nonpharmacologic OA treatment therapies include: weight reduction for overweight individuals, physical/occupational therapy, muscle-strengthening exercises, use of appropriate footwear and assistive devices, heat application to affected joints, surgery, and regular patient contact with a provider.
- Pharmacologic agents include: oral and topical analgesics, NSAIDs, intra-articular corticosteroids and HA, opioids, duloxetine, and nutritional supplements.

- First-line therapy for OA is acetaminophen.
- Nonselective NSAIDs and nonacetylated salicylates are used when acetaminophen is contraindicated or ineffective.
- Selective NSAIDs (COX-2 inhibitors) can be used in place of nonselective NSAIDs.
- If other analgesics are ineffective, tramadol can be trialed for pain relief. Opiates should be a final alternative due to their addictive and respiratory depression effects.
- Patients at risk for GI bleeding should avoid nonselective NSAIDs, if possible. If unavoidable, a gastroprotective agent should be added.
- NSAID (nonselective and selective) should be used cautiously in patients with HTN, congestive heart failure, renal insufficiency, or advanced age.
- Topical analgesic creams are an option for patients who do not wish to take systemic treatment or as an adjunct to drug therapy.
- Intra-articular corticosteroids are an option during OA exacerbations or in those who are not NSAID candidates.
- Intra-articular HA can be used in place of intra-articular corticosteroids for chronic inflammation.
- Glucosamine and chondroitin are dietary supplements used solely or as an adjunct in OA. Studies do not show a statistically significant difference in pain improvement.

BIBLIOGRAPHY

Buys LM, Elliott M. Osteoarthritis. In: Linn WD, Wofford MR, O'Keefe M, Posey L, eds. *Pharmacotherapy in Primary Care.* New York, NY: McGraw-Hill; 2009:chap 35.

Buys LM, Wiedenfeld SA. Osteoarthritis. In: DiPiro JT, Talbert RL, Yee GC, Matzke GR, Wells BG, Posey L, eds. *Pharmacotherapy: A Pathophysiologic Approach.* 10th ed. New York, NY: McGraw-Hill; 2017.

Felson DT. Osteoarthritis. In: Longo DL, Fauci AS, Kasper DL, Hauser SL, Jameson J, Loscalzo J, eds. *Harrison's Principles of Internal Medicine.* 18th ed. New York, NY: McGraw-Hill; 2012:chap 332.

Grosser T, Smyth E, FitzGerald GA. Anti-inflammatory, antipyretic, and analgesic agents; pharmacotherapy of gout. In: Brunton LL, Chabner BA, Knollmann BC, eds. *Goodman & Gilman's The Pharmacological Basis of Therapeutics.* 12th ed. New York, NY: McGraw-Hill; 2011:chap 34.

KEY ABBREVIATIONS

CNS = central nervous system
GI = gastrointestinal
HTN = hypertension
NSAID = nonsteroidal anti-inflammatory drug

OA = osteoarthritis
OTC = over-the-counter
PMH = past medical history

8

Neurologic Disorders

52

Parkinson Disease

Michele Faulkner

FOUNDATION OVERVIEW

Parkinson disease (PD) also called Parkinson's disease, is a slow, progressive neurodegenerative disease of the extrapyramidal motor system for which there is presently no cure. The neurodegenerative disorder results from the loss of nigrostriatal neurons in the substantia nigra pars compacta and lewy body formation (misfolded proteins). By the time symptoms emerge and a diagnosis is made, it is estimated that 80% of nigrostriatal neurons have been lost. Due to a resultant deficiency in the neurotransmitter dopamine, there is less inhibitory output from the basal ganglia allowing for overactivity of acetylcholine. The neurotransmitter imbalance is responsible for the motor function abnormalities that characterize PD. The cardinal features of PD include tremor, bradykinesia, rigidity, and postural instability (though this symptom is rare in the early stages of the disease). PD symptoms typically begin unilaterally and spread to the opposite side as the disease progresses. Presentation varies among individuals and can differ substantially from person to person.

Tremor is the most common PD symptom, however it is not universal. It may be described as a feeling of an internal vibration that is not outwardly apparent. Pill rolling (fingers and thumb moving in opposing directions) is a term used to describe the symptom. In mild disease, the tremor usually disappears with purposeful movement and during sleep. In some cases, tremor may also be present in the lips, chin, and jaw.

Bradykinesia (slow movement) may result in difficulty with tasks requiring repetitive movements and fine motor control (eg, teeth brushing). Arm swinging when walking may be diminished or absent and spontaneous gesturing and facial expression are often blunted. Shuffling gait may become apparent and difficulty in turning in bed or rising from a chair may affect the patient's ability to function. Handwriting frequently becomes smaller (micrographia) and difficult to read. Eventually, all voluntary movement will be affected to some degree.

Rigidity is resistance in the muscles upon initiation of passive movement and is described as "jerky" or "cogwheeling." Vague muscle aches may be the first sign of rigidity and often occur in the back, shoulder, or arm. Some patients experience painful dystonias and cramping in the feet.

Postural instability (or postural reflex impairment) typically appears later in the disease process and is connected with advancing rigidity. Patients may be observed in a stooped position with flexion at the knees, hips, and waist. Patients may also be observed walking on the balls of their feet. Impairment of posture contributes substantially to the risk of injury secondary to falling.

PD is a diagnosis of exclusion. There are no biological or laboratory tests that can confirm PD (although a radiopharmaceutical indicated for striatal dopamine transporter visualization can be used to differentiate PD from other movement disorders). In general, if two of the cardinal features are present and characteristics of another movement disorder are absent, the diagnosis is made. A positive response to administration of the drug levodopa (which will temporarily increase dopamine levels in the central nervous system [CNS]) may be considered confirmatory. Medication-induced parkinsonism (associated most often with phenothiazine antiemetics, metoclopramide and neuroleptic medications) should be evaluated in patients with PD symptoms, especially if onset is sudden.

TREATMENT

The goal of PD treatment is to maintain the patient's functional ability by controlling motor symptoms. The optimal time to start drug therapy in PD varies, but in general, treatment should be initiated when the disease begins to interfere with activities of daily living, employment, or quality of life. Specific objectives to consider when selecting an intervention include preservation of the ability to perform activities of daily living; employment; improvement of mobility; minimization of adverse effects and treatment complications; and improvement of nonmotor features. To accomplish these objectives, an interprofessional approach is helpful (eg, neurology, pharmacotherapy, physical/occupational/speech therapy, psychiatry, and sleep medicine). Exercise helps delay functional decline, and improve gait, balance, and strength. Ultimately, therapy should be tailored to the individual needs of the patient (Figure 52-1). Tables 52-1 and 52-2 summarize medications used for treatment and the monitoring for potential adverse reactions.

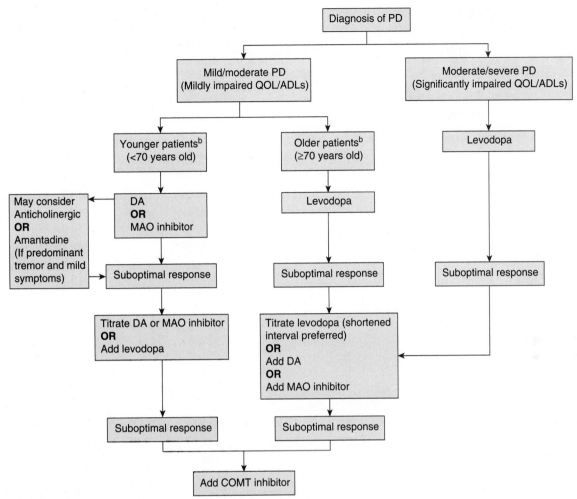

FIGURE 52-1 General approach to pharmacologic management of Parkinson disease.
Abbreviations: ADL, activities of daily living; COMT, catechol-o-methyltransferase; DA, dopamine agonist; MAO, monoamine oxidase; PD, Parkinson disease; QOL, quality of life.
aChoice of pharmacologic agents and order of introduction should be tailored according to individual patient needs and characteristics.
bConsider physiological, not chronological age.

Levodopa/Carbidopa

Levodopa is the primary agent for controlling PD motor symptoms. Levodopa is converted to dopamine leading to a decrease in the neurotransmitter imbalance. Carbidopa is utilized to inhibit the activity of the enzyme dopa decarboxylase, thus preventing the conversion of levodopa to dopamine in the periphery. Without carbidopa, levels of dopamine in the CNS would be diminished and the patient would be subject to nausea and orthostatic hypotension. A minimum daily dose of 75 to 100 mg of carbidopa is recommended to prevent peripheral conversion, and carbidopa supplementation may be given without an increase in the levodopa dose if necessary. The typical starting dose of carbidopa/levodopa is 25/100 mg orally given three times daily (Table 52-1). Oral formulations are best taken on an empty stomach, but if side effects necessitate that they be taken with food, a low protein meal is preferred as dietary amino acids compete with levodopa (also an amino acid) for transport into the CNS. Immediate-release, controlled-release, extended-release and orally dissolving tablet formulations of carbidopa/levodopa are available, as is an enteral suspension that is continuously delivered via pump through a gastrointestinal tube. The controlled-release formulation is not absorbed as well, and may require a 30% increase in daily dose if a conversion from the immediate-release form is desired. The extended-release formulation is not intended for initial therapy, and cannot be converted on a 1:1 basis due to unique capsule strengths.

Carbidopa/levodopa works for the entire range of motor symptoms and most patients can be maintained on 600 mg of levodopa or less for the first several years. However, the efficacy of levodopa will eventually decrease because of a decline in the ability of the brain to store dopamine. The result is a return of symptoms prior to the next administration time known as "wearing off." In contrast, "on-off" phenomena begins to appear after extended use of levodopa, but the return of symptoms occurs in an unpredictable manner, typically lasting seconds to minutes. This unpredictability can be distressing for patients, particularly as symptom breakthrough begins to occur with increasing frequency.

Dyskinesias, primarily dystonia and chorea, are involuntary movements that may occur in a patient taking levodopa.

TABLE 52-1   **Dosing of Medications Used in the Treatment of Parkinson Disease[a]**

Generic Name	Trade Name	Starting Dose[b](mg/d)	Maintenance Dose[b] (mg/d)	Dosage Forms (mg)
Anticholinergic Drugs				
Benztropine	Cogentin	0.5-1	1-6	0.5, 1, 2
Trihexyphenidyl	Artane	1-2	6-15	2, 5, 2/5 mL
Carbidopa/Levodopa Products				
Carbidopa/L-dopa	Sinemet	300[c]	300-2,000[c]	10/100, 25/100, 25/250
Carbidopa/L-dopa ODT	Parcopa	300[c]	300-2,000[c]	10/100, 25/100, 25/250
Carbidopa/L-dopa CR	Sinemet CR	400[c]	400-2,000[c]	25/100, 50/200
Carbidopa/L-dopa IR/ER	Rytary	435[c]	435-2,450[c]	23.75/95, 36.25/145, 48.75/195, 61.25/245[d]
Carbidopa/L-dopa enteral suspension	Duopa	1,000[c]	1,000-2,000[c]	4.63/20 per mL
Carbidopa/L-dopa/ entacapone	Stalevo	600[e]	varies	12.5/50/200, 18.75/75/200, 25/100/200, 31.25/125/200, 37.5/150/200, 50/200/200
Carbidopa	Lodosyn	25	25-75	25
Dopamine Agonists				
Apomorphine	Apokyn	1-3	3-12	30/3 mL[f]
Bromocriptine	Parlodel	2.5-5	15-40	2.5, 5
Pramipexole	Mirapex	0.125	1.5-4.5	0.125, 0.25, 0.5, 1, 1.5
Pramipexole ER	Mirapex ER	0.375	1.5-4.5	0.375, 0.75, 1.5, 3, 4.5
Ropinirole	Requip	0.75	9-24	0.25, 0.5, 1, 2, 3, 4, 5
Ropinirole XL	Requip XL	2	8-24	2, 4, 6, 8, 12
Rotigotine	Neupro	2	2-8	1, 2, 3, 4, 6, 8
COMT Inhibitors				
Entacapone	Comtan	200-600	200-1,600	200
Tolcapone	Tasmar	300	300-600	100, 200
MAO-B Inhibitors				
Rasagiline	Azilect	0.5-1	0.5-1	0.5, 1
Selegiline	Eldepryl	5-10	5-10	5
Selegiline ODT	Zelapar	1.25	1.25-2.5	1.25, 2.5
Miscellaneous				
Amantadine	Symmetrel	100	200-300	100, 50/5 mL

Abbreviations: COMT, catechol-o-methyltransferase; CR, controlled release; IR/ER, immediate-release/extended-release; L-dopa, levodopa; MOA-B, monoamine oxidase-B; ODT, orally disintegrating tablet.

[a]Marketed in the United States for Parkinson disease.

[b]Dosages may vary.

[c]Dosages expressed as L-dopa component.

[d]Dosages of Rytary were developed to avoid confusion with other oral carbidopa/L-dopa products that contain L-dopa in multiples of 50 mg.

[e]The optimum daily dosage of Stalevo must be determined by careful titration in each patient. Clinical experience with daily doses above 1,600 mg of entacapone is limited. The maximum recommended daily dose of Stalevo depends on the strength used. The maximum number of tablets to be used in a 24-hour period is less with the highest strength (Stalevo 200) than with lower strengths.

[f]Sterile solution of subcutaneous injection with supplied pen injector.

Reproduced with permission from DiPiro JT, Talbert RL, Yee GC, et al: *Pharmacotherapy: A Pathophysiologic Approach*, 10th ed: New York, NY: McGraw-Hill; 2017.

These movements appear when the motor symptoms of PD are controlled (sometimes referred to as "peak dose" dyskinesias). Practitioners may elect to delay the use of levodopa, especially in younger patients, in an effort to delay the onset of these motor fluctuations as data suggest onset corresponds to total daily dose.

Adverse effects associated with carbidopa/levodopa include confusion, changes in bowel habits, depression, dizziness, and nausea. The drug should be tapered when discontinued to avoid neuroleptic malignant syndrome which may result in delirium, fevers, and muscular rigidity. (This is true of all dopaminergic agents used to treat PD.)

TABLE 52-2 Monitoring of Potential Adverse Reactions to Drug Therapy for Parkinson Disease

Generic Name	Adverse Drug Reaction	Monitoring Parameter	Comments
Amantadine	Confusion	Mental status, renal function	Reduce dosage, adjust dose for renal impairment
	Livedo reticularis	Lower extremity examination, ankle edema	Reversible upon drug discontinuation
Benztropine	Anticholinergic effects, confusion, drowsiness	Dry mouth, mental status, constipation, urinary retention, vision	Reduce dosage, avoid in elderly and in those with a history of constipation, memory impairment, urinary retention
Trihexyphenidyl	See benztropine	See benztropine	See benztropine
Carbidopa/L-dopa	Drowsiness Dyskinesias Nausea	Mental status Abnormal involuntary movements Nausea	Reduce dose Reduce dose, add amantadine Take with food
COMT Inhibitors			
Entacapone	Augmentation of L-dopa side effects, also diarrhea	See carbidopa/L-dopa, also bowel movements	Reduce dose of L-dopa, antidiarrheal agents
Tolcapone	See entacapone, also liver toxicity	See carbidopa/L-dopa, also ALT/AST	See carbidopa/L-dopa, also at start of therapy and for every dose increase, ALT and AST levels at baseline and every 2-4 week for the first 6 months of therapy; afterward monitor based on clinical judgment
Dopamine Agonists			
Apomorphine	Drowsiness Nausea Orthostatic hypotension	Mental status Nausea Blood pressure, dizziness upon standing	Reduce dose Premedicate with trimethobenzamide Reduce dose
Bromocriptine	See pramipexole, also pulmonary fibrosis	Mental status, also chest radiograph	Reduce dose, chest radiograph at baseline and once yearly
Pramipexole	Confusion Drowsiness Edema Hallucinations/delusions Impulsivity Nausea Orthostatic hypotension	Mental status Mental status Lower extremity swelling Behavior, mental status Behavior Nausea Blood pressure, dizziness upon standing	Reduce dose Reduce dose Reduce dose or discontinue medication Reduce dose or discontinue medication Discontinue medication Titrate dose upward slowly; take with food Reduce dose
Ropinirole	See pramipexole	See pramipexole	See pramipexole
Rotigotine	See pramipexole, also skin irritation at site of patch application	See pramipexole, also skin examination	See pramipexole, rotate patch application site
MAO-B Inhibitors			
Rasagiline	Nausea	Nausea	Take with food
Selegiline	Agitation/confusion Insomnia Hallucinations Orthostatic hypotension	Mental status Sleep Behavior, mental status Blood pressure, dizziness upon standing	Reduce dose Administer dose earlier in day Reduce dose Reduce dose

Abbreviations: ALT/AST, aspartate transaminase/alanine transaminase; COMT, catechol-o-methyltransferase; L-dopa, levodopa; MOA-B, monoamine oxidase-B.
Reproduced with permission from DiPiro JT, Talbert RL, Yee GC, et al: *Pharmacotherapy: A Pathophysiologic Approach*, 10th ed: New York, NY: McGraw-Hill; 2017.

Dopamine Agonists

Dopamine agonists (DA) are indicated for the treatment of PD as initial therapy or add-on therapy. The DAs work by bypassing nigrostriatal neurons and directly stimulating postsynaptic dopamine receptors. The efficacy of the DAs is slightly less than levodopa; however, as monotherapy they are less likely to cause dyskinesias. Most patients on DA monotherapy experience symptom control for a year or more. If a DA is added to levodopa therapy when wearing off has begun to occur, the dose of the latter should be decreased by one-fourth to one-third to help avoid dyskinesias. Three of the DAs (rotigotine, pramipexole, and ropinirole) are nonergolines and bind to D2 and D3 receptors, both of which are inhibitory. Bromocriptine is an ergot derivative which binds to D2 receptors, but also to excitatory D1 receptors. The oldest of the DAs, apomorphine, is used in the treatment of severe off periods. See Table 52-1 for dosing of PD medications. Like levodopa, DA doses should be slowly tapered when therapy is being discontinued.

DA side-effects are similar to levodopa side-effects including nausea, somnolence, and hypotension. DAs cause psychiatric side effects (primarily visual hallucinations) three times more often than levodopa. Edema of the lower extremities and impulsive behavior (eg, gambling, shopping, eating, hypersexuality) has been noted with the DAs. Some users claim to have experienced sleep attacks described as being akin to narcolepsy. The ergot derivatives have been associated with pulmonary and retroperitoneal fibrosis which has limited use.

Monoamine Oxidase Inhibitors

Selegiline and rasagiline work by hindering dopamine breakdown by monoamine oxidase (MAO) in the brain. At normal doses, the inhibitors are selective for MAO type B, the primary type present in the basal ganglia. As MOA inhibition by these agents is irreversible, it may take weeks before levels of MAO are back to normal after an inhibitor is discontinued. The older of the MAO inhibitors, selegiline, is only approved for add-on therapy. Traditional dosing is 5 mg orally given twice daily, but a single 10 mg daily dose may be given. An orally disintegrating selegiline tablet with a quicker onset of action is available, and is initiated at a dose of 1.25 mg daily. After 6 weeks of therapy, the dose may be increased to a maximum of 2.5 mg daily if necessary. Rasagiline, is approved as both monotherapy and as add-on therapy. When given alone, the dose is 1 mg daily. However, if the drug is being added to levodopa, the starting dose is 0.5 mg daily. There is some evidence that rasagiline may slow the advancement of PD, but this supposition is controversial. The question of whether MAO inhibitors possess neuroprotective properties remains unanswered.

MAO inhibitors side effects include nausea, headache, and dizziness. Selegiline in particular is associated with insomnia due to its amphetamine metabolite. Doses of selegiline should be given no later than early afternoon in order to avoid sleep disturbances. The orally disintegrating tablet is less likely to cause insomnia because it avoids first pass metabolism. Due to their selectivity, selegiline and rasagiline are less likely to lead to serotonin toxicity when given in conjunction with other drugs; however, caution should be used when administering them in conjunction with other medications including selective serotonin and norepinephrine reuptake inhibiting antidepressants, sympathomimetics, dextromethorphan, meperidine, and tramadol. Similarly, tyramine interactions that increase levels of norepinephrine leading to sympathomimetic effects such as hypertension and tachycardia are unlikely when selegiline and rasagiline are used at normal doses. There have, however, been rare reports of this interaction (sometimes referred to as the "cheese effect") occurring with selegiline when users have ingested foods such as aged cheese, and pickled or fermented foods and drinks.

Amantadine

Amantadine is an antiviral drug that was serendipitously found useful for the treatment of PD. Because its effects are mild and transient, its place in therapy is limited. The drug is typically employed near the time of diagnosis and is best used when tremor is a predominant symptom (though it has efficacy in decreasing rigidity). When used early in the treatment of PD, amantadine's effectiveness wanes after several months. The usual dose is 100 mg twice daily, and adjustment for renal disease is recommended. Amantadine's mechanism of action is not well understood, but the drug is an N-methyl-D-aspartate (NMDA) receptor antagonist, and may decrease the activity of the excitatory neurotransmitter glutamate. Additionally, it has anticholinergic properties. Constipation, leg edema, nightmares, hallucinations, and confusion may occur with amantadine. Amantadine should be slowly tapered when discontinuing use as rebound symptoms have occurred. Later in therapy, amantadine may be useful in controlling levodopa-induced dyskinesias.

Anticholinergics

Multiple anticholinergic agents have been used in the treatment of PD, but the most common are benztropine and trihexyphenidyl. These drugs act primarily to correct the relative overactivity of acetylcholine that occurs due to diminished levels of dopamine. Anticholinergics are used primarily to control tremor. Use in older patients is limited due to frequent side effects which include dry mucous membranes, tachycardia, memory impairment, inhibition of perspiration, and orthostatic hypotension. Caution is also warranted in individuals with pre-existing constipation, benign prostatic hyperplasia, closed-angle glaucoma, and cardiac arrhythmias. Anticholinergic drugs should be tapered to avoid rebound PD symptoms. Of note, the use of anticholinergics has largely fallen out of favor due to a possible link to an increased incidence of dementia.

Catechol-O-Methyltransferase Inhibitors

Two catechol-o-methyltransferase (COMT) inhibitors are currently available for PD treatment. These enzyme inhibiting drugs help prevent the breakdown of both levodopa and dopamine by COMT. Though it is normally a secondary enzymatic pathway, COMT predominates when dopa decarboxylase activity is being inhibited by carbidopa. COMT inhibitors should only be used as an adjunct to levodopa therapy. They are particularly useful for PD patients who are experiencing "off time."

Tolcapone works in both the periphery and the brain. However, due to several cases of liver failure it is reserved for patients who do not respond adequately to other agents. The normal dose for therapy initiation is 100 mg three times daily. Liver function tests are recommended every 2 to 4 weeks for 6 months, and then periodically thereafter when tolcapone is used. The drug may be given independent of the timing of levodopa administration, and should be discontinued if no improvement is noted within 3 weeks of initiation. In contrast, entacapone is administered simultaneously with levodopa, usually at a dose of 200 mg. It exerts its action in the periphery only. A combination drug containing carbidopa/levodopa and entacapone is available for use when appropriate doses of the individual ingredients have been established.

Some data suggest that early use of COMT inhibitors may hasten the development of dyskinesias. Decreasing the levodopa dose when the drugs are initially added (typically by approximately 25%) can help avoid dyskinesia when a COMT inhibitor is added to therapy. Patient counseling should include a discussion regarding diarrhea, the onset of which might not occur until weeks after the drug has been started. In some cases, the problem is significant enough that the drug must be discontinued. Patients may also experience orange discoloration of body fluids.

SPECIAL CONSIDERATIONS

Though the primary neurotransmitter derangement associated with PD is dopamine deficiency, serotonergic, adrenergic and cholinergic pathways may also be affected. As a result, there are several comorbid conditions that frequently exist with PD. Some of these conditions are neuropsychiatric in nature. Depression is estimated to occur in up to 60% of patients, and may be part of the disease itself. No class of antidepressant is preferred over another, but other comorbidities (insomnia, hypersomnia, and sexual dysfunction) must be taken into consideration when choosing a therapeutic agent. Select antidepressant classes have been associated with drug-induced tremor, and these drugs should be evaluated as a possible cause if symptoms worsen. Additionally, caution is warranted when using select antidepressants in conjunction with medications used to treat PD (such as the MAO inhibitors). Psychosis and dementia also commonly exist in the PD population. If antipsychotic therapy is warranted, the more antidopaminergic drugs should be avoided. Pimavanserin, an inverse agonist of serotonin receptors 5HT2A and 5HT2C, is the only medication approved specifically for the treatment of PD psychosis. Because of its receptor selectivity, it does not exacerbate motor symptoms. Additional choices are limited to quetiapine and clozapine, as other antipsychotics may induce or worsen symptoms. Rivastigmine is indicated for PD dementia, but because it inhibits cholinesterase, it has the potential to make PD symptoms worse by potentiating the relative overactivity of acetylcholine. Bladder dysfunction, sexual dysfunction, sialorrhea, constipation, hypotension (both medication-induced and disease-related), and falls predisposing patients to fracture are also common in the PD patient and frequently warrant intervention with drug therapy.

CASE Application

1. What is the primary neurotransmitter deficiency in PD?

   a. Acetylcholine
   b. Dopamine
   c. Norepinephrine
   d. Serotonin

2. What is the primary goal of PD treatment?

   a. Cessation of disease progression
   b. Facilitate an increase in the storage capacity of dopamine
   c. Maintenance of functional ability
   d. Reversal of neuronal loss

3. What is the role of carbidopa in the treatment of PD?

   a. It inhibits acetylcholine.
   b. It inhibits dopa decarboxylase.
   c. It inhibits COMT.
   d. It inhibits MAO.

4. KJ is a young-onset Parkinson disease patient who was started on therapy approximately 1 month ago. Her husband is on the phone to your clinic concerned about his wife's behavior. He claims that KJ has been shopping online almost continuously over the previous few weeks, and recently went out and purchased a new vehicle without his knowledge. Assuming this is a medication-induced phenomenon, which medication are you most likely to discover when you view KJ's medication profile? Select all that apply.

   a. Amantadine
   b. Pramipexole
   c. Rasagiline
   d. Rotigotine

5. SP was diagnosed with PD 7 years ago. Originally, she was taking carbidopa/levodopa 25/100 mg po tid, which has since been increased to 50/250 mg po qid. Nonmotor symptoms include constipation and insomnia, and she also has arthritis for which she takes acetaminophen 650 mg po tid. Assuming another medication is to be added at this time, which medication would you suggest avoiding based on her history of present illness?

   a. Pramipexole
   b. Rasagiline
   c. Ropinirole
   d. Selegiline

6. For which PD symptom are anticholinergics primarily used?"

   a. Bradykinesia
   b. Postural instability
   c. Rigidity
   d. Tremor

7. AB is a long-term PD patient. His neurologist has written a new prescription for tolcapone 100 mg po tid. What laboratory values need to be monitored with the addition of this medication?

   a. Hematocrit
   b. Liver function tests
   c. Platelet count
   d. Serum glucose

8. Which drug should be dosed simultaneously with levodopa?

    a. Amantadine
    b. Entacapone
    c. Pramipexole
    d. Rasagiline

9. EF is a new patient at your clinic. He presents with tremor and rigidity, the onset of which he claims was "overnight." His symptoms appear to be parkinsonian in nature. In order to rule out drug-induced symptoms, his medication profile should be screened for which of the following? Select all that apply.

    a. Haloperidol
    b. Metoclopramide
    c. Prochlorperazine
    d. Risperidone

10. What is the mechanism of action of ropinirole?

    a. Direct replacement of dopamine in the CNS
    b. Direct stimulation of postsynaptic dopamine receptors
    c. Inhibition of the enzymatic breakdown of dopamine in the CNS
    d. Inhibition of the enzymatic breakdown of dopamine in the periphery

11. One of your long-term PD patients, WO, is complaining of hallucinations. She has experienced no recent additions to her medication regimen, or changes in medication doses. Her symptoms include visual hallucinations which are frightening to her, and the decision is made to initiate antipsychotic therapy. Which medication is the best initial choice for the treatment of PD associated psychosis?

    a. Chlorpromazine
    b. Haloperidol
    c. Olanzapine
    d. Pimavanserin

12. PY is a patient with PD who has a difficult time in swallowing medications. His family states he sometimes chokes on his medications and when he drinks more than just a sip of liquid. Which medication used for the treatment of PD is available in an oral formulation that might be a safer option for PY? Select all that apply.

    a. Carbidopa/levodopa
    b. Pramipexole
    c. Selegiline
    d. Trihexyphenidyl

13. Which medication can cause rebound PD symptoms, if stopped abruptly?

    a. Amantadine
    b. Carbidopa/levodopa
    c. Pramipexole
    d. Rasagiline

14. GR was recently diagnosed with PD. His family practitioner initiated therapy with carbidopa/levodopa 10/100 mg three times daily. He has been taking the medication with meals, but he is experiencing significant nausea. GR has noticed very little difference in his symptoms. What is the most probable reason GR is experiencing such significant nausea?

    a. Carbidopa/levodopa should be taken on an empty stomach.
    b. Carbidopa/levodopa should be taken with a meal high in protein.
    c. The levodopa component is being converted to dopamine in the periphery.
    d. Carbidopa/levodopa always causes nausea.

15. Comorbid conditions frequently present in persons with PD include which of the following? Select all that apply.

    a. Constipation
    b. Dementia
    c. Depression
    d. Hypotension

16. You receive a communication from a pulmonologist about your patient, JL. JL has been experiencing shortness of breath upon exertion with increasing severity. The pulmonologist is inquiring as to JL's PD medications. Which is likely to be the cause of JL's symptoms?

    a. Bromocriptine
    b. Pramipexole
    c. Ropinirole
    d. Rotigotine

17. What is the trade name of rasagiline?

    a. Azilect
    b. Comtan
    c. Mirapex
    d. Zelapar

18. WR was diagnosed with PD 12 years ago. He has developed dementia which has progressively worsened over the last year. It has become difficult for his caregiver to administer oral medications as he is resistant to swallowing them, and frequently spits them out. Which DA is available in a dosage form that bypasses this problem?

    a. Bromocriptine
    b. Pramipexole
    c. Ropinirole
    d. Rotigotine

19. NE is a PD patient who is nonadherent with her medications because she has difficulty in remembering to take all but her morning doses. Which medications are available in formulations that might increase NE's success

in taking her medications as prescribed? Select all that apply.

   a. Carbidopa/levodopa

   b. Pramipexole

   c. Rasagiline

   d. Rotigotine

20. MV has been taking carbidopa/levodopa for 6 years. He has begun to develop involuntary movements of his trunk and extremities which include tics and chorea. Which of the following is a true statement about the symptoms MV is experiencing? Select all that apply.

   a. The symptoms often appear when the cardinal motor symptoms of PD are under good control.

   b. Decreasing the dose of levodopa might alleviate the symptoms.

   c. They rarely occur early in the disease process.

   d. They are more likely to occur with DA monotherapy.

21. TS lives in a rural community where there is no neurology practice. For the last several years, he has been experiencing tremors, rigidity, and bradykinesia that began on his left side, but has since migrated and become bilateral, though his left side is still affected more than his right. He is diagnosed with PD and his motor symptoms are graded as moderate (tremor and bradykinesia), and moderate-severe (rigidity). What is the most appropriate order for the initiation and progression of treatment for his PD?

   a. Benztropine, rasagiline, carbidopa/levodopa

   b. Pramipexole, entacapone, carbidopa/levodopa

   c. Ropinirole, levodopa/carbidopa, tolcapone

   d. Carbidopa/levodopa, rotigotine, rasagiline

TAKEAWAY POINTS »

- There are currently no medications proven to slow, halt, or reverse disease progression.
- The pathological hallmarks of PD are loss of nigrostriatal neurons in the substantia nigra which leads to dopamine deficiency and the formation of lewy bodies.
- The decrease in dopamine concentration in the brain causes a relative overactivity of acetylcholine. It is this neurotransmitter imbalance that is responsible for the movement derangements that are the primary symptoms of PD.
- The cardinal features of the disease are bradykinesia, rigidity, tremor, and postural instability.
- Carbidopa/levodopa administration results in the direct replacement of dopamine. The carbidopa component prevents peripheral conversion of levodopa to dopamine prior to its entrance into the brain.
- Carbidopa/levodopa efficacy wanes after several years of use resulting in periods of off-time. Dyskinesias, particularly dystonia and chorea, often appear after several years as well.
- The DAs bypass the nigrostriatal neurons directly stimulating postsynaptic dopamine receptors.
- The MAO inhibitors used for the treatment of PD are selective for MAO type B. At normal doses, they are much less likely to interact with tyramine or contribute to serotonin toxicity than nonselective agents.
- Amantadine is an antiviral agent that is helpful for the control of tremor in PD. Its effects are mild and typically wane after several months of use. Amantadine may be employed to treat dyskinesias associated with levodopa use.
- The anticholinergic medications are used primarily for tremor. They serve to offset the imbalance between dopamine and acetylcholine activity. Use is limited in older patients due to the high frequency of side effects.
- The COMT inhibitors prevent the breakdown of both levodopa and carbidopa in the periphery allowing levodopa to cross the blood brain barrier for conversion.
- The COMT inhibitor tolcapone has been associated with liver failure and its use requires monitoring of liver function tests.
- The COMT inhibitor entacapone should be dosed simultaneously with levodopa, while tolcapone may be dosed independently.
- Multiple comorbidities are associated with PD. The selection of medications used to treat them must be done with care so as to avoid significant drug interactions or exacerbation of Parkinsonian symptoms.

BIBLIOGRAPHY

Aminoff MJ. Pharmacologic management of parkinsonism and other movement disorders. In: Katzung BG, Masters SB, Trevor AJ. *Basic and Clinical Pharmacology*. 12th ed. New York, NY: McGraw-Hill; 2012.

Chen JJ, Dashtipour K. Parkinson disease. In: DiPiro JT, Talbert RL, Yee GC, Matzke GR, Wells BG, Posey L, eds. *Pharmacotherapy: A Pathophysiologic Approach*. 10th ed. New York, NY: McGraw-Hill; 2017.

Fox SH, Katzenschlager R, Lim SY, et al. The Movement Disorder Society Evidence-Based Medicine Review Update: Treatments for the motor symptoms of Parkinson's disease. *Mov Disord.* 2011;26(Suppl 3):S2-S41.

Movement disorders. In: Greenberg DA, Aminoff MJ, Simon RP, eds. *Clinical Neurology*. 8th ed. New York, NY: McGraw-Hill; 2012.

Standaert DG, Roberson ED. Treatment of central nervous system degenerative disorders. In: Brunton L, Chabner B, Knollman B. *Goodman and Gilman's The Pharmacological Basis of Therapeutics*. 12th ed. New York, NY: McGraw-Hill; 2011.

KEY ABBREVIATIONS

CNS = central nervous system
COMT = catechol-o-methyltransferase
DA = dopamine agonist

MAO = monoamine oxidase
NMDA = N-methyl-D-aspartate
PD = Parkinson disease

53

Epilepsy

McKenzie C. Ferguson

FOUNDATION OVERVIEW

Epilepsy is a chronic disease of disturbed electrical activity in the brain, resulting in recurrent seizures with or without convulsions. Epilepsy is a disorder with profound impact on lifestyle and patients are often dependent upon caregivers to assist with medications and transportation. All states impose limitations on driving for individuals who have recently had a seizure with impaired consciousness.

The pathophysiology of a seizure is due to an unstable cell membrane in the gray matter of the brain. The cause of the unstable cell membrane has been linked to three causes: an abnormality in potassium conductance, an abnormality in voltage-sensitive ion channels, or a deficiency in membrane ATPases linked to ion transport. Excitatory neurotransmitters (glutamate, aspartate, acetylcholine, norepinephrine) enhance the propagation of seizures while inhibitory neurotransmitters (gamma-aminobutyric acid [GABA], dopamine) decrease the propagation of seizure activity in the brain. The spread can be local (partial seizure) or throughout the entire brain (generalized seizure). The different types of epilepsies are due to the different pathophysiologic abnormalities.

Epilepsy is classified by the seizure presentation (Table 53-1). The classification system is based on how the seizure begins; therefore, obtaining an adequate description from a third party is important. The classifications of epilepsy are:

- *Absence* seizures (petit mal)—sudden interruption of activities and a blank stare.
- Myoclonic seizures—brief shock-like contraction of a muscle group.
- Clonic seizures—jerking motion while tonic seizures involve a sustained muscle contraction.
- Tonic-clonic seizures (grand mal)—alternating muscle contraction and jerking.
- Atonic seizures involve a sudden loss of muscle tone known as drop attacks.

Epilepsy syndromes are another classification system of epilepsies based on seizure type and etiology. The syndrome approach provides a tool to aid clinical management and provide prognosis.

- *Idiopathic* epilepsy—no underlying etiology and is presumed genetic.

- *Symptomatic* epilepsy—an underlying cause which is usually brain damage.
- *Cryptogenic* epilepsy—presumed to have an underlying etiology that cannot be identified.

Epilepsy is a clinical diagnosis made when the patient has recurrent seizures. An isolated seizure does not justify the diagnosis of epilepsy. Laboratory tests are evaluated to rule out treatable causes of seizures such as hypoglycemia, altered electrolytes, and infections. A seizure produced by treatable causes does not represent epilepsy. Electroencephalogram (EEG) can be useful to confirm a seizure and identify seizure types based on the spike and wave pattern generated; however, the EEG may be normal in some patients.

The underlying etiology of epilepsy is unknown in 80% of patients. The most common recognized causes of epilepsy are head trauma and stroke. Developmental and genetic defects represent 5% of epilepsy cases. Central nervous system tumors, infections, metabolic disturbances (hyponatremia and hypoglycemia), neurodegenerative diseases, and medications represent other causes. Medications associated with development of seizures include tramadol, bupropion, theophylline, some antidepressants, some antipsychotics, amphetamines, cocaine, imipenem, lithium, excessive doses of penicillins or cephalosporins, sympathomimetics, and stimulants. Cefepime has been linked to seizures and non-convulsive status epilepticus (SE), a risk that is increased in patients with renal impairment and in patients with a history of a seizure disorder.

PREVENTION

Epilepsy cannot be prevented, but the seizures experienced by the patient can be minimized in both number and duration. There is a positive association between early initiation of antiepileptic drug (AED) therapy and seizure control. The inability to control seizures early can lead to increased frequency in seizure activity and the generation of other seizure types. External factors known to precipitate seizures in patients with epilepsy include hyperventilation, sleep deprivation, sensory stimuli, emotional stress, and hormonal fluctuations during pregnancy/menses/puberty. These external factors should be minimized in the epilepsy population.

To access your complimentary online question exams, visit https://accesspharmacy.mhmedical.com/NAPLEX.aspx

TABLE 53-1	Classification and Management of Seizure Disorders			
Seizure Type	**Features**		**Conventional Antiseizure Drugs**	**Recently Developed Antiseizure Drugs**
Partial Seizures				
Simple partial	Diverse manifestations determined by the region of cortex activated by the seizure (eg, if motor cortex representing left thumb, clonic jerking of left thumb results; if somatosensory cortex representing left thumb, paresthesia of left thumb results), lasting approximating 20-60 s. *Key feature is preservation of consciousness.*		Carbamazepine, phenytoin, valproate	Gabapentin, lacosamide, lamotrigine, levetiracetam, rufinamide, tiagabine, topiramate, zonisamide
Complex partial	Impaired consciousness lasting 30 s to 2 min, often associated with purposeless movements such as lip smacking or hand wringing.			
Partial with secondarily generalized tonic-clonic seizure	Simple or complex partial seizure evolves into a tonic-clonic seizure with loss of consciousness and sustained contractions (tonic) of muscles throughout the body followed by periods of muscle contraction alternating with periods of relaxation (clonic), typically lasting 1-2 min.		Carbamazepine, phenobarbital, phenytoin, primidone, valproate	
Generalized Seizures				
Absence seizure	Abrupt onset of impaired consciousness associated with staring and cessation of ongoing activities typically lasting less than 30 s.		Ethosuximide, valproate, clonazepam	Lamotrigine
Myoclonic seizure	A brief (perhaps a second), shock-like contraction of muscles that may be restricted to part of one extremity or may be generalized.		Valproate, clonazepam	Levetiracetam
Tonic-clonic seizure	As described earlier in table for partial with secondarily generalized tonic-clonic seizures except that it is not preceded by a partial seizure.		Carbamazepine, phenobarbital, phenytoin, primidone, valproate	Lamotrigine, levetiracetam, topiramate

Reproduced with permission from Brunton LL, Chabner BA, Knollmann BC: *Goodman & Gilman's The Pharmacological Basis of Therapeutics*, 12th ed. New York, NY: McGraw-Hill; 2011.

TREATMENT

The goal of epilepsy treatment is complete elimination of seizures with no drug side effects. This is not always possible and the patient should be involved in deciding the balance between frequency of seizures and occurrence of side effects. In certain situations, some seizure control may be sacrificed to improve the patient's day to day functioning. Optimal quality of life requires balancing seizures, side effects, and addressing life issues (eg, driving, safety, relationships, and social stigma). Epilepsy patients may have neuropsychiatric diseases such as depression, anxiety, and sleep disturbances which require treatment to optimize quality of life.

Initial therapy is initiated with one AED and up to 70% of patients are controlled on monotherapy. Management of seizure disorders depends upon the type of seizure (Table 53-1). Combination AED therapy is required in 30% of patients in order to achieve seizure control; however, combination therapy increases the chance of side effects and drug interactions. Combination AED therapy is achieved by combining seizure medications with different mechanisms of action. Table 53-2 lists key AED properties that impact medication selection, dosing, and adverse reactions.

SPECIAL CONSIDERATIONS

Complications of Therapy

Adverse effects of AEDs are often dose limiting or cause a drug to be discontinued. AED adverse reactions are classified as dose related or idiosyncratic (Table 53-3). Dose-related adverse reactions are associated with the dose or concentration. Dose-related adverse effects include sedation, ataxia, and diplopia. Idiosyncratic adverse reactions are not related to the dose of the AED and often lead to discontinuation of the AED. Examples of idiosyncratic reactions include rash, hepatotoxicity, and hematologic toxicities. Because idiosyncratic reactions may be life threatening, the AED should be discontinued. Idiosyncratic reactions are associated with an immunologic reaction; therefore, cross-reactivity among AEDs is possible.

Switching Antiepileptic Drugs

Switching AEDs requires a titration process, because abrupt discontinuation of an AED may lead to breakthrough seizures. The process requires starting the new AED at a low dose and titrating up to the minimal effective dose. Once the minimal

TABLE 53-2 Antiepileptic Drug Dosing and Target Serum Concentrations

Drug	Brand Name	Initial or Starting Dose	Usual Range or Maximum Dose	Comments Target Serum Concentration Range
Barbiturates				
Phenobarbital	Various	1-3 mg/kg/d (10-20 mg/kg LD)	180-300 mg	10-40 mcg/mL[a] (43-172 µmol/L)
Primidone	Mysoline	100-125 mg/d	750-2000 mg	5-10 mcg/mL (23-46 µmol/L)
Benzodiazepines				
Clobazam	Onfi	≤30 kg 5 mg/d; >30 kg 10 mg/d	≤30 kg up to 20 mg; >30 kg up to 40 mg	0.03-0.3 ng/mL (0.1-1.0 nmol/L)
Clonazepam	Klonopin	1.5 mg/d	20 mg	20-70 ng/mL (67-233 pmol/L)
Diazepam	Valium	po: 4-40 mg IV: 5-10 mg	po: 4-40 mg IV: 5-30 mg	100-1000 ng/mL (0.4-3.5 µmol/L)
Lorazepam	Ativan	po: 2-6 mg IV: 0.05 mg/kg IM: 0.05 mg/kg	po: 10 mg IV: 0.05 mg/kg	10-30 ng/mL (31-93 nmol/L)
Hydantoin				
Phenytoin	Dilantin	po: 3-5 mg/kg (200-400 mg) (15-20 mg/kg LD)	po: 300-600 mg	Total: 10-20 mcg/mL (40-79 µmol/L) Unbound: 0.5-3 mcg/mL (2-12 µmol/L)
Succinimide				
Ethosuximide	Zarontin	500 mg/d	500-2000 mg	40-100 mcg/mL (282-708 µmol/L)
Other				
Carbamazepine	Tegretol Tegretol XR	400 mg/d	400-2400 mg	4-12 mcg/mL (17-51 µmol/L)
Eslicarbazepine	Aptiom	400 mg/d	800-1600 mg	Not defined
Ezogabine	Potiga	300 mg/d	1200 mg	Not defined
Felbamate	Felbatol	1200 mg/d	3600 mg	30-60 mcg/mL (126-252 µmol/L)
Gabapentin	Neurontin	300-900 mg/d	4800 mg	2-20 mcg/mL (12-117 µmol/L)
Lacosamide	Vimpat	100 mg/d	400 mg	Not defined
Lamotrigine	Lamictal Lamictal XR	25 mg every other d if on VPA; 25-50 mg/d if not on VPA	100-150 mg if on VPA; 300-500 mg if not on VPA	4-20 mcg/dL (16-78 µmol/L)
Levetiracetam	Keppra Keppra XR	500-1000 mg/d	3000-4000 mg	12-46 mcg/mL (70-270 µmol/L)
Oxcarbazepine	Trileptal Oxtellar XR	300-600 mg/d	1200-2400 mg	3-35 mcg/mL (MHD) (12-139 µmol/L)
Perampanel	Fycompa	2 mg/d	8-12 mg	Not defined
Pregabalin	Lyrica	150 mg/d	600 mg	Not defined
Rufinamide	Banzel	400-800 mg/d	3200 mg	Not defined
Tiagabine	Gabitril	4-8 mg/d	80 mg	0.02-0.2 mcg/mL (0.05-0.5 µmol/L)
Topiramate	Topamax Trokendi XR	25-50 mg/d	200-1000 mg	5-20 mcg/mL (15-59 µmol/L)
Valproic acid	Depakene Depakote DR/ER Depacon	15 mg/kg (500-1000 mg)	60 mg/kg (3000-5000 mg)	50-100 mcg/mL (347-693 µmol/L)
Vigabatrin	Sabril	1000 mg/d	3000 mg	0.8-36 mcg/mL (6-279 µmol/L)
Zonisamide	Zonegran	100-200 mg/d	600 mg	10-40 mcg/mL (47-188 µmol/L)

Abbreviations: IM, intramuscular; LD, loading does; MHD, 10-monohydroxy-derivative; po, orally; VPA, valproic acid.

[a]Units mcg/mL and mg/L are numerically equivalent, and units of ng/mL and mcg/L are numerically equivalent.

Reproduced with permission from DiPiro JT, Talbert RL, Yee GC, et al: *Pharmacotherapy: A Pathophysiologic Approach*, 10th ed: New York, NY: McGraw-Hill; 2017.

TABLE 53-3   **Adverse Reactions of Antiepileptic Drugs**

Drug	Adverse Drug Reaction Acute Side Effects		Chronic Side Effects
	Concentration Dependent	**Idiosyncratic**	**Chronic Side Effects**
Carbamazepine	Diplopia Dizziness Drowsiness Nausea Unsteadiness Lethargy	Blood dyscrasias Rash (HLA antigen testing may be relevant to avoid Stevens-Johnson or toxic epidermal necrolysis)	Hyponatremia Metabolic bone disease (monitor Vit D and serum calcium)
Clobazam	Somnolence Sedation Pyrexia Ataxia	Drooling Aggression Irritability Constipation	
Eslicarbazepine	Dizziness Ataxia Somnolence/fatigue Cognitive changes Visual changes	Rash	Hyponatremia
Ethosuximide	Ataxia Drowsiness GI distress (avoid by multiple daily dosing) Unsteadiness Hiccoughs	Blood dyscrasias Rash	Behavior changes Headache
Ezogabine	Dizziness Somnolence Fatigue Confusion Vertigo Tremors Blurred vision	Urinary retention QT prolongation (get baseline ECG and during treatment) Euphoria	Blue gray skin discoloration Retinal abnormalities
Felbamate	Anorexia Nausea Vomiting Insomnia Headache	Aplastic anemia (follow CBC) Acute hepatic failure (follow liver enzymes)	Not established
Gabapentin	Dizziness Fatigue Somnolence Ataxia	Pedal edema	Weight gain
Lacosamide	Dizziness Vertigo Headache Nausea Vomiting PR interval increase (get baseline ECG and during treatment)	Liver enzyme elevation	Not established
Lamotrigine	Diplopia Dizziness Unsteadiness Headache	Rash (slower titration of dose may decrease chance of occurrence)	Not established
Levetiracetam	Sedation Behavioral disturbance	Psychosis (rare but more common in elderly or persons with mental illness)	Not established
Oxcarbazepine	Sedation Dizziness Ataxia Nausea	Rash	Hyponatremia

TABLE 53-3 | **Adverse Reactions of Antiepileptic Drugs** *(Continued)*

| Drug | Adverse Drug Reaction Acute Side Effects | | Chronic Side Effects |
	Concentration Dependent	Idiosyncratic	
Perampanel	Severe behavior changes Dizziness Ataxia/falls Somnolence/fatigues	Rash	Weight gain
Phenobarbital	Ataxia Hyperactivity Headache Unsteadiness Sedation Nausea	Blood dyscrasias Rash	Behavior changes Connective tissue disorders Intellectual blunting Metabolic bone disease Mood change Sedation
Phenytoin	Ataxia Nystagmus Behavior changes Dizziness Headache Incoordination Sedation Lethargy Cognitive impairment Fatigue Visual blurring	Blood dyscrasias Rash (HLA antigen testing may be relevant to avoid Stevens-Johnson or toxic epidermal necrolysis) Immunologic reaction	Behavior changes Cerebellar syndrome (occurs high serum levels) Connective tissue changes Skin thickening Folate deficiency Gingival hyperplasia Hirsutism Coarsening of facial features Acne Cognitive impairment Metabolic bone disease (monitor Vit D and serum calcium) Sedation
Pregabalin	Dizziness Somnolence Incoordination Dry mouth Blurred vision	Pedal edema Creatine kinase elevation Decrease platelets	Weight gain
Primidone	Behavior changes Headache Nausea Sedation Unsteadiness	Blood dyscrasias Rash	Behavior change Connective tissue disorders Cognitive impairment Sedation
Rufinamide	Dizziness Nausea Vomiting Somnolence	Multiorgan hypersensitivity Status epilepticus Leukopenia QT shortening	Not established
Tiagabine	Dizziness Fatigue Difficulties concentrating Nervousness Tremor Blurred vision Depression Weakness	Spike-wave stupor	Not established
Topiramate	Difficulties concentrating Psychomotor slowing Speech or language problems Somnolence, fatigue Dizziness Headache	Metabolic acidosis Acute angle glaucoma Oligohydrosis	Kidney stones Weight loss
Valproic acid	GI upset Sedation Unsteadiness Tremor Thrombocytopenia	Acute hepatic failure Acute pancreatitis Alopecia	Polycystic ovary-like syndrome (increase incidence in females <20 year or overweight) Weight gain Hyperammonemia Menstrual cycle irregularities

(Continued)

TABLE 53-3 **Adverse Reactions of Antiepileptic Drugs (*Continued*)**

| Drug | Adverse Drug Reaction Acute Side Effects | | Chronic Side Effects |
	Concentration Dependent	Idiosyncratic	
Vigabatrin	Permanent vision loss Fatigue Somnolence Weight gain Tremor Blurred vision	Abnormal MRI brain signal changes (infants with infantile spasms) Peripheral neuropathy Anemia	Permanent vision loss (greater frequency, adults vs children vs infants)
Zonisamide	Sedation Dizziness Cognitive impairment Nausea	Rash (is a sulfa drug) Metabolic acidosis Oligohydrosis	Kidney stones Weight loss

Reproduced with permission from DiPiro JT, Talbert RL, Yee GC, et al: *Pharmacotherapy: A Pathophysiologic Approach*, 10th ed: New York, NY: McGraw-Hill; 2017.

effective dose is reached, the drug to be discontinued is gradually tapered, while the dose of the new AED continues to be increased to the target dose.

Discontinuing Antiepileptic Drugs

Epilepsy is considered a lifelong disorder; however, patients who are seizure-free may desire to discontinue their medication. Factors favoring successful withdrawal of AEDs include a seizure-free period of 2 to 4 years, complete seizure control within 1 year of onset, an onset of seizures after age 2 but before age 35, and a normal neurologic examination and EEG. Withdrawal of AEDs is done slowly with a dose tapered over at least 3 months.

Drug Interactions

AEDs are associated with numerous drug interactions related to absorption, metabolism, and protein binding. Tube feedings and antacids reduce the absorption of phenytoin and carbamazepine. Phenytoin, carbamazepine, and phenobarbital are potent inducers of the cytochrome P-450 (CYP-450) isoenzyme system and valproic acid is an inhibitor of the P-450 isoenzyme system (Table 53-4).

Special Populations

Children require prompt control of seizures to avoid interference with development of the brain and cognition. AED doses are increased rapidly and frequent changes in the regimen are made to maximize control of seizures. Due to high metabolic rates in children, doses of AEDs are higher on a milligram per kilogram basis compared to adults.

Women of child-bearing potential or who are pregnant have recommendations for AED management (Table 53-5). Several AEDs have been implicated in minor and serious birth defects. Valproic acid and carbamazepine are associated with neural tube defects (eg, spina bifida). The majority of pregnant epileptic patients receiving AEDs produce a normal infant, but special recommendations must be followed. AEDs induce hepatic CYP-450 isoenzymes and decrease the effectiveness of hormonal contraceptives. Epileptic women taking AEDs and hormonal contraceptives are recommended to use other forms of birth control.

Michaelis-Menten Metabolism

Phenytoin exhibits dose-dependent capacity-limited (Michaelis-Menten) pharmacokinetics, meaning the maximum capacity of hepatic enzymes to metabolize the drug is reached within the normal dosage range. Therefore, small changes in doses result in disproportionate and large changes in serum concentrations. Due to individual differences in metabolism, each patient follows a different curve in the relationship between dose and serum concentrations.

Protein Binding

Phenytoin and valproic acid are highly protein bound and only unbound medication is able to produce clinical and adverse effects. When interpreting serum concentrations for highly protein-bound AEDs, it is important to remember that the value represents the total concentration (bound and unbound). Patients with decreased protein (albumin) will have the same total concentration of AEDs, but the unbound concentration (active component) will be increased. Also, certain diseases states and medications may displace AEDs from protein, thereby increasing the unbound concentration. Examples of patients with low protein or disease states/medications that increase the unbound concentration of AEDs include:

- Patients with renal failure
- Patients with hypoalbuminemia
- Neonates
- Pregnant women
- Patients taking other highly protein bound medications
- Critical care patients

Alterations in protein binding of phenytoin will result in increased dose-related side effects. In patients with suspected changes in protein binding, it is useful to measure or calculate unbound (free) phenytoin concentrations.

Autoinduction

Carbamazepine is a potent inducer of the CYP-450 isoenzyme system, leading to increased clearance of many medicines and itself. Carbamazepine displays autoinduction of its own metabolism.

TABLE 53-4 Drug Interaction Properties with Antiepileptic Drugs

Antiepileptic Drugs	Major Hepatic Enzymes	Renal Elimination (%)	Induced	Inhibited
Carbamazepine	CYP3A4; CYP1A2; CYP2C8	<1	CYP1A2; CYP2C; CYP3A; GT	None
Clobazam	CYP3A4; CYP2C19; CYP2B6	0	CYP3A4 (weak)	CYP2D6
Eslicarbazepine	Undergoes hydrolysis	<90% parent drug >60% active metabolite	GT (mild)	CYP2C19
Ethosuximide	CYP3A4	12-20	None	None
Ezogabine	GT; acetylation	85	None	None
Felbamate	CYP3A4; CYP2E1; other	50	CYP3A4	CYP2C19; β-oxidation
Gabapentin	None	Almost completely	None	None
Lacosamide	CYP2C19	70	None	None
Lamotrigine	GT	10	GT	None
Levetiracetam	None (undergoes nonhepatic hydrolysis)	66	None	None
Oxcarbazepine (MHD is active oxcarbazepine metabolite)	Cytosolic system	1 (27 as MHD)	CYP3A4; CYP3A5; GT	CYP2C19
Perampanel	CYP3A4/5; CYP1A2; CYP2B6	Undefined	CYP3A4/5; GT	CYPA3A4/5
Phenobarbital	CYP2C9; other	25	CYP3A; CYP2C; GT	None
Phenytoin	CYP2C9; CYP2C19	5	CYP3A; CYP2C; GT	None
Pregabalin	None	100	None	None
Rufinamide	Hydrolysis	2	CYP3A4 (weak)	CYP2E1 (weak)
Tiagabine	CYP3A4	2	None	None
Topiramate	Not known	70	CYP3A (dose dependent)	CYP2C19
Valproate	GT; β-oxidation	2	None	CYP2C9; GT epoxide hydrolase
Vigabatrin	None	Almost completely	CYP2C9	None
Zonisamide	CYP3A4	35	None	None

Abbreviations: CYP, cytochrome P450 isoenzyme system; GT, glucuronyltransferase.
Reproduced with permission from DiPiro JT, Talbert RL, Yee GC, et al: *Pharmacotherapy: A Pathophysiologic Approach*, 10th ed: New York, NY: McGraw-Hill; 2017.

Serum Concentration Monitoring

A therapeutic range should be established for each patient and this range should define concentrations that result in minimal side effects and optimal seizure control. Table 53-2 lists usual serum concentrations for the AEDs.

Status Epilepticus

SE is a neurologic emergency that can lead to permanent brain damage or death. SE is defined as any seizure lasting more than

TABLE 53-5 Management of Antiepileptic Drugs During Pregnancy

- Give supplemental folic acid 1-4 mg daily to all women of child-bearing potential
- Use monotherapy when possible
- Use lowest dose possible to control seizures
- Monitor AED serum concentrations at the start of pregnancy and monthly thereafter
- Administer supplemental vitamin K during the eighth month of pregnancy to women receiving enzyme-inducing AEDs

30 minutes, with or without a loss of consciousness or having recurrent seizures without regaining consciousness between seizure episodes. The goals for treatment of SE include the cessation of any seizure activity and the prevention of further seizures. Ideally, this is accomplished through directed pharmacotherapy with minimization of adverse reactions. Treatment of SE includes benzodiazepines and anticonvulsants (Tables 53-6 and 53-7).

Phenytoin and Fosphenytoin in Status Epilepticus

Phenytoin is administered intravenously as a loading dose (for patients not previously on phenytoin) of 15 to 20 mg/kg. The loading dose is infused no faster than 50 mg/min due to risks of hypotension and arrhythmias. Continuous monitoring of electrocardiogram (ECG) and blood pressure is recommended. Maintenance dosing can be started in 12 hours after the loading dose. Phenytoin should not be administered via the intramuscular route due to alkaline nature. Extravasation of the drug can cause local discoloration, edema, pain, and sometimes necrosis.

Fosphenytoin is a water-soluble, prodrug of phenytoin that is rapidly converted to phenytoin in the body. Unlike

TABLE 53-6 | **Parenteral Medications Used in Status Epilepticus in Adults**

Drug (Route)	Brand Name	Initial Dose (Maximum Dose)	Maintenance Dose	Comments
Diazepam (IV)	Valium plus generic			
Adult		0.25 mg/kg[a,b,c] (20 mg)	Not used	Given IV at a rate not to exceed 5 mg/min
Pediatric		0.25-0.5 mg/kg[a,c] (20 mg)	Not used	
Fosphenytoin (IV)	Cerebyx plus generic			
Adult		20-25 mg PE/kg	4-5 mg PE/kg/d	Given IV at a rate not to exceed 150 mg PE/min in
Pediatric		20-25 mg PE/kg	5-10 mg PE/kg/d	adults and 3 mg PE/kg/min in pediatric patients
Lorazepam (IV)	Ativan plus generic			
Adult		4 mg[b,c] (6 mg)	Not used	Given IV at a rate not to exceed 2 mg/min in adult
Pediatric		0.1 mg/kg[a,c] (6 mg)	Not used	and pediatric patients
Midazolam (IV, IM)	Versed plus generic			
Adult		200 mcg/kg[a,d] (10 mg)	50-500 mcg/kg/h[e]	Given IV at a rate 0.5-1 mg/min in adults and
Pediatric		150 mcg/kg[a,d] (10 mg)	60-120 mcg/kg/h[e]	over 2-3 minutes in pediatric patients
Phenobarbital (IV)	Generic			
Adult		10-20 mg/kg[e]	1-4 mg/kg/d[e]	Given IV at a rate not to exceed 100 mg/min in
Pediatric		15-20 mg/kg[e]	3-5 mg/kg/d[e]	adults and 30 mg/min in pediatric patients
Phenytoin (IV)	Dilantin plus generic			
Adult		20-25 mg/kg[f]	4-5 mg/kg/d[e]	Given IV at a rate not to exceed 50 mg/min[g] in
Pediatric		20-25 mg/kg[f]	5-10 mg/kg/d[e]	adults and 3 mg/kg/min (max 50 mg/min) in pediatric patients

Abbreviations: GCSE, generalized convulsive status epilepticus; PE, phenytoin equivalents.

[a]Doses can be repeated every 10 to 15 minutes until the maximum dosage is given.

[b]Initial doses in the elderly are 2 to 5 mg.

[c]Larger doses can be required if patients chronically on a benzodiazepine (eg, clonazepam).

[d]Can be given by the intramuscular, rectal, or buccal routes.

[e]Titrate dose as needed.

[f]Administer additional loading dose based on serum concentration.

[g]The rate should not exceed 25 mg/min in elderly patients and those with known atherosclerotic cardiovascular disease.

Reproduced with permission from DiPiro JT, Talbert RL, Yee GC, et al: *Pharmacotherapy: A Pathophysiologic Approach*, 10th ed: New York, NY: McGraw-Hill; 2017.

TABLE 53-7 | **Adverse Drug Reactions and Monitoring of Patients Receiving Drugs for GCSE**

Drug	Adverse Drug Reaction	Monitoring Parameters	Comments
Diazepam	Hypotension and cardiac arrhythmias	Vital signs and ECG during administration	Propylene glycol causes hypotension and cardiac arrhythmias when administered too rapidly; hypotension may occur with large doses
Fosphenytoin	Hypotension and cardiac arrhythmias; paresthesia, pruritus	Vital signs and ECG during administration	Hypotension is less than that noted with phenytoin, as this product does not contain propylene glycol; pruritus generally involves the face and groin areas, is dose and rate related, and subsides 5-10 min after infusion
Lidocaine	Fasciculations, visual disturbances, tinnitus, seizures		Occur at serum concentrations between 6 and 8 mg/L (25.6-34.1 μmol/L); seizures >8 mg/L (>34.1 μmol/L)
Lorazepam	Apnea, hypotension, bradycardia, cardiac arrest, respiratory depression, metabolic acidosis, and renal toxicity	Vital signs and ECG during administration; HCO_3 and serum creatinine; cumulative dose of propylene glycol	Accumulation of propylene glycol during prolong continuous infusions may cause acidosis
Pentobarbital	Hypotension	Vital signs and ECG during administration	Rate of infusion should be slower or dopamine should be added if hypotension occurs
Phenytoin	Hypotension and cardiac arrhythmia; nystagmus	Vital signs and ECG during administration	Propylene glycol causes hypotension and cardiac arrhythmias when administered too rapidly. Large loading doses are generally not given to elderly individuals with preexisting cardiac disease or in critically ill patients with marginal blood pressure. The infusion rate should be slowed if the QT interval widens or if hypotension or arrhythmias develop; horizontal nystagmus suggests serum concentration above the reference range and toxicity; if a serum phenytoin concentration validates this, the dose should be decreased

TABLE 53-7	Adverse Drug Reactions and Monitoring of Patients Receiving Drugs for GCSE *(Continued)*		
Drug	**Adverse Drug Reaction**	**Monitoring Parameters**	**Comments**
Phenobarbital	Hypotension, respiratory, and CNS depression	Vital signs and mental status; EEG if used in anesthesia doses	Contains propylene glycol; if hypotension occurs, slow the rate of administration or begin dopamine; apnea and hypopnea can be more profound in patients treated initially with benzodiazepines
Propofol	Progressive metabolic acidosis, hemodynamic instability, and bradyarrhythmias	Vital signs, ECG, osmolar gap; EEG if used in anesthesia doses	Referred to as propofol-related infusion syndrome, which can be fatal
Topiramate	Metabolic acidosis	Acid base status (serum bicarbonate)	Extremely rare

Abbreviations: CNS, central nervous system; ECG, electrocardiogram; EEG, electroencephalogram; GCSE, generalized convulsive status epilepticus.
Reproduced with permission from DiPiro JT, Talbert RL, Yee GC, et al: *Pharmacotherapy: A Pathophysiologic Approach*, 10th ed: New York, NY: McGraw-Hill; 2017.

phenytoin, fosphenytoin is compatible with most intravenous solutions and is tolerated as an intramuscular injection. Fosphenytoin is dosed on phenytoin equivalents (PE), and it can be infused up to 150 mg PE/min. The loading dose for patients not taking phenytoin is 15 to 20 mg PE/kg. Although fosphenytoin has fewer cardiovascular side effects compared to phenytoin, blood pressure and ECG should still be monitored.

CASE Application

1. Select the treatable cause(s) of seizures. Select all that apply.

    a. Hypoglycemia
    b. Altered electrolytes
    c. Infections
    d. Genetic defects

2. WW is a 56-year-old hospitalized patient taking the following medications: cefepime, metoprolol succinate, levothyroxine, and acetaminophen. The patient developed seizures. Select the possible drug-induced cause(s) of seizures.

    a. Levothyroxine
    b. Acetaminophen
    c. Cefepime
    d. Metoprolol

3. JW is a 29-year-old woman presenting to the pharmacy with a new prescription for phenytoin. She is currently not taking any other medications. What should this patient be counseled about in relation to her new drug therapy? Select all that apply.

    a. Avoid alcohol while taking this medication.
    b. Use appropriate barrier methods of contraception.
    c. Wear sunscreen. This medication is associated with increased photosensitivity.
    d. Take this medication with food at the same time every day.

4. Select the goal therapeutic level for phenytoin in this patient.

    a. 4 to 12 mcg/mL
    b. 10 to 20 mcg/mL
    c. 50 to 100 mcg/mL
    d. No therapeutic drug monitoring is required with this drug.

5. A year later, JW tells you that she wants to become pregnant and would like to change to a different AED that might be safer during pregnancy. What is important to discuss with her and her physician in regards to switching therapy?

    a. Her current medication should be stopped immediately in order to ensure that the current AED has been fully removed out of her system prior to getting pregnant.
    b. Her existing AED can be stopped abruptly and the new AED should be started at a low dose and titrated up to the target dose.
    c. Her new AED should be initiated at a low dose and titrated up to become minimally effective at which time the existing AED can be gradually tapered.
    d. She should avoid pregnancy altogether and remain on her current AED therapy.

The following case pertains to questions 6 and 7.

6. A patient is admitted to the hospital with seizures that result in a sudden interruption of activities and a blank stare. What type of seizure disorder is this?

    a. Absence seizures
    b. Tonic-clonic
    c. Myoclonic
    d. Atonic

7. What is the recommended first-line treatment for this type of seizure disorder?

    a. Phenytoin
    b. Felbamate
    c. Levetiracetam
    d. Ethosuximide

The following case pertains to questions 8 and 9.

8. BH is a 47-year-old man in SE in need of drug therapy. Intravenous dosing of phenytoin cannot be infused faster than 50 mg/min. Select the adverse reactions that are associated with infusions faster than 50 mg/min.

    a. Hypotension
    b. Gingival hyperplasia

c. Anemia

d. Rash

9. What is the water-soluble prodrug of phenytoin that is rapidly converted to phenytoin in the body and can be used as an alternate?

a. Trileptal

b. Tegretol

c. Cerebyx

d. Dilantin

10. GG is a 67-year-old woman on carbamazepine for her seizure disorder. Her family is worried about serious side effects because of her age. Which of the following are idiosyncratic adverse reaction(s) associated with use of carbamazepine?

a. Aplastic anemia

b. Hyponatremia

c. Rash

d. Colitis

11. Select the patient population or condition that often leads to fast titration of AEDs.

a. Switching AEDs

b. Discontinuing AEDs

c. Children

d. Women of child-bearing potential

The following case pertains to questions 12 and 13.

12. DD is an elderly man currently on phenytoin. He has begun experiencing confusion and nystagmus in the past week. His last serum creatinine was 3.6 mg/dL and albumin 2.4 g/dL. His only other medications are aspirin and omeprazole. What could this be a symptom of?

a. Aura before seizure onset

b. Lack of seizure control

c. Phenytoin toxicity

d. Normal side effects of the drug

13. What could be contributing to the development of these symptoms? Select all that apply.

a. Drug interaction

b. Low albumin

c. Renal impairment

d. Not taking the medication

14. A physician tells you that she would like to begin lamotrigine in a patient in order to avoid some drug interactions with other AEDs, but she would like to know if there are any other adverse effects she should educate the patient about. Which of the following should be addressed with the patient?

a. Rash

b. Edema

c. Pancreatitis

d. Alopecia

The following case pertains to questions 15 and 16.

15. SB is a patient with newly diagnosed complex seizure disorder. His physician has noted that he is taking warfarin for atrial fibrillation and also has restless leg syndrome. For this reason, he would like to avoid an AED that is a substrate and inducer of the CYP-450 2C9. Which of the following should be avoided in this patient? Select all that apply.

a. Phenytoin

b. Phenobarbital

c. Carbamazepine

d. Primidone

16. Which of the following would be the best option for this patient based on the information presented?

a. Gabapentin

b. Levetiracetam

c. Carbamazepine

d. Ethosuximide

17. Select the dose-related adverse reaction(s) of AEDs. Select all that apply.

a. Neutropenia

b. Sedation

c. Thrombocytopenia

d. Ataxia

18. Select the AED that is associated with the idiosyncratic adverse effect of gingival hyperplasia.

a. Phenobarbital

b. Primidone

c. Tiagabine

d. Phenytoin

19. Select the AED that is available in oral and parenteral formulations. Select all that apply.

a. Neurontin

b. Dilantin

c. Keppra

d. Trileptal

20. Which drug(s) for SE can be given intramuscularly?

a. Phenytoin

b. Lamotrigine

c. Diazepam

d. Fosphenytoin

21. You read a clinical study for a new antiepileptic medication that has strong data to support its efficacy against other AEDs. The treatment duration studied was 18 weeks. However, clinical studies have shown the following data related to safety:

Adverse Effect	Placebo %	New Drug %
Nausea	14	16
Diarrhea	12	11
Serious Arrhythmia	1	5

What is the number needed-to-harm (NNH) related to arrhythmia?

a. 1
b. 4
c. 20
d. 25

The following case pertains to questions 22 and 23.

22. You get a call from a provider asking about the occurrence of vision loss with Sabril®. They tell you that they suspect this serious adverse drug event has occurred in a patient. Where should this event be reported?

a. FDA MedWatch
b. Centers for Disease Control
c. PubMed
d. National Library of Medicine

23. You are asked to substitute the oral solution packets for the tablets because your patient has a hard time swallowing tablets. You look in the FDA Orange Book for information and this is what you find. What do you do based on this information?

Appl No	N022006	N020427
TE Code		
RLD	Yes	Yes
Active Ingredient	Vigabatrin	Vigabatrin
Dosage Form; Route	For solution; oral	Tablet; oral
Strength	500 mg/packet	500 mg
Proprietary Name	Sabril	Sabril
Applicant	Lundbeck LLC	Lundbeck LLC

a. Substitute the product without calling the physician; the products are therapeutic equivalents.
b. Call the physician to ask about switching products; they are not therapeutic equivalents.
c. Substitute the product without calling the physician; the products are pharmaceutical equivalents.
d. Call the physician to ask about switching products; they are therapeutic equivalents.

TAKEAWAY POINTS »

- Epilepsy is a chronic disease of disturbed electrical activity in the brain resulting in recurrent seizures with or without convulsions.
- The classifications of epilepsy are: absence seizures (petit mal)—sudden interruption of activities and a blank stare; myoclonic seizures—brief shock-like contraction of a muscle group; clonic seizures—jerking motion while tonic seizures involve a sustained muscle contraction; tonic-clonic seizures (grand mal)—alternating muscle contraction and jerking; and atonic seizures involve a sudden loss of muscle tone known as "drop attacks."
- Laboratory tests are evaluated to rule out treatable causes of seizures, such as hypoglycemia, altered electrolytes, and infections. A seizure produced by treatable causes does not represent epilepsy.
- Medications associated with causing seizures include tramadol, bupropion, theophylline, some antidepressants, some antipsychotics, amphetamines, cocaine, imipenem, lithium, excessive doses of penicillins or cephalosporins, sympathomimetics, and stimulants.
- Pharmacotherapy of epilepsy is highly individualized and requires titration of the dose to optimize AED therapy (maximal seizure control with minimal or no side effects). Approximately, 50% to 70% of patients can be maintained on one AED.
- Adverse effects of AEDs are often dose limiting or cause a drug to be discontinued. AED adverse reactions are classified as dose related or idiosyncratic.
- Dose-related adverse effects include sedation, ataxia, and diplopia. Idiosyncratic adverse reactions are not related to the dose of the AED and often lead to discontinuation of the AED.
- AEDs are associated with numerous drug interactions related to absorption, metabolism, and protein binding.
- Phenytoin exhibits dose-dependent capacity-limited (Michaelis-Menten) pharmacokinetics, meaning the maximum capacity of hepatic enzymes to metabolize the drug is reached within the normal dosage range.
- Phenytoin and valproic acid are highly protein bound and only unbound medication is able to produce clinical and adverse effects.
- A therapeutic range should be established for each patient and this range should define concentrations that result in minimal side effects and optimal seizure control.
- SE is a neurologic emergency that can lead to permanent brain damage or death.

BIBLIOGRAPHY

French JA, Kanner AM, Bautista J, et al. Efficacy and tolerability of the new antiepileptic drugs I: treatment of new onset epilepsy, report of the Therapeutics and Technology Assessment Subcommittee and Quality Standards Subcommittee of the American Academy of Neurology and the American Epilepsy Society. *Neurology.* 2005;62:1252-1260.

French JA, Kanner AM, Bautista J, et al. Efficacy and tolerability of the new antiepileptic drugs II: treatment of new onset epilepsy, report of the Therapeutics and Technology Assessment Subcommittee and Quality Standards Subcommittee of the American Academy of Neurology and the American Epilepsy Society. *Neurology.* 2005;62:1261-1273.

McNamara JO. Pharmacotherapy of the epilepsies. In: Brunton LL, Chabner BA, Knollmann BC, eds. *Goodman & Gilman's The Pharmacological Basis of Therapeutics.* 12th ed. New York, NY: McGraw-Hill; 2011:chap 21.

Meierkord H, Boon P, Engelsen B, et al.; European Federation of Neurological Societies. EFNS guideline on the management of status epilepticus in adults. *Eur J Neurol.* 2010;17(3): 348-355.

Nguyen VV, Baca CB, Chen JJ, Rogers SJ. Epilepsy. In: DiPiro JT, Talbert RL, Yee GC, Matzke GR, Wells BG, Posey L, eds. *Pharmacotherapy: A Pathophysiologic Approach.* 10th ed. New York, NY: McGraw-Hill; 2017.

Phelps SJ, Wheless JW. Status epilepticus. In: DiPiro JT, Talbert RL, Yee GC, Matzke GR, Wells BG, Posey L, eds. *Pharmacotherapy: A Pathophysiologic Approach.* 10th ed. New York, NY: McGraw-Hill; 2017.

Quality Standards Subcommittee of the American Academy of Neurology. Practice parameter: a guideline for discontinuing antiepileptic drugs in seizure free patients [summary statement]. *Neurology.* 1996;47:600-602.

KEY ABBREVIATIONS

AED = antiepileptic drug
ECG = electrocardiogram
EEG = electroencephalogram
GABA = gamma-aminobutyric acid

IV = intravenous
PE = phenytoin equivalents
SE = status epilepticus

54 Headache

Carrie Koenigsfeld, Anisa Fornoff, and Darla Klug Eastman

FOUNDATION OVERVIEW

Headaches are a common chief complaint of patients seeking advice from a pharmacist. The three main categories of primary headache disorder are migraine, tension-type, and cluster headaches.

The pathophysiologic and etiologic mechanisms of migraine are not known. The sensory sensitivity may be due to a dysfunction of monoaminergic sensory control systems of the brainstem and thalamus. It is speculated that the trigeminovascular input from the meningeal vessels is a pathway for pain recognized in migraine headaches. There is a release of vasoactive neuropeptides, specifically calcitonin gene-related peptide (CGRP), when the cells in the trigeminal nucleus are activated. There is a deficiency of serotonin levels in the plasma during a migraine attack. The use of serotonin agonists, triptans, in migraine therapy has demonstrated the role of serotonin in treatment, being potent agonists of 5-HT_{1B}, 5-HT_{1D}, and 5-HT_{1F}. Dopamine may also play a role in migraine headaches as dopamine receptor antagonists are effective treatments administered as monotherapy or with other antimigraine medications; however, there is a lack of clinical data to support this theory.

The pathophysiology behind tension headache also remains unknown, but one hypothesis is that stress is an important stimulus. Cluster headaches may be precipitated by hypothalamic-related changes in cortisol, prolactin, testosterone, growth hormone, luteinizing hormone, endorphins, or melatonin.

When considering the diagnosis of headaches, a comprehensive history of present illness and physical examination are critical. A thorough history will include time of onset, attack frequency, duration, aggravating and relieving factors, characteristics of pain, associated signs and symptoms, and treatment history. History and physical examination findings that may be suggestive of a secondary headache disorder include the worst headache ever, head pain with exercise, sneezing or coughing, headache that wakes patient from sleep, ataxia, history of head trauma, and changes in mental status. Headaches beginning after the age of 50 suggest underlying issues such as a mass lesion or cerebrovascular disease. Any of these findings are considered red flags that warrant a referral to the physician.

The types of headaches are differentiated based upon duration, location, frequency, severity, and quality of pain. Tension headaches last 30 minutes to 7 days and are located in the occipital or frontal region of the head with a band-like tightness. Pain associated with cluster headaches is unilateral and the headaches are vascular in nature, producing pain around the eye, temple, or forehead. Cluster headaches resolve within 3 hours and are accompanied with nasal congestion, watering eyes, eyelid edema, or ptosis. There is clinical variability among migraine headaches. Onset of migraine pain is gradual with the peak occurring in minutes to hours. In adults, pain lasts 4 to 72 hours and located in the frontal or temporal region of the head. Patients describe the headache as moderate to severe, pulsating, and aggravated by physical activity. A combination of nausea, vomiting, photophobia, and phonophobia accompany the headache. Migraine headaches occur with or without an aura. An aura refers to neurologic symptoms that precede an attack and include diplopia, scotomas, blurry vision, ataxia, and vertigo.

PREVENTION

Headaches are triggered by a variety of patient-specific factors. Possible triggers include emotional stress; changes in sleeping habits; physical activity; environmental factors such as flickering lights and loud noises; ingestion of chocolate, red wine, caffeine, alcohol, nitrates, aspartame, and medications including oral contraceptives. Patients should avoid possible triggers. Encouraging patients to keep a headache diary can be helpful in tracking the duration and frequency of symptoms, triggers, and responses to treatment interventions.

Nonpharmacologic treatment may be considered for prevention and adjunctive treatment for alleviating headaches. Headache sufferers may find relief by reducing activity and sensory input and by sleep. Some patients have used relaxation therapy, including biofeedback, hypnosis, or acupuncture to alleviate the pain. Patients should avoid identified triggers and consider a wellness program focused on a consistent sleep pattern, exercise, healthy diet, and limited caffeine and nicotine intake.

TREATMENT

Migraine Headache

Acute Therapy

The goals for treatment of an acute migraine headache are to treat attacks quickly and consistently while avoiding recurrence, restore the patient's ability to function, optimize self-care, minimize adverse effects, and be cost-effective. Several medications may be used during an acute migraine attack, including nonsteroidal anti-inflammatory drugs (NSAIDs), analgesic combination products, ergot derivatives, serotonin agonists (triptans), and opiates (Table 54-1). A stratified approach to treatment of an acute migraine attack is employed, although a step-wise approach may be used at times. The stratified approach tailors therapy to the severity and disability of the headache using a migraine-specific medication. A patient would have multiple medications available to select appropriate drug therapy based on headache severity.

TABLE 54-1 Medication Therapy for Headache

Class	Generic (Brand)	Route	Mechanism of Action	Adverse Reactions	Contraindications
NSAID	Ibuprofen (Advil/Motrin)	po	Inhibit prostaglandin synthesis, which may prevent inflammation in the trigeminovascular system	GI upset, somnolence, dizziness	Caution with peptic ulcer disease, renal dysfunction, hypersensitivity to aspirin or NSAIDs
	Aspirin	po			
	Naproxen (Naprosyn, Aleve)	po			
	Ketorolac (Toradol)	IV			
	Diclofenac (Voltaren)	po			
Analgesic	Acetaminophen (Tylenol)	po, PR	Inhibition of prostaglandins	Rash, increased LFTs or bilirubin	Cautious use along with alcohol or other products containing acetaminophen
Combination product	Acetaminophen/aspirin/ caffeine (Excedrin Extra Strength, Excedrin Migraine, Excedrin Tension Headache)	po	Inhibition of prostaglandins	Overuse, medication-overuse headache, withdrawal	Cautious use along with alcohol or other products containing acetaminophen
	Butalbital/caffeine + aspirin (Fiorinal) or acetaminophen (Fioricet)	po			
	Isometheptene/ dichloralphenazone/ acetaminophen (Midrin)	po			
Opioid	Meperidine (Demerol)	IV, po	Binds to opiate receptors altering perception and response to pain	Dependence, medication-overuse headache, constipation, nausea/vomiting	
	Butorphanol (Stadol)	IV, intranasal			
	Oxycodone	IV, po			
	Hydromorphone	IV, po			
Serotonin agonist (Triptan)	Sumatriptan (Imitrex, Zembrace SymTouc, Sumavel DosePro, Onzetra Xsail Nasal)—t1/2 2-2.5 h	Imitrex (po, nasal, SQ) Zembrace SymTouch (SQ autoinjector) Sumavel DosePro (SQ jet injector) Onzetra Xsail Nasal (exhaler powder)	Vasoconstriction of dilated intracranial arteries	Parasthesias, fatigue, dizziness, flushing warmth, somnolence, chest tightness, pain in the chest or neck	Ischemic heart disease, uncontrolled hypertension, cerebrovascular disease, hemiplegic or basilar migraine, use of ergot derivative within 24 h, use of SSRI or SNRI
	Sumatriptan/naproxen (Treximet)				
	Rizatriptan (Maxalt, Maxalt MLT)—t1/2 2-3 h	po, oral disintegrating			
	Zolmitriptan (Zomig, Zomig ZMT)—t1/2 2-3 h	po, oral disintegrating, intranasal			
	Naratriptan (Amerge)—t1/2-6 h	po			
	Frovatriptan (Frova)—t1/2-26 h	po			

TABLE 54-1 | **Medication Therapy for Headache** (*Continued*)

Class	Generic (Brand)	Route	Mechanism of Action	Adverse Reactions	Contraindications
	Eletriptan (Relpax)—t1/2-4 h	po			
	Almotriptan (Axert)—t1/2-3 h	po			
Ergot derivative	Ergotamine (Ergomar)	Sublingual	Constriction of intracranial blood vessels that decreases neurogenic inflammation in the trigeminovascular system	Nausea/vomiting, vasoconstriction, retroperitoneal fibrosis, ergotism or intense vasoconstriction resulting in peripheral vascular ischemia or gangrene	Peripheral vascular disease, hepatic or renal failure, coronary artery disease, sepsis, uncontrolled hypertension, concomitant use of strong inhibitors of CYP 3A4, pregnancy, triptan use within 24 h
	Dihydroergotamine (Migranal)	IM, SQ, intranasal			
Antiemetic	Metoclopramide (Reglan)	IV	Blocks dopamine and serotonin receptors in the CNS, enhances acetylcholine in the GI tract	Drowsiness, fatigue, EPS	Seizure history
	Prochlorperazine (Compro)	IV, IM, PR	Blocks dopamine receptors in the CNS	Sedation, hypotension, anticholinergic effects	Reye syndrome, children less than 2 y old
Miscellaneous	100% oxygen	IH	Unknown but likely vasoconstriction	None	Caution in COPD and smokers
	Lidocaine	Intranasal	Blocks pain impulses	Local irritation	

Abbreviations: CNS, central nervous system; COPD, chronic obstructive pulmonary disease; EPS, extrapyramidal syndrome; GI, gastrointestinal; IH, inhalation; IM, intramuscular; IV, intravenous; LFT, liver function test; NSAID, nonsteroidal anti-inflammatory drugs; po, per oral; PR, per rectum; SNRI, serotonin-norepinephrine reuptake inhibitor; SQ, subcutaneous; SSRI, selective serotonin reuptake inhibitor.

A step-wise approach initiates a safe, effective, and inexpensive medication as first-line therapy. Examples of initial pharmacotherapy in a step-wise approach would be NSAIDs or analgesic combination products. If the first agent does not work, a second agent which is more specific for migraine, such as a triptan or ergot derivative, is selected.

Many factors must be taken into consideration when choosing an appropriate abortive agent for acute headache therapy. The severity of headache and its effect on patient function should be taken into account. Past response of headaches to treatment is an important factor in selecting an option. Route of administration should be considered due to patient preference, necessity of a certain route, and differences in the onset of action. Duration of action of medications is also important as medications with longer half-lives may require less frequent dosing and may limit headache recurrence.

NSAIDs and analgesic combination products are appropriate for mild to moderate migraine headaches. Caution should be taken to avoid medication overuse when these drugs are employed. Many of these medications are available over the counter, which makes them convenient, less expensive choices for some patients. Acetaminophen monotherapy has not been shown to provide adequate relief and is not recommended.

Ergot derivatives, including ergotamine tartrate and dihydroergotamine, are migraine-specific medications used for moderate to severe migraine headaches. Individual dosage forms have specific guidelines for repeating doses. Dihydroergotamine nasal spray (Migranal) once assembled must be used within 8 hours and the remaining solution must be discarded. Also noteworthy is the risk of ergotism. Ergotism is severe peripheral ischemia that may present as cold and painful extremities, paresthesias, decreased peripheral pulses, and claudication that may ultimately result in gangrene. There are several contraindications to use of ergot derivatives including peripheral vascular disease, coronary artery disease, uncontrolled hypertension, hepatic or renal failure, sepsis, pregnancy or lactation, and use of a triptan within 24 hours.

Triptans are also migraine-specific and should be used for moderate to severe migraines. Triptan medications have specific guidelines related to repeating doses as needed for full effect. Important considerations about triptans include:

- The risk of serotonin syndrome when combined with other agents affecting serotonin.

- Triptans and ergot derivatives should not be used within 24 hours of each (vasoconstrictive effects).

- Patients with ischemic heart disease, uncontrolled hypertension, cerebrovascular disease, or hemiplegic or basilar migraine should not receive a triptan as these are contraindications to therapy.

Due to the risk of causing medication-overuse headaches, opioid use is limited to patients requiring rescue therapy or contraindications to other options. Patients should be counseled on medication-overuse headache potential. Medication-overuse headaches occur as the acute treatment wears off resulting in additional medication use to provide relief for the new headache pain. This results in a cycle of increased headaches and use of acute therapy.

In addition to abortive therapy, patients may require adjuvant therapy with antiemetic medications (metoclopramide or prochlorperazine). An antiemetic given 15 to 30 minutes prior to an oral abortive medication limits nausea and vomiting and improves absorption of migraine medication.

Preventative Therapy

Preventative therapy should be evaluated in patients treated for acute migraine attacks. Considerations for prophylactic therapy include frequency of attacks, impact on activities of daily living, ability to use abortive medications, and complexity of medical condition.

Agents used for preventative therapy include β-blockers, antidepressants, anticonvulsants, NSAIDs, calcium-channel blockers, and serotonergic agents, including the ergot derivatives (Tables 54-1 and 54-2).

When selecting an agent for preventative therapy, it is important to consider a patient's medical history. It is preferable to select an agent that is indicated for a comorbid condition whenever possible. For example, a β-blocker or calcium-channel blocker would be preferred in a patient with hypertension. Although the data are limited for herbal or vitamin alternatives, the American Academy of Neurology recognizes feverfew, riboflavin, and magnesium as possible preventative treatment options.

Cluster Headache

The goal for treatment of an acute cluster headache is to abort an attack as quickly as possible. It is important for treatment to have a fast onset of action due to the rapid and short-lived nature of cluster headaches. As a result, oral medications have a limited role in the treatment of an acute attack, while subcutaneous injections, intranasal, or inhaled products are useful. Subcutaneous sumatriptan or inhaled 100% oxygen via a non-rebreather mask are the treatments of choice for acute cluster headaches. Other triptans or ergotamine derivatives may also be considered.

Preventative therapy may be considered for cluster headache patients when individuals suffer two or more daily

TABLE 54-2 **Medication Therapy for Headache Prevention[a]**

Class	Generic (Brand)	Mechanism of Action	Adverse Reactions	Contraindications
β-Antagonist	Atenolol	Unknown but may raise the migraine threshold by modulating adrenergic or serotonergic neurotransmission	Fatigue, depression, nausea, dizziness, insomnia, bradycardia, impotence	Caution in CHF, PVD, atrioventricular conduction disturbances, asthma, depression, and diabetes
	Metoprolol Nadolol Propranolol Timolol			
Antidepressant	Amitriptyline	Unknown but may cause downregulation of central serotonin and adrenergic receptors	Sedation, urinary retention, dry eyes, increased appetite	Concurrent use of MAOI Caution with BPH, glaucoma, hypotension
	Doxepin Imipramine Nortriptyline Protriptyline Fluoxetine Venlafaxine		Fewer side effects than TCAs but increased risk of serotonin syndrome	Concurrent use of MAOI Caution with triptan use and risk for serotonin syndrome
Anticonvulsant	Gabapentin (Neurontin)	Inhibition of GABA, glutamate modulation, inhibition of sodium and calcium ion channels	Somnolence, dizziness, asthenia	Avoid abrupt withdrawal
	Topiramate (Topamax) Valproic acid (Depakote/ Depakote ER)		Paresthesia, fatigue, anorexia, diarrhea, weight loss, nausea Nausea/vomiting, alopecia, tremor, asthenia, somnolence, weight gain	Pregnancy
Calcium channel antagonist	Verapamil	Inhibition of calcium ions from entering areas of the vascular smooth muscle	Gingival hyperplasia, constipation, edema, hypotension, dizziness, nausea	Left ventricular dysfunction, hypotension
Other	Lithium	Alters cation transport in nerve and muscle cells; influences reuptake of serotonin	Tremor, lethargy, nausea, diarrhea, GI upset	Use with severe renal or cardiovascular disease, dehydration, pregnancy, or concomitant diuretic use
	Onabotulinumtoxin A (Botox)	Prevents calcium-dependent release of acetylcholine in the neuromuscular junction	Hypertension, injection site pain, neck pain, blepharoptosis	

Abbreviations: BPH, benign prostatic hypertrophy; CHF, congestive heart failure; GABA, gamma-aminobutyric acid; GI, gastrointestinal; MAOI, monoamine oxidase inhibitor; PVD, peripheral vascular disease; TCA, tricyclic antidepressant.

[a]Please note that NSAIDs and ergot derivatives may also be used for preventative therapy.

attacks or when acute treatment is ineffective or is limited by adverse effects. The prophylactic medication should be started early in the cluster headache cycle and continued through the cycle until the patient is headache free for at least 2 weeks. The calcium-channel blocker verapamil, ergot derivative ergotamine, lithium, corticosteroids, or anticonvulsant valproic acid may be considered. Comorbid conditions, adverse effects, and drug interaction potential should guide agent selection.

Tension Headache

The goal of treatment for tension headache is to alleviate symptoms while avoiding recurrence. Tension headaches can be treated with medications available over the counter, including NSAIDs or combination analgesic products with aspirin, acetaminophen, and/or caffeine. Failure of these agents to provide adequate relief may warrant prescription therapy. Preventative therapy may be considered in patients who have two or more headaches weekly, headaches exceeding 3 to 4 hours, or headache severity resulting in medication overuse or disability. Tricyclic antidepressants or botulinum toxin injections may be considered.

CASE Application

1. Which of the following plays a role in migraine pathogenesis? Select all that apply.
   a. Norepinephrine
   b. Serotonin
   c. Dopamine
   d. Substance P

2. A patient presents to your community pharmacy complaining of a headache. She rates the headache as a 7 on a scale of 1 to 10, and the pulsating worsens as the headache progresses. She experiences nausea and sensitivity to light until the headache dissipates after about 12 hours. She is unable to function during the headache. Which of the following headache types is this patient experiencing?
   a. Migraine
   b. Tension
   c. Cluster
   d. Caffeine

3. Which of the following signs/symptoms are classified as red flags, indicating need for physician referral and diagnostic evaluation? Select all that apply.
   a. "Worst headache of my life"
   b. Acute headache that occurs after coughing/sneezing
   c. Headache onset age ≥40 years
   d. Blood pressure of 150/80 mm Hg

4. LK suffers from chronic migraines and is currently experiencing an acute attack. She calls your community pharmacy and asks your professional advice. In talking with her you learn that she stopped drinking regular coffee, joined a gym, and started a monophasic oral contraceptive in the past two weeks. She attended a wine and cheese party last night with friends she met at the gym. Which recommendation would be best to provide that may help prevent migraines in the future?
   a. Avoid intake of wine and cheese.
   b. She should resume drinking regular coffee.
   c. She may benefit from switching to a triphasic oral contraceptive.
   d. She should avoid physical activity.

5. Which of the following would be an absolute contraindication for receiving a selective 5-HT$_1$ receptor agonist (triptan)?
   a. Diabetes
   b. Ischemic heart disease
   c. Anemia
   d. Controlled hypertension

6. Which of the following is the brand name for rizatriptan?
   a. Imitrex
   b. Maxalt
   c. Amerge
   d. Frova

7. A patient is taking Zomig ZMT. Which of the following is true regarding this medication? Select all that apply.
   a. It is a subcutaneous injection.
   b. Liquid is not required for administration.
   c. It is an orally disintegrating tablet.
   d. It is a transdermal patch.

8. A patient who currently takes oral sumatriptan often experiences headache recurrence, where the headache comes back within 24 hours after a positive response to the medication. Her physician would like a recommendation of a selective 5-HT$_1$ receptor agonist (triptan) with a longer half-life. Which of the following would you recommend?
   a. Frovatriptan
   b. Rizatriptan
   c. Zolmitriptan
   d. Almotriptan

9. Which of the following are correct repeat dose instructions for the migraine medication?
   a. Zomig tablets: take one tablet now; may repeat in 2 hours
   b. Imitrex subcutaneous injection: use one injection now; may repeat in 30 minutes
   c. Amerge tablets: take one tablet now; may repeat in 2 hours
   d. Imitrex subcutaneous injection: use one injection now; may repeat in 30 minutes and then again at hour 2

10. Treximet is a combination headache medication made up of which of the following?

    a. Sumatriptan and naproxen
    b. Acetaminophen, aspirin, and caffeine
    c. Acetaminophen, isometheptene mucate, and dichloralphenazone
    d. Acetaminophen, butalbital, and caffeine

11. CJ is a 30-year-old patient admitted to the hospital with an unremitting migraine headache. She has tried two doses of naratriptan in the past 12 hours. She also takes lisinopril 10 mg once daily for her blood pressure and terbinafine for her onychomycosis. Her vital signs are BP 132/88 mm Hg, heart rate 70 beats/min, height 5 feet 5 inches, and weight 130 lb. The physician plans to administer dihydroergotamine. Which of the following are contraindications for CJ receiving this treatment?

    a. Uncontrolled hypertension
    b. Elevated heart rate
    c. Terbinafine
    d. Naratriptan

12. Which of the following represent a severe adverse effect that may result from taking ergotamine tartrate? Select all that apply.

    a. Purple toe syndrome
    b. Ergotism
    c. Pruritus
    d. Nausea

13. JB is a 55-year-old woman who has suffered from migraines for many years. Her zolmitriptan 5 mg works well to abort her headaches when they occur. Over the past few months, her headaches have increased in frequency to one every 2 weeks. She also complains of difficulty sleeping. Her vital signs today upon physical examination are height 5 feet 6 inches, weight 140 lb, blood pressure 120/80 mm Hg, and heart rate 60 beats/min. Her physician would like to start her on prophylactic drug therapy. Which of the following drug therapy would be a best next step for prophylaxis for this patient? Select all that apply.

    a. Propranolol
    b. Botulinum toxin type A
    c. Amitriptyline
    d. Phenelzine

14. Which of the following are prophylactic treatment options for migraine headache? Select all that apply.

    a. Verapamil
    b. Topiramate
    c. Valproic acid
    d. Ergotamine

15. JJ is a 49-year-old man who experiences headache cycles two times a year, usually in the spring and fall. The headaches occur for about 3 to 4 weeks and he may have up to 5 headaches daily. The headaches are an unbearable type of pain that comes suddenly, located in his left eye, and stops within 1 to 2 hours. He experiences severe ocular and nasal symptoms, such as nasal stuffiness or rhinorrhea, ocular lacrimation, and ptosis. He tells you that in order to attempt to stop the pain, he sometimes rubs the areas of pain or even beats his head against objects. Which of the following are appropriate abortive treatment options for this patient's headache?

    a. Oxygen
    b. Imitrex (sumatriptan) tablets
    c. Amitriptyline
    d. Topiramate

16. AB is a 25-year-old college student who has been having headaches 3 to 4 times a month that last for 12 to 24 hours for the past couple of months. He describes them as having a gripping quality with pressure on both sides of his head, as if someone is squeezing his head with a rubber band. He does not experience nausea or vomiting. His headaches do not stop him from going to class, but sometimes he finds himself having to turn off his radio when studying since he just can't handle any noise. Light does not bother him during his headaches. Which of the following abortive treatment options would be appropriate recommendations for AB's headache?

    a. NSAIDS
    b. Imitrex (sumatriptan)
    c. Amitriptyline
    d. Metoclopramide

17. DT is a 31-year-old woman who is 36 weeks pregnant. She currently has a headache with presentation most like a tension-type headache. She is requesting a recommendation for treatment. Which of the following is the best recommendation?

    a. Naproxen
    b. Ergotamine
    c. Acetaminophen
    d. Ibuprofen

18. MM presents to the emergency room (ER) with a severe migraine headache and nausea and vomiting. He has taken one dose of zolmitriptan 5 mg orally within the past 6 hours, but vomited within 10 minutes. Which of the following would be the most appropriate next step for treatment?

    a. Metoclopramide 10 mg IV
    b. Biofeedback
    c. Three days of inpatient dihydroergotamine IV
    d. Acetaminophen 650 mg per rectum (PR)

19. A physician you work with at your ambulatory care practice site asks your advice. He would like to know which serotonin receptor agonist migraine medication(s) is available as a nasal spray. You respond: (Select all that apply)

    a. Sumatriptan
    b. Rizatriptan

c. Zolmitriptan

d. Naratriptan

20. A patient is picking up a prescription for Migranal (dihydroergotamine) at your community pharmacy counter. She has not used this medication before. Which of the following is an important counseling point to provide?

a. Remove the foil wrapper before inserting PR

b. Once prepared, use within 8 hours

c. Wear latex-free gloves to apply

d. Take with a full glass of water

21. Select the brand name for eletriptan.

a. Maxalt

b. Zomig

c. Ergomar

d. Relpax

22. Which of the following herbal medications has evidence of support for the treatment of migraine?

a. Glucosamine

b. Black cohosh

c. Feverfew

d. Saw palmetto

23. A patient presents to pick up a new prescription for sumatriptan tablets. When verifying the prescription, the computer alerts you of a contraindication with a current prescription: Paxil 20 mg. Which of the following is the reason for this contraindication?

a. Stevens-Johnson syndrome

b. Serotonin syndrome

c. Neuroleptic malignant syndrome

d. Computer error—there is no contraindication

TAKEAWAY POINTS ❯❯

- Headaches are a common, disabling disorder that pharmacists encounter.
- A thorough history and physical examination is useful in determining the types of headache and appropriate therapy.
- Migraine headaches have gradual onset of pain in the frontal or temporal region of the head, last 4 to 72 hours, and may or may not present with an aura.
- Tension headaches are a band-like pressure in the occipital or frontal region of the head lasting 30 minutes to 1 week.
- Cluster headaches present as unilateral pain around the eye, temple, or forehead lasting for less than 3 hours.
- A headache diary may help patients identify and avoid headache triggers.
- Acute therapy for a mild to moderate migraine headache may include NSAIDs or analgesics.

- Ergot derivatives may be used for a moderate to severe acute migraine attack but use should be avoided in patients with peripheral vascular disease, coronary artery disease, uncontrolled hypertension, or within 24 hours of triptan use.
- Triptans, or serotonin agonists, are used for moderate to severe migraine headaches. Triptans should not be used in patients with coronary artery disease, uncontrolled hypertension, or within 24 hours of ergot administration.
- β-Blockers, antidepressants, anticonvulsants, NSAIDs, calcium-channel blockers, or serotonergic agents may be considered as preventative therapy for migraine sufferers.
- Subcutaneous sumatriptan or inhaled 100% oxygen are first-line options for cluster headaches.
- Tension headaches can typically be treated with NSAIDs or simple analgesics.

BIBLIOGRAPHY

Chu J. Antimigraine medications. In: Nelson LS, Lewin NA, Howland M, Hoffman RS, Goldfrank LR, Flomenbaum NE, eds. *Goldfrank's Toxicologic Emergencies*. 9th ed. New York, NY: McGraw-Hill; 2011:chap 51.

Goadsby PJ, Raskin NH. Headache. In: Longo DL, Fauci AS, Kasper DL, Hauser SL, Jameson J, Loscalzo J, eds. *Harrison's Principles of Internal Medicine*. 18th ed. New York, NY: McGraw-Hill; 2012:chap 14.

Katzung BG. Histamine, serotonin, & the ergot alkaloids. In: Katzung BG, Masters SB, Trevor AJ, eds. *Basic &*

Clinical Pharmacology. 12th ed. New York, NY: McGraw-Hill; 2012:chap 16.

Minor DS, Harrell T. Headache disorders. In: DiPiro JT, Talbert RL, Yee GC, Matzke GR, Wells BG, Posey L, eds. *Pharmacotherapy: A Pathophysiologic Approach*. 10th ed. New York, NY: McGraw-Hill; 2017.

Minor DS, Jackson D. Headache disorders. In: Linn WD, Wofford MR, O'Keefe M, Posey L, eds. *Pharmacotherapy in Primary Care*. New York, NY: McGraw-Hill; 2009:chap 19.

KEY ABBREVIATIONS

CGRP = calcitonin gene-related peptide

ER = emergency room

NSAIDs = nonsteroidal anti-inflammatory drugs

PR = per rectum

55

Pain Management

Justin Kullgren

FOUNDATION OVERVIEW

Pain is an unpleasant sensation that negatively affects a person's life, including comfort, sleep, emotion, and daily activity. Pain is an unpleasant sensory and emotional experience associated with actual or potential tissue damage or described in terms of such damage. Additionally, pain is always subjective. Because pain is a variable and personal experience, it is difficult to describe and measure objectively. The clinician must guard against personal biases, which can interfere with treatment. One must also rely on tools such as pain scales to communicate with patients and understand the extent of their pain.

Types of Pain

Pain is categorized according to its cause, location, duration, and clinical features. Pain categorization involves differentiating brief-duration (acute) pain from long-lasting (chronic) pain and malignant (cancer) versus nonmalignant pain (noncancer). Other types of pain include nociceptive (visceral and somatic) and neuropathic.

Acute Pain

Acute pain results from injury or surgery. Acute pain is limited in duration and associated with objective features, such as increased heart rate, pulse pressure, anxiety, and/or sweating. Acute pain is intense at the beginning and decreases in intensity over time or becomes intermittent depending on the individual's activities.

Chronic Pain

Chronic pain is a long-term experience, and sometimes subjective. A chronic disease that is characteristically painful for which there is no cure may lead to chronic pain, examples include: arthritis, cancer, migraine headaches, fibromyalgia, and diabetic neuropathy. Psychological conditions such as depression may exacerbate or contribute to chronic pain. Managing chronic pain should focus on improving the patient's day to day function.

Visceral Pain

Visceral pain results from stimulation of internal organ pain receptors. Examples are pancreatic cancer pain or cancer metastases. The painful stimuli from the internal organ receptors enter the spinal cord at multiple levels along with somatic fibers; therefore, patients describe the sensation as pressure-like, deep squeezing, and usually not very well localized or defined. In general, the patients often cannot pinpoint the source of the pain.

Somatic Pain

Somatic pain originates from irritation of pain fibers in the body surface or deep tissues. Examples are surgical incisional pain or bone pain. Painful stimuli enter spinal cord at a single level, and the painful stimuli can be mapped on parietal cortex. The patient describes the pain as sharp, piercing from body surface or dull aching from deep tissues, and the individual can usually pinpoint the precise location of the painful origin.

Neuropathic Pain

Neuropathic pain is initiated or caused by a primary lesion, dysfunction, or transitory alteration in the peripheral or central nervous system (CNS) resulting in sensations of burning, tingling, knife-like, or electric shock-like quality. These sensations are triggered by slight touches that are normally tolerated, and result in an exaggerated painful sensation. Common causes of neuropathic pain include diabetes mellitus, cancer, and chemotherapy.

TREATMENT

Effective treatment considers the cause, duration, and intensity of pain and matches the appropriate intervention to the situation. The goal of therapy is to reduce pain perception to the lowest tolerable intensity and prevent it from recurring. Clinically, an improvement in pain should translate to improved functionality for the patient. The clinical situation must be considered when selecting analgesics, for example:

- Reducing chronic pain is best accomplished by using analgesics at fixed time intervals rather than on an as-needed basis.

- Patients with severe acute or malignant pain may require additional analgesics for breakthrough pain, as the scheduled analgesics alone may not be adequate.

Drug selection, doses, routes of administration, and dosing frequency should be adjusted as needed until the goals

TABLE 55-1	Mechanism of Action of Analgesics (Drugs That Modify the Source of Pain)	
Effect	**Agents**	
↓Pain stimulus	NSAIDs, antihistamines, sympatholytics	
↓Pain transmission	Membrane stabilizers, antidepressants	
Alter central perception	Opioids, antidepressants	

of therapy are met. Until the dosage is stabilized, all patients who are receiving analgesics should be monitored for efficacy of analgesia as well as untoward side effects. Successful pain management may also include the use of nonpharmacological measures, such as ensuring that the patient receives adequate rest and emotional support. Table 55-1 is a summary of the mechanism of action of analgesics.

Opioids are the standard for management of moderate to severe pain related to acute, traumatic, and some types of chronic painful conditions (nociceptive) and nonsteroidal anti-inflammatory drugs (NSAIDs) are useful for musculoskeletal pain syndromes. However, some painful conditions, particularly those associated with chronic or neuropathic pain, are poorly responsive to opioids and NSAIDs. In addition, opioids may have limited benefits in chronic neuropathic pain syndromes due to dose-limiting side effects. Adjunct medications are often synergistic with other analgesics. Tricyclic antidepressants (TCAs), anticonvulsants, and serotonin/norepinephrine reuptake inhibitors have demonstrated utility in managing neuropathic pain as well as other conditions such as migraine headache.

Acetaminophen

Acetaminophen has central (spinal cord) prostaglandin inhibition similar to NSAIDs. The dosing of acetaminophen is similar to aspirin (eg, 325-650 mg q 4-6 hours as needed for pain), and should not exceed 3 g/d (varies some depending on formulation). Acetaminophen is used as monotherapy for mild to moderate nociceptive pain such degenerative joint disease. It is used in combination with opioids for moderate to severe nociceptive pain (in a fixed product such as acetaminophen 325 mg/oxycodone 5 mg or added to an existing opioid regimen). Acetaminophen has no clinically significant anti-inflammatory activity and is less effective than full doses of NSAIDs, but has fewer adverse reactions. Advantages of acetaminophen include multiple formulations, including rectal and intravenous, combination with other pain medications, and no tolerance to the analgesic effects. Acetaminophen overdose can cause fatal hepatotoxicity and risk factors include heavy alcohol users, concurrent isoniazid, zidovudine, or barbiturate therapy.

Salicylates

Aspirin is effective for mild to moderate nociceptive pain, but is usually reserved for antiplatelet indications (baby aspirin for stroke prevention). Unlike other NSAIDs, aspirin irreversibly inhibits platelet function for the life of the platelet. Additionally, key characteristics regarding aspirin include:

- Precipitate asthma symptoms in aspirin sensitive patients
- Cause a gastrointestinal (GI) bleed
- Taking buffered or enteric coated formulations reduces GI upset, but does not reduce GI bleed risk
- Should not be used during viral syndromes in children and teenagers because of the development of Reye syndrome.

Nonacetylated salicylates do not interfere with platelet aggregation, are rarely associated with a GI bleed, and well tolerated in asthma patients. Examples include diflunisal and salsalate.

Nonsteroidal Anti-Inflammatory Agents

NSAIDs are valuable in the management of postprocedural, acute, and chronic nociceptive pain. They are also used for symptom management of autoimmune inflammatory disorders (eg, rheumatoid arthritis). NSAIDs exhibit highly individual responses with respect to efficacy and side effects. NSAIDs have two key pharmacologic properties:

1. Anti-inflammatory: Peripheral prostaglandin inhibition
2. Analgesia: Central inhibition of prostaglandins/other neuroactive chemicals

Note: The anti-inflammatory duration (but not analgesic duration of action) correlates to serum half-life.

The properties of NSAIDs are due to inhibition of the two isoforms of cyclooxygenase, COX-1 and COX-2. COX-1 protects the gastric mucosa and COX-2 is expressed in the various tissues (including the kidneys to help maintain perfusion). Inhibition of COX-1 interferes with platelet aggregation and inhibition of COX-2 is responsible for the anti-inflammatory effects. NSAIDs are more effective than acetaminophen and salicylates for acute pain treatment. Diclofenac is available for topical use as a patch (Flector), a topical gel (Voltaren 1% gel), and a topical solution (Pennsaid 1.5% solution) for management of degenerative joint disease and musculoskeletal pain. Topical diclofenac is effective in reducing localized pain with a low risk of systemic side effects.

The advantages of NSAIDs include: minimal CNS side effects, they do not slow intestinal motility (eg, not constipating), and they provide synergism with opioid analgesics. The disadvantages of NSAIDs include:

- They have a ceiling analgesic effect (eg, higher doses do not provide better pain relief, but do provide a slightly longer duration of analgesic action).
- Analgesic duration is shorter than predicted by half-life of drug.
- GI irritation and bleeding.
    - Celecoxib is a COX-2 selective NSAID and appears to cause less GI toxicity compared to nonselective NSAIDs. Diclofenac, etodolac, and meloxicam have some degree of COX-2 selectivity *in vitro*. However, there are no clinical data to evaluate the outcome in patients.

- Concurrent use of a proton pump inhibitor, H2-receptor antagonist, or prostaglandin analog misoprostol (Cytotec) decreases the GI bleeding risk. There are coformulations of these products: diclofenac/misoprostol (Arthrotec); ibuprofen/famotidine (Duexis), and naproxen/esomeprazole (Vimovo).

- Antiplatelet effects: For nonaspirin NSAIDs, duration approximates analgesic duration, although antiplatelet activity increases with chronic dosing.

- Decreased renal function: Decreased glomerular filtration rate (GFR), analgesic nephropathy, acute tubular necrosis (ATN). Patients with hypovolemia, compromised circulation, or dehydration are at greater risk.

- Other effects: Fluid retention; agranulocytosis; dermatologic/photosensitivity; asthma exacerbation; tinnitus, headache, cognitive dysfunction; mild reversible hepatic enzyme elevation.

- Increase cardiovascular events with chronic use or immediately after cardiovascular bypass surgery. With the exception of aspirin, it is best to avoid NSAIDs in patients with known heart disease.

NSAID drug interactions reduce or increase the effect of certain medications. NSAIDs reduce the effects of angiotensin-converting enzyme (ACE) inhibitors, β-blockers, loop diuretics, and thiazide diuretics, and increase the effects of anticoagulants, cyclosporine (nephrotoxicity), digoxin, phenytoin, lithium, methotrexate, and probenecid.

Adjunct Analgesics/Neuropathic Pain

Antidepressants and antiepileptics are used for neuropathic pain including postherpetic neuralgia, diabetic neuropathy, and fibromyalgia; however, some are not approved for these pain indications. Table 55-2 lists key characteristics of first-line neuropathic pain agents. Commonly used first-line medications for neuropathic pain include desipramine, nortriptyline, amitriptyline (most side effects of TCAs so less commonly used), gabapentin, pregabalin, and duloxetine.

Tricyclic Antidepressants

TCAs exert analgesic effects by working in the spinal cord to reduce trafficking of pain signals by enhancing serotonin and/or norepinephrine. TCAs also potentiate opioid analgesia. The starting dose is 10 to 25 mg at bedtime and the dose is titrated to pain relief. The dose should be titrated slowly (every 7-14 days). In general, TCAs should be avoided in the elderly patient population due to side effects. Side effects associated with TCAs include:

- Anticholinergic (eg, dry mouth, blurred vision, constipation)

- Cardiovascular (eg, tachycardia, heart blockade, orthostasis)

- CNS (eg, dizziness, drowsiness, confusion, tremor, seizure)

- Dermatological (eg, photosensitivity)

Antiepileptics

Antiepileptics prolong the depolarization of nerves causing reduced neuronal excitability and decrease in pain signaling. Examples of commonly used anticonvulsants used in pain include gabapentin and pregabalin. Less commonly used anticonvulsants for neuropathic pain include carbamazepine, valproate, topiramate, lamotrigine, and other newer anticonvulsants. Some key points are below.

- Gabapentin and pregabalin: Used for chronic neuropathic pain and postherpetic neuralgia. Side effects include somnolence, ataxia, dizziness, fatigue,

TABLE 55-2	Summary of First-Line Neuropathic Pain Agents			
Drug	**Dose**	**Mechanism of Action**	**Side Effects**	**Comments**
Desipramine Nortriptyline	Start 25 mg QHS, 10 mg if geriatric or sensitive Max dose 100-150 mg daily	Inhibits serotonin and norepinephrine reuptake. Blocks sodium and calcium channel and NMDA receptors	Anticholinergic effects, sedation, orthostatic hypotension	Use with caution in patients with cardiovascular disease Analgesic dose typically less than antidepressant dose Slow titrations recommended
Gabapentin	2400-4800 mg/d	Binds to the α2-δ subunit of voltage gated calcium channels to reduce calcium dependent release of neurotransmitters	Somnolence, dizziness, depression, tremor, peripheral edema	Can be expensive Caution use in renal impairment Relative "good" side effect profile Minimal drug-drug interactions Slow titrations recommended
Pregabalin	50 mg tid or 75 mg bid, max 300-600 mg/d		Somnolence, dizziness, peripheral edema	
Duloxetine	60 mg once daily	Selective NE and 5-HT reuptake inhibitor	Nausea, insomnia, constipation/diarrhea	Caution with use in hepatic or renal impairment Avoid abrupt discontinuation May benefit patients with depression

nystagmus, tremor, diplopia, and rhinitis. Additionally, pregabalin is used for fibromyalgia.

- Carbamazepine: Used for trigeminal neuralgia and neuropathies. Side effects include sedation, ataxia, and rare blood dyscrasias (anemia, neutropenia, and thrombocytopenia). Additionally, carbamazepine is associated with CYP-450 drug interactions and auto-induces its own metabolism initially.

Systemic Local Anesthetics

Systemic local anesthetics prolong nerve depolarization via sodium channels in the nerve membranes. Examples include lidocaine and mexiletine. Lidocaine is used for regional nerve blocks and local anesthesia applications. Lidocaine may need to be repeated or infused via a regional nerve catheter.

Other Agents

- Capsaicin: Topical 0.025% and 0.075% used for diabetic and other neuropathies. Alters function of pain-sensitive nerve endings (nociceptors) through substance-P depletion as well as alter the activities of the nociceptors. There are reports of skin burns. There is an 8% capsaicin patch (Qutenza) available by prescription for postherpetic neuralgia.

- Lidocaine 5% patches (Lidoderm): Approved for the treatment of postherpetic neuralgia. Analgesic effect due to decrease in sensory activities of the pain receptors through local anesthetic effects. Tachyphylaxis can occur with continuous use; therefore, patients require a 12-hour break between the patch changes daily.

- Skeletal muscle relaxants: Cyclobenzaprine has tricyclic structure and is primarily used for acute musculoskeletal conditions (back pain). Baclofen and benzodiazepines are gamma-aminobutyric acid (GABA) agonists. Tizanidine, a congener of clonidine, has antinociceptive (pain relieving) properties. These agents are used for spasms from spinal origin such as nerve root impingement or spinal cord compression and irritation.

Opioid Analgesics

Opioids are more potent than nonopioid analgesics such as NSAIDs, although the range of potencies is wide with this class of medicines. They are recommended for moderate to severe pain and used in acute and chronic pain syndromes refractory to other classes. The administration of opioid analgesics is complicated by the need to convert between different routes of administration or different opioid formulations. The equianalgesic doses of parenteral and oral opioid analgesics are listed in Table 55-3. Rational use of opioid analgesics starts with patient and technology assessment. Opioid dosing has

TABLE 55-3	**Common Opioid Analgesics**						
Receptor Effects[1]							
Generic Name	**μ**	**δ**	**κ**	**Approximately Equivalent Dose (mg)**	**Oral:Parenteral Potency Ratio**	**Duration of Analgesia (hours)**	**Maximum Efficacy**
Morphine[2]	+++		+	10	Low	4-5	High
Hydromorphone	+++			1.5	Low	4-5	High
Oxymorphone	+++			1.5	Low	3-4	High
Methadone	+++			10	High	4-6	High
Meperidine	+++			60-100	Medium	2-4	High
Fentanyl	+++			0.1	Low	1-1.5	High
Sufentanil	+++	+	+	0.02	Parenteral only	1-1.5	High
Alfentanil	+++			Titrated	Parenteral only	0.25-0.75	High
Remifentanil	+++			Titrated[3]	Parenteral only	0.05[4]	High
Levorphanol	+++			2-3	High	4-5	High
Codeine	±			30-60	High	3-4	Low
Hydrocodone[5]	±			5-10	Medium	4-6	Moderate
Oxycodone[2,6]	++			4.5	Medium	3-4	Mod-High
Pentazocine	±		+	30-50	Medium	3-4	Moderate
Nalbuphine	—		++	10	Parenteral only	3-6	High
Buprenorphine	±	—	—	0.3	Low	4-8	High
Butorphanol	±		+++	2	Parenteral only	3-4	High

[1]+++, ++, +, strong agonist; ±, partial agonist; —, antagonist.

[2]Available in sustained-release forms, morphine (MS Contin); oxycodone (Oxy Contin).

[3]Administered as an infusion at 0.025-0.2 mcg/kg/min.

[4]Duration is dependent on a context-sensitive half-time of 3-4 minutes.

[5]Available in tablets containing acetaminophen (Norco, Vicodin, Lortab, others).

[6]Available in tablets containing acetaminophen (Percocet); aspirin (Percodan).

Reproduced with permission from Katzung BG: *Basic & Clinical Pharmacology*, 14th ed. New York, NY: McGraw-Hill; 2018.

to be based on the patient's history of opioid analgesic used, the specific patient's needs, and on the delivery system being utilized. Depending on the delivery system and the route, the dose of opioid can vary by a factor of 10 to 100. Therefore, changes in the route of opioid delivery can result in significant changes in the patient's clinical response or toxicity. Often, the concept of equianalgesic dosing is the source of confusion and misunderstanding. Tolerance to most of the opioid adverse effects develops quickly while tolerance to the analgesic effect occurs very slowly.

Key properties of opioid analgesics are listed below.

1. Morphine
   a. At large doses and renal impairment, metabolite can cause CNS excitability and results in increased anxiety, restlessness, or pain.
   b. Morphine is a smooth muscle relaxant, which can cause vasodilatation and hypotension which is often associated with intravenous administration.
   c. Undergoes significant first-pass metabolism.
2. Meperidine (*Not recommended without good justification*)
   a. Active metabolite (Normeperidine) is renally excreted and can accumulate and cause CNS irritability and myoclonic seizures, if the dose of meperidine is pushed too high or if the patient's renal function is decreased.
   b. Widely variable intramuscular absorption from injection site after repeated injections.
3. Hydromorphone
   a. Pharmacologically it is similar to morphine, except it is more potent than morphine on milligram per milligram basis.
4. Methadone
   a. 24-Hour average half-life, dosage must be carefully adjusted because frequent dosing can lead to drug accumulation. Avoid rapid dose escalation when initiating methadone therapy, especially in opiate naïve patients.
   b. Good oral bioavailability due to low first-pass effect and extraction ratio.
   c. Metabolism by CYP-450 3A4 and CYP inducers can increase metabolism significantly to decrease effectiveness.
   d. Can prolong the QT interval.
5. Oxymorphone
   a. Rapid onset with IV administration because it is highly lipophilic
   b. Less pharmacokinetic drug interactions
6. Fentanyl
   a. Passive diffusion fentanyl patch has a slow onset, but has a long 72-hour duration of action. Patches are most often used in chronic pain. In acute pain patients with rapidly changing needs, the patches are not responsive or sensitive enough to be useful. In patients with rapidly changing analgesic needs, IV, transmucosal, or iontophoresis active transdermal routes might be more appropriate.

   b. Less hypotensive effect than morphine or hydromorphone at equianalgesic doses, especially when it is administered intravenously.
   c. Transdermal patches need to be disposed and discarded carefully to prevent accidental poisoning of animals or children. It is only recommended for use in opiate tolerant patients. Tolerance is defined by taking more than 60 mg or oral morphine daily for more than 2 weeks.
   d. Transmucosal use is in opioid tolerant cancer pain patients for breakthrough pain.
7. Codeine
   a. Requires metabolic conversion by CYP 2D6 to active metabolite, morphine.
   b. CYP-450 2D6 inhibition can reduce efficacy thus not routinely used for pain management.
   c. Not effective for severe pain.
8. Hydrocodone
   a. Recently reschedule to schedule II
   b. Frequently used in combination with acetaminophen for pain
   c. Causes less emesis than codeine, and no cross sensitivity in nausea, vomiting, or itching with codeine
9. Tramadol
   a. It is a mu$_1$-specific agonist and very weak opiate analgesic, can help with mild to moderate nociceptive pain.
   b. Should start with lower doses in elderly.
   c. Tramadol also has properties that make it a consideration for neuropathic pain.
   d. Tramadol can produce either CNS excitation or sedation depending on the specific patient during initiation of therapy.
   e. A consideration when used for the management of acute mild neuropathic pain.

Adverse effects of opioid analgesics associated include:

- Slowed mentation: Most often associated with morphine in elderly patients. Effect may be reduced with an alternative opioid analgesic.

- Urinary retention: May be managed with bethanechol or terazosin if symptoms are severe. Consider opioid rotation.

- Constipation: Tolerance to constipation does not develop. Should always be therapeutically prevented while receiving opioid analgesics. Treat with stimulant laxatives such as senna or bisacodyl and consider adding stool softeners. Polyethylene glycol is a good consideration for those who do not tolerate a stimulant. Newer peripheral opioid antagonists are available though use is limited by expense (naloxegol and methylnaltrexone).

- Unavoidable sedation: Can be managed with amphetamine 5 mg at 8 AM and 12 noon for chronic malignant pain. Consider opioid rotation.

- CNS irritability: Frequently associated with meperidine due to its metabolite normeperidine, but can also occur with high doses of morphine and hydromorphone analogs secondary to the 3 and 6-glucuronide metabolites, which is centrally active.

- Hypotension: Most pronounced immediately following general anesthesia or in volume-depleted patients. Most frequently associated with intravenous opioid boluses. Fentanyl is frequently used in critical care situations because it has the least amount of hypotensive effect.

- Respiratory depression: Occurs only occasionally at therapeutic doses, most often is associated with rapid IV boluses, and can be reversed easily with naloxone if it is identified early. The patients are especially at risk when opiates are given together with other CNS depressants. Managed with naloxone.

- Opioid abstinence symptoms: This may occur after patient is abruptly discontinued of chronic opioids. Opiate abstinence may occur in opioid dependent patients whose pain is managed with spinal analgesia alone. These abstinence symptoms may be relieved by systemic opioids or clonidine.

Dosing regimens and delivery systems for opioid analgesics include:

1. Intermittent on demand dosing (prn): The preferred regimen for patients who are neurologically or hemodynamically unstable.

2. Scheduled dosing (round-the-clock): The preferred method for controlling severe pain or chronic pain. This method should also be used for the oral regimen when transitioning a patient from patient-controlled IV analgesia (PCA) to the oral route.

3. Continuous infusion: Used only for patients when other routes of analgesic administration is either unavailable or impractical. Not recommended outside of the critical care or monitored environment. May be used for managing cancer pain.

4. Patient-controlled IV analgesia: The preferred method for controlling moderate to severe postoperative pain. It allows the patient to control the pain on their own.

5. Spinal analgesia (epidural or intrathecal): Duration of analgesia depends on the lipophilicity of the opioid used. Less lipophilic opioids have a longer duration of action. More lipophilic opioids have a shorter duration of analgesia. The analgesic effect of epidural or intrathecal morphine may last 12 to 24 hours. Dosing basics: intrathecal >> epidermal > IV > PO. (Use of low molecular weight heparins are **contraindicated** within 12 hours before spinal analgesia administration or spinal catheter insertion or within 2 hours after spinal analgesia administration or spinal catheter removal.)

6. Regional analgesia (nerve plexus blocks or nerve blocks): This is different from spinal analgesia, because local anesthetic and opioid are administered around the peripheral nerve outside the spine. (Low molecular weight heparin is also contraindicated within 12 hours of catheter placement or 2 hours after removal.)

7. Sustained-release opioids: Used for controlling chronic pain after the patient is stabilized by the immediate release preparation. It has a slower onset, but a long lasting duration of action of 8 to 24 hours. The use of sustained-release opioid is not appropriate for the management of acute pain immediately after surgery or trauma, because the delayed onset and exceptionally long duration of opiate effect can lead to delay in pain control or unforeseen toxicity. Patients receiving sustained-release opioids should also receive immediate release opioids for breakthrough pain.

8. Transdermal fentanyl: Should only be used for constant, but stable persistent pain where the patient cannot take oral medications. It should not be used in patients with rapidly escalating or unstable pain because of delayed maximum effects of at least 8 hours. Fentanyl transdermal use should be limited to patients who are opioid tolerant. Transdermal fentanyl is not recommended in opiate-naive patients. One should always treat the patient with other short-acting opioid analgesics during the first 8 hours after patch application. Must tell the patient to discard the used patch carefully to prevent accidental poisoning of either children or pets. It is primarily used for the management of persistent chronic pain. Usually, oral sustained-release opioids can be just as effective. (Opiate tolerance is defined by taking equivalent to 60 mg of oral morphine daily for 2 weeks.)

CASE Application

Use the following case for questions 1 and 2:

KK is a 65-year-old woman with a chief complaint of left arm, shoulder, and axillary pain. She underwent a left subtotal mastectomy, radiation, and chemotherapy for breast cancer. KK has currently no evidence of cancer, but complains of two types of pain. The first in her chest is a dull achy pain; the second is a burning and stinging pain down her left arm and nothing has worked well for this pain. She is also complaining of severe constipation. Her current medications are bupropion 150 mg bid, ibuprofen 600 mg one tablet tid, morphine sulfate extended release (ER) 30 mg bid, atenolol 50 mg every morning, and tamoxifen 10 mg bid. All medications are taken by mouth.

1. What is best therapeutic plan of this patient's analgesic regimen?

    a. Analgesic regimen should be discontinued, because long-acting opiate is not appropriate for this patient's pain.

    b. Increase morphine ER to 30 mg po every 4 hours since it is not providing adequate analgesia.

    c. Increase morphine ER to 60 mg po tid since it is not optimally controlling patient's pain.

    d. Add pain medication to focus on neuropathic symptoms.

2. What is the best approach for the burning pain in this patient?

   a. Add amitriptyline low dose at bedtime and titrate
   b. Add duloxetine low dose at bedtime and titrate
   c. Add nortriptyline high dose at bedtime and titrate
   d. Add gabapentin low dose at bedtime and titrate

3. A patient with chronic pain from a long-standing back injury presents with worsening mild to moderate dull, achy, pressure like pain. The patient works many long and stressful hours. The patient currently takes ibuprofen 800 mg tid for his back pain. Which of the following recommendations would be least preferred?

   a. Increasing dose of ibuprofen
   b. Addition of scheduled acetaminophen
   c. Ensuring the patient is receiving adequate rest
   d. Ensuring the patient is receiving adequate emotional support

4. TP is a 67-year-old man with newly diagnosed degenerative joint disease. He is prescribed an NSAID for management of the pain. TP has concerns about the NSAID causing side effects. Select the potential side effect(s) associated with using NSAIDs for pain management. Select all that apply.

   a. GI bleeding
   b. Antiplatelet effects
   c. Decreased renal function
   d. Fluid retention
   e. Somnolence

5. AO is a patient with osteoarthritis that presents to the orthopedic clinic. AO has a past medical history (PMH) of hypertension, chronic obstructive pulmonary disease, and reflux. Medications include lisinopril, as needed albuterol, metoprolol, chlorthalidone, meloxicam, and pantoprazole. The doctor at the clinic is worried about potential drug interactions. Select the medication(s) that AO is receiving that may have reduced effectiveness when used with their pain medication. Select all that apply.

   a. Lisinopril
   b. Albuterol
   c. Metoprolol
   d. Chlorthalidone

6. QP is a 71-year-old patient diagnosed with severe diabetic neuropathy. He is currently being treated with an alpha-blocker (terazosin) for an enlarged prostate. Terazosin has significantly improved the symptoms of the enlarged prostate, but the patient is having orthostatic hypotension episodes. Select the medication that would be most appropriate for QP's diabetic neuropathy.

   a. Naproxen
   b. Morphine
   c. Nortriptyline
   d. Gabapentin

7. HA is a 53-year-old patient with chronic pain from cancer. In addition to the cancer, HA has a PMH of gout, hypertension, and anemia. HA is currently taking desipramine, allopurinol, HCTZ, lisinopril, and iron. Select the potential side effect(s) associated with HA's pain medication. Select all that apply.

   a. Drowsiness
   b. Dry mouth
   c. Constipation
   d. Hyperkalemia

8. Select the medication(s) that may cause CNS side effects. Select all that apply.

   a. Gabapentin
   b. Morphine
   c. Amitriptyline
   d. Duloxetine
   e. Naproxen

9. KL is a 69-year-old patient with a burning, stinging, and knife-like pain. KL's diagnoses include hypertension, diabetes mellitus II, multiple myeloma with recent chemotherapy, and depression. Which of the following is the most appropriate for the treatment of KL's pain?

   a. Valproate
   b. Pregabalin
   c. Topiramate
   d. Carbamazepine
   e. Amitriptyline

10. A patient presents to the pharmacy that has chronic neuropathic pain. The patient prefers to use a topical product for their pain. Select the best medication for this patient's pain.

   a. Capsaicin
   b. Amitriptyline
   c. Carbamazepine
   d. Topiramate

11. VI is a 79-year-old female patient in the intensive care unit for sepsis. The cause of the sepsis is from a decubitus ulcer. The ulcer is very painful and the first year medical resident ordered meperidine for dressing changes. The patient has a PMH for hypertension, angina, chronic kidney disease, and osteoporosis. VI is anticipated to use the meperidine frequently. Select the potential side

effect(s) associated with meperidine use in VI. Select all that apply.

a. Seizures
b. GI bleeding
c. Respiratory depression
d. Anemia

12. LD is a 62-year-old patient with chronic pain from an automobile accident several years ago. LD has chronic moderate to severe nociceptive pain. Additional PMH includes diabetes and CKD. The patient does not like to take pills or tablets. What is the BEST medication for LD's chronic pain?

a. Morphine
b. Oxycodone
c. Meperidine
d. Fentanyl

13. IT is a 74-year-old man with severe chronic nociceptive pain. He has been previously treated with scheduled acetaminophen, but is prescribed morphine today. The patient will be receiving morphine chronically. Select the medication that IT should receive in addition to the acetaminophen and morphine.

a. Ibuprofen
b. Gabapentin
c. Capsaicin
d. Bisacodyl

14. SQ is a patient from a motor vehicle collision. She suffered a broken leg during the accident and was given opioids for pain management. SQ's pain has gone completely away but now has developed respiratory depression. Select the BEST medication to give SQ for her current symptoms.

a. Flumazenil
b. Naloxone
c. Acetylcysteine
d. Albuterol
e. Ipratropium

15. A patient is involved in a severe car accident and is going to require several surgeries to fix multiple broken bones. The patient is expected to have severe acute pain. Select the dosing method that should be employed for this patient.

a. Intermittent
b. Scheduled dosing
c. Directly observed therapy
d. As needed

16. A patient presents with acute mild to moderate dull and achy pain from doing too much hard work. The patient is otherwise healthy and currently takes no medication. What is the best medication to treat the patient's pain?

a. Naproxen
b. Carbamazepine

c. Oxycodone
d. Capsaicin

17. Which of the following medications would be appropriate for a patient experiencing moderate to severe nociceptive pain that has high dose opioid requirements and cannot tolerate morphine due to side effects? Assume each of the medications used below will be used as monotherapy. Select all that apply.

a. Fentanyl
b. Diclofenac
c. Hydromorphone
d. Duloxetine

18. MS is a 32-year-old patient that presents to the doctor with new onset nociceptive back pain from playing back-yard football. At times the pain feels like back spasms. MS has tried heat and ibuprofen with no success. Recommend a nonopioid for MS's back pain.

a. Mexiletine
b. Cyclobenzaprine
c. Tapentadol
d. Hydrocodone

19. QY is a 41-year-old accountant with an acute pain issue. He would like to receive a medication that will not affect his ability to work, but will effectively treat his pain. Select the analgesic that is minimally associated with CNS side effects and does not slow intestinal motility.

a. Naproxen
b. Hydrocodone
c. Meloxicam
d. Amitriptyline

20. A patient is experiencing a mild to moderate mixed nociceptive and neuropathic pain from acute shingles. The patient has no other significant PMH or other medications. Select the BEST pain medication for this patient.

a. Ibuprofen
b. Amitriptyline
c. Carbamazepine
d. Tramadol
e. Morphine

21. Rank the following opioid analgesics in order from least potent analgesic effect to most potent analgesic effect.

Unordered options	Ordered response
Hydrocodone	
Codeine	
Hydromorphone	
Fentanyl	

TAKEAWAY POINTS »

- Pain is an unpleasant sensation that can negatively affect a person's life, including comfort, thought, sleep, emotion, and normal daily activity.

- Pain is categorized according to its cause, location, duration, and clinical features. The most simplistic categorization involves differentiating brief-duration (acute) pain from long-lasting (chronic) pain.

- Effective treatment considers the cause, duration, and intensity of pain and matches the appropriate intervention to the situation. The goal of therapy is to eliminate or reduce the pain to the lowest tolerable intensity, prevent it from recurring, and restore patient functionality. The clinical situation must be considered when selecting analgesics.

- Drug selection, doses, routes of administration, and dosing frequency should be adjusted as needed until the goals of therapy are met. Until the dosage is stabilized, all patients who are receiving analgesics should be monitored for efficacy of analgesia as well as side effects.

- Opioids remain the standard for management of acute, traumatic, and many types of chronic painful conditions, while NSAIDs are useful for musculoskeletal pain syndromes.

- Some painful conditions, particularly those associated with chronic or neuropathic pain, are poorly responsive to opioids and NSAIDs.

- TCAs, anticonvulsants, and other membrane stabilizers have demonstrated utility in managing neuropathic pain as well as other conditions such as migraine headache.

- The advantages of NSAIDs include: minimal CNS side-effects, they do not slow intestinal motility (eg, not constipating), and they provide synergism with opioid analgesics.

- Side effects associated with TCAs include anticholinergic, cardiovascular, CNS, and dermatological.

- Anticonvulsants prolong the depolarization of nerves causing reduced neuronal excitability and decrease in pain signaling.

- Opioids are more potent than nonopioid analgesics such as NSAIDs, although the range of potencies is wide with this class of medicines.

- Opioids are recommended for moderate to severe pain intensity and are used in acute and chronic pain syndromes that are refractory to other classes of agents.

BIBLIOGRAPHY

Herndon CM, Strickland JM, Ray JB. Pain management. In: DiPiro JT, Talbert RL, Yee GC, Matzke GR, Wells BG, Posey L, eds. *Pharmacotherapy: A Pathophysiologic Approach.* 10th ed. New York, NY: McGraw-Hill; 2017:chap 60.

Schumacher MA, Basbaum AI, Naidu RK. Opioid agonists & antagonists. In: Katzung BG, Trevor AJ, eds. *Basic & Clinical Pharmacology.* 13th ed. New York, NY: McGraw-Hill; 2015.

Scullion B, Ryan L. Pain management. In: Attridge RL, Miller ML, Moote R, Ryan L, eds. *Internal Medicine: A Guide to Clinical Therapeutics.* New York, NY: McGraw-Hill; 2013:chap 45.

Yaksh TL, Wallace MS. Opioids, analgesia, and pain management. In: Brunton LL, Chabner BA, Knollmann BC, eds. *Goodman & Gilman's The Pharmacological Basis of Therapeutics.* 12th ed. New York, NY: McGraw-Hill; 2011:chap 18.

KEY ABBREVIATIONS

ACE = angiotensin-converting enzyme
CNS = central nervous system
GABA = gamma-aminobutyric acid
GI = gastrointestinal

NSAIDs = nonsteroidal anti-inflammatory drugs
PCA = patient-controlled IV analgesia
TCAs = Tricyclic antidepressants

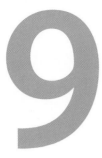

Psychiatric Disorders

56

Schizophrenia

Krina H. Patel

FOUNDATION OVERVIEW

Schizophrenia is a psychiatric illness representing a heterogeneous syndrome of disorganized and bizarre thoughts, delusions, hallucinations, inappropriate affect, and impaired psychosocial function. The etiology of schizophrenia is unknown, but genetics and alteration of neurotransmitters, such as dopamine, have a significant role in the development of schizophrenia.

Symptoms

A common misconception is that schizophrenia means split personalities or multiple personalities. Schizophrenia is an illness associated with various types of symptoms and is not a split personality disorder. Positive, negative, and cognitive symptoms are the different types of symptoms associated with schizophrenia. Positive symptoms are an excess of normal functions or are added to normal functions. Delusions, defined as false, fixed beliefs and hallucinations, defined as real perception of senses in the absence of external stimuli, are examples of positive symptoms. Hallucinations may affect all five senses and are primarily categorized as visual, auditory, olfactory, tactile, and gustatory depending on the sensation alteration. Other positive symptoms may also include: disorganized speech, tangentiality, disorganized behavior, and catatonic behavior. Negative symptoms are loss of normal functions or qualities that subtract from an individual's personality. Examples of negative symptoms include alogia, avolition, and anhedonia. Negative symptoms are difficult to assess as compared to positive symptoms, because they are also associated with other psychiatric disorders. Examples of cognitive symptoms are impaired attention or memory. Additionally, individuals with schizophrenia may present with social and occupational dysfunction. For example, patients may have difficulty with self-care, maintaining employment, or maintaining relationships.

Diagnosis

No objective measures exist to confirm the diagnosis of schizophrenia. Schizophrenia is diagnosed by evaluating the patient and the patient's symptoms. The Diagnostic and Statistical Manual of Mental Disorders, fifth edition (DSM-5) is a diagnostic reference that provides criteria for schizophrenia diagnosis. Characteristic symptoms, social and occupational dysfunction, duration and the ruling out of other disorders are key components of the DSM-5 criteria for schizophrenia.

TREATMENT

The goal is to develop a treatment plan that decreases symptoms, improves quality of life, improves patient functioning, and minimizes medication side effects. Treatment options for schizophrenia include nonpharmacologic therapy and pharmacologic therapy, and both are beneficial for the treatment of schizophrenia. Nonpharmacologic therapy includes psychosocial support groups and programs that focus on enhancing patient functioning, though these are utilized in conjunction to pharmacologic therapy. Antipsychotics are the mainstay of treatment for schizophrenia. There are two classes of antipsychotics: first-generation antipsychotics (FGAs) and second-generation antipsychotics (SGAs), also known as typical and atypical antipsychotics, respectively. Both antipsychotic classes are effective for improving positive symptoms; however, SGAs are more likely to control negative symptoms when compared to FGAs. Tables 56-1 to 56-3 provide a list of FGAs and SGAs including formulations and dosing.

Pharmacologic Treatment

FGAs are high-affinity dopamine-2 (D_2) receptor antagonists. FGAs are classified as high, medium, and low-potency agents (Table 56-4); however, they are equally effective in equipotent doses. FGAs are not considered first-line therapy due to safety and tolerability concerns. For example, FGAs are likely to cause extrapyramidal symptoms (EPS). EPS are movement disorders such as dystonia, akathisia, pseudoparkinsonism, and tardive dyskinesia (Table 56-5). *Note*: Low, medium, and high-potency FGAs can cause EPS; additionally, SGAs can cause EPS, just not as commonly as FGAs.

The SGAs are also D_2 receptor antagonists; however, the affinity for the D_2 receptor is less than that seen with FGAs (Table 56-4). The SGAs exhibit greater affinity toward serotonin 5-HT_2 when compared to D_2 receptor. The SGAs differ in their D_2 and $5HT_2$ activity along with variable affinity for histamine, muscarinic and alpha receptors. This variation in mechanism of action among SGAs is why each displays a slightly different adverse effect profile. SGAs are considered as first-line treatment (with the exception of clozapine) and are advantageous because of a lower EPS risk as compared to FGAs. Key concepts about select SGAs include:

1. Clozapine is the only SGA with superior efficacy in the management of treatment-resistant patients; however, it is not considered as first-line due to its safety profile.
2. Risperidone loses its atypical profile and resembles an FGA at doses more than 6 mg.
3. Aripiprazole exhibits both D_2 antagonism and agonism activities depending on the current dopaminergic status.
4. Paliperidone is an extended-release formulation of the active metabolite of risperidone.
5. Asenapine, brexpiprazole, cariprazine, and lurasidone are a few of the newer SGAs on the market.

Additionally, antipsychotics cause adverse effects such as sedation, metabolic abnormalities, orthostasis, QTc prolongation, and prolactin elevation. The likelihood of antipsychotics causing these adverse effects varies based on the class of antipsychotic and, many times, varies between agents. For example, patients treated with FGAs are at a higher risk for

TABLE 56-1 Antipsychotic Medications Classified by Generation

First-Generation Antipsychotics (FGAs)[1]	Second-Generation Antipsychotics (SGAs)[2]
[a]Haloperidol	Clozapine
[b]Chlorpromazine	Risperidone
[a]Fluphenazine	Olanzapine
Loxapine	Quetiapine
Molindone	Ziprasidone
Perphenazine	Aripiprazole
[a]Pimozide	Paliperidone
[b]Thioridazine	Iloperidone
[a]Thiothixene	Asenapine
Trifluoperazine	Lurasidone
	Brexpiprazole
	Cariprazine

[1]Also referred to as typical or conventional antipsychotics
[2]Also referred to as atypical antipsychotics
[a]High-potency agents.
[b]Low-potency agents.

TABLE 56-2 Available Antipsychotics and Dosage Ranges

Generic Name	Trade Name	Starting Dose (mg/d)	Usual Dosage Range (mg/d)	Comments
First-Generation Antipsychotics				
Chlorpromazine	Thorazine	50-150	300-1000	Most weight gain among FGAs
Fluphenazine	Prolixin	5	5-20	
Haloperidol	Haldol	2-5	2-20	Higher dropout rate in first episode
Loxapine	Loxitane	20	50-150	
Loxapine inhaled	Adasuve	10	10	Maximum 10 mg per 24 hours Approved REMS program only
Perphenazine	Trilafon	4-24	16-64	
Thioridazine	Mellaril	50-150	100-800	Significant QTc prolongation
Thiothixene	Navane	4-10	4-50	
Trifluoperazine	Stelazine	2-5	5-40	
Second-Generation Antipsychotics				
Aripiprazole	Abilify	5-15	15-30	
Asenapine	Saphris	5	10-20	Sublingual only, no food or drink for 10 minutes after administration of the dose
Brexpiprazole	Rexulti	1	2-4	
Cariprazine	Vraylar	1.5	1.5-6	Due to long half-life, steady-state is not reached for several weeks
Clozapine	Clozaril	25	100-800	Check plasma level before exceeding 600 mg
Iloperidone	Fanapt	1-2	6-24	Care with dosing in CYP2D6 slow metabolizers
Lurasidone	Latuda	20-40	40-120	Take with food; ≥350 calories (≥1,460 J)
Olanzapine	Zyprexa	5-10	10-20	Avoid in first episode because of weight gain
Paliperidone	Invega	3-6	3-12	Bioavailability increased when administered with food
Quetiapine	Seroquel	50	300-800	
Quetiapine XR	Seroquel XR	300	400-800	
Risperidone	Risperdal	1-2	2-8	
Ziprasidone	Geodon	40	80-160	Take with food, ≥500 calories (≥2,100 J)

Data from Hasan A, et al: World J Biol Psychiatry 2012;13:318–378; Initial REMS Approval. NDA 022549, ADASUVE (Loxapine) Inhalation Powder. Approved Risk and Mitigation Strategies (REMS). U.S. Food and Drug Administration; Citrome L: Int J Clin Pract 2009;63:1237–1248; Citrome L: Int J Clin Pract 2009;63:1762–1784; McCormack PL: Drugs 2015;75:2035–2043; Prescribing information. Rexulti. Tokyo, Japan: Otsuka pharmaceutical Co, Ltd July, 2015; Citrome L: Int J Clin Pract 2011;65:189–210; Clozapine FDA prescribing information. Teva Pharmaceuticals, revised 11/2015.

TABLE 56-3	Long Acting Injectable Antipsychotics		
First-Generation Antipsychotics	**Brand Name**	**Dose Range (mg)**	**Frequency**
Fluphenazine Decanoate	Prolixin Decanoate®	12.5-100	2-4 wk
Haloperidol Decanoate	Haldol Decanoate®	50-200	4 wk
Second-Generation Antipsychotics			
Risperidone long-acting injectable	Risperidone Consta®	12.5-50	2 wk
Paliperidone Palmitate	Invega Sustenna®	39-234	4 wk
Paliperidone Palmitate	Invega Trinza®	273-819	3 mo
Olanzapine Pamoate	Zyprexa Relprevv®	150-405	*2 or 4 wk
Aripiprazole Monohydrate	Abilify Maintena®	160-400	4 wk
Aripiprazole Lauroxil	Aristada®	441-882	*4 or 6 wk

*Dose dependent

Data from DiPiro JT, Talbert RL, Yee GC, et al: *Pharmacotherapy: A Pathophysiologic Approach*, 10th ed: New York, NY: McGraw-Hill; 2017.

developing EPS, prolactin elevation, and neuroleptic malignant syndrome (NMS). Signs and symptoms associated with NMS include autonomic instability, altered level of consciousness, muscle rigidity, and an elevated creatine kinase.

Patients treated with SGAs are at a higher risk for metabolic abnormalities (glucose dysregulation, lipid abnormalities, and weight gain). Clozapine and olanzapine are most likely to induce metabolic abnormalities, while aripiprazole, ziprasidone, and lurasidone are least likely. Prolactin elevation is associated with FGAs; however, risperidone and paliperidone also cause elevated prolactin levels. Finally, clozapine is associated with an increased risk of seizures and agranulocytosis.

Monitoring

Patients receiving SGA treatment should regularly monitor their weight, fasting lipids, fasting glucose, and blood pressure. Frequent monitoring of these parameters will allow early detection of metabolic abnormalities. Patients receiving clozapine should have their absolute neutrophil count (ANC) strictly monitored (Table 56-6). If a patient's ANC falls below

the recommended values, additional monitoring and clozapine discontinuation may be necessary. QTc monitoring is recommended with ziprasidone and iloperidone. Patients receiving treatment with FGAs, risperidone, or paliperidone should have their prolactin levels monitored. All patients should also be monitored for any signs of EPS. If EPS is suspected, benzodiazepines, dopamine agonists, and anticholinergic agents such as diphenhydramine and benztropine may be utilized (Table 56-5).

Treatment Algorithm

The treatment algorithm provides guidance for making pharmacotherapeutic recommendations for the treatment of schizophrenia (Figure 56-1). The algorithm indicates that SGAs are first-line treatment and FGAs are initiated if treatment failure occurs with an SGA. The algorithm also indicates that clozapine may be used if a patient has no response with SGAs or FGAs. Combination therapy may also be utilized in later stages if no response to monotherapy is observed; however, data supporting combination therapy is inconsistent and

TABLE 56-4	Antipsychotic Drugs: Relation of Chemical Structure to Potency and Toxicities					
Chemical Class	**Drug**	**D_2/5-HT$_{2A}$Ratio[1]**	**Clinical Potency**	**Extrapyramidal Toxicity**	**Sedative Action**	**Hypotensive Actions**
Phenothiazines						
Aliphatic	Chlorpromazine	High	Low	Medium	High	High
Piperazine	Fluphenazine	High	High	High	Low	Very low
Thioxanthene	Thiothixene	Very high	High	Medium	Medium	Medium
Butyrophenone	Haloperidol	Medium	High	Very high	Low	Very low
Dibenzodiazepine	Clozapine	Very low	Medium	Very low	Low	Medium
Benzisoxazole	Risperidone	Very low	High	Low[2]	Low	Low
Thienobenzodiazepine	Olanzapine	Low	High	Very low	Medium	Low
Dibenzothiazepine	Quetiapine	Low	Low	Very low	Medium	Low to medium
Dihydroindolone	Ziprasidone	Low	Medium	Very low	Low	Very low
Dihydrocarbostyril	Aripiprazole	Medium	High	Very low	Very low	Low

[1]Ratio of affinity for D_2 receptors to affinity for 5-HT2$_A$ receptors.

[2]At dosages below 8 mg/d.

Reproduced with permission from Katzung BG, Masters SB, Trevor AJ: *Basic & Clinical Pharmacology*, 12th ed. New York, NY: McGraw-Hill; 2012.

TABLE 56-5	Neurological Side Effects of Antipsychotic Drugs			
Reaction	Features	Time of Onset and Risk Info	Proposed Mechanism	Treatment
Acute dystonia	Spasm of muscles of tongue, face, neck, back	Time: 1-5 days Young, antipsychotic naïve patients at highest risk	Acute DA antagonism	Anti-parkinsonian agents are diagnostic and curative[a]
Akathisia	Subjective and objective restlessness; *not* anxiety or "agitation"	Time: 5-60 days	Unknown	Reduce dose or change drug; clonazepam, propranolol more effective than anti-parkinsonian agents[b]
Parkinsonism	Bradykinesia, rigidity, variable tremor, mask facies, shuffling gait	Time: 5-30 days Elderly at greatest risk	DA antagonism	Dose reduction; change medication; anti-parkinsonian agents[c]
Neurolepticmalignant syndrome	Extreme rigidity, fever, unstable BP, myoglobinemia; can be fatal	Time: weeks–months. Can persist for days after stopping antipsychotic	DA antagonism	Stop antipsychotic immediately; supportive care; dantrolene and bromocriptine[d]
Perioral tremor ("rabbit syndrome")	Perioral tremor (may be a late variant of parkinsonism)	Time: months or years of treatment	Unknown	Anti-parkinsonian agents often help[c]
Tardive dyskinesia	Orofacial dyskinesia; rarely widespread choreoathetosis or dystonia	Time: months, years of treatment. Elderly at 5-fold greater risk. Risk ∝ potency of D_2 blockade	Postsynaptic DA receptor supersensitivity, up-regulation	Prevention crucial; treatment unsatisfactory. May be reversible with early recognition and drug discontinuation

[a]Treatment: diphenhydramine 25-50 mg IM, or benztropine 1-2 mg IM. Due to long antipsychotic $t_{1/2}$, may need to repeat, or follow with oral medication.

[b]Propranolol often effective in relatively low doses (20-80 mg/d in divided doses). β_1-Selective adrenergic receptor antagonists are less effective. Non-lipophilic β-adrenergic antagonists have limited CNS penetration and are of no benefit (eg, atenolol).

[c]Use of amantadine avoids anticholinergic effects of benztropine or diphenhydramine.

[d]Despite the response to dantrolene, there is no evidence of abnormal Ca^{2+} transport in skeletal muscle; with persistent antipsychotic effects (eg, long-acting injectable agents), bromocriptine may be tolerated in large doses (10-40 mg/d). Anti-parkinsonian agents are not effective.

Reproduced with permission from Brunton LL, Chabner BA, Knollmann BC: *Goodman & Gilman's The Pharmacological Basis of Therapeutics*, 12th ed. New York, NY: McGraw-Hill; 2011.

limited. Selection of a specific antipsychotic agent should be based on cost, adverse effect profile, monitoring parameters, patient response, and adherence to treatment.

Treatment Adherence

Schizophrenia is a chronic disorder that requires maintenance treatment, and treatment adherence among this population may be a challenge. Reasons for non-adherence include presence of paranoid symptoms, medication adverse effects, and lack of insight. Providing patient education, as well as using long-acting formulations (Table 56-3), may be

plausible options for patients who have problems with treatment adherence.

Special Populations

The use of antipsychotics during pregnancy is complex. Risks and benefits of continuing antipsychotics during pregnancy should be evaluated for each individual patient. Discontinuing antipsychotics may put the female at risk for relapse, potentially causing complications during pregnancy. Currently, the teratogenicity of antipsychotics is unclear. Most antipsychotics were previously classified as pregnancy category C in the retired FDA pregnancy category system and are also excreted in breast milk. A discussion with the patient to determine a treatment plan during pregnancy is the best option.

The use of antipsychotics in elderly patients with dementia-related psychosis requires extreme caution. A black box warning is assigned to all antipsychotics due to an increased risk of death associated with the use of antipsychotics for the treatment of dementia-related psychosis. Nonpharmacologic treatment may be an option for certain patients; however, those who are nonresponsive to nonpharmacologic treatment or present with severe symptoms may require antipsychotic treatment. A careful assessment of the risks and benefits of antipsychotic treatment in this population should be considered prior to the treatment. When antipsychotic treatment is a must, using lower doses and carefully monitoring for adverse effects are essential.

TABLE 56-6	Clozapine Monitoring	
Therapy	Frequency of Monitoring	ANC Values
First 6 mo of clozapine treatment	Weekly	
		ANC >1500/mm³
6-12 mo of clozapine treatment	Every 2 wk	
		ANC >1500/mm³
After 12 mo of clozapine treatment	Every 4 wk	
		ANC >1500/mm³

* Patients with Benign Ethnic Neutropenia (BEN) will have different ANC parameters.

Choice of antipsychotic (AP) should be guided by considering the clinical characteristics of the patient and the efficacy and side effect profiles of the medication.

Any stage(s) can be skipped depending on clinical picture or history of antipsychotic failure and returning to an earlier stage may be justified by history of past response.

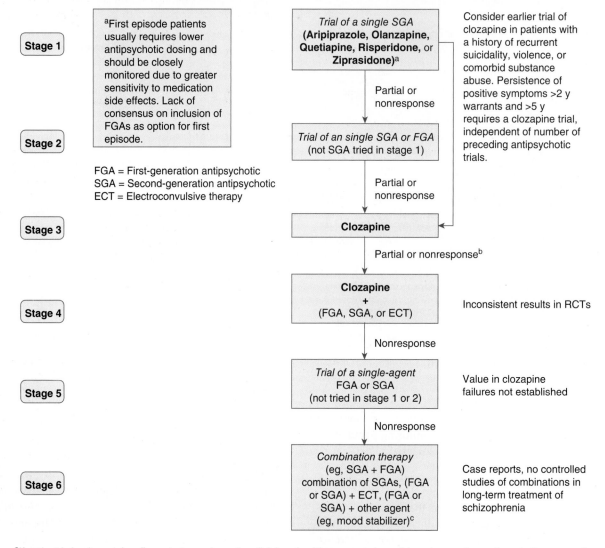

FIGURE 56-1   Algorithm for the treatment of schizophrenia.

*a*First episode patients usually requires lower antipsychotic dosing and should be closely monitored due to greater sensitivity to medication side effects. Lack of consensus on inclusion of FGAs as option for first episode.

FGA = First-generation antipsychotic
SGA = Second-generation antipsychotic
ECT = Electroconvulsive therapy

*a*If patient is inadequately adherent at any stage, the clinician should assess and consider a long-acting antipsychotic preparation, such as risperidone microspheres, haloperidol decanoate, or fluphenazine decanoate.

*b*A treatment refractory evaluation should be performed to reexamine diagnosis, substance abuse, medication adherence, and psychosocial stressors. Cognitive behavioral therapy (CBT) or psychosocial augmentations should be considered.

*c*Whenever a second medication is added to an antipsychotic (other than clozapine) for the purpose of improving **psychotic** symptoms, the patient is considered to be in stage 6.

CASE Application

1. Which of the following symptoms is/are associated with schizophrenia? Select all that apply.

   a. Tangentiality and disorganized speech
   b. Flat affect and alogia
   c. Impaired memory and attention
   d. Hallucinations and delusions

2. Which of the following is/are accepted and reliable when diagnosing a patient with schizophrenia?

   a. Diagnosis can be confirmed by a laboratory measure such as a blood test.
   b. Diagnosis can be confirmed if the patient meets the Diagnostic and Statistical Manual-5 (DSM-5) criteria for schizophrenia.

c. Diagnosis can be confirmed by conducting a brain imaging study on the patient.

d. Diagnosis can be confirmed by a physical examination.

3. Which of the following is the best way to reduce the risk of relapse?

a. Acute treatment with antipsychotic therapy

b. Acute treatment with nonpharmacologic therapy

c. Maintenance treatment with nonpharmacologic therapy

d. Maintenance treatment with antipsychotic therapy

4. MY is a 27-year-old man who presents to his psychiatrist with symptoms associated with schizophrenia. MY reports to the psychiatrist that over the past several months he has experienced auditory hallucinations. During the evaluation the psychiatrist noted that MY also displays negative and cognitive symptoms. The psychiatrist would like to initiate MY on an antipsychotic in order to improve positive symptoms, negative symptoms, and cognitive symptoms. Which of the following is the best option for MY?

a. Fluphenazine

b. Haloperidol

c. Perphenazine

d. Paliperidone

5. Which of the following antipsychotics exhibits a mechanism of action with greater affinity for D_2 receptors as compared to serotonin receptors? Select all that apply.

a. Cariprazine

b. Asenapine

c. Haloperidol

d. Fluphenazine

6. Which of the following is the generic name for Rexulti®?

a. Iloperidone

b. Brexpiprazole

c. Lurasidone

d. Asenapine

7. JL is a 34-year-old man who is admitted to the hospital for having visual and auditory hallucinations. JL has been experiencing these symptoms for several months. Upon admission, JL is diagnosed with schizophrenia. JL has no family history of psychiatric illnesses. JL does not have any other medical conditions and is not taking any medications. All of JL's labs are within normal limits. What is the best treatment for JL?

a. Risperidone

b. Clozapine

c. Thiothixene

d. Haloperidol

8. YR is a 29-year-old woman newly diagnosed with schizophrenia. The treating psychiatrist has told YR that she will be started on an antipsychotic for the management of her schizophrenia. YR is having a very difficult time accepting her diagnosis and treatment and is seeking more information regarding her treatment. YR would like to know what adverse effects she can expect. YR should be counseled on which of the following adverse effects associated with antipsychotic use? Select all that apply.

a. Dystonia

b. Orthostasis

c. Sedation

d. Cholinergic effects

9. AC is a 33-year-old woman with a 9-year history of schizophrenia. AC has a past medical history of asthma and chronic pain resulting from a motor vehicle accident. AC's current medications are an albuterol MDI and acetaminophen. GB has previously failed treatment with several SGAs and FGAs. The plan for AC is to initiate clozapine treatment. Which of the following parameter(s) are required to be monitored while AC is on clozapine? Select all that apply.

a. Absolute neutrophil count

b. Prolactin

c. White blood cell

d. Weight

10. CX is a 26-year-old man who has been diagnosed with schizophrenia. CX has a significant family history of schizophrenia. Family history includes father, paternal uncle, and brother diagnosed with schizophrenia. CX shows concerns regarding the use of antipsychotics, because his father has developed EPS while on antipsychotic treatment. CX would like to be educated on the types of EPS associated with antipsychotic use and should be counseled on movement disorders associated with the use of antipsychotics. Which of the following is a movement disorder that may occur with antipsychotic use? Select all that apply.

a. Tardive dyskinesia

b. Pseudoparkinsonism

c. Akathisia

d. Dystonia

11. LZ is a 31-year-old man with a 5-year history of schizophrenia. LZ has tried SGAs in the past; however, he has not had adequate response. LZ continues to present with severe positive symptoms such as delusions and auditory hallucinations. LZ was initiated on an FGA today. Which of the following adverse effects are most commonly associated with FGAs and should be discussed with LZ?

a. Prolactin elevation and tardive dyskinesia

b. Weight gain and hyperlipidemia

c. Nephrotoxicity and toxic epidermal necrolysis

d. Anxiety and depression

12. HN is a 33-year-old woman with a recent diagnosis of schizophrenia. She is refusing to take any antipsychotics, because she has read on the internet that these types of medications can cause weight gain and diabetes. After encouragement from the psychiatrist, she has agreed to try an antipsychotic. The attending psychiatrist would like to initiate HN on an antipsychotic that is least likely to cause weight gain and metabolic disturbances. Which of the following is the best option for HN? Select all that apply.

    a. Iloperidone
    b. Olanzapine
    c. Aripiprazole
    d. Ziprasidone

13. ZN is a 60-year-old man with a 25-year history of schizophrenia. He has a significant history of stopping his medications. ZN's reasons for non-adherence are that he does not like to take medications daily and he tends to skip his doses scheduled during the time that he is at work. ZN also has a history of not getting his antipsychotic medication refilled on time. Additionally, ZN has been hospitalized 4 times over the past 2 years as a result of nonadherence. Which of the following may be a potential option for ZN? Select all that apply.

    a. Haloperidol decanoate
    b. Asenapine
    c. Paliperidone palmitate
    d. Aripiprazole lauroxil

14. Rank the following antipsychotics from the highest likelihood of causing weight gain to the lowest likelihood of causing weight gain. Aripiprazole, Clozapine, Iloperidone, and Ziprasidone.

    a. Aripiprazole < Clozapine < Iloperidone < Ziprasidone
    b. Clozapine < Iloperidone < Ziprasidone < Aripiprazole
    c. Iloperidone = Clozapine < Ziprasidone < Aripiprazole
    d. Ziprasidone = Aripiprazole < Iloperidone < Clozapine

15. BC is a 31-year-old woman who presents to her psychiatrist today with negative and positive symptoms. Past medical history includes hypertension, seasonal allergies, and gastroesophageal reflux disease. Medications include atenolol, loratadine, and omeprazole. BC has been experiencing psychotic symptoms for several months now. Her psychiatrist has decided to start her on an SGA today. Which of the following should be monitored while BC is receiving treatment with an SGA? Select all that apply.

    a. Fasting glucose
    b. Blood pressure
    c. Fasting plasma lipids
    d. Weight

16. TM is a 34-year-old Caucasian man with a 3-year history of schizophrenia. TM has been on numerous antipsychotics in the past. One week ago, TM was admitted to the hospital due to worsening psychiatric symptoms while adherent to antipsychotic treatment. TM was started on clozapine treatment. It is now 1 week later and ANC values for TM have been drawn. The recommended ANC values during clozapine treatment should be:

    a. ANC <2000/mm³
    b. ANC >1000/mm³
    c. ANC >1500/mm³
    d. ANC >2000/mm³

17. SW is a 45-year-old woman with a 15-year history of schizophrenia. SW was on antipsychotic treatment; however, about 2 weeks ago she stopped taking her antipsychotic, because she lost her job and could not afford her medication. SW's psychiatrist has now prescribed haloperidol which she started taking 2 days ago. SW presents today with a stiff neck and muscle spasms. Her psychiatrist has identified this reaction as dystonia. Which of the following agents may be used to treat SW's EPS?

    a. Cyclobenzaprine
    b. Loxapine
    c. Benztropine
    d. Bromocriptine

18. NK was recently started on Paliperidone for the treatment of schizophrenia. He has been taking the Paliperidone for 3 days now and is not feeling well on this treatment. NK is experiencing muscle rigidity, hyperthermia, hypertension, and presents with an altered level of consciousness. Which of the following is NK experiencing?

    a. Tardive dyskinesia
    b. Dystonia
    c. Neuroleptic malignant syndrome
    d. Serotonin syndrome
    e. Hypertensive crisis

19. CJ is a 55-year-old man who was diagnosed with schizophrenia 30 years ago. Since his diagnosis, CJ has always been on an FGA; however, over the past several months, he has started to show signs of tardive dyskinesia. CJ's treating psychiatrist feels that it may be best for CJ to try an SGA at this point. CJ has a history of cardiac disease, and, therefore, his psychiatrist would like to avoid medications that may be associated with QTc prolongation. Which of the following antipsychotics should be avoided due to the risk of QTc prolongation?

    a. Cariprazine
    b. Brexpiprazole
    c. Ziprasidone
    d. Lurasidone

20. The blockade of which of the following receptors is responsible for inducing EPS?

    a. Serotonin
    b. Dopamine-2 (D_2)
    c. Norepinephrine
    d. Histamine

21. TL is a 39-year-old man with a 9-year history of schizophrenia who is being switched to an FGA. TL has tried asenapine, lurasidone, and aripiprazole in the past; however, his positive symptoms have been uncontrolled on these medications. The psychiatrist would now like to try TL on an FGA. TL has a history of unwanted side effects such as extreme dry mouth, constipation, and urinary incontinence. The treating psychiatrist would like to find a medication with the *least risk* of these adverse effects. Which of the following is the best option for TL?

    a. Haloperidol
    b. Chlorpromazine
    c. Loxapine
    d. Thioridazine

22. TS is a 30-year-old woman with a 2-year history of schizophrenia. She has been on a few FGAs in the past, and they have all caused her prolactin levels to rise. The psychiatrist treating TS would like to avoid any agents likely to elevate prolactin levels. Which of the following agents should be avoided? Select all that apply.

    a. Aripiprazole
    b. Risperidone
    c. Ziprasidone
    d. Paliperidone

23. Which of the following is the brand name for lurasidone?

    a. Vraylar
    b. Latuda
    c. Fanapt
    d. Saphris

24. Which of the following is commercially available in a long-acting injection formulation? Select all that apply.

    a. Risperidone
    b. Paliperidone
    c. Olanzapine
    d. Fluphenazine
    e. Aripiprazole

25. RI is a 34-year-old man who has an 8-year history of schizophrenia. RI has a history of medication nonadherence. RI was initiated on Invega Trinza® last month. How often should RI receive his Invega Trinza® injection?

    a. Every 2 weeks
    b. Monthly
    c. Every 6 weeks
    d. Every 3 months

26. BJ is a 39-year-old woman who has a 10-year history of schizophrenia. BJ over the past 10 years has tried many antipsychotics for the treatment of schizophrenia. BJ has no significant medical conditions and is not on any prescription medications. She does state that she uses acetaminophen on occasion for back pain and also uses loratadine during allergy season. BJ's psychiatrist would like to initiate her on cariprazine for the treatment of her schizophrenia. BJ is requesting additional information regarding adverse effects associated with this medication. Which of the following adverse effect is most likely to occur with cariprazine?

    a. Akathisia
    b. Hyperprolactinemia
    c. Increased risk of seizures
    d. QTc prolongation

TAKEAWAY POINTS ≫

- Schizophrenia is a chronic and complex disorder of thought and affect.
- Patients with schizophrenia may present with positive, negative, and cognitive symptoms.
- The Diagnostic and Statistical Manual of Mental Disorders, fifth edition (DSM-5) provides the criteria for schizophrenia.
- The goal of treatment is to decrease symptoms, improve quality of life, improve patient functioning, and minimize adverse effects.
- FGAs and SGAs are the two classes of antipsychotics that are used for the treatment of schizophrenia.
- SGAs, with the exception of clozapine, are considered first-line therapy for the treatment of schizophrenia.

- FGAs and SGAs are effective for the treatment of schizophrenia; however, adverse effects and monitoring parameters vary among the two classes. FGAs are likely to cause EPS and prolactin elevation while SGAs are likely to cause metabolic effects. Other common adverse effects associated with antipsychotics include sedation, anticholinergic effects, and orthostasis.
- Patients receiving clozapine treatment should have their ANC monitored on a regular basis due to the risk of agranulocytosis which may occur with clozapine treatment.
- When making pharmacotherapeutic recommendations, adverse effects, monitoring parameters, cost, patient response, and adherence to treatment are all factors which should be considered.

BIBLIOGRAPHY

American Psychiatric Association. Schizophrenia and other psychotic disorders. In: *Diagnostic and Statistical Manual of Mental Disorders.* 5th ed. Arlington, VA: American Psychiatric Association; 2013.

Crismon L, Argo TR, Buckley PF. Schizophrenia. In: DiPiro JT, Talbert RL, Yee GC, Matzke GR, Wells BG, Posey L, eds. *Pharmacotherapy: A Pathophysiologic Approach.* 9th ed. New York, NY: McGraw-Hill; 2014:chap 50.

Lehman AF, Lieberman JA, Dixon LB, et al. Practice guidelines for the treatment of patients with schizophrenia, 2nd ed. *Am J Psychiatry.* 2004;161:1-56.

Meltzer H. Antipsychotic Agents & Lithium. In: Katzung BG, Masters SB, Trevor AJ, eds. *Basic & Clinical Pharmacology.* 12th ed. New York, NY: McGraw-Hill; 2012:chap 29.

Meyer JM. Pharmacotherapy of psychosis and mania. In: Brunton LL, Chabner BA, Knollmann BC, eds. *Goodman & Gilman's The Pharmacological Basis of Therapeutics.* 12th ed. New York, NY: McGraw-Hill; 2011:chap 16.

KEY ABBREVIATIONS

ANC = absolute neutrophil count
EPS = extrapyramidal symptoms
FGAs = first-generation antipsychotics

NMS = neuroleptic malignant syndrome
SGAs = second-generation antipsychotics

57

Anxiety Disorders

Patricia A. Pepa and Kelly C. Lee

FOUNDATION OVERVIEW

Anxiety disorders include panic disorder (PD), generalized anxiety disorder (GAD), social anxiety disorder (SAD), and specific phobic disorders. Until the publication of the Diagnostic and Statistical Manual of Mental Disorders, 5th Edition (DSM-5), obsessive-compulsive disorder (OCD) and post-traumatic stress disorder (PTSD) were classified as anxiety disorders. Now, OCD and PTSD are classified separately from anxiety disorders; however, they will be discussed in this chapter due to significant overlap in medications used to treat these disorders. Specific phobias will not be addressed in this chapter, because pharmacotherapy has only a limited role in phobia treatment. For patients to be diagnosed with an anxiety disorder, the symptoms must cause significant impairment in social or occupational functioning and cannot be due to a general medical condition or substance.

Panic Disorder

PD is characterized by recurrent unexpected panic attacks with associated anticipatory anxiety for at least 1 month. PD may be associated with agoraphobia, which is the fear of being in a place or situation where escape may be difficult. A panic attack is a discrete period of fear or discomfort, and characterized by somatic or cognitive symptoms such as chest pain, palpitations, sweating, shortness of breath, fear of dying, dizziness, or hot flashes. These symptoms appear suddenly and last about 10 minutes. Patients can have multiple panic attacks in their lifetime; therefore, panic attacks alone do not constitute a diagnosis of PD.

Generalized Anxiety Disorder

GAD is characterized by chronic excessive worry and anxiety about life events, difficulty controlling the worry, and lasting at least 6 months. Additional symptoms include feeling restless, difficulty concentrating, muscle tension, sleep disturbance, and being easily fatigued. A high incidence of comorbidity exists with major depressive disorder.

Obsessive-Compulsive Disorder

Patients with OCD have either obsessions, compulsions, or both. Obsessions are marked by recurrent and persistent thoughts that are intrusive and cause significant anxiety. Compulsions are characterized by repetitive behaviors that a person feels driven to perform to reduce anxiety. Adults who have either obsessions or compulsions recognize that these feelings are excessive, but they are unable to control these thoughts or actions. To meet criteria for a diagnosis of OCD, the symptoms must cause significant distress and must be time consuming (>1 h/d).

Post-traumatic Stress Disorder

PTSD is characterized by symptoms that occur after exposure to a traumatic event such as military combat or violent personal attack. Symptoms must be present for at least 1 month and include the following types of indicators: re-experiencing (flashbacks, dreams), avoidance (of activities or people associated with the trauma), and increased arousal (sleep disturbance, exaggerated startle response). Comorbidity with another psychiatric illness such as major depressive disorder is common among patients with PTSD. Most symptoms of PTSD occur within 3 months of exposure to the trauma, but they can appear at any time during a patient's lifetime.

Social Anxiety Disorder

Patients with SAD have a persistent fear of at least one or more social or performance situations. The fear is usually of embarrassment, scrutiny, or humiliation. They may have a fear of performing tasks in public (speaking, eating, or writing). For these patients, social exposure produces significant anxiety to the point that they may precipitate a panic attack or lead to avoidance of public situations altogether. Patients with SAD tend to self-treat with alcohol or drugs; comorbidity with substance use disorders or depression is very common.

TREATMENT

The goals of treatment for anxiety disorders are to reduce symptoms, prevent recurrence of symptoms or episodes and improve functioning. Anxiety disorders are difficult to treat because of the chronic nature of the illness. Medications need to be titrated to an effective dose and are most effective when combined with cognitive behavioral therapy. Cognitive behavioral therapy is considered first line for treating most anxiety

To access your complimentary online question exams, visit https://accesspharmacy.mhmedical.com/NAPLEX.aspx

TABLE 57-1   FDA-Approved Medications for Anxiety Disorders*

Anxiety Disorder	Panic Disorder	Generalized Anxiety Disorder	Obsessive-compulsive Disorder	Post-traumatic Stress Disorder	Social Anxiety Disorder
Buspirone		X			
Clomipramine			X		
Duloxetine		X			
Escitalopram		X			
Fluoxetine	X		X		
Fluvoxamine			X		
Paroxetine	X	X	X	X	X
Sertraline	X		X	X	X
Venlafaxine XR	X	X			X

*Per DSM-5, obsessive-compulsive disorder and post-traumatic stress disorder are no longer classified as anxiety disorders.
Abbreviation: FDA, Food and Drug Administration.

disorders either as monotherapy or in combination with pharmacologic treatment, depending on the severity and duration of illness.

There are two major classes of medications utilized to treat anxiety disorders: antidepressants and benzodiazepines as well as buspirone. Antidepressants include selective serotonin reuptake inhibitors (SSRIs), serotonin norepinephrine reuptake inhibitors (SNRIs) and tricyclic antidepressants (TCAs). While other antidepressants, such as bupropion, mirtazapine, and monoamine oxidase inhibitors (MAOIs), may be used for select anxiety disorders, their limited effectiveness and tolerability make them third- or fourth-line agents. Table 57-1 lists medications approved for use in anxiety disorders. In patients with anxiety disorders, antidepressants may increase anxiety or restlessness at the initiation of therapy; therefore, the lowest effective dose should be used and doses should be titrated slowly.

Selective Serotonin Reuptake Inhibitors

SSRIs are effective and first-line options for all anxiety disorders except phobia disorders (which are treated with nonpharmacologic modalities). SSRIs work by preventing the reuptake of serotonin by the presynaptic neuron, thereby leaving serotonin in the synaptic cleft. The mechanism of action specific for anxiety disorders is unknown. SSRIs are first-line options for treating anxiety disorders due to tolerability, safety, decreased risk for dependence and/or withdrawal. SSRIs are also preferable in patients with comorbid depression. Not all SSRIs are FDA approved for major anxiety disorders; however, any SSRI would be appropriate to use. SSRIs are generally available orally in tablet/capsule and liquid formulation.

Common adverse effects of SSRIs include sleep disturbances, gastrointestinal upset, headache, and sexual dysfunction. With the exception of sexual dysfunction, these adverse effects are generally limited to the first 1 to 2 weeks of therapy. SSRIs are metabolized by the liver and caution should be exercised in patients with significant liver function impairment. The use of SSRIs is contraindicated in patients receiving MAOIs and caution should be used when combined with

other agents that increase serotonin (eg, TCAs, venlafaxine, and duloxetine). Upon discontinuation of SSRIs, patients must wait 2 weeks before starting therapy with MAOIs. SSRIs may also interact with nonpsychiatric medications (eg, linezolid, serotonin 1A agonists, tramadol), increasing the risk of serotonin syndrome. Pharmacokinetic drug interactions are common, and many SSRIs inhibit the cytochrome P450 enzymes. Most notably, fluoxetine inhibits CYP2C9/2C19 and CYP2D6 enzymes; fluvoxamine inhibits CYP1A2 and CYP2C9/2C19 enzymes; and paroxetine is a potent inhibitor of CYP2D6 enzyme. Drugs that undergo metabolism by these enzymes may have elevated concentrations if given concomitantly with these SSRIs. Discontinuation symptoms, such as flu-like symptoms or paresthesias, may occur upon abrupt cessation of SSRIs with short half-lives such as paroxetine. SSRIs and SNRIs are considered superior to other classes of agents for use in PTSD. While many adjunctive agents may be used to treat specific symptoms of PTSD, antidepressants should be the treatment of choice for long-term management of PTSD.

Serotonin Norepinephrine Reuptake Inhibitors

Venlafaxine is an SNRI that is used for multiple anxiety disorders (Table 57-1). Unlike TCAs, venlafaxine lacks anticholinergic, alpha-adrenergic blocking, and anti-histaminic properties. Common adverse effects of venlafaxine include gastrointestinal upset, sedation, sexual dysfunction, and dose-related hypertension (at doses >150 mg/d). Dosing in anxiety disorders is similar to that used for depression. Venlafaxine has a short half-life, potentially predisposing patients to discontinuation symptoms if the medication is stopped abruptly. As with SSRIs, discontinuation symptoms may include agitation, dizziness, sensory disturbances, sweating, and tremor. Duloxetine is another SNRI that is approved for use in GAD. Duloxetine is associated with nausea, dry mouth, constipation, and sexual dysfunction. Venlafaxine and duloxetine should not be used in combination with MAOIs and, similar to SSRIs, caution should be exercised when used with other serotonergic agents. Duloxetine inhibits CYP2D6 and may interact with drugs metabolized by this isoenzyme. Both drugs are available orally in tablet and/or capsule formulations. Newer SNRIs, desvenlafaxine and levomilnacipran, have limited data for anxiety disorders.

Tricyclic Antidepressants

TCAs are effective in managing anxiety disorders; however, they are second line due to the potential side effects and their potential for toxicity in overdose. Similar to SNRIs, TCAs block the reuptake of serotonin and norepinephrine. They also inhibit muscarinic, histaminic, and alpha-adrenergic receptors. These additional receptor activities are responsible for adverse effects such as sedation, dry mouth, weight gain, and orthostasis. TCAs have the potential to lower seizure threshold, cause sexual dysfunction, and induce cardiac arrhythmias in overdose situations. Of the TCAs, imipramine and clomipramine have been widely studied in PD. TCAs have minimal or conflicting evidence for use in PTSD and SAD. One of the advantages of TCAs is that serum drug levels can be measured. These levels may be useful in situations of overdose, non-adherence, and toxicity. Most of the TCAs undergo metabolism by the cytochrome P450 2D6 enzyme; therefore, concomitant drugs that inhibit or induce this enzyme may elevate or lower the TCA concentration. The use of TCAs with MAOIs is contraindicated. Concurrent use with alcohol and other central nervous system depressants should also be avoided.

Benzodiazepines

Benzodiazepines act at GABA-A receptors and cause a shift in chloride ions resulting in hyperpolarization (a less excitable state) and membrane stabilization. Benzodiazepines may be used on a short-term basis during the period when an antidepressant is initiated for anxiety disorders since the expected time to response with antidepressants is delayed. Additionally, they may be used on a scheduled basis in a patient who cannot tolerate or do not respond to antidepressants, or on an as needed basis in combination with antidepressants. The utility of benzodiazepines in other anxiety disorders is as second- or third-line agents due to the potential for physical dependence and abuse. Another reason they are not considered first-line options is that they have no efficacy in depressive disorders

and many patients with anxiety disorders also suffer from depression. Benzodiazepines are not recommended for PTSD as it may worsen recovery from trauma. Benzodiazepines have a rapid onset of effect compared to antidepressants and may therefore be preferred by patients. Common adverse effects of benzodiazepines are sedation, cognitive impairment, anterograde amnesia, respiratory depression, and dependence. Paradoxical effects such as excitation and disinhibition may occur, especially in elderly and younger patients. Abrupt discontinuation of benzodiazepine treatment should be avoided to minimize the risk of withdrawal symptoms and seizures. Benzodiazepines that have short durations of action have the highest potential for withdrawal symptoms and risk for physical dependence (Table 57-2). Patients taking benzodiazepines should avoid use of other CNS depressants including opioids, alcohol, and barbiturates due to the potential for additive effects. Benzodiazepines that undergo conjugative metabolism (lorazepam, oxazepam) are preferred in patients who have liver dysfunction, are elderly, or are on concomitant medications that induce or inhibit cytochrome P450 enzymes. Triazolobenzodiazepines (alprazolam, triazolam, and midazolam) are significantly affected by CYP3A4 inhibitors and inducers; caution should be used when these drugs are combined. Benzodiazepines are available in oral, intramuscular, and intravenous formulations. Intramuscular lorazepam produces reliable absorption, whereas intramuscular diazepam is less reliable.

Buspirone

The primary pharmacologic activity of the oral tablet buspirone is theorized as a serotonin 1A partial agonist. Buspirone is indicated for GAD and has an onset of effect that takes at least 2 weeks. The full therapeutic effect may not be observed until 4 to 6 weeks. Buspirone is an option for those who have not responded to or cannot tolerate antidepressants. In addition, buspirone may be desirable in patients with a substance use history since benzodiazepines should be avoided. Common adverse effects of buspirone include nausea, headache, and jitteriness. Buspirone must be taken two to three times daily due to its short half-life. Drug interactions may occur with buspirone and CYP450 3A4 inhibitors or inducers, other serotonergic agents, and MAOIs.

TABLE 57-2	Pharmacokinetic Properties and Formulations of Benzodiazepines			
Benzodiazepine	Onset	Duration	Metabolism	Formulations
Alprazolam (Xanax)	Intermediate	Short	Oxidation	ER tablet, ODT, solution, tablet
Clonazepam (Klonopin)	Intermediate	Long	Nitroreduction	ODT, tablet
Diazepam (Valium)	Very fast	Short (single dose) Long (chronic dose)	Oxidation	Intravenous, rectal gel, solution, tablet
Lorazepam (Ativan)	Intermediate (single dose)	Intermediate	Conjugation	Intravenous, solution, tablet
Oxazepam (Serax)	Slow	Intermediate	Conjugation	Capsule
Temazepam (Restoril)	Slow	Intermediate	Conjugation	Capsule
Triazolam (Halcion)	Intermediate	Very short	Oxidation	Tablet

Abbreviations: ER, extended release; ODT, orally disintegrating tablet.

Special Populations

General

Antidepressants have the potential to exacerbate anxiety symptoms when initiated in patients with anxiety disorders (eg, SSRIs can precipitate panic attacks). Caution should be used when initiating these agents and the lowest dose should be used with slow titration to minimize this risk. TCAs should be avoided in patients with active suicidality due to potential for death in an overdose situation. TCAs should also be avoided in elderly or others who may be sensitive to anticholinergic effects.

Benzodiazepines should be avoided in patients with active or past history of substance use disorder. Benzodiazepines should be avoided in elderly patients due to the increased risk for impaired cognition, falls, and hip fractures.

Pregnancy

The decision to use anxiety medications during pregnancy should be based upon the risks and benefits to both the mother and fetus. While some women may want to avoid any medications during pregnancy, the severity of the anxiety disorder and the potential risks of not treating the illness should be considered.

The safety of SSRIs during pregnancy has been studied extensively and has led to labeling changes by the manufacturer. Paroxetine may be associated with fetal heart defects when taken during the first trimester. First trimester use of other SSRIs have not shown an increased risk of major malformations. Use of SSRIs in the third trimester have been associated with persistent pulmonary hypertension (PPHN) in newborns in some studies but not others. While pregnancy categories are no longer valid, the related risks of these agents should still be regarded. Poor neonatal adaptation syndrome (or neonatal withdrawal syndrome) has been reported in 15% to 30% of women with major depression who took SSRIs in late pregnancy. Symptoms include hypoglycemia, irritability, temperature instability, and seizures in the infant. Symptoms are transient and usually resolve within 2 weeks after delivery.

First trimester use of benzodiazepines has been associated with increased risk of cleft lip/palate, although this association has been challenged in recent studies. When used in the third trimester, they may result in sedation, atonicity ("floppy baby" syndrome), and withdrawal symptoms in the newborn. Benzodiazepines have a pregnancy category D and should be avoided during pregnancy unless benefits outweigh the risks. Experience with buspirone in pregnancy is limited.

Lactation

Benzodiazepines should be avoided during lactation, as they pass into the breast milk and can cause lethargy and temperature dysregulation in the infant. SSRIs pass into the breast milk and have been rarely associated with various symptoms in the infant such as irritability, crying, poor feeding, and colic-like symptoms. Individual risks and benefits should be considered in women who wish to breastfeed while taking these medications.

Children and Adolescents

The use of antidepressants in children and adolescents is controversial in anxiety disorders. Fluoxetine is FDA-indicated for use in children 7 years or more and adolescents with OCD, and sertraline is FDA-indicated for OCD in children 6 years or more and adolescents. Fluvoxamine is FDA-indicated for OCD in children 8 years or more and adolescents. Antidepressants are labeled with a black box warning for suicidality in children and young adults (up to age 24 years old). A medication guide should be dispensed with all prescriptions for these medications. Patients should be monitored for signs and symptoms of increased agitation, anxiety, or changes in mood/behavior, especially at the initiation of therapy or with dose changes.

CASE Application

Please use the following case for Questions 1 and 2.

A 27-year-old woman complains of excessive worrying, poor concentration, back and neck pain, and difficulty sleeping through the night. She constantly worries about losing her job as a data analyst despite the fact that she recently received a promotion. These symptoms have progressively worsened in the past 7 months and have negatively affected her relationship with her friends.

1. The psychiatrist is seeking a recommendation for this new diagnosis of generalized anxiety disorder. Which medication has an FDA indication for this disorder?

   a. Levomilnacipran
   b. Amitriptyline
   c. Bupropion
   d. Buspirone
   e. Fluvoxamine

2. The mechanism of action of buspirone is:

   a. Dopamine 2A partial agonist
   b. Selective serotonin reuptake inhibitor
   c. Serotonin and norepinephrine reuptake inhibitor
   d. Serotonin 1A partial agonist
   e. Serotonin and dopamine antagonist

3. Which of the following benzodiazepines has the longest duration of action at steady state?

   a. Alprazolam
   b. Oxazepam
   c. Diazepam
   d. Triazolam
   e. Lorazepam

Please use the following case for Questions 4 and 5.

A 20-year-old man admits excessive anxiety when meeting new people or when he is in large crowds since middle school. While giving a speech for his college public speaking class, he fears being humiliated and worries when he will have to do it again. After 1 month, he dropped the class and avoids any future classes that involve oral presentations.

4. Which of the following antidepressants is the most appropriate initial treatment for this young man with newly diagnosed social anxiety disorder?

    a. Wellbutrin
    b. Cymbalta
    c. Remeron
    d. Oleptro
    e. Effexor XR

5. The patient has had concerns with Effexor and side effects. The most significant dose-related adverse effect of Effexor is:

    a. Sedation
    b. Seizures
    c. Increased blood pressure
    d. Hepatotoxicity
    e. Renal dysfunction

6. What is a significant concern for patients with panic disorder when starting an SSRI?

    a. Anxiety
    b. Bruxism
    c. Gastrointestinal upset
    d. Headache
    e. Sexual dysfunction

7. Select the generic name for Cymbalta.

    a. Duloxetine
    b. Citalopram
    c. Mirtazapine
    d. Sertraline
    e. Venlafaxine

8. A 25-year-old woman presents to your community pharmacy explaining that she was recently diagnosed with obsessive-compulsive disorder. She has been consumed with disturbing thoughts that she will get the Zika virus. She has begun washing her hands after touching anything that is not her own property. This washing is so frequent that she cannot complete her tasks until she has washed her hands. Which of the following medications might be on her medication profile to help manage the issue? Select all that apply.

    a. Phenelzine
    b. Sertraline
    c. Clomipramine
    d. Paroxetine
    e. Clonazepam

9. For the treatment of anxiety disorders, which of the following is an advantage of an SSRI compared to a tricyclic antidepressant? Select all that apply.

    a. Safer in overdose
    b. Can measure drug levels

    c. No seizure risk
    d. No gastrointestinal upset
    e. No sexual dysfunction

10. The SSRIs are effective for treating which of the following anxiety disorders? Select all that apply.

    a. Generalized anxiety disorder
    b. Obsessive-compulsive disorder
    c. Post-traumatic stress disorder
    d. Panic disorder
    e. Social anxiety disorder

11. A 50-year-old man with a history of alcohol abuse and cirrhosis presents to your clinic, and your attending physician wants to initiate a benzodiazepine for his panic attacks. Which of the following benzodiazepines would be most appropriate to minimize risk of adverse effects?

    a. Alprazolam, clonazepam, estazolam
    b. Chlordiazepoxide, clorazepate, diazepam
    c. Lorazepam, oxazepam, temazepam
    d. Lorazepam, clonazepam, triazolam
    e. Diazepam, clonazepam, lorazepam

12. A mother comes to pick up a new prescription for fluoxetine for her 10-year-old son who has been diagnosed with major depression and obsessive-compulsive disorder. Her son has never received an antidepressant. Along with medication counseling, what is the pharmacist required to provide? Select all that apply.

    a. Medication guide
    b. Package insert
    c. Brochure about depression
    d. List of educational websites for obsessive-compulsive disorder
    e. Depression Guideline

13. A patient brings in a new prescription for alprazolam today and asks if it will interact with any of his medications. He is currently taking phenytoin and carbamazepine for seizures, citalopram for depression, acetaminophen with codeine for low back pain and warfarin for a recent DVT. Which of the following is most likely to have a clinically significant pharmacokinetic drug-drug interaction with the new prescription?

    a. Citalopram
    b. Carbamazepine
    c. Codeine
    d. Phenytoin
    e. Warfarin

14. Which of the following benzodiazepines are available in orally disintegrating tablet formulation?

    a. Clonazepam
    b. Diazepam
    c. Oxazepam
    d. Lorazepam
    e. Alprazolam

15. PP is a 38-year-old man with panic disorder who needs treatment. He also has a history of substance abuse with opioids and alcohol. Which of the following treatments is most appropriate for PP?

    a. Alprazolam
    b. Diazepam
    c. Imipramine
    d. Phenelzine
    e. Sertraline

Please use the following case for Questions 16 and 17.

A 32-year-old pregnant woman in her first trimester presents with worsening of her obsessive-compulsive symptoms. Due to the potential risk of her compulsive behaviors on her fetus, she has agreed to start pharmacologic treatment.

16. Which of the following agents should be avoided?

    a. Citalopram
    b. Fluoxetine
    c. Fluvoxamine
    d. Paroxetine
    e. Sertraline

17. She was previously prescribed clonazepam at the start of her pregnancy, but it was discontinued. Which of the following was the reason for this discontinuation?

    a. Cleft palate
    b. Heart defects
    c. Limb abnormalities
    d. Pulmonary hypertension
    e. Renal defects

18. Which of the following medications has the lowest risk of causing serotonin syndrome when combined with sertraline?

    a. Clonazepam
    b. Fluoxetine
    c. Desipramine
    d. Phenelzine
    e. Desvenlafaxine

19. The brand name for escitalopram is:

    a. Celexa
    b. Effexor
    c. Lexapro
    d. Paxil
    e. Zoloft

20. Place the following benzodiazepines in order of duration: alprazolam, oxazepam, triazolam, clonazepam. Start with the shortest duration and end with the longest duration.

    a. Alprazolam, oxazepam, triazolam, clonazepam
    b. Triazolam, alprazolam, oxazepam, clonazepam
    c. Clonazepam, triazolam, alprazolam, oxazepam
    d. Oxazepam, clonazepam, triazolam, alprazolam

21. CD is a 34-year-old man experiencing frequent flashbacks and nightmares of a very traumatic event that occurred a few years ago. He feels constantly "on edge" and easily startled. His primary care provider diagnosed CD with PTSD. Which of the following medications should be avoided?

    a. Clonazepam
    b. Sertraline
    c. Prazosin
    d. Citalopram

TAKEAWAY POINTS »

- Anxiety disorders are common psychiatric disorders and include panic disorder, generalized anxiety disorder, obsessive-compulsive disorder.
- SSRIs are first-line agents to treat anxiety disorders and can treat acute symptoms as well as prevent recurrent symptoms.
- SSRIs can be recommended during pregnancy if benefits outweigh the risks to the fetus; paroxetine should be avoided if possible.
- SNRIs such as venlafaxine and duloxetine are effective for selected anxiety disorders and are preferred over TCAs and benzodiazepines.

- TCAs are reserved as third- or fourth-line agents to treat anxiety disorders due to their tolerability and safety profiles.
- Benzodiazepines may be used as sole treatment or as adjunctive agents to treat anxiety disorders; however, caution should be used in high-risk populations such as patients with substance use problems, elderly patients, and patients who are pregnant.
- Buspirone is reserved for use in generalized anxiety disorder and does not have any risk for physical dependence or abuse.

BIBLIOGRAPHY

American Psychiatric Association. *Diagnostic and Statistical Manual of Mental Disorders: DSM-5*, 5th ed. Arlington: American Psychiatric Association, 2013.

Bandelow B, Sher L, Bunevicius R, et al. Guidelines for the pharmacological treatment of anxiety disorders, obsessive-compulsive disorder and post-traumatic stress disorder in primary care. *International Journal of Psychiatry in Clinical Practice.* 2012;16(2):77-84.

Koran LM, Hanna GL, Hollander E, Nestadt G, Simpson HB. Practice guideline for the treatment of patients with obsessive-compulsive disorder. *Am J Psychiatry.* 2007;164(7 Suppl):5-53.

Locke AB, Kirst N, Shultz CG. Diagnosis and management of generalized anxiety disorder and panic disorder in adults. *Am Fam Physician.* 2015;91(9):617-624.

Melton ST, Kirkwood CK. Anxiety disorders I: generalized anxiety, panic, and social anxiety disorders. In: DiPiro JT, Talbert RL, Yee GC, Matzke GR, Wells BG, Posey L, eds. *Pharmacotherapy: A Pathophysiologic Approach*, 10th ed. New York, NY: McGraw-Hill; 2016:chap 53.

Mihic S, Harris R. Hypnotics and sedatives. In: Brunton LL, Chabner BA, Knollmann BC, eds. *Goodman & Gilman's The Pharmacological Basis of Therapeutics*, 12th ed. New York, NY: McGraw-Hill; 2011:chap 17.

Trevor AJ, Way WL. Sedative-Hypnotic drugs. In: Katzung BG, Masters SB, Trevor AJ, eds. *Basic & Clinical Pharmacology*, 13th ed. New York, NY: McGraw-Hill; 2014:chap 22.

Ursano RJ, Bell C, Eth S, et al. Practice guideline for the treatment of patients with acute stress disorder and posttraumatic stress disorder. *Am J Psychiatry.* 2004;161(11 Suppl):3-31.

KEY ABBREVIATIONS

DSM-5 = Diagnostic and Statistical Manual of Mental Disorders, 5th Edition
GAD = generalized anxiety disorder
MAOIs = monoamine oxidase inhibitors
OCD = obsessive-compulsive disorder
PD = panic disorder

PPHN = persistent pulmonary hypertension
PTSD = post-traumatic stress disorder
SAD = social anxiety disorder
SNRIs = serotonin norepinephrine reuptake inhibitors
SSRIs = selective serotonin reuptake inhibitors
TCAs = tricyclic antidepressants

58

Bipolar Disorders

Susie H. Park

FOUNDATION OVERVIEW

Bipolar disorder is a recurrent psychiatric illness characterized by recurring episodes of mania and depression. Individuals diagnosed with bipolar disorder display extreme shifts in mood, energy level, thinking, and activities of daily living. Patients require lifelong treatment to control symptoms.

Pathophysiology

The cause of bipolar disorder is unknown; however, evidence exists that indicates a chemical imbalance with neurotransmitters is involved. Excess norepinephrine and dopamine may be present in mania, whereas a deficiency of serotonin, norepinephrine, and dopamine may be present in depression. Medications used to manage the symptoms of bipolar disorder alter the transmission of serotonin, dopamine, norepinephrine, as well as gamma-aminobutyric acid (GABA), glutamate, and aspartate. Additionally, family studies provide evidence for a genetic association of developing bipolar disorder.

Clinical Presentation and Diagnosis

Discrete types of mood episodes are classified as manic, hypomanic, depressive, or mixed type. Mania is the hallmark of bipolar disorder. The signs and symptoms of *mania* include an elated, euphoric, expansive, or irritable mood; increased self-esteem or grandiosity; a decreased need for sleep; talkative or pressured speech; racing thoughts or flight of ideas; distractibility; increased goal-directed activities; and psychomotor agitation. The patient may also report an increase in risk-taking behaviors or excessive involvement in pleasurable activities (eg, sexual promiscuity, unrestrained buying sprees). Three or more of these symptoms must be present in a patient if his/her mood is euphoric or expansive; four or more if the mood is irritable. These symptoms must last at least 1 week or any duration, if hospitalization was required. Psychosis may accompany a manic episode. *Hypomania* is a less severe form of mania, lasting at least four consecutive days and not requiring hospitalization. Patients state that they are more creative, feel more important, become extremely productive and that they do not need medical treatment. If a *depressive* episode alternates with the manic episodes, the patient is classified as having bipolar depression (as opposed to unipolar depression, otherwise known as major depressive disorder (MDD);

see Chapter "Depression"). An example of the episodic course of bipolar disorder includes one manic episode followed by three depressive episodes over several years, with or without a return to mania. Another example may include an initial depressive episode lasting a few months followed by a manic episode, then a return to a depressive episode several months to years later. *Mixed* (or dysphoric) type includes episodes of both mania and major depression occurring at the same time for at least 1 week. Agitation, psychosis, and suicidality are symptoms associated with mixed episodes. Rapid cycling is a term to describe when a patient experiences four or more episodes of depression or mania within a 12-month period.

There are different types of bipolar disorder diagnoses. *Bipolar I disorder* includes manic or mixed episodes usually accompanied by major depressive episodes. *Bipolar II disorder* includes major depressive episodes in addition to hypomanic episodes. *Cyclothymic disorder* involves recurring hypomania with additional depressive symptoms that recur for a minimum of 2 years. *Substance/medication-induced bipolar disorder* and *bipolar disorder due to another medical condition* are associated with manic-like phenomena.

TREATMENT

The goal of treating an acute manic episode is to control agitation, reduce risk of self-harm or harm to others, and an eventual return to normal functioning. This may require sedation and sleep-induction, especially if the patient has not slept for several days. A mood stabilizer (eg, lithium or divalproex sodium) with or without an antipsychotic or benzodiazepine is used for the treatment of *acute* manic episodes. Benzodiazepines (eg, clonazepam or lorazepam) can be used as an adjunctive treatment to promote sleep in agitated and overactive patients. The goal of *maintenance* treatment is to prevent or minimize future episodes, prevent rehospitalizations, and maximize the patient's functioning ability and quality of life. Maintenance treatment options include lithium, divalproex sodium, carbamazepine (CBZ), or lamotrigine with or without atypical antipsychotics (AAPs) and antidepressants. Table 58-1 lists the medications used for treating bipolar disorder. Multiple medication combinations may be used at one time to manage the symptoms. In the case of treating bipolar depression, the goal is to relieve the depression without

TABLE 58-1 Medications Used for the Treatment of Bipolar Disorder

Agent	Dosage Forms and Strengths	Brand Name	Daily Dosing Range (mg)	Comments

Lithium carbonate	150 mg, 600 mg capsules
	300 mg tablets
	300 mg capsules
	450 mg ER tablets
	300 mg ER tablets
		Eskalith
		Eskalith CR
		Lithobid slow-release
			600-2400	Therapeutic range:
				  Acute: 0.5-1.2 mEq/L
				  Maintenance: 0.6-0.8 mEq/L

Lithium citrate	300 mg/5 mL oral solution	Cibalith-S		
Valproic acid	250 mg capsules 250 mg/5 mL	Depakene	750-3500	Therapeutic range: 50-125 mcg/mL Loading dose in acute manic or mixed episodes: 20-30 mg/kg/d
Divalproex sodium	125, 250, 500 mg tabs	Depakote		
Divalproex sodium ER	250, 500 mg tablets	Depakote ER		
Carbamazepine[a]	100 mg chewable tablets 200 mg tablets 100 mg/5 mL oral suspension 100, 200, 400 mg ER tablets 100, 200, 300 mg ER caps	Tegretol Tegretol XR Equetro	200-1600	Therapeutic range: 4-12 mcg/mL to avoid toxicity
Oxcarbazepine	150, 300, 600 mg tablets 300 mg/5 mL oral suspension	Trileptal	600-2400	Not FDA-approved for BPD
Lamotrigine	25, 100, 150, 200 mg tablets 25, 50, 100, 200 mg ODT 2, 5, 25 mg chewable dispersible tablets	Lamictal Lamictal ODT	100-400	Indicated for maintenance treatment of BDI Dosing is based on concomitant medications
Lamotrigine XR	25, 50, 100, 200, 250, 300 mg tablets	Lamictal XR		Not FDA-approved for BPD
Olanzapine/fluoxetine combination	3/25, 6/25, 6/50, 12/25, 12/50 mg capsules	Symbyax	6/25-12/50	Bipolar depression
Quetiapine	25, 50, 100, 200, 300, 400 mg tablets	Seroquel	200-800	Bipolar depression Acute mania Maintenance
Quetiapine XR	50, 150, 200, 300, 400 mg ER tablets	Seroquel XR		
Olanzapine[b]	2.5, 5, 7.5, 10, 15, 20 mg tablets 5, 10, 15, 20 mg ODT	Zyprexa Zydis	5-20	Acute mania Maintenance
Aripiprazole[b]	2, 5, 10, 15, 20, 30 mg tablets 1 mg/mL oral solution 10, 15 mg ODT	Abilify Discmelt	10-30	Acute mania Maintenance
Risperidone long-acting injection	12.5, 25, 37.5, 50 mg vial kits for IM injection	Consta	25-50	Maintenance
Risperidone	0.25, 0.5, 1, 2, 3, 4 mg tablets 1 mg/mL oral solution 0.5, 1, 2, 3, 4 mg ODT	Risperdal M-Tab	2-6	Acute mania
Ziprasidone	20, 40, 60, 80 mg caps	Geodon	40-160	Acute mania Maintenance
Asenapine	5, 10 mg sublingual tablets	Saphris	10-20	Acute mania
Paliperidone Paliperidone long-acting injection Lurasidone Cariprazine	1.5, 3, 6, 9 mg tabs 39, 78, 117, 156, 234 mg IM injection 20, 40, 60, 80, 120 mg caps 1.5, 3, 4.5, 6 mg caps	Invega Sustenna Latuda Vraylar	3-12 78-234 20-120 3-6	Acute treatment of schizoaffective disorder Schizoaffective disorder Bipolar depression Acute mania

Abbreviations: BPD, bipolar disorder; BDI, bipolar I disorder; ER & XR, extended-release; IM, intramuscular; ODT, orally disintegrating tablet (to be placed on top of the tongue with dry hands).

[a]Other brand name products of carbamazepine include Carbatrol and Epitol. Equetro is the only FDA-approved brand for BPD treatment.

[b]Olanzapine and aripiprazole are available in IM formulations FDA-approved for acute agitation associated with bipolar I mania in adults.

inducing a manic episode. This requires treatment with an antidepressant and a concomitant mood stabilizer or antipsychotic. Antidepressants should not be used as monotherapy, even when treating the depressive episode in bipolar disorder due to their ability to precipitate mania.

Lithium

Lithium is an effective antimanic medication used for initial treatment in acute manic, mixed episodes and maintenance treatment. It is an alternative to lamotrigine for bipolar depressive episodes. Lithium has a therapeutic advantage of decreasing suicidality in bipolar patients; however, it has a slow onset of action, which may limit its use in acute manic episodes. Lithium is a cation eliminated through the kidneys and exhibits a narrow therapeutic/safety effect. Serum concentration monitoring is required (0.5-1.2 mEq/L for acute manic treatment; 0.6-0.8 mEq/L for maintenance treatment). Lithium serum concentrations more than 1.5 mEq/L can lead to lithium toxicity. Lithium toxicity may manifest as coarse hand tremor, persistent diarrhea, uncoordinated motor movements (ataxia), slurred speech, and confusion. Levels more than 2.5 mEq/L may result in renal failure, seizure, and coma. Table 58-2 lists required monitoring and Table 58-3 lists key

drug interactions for lithium. The recommended starting dose is 300 mg three times per day or less, depending on patient's age and weight (maximum dose 2400 mg/d). Select adverse effects of lithium include nausea, vomiting, diarrhea, hand tremor, polyuria, polydipsia, sedation, weight gain, acne, and hypothyroidism. Patients should be counseled to maintain adequate water intake (dehydration increases lithium concentrations) and consistent sodium intake (low sodium can increase lithium). Patients should also be made aware that large amounts of caffeine can decrease lithium concentrations via increased diuresis. Lithium should not be used in renal failure or pregnant women in their first trimester. Lithium is a known teratogen and has been associated with causing Ebstein anomaly, a cardiac abnormality.

Valproic Acid/Divalproex Sodium

Valproate (divalproex sodium, Depakote or Depakote ER and valproic acid, Depakene; VPA) is an option for initial management of acute manic episodes. Valproate has two advantages compared to lithium: (1) a wider safety margin (therapeutic range of VPA is 50-125 mcg/mL) and (2) a faster onset of action. Valproate is the preferred agent for mixed episodes of bipolar disorder. The recommended starting dose is 250 mg

TABLE 58-2	Lithium Monitoring
Baseline Laboratory/ Ongoing Monitoring	**Explanation**
SCr, BUN	Renal excretion of lithium
Urine-specific gravity	Polyuria caused by lithium Lithium decreases the kidney's ability to concentrate the urine
Electrolytes	Hyponatremia and dehydration can lead to ↑ renal reabsorption of lithium; ↑ lithium levels; lithium toxicity Hypokalemia may ↑ the risk of lithium-induced cardiac toxicity
CBC with differential	Lithium can ↑ WBC (except basophils) Lithium can ↑ platelets
TSH; T$_4$	Hyperthyroidism can mimic mania Lithium can induce hypothyroidism with long-term treatment
ECG (in patients with cardiovascular disease risk; age >40)	Lithium can worsen cardiac disease Lithium can cause cardiac conduction abnormalities
Weight	Lithium causes weight gain
Pregnancy test	Lithium is pregnancy category D Lithium can cause teratogenicity: Ebstein anomaly
Lithium levels	Lithium is a narrow-therapeutic index drug; avoid toxicity Levels assist in determining therapeutic response

Abbreviations: BUN, blood urea nitrogen; CBC, complete blood count; ECG, electrocardiography; SCr, serum creatinine; TSH, thyroid-stimulating hormone; WBC, white blood cell.

TABLE 58-3	Lithium Drug Interactions
Drugs That Increase (↑) Lithium	
ACE inhibitors result in volume depletion and a reduction in glomerular filtration rate → reduced Li$^+$ excretion → increased Li$^+$ levels	
▪ Reports exist of ARBs (eg, losartan) also increasing Li$^+$	
Diuretics, especially thiazide diuretics cause the greatest ↑ in Li$^+$; all diuretics can cause sodium depletion → Na$^+$ depletion causes an ↑ in proximal tubular reabsorption of both Na$^+$ and Li$^+$	
▪ Loop diuretics and potassium-sparing diuretics appear less interacting	
NSAIDs can increase Li$^+$ by up to 50%; most likely due to enhanced reabsorption of sodium and lithium secondary to inhibition of prostaglandin synthesis	
▪ Not likely to occur with aspirin or sulindac (Clinoril)	
Drugs That Decrease (↓) Lithium	
Acetazolamide may impair the proximal tubular reabsorption of Li$^+$	
Sodium promotes the renal clearance of lithium	
Theophylline and *caffeine* will ↑ the renal clearance of lithium and can ↓ Li$^+$ by 20%	
Drugs That Increase Lithium Toxicity	
Carbamazepine can cause an increase in neurotoxicity	
▪ No change in lithium levels	
Calcium channel blockers cause an increase in neurotoxicity; mostly caused by nondihydropyridine CCBs (eg, diltiazem, verapamil)	
▪ No change in lithium levels	
Methyldopa may increase neurotoxicity	
Phenytoin may increase neurotoxicity	

Abbreviations: ACE, angiotensin-converting enzyme; ARB, angiotensin II receptor blocker; CCB, calcium channel blockers; NSAID, nonsteroidal anti-inflammatory drugs.

three times a day with a maximum daily dose of 60 mg/kg. During an acute episode, VPA can be given in divided doses as a loading dose of 20 to 30 mg/kg. The following baseline laboratory monitoring tests should be performed: complete blood count (CBC) with differential including platelets, liver function tests, and a pregnancy test in women of childbearing age. Adverse effects include nausea, vomiting, dyspepsia, sedation, tremor, alopecia, weight gain, elevated liver enzymes, and thrombocytopenia. VPA has also been associated with causing polycystic ovary syndrome (PCOS) in women, hyperammonemia, and pancreatitis. Patients should be counseled to take VPA with food to minimize adverse gastrointestinal effects. Patients may take selenium and zinc to treat hair loss; however, the dose of VPA and these supplements should be separated by at least 4 hours. VPA is involved in multiple cytochrome P450 isoenzyme 2C9 drug-drug interactions, and it is also highly protein bound. VPA is a known teratogen and may significantly increase the risk of causing spina bifida. If the mother uses VPA or any other anticonvulsants during pregnancy, she should be counseled to take a folic acid supplement.

Carbamazepine

CBZ (Tegretol, Equetro) is effective in manic, mixed episodes (Food and Drug Administration [FDA]-approved indication), and maintenance treatment of bipolar disorder. CBZ may be used as an alternative agent when lithium, VPA, or AAPs fail. The recommended starting dose is 200 mg twice daily, up to 1600 mg/d if needed. CBZ is a cytochrome P450 enzyme inducer, potentially lowering the blood concentrations of concomitantly administered P450 substrates, such as oral contraceptives. Other select P450 3A4 substrates include haloperidol, midazolam, valproate, and warfarin. Dosage adjustments would be required of these agents when used with CBZ. Also an autoinducer, CBZ induces its own metabolism. Blood concentration monitoring is required of CBZ. Therapeutic levels are 4 to 12 mcg/mL, and levels more than 12 mcg/mL are associated with toxicity. CBZ may cause Stevens-Johnson syndrome (SJS) or toxic epidermal necrolysis (TEN), two potentially fatal dermatologic reactions. The allelic variation of the human leukocyte antigen type B (HLA-B) gene (HLA-B*1502) has been linked to these dermatologic reactions. Testing positive for HLA-A*3101 may also be associated with dermatologic reactions. Genotyping susceptible patients is advised prior to starting CBZ. Adverse effects of CBZ include sedation, dizziness, weight gain, nausea, diplopia, elevated liver enzymes, and hyponatremia. Additionally, rare adverse effects are agranulocytosis and aplastic anemia. Like VPA, CBZ is also associated with causing spina bifida if the fetus is exposed.

Lamotrigine

Lamotrigine (Lamictal) is FDA-approved for maintenance treatment of bipolar I disorder and may be used as an alternative to lithium for bipolar depressive episodes. Lamotrigine is an effective treatment for bipolar depressive episodes but is not effective for treating manic episodes. Treatment of acute manic or mixed episodes is not recommended with lamotrigine. The starting dose of lamotrigine is dependent upon concomitant medications. For patients taking lamotrigine alone, the initial dose is 25 mg/d for weeks 1 to 2, followed by 50 mg/d for weeks 3 to 4, 100 mg/d for week 5, and then is increased to 200 mg/d beginning week 6. If lamotrigine is taken with valproate, the starting dose is 25 mg every *other* day with a target dose of 100 mg at week 6. If lamotrigine is taken with CBZ, an enzyme inducer, start 50 mg/d with a target dose of 300 mg/d by week 6; may be up to 400 mg/d. Higher doses are usually given twice daily and titrated slowly in order to avoid potentially life-threatening *rashes*. Factors that may increase the risk of rash include coadministration with valproate, exceeding recommended initial doses of lamotrigine, or accelerating the recommended dose escalation schedule. It is also recommended that lamotrigine be discontinued at the first sign of rash, unless the rash does not appear to be drug-related. Other adverse drug reactions of lamotrigine include headache, dizziness, sedation, blurred vision, and gastrointestinal distress. Women taking an estrogen-containing oral contraceptive may need increased doses of lamotrigine by as much as twofold in order to maintain a consistent lamotrigine plasma level.

Other Anticonvulsants

Oxcarbazepine (Trileptal), topiramate (Topamax), gabapentin (Neurontin), phenytoin (Dilantin), zonisamide (Zonegran), and levetiracetam (Keppra) have been studied for use in bipolar disorders with mixed evidence of efficacy and safety. These agents are not standard treatments and are not FDA-approved for treatment of bipolar disorders. They may be used as adjunctive treatment or for refractory cases.

Atypical Antipsychotics

The role of AAPs (second-generation antipsychotics) in the treatment of bipolar disorder is growing. These agents are indicated as monotherapy or adjunct therapy with lithium or divalproex. Olanzapine (Zyprexa), aripiprazole (Abilify), quetiapine (Seroquel), quetiapine XR (Seroquel XR for once-daily dosing), ziprasidone (Geodon), and asenapine (Saphris) are AAP agents FDA-approved for the treatment of acute manic or mixed episodes, as well as for maintenance treatment in bipolar I disorder. Risperidone (Risperdal) and cariprazine (Vraylar) are approved for the treatment of acute manic or mixed episodes. Quetiapine, quetiapine XR, and lurasidone (Latuda) are approved for bipolar depression, specifically. When AAPs are used during the depressive phase, the doses are lower than those used for mania. The olanzapine plus fluoxetine combination (OFC) product (Symbyax) is also indicated for bipolar depression. Risperidone long-acting injection (LAI; Consta) is approved for maintenance treatment of bipolar I disorder. This agent is administered intramuscularly (IM) every 2 weeks. Oral risperidone (or other oral antipsychotic) should be given with the first IM injection for the first 3 weeks in order to ensure an adequate therapeutic plasma concentration, tolerability, and safety. Paliperidone (Invega), the active metabolite of risperidone, is indicated for the acute treatment of schizoaffective disorder, as is the LAI formulation, paliperidone palmitate extended-release injectable (Invega Sustenna). This preparation is administered every 4 weeks and does not require concomitant oral paliperidone. The presence of psychosis (eg, hallucinations, delusions) accompanying the manic or depressive episode warrants the use of an antipsychotic medication until the mood episode is well-controlled. In schizoaffective disorder, however, the antipsychotic may be used as long as the psychotic symptoms persist concurrent to the depressive, manic, or mixed episode. A major limitation to the use of AAPs is the metabolic side effects associated with their long-term use, including weight gain, dyslipidemia, and glucose intolerance, which require regular monitoring during treatment.

Antidepressants

Antidepressants are used to treat the depressive episode in bipolar disorder; however, they should be used in combination treatment with a mood stabilizer. If used as monotherapy, antidepressants can precipitate a manic episode. Selective serotonin reuptake inhibitors (SSRIs) such as fluoxetine (Prozac), paroxetine (Paxil), and sertraline (Zoloft) and the dopamine/norepinephrine reuptake inhibitor, bupropion (Wellbutrin) are less likely to cause a conversion into mania compared to tricyclic antidepressants (TCAs). Other SSRIs safe to use are citalopram (Celexa) and escitalopram (Lexapro).

Other Treatments for Bipolar Disorder

Calcium channel blockers, such as verapamil, have been used for treating bipolar mania. Unfortunately, results are conflicting regarding the efficacy of this class of agents. Additionally, research has demonstrated positive outcomes utilizing omega-3 fatty acids for the treatment of bipolar disorder.

Special Populations

Bipolar disorder is challenging to treat during pregnancy. Lithium, VPA, and CBZ when used during pregnancy are associated with causing fetal harm and are, therefore, often avoided. Typical, high-potency antipsychotics, such as haloperidol, have been used to manage acute mania. Patients taking lithium or an anticonvulsant may switch to a first-generation antipsychotic either for the first trimester or the entire pregnancy. Growing evidence exists for the use of atypical, second-generation antipsychotics during pregnancy. Electroconvulsive therapy (ECT) is also effective and safe in managing bipolar disorder in pregnancy.

CASE Application

1. Which of the following are signs and symptoms of a manic episode? Select all that apply.

   a. Irritable mood
   b. Anhedonia
   c. Racing thoughts
   d. Psychomotor agitation
   e. Decreased need for sleep

2. VV is a patient who was recently diagnosed with bipolar disorder before being discharged for a related hospitalization. VV reports a positive family history of mood disorders but denies hospitalizations of any family members. You explain to VV that it is possible that the family members were never hospitalized due to prominent symptoms of hypomania, characterized by which of the following?

   a. Multiple hospitalizations
   b. Psychotic episodes
   c. Impairment in social functioning
   d. Impairment in occupational functioning
   e. An inflated self-esteem

3. The treatment team asks you, the clinical pharmacist, for a consult on a patient with bipolar disorder. There is a question regarding whether or not the patient meets criteria for rapid cycling. You explain to the team that there needs to be a confirmed history of ____ or more manic or depressive episodes within a _____ time period.

   a. 2; 6-month
   b. 2; 1-year
   c. 3; 2-year
   d. 4; 1-year
   e. 4; 2-year

4. Patient LC requires treatment for bipolar disorder, and is currently in a depressive episode. The patient has a history of predominantly depressive episodes in the last 3 years. The patient refuses to take more than one medication at a time for management of symptoms and relapse prevention. Which medication will you recommend for LC, confident that it can be used as monotherapy for managing the associated symptoms? Select all that apply.

   a. Lithium
   b. Lamotrigine
   c. Olanzapine
   d. Quetiapine
   e. Citalopram

5. JA is being transitioned from olanzapine to lithium for the management of bipolar disorder. You have been asked to provide a counseling session on medication adverse drug reactions after JA inquired about common and expected adverse drug reactions of lithium. Select the counseling point that should be discussed.

   a. Alopecia
   b. Increased urination
   c. Hyperammonemia
   d. Hyperthyroidism
   e. Diplopia

6. You are asked to start a 24-year-old patient on lithium for the maintenance treatment of bipolar disorder. The patient's renal function is within normal limits and body mass index (BMI) is 22. What is the starting dose and

frequency of lithium that you will recommend for this patient?

a. 300 mg tid
b. 15 mg qhs
c. 200 mg bid
d. 500 mg bid
e. 50 mg every day

7. Which of the following is the teratogenicity associated with lithium use in the first trimester of pregnancy?

a. Cardiovascular
b. Renal
c. Hepatic
d. Neuromuscular
e. Dermatological

8. Which of the following are appropriate counseling points to mention to a patient starting lithium? Select all that apply.

a. "You should avoid dehydration, so maintain your water intake."
b. "Stop your medication if you experience persistent diarrhea."
c. "Use caution while operating machinery or driving a car."
d. "Ask your pharmacist before starting any new pain medications."
e. "You should reduce your sodium intake while taking lithium."

9. A patient has been taking lithium for 3 years and has been stable on it without relapse of symptoms. There has been no change in renal function or other laboratory monitoring parameters. The patient is also being monitored by another health care professional. Together, you both agree that the patient's target therapeutic concentration should be which of the following ranges?

a. 4 to 12 mcg/mL
b. 4 to 12 mEq/L
c. 50 to 125 mcg/mL
d. 0.6 to 0.8 mEq/L
e. 1 to 1.8 mEq/L

10. Your 39-year-old patient with bipolar disorder is on several medications, reporting the following during your clinic visit:
Aleve (naproxen sodium) 1 tablet twice daily for back pain when working, Motrin (ibuprofen) 400 mg 1 tablet every 8 hours as need for headache occurring three times per month, Cozaar (losartan) 50 mg 1 tablet bid, Glucophage (metformin) 850 mg 1 tablet bid. The patient smokes six to seven cigarettes per day, drinks alcohol occasionally, and has five large cups of coffee every morning except Fridays and Saturdays.

Which of the following factors can affect the level of lithium when blood is drawn at the next clinic visit? Select all that apply.

a. Aleve
b. Cozaar

c. Glucophage
d. Smoking
e. Coffee

11. The physician wants to know what extended-release preparations of lithium are available, if any. You advise that a prescription be written for which of the following?

a. Lithium citrate
b. Lithium carbonate tablets
c. Lithium carbonate capsules
d. Eskalith
e. Lithobid

12. A patient on the psychiatry ward is being considered for lithium treatment. You recommend which of the following laboratory parameters be checked prior to starting treatment? Select all that apply.

a. Serum creatinine (SCr)
b. Electrocardiogram (ECG)
c. Thyroid function tests
d. Liver enzyme tests
e. Electrolytes

13. PCOS has been associated with which of the following medications? Select all that apply.

a. Cariprazine
b. Divalproex sodium
c. Lithium
d. Lamotrigine
e. Olanzapine

14. A patient was just admitted into the psychiatry emergency department for an acute manic episode presenting with a flight of ideas and hypersexuality toward staff, reporting "I am the best lover you will ever have in your entire life- that's what all of my partners say, and there are lots of them!" The patient is accompanied by a family member who reports a past medication history of divalproex sodium. What recommended loading dose (in kg/d) do you recommend for this individual?

a. 5 mg
b. 10 to 15 mg
c. 20 to 30 mg
d. 40 mg
e. 50 to 55 mg

15. A patient with bipolar disorder is concerned about using certain medications for her psychiatric condition. She heard that some medications are associated with causing a neural tube defect if taken during pregnancy. You confirm her suspicion and tell her that some agents are associated with causing this condition in the newborn when used by the mother during pregnancy. You proceed to counsel her about which of the following agent? Select all that apply.

a. Lithium
b. Divalproex sodium
c. CBZ

d. Paliperidone

e. Risperidone

16. It is recommended that the human leukocyte antigen type B, *HLA-B*1502*, allele is genotyped in Asian patients prior to taking which of the following medications? Select all that apply.

    a. Lithium

    b. CBZ

    c. Lorazepam

    d. Haloperidol

    e. Quetiapine

17. You discover that a bipolar patient in the hospital ward has been "cheeking" medication for the past 4 days. You decide to recommend the same medication in an orally disintegrating tablet (ODT) formulation. Which of the following medications is available in an ODT dosage form?

    a. CBZ

    b. Haloperidol

    c. Lithium

    d. Quetiapine

    e. Risperidone

18. Which of the following factors is likely to increase the risk of lamotrigine-related rash? Select all that apply.

    a. Coadministration with another anticonvulsant, valproate

    b. Coadministration with another anticonvulsant, CBZ

    c. Exceeding the recommended initial dose of lamotrigine

    d. Exceeding the recommended maximum dose of lamotrigine

    e. Exceeding the recommended dose escalation schedule of lamotrigine

19. The psychiatric treatment team decides to start Risperdal Consta on a patient who has a history of nonadherence to the current mood stabilizer for bipolar disorder in the past 6 years. They ask you, the clinical pharmacist, for the recommended starting dose and directions for administration. You reply with the following:

    a. 2 mg tablet, 1 tab po bid

    b. 3 mg ODT, 1 tab on top of the tongue everyday

    c. 25 mg subcutaneously (SQ) every 2 weeks

    d. 25 mg IM every 2 weeks

    e. 50 mg IM every 2 weeks

20. Which agent is considered the safest option for treating a pregnant female with acute bipolar mania?

    a. CBZ

    b. Chlorpromazine

    c. Haloperidol

    d. Lithium

    e. VPA

21. Symbyax is a combination product with several therapeutic indications. This product contains fixed doses of which of the following agents for treating bipolar depression?

    a. Lithium + divalproex sodium

    b. Risperidone + fluoxetine

    c. Olanzapine + fluoxetine

    d. Risperidone + sertraline

    e. Lurasidone + sertraline

22. Which antidepressant is most likely to cause a switch into mania when used in a patient with bipolar disorder?

    a. Amitriptyline

    b. Bupropion

    c. Citalopram

    d. Escitalopram

    e. Sertraline

23. Which of the following medication classes can be used for a patient with bipolar disorder, even if some of them are used off-label? Select all that apply.

    a. ACE-Inhibitors

    b. Anticonvulsants

    c. Antidepressants

    d. Antipsychotics

    e. Calcium channel blockers

24. You are providing a literature review grand rounds presentation of pharmacological treatments for bipolar disorder management. Which agent will you describe as effective for the treatment of bipolar I disorder and possibly more effective than lithium for bipolar depression?

    a. Dilantin

    b. Lamictal

    c. Lamisil

    d. Neurontin

    e. Trileptal

25. You are the pharmacist on a Pharmacy and Therapeutic committee at your hospital. The committee has asked you to present on alternatives to lithium and lamotrigine for managing bipolar depression in patients with bipolar disorder. Which of the following agents will you present data on, based on their FDA-approved indication for this therapeutic use? Select all that apply.

    a. Asenapine

    b. Iloperidone

    c. Lurasidone

    d. Paliperidone

    e. Quetiapine

26. Which of the following counseling points will you provide to a patient who is taking asenapine for managing a manic episode in bipolar disorder? Select all that apply.

    a. "Use this medication as directed, once daily at bedtime."

b. "Inject all of the contents from the syringe to ensure the full dose."

c. "Carefully and gently remove the tablet from its original package."

d. "Do not eat or drink for 10 minutes after taking the dose."

e. "Place tablet under tongue and allow it to dissolve completely."

27. You receive a prescription for cariprazine 1.5 mg po qd. You ask your pharmacy technician to fill which of the following products?

a. Carbatrol

b. Equetro

c. Sinemet

d. Tegretol

e. Vraylar

TAKEAWAY POINTS »

- The clinical presentation of bipolar disorder includes mania, hypomania, mixed (or dysphoric) mania, major depression, and rapid cycling.
- Mood stabilizers such as lithium and divalproex sodium (valproate) are used as monotherapy or in combination treatment for treating bipolar disorder.
- AAPs (monotherapy or in combination with mood stabilizers) are used in the treatment of bipolar disorders.
- Antidepressant *monotherapy* should be avoided during bipolar disorder treatment.

- Lithium has a narrow therapeutic window and requires careful monitoring during treatment.
- Lithium is implicated in numerous drug-drug interactions.
- Lamotrigine is effective for treating bipolar depression but not for acute manic episodes.
- Lithium, valproate, and CBZ should be avoided during the first trimester of pregnancy.
- Treatment adherence is important in preventing relapse, suicidal behavior, and rehospitalization.

BIBLIOGRAPHY

Drayton SJ, Pelic CM. Bipolar disorder. In: DiPiro JT, Talbert RL, Yee GC, Matzke GR, Wells BG, Posey L, eds. *Pharmacotherapy: A Pathophysiologic Approach.* 9th ed. New York, NY: McGraw-Hill; 2014:chap 52.

Goodwin GM, Haddad PM, Ferrier IN, et al. Evidence-based guidelines for treating bipolar disorder: Revised third edition recommendations from the British Association for Psychopharmacology. *J Psychopharmacol.* 2016;30(6):495-553.

Hirschfeld RMA, Bowden CL, Gitlin MJ, et al. Practice guideline for the treatment of patient with bipolar disorder (revision). *Am J Psychiatry.* 2002;159:1-50.

Meltzer H. Antipsychotic agents & lithium. In: Katzung BG, Masters SB, Trevor AJ, eds. *Basic & Clinical Pharmacology.* 12th ed. New York, NY: McGraw-Hill; 2012:chap 29.

Meyer JM. Pharmacotherapy of psychosis and mania. In: Brunton LL, Chabner BA, Knollmann BC, eds. *Goodman & Gilman's The Pharmacological Basis of Therapeutics.* 12th ed. New York, NY: McGraw-Hill; 2011:chap 16.

Yatham LN, Kennedy SH, Parikh SV, et al. Canadian Network for Mood and Anxiety Treatments (CANMAT) and International Society for Bipolar Disorders (ISBD) collaborative update of CANMAT guidelines for the management of patients with bipolar disorder: update 2013. *Bipolar Disord.* 2013;15(1):1-44.

KEY ABBREVIATIONS

AAP = atypical antipsychotic
BMI = body mass index
BUN = blood urea nitrogen
CBC = complete blood count
CBZ = carbamazepine
CNS = central nervous system
ECT = electroconvulsive therapy
FDA = Food and Drug Administration
GABA = gamma-aminobutyric acid
HLA-B = human leukocyte antigen type B

LAI = long-acting injection
MDD = major depressive disorder
NSAIDs = Nonsteroidal anti-inflammatory drugs
ODT = orally disintegrating tablet
OFC = olanzapine plus fluoxetine combination
PCOS = polycystic ovary syndrome
SJS = Stevens-Johnson syndrome
SSRI = selective serotonin reuptake inhibitor
TEN = toxic epidermal necrolysis
VPA = valproate

59

Post-Traumatic Stress Disorder

Joshua Caballero and Jennifer E. Thomas

FOUNDATION OVERVIEW

Post-traumatic stress disorder (PTSD) has traditionally been classified as an anxiety disorder; however, it is now considered a trauma- and stressor-related disorder under the latest diagnostic criteria. PTSD develops as a result of emotional or psychological trauma, or physical harm (eg, unwanted sexual act, physical injury). PTSD may also develop after experiencing a life-threatening event such as a war or hurricane, or learning about a traumatic event that occurred to a close family member or friend.

Risk Factors

Intense or repeated traumatic events increase the risk of PTSD. Genetic factors may predispose a person's susceptibility to experience an episode. Neurobiologic changes, such as decreased hippocampus size, hypocortisolism, or a hyperactive amygdala, increase the risk. Additionally, preexisting mental disorders (eg, depression, anxiety), poor socioeconomic or educational status, and substance use disorders enhance the risk of developing PTSD.

Pathophysiology

The development of PTSD may be due to a dysregulation of the hypothalamus-pituitary-adrenal (HPA) axis. The HPA axis is responsible for regulating responses to stress. Dysregulation of the HPA axis causes elevated glucocorticoid negative feedback sensitivity of the HPA axis which results in hypocortisolism. Since cortisol is a glucocorticoid that reduces stress, below normal concentrations cause an elevated stress response.

Several neurotransmitters play a role in the pathophysiology of PTSD. The two most common neurotransmitters are serotonin (5-HT) and norepinephrine (NE). Gamma aminobutyric acid (GABA) and dopamine (DA) may indirectly play a role as well. The primary neurotransmitters (ie, 5-HT, NE) are implicated in PTSD in the following way:

1. Serotonin affects sleep, motor function, impulsivity, and aggression. Patients with PTSD have decreased 5-HT concentrations and neurotransmission which may result in insomnia, abnormal motor function, and aggressive behavior.
2. NE may be involved in regulating fear, arousal, emotional memories, and vigilance. Alpha receptors are

autoreceptors which inhibit NE release. Therefore, PTSD downregulation of α_2 receptors results in increased NE concentrations and overactivity in the noradrenergic system.

Clinical Presentation

PTSD typically occurs within 3 months after a traumatic event, but may be deferred until month 6 or beyond. After the initial onset, patients experience four core symptom clusters. The four clusters include: (1) symptoms of intrusion related to the traumatic event, (2) avoidance, (3) negative changes in cognitions and emotions in relation to the event, and (4) hyperarousal symptoms. Patients with PTSD may suffer from sleep disturbances such as insomnia. Additionally, patients may present with general psychiatric distress, poor physical health, and social dysfunction.

Diagnosis

According to the Diagnostic and Statistical Manual of Mental Disorders, Fifth Edition (DSM-5) criteria, a patient with a diagnosis of PTSD must have all of the following symptoms lasting for more than or equal to 1 month:

1. Exposure to traumatic event
2. Occurrence of intrusive symptoms related to the traumatic event:
   - May appear as a recurrent memory, dream, thought, or feeling
   - May involve dissociative reactions in which the individual feels as if they are re-experiencing the traumatic event
3. Persistence of one or more avoidance symptoms including:
   - Avoids activities linked to the trauma, such as thoughts, memories, or emotions
   - Avoids people, places, objects, situations, conversations and events that will stimulate thoughts of the trauma
4. Two or more negative changes in cognitions and emotions related to the traumatic event such as:
   - Inability to recall an important aspect of the trauma
   - Persistent and excessive negative feelings about oneself or others

TABLE 59-1	Pharmacologic Treatments for PTSD					
Drug (Brand)	FDA Approved[a]	Initial Dose (mg/d)	Dosage Range (mg/d)	Schedule[b]	Formulations[c]	Comments/Class Side Effects
SSRIs						
Citalopram (Celexa)	N	20	20-60	qd	S, T	SSRIs are first line
Escitalopram (Lexapro)	N	10	10-20	qd	S, T	Need 8-12 wk for improvement
Fluoxetine (Prozac)	N	10-20	10-80	qd	C, S, SY, T, EC	Sertraline and paroxetine are FDA approved for PTSD
Fluvoxamine (Luvox)	N	50	100-250	qd, bid	EC, T	
Paroxetine (Paxil)	Y	10-20	20-50	qd	ET, OS, T	Paroxetine is most sedating
Sertraline (Zoloft)	Y	25-50	50-200	qd	S, T	CYP-450 interactions with fluoxetine (3A4, 2D6), paroxetine (2D6), and fluvoxamine (2D6, 1A2, 2C19)
						Paroxetine is pregnancy category D. All other SSRIs are pregnancy category C
						Nausea/vomiting
						Sexual dysfunction
						Diarrhea/constipation
						Headaches
Other Agents						
Venlafaxine extended-release (Effexor XR)	N	37.5	37.5-225	qd, bid, tid	EC, ET, T	First/second line
						Increased blood pressure at high doses
						Nausea/vomiting
						Sexual dysfunction
Amitriptyline (Elavil)	N	25-50	50-300	qd, bid, tid	T	Third line due to intolerable adverse events
Imipramine (Tofranil)	N	25-50	50-300	qd, bid, tid	T, C	Anticholinergic symptoms (eg, constipation, blurred vision, dry mouth)
						Sedation
						Sexual dysfunction
Mirtazapine (Remeron)	N	15	15-45	qhs	D, T	Third line due to limited evidence and adverse events
						Increased appetite/weight gain
						Sedation
Phenelzine (Nardil)	N	15	15-90	tid, qid	T	Last line due to drug-food interactions and adverse events
						Avoid eating foods high in tyramine
						Orthostatic hypotension
						Sedation
						Edema, weight gain
						Sexual dysfunction
Prazosin (Minipress)	N	1	1-14	qd, bid, tid	C	Mostly used adjunctively
						Preferably for nightmares
						High doses may be necessary
						Orthostatic hypotension
						Angina, tachycardia

[a]N, No; Y, Yes.

[b]bid, twice daily; qd, daily; qid, four times daily; qhs, at bedtime; tid, three times daily.

[c]C, capsule; D, (oral tablet) disintegrating; EC, extended-release capsule; ET, extended-release tablet; OS, oral suspension; S, oral solution; SY, oral syrup; T, tablet.

- Poor emotional state
- Distorted beliefs about the traumatic event, in which the individual blames himself/herself or others
- Decreased interest in significant events
- Minimal feelings expressed toward people

5. Persistence of two or more hyperarousal symptoms including:
   - Exaggerated startle response
   - Irritability or anger
   - Hypervigilance
   - Difficulty falling or staying asleep
   - Difficulty concentrating
   - Self-destructive behavior

6. All symptoms cause distress and impair social or occupational functioning.

7. The symptoms are not caused by another medical condition or the use of a substance such as medication or alcohol.

PREVENTION

Cognitive behavioral therapy (CBT) may be utilized in the prevention and management of PTSD. This includes an emphasis on return to normalcy and normal daily routine with trauma focused anxiety management. Additionally, medications have been studied for the prevention of PTSD. One example includes the use of propranolol, administered within 3 months of trauma, given for a 10-day course to block memory consolidation. While the use of propranolol may be controversial, recent data have shown possible effectiveness (propranolol with CBT) in this population when administered soon after trauma.

TREATMENT

The primary short-term goal of PTSD treatment is reduction in symptom severity. The long-term goals emphasize quality of life improvement, including adaptive functioning improvement and overall remission, as well as preventing trauma-based comorbid conditions and relapse. The ultimate outcome of the various methods of intervention is to return the patient to the pretraumatic state. The goal for duration of treatment for PTSD is a minimum of 12 months. It is important to discuss idealistic treatment goals with the patient, since complete resolution of symptoms is very difficult to accomplish. Also, because of black box warnings regarding a possible increase in suicidality or worsening of symptoms, patients (especially 24 years old or younger) should be monitored (eg, early follow-up, phone communication) when beginning antidepressant therapy.

Nonpharmacologic Treatment

Nonpharmacologic treatment includes CBT, eye movement desensitization and reprocessing (EMDR), exposure desensitization, stress training, communication therapy, coping skills, and relaxation training. However, most of the published data support the use of CBT.

Pharmacologic Treatment

Antidepressants are the major pharmacotherapeutic treatment for PTSD. In addition to their efficacy in PTSD, these agents are also effective for concurrent depression and anxiety disorders. Selective serotonin reuptake inhibitors (SSRIs) and venlafaxine are the first-line pharmacotherapy of PTSD. The tricyclic antidepressants (TCAs) and monoamine oxidase inhibitors (MAOIs) can also be effective, but they have less favorable side-effect profiles. Both sertraline and paroxetine are approved for the acute treatment of PTSD and sertraline is approved for the long-term (eg, 52 weeks) management of PTSD. A number of drugs can be used as augmentation agents (eg, antiadrenergic drugs and second generation antipsychotics). Benzodiazepines are not effective for PTSD.

First-Line Agents

Consensus guidelines state that SSRIs or venlafaxine should be recommended as first-line treatment since they have been found to be effective and provide a safe adverse event profile compared to other agents. Overall, SSRIs are effective in reducing several symptoms (numbing/avoidance, hyperarousal, re-experiencing). Among the SSRIs, paroxetine and sertraline are Food and Drug Administration (FDA) approved and most commonly used (Table 59-1). Paroxetine is dosed 20 to 60 mg per day and is efficacious. However, paroxetine is among the highest anticholinergic SSRIs, with excessive sedation and weight gain being the most common adverse effects. Other SSRIs such as fluoxetine, citalopram, escitalopram, and fluvoxamine have also shown benefits. Data suggest sertraline may be better than citalopram in reducing numbing symptoms. Finally, long-term studies have shown efficacy for fluoxetine (9 months) and sertraline (16 months). All SSRIs should be initiated at low doses and titrated over several weeks to average dosing ranges (see Table 59-1). It is important to note that clinical response may not be evident until 8 to 12 weeks of treatment. Common adverse events associated with SSRIs include headaches, diarrhea, sexual dysfunction, insomnia, and agitation (paroxetine minimizes these symptoms as it is sedating). SSRIs are pregnancy category C, except for paroxetine (category D). Tapering for all SSRIs (possible exception may be fluoxetine) is recommended since withdrawal symptoms (eg, nausea/vomiting, sweating, dizziness) may occur with abrupt discontinuation.

Venlafaxine is a 5-HT/NE reuptake inhibitor (SNRI). Venlafaxine extended release (mean dose: 221 mg/d) has benefits lasting for 6 months. Venlafaxine extended release (mean dose: 225 mg/d) had similar efficacy to sertraline (mean dose: 151 mg/d) over 12 weeks. Unlike SSRIs, data are unclear on the efficacy of venlafaxine for hyperarousal symptoms. While both venlafaxine and SSRIs are first-line agents, SSRIs may be preferred since they appear to target more symptoms.

Second-Line Agents

Second-line agents include another SSRI not previously used or venlafaxine (if not used initially).

Third-Line Agents

Third-line agents include mirtazapine or TCAs. Mirtazapine enhances serotonergic activity, while TCAs increase both 5-HT and NE. In two small studies, mirtazapine demonstrated efficacy in doses up to 45 mg/d over 8 to 12 weeks. Due to its pharmacologic profile, mirtazapine exhibits greater sedation and weight gain at lower doses; however, as the dose is increased the medication becomes less sedating. Among TCAs, imipramine and amitriptyline may be used, as they have demonstrated effectiveness over 8 weeks. However, TCAs are reserved as third-line agents because of cardiovascular adverse events. Phenelzine is an MAOI with greater efficacy compared to imipramine. However, phenelzine is a last-line treatment option due to drug-food interactions and adverse events. Additionally, TCAs and MAOIs are lethal in overdose, which may be an issue in those who have suicidal ideations.

Other Agents

Prazosin may also play a role in the treatment of PTSD. This α₁ adrenergic antagonist has demonstrated benefits especially in patients with night time complications (eg, nightmares). A large 15-week study involving active-duty soldiers with PTSD demonstrated a reduction in nightmares and improved sleep with prazosin. Prazosin is considered in PTSD with nightmares and sleep disturbances; however, caution is warranted in patients with cardiac disease.

Second-generation antipsychotics (SGAs) may be recommended as adjunctive therapy to antidepressants or those experiencing psychotic symptoms (eg, aggressiveness, hallucinations). Risperidone, olanzapine, and quetiapine have been used with favorable results in small studies. A large randomized trial with risperidone was not effective in reducing the overall Clinician-Administered PTSD Scale (CAPS) score when compared to placebo; however, risperidone may have some use in reducing symptoms of re-experiencing and hyperarousal. Metabolic syndrome is one of the major complications with SGAs, especially with olanzapine and quetiapine. Proper monitoring (eg, weight, body mass index, fasting blood glucose) should be done in patients receiving these agents.

Benzodiazepines are not effective in PTSD and recent data suggest that they should be contraindicated since they may worsen PTSD symptoms. Additionally, bupropion lacks supporting evidence for use. Duloxetine showed some benefits in one case report, but exacerbated symptoms in another. However, these case reports are confounded by comorbid illnesses and concomitant psychotropic agents. A small open-label study found that duloxetine was effective at improving CAPS scores in patients with PTSD. Mood stabilizers (eg, topiramate, divalproex, tiagabine) have been studied but have limited or no efficacy.

SPECIAL POPULATIONS

Children and adolescents can be treated with nonpharmacologic and pharmacologic treatments. Examples of nonpharmacologic treatment includes CBT, psychotherapy, debriefing, and supportive therapy. However, CBT is the most studied and may be the preferred treatment.

Medications for children and adolescents are focused on the use of antidepressants primarily with SSRIs. However, there is a black box warning for suicide in this population (mainly patients 24 years old or younger) and caution is warranted. First-line pharmacologic treatment for elderly patients includes SSRIs due to a safer side effect profile compared to TCAs.

RELAPSE PREVENTION

Long-term treatment has been studied with fluoxetine and sertraline. One trial demonstrated efficacy of fluoxetine (mean dose: 53 mg/d) over an additional 24 weeks of treatment after patients had initially completed 12 weeks of therapy. Another study showed benefits with sertraline (mean dose: 137 mg/d) over an additional 28 weeks of treatment after patients had initially completed 36 weeks of therapy.

CASE Application

1. Which are core symptoms of PTSD? Select all that apply.

   a. Recurrent, intrusive, distressing memories of the trauma
   b. Ability to recall an important aspect of the trauma
   c. Avoidance of conversations about the trauma
   d. Hypervigilance

The following case pertains to questions 2 and 3.

LH is a 34-year-old woman who has experienced persistent flashbacks and nightmares after being robbed at gunpoint while leaving a restaurant several months ago. She finds it difficult to talk about the experience, and avoids situations that remind her of the event. She was recently diagnosed with PTSD.

2. Which agent should be used as a first-line treatment for PTSD in this patient?

   a. Phenelzine
   b. Paroxetine
   c. Amitriptyline
   d. Bupropion

3. In addition to medication therapy, LH would like to receive some type of nonpharmacologic treatment. Which nonpharmacologic treatment for PTSD has the most evidence supporting its use and is often utilized in the management of PTSD?

   a. Group counseling
   b. Stress inoculation treatment
   c. Psychoeducation
   d. CBT

4. Which SSRIs is/are approved by the FDA for the treatment of PTSD? Select all that apply.

   a. Sertraline
   b. Fluoxetine

c. Paroxetine
d. Citalopram

5. TW is a 43-year-old man with PTSD. He has tried several medications in the past, including sertraline, escitalopram, and venlafaxine; however, he has not experienced significant improvement of symptoms with any of these agents. The physician wants to start alprazolam 1 mg twice daily and asks if this is appropriate. How do you correctly respond to the physician?

    a. Alprazolam is not effective in the treatment of PTSD and may worsen symptoms.
    b. Alprazolam is effective; however, dose should be started at 0.5 mg twice daily.
    c. Alprazolam is effective and dosing is appropriate.
    d. Alprazolam is not the most appropriate benzodiazepine to use. It is best to initiate clonazepam 0.5 mg twice daily.

6. RB is a 27-year-old male combat veteran who was diagnosed with PTSD 1 year ago. He was originally prescribed fluoxetine, but did not experience any improvement while taking the medication. He has been taking sertraline 200 mg daily for the past 2 months; however, he still experiences symptoms. His psychiatrist would like to change his medication regimen and asks for your recommendation. Which medication(s) has demonstrated a favorable response in the management of PTSD? Select all that apply.

    a. Risperidone
    b. Venlafaxine
    c. Bupropion
    d. Prazosin

7. What is the *correct* dosing range for sertraline recommended for the treatment of PTSD?

    a. 2 to 8 mg/d
    b. 20 to 60 mg/d
    c. 50 to 200 mg/d
    d. 200 to 800 mg/d

8. Which of the following generic-brand name matches are correct?

    a. Sertraline—Zoloft
    b. Paroxetine—Prozac
    c. Citalopram—Celexa
    d. Imipramine—Tofranil

9. AB is a 32-year-old woman diagnosed with PTSD. She asks the pharmacist how long she needs to take the medication for the prevention of symptom recurrence. What is the goal for duration of treatment for PTSD?

    a. 1 month
    b. 6 months
    c. 12 months
    d. 5 years

10. CR is a 42-year-old man who was diagnosed with PTSD. He was prescribed citalopram 20 mg daily. He returns for a refill 1 month later and states, "I feel somewhat better, but still have flashbacks." How would you counsel this patient?

    a. Call the MD to change the medication to another SSRI, such as paroxetine.
    b. Call the MD to change the medication to venlafaxine.
    c. Remind the patient, it may take 8 to 12 weeks for the medication to show full benefits.
    d. Advise the patient that according to Federal laws, it is not your responsibility to counsel.

11. MN is a 23-year-old obese female diagnosed with PTSD after a car accident several years ago. Although MN has been treated with an SSRI and other agents, she still has recurrent, disturbing dreams of the event with minor daytime hallucinations. Her psychiatrist wants to prescribe a second generation antipsychotic for augmentation therapy and would like to avoid a medication with weight gain. Which agent do you *most* appropriately recommend as a pharmacist?

    a. Risperidone
    b. Olanzapine
    c. Quetiapine
    d. Haloperidol

12. PK is a 32-year-old woman diagnosed with PTSD. She would like to start a family soon, and plans on becoming pregnant in the next year. Which of the following medications has a pregnancy rating of category D?

    a. Paroxetine
    b. Fluoxetine
    c. Citalopram
    d. Sertraline

13. Which medication would you counsel a patient regarding drug-food interactions, especially avoiding tyramine containing foods?

    a. Prazosin
    b. Phenelzine
    c. Venlafaxine
    d. Zoloft

14. Which neurotransmitters are primarily implicated in PTSD? Select all that apply.

    a. Acetylcholine
    b. GABA
    c. 5-HT
    d. NE

15. MR is a 14-year-old boy recently diagnosed with PTSD. Which medication has a Black Box Warning for increased risk of suicidal ideations in pediatrics, and if used in this patient, would require that the patient be monitored closely for this adverse effect? Select all that apply.

    a. Venlafaxine
    b. Lorazepam

c. Sertraline

d. Fluoxetine

16. PT is a 57-year-old man with PTSD. He has not received any treatment for the disorder in the past. You are asked to provide a recommendation for initial medication therapy. Rank the following medication options in the order that they would be preferred.

Unordered Response	Ordered Response
Venlafaxine	
Sertraline	
Topiramate	
Amitriptyline	

17. SB is a 23-year-old woman with PTSD and presents to the outpatient clinic with complaints of nightmares and difficulty in sleeping. She is currently on paroxetine 40 mg daily and cannot tolerate higher dosages. Which medication can be most appropriately used as adjunctive therapy?

a. Olanzapine

b. Prazosin

c. Bupropion

d. Alprazolam

18. SSRIs have demonstrated effectiveness in which of the following core symptoms?

a. Re-experiencing

b. Numbing

c. Avoidance

d. Hyperarousal

19. Which agent(s) is/are available in extended-release formulations? Select all that apply.

a. Citalopram

b. Venlafaxine

c. Paroxetine

d. Sertraline

20. Place the SSRIs in order of maximum dose. Start with highest maximum dose.

Unordered Response	Ordered Response
Sertraline	
Escitalopram	
Paroxetine	
Fluoxetine	

TAKEAWAY POINTS »

- CBT may be the preferred nonpharmacologic treatment used in PTSD.
- SSRIs remain first-line treatment for PTSD in any population.
- Response may not be observed until 8 to 12 weeks of treatment.
- Sertraline and paroxetine are the only SSRIs that are FDA approved for PTSD.
- Paroxetine may carry more sedative properties and weight gain among the SSRIs.
- Venlafaxine may be used first-line or may be used as a second-line agent if patient fails to respond to SSRIs.

- Mirtazapine or TCAs (eg, imipramine, amitriptyline) may be used as third-line agents.
- Prazosin may play a role in reducing nightmare severity in this population.
- Second-generation antipsychotics may be used as adjunctive therapy to antidepressants, if partial response or psychotic features are present.
- Benzodiazepines and bupropion have not demonstrated any effectiveness in PTSD.
- Mood stabilizers and duloxetine have very limited evidence in treating PTSD.

BIBLIOGRAPHY

DeBattista C. Antidepressant agents. In: Katzung BG, Masters SB, Trevor AJ, eds. *Basic & Clinical Pharmacology*. 12th ed. New York, NY: McGraw-Hill; 2012:chap 30.

Kirkwood CK, Melton ST, Wells BG. Posttraumatic stress disorder and obsessive-compulsive disorder. In: DiPiro JT, Talbert RL, Yee GC, Matzke GR, Wells BG, Posey L, eds. *Pharmacotherapy: A Pathophysiologic Approach*. 10th ed. New York, NY: McGraw-Hill; 2017.

Molinoff PB. Neurotransmission and the central nervous system. In: Brunton LL, Chabner BA, Knollmann BC, eds. *Goodman & Gilman's The Pharmacological Basis of Therapeutics*. 12th ed. New York, NY: McGraw-Hill; 2011:chap 14.

O'Donnell JM, Shelton RC. Drug therapy of depression and anxiety disorders. In: Brunton LL, Chabner BA, Knollmann BC, eds. *Goodman & Gilman's The Pharmacological Basis of Therapeutics*. 12th ed. New York, NY: McGraw-Hill; 2011:chap 15.

Porter RJ, Meldrum BS. Antiseizure drugs. In: Katzung BG, Masters SB, Trevor AJ, eds. *Basic & Clinical Pharmacology*. 12th ed. New York, NY: McGraw-Hill; 2012:chap 24.

KEY ABBREVIATIONS

CAPS = Clinician-Administered PTSD Scale
DA = dopamine
DSM-5 = Diagnostic and Statistical Manual of Mental
  Disorders, Fifth Edition
EMDR = eye movement desensitization and reprocessing
FDA = Food and Drug Administration
GABA = gamma aminobutyric acid
HPA = hypothalamus-pituitary-adrenal

MAOI = monoamine oxidase inhibitor
NE = norepinephrine
PTSD = post-traumatic stress disorder
SGAs = second-generation antipsychotics
SNRIs = serotonin–norepinephrine reuptake inhibitors
SSRI = selective serotonin reuptake inhibitors
TCA = tricyclic antidepressant

60

Depression

Patricia A. Pepa and Kelly C. Lee

FOUNDATION OVERVIEW

Major depressive disorder (MDD) is diagnosed when an individual experiences one or more major depressive episodes without a history of manic or hypomanic episodes. An MDD episode is defined by the criteria listed in the *Diagnostic and Statistical Manual of Mental Disorders*, fifth edition (DSM-5). Depression is associated with significant functional disability, morbidity, and mortality. Individuals with MDD experience symptoms that can affect mood, thinking, physical health, work, and relationships. Unfortunately, suicide may be a result of MDD that has not been diagnosed or treated adequately.

Pathophysiology

The exact cause of MDD is unknown, but appears to be multifactorial. There are many biologic, psychological, and social theories that attempt to explain depressive disorders, but none of them do so completely. Most individuals have a variety of factors that contribute to the onset and severity of their symptoms.

1. *Genetics*: The occurrence of MDD exhibits a genetic pattern. First-degree relatives of MDD patients are more likely to develop MDD compared to first-degree relatives of control individuals.
2. *Stress/Environmental*: Depression can occur in the absence or presence of major life stressors or environmental and household stressors. In addition, when a genetic predisposition accompanies significant life stressors, chances for depressive episodes increase.
3. *Neurotransmitter and receptor*: Classic views for the cause of MDD focus on the neurotransmitters such as norepinephrine (NE), serotonin (5-HT), and dopamine (DA). The neurotransmitter hypothesis asserts that depression is due to a deficiency of neurotransmitters. The supporting evidence for this hypothesis is that existing antidepressants increase neurotransmitters concentrations. The neurotransmitter receptor hypothesis suggests that depression is related to abnormal functioning of neurotransmitter receptors. In this model, antidepressants exert therapeutic effects by altering receptor sensitivity. Chronic administration of antidepressants causes desensitization (downregulation) of β-adrenergic receptors and various 5-HT receptors. Importantly, the time required for changes in receptor sensitivity corresponds to the onset of action of antidepressant therapy.

While such models of depression are useful in conceptualizing the mechanisms behind antidepressant activity, they most likely represent an oversimplification of the actual pathophysiological process of the disorder. Depression likely involves a complex dysregulation of neurotransmitter systems, and these systems modulate or are modulated by other biologic systems. Thus, the underlying cause of depression may extend beyond dysfunction of the neurotransmitter system.

Clinical Presentation and Diagnosis

Patients with MDD present with a combination of emotional, physical, and cognitive symptoms. Table 60-1 lists the clinical presentation of patients with depression. Symptoms of a major depressive episode develop over days to weeks, but mild depressive and anxiety symptoms may be present for weeks to months prior to the onset of the full syndrome. Left untreated, major depressive episodes may last 6 months or more. A minority of patients experience chronic episodes that can last for at least 2 years. Approximately two-thirds of patients recover fully from major depressive episodes and return to usual mood and functioning, whereas the other third will have partial remission and may continue to experience various degrees of symptoms.

The diagnosis of MDD requires the presence of at least five depressive symptoms present nearly every day for a minimum of a 2-week period. These symptoms must cause clinically significant impairment in one's ability to function at home, work, or school. One of these symptoms must include depressed mood or loss of interest or pleasure. Other examples of depressive symptoms include: diminished interest in usual activities, change in appetite or weight, change in psychomotor activity, change in amount of sleep, loss of energy, feelings of worthlessness or guilt, diminished ability to think or concentrate, or recurrent thoughts of death or suicide.

When a patient presents with depressive symptoms, it is necessary to rule out the possibility of a contributing medical or drug-induced condition. For example:

- Patients with neurological disorders (eg, stroke, Alzheimer disease, or Parkinson disease) may develop

TABLE 60-1 | **Clinical Presentation of Major Depression**[a]

- Depressed mood
- Sleep disturbances
- Changed in appetite
- Decreased interest in activities previously enjoyed (anhedonia)
- Excessive guilt and feelings of worthlessness
- Decreased energy/increased fatigue
- Difficult/impaired concentration and memory
- Psychomotor changes (excitation or retardation)
- Suicidal thoughts or ideation

[a]Severely depressed patients may also present with psychotic symptoms (hallucinations or delusions) that resolve once the depressive symptoms are adequately treated.

depressive symptoms in the course of their medical illness.

- Individuals experiencing withdrawal from substances of abuse (eg, cocaine, heroin) can present with depressive symptoms.

Depressed patients should have a complete physical examination, mental status examination, and basic laboratory workup, including a complete blood count, thyroid function tests, and electrolyte assessments to identify potential medical problems. A complete medication review should be performed, as several medications can contribute to depressive symptoms. Table 60-2 lists examples of conditions and medications associated with depressive symptoms. Once medical conditions or concomitant medications have been ruled out as the cause of depressive symptoms, the patient should be evaluated for MDD.

TABLE 60-2 | **Medical Conditions, Substance Use Disorders, and Medications Associated With Depressive Symptoms**

- **Medical conditions**
  - Endocrine diseases (hypothyroidism, Addison, Cushing)
  - Deficiency states (severe anemia, Wernicke encephalopathy)
  - Infections (encephalitis, human immunodeficiency virus, tuberculosis, mononucleosis)
  - Collagen disorder (systemic lupus erythematosus)
  - Cardiovascular disease (coronary artery disease, heart failure, myocardial infarction)
  - Neurologic disorders (Alzheimer disease, epilepsy, Parkinson disease, multiple sclerosis, Huntington disease)
  - Malignant disease
- **Substance use disorders (intoxication, withdrawal, or chronic use)**
  - Alcohol
  - Marijuana
  - Nicotine
  - Opiate
  - Psychostimulant (eg, cocaine)
- **Drug therapy**
  - Antihypertensives (clonidine, diuretics, guanethidine, hydralazine, methyldopa, propranolol, reserpine)
  - Hormonal therapy (oral contraceptives, steroids)
  - Acne therapy (isotretinoin)
  - Interferon

TREATMENT

The goals of treatment are to reduce the symptoms of acute depression, facilitate the patient's return to their previous level of functioning, and prevent further episodes of depression. Additionally, one should also closely monitor the patient for suicidal thoughts or behaviors. An extremely important outcome in the treatment of MDD is the prevention of suicide attempts.

Antidepressants can be classified in several ways, including classification by chemical structure and mechanism of antidepressant activity. Although the link between the mechanism of action and antidepressant response is tenuous, the classification has the advantage of being based on established pharmacology and explains some of the common and predictable adverse effects. Historically, studies have found that antidepressants are of equivalent efficacy when given in equipotent doses. Because one cannot predict which antidepressant will be the most effective in an individual patient, the initial choice is made empirically. Factors that influence the choice of an antidepressant include the patient's history of response, pharmacogenetics (history of familial antidepressant response), patient's concurrent medical history, presenting symptoms, potential for drug–drug interactions, adverse events profile, patient preference, and drug cost.

Selective Serotonin Reuptake Inhibitors

The efficacy of selective serotonin reuptake inhibitors (SSRIs) is superior to placebo and comparable to other classes of antidepressants. SSRIs are generally chosen as first-line antidepressants due to their improved tolerability and side effect profile, as well as their safety in overdose when compared to other available medications. The SSRIs have a low affinity for histaminergic, α_1-adrenergic, and muscarinic receptors; therefore, they produce fewer anticholinergic and cardiovascular side effects. Side effects associated with SSRIs are usually mild but common and include gastrointestinal effects (nausea, vomiting, and diarrhea), sexual dysfunction, and headache. To mitigate potential insomnia, SSRIs (with the exception of paroxetine [Paxil]) are most frequently administered in the morning. Paroxetine is the most sedating of the SSRIs and usually requires dosing at bedtime to improve tolerability. A withdrawal syndrome can occur if an SSRI is abruptly discontinued (particularly shorter-acting paroxetine). Tables 60-3 and 60-4 list key parameters for SSRIs.

Serotonin/Norepinephrine Reuptake Inhibitors

Venlafaxine (Effexor), desvenlafaxine (Pristiq), duloxetine (Cymbalta), and levomilnacipran (Fetzima) are serotonin/norepinephrine reuptake inhibitors (SNRIs). These medications may be used first-line, especially in patients with comorbid neuropathic pain or fibromyalgia. Venlafaxine inhibits 5-HT reuptake at low doses, with additional NE reuptake inhibition at higher doses ($\geq$150 mg). Duloxetine inhibits reuptake of 5-HT and NE at initial doses and levomilnacipran

TABLE 60-3 Antidepressant Dosing and Available Dosage Forms

Antidepressant	Brand Name	Usual Dosing	Dosage Form
Selective Serotonin Reuptake Inhibitors			
Citalopram	Celexa	20-40 mg	Tablets, oral solution
Escitalopram	Lexapro	10-20 mg	Tablets, oral solution
Fluoxetine	Prozac, Prozac weekly	20-60 mg	Tablet, capsule (immediate and delayed-release), oral solution
Paroxetine	Paxil, Paxil CR, Pexeva	20-60 mg	Extended-release tablet, tablet, capsule, oral suspension (CR product should not be broken or crushed)
Sertraline	Zoloft	50-200 mg	Tablets, oral solution
Serotonin and Norepinephrine Reuptake Inhibitors			
Desvenlafaxine	Pristiq	50-100 mg	Extended release tablet
Duloxetine	Cymbalta	60-90 mg	Delayed-release capsules (should not be opened per manufacturer)
Levomilnacipran	Fetzima	40-120 mg	Extended-release capsules (should not be opened per manufacturer)
Venlafaxine	Effexor, Effexor XR	37.5-225 mg	Extended-release capsules, extended-release tablet, tablet (XR capsules may be opened and sprinkled on food)
Tricyclic Antidepressants			
Amitriptyline	Elavil	100-300 mg	Tablets
Desipramine	Norpramin	100-300 mg	Tablets
Doxepin	Silenor	100-300 mg	Capsule, tablet, oral solution
Imipramine	Tofranil	100-300 mg	Capsules, tablet
Nortriptyline	Pamelor	50-200 mg	Capsules, oral solution
Monoamine Oxidase Inhibitors			
Phenelzine	Nardil	30-90 mg	Tablets
Selegiline	Emsam	6-12 mg	Transdermal Patch
Tranylcypromine	Parnate	20-60 mg	Tablets
Isocarboxazid	Marplan	10-40 mg	Tablet
Other Antidepressants			
Trazodone	Oleptro	100-600 mg	Tablets, extended-release tablet (XR product should be taken on an empty stomach and may be broken along score line or swallowed whole)
Nefazodone	Serzone	150-300 mg	Tablets
Bupropion	Wellbutrin Wellbutrin SR Wellbutrin XL Aplenzin	150-450 mg 150-400 mg 150-450 mg 174-522 mg	Immediate-release, sustained-release, and extended-release tablets (SR and XL products should not be crushed or broken)
Mirtazapine	Remeron	7.5-45 mg	Tablets, orally disintegrating tablet
Vilazodone	Viibryd	10-40 mg	Tablets
Vortioxetine	Trintellix	10-20 mg	Tablets

inhibits NE at low doses and 5-HT at higher doses. The most commonly reported adverse effects associated with SNRIs are dose related and include headache, nausea, dry mouth, sweating, sexual dysfunction, insomnia, and anxiety. Venlafaxine can also cause dose-related increases in systolic and diastolic blood pressure. Blood pressure should be monitored regularly during therapy. Tables 60-3 and 60-4 list key parameters for SNRIs. A withdrawal syndrome is also common with short-acting venlafaxine.

Tricyclic Antidepressants

Tricyclic antidepressants (TCAs) are effective in treating all depressive subtypes; however, the use of TCAs has diminished due to the availability of equally effective therapies that are safer and better tolerated. TCAs potentiate the activity of NE and 5-HT by blocking their reuptake into presynaptic terminals. Because TCAs have activities on many other receptor systems, adverse events are varied and frequently reported. The most common side effects are dose related and associated with blockade of cholinergic receptors (anticholinergic effects) and affinity for adrenergic receptors (often resulting in orthostatic hypotension). TCAs may also cause cardiac conduction delays and can induce heart block and produce arrhythmias, particularly in overdose. Abrupt withdrawal of TCAs is associated with symptoms of cholinergic rebound (eg, dizziness, nausea, diarrhea, insomnia, and restlessness), so it is recommended that doses be tapered over several days. The tertiary amine TCAs (such as amitriptyline and doxepin) are highly sedating,

TABLE 60-4 Antidepressant Characteristics

Antidepressant	Mechanism of Action	Contraindications (C) & Warnings (W)[a]	Adverse Reactions	General Information
Fluoxetine, Citalopram, Escitalopram, Sertraline, Paroxetine	Inhibits reuptake of 5-HT	C: Hypersensitivity to SSRI W: All SSRIs carry a risk of hyponatremia as well as bleeding associated with impaired platelet aggregation; citalopram should not be used in patients with hypokalemia, hypomagnesemia, recent myocardial infarction, or heart failure	Headache, nausea, vomiting, diarrhea, insomnia, sexual dysfunction, decreased appetite (fluoxetine), sedation, dizziness, dry mouth (paroxetine)	All agents pregnancy category C (except paroxetine: category D); withdrawal symptoms with abrupt discontinuation; individual agents have varying activity at CYP450 enzymes (and should be reviewed individually)
Venlafaxine, Desvenlafaxine, Duloxetine, Levomilnacipran	Inhibits reuptake of 5-HT and NE	C: Hypersensitivity to SNRI; uncontrolled narrow angle glaucoma W: All SNRIs carry a risk of hyponatremia as well as increased bleeding due to impaired platelet aggregation; duloxetine should not be used in patients with substantial alcohol use or chronic liver disease due to risk of hepatotoxicity; risk of orthostatic hypotension and syncope with duloxetine	Headache, nausea, vomiting, constipation, dizziness, insomnia, sexual dysfunction, diaphoresis, increased blood pressure, hypercholesterolemia	Pregnancy category C; withdrawal symptoms with abrupt discontinuation; metabolized via CYP450 2D6 (venlafaxine, duloxetine) 3A4 (venlafaxine, desvenlafaxine) and 1A2 (duloxetine)
Tertiary amines: Amitriptyline, Clomipramine, Doxepin, Imipramine Secondary amines: Desipramine, Nortriptyline	Inhibits reuptake of 5-HT and NE; affinity for reuptake inhibition depends on medication	C: Hypersensitivity to TCAs; should not be given to patients in acute recovery of a myocardial infarction W: May be fatal if taken in overdose; may cause cardiac conduction abnormalities (including Torsades de Pointes at high doses)	Sedation, dry mouth, orthostatic hypotension, seizures (high doses), weight gain, sexual dysfunction	Withdrawal symptoms with abrupt discontinuation; pregnancy category C; individual agents have varying activity at CYP450 enzymes (and should be reviewed individually); most agents metabolized via 2D6, 3A4, and 2C19
Phenelzine Tranylcypromine Selegiline	Increases endogenous concentrations of NE, 5-HT, and DA through inhibition of monoamine oxidase	C: Hypersensitivity to MAOI; heart failure, abnormal liver function tests, renal disease, use of sympathomimetics, foods high in tyramine content W: Risk of hypertensive crisis with foods and supplements high in tyramine; risk of orthostatic hypotension	Orthostatic hypotension, weight gain, sexual dysfunction, hypertensive crisis	Pregnancy category C; 2 wk should elapse between discontinuation of MAOI and start of new antidepressant or vice versa; washout of 3 wk (for vortioxetine) or 5 wk (for fluoxetine) required before starting MAOI; see Table 60-5 for dietary restrictions
Trazodone, Nefazodone	Inhibits 5-HT reuptake; 5-HT₂ receptor antagonist; blocks α₁-adrenergic and histaminergic receptors	C: Hypersensitivity to trazodone or nefazodone; liver disease or elevated serum transaminases W: Risk of priapism (trazodone); risk of hepatotoxicity (nefazodone)	Dizziness, orthostatic hypotension, sedation, somnolence, dry mouth, nausea, diarrhea	Pregnancy category C; both medications metabolized via CYP450 3A4 and 2D6 enzymes; doses of nefazodone should be reduced in patients on concomitant triazolam or alprazolam
Bupropion	Inhibits reuptake of dopamine and NE	C: Hypersensitivity to bupropion or any component of the formulation; seizure disorder; anorexia or bulimia; patients with electrolyte abnormalities; W: Risk of dose-related seizures	Headache, insomnia, tachycardia, tremor, dry mouth, weight loss	Pregnancy category C; doses >450 mg associated with seizures; metabolized via CYP450 2B6 enzyme, but also potent inhibitor of 2D6
Mirtazapine	Presynaptic α₂-adrenergic antagonist leading to increased release of NE and 5-HT; antagonist of 5-HT₂&₃ and H₁ receptors	C: Hypersensitivity to mirtazapine W: Risk of hyponatremia	Somnolence, increased appetite, sedation, weight gain, dry mouth, constipation, hyperlipidemia	Pregnancy category C; may increase appetite, leading to weight gain; metabolized via CYP450 2D6, 1A2, and 3A4 enzymes
Vilazodone	Inhibits reuptake of 5-HT and is a partial agonist at 5-HT₁ₐ	C: Hypersensitivity to vilazodone W: Risk of hyponatremia as well as increased bleeding due to impaired platelet aggregation; risk of seizures—should be avoided in patients with epilepsy	Sedation, dizziness, nausea, diarrhea, dry mouth, insomnia	Pregnancy category C; requires fixed titration schedule upon initiation; dosing requires adjustment if given with strong 3A4 inhibitors or inducers
Vortioxetine	Inhibits 5-HT reuptake; 5-HT₁ₐ, 5-HT₁ᵦ, 5-HT₇ antagonist; 5-HT₁ₐ agonist, 5-HT₁ᵦ partial agonist	C: Hypersensitivity to vortioxetine, concurrent use of linezolid or methylene blue W: Risk of hyponatremia as well as increased bleeding due to impaired platelet aggregation	Sexual dysfunction, nausea, dizziness, abnormal dreams, diarrhea, dry mouth, constipation, vomiting	Pregnancy category C; withdrawal symptoms with abrupt discontinuation; metabolized via CYP450 3A4 and 2D6 enzymes

[a]All antidepressants have a black box warning for increased risk of suicidal behaviors and ideation ≤24 years old; patients should be closely monitored for worsening of symptoms, suicidal behaviors, and changes in behavior when starting antidepressants. These medications also have a warning to avoid overlap of therapy with an MAOI. All patients should be given a 14-day washout period before starting on a new antidepressant if previously treated with an MAOI. Likewise, patients starting on an MAOI should be given a minimum of a 14-day washout period when discontinuing treatment with another antidepressant. Patients who were previously taking vortioxetine should be given a 3-week washout, while patients previously taking fluoxetine should be given a 5-week washout period prior to starting an MAOI.

usually requiring bedtime administration and commonly used as hypnotics due to their sedating properties. Tables 60-3 and 60-4 list key parameters for TCAs.

Monoamine Oxidase Inhibitors

Monoamine oxidase inhibitors (MAOIs) increase the concentration of NE, 5-HT, and DA within the neuronal synapse through inhibition of the MAO enzyme. The most common MAOI side effect is orthostatic hypotension. Other common adverse effects include weight gain and sexual side effects. Hypertensive crisis is a rare but serious, life-threatening reaction that may occur when MAOIs are taken concurrently with foods high in tyramine content or sympathomimetic medications. These incidents can culminate in cerebrovascular accidents and death if undiagnosed or untreated. Patients must be thoroughly counseled on dietary requirements while taking MAOIs and alert their provider to any new medications that are started. Tables 60-3 and 60-4 list key parameters for MAOIs; Table 60-5 reviews dietary restrictions with the use of MAOI medications.

Other Antidepressants

Trazodone and Nefazodone

Trazodone (Oleptro) and nefazodone (Serzone) are effective in treating depression; however, they both carry risks and side effects that limit their use as antidepressants. Trazodone and nefazodone have dual actions on serotonergic neurons, acting as $5\text{-}HT_2$ receptor antagonists and 5-HT reuptake inhibitors. Tables 60-3 and 60-4 list key parameters for trazodone and nefazodone.

The use of nefazodone as an antidepressant has declined following reports of medication-related hepatotoxicity. Labeling information for nefazodone includes a black box warning describing rare cases of liver failure. Because of the potential for hepatic injury associated with nefazodone use, treatment should not be initiated in individuals with active liver disease or with elevated baseline serum transaminases. Common adverse effects associated with nefazodone include dizziness, orthostatic hypotension, sedation, dry mouth, nausea, and weakness.

In addition to the $5\text{-}HT_2$ receptor, trazodone blocks α_1-adrenergic and histaminergic receptors leading to increased side effects that limit its tolerability as an antidepressant. Sedation and dizziness are the most common dose-limiting side effects associated with trazodone. Due to these sedating effects, trazodone is used more commonly to treat insomnia than depression. Though trazodone does not carry a risk of hepatotoxicity, it does have a small but potentially serious risk of priapism, which is reported to occur in 1 in 6000 male patients.

Bupropion

Bupropion (Wellbutrin) is a DA and NE reuptake inhibitor used in the treatment of MDD. Adverse effects associated with bupropion include headache, nausea, tremor, insomnia, dry mouth, and decreased appetite. Sexual side effects are minimal with bupropion, and it may be used as monotherapy or in combination with other antidepressants to minimize medication-induced sexual dysfunction. The occurrence of seizures with bupropion is dose-related (max doses are ≤450 mg) and may be increased in patients with electrolyte abnormalities. Due to its stimulating properties, bupropion should be dosed in the morning or in the morning and early afternoon (if given twice daily) to avoid sleep disturbances.

Mirtazapine

Mirtazapine (Remeron) enhances noradrenergic and serotonergic activity through the antagonism of central presynaptic α_2-adrenergic autoreceptors and heteroreceptors. Mirtazapine also antagonizes $5\text{-}HT_2$ and $5\text{-}HT_3$, leading to lower rates of gastrointestinal, sexual dysfunction, and anxiety side effects, as well as histamine receptors, leading to sedation. The most common adverse effects of mirtazapine are sedation, increased appetite and subsequent weight gain, dry mouth, and constipation. Several side effects of mirtazapine are dose dependent and more common at low doses, such as sedation and increased appetite. These side effects will often dissipate as the dose is increased. Tables 60-3 and 60-4 list key parameters for mirtazapine.

Vilazodone

Vilazodone (Viibryd) is primarily a 5-HT reuptake inhibitor, similar to the SSRI medications; however, it also binds selectively to the $5\text{-}HT_{1a}$ receptor and acts as a partial $5\text{-}HT_{1a}$ agonist. This activity is believed to help minimize anxiety symptoms that are commonly seen with initiation of antidepressant medications. Vilazodone is also unique in its administration, requiring a specific dose titration for all patients in the first 2 weeks of treatment. The most common adverse effects of vilazodone are diarrhea, nausea, sedation, dry mouth, dizziness, and insomnia. Tables 60-3 and 60-4 list key parameters for vilazodone.

Vortioxetine

Vortioxetine (Trintellix) has a multimodal mechanism of action. It is a 5-HT reuptake inhibitor, similar to SSRI medications; however, it is also a full $5\text{-}HT_{1A}$ receptor agonist and $5\text{-}HT_3$ receptor antagonist. It is also a $5\text{-}HT_7$ and $5\text{-}HT_{1D}$ receptor antagonist and partial $5\text{-}HT_{1B}$ receptor agonist. As a result of its multimodal action, it causes a downstream increase in DA, NE, and acetylcholine activity in the prefrontal cortex. This activity is believed to help restore some cognitive deficits

TABLE 60-5	Dietary Restrictions for Patients Taking Monoamine Oxidase Inhibitors
Dairy	Aged cheese, especially blue cheese, cheddar, Gouda, Parmesan, and provolone
Beverages	Wine (especially Chianti), sherry, beer
Meat	Herring (pickled, salted, dry), sardines, caviar, liver (chicken or beef), salami, dried/salted meats
Vegetables	Chinese pea pods, Fava beans, soybean products
Condiments/other	Yeast extract, marmite, soy sauce, sauerkraut, monosodium glutamate (MSG)

associated with depression. The most common adverse effects of vortioxetine are headache and nausea.

Second-Generation Antipsychotics

Aripiprazole (Abilify), brexpiprazole (Rexulti), olanzapine + fluoxetine (Symbyax), and quetiapine extended release (Seroquel XR) are indicated for adjunctive treatment to antidepressants for MDD. Their efficacy as adjunctive medications for MDD are hypothesized to be due to their serotonergic, noradrenergic and dopaminergic properties. Refer to Schizophrenia Chapter for further medication details.

SPECIAL CONSIDERATIONS

Black Box Warning

All antidepressants carry a black box warning for increased risk of suicidality in children, adolescents, and young adults age 24 and younger. Patients who are started on antidepressant therapy should be educated and monitored closely for clinical worsening, suicidality, or unusual changes in behavior. If this occurs, the patient's physician should be contacted immediately.

Drug Interactions

Antidepressants can cause pharmacodynamic (eg, additive pharmacologic effects) and pharmacokinetic (eg, changes in drug levels) interactions with other medications. The pharmacodynamic interactions involve receptor blockade by the antidepressants. For example:

- TCAs can cause significant additive effects with other medications that cause sedation, hypotension, or anticholinergic effects.

- Nefazodone and mirtazapine can interact with other drugs that cause hypotension and sedation effects, respectively.

The most concerning pharmacodynamic interactions are hypertensive crisis and serotonin syndrome. Hypertensive crisis is characterized by sharply elevated blood pressure, headache, nausea, vomiting, and sweating. It may result during MAOI therapy if the patient takes a sympathomimetic medication (eg, ephedrine and pseudoephedrine) or if the patient consumes foods rich in tyramine (Table 60-5). Since many over-the-counter cough and cold products contain sympathomimetics, patients should always be told to consult their pharmacist prior to using any new medications.

Serotonin syndrome is characterized by confusion, nausea, vomiting, fever, myoclonic spasms, hyperreflexia, sweating, diarrhea, and tachycardia. This reaction most often occurs when serotonergic agents are added to a serotonergic antidepressant. MAOIs are associated with severe cases of serotonin syndrome, but all antidepressants that increase 5-HT may contribute to serotonin syndrome. Certain medications may increase the risk of serotonin syndrome when used with antidepressants because their serotonergic properties are often overlooked (eg, dextromethorphan, meperidine, tramadol).

TABLE 60-6   Select Drug Interactions of Antidepressants

Antidepressant	Type of Interaction	Examples of Interacting Drugs
TCAs Trazodone Mirtazapine	Pharmacodynamic-additive sedation	Benzodiazepines Opioid and opiate analgesics Alcohol Antihistamines
TCAs Trazodone	Pharmacodynamic-additive hypotensive effects	Prazosin (α-blockers) Antipsychotics
TCAs	Pharmacodynamic-additive anticholinergic effects	Phenothiazines Benztropine Antipsychotics
TCAs	Pharmacodynamic-additive cardiac toxicity	Thioridazine Quinidine Methadone
TCAs	Pharmacodynamic-decreased antihypertensive effect	Guanethidine Clonidine Methyldopa
Bupropion	Pharmacodynamic-increased seizure risk	TCAs Phenothiazines
MAOIs	Pharmacodynamic-hypertensive crisis	Tyramine-rich foods Sympathomimetics
MAOIs TCAs SSRIs SNRIs	Pharmacodynamic-serotonin syndrome	Serotonergic antidepressants Meperidine Dextromethorphan Tramadol
Fluvoxamine	Pharmacokinetic-CYP1A2 inhibition	TCAs Clozapine Olanzapine Theophylline
Fluoxetine Fluvoxamine Sertraline	Pharmacokinetic-CYP2C inhibition	TCAs Phenytoin Warfarin
Fluoxetine Paroxetine Duloxetine Sertraline Bupropion	Pharmacokinetic-CYP2D6 inhibition	TCAs Haloperidol Risperidone Codeine Propranolol
Nefazodone Fluoxetine Fluvoxamine	Pharmacokinetic-CYP3A4 inhibition	TCAs Alprazolam Verapamil Aripiprazole Carbamazepine Lovastatin

Abbreviations: MAOI, monoamine oxidase inhibitor; SNRI, serotonin norepinephrine reuptake inhibitor; SSRI, selective serotonin reuptake inhibitor; TCAs, tricyclic antidepressant.

*List is not all-inclusive

Reproduced with permission from Jann MW, Penzak SR, Cohen LJ: *Applied Clinical Pharmacokinetics and Pharmacodynamics of Psychopharmacological Agents.* New York, NY: Springer International Publishing Switzerland; 2016.

Several antidepressants are known to inhibit various cytochrome P450 isoenzymes, thereby preventing the metabolism of other medications and leading to elevated plasma levels of substrates. These interactions may cause increased adverse effects or toxicities of the medications. The propensity to cause these interactions varies with the antidepressant. Table 60-6 lists select antidepressant interactions.

Efficacy

Antidepressants, when dosed properly and given for an appropriate period of time, have a response rate of 60% to 80%. Various factors must be taken into account when selecting antidepressant activity to optimize efficacy. Examples include patient's past history of response, family history of antidepressant response, side effects, comorbid conditions, drug interactions, and cost.

Despite their efficacy, antidepressants do not produce a clinical response immediately. Improvement in physical symptoms (sleep, appetite, energy) can occur within the first week or two of treatment. Improvement of emotional symptoms of depression may take as long as 6 to 8 weeks to see full effects of the medication. For patients who do not see improvement, the provider should consider titrating the medication to higher doses, augmenting improvement with an additional medication, or switching to a new agent.

CASE Application

Use the following case to answer questions 1 through 5.

Sebastian W is a 30-year-old man with chronic neuropathic pain and just lost his job due to consistently missing deadlines. He presents to his physician with troubling symptoms of decreased appetite and sleep, increased feelings of guilt and worthlessness, impaired concentration, and decreased interest in his usual hobbies. Sebastian's mother was diagnosed with MDD when she was 30. Sebastian's physician diagnoses him with MDD.

1. The cause of Sebastian's MDD is most likely associated with which of the following? Select all that apply.

   a. Genetic factors
   b. Stress/environmental factors
   c. Deficiency in neurotransmitters
   d. Cultural factors

2. Which of the following neurotransmitter(s) may be involved in the pathophysiology of Sebastian's depression? Select all that apply.

   a. NE
   b. 5-HT
   c. DA
   d. Acetylcholine

3. What other symptom(s) of MDD would you ask Sebastian about? Select all that apply.

   a. Depressed mood
   b. Sleep duration and quality
   c. Suicidal thoughts or behaviors
   d. Psychomotor changes

4. Sebastian's doctor decides to start him on a medication with dual neurotransmitter effects to target his neuropathic pain and MDD. Which of the following

antidepressants inhibit the reuptake of both NE and 5-HT? Select all that apply.

   a. Desipramine
   b. Venlafaxine
   c. Escitalopram
   d. Phenelzine
   e. Bupropion

5. Three months later Sebastian returns to his doctor and mentions he is still having difficulty sleeping. Sebastian's doctor starts him on trazodone due to its sedating properties. Select the mechanism of action of trazodone that leads to the side effects of dizziness and sedation.

   a. 5-HT receptor antagonist
   b. 5-HT reuptake inhibitor
   c. α_1-Adrenergic and histaminergic antagonism
   d. Angiotension receptor blockade

6. Select the antidepressant that has a black box warning for rare cases of liver failure.

   a. Mirtazapine
   b. Bupropion
   c. Amitriptyline
   d. Nefazodone

7. Which of the following antidepressants is classified as a DA and NE reuptake inhibitor?

   a. Wellbutrin
   b. Elavil
   c. Viibryd
   d. Cymbalta

8. Utilization of which of the following medications would result in the highest risk of developing the side effect of hypertensive crisis?

   a. Phenelzine plus lisinopril
   b. Imipramine plus sertraline
   c. Tranylcypromine plus pseudoephedrine
   d. Venlafaxine plus lorazepam

9. Mia is a 49-year-old patient who suffered a myocardial infarction 1 week ago. Upon discharge, it was noted that Mia appeared depressed. At a follow-up visit with her physician a week later, Mia met criteria for a diagnosis of MDD. Her past medical history includes: treatment-refractory hypertension, diabetes mellitus (type II), and severe uncontrolled narrow angle glaucoma. Select the antidepressant that would be the safest and most effective pharmacotherapy option for Mia.

   a. Elavil
   b. Fetzima
   c. Zoloft
   d. Pamelor

10. A month later, Mia has fully recovered from her myocardial infarction and is feeling much better since initiation of her antidepressant 4 weeks ago. Mia presents for a follow-up

today and states that while she is happy with the results of her antidepressant, she is concerned about her acquired sexual dysfunction. Which antidepressant can be administered to Mia to avoid a sexual dysfunction side effect?

a. Wellbutrin
b. Pamelor
c. Prozac
d. Cymbalta

11. Harry is a 49-year-old patient diagnosed with major depressive disorder. His past medical history is significant for alcohol-induced liver damage (with increased liver function tests), hypertension, and hyperlipidemia. Which of the following antidepressants would be safe and appropriate for him? Select all that apply.

a. Nefazodone
b. Sertraline
c. Vilazodone
d. Duloxetine

12. Felicia is a 44-year-old patient with a history of bulimia and multiple recent hospitalizations for electrolyte abnormalities that have caused seizures. Felicia has recently been diagnosed with MDD. Which of the following antidepressants is contraindicated in Felicia due to her comorbid condition?

a. Wellbutrin
b. Prozac
c. Cymbalta
d. Remeron

13. On her most recent hospitalization, Felicia was found to have atrial fibrillation. Which of the following medications can be used safely in patients with cardiac conduction abnormalities and avoids alterations in the QTc interval? Select all that apply.

a. Celexa
b. Norpramin
c. Zoloft
d. Elavil

14. Which of the following would cause a clinically significant drug interaction if taken with a TCA antidepressant?

a. Alcohol
b. Thioridazine
c. Meperidine
d. Fluoxetine

Use the following case to answer questions 15 and 16.

15. Laura is a patient with MDD currently taking phenelzine. She has been experiencing painful sinus pressure, headaches, and congestion. She approaches your pharmacy and asks if she can take a decongestant for

the congestion. You inform her that she cannot take the decongestant with her antidepressant medication due to the risk of what side effect?

a. Serotonin syndrome
b. Hypertensive crisis
c. Sexual dysfunction
d. Orthostatic hypotension

16. While Laura is at the pharmacy counter, you notice that she has been doing some grocery shopping before asking about the decongestant. Which of the following food items would result in a clinically significant interaction with her antidepressant? Select all that apply.

a. Sauerkraut
b. Eggs
c. Blue cheese
d. Whole milk

17. Select the drug interaction(s) associated with Prozac. Select all that apply.

a. Verapamil
b. Carbamazepine
c. Codeine
d. Azithromycin

18. Select the brand name of paroxetine.

a. Paxil
b. Remeron
c. Prozac
d. Effexor

19. Select the generic name of Pristiq.

a. Desvenlafaxine
b. Vortioxetine
c. Duloxetine
d. Vilazodone

20. Which of the following antidepressants is available as a once-weekly formulation?

a. Fluvoxamine
b. Duloxetine
c. Venlafaxine
d. Fluoxetine

21. Mary Lou is a 76-year-old who has recently been diagnosed with depression. Mary Lou also has early stages of dementia and has difficulty swallowing tablets and capsules. Which of the following medications is available in a liquid formulation?

a. Sertraline
b. Venlafaxine
c. Amitriptyline
d. Duloxetine

22. Mary Lou's daughter returns to the doctor and asks for a new medication, saying Mary Lou doesn't like the taste of the liquid medication. The daughter would like to

switch to a medication she can crush or open and put in applesauce. Which of the following medications can be crushed or opened due to its formulation or delivery mechanism? Select all that apply.

a. Phenelzine
b. Zoloft
c. Cymbalta
d. Paxil CR

23. Two months later, Mary Lou presents with decreased appetite and weight loss and continues to have difficulty swallowing. Which of the following medications is available as an orally disintegrating tablet?

a. Bupropion
b. Duloxetine
c. Mirtazapine
d. Fluoxetine

24. Which of the following counseling point(s) apply to Wellbutrin SR? Select all that apply.

a. Take this at bedtime because it can cause significant sedation.
b. Do not take more than prescribed dose at once to minimize risk of seizure.
c. This medication can cause significant sexual side effects.
d. Improvement of depression symptoms may not occur for a few weeks, so it is important to continue to take the medication on a daily basis.

TAKEAWAY POINTS »

- MDD is diagnosed when an individual experiences one or more major depressive episodes without a history of manic, mixed, or hypomanic episodes. Individuals must have five or more depressive symptoms that last a minimum of 2 weeks and cause clinically significant impairment in mood, thinking, physical health, work, and relationships.

- The exact cause of MDD is unknown, but appears to be multifactorial. Genetic, psychological, and environmental factors appear to work in combination and may precipitate depressive episodes.

- Classic views for the cause of MDD focus on the neurotransmitters 5-HT, NE, and DA.

- Goals of treatment are to reduce the symptoms of acute depression, facilitate the patient's return to a level of functioning before the onset of illness, and prevent further episodes of depression. An extremely important outcome in the treatment of MDD is the prevention of suicide attempts.

- The efficacy of SSRIs is superior to placebo and comparable to other classes of antidepressants. SSRIs are generally chosen first-line due to improved tolerability and a better safety profile in overdose.

- Venlafaxine (Effexor), desvenlafaxine (Pristiq), levomilnacipran (Fetzima), and duloxetine (Cymbalta) are SNRIs.

- Trazodone (Oleptro) and nefazodone (Serzone) are effective in treating depression; however, they both carry risks that limit their utility as antidepressants. Trazodone and nefazodone have dual actions on serotonergic neurons, acting as 5-HT$_2$ receptor antagonists and 5-HT reuptake inhibitors. Trazodone's primary use is as a sedative/hypnotic.

- Bupropion (Wellbutrin) is a DA and NE reuptake inhibitor used in the treatment of MDD. Bupropion has a lower incidence of sexual dysfunction than other antidepressants, allowing it to be used as monotherapy or in combination with other antidepressants to minimize sexual side effects.

- Mirtazapine (Remeron) enhances noradrenergic and serotonergic activity through the antagonism of central presynaptic α$_2$-adrenergic autoreceptors and heteroreceptors. Mirtazapine also antagonizes 5-HT$_2$ and 5-HT$_3$, leading to fewer gastrointestinal effects and antianxiety properties. The antagonism of histamine receptors leads to sedative properties.

- TCAs are effective in treating all depressive subtypes, but their use has diminished greatly due to the availability of therapies that are safer in overdose and better tolerated. TCAs potentiate the activity of NE and 5-HT by blocking their reuptake; however, the potency and selectivity of TCAs for the reuptake inhibition varies greatly within in the class.

- MAOIs increase the concentration of NE, 5-HT, and DA within the neuronal synapse through inhibition of the MAO enzyme. The most common MAOI side effect is postural hypotension.

- Hypertensive crisis is a rare but serious, life-threatening reaction that may occur when MAOIs are taken concurrently with sympathomimetic medications or food and/or drinks that are high in tyramine.

- Antidepressants may cause pharmacodynamic (eg, additive pharmacologic effects) and pharmacokinetic (eg, changes in drug levels) interactions with other medications and must be carefully selected based on a patient's current medication regimen.

- Antidepressants do not produce an immediate clinical response. Improvement in physical symptoms (sleep, appetite, energy) can occur within the first 2 weeks of treatment, but improvement in emotional symptoms may take 6 to 8 weeks for full effects. However, when dosed properly over an appropriate period of time, antidepressants have a response rate of 60% to 80%.

BIBLIOGRAPHY

Aan het Rot M, Mathew SJ, Charney DS. Neurobiological mechanisms in major depressive disorder. *CMAJ*. 2009;180(3):305-313.

Alvarez W, Pickworth KK. Safety of antidepressant drugs in the patient with cardiac disease: a review of the literature. *Pharmacotherapy: The Journal of Human Pharmacology and Drug Therapy*. 2003;23:754-771.

American Psychiatric Association. Practice guideline for the treatment of patients with major depressive disorder, 3rd ed. Arlington, Virginia: American Psychiatric Association, 2010.

American Psychiatric Association. Diagnostic and Statistical Manual of Mental Disorders: DSM-5. 5th ed. Arlington: American Psychiatric Association, 2013.

Blanco C, Okuda M, Markowitz JC, Liu S-M, Grant BF, Hasin DS. The epidemiology of chronic major depressive disorder and dysthymic disorder: results from the National Epidemiologic Survey on Alcohol and Related Conditions. *The Journal of Clinical Psychiatry*. 2010;71(12):1645-1656.

Boland RJ, Gaud KG, Keller MB. Antidepressants. In: Tasman A, Kay J, Lieberman JA, eds. *Psychiatry*. 4th ed. Chichester, UK: John Wiley & Sons; 2015:2052-2087.

Boyer EW, Shannon M. The serotonin syndrome. *N Engl J Med*. 2005;352:1112-1120.

Cipriani A, Furukawa TA, Salanti G, et al. Comparative efficacy and acceptability of 12 new-generation antidepressants: a multiple-treatment meta-analysis. *Lancet*. 2009;373:746-758.

Masand PS, Gupta S. Long term side effects of newer generation antidepressants: SSRIs, venlafaxine, nefazodone, bupropion, and mirtazapine. *Ann Clin Psychiatry*. 2002;14:175-182.

Mørk A, Pehrson A, Brennum LT, et al. Pharmacological effects of Lu AA21004: a novel multimodal compound for the treatment of major depressive disorder. *J Pharmacol Exp Ther*. 2012;340(3):666-675.

Pierz KA, Thase ME. A review of vilazodone, serotonin, and major depressive disorder. *The Primary Care Companion for CNS Disorders*. 2014;16(1):PCC.13r01554.

Renoir T. Selective serotonin reuptake inhibitor antidepressant treatment discontinuation syndrome: a review of the clinical evidence and the possible mechanisms involved. *Frontiers in Pharmacology*. 2013;4:45.

Spina E, Scordo MG. Clinically significant drug interactions with antidepressants in the elderly. *Drug Aging*. 2002;19:299-320.

Spina E, Trifirò G, Caraci F. Clinically significant drug interactions with newer antidepressants. *CNS Drugs*. 2012;26(1):39-67.

Stahl SM. *Essential Psychopharmacology: Neuroscientific Basis and Practical Applications*. 4th ed. New York, NY: Cambridge University Press; 2013.

Stahl SM, Grady MM, Moret C, Briley M. SNRIs: their pharmacology, clinical efficacy, and tolerability in comparison with older classes of antidepressants. *CNS Spectr*. 2005;10:732-747.

Stahl SM, Pradko JF, Haight BR, Modell JG, Rockett CB, Learned-Coughlin S. A review of the neuropharmacology of bupropion, a dual norepinephrine and dopamine reuptake inhibitor. *Primary Care Companion to The Journal of Clinical Psychiatry*. 2004;6(4):159-166.

KEY ABBREVIATIONS

5-HT = serotonin	NE = norepinephrine
DA = dopamine	REM = rapid eye movement
MAOI = monoamine oxidase inhibitor	SNRI = serotonin norepinephrine reuptake inhibitor
MDD = major depressive disorder	

Endocrinologic Disorders

CHAPTER 61

Diabetes Mellitus

Jessica L. Kerr

FOUNDATION OVERVIEW

Diabetes mellitus (DM) is a group of metabolic disorders characterized by high blood glucose as well as altered fat and protein metabolism that results from defects in insulin secretion, insulin action (sensitivity), or both. Type 1 diabetes mellitus (T1DM) characterized by insulin deficient and type 2 diabetes mellitus (T2DM) characterized by insulin resistance combined with beta cell dysfunction. Additional subclasses include gestational diabetes mellitus (GDM) and secondary diabetes associated with hormonal syndromes, medications, and diseases of the pancreas. The key differences between T1DM and T2DM are the pathophysiology, etiology of hyperglycemia, and clinical presentation; however, both are associated with microvascular and macrovascular complications.

T1DM is a cellular-mediated autoimmune process that destroys pancreatic β-cells resulting in insulin deficiency. Due to the lack of insulin, glucose is not able to be used as energy. The onset of symptoms leading to the diagnosis of T1DM is abrupt and includes polydipsia, polyuria, polyphagia, weight loss, or ketoacidosis. T2DM is impaired insulin secretion and insulin resistance at sites such as the liver, muscles, and adipocytes. Patients with T2DM can produce insulin, but the amount may not be sufficient to keep up with the body's glucose metabolism, or the insulin that is produced may not work appropriately at its receptor sites. There are multiple risk factors for the development of T2DM, including family history; obesity (ie, ≥20% over ideal body weight, or body mass index [BMI] ≥25 kg/m²); chronic physical inactivity; history of impaired glucose tolerance (IGT), impaired fasting glucose (IFG), or hemoglobin A1c (HbA1c) 5.7% to 6.4%; hypertension (≥140/90 mm Hg in adults); high-density lipoprotein (HDL) cholesterol less than or equal to 35 mg/dL (≤0.91 mmol/L) and/or a triglyceride level more than or equal to 250 mg/dL (≥2.83 mmol/L); history of vascular disease; presence of acanthosis nigricans; and polycystic ovary disease. Additionally, the prevalence of T2DM increases with age and varies widely among racial and ethnic populations. The prevalence of T2DM is especially high in Native Americans, Hispanic Americans, African Americans, Asian Americans, and Pacific Islanders. While the prevalence of T2DM increases with age, the disorder is increasingly being diagnosed in adolescence. The increased incidence of T2DM in adolescence and young adults has been attributed to an increase in overweight/obesity and sedentary lifestyle, in addition to genetic predisposition.

The clinical presentations of T1DM and T2DM are different. Most patients (75%) develop T1DM before age 20 years, but it can develop at any age. Individuals with T1DM are often thin and are prone to ketoacidosis if insulin is withheld or under conditions of severe physiological stress. Symptoms, such as polyuria, polydipsia, polyphagia, weight loss, and lethargy, are common at the time of initial presentation. In the outpatient setting, some patients present with vague complaints of weight loss and fatigue but other symptoms may not be apparent unless a comprehensive history is taken. Twenty percent to forty percent of patients with T1DM present with diabetic ketoacidosis (DKA) after several days of polyuria, polydipsia, polyphagia, and weight loss. Patients with T2DM often present without symptoms, but the presence of microvascular complications at the time of diagnosis suggests that many patients have had hyperglycemia for years. Often patients with T2DM are diagnosed during routine blood testing or screening. Lethargy, polyuria, nocturia, and polydipsia can be seen at diagnosis in some patients with T2DM, but significant weight loss is less common. Most patients with T2DM are overweight or obese.

SCREENING AND DIAGNOSIS

The prevalence of T1DM is low in the general population. Due to the acute onset of symptoms in most individuals, screening for T1DM in the asymptomatic general population is not recommended. Pregnant women, overweight adults, children who are at risk for diabetes be screened (Table 61-1). Screening identifies patients likely to develop or have diabetes. The American Diabetes Association (ADA) does not recommend fasting glucose levels as a measure of screening every patient. Patients at risk complete the ADA Diabetes Risk Screening Test. If a patient scores a 10 or greater a finger stick blood sample is recommended. The online version of this screening tool is available at http://www.diabetes.org/are-you-at-risk/diabetes-risk-test/. The diagnosis of diabetes or prediabetes is via evaluation of HbA1c, fasting, or random plasma glucose level, or with the oral glucose tolerance test (OGTT) (Table 61-2). The HbA1c evaluates glucose control over the last 2 to 3 months and can be expressed as the estimated average glucose (eAG)

To access your complimentary online question exams, visit https://accesspharmacy.mhmedical.com/NAPLEX.aspx

TABLE 61-1	Screening Recommendations for Diabetes in Adults, Children, and Pregnancy (GDM)		
Adults[a]		**Children[b]**	**Pregnancy[c]**
All adults who have a BMI ≥25 kg/m² and at least one additional risk factor below: ■ Physical inactivity ■ First-degree relative with diabetes ■ Ethnic population—African-American, Asian-American, Latino, Native American, Pacific islander ■ IFG or IGT or A1c ≥5.7% ■ HTN (≥140/90 mm Hg or on antihypertensive agents) ■ HDL-C <35 mg/dL and/or TG >250 mg/dL ■ Women with PCOS ■ GDM ■ History of CVD ■ Acanthosis nigricans		All children who have a BMI >85th percentile for age and sex, weight for height >85th percentile or weight >120% of ideal height plus at least two risk factors below: ■ Ethnic population—African-American, Asian-American, Latino, Native American, Pacific islander ■ Family history of T2DM in first- or second-degree relative ■ Signs of insulin resistance or condition associated with insulin resistance (PCOS, HTN, dyslipidemia, small-for-gestational-age birth weight, acanthosis nigricans)	All women should be screened for T2DM at first prenatal visit us general screening criteria. All women during wk 24-28 of pregnancy not known to have T2DM.

Abbreviations: BMI, body mass index; CVD, cardiovascular disease; GDM, gestational diabetes mellitus; HDL-C, high-density lipoprotein cholesterol; HTN, hypertension; IFG, impaired fasting glucose; IGT, impaired glucose tolerance; PCOS, polycystic ovarian syndrome; TG, triglycerides.

[a]Screening for prediabetes and diabetes should begin at the age of 45, if the patient lacks the above criteria. If the results are normal, repeat at least every 3 y.

[b]Screening should occur at age 10 or at the onset of puberty, if puberty occurs at a younger age. These recommendations are specifics for Type 2 diabetes and ≤18 y.

[c]Women with the diagnosis of GDM should be screened 4 to 12 wk postpartum for prediabetes or diabetes.

level. The eAG is expressed as measures of blood glucose levels. The eAG equation is: eAG (mg/dL) = 28.7 × A1c − 46.7.

PREVENTION

Lifestyle modifications can have a significant impact on diabetes development and reduce insulin resistance. For example, in the Diabetes Prevention Program (DPP) study patients were randomized to lifestyle modifications, metformin, or placebo. The lifestyle interventions cohort (physical activity for 150 min/wk and a healthy diet) reduced diabetes development by 58%, while the metformin cohort had a 31% reduction. Additionally, the ADA Consensus Development Panel recommends lifestyle interventions for patients at risk for diabetes. Oral medications including metformin, glucagon-like peptide 1 (GLP-1), acarbose, orlistat and thiazolidinediones are effective for diabetes prevention, however none of these agents are FDA approved for this indication. However, metformin is the only recommended medication because of the side effect profile of the other medications. Metformin is recommended for the prevention of diabetes in obese patients with IFG, IGT, and age less than 60 with an additional risk factor for diabetes.

Diabetes is associated with microvascular, macrovascular, and neuropathic complications (Table 61-3). The ADA recommends:

■ goal attainment for blood pressure and cholesterol,
■ antiplatelet therapy,

TABLE 61-2	Diagnosis of Diabetes or Classification of Prediabetes	
	Plasma Glucose Levels	**Methods for Diagnosis**
Prediabetes (At risk)	FPG: 100 mg/dL-125 mg/dL *or* 2-h plasma glucose 140 mg/dL-199 mg/dL *or* Hemoglobin A1c 5.7-6.4%	Fasting defined as no caloric intake for at least 8 h prior to blood sample 2-h plasma glucose level should be obtained after a 75-g anhydrous glucose OGTT Random plasma glucose defined as a glucose sample obtained at any time of the day without regard to meals Symptoms of hyperglycemia include polyuria, polydipsia, and unexplained weight loss
Diabetes	FPG: ≥126 mg/dL[a] *or* 2-h plasma glucose ≥200 mg/dL[a] *or* Random plasma glucose ≥200 mg/dL plus symptoms of hyperglycemia *or* Hemoglobin A1c ≥6.5%	

Abbreviations: FPG, fasting plasma glucose; OGTT, oral glucose tolerance test.

[a]In the absence of unequivocal hyperglycemia, these criteria should be confirmed by repeating a test on a different day.

- smoking cessation,
- screening and treatment for nephropathy, retinopathy, and neuropathy,
- proper foot and dental care,
- appropriate vaccinations.

TREATMENT

The primary goals of DM management are to reduce the risk for microvascular and macrovascular disease complications, to ameliorate symptoms, to reduce mortality, and to improve quality of life. Early diagnosis and treatment to near-normal glycemia reduces the risk for developing microvascular disease complications, but aggressive management of cardiovascular risk factors including smoking cessation, treatment of dyslipidemia, intensive blood pressure control, and antiplatelet therapy are needed to reduce the likelihood for developing macrovascular disease (Table 61-4). Hyperglycemia also contributes to poor wound healing by compromising white blood cell function and altering capillary function. Diabetic DKA and hyperosmolar hyperglycemic state (HHS) are severe manifestations of poor diabetes control, almost always requiring hospitalization. Minimizing weight gain and hypoglycemia, especially severe hypoglycemia, are also therapeutic goals and may necessitate altering glycemic goals. Patients are encouraged to self-monitor blood glucose and follow-up with their health care provider to address issues of hyperglycemia or hypoglycemia (Table 61-5).

The approved pharmacologic agents for glycemic control in T1DM are insulin and amylin analogs. T2DM glycemic control is obtained with oral antihyperglycemic agents, GLP-1 receptor agonists, or pramlintide with or without insulin. Antihyperglycemic agents should be selected based on their effectiveness in lowering glucose, extra glycemic effects that may reduce diabetes complications, safety profiles, tolerability, ease of use, and cost.

Injectable Therapy

Insulins

Insulin is classified by three parameters: (1) onset and duration of action, (2) purity, and (3) concentration. Beef and pork insulin are no longer used in the United States as all animal products have been discontinued. Two types of human insulins are available: (1) biosynthetic human insulin produced with recombinant DNA technology by genetically altering microorganisms and (2) biosynthetic human insulin produced with recombinant DNA technology in baker's yeast cells. Human insulin is less antigenic; therefore, the risk of allergy is reduced compared to animal insulin. Insulin is available in several concentrations containing 100 units/mL (U-100), 200 units/mL (U-200), 300 units/mL (U-300), or 500 units/mL (U-500) (this represents the number of insulin units per milliliter). The most commonly used insulin preparation is the U-100 concentration. Insulin U-500 and insulin analogues (lispro, aspart, glulisine, glargine, and detemir) are available

by prescription only. The mechanism of action for insulin is multifactorial (Table 61-6). It is recommended to choose a regimen that mimics normal physiological release of insulin. Therefore, the use of basal and bolus insulin is recommended for patients with T1DM and in select patients with T2DM requiring insulin therapy. There are currently four pharmacokinetic profiles available: (1) rapid, (2) short, (3) intermediate, and (4) long-acting insulin (Table 61-7). Insulin adverse effects include hypoglycemia and weight gain (anabolic effect of insulin and peripheral edema due to sodium retention). Local allergies may occur presenting with erythema, swelling, and urticaria at the injection site. Systemic allergies are not common; however, allergic reactions may occur with all forms of insulin. Patients may develop injection site reactions including lipohypertrophy (thickening of adipose tissue) and lipoatrophy (thinning of adipose tissue). These reactions may be reduced by rotating injection sites.

The dose of insulin must be individualized. In T1DM, the average daily requirement for insulin is 0.5 to 0.6 units/kg, with approximately 50% being delivered as basal insulin, and the remaining 50% dedicated to meal coverage. During the honeymoon phase, it may fall to 0.1 to 0.4 units/kg. During acute illness or with ketosis or states of relative insulin resistance, the need for higher dosages is common. In T2DM, a higher dosage is required for those patients with significant insulin resistance. Dosages vary widely depending on degree of insulin resistance and concomitant antihyperglycemic medication use.

Amylin Analog

Amylin is a neurohormone that is cosecreted with insulin in the secretory granules of pancreatic β-cells. Pramlintide is a synthetic analog of amylin used to reduce postprandial blood glucose levels. This occurs by suppressing postprandial glucagon release via limiting gluconeogenesis, slowing gastric emptying and inducing postprandial satiety. Pramlintide is indicated for use in T1DM and T2DM. Gastrointestinal adverse effects are common and include nausea (20% in T2DM; 40% in T1DM), vomiting (10%) and anorexia. These adverse effects may be limited by commencing therapy at a low dose and titrate upward once the adverse effects from the previous dose have subsided. In monotherapy, hypoglycemia is not a concern due to the glucose-dependent mechanism of action. However, if used in combination with preprandial rapid or short-acting insulin, the insulin dose should be reduced by 50%. Promotility medications may interact with pramlintide. If rapid absorption of the promotility medication is necessary, it is recommended to take the medication 1 hour before or 3 hours after administration of pramlintide. Table 61-8 lists key characteristics for pramlintide.

Glucagon-Like Peptide (GLP-1) Receptor Agonists

GLP-1 is released from the bowel to stimulate glucose-dependent insulin release. Circulating endogenous GLP-1 is degraded within minutes by the dipeptidyl peptidase IV enzyme (DPP-IV). The mechanism for lowering fasting and postprandial blood glucose level is glucose-dependent. GLP-1

TABLE 61-3	Prevention and Management of Complications for Adults		
	Goals	**Screening/Diagnosis**	**Treatment**
Macrovascular Complications			
Hypertension[a]	SBP <140 mm Hg DBP <90 mm Hg	Screening: Measure BP at every visit BP should be assessed every routine visit Patients with BP >120/80 should engage in LSM of weight control, DASH diet, moderation of alcohol and increased physical activity	LSM ACEi or ARB is recommended for patient with diabetes + increased urine albumin excretion Additional BP medications may be added to gain control. Use appropriate agents for patient with multiple comorbidities Review special populations to make sure no contraindications or unwanted side effects occur
Hyperlipidemia[b]	TC <200 mg/dL TG <150 mg/dL HDL-C >50 mg/dL in women HDL-C >40 mg/dL in men	Screening: Yearly fasting lipid panel for most patients. In patients with low-risk lipid profiles (LDL-C <100 mg/dL, HDL-C >50 mg/dL, and TG <150 mg/dL) at least every 2 y	LSM focusing on reduced saturated fats, trans fats, cholesterol and n-3 fatty acids, fiber, and plant stanols/sterol intake in addition to physical activity *Statin* therapy, regardless of baseline lipid levels, for patients <40 y + atherosclerotic CVD risk factors, consider using moderate/high intensity statin + LSM Patients 40-75 y without atherosclerotic CVD risk factors consider using moderate-intensity statin + LSM Patients >75 y +/− CVD risk factors should be evaluation for consideration of at least moderate intensity statin Review special populations to make sure no contraindications or unwanted side effects occur, may consider following other cholesterol guidelines
Antiplatelet therapy	To be on therapy if no contraindications or specific population concerns are present	Screening: Advised to assess each visit for antiplatelet therapy	Aspirin therapy 75-162 mg/d for secondary prevention Consider aspirin therapy 75-162 mg/d as primary prevention in those who are increase risk with at least one addition major risk factor for CVD Aspirin should not be recommended for those with low atherosclerotic CVR (women/men <50 y)
Smoking cessation	Complete cessation	Screening: Advised to assess smoking status at each visit	Include smoking cessation counseling and forms of treatment for cessation
Microvascular Complications			
Nephropathy	Reduce the risk or slow the progression leading to chronic kidney disease or dialysis Achieve BP and glucose goals	Screening: Obtain annual test to assess excretion of urine albumin in patients with T1DM with duration of diabetes ≥5 y and in all T2DM at diagnosis	ACEi or ARBs should be used in nonpregnant patients who have an elevated urine albumin-to-creatinine ratio of >30mg/g When eGFR is <60 mL/min/1.73 m² evaluate renal function and monitor for CKD
Retinopathy	Reduce the risk or slow progression leading to blindness or other complications Achieve BP and glucose goals	Screening: 1. All T1DM within 5 y after diagnosis should have a dilated/comprehensive examination 2. All T2DM shortly after diagnosis of diabetes. Further follow-up examinations should be performed yearly[c] 3. Women with preexisting diabetes who are planning pregnancy or to become pregnant should have an examination within the first trimester	Laser photocoagulation may be an option Retinopathy is NOT a contraindication to a cardioprotective dose of aspirin
Neuropathy	Reduce the risk or slow progression leading to DPN Obtain glucose goals	Screening: 1. All patients should be assessed starting at diagnosis for T2DM and 5 y after diagnosis for T1DM, with at least annual follow-up	Medical relief of symptoms related to DPN and autonomic neuropathies are recommended: TCA (amitriptyline, nortriptyline, imipramine), gabapentin, carbamazepine, pregabalin,[d]), tramadol, tapentadol[d], capsaicin cream, duloxetine[d] or capsaicin cream Surgical options

(Continued)

TABLE 61-3	Prevention and Management of Complications for Adults (Continued)		
	Goals	**Screening/Diagnosis**	**Treatment**
		2. Assess annually using simple clinical tests (pinprick sensation, vibration perception [128-Hz tuning fork], and 10-g monofilament pressure sensation at the distal plantar region of both great toes and metatarsal joints for DPN)	Smoking cessation
Foot care	Reduce the risk of infection or amputation	Screening: All patients with diabetes should have an annual comprehensive foot examination/inspection which includes screening recommendations for neuropathies	Provide education to patients
	Achieve glucose goals	Initial screening for PAD is recommended; possible ABI should be performed if symptoms are present	Smoking cessation
Dental care	Reduce the risk of infection or gingival disorders	Screening: Yearly to twice yearly	Preventative measures
	Achieve glucose goals		Good oral hygiene
Infectious Disease			
Influenza vaccination	Reduce the risk of infection or death	Screening: Identify those who have not received the vaccine. It is important to start talking with patients about this in the summer and throughout influenza season	Provide influenza vaccine yearly during influenza season
Pneumococcal vaccination	Reduce the risk of infection or death	Screening: Identify those who have not received the vaccine	Provide vaccine up to three times throughout the lifetime. Revaccinate patients who are >65 y of age and received initial dose ≥5 y ago and were <65 y of age at that time. Recommended to provide the PCV13 vaccine first after the age of 65 then 1 y post to be followed up with PPSV23. Patients with diabetes under the age of 65 y of age should have the PPSV23 vaccine.
Hepatitis B	Reduce the risk of infection or death	Screening: Identify those who have not received the vaccine	Vaccinate those who are 19-59 y of age. Clinical judgment can be used once patient is ≥60 y old due to limited risk old

Abbreviations: ABI, ankle brachial index; ACEi, angiotensin-converting enzyme inhibitor; ARB, angiotensin receptor blocker; BP, blood pressure; CKD, chronic kidney disease; CrCl, creatinine clearance; CVD, cardiovascular disease; CVR, cardiovascular risk; DBP, diastolic blood pressure; DPN, distal symmetric polyneuropathy; eGFR, estimated glomerular filtration rate; HDL-C, high-density lipoprotein cholesterol; HTN, hypertension; LDL-C, low-density lipoprotein cholesterol; LSM, lifestyle modifications; PAD, peripheral arterial disease; PCV13, pneumaticallyonjugate vaccine; PSV23, pnpneumaticallyysaccharide vaccine; SBP, systolic blood pressure; TC, total cholesterol; TCA, tricyclic antidepressants; TG, triglycerides.

[a]Lower blood pressure targets may be acceptable due to other comorbid conditions or patient character specifics (younger patients, shorter duration of diabetes diagnosis).

[b]Recent 2013 AHA/ACC Hyperlipidemia management guidelines no longer recommend specific LDL-C goals and indicate that statin dose-intensity should be moderate to high.

[c]Less frequent examination may be appropriate following one or more normal eye examination.

[d]FDA-approved treatment for painful diabetic neuropathy.

analogs can suppress glucagon release, reduce hepatic glucose production, improve first-phase insulin release, slow gastric emptying, and decrease appetite. Due to the alteration of gastric emptying, many adverse effects are like pramlintide. Newer generations of GLP-1 analogs have an improved tolerability profile and A1c lowering. Patients should be instructed to eat slowly and limit portion sizes as satiety will occur. Hypoglycemic reactions may be increased when used in combination with oral insulin secretagogues or insulin. Adverse effects for this class can include pancreatitis, gastrointestinal symptoms. Patients with self/family-history of thyroid cancers should not

be consider candidate to use once daily liraglutide or once weekly formulations of dulaglutide, exenatide or semaglutide. Table 61-8 lists key characteristics for GLP-1 analogs.

Oral Therapies

Sulfonylureas

Sulfonylureas are classified as first- or second-generation agents. This classification differentiates side effects, protein binding, and potency. Second-generation sulfonylureas (glyburide, glipizide, and glimepiride) are 100 to 200 times

TABLE 61-4	Selected American Diabetes Association Recommendations
Recommendation Area	**Specific Recommendation**
Screening for diabetes	Screen overweight or obese at any age; screen those without risk factors beginning at age 45 y
	To screen for diabetes an FPG, 2-h 75-g OGTT, or HbA1c are appropriate
	Interval between screenings should be individualized based on risk, or every 3 y
Monitoring	Home blood glucose monitoring is recommended for patients on multidose insulin or pump therapy at least prior to meals and snacks, and before events such as driving
	Patients on other therapeutic interventions, including oral agents may perform home blood glucose monitoring, but ongoing instruction to patient on how to adjust therapy based on monitoring must be in place
	Quarterly HbA1c in individuals not meeting glycemic goals, twice yearly in individuals meeting glycemic goals, should be performed
	In adults, measure fasting lipid profile at least annually
	At least once a year, quantitatively assess urinary albumin (eg, urine albumin-to-creatinine ratio [UACR]) and estimated glomerular filtration rate (eGFR) in patients with type 1 diabetes duration of ≥5 y and in all patients with type 2 diabetes
	All patients should be screened for diabetic peripheral neuropathy (DPN) starting at diagnosis of type 2 diabetes and 5 y after the diagnosis of type 1 diabetes, at least annually thereafter, using simple clinical tests, such as a 10-g monofilament
	A dilated eye examination should be performed within 5 y of diagnosis in type 1 DM, and shortly after diagnosis in type 2 DM, with follow-up every year, or every 2-3 y as recommended by an eye specialist
Glycemic goals	HbA1c goal for nonpregnant adults in general is <7% (<0.07; <53 mmol/mol Hb)
	HbA1c goal should be individualized, with <6.5% (<0.065; <48 mmol/mol Hb) if achieved without significant hypoglycemia or adverse effects in younger, long-life expectancy, and no CVD patients
	Less stringent HbA1c goal (<8% [<0.08; <64 mmol/mol Hb]) may be appropriate in patients with a history of severe hypoglycemia, limited life expectancy, advanced micro/macrovascular complications or comorbidities, or in difficult to reach goal patients despite adequate therapy
	Hospitalized patients:
	Critically ill: 140-180 mg/dL (7.8-10.0 mmol/L) (A), or more stringent guidelines down to 110-140 mg/dL (6.1-7.8 mmol/L) if without hypoglycemia (C)
	Noncritically ill: No clear evidence but in general premeal BG <140 mg/dL (<7.8 mmol/L) and random BG <180 mg/dL (<10.0 mmol/L) (C)
	A basal plus correction insulin regimen is the preferred treatment for patients with poor oral intake or who are taking nothing by mouth (NPO). An insulin regimen with basal, nutritional, and correction components is the preferred treatment for patients with good nutritional intake (A)
Treatment	
Prevention of type 2 diabetes	Patients with IGT (A), IFG (E), or an A1c of 5.7%-6.4% (0.057-0.064; 39-46 mmol/mol Hb) (E) should be referred to an intensive diet and physical activity behavioral counseling program targeting loss of 7% of body weight and increasing moderate-intensity physical activity (such as brisk walking) to at least 150 min/wk
	Metformin may be considered with IGT (A), IFG (E), or an A1c 5.7%-6.4% (0.057-0.064; 39-46 mmol/mol Hb) (E), especially in obese, <60-year-old patients, and women with prior GDM
Medical nutrition therapy	Weight loss is recommended for all insulin-resistant/overweight or obese individuals. Either low-carbohydrate, low-fat calorie restricted diets, or Mediterranean diets may work
	In individuals with type 2 diabetes, ingested protein appears to increase insulin response without increasing plasma glucose concentrations. Therefore, carbohydrate sources high in protein should not be used to treat or prevent hypoglycemia
	Saturated fat should be <7% (<0.07; <53 mmol/mol Hb) of total calories
	Monitoring carbohydrate intake by carbohydrate counting, exchanges, or experienced estimation is recommended to achieve glycemic goals
	Routine supplementation with antioxidants, such as vitamins E and C is not advised due to lack of efficacy
	A Mediterranean-style eating pattern, rich in monounsaturated fatty acids, may benefit glycemic control and CVD risk factors and can therefore be recommended as an effective alternative to a lower-fat, higher-carbohydrate eating pattern
Physical activity	150 min/wk of moderate intensity exercise spread over at least 3 d and with no more than 2 d without exercise
	Resistance training of large muscle groups should be ≥2 times/wk
Blood pressure	Systolic blood pressure should be treated to <140 mm Hg
	Diastolic blood pressure should be treated to <90 mm Hg
	Lower goals systolic blood pressure <130 mm Hg and/or diastolic blood pressure <80 mm Hg may be appropriate for some, such as younger patients, if attained without undue treatment burden

(Continued)

TABLE 61-4	Selected American Diabetes Association Recommendations (*Continued*)
Recommendation Area	**Specific Recommendation**
	Lifestyle intervention for elevated blood pressure consists of weight loss, if overweight or obese; a Dietary Approaches to Stop Hypertension (DASH)-style dietary pattern including reducing sodium and increasing potassium
	Initial drug therapy should be with an ACEi or ARB; if intolerant to one, the other should be tried
Nephropathy	In treatment of nonpregnant patients with modest (30-299 mg/d) (C), or higher levels (≥300 mg/d) (A) of urinary albumin excretion, either ACE inhibitors or ARBs are recommended
Dyslipidemia	If lipids are abnormal, annual monitoring is reasonable; if the LDL-C ≥100 mg/dL (≥2.59 mmol/L) upon screening, recheck every 5 y at a minimum is reasonable
	Lifestyle modification focusing on the reduction of saturated fat, trans fat, and cholesterol intake; increase omega-3 acids, viscous fiber, and plant stanols/sterols; weight loss if indicated, and increased physical activity should be recommended
	For patients with diabetes aged <40 y with additional CVD risk factors, consider using moderate or high-intensity statin (C)
	For patients with diabetes aged 40-75 y without additional CVD risk factors, consider using moderate-intensity statin (A); if with additional risk factors, high-intensity statin (B)
	For patients with diabetes aged 75 y without additional risk factors consider using moderate intensity statin (B); if with additional risk factors, high-intensity statin (B)
Antiplatelet therapy	Use aspirin (75-162 mg daily) for secondary cardioprotection
	Use aspirin (75-162 mg) for primary prevention in type 1 or 2 DM if the 10-y risk of CVD is ≥10%, the patient is >50 (men) or >60 (women) with at least one additional major CVD risk factor is present
Hospitalized patients	Critically ill: by IV insulin protocol (E); noncritically ill: scheduled subcutaneous insulin with basal, nutritional, and correction coverage (A)
Psychosocial	Include assessment of the patient's psychological and social situation as an ongoing part of the medical management of diabetes

Reproduced with permission from DiPiro JT, Talbert RL, Yee GC, et al: *Pharmacotherapy: A Pathophysiologic Approach*, 10th ed: New York, NY: McGraw-Hill; 2017.

more potent than first-generation sulfonylureas (acetohexamide, chlorpropamide, tolazamide, and tolbutamide). However, when prescribed in equipotent doses, sulfonylureas are equally effective at glucose lowering. Sulfonylureas bind to the sulfonylurea receptor 1 (SUR1) on pancreatic β-cells and block the ATP-sensitive K$^+$ channel causing a decrease in potassium efflux and depolarization of the membrane. Calcium channels open allowing an influx of Ca^{2+}. This increase of intracellular Ca^{2+} relocates the secretory granules of insulin to the cell surface and results in exocytosis of insulin. Additionally, sulfonylureas reduce the secretion of glucagon due to their ability to stimulate the release of somatostatin. Sulfonylureas are metabolized by the liver to active and inactive metabolites. Sulfonylureas with parent drugs or active metabolites that are renally excreted require dosage adjustments in the presence of renal dysfunction to reduce the risk of hypoglycemia. Hypoglycemia is more common in sulfonylureas with longer half-lives (chlorpropamide and glyburide). Other adverse effects

include skin rash, erythema, urticaria, pruritus, dyspepsia, nausea and vomiting, and weight gain. A disulfiram-like reaction may be noted with the usage of the first-generation sulfonylureas, chlorpropamide, and tolbutamide. Chlorpropamide may induce hyponatremia by enhancing the effects of antidiuretic hormone on the collecting ducts in the kidney causing a syndrome of inappropriate antidiuretic hormone (SIADH) reaction. Drug interactions involving sulfonylureas include alterations in protein binding and coadministration of drugs that induce or inhibit cytochrome P-450 (CYP) 2C9. Due to increased side effects with first-generation agents, it is recommended to use second-generation sulfonylureas. Table 61-8 lists key characteristics for sulfonylureas.

Short-Acting Secretagogues

Meglitinides Nateglinide, a phenylalanine amino acid derivative, and repaglinide, a benzoic acid derivative, have a mechanism of action similar to sulfonylureas except that the

TABLE 61-5	Glucose Goals^{a,b}
A1c	<7%
Fasting SMBGs	80-130 mg/dL
Postprandial SMBGs	<180 mg/dL, 1-2 h after the start of the meal

Abbreviation: SMBGs, self-monitoring blood glucose.
^{a}For nonpregnant adults.
^{b}Select populations may not choose to target these goals due to increased risk for complications or hypoglycemia.

TABLE 61-6	Mechanism of Action for Insulin

- Stimulates glucose uptake into muscles and adipose tissue
- Stimulates hepatic glucose uptake
- Stimulates amino acid uptake and protein synthesis
- Inhibits hepatic glucose production
- Inhibits breakdown of triglycerides in adipose tissue
- Inhibits protein degradation

TABLE 61-7	Pharmacokinetic Profile of Insulin				
Insulin	**Trade Name (Manufacturer)**	**Onset (h)**	**Peak (h)**	**Duration (h)**	**Comments**
Rapid-Acting					

Insulin aspart	NovoLog (Novo Nordisk), Fiasp, (Novo Nordisk)	≤0.25	0.5-1.5	3-4	▪ Bolus-type insulin
					▪ Route of administration: SC, IV, CSII
					▪ Available in insulin-delivery devices (pens)
					▪ Concentration: U-100
					▪ Formulations:
					  1. NovoLog
					  2. Fiasp
					  3. NovoLog 70/30 (insulin aspart protamine/aspart)
					▪ Unopened refrigerated vial/pen device: good until expiration date
					▪ Opened vial/pen device: good for 28 d regardless of refrigeration (once device is open, should not be refrigerated)
					▪ Lactation: unknown if excreted in human milk

Insulin lispro	Humalog (Eli Lilly)	≤0.25	0.5-1.5	3-4	▪ Bolus-type insulin
					▪ Route of administration: SC, IV, CSII
					▪ Available in insulin-delivery devices (pens)
					▪ Concentration: U-100, U-200
					▪ Formulations:
					  1. Humalog
					  2. Humalog 50/50 (insulin lispro protamine/lispro)
					  3. Humalog 75/25 (insulin lispro protamine/lispro)
					▪ Unopened refrigerated vial/pen device: good until expiration date
					▪ Opened vial/pen device: good for 28 d regardless of refrigeration (once device is open, should not be refrigerated)
					▪ Lactation: unknown if excreted in human milk

Insulin glulisine	Apidra (Sanofi-aventis)	≤0.25	0.5-1.75	1-3	▪ Bolus-type insulin ▪ Administered: SC, IV, CSII ▪ Available in insulin-delivery device (pens) ▪ Concentration: U-100 ▪ Mix only with NPH ▪ Unopened refrigerated vial/pen device: good until expiration date ▪ Opened vial/pen device: good for 28 d regardless refrigeration (once device is open, should not be refrigerated) ▪ Lactation: unknown if excreted in human milk
Short-Acting					

Regular	Humulin R (Eli Lilly), Novolin R (Novo Nordisk)[a]	0.5-1	2-3	3-6	▪ Bolus-type insulin
					▪ Administered: SC, IV, CSII
					▪ Concentration: U-100 and U-500 (only Humulin R)
					▪ Formulations:
					  1. Humulin R
					  2. Humulin 70/30 (insulin isophane suspension/regular)
					  3. Novolin R
					  4. Novolin 70/30 (insulin isophane suspension/regular)
					  5. ReliOn R
					  6. ReliOn 70/30 (insulin isophane suspension/regular)
					▪ Unopened refrigerated vial/device: good until expiration date
					▪ Opened vial/pen device: see individual package inserts (once device is open, should not be refrigerated)
					▪ Lactation: unknown if excreted in human milk

(Continued)

TABLE 61-7   **Pharmacokinetic Profile of Insulin** (*Continued*)

Insulin	Trade Name (Manufacturer)	Onset (h)	Peak (h)	Duration (h)	Comments
Intermediate-Acting					

NPH	Humulin N (Eli Lilly), Novolin N (Novo Nordisk)	1-4	4-10	10-16	▪ Basal-type insulin
					▪ Administered: SC
					▪ Formulation:
					  1. Humulin N
					  2. Humulin 70/30 (insulin isophane suspension/regular)
					  3. Novolin N
					  4. Novolin 70/30 (insulin isophane suspension/regular)
					  5. ReliOn N
					  6. ReliOn 70/30 (insulin isophane suspension/regular)
					▪ Concentration: U-100
					▪ Mix only with short or rapid-acting insulin.
					▪ Unopened refrigerated vial/pen device: good until expiration date
					▪ Opened vial/pen device: see individual package inserts (once device is open, should not be refrigerated)
					▪ Lactation: unknown if excreted in human milk

Long-Acting					
Insulin glargine	Lantus (Sanofi-aventis), Basaglar (Eli Lilly), Toujeo (Sanofi-aventis)[b], Toujeo Max	1.5	None	20-24	▪ Basal-type insulin ▪ Administered: SC ▪ Concentration: U-100, U-300 ▪ Do *not* mix with any other insulins/solutions ▪ Unopened refrigerated vial/device: good until expiration date ▪ Opened vial/device: good for 28 d regardless of refrigeration (once device is open, should not be refrigerated)[b] ▪ Lactation: unknown if excreted in human milk
Insulin detemir	Levemir (Novo Nordisk)	1.5	Relatively none	12-24	▪ Basal-type insulin ▪ Administered: SC ▪ Concentration: U-100 ▪ Do *not* mix with any other insulins/solutions ▪ Unopened refrigerated vial/pen device: good until expiration date ▪ Opened vial/pen device: good for up to 42 d regardless of refrigeration (once device is open, should not be refrigerated)
Insulin Degludec	Tresiba (Novo Nordisk)	1.5		42	▪ Lactation: unknown if excreted in human milk ▪ Basal type insulin ▪ Administered SC ▪ Available only in pen device ▪ Concentration U-100 and U-200 ▪ Do not mix with any other insulins/solutions ▪ Unopened device: good for up to 56 d ▪ Lactation: unknown if excreted in human milk

Abbreviations: CSII, continuous subcutaneous insulin infusion; IV, intravenously; SC, subcutaneously.

[a]Time curves are based on the U-100 concentration. U-500 concentration has a much different and possibly prolonged peak and duration of action.

[b]U-300 insulin by trade name U-300 is only available by pen device and has an in use expiration date of 42 days at room temperature. U-100 insulin glargine by trade name of Basaglar is only available in pen device.

stimulation of insulin release from the β-cells is glucose dependent. Therefore, a lowering of postprandial glucose occurs. This glucose-dependent mechanism allows glucose levels to reduce to normal while also decreasing the release of insulin. This mechanism and short duration of action are responsible for the low incidence of hypoglycemia as compared to sulfonylureas. Weight gain may occur with meglitinides. Due to the short duration of action, meglitinides should be taken 30 minutes preprandial. Drug interactions may occur because of metabolism by CYP450 3A4. Concomitant use of gemfibrozil and repaglinide may cause excessive hypoglycemia and is contraindicated. Nateglinide is metabolized by the cytochrome P-450 pathway with approximately 70% being metabolized by CYP 2C9 and 30% by CYP 3A4. Short-acting secretagogues

Generic Name	Trade Name	Class	FDA Indication	Dose	Pharmacokinetics	Monitoring	Clinical Concerns
Pramlintide	Symlin	Amylin analog	T1DM T2DM	**T1DM:** starting dose of 15 mcg tid with meals titrated to maximum dose of 60 mcg tid with meals **T2DM:** starting dose of 60 mcg tid with meals titrated to maximum dose of 120 mcg tid with meals	**A:** 30%-40% BA **D:** not extensively PPB **M:** Renal **E:** Renal	Renal function A1c; signs and symptoms of hypoglycemia, excessive weight loss	1. Reduce preprandial insulin by 50% if started on pramlintide 2. Use caution in patients with GI motility disorders 3. Use caution in patients receiving oral medication requiring rapid GI absorption 4. Should not be considered in patients with A1c >9%
Exenatide	Byetta (bid)	Incretin	T2DM	Starting dose of 5 mcg bid for 4 wk titrated to maximum dose of 10 mcg bid Dosing should be spaced 6 h apart, normally given before the morning and evening meals up to 60 min before meals	**A:** 65%-76% BA **D:** ND **M:** ND **E:** Renal	Renal function A1c Signs and symptoms of acute pancreatitis, risk of thyroid cancers of self and known family history	1. No dosage adjustments indicated in mild-moderate renal or hepatic insufficiency 2. Not recommended for use in CrCl <30 m/min (specific for exenatide products) 3. Use caution in patients with GI motility disorders 4. Use caution in patients receiving oral medication requiring rapid GI absorption 5. Positive outcomes with weight loss (reduction 0.3-2.6 kg) 6. Postmarketing cases of acute pancreatitis. Screen for thyroid cancers
	Bydureon (qwk)			Starting and final titration dose of 2 mg once weekly	*Bydureon may take 6-7 wk to get to steady state due to the slow release of microspheres		
Liraglutide	Victoza	Incretin	T2DM	Starting subcutaneous administration dose of 0.6 mg qd × 7 d titrated to 1.2 mg qd × 7 d then if necessary for glucose control titrated to max dose of 1.8 mg qd	**A:** 55% BA **D:** extensively PPB **M:** ND **E:** <6% found in urine/feces		
Dulaglutide	Trulicity	Incretin	T2DM	Starting dose of 0.75 mg once weekly, may increase to maximum dose of 1.5 mg weekly	**A:** 47-65% **D:** Volume of distribution is 17-19 L **M:** ND **E:** elimination t1/2 5 d		
Semaglutide	Ozempic	Incretin	T2DM	Dosing: 0.25 mg once weekly for 4 wk. Dose can be increase to 0.5 mg once weekly for 4 wk. If further efficacy is needed then increase to 1.0 mg weekly	**A:** 89% BA **D:** >99% PPB, volume of distribution 12.5L **M:** proteolytic cleavage of peptide backbone and beta-oxidation of fatty acid side chain **E:** 3% found in urine/primary route is urine/feces		

(Continued)

TABLE 61-8   Noninsulin Agents for Use in the Management of T1DM and T2DM (*Continued*)

Generic Name	Trade Name	Class	FDA Indication	Dose	Pharmacokinetics	Monitoring	Clinical Concerns
Lixisenatide	Adlyxin	Incretin	T2DM	Dosing: 10 mcg daily x 14 d, then increase to 20 mcg daily	**A:** ND **D:** Volume of distribution ~100L **M:** ND **E:** through glomerular filtration, proteolytic degradation		
Acetohexamide	Dymelor	Sulfonylurea (first generation)	T2DM	Starting dose of 250 mg qd-bid titrated to maximum dose of 1500 mg daily	**A:** ND **D:** 60%-90% PPB **M:** Liver, (inactive/active metabolites) **E:** Renal 80%	Renal and hepatic function, A1c, Electrolytes	1. Should not be used in renal dysfunction due to renal clearance of parent drug and active metabolites 2. Dosage adjustment may be needed for hepatic impairment 3. Should not be used due to side-effect profile and risk of hypoglycemia compared to second-generation sulfonylureas
Chlorpropamide	Diabinese	Sulfonylurea (first generation)	T2DM	Starting dose of 250 mg qd titrated to maximum dose of 750 mg daily Plateau effect: 500 mg daily for most patients	**A:** ND **D:** 60%-90% PPB **M:** Liver, moderate **E:** Renal 80%-90% (unchanged in urine)	Renal and hepatic function, A1c, Electrolytes	1. Use caution with renal and hepatic dysfunction; dosage recommendations are not provided 2. Should not be used due to side-effect profile and risk of hypoglycemia compared to second-generation sulfonylureas
Tolazamide	Tolinase	Sulfonylurea (first generation)	T2DM	Starting dose of 100 mg daily and titrated to maximum dose of 1000 mg daily	**A:** ND **D:** ND **M:** Liver, extensive (active metabolites) **E:** Renal 85% Feces 7%	Renal and hepatic function, A1c, Electrolytes	1. Caution use in renal and hepatic dysfunction; dosage recommendations are not provided 2. Should not used due to side-effect profile and risk of hypoglycemia compared to second-generation sulfonylureas

Tolbutamide	Orinase	Sulfonylurea (first generation)	T2DM	Starting dose of 1-2 g qd or in divided doses titrated to maximum dose of 3 g daily	**A:** ND **D:** 80%-99% PPB **M:** Liver, extensive (inactive metabolites) **E:** Renal, extensive	Renal and hepatic function, A1c, Electrolytes	1. Caution use in renal and hepatic dysfunction; dosage recommendations are not provided 2. Should not be used due to side-effect profile and risk of hypoglycemia compared to second-generation sulfonylureas
Glipizide	Glucotrol	Sulfonylurea (second generation)	T2DM	Starting dose of 2.5-5 mg qd-bid titrated to maximum dose of 40 mg daily (qd or divided doses)	**A:** 100% BA **D:** 97%-99% PPB **M:** Liver, extensive (inactive metabolites) **E:** Renal 63%-89% Feces 11%	Renal and hepatic function, A1c,	1. Possibly less hypoglycemic reactions with glipizide than with glyburide and similar hypoglycemic reactions with glimepiride 2. First choice of sulfonylurea therapy in renal dysfunction 3. Good agent to use early in disease progression due to MOA
Glipizide	Glucotrol XL	Sulfonylurea (second generation)	T2DM	Starting dose of 5-10 mg daily titrated to maximum dose of 20 mg daily	**A:** 100% BA **D:** 97%-99% PPB **M:** Liver, extensive (inactive metabolites) **E:** Renal 63%-89% Feces 11%	Renal and hepatic function, A1c,	1. Possibly less hypoglycemic reactions with glipizide than with glyburide and similar hypoglycemic reactions with glimepiride 2. First choice of sulfonylurea therapy in renal dysfunction 3. Good agent to use early in disease progression due to MOA
Glyburide	DiaBeta Micronase	Sulfonylurea (second generation)	T2DM	Starting dose of 1.25-5 mg qd-bid titrated to maximum of 20 mg daily (qd or in divided doses)	**A:** ND **D:** 99% PPB **M:** Liver, extensively (active metabolites) **E:** Renal 50%	Renal and hepatic function, A1c,	1. Not recommended with CrCl <50 mL/min because as much as 50% of dose may be eliminated unchanged in the urine
Micronized glyburide	Glynase	Sulfonylurea (second generation)	T2DM	Starting dose of 1.5-3 mg qd-bid titrated to maximum of 12 mg daily (qd or in divided doses)	**A:** ND **D:** 99% PPB **M:** Liver, extensively (active metabolites) **E:** Renal 50%	Renal and hepatic function, A1c,	1. Not recommended with CrCl <50 mL/min because as much as 50% of a dose may be eliminated unchanged in the urine

(Continued)

TABLE 61-8 Noninsulin Agents for Use in the Management of T1DM and T2DM (*Continued*)

Generic Name	Trade Name	Class	FDA Indication	Dose	Pharmacokinetics	Monitoring	Clinical Concerns
Glimepiride	Amaryl	Sulfonylurea (second generation)	T2DM	Starting dose of 1–2 mg daily titrated to maximum dose of 8 mg daily	**A:** 100% BA **D:** >99% PPB **M:** Liver (CYP 2C9) **E:** Renal 60%	Renal and hepatic function, A1c,	1. Caution use with renal and hepatic dysfunction; dosage recommendations are not provided
Nateglinide	Starlix	Meglitinides	T2DM	Starting and maximum dose of 120 mg tid Do not take if not administering a meal	**A:** 72%–75% BA **D:** 97%–99% PPB **M:** Liver, extensively (CYP 3A4/2C9) **E:** Renal (13%–14% unchanged in urine)	Renal and hepatic function, A1c,	1. Not recommended to be used with sulfonylureas due to similar MOA 2. Caution with moderate-to-severe hepatic impairment 3. Displacement of protein-bound drugs may cause interactions and complications
Repaglinide	Prandin	Meglitinides	T2DM	A1c, <8%: starting dose of 0.5 mg with each meal titrated to maximum dose of 16 mg daily A1c, >8%: starting dose of 1–2 mg with each meal titrated to maximum dose of 16 mg daily Do not take if not administering a meal	**A:** 56% BA **D:** > 98% PPB **M:** Liver, extensively (CYP 3A4/2C8) **E:** Fecal 90%; renal 8% (0.1% unchanged in urine)	Renal and hepatic function, A1c,	1. Not recommended to be used with sulfonylureas due to similar MOA 2. Caution with moderate-to-severe hepatic impairment 3. Displacement of protein-bound drugs may cause interactions and complications
Acarbose	Precose	α-Glucosidase inhibitors	T2DM	Starting dose of 25 mg qd-tid with meals titrated up to maximum dosage of 50 mg tid[a] Do not take if not administering a meal	**A:** <2% BA **D:** ND **M:** Exclusively GI: intestinal bacteria **E:** Fecal 51%; renal 34%	Renal and hepatic function, A1c,	1. Treatment of hypoglycemia must be with simple glucose 2. Use in patients with SCr >2 mg/dL has not been studied, therefore not recommended 3. May not be drug of choice for reduction in postprandial blood glucose in patients with GI issues due to side-effect profile
Miglitol	Glyset	α-Glucosidase inhibitors	T2DM	Starting dose of 25 mg qd-tid with meals titrated to maximum dose of 100 mg tid Do not take if not administering a meal	**A:** 50%–100% BA; depending on dose **D:** <4% PPB **M:** Not metabolized **E:** Renal >95% (unchanged in urine)	Renal function, A1c,	1. Treatment of hypoglycemia must be with simple glucose 2. Plasma miglitol levels had a two-fold increase in patients with CrCl <25 mL/min 3. May not be drug of choice for reduction in postprandial blood glucose in patients with GI issues due to side-effect profile

				Starting dose of 500 mg twice daily or 850 mg daily titrated to maximum dose of 2550 mg daily	A: 50%-60% BA D: 90% PPB M: Not metabolized E: Renal 90%	Renal and hepatic function, A1c, signs and symptoms of lactic acidosis	1. Due to the risk of lactic acidosis, metformin is contraindicated in females with SCr ≥1.4 mg/dL and males with SCr ≥1.5 mg/dL 2. Other conditions or medications causing hypoprofusion and concomitant use of metformin may increase the risk of lactic acidosis and caution should be exercised
Metformin	Glucophage Riomet (solution)	Biguanide	T2DM				
Extended-release metformin	Glucophage XR Fortamet Glumetza	Biguanide	T2DM	Starting dose of 500 mg daily titrated to maximum dose of 2500 mg daily			1. Metallic taste 2. Do not use in estimated GFR <30 mL/min 3. Comes in a liquid formulation (Riomet)
Pioglitazone	Actos	TZD	T2DM	Starting dose of 15-30 mg daily titrated to maximum dose of 45 mg daily	A: ND BA D: >90% PPB M: Hepatic (CYP 2C8/3A4; active metabolites) E: Fecal metabolite/ unchanged Renal 15%-30%: Metabolites/conjugates	Liver function Edema Signs/ symptoms of HF	1. May cause or exacerbate HF 2. Not recommended in patients with symptomatic HF 3. Contraindicated in NYHA III/IV 4. Pioglitazone provides a more positive lipid-profile effect than rosiglitazone 5. Associated risk for bladder cancer after 1 year of use
Rosiglitazone	Avandia	TZD	T2DM	Starting dose of 4 mg qd or in divided doses titrated to maximum dose of 8 mg daily	A: 99% BA D: 99.8% PPB M: Liver, extensive (CYP 2C8/9) E: Renal 64%, (no unchanged drug in urine) Feces: 23%	Liver function Edema Signs/ symptoms of HF	1. May cause or exacerbate HF 2. Not recommended in patients with symptomatic HF 3. Contraindicated in NYHA III/IV

(Continued)

TABLE 61-8   Noninsulin Agents for Use in the Management of T1DM and T2DM (Continued)

Generic Name	Trade Name	Class	FDA Indication	Dose	Pharmacokinetics	Monitoring	Clinical Concerns
Sitagliptin	Januvia	DPP-IV inhibitor	T2DM	Starting and maximum dose of 100 mg daily Renal adjustments: 1. 50 mg daily. CrCl ≥30 mL/min–<50 mL/min or SCr in men >1.7 mg/dL–≤3.0 mg/dL or in women >1.5 mg/dL–≤2.5 mg/dL 2. 25 mg daily: Severe and ESRD CrCl <30 mL/min or SCr in men >3.0 mg/dL or in women >2.5 mg/dL or on dialysis	**A:** 87% BA **D:** 38% PPB **M:** Liver, minimal (CYP3A4/2C8) **E:** ~ Renal 87% (79% unchanged in urine)	Renal function, A1c	1. Lower dosage of sulfonylurea if used in combination 2. SJS, angioedema, anaphylaxis has been documented 3. Renal adjustments necessary 4. Pancreatitis risk
Saxagliptin	Onglyza	DPP-IV inhibitor	T2DM	Starting dose of 2.5 mg or 5 mg daily titrated to maximum dose of 5 mg daily Renal adjustments: 1. 2.5 mg daily: CrCl <50 mL/min	**A:** ND **D:** Negligible PPB **M:** Liver (CYP 3A4/5, active metabolite) **E:** Renal/hepatic	Renal function, A1c	1. Lower dosage of sulfonylurea if used in combination 2. SJS, angioedema, anaphylaxis has been documented 3. Combination use with CYP450 inhibitor may require use of saxagliptin 2.5 mg dose 4. Renal adjustments necessary 5. Pancreatitis risk
Linagliptin	Tradjenta	DPP-IV inhibitor	T2DM	5 mg daily	**A:** ND **D:** PPB is concentration dependent **M:** ND **E:** Renal 5% (90% unchanged in urine)	A1c	1. Lower dosage of sulfonylurea if used in combination 2. No renal adjustments needed 3. Pancreatitis risk
Alogliptin	Nesina	DPP-IV inhibitor	T2DM	25 mg daily Renal adjustments: 1. 12.5 mg daily if CrCl ≥30 to <60 mL/min 2. 6.25 mg if CrCl <30 mL/min	**A:** 100% BA **D:** 20% PPB **M:** some CYP2D6/CYP3A4) **E:** 75% renal; 13% feces	Renal function, A1c	1. Lower dosage of sulfonylurea if used in combination 2. SJS, angioedema, anaphylaxis has been documented 3. Renal adjustments necessary 4. Pancreatitis risk

Drug	Brand	Class	Indication	Dosing	Pharmacokinetics	Monitoring	Notes
Canagliflozin	Invokana	SGLT2 inhibitor	T2DM	Starting dose of 100 mg daily with first meal of day, may increase to 300 mg daily. Do not exceed 100 mg daily if eGFR <60 mL/min/1.73 m². Do not use product if eGFR <45 mL/min/1.73 m²	**A:** 65% BA **D:** extensively PPB (99%) **M:** O-glucuronidation/minimal 3A4 (7%) **E:** Renal	Renal function, A1c, Lipid panel, Blood pressure	1. Renal dosing needed 2. Genital mycotic infections may occur 3. Hyperkalemia and hyponatremia noted, monitor fluid status 4. Hypotension 5. An imbalance in bladder cancers was observed in clinical trials (Dapagliflozin) 6. Possible increase risk for amputations was observed (Canagliflozin) 7. Increase risk of euglycemia DKA
Dapagliflozin	Farxiga	SGLT2 inhibitor	T2DM	Starting dose of 5 mg daily in the morning, may increase to 10 mg daily in the morning. Do not use if < 60 mL/min/1.73 m²	**A:** ~78% for 10 mg dose **D:** 91% PPB **M:** UGT1A9 with minor CYP450 **E:** Renal 75% Feces 21%		
Empagliflozin	Jardiance	SGLT2 inhibitor	T2DM	Starting dose of 10 mg daily. May be increased to 25 mg daily. Do not use if eGFR is below 45 mL/min/1.73 m². Discontinue if eGFR falls below 45 mL/min/1.73 m²	**A:** first order absorption **D:** Vd = 73 L, PPB 86% **M:** uridine 5'-diphospho-glucuronosyltransferases UGT2B7, UGT1A3, UGT1A8, and UGT1A9 **E:** feces = 41%; urine = 54%		
Bromocriptine	Cycloset	Dopamine receptor agonist	T2DM	Starting dose of 0.8 mg daily titrated weekly to maximum dose of 1.6–4.8 mg daily	**A:** 65%–95% BA **D:** 90%–96% PPB **M:** Extensively by GI and liver (CYP 3A4) **E:** Bile	Renal/hepatic function A1c, BP	1. Hypotension 2. Somnolence 3. Psychiatric disorders treated with a bromocriptine may exacerbate the disorder or diminish the effectiveness of drugs used to treat the disorder 4. Interaction with dopamine receptor antagonists 5. Caution with renal/hepatic impairment—no dosage adjustment recommendations 6. Neutral effects on lipids

Abbreviations: A, absorption; BA, bioavailability; bid, twice daily; CrCl, creatinine clearance; CYP, cytochrome P450; D, distribution; DKA, diabetic ketoacidosis; eGFR, estimated glomerular filtration rate; E, elimination; ESRD, end-stage renal disease; GI, gastrointestinal; HF, heart failure; M, metabolism; MI, myocardial infarction; MOA, mechanism of action; ND, not documented; NYHA, New York Heart Associations; PPB, plasma protein binding; qd, once daily; SCr, serum creatinine; SJS, Stevens-Johnson syndrome; tid, three times daily; T1DM, type 1 diabetes mellitus; T2DM, type 2 diabetes mellitus; UGT, uridine diphosphate glucuronosyltransferase.

ªIf the patient is >60 kg, then maximum dose is 100 mg tid.

should not be used in combination with sulfonylurea therapy. Nateglinide and repaglinide are beneficial for patients who are close to the A1c goal of less than 7% and who have elevated postprandial blood glucose. Table 61-8 lists key characteristics for meglitinides.

α-Glucosidase Inhibitors Acarbose and miglitol delay the breakdown of sucrose and complex carbohydrates in the intestinal brush border by competitively inhibiting enzymes such as maltase, isomaltase, sucrose, and glucoamylase. Their place in therapy is reducing postprandial blood glucose. Hypoglycemia is not common with monotherapy because insulin release is not stimulated. If hypoglycemia occurs during monotherapy or in combination with other antihyperglycemic agents, it is recommended to treat the hypoglycemic reaction with oral glucose or milk with lactose sugar. Side effects include gastrointestinal such as abdominal bloating, diarrhea, and flatulence. Starting with a low dose and titrating slowly may decrease or eliminate gastrointestinal symptoms. These agents are poorly absorbed; therefore, drug interactions are minimal. Table 61-8 lists key characteristics for α-glucosidase inhibitors.

Biguanide Metformin is an insulin sensitizer that increases insulin action at the site of muscle and adipose tissue. Additionally, metformin decreases hepatic glucose production. Metformin is renally eliminated by tubular secretion and glomerular filtration and contraindicated in renal insufficiency with creatinine clearance of less than 30 mL/min. Dosage adjustments or other considerations for metformin use need to be evaluated whenever the creatinine clearance falls below 60 mL/min. Administration of metformin in renal insufficiency may cause lactic acidosis. Although lactic acidosis is rare, conditions that affect the production or accumulation of lactic acid (shock, heart failure, recent myocardial infarction, chronic obstructive lung disease) increase the risk. Approximately 30% of patients using metformin complain of gastrointestinal side effects including diarrhea and abdominal discomfort. Administration after a meal, commence with lower doses, titrate over several weeks, or the extended-release formulation may decrease the gastrointestinal side effects. Metformin is recommended as first line in the treatment of T2DM for most patients. Table 61-8 lists key characteristics for metformin.

Thiazolidinediones Thiazolidinediones (TZDs) are insulin sensitizers due to their indirect effect at muscle, liver, and adipose tissue. Second-generation TZDs, pioglitazone and rosiglitazone bind to the peroxisome proliferator-activated receptor-γ (PPAR-γ) located on adipose and vascular cells. These receptors regulate carbohydrate and lipid metabolism. Pioglitazone is beneficial on triglycerides and high density lipoprotein cholesterol (HDL-C) levels due to increased activity of PPAR-α. Both agents cause fluid retention and edema initiating or exacerbating heart failure. TZDs are contraindicated in patients with New York Heart Association (NYHA) class III and IV heart failure and should be used with caution in patients with NYHA class I and II heart failure or other

cardiac diseases. Weight gain of 2 to 4 kg is common and positively predicts a larger reduction in A1c. In postmenopausal women, TZDs increase fracture rate in the upper and lower limbs. Patient treated with pioglitazone may be at increased risk for bladder cancer. Hepatotoxicity is rare with the second-generation TZDs, but a baseline and periodic aminotransferase monitoring is recommended. Table 61-8 lists key characteristics for TZDs.

Dipeptidyl Peptidase-IV (DPP-IV) Inhibitors

Alogliptin, linagliptin, sitagliptin, and saxagliptin are DPP-IV inhibitors. These agents block the DPP-IV enzymes activity and in a glucose-dependent manner prolong the half-life of endogenous glucagon-like peptide 1 (GLP-1). This enhances insulin secretion and reduces postprandial glucagon. While the mechanism of action is similar to amylin analogs and incretin mimetics, it does not alter gastric emptying. Mild hypoglycemia may occur. Adverse effects consist of upper respiratory tract infections, nasopharyngitis, headache, and urinary tract infections. Cases of pancreatitis, urticaria, and angioedema have been documented. Due to the hepatic metabolism, the saxagliptin dose should be reduced when used with strong inhibitors of CYP 3A4/3A5. Dose modification is required for select DPP-IV inhibitors in renal dysfunction. Table 61-8 lists key characteristics for DPP-IV inhibitors.

Sodium Glucose Transport 2 Protein Inhibitors

Canagliflozin, dapagliflozin, and empagliflozin inhibit the SGLT-2 resulting in a decrease of blood glucose by enhancing renal excretion of glucose at the S1 segment of the proximal tubule. Side effects include hyperkalemia and hyponatremia, hypotension, and dehydration. Additional effects include genital mycotic infections, weight loss, decrease in blood pressure, and bladder cancer (dapagliflozin). It is important to monitor for sign and symptoms of euglycemic DKA and appropriate foot care to limit the risk of amputations. Table 61-8 lists key characteristics for SGLT-2 inhibitors.

Dopamine Receptor Agonist

Bromocriptine is a sympatholytic dopamine D_2 subtype receptor agonist approved for diabetes. The mechanism of action is unknown. It is postulated that bromocriptine provides inhibitory effects on serotonin turnover in the central nervous system resulting in alterations in hypothalamic circadian activity, thereby improving insulin sensitivity. Side effects include headache, dizziness, and gastrointestinal intolerance (nausea). Hypoglycemia may occur with monotherapy and is increased when used in combination with sulfonylureas. Orthostatic hypotension may be observed upon the initiation of therapy and with escalating dosage. Bromocriptine is not recommended in patients with psychotic disorders due to its mechanism of action (increase in dopamine). Patients on potent inhibitors or inducers of CYP 3A4 may have increased levels of bromocriptine. Table 61-8 lists key characteristics for bromocriptine.

SPECIAL CONSIDERATIONS

The ADA recommends screening for complications at the time of diagnosis of DM. Current recommendations continue to advocate yearly dilated eye examinations in T2DM and an initial dilated eye examination in the first 3 to 5 years in T1DM, then yearly thereafter. Less frequent eye examinations, every 2 to 3 years, may be appropriate if the patient has no evidence of retinopathy and is at low risk of developing eye disease. The patient's blood pressure should be assessed at each visit. The feet should be examined at each visit including palpation of distal pulses and a visual inspection for skin integrity, calluses, and deformities. Screening for nephropathy should be done at the time diagnosis in patients T2DM and 5 years after diagnosis if the patient has T2DM with urine microalbumin. Yearly testing for lipid abnormalities is appropriate if the patient is on lipid lowering therapy. It is generally accepted that a thyroid stimulating hormone concentration be measured in patients with T2DM as thyroid abnormalities are more common in DM.

CASE Application

Use the following patient profile to answer questions 1 to 4.

JR is a 68-year-old African American man with a new diagnosis of T2DM. He was classified as having prediabetes (at risk for developing diabetes) 5 years before the diagnosis and has a strong family history of T2DM. JR's blood pressure was 150/92 mm Hg. His laboratory results revealed an A1c of 9.2%, glucose of 279 mg/dL, cholesterol panels renal/hepatic function were normal today.

Past Medical History	Hypertension (diagnosed 4 years ago) Hyperlipidemia (diagnosed 2 years ago) Pancreatitis [idiopathic] (acute hospitalization 3 years ago)
Family History	T2DM
Medication	HCTZ 25 mg daily, Simvastatin 10 mg daily
Vitals	BP: 150/92 mm Hg, P: 78 beats/min, RR: 12 Waist circumference 46 inches Weight: 267 lb Height: 5′6″ BMI: 43.1 kg/m^2

1. What known risk factor(s) does JR display for the development of diabetes? Select all that apply.

   a. Obesity
   b. African American
   c. Family history of diabetes
   d. Prediabetes

2. Six weeks later, JR returns to obtain new labs results. He tests his blood glucose and blood pressures at home. Within the last 4 weeks he has started an exercise program 4 times per week consisting of cardio/resistant

training for 40 minutes per session. JR indicates he is motivated to beat this and has reviewed a lot of educational material about diabetes.

Home blood pressure (mm Hg): [electronic cuff/sitting/ right arm]	150/85, 161/74, 152/82, 148/83, 156/71, 150/74
Home fasting blood glucose readings (mg/dL)	278, 218, 219, 119, 156, 193

Today's Labs and Vitals

A1c → 8.1%	Fasting glucose → 176 mg/dL
Total cholesterol → 201 mg/dL	LDL cholesterol → 124 mg/dL
SCr → 0.98 mg/dL	Na → 138 mEq/L, K → 4.3 mEq/L
Albumin-to-creatinine ratio: 152 mg/g creatinine	
BP: 148/92 mm Hg	P: 75 beats/min

Due to elevated home and clinic blood pressure readings it has been decided a second blood pressure medication is needed. Which agent would be the best to start in order to achieve blood pressure control and prevent microvascular complications?

   a. Clonidine 0.1 mg twice daily
   b. Isosorbide mononitrate 60 mg daily
   c. Lisinopril 5 mg daily
   d. Terazosin 10 mg at bedtime

3. Today, JR's A1c value was an 8.1%, which is down from 6 weeks ago. Despite improvements in lifestyle choices, he has met the diagnosis for diabetes. As the clinical pharmacist in charge of the diabetes management clinic, you provide him options of lifestyle, medications or both. He would like to start a drug therapy in addition to more stringent lifestyle modifications. Which drug therapy would be the best for JR to trial?

   a. Pramlintide subcutaneously 15 mcg twice daily.
   b. Liraglutide subcutaneously 0.6 mg daily for 1 week with an upward titration until glycemic goals have been met (do not exceed more than 1.8 mg daily).
   c. Metformin 500 mg daily by mouth with an upward titration to 2000 mg/d (qd or bid) over several days to weeks.
   d. Acarbose 100 mg three times daily by mouth with each meal.

4. What preventative measures should JR be educated on to reduce the risk of complications associated with diabetes? Select all that apply.

   a. Perform daily foot inspections.
   b. See a dentist/dental hygienist routinely throughout the year.
   c. Receive the pneumococcal vaccine yearly.
   d. Assuming no contraindications, take an aspirin daily for cardioprotection.

5. What counseling information should a pharmacist provide to a patient taking a diuretic and ARB therapy in order to reduce the risk of side effects? Select all that apply.

   a. Avoid/limit salt substitutes.
   b. Stop exercising because these blood pressure medications will cause your blood pressure to drop significantly resulting in falls.
   c. Stay hydrated.
   d. Do not take an HMG-CoA Reductase inhibitor (statin) while on blood pressure medications.

Use the following patient profile for questions 6 and 7.

PT is a 58-year-old white woman with a BMI of 32 kg/m². She was recently referred to a dietitian for weight reduction and lost 40 lb over the past 8 months. She is very dedicated to getting her blood glucose under control. At this time she is not willing to go on insulin therapy. She tests her blood glucose at home: fasting blood glucose readings are all less than 130 mg/dL and her 2-hour postprandial glucose readings are in the range of 190 to 200 mg/dL. Her past medical history (PMH) is hypertension, hyperlipidemia, T2DM, sleep apnea, and depression; family history (FHx) is unknown (patient was adopted); and social history (SHx) is (+) tobacco use—1.5 packs per day for 42 years, (+) alcohol use—2 sifters (6 oz) of gin and tonic daily. Her medications are metformin 1000 mg twice daily, enalapril 10 mg twice daily, hydrochlorothiazide 25 mg daily, citalopram 40 mg daily, rosuvastatin 5 mg daily. Her laboratory results revealed normal electrolyte and cholesterol panels, normal renal and hepatic function A1c 7.9%.

6. What therapy is the best option to help lower her A1c and improve glycemic control considering her specific patient profile concerns?

   a. Exenatide twice daily with meals
   b. Chlorpropamide 250 mg daily
   c. Increase metformin to 2000 mg twice daily
   d. Start insulin NPH 10 units at bedtime

7. Which of the following is/are common side effect(s) of glucophage?

   a. Weight gain
   b. Diarrhea
   c. Lactic acidosis
   d. Pancreatitis

8. Commercially available Symlin should be administered by which route?

   a. Intravenously
   b. Intramuscularly
   c. Subcutaneously
   d. Via insulin pump

9. Which insulin can be mixed with insulin glargine in one syringe in order to decrease daily insulin injections?

   a. Insulin aspart

   b. Insulin regular
   c. Insulin detemir
   d. Insulin glargine cannot be mixed with any insulin in a given syringe/pen/insulin pump

10. Due to acarbose mechanism of action to lower blood glucose, what is the most appropriate way to treat a hypoglycemic reaction in a patient taking acarbose?

   a. 1 candy bar
   b. 3 to 4 glucose tablets
   c. 2-ounces of mash potatoes
   d. Inject 2 units of rapid-acting insulin at the time of episode

11. Which drug would not be recommended for a patient with an ejection fraction of 32% and in symptomatic heart failure documented by a NYHA class III?

   a. Starlix
   b. Invokana
   c. Pioglitazone
   d. Victoza

Use the following patient profile for questions 12 to 14.

EP is a 38-year-old female patient that comes in for diabetes education and management. She was diagnosed 12 years ago and states lately she is not able to control her diet although she continues a 1600 calorie diet with appropriate daily carbohydrate intake (per dietitian prescription) and walks 40 minutes every day of the week. She states compliance with all medications. She denies any history of hypoglycemia despite being able to identify signs and symptoms and describe appropriate treatment strategies.

PMH	T2DM, HTN, obesity, depression, s/p thyroidectomy due to thyroid cancer
FHx	Noncontributory
SHx	(-) Smoking, alcohol use, past marijuana use while in high school
Medications	Metformin 850 mg tid, Glipizide 20 mg bid, Lisinopril 20 mg daily, Sertraline 100 mg daily, Multivitamin daily
Vitals	BP: 128/82 mg Hg, P: 72, BMI: 31 m/kg²
Labs	Na: 134 mEq/L, K: 5.4 mEq/L, Cl: 106 mEq/L, BUN: 16 mg/dL SCr: 0.89 mg/dL, Glucose: 128 mg/dL, A1c: 7.8%

12. In order to reduce the risk of side effects or to eliminate contraindications to therapy, what objective measure(s) of EP do you need to assess before you recommend canagliflozin? Select all that apply.

   a. Blood pressure
   b. CrCl or SCr
   c. Potassium concentration
   d. Sodium concentration

13. EP states that she is not ready to start insulin, but has heard about newer drug therapies that help limit weight gain or actually cause weight loss. Which drugs might EP be referring to? Select all that apply.

    a. Alogliptin
    b. Canagliflozin
    c. Exenatide once weekly
    d. Rosiglitazone

14. Based on EP's profile above, which of the agents would be able to obtain an A1c goal of less than 7% with limited side effects projected to occur?

    a. Bydureon
    b. Farxiga
    c. Januvia
    d. Precose

15. How many minutes before a meal should a patient administer glulisine insulin?

    a. 15 minutes before the start of a meal.
    b. 30 minutes before the start of a meal.
    c. 60 minutes before the start of a meal.
    d. Glulisine is a basal insulin and administration should be regardless of the mealtime.

16. Which of the following is true regarding the action of insulin?

    a. Enhances ketone production
    b. Stimulates glucose uptake in the periphery
    c. It activates peroxisome-proliferator-activated receptor-γ (PPAR-γ)
    d. Increases amylin production

17. Adjustments or selection of antihyperglycemic drug therapy should be based on which of the following concerns? Select all that apply.

    a. Blood glucose levels
    b. History of genital mycotic infections
    c. Frequency of hypoglycemic reactions
    d. Liver function tests if the patient is on a TZD

18. Which of the following statements are true of repaglinide? Select all that apply.

    a. Dosage of repaglinide should be administered regardless of meal.
    b. Normal treatment of hypoglycemia is recommended for patients on repaglinide.
    c. Caution for hypoglycemic in concomitant therapy with gemfibrozil.
    d. Maximum dose of repaglinide is 16 mg daily (divided with meals).

19. Which drug therapy may mask the signs of hypoglycemia?

    a. Atenolol
    b. Valsartan
    c. Hydrochlorothiazide
    d. Pioglitazone

20. Place the following insulin products in order of onset. Start with the fastest onset.

Unordered Response	Ordered Response
NPH	
Detemir	
Regular	
Aspart	

TAKEAWAY POINTS »

- Type 1 diabetes mellitus (T1DM) is an autoimmune disorder that results in insulin deficiency.
- T2DM is impaired insulin secretion and insulin resistance at sites such as the liver, muscles, and adipocytes.
- Diabetes management consists of glycemic control, blood pressure, and cholesterol management to reduce the risk of microvascular, macrovascular, and neuropathic complications.
- An A1c test is recommended on a quarterly basis to reflect the status of long-term glucose control (until glucose control is achieved at which time biannual measurement of A1c is recommended).
- The eAG is recommended to be used when educating patient about the result of the A1c.
- Lifestyle modification and metformin therapy have been recommended by the ADA for the treatment of prediabetes in select patients.

- There are different pharmacokinetic profiles of available insulin products which aid in mimicking normal physiologic release of insulin.
- Patients on metformin need to be educated about diarrhea and the signs and symptoms of lactic acidosis. These patients need to have continual monitoring for renal dysfunction or signs and symptoms of organ hypoprofusion.
- Patients on TZDs should have liver function tests periodically and should be educated about possible signs and symptoms for heart failure.
- New agents, such as DPP-IV inhibitors, GLP-1 analog, SGLT2-inhibitors have positive nonglycemic parameters. Their limited risk for hypoglycemia and weight neutral/loss effects can be viewed as a positive for providers and patients.

BIBLIOGRAPHY

American Diabetes Association. Standards of medical care in diabetes. *Diabetes Care.* 2014;37(suppl 1):S5-S80.

Nolte Kennedy MS. Pancreatic hormones & antidiabetic drugs. In: Katzung BG, Masters SB, Trevor AJ, eds. *Basic & Clinical Pharmacology.* 12th ed. New York, NY: McGraw-Hill; 2012:chap 41.

Powers AC, D'Alessio D. Endocrine pancreas and pharmacotherapy of diabetes mellitus and hypoglycemia. In: Brunton LL, Chabner BA, Knollmann BC, eds. *Goodman & Gilman's The Pharmacological Basis of Therapeutics.* 12th ed. New York, NY: McGraw-Hill; 2011:chap 43.

Triplitt CL, Repas T, Alvarez C. Diabetes Mellitus. In: DiPiro JT, Talbert RL, Yee GC, Matzke GR, Wells BG, Posey L, eds. *Pharmacotherapy: A Pathophysiologic Approach.* 10th ed, New York, NY: McGraw-Hill.

Ulbrich TR, Krinsky DL. Self-care concepts of selected chronic disorders. In: Krinsky DL, Berardi RR, Ferreri SP, et al., eds. *Handbook of Nonprescription Drugs: An Interactive Approach to Self Care.* 17th ed. Washington, DC: American Pharmacists Association; 2012:825-841.

KEY ABBREVIATIONS

ADA = American Diabetes Association
BMI = body mass index
DKA = diabetic ketoacidosis
DM = diabetes mellitus
DPP = Diabetes Prevention Program
DPP-IV = dipeptidyl peptidase IV enzyme
eAG = estimated average glucose
GDM = gestational diabetes mellitus
GLP-1 = glucagon-like peptide 1
HbA1c = hemoglobin A1c
HDL = high-density lipoprotein
HDL-C = high density lipoprotein cholesterol

HHS = hyperosmolar hyperglycemic state
IFG = impaired fasting glucose
IGT = impaired glucose tolerance
NYHA = New York Heart Association
OGTT = oral glucose tolerance test
PPAR-γ = peroxisome proliferator-activated receptor-γ
SIADH = syndrome of inappropriate antidiuretic hormone
SUR1 = sulfonylurea receptor 1
T1DM = Type 1 diabetes mellitus
T2DM = Type 2 diabetes mellitus
TZDs = thiazolidinediones

62

Thyroid Disorders

Elizabeth W. Blake

FOUNDATION OVERVIEW

The thyroid gland is located in the front of the neck and operates via negative feedback to synthesize thyroid hormones. The hypothalamus produces thyrotropin-releasing hormone (TRH) which stimulates the pituitary to release thyroid-stimulating hormone (TSH). TSH, also known as thyrotropin, stimulates the synthesis and release of thyroid hormones from the thyroid gland. Formation of thyroid hormones requires iodination of tyrosine residues by thyroid peroxidase to produce monoiodinated and diiodinated residues that couple to form triiodothyronine (T_3) and levothyroxine (T_4). Circulating levels of T_3 and T_4 regulate TSH secretion via negative feedback. The thyroid gland is responsible for the production of T_4 and less than 20% of T_3. Peripheral conversion of T_4 to T_3 forms the majority of T_3. Compared to T_4, T_3 is more potent, less bound to plasma proteins, and has a shorter half-life. Thyroid hormones affect multiple organ systems throughout the body and alterations in hormone concentrations and TSH lead to hyper- or hypothyroidism (Tables 62-1 and 62-2).

Thyrotoxicosis occurs when excessive thyroid hormones are present, and the majority of cases are caused by hyperthyroidism due to Graves disease. Graves disease is an autoimmune condition in which antibodies form against the thyrotropin receptor and stimulate the production of thyroid hormones. The remaining causes of hyperthyroidism are toxic nodular goiter, adenomas or tumors, and drug induced. Thyrotoxicosis presents with nervousness, anxiety, palpitations and tachycardia, weight loss, sleep disturbances, frequent bowel movements, and heat intolerance. Women experience irregular menses or decreased fertility and men have decreased libido or gynecomastia. Graves disease may induce ophthalmopathies including exophthalmos. Select patients present with a thyroid storm, a rare and life-threatening form of hyperthyroidism.

Hyperthyroidism diagnosis includes a thorough evaluation including a comprehensive history and physical examination and laboratory evaluation of thyroid hormones. TSH concentrations will be decreased to less than 0.01 mIU/L and unbound T_3 and T_4 concentrations will be elevated. Subclinical hyperthyroidism results when T_4 concentrations remain within the normal reference range but serum TSH is decreased. Though rarely needed for diagnosis, the presence of thyrotropin-receptor antibodies (TRAb) or thyroid-stimulating immunoglobulins may indicate Graves disease. Radioactive iodine uptake tests may further indicate thyrotoxicosis.

Hypothyroidism occurs when there are insufficient amounts of thyroid hormones detected in the body. Hashimoto thyroiditis is a chronic autoimmune disorder and the most common cause of hypothyroidism in the United States (congenital hypothyroidism occurs frequently in other parts of the world due to iodine deficiency). Hypothyroidism develops slowly, and signs and symptoms include fatigue, cold intolerance, constipation, dry skin, weight gain, goiter, or hoarseness. Depression and slow mental cognition also occur. Additionally, patients may experience bradycardia, dyslipidemia, edema, irregular or heavy menses, and infertility. Rarely, coma, seizure, or hypothermia occur.

Primary hypothyroidism is diagnosed by elevated TSH concentrations with a decrease in serum free T_4 concentrations. Overt symptomatic hypothyroidism will have TSH levels greater than 10 mIU/L. Patients with autoimmune thyroiditis may test positive for thyroid antibodies such as antithyroid peroxidase antibodies or other antithyroid antibodies. Subclinical hypothyroidism may be diagnosed by slightly elevated TSH concentrations between 4.5 mIU/L and 10 mIU/L while T_4 concentrations remain within the normal reference range. Additionally, a 40% diurnal variation in TSH concentrations occurs with the lowest levels occurring late afternoon, further confounding the diagnosis of hypothyroidism. Nonthyroidal illnesses and drugs may also affect TSH concentrations. Even in the presence of hypothyroidism, certain drugs including glucocorticoids and dopamine suppress TSH concentrations.

TREATMENT

Hyperthyroidism

General Overview

Since Graves disease is the most common cause of hyperthyroidism, treatment recommendations focus on this disease state. Treatment options include thyroidectomy, radioiodine therapy, and antithyroid medications (Tables 62-3 and 62-4). Clinical judgment and patient preference should be considered when determining a treatment plan.

TABLE 62-1	**Physiologic Effects of Thyroid Hormones**	
Target Tissue	**Effect**	**Mechanism**
Heart	Chronotropic	Increase number and affinity of β-adrenergic receptors
	Inotropic	Enhance responses to circulating catecholamines
		Increase proportion of α-myosin heavy chain (with higher ATPase activity)
Adipose tissue	Catabolic	Stimulate lipolysis
Muscle	Catabolic	Increase protein breakdown
Bone	Developmental and metabolic	Promote normal growth and skeletal development; accelerate bone turnover
Nervous system	Developmental	Promote normal brain development
Gut	Metabolic	Increase rate of carbohydrate absorption
Lipoprotein	Metabolic	Stimulate formation of LDL receptors
Other	Calorigenic	Stimulate oxygen consumption by metabolically active tissues (exceptions: adult brain, testes, uterus, lymph nodes, spleen, anterior pituitary) Increase metabolic rate

Reproduced with permission from Hammer GD, McPhee SJ: *Pathophysiology of Disease: An Introduction to Clinical Medicine*, 7th ed. New York, NY: McGraw-Hill; 2014.

Specific Agents

Antithyroid Drugs The thioamides (methimazole, propylthiouracil) are given as monotherapy for hyperthyroidism or in preparation for radioactive iodine therapy or surgery. These agents block the formation of thyroid hormones by preventing the incorporation of iodine into tyrosine residues by thyroid peroxidase. Additionally, propylthiouracil blocks the peripheral conversion of T_4 to T_3. Over the course of therapy, thioamides provide immunosuppressive effects including a reduction in the concentrations of TRAb. Although the two drugs are similar in action, methimazole is preferred due to a better side effect profile. Propylthiouracil is only preferred during the first trimester of pregnancy. As propylthiouracil binds to plasma protein in much greater amounts than methimazole, less drug then crosses the placenta.

Methimazole and propylthiouracil are given orally with rapid gastrointestinal absorption. Higher starting doses with multiple daily dosing may be required, but doses may be reduced as symptoms of thyrotoxicosis improve (Table 62-3).

TABLE 62-2	**Overview of Thyroid Disorders**	
Disorder	**TSH**	**T_4 and T_3**
Thyrotoxicosis or hyperthyroidism	Low or undetectable	Increased
Subclinical hyperthyroidism	Low or undetectable	Normal
Hypothyroidism	Elevated	Decreased
Subclinical hypothyroidism	Elevated	Normal

TABLE 62-3	**Antithyroid Medications**	
	Methimazole	**Propylthiouracil**
Mechanism of action	Blocks formation of T_4 and T_3	Blocks formation of T_4 and T_3
		Blocks peripheral conversion of T_4 to T_3
Starting dose	30-60 mg divided into 2-3 daily doses	300-600 mg divided into 2-3 daily doses
Maintenance dose	5-10 mg daily	100-300 mg divided in 2-3 daily doses
Half-life	6-9 h	1-2.5 h
Protein binding	None	60%-80%
Major side effects	Agranulocytosis, rash, cholestasis, arthralgias	Agranulocytosis, vasculitis, hepatotoxicity (black box warning), arthralgias, rash

Due to a long duration of action, methimazole is administered once daily, while propylthiouracil requires dosing two to three times daily. Both are actively concentrated in the thyroid gland. Inadequate dosing of antithyroid medications leads to continuation of hyperthyroidism or development of hypothyroidism.

The goal of monotherapy is to achieve remission and is defined as the ability to maintain normal thyroid function for 1 year without antithyroid medication. Remission is achieved in 30% to 50% of patients within 18 to 24 months; however, relapse occurs frequently. Most relapses occur within the first year of stopping therapy. Factors such as male sex, age less than 40 years, a large goiter, higher baseline T_4 and T_3 concentrations, longer duration of disease , and higher levels of TRAb reduce the likelihood of remission. Strategies to improve remission rates, such as longer duration of therapy (>1 year) or addition of thyroxine, have not proven to be successful. Radioactive iodine therapy remains an alternative for patients who fail antithyroid medications versus retrial with medications.

Symptom and laboratory improvement is seen in 3 to 8 weeks after initiation of antithyroid medication. While T_4 and T_3 normalize quickly, serum concentrations of TSH takes months to normalize. Thyroid function tests should be assessed every 4 to 8 weeks until euthyroid levels are reached. As symptoms improve and thyroid function returns to normal, doses of antithyroid medications may be reduced. Monotherapy should be continued for 12 to 18 months to induce remission, then tapered or discontinued once TSH is normal. After discontinuation of antithyroid medications, thyroid function tests should be evaluated every 1-3 months for the first year to monitor for relapse.

Side effects of antithyroid medications occur in 5% to 25% of patients and include cutaneous reactions, gastrointestinal upset, and arthralgias. The occurrence of arthralgias must be taken seriously, and antithyroid medication must be stopped as it may signal the development of a severe polyarthritis. Other side effects occur infrequently but produce severe reactions. A complete blood count and liver function tests (LFTs) should be drawn prior to starting antithyroid medications to aid in evaluation of side effects. Agranulocytosis occurs in 0.5% of patients treated with antithyroid medications. Most cases occur

TABLE 62-4	Medications Used in the Management of Thyroid Disorders		
Class	**Mechanism of Action and Effects**	**Indications**	**Pharmacokinetics, Toxicities, Interactions**
Thyroid Preparations			
Levothyroxine (T$_4$) Liothyronine (T$_3$)	Activation of nuclear receptors results in gene expression with RNA formation and protein synthesis	Hypothyroidism	Oral ▪ Duration of action: Half-life of 7 days, 80% oral absorption (Levothryoxine); Half-life of 1 day, 95% oral absorption (Liothyroinine) ▪ Maximum effect seen after 6-8 weeks of therapy ▪ *Toxicity:* Sweating, heat intolerance, tachycardia, diarrhea, nervousness, menstrual irregularities, increased basal metabolic rate are
Antithyroid Agents			
Thioamides Methimazole Propylthiouracil (PTU)	Inhibit thyroid peroxidase reactions ▪ Block iodine organification ▪ Inhibit peripheral deiodination of T$_4$ and T$_3$ (primarily PTU)	Hyperthyroidism	Oral ▪ Duration of action: 24 h (methimazole), 6-8 h (PTU) ▪ Delayed onset of action ▪ *Toxicity:* Nausea, gastrointestinal distress, rash, agranulocytosis, hepatitis (PTU black box), hypothyroidism
β-BLOCKERS			
Propranolol	Inhibition of β adrenoreceptors ▪ Inhibit T$_4$ to T$_3$ conversion (only propranolol)	Hyperthyroidism, especially thyroid storm ▪ Adjunct to control tachycardia, hypertension, and atrial fibrillation	Onset within hours ▪ Duration of 4-6 h (oral propranolol) ▪ *Toxicity:* Asthma, AV blockade, hypotension, bradycardia
RADIOACTIVE IODINE I (RAI)[131]			
	Radiation destruction of thyroid parenchyma	Hyperthyroidism ▪ Patients should be euthyroid or on β-blockers before RAI ▪ Avoid in pregnancy or in nursing mothers	Oral ▪ Half-life 5 days ▪ Onset of 6-12 weeks ▪ Maximum effect in 3-6 months ▪ *Toxicity:* Sore throat, sialadenitis, hypothyroidism

Reproduced with permission from Katzung BG, Masters SB, Trevor AJ: *Basic & Clinical Pharmacology, 12th ed. New York,* NY: McGraw-Hill; 2012.

within 3 months, but may develop after more than a year. Routine monitoring of white blood cells is not recommended as agranulocytosis usually develops rapidly. Patients should be advised to discontinue antithyroid medications and seek medical attention if they develop fever, sore throat, or mouth ulcers. Cross-reactivity between methimazole and propylthiouracil for agranulocytosis can occur. As a result, patients must pursue an alternative therapy for the treatment of hyperthyroidism.

Hepatotoxicity may occur with methimazole and propylthiouracil. Propylthiouracil, however, can induce liver failure that may be fatal in a small portion of patients, typically developing in the first 6 months of therapy. Routine monitoring of LFTs is not recommended but the development of hepatotoxicity symptoms including fatigue, jaundice, dark urine, and bruising should prompt patients to seek medical attention with evaluation of LFTs. Discontinuation of propylthiouracil is required. The development of any life-threatening side effects including agranulocytosis, vasculitis, or hepatotoxicity precludes future use of antithyroid medications.

Radioactive Iodine Radioactive iodine may be the initial choice of therapy for hyperthyroidism or may be initiated once a patient relapses after a trial with antithyroid medications. Effects occur by destruction of thyroid cells over time. This treatment, however, induces permanent hypothyroidism within months to years. Radioactive iodine may be administered as a fixed dose or as a calculated dose based on the size of the thyroid gland, anticipated uptake of radioactive iodine, and iodine turnover. Rarely, patients require retreatment with radioactive iodine. For patients with underlying cardiovascular disease or serious chronic diseases as well elderly patients, pretreatment with methimazole reduces the risk of cardiovascular events associated with post-treatment exacerbation of hyperthyroidism. If used, methimazole must be discontinued 3 to 5 days prior to radioiodine therapy, restarted 3 to 5 days later, then tapered over the next few weeks to minimize the risk of treatment failure. Free T$_4$ concentrations should be assessed within 1 to 2 months after treatment. Assessment of thyroid function is recommended annually once thyroid concentrations normalize. Should hypothyroidism develop, replacement with T$_4$ should be based on free T$_4$ levels.

Patients must take several precautions after treatment with radioactive iodine to prevent transference of radioactive iodine to others. Pregnancy contraindicates the use of radioactive iodine as it crosses the placenta and can be taken up by the fetal thyroid hormone. Additionally, women of childbearing age should avoid becoming pregnant for 6 to 12 months after treatment.

β-Adrenergic Blocking Drugs β-Adrenergic blocking agents are used as adjunctive therapy to minimize the symptoms of hyperthyroidism (anxiety, palpitations, tremor) until thyroid hormone levels normalize. Propranolol and nadolol minimally inhibit the conversion of T_4 to T_3. Choice of β-adrenergic blocking agent will depend on frequency of dosing and concomitant disease states with consideration of β-selectivity of the chosen agent.

Special Considerations

Pregnancy and Lactation

Hyperthyroidism can develop during pregnancy. Due to the risk of miscarriage, preeclampsia, and preterm delivery, treatment must be started. The use of radioactive iodine is contraindicated and surgery should be avoided; therefore, antithyroid drugs are recommended. Propylthiouracil is preferred over methimazole during the first trimester because methimazole is associated with congenital abnormalities (aplasia cutis and gastrointestinal defects). However, due to the risk of hepatotoxicity with propylthiouracil, therapy should be changed to methimazole from the second trimester forward. Thyroid hormone levels should be maintained at the upper limit of normal with the lowest dose possible to reduce the risk of neonatal hypothyroidism. In some patients, symptoms improve during the third trimester such that antithyroid medications can be discontinued, but hyperthyroidism may worsen during the postpartum period. Both antithyroid drugs are secreted in breast milk in low concentrations, but may be safe in nursing mothers.

Thyroid Storm

Thyroid storm is a life-threatening event resulting from the exaggerated effects of elevated thyroid hormones. The condition occurs rarely but has a 20% to 30% mortality rate. Contributing factors include infection, trauma, diabetic ketoacidosis, certain medications, and inappropriate administration of antithyroid hormones or T_4. Patients present with exaggerated symptoms of hyperthyroidism, fever, tachycardia, confusion or coma, and gastrointestinal disturbances. Treatment recommendations include high-dose β-adrenergic blocking agents administered concomitantly with propylthiouracil, glucocorticoids, stable iodide, and supportive care. Propylthiouracil is recommended preferentially over methimazole due to its ability to block the peripheral conversion of T_4 to T_3. The precipitating event should also be managed appropriately.

TREATMENT

Hypothyroidism

General Overview

The combination of T_4 and liothyronine (T_3) produces no significant benefit compared to T_4 alone. Since synthetic T_4 undergoes peripheral conversion to T_3 in the body, the treatment of choice for hypothyroidism is T_4 (Table 62-4). Treatment goals revolve around improvement in patient's symptoms and maintaining TSH concentrations within the reference range.

Specific Agents

Levothyroxine Replacement therapy with T_4 requires individualized dosing. Initial doses of oral T_4 should start low (25-50 mcg daily) and be titrated gradually (especially in patients >60 or with ischemic heart disease). Initial therapy may begin with full treatment doses of T_4 1.6 mcg/kg/d of ideal body weight in most healthy patients and titrated to optimal TSH levels. Dose adjustments should occur in 12.5 to 25 mcg increments. The total weekly T_4 dose may be given in once weekly doses (or divided into twice weekly doses) for those patients who have difficulty in adhering to a daily dosage regimen. Due to the long half-life of T_4 (7 days), TSH concentrations should be assessed every 4 to 6 weeks to allow medication to reach steady state. Once optimal TSH concentrations have been achieved, follow-up assessments can occur every 6 to 12 months. Patients should be reminded that it may take months for symptoms of hypothyroidism to resolve and that treatment continues indefinitely.

Thyroid hormone replacement is complicated by many factors. Age and celiac disease affect absorption. Taking T_4 alone on an empty stomach maximizes absorption. Certain drugs, including calcium salts, ferrous sulfate, aluminum hydroxide, and cholestyramine, prevent the absorption of T_4. Other medications, particularly anticonvulsants and rifampin, increase the clearance of T_4.

Most patients require oral replacement with T_4, but parenteral administration (intravenous, intramuscular) may be needed if the patient cannot take oral medication for an extended time or for the treatment of myxedema coma. The parenteral replacement dose should be 70% to 80% of the oral dose due to bioavailability differences. Reconstituted parenteral doses must be given immediately due to poor stability.

Due to a narrow therapeutic index, inadequately dosed T_4 increases the risk of adverse effects. Excessive T_4 may precipitate atrial fibrillation and worsen bone loss. Consequently, patients with cardiac disease should start T_4 at low doses with a slow titration to normal TSH concentrations. Unresolved symptoms of hypothyroidism will continue with subtherapeutic doses of T_4. Use of T_4 for nontoxic diffuse goiter or nodular thyroid disease may precipitate thyrotoxicosis. Additionally, T_4 should be avoided in patients with acute myocardial infarction, thyrotoxicosis, and adrenal insufficiency. Inappropriate use of T_4 for the treatment of obesity or for weight reduction should also be avoided.

Special Considerations

Pregnancy

Serious consequences can occur in the mother and fetus, if overt hypothyroidism remains untreated. As T_4 has been determined safe and effective during pregnancy, hypothyroidism should be treated with thyroid replacement hormone. T_4 requirements are considerably higher during pregnancy as pregnancy changes thyroid function. TSH concentrations should be assessed every 4 to 6 weeks and tightly controlled. Free T_4 concentrations should be maintained in the normal range as designated by trimester-specific TSH levels.

Bioequivalency of Oral Levothyroxine Preparations

T_4 first became available in 1962, without a new drug application through the Food and Drug Administration (FDA).

In 1997, the FDA mandated that all marketed T_4 products submit a new drug application. At that time, the FDA did not recognize these products to be safe and effective due to lack of data showing consistent potency and stability. T_4 products were not considered therapeutically interchangeable, as well. In July 2001, the FDA determined standards for bioequivalency of T_4 products, based on the absorption of T_4 rather than the more reliable effect on TSH concentrations. Regardless of the product used, patients should be maintained on one particular brand of T_4. TSH concentrations should be monitored frequently, if a patient changes brands of T_4.

AMIODARONE AND THE THYROID

Amiodarone can induce thyroid dysfunction in 4% to 18% of treated patients. Amiodarone contains a significant amount of iodine (about 75 mg iodine per a 200-mg dose) and inhibits thyroid function. Additionally, amiodarone blocks the conversion of T_4 to T_3 and may induce hypothyroidism or hyperthyroidism. Baseline TSH levels should be obtained prior to starting amiodarone and should be reassessed every 6 months during treatment. Even after discontinuation, amiodarone may continue to exert its effect on the thyroid due to its long half-life and storage in adipose tissue.

In iodine-sufficient areas of the world, amiodarone-induced hypothyroidism is common and occurs after 6 to 12 months of treatment with amiodarone. Similar to other forms of hypothyroidism, treatment with T_4 remains the therapy of choice. Evaluation of therapy should be based on TSH concentrations rather than T_4 levels. Although amiodarone may be continued if needed for treatment of cardiac disease, once it has been discontinued, thyroid levels may return to normal in 2 to 4 months.

Amiodarone-induced hyperthyroidism can occur in two forms (type 1 and type 2) and is common in iodine-deficient areas of the world. Type 1 occurs at any time in patients treated with amiodarone who have underlying thyroid disease. Thyroid hormone levels increase due to increased exposure to iodine. Radioactive iodine cannot be used due to low radioiodine uptake associated with this form. Antithyroid medications offer some benefit, but resumption of a euthyroid state takes time and discontinuation of amiodarone. Type 2 amiodarone-induced hyperthyroidism is caused by an inflammatory process resulting in a destructive thyroiditis that lasts for 1 to 3 months. Patients may be treated with corticosteroids, and amiodarone may be continued. Rarely, surgery to remove the thyroid gland may be necessary.

CASE Application

1. BS is a 36-year-old woman who presents to her doctor with symptoms of anxiety, sleep disturbances, and recent weight loss. Her doctor suspects hyperthyroidism. Which of the following lab results would be consistent with overt hyperthyroidism?

   a. Increased TSH, increased thyroid hormones
   b. Decreased TSH, increased thyroid hormones
   c. Increased TSH, decreased thyroid hormones
   d. Decreased TSH, decreased thyroid hormones

2. MM is a pregnant 27-year-old woman who has just been diagnosed with hyperthyroidism. Which symptoms might MM be experiencing due to her diagnosis?

   a. Bradycardia and cold intolerance
   b. Tachycardia and heat intolerance
   c. Depression and cognition difficulties
   d. Weight gain and constipation

3. MM is currently in first trimester of her pregnancy, but her doctor consults you for treatment options for hyperthyroidism throughout MM's pregnancy. Select all that apply.

   a. Surgery
   b. Radioactive iodine
   c. Methimazole
   d. Propylthiouracil

4. Dr. M wants to know which antithyroid medication would be preferred in a nonpregnant patient with hyperthyroidism without thyroid storm and why. What is your response?

   a. Propylthiouracil is preferred due to fewer side effects and less frequent dosing.
   b. Methimazole is preferred due to fewer side effects and less frequent dosing.
   c. Methimazole is preferred since it blocks the peripheral conversion of T_4 to T_3.
   d. Propylthiouracil is preferred since it blocks the peripheral conversion of T_4 to T_3.

5. TS is a 35-year-old woman started on propylthiouracil for treatment of hyperthyroidism. Which of the following side effects might she experience that would require discontinuation of her medication? Select all that apply.

   a. Agranulocytosis
   b. Insomnia
   c. Gastrointestinal upset
   d. Hepatotoxicity

6. LR is a 32-year-old woman who is still experiencing symptoms of hyperthyroidism despite treatment with methimazole. Which medication can be added to provide additional symptomatic relief?

   a. Nifedipine
   b. Prednisone
   c. Propranolol
   d. Ibuprofen

7. YD presents to the emergency room in coma with fever and tachycardia. Based on results of his thyroid function tests, YD is diagnosed with thyroid storm. Which therapy would be preferred as initial treatment for YDs symptoms? Select all that apply.

   a. Radioactive iodine
   b. Propylthiouracil

c. Methimazole

d. Glucocorticoids

8. You are consulted by Dr. X to determine the plan for a patient's methimazole dose. She has been taking methimazole for 3 months. What is your response?

TSH	1.5	(0.4-4.0 mIU/L)
Free T$_4$	6.2	(4.5-11.2 mcg/dL)
Free T$_3$	125	(100-200 ng/dL)

a. Begin reducing the dose of methimazole since thyroid function tests are within normal range.

b. Stop methimazole now since thyroid function tests are within normal range.

c. Methimazole will need to be continued indefinitely to maintain thyroid levels in the normal range.

d. Gradually transition patient from methimazole to levothyroxine since the patient will become hypothyroid due to treatment from methimazole.

9. You have been asked to counsel a 72-year-old patient with a history of heart disease about her upcoming treatment with radioactive iodine. Which of the following should be included in your counseling recommendations? Select all that apply.

a. The patient does not need to take any extra precautions due to exposure to radioactive iodine.

b. The patient should be treated with methimazole up to 3 to 7 days prior to treatment with radioactive iodine to reduce the risk of cardiovascular events associated with post-treatment exacerbation of hyperthyroidism.

c. Once the patient's thyroid function returns to normal after radioactive iodine therapy, she will no longer need to have her thyroid function monitored.

d. The patient should anticipate a change to a hypothyroid state over time after treatment with radioactive iodine that will require treatment with levothyroxine.

10. GB is a 55-year-old woman recently diagnosed with hypothyroidism. Which symptoms might she be experiencing?

a. Bradycardia and cold intolerance

b. Anxiety and nervousness

c. Weight loss and insomnia

d. Frequent bowel movements and edema

11. Which of the following lab results would indicate hypothyroidism in GB?

a. Increased TSH, increased thyroid hormones

b. Decreased TSH, increased thyroid hormones

c. Increased TSH, decreased thyroid hormones

d. Decreased TSH, decreased thyroid hormones

12. GBs doctor has been concerned about new trends in the treatment of hypothyroidism. He requests your recommendation for the most appropriate therapy for GB.

a. Desiccated thyroid hormone

b. Liothyronine

c. Levothyroxine

d. The combination of liothyronine and levothyroxine

13. Which of the following patient counseling tips would be appropriate for GB? Select all that apply.

a. Levothyroxine will need to be continued lifelong.

b. Levothyroxine should be taken on an empty stomach to maximize absorption.

c. Levothyroxine should be taken with food to maximize absorption.

d. Levothyroxine produces immediate symptomatic relief of hypothyroidism.

14. As KM picks up her first prescription of levothyroxine, she asks you when she should have her thyroid function tests rechecked. What is your response?

a. 1 week

b. 1 month

c. 3 months

d. 6 months

15. Dr. Z in your clinic asks you what the most recent dosing recommendations are for initiating levothyroxine for the treatment of hypothyroidism. Which of the following responses are correct? Select all that apply.

a. Full treatment doses of levothyroxine may be started in some patients.

b. Levothyroxine must be started at low doses and titrated up slowly in all patients.

c. Patients with ischemic heart disease may begin levothyroxine at full treatment doses.

d. Full treatment doses of levothyroxine should be started only in younger healthy patients.

16. Calculate an appropriate starting dose of levothyroxine in an otherwise healthy 42-year-old woman recently diagnosed with hypothyroidism. Her vitals are:

Height 5' 2" Weight 235 lb

Answer = _____

Calculate based on ideal body weight (equals 50.1 kg) and starting dose of 1.6 mcg/kg/d since she is young and healthy. Round to nearest available tablet size.

17. PR is a 35-year-old woman admitted for uncontrollable nausea and vomiting during the first trimester of her pregnancy. Her past medical history is significant for hypothyroidism and GERD. How should her hypothyroidism be managed during her hospitalization?

a. Levothyroxine should be held until PR can restart her oral medication.

b. Levothyroxine should be given intravenously until PR can restart her oral medication.

c. Levothyroxine should be given orally at a lower dose to reduce nausea and vomiting.

d. Levothyroxine should be changed to liothyronine to reduce nausea and vomiting.

18. FN is diagnosed with Hashimoto disease during the second trimester of her pregnancy. Which medication would be preferred for FN?

    a. Desiccated thyroid hormone
    b. Liothyronine alone
    c. Levothyroxine alone
    d. Levothyroxine in combination with liothyronine

19. TC has been on amiodarone for 2 months and has now been diagnosed with amiodarone-induced hypothyroidism. What is the treatment of choice for amiodarone-induced hypothyroidism?

    a. Discontinuation of amiodarone
    b. Liothyronine alone

    c. Levothyroxine alone
    d. Levothyroxine in combination with liothyronine

20. Which of the following is true?

    a. Radioactive iodine will adequately treat type 1 amiodarone-induced hyperthyroidism.
    b. Amiodarone must be discontinued to adequately treat type 1 amiodarone-induced hyperthyroidism.
    c. Amiodarone must be discontinued to adequately treat type 2 amiodarone-induced hyperthyroidism.
    d. Antithyroid medications may offer some benefit in type 2 amiodarone-induced hyperthyroidism.

TAKEAWAY POINTS »

- A negative feedback system based on circulating thyroid hormone concentrations affects production of TSH.
- T_4 is produced in the thyroid gland while the majority of T_3 is produced by peripheral conversion of T_4 to T_3.
- Symptoms of hyperthyroidism include tachycardia, weight loss, nervousness, heat intolerance, and exophthalmos.
- In hyperthyroidism, TSH concentrations may be undetectable while free thyroid concentrations are elevated above the normal reference range.
- Treatment options for hyperthyroidism include surgery, radioactive iodine, and antithyroid medications.
- Methimazole and propylthiouracil block the formation of thyroid hormones, but propylthiouracil also blocks the peripheral conversion of T_4 to T_3. Methimazole is preferred due to higher potency and fewer side effects. Serious side effects associated with antithyroid medications include agranulocytosis, hepatotoxicity, and vasculitis. Treatment should continue for 12 to 18 months then gradually discontinued.
- β-Adrenergic blocking drugs may be given as adjunctive therapy to provide symptomatic relief.
- Treatment recommendations for thyroid storm include propylthiouracil, β-adrenergic blocking agents, glucocorticoids, stable iodide, and supportive care.

- Symptoms of hypothyroidism include cold intolerance, weight gain, depression, and fatigue.
- Serum TSH concentrations are elevated in hypothyroidism while free T_4 concentrations are decreased.
- The treatment of choice for hypothyroidism is T_4 though it may take 4 to 6 weeks to reach steady state with T_4 due to the long half-life of 7 days.
- Full treatment doses of T_4 should be started as initial therapy in most healthy patients. T_4 should be initiated at lower doses to prevent adverse effects in patients over the age of 60 and those with ischemic heart disease.
- T_4 is safe and effective for the treatment of hypothyroidism in pregnancy.
- Amiodarone may induce hypo- or hyperthyroidism due to a significant iodine content that inhibits thyroid function and by blocking conversion of T_4 to T_3.
- Amiodarone-induced hypothyroidism may be treated with T_4 along with discontinuation of amiodarone.
- Amiodarone may induce two types of hyperthyroidism. Type 1 may be treated with antithyroid medication, but may require discontinuation of amiodarone. Type 2 may be treated with glucocorticoids, and therapy with amiodarone may continue.

BIBLIOGRAPHY

Alexander EK, Pearce EN, Brent GA, et al. 2017 Guidelines of the American Thyroid Association for the diagnosis and management of thyroid disease during pregnancy and the postpartum. *Thyroid.* 2017;27(3):315-389.

Bahn RS, Burch HB, Cooper DS, et al. Hyperthyroidism and other causes of thyrotoxicosis: Management guidelines of the American Thyroid Association and American Association of Clinical Endocrinologists. *Thyroid.* 2011;21(6):593-646.

Bauer DC, McPhee SJ. Thyroid disease. In: McPhee SJ, Hammer GD, eds. *Pathophysiology of Disease.* 6th ed. New York, NY: McGraw-Hill; 2010:chap 20.

Brent GA, Koenig RJ. Thyroid and anti-thyroid drugs. In: Brunton LL, Chabner BA, Knollmann BC, eds. *Goodman & Gilman's The Pharmacological Basis of Therapeutics.* 12th ed. New York, NY: McGraw-Hill; 2011:chap 39.

Dong BJ, Greenspan FS. Thyroid and antithyroid drugs. In: Katzung BG, Masters SB, Trevor AJ, eds. *Basic & Clinical Pharmacology.* 12th ed. New York, NY: McGraw-Hill; 2012:chap 38.

Garber JR, Cobin RH, Gharib H, et al. Clinical practice guidelines for hypothyroidism in adults: Cosponsored by the American Association of Clinical Endocrinologists and the American Thyroid Association. *Thyroid.* 2012;22(12):1200-1235.

Jameson J, Weetman AP. Disorders of the thyroid gland. In: Longo DL, Fauci AS, Kasper DL, Hauser SL, Jameson J, Loscalzo J, eds. *Harrison's Principles of Internal Medicine.* 18th ed. New York, NY: McGraw-Hill; 2012:chap 341.

Jonklaas J, Bianco, AC, Bauer AJ, et al. Guidelines for the treatment of hypothyroidism. *Thyroid.* 2014;24(12):1670-1751.

Jonklaas J, Kane MP. Thyroid disorders. In: DiPiro JT, Talbert RL, Yee GC, Matzke GR, Wells BG, Posey L, eds. *Pharmacotherapy: A Pathophysiologic Approach.* 10th ed. New York, NY: McGraw-Hill; 2017.

KEY ABBREVIATIONS

FDA = Food and Drug Administration	TRAb = thyrotropin-receptor antibodies
LFT = liver function test	TRH = thyrotropin-releasing hormone
T_3 = triiodothyronine	TSH = thyroid-stimulating hormone
T_4 = levothyroxine	

Health and Wellness and Other Topics

Contraception

Shareen El-Ibiary

FOUNDATION OVERVIEW

Contraception implies the prevention of pregnancy following sexual intercourse by inhibiting viable sperm from coming into contact with a mature ovum or by preventing a fertilized ovum from implanting successfully in the endometrium. Additional benefits of contraception include improvements in menstrual cycle regularity, prevention of sexually transmitted diseases, and management of perimenopause. Contraceptive methods are available nonprescription or by prescription. Nonprescription contraceptives include condoms, spermicides, emergency contraception (EC), and in some states hormonal contraception is provided by pharmacists without a prescription. Prescription contraceptives are generally hormone based. There are a variety of factors that go into method selection and include effectiveness, cost, accessibility, side effects, return to fertility rate, frequency of sexual activity, STI prevention, past medical history, and concomitant medications.

PRODUCT OVERVIEW

Nonhormonal Contraception

A condom is the most common nonhormonal contraceptive and is available over the counter (OTC). Male latex condoms protect against sexually transmitted infections (STIs); however, oil-based lubricants breakdown latex condoms and should not be used concurrently. Latex allergic individuals may use polyurethane, polyisoprene and lamb cecum condoms. Nonlatex condoms increase heat conduction, increase sensitivity, and can be used with water or oil-based lubricants. Additionally, polyurethane condoms break easier than latex condoms and lamb cecum condoms are porous, expensive, and do not protect against select STIs. Overall, male condoms have an 18% failure rate in preventing pregnancy. This percentage may decrease if spermicides are used in conjunction.

The female condom (FC2) is an option for contraception and prevention of STIs. The female condom is inserted vaginally and may be worn up to 8 hours prior to intercourse. The condom should be discarded by closing the bottom of the condom and removing it from the vagina. Disadvantages include squeaking during intercourse, appearance, irritation, decreased sensitivity, difficulty in inserting the condom, and

a 21% failure rate in preventing pregnancy. Male and female condoms may not be used together because they stick together causing friction and may break.

Spermicides are also available OTC in a variety of formulations including jellies, gels, foams, suppositories, and films. The active ingredient in spermicides available in the United States is nonoxynol-9. Nonoxynol-9 is a nonionic detergent that inhibits sperm motility and function. The failure rate of spermicides when used alone is 18% to 29%. Nonoxynol-9 is *not* a microbicide and does *not* kill viruses such as human immunodeficiency virus (HIV). In some reports, it has been shown to increase the risk of HIV transmission by causing irritation to the mucosal lining of the vagina or rectum, which may allow passage of the virus into the bloodstream. Key counseling points for spermicides include: no douching within 6 hours of use, apply within 1 hour of intercourse, and each application only works for one act of intercourse. In addition, the vaginal film and suppository must dissolve completely for at least 15 minutes before intercourse. The film is activated by the female secretions; therefore, it is not best for women who have trouble with lubrication. Nonoxynol-9 may be irritating to the skin. If irritation occurs, another product with lower concentration of nonoxynol-9 is recommended. The highest concentration is found in the film (28%), foams (8%-12%), suppository (2.3%-5.6%), and jelly/gels (2%-5%).

The sponge is a form of OTC contraception containing polyurethane foam and 1 g of nonoxynol-9. After moistening the sponge with two teaspoons of water, it is inserted vaginally, placed against the cervix, and may be worn up to 24 hours. After intercourse, the sponge should remain in place for 6 hours. It acts as a spermicide, mechanical barrier, and absorbs semen. The typical failure rate reported is 12% to 18% for nulliparous women and 24% to 36% for parous women. Side effects may include irritation or ulceration of the cervix and vaginal mucosa. In addition, toxic shock syndrome may be a concern if the sponge is not removed within 24 to 30 hours or if particles remain after removal.

Other nonhormonal contraceptives include the *prescription* copper-T intrauterine device (IUD) and diaphragm. The copper-T IUD is a device that is placed in the uterus and prevents implantation. The copper in the IUD has an acrosomal enzyme that stops the sperm from moving. The copper-T may be used for up to 10 years. It is very effective with a typical use failure rate of 0.8%. Select side effects include breakthrough bleeding, cramping, pain, and expulsion. The diaphragm is inserted vaginally and acts as a barrier device to sperm. It has a typical use failure rate of 12% to 16%.

Hormonal Contraception

Combined Hormonal Contraception

There are two main types of hormonal contraceptives, progestin-only (progestin) and combined (estrogen and progestin). Ethinyl estradiol (EE) is the main estrogen used in most products. Combined hormonal contraceptives (CHCs) work by inhibiting ovulation. CHCs are Food and Drug Administration (FDA)-indicated for the prevention of pregnancy, have a failure rate of 9%. Select CHCs are indicated for uses other than preventing pregnancy. YAZ (EE/drospirenone), Yasmin (EE/drospirenone), Beyaz (EE/drospirenone/levomefolate), Ortho Tri-Cyclen (EE, norgestimate), and Estrostep (EE/norethindrone) are FDA approved for acne treatment. YAZ and Beyaz are also FDA-approved for premenstrual dysphoric disorder (PMDD). Safyral (EE/drospirenone/levomefolate) and Beyaz are indicated to raise folate levels and Natazia (estradiol valerate/dienogest) is indicated to treat heavy menstrual bleeding without organic pathology. Off-label uses for most CHCs include regulation of menstrual cycle, iron deficiency anemia, polycystic ovary syndrome, hirsutism, dysmenorrhea, and decreased risk of ovarian cancer.

Unfortunately, CHCs are not without side effects. Select side effects may be attributed to the estrogen or the progestin component (Table 63-1). Common side effects include: nausea, breakthrough bleeding, mood changes, and weight gain. It is recommended that a woman try a product for at least 3 months before changing because it takes a few months for the body to adjust to the CHC. If side effects continue after 3 months, a product switch is recommended.

Estrogens and progestins are metabolized by the cytochrome P450 (CYP-450) enzymes and concomitant medications that affect these enzymes alter the effectiveness of hormonal contraceptives (Table 63-2). Well known interactions that decrease the effectiveness of CHCs include antiepileptics, antibiotics, antiretrovirals, protease inhibitors, and herbal products such as St. John's wort. Depending on the interaction, higher doses of hormonal contraceptives may be needed or alternate forms of contraception may be recommended. In particular, controversies surround the use of antibiotics and hormonal contraceptives. Most conservative approaches suggest using a backup method while using antibiotics and for a week following the discontinuation of antibiotics.

CHCs are available in oral tablets, transdermal patch, and vaginal ring. Oral tablets are offered in four types of formulations: monophasic, biphasic, triphasic, and quadriphasic (Table 63-3). Monophasic regimens contain the same strength of the hormones in the active tablets throughout the pack. Biphasic regimens contain 10 days of hormones and 11 days of an increased amount of hormones. Triphasic regimens vary

TABLE 63-1 Side Effects of Hormones[a]

Adverse Effects	Management
Estrogen excess	
Nausea, breast tenderness, headaches, cyclic weight gain due to fluid retention	Decrease estrogen content in CHC Consider progestin-only methods or IUD
Dysmenorrhea, menorrhagia, uterine fibroid growth	Decrease estrogen content in CHC Consider extended-cycle or continuous regimen OC Consider progestin-only methods or IUD NSAIDs for dysmenorrhea
Estrogen deficiency	
Vasomotor symptoms, nervousness, decreased libido	Increase estrogen content in CHC Increase estrogen content in CHC
Early-cycle (days 1–9) breakthrough bleeding and spotting	Exclude pregnancy Increase estrogen content in CHC if menses is desired
Absence of withdrawal bleeding (amenorrhea)	Continue current CHC if amenorrhea acceptable
Progestin excess	
Increased appetite, weight gain, bloating, constipation	Decrease progestin content in CHC Decrease progestin content in CHC
Acne, oily skin, hirsutism	Choose less androgenic progestin in CHC
Depression, fatigue, irritability	Decrease progestin content in CHC
Progestin deficiency	
Dysmenorrhea, menorrhagia	Increase progestin content in CHC
Late-cycle (days 10–21) breakthrough bleeding and spotting	Consider extended-cycle or continuous regimen OC Consider progestin-only methods or IUD NSAIDs for dysmenorrhea Increase progestin content in CHC

Abbreviations: CHC, combined hormonal contraceptive; IUD, intrauterine device; NSAID, nonsteroidal antiinflammatory drug; OC, oral contraceptive.

[a]CHC regimens should be continued for at least 3 months before adjustments are made based on adverse effects.

Reproduced with permission from DiPiro JT, Talbert RL, Yee GC, et al: *Pharmacotherapy: A Pathophysiologic Approach*, 8th ed. New York, NY: McGraw-Hill; 2011.

each week of the cycle with different amount of hormones and quadriphasic regimens have four different hormone amounts. For most formulations, the estrogen dose stays the same while progestin dose increases each week. The benefit of these formulations was *thought* to decrease the exposure to progestins. Some products such as Cyclessa (EE/desogestrel) and Estrostep (EE/norethindrone) have varying estrogen doses each week while the progestin remains the same. Natazia (estradiol valerate/dienogest), a quadriphasic product, has both varying estrogen and progestin levels throughout the cycle. The benefits of these products decrease the exposure to estrogens and their side effects. All prevent pregnancy with equal effectiveness.

There are various doses of CHCs based on the estrogen content. They are classified as very low dose (10-25 mcg EE), low dose (30-35 mcg EE), and high dose (50 mcg EE). The low dose and very low dose are prescribed more frequently due

TABLE 63-2   Selected CHCs Drug Interactions[a]

Drugs That Decrease the Effect of CHCs	Drugs That *May* Decrease the Effect of CHCs (Controversial)	Drugs That Increase Effect of CHCs	CHC Alter Metabolism or Clearance of These Agents
Amprenavir	Ampicillin	Atorvastatin	Acetaminophen
Barbiturates	Amoxicillin	Atazanavir	Antidepressants, tricyclic
Carbamazepine	Ciprofloxacin	Indinavir	Aspirin
Felbamate	Clarithromycin		Benzodiazepines
Griseofulvin	Doxycycline		β-blockers
Lopinavir	Erythromycin		Caffeine
Modafinil	Fluconazole		Corticosteroids
Nelfinavir	Metronidazole		Cyclosporine
Nevirapine	Minocycline		Lamotrigine
Oxcarbazepine	Ofloxacin		Theophyllines
Phenobarbital	Tetracycline		
Phenytoin	Topiramate		
Primidone			
Rifamycins			
Ritonavir			
Saquinavir			
St. John's wort			
Tipranavir			

[a]Drug list is not all inclusive. Some drug interactions may exist that are not cited in this table.

TABLE 63-3   Composition of Commonly Prescribed Oral Contraceptives[a]

Product	Estrogen	Micrograms[b]	Progestin	Milligrams[b]	Spotting and Breakthrough Bleeding
50 mcg estrogen					
Necon 1/50, Norinyl 1+50, Ortho-Novum 1/50	Mestranol	50	Norethindrone	1	10.6
Ovcon 50	Ethinyl estradiol	50	Norethindrone	1	11.9
Ovral, Ogestrel 0.5/50	Ethinyl estradiol	50	Norgestrel	0.5	4.5
Demulen 1/50, Zovia 1/50	Ethinyl estradiol	50	Ethynodiol diacetate	1	13.9
Sub-50 mcg estrogen monophasic					
Aviane, Lessina, Levlite, Lutera, Sronyx	Ethinyl estradiol	20	Levonorgestrel	0.1	26.5
Brevicon, Modicon, Necon 0.5/35, Nortrel 0.5/35	Ethinyl estradiol	35	Norethindrone	0.5	24.6
Demulen 1/35, Zovia 1/35, Kelnor	Ethinyl estradiol	37.4	Ethynodiol diacetate	1	37.4
Apri, Desogen, Ortho-Cept, Reclipsen, Solia	Ethinyl estradiol	30	Desogestrel	0.15	13.1
Levlen, Levora, Nordette, Portia	Ethinyl estradiol	30	Levonorgestrel	0.15	14
Junel 1/20, Junel Fe 1/20, Loestrin 1/20; Fe 1/20, Microgestin 1/20; Fe 1/20	Ethinyl estradiol	20	Norethindrone 1 mg	1	26.5
Junel 1.5/30, Junel Fe 1.5/30, Loestrin Fe 1.5/30, Microgestin 1.5/30, Microgestin Fe 1.5/30	Ethinyl estradiol	30	Norethindrone acetate	1.5	25.2
Cryselle, Lo-Ovral, Low-Ogestrel	Ethinyl estradiol	30	Norgestrel	0.3	9.6
Necon 1/35, Norinyl 1+35, Norethin 1/35, Nortrel 1/35, Ortho-Novum 1/35	Ethinyl estradiol	35	Norethindrone	1	14.7
Ortho-Cyclen, Mononessa, Previfem, Sprintec	Ethinyl estradiol	35	Norgestimate	0.25	14.3
Ovcon-35, Balziva, Femcon Fe chewable, Zenchent	Ethinyl estradiol	35	Norethindrone	0.4	11
Yasmin	Ethinyl estradiol	30	Drospirenone	3	14.5

TABLE 63-3	**Composition of Commonly Prescribed Oral Contraceptives**[a] *(Continued)*					

Product	Estrogen	Micrograms[b]	Progestin	Milligrams[b]	Spotting and Breakthrough Bleeding
Sub-50 mcg estrogen monophasic extended cycle					
Loestrin-24 FE[c]	Ethinyl estradiol	20	Norethindrone	1	50[e]
Lybrel	Ethinyl estradiol	20	Levonorgestrel	0.09	52[e]
Seasonale, Jolessa, Quasense[d]	Ethinyl estradiol	30	Levonorgestrel	0.15	58.5[e]
Yaz[c]	Ethinyl estradiol	20	Drospirenone	3	52.5[e]
Beyaz[f]	Ethinyl estradiol	20	Drospirenone	3	52.5[e]
Sub-50 mcg estrogen multiphasic					
Cyclessa, Cesia, Velivet	Ethinyl estradiol	25 (7)	Desogestrel	0.1 (7)	11.1
		25 (7)		0.125 (7)	
		25 (7)		0.15 (7)	
Estrostep Fe, Tilia Fe, Tri-Legest Fe	Ethinyl estradiol	20 (5)	Norethindrone acetate	1 (5)	21.7
	Ethinyl estradiol	30 (7)	Norethindrone acetate	1 (7)	
	Ethinyl estradiol	35 (9)	Norethindrone acetate	1 (9)	
Kariva, Mircette	Ethinyl estradiol	20 (21)	Desogestrel	0.15 (21)	19.7
	Ethinyl estradiol	10 (5)	Desogestrel		
Gencept 10/11, Necon 10/11, Ortho-Novum 10/11	Ethinyl estradiol	35 (10)	Norethindrone	0.5 (10)	17.6
	Ethinyl estradiol	35 (11)	Norethindrone	1 (11)	
Ortho-Novum 7/7/7, Nortrel 7/7/7, Necon 7/7/7	Ethinyl estradiol	35 (7)	Norethindrone	0.5 (7)	14.5
	Ethinyl estradiol	35 (7)	Norethindrone	0.75 (7)	
	Ethinyl estradiol	35 (7)	Norethindrone	1 (7)	
Ortho Tri-Cyclen, Trinessa, Tri-Previfem, Tri-Sprintec	Ethinyl estradiol	35 (7)	Norgestimate	0.18 (7)	17.7
	Ethinyl estradiol	35 (7)	Norgestimate	0.215 (7)	
	Ethinyl estradiol	35 (7)	Norgestimate	0.25 (7)	
Ortho Tri-Cyclen Lo	Ethinyl estradiol	25 (7)	Norgestimate	0.18 (7)	11.5
	Ethinyl estradiol	25 (7)	Norgestimate	0.215 (7)	
	Ethinyl estradiol	25 (7)	Norgestimate	0.25 (7)	
Aranelle, Leena, Tri-Norinyl	Ethinyl estradiol	35 (7)	Norethindrone	0.5 (7)	25.5
	Ethinyl estradiol	35 (9)	Norethindrone	1 (9)	
	Ethinyl estradiol	35 (5)	Norethindrone	0.5 (5)	
Enpresse, Tri-Levlen, Triphasil, Trivora	Ethinyl estradiol	30 (6)	Levonorgestrel	0.05 (6)	
	Ethinyl estradiol	40 (5)	Levonorgestrel	0.075 (5)	
	Ethinyl estradiol	30 (10)	Levonorgestrel	0.125 (10)	
Sub-50 mcg estrogen multiphasic extended cycle					
Seasonique	Ethinyl estradiol	30 (84)	Levonorgestrel	0.15 (84)	42.5[e]
	Ethinyl estradiol	10 (7)	Levonorgestrel	0.15 (7)	
Progestin only					
Camila, Errin, Jolivette, Micronor, Nor-QD, Nora-BE	Ethinyl estradiol	—	Norethindrone	0.35	42.3

[a]28-day regimens (21-day active pills, then 7-day pill-free interval) unless otherwise noted.
[b]Number in parentheses refers to the number of days the dose is received in multiphasic oral contraceptives.
[c]28-day regimen (24-day active pills, then 4-day pill-free interval).
[d]91-day regimen (84-day active pills, then 7-day pill-free interval).
[e]Percentage reporting after 6-12 months of use.
[f]Contains folate supplementation (levomefolate calcium 0.451 mg).
Reproduced with permission from DiPiro JT, Talbert RL, Yee GC, et al: *Pharmacotherapy: A Pathophysiologic Approach,* 10th ed: New York, NY: McGraw-Hill; 2017.

to fewer side effects associated with estrogen. The high-dose CHCs are generally prescribed when there are drug interactions or breakthrough bleeding issues that require higher levels of estrogen.

There are varying regimens with the number of active pills as well. Most combined oral contraceptives (COCs) are formulated for 21 days of active tablets with 7 days of placebo. COCs such as YAZ (EE/drospirenone), Loestrin 24

TABLE 63-4 | **Initiation of CHC Products**

Initiation Method	Description
First day	Woman starts method the first day of her menses and uses a backup method for 7 days (some sources say no backup method is necessary, however, this is most conservative approach)
Sunday start	Woman starts method the Sunday after her menses begin (for ring best if within 5 days of menses), uses a backup method for 7 days
Quick start	Woman starts method in the clinic regardless of date of the menses, uses a backup method for 7 days

(EE/norethindrone) have 24 days of active tablets and 4 days of placebo to decrease breakthrough bleeding and minimize bleeding at menses. Other products first marketed as Seasonale and Seasonique (EE/levonorgestrel) contain 84 active tablets allowing for four menses per year. Monophasic formulations, the vaginal ring and transdermal patch, may be used by continuing on active hormones without a hormone-free interval. Benefits of extended regimens include decreased menstrual migraines during the hormone-free interval, less bleeding, and decreased premenstrual syndrome (PMS) symptoms.

Counseling is very important to ensure maximum effectiveness. There are three ways of initiating COCs (Table 63-4). Ideally, COCs should be taken at the same time everyday. If nausea occurs, it is recommended to take the COCs at bedtime. If more than 24 hours have passed since the last dose of a COC, it is considered a missed dose (Table 63-5). For products that contain less than 30 mcg of EE, missing two tablets anytime in the cycle should be treated as if missing more than two tablets. If unprotected intercourse occurred within the last 7 days, EC is also an option for any doses missed.

Transdermal Patch The contraceptive patch (Xulane formerly marketed as Ortho Evra) is an adhesive square applied

to skin once weekly that was thought to deliver norelgestromin 0.15 mg/d and EE 20 mcg/d; however, it is now known to deliver 60% more EE than a 35 mcg EE oral tablet. The transdermal patch has a typical use failure rate of 9%; however, the failure rate increases in obese women weighing more than 90 kg. The patch should be placed on a clean, dry, hairless area on the shoulder, upper arm, or abdomen and rotated *weekly* to prevent irritation. The patch may be worn while taking showers, swimming, exercising, or sitting in a sauna. A backup birth control method should be used for the first 7 days after applying the patch if the patch was not started on the first day of the woman's menses (new start). The patch is removed at the start of the fourth week and menses generally occur at that time. If the patch falls off for more than 24 hours, then a new patch should be applied. This is considered a new cycle; therefore, a backup birth control method for 7 days is recommended. EC is also a consideration if unprotected intercourse occurred in the last 5 days. If the patch falls off for less than 24 hours, it should be reapplied as soon as possible and no backup birth control method is necessary.

Vaginal Ring The contraceptive ring (NuvaRing) is inserted vaginally and left in place for 3 weeks releasing etonogestrel

TABLE 63-5 | **Missed Doses**[a]

Product	Missed Dose	Remedy
Birth control pills (combined)	Missed one dose (over 24 h)	Take two tablets the next day, no backup necessary, but best if used
	Missed two doses	Take missed dose with today's dose, backup method for 7 days, if less than 7 active tablets remain after the missed dose, skip placebo week and start a new pack, may also use EC if had unprotected sex during those days
		If taking a very low dose COC (<30 mcg EE), treat two missed doses as missing three doses.
	Missed more than two doses in pack	Discard pack, start new pack, and use backup method for 7 days, may use EC if had unprotected sex during those days, alternatively, continue same pack if there are 7 active tablets left, skip placebo week, start new pack and use a backup method for 7 days, may use EC if had unprotected sex during those days
	Missed three doses in extended cycle	Skip missed pills and start taking active pills for current day. Continue taking active pills until pack is finished and use a backup method for 7 days. May use EC if had unprotected sex during those days.
Progestin-only	Missed dose is considered 3 h overdue	Continue to take tablets as scheduled, use a backup method for 2 days
Transdermal patch	Detached <24h	Reapply patch, no backup is necessary
	Off >24 h	Apply new patch, start new patch day and use backup method for 7 days
Vaginal ring	Left out <3 h	Wash with warm water and reinsert, no backup is needed
	Left out >3 h	Reinsert new ring, use backup method for 7 days
DMPA injection	Missed dose is considered >13 wk since last injection	Use backup method until injection is given and continue to use a backup method for 7 days after injection

[a]Recommendations are according to the product manufacturer.

0.120 mg/d and EE 0.015 mg/d. It has a typical use failure rate of 9%. The exact location of the ring is not important as long as it rests inside the vagina. During the fourth week, the ring is removed and menses will begin in 2 to 3 days. Douching or use of a diaphragm is not recommended with the ring. The ring may be left in place during sexual intercourse, while using a tampon for breakthrough bleeding, and with use of antifungal creams or spermicides. The ring is removed by grasping the ring with the index and middle fingers and pulling it out. Initiation of the ring should be within the first 5 days of the menstrual cycle and a backup birth control method should be used for at least 7 days after insertion of the ring. Side effects include those of CHCs but may also include vaginitis, headache, and sensation of the ring.

If removed or expelled, the ring should be rinsed with cool to lukewarm water and reinserted as soon as possible within 3 hours (Table 63-5). If the ring is left out of the vagina for longer than 3 hours, a backup birth control method should be used until the ring has been in place for at least 7 days. EC could be considered if a woman had unprotected intercourse in the last 5 days.

Progestin-Only Hormonal Contraceptives

For patients who cannot use estrogen containing hormonal contraception, there are alternatives such as progestin-only hormonal contraceptives. Progestin-only contraceptives work by thickening cervical mucus, altering the environment in the uterus making it less suitable for implantation, and at times preventing ovulation. There are different formulations available which include a tablet, injection, IUD, and implant.

The progestin is an oral tablet taken once daily, also known as the mini-pill. There are no placebo pills with the progestin-only tablets. They should be taken at the same time everyday and a missed dose is considered 3 hours after the scheduled dose (Table 63-5). The missed tablet should be taken as soon as possible and a backup method is recommended for 48 hours. Side effects include progestin-associated adverse effects such as acne, weight gain, depression, and male pattern balding. The return to fertility with progestin is rapid with ovulation occurring within 1 to 3 months after discontinuation.

The progestin-only injection (Depo-Provera) is depot medroxyprogesterone acetate (DMPA) available as 150 mg intramuscular injection or 104 mg subcutaneous injection. The injection is given every 12 weeks + 1 week. Side effects are similar to other progestins; however, it is thought that there is more weight gain associated with DMPA. In addition, there is a FDA black box warning indicating that women may be at risk for low bone density and that DMPA should only be used for long periods of time (>2 years) if an alternate method is not available. A calcium supplement of 1000 to 1200 mg should be recommended while using DMPA. Other side effects include amenorrhea, depression, pain at injection site, and long return of fertility (up to 10 months).

Another progestin-only contraceptive available is the levonorgestrel (Mirena, Kyleena, Liletta, Skyla) intrauterine device/system (IUD/IUS). The IUS provides 20 mcg/d, 17.5 mcg/d, 18 mcg/d, and 14 mcg/d of levonorgestrel,

respectively. The IUS is a T-shaped device inserted into the uterus by a health care provider and may be left inside for up to 5 years (Mirena, Kyleena), 4 years (Liletta), or 3 years (Skyla). The IUS works by blocking implantation and thinning the endometrial lining of the uterus. Side effects are similar to those seen with other progestin agents but may cause more breakthrough bleeding. There is a rapid return to fertility of 1 to 3 months after removal of the IUS.

The progestin implant (Nexplanon) is a rod inserted by a health care provider underneath the skin of the upper arm. It may be left in for up to 3 years and helps prevent pregnancy by suppressing ovulation, thickening cervical mucus, and altering the endometrium. After removal of the rod, return to fertility is relatively short with 24% of women conceiving within 4 months. Side effects of the implant include fibrosis around the device, difficulty in removing the device, pain at site, and other side effects associated with progestins (Table 63-1). Nexplanon is made of radiopaque material that may be seen by x-ray to pinpoint the exact location of the rod.

Special Populations

Hormonal contraceptives are contraindicated in special populations (Table 63-6). Because estradiol can increase blood pressure and clotting factors, women with a history of venous thromboembolism (VTE), uncontrolled hypertension, history of migraine with aura, stroke, or cardiovascular disease should avoid the use of CHCs. In addition, women who are older than 35 years and smoke more than 15 cigarettes per day should not use CHCs due to an increased risk of stroke, heart attack, and blood clots.

Women who are 6 weeks postpartum or less should also avoid the use of CHCs, since the risk of blood clots is higher for postpartum women. CHC's may be initiated at 3 weeks postpartum if the patient is not breastfeeding or lacks VTE risk factors. Estradiol may decrease milk production, though waiting 6 weeks postpartum may be best. Currently, the American College of Obstetrics and Gynecology (ACOG) states that a CHC may be used while breastfeeding if there is adequate milk production. However, for women who have low milk production or are struggling to produce milk on

TABLE 63-6 Contraindications to Estrogen

- Older than 35 years and smokes 15 cigarettes per day
- History of VTE
- Migraine with aura
- Cardiovascular disease
- Less than 4-6 wk postpartum
- Liver disease
- Blood pressure >160/100 mm Hg
- Pregnancy
- Breast cancer
- Surgery within 4 wk
- Gallbladder disease
- Diabetes with retinopathy, neuropathy, or vascular disease
- Lactation
- Coagulopathies (eg, antiphospholipid syndrome, factor V Leiden)
- Stroke
- Complicated solid organ transplant

CHCs, a progestin-only or nonhormonal contraceptive may be more appropriate. Active liver disease is also a contraindication for CHCs since metabolism through the liver is required. Women with a history of breast cancer or other cancer that may be hormone-mediated should also avoid the use of CHCs and possibly progestin-only products. A common pneumonic used to help remember the serious side effects of CHCs is ACHES, where A = abdominal pain (liver), C = chest pain (pulmonary embolism), H = headache (stroke or clot), E = eye pain (stroke), S = swelling in legs (deep vein thrombosis [DVT]).

EMERGENCY CONTRACEPTION

EC is therapy for women who have had unprotected intercourse. Indications include contraceptive failure, exposure to a teratogen, sexual assault, and unprotected intercourse within 72 to 120 hours. There are different types of EC. The copper IUD and RU-486 must be provided by a licensed prescriber and are not used that frequently. Although, RU-486 may be used for EC, it is considered an abortifacient. High-dose hormones are most commonly known and referred to as the "morning after pill" and "EC" to the lay public. The use of high-dose hormones is not considered as an abortifacient and works primarily by preventing ovulation, increasing cervical mucus, and preventing implantation. It does not disrupt an implanted fertilized egg.

Two hormone methods exist, the Yuzpe method which contains two doses of high-dose estrogen (100 mcg) and high-dose progestin (0.5 mg levonorgestrel) and progestin-only (1.5 mg × 1 dose). Currently, the one tablet of levonorgestrel 1.5 mg is marketed OTC for all ages. Both methods are highly effective in preventing pregnancy (Yuzpe 75% effective and progestin-only 89% effective). EC should be taken within 72 hours of unprotected intercourse; however, EC may be effective up to 120 hours post-coitus.

Common side effects for both regimens (Yuzpe and levonorgestrel) include headache, breast tenderness, nausea, fatigue, and breakthrough bleeding. The incidence of nausea and vomiting is higher with the Yuzpe method. To mediate this side effect, antiemetics such as meclizine, dimenhydrinate, and diphenhydramine may be given 1 hour prior to the EC dose. For women who vomit within 1 to 2 hours of taking an EC dose, another dose should be administered. If a woman does not have her menses within 3 weeks, she should see her provider as pregnancy may have occurred.

Another product approved for EC is ella (ulipristal). Ella is a progesterone-receptor modulator and may be taken by mouth within 120 hours of unprotected intercourse. It is available by prescription only though in some states pharmacists may initiate prescriptions under collaborative agreements.

CASE Application

1. TK is a 23-year-old woman who comes to your pharmacy stating that she is taking the mini-pill and missed her dose yesterday. Based on this information, what is the best remedy in this situation?

   a. She should take two tablets today as soon as possible, no backup method is needed.
   b. She should start taking her tablets as scheduled and use a backup method for the next 48 hours.
   c. She should take two tablets today as soon as possible and use a backup method until she gets her period.
   d. She should start taking her tablets as scheduled and use a backup method until she gets her period.

2. AC is a 26-year-old woman who presents to the pharmacy asking to buy emergency contraceptive (Plan B One-Step) and says she had unprotected intercourse 3 days ago. Based on the information, select the best statement as it relates to EC.

   a. EC will not be effective for AC because it has been longer than 24 hours since she has had unprotected sex.
   b. EC will not be effective for AC because it has been longer than 48 hours since she has had unprotected sex.
   c. EC cannot be provided to AC without a prescription from her doctor.
   d. EC may still work for AC because it is still within 72 hours since she has had unprotected sex.
   e. EC may still work for AC because it is still within 120 hours since she has had unprotected sex, but she will require a prescription.

3. Please select the appropriate ranked products based on EE content from highest to lowest.

   a. Contraceptive vaginal ring> contraceptive patch> oral combined contraceptive (30 mcg EE)
   b. Contraceptive patch> oral combined contraceptive (30 mcg EE)> contraceptive vaginal ring
   c. Oral combined contraceptive (30 mcg EE)> contraceptive vaginal ring> contraceptive patch
   d. All of the above provide the same amount of EE.

4. GT is a 21-year-old woman who has a history of acne. Her acne has been refractory to doxycycline and topical agents. She is otherwise healthy. Her physician would like prescribe a hormonal treatment that has an FDA indication for acne. Which of the following could be recommended to GT? Select all that apply.

   a. Depo-Provera
   b. NuvaRing
   c. YAZ
   d. Estrostep

5. JK is a 32-year-old woman who weighs 75 kg and is 5'1". Which of the following is best to avoid in overweight/obese patients due to the side effects of weight gain?

   a. Depo-Provera
   b. NuvaRing

c. Xulane
d. Yasmin

6. How often is one NuvaRing inserted vaginally?

   a. 1 week
   b. 3 weeks
   c. 2 weeks
   d. 4 weeks

7. BD is a 28-year-old obese, woman who delivered a baby 1 week ago via C-section. She does not plan to breast-feed and would like to start a COC as soon as possible. When is the earliest she can start taking COCs without an increased risk of blood clots?

   a. Immediately
   b. 2 weeks postpartum
   c. 6 weeks postpartum
   d. 6 months postpartum

8. AJ is a 22-year-old woman who weighs 220 lb and would like to start hormonal contraception. Which of the following products would not be as effective in preventing pregnancy for AJ? Select all that apply.

   a. Depo-Provera
   b. NuvaRing
   c. Xulane
   d. Yasmin

9. Which of the following products contains drospirenone and may increase potassium levels? Select all that apply.

   a. Safyral
   b. YAZ
   c. Cyclessa
   d. Nor-QD

10. RS just started a new COC 2 weeks ago and has had some mild nausea when she takes the pill. What is the best recommendation for RS with respect to changing products?

    a. Change the oral combined contraceptive to another agent this week
    b. Wait for 3 months to see if side effects improve, if not change products
    c. Wait for 2 months to see if side effects improve, if not change products
    d. Wait for 6 months to see if side effects improve, if not change products

11. Select the name for levonorgestrel emergency contraceptive products. Select all that apply.

    a. Plan B One-Step
    b. Ortho Tri-Cyclen Lo
    c. My Way
    d. Xulane
    e. Next Choice One Dose

12. Select the contraceptive agent that is formulated as an injection.

    a. Desogen
    b. Mirena
    c. Estrostep
    d. Xulane
    e. Depo-Provera

13. JS is a 21-year-old man who comes to your pharmacy and states, "What can my girlfriend and I use to make sure she doesn't get pregnant and protect ourselves from, you know...diseases?" Select the best regimen to recommend from the following choices below.

    a. Water-based lubricant + male latex condom
    b. Oil-based lubricant + male latex condom
    c. Female condom + male latex condom
    d. Female condom + male lamb cecum condom
    e. Oil-based lubricant + male lamb cecum condom

14. Which of the following condoms conducts heat very well and protects against STIs? Select all that apply.

    a. Polyurethane
    b. Latex
    c. Lamb cecum
    d. Polyisoprene

15. QS is a 32-year-old woman who suffers from migraines without aura during her menses every time she takes the placebo pills in her oral contraceptive pack. The physician recommends that she switch to an extended cycle oral contraceptive to reduce the placebo pill weeks and number of menses to four per year. What is the appropriate number of active tablets contained in an extended cycle oral contraceptive product for QS to have four menses per year?

    a. 24
    b. 21
    c. 44
    d. 84
    e. 352

16. CS is a 36-year-old woman who admits to smoking one pack of cigarettes per day. She is getting married and would like to start hormonal contraception. Which of the following products is most appropriate for CS?

    a. NuvaRing
    b. Xulane
    c. Mircette
    d. Tri-Levlen
    e. Nor-QD

17. Which of the following drugs may decrease the effectiveness of Ortho-Tri Cyclen? Select all that apply.

    a. Atorvastatin
    b. Carbamazepine
    c. Lamotrigine

d. Acetaminophen

e. Phenytoin

18. DL is a 19-year-old woman who calls you and states that she forgot to take her Desogen (EE 30 mcg/0.15 mg desogestrel) tablets for the last 2 days. She says she is in her second week of the cycle. Select the following statement that is most appropriate for missed tablets.

a. DL should take two tablets the next day and use a backup method for 7 days

b. DL should continue taking her tablets as scheduled, one per day, no backup method is necessary

c. DL should discard her pill pack and start a new one, use a backup method for 7 days

d. DL should take two tablets for 2 days, no backup method is necessary

19. Combined hormonal contraception is contraindicated in which of the following conditions? Select all that apply.

a. History of DVT

b. Migraine with aura

c. Active liver disease

d. Uncontrolled hypertension

20. RR is a 26-year-old woman who has just been diagnosed with PMDD and is also seeking contraception. She is otherwise healthy and is not obese or overweight. Which of the following products is best to recommend for RR?

a. YAZ

b. Ortho Tri-Cyclen

c. Estrostep

d. Mircette

e. Yasmin

TAKEAWAY POINTS »

- Latex is the best choice of condoms for the prevention of STIs and pregnancy, but should not be used with oil-based lubricants.
- The female condom and male condom should not be used together at the same time, otherwise breakage may occur.
- Factors such as effectiveness, cost, accessibility, return to fertility, side effects, adherence, and comfort need to be considered when selecting a contraceptive agent for a patient.
- The contraceptive patch is less effective in women who weigh more than 198 lb.
- The contraceptive patch provides 60% more estrogen than a 35 mcg oral tablet of EE which may increase the risk of VTE.

- The vaginal ring is inserted vaginally for 3 weeks at a time and provides the least amount of estrogen compared to all other forms of combined hormonal contraception.
- DMPA is an injectable contraceptive agent administered subcutaneously or intramuscularly every 12 weeks.
- Calcium supplements of 1000 to 1200 mg daily should be taken when using DMPA.
- CHCs should not be used in patients who have a history of DVT, migraine with aura, stroke, who are 35 years old and smoke more than 15 cigarettes per day, cardiovascular disease, uncontrolled hypertension, or liver disease.
- Hormonal EC is also known as the morning after pill, but works up to 5 days after unprotected intercourse.

BIBLIOGRAPHY

Carroll S, Dean WS. Contraception. In: Linn WD, Wofford MR, O'Keefe M, Posey L, eds. *Pharmacotherapy in Primary Care.* New York, NY: McGraw-Hill; 2009:chap 28.

Contraception. In: DiPiro CV, Schwinghammer TL, eds. *Quick Answers: Pharmacy.* New York, NY: McGraw-Hill; 2013.

Hall JE. The female reproductive system, infertility, and contraception. In: Longo DL, Fauci AS, Kasper DL, Hauser SL, Jameson J, Loscalzo J, eds. *Harrison's Principles of Internal Medicine.* 18th ed. New York, NY: McGraw-Hill; 2012:chap 347.

Levin ER, Hammes SR. Estrogens and progestins. In: Brunton LL, Chabner BA, Knollmann BC, eds. *Goodman & Gilman's The Pharmacological Basis of Therapeutics.* 12th ed. New York, NY: McGraw-Hill; 2011:chap 40.

Shrader SP, Ragucci KR. Contraception. In: DiPiro JT, Talbert RL, Yee GC, Matzke GR, Wells BG, Posey L, eds. *Pharmacotherapy: A Pathophysiologic Approach.* 9th ed. New York, NY: McGraw-Hill; 2014:chap 62.

KEY ABBREVIATIONS

ACOG = American College of Obstetrics and Gynecology
CHCs = combined hormonal contraceptives
COCs = combined oral contraceptives
DMPA = depot medroxyprogesterone acetate
EC = emergency contraception
EE = ethinyl estradiol
FDA = Food and Drug Administration

HIV = human immunodeficiency virus
IUD = intrauterine device
IUS = intrauterine system
OTC = over the counter
PMDD = premenstrual dysphoric disorder
PMS = premenstrual syndrome
STIs = sexually transmitted infections

64

Allergic Rhinitis

Nancy Borja-Hart and Karen Whalen

FOUNDATION OVERVIEW

Allergic rhinitis is a chronic inflammatory disease of the upper airways. It is characterized by one or more of the following symptoms: nasal congestion, rhinorrhea, sneezing, and itching. Allergic rhinitis can impact quality of life and can lead to sleep disturbance and missed work and school.

Allergic nasal reactions are mediated by immunoglobulin E (IgE). Airborne allergens react with antigen-specific IgE bound to mast cells, triggering a release of inflammatory mediators such as histamine and leukotrienes. Both early (immediate) and late-phase allergic reactions occur following allergen exposure. Early-phase reactions happen within seconds to minutes and are due to the release of histamine, leukotrienes, tryptase, and cytokines. Sneezing, itching, rhinorrhea, and congestion are typical symptoms. The release of cytokines results in the infiltration of inflammatory cells such as basophils and eosinophils. This produces a late-phase reaction occurring 4 to 8 hours after allergen exposure. With continued exposure to the allergen, the late-phase inflammatory response results in chronic symptoms of allergic rhinitis.

Patients with allergic rhinitis may present with the following symptoms: clear rhinorrhea, nasal congestion, allergic conjunctivitis, sneezing, postnasal drip, and itchiness in the nose, ears, and/or eyes. Allergic shiners (swelling and darkening of circles under the eyes due to nasal obstruction and venous congestion) and allergic salute (upward rubbing of the nose) are less common signs.

Allergic rhinitis is differentiated from other types of rhinitis by a thorough medical history, complete medication history, and physical examination. Chief concerns, symptoms, patterns, and triggers of nasal and related symptoms should be obtained from the patient. Allergy skin testing or blood tests to identify allergen-specific IgE antibodies may be used to confirm the diagnosis of allergic rhinitis.

Depending on the frequency and severity of symptoms, allergic rhinitis is classified as mild intermittent, mild persistent, moderate-severe intermittent, and moderate-severe persistent. Patients who experience symptoms less than 4 days per week or for less than 4 consecutive weeks meet the criteria for *intermittent* allergic rhinitis. The *persistent* classification applies to patients whose allergic rhinitis symptoms occur more than 4 days per week and for more than 4 consecutive weeks. If symptoms do not impact daily activities, sleep patterns, work, or school, then the disease is considered *mild*. If these activities are impacted by allergic rhinitis, then the patient has a *moderate-severe* form. Other descriptors for allergic rhinitis include *seasonal*, *perennial*, or *episodic*. *Seasonal* allergic rhinitis refers to those patients with symptoms primarily during the spring and fall (high pollen seasons). Patients with *perennial* allergic rhinitis have symptoms throughout the year. Patients with *episodic* allergic rhinitis experience symptoms with sporadic exposures to aeroallergens.

PREVENTION

Patients should be advised to try and avoid offending allergens (pollen, fungi, mold, dust mites, and animals) if possible. During high pollen seasons, patients should limit outside exposure. To further assist with allergen avoidance, patients may take the following additional precautions to minimize exposure to indoor allergens: use a high-efficiency particulate air (HEPA) filter, vacuum with a HEPA filter (or remove carpets), wash laundry in hot water, use barrier protection on pillows and mattresses, use a pest control system to avoid insect emanations, and reduce indoor humidity to prevent growth of mold.

TREATMENT

The management of allergic rhinitis includes allergen avoidance, pharmacotherapy, and, if needed, immunotherapy. Six classes of medication are available for the management of allergic rhinitis. These include antihistamines, decongestants, intranasal corticosteroids, intranasal mast cell stabilizers, intranasal anticholinergic agents and leukotriene receptor antagonists (Table 64-1). The goals of therapy for patients with allergic rhinitis are to improve symptoms, improve quality of life, and provide a medication (if needed) with minimal adverse effects (Table 64-2). When considering pharmacotherapy, presenting symptoms, severity of symptoms, patient age, and comorbidities are important considerations.

Antihistamines

Antihistamines are histamine (H_1)-receptor antagonists. Oral, intranasal, and ophthalmic dosage forms are available for the

To access your complimentary online question exams, visit https://accesspharmacy.mhmedical.com/NAPLEX.aspx

TABLE 64-1   **Available Medications for Allergic Rhinitis**

Medication (Brand Name)	Normal Adult Dosage
Antihistamines	
Oral first-generation	
Brompheniramine[a]	4 mg po every 4-6 h as needed
(LoHist-12 extended-release tablet)[b]	6-12 mg po every 12 h
(Bromax extended-release tablet)[b]	11 mg po every 12 h as needed
Chlorpheniramine[a] (Aller-Chlor, Chlor-Trimeton Allergy)	4 mg po every 4-6 h
(Chlor-Trimeton Allergy 12 h 12 mg extended-release tablet)	12-18 mg po twice daily
(Chlorphen SR12 mg extended-release tablet)	
Clemastine[a] (Tavist Allergy)	1.34 mg po every 12 h
Diphenhydramine[a] (Benadryl, Diphenhist)	25-50 mg po every 4-6 h as needed
Triprolidine[a] (HISTEX)	2.5 mg po every 4-6 h
Oral second-generation	
Cetirizine[a] (Zyrtec)	5-10 mg po once daily
Desloratadine (Clarinex)[b]	5 mg po once daily
Fexofenadine[a]	
(Allegra 12 h)	60 mg po twice daily
(Allegra 24 h)	180 mg po once daily
Levocetirizine (Xyzal Allergy 24 h)	5 mg po once daily in the evening
Loratadine[a] (Claritin, Alavert)	10 mg po once daily
Intranasal	
Azelastine 0.1%[b,c]	1-2 sprays per nostril twice daily
Azelastine 0.15% (Astepro 0.15%)[b]	1-2 sprays per nostril twice daily *or* 2 sprays per nostril once daily
Olopatadine 665 mcg/spray (Patanase)[b]	2 sprays per nostril twice daily
Ophthalmic	
Azelastine 0.05%[b]	1 drop in affected eye twice daily
Bepotastine 1.5% (Bepreve)[b]	1 drop in affected eye twice daily
Ketotifen fumarate 0.025% (Alaway, Zaditor)	1 drop in affected eye every 8-12 h
Olopatadine 0.1% (Patanol)[b]	1 drop in affected eye twice daily
Olopatadine 0.2% (Pataday)[b]	1 drop in affected eye once daily
Olopatadine 0.7% (Pazeo)[b]	1 drop in affected eye once daily
Decongestants	
Oral	
Phenylephrine (Sudafed PE)	10-20 mg po every 4-6 h
Pseudoephedrine (Sudafed)	60 mg po every 4-6 h
(Sudafed 12 h extended-release tablet)	120 mg po every 12 h
(Sudafed 24 h extended-release tablet)	240 mg po every 24 h
Topical	
Oxymetazoline 0.05% (Afrin, Vicks Sinex)	2-3 sprays per nostril twice daily
Phenylephrine 0.25%, 0.5%, 1% (Neo-Synephrine, 4-Way Fast Acting)	2-3 sprays per nostril every 4 h
Intranasal Corticosteroids	
Beclomethasone 42 mcg/spray (Beconase AQ)[b]	1-2 sprays per nostril twice daily
Beclomethasone 80 mcg/spray (Qnasl)[b]	2 sprays per nostril once daily
Budesonide 32 mcg/spray (Rhinocort Allergy, Rhinocort Aqua[b])	1-2 sprays per nostril daily
Ciclesonide 37 mcg/spray (Zetonna)[b]	1 spray per nostril once daily
Ciclesonide 50 mcg/spray (Omnaris)[b]	2 sprays per nostril once daily
Flunisolide 25 mcg/spray[b]	2 sprays per nostril twice daily
Fluticasone furoate 27.5 mcg/spray (Flonase Sensimist)	2 sprays per nostril once daily; may reduce to 1 spray per nostril once daily
Fluticasone propionate 50 mcg/spray (Flonase, ClariSpray)	2 sprays per nostril once daily; may reduce to 1 spray per nostril once daily
Mometasone furoate 50 mcg/spray (Nasonex)[b]	2 sprays per nostril once daily
Triamcinolone acetonide 55 mcg/spray (Nasacort Allergy)	2 sprays per nostril once daily; may reduce to 1 spray per nostril once daily

TABLE 64-1	Available Medications for Allergic Rhinitis *(Continued)*
Medication (Brand Name)	**Normal Adult Dosage**
Mast Cell Stabilizer	
Intranasal	
Cromolyn sodium 5.2 mg/spray (Nasalcrom)	1 spray per nostril 3-4 times daily
Ophthalmic	
Cromolyn sodium 4%[b]	1-2 drops in each eye 4-6 times daily
Intranasal Anticholinergic	
Ipratropium bromide 0.03%[b]	2 sprays per nostril 2-3 times daily
Ipratropium bromide 0.06%[b]	2 sprays per nostril 4 times daily
Leukotriene Receptor Antagonist	
Montelukast (Singulair)[b]	10 mg po once daily

Abbreviations: h, hours; po (per os), by mouth; prn (pro re nata), as needed.
[a]Antihistamines are also available as a combination product with a decongestant.
[b]Product available by prescription only (Rx).
[c]Available in combination with intranasal fluticasone propionate 50 mcg as Dymista

TABLE 64-2	Side Effects and Monitoring of Medications for Allergic Rhinitis		
Drug	**Adverse Reaction**	**Monitoring Parameter**	**Comments**
Antihistamines	Drowsiness	Caution patient about the potential for drowsiness, even with nonsedating and intranasal products	Do not mix with alcohol or other CNS depressants
	Gastrointestinal effects	Counsel patient to take with a meal or full glass of water	
	Anticholinergic effects	Watch for dry mouth and difficulty with urination. Caution patient about other medications with anticholinergic effects	Switching to an antihistamine with less anticholinergic effects may be necessary
Decongestants			
■ Topical	■ Rebound vasodilation ■ Local irritation	■ Watch for decreased response to topical agent ■ Watching for burning, stinging, sneezing, and dryness of mucosa	■ Avoid prolonged use (>3-5 d) ■ Self-limiting due to short-term use. May try nasal saline for dryness
■ Systemic	■ Hypertension ■ CNS stimulation	■ If used in a patient with hypertension, monitor blood pressure regularly and discontinue if the pressure increases ■ Usually mild but discuss with patient	■ Usually not an issue for patients without pre-existing hypertension. Use lowest effective dose ■ Use lowest effective dose
Nasal steroids	■ Local effects such as sneezing, stinging, and epistaxis	■ These effects may vary among products	
Other intranasal agents			
■ Cromolyn	■ Local effects such as sneezing, burning, or coughing	■ Usually mild but tell patient to report bothersome symptoms	If patient cannot tolerate local reactions, choose an alternative agent
■ Ipratropium	■ Headache, nosebleeds, and nasal dryness		
Montelukast	■ Headache, diarrhea, abdominal pain ■ Behavioral changes rare	■ Monitor for mood and behavioral changes including suicidal ideation	■ Rare but should be monitored
Immunotherapy, SubQ	■ Local reactions	■ Watch for induration or swelling at site of injection	■ Anaphylaxis rare, but should only be given under direct medical supervision with epinephrine available
Immunotherapy, SL	■ Allergic reactions ■ Pruritus of ear, oral itching, mouth edema, throat irritation	■ Monitor for signs of anaphylaxis ■ Caution patient about these reactions as they are fairly common	■ First dose given in physician's office so patient can be observed for 30 min. Treatment must be accompanied by a prescription for an epinephrine autoinjector

treatment of allergic rhinitis. Oral antihistamines are efficacious for management of rhinorrhea, sneezing, itching, and allergic conjunctivitis. These agents are more effective at preventing symptoms of allergic rhinitis than alleviating symptoms once they have occurred. As such, they are best taken prior to anticipated allergen exposure.

Among the oral antihistamines, the second-generation agents (eg, desloratadine, fexofenadine) are preferred. In general, the first-generation antihistamines are nonselective and more sedating than the second-generation antihistamines. In children, the first-generation oral antihistamines can cause paradoxical agitation rather than sedation. Additionally, the first-generation antihistamines have more anticholinergic adverse effects (dry mouth, constipation) compared to the second-generation agents. Some of the second-generation antihistamines can be sedating at usual doses (eg, cetirizine and intranasal azelastine) or when usual doses are exceeded (eg, loratadine and desloratadine). Intranasal antihistamines (azelastine and olopatadine) are effective in patients with seasonal allergic rhinitis. Azelastine has a rapid onset of action, which allows patients to administer the dose shortly before contact with a known allergen. Intranasal antihistamines do not target ocular symptoms. Thus, topical ocular antihistamines (bepotastine and olopatadine) may be needed for management of allergic conjunctivitis. Ketotifen is an over-the-counter (OTC) ophthalmic antihistamine and mast cell stabilizer that provides ocular itch relief. It is indicated for children as young as 3 years of age.

Decongestants

Decongestants produce vasoconstriction due to sympathomimetic effects. In allergic rhinitis, decongestants are most effective for patients with nasal congestion. These agents should be used on a short-term as-needed basis. For years, pseudoephedrine was the most common oral decongestant; however, misuse of the medication in the illegal production of methamphetamine resulted in substitution of phenylephrine as the decongestant in many OTC products. Because of the concern for misuse, pseudoephedrine is only available behind the counter. Pseudoephedrine, especially at higher than recommended doses, may increase blood pressure. Additional adverse effects include insomnia and irritability. Phenylephrine is a less effective oral decongestant with a similar adverse effect profile. Oral decongestants should be avoided in patients with uncontrolled hypertension, coronary artery disease, angle-closure glaucoma, and urinary retention. These agents may be used cautiously in patients with diabetes, controlled hypertension, and renal impairment.

Topical decongestants work quickly and are available as nasal sprays or nasal drops. Adverse effects include burning, stinging, sneezing, or dryness of the nasal mucosa. Patients should be advised to use topical decongestants infrequently and to avoid use for greater than 3 to 5 days, which may lead to the development of *rhinitis medicamentosa* or rebound nasal congestion.

Intranasal Corticosteroids

Intranasal corticosteroids inhibit allergic inflammation in the nose. These agents target the four hallmark symptoms of allergic rhinitis including sneezing, itching, rhinorrhea, and nasal congestion. Intranasal corticosteroids are the most effective medications for allergic rhinitis. Maximum effects of these agents may take several days to a few weeks. Following application, patients should be instructed to avoid blowing the nose or sneezing for at least 10 minutes to ensure the medication remains on the nasal mucosa. The likelihood of significant systemic absorption and hypothalamic-pituitary-adrenal (HPA) axis suppression with intranasal corticosteroids is minimal. Slight growth suppression has been associated with use of intranasal steroids, and the labeling for OTC intranasal steroids contains a statement that growth may be slower in children using these products. Local irritation of nasal mucosa (burning, drying, and irritation) is common with intranasal corticosteroids.

Mast Cell Stabilizer

Cromolyn sodium is an intranasal mast cell stabilizer that is modestly effective in the prevention and treatment of allergic rhinitis. Cromolyn works by inhibiting mast cell degranulation and release of inflammatory leukotrienes. For prevention of seasonal allergies, cromolyn should be initiated 1 week prior to allergen exposure. For perennial rhinitis, effects may take 2 weeks or more. It should be administered intranasally four times a day and must cover the entire nasal lining to be most effective. Therefore, patients should be instructed to blow the nose prior to administration. Cromolyn sodium is also available as an ophthalmic solution for allergic conjunctivitis; however, it needs to be administered four to six times daily for maximum effect.

Intranasal Anticholinergic Agent

Ipratropium is an intranasal anticholinergic agent that provides relief of rhinorrhea. It may be useful for patients who still experience rhinorrhea with an intranasal corticosteroid. Intranasal ipratropium is dosed two to four times daily, depending on symptoms. Efficacy beyond 3 weeks has not been established.

Leukotriene Receptor Antagonists

Montelukast is the only antileukotriene agent approved for management of allergic rhinitis. Although it is not a first-line agent for allergic rhinitis, it may be a good choice in patients with coexisting asthma. Montelukast is available as an oral tablet, chewable tablet, or granule formulation and can be used in children as young as 6 months of age.

Nasal Saline

Nasal saline is effective for removing mucus from the nose and clearing blocked nasal passages prior to the administration of other intranasal medications.

Allergen Immunotherapy

Immunotherapy is the gradual administration of antigens to induce tolerance and reduce symptoms with subsequent allergen exposure. Immunotherapy should be considered for patients whose symptoms are not relieved with pharmacologic management and for those who are experiencing undesirable adverse effects. Patients with specific IgE antibodies to clinically relevant allergens are optimal candidates for immunotherapy.

Special Populations

Infants and children older than 6 months of age can use cetirizine, levocetirizine, desloratadine, or montelukast for mild allergic rhinitis symptoms. Loratadine and fexofenadine are also approved for use in children 2 years of age and up. If symptoms become more severe, this population may benefit from intranasal corticosteroids, some of which are approved for children 2 years of age or older.

First-generation antihistamines should not be used in geriatric patients due to increased fall risk. At usual doses, second generation antihistamines are nonsedating and are appropriate for this population. The dose of cetirizine should be limited to 5 mg in patients who are 77 years of age or older.

Self-treatment of allergic rhinitis with nonprescription therapy is not recommended in pregnancy unless approved by a health care prescriber. Antihistamines, particularly cetirizine and levocetirizine, can be used in pregnant patients with approval from a health care prescriber. Intranasal cromolyn may be used for mild allergic rhinitis in pregnancy, and intranasal corticosteroids such as budesonide are first-line therapy for moderate-to-severe symptoms. Oral decongestants can be used following the first trimester though they are not highly recommended due to vasoconstriction of uterine blood vessels. Topical decongestants have limited systemic absorption and are appropriate for short-term use. Women should not initiate immunotherapy during pregnancy; however, it may be continued during pregnancy.

CASE Application

1. Which of the following are classic symptoms of allergic rhinitis? Select all that apply.

    a. Rhinorrhea
    b. Congestion
    c. Sneezing
    d. Fever

2. Which of the following is a potential adverse effect when using oral antihistamines for the management of allergic rhinitis in a 3-year-old child?

    a. HPA axis suppression
    b. Paradoxical agitation
    c. Rebound congestion
    d. Medication tolerance

3. MH is a 37-year-old man with a history of chronic nasal stuffiness. He reports symptoms all year round. His only other medical condition is high blood pressure. In addition to stuffiness, he has been sneezing a lot at work (which he finds very embarrassing). Also, his allergies have caused him to cancel park outings with his family. Which of the following best classifies MH's symptoms?

    a. Mild intermittent
    b. Moderate-to-severe intermittent
    c. Mild persistent
    d. Moderate-to-severe persistent

4. Which therapeutic option would be best for MH?

    a. Oral decongestant
    b. First-generation antihistamine
    c. Intranasal corticosteroid
    d. Intranasal decongestant

5. CF is a 25-year-old pregnant female (first trimester) who presents to the pharmacy complaining of constant sneezing, congestion, and a runny nose. Which therapeutic option would be best for CF?

    a. Intranasal corticosteroid
    b. Nonselective antihistamine
    c. Oral decongestant
    d. Mast cell stabilizer

6. Select the brand name for levocetirizine.

    a. Clarinex
    b. Zaditor
    c. Xyzal
    d. Singulair

7. The use of pseudoephedrine is concerning in a patient with which of the following disease states? Select all that apply.

    a. Diabetes mellitus
    b. Chronic kidney disease
    c. Hypertension
    d. Osteoarthritis

8. Which of the following antihistamines is available by over-the-counter? Select all that apply.

    a. Desloratadine
    b. Diphenhydramine
    c. Ketotifen
    d. Levocetirizine

9. Which of the following classes of medication can be used for management of allergic rhinitis in pregnancy? Select all that apply.

    a. Oral antihistamines
    b. Intranasal corticosteroids
    c. Oral decongestants
    d. Topical decongestants

10. JS is a 23-year-old man with a history of seasonal allergic rhinitis. He complains of bothersome nasal stuffiness each year during the fall when ragweed pollen is prevalent. Which of the following medications is most appropriate to provide immediate relief of his nasal congestion?

    a. Cetirizine
    b. Chlorpheniramine
    c. Fluticasone
    d. Oxymetazoline

11. Which of the following allergen avoidance techniques would be appropriate to help reduce JS's allergic symptoms caused by ragweed pollen?

    a. Encase pillow and mattress in allergen-proof cover.
    b. Keep windows closed and minimize outdoor activities.
    c. Reduce indoor humidity to <50%.
    d. Wash bedding in hot water.

12. Which of the following medications would be beneficial to JS in reducing symptoms of seasonal allergic rhinitis when started prior to allergen exposure? Select all that apply.

    a. Intranasal corticosteroid
    b. Leukotriene antagonist
    c. Oral antihistamine
    d. Topical decongestant

13. CW is an 8-year-old boy with seasonal allergic rhinitis and mild persistent asthma. Which of the following medications would be appropriate to manage symptoms of both his asthma and allergic rhinitis?

    a. Intranasal beclomethasone
    b. Intranasal cromolyn
    c. Cetirizine
    d. Montelukast

14. Sedation would most likely occur with which of the following antihistamines when used at recommended dosages for adult patients?

    a. Desloratadine
    b. Diphenhydramine
    c. Fexofenadine
    d. Olopatadine

15. Which of the following antihistamines is available in an intranasal formulation?

    a. Azelastine
    b. Ketotifen
    c. Levocetirizine
    d. Loratadine

16. Which of the following categories of allergic rhinitis medications is most likely to be associated with rhinitis medicamentosa (rebound nasal congestion) with prolonged use?

    a. Intranasal corticosteroid
    b. Intranasal decongestant
    c. Intranasal antihistamine
    d. Oral decongestant

17. Which of the following medications must be kept behind the pharmacy counter, since it may be used in the production of methamphetamine?

    a. Brompheniramine
    b. Chlorpheniramine
    c. Phenylephrine
    d. Pseudoephedrine

18. NH is a 35-year-old woman who is taking a combination of cetirizine, intranasal fluticasone, pseudoephedrine, and montelukast to manage symptoms of persistent allergic rhinitis. She complains of feeling jittery and having palpitations after taking all of her medications in the morning. Which of the following medications is most likely causing her complaints?

    a. Cetirizine
    b. Fluticasone
    c. Montelukast
    d. Pseudoephedrine

19. TR is a 6-year-old boy with persistent allergic rhinitis. He is experiencing symptoms despite the use of an oral antihistamine, and the physician would like to add an intranasal corticosteroid. Which of the following is correct regarding the use of an intranasal corticosteroid for TR?

    a. Intranasal corticosteroids should not be combined with oral antihistamines in pediatric patients.
    b. Growth may be slower in children while using intranasal corticosteroids.
    c. The use of intranasal corticosteroids is contraindicated in children less than 12 years of age.
    d. TR should obtain relief of his symptoms within minutes of using the intranasal corticosteroid.

20. KW is a 45-year-old woman who experiences daily rhinorrhea despite the use of loratadine and intranasal fluticasone. Addition of which of the following medications would best target the symptoms of rhinorrhea?

    a. Azelastine
    b. Ipratropium
    c. Oxymetazoline
    d. Phenylephrine

TAKEAWAY POINTS »

- Allergic rhinitis is a common inflammatory disorder of the nasal mucosa characterized by one or more of the following nasal symptoms: rhinorrhea, itching, sneezing, and nasal congestion. Symptoms of allergic conjunctivitis often accompany allergic rhinitis.

- Avoidance of allergens (eg, encasing mattresses and pillows, getting rid of carpets, using HEPA filters) may help reduce or prevent symptoms of allergic rhinitis.

- Selection of pharmacotherapy for allergic rhinitis should be based on the presenting symptoms, age of the patient, and coexisting medical conditions.

- Overall, intranasal corticosteroids are the most effective medication for allergic rhinitis. They target multiple symptoms of allergic rhinitis including rhinorrhea, itching, sneezing, and nasal congestion. Intranasal corticosteroids may also be beneficial in reducing ocular symptoms.

- Growth may be slower in children using intranasal corticosteroids.

- Oral antihistamines target multiple symptoms of allergic rhinitis, although they are less effective than intranasal corticosteroids for managing nasal congestion. For optimal efficacy, antihistamines should be taken prior to exposure to the allergen.

- In general, first-generation antihistamines have more anticholinergic and sedative properties than the second-generation antihistamines.

- Intranasal topical antihistamines have a rapid onset of action and are an alternative to oral antihistamines. They do not target ocular symptoms. Thus, the addition of topical ocular antihistamines may be needed for management of allergic conjunctivitis.

- Oral and topical decongestants are only effective for management of the nasal congestion aspect of allergic rhinitis. Patients should be advised not to use topical decongestants for greater than 3 to 5 days due to the possibility of developing rhinitis medicamentosa.

- The leukotriene antagonist montelukast is indicated for seasonal allergic rhinitis and is a reasonable choice for patients with allergic rhinitis and asthma.

- Intranasal ipraptropium may be considered for patients with persistent rhinorrhea despite other therapies, or those intolerant of other treatments.

- Effective agents for seasonal allergic rhinitis include oral and topical antihistamines, intranasal corticosteroids, leukotriene antagonists (montelukast), and intranasal cromolyn. For maximal efficacy, these agents should be started prior to the expected onset of allergic symptoms.

BIBLIOGRAPHY

Bousquet J, Khaltaev N, Cruz AA, et al. Allergic rhinitis and its impact on asthma (ARIA) 2008. *Allergy.* 2008;63(Suppl 86):8-160.

Boyce A, Austen K. Allergies, anaphylaxis, and systemic mastocytosis. In: Kasper D, Fauci A, Hauser S, Longo D, Jameson J, Loscalzo J, eds. *Harrison's Principles of Internal Medicine.* 19th ed. New York, NY: McGraw-Hill; 2014.

Inamdar S. Allergic and nonallergic rhinitis. In: Linn WD, Wofford MR, O'Keefe M, Posey L, eds. *Pharmacotherapy in Primary Care.* New York, NY: McGraw-Hill; 2009:chap 37.

May J. Allergic rhinitis. In: DiPiro JT, Talbert RL, Yee GC, Matzke GR, Wells BG, Posey L, eds. *Pharmacotherapy: A Pathophysiologic Approach.* 10th ed. New York, NY: McGraw-Hill;

http://accesspharmacy.mhmedical.com.lp.hscl.ufl.edu/content.aspx?bookid=1861&sectionid=134128639. May 25, 2017.

Skidgel RA, Kaplan AP, Erdös EG. Histamine, bradykinin, and their antagonists. In: Brunton LL, Chabner BA, Knollmann BC, eds. *Goodman & Gilman's The Pharmacological Basis of Therapeutics.* 12th ed. New York, NY: McGraw-Hill; 2011:chap 32.

Wallace DV, Dykewicz MS, Bernstein DI, et al; Joint Task Force on Practice; American Academy of Allergy; Asthma & Immunology; American College of Allergy; Asthma and Immunology; Joint Council of Allergy, Asthma and Immunology. The diagnosis and management of rhinitis: an updated practice parameter. *J Allergy Clin Immunol.* 2008;122(2 suppl):S1-S84.

KEY ABBREVIATIONS

HEPA = high-efficiency particulate air
HPA = hypothalamic-pituitary-adrenal

IgE = immunoglobulin E
OTC = over-the-counter

Matthew Cantrell, Michael W. Kelly, and Scott M. Vouri

FOUNDATION OVERVIEW: BENIGN PROSTATIC HYPERPLASIA

Benign prostatic hyperplasia (BPH) is an enlarged prostate gland. The prostate gland surrounds the urethra, the tube that carries urine from the bladder out of the body. As the prostate gets bigger, it may squeeze or partly block the urethra causing problems with urinating. The prostate begins to grow as men age, increasing the risk for BPH. Patients with BPH have increased smooth muscle tissue in the prostate containing α_1-adrenergic receptors resulting in vasoconstriction and narrowing of the urethral lumen. Additionally, patients have physical obstruction symptoms resulting from an enlarged prostate.

Lower urinary tract symptoms (LUTS) suggestive of BPH alter bladder emptying or storage. Voiding symptoms are found early in the disease course and include urinary hesitancy, weak urinary stream, and the sensation of incomplete bladder emptying. Storage symptoms include urinary frequency, nocturia, urinary urgency, and urge incontinence. These symptoms occur after several years as the bladder smooth muscle hypertrophies and weaken. BPH increases the risk of urinary tract infections, bladder stones secondary to urinary stasis, and renal impairment. A serious complication of BPH is acute urinary retention, which often requires immediate catheterization.

Patients with LUTS should be referred to their physician as a detailed history and physical examination are necessary to exclude other possible etiologies, including prostate cancer, urinary tract infections, and neurological or endocrine disorders. A digital rectal examination (DRE) determines the prostate size and can identify nodules suggestive of malignancy. A urinalysis excludes urinary tract infections or bladder stones. Pharmacists should be aware of medications that worsen LUTS. Examples include medications with anticholinergic properties such as antihistamines, tricyclic antidepressants, and opiates. Furthermore, as prostate tissue contains α_1-adrenergic receptors, α-agonists such as pseudoephedrine or other decongestants exacerbate symptoms or attenuate therapy with α_1-adrenergic antagonists.

TREATMENT

BPH treatment depends on multiple factors: LUTS severity, concurrent medical illness that affects hemodynamic stability, prostate size, and presence of BPH-related complications. The American Urological Association (AUA) has a scoring system to rate BPH symptoms. Patients with mild BPH (AUA score of 0-7) are candidates for watchful waiting (if symptoms are not bothersome). This is a reasonable strategy as symptoms of BPH wax and wane and treatment may not be needed. If this strategy is used, patients should be monitored for worsening of symptoms indicating the need for pharmacologic treatment. The goals of treatment are to control symptoms, as evidenced by a minimum of a 3-point decrease in the AUA symptom index, prevent progression of BPH disease by reducing the risk of developing complications, and delay the need for surgical intervention. Drug therapy for BPH can be categorized into three types: agents that relax prostatic smooth muscle (reducing the dynamic factor), agents that interfere with testosterone's stimulatory effect on prostate gland enlargement (reducing the static factor), and agents that relax bladder detrusor muscle (improving the urine storage capacity of the bladder). Of the agents that relax prostatic smooth muscle, second- and third-generation α_1-adrenergic antagonists have been most widely used. These agents relax the intrinsic urethral sphincter and prostatic smooth muscle, thereby enhancing urinary outflow from the bladder. PDE-5 also relax bladder neck and prostatic smooth muscle. α_1-Adrenergic antagonists and PDE-5 do not reduce prostate size. Of the agents that interfere with testosterone's stimulatory effect on prostate gland size, the only agents approved by the FDA are 5α-reductase inhibitors (eg, finasteride, dutasteride). Antimuscarinic agents relax detrusor muscle contraction, which reduces irritable voiding symptoms in some patients with BPH. Antimuscarinic agents and mirabegron both reduce irritative voiding symptoms, improve urine storage capacity of the bladder, and increase the interval between voidings. Tables 65-1 to 65-3 describe key treatment parameters for BPH medications.

α_1-Adrenergic Antagonists

For patients with moderate to severe BPH (AUA score 8-35), α_1-adrenergic antagonists are effective in reducing LUTS. This class of medications improves voiding symptoms by relaxing prostatic smooth muscle tissue, thereby allowing passage of urine through the urethra. However, they do not reduce the prostate size or prevent progression of BPH. The primary distinction between α_1-adrenergic antagonists is their selectivity for the α_{1A}-adrenergic receptor, which ultimately

TABLE 65-1	Comparison of α₁-Adrenergic Antagonists, 5α-Reductase Inhibitors, Phosphodiesterase Inhibitors, and Anticholinergic Agents for Benign Prostatic Hyperplasia	
	α₁-Adrenergic Antagonists	**5α-Reductase Inhibitors**
Relaxes prostatic smooth muscle	Yes	No
Decreases prostate size	No	Yes
Halts disease progression	No	Yes
Peak onset	1-6 wk	3-6 mo
Efficacy in relieving BOO	++	++ (for patients with enlarged prostates)
Frequency of dosing	One to two times per day, depending on the agent and dosage formulation	Once per day
Decreases PSA	No	Yes
Sexual dysfunction adverse effects	EJD	Decreased libido, ED, EJD
Cardiovascular adverse effects	Yes	No
	Phosphodiesterase Inhibitors	**Anticholinergic Agents**
Relaxes prostatic smooth muscle	Yes	No
Decreases prostate size	No	No
Halts disease progression	No	No
Peak onset	4 wk	1-2 wk
Efficacy in relieving BOO	+	0 (irritative symptoms only)
Frequency of dosing	Once per day	Once per day
Decreases prostate-specific antigen	No	No
Sexual dysfunction adverse effects	No	ED
Cardiovascular adverse effects	Yes (mild hypotension)	Yes (tachycardia)
	β₃-Adrenergic Agonists	
Relaxes prostatic smooth muscle	No	
Decreases prostate size	No	
Halts disease progression	No	
Peak onset	2 wk, but may take up to 8 wk	
Efficacy in relieving BOO	0 (irritative symptoms only)	
Frequency of dosing	Once per day	
Decreases prostate-specific antigen	No	
Sexual dysfunction adverse effects	No	
Cardiovascular adverse effects	Yes (hypertension)	

Abbreviations: BOO, bladder outlet obstruction; ED, erectile dysfunction; EJD, ejaculation disorder; PSA, prostate-specific antigen.
⁺Notation is a quantitative assessment.
Reproduced with permission from DiPiro JT, Talbert RL, Yee GC, et al: *Pharmacotherapy: A Pathophysiologic Approach,* 10th ed: New York, NY: McGraw-Hill; 2017.

affects tolerability. Efficacy of α₁-adrenergic antagonists is comparable.

Prazosin (Minipress) is not recommended because of multiple daily dosing, quick onset, and lipophilic structure (increases orthostatic hypotension and syncope). Terazosin (Hytrin) and doxazosin (Cardura) are second generation α₁-adrenergic receptor antagonists. Immediate-release terazosin and doxazosin require dose titration to prevent cardiovascular side effects, thus delaying the time to reach an effective dose. Doxazosin is available as an extended-release formulation which may improve tolerability. Side effects include orthostatic hypotension, syncope, muscle weakness, and fatigue. Patients should be cautioned about decreases in blood pressure if they also use PDE-5 for erectile dysfunction (ED).

Tamsulosin (Flomax) and silodosin (Rapaflo) are uroselective based on their affinity for α₁ₐ-receptors and alfuzosin

(Uroxatral) is functionally uroselective based on its extended-release formulation preventing peaks in serum concentrations. These agents target α₁ₐ-receptors in the prostate and are less likely to cause hypotension or syncope. These agents improve urinary symptoms within 1 week because they do not require dose titration. Additional effects include ejaculatory disturbances and intraoperative floppy iris syndrome (IFIS). Pharmacists should counsel patients to inform their ophthalmologist prior to cataract surgery, if they take this class of medications.

5-α-Reductase Inhibitors

The conversion of testosterone to dihydrotestosterone (DHT) mediated by the enzyme 5-α-reductase stimulates prostate growth. Inhibiting 5-α-reductase decreases symptoms of BPH by reducing prostate size and decrease prostate specific antigen by 25%. Two 5-α-reductase inhibitors (5ARIs) include

TABLE 65-2 Dosing of Drugs Used in Treatment of Benign Prostatic Hyperplasia

Drug	Brand Name	Initial Dose	Usual Dose	Special Population Dose
α-Adrenergic Antagonists				
Prazosin	Minipress	0.5 mg twice a day orally	1-5 mg twice a day orally	For uptitrating the dose, double the dose every 2 wk
Terazosin	Hytrin	1 mg at bedtime orally	10-20 mg daily orally	For uptitrating the dose, increase slowly to 2 mg, 5 mg, and then 10 mg daily in a stepwise fashion. Take extra care if the patient is taking other drugs that lower blood pressure
Doxazosin	Cardura Cardura XL	1 mg daily orally 4 mg daily orally	8 mg daily orally 4-8 mg daily	For the immediate-release formulation, doses of 16 mg daily have been used for hypertension. For the XL formulation, increase from 4-8 mg daily after a 3- to 4-wk interval. When switching from the immediate- to the extended-release formulation, start at 4 mg of the extended-release formulation no matter what maintenance dose of immediate-release doxazosin the patient is taking
Alfuzosin	Uroxatral	10 mg daily orally	10 mg daily orally (no dose titration)	This is an extended-release formulation, and it should not be chewed or crushed. The drug should be taken after meals and used cautiously in patients with creatinine clearance less than 30 mL/min (0.5 mL/s)
Tamsulosin	Flomax	0.4 mg daily orally	0.4-0.8 mg daily orally	This is an extended-release formulation, and it should not be chewed or crushed. The drug should be taken after meals. No dosage adjustment is needed in patients with renal or liver dysfunction. Allow several weeks after starting a dose before increasing to a higher dose
Silodosin	Rapaflo	8 mg daily orally	8 mg daily orally (no dose titration)	This drug is contraindicated when creatinine clearance is less than 30 mL/min (0.5 mL/s). If creatinine clearance is 30-50 mL/min (0.5-0.83 mL/s), use 4 mg daily orally, preferably after the same meal each day. Should not be given to patients on potent CYP 3A4 inhibitors or to patients known to be poor metabolizers of CYP 2D6
5α-Reductase Inhibitors				
Finasteride	Proscar	5 mg daily orally	5 mg daily orally	No dosage adjustment in patients with renal impairment. Use cautiously in patients with hepatic impairment
Dutasteride	Avodart	0.5 mg daily orally	0.5 mg daily orally	No dosage adjustment in patients with renal impairment. Use cautiously in patients with hepatic impairment
Dutasteride + tamsulosin	Jalyn	1 tablet (equivalent to 0.5 mg dutasteride + 0.4 mg tamsulosin) daily orally	1 tablet daily orally	No dosage adjustment needed in patients with renal or hepatic impairment
Phosphodiesterase Inhibitor				
Tadalafil	Cialis	5 mg daily orally	5 mg daily orally	If creatinine clearance is 30-50 mL/min (0.5-0.83 mL/s), use 2.5 mg daily orally. Do not use if creatinine clearance is less than 30 mL/min (0.5 mL/s)
Anticholinergic Agents				
Darifenacin	Enablex	7.5 mg daily orally	7.5-15 mg daily orally	For uptitrating the dose, double the dose after 2 wk. If the patient is taking a potent CYP3A4 inhibitor (eg, ketoconazole, itraconazole, ritonavir, nelfinavir, and clarithromycin), do not exceed 7.5 mg daily orally
Fesoterodine	Toviaz	4 mg daily orally	4-8 mg daily orally	This is an extended-release formulation, and it should not be chewed or crushed. If the patient is taking a potent CYP3A4 inhibitor (eg, ketoconazole, itraconazole, ritonavir, nelfinavir, and clarithromycin), do not exceed 4 mg daily orally. If the creatinine clearance is less than 30 mL/min (0.5 mL/s), do not exceed 4 mg daily orally
Oxybutynin	Ditropan	5 mg two to three times a day orally	5-10 mg two to three times a day orally	Increase daily dose at 5-mg increments at weekly intervals. No specific dosing modifications available for patients with renal impairment, however use cautiously in these patients
	Ditropan XL	5 mg daily orally	5-30 mg daily orally	This is an extended release formulation, and it should not be crushed or chewed. Increase daily dose at 5-mg increments at weekly intervals. No specific dosing modifications available for patients with renal impairment, but use cautiously in these patients

Drug	Brand Name	Initial Dose	Usual Dose	Special Population Dose
	Oxytrol TDS	1 patch (3.9 mg oxybutynin) twice weekly	1 patch (3.9 mg) twice weekly	This is a transdermal patch. Apply to abdomen, hip, or buttock. Rotate application site. Do not expose patch to sunlight. No specific dosing modifications available for patients with renal impairment, however use cautiously in these patients
	Gelnique 10% gel	1 g gel (100 mg oxybutynin) daily	1 g gel (100 mg oxybutynin) daily	This is available as premeasured dose packets. Apply to abdomen, thighs, upper arms, or shoulders. Wash hands after application. Do not bathe, shower, or swim for 1 h after application. Cover application site with clothing until medication dries on skin. Rotate application site daily. No specific dosing modifications available for patients with renal impairment, but use cautiously in these patients
Solifenacin	Vesicare	5 mg daily orally	5-10 mg daily orally	If the creatinine clearance is less than 30 mL/min (0.5 mL/s) or the patient has moderate hepatic impairment, do not exceed 5 mg daily orally. If the patient is taking a potent CYP3A4 inhibitor (eg, ketoconazole, itraconazole, ritonavir, nelfinavir, and clarithromycin), do not exceed 5 mg daily orally
Tolterodine	Detrol	2 mg twice daily orally	2 mg twice daily orally	If the patient has significant renal impairment, limit dose to 1 mg twice a day
	Detrol LA	4 mg daily orally	4 mg daily orally	The LA formulation is an extended-release formulation, and it should not be chewed or crushed. If the creatinine clearance is 10-30 mL/min (0.17-0.5 mL/s) or the patient has mild/moderate hepatic impairment, do not exceed 2 mg daily orally. If the creatinine clearance is less than 10 mL/min (0.17 mL/s), do not use Detrol LA
Trospium	Sanctura	20 mg twice daily orally	20 mg twice daily orally	Avoid alcohol ingestion for 2 h after a dose. Use cautiously in patients with moderate or severe hepatic impairment. In patients older than 75 y, use the immediate-release formulation and start with 20 mg daily orally. If the creatinine clearance is less than 30 mL/min (0.5 mL/s), use 20-mg immediate-release formulation
	Sanctura XR	60 mg daily orally	60 mg daily orally	The XR is an extended-release formulation, and it should not be chewed or crushed. This is not recommended in patients with creatinine clearance less than 30 mL/min (0.5 mL/s)
β₃-Adrenergic Agonist				
Mirabegron	Myrbetriq	25 mg daily orally	25-50 mg daily orally	This is an extended-release formulation. Do not chew, crush, or divide tablet. In patients with a creatinine clearance of 15-29 mL/min (0.25-0.48 mL/s) or those with moderate hepatic impairment, the maximum daily dose should be 25 mg daily. This drug is not recommended in patients with creatinine clearance less than 15 mL/min (0.25 mL/s)

TABLE 65-2 Dosing of Drugs Used in Treatment of Benign Prostatic Hyperplasia (*Continued*)

finasteride (Proscar) and dutasteride (Avodart) (Table 65-1). The difference between agents is that finasteride inhibits type II 5-α-reductase while dutasteride inhibits type I and II. This mechanism results in a faster, complete decrease in intraprostatic DHT; however, there is no known clinical advantage compared to finasteride. A 5ARI trail should last 6 to 12 months because they do not result in immediate symptom relief. To retain clinical utility of using prostate-specific antigen (PSA) as a screening tool for prostate cancer, patients should have a baseline PSA measured prior to initiating therapy. Additionally, subsequent PSA values should be interpreted twofold higher to account for the reduction that occurs from the 5ARIs. Side effects include reduced libido and rarely gynecomastia. Finasteride and dutasteride are pregnancy category X, so women who are pregnant or of child-bearing age should not handle these medications. Monotherapy with a 5ARI should be considered in patients with BPH due to an enlarged prostate. Combination therapy with a 5ARI and an α-1-adrenergic antagonist improves urinary flow rates and prevents progression of BPH in patients with moderate to severe BPH with evidence of an enlarged prostate (>40 g).

Phosphodiesterase Inhibitors

Tadalafil is approved for LUTS secondary to BPH. The recommended dose is 5 mg once daily. Most studies have examined use of tadalafil as monotherapy and there is limited long-term data with this agent. Tadalafil may be best reserved as an alternative to α₁-adrenergic antagonists and 5ARI or in patients with comorbid ED which is a rather common comorbidity.

Anticholinergic

Treatment with an α₁-adrenergic antagonist, 5α-reductase inhibitor, or surgery may improve urinary flow rate and bladder emptying; however, the patient may still complain of irritative voiding symptoms (eg, urinary frequency, urgency, and

TABLE 65-3   **Monitoring of Drugs Used in Treatment of Benign Prostatic Hyperplasia**

Drug	Adverse Reaction	Monitoring Parameter	Comment
α-Adrenergic antagonists	Syncope Lightheadedness Orthostatic hypotension Tachycardia Nasal congestion Ejaculatory dysfunction Priapism Floppy iris syndrome	Blood pressure Heart rate	If prescribing an immediate-release formulation, start the patient on the lowest possible dose and instruct the patient to take the first dose at bedtime. Slowly uptitrate the dose over several weeks. Stabilize the patient's blood pressure on the α-adrenergic antagonist before adding any other hypotensive agent. If the patient needs cataract surgery, instruct the patient to inform the ophthalmologist so that appropriate measures can be taken during the procedure to prevent intraoperative complications. If the patient has a painful erection lasting longer than 4 h, the patient should seek immediate medical attention
5α-Reductase inhibitors	ED Decreased libido Ejaculatory dysfunction Gynecomastia	PSA	The patient's PSA level should decrease by 50% if he is adherent to therapy
Phosphodiesterase inhibitor	Headache Dizziness Nasal congestion Dyspepsia Back pain Myalgia Hearing loss	Blood pressure Pulse Hearing loss	If the patient experiences hearing loss, discontinue tadalafil
Anticholinergic agents	Dry mouth Constipation Headache Tachycardia Blurry vision Acute urinary retention Drowsiness Confusion Angioedema Anaphylaxis ED	Mental status Bowel habits Ability to urinate	Adverse effects are dose-related and generally reversible. Patients with signs of severe allergic reaction need immediate medical attention
β$_3$ Adrenergic agonist	Hypertension Tachycardia Dry mouth Nausa Constipation Diarrhea Headache Nasopharyngitis Impaired cognition	Blood pressure Bowel habits	Adverse effects are dose-related and generally reversible

Abbreviations: ED, erectile dysfunction; PSA, prostate-specific antigen.

Reproduced with permission from DiPiro JT, Talbert RL, Yee GC, et al: *Pharmacotherapy: A Pathophysiologic Approach,* 10th ed: New York, NY: McGraw-Hill; 2017.

nocturia), which mimic those of overactive bladder (OAB) syndrome. A variety of anticholinergic agents, including oxybutynin or tolterodine, have been added to an α-adrenergic antagonist regimen to relieve these symptoms. By blocking muscarinic receptors in the detrusor muscle, anticholinergic agents can reduce uninhibited detrusor contractions, a sequela of prolonged bladder outlet obstruction. Thus, irritative voiding symptoms are reduced. Because older patients are sensitive to the central nervous system adverse effects and dry mouth, such patients should be started on the lowest effective dose and then slowly titrated up. Anticholinergic agents are contraindicated in patients with narrow angle glaucoma, urinary or gastric retention, or severely decreased intestinal motility. The total anticholinergic burden should be considered prior to making the decision to initiate an anticholinergic agent if the patient is already taking other anticholinergic agents (eg, antipsychotic, antidepressant, antihistamine, antiparkinsonian agents). When multiple anticholinergic agents are taken concurrently, anticholinergic adverse effects, including dry mouth, nausea, constipation, blurred vision, and confusion, will more likely occur and be more severe. Uroselective anticholinergic agents, which preferentially inhibit M$_3$ receptors (eg, darifenacin or solifenacin), or transdermal (oxybutynin), or extended-release formulations of anticholinergic agents (eg, tolterodine) are recommended for patients who poorly tolerate systemic adverse effects of other anticholinergic agents. In the presence of BPH, anticholinergic agents can cause acute urinary retention in patients with poor detrusor contractility.

Mirabegron

Mirabegron is a β_3-adrenergic agonist and relaxes the detrusor muscle during the storage phase of the micturition cycle. Mirabegron reduces irritative voiding symptoms, increases urinary bladder capacity, and increases the interval between voidings. Mirabegron does not inhibit voiding or reduce urinary flow rate or cause acute urinary retention. The clinical effect of mirabegron for LUTS is similar to that of anticholinergic agents, but mirabegron is better tolerated. Mirabegron does not produce anticholinergic adverse effects, nor does it cause acute urinary retention.

Herbal

Saw palmetto (*Serenoa repens)* is a herbal agent with mixed clinical results. Saw palmetto has a modest effect at reducing BPH symptoms; however, a large trial found no difference compared to placebo. Based on a lack of clinical studies demonstrating improvement in symptoms, the AUA does not recommend this product. If patients decide to take saw palmetto, the recommended dose is 160 mg twice daily of the standardized extract. Patients taking saw palmetto along with antiplatelet agents or anticoagulants should be counseled on possible bleeding side effects.

FOUNDATION OVERVIEW: ERECTILE DYSFUNCTION

ED is the inability to achieve and sustain an erection of sufficient rigidity for intercourse. The risk of ED is increased in men with diabetes, heart disease, hypertension, and smokers. ED results from organic or psychological factors leading to decreased penile blood flow. Examples include vascular (eg, heart disease, hypertension, dyslipidemia), neurologic (eg, spinal cord injury, Parkinson disease), endocrine disorders (eg, diabetes, hypogonadism), miscellaneous causes (eg, Peyronie disease, prostatic hyperplasia), and psychogenic causes (eg, depression, anxiety, and stress). Use of prescription medications (eg, antihypertensives, antipsychotics, hormones) as well as alcohol and drugs of abuse (eg, cocaine, amphetamine) can also lead to ED.

Evaluation of patients with ED includes a medical history, physical examination, and laboratory tests to exclude conditions associated with ED and to identify risk factors. A sexual history should be obtained from the patient and his partner focusing on the nature of the problem (frequency, duration, quality, and duration of erections) and psychosocial factors that may suggest potential causes and the most appropriate approach to treatment. Standardized questionnaires such as the Sexual Health Inventory for Men are also helpful.

TREATMENT

A treatment goal is to identify and treat medical or psychological conditions contributing to ED. This includes management of risk factors such as diabetes, hypertension, dyslipidemia, and hypogonadism. If these causes have been excluded or managed, the goal is treatment response (consisting of efficacy and tolerability) and treatment satisfaction (how well the treatment meets or exceeds the expectations of the patient and his partner).

Phosphodiesterase Type 5 Inhibitors

Sildenafil (Viagra), vardenafil (Levitra), tadalafil (Cialis), and avanafil (Stendra) enhance the effect of nitrous oxide by selectively inhibiting the PDE-5 enzyme. Clinical trials demonstrate a response to these agents regardless of cause (organic, psychogenic, or mixed), duration, age, race, or severity. When PDE-5 inhibitors are not effective, secondary causes of ED should be considered (incorrect dose, hypogonadism, psychological component, comorbidities). There is no convincing evidence that one agent is superior; however, patients unresponsive to on-demand or as needed dosing schedules, daily use of tadalafil 2.5 to 5 mg may improve ED. The serum half-life of tadalafil (17.5 hours) is longer than sildenafil (3.7 hours), vardenafil (3.9 hours), and avanavil (5 hours) providing extended activity. As such, tadalafil is effective for up to 36 hours following administration, while both sildenafil and vardenafil should be taken 30 to 60 minutes before anticipated intercourse. Additionally, tadalafil is indicated for the management of the signs and symptoms of BPH.

PDE-5 inhibitor adverse effects include headache, flushing, dyspepsia, and rhinitis. Patients receiving concomitant α-adrenergic blockers may experience postural hypotension and dizziness. Since blood pressure is significantly lowered in patients taking concomitant nitrates and PDE-5 inhibitors, the combination is contraindicated. Serious cardiovascular events have been associated with PDE-5 inhibitors; therefore, they should not be used in patients in whom sexual intercourse is inadvisable because of poor cardiac status. These drugs have been associated with temporary difficulty in distinguishing blue and green colors. Sudden vision and hearing loss has been observed in a few patients. Prolonged erections and priapism have been reported infrequently. Patients should seek medical attention for erections lasting more than 4 hours. The PDE-5 inhibitors are metabolized by cytochrome P450 (CYP) 3A4 enzymes. The PDE-5 inhibitor dose should be reduced if coadministered with medications affecting this enzyme system (eg, erythromycin, ketoconazole, ritonavir).

Vasoactive Agents

These agents mimic vascular response in erection and are used when PDE-5 inhibitors fail or are not tolerated. Alprostadil is synthetic prostaglandin E_1 and exerts its activity by relaxing vascular smooth muscle. It is administered by injection into the corpus cavernosa of the penis (Caverject, Edex) or via a medicated transurethral suppository (Muse). Two other vasoactive agents used in ED are phentolamine, an α_1-adrenergic antagonist, and papaverine, a nonspecific PDE-5. They are administered by intracavernosal injection usually in combination with alprostadil in patients not responding to alprostadil alone. Use of these agents can be very effective with response

TABLE 65-4   Medications That Influence Lower Urinary Tract Function

Medication	Effect
Diuretics, acetylcholinesterase inhibitors	Polyuria resulting in urinary frequency, urgency
α-Receptor antagonists	Urethral muscle relaxation and stress urinary incontinence
α-Receptor agonists	Urethral muscle contraction (increased urethral closure forces) resulting in urinary retention (more common in men)
Calcium channel blockers	Urinary retention due to reduced bladder contractility
Narcotic analgesics	Urinary retention due to reduced bladder contractility
Sedative hypnotics	Functional incontinence caused by delirium, immobility
Antipsychotic agents	Anticholinergic effects resulting in reduced bladder contractility and urinary retention
Anticholinergics	Urinary retention due to reduced bladder contractility
Antidepressants, tricyclic	Anticholinergic effects resulting in reduced bladder contractility, and α-antagonist effects resulting in urethral smooth muscle contraction (increased urethral closure forces) both contributing to urinary retention
Alcohol	Polyuria resulting in urinary frequency, urgency
ACEIs	Cough as a result of ACEIs may aggravate stress urinary incontinence

Abbreviation: ACEIs, angiotensin-converting enzyme inhibitors.
Reproduced with permission from DiPiro JT, Talbert RL, Yee GC, et al: Pharmacotherapy: A Pathophysiologic Approach, 10th ed: New York, NY: McGraw-Hill; 2017.

rates more than 70% for alprostadil alone and approaching 90% for the combination.

Pain may be a particular problem with the use of alprostadil and may lead to treatment failure. The combination allows for lower doses of all three agents and better tolerability. Penile fibrosis can occur with intracavernosal injection. Priapism is an adverse effect and patients should seek medical attention for erections lasting longer than 6 hours. These agents are contraindicated in individuals prone to priapism (patients with sickle cell anemia, multiple myeloma, or leukemia).

Other Treatments

When PDE-5 inhibitors and vasoactive agents fail separately, they have been tried in combination with success. Vacuum erection devices, which draw blood into the penis with negative pressure to create an erection that is maintained by a constriction ring, may also be effective. Implantation of penile prosthetic devices is another treatment option.

FOUNDATION OVERVIEW: URINARY INCONTINENCE

Urinary incontinence (UI) is an involuntary loss of urine occurring in the absence of stones or infection. There are five types of UI which include stress urinary incontinence (SUI), urge urinary incontinence (UUI) also known as OAB, overflow incontinence (OI), mixed incontinence, and functional incontinence. SUI occurs during increased intra-abdominal pressure on the bladder in a patient with a weakened urethral sphincter after exertion (sneezing, coughing). OAB results from premature contraction of the bladder detrusor muscle prior to normal maximum filling capacity. Patients with OAB suffer from urinary urgency, frequency, and nocturia. OI is caused by urinary obstruction (LUTS caused by BPH, bladder underactivity from neurological dysfunction). Mixed incontinence is a combination of any of the three previous types of incontinence. Functional incontinence occurs when patients with functional or cognitive impairment such as decreased mobility or low physical functioning leads to urine leakage. Overall, patients presenting with any type of incontinence should undergo tests to rule out bladder or kidney infections, bladder cancer, prostate cancer, diabetes, and medication related causes (Table 65-4).

TREATMENT

Nonpharmacologic Treatments

Nonpharmacologic treatment is first line and can be used in combination with pharmacologic treatment. A voiding diary is recommended to assess the severity of UI as it documents the frequency of voiding and incontinent episodes. Fluid management and avoidance of caffeine and other bladder irritants will correct UI. Obesity is a contributing factor to SUI and weight loss can provide significant improvements. The most common nonpharmacologic approaches to UI are bladder training, which includes scheduled urination and urge-suppression techniques (beneficial in OAB), and pelvic floor exercises, which include voluntary contraction and relaxation of muscles used to help control urination (helpful in OAB and SUI). Patients with functional incontinence may benefit from the assistance of caregivers, scheduled bathroom visits, and absorbent pads or garments.

Antimuscarinic Agents

Antimuscarinic agents (Tables 65-5 and 65-6) are the most widely prescribed class of drugs for OAB and are first line unless a patient has contraindications (urinary retention, gastric retention, narrow-angle glaucoma, or hypersensitivity). Antimuscarinics are divided into two classes, tertiary amines and quaternary amines. The tertiary amine antimuscarinics are uncharged, lipophilic entities that cause central nervous system side event. Quaternary amines are charged molecules

TABLE 65-5	**Dosing of Medications Approved for OAB or UUI**				
Drug	**Brand Name**	**Initial Dose**	**Usual Range**	**Special Population Dose**	**Comments**
Anticholinergics/Antimuscarinics					
Oxybutynin IR	Ditropan	2.5 mg twice daily	2.5-5 mg two to four times daily		Titrate in increments of 2.5 mg/d every 1-2 mo; available in oral solution
Oxybutynin XL	Ditropan XL	5-10 mg once daily	5-30 mg once daily		Adjust dose in 5-mg increments at weekly interval; swallow whole
Oxybutynin TDS	Oxytrol Oxytrol for Women (OTC)		3.9 mg/d apply one patch twice weekly		Apply every 3-4 d rotate application site
Oxybutynin gel 10%	Gelnique		One sachet (100 mg) topically daily		Apply to clean and dry, intact skin on abdomen, thighs or upper arms/shoulders; contains alcohol
Oxybutynin gel 3%	Gelnique 3%		Three pumps (84 mg) topically daily		Same as above
Tolterodine IR	Detrol		1-2 mg twice daily	1 mg twice daily if patient is taking CYP3A4 inhibitors, or with renal/hepatic impairment	
Tolterodine LA	Detrol LA		2-4 mg once daily	2 mg once daily in those who are taking CYP3A4 inhibitors or with renal/hepatic impairment	Swallow whole; avoid in patients with creatinine clearance ≤10 mL/min (≤0.17 mL/s)
Trospium chloride IR	Sanctura		20 mg twice daily	20 mg once daily in patient age ≥75 y or creatinine clearance ≤30 mL/min (≤0.5 mL/s)	Take 1 h before meals or on empty stomach; patient age ≥75 y should take at bedtime
Trospium chloride ER	Sanctura XR		60 mg once daily	Avoid in patient age ≥75 y or creatinine clearance ≤30 mL/min (≤0.5 mL/s)	Take 1 h before meals or on empty stomach; swallow whole
Solifenacin	VESIcare	5 mg daily	5-10 mg once daily	5 mg daily if patient is taking CYP3A4 inhibitors or with creatinine clearance ≤30 mL/min (≤0.5 mL/s) or moderate hepatic impairment; avoid in severe hepatic impairment	Swallow whole
Darifenacin ER	Enablex	7.5 mg once daily	7.5-15 mg once daily	7.5 mg daily if patient is taking potent CYP3A4 inhibitors or with moderate hepatic impairment; avoid in severe hepatic impairment	Titrate dose after at least 2 wk; swallow whole
Fesoterodine ER	Toviaz	4 mg once daily	4-8 mg once daily	4 mg daily if patient is taking potent CYP3A4 inhibitors or with creatinine clearance ≤30 mL/min (≤0.5 mL/s); avoid in severe hepatic impairment	Prodrug (metabolized to 5-hydroxymethyl tolterodine); swallow whole
β₃-Adrenergic Agonist					
Mirabegron ER	Myrbetriq	25 mg once daily	25-50 mg once daily	25 mg once daily if creatinine clearance 15-29 mL/min (0.25-0.49 mL/s) or moderate hepatic impairment; avoid in patients with ESRD or severe hepatic impairment	Swallow whole

Abbreviations: CYP, cytochrome P450 enzyme; ER, extended-release; ESRD, end-stage renal disease; IR, immediate release; LA, long acting; OAB, overactive bladder; OTC, over-the-counter; TDS, transdermal system; UUI, urge urinary incontinence; XL, extended release.
Reproduced with permission from DiPiro JT, Talbert RL, Yee GC, et al: *Pharmacotherapy: A Pathophysiologic Approach,* 10th ed: New York, NY: McGraw-Hill; 2017.

that do not readily penetrate the blood–brain barrier. Patients taking antimuscarinics experience half the number of incontinent episodes compared to placebo and efficacy is comparable within the class. For relief of OAB symptoms, antimuscarinics antagonize the M_3 receptors; however, M_3 muscarinic receptors are also located in the salivary glands, lower bowel, and ciliary smooth muscle. Therefore, they are associated with dry mouth, constipation, and blurred vision.

Antimuscarinic agents also antagonize other muscarinic receptors (M_1 muscarinic receptors) leading to central nervous system side effects (delirium). Key concepts about antimuscarinic agents include:

- Oxybutynin has a higher incidence of dry mouth in the immediate release (IR) formulation due to a higher rate of conversion to the active metabolite, *N*-desethyloxybutynin, as compared to the extended release (ER) formulation.

- Oxybutynin transdermal patch can be applied to abdomen, hip, or buttock while the gel can also be applied to the upper arm, shoulder, or thigh.

- Oxybutynin transdermal patch is available as an over-the-counter product for women only.

- Tolterodine is highly selective for the M_3 receptor but has shown to be equally effective when compared to oxybutynin in clinical trials.

- Darifenacin is the most selective agent for the M_3 receptor. Because of the higher selectivity ratio for M_3 receptors over M_1 receptors, there are few cognitive function side effects.

- Fesoterodine is a prodrug which is hydrolyzed via esterases, thus avoiding the CYP system, into the active ingredient, 5-hydroxymethyl tolterodine.

- Trospium chloride is derived from atropine and has a lower risk for side effects and drug–drug interactions due to its quaternary amine properties and lack of CYP hepatic metabolism.

Miscellaneous Agents

Mirabegron (Tables 65-5 and 65-6) is a nonantimuscarinic medication approved for the treatment of OAB. The mechanism of action of mirabegron is stimulation of the β-3 agonist causing increased sympathetic action on the bladder resulting in increased bladder compliance and reducing urinary frequency. The β-3 agonist is associated with an increase in blood pressure and heart rate; therefore, appropriate monitoring is recommended.

OnabotulinumtoxinA is a potent neurotoxin approved for use in OAB. OnabotulinumtoxinA is administered via intravesical injection every 12 weeks. Dosing ranges from 50 to 300 units per session and is adjusted based on efficacy and safety. OnabotulinumtoxinA has equal efficacy, less anticholinergic effects, and a higher risk of urinary tract infections compared to antimuscarinics. Therefore, it is second-line treatment for OAB after failing antimuscarinic therapy.

Duloxetine (Cymbalta) is a nonapproved treatment option for SUI. Duloxetine increases the urethral striated sphincter-muscle tone leading to a decrease in frequency and improved quality of life. Duloxetine is dosed 40 mg orally twice daily and common side effects include mild to moderate nausea and increased blood pressure.

Vaginal atrophy is a condition seen in postmenopausal women with symptoms of dryness, burning, itching, and an increase in SUI. The vaginal application of micronized 17-β estradiol (Vagifem) daily for 2 weeks then twice weekly decreases vaginal atrophy symptoms including UI. The deficiency of estrogen in postmenopausal women was once thought to contribute to OAB; however, an increase in OAB

TABLE 65-6	**Monitoring of Medications Approved for OAB or UUI**		
Drug	**Adverse Drug Reaction**	**Monitoring Parameters**	**Comments**
Antimuscarinic			
Oxybutynin IR Oxybutynin XL Oxybutynin TDS Oxybutynin gel 10% Oxybutynin gel 3% Tolterodine IR Tolterodine LA Trospium chloride IR Trospium chloride ER Solifenacin Darifenacin ER Fesoterodine ER	Anticholinergic adverse effects: dry mouth, constipation, headache, dyspepsia, dry eyes, blurred vision, cognitive impairment, tachycardia, sedation, orthostatic hypotension Application site reactions (topical agents): pruritus, erythema	Contraindications and precautions: urinary retention, gastric retention, severely decreased GI motility, angioedema, myasthenia gravis, uncontrolled narrow-angle glaucoma Worsening of renal/hepatic condition or concomitant drug therapy, which may necessitate dosage reduction or drug cessation Mental status change or risk for falls in elderly or frail patients	In general, ER, LA, XL, and topical products are associated with fewer anticholinergic adverse effects, particularly dry mouth Possible transference of drug from topical application Avoid open fire or smoke until alcohol-based gel has dried
β₃-Adrenergic Agonist			
Mirabegron ER	Hypertension, nasopharyngitis, urinary tract infection, headache	Precautions: urinary retention, severe uncontrolled hypertension Worsening of renal/hepatic condition, which may necessitate dosage reduction or drug cessation Increased effect of narrow therapeutic index drugs that are CYP2D6 substrates QT prolongation	Mirabegron is a CYP2D6 inhibitor

Abbreviations: CYP, cytochrome P450 enzyme; ER, extended-release; GI, gastrointestinal; IR, immediate release; LA, long acting; OAB, overactive bladder; TDS, transdermal system; UUI, urge urinary incontinence; XL, extended release.
Reproduced with permission from DiPiro JT, Talbert RL, Yee GC, et al: *Pharmacotherapy: A Pathophysiologic Approach,* 10th ed: New York, NY: McGraw-Hill; 2017.

symptoms has been seen in patients taking oral estrogen; therefore, oral estrogen is not recommended.

There are many medications previously used for UI that are no longer recommended due to lack of efficacy or poor tolerance. These medications include antimuscarinic agents (propantheline, methantheline, emepronium, dicyclomine, terodiline), antispasmodic agents (flavoxate), tricyclic antidepressants (imipramine), and prostaglandin synthetase inhibitors (indomethacin).

CASE Application

1. Which of the following is the brand name for dutasteride?

   a. Hytrin®
   b. Flomax®
   c. Proscar®
   d. Avodart®
   e. Cardura®

2. An 82-year-old patient, taking 2 mg of terazosin for BPH, comes into the pharmacy complaining of dizziness and generalized muscle weakness and persistent LUTS. What would you recommend to his physician?

   a. Add finasteride 5 mg daily to his regimen
   b. Switch his terazosin to doxazosin 4 mg
   c. Switch his terazosin to tamsulosin 0.4 mg daily
   d. Lower the dose of his terazosin to 1 mg
   e. Add saw palmetto twice daily

3. What pregnancy category is finasteride?

   a. A
   b. B
   c. C
   d. D
   e. X

4. A patient reports that he has been taking his finasteride daily for the last 6 months for BPH. His last PSA was 2.6 ng/mL. Today it is 1.3 ng/mL. This can be best explained by which of the following:

   a. Finasteride stops the prostate from producing PSA.
   b. Finasteride can cause erroneous results in laboratory testing for PSA.
   c. PSA levels are often significantly decreased in patients taking 5ARI.
   d. Finasteride has no effect on the PSA level.

5. A patient planning on having cataract surgery next week presents with a prescription for tamsulosin. His symptoms are not bothersome but reports urinary hesitancy and straining. You decide to:

   a. Fill the prescription and counsel the patient on risk of sexual side effects.
   b. Call his physician and ophthalmologist and get his order changed to finasteride.
   c. Call his physician and ophthalmologist to determine if treatment with tamsulosin should be deferred until after his cataract surgery.
   d. Fill the prescription and counsel on risk of dizziness and orthostatic hypotension.
   e. Call his physician and get his order changed to terazosin.

6. Which of the following is an advantage of tamsulosin when compared to doxazosin? Select all that apply.

   a. Increased efficacy in reducing LUTS
   b. Decreased orthostatic hypotension
   c. Quicker onset of action in lowering symptoms
   d. Decreased syncope

7. Which of the following is responsible for increased prostate growth?

   a. PSA
   b. DHT
   c. 5-α reductase
   d. Testosterone

8. Select the statement that correctly describes ED.

   a. Individuals with diabetes are at higher risk.
   b. It is uncommon in the United States.
   c. It generally afflicts younger men.
   d. Individuals with above normal blood pressure are protected.
   e. Smokers are less likely to develop the condition.

9. Select a vascular cause of ED.

   a. Depression
   b. Parkinson disease
   c. Hypogonadism
   d. Anxiety
   e. Dyslipidemia

10. Select the item that should be part of an evaluation of ED. Select all that apply.

   a. A sexual history from the patient and partner
   b. A medical history
   c. A physical examination
   d. A psychosocial assessment

11. KR is a 62-year-old Hispanic male with a history of hypertension. He complains of ED for which he seeks treatment. There is no identifiable organic cause for his ED. Select the statement that correctly describes the approach to treatment in this patient.

   a. PDE5 inhibitors would not be the treatment of choice in this patient.
   b. PDE5 inhibitors are less efficacious in Hispanics.
   c. The use of a PDE5 inhibitor is not likely to be effective in this patient with hypertension.
   d. A PDE5 inhibitor would exert its activity by enhancing the effect of nitric oxide.
   e. He should not receive a PDE5 inhibitor because sexual intercourse would not be advisable because of his cardiac status.

12. DL is a 59-year-old Caucasian male with a history of BPH that is adequately managed with doxazosin who comes to the office with concerns about ED. His workup is unremarkable and a decision is made to start treatment with a PDE5 inhibitor. Select the statement that correctly describes treatment in this patient.

    a. DL should be advised to take the medication immediately prior to sexual intercourse.
    b. Use of a PDE5 inhibitor could lead to postural hypotension.
    c. PDE5 inhibitors are contraindicated in patients with BPH.
    d. The medication of choice would be sildenafil because of its greater efficacy.
    e. The use of a PDE5 inhibitor is contraindicated in a patient receiving doxazosin.

13. JC is a 72-year-old African-American male with ED and no contraindication to the use of a PDE5 inhibitor. Which of the following medications could potentially interact and lead to increased serum concentrations of the PDE5 inhibitor?

    a. Erythromycin
    b. Aspirin
    c. Ampicillin
    d. Haloperidol
    e. Influenza vaccine

14. Select the brand name for tadalafil.

    a. Relenza®
    b. Viagra®
    c. Enzyte®
    d. Cialis®
    e. Levitra®

15. Which statement best describes alprostadil?

    a. It should be the first agent tried for the treatment of ED.
    b. It is a nonspecific PDE5 inhibitor.
    c. It can be administered via a medicated transurethral suppository.
    d. Priapism has not been reported with the use of alprostadil.
    e. It exerts its activity by constricting smooth muscle in the penis.

16. LT, a 75-year-old woman, has severe renal impairment (CrCl <30 mL/min). Which of the following are options for UUI? Select all that apply.

    a. Oxybutynin transdermal patch
    b. Tolterodine ER

    c. Solifenacin
    d. Oxybutynin IR
    e. Trospium chloride ER

17. Which subtype of muscarinic receptor is the primary target of antimuscarinics in patients with OAB?

    a. M_1
    b. M_2
    c. M_3
    d. M_4
    e. M_5

18. TV, a 55-year-old woman, is postmenopausal. Along with UI, this patient is also suffering from symptoms of vaginal dryness, burning, and itching. Which of the following would be the best pharmacologic option for her?

    a. Oral estrogen
    b. Duloxetine
    c. OnabotulinumtoxinA
    d. Topical estrogen

19. Which of the following are nonpharmacologic options for a patient with UI?

    a. Weight reduction
    b. Decrease fluid intake
    c. Increase intake of caffeine
    d. Pelvic floor exercises

20. What type of incontinence can be described as having urinary urgency, frequency, and nocturia along with leakage during exercise?

    a. SUI
    b. UUI
    c. OI
    d. Mixed incontinence
    e. Functional incontinence

21. What is the brand name for mirabegron?

    a. Detrol LA
    b. Ditropan
    c. Myrbetriq
    d. Vesicare
    e. Sanctura XR

TAKEAWAY POINTS »

- BPH is a common urological condition in older men although not all patients will exhibit bothersome LUTS.

- Symptoms of BHP may include urinary hesitancy, weak urinary stream, urinary frequency, nocturia, and incontinence.

- Complications of BPH include urinary retention, urinary tract infections, bladder stones, and renal failure.

- α-Adrenergic antagonists including terazosin, doxazosin, tamsulosin, alfuzosin, and silodosin are effective at reducing LUTS suggestive of BPH.

- In patients with evidence of enlarged prostate (>40 g), 5-α-reductase therapy is used to shrink the prostate, slow disease progression, and reduce the need for urgency.

- A therapeutic trial of a 5ARI should last at least 6 to 12 months.

- Phytotherapy with saw palmetto is not recommended by the AUA based on a lack of clinical data.

- ED is the inability to achieve and sustain an erection of sufficient rigidity for intercourse.

- Evaluation of an individual with ED is directed at identifying treatable organic and psychological causes.

- PDE-5 inhibitors are first-line agents for ED and work by enhancing the effect of nitric oxide on smooth muscle in the penis, resulting in arterial vasodilation and erection.

- Sildenafil and vardenafil should be taken 30 to 60 minutes before anticipated intercourse.

- PDE-5 inhibitors may cause dizziness and postural hypotension in patients receiving α-blockers. PDE-5 inhibitors are contraindicated in patients receiving nitrates because of potential for significant blood pressure reduction.

- PDE-5 inhibitors are metabolized by the CYP 3A4 hepatic enzyme system and may interact with inhibitors of this enzyme.

- The vasoactive agents, alprostadil, phentolamine, and papaverine, work by relaxing vascular smooth muscle and are injected directly into the penis.

- Pain and priapism may occur with the use of the vasoactive agents and they are contraindicated in patients prone to priapism.

- The five types of UI include SUI, UUI, OI, mixed incontinence, and functional incontinence.

- Nonpharmacologic treatment is first line and can be used in combination with pharmacologic treatment.

- Antimuscarinics antagonize the M_3 muscarinic receptor in the bladder reduce urgency and frequency.

- Antimuscarinic agents are the first line of therapy unless contraindicated.

- Adverse effects of antimuscarinics are dry mouth, constipation, and blurred vision.

- There are several other pharmacologic agents for the other types of UI including mirabegron, onabotulinumtoxinA A, duloxetine, and micronized 17-β estradiol.

BIBLIOGRAPHY

Lee M, Sharifi R. Benign prostatic hyperplasia. In: DiPiro JT, Talbert RL, Yee GC, Matzke GR, Wells BG, Posey L, eds. *Pharmacotherapy: A Pathophysiologic Approach.* 10th ed. New York, NY: McGraw-Hill; 2017.

Lee M, Sharifi R. Erectile dysfunction. In: DiPiro JT, Talbert RL, Yee GC, Matzke GR, Wells BG, Posey L, eds. *Pharmacotherapy: A Pathophysiologic Approach.* 10th ed. New York, NY: McGraw-Hill; 2017.

Linnebur SA, Wallace JI. Erectile dysfunction. In: Linn WD, Wofford MR, O'Keefe M, Posey L, eds. *Pharmacotherapy in Primary Care.* New York, NY: McGraw-Hill; 2009:chap 30.

Martin CP, Talbert RL. Section 15. Urology. In: Martin CP, Talbert RL, eds. *Pharmacotherapy Bedside Guide.* New York, NY: McGraw-Hill; 2013.

Rovner ES, Wyman J, Lam S. Urinary incontinence. In: DiPiro JT, Talbert RL, Yee GC, Matzke GR, Wells BG, Posey L, eds. *Pharmacotherapy: A Pathophysiologic Approach.* 10th ed. New York, NY: McGraw-Hill; 2017.

KEY ABBREVIATIONS

5ARI = 5-α-reductase inhibitor
AUA = American Urological Association
BPH = benign prostatic hyperplasia
DHT = dihydrotestosterone
DRE = digital rectal examination
ER = extended release
IR = immediate release
LUTS = lower urinary tract symptom

OAB = overactive bladder
OI = overflow incontinence
PDE-5 = phosphodiesterase inhibitor
PSA = prostate-specific antigen
SUI = stress urinary incontinence
UI = urinary incontinence
UUI = urge urinary incontinence

66

Vaccines and Immunizations

Patricia H. Fabel and Catherine H. Kuhn

FOUNDATION OVERVIEW

Rates of vaccine preventable diseases in the United States are at an all-time low due to the routine vaccination of infants, children, and adults. Unfortunately, gaps in coverage still exist. Providers are responsible for the appropriate administration of vaccines and for ensuring patients receive vaccinations as recommended by the Advisory Committee on Immunization Practices (ACIP). Routine childhood, adolescent, and adult vaccines are covered in this chapter. Readers are encouraged to visit the Centers for Disease Control and Prevention (CDC) vaccines website (http://www.cdc.gov/vaccines/) for information regarding travel and bioterrorism vaccines.

Indications

Indications and target populations for the vaccines available for use in the United States are listed in Table 66-1.

Diphtheria, Tetanus, and Pertussis (DTaP, DT, Td, and Tdap)

Diphtheria is a disease caused by a toxin produced by *Corynebacterium diphtheriae*. The bacterium is transmitted person-to-person through respiratory droplets and most commonly infects the pharynx and tonsils. Symptoms include fever, sore throat, and a bluish-white membrane on the soft palate. The membrane can grow leading to respiratory obstruction. Systemic absorption of the toxin can occur and causes tachycardia, stupor, coma, and death. Serious complications (myocarditis, neuritis, thrombocytopenia, proteinuria) are caused by the toxin produced by certain strains of diphtheria. A diphtheria toxoid is available in different combinations with tetanus toxoid and pertussis vaccine. Diphtheria toxoid, tetanus toxoid, and acellular pertussis (DTaP) and diphtheria-tetanus toxoid (DT) vaccines contain a larger amount of diphtheria toxoid and are indicated in children less than 7 years of age. Children who have had an anaphylactic reaction to the pertussis vaccine should receive DT as their primary diphtheria-tetanus vaccine. Adults receive adult tetanus-diphtheria toxoid vaccine (Td) or tetanus, diphtheria toxoids, and acellular pertussis vaccine (Tdap) because these products contain a smaller dose of the diphtheria toxoid.

Tetanus is a disease caused by an exotoxin produced by *Clostridium tetani*. The spores are found in soil and generally enter the body through a wound. Tetanus commonly presents with trismus (lockjaw) and difficulty in swallowing which progresses as descending paralysis, muscle rigidity, and convulsions. Major complications include laryngospasm and spine or hip fractures due to the convulsions. A tetanus toxoid was developed in the 1920s and is currently available in combination with diphtheria toxoid and pertussis vaccine.

Pertussis (whooping cough) is a highly contagious respiratory infection caused by *Bordetella pertussis*. Patients present with a deep cough that makes it difficult to breathe and the cough can last for more than 3 weeks. Since antibiotics do little to decrease the duration of symptoms, routine vaccination is the primary method used to decrease incidence. The number of cases of pertussis in adolescents and adults has increased because immunity to pertussis decreases 5 to 10 years after vaccination. For this reason, ACIP recommends routine vaccination with Tdap for 11-12 year olds and for adults 65 years and older. Adults should obtain one booster dose of the Tdap vaccine to replace a single dose of Td. Pregnant females should receive one dose of Tdap during the third trimester of every pregnancy.

Haemophilus Influenzae Type b (Hib)

Haemophilus influenza is a bacterium that enters the body through the nasopharynx. There are six different serotypes (a-f), the majority of which remain locally and cause flu-like symptoms. In some cases, the organism enters the bloodstream and causes invasive disease, such as meningitis. Type b was the leading cause of meningitis in children less than 5 years of age before routine vaccination was recommended. Refer to Table 66-2 for the dosing differences between the three Haemophilus Influenzae Type b (Hib) vaccines available for use in the United States.

Hepatitis A (Hep A)

Infection with the hepatitis A (Hep A) virus presents as fever, malaise, anorexia, nausea, dark urine, and jaundice. Symptoms are generally worse in adults than in children. The Hep A virus replicates in the liver, is excreted in the bile, and shed in the stool. Primary mode of transmission is through the fecal-oral route. Those at greatest risk for Hep A infection

TABLE 66-1	Vaccine Indications	
Vaccine	**Indication**	**Target Population**
DTaP	Prevention of diphtheria, tetanus, and pertussis	Children <7 y of age
Td	Booster immunization against tetanus and diphtheria as well as tetanus prophylaxis in wound management	Adolescents and adults >7 y of age
Tdap	Booster immunization against tetanus, diphtheria, and pertussis	Adolescents and adults ≥11 y of age
DT	Prevention of diphtheria and tetanus	Children <7 y of age who are allergic to the pertussis vaccine
Hep A	Prevention of hepatitis A infection	Children >12 mo of age Adults at high risk for Hep A infection
Hep B	Prevention of hepatitis B infection	All infants beginning at birth Unvaccinated children and adolescents Adults at high risk for Hep B infection
Hib	Prevention of invasive bacterial disease caused by *Haemophilus influenzae* type b	Children <5 y of age Adults with sickle cell disease, asplenia, leukemia, stem cell transplant, or HIV infection
HPV-4	Prevention of cervical cancer, precancerous or dysplastic lesions, and genital warts caused by the human papillomavirus types 6, 11, 16, 18	Females aged 9-26 y Males 9-26 y[a]
HPV-2	Prevention of cervical cancer, cervical intraepithelial neoplasia, and adenocarcinoma in situ caused by HPV types 16 and 18	Females aged 10-26 y
HPV-9	Prevention of cervical, vulvar, vaginal, and anal cancer, precancerous or dysplastic lesions, and genital warts caused by HPV types 6, 11, 16, 18, 31, 33, 45, 52, and 58.	Females aged 9-26 y Males 9-26 y[a]
IPV	Prevention of poliomyelitis cause by poliovirus types 1,2,3	All children
MCV, MPSV	Prevention of invasive meningococcal disease caused by *N. meningitides* serogroups A, C, Y, W135	Adolescents 11-12 y of age Adults at high risk for meningococcal disease
MenB-FHbp, MenB-4C	Prevention of invasive disease caused by *N. meningitides* serogroup B	High-risk children and adults ≥10 y of age at high risk (persistent complement component deficiencies, asplenia, microbiologists, outbreaks)[b]
MMR	Prevention of measles, mumps, rubella, and congenital rubella syndrome	Children >12 mo of age
PCV	Prevention of invasive pneumococcal disease caused by *S. pneumoniae*	Children <2 y of age High-risk adults (cochlear implant, asplenia, cerebrospinal fluid leaks, immunocompromising condition, or immunosuppressive therapy) ≥19 y of age[c]
PPSV	Prevention of invasive pneumococcal disease caused by *S. pneumoniae*	Adults ≥65 y of age Aged 2-64 y with chronic heart disease (excluding hypertension), chronic lung disease, diabetes mellitus, cerebrospinal fluid leaks, cochlear implant, alcoholism, chronic liver disease, asplenia, immunocompromising condition or therapy, or those who smoke
RV	Prevention of gastroenteritis caused by rotavirus	Infants aged 6 wk to 8 mo
Varicella	Prevention of varicella caused by varicella-zoster	Children >12 mo
Zoster	Prevention of shingles and reducing the pain associated with shingles caused by herpes zoster	Adults over the age of 60 y[d]

[a]HPV-4 vaccine used in males to prevent genital warts.

[b]MenB-FHbp and MenB-4C vaccines are FDA approved for children and young adults aged 10 to 25 years.

[c]PCV vaccine is FDA approved for children <5 years and adults 50 years and older.

[d]Zoster vaccine is FDA approved for adults aged 50 years and older; however, ACIP still only recommends it for those 60 years and older.

are travelers to developing countries, injection drug users, patients with clotting factor disorders, and close contacts of a child recently adopted from a developing country. It is recommended that all children receive the Hep A vaccine series at 1 year of age; children and adolescents over the age of 2 years living in states with specific vaccination programs or those at high risk for infection should be offered the Hep A series. Adults not previously vaccinated, who remain at high risk for infection, should also be offered the series. Currently, it is not recommended that food-service workers receive the Hep A vaccine.

Hepatitis B (Hep B)

Hepatitis B (Hep B) is a bloodborne and sexually transmitted virus that replicates in the liver. Symptoms of Hep B infection, if present, are jaundice, anorexia, nausea, vomiting, and malaise.

TABLE 66-2	Vaccine Dose and Administration			
Vaccine	**Brand Name (Manufacturer)**	**Dose**	**Route**	**Series**
DtaP	Daptacel (SP) Infanrix (GSK)	0.5 mL	IM	Five-dose series given at 2, 4, 6, 15-18 mo, and 4-6 y of age
Td	Decavac (SP) *Available generic*	0.5 mL	IM	Booster dose every 10 y As needed in wound management[a]
Tdap	Boostrix (GSK) Adacel (SP)	0.5 mL	IM	Single dose as a substitute for *one* Td booster for those 11 y and older[b] As needed in wound management[a]
DT	*Available generic*	0.5 mL	IM	Five-dose series given at 2, 4, 6, 15-18 mo, and 4-6 y of age
Hep A	Havrix (GSK) Vaqta (Merck)	≤18 y: 0.5 mL ≥ 19 y: 1.0 mL	IM	Two-dose series given 6 mo apart
Hep B	Engerix-B (GSK) Recombivax HB (Merck)	≤19 y: 0.5 mL ≥20 y: 1.0 mL	IM	Three-dose series given 0, 1, and 6 mo apart
Hib	ActHIB (SP)	0.5 mL	IM	Three-dose series given at 2, 4, and 6 mo of age *plus* one booster dose at 12-15 mo of age
Hib	PedvaxHIB (Merck)	0.5 mL	IM	Two-dose series given at 2 and 4 mo of age *plus* one booster dose at 12-15 mo of age
Hib	Hiberix (GSK)	0.5 mL	IM	Substitute for booster dose at 12-15 mo of age and children aged 15 mo to 4 y who have not received a booster dose
HPV-9	Gardasil-9 (Merck)	0.5 mL	IM	Three-dose series given 0, 2, and 6 mo apart[c]
IPV	Ipol (SP)	0.5 mL	IM or SC	Four-dose series given at 2, 4, 6-18 mo, and 4-6 y
MCV	Menactra (SP)[d] Menveo (Novartis)[e]	0.5 mL 0.5 mL	IM IM	One dose at 11-12 y plus a booster dose at age 16 y One dose every 5 y for high-risk patients Same as Menactra
MenB-4C	Bexsero (Novartis)	0.5 mL	IM	Two-dose series given at least 1 mo apart
MenB-FHbp	Trumenba (Wyeth)	0.5 mL	IM	Three-dose series given 0, 1-2, and 6 mo apart[f]
MMR	M-M-R II (Merck)	0.5 mL	SC	Two-dose series given at 12-15 mo and 4-6 y
PCV	Prevnar-13 (Wyeth)	0.5 mL	IM	Four-dose series given at 2, 4, 6, and 12-15 mo of age One dose for high-risk adults aged 19 y and older
PPSV	Pneumovax 23 (Merck)	0.5 mL	IM or SC	Single dose[g]
RV	RotaTeq (Merck)	2 mL	Oral	Three-dose series given at 2, 4, and 6 mo[h]
RV	Rotarix (GSK)	1 mL	Oral	Two-dose series given at 2 and 4 mo[h]
Varicella	Varivax (Merck)	0.5 mL	SC	Two-dose series given at 12-15 mo and 4-6 y
ZVL	Zostavax (Merck)	0.65 mL	SC	Single dose
RZV	Shingrix (GSK)	0.5 mL	IM	Two-dose series given 2 to 6 mo apart

[a]Administration of Td or Tdap is recommended as part of proper wound management; however, this use is not discussed in this chapter.

[b]Pregnant females are the only group of patients who receive repeat dosing of Tdap. They receive one dose in the third trimester of every pregnancy.

[c]Adolescents ages 9 through 14 years can receive a two-dose series of any HPV vaccine given 0 and 6 months apart. All other ages require a three-dose series.

[d]Menactra is approved for patients aged 9 months through 55 years.

[e]Menveo is approved for patients aged 2 months through 55 years.

[f]MenB-FHbp may be given as a two-dose series given at least 6 months apart.

[g]A second dose is recommended at least 5 years after the first for patients ≥2 years who are immunocompromised, have sickle cell disease, asplenia, or received their first dose prior to age 65.

[h]First dose of RV vaccine cannot be administered after 14 weeks and 6 days of age; maximum age to receive any RV vaccine dose is 8 months.

Routine vaccination of all infants beginning at birth is recommended. In addition to all infants, patients at risk for Hep B infection should receive the vaccine. Patients who engage in risky sexual behavior, use injection drugs, live with someone who has chronic Hep B infection, are at risk for occupational exposure, are on dialysis, and who travel to Hep B–endemic regions are at the greatest risk of contracting Hep B. Diabetic patients are also considered at risk for Hep B infection; it is now recommended that previously unvaccinated diabetic adults aged 19 to 59 years receive the Hep B vaccine series.

Human Papillomavirus (HPV)

Human papillomavirus (HPV) is the most common sexually transmitted infection in the United States. Most infections do not cause symptoms; however, persistent infection can lead to genital warts in both men and women as well as cervical, vaginal, and vulvar cancers. Of the cervical cancer cases that are caused by HPV, 70% are caused by HPV types 16 and 18. Ninety percent of HPV-related genital warts cases are caused by HPV types 6 and 11. One 9 valent HPV vaccine (HPV-9) is available in the United States. The HPV-9 vaccine provides coverage against HPV types 6, 11, 16, 18, and an additional 5 types (31, 33, 45, 52, and 58). These additional types cause about 15% of the HPV-related cervical cancer cases. Routine vaccination is recommended for adolescents, regardless of gender, at age 11 to 12 years. Postmarketing safety analysis has shown an increased incidence in syncope following administration of the HPV vaccine. It is recommended that patients remain seated or lie down for at least 15 minutes right after receiving the vaccine.

Measles, Mumps, and Rubella (MMR)

The measles rash generally appears 14 days after exposure. Measles can cause diarrhea, otitis media, encephalitis, mental retardation, and death. Mumps cause bilateral or unilateral parotitis (swollen parotid gland). Mumps can lead to permanent sequelae, including paralysis, seizures, and deafness. Rubella can cause an erythematous, pruritic rash, arthralgia, and low-grade fever. Most severe complications of rubella occur when pregnant women become infected in the first trimester. Congenital rubella syndrome (CRS) can lead to deafness, cataracts, and mental retardation. Routine vaccination is recommended for all children at least 1 year of age. A second dose at age 4 to 6 years is recommended for all children. If necessary, the second dose of the measles, mumps, and rubella (MMR) vaccine may be administered 28 days after the first dose.

Meningococcal Infection (MCV, MenB)

Neisseria meningitides is transmitted through respiratory droplets and is the leading cause of bacterial meningitis in the United States. The fatality rate is 10% to 14% despite the availability of effective antibiotics. Persons at risk for meningococcal disease are college freshmen living in dormitories, military recruits, travelers to countries in which infection is widespread, and patients with functional or anatomical asplenia. There are five serogroups of meningococcal disease (A, C, W, Y, and B). Two quadrivalent (serogroups A,C,W,Y) conjugate vaccines (MCV) are available. Current recommendations are to routinely vaccinate all children at the age of 11 or 12 years of age with a booster dose given at the age of 16 years. Vaccination with one dose every 5 years is also recommended for adults who are (and remain) at high risk for infection. Two serogroup B meningococcal vaccines are available (MenB-FHbp and MenB-4C). Current recommendations are to vaccinate children and adults at least 10 years of age who are at increased risk for serogroup B meningococcal disease (persistent complement component deficiencies, asplenia, microbiologists routinely exposed to *N. meningitides*, or those at risk due to an outbreak).

Pneumococcal Infection (PCV, PPSV)

Streptococcus pneumoniae, a bacterial pathogen, can cause upper respiratory tract infections (otitis media, sinusitis), lower respiratory tract infections (pneumonia), and invasive disease (bacteremia, meningitis). Persons at greatest risk for invasive disease are children less than 5 years of age, adults more than 65 years, patients with chronic lung disease, chronic cardiovascular disease, diabetes mellitus, chronic liver disease, functional or anatomic asplenia, and smokers. Two vaccines are licensed for use in the United States—a pneumococcal conjugate vaccine (PCV) and a pneumococcal polysaccharide vaccine (PPSV). See Tables 66-1 and 66-2 for differences between the two pneumococcal vaccines.

Poliomyelitis (IPV)

Poliomyelitis is a highly contagious disease caused by the poliovirus that is mainly transmitted by the fecal-oral route. Symptoms of polio range from a fever to meningitis and paralysis. Poliovirus replicates in the motor neurons and may cause asymmetric paralysis. However, the majority of polio infections are asymptomatic. The ratio of asymptomatic to paralytic illness ranges from 100:1 to 1000:1 (usually 200:1). Several decades after infection, patients can develop post-polio syndrome which is characterized by muscle pain and weakness and even paralysis. Due to routine vaccination, the United States is free from indigenous polio. Therefore, the oral polio vaccine is no longer included in the recommendations. All children should receive four doses of the inactivated polio vaccine (IPV) starting at age 2 months.

Rotovirus (RV)

Rotovirus is the most common cause of severe gastroenteritis in infants and young children and is responsible for over 50,000 hospitalizations every year. It infects the small intestine causing diarrhea, vomiting, and fever leading to dehydration. Two RV vaccines are available in the United States—a monovalent human vaccine (Rotarix®) and a pentavalent human-bovine reassortant vaccine (RotaTeq). A previous RV vaccine (Rotashield®) was removed from the market due to an increased incidence of intussusception. Currently licensed RV vaccines have not been shown to increase the risk of intussusception. It is recommended that the first dose of the RV vaccine be administered to all infants before the age of 14 weeks and 6 days. The last dose in the RV vaccine series should be administered before the age of 8 months.

Varicella Zoster Virus (Varicella, Zoster)

The varicella zoster virus (VZV) causes two conditions—varicella (chickenpox) and herpes zoster (shingles). The VZV enters the respiratory tract and replicates in the nasopharynx. Varicella, the primary infection, is a contagious rash that is common among children. It can present with fever and general malaise before the characteristic rash appears. Varicella is generally mild and self-limiting, but complications can occur. They include bacterial skin infections, pneumonia, meningitis, and encephalopathy.

The VZV can lie dormant in the sensory dorsal root ganglia of the spine. It can reactivate years later to cause herpes zoster, a localized painful rash. The rash occurs unilaterally and does not cross the center of the body. The pain is described as aching and shock-like. The rash will typically disappear within 4 weeks, but postherpetic neuralgia (PHN), a complication of herpes zoster, can last for weeks to months or even years. PHN is a debilitating pain that persists after the rash dissipates.

Three live attenuated viral vaccines for the VZV are available for use in the United States—a varicella vaccine, a combination vaccine with MMR and varicella, and a vaccine to prevent herpes zoster infection (ZVL). See Table 66-1. A recombinant zoster vaccine (RZV) was approved for the prevention of herpes zoster infection in 2017. ACIP recommends adults aged 50 years and older receive 2 doses of RZV 2 to 6 months apart regardless of past episode of herpes zoster or receipt of zoster vaccine live (ZVL).

VACCINE ADMINISTRATION

Injection Route and Site

Most vaccines are administered intramuscularly (IM) or subcutaneously (SC). A 1-inch needle should be used for IM injections in most adults. Intramuscular injections are administered at a 90° angle in the deltoid muscle of the arm for adults and children or the anterolateral thigh for infants. A 5/8-inch needle should be used for subcutaneous injections. Subcutaneous injections are administered at a 45° angle in the outer aspect of the triceps. Table 66-2 lists the dosages and routes of administration for most of the vaccines available in the United States.

Simultaneous Administration

Simultaneously administering all vaccines a patient is eligible for in one office visit has been shown to increase vaccination rates without decreasing vaccine efficacy. Therefore, it is recommended that all age-appropriate vaccinations be administered on the same day unless contraindications/precautions are present. Whether the vaccine is live or inactivated does not affect simultaneous administration. Inactivated vaccines can be administered without regard to spacing. A live and inactivated vaccine may be administered without regard to spacing, as well. There is evidence suggesting that the varicella vaccine is not effective when administered less than 28 days after the MMR vaccine, but is effective if administered on the same day as the MMR vaccine. Therefore, it is recommended to administer two live vaccines on the same day or separated by at least 28 days. The exception to this

TABLE 66-3	Inactivated and Live Vaccines
Inactivated	**Live Attenuated**
DTaP, DT, Td, Tdap	MMR
Hep B	Varicella
Hib	ZVL
Hep A	RV
HPV	LAIV[a]
PCV	Yellow fever[a]
PPSV	Oral typhoid[a]
IPV	
MCV	
MPSV	
MenB	
Influenza[a]	

Abbreviation: LAIV, live attenuated influenza vaccine.
[a]Vaccines not covered in this chapter.

recommendation is with oral live vaccines—they may be administered at any interval from previous vaccination with either live or inactivated vaccines. Vaccines that require a series of doses have specific recommendations regarding spacing intervals. Administering a dose in a series earlier than recommended may decrease vaccine efficacy and should be avoided. Table 66-3 lists the inactivated and live vaccines available for use in the United States.

Contraindications and Precautions

Prior to administering a vaccine, it is important to screen the patient for potential contraindications and precautions. A contraindication is a patient condition that greatly increases the likelihood that a serious adverse reaction will occur if the vaccine is administered. Vaccines are contraindicated in a patient who has experienced an anaphylactic reaction to a prior dose or any component of that vaccine. A precaution is a condition that might increase the risk of a serious adverse reaction or decrease the effectiveness of the vaccine. Generally, the vaccination should be withheld until the precaution has resolved. In some instances, the benefit of administering the vaccine outweighs the risk and can be administered. Administration of any vaccine should be cautioned in patients with moderate to severe acute illness with or without a fever. Contraindications and precautions for most of the vaccines available in the United States are listed in Table 66-4. Health care professionals are encouraged to visit the CDC vaccine website for the latest safety information on vaccines.

Adverse Events

Adverse events for most vaccines available in the United States are listed in Table 66-5. Health care professionals administering vaccinations are required to report any adverse event that occurs after vaccine administration. The CDC requires that the provider complete the Vaccine Adverse Event Reporting System (VAERS) form. The form is available from http://vaers

TABLE 66-4 Vaccine Contraindications and Precautions

Vaccine	Contraindication	Precautions
DTaP, Tdap	Encephalopathy within 7 d of a previous dose Progressive neurologic disorder—infantile spasms, uncontrolled epilepsy, encephalopathy	Seizure within 3 d of receiving a previous dose Guillain-Barre syndrome within 6 wk after previous dose Any of the following within 48 h of a previous dose: Fever >40.5°C Collapse or shock-like state Persistent, inconsolable crying for >3 h
Hep B		Infant weighing <2000 g
Hib	Age <6 wk	
HPV	Pregnancy	
IPV	Allergy to neomycin, streptomycin, or polymyxin B	Pregnancy
MMR	Allergy to gelatin or neomycin Pregnancy Severe immunodeficiency	Receipt of antibody-containing blood product within 11 mo History of thrombocytopenia or thrombocytopenic purpura
RV	Severe latex allergy (Rotarix only) History of intussusception Severe combined immunodeficiency	Immunodeficiency Acute gastroenteritis Preexisting chronic gastrointestinal disease Spinal bifida or bladder exstrophy
Varicella	Pregnancy Immunodeficiency Untreated active tuberculosis Allergy to gelatin or neomycin	Receipt of antibody-containing blood product within 11 mo
ZVL	Pregnancy Immunodeficiency Allergy to gelatin or neomycin	Receipt of antivirals (ie, acyclovir, famciclovir) 24 h before vaccination; avoid use 14 d post vaccination

TABLE 66-5 Vaccine Adverse Events

Vaccine	Adverse Events
DTaP	Injection site reactions (pain, swelling, erythema), fever, fatigue, vomiting, anorexia, febrile seizures (rare)
Td, Tdap	Injection site reactions, headache, myalgias, fatigue, neuropathy (rare), and paralysis (rare)
Hep A	Injection site reactions, headache, malaise, fever, Guillain-Barré syndrome(GBS)
Hep B	Injection site reactions, fever, GBS
Hib	Injection site reactions, fever
HPV	Injection site reactions, syncope, fever, nausea, headache, GBS, thromboembolism
IPV	Injection site reactions, fever
MCV	Injection site reactions, fever, diarrhea, anorexia, drowsiness, GBS[a]
MMR[b]	Injection site reactions, thrombocytopenia, febrile seizures, GBS
PCV	Injection site reactions, fever, febrile seizures
PPSV	Injection site reactions, fever, myalgias
RV	Mild diarrhea and vomiting, irritability
Varicella	Injection site reactions, varicella-like rash
ZVL	Injection site reactions, fever, arthralgias, varicella-like reactions

[a]MCV has a higher incidence of GBS than MPSV.
[b]MMR is not associated with an increased risk of autism.

.hhs.gov. Personnel administering vaccinations should be prepared to handle emergency situations that may arise from vaccine administration. Epinephrine, diphenhydramine, and cardiopulmonary resuscitation (CPR) may need to be administered if a patient has an anaphylactic reaction. Practitioners will need to be CPR and first aid certified.

Combination Vaccines

Combination vaccines approved for use in the United States are listed in Table 66-6. The main advantage of using combination vaccines is the decrease in the number of injections. The ACIP recommends the use of combination vaccines whenever possible based upon provider assessment, patient preference, safety, availability, and cost.

TABLE 66-6 Combination Vaccines

Brand Name (Manufacturer)	Vaccines	Dose	Route
Pediarix (GSK)	DTaP/IPV/Hep B	0.5 mL	IM
Pentacel (SP)	DTaP/IPV/Hib	0.5 mL	IM
Kinrix (GSK)	DTaP/IPV	0.5 mL	IM
Twinrix (GSK)	Hep A/Heb B	1 mL	IM
Comvax (Merck)	Hep B/Hib	0.5 mL	IM
ProQuad (Merck)	MMR/Varicella	0.5 mL	SC

Vaccine Storage

Proper storage is important to maintain vaccine potency. Package inserts contain recommended storage temperatures as well as instructions for reconstitution (if necessary). Most vaccines require refrigeration; however, some need to be kept frozen (eg, ZVL). Recommended storage temperature for refrigerated vaccines is 35°F to 46°F (2°C-8°C). Frozen vaccines should be stored at less than or equal to 5°F (≤15°C).

VACCINE SCHEDULES

The 2017 recommended vaccination schedule for children, adolescents, and adults are provided in Appendices 66-1 and 66-2. Changes to vaccine schedules are made annually. Readers are encouraged to visit the CDC vaccines website for the most current vaccination schedule (http://www.cdc.gov/vaccines/schedules/index.html).

CASE Application

1. Which of the following can safely be given to a 6-month-old child who had an allergic reaction to the pertussis vaccine?

    a. DTaP
    b. Tdap
    c. Td
    d. DT

2. KS, a 5-year-old girl, has an appointment today with her pediatrician to receive vaccines. Her vaccination record shows the following: Hep B at birth, 2 months, and 6 months; RV at 2, 4, and 6 months; DTaP at 2, 4, 6, and 15 months; Hib (ActHIB®) at 2, 4, 6, and 15 months; PCV at 2, 4, 6, and 15 months; IPV at 2, 4, and 6 months; MMR at 15 months; Varicella at 15 months; and Hep A at 15 months. She does not have any medical conditions and is not allergic to any medications or vaccines. What vaccines should KS receive today?

    a. DT, PPSV, IPV, MMR, MCV, and Hep A
    b. DTaP, IPV, MMR, Varicella, and Hep A
    c. Tdap, IPV, MMR, Varicella, and Hep A
    d. DTaP, PPSV, IPV, MMR, Varicella, and Hep A

3. Which of the following vaccines is only given as a single dose?

    a. PCV
    b. Zoster
    c. RV
    d. Td

4. Which of the following pediatric vaccines is administered orally?

    a. IPV
    b. PCV

    c. RV
    d. Varicella

5. A 69-year-old man comes into your pharmacy after receiving a letter advertising your immunization program. He has diabetes and hypertension and smokes a pack of cigarettes a day. He does not have any medication or vaccine allergies. His vaccination record shows that he completed all of his childhood vaccinations (DTaP, Hib, PCV, IPV, and MMR) as well as the Hep B series, he had the chickenpox when he was 5 years old, and received his last Td booster 11 years ago. Which vaccines should this patient receive TODAY?

    a. Td, Zoster, PPSV, and Hep A
    b. Tdap, Varicella, and PPSV
    c. Td, Zoster, and PPSV
    d. Tdap, RZV, and PCV

6. Which of the following diphtheria and tetanus vaccines should be used in adults as a one-time booster dose?

    a. Td
    b. DT
    c. Tdap
    d. DTaP

7. Which of the following adults under the age of 65 would require a PPSV? Select all that apply.

    a. Pregnant women
    b. Smokers
    c. Heart failure patients
    d. Hypertensive patients

8. How should the Hep B vaccine be administered?

    a. In the deltoid muscle at a 90° angle
    b. In the deltoid muscle at a 45° angle
    c. In the outer aspect of the triceps at a 45° angle
    d. In the anterolateral thigh at a 45° angle

9. EP is pregnant and in her third trimester. Which of the following vaccines can EP receive? Select all that apply.

    a. HPV
    b. Hep B
    c. MMR
    d. Tdap

10. An 11-year-old girl fainted after receiving her 11 to 12-year-old routine vaccinations. Which of the following vaccines most likely caused her to faint?

    a. Tdap
    b. HPV
    c. MCV
    d. Hep B

11. The live herpes zoster vaccine (ZVL) should be stored at what temperature?

    a. ≤5°F
    b. 6°F to 35°F

c. 36°F to 46°F

d. 47°F to 77°F

12. JM, a 6-month-old infant is seeing his pediatrician today in order to receive his 6-month vaccinations. His vaccination records are as follows: Hep B at birth and 2 months; DTaP at 2 and 4 months; Hib (PedvaxHIB®) at 2 and 4 months; PCV at 2 and 4 months; and IPV at 2 and 4 months. JM does not have any medical conditions or allergies to medications or vaccines. Which vaccines should JM receive today?

a. Hep B, RV, DTaP, Hib, PCV, and IPV

b. Hep B, RV, DTaP, PCV, and IPV

c. Hep B, DTaP, Hib, PCV, and IPV

d. Hep B, DTaP, PCV, and IPV

13. A 68-year-old female patient calls your pharmacy complaining of a rash on the left side of her midsection. It wraps around her side; however, it doesn't cross her spine or belly button. She informs you that it doesn't itch; however, it is very painful. It started to appear 2 days ago. She thinks it is shingles and remembers having chickenpox as a child. She would like to know how she got this infection since she doesn't remember being around anyone recently who has had shingles. Which of the following statements should be included in your consultation with her regarding how she got the herpes zoster infection?

a. The VZV causes shingles. It originally presents as the chickenpox rash, then lays dormant in the spine and can reemerge years later presenting as shingles.

b. The VZV causes shingles. She had to have come into contact with someone who had an active case of shingles in order to get it herself.

c. The VZV causes shingles. She had to have come into contact with someone who had an active case of chickenpox. She got shingles from it since she has already had chickenpox.

d. The VZV only causes chickenpox. She had to have come into contact with another virus that causes shingles.

14. Which of the following patients can receive the Hib vaccine? (Select all that apply.)

a. A 4-month-old child

b. A 20-year-old smoker

c. A 58-year-old man with leukemia

d. A 26-year-old with asplenia

15. How should the live herpes zoster vaccine (ZVL) be administered?

a. In the deltoid muscle at a 90° angle

b. In the deltoid muscle at a 45° angle

c. In the outer aspect of the triceps at a 45° angle

d. In the anterolateral thigh at a 45° angle

16. LM is an 18-year-old woman who is leaving for her first semester of college next month. She would like to know what vaccinations she needs before going to college. Her vaccination record shows the following: DTaP at 2, 4, 6, and 15 months, and 5 years; Hib (ActHIB®) at 2, 4, and 6 months; PCV at 2, 4, 6, and 15 months; IPV at 2, 4, and 6 months, and 5 years; MMR at 15 months and 5 years; Varicella at 15 months and 5 years; Hep A at 12 and 18 months; Hep B at 11 years, 11 years 2 months, and 11 years 6 months; and Tdap at 15 years. LM does not have any medical conditions and is not allergic to any medications or vaccines. What vaccines should LM receive today?

a. MCV and HPV

b. Tdap, MCV, and HPV

c. Tdap and MCV

d. PPSV and HPV

17. TR, a 4-year-old girl, is in the doctor's office for her 4 to 6-year-old vaccinations. She has completed her Hep B, Hib, PCV, and Hep A series. She has no medical conditions and is not allergic to any medications or vaccines. Five days ago she received the influenza vaccine. Which vaccines should TR receive today?

a. DTaP, IPV, MMR, and Varicella

b. DTaP, PPSV, IPV, and MMR

c. IPV only

d. DTaP and IPV

18. When should the second dose of the Hep A vaccine be administered?

a. 28 days after the first dose

b. 2 months after the first dose

c. 6 months after the first dose

d. 30 days after the first dose

19. Which of the following patients are at risk for Hep B infection and should be counseled to receive the Hep B vaccine to protect themselves? Select all that apply.

a. A 23-year-old man who has sex with men

b. A 58-year-old woman diabetic

c. A 63-year-old man with hypertension

d. A 34-year-old woman wound-care nurse

20. Which of the following patients should receive the herpes zoster vaccine?

a. A 58-year-old diabetic

b. A 37-year-old without a spleen

c. A 68-year-old with hypertension

d. A 72-year-old allergic to neomycin

TAKEAWAY POINTS »

- DTaP is indicated for the prevention of diphtheria, tetanus, and pertussis in children less than 7 years of age. DT is indicated for the prevention of diphtheria and tetanus in children less than 7 years of age who have a history of anaphylactic or neurologic reaction to the pertussis vaccine.

- Adults should receive one Td booster every 10 years. Patients aged 11 to 12 years should receive one Tdap dose. Adults should replace one Td booster with a Tdap dose once in their lifetime. Pregnant females receive one Tdap dose in the third trimester of every pregnancy.

- The three Hib vaccines available in the United States have different dosing guidelines and are not interchangeable.

- Hep B is given in a three-dose series at 0, 1, and 6 months. It is the only vaccine that can be given at birth.

- Administration of the HPV vaccine can cause syncope. Therefore, patients should remain seated for at least 15 minutes after receiving the vaccine.

- Adolescents should receive one dose of MCV at 11 to 12 years of age and booster dose at age 16 years. Patients at high risk (college freshman living in dormitories, military recruits, travelers to countries with wide-spread meningococcal disease, and asplenic patients) should receive one dose of MCV every 5 years as long as they remain at high risk. Those patients at least 10 years of age who are at increased risk for serogroup B meningococcal disease should receive MenB.

- PCV is recommended in all children less than 5 years of age. Adults 19 years of age and older should receive one dose of PCV if they are considered at high risk (cochlear implant, asplenia, cerebrospinal fluid leaks, immunocompromising condition, immunosuppressive therapy, or over the age of 65 years).

- PPSV is recommended in patients more than 2 years who are at high risk for invasive disease: adults more than 65 years, patients with chronic heart disease (excluding hypertension), chronic lung disease, diabetes mellitus, cerebrospinal fluid leaks, cochlear implant, alcoholism, chronic liver disease, asplenia, immunocompromising condition or therapy, or those who smoke.

- A second dose of PPSV is recommended at least 5 years after the first for patients more than or equal to 2 years who are immunocompromised, have sickle cell disease, asplenia, or received their first dose prior to age 65.

- Several patients may require both the PCV and PPSV vaccines. For adults less than 65 years, it is preferred to give PCV first followed by PPSV 8 weeks later. For adults more than 65 years, it is preferred to give PCV first followed by PPSV 12 months later. Regardless of age, if PPSV is given first, the patient must wait 12 months to receive PCV.

- The first dose of the RV vaccine should be given before 14 weeks and 6 days. The last dose should be administered before 8 months.

- IM vaccines are administered in adults at a 90° angle in the deltoid muscle using a 1-inch needle. SC vaccines are given at a 45° angle in the outer aspect of the triceps using a 5/8-inch needle.

- Most vaccines may be administered without regard to spacing. However, two live vaccines should be given on the same day or 28 days apart.

- Administration of any vaccine should be cautioned in patients with moderate to severe acute illness.

- The CDC requires that immunizing practitioners report any adverse event that occurs after vaccine administrations using the VAERS form.

- Refrigerated vaccines should be stored at 35°F to 46°F (2°C-8°C). Frozen vaccines should be stored at less than or equal to 5°F (−15°C)

BIBLIOGRAPHY

Hayney MS. Vaccines and immunoglobulins. In: DiPiro JT, Talbert RL, Yee GC, Matzke GR, Wells BG, Posey L, eds. *Pharmacotherapy: A Pathophysiologic Approach.* 10th ed. New York, NY: McGraw-Hill; 2017.

Lampiris HW, Maddix DS. Vaccines, immune globulins, & other complex biologic products. In: Katzung BG, Masters SB, Trevor AJ, eds. *Basic & Clinical Pharmacology.* 12th ed. New York, NY: McGraw-Hill; 2012.

Schuchat A, Jackson LA. Immunization principles and vaccine use. In: Longo DL, Fauci AS, Kasper DL, Hauser SL, Jameson J, Loscalzo J, eds. *Harrison's Principles of Internal Medicine.* 18th ed. New York, NY: McGraw-Hill; 2012:chap 122.

Tovar J, Farrell N. Immunizations. In: Attridge RL, Miller ML, Moote R, Ryan L, eds. *Internal Medicine: A Guide to Clinical Therapeutics.* New York, NY: McGraw-Hill; 2013.

KEY DEFINITIONS

ACIP = Advisory Committee on Immunization Practices

CDC = Centers for Disease Control and Prevention

DTaP = pediatric diphtheria toxoid, tetanus toxoid, and acellular pertussis vaccine

DT = pediatric diphtheria-tetanus toxoid vaccine

FDA = Food and Drug Administration

GBS = Guillain-Barré syndrome

GSK = GlaxoSmithKline

Hep A = hepatitis A

Hep B = hepatitis B

Hib = *Haemophilus influenzae* type b

HIV = Human Immunodeficiency Virus

HPV = Human Papillomavirus

IM = intramuscularly

IPV = inactivated polio vaccine

MCV = meningococcal conjugate vaccine

MenB = serogroup B meningococcal vaccine

MMR = measles, mumps, rubella

MMWR = *Morbidity and Mortality Weekly Report*

PCV = pneumococcal conjugate vaccine

PHN = postherpetic neuralgia

PPSV = pneumococcal polysaccharide vaccine

RV = rotavirus

RZV = recombinant zoster vaccine

SC = subcutaneously

SP = Sanofi Pasteur

Td = adult tetanus-diphtheria toxoid vaccine

Tdap = tetanus, diphtheria toxoids, and acellular pertussis vaccine

VAERS = Vaccine Adverse Event Reporting System

VZV = varicella zoster virus

ZVL = zoster vaccine live

Recommended Immunization Schedule for Children and Adolescents Aged 18 Years or Younger, United States, 2017

This schedule includes recommendations in effect as of January 1, 2017. Any dose not administered at the recommended age should be administered at a subsequent visit, when indicated and feasible. The use of a combination vaccine generally is preferred over separate injections of its equivalent component vaccines. Vaccination providers should consult the relevant Advisory Committee on Immunization Practices (ACIP) statement for detailed recommendations, available online at www.cdc.gov/vaccines/hcp/acip-recs/index.html. Clinically significant adverse events that follow vaccination should be reported to the Vaccine Adverse Event Reporting System (VAERS) online (www.vaers.hhs.gov) or by telephone (800-822-7967). Suspected cases of vaccine-preventable diseases should be reported to the state or local health department. Additional information, including precautions and contraindications for vaccination, is available from CDC online (www.cdc.gov/vaccines/hcp/admin/contraindications.html) or by telephone (800-CDC-INFO [800-232-4636]).

The Recommended Immunization Schedule for Children and Adolescents Aged 18 Years or Younger are approved by the

Advisory Committee on Immunization Practices
(www.cdc.gov/vaccines/acip)

American Academy of Pediatrics
(www.aap.org)

American Academy of Family Physicians
(www.aafp.org)

American College of Obstetricians and Gynecologists
(www.acog.org)

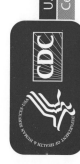

U.S. Department of Health and Human Services
Centers for Disease Control and Prevention

FIGURE 1. Recommended immunization schedule for children and adolescents aged 18 years or younger—United States, 2017.

(FOR THOSE WHO FALL BEHIND OR START LATE, SEE THE CATCH-UP SCHEDULE [FIGURE 2]).

These recommendations must be read with the footnotes that follow. For those who fall behind or start late, provide catch-up vaccination at the earliest opportunity as indicated by the green bars in Figure 1. To determine minimum intervals between doses, see the catch-up schedule (Figure 2). School entry and adolescent vaccine age groups are shaded in gray.

NOTE: The above recommendations must be read along with the footnotes of this schedule.

FIGURE 2. Catch-up immunization schedule for persons aged 4 months through 18 years who start late or who are more than 1 month behind—United States, 2017.

The figure below provides catch-up schedules and minimum intervals between doses for children whose vaccinations have been delayed. A vaccine series does not need to be restarted, regardless of the time that has elapsed between doses. Use the section appropriate for the child's age. Always use this table in conjunction with Figure 1 and the footnotes that follow.

Vaccine	Minimum Age for Dose 1	Minimum Interval Between Doses			
		Dose 1 to Dose 2	Dose 2 to Dose 3	Dose 3 to Dose 4	Dose 4 to Dose 5
Children age 4 months through 6 years					
Hepatitis B[1]	Birth	4 weeks	8 weeks *and* at least 16 weeks after first dose. Minimum age for the final dose is 24 weeks.		
Rotavirus[2]	6 weeks	4 weeks	4 weeks[2]		
Diphtheria, tetanus, and acellular pertussis[3]	6 weeks	4 weeks	4 weeks	6 months	6 months[3]
Haemophilus influenzae type b[4]	6 weeks	4 weeks if first dose was administered before the 1st birthday. 8 weeks (as final dose) if first dose was administered at age 12 through 14 months. No further doses needed if first dose was administered at age 15 months or older.	4 weeks[4] if current age is younger than 12 months **and** first dose was administered at younger than age 7 months, **and** at least 1 previous dose was PRP-T (ActHib, Pentacel, Hiberix) or unknown. 8 weeks *and* age 12 through 59 months (as final dose)[4] • if current age is younger than 12 months **and** first dose was administered at age 7 through 11 months; OR • if current age is 12 through 59 months **and** first dose was administered before the 1st birthday, **and** second dose administered at younger than 15 months; OR • if both doses were PRP-OMP (PedvaxHIB; Comvax) **and** were administered before the 1st birthday. No further doses needed if previous dose was administered at age 15 months or older.	8 weeks (as final dose) This dose only necessary for children age 12 through 59 months who received 3 doses before the 1st birthday.	
Pneumococcal[5]	6 weeks	4 weeks if first dose administered before the 1st birthday. 8 weeks (as final dose for healthy children) if first dose was administered at the 1st birthday or after. No further doses needed for healthy children if first dose was administered at age 24 months or older.	4 weeks if current age is younger than 12 months and previous dose given at <7 months old. 8 weeks (as final dose) if previous dose given between 7-11 months (wait until at least 12 months old); OR if current age is 12 months or older and at least 1 dose was given before age 12 months. No further doses needed for healthy children if previous dose administered at age 24 months or older.	8 weeks (as final dose) This dose only necessary for children aged 12 through 59 months who received 3 doses before age 12 months or for children at high risk who received 3 doses at any age.	
Inactivated poliovirus[6]	6 weeks	4 weeks[6]	4 weeks[6]	6 months[6] (minimum age 4 years for final dose).	
Measles, mumps, rubella[8]	12 months	4 weeks			
Varicella[9]	12 months	3 months			
Hepatitis A[10]	12 months	6 months			
Meningococcal[11] (Hib-MenCY ≥6 weeks; MenACWY-D ≥9 mos; MenACWY-CRM ≥2 mos)	6 weeks	8 weeks[11]	See footnote 11	See footnote 11	
Children and adolescents age 7 through 18 years					
Meningococcal[11] (MenACWY-D ≥9 mos; MenACWY-CRM ≥2 mos)	Not Applicable (N/A)	8 weeks[11]			
Tetanus, diphtheria; tetanus, diphtheria, and acellular pertussis[12]	7 years[12]	4 weeks	4 weeks if first dose of DTaP/DT was administered before the 1st birthday. 6 months (as final dose) if first dose of DTaP/DT or Tdap/Td was administered at or after the 1st birthday.	6 months if first dose of DTaP/DT was administered before the 1st birthday.	
Human papillomavirus[13]	9 years	Routine dosing intervals are recommended.[13]			
Hepatitis A[10]	N/A	6 months			
Hepatitis B[1]	N/A	4 weeks	8 weeks **and** at least 16 weeks after first dose.		
Inactivated poliovirus[6]	N/A	4 weeks	4 weeks[6]	6 months[6]	
Measles, mumps, rubella[8]	N/A	4 weeks			
Varicella[9]	N/A	3 months if younger than age 13 years. 4 weeks if age 13 years or older.			

NOTE: The above recommendations must be read along with the footnotes of this schedule.

FIGURE 3. Vaccines that might be indicated for children and adolescents aged 18 years or younger based on medical indications

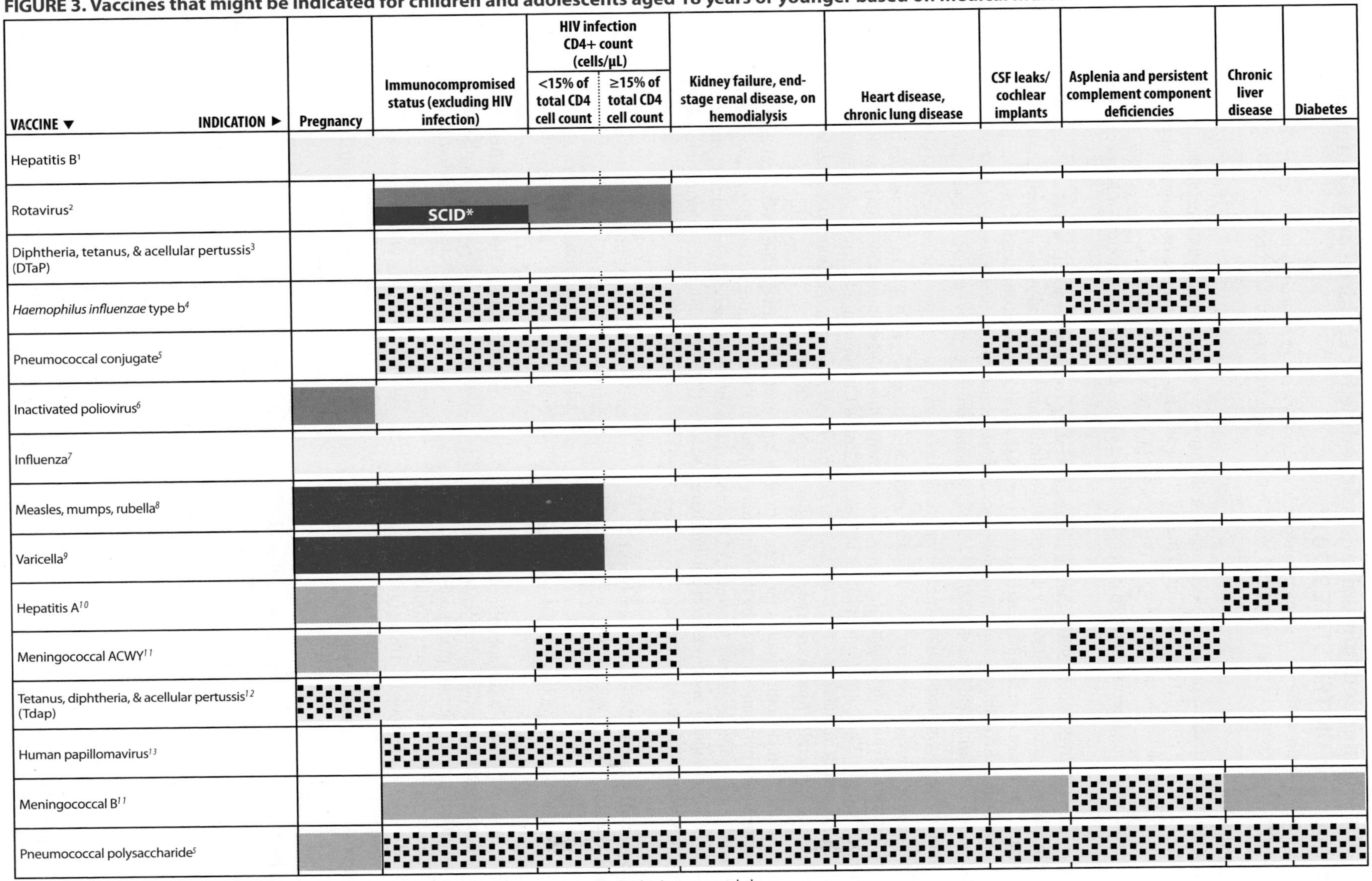

645

Footnotes—Recommended Immunization Schedule for Children and Adolescents Aged 18 Years or Younger, UNITED STATES, 2017

For further guidance on the use of the vaccines mentioned below, see: www.cdc.gov/vaccines/hcp/acip-recs/index.html. For vaccine recommendations for persons 19 years of age and older, see the Adult Immunization Schedule.

Additional information

- For information on contraindications and precautions for the use of a vaccine and for additional information regarding that vaccine, vaccination providers should consult the ACIP General Recommendations on Immunization and the relevant ACIP statement, available online at www.cdc.gov/vaccines/hcp/acip-recs/index.html.

- For purposes of calculating intervals between doses, 4 weeks = 28 days. Intervals of 4 months or greater are determined by calendar months.

- Vaccine doses administered ≤4 days before the minimum interval are considered valid. Doses of any vaccine administered ≥5 days earlier than the minimum interval or minimum age should not be counted as valid doses and should be repeated as age-appropriate. The repeat dose should be spaced after the invalid dose by the recommended minimum interval. For further details, see Table 1, *Recommended and minimum ages and intervals between vaccine doses, in MMWR, General Recommendations on Immunization and Reports / Vol. 60 / No. 2*, available online at www.cdc.gov/mmwr/pdf/rr/rr6002.pdf.

- Information on travel vaccine requirements and recommendations is available at wwwnc.cdc.gov/travel/.

- For vaccination of persons with primary and secondary immunodeficiencies, see Table 13, *Vaccination of persons with primary and secondary immunodeficiencies, in General Recommendations on Immunization (ACIP)*, available at www.cdc.gov/mmwr/pdf/rr/rr6002.pdf.; and Immunization in Special Clinical Circumstances, (American Academy of Pedatrics). In: Kimberlin DW, Brady MT, Jackson MA, Long SS, eds. *Red Book: 2015 report of the Committee on Infectious Diseases. 30th ed.* Elk Grove Village, IL: American Academy of Pediatrics, 2015:68-107.

- The National Vaccine Injury Compensation Program (VICP) is a no-fault alternative to the traditional legal system for resolving vaccine injury petitions. Created by the National Childhood Vaccine Injury Act of 1986, it provides compensation to people found to be injured by certain vaccines. All vaccines within the recommended childhood immunization schedule are covered by VICP except for pneumococcal polysaccharide vaccine (PPSV23). For more information; see www.hrsa.gov/vaccinecompensation/index.html.

1. **Hepatitis B (HepB) vaccine. (Minimum age: birth)**
   Routine vaccination:

   At birth:
   - Administer monovalent HepB vaccine to all newborns within 24 hours of birth.
   - For infants born to hepatitis B surface antigen (HBsAg)- positive mothers, administer HepB vaccine and 0.5 mL of hepatitis B immune globulin (HBIG) within 12 hours of birth. These infants should be tested for HBsAg and antibody to HBsAg (anti-HBs) at age 9 through 12 months (preferably at the next well-child visit) or 1 to 2 months after completion of the HepB series if the series was delayed.
   - If mother's HBsAg status is unknown, within 12 hours of birth, administer HepB vaccine regardless of birth weight. For infants weighing less than 2000 g, administer HBIG in addition to HepB vaccine within 12 hours of birth. Determine mother's HBsAg status as soon as possible and, if mother is HBsAg-positive, also administer HBIG to infants weighing 2000 g or more as soon as possible, but no later than age 7 days.

   Doses following the birth dose:
   - The second dose should be administered at age 1 or 2 months. Monovalent HepB vaccine should be used for doses administered before age 6 weeks.
   - Infants who did not receive a birth dose should receive 3 doses of a HepB-containing vaccine on a schedule of 0, 1 to 2 months, and 6 months, starting as soon as feasible (see figure 2).
   - Administer the second dose 1 to 2 months after the first dose (minimum interval of 4 weeks); administer the third dose at least 8 weeks after the second dose AND at least 16 weeks after the **first** dose. The final (third or fourth) dose in the HepB vaccine series should be administered **no earlier than age 24 weeks**.
   - Administration of a total of 4 doses of HepB vaccine is permitted when a combination vaccine containing HepB is administered after the birth dose.

   Catch-up vaccination:
   - Unvaccinated persons should complete a 3-dose series.
   - A 2-dose series (doses separated by at least 4 months) of adult formulation Recombivax HB is licensed for use in children aged 11 through 15 years.
   - For other catch-up guidance, see Figure 2.

2. **Rotavirus (RV) vaccines. (Minimum age: 6 weeks for both RV1 [Rotarix] and RV5 [RotaTeq])**
   Routine vaccination:
   Administer a series of RV vaccine to all infants as follows:
   1. If Rotarix is used, administer a 2-dose series at ages 2 and 4 months.
   2. If RotaTeq is used, administer a 3-dose series at ages 2, 4, and 6 months.

3. If any dose in the series was RotaTeq or vaccine product is unknown for any dose in the series, a total of 3 doses of RV vaccine should be administered.

Catch-up vaccination:

- The maximum age for the first dose in the series is 14 weeks, 6 days; vaccination should not be initiated for infants aged 15 weeks, 0 days, or older.
- The maximum age for the final dose in the series is 8 months, 0 days.
- For other catch-up guidance, see Figure 2.

3. **Diphtheria and tetanus toxoids and acellular pertussis (DTaP) vaccine. (Minimum age: 6 weeks. Exception: DTaP-IPV [Kinrix, Quadracel]: 4 years)**

Routine vaccination:

- Administer a 5-dose series of DTaP vaccine at ages 2, 4, 6, 15 through 18 months, and 4 through 6 years. The fourth dose may be administered as early as age 12 months, provided at least 6 months have elapsed since the third dose.
- Inadvertent administration of fourth DTaP dose early: If the fourth dose of DTaP was administered at least 4 months after the third dose of DTaP and the child was 12 months of age or older, it does not need to be repeated.

Catch-up vaccination:

- The fifth dose of DTaP vaccine is not necessary if the fourth dose was administered at age 4 years or older.
- For other catch-up guidance, see Figure 2.

4. *Haemophilus influenzae* **type b (Hib) conjugate vaccine. (Minimum age: 6 weeks for PRP-T [ActHIB, DTaP-IPV/Hib (Pentacel), Hiberix, and Hib-MenCY (MenHibrix)], PRP-OMP [PedvaxHIB])**

Routine vaccination:

- Administer a 2- or 3-dose Hib vaccine primary series and a booster dose (dose 3 or 4, depending on vaccine used in primary series) at age 12 through 15 months to complete a full Hib vaccine series.
- The primary series with ActHIB, MenHibrix, Hiberix, or Pentacel consists of 3 doses and should be administered at ages 2, 4, and 6 months. The primary series with PedvaxHIB consists of 2 doses and should be administered at ages 2 and 4 months; a dose at age 6 months is not indicated.
- One booster dose (dose 3 or 4, depending on vaccine used in primary series) of any Hib vaccine should be administered at age 12 through 15 months.
- For recommendations on the use of MenHibrix in patients at increased risk for meningococcal disease, refer to the meningococcal vaccine footnotes and also to *MMWR* February 28, 2014 / 63(RR01):1-13, available at www.cdc.gov/mmwr/PDF/rr/rr6301.pdf.

Catch-up vaccination:

- If dose 1 was administered at ages 12 through 14 months, administer a second (final dose at least 8 weeks after dose 1, regardless of Hib vaccine used in the primary series.

- If both doses were PRP-OMP (PedvaxHIB or COMVAX) and were administered before the first birthday, the third (and final dose should be administered at age 12 through 59 months and at least 8 weeks after the second dose.
- If the first dose was administered at age 7 through 11 months, administer the second dose at least 4 weeks later and a third (and final dose at age 12 through 15 months or 8 weeks after second dose, whichever is later.
- If first dose is administered before the first birthday and second dose administered at younger than 15 months, a third (and final dose should be administered 8 weeks later.
- For unvaccinated children aged 15-59 months, administer only 1 dose.
- For other catch-up guidance, see Figure 2. For catch-up guidance related to MenHibrix, see the meningococcal vaccine footnotes and also *MMWR* February 28, 2014/63(RR01):1-13, available at www.cdc.gov/mmwr/PDF/rr/rr6301.pdf.

Vaccination of persons with high-risk conditions:
Children aged 12 through 59 months who are at increased risk for Hib disease, including chemotherapy recipients and those with anatomic or functional asplenia (including sickle cell disease), human immunodeficiency virus (HIV) infection, immunoglobulin deficiency, or early component complement deficiency, who have received either no doses or only 1 dose of Hib vaccine before age 12 months, should receive 2 additional doses of Hib vaccine, 8 weeks apart; children who received 2 or more doses of Hib vaccine before age 12 months should receive 1 additional dose.

- For patients younger than age 5 years undergoing chemotherapy or radiation treatment who received a Hib vaccine dose(s) within 14 days of starting therapy or during therapy, repeat the dose(s) at least 3 months following therapy completion.
- Recipients of hematopoietic stem cell transplant (HSCT) should be revaccinated with a 3-dose regimen of Hib vaccine starting 6 to 12 months after successful transplant, regardless of vaccination history; doses should be administered at least 4 weeks apart.
- A single dose of any Hib-containing vaccine should be administered to unimmunized* children and adolescents 15 months of age and older undergoing an elective splenectomy; if possible, vaccine should be administered at least 14 days before procedure.
- Hib vaccine is not routinely recommended for patients 5 years or older. However, 1 dose of Hib vaccine should be administered to unimmunized* persons aged 5 years or older who have anatomic or functional asplenia (including sickle cell disease) and unimmunized* persons 5 through 18 years of age with HIV infection.

Patients who have not received a primary series and booster dose or at least 1 dose of Hib vaccine after 14 months of age are considered unimmunized.

5. **Pneumococcal vaccines. (Minimum age: 6 weeks for PCV13, 2 years for PPSV23)**

   Routine vaccination with PCV13:
   - Administer a 4-dose series of PCV13 at ages 2, 4, and 6 months and at age 12 through 15 months.

   Catch-up vaccination with PCV13:
   - Administer 1 dose of PCV13 to all healthy children aged 24 through 59 months who are not completely vaccinated for their age.
   - For other catch-up guidance, see Figure 2.

   Vaccination of persons with high-risk conditions with PCV13 and PPSV23:
   - All recommended PCV13 doses should be administered prior to PPSV23 vaccination if possible.
   - For children aged 2 through 5 years with any of the following conditions: chronic heart disease (particularly cyanotic congenital heart disease and cardiac failure); chronic lung disease (including asthma if treated with high-dose oral corticosteroid therapy); diabetes mellitus; cerebrospinal fluid leak; cochlear implant; sickle cell disease and other hemoglobinopathies; anatomic or functional asplenia; HIV infection; chronic renal failure; nephrotic syndrome; diseases associated with treatment with immunosuppressive drugs or radiation therapy, including malignant neoplasms, leukemias, lymphomas, and Hodgkin disease; solid organ transplantation; or congenital immunodeficiency:
     1. Administer 1 dose of PCV13 if any incomplete schedule of 3 doses of PCV13 was received previously.
     2. Administer 2 doses of PCV13 at least 8 weeks apart if unvaccinated or any incomplete schedule of fewer than 3 doses of PCV13 was received previously.
     3. The minimum interval between doses of PCV13 is 8 weeks.
     4. For children with no history of PPSV23 vaccination, administer PPSV23 at least 8 weeks after the most recent dose of PCV13.
   - For children aged 6 through 18 years who have cerebrospinal fluid leak; cochlear implant; sickle cell disease and other hemoglobinopathies; anatomic or functional asplenia; congenital or acquired immunodeficiencies; HIV infection; chronic renal failure; nephrotic syndrome; diseases associated with treatment with immunosuppressive drugs or radiation therapy, including malignant neoplasms, leukemias, lymphomas, and Hodgkin disease; generalized malignancy; solid organ transplantation; or multiple myeloma:
     1. If neither PCV13 nor PPSV23 has been received previously, administer 1 dose of PCV13 now and 1 dose of PPSV23 at least 8 weeks later.
     2. If PCV13 has been received previously but PPSV23 has not, administer 1 dose of PPSV23 at least 8 weeks after the most recent dose of PCV13.
     3. If PPSV23 has been received but PCV13 has not, administer 1 dose of PCV13 at least 8 weeks after the most recent dose of PPSV23.
   - For children aged 6 through 18 years with chronic heart disease (particularly cyanotic congenital heart disease and cardiac failure), chronic lung disease (including asthma if treated with high-dose oral corticosteroid therapy), diabetes mellitus, alcoholism, or chronic liver disease, who have not received PPSV23, administer 1 dose of PPSV23. If PCV13 has been received previously, then PPSV23 should be administered at least 8 weeks after any prior PCV13 dose.
   - A single revaccination with PPSV23 should be administered 5 years after the first dose to children with sickle cell disease or other hemoglobinopathies; anatomic or functional asplenia; congenital or acquired immunodeficiencies; HIV infection; chronic renal failure; nephrotic syndrome; diseases associated with treatment with immunosuppressive drugs or radiation therapy, including malignant neoplasms, leukemias, lymphomas, and Hodgkin disease; generalized malignancy; solid organ transplantation; or multiple myeloma.

6. **Inactivated poliovirus vaccine (IPV). (Minimum age: 6 weeks)**

   Routine vaccination:
   - Administer a 4-dose series of IPV at ages 2, 4, 6 through 18 months, and 4 through 6 years. The final dose in the series should be administered on or after the fourth birthday and at least 6 months after the previous dose.

   Catch-up vaccination:
   - In the first 6 months of life, minimum age and minimum intervals are only recommended if the person is at risk of imminent exposure to circulating poliovirus (ie, travel to a polio-endemic region or during an outbreak).
   - If 4 or more doses are administered before age 4 years, an additional dose should be administered at age 4 through 6 years and at least 6 months after the previous dose.
   - A fourth dose is not necessary if the third dose was administered at age 4 years or older and at least 6 months after the previous dose.
   - If both oral polio vaccine (OPV) and IPV were administered as part of a series, a total of 4 doses should be administered, regardless of the child's current age. If only OPV was administered, and all doses were given prior to age 4 years, 1 dose of IPV should be given at 4 years or older, at least 4 weeks after the last OPV dose.
   - IPV is not routinely recommended for U.S. residents aged 18 years or older.
   - For other catch-up guidance, see Figure 2.

7. **Influenza vaccines. (Minimum age: 6 months for inactivated influenza vaccine [IIV], 18 years for recombinant influenza vaccine [RIV])**

   Routine vaccination:
   - Administer influenza vaccine annually to all children beginning at age 6 months. For the 2016–17 season, use of live attenuated influenza vaccine (LAIV) is not recommended.

   For children aged 6 months through 8 years:
   - For the 2016–17 season, administer 2 doses (separated by at least 4 weeks) to children who are receiving influenza vaccine for the first time or who have not previously received ≥2 doses of trivalent or quadrivalent influenza vaccine before July 1, 2016. For additional guidance, follow dosing guidelines in the 2016–17 ACIP influenza vaccine recommendations (see *MMWR* August 26, 2016;65(5):1-54, available at www.cdc.gov/mmwr/volumes/65/rr/pdfs/rr6505.pdf).
   - For the 2017–18 season, follow dosing guidelines in the 2017–18 ACIP influenza vaccine recommendations.

   For persons aged 9 years and older:
   - Administer 1 dose.

8. **Measles, mumps, and rubella (MMR) vaccine. (Minimum age: 12 months for routine vaccination)**

   Routine vaccination:
   - Administer a 2-dose series of MMR vaccine at ages 12 through 15 months and 4 through 6 years. The second dose may be administered before age 4 years, provided at least 4 weeks have elapsed since the first dose.
   - Administer 1 dose of MMR vaccine to infants aged 6 through 11 months before departure from the United States for international travel. These children should be revaccinated with 2 doses of MMR vaccine, the first at age 12 through 15 months (12 months if the child remains in an area where disease risk is high), and the second dose at least 4 weeks later.
   - Administer 2 doses of MMR vaccine to children aged 12 months and older before departure from the United States for international travel. The first dose should be administered on or after age 12 months and the second dose at least 4 weeks later.

   Catch-up vaccination:
   - Ensure that all school-aged children and adolescents have had 2 doses of MMR vaccine; the minimum interval between the 2 doses is 4 weeks.

9. **Varicella (VAR) vaccine. (Minimum age: 12 months) Routine vaccination:**
   - Administer a 2-dose series of VAR vaccine at ages 12 through 15 months and 4 through 6 years. The second dose may be administered before age 4 years, provided at least 3 months have elapsed since the first dose. If the second dose was administered at least 4 weeks after the first dose, it can be accepted as valid.

   Catch-up vaccination:
   - Ensure that all persons aged 7 through 18 years without evidence of immunity (see *MMWR* 2007;56[No. RR-4], available at www.cdc.gov/mmwr/pdf/rr/rr5604.pdf) have 2 doses of varicella vaccine. For children aged 7 through 12 years, the recommended minimum interval between doses is 3 months (if the second dose was administered at least 4 weeks after the first dose, it can be accepted as valid); for persons aged 13 years and older, the minimum interval between doses is 4 weeks.

10. **Hepatitis A (HepA) vaccine. (Minimum age: 12 months) Routine vaccination:**
    - Initiate the 2-dose HepA vaccine series at ages 12 through 23 months; separate the 2 doses by 6 to 18 months.
    - Children who have received 1 dose of HepA vaccine before age 24 months should receive a second dose 6 to 18 months after the first dose.
    - For any person aged 2 years and older who has not already received the HepA vaccine series, 2 doses of HepA vaccine separated by 6 to 18 months may be administered if immunity against hepatitis A virus infection is desired.

    Catch-up vaccination:
    - The minimum interval between the 2 doses is 6 months.

    Special populations:
    - Administer 2 doses of HepA vaccine at least 6 months apart to previously unvaccinated persons who live in areas where vaccination programs target older children, or who are at increased risk for infection. This includes persons traveling to or working in countries that have high or intermediate endemicity of infection; men having sex with men; users of injection and non-injection illicit drugs; persons who work with HAV-infected primates or with HAV in a research laboratory; persons with clotting-factor disorders; persons with chronic liver disease; and persons who anticipate close, personal contact (eg, household or regular babysitting) with an international adoptee during the first 60 days after arrival in the United States from a country with high or intermediate endemicity. The first dose should be administered as soon as the adoption is planned, ideally, 2 or more weeks before the arrival of the adoptee.

11. **Meningococcal vaccines. (Minimum age: 6 weeks for Hib-MenCY [MenHibrix], 2 months for Men-ACWY-CRM [Menveo], 9 months for MenACWY-D [Menactra], 10 years for serogroup B meningococcal [MenB] vaccines: MenB- 4C [Bexsero] and MenB-FHbp [Trumenba])**

    Routine vaccination:
    - Administer a single dose of Menactra or Menveo vaccine at age 11 through 12 years, with a booster dose at age 16 years.

- For children aged 2 months through 18 years with high-risk conditions, see "Meningococcal conjugate ACWY vaccination of persons with high-risk conditions and other persons at increased risk" and "Meningococcal B vaccination of persons with high-risk conditions and other persons at increased risk of disease" below.

Catch-up vaccination:

- Administer Menactra or Menveo vaccine at age 13 through 18 years if not previously vaccinated.
- If the first dose is administered at age 13 through 15 years, a booster dose should be administered at age 16 through 18 years, with a minimum interval of at least 8 weeks between doses.
- If the first dose is administered at age 16 years or older, a booster dose is not needed.
- For other catch-up guidance, see Figure 2.

Clinical discretion:

- Young adults aged 16 through 23 years (preferred age range is 16 through 18 years) who are not at increased risk for meningococcal disease may be vaccinated with a 2-dose series of either Bexsero (0, ≥1 month) or Trumenba (0, 6 months) vaccine to provide short-term protection against most strains of serogroup B meningococcal disease. The two MenB vaccines are not interchangeable; the same vaccine product must be used for all doses.
- If the second dose of Trumenba is given at an interval of <6 months, a third dose should be given at least 6 months after the first dose; the minimum interval between the second and third doses is 4 weeks.

Meningococcal conjugate ACWY vaccination of persons with high-risk conditions and other persons at increased risk:

Children with anatomic or functional asplenia (including sickle cell disease), children with HIV infection, or children with persistent complement component deficiency (includes persons with inherited or chronic deficiencies in C3, C5-9, properdin, factor D, factor H, or taking eculizumab [Soliris]):

- **Menveo**
  - *Children who initiate vaccination at 8 weeks.* Administer doses at ages 2, 4, 6, and 12 months.
  - *Unvaccinated children who initiate vaccination at 7 through 23 months.* Administer 2 primary doses, with the second dose at least 12 weeks after the first dose AND after the first birthday.
  - *Children 24 months and older who have not received a complete series.* Administer 2 primary doses at least 8 weeks apart.
- **MenHibrix**
  - *Children who initiate vaccination at 6 weeks.* Administer doses at ages 2, 4, 6, and 12 through 15 months.
  - If the first dose of MenHibrix is given at or after age 12 months, a total of 2 doses should be given

at least 8 weeks apart to ensure protection against serogroups C and Y meningococcal disease.

- **Menactra**
  - **Children with anatomic or functional asplenia or HIV infection**
    - *Children 24 months and older who have not received a complete series.* Administer 2 primary doses at least 8 weeks apart. If Menactra is administered to a child with asplenia (including sickle cell disease) or HIV infection, do not administer Menactra until age 2 years and at least 4 weeks after the completion of all PCV13 doses.
  - **Children with persistent complement component deficiency**
    - *Children 9 through 23 months.* Administer 2 primary doses at least 12 weeks apart.
    - *Children 24 months and older who have not received a complete series.* Administer 2 primary doses at least 8 weeks apart.
  - **All high-risk children**
    - If Menactra is to be administered to a child at high risk for meningococcal disease, it is recommended that Menactra be given either before or at the same time as DTaP.

Meningococcal B vaccination of persons with high-risk conditions and other persons at increased risk of disease: Children with anatomic or functional asplenia (including sickle cell disease) or children with persistent complement component deficiency (includes persons with inherited or chronic deficiencies in C3, C5-9, properdin, factor D, factor H, or taking eculizumab [Soliris]):

- **Bexsero or Trumenba**
  - *Persons 10 years or older who have not received a complete series.* Administer a 2-dose series of Bexsero, with doses at least 1 month apart, or a 3-dose series of Trumenba, with the second dose at least 1-2 months after the first and the third dose at least 6 months after the first. The two MenB vaccines are not interchangeable; the same vaccine product must be used for all doses.

For children who travel to or reside in countries in which meningococcal disease is hyperendemic or epidemic, including countries in the African meningitis belt or the Hajj:

- Administer an age-appropriate formulation and series of Menactra or Menveo for protection against serogroups A and W meningococcal disease. Prior receipt of MenHibrix is not sufficient for children traveling to the meningitis belt or the Hajj because it does not contain serogroups A or W.

For children at risk during an outbreak attributable to a vaccine serogroup:

- For serogroup A, C, W, or Y: Administer or complete an age- and formulation-appropriate series of MenHibrix, Menactra, or Menveo.

- For serogroup B: Administer a 2-dose series of Bexsero, with doses at least 1 month apart, or a 3-dose series of Trumenba, with the second dose at least 1-2 months after the first and the third dose at least 6 months after the first. The two MenB vaccines are not interchangeable; the same vaccine product must be used for all doses.

For MenACWY booster doses among persons with high-risk conditions, refer to *MMWR* 2013;62(RR02):1-22, at www.cdc.gov/mmwr/preview/mmwrhtml/rr6202a1.htm, *MMWR* June 20, 2014/63(24):527-530, at www.cdc.gov/mmwr/pdf/wk/mm6324.pdf, and *MMWR* November 4, 2016;65(43):1189-1194, at www.cdc.gov/mmwr/volumes/65/wr/pdfs/mm6543a3.pdf.

For other catch-up recommendations for these persons and complete information on use of meningococcal vaccines, including guidance related to vaccination of persons at increased risk of infection, see meningococcal *MMWR* publications, available at: www.cdc.gov/vaccines/hcp/acip-recs/vacc-specific.html.

12. **Tetanus and diphtheria toxoids and acellular pertussis (Tdap) vaccine. (Minimum age: 10 years for both Boostrix and Adacel)**

Routine vaccination:
- Administer 1 dose of Tdap vaccine to all adolescents aged 11 through 12 years.
- Tdap may be administered regardless of the interval since the last tetanus and diphtheria toxoid-containing vaccine.
- Administer 1 dose of Tdap vaccine to pregnant adolescents during each pregnancy (preferably during the early part of gestational weeks 27 through 36), regardless of time since prior Td or Tdap vaccination.

Catch-up vaccination:
- Persons aged 7 years and older who are not fully immunized with DTaP vaccine should receive Tdap vaccine as 1 dose (preferably the first in the catch-up series; if additional doses are needed, use Td vaccine. For children 7 through 10 years who receive a dose of Tdap as part of the catch-up series, an adolescent Tdap vaccine dose at age 11 through 12 years may be administered.
- Persons aged 11 through 18 years who have not received Tdap vaccine should receive a dose, followed by tetanus and diphtheria toxoids (Td) booster doses every 10 years thereafter.
- Inadvertent doses of DTaP vaccine:
    - If administered inadvertently to a child aged 7 through 10 years, the dose may count as part of the catch-up series. This dose may count as the adolescent Tdap dose, or the child may receive a Tdap booster dose at age 11 through 12 years.
    - If administered inadvertently to an adolescent aged 11 through 18 years, the dose should be counted as the adolescent Tdap booster.
- For other catch-up guidance, see Figure 2.

13. **Human papillomavirus (HPV) vaccines. (Minimum age: 9 years for 4vHPV [Gardasil] and 9vHPV [Gardasil 9]) Routine and catch-up vaccination:**
- Administer a 2-dose series of HPV vaccine on a schedule of 0, 6-12 months to all adolescents aged 11 or 12 years. The vaccination series can start at age 9 years.
- Administer HPV vaccine to all adolescents through age 18 years who were not previously adequately vaccinated. The number of recommended doses is based on age at administration of the first dose.
- For persons initiating vaccination before age 15, the recommended immunization schedule is 2 doses of HPV vaccine at 0, 6-12 months.
- For persons initiating vaccination at age 15 years or older, the recommended immunization schedule is 3 doses of HPV vaccine at 0, 1-2, 6 months.
- A vaccine dose administered at a shorter interval should be readministered at the recommended interval.
    - In a 2-dose schedule of HPV vaccine, the minimum interval is 5 months between the first and second dose. If the second dose is administered at a shorter interval, a third dose should be administered a minimum of 12 weeks after the second dose and a minimum of 5 months after the first dose.
    - In a 3-dose schedule of HPV vaccine, the minimum intervals are 4 weeks between the first and second dose, 12 weeks between the second and third dose, and 5 months between the first and third dose. If a vaccine dose is administered at a shorter interval, it should be readministered after another minimum interval has been met since the most recent dose.

Special populations:
- For children with history of sexual abuse or assault, administer HPV vaccine beginning at age 9 years.
- Immunocompromised persons*, including those with human immunodeficiency virus (HIV) infection, should receive a 3-dose series at 0, 1-2, and 6 months, regardless of age at vaccine initiation.
- Note: HPV vaccination is not recommended during pregnancy, although there is no evidence that the vaccine poses harm. If a woman is found to be pregnant after initiating the vaccination series, no intervention is needed; the remaining vaccine doses should be delayed until after the pregnancy. Pregnancy testing is not needed before HPV vaccination.

*See *MMWR* December 16, 2016;65(49):1405-1408, available at www.cdc.gov/mmwr/volumes/65/wr/pdfs/mm6549a5.pdf.

APPENDIX 66-2 | **2017 Adult Immunization Schedule**

Recommended Immunization Schedule for Adults Aged 19 Years or Older, United States, 2017

In February 2017, the *Recommended Immunization Schedule for Adults Aged 19 Years or Older, United States, 2017* became effective, as recommended by the Advisory Committee on Immunization Practices (ACIP) and approved by the Centers for Disease Control and Prevention (CDC). The 2017 adult immunization schedule was also reviewed and approved by the following professional medical organizations:

- American College of Physicians (www.acponline.org)
- American Academy of Family Physicians (www.aafp.org)
- American College of Obstetricians and Gynecologists (www.acog.org)
- American College of Nurse-Midwives (www.midwife.org)

CDC announced the availability of the 2017 adult immunization schedule at www.cdc.gov/vaccines/schedules/hcp/index.html in the *Morbidity and Mortality Weekly Report* (*MMWR*).[1] The schedule is published in its entirety in the *Annals of Internal Medicine*.[2]

The adult immunization schedule describes the age groups and medical conditions and other indications for which licensed vaccines are recommended. The 2017 adult immunization schedule consists of:

- Figure 1. Recommended immunization schedule for adults by age group
- Figure 2. Recommended immunization schedule for adults by medical condition and other indications
- Footnotes that accompany each vaccine containing important general information and considerations for special populations
- Table. Contraindications and precautions for vaccines routinely recommended for adults

Consider the following information when reviewing the adult immunization schedule:

- The figures in the adult immunization schedule should be read with the footnotes that contain important general information and information about vaccination of special populations.
- When indicated, administer recommended vaccines to adults whose vaccination history is incomplete or unknown.
- Increased interval between doses of a multi-dose vaccine does not diminish vaccine effectiveness;

therefore, it is not necessary to restart the vaccine series or add doses to the series because of an extended interval between doses.

- Adults with immunocompromising conditions should generally avoid live vaccines, eg, measles, mumps, and rubella vaccine. Inactivated vaccines, eg, pneumococcal or inactivated influenza vaccines, are generally acceptable.
- Combination vaccines may be used when any component of the combination is indicated and when the other components of the combination vaccine are not contraindicated.
- The use of trade names in the adult immunization schedule is for identification purposes only and does not imply endorsement by the ACIP or CDC.

Details on vaccines recommended for adults and complete ACIP statements are available at www.cdc.gov/vaccines/hcp/acip-recs/index.html. Additional CDC resources include:

- A summary of information on vaccination recommendations, vaccination of persons with immunodeficiencies, preventing and managing adverse reactions, vaccination contraindications and precautions, and other information can be found in *General Recommendations on Immunization* at www.cdc.gov/mmwr/preview/mmwrhtml/rr6002a1.htm.
- Vaccine Information Statements that explain benefits and risks of vaccines are available at www.cdc.gov/vaccines/hcp/vis/index.html.
- Information and resources regarding vaccination of pregnant women are available at www.cdc.gov/vaccines/adults/rec-vac/pregnant.html.
- Information on travel vaccine requirements and recommendations is available at wwwnc.cdc.gov/travel/destinations/list.
- *CDC Vaccine Schedules App* for clinicians and other immunization service providers to download is available at www.cdc.gov/vaccines/schedules/hcp/schedule-app.html.
- *Recommended Immunization Schedule for Children and Adolescents Aged 18 Years or Younger* is available at www.cdc.gov/vaccines/schedules/hcp/index.html.

Report suspected cases of reportable vaccine-preventable diseases to the local or state health department.

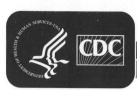

U.S. Department of Health and Human Services
Centers for Disease Control and Prevention

Report all clinically significant post-vaccination reactions to the Vaccine Adverse Event Reporting System at www.vaers.hhs.gov or by telephone, 800-822-7967. All vaccines included in the 2017 adult immunization schedule except herpes zoster and 23-valent pneumococcal polysaccharide vaccines are covered by the Vaccine Injury Compensation Program. Information on how to file a vaccine injury claim is available at www.hrsa.gov/vaccinecompensation or by telephone, 800-338-2382.

Submit questions and comments regarding the 2017 adult immunization schedule to CDC through www.cdc.gov/cdc-info or by telephone, 800-CDC-INFO (800-232-4636), in English and Spanish, 8:00 am–8:00 pm ET, Monday–Friday, excluding holidays.

The following acronyms are used for vaccines recommended for adults:

HepA	hepatitis A vaccine
HepA-HepB	hepatitis A and hepatitis B vaccines
HepB	hepatitis B vaccine
Hib	*Haemophilus influenza* type b conjugate vaccine
HPV vaccine	human papillomavirus vaccine

HZV	herpes zoster vaccine
IIV	inactivated influenza vaccine
LAIV	live attenuated influenzae vaccine
MenACWY	serogroups A, C, W, and Y meningococcal conjugate vaccine
MenB	serogroup B meningococcal vaccine
MMR	measles, mumps, and rubella vaccine
MPSV4	serogroups A, C, W, and Y meningococcal polysaccharide vaccine
PCV13	13-valent pneumococcal conjugate vaccine
PPSV23	23-valent pneumococcal polysaccharide vaccine
RIV	recombinant influenza vaccine
Td	tetanus and diphtheria toxoids
Tdap	tetanus toxoid, reduced diphtheria toxoid, and acellular pertussis vaccine
VAR	varicella vaccine

[1]MMWR Morb Mortal Wkly Rep. 2017;66(5). Available at www.cdc.gov/mmwr/volumes/66/wr/mm6605e2.htm?s_cid=mm6605e2_w.

[2]Ann Intern Med. 2017;166:209-218. Available at annals.org/aim/article/doi/10.7326/M16-2936.

Footnotes—Recommended immunization schedule for adults aged 19 years or older, United States, 2017

1. **Influenza vaccination**

   General information

   - All persons aged 6 months or older who do not have a contraindication should receive annual influenza vaccination with an age-appropriate formulation of inactivated influenza vaccine (IIV) or recombinant influenza vaccine (RIV).
   - In addition to standard-dose IIV, available options for adults in specific age groups include: high-dose or adjuvanted IIV for adults aged 65 years or older, intradermal IIV for adults aged 18 through 64 years, and RIV for adults aged 18 years or older.
   - Notes: Live attenuated influenza vaccine (LAIV) should not be used during the 2016–2017 influenza season. A list of currently available influenza vaccines is available at www.cdc.gov/flu/protect/vaccine/vaccines.htm.

   Special populations

   - Adults with a history of egg allergy who have only hives after exposure to egg should receive age-appropriate IIV or RIV.
   - Adults with a history of egg allergy other than hives, eg, angioedema, respiratory distress, lightheadedness, or recurrent emesis, or who required epinephrine or another emergency medical intervention, may receive age-appropriate IIV or RIV. The selected vaccine should be administered in an inpatient or outpatient medical setting and under the supervision of a healthcare provider who is able to recognize and manage severe allergic conditions.
   - Pregnant women and women who might become pregnant in the upcoming influenza season should receive IIV.

2. **Tetanus, diphtheria, and acellular pertussis vaccination**

   General information

   - Adults who have not received tetanus and diphtheria toxoids and acellular pertussis vaccine (Tdap) or for whom pertussis vaccination status is unknown should receive 1 dose of Tdap followed by a tetanus and diphtheria toxoids (Td) booster every 10 years. Tdap should be administered regardless of when a tetanus or diphtheria toxoid-containing vaccine was last received.
   - Adults with an unknown or incomplete history of a 3-dose primary series with tetanus and diphtheria toxoid-containing vaccines should complete the primary series that includes 1 dose of Tdap. Unvaccinated adults should receive the first 2 doses at least 4 weeks apart and the third dose 6-12 months after the second dose.
   - Notes: Information on the use of Td or Tdap as tetanus prophylaxis in wound management is available at www.cdc.gov/mmwr/preview/mmwrhtml/rr5517a1.htm.

Figures 1 and 2 should be read with the footnotes that contain important general information and considerations for special populations.

Figure 1. Recommended immunization schedule for adults aged 19 years or older by age group, United States, 2017

Vaccine	19–21 years	22–26 years	27–59 years	60–64 years	≥65 years
Influenza[1]	1 dose annually				
Td/Tdap[2]	Substitute Tdap for Td once, then Td booster every 10 yrs				
MMR[3]	1 or 2 doses depending on indication				
VAR[4]	2 doses				
HZV[5]				1 dose	
HPV–Female[6]	3 doses				
HPV–Male[6]	3 doses				
PCV13[7]				1 dose	
PPSV23[7]	1 or 2 doses depending on indication				1 dose
HepA[8]	2 or 3 doses depending on vaccine				
HepB[9]	3 doses				
MenACWY or MPSV4[10]	1 or more doses depending on indication				
MenB[10]	2 or 3 doses depending on vaccine				
Hib[11]	1 or 3 doses depending on indication				

Legend:
- Recommended for adults who meet the age requirement, lack documentation of vaccination, or lack evidence of past infection
- Recommended for adults with additional medical conditions or other indications
- No recommendation

Figure 2. Recommended immunization schedule for adults aged 19 years or older by medical condition and other indications, United States, 2017

Vaccine	Pregnancy[1-6,9]	Immuno-compromised (excluding HIV infection)[3-7,11]	HIV infection CD4+ count (cells/µL)[3-7,9-11] <200	HIV infection CD4+ count (cells/µL)[3-7,9-11] ≥200	Asplenia, persistent complement deficiencies[7,10,11]	Kidney failure, end-stage renal disease, on hemodialysis[7,9]	Heart or lung disease, chronic alcoholism[7]	Chronic liver disease[7,9]	Diabetes[7,9]	Healthcare personnel[3,4,9]	Men who have sex with men[6,8,9]
Influenza[1]	1 dose annually										
Td/Tdap[2]	1 dose Tdap each pregnancy	Substitute Tdap for Td once, then Td booster every 10 yrs									
MMR[3]	contraindicated	contraindicated	contraindicated	1 or 2 doses depending on indication							
VAR[4]	contraindicated	contraindicated	contraindicated	2 doses							
HZV[5]	contraindicated	contraindicated	contraindicated		1 dose						
HPV-Female[6]		3 doses through age 26 yrs	3 doses through age 26 yrs		3 doses through age 26 yrs						
HPV-Male[6]		3 doses through age 26 yrs	3 doses through age 26 yrs		3 doses through age 21 yrs						3 doses through age 26 yrs
PCV13[7]					1 dose	1 dose					
PPSV23[7]					1, 2, or 3 doses depending on indication						
HepA[8]							2 or 3 doses depending on vaccine				
HepB[9]							3 doses				
MenACWY or MPSV4[10]					1 or more doses depending on indication						
MenB[10]					2 or 3 doses depending on vaccine						
Hib[11]		3 doses post-HSCT recipients only			1 dose						

Legend:

Recommended for adults who meet the age requirement, lack documentation of vaccination, or lack evidence of past infection

Recommended for adults with additional medical conditions or other indications

Contraindicated

No recommendation

Special populations

- Pregnant women should receive 1 dose of Tdap during each pregnancy, preferably during the early part of gestational weeks 27-36, regardless of prior history of receiving Tdap.

3. **Measles, mumps, and rubella vaccination**

General information

- Adults born in 1957 or later without acceptable evidence of immunity to measles, mumps, or rubella (defined below) should receive 1 dose of measles, mumps, and rubella vaccine (MMR) unless they have a medical contraindication to the vaccine, eg, pregnancy or severe immunodeficiency.
- Notes: Acceptable evidence of immunity to measles, mumps, or rubella in adults is: born before 1957, documentation of receipt of MMR, or laboratory evidence of immunity or disease. Documentation of healthcare provider-diagnosed disease without laboratory confirmation is not acceptable evidence of immunity.

Special populations

- Pregnant women who do not have evidence of immunity to rubella should receive 1 dose of MMR upon completion or termination of pregnancy and before discharge from the healthcare facility; non-pregnant women of childbearing age without evidence of rubella immunity should receive 1 dose of MMR.
- Adults with primary or acquired immunodeficiency including malignant conditions affecting the bone marrow or lymphatic system, systemic immunosuppressive therapy, or cellular immunodeficiency should not receive MMR.
- Adults with human immunodeficiency virus (HIV) infection and CD4+ T-lymphocyte count $\geq$200 cells/μL for at least 6 months who do not have evidence of measles, mumps, or rubella immunity should receive 2 doses of MMR at least 28 days apart. Adults with HIV infection and CD4+ T-lymphocyte count <200 cells/μL should not receive MMR.
- Adults who work in healthcare facilities should receive 2 doses of MMR at least 28 days apart; healthcare personnel born before 1957 who are unvaccinated or lack laboratory evidence of measles, mumps, or rubella immunity, or laboratory confirmation of disease should be considered for vaccination with 2 doses of MMR at least 28 days apart for measles or mumps, or 1 dose of MMR for rubella.
- Adults who are students in postsecondary educational institutions or plan to travel internationally should receive 2 doses of MMR at least 28 days apart.
- Adults who received inactivated (killed) measles vaccine or measles vaccine of unknown type during years 1963–1967 should be revaccinated with 1 or 2 doses of MMR.
- Adults who were vaccinated before 1979 with either inactivated mumps vaccine or mumps vaccine of unknown type who are at high risk for mumps

infection, eg, work in a healthcare facility, should be considered for revaccination with 2 doses of MMR at least 28 days apart.

4. **Varicella vaccination**

General information

- Adults without evidence of immunity to varicella (defined below) should receive 2 doses of single-antigen varicella vaccine (VAR) 4-8 weeks apart, or a second dose if they have received only 1 dose.
- Persons without evidence of immunity for whom VAR should be emphasized are: adults who have close contact with persons at high risk for serious complications, eg, healthcare personnel and household contacts of immunocompromised persons; adults who live or work in an environment in which transmission of varicella zoster virus is likely, eg, teachers, childcare workers, and residents and staff in institutional settings; adults who live or work in environments in which varicella transmission has been reported, eg, college students, residents and staff members of correctional institutions, and military personnel; non-pregnant women of childbearing age; adolescents and adults living in households with children; and international travelers.
- Notes: Evidence of immunity to varicella in adults is: U.S.-born before 1980 (for pregnant women and healthcare personnel, U.S.-born before 1980 is not considered evidence of immunity); documentation of 2 doses of VAR at least 4 weeks apart; history of varicella or herpes zoster diagnosis or verification of varicella or herpes zoster disease by a healthcare provider; or laboratory evidence of immunity or disease.

Special populations

- Pregnant women should be assessed for evidence of varicella immunity. Pregnant women who do not have evidence of immunity should receive the first dose of VAR upon completion or termination of pregnancy and before discharge from the healthcare facility, and the second dose 4-8 weeks after the first dose.
- Healthcare institutions should assess and ensure that all healthcare personnel have evidence of immunity to varicella.
- Adults with malignant conditions, including those that affect the bone marrow or lymphatic system or who receive systemic immunosuppressive therapy, should not receive VAR.
- Adults with human immunodeficiency virus (HIV) infection and CD4+ T-lymphocyte count $\geq$200 cells/μL may receive 2 doses of VAR 3 months apart. Adults with HIV infection and CD4+ T-lymphocyte count <200 cells/μL should not receive VAR.

5. **Herpes zoster vaccination**

General information

- Adults aged 60 years or older should receive 1 dose of herpes zoster vaccine (HZV), regardless of whether they had a prior episode of herpes zoster.

Special populations

- Adults aged 60 years or older with chronic medical conditions may receive HZV unless they have a medical contraindication, eg, pregnancy or severe immunodeficiency.
- Adults with malignant conditions, including those that affect the bone marrow or lymphatic system or who receive systemic immunosuppressive therapy, should not receive HZV.
- Adults with human immunodeficiency virus (HIV) infection and CD4+ T-lymphocyte count <200 cells/μL should not receive HZV.

6. **Human papillomavirus vaccination**

General information

- Adult females through age 26 years and adult males through age 21 years who have not received any human papillomavirus (HPV) vaccine should receive a 3-dose series of HPV vaccine at 0, 1-2, and 6 months. Males aged 22 through 26 years may be vaccinated with a 3-dose series of HPV vaccine at 0, 1–2, and 6 months.
- Adult females through age 26 years and adult males through age 21 years (and males aged 22 through 26 years who may receive HPV vaccination) who initiated the HPV vaccination series before age 15 years and received 2 doses at least 5 months apart are considered adequately vaccinated and do not need an additional dose of HPV vaccine.
- Adult females through age 26 years and adult males through age 21 years (and males aged 22 through 26 years who may receive HPV vaccination) who initiated the HPV vaccination series before age 15 years and received only 1 dose, or 2 doses less than 5 months apart, are not considered adequately vaccinated and should receive 1 additional dose of HPV vaccine.
- Notes: HPV vaccination is routinely recommended for children at age 11 or 12 years. For adults who had initiated but did not complete the HPV vaccination series, consider their age at first HPV vaccination (described above) and other factors (described below) to determine if they have been adequately vaccinated.

Special populations

- Men who have sex with men through age 26 years who have not received any HPV vaccine should receive a 3-dose series of HPV vaccine at 0, 1-2, and 6 months.
- Adult females and males through age 26 years with immunocompromising conditions (described below), including those with human immunodeficiency virus (HIV) infection, should receive a 3-dose series of HPV vaccine at 0, 1-2, and 6 months.
- Pregnant women are not recommended to receive HPV vaccine, although there is no evidence that the vaccine poses harm. If a woman is found to be pregnant after initiating the HPV vaccination series, delay the remaining doses until after the pregnancy.

No other intervention is needed. Pregnancy testing is not needed before administering HPV vaccine.
- Notes: Immunocompromising conditions for which a 3-dose series of HPV vaccine is indicated are primary or secondary immunocompromising conditions that might reduce cell-mediated or humoral immunity, eg, B-lymphocyte antibody deficiences, complete or partial T-lymphocyte defects, HIV infection, malignant neoplasm, transplantation, autoimmune disease, and immunosuppressive therapy.

7. **Pneumococcal vaccination**

General information

- Adults who are immunocompetent and aged 65 years or older should receive 13-valent pneumococcal conjugate vaccine (PCV13) followed by 23-valent pneumococcal polysaccharide vaccine (PPSV23) at least 1 year after PCV13.
- Notes: Adults are recommended to receive 1 dose of PCV13 and 1, 2, or 3 doses of PPSV23 depending on indication. When both PCV13 and PPSV23 are indicated, PCV13 should be administered first PCV13 and PPSV23 should not be administered during the same visit. If PPSV23 has previously been administered, PCV13 should be administered at least 1 year after PPSV23. When two or more doses of PPSV23 are indicated, the interval between PPSV23 doses should be at least 5 years. Supplemental information on pneumococcal vaccine timing for adults aged 65 years or older and adults aged 19 years or older at high risk for pneumococcal disease (described below) is available at www.cdc.gov/vaccines/vpd-vac/pneumo/downloads/adult-vax-clinician-aid.pdf. No additional doses of PPSV23 are indicated for adults who received PPSV23 at age 65 years or older. When indicated, PCV13 and PPSV23 should be administered to adults whose pneumococcal vaccination history is incomplete or unknown.

Special populations

- Adults aged 19 through 64 years with chronic heart disease including congestive heart failure and cardiomyopathies (excluding hypertension); chronic lung disease including chronic obstructive lung disease, emphysema, and asthma; chronic liver disease including cirrhosis; alcoholism; or diabetes mellitus; or who smoke cigarettes should receive PPSV23. At age 65 years or older, they should receive PCV13 and another dose of PPSV23 at least 1 year after PCV13 and at least 5 years after the most recent dose of PPSV23.
- Adults aged 19 years or older with immunocompromising conditions or anatomical or functional asplenia (described below) should receive PCV13 and a dose of PPSV23 at least 8 weeks after PCV13, followed by a second dose of PPSV23 at least 5 years after the first dose of PPSV23. If the most recent dose of PPSV23 was administered before age 65 years, at age 65 years

or older, administer another dose of PPSV23 at least 8 weeks after PCV13 and at least 5 years after the most recent dose of PPSV23.

- Adults aged 19 years or older with cerebrospinal fluid leak or cochlear implant should receive PCV13 followed by PPSV23 at least 8 weeks after PCV13. If the most recent dose of PPSV23 was administered before age 65 years, at age 65 years or older, administer another dose of PPSV23 at least 8 weeks after PCV13 and at least 5 years after the most recent dose of PPSV23.

- Notes: Immunocompromising conditions that are indications for pneumococcal vaccination are congenital or acquired immunodeficiency including B- or T-lymphocyte deficiency, complement deficiencies, and phagocytic disorders excluding chronic granulomatous disease; human immunodeficiency virus (HIV) infection; chronic renal failure and nephrotic syndrome; leukemia, lymphoma, Hodgkin disease, generalized malignancy, and multiple myeloma; solid organ transplant; and iatrogenic immunosuppression including long-term systemic corticosteroid and radiation therapy. Anatomical or functional asplenia that are indications for pneumococcal vaccination are sickle cell disease and other hemoglobinopathies, congenital or acquired asplenia, splenic dysfunction, and splenectomy. Pneumococcal vaccines should be given at least 2 weeks before immunosuppressive therapy or an elective splenectomy, and as soon as possible to adults who are diagnosed with HIV infection.

8. Hepatitis A vaccination

General information

- Adults who seek protection from hepatitis A virus infection may receive a 2-dose series of single antigen hepatitis A vaccine (HepA) at either 0 and 6-12 months (Havrix) or 0 and 6-18 months (Vaqta). Adults may also receive a combined hepatitis A and hepatitis B vaccine (HepA-HepB) (Twinrix) as a 3-dose series at 0, 1, and 6 months. Acknowledgment of a specific risk factor by those who seek protection is not needed.

Special populations

- Adults with any of the following indications should receive a HepA series: have chronic liver disease, receive clotting factor concentrates, men who have sex with men, use injection or non-injection drugs, or work with hepatitis A virus-infected primates or in a hepatitis A research laboratory setting.

- Adults who travel in countries with high or intermediate levels of endemic hepatitis A infection or anticipate close personal contact with an international adoptee, eg, reside in the same household or regularly babysit, from a country with high or intermediate level of endemic hepatitis A infection within the first 60 days of arrival in the United States should receive a HepA series.

9. Hepatitis B vaccination

General information

- Adults who seek protection from hepatitis B virus infection may receive a 3-dose series of single-antigen hepatitis B vaccine (HepB) (Engerix-B, Recombivax HB) at 0, 1, and 6 months. Adults may also receive a combined hepatitis A and hepatitis B vaccine (HepA-HepB) (Twinrix) at 0, 1, and 6 months. Acknowledgment of a specific risk factor by those who seek protection is not needed.

Special populations

- Adults at risk for hepatitis B virus infection by sexual exposure should receive a HepB series, including sex partners of hepatitis B surface antigen (HBsAg)-positive persons, sexually active persons who are not in a mutually monogamous relationship, persons seeking evaluation or treatment for a sexually transmitted infection, and men who have sex with men (MSM).

- Adults at risk for hepatitis B virus infection by percutaneous or mucosal exposure to blood should receive a HepB series, including adults who are recent or current users of injection drugs, household contacts of HBsAg-positive persons, residents and staff of facilities for developmentally disabled persons, incarcerated, healthcare and public safety workers at risk for exposure to blood or blood-contaminated body fluids, younger than age 60 years with diabetes mellitus, and age 60 years or older with diabetes mellitus at the discretion of the treating clinician.

- Adults with chronic liver disease including, but not limited to, hepatitis C virus infection, cirrhosis, fatty liver disease, alcoholic liver disease, autoimmune hepatitis, and an alanine aminotransferase (ALT) or aspartate aminotransferase (AST) level greater than twice the upper limit of normal should receive a HepB series.

- Adults with end-stage renal disease including those on pre-dialysis care, hemodialysis, peritoneal dialysis, and home dialysis should receive a HepB series. Adults on hemodialysis should receive a 3-dose series of 40 mcg Recombivax HB at 0, 1, and 6 months or a 4-dose series of 40 mcg Engerix-B at 0, 1, 2, and 6 months.

- Adults with human immunodeficiency virus (HIV) infection should receive a HepB series.

- Pregnant women who are at risk for hepatitis B virus infection during pregnancy, eg, having more than one sex partner during the previous 6 months, been evaluated or treated for a sexually transmitted infection, recent or current injection drug use, or had an HBsAg-positive sex partner, should receive a HepB series.

- International travelers to regions with high or intermediate levels of endemic hepatitis B virus infection should receive a HepB series.
- Adults in the following settings are assumed to be at risk for hepatitis B virus infection and should receive a HepB series: sexually transmitted disease treatment facilities, HIV testing and treatment facilities, facilities providing drug-abuse treatment and prevention services, healthcare settings targeting services to persons who inject drugs, correctional facilities, healthcare settings targeting services to MSM, hemodialysis facilities and end-stage renal disease programs, and institutions and nonresidential day care facilities for developmentally disabled persons.

10. **Meningococcal vaccination**

    Special populations
    - Adults with anatomical or functional asplenia or persistent complement component deficiencies should receive a 2-dose primary series of serogroups A, C, W, and Y meningococcal conjugate vaccine (MenACWY) at least 2 months apart and revaccinate every 5 years. They should also receive a series of serogroup B meningococcal vaccine (MenB) with either a 2-dose series of MenB-4C (Bexsero) at least 1 month apart or a 3-dose series of MenB-FHbp (Trumenba) at 0, 1–2, and 6 months.
    - Adults with human immunodeficiency virus (HIV) infection who have not been previously vaccinated should receive a 2-dose primary series of MenACWY at least 2 months apart and revaccinate every 5 years. Those who previously received 1 dose of MenACWY should receive a second dose at least 2 months after the first dose. Adults with HIV infection are not routinely recommended to receive MenB because meningococcal disease in this population is caused primarily by serogroups C, W, and Y.
    - Microbiologists who are routinely exposed to isolates of *Neisseria meningitidis* should receive 1 dose of MenACWY and revaccinate every 5 years if the risk for infection remains, and either a 2-dose series of MenB- 4C at least 1 month apart or a 3-dose series of MenB-FHbp at 0, 1-2, and 6 months.
    - Adults at risk because of a meningococcal disease outbreak should receive 1 dose of MenACWY if the outbreak is attributable to serogroup A, C, W, or Y, or either a 2-dose series of MenB-4C at least 1 month apart or a 3-dose series of MenB-FHbp at 0, 1-2, and 6 months if the outbreak is attributable to serogroup B.
    - Adults who travel to or live in countries with hyperendemic or epidemic meningococcal disease should receive 1 dose of MenACWY and revaccinate every 5 years if the risk for infection remains. MenB is not routinely indicated because meningococcal disease in these countries is generally not caused by serogroup B.
    - Military recruits should receive 1 dose of MenACWY and revaccinate every 5 years if the increased risk for infection remains.
    - First-year college students aged 21 years or younger who live in residence halls should receive 1 dose of MenACWY if they have not received MenACWY at age 16 years or older.
    - Young adults aged 16 through 23 years (preferred age range is 16 through 18 years) who are healthy and not at increased risk for serogroup B meningococcal disease (described above) may receive either a 2-dose series of MenB-4C at least 1 month apart or a 2-dose series of MenB- FHbp at 0 and 6 months for short-term protection against most strains of serogroup B meningococcal disease.
    - For adults aged 56 years or older who have not previously received serogroups A, C, W, and Y meningococcal vaccine and need only 1 dose, meningococcal polysaccharide serogroups A, C, W, and Y vaccine (MPSV4) is preferred. For adults who previously received MenACWY or anticipate receiving multiple doses of serogroups A, C, W, and Y meningococcal vaccine, MenACWY is preferred.
    - Notes: MenB-4C and MenB-FHbp are not interchangeable, ie, the same vaccine should be used for all doses to complete the series. There is no recommendation for MenB revaccination at this time. MenB may be administered at the same time as MenACWY but at a different anatomic site, if feasible.

11. *Haemophilus influenzae* **type b vaccination**

    Special populations
    - Adults who have anatomical or functional asplenia or sickle cell disease, or are undergoing elective splenectomy should receive 1 dose of *Haemophilus influenzae* type b conjugate vaccine (Hib) if they have not previously received Hib. Hib should be administered at least 14 days before splenectomy.
    - Adults with a hematopoietic stem cell transplant (HSCT) should receive 3 doses of Hib in at least 4 week intervals 6-12 months after transplant regardless of their Hib history.
    - Notes: Hib is not routinely recommended for adults with human immunodeficiency virus infection because their risk for *Haemophilus influenzae* type b infection is low.

Table—Contraindications and precautions for vaccines recommended for adults aged 19 years or older*

The Advisory Committee on Immunization Practices (ACIP) recommendations and package inserts for vaccines provide information on contraindications and precautions related to vaccines. Contraindications are conditions that increase chances of a serious adverse reaction in vaccine recipients and the vaccine should not be administered when a contraindication is present. Precautions should be reviewed for potential risks and benefits for vaccine recipient. For a person with a severe allergy to latex, eg, anaphylaxis, vaccines supplied in vials or syringes that contain natural rubber latex should not be administered unless the benefit of vaccination clearly outweighs the risk for a potential allergic reaction. For latex allergies other than anaphylaxis, vaccines supplied in vials or syringes that contain dry, natural rubber or natural rubber latex may be administered.

Contraindications and precautions for vaccines routinely recommended for adults

Vaccine	Contraindications	Precautions
All vaccines routinely recommended for adults	▪ Severe reaction, eg, anaphylaxis, after a previous dose or to a vaccine component	▪ Moderate or severe acute illness with or without fever

Additional contraindications and precautions for vaccines routinely recommended for adults

Vaccine	Additional Contraindications	Additional Precautions
IIV[1]		▪ History of Guillain-Barré Syndrome within 6 wk after previous influenza vaccination ▪ Egg allergy other than hives, eg, angioedema, respiratory distress, lightheadedness, or recurrent emesis; or required epinephrine or another emergency medical intervention (IIV may be administered in an inpatient or outpatient medical setting and under the supervision of a healthcare provider who is able to recognize and manage severe allergic conditions)
RIV[1]		▪ History of Guillain-Barré Syndrome within 6 wk after previous influenza vaccination
LAIV[1]	▪ LAIV should not be used during 2016–2017 influenza season	▪ LAIV should not be used during 2016–2017 influenza season
Tdap/Td	▪ For pertussis-containing vaccines: encephalopathy, eg, coma, decreased level of consciousness, or prolonged seizures, not attributable to another identifiable cause within 7 d of administration of a previous dose of a vaccine containing tetanus or diphtheria toxoid or acellular pertussis	▪ Guillain-Barré Syndrome within 6 wk after a previous dose of tetanus toxoid-containing vaccine ▪ History of Arthus-type hypersensitivity reactions after a previous dose of tetanus or diphtheria toxoid-containing vaccine. Defer vaccination until at least 10 y have elapsed since the last tetanus toxoid-containing vaccine ▪ For pertussis-containing vaccine, progressive or unstable neurologic disorder, uncontrolled seizures, or progressive encephalopathy (until a treatment regimen has been established and the condition has stabilized)
MMR[2]	▪ Severe immunodeficiency, eg, hematologic and solid tumors, chemotherapy, congenital immunodeficiency or long-term immunosuppressive therapy[4], human immunodeficiency virus (HIV) infection with severe immunocompromise ▪ Pregnancy	▪ Recent (within 11 mo) receipt of antibody-containing blood product (specific interval depends on product)[4] ▪ History of thrombocytopenia or thrombocytopenic purpura ▪ Need for tuberculin skin testing[5]
VAR[2]	▪ Severe immunodeficiency, eg, hematologic and solid tumors, chemotherapy, congenital immunodeficiency or long-term immunosuppressive therapy[3], HIV infection with severe immunocompromise ▪ Pregnancy	▪ Recent (within 11 mo) receipt of antibody-containing blood product (specific interval de pends on product)[4] ▪ Receipt of specific antiviral drugs (acyclovir, famciclovir, or valacyclovir) 24 h before vaccination (avoid use of these antiviral drugs for 14 d after vaccination)
HZV[2]	▪ Severe immunodeficiency, eg, hematologic and solid tumors, chemotherapy, congenital immunodeficiency or long-term immunosuppressive therapy[3], HIV infection with severe immunocompromise ▪ Pregnancy	▪ Receipt of specific antiviral drugs (acyclovir, famciclovir, or valacyclovir) 24 h before vaccination (avoid use of these antiviral drugs for 14 d after vaccination)

(Continued)

Vaccine	Additional Contraindications	Additional Precautions
HPV vaccine		▪ Pregnancy
PCV13	▪ Severe allergic reaction to any vaccine containing diphtheria toxoid	

[1]For additional information on use of influenza vaccines among persons with egg allergy, see: CDC. Prevention and control of seasonal influenza with vaccines: recommendations of the Advisory Committee on Immunization Practices–United States, 2016–17 influenza season. MMWR 2016;65(RR-5):1–54. Available at www.cdc.gov/mmwr/volumes/65/rr/rr6505a1.htm.

[2]MMR may be administered together with VAR or HZV on the same day. If not administered on the same day, separate live vaccines by at least 28 days.

[3]Immunosuppressive steroid dose is considered to be daily receipt of 20 mg or more prednisone or equivalent for two or more weeks. Vaccination should be deferred for at least 1 month after discontinuation of immunosuppressive steroid therapy. Providers should consult ACIP recommendations for complete information on the use of specific live vaccines among persons on immune-suppressing medications or with immune suppression because of other reasons.

[4]Vaccine should be deferred for the appropriate interval if replacement immune globulin products are being administered. See: CDC. General recommendations on immunization: recommendations of the Advisory Committee on Immunization Practices (ACIP). MMWR 2011;60(No. RR-2). Available at www.cdc.gov/mmwr/preview/mmwrhtml/rr6002a1.htm.

[5]Measles vaccination may temporarily suppress tuberculin reactivity. Measles-containing vaccine may be administered on the same day as tuberculin skin testing, or should be postponed for at least 4 weeks after vaccination.

*Adapted from: CDC. Table 6. Contraindications and precautions to commonly used vaccines. General recommendations on immunization: recommendations of the Advisory Committee on Immunization Practices. MMWR 2011;60(No. RR-2):40–41 and from: Hamborsky J, Kroger A, Wolfe S, eds. Appendix A. Epidemiology and prevention of vaccine preventable diseases. 13th ed. Washington, DC: Public Health Foundation, 2015. Available at www.cdc.gov/vaccines/pubs/pinkbook/index.html.

Acronyms of vaccines recommended for adults

HepA	hepatitis A vaccine
HepA-HepB	hepatitis A and hepatitis B vaccines
HepB	hepatitis B vaccine
Hib	*Haemophilus influenzae* type b conjugate vaccine
HPV vaccine	human papillomavirus vaccine
HZV	herpes zoster vaccine
IIV	inactivated influenza vaccine
LAIV	live attenuated influenza vaccine
MenACWY	serogroups A, C, W, and Y meningococcal conjugate vaccine
MenB	serogroup B meningococcal vaccine
MMR	measles, mumps, and rubella vaccine
MPSV4	serogroups A, C, W, and Y meningococcal polysaccharide vaccine
PCV13	13-valent pneumococcal conjugate vaccine
PPSV23	23-valent pneumococcal polysaccharide vaccine
RIV	recombinant influenza vaccine
Td	tetanus and diphtheria toxoids
Tdap	tetanus toxoid, reduced diphtheria toxoid, and acellular pertussis vaccine
VAR	varicella vaccine

67

Smoking Cessation

Daniel S. Longyhore

FOUNDATION OVERVIEW

Nicotine dependence, also called tobacco dependence, is an addiction to tobacco products caused by the drug nicotine. Cigarette smoking is the most prevalent type of tobacco use; additional options include smokeless products (chew and snuff) and other smoke products (pipes, cigars, bidis, and hookah pipes). Cigarette smoking increases the risk of cardiovascular disease (stroke, sudden death, heart attack), respiratory diseases (emphysema, asthma, chronic obstructive pulmonary disease), lung cancer, and other cancers.

Nicotine is a ganglionic agonist with pharmacologic effects that are dose dependent. Pharmacologic effects include central and peripheral nervous systems stimulation and depression, respiratory stimulation, skeletal muscle relaxation, catecholamine release by the adrenal medulla, peripheral vasoconstriction, increased blood pressure, heart rate, cardiac output, and oxygen consumption. Nicotine dependence entails a physiologic and psychological process. *Physiologic dependence:* Nicotine stimulates the neurotransmitter dopamine activating the reward pathway in the brain. Initially, the person is rewarded for using tobacco with pleasure or a perceived relief from stress. However, the pleasurable effects diminish with continued use, but smoking continues to avoid nicotine withdrawal. *Psychological addiction:* In the absence of a physical reward for smoking, persons experience cravings with certain activities, stimuli, or times throughout the day. Unlike the physical component to addiction, the psychological component persists indefinitely. Therefore, there is always a chance of relapsing. Physiologic and psychological withdrawal processes manifest as a variety of symptoms lasting 2 to 4 weeks. Nicotine withdrawal symptoms may include: irritability, insomnia, hunger, fatigue, dizziness, difficulty in concentrating, depressed mood, and chest tightness. While nicotine replacement therapy (NRT) may diminish or alleviate nicotine withdrawal, symptoms may persist to some degree.

TREATMENT

The best smoking cessation treatment is prevention through public health education and abstinence. However, the availability of prescription and over-the-counter medications offers an array of options for those attempting to quit tobacco.

Additionally, cognitive behavioral therapy and increased provider contact increases the chance of quitting tobacco products. Health care providers should utilize the five A's each time they come in contact with a person who smokes (Table 67-1).

NRT has proven successful for tobacco cessation. NRT is available in multiple dosage forms and delivery devices, allowing for various cessation strategies. A compilation of NRT products, doses, and special considerations are provided in Table 67-2. NRT may be combined with each other and/or bupropion to increase long-term abstinence rates. Common symptoms of nicotine toxicity include nausea, vomiting, abdominal pain, hypertension, and tachycardia.

Nicotine Transdermal Patch

Nicotine transdermal patches provide a controlled release of nicotine over 16 to 24 hours. The patch is utilized to control long-term cravings and diminish the severity of breakthrough cravings. The 24-hour patch may be left on overnight; however, it may cause insomnia or abnormal dreaming. If the central nervous system (CNS) effects occur, changing to the 16-hour patch or removing the patch 60 minutes before bedtime will minimize CNS side effects. Plasma nicotine levels begin to decline 60 to 120 minutes after removing the patch.

Patients should receive counseling on proper administration. The patch should be applied to a clean, relatively hairless portion of the upper body. Additionally, the patch application site should be rotated daily. When removing patches, patients should fold the patch over itself to avoid others from coming into contact with nicotine. Patches should not be cut as a method of reducing the dose.

Nicotine Gum

Nicotine polacrilex gum provides an *immediate* release of nicotine to control cravings. The dose is absorbed transbuccally after a vigorous chewing of the gum. After chewing and a distinguishable taste change, the gum should be placed between the gums and the cheek until a tingling sensation subsides. Patients should avoid coffee, juice, or other products that would acidify the mouth pH for at least 15 minutes before using the gum. Acidification will decrease the absorption of the nicotine. The 2-mg gum is recommended for patients smoking fewer than 25 cigarettes per day and the 4-mg is

To access your complimentary online question exams, visit https://accesspharmacy.mhmedical.com/NAPLEX.aspx

TABLE 67-1	The Five A's of Smoking Cessation

Ask—Ask the patient about current use of tobacco products.

Advise—Let the patient know about the harms associated with tobacco use.

Assess—Evaluate the patient's readiness to quit tobacco use. If patient is not ready to quit here, continue to use the 5 A's with each additional encounter.

Assist—Work with the patient to identify barriers to cessation and develop a treatment regimen.[a]

Arrange—Create a follow-up plan for patient to facilitate complete cessation.

[a]For most patients who smoke, it will take multiple attempts to quit before complete success is accomplished.

recommended for patients smoking 25 or more cigarettes per day. The gum should be used for up to 12 weeks and no more than 24 pieces chewed per day. Chewing the gum on a fixed schedule (eg, at least one piece every 1-2 hours) for at least 1 to 3 months may be more beneficial than as needed use.

Nicotine Lozenges

Nicotine polacrilex lozenges are an acceptable option for individuals with limitations to using gum (orthodontics, temporomandibular joint [TMJ] disorder, social or professional situations, personal preference). The lozenge should be placed (not chewed) between the gums and cheek and rotated to a new site in the mouth periodically to avoid mucosal irritation. Patients should avoid coffee, juice, or other products that would acidify the mouth pH for at least 15 minutes before use. Acidification will decrease the absorption of the nicotine. The nicotine lozenge is available as a 2-mg and a 4-mg dose. The 2-mg lozenge is recommended for patients who smoke later than 30 minutes after awakening and the 4-mg lozenge is for smokers who smoke within 30 minutes of waking. The duration of treatment is 12 weeks and no more than 20 lozenges should be used in 1 day.

Nicotine Oral Inhaler

A nicotine inhaler mimics the nicotine delivery system of a cigarette, without the other caustic inert ingredients. A cartridge is loaded into the inhalation device and puffed for the duration of the cartridge (approximately 20 minutes) or until the craving subsides. Persons using the nicotine inhaler should start using 6 cartridges daily and increase as needed up to 16 cartridges daily for up to 12 weeks. An additional 12 weeks may be needed to taper off the inhaler.

Nicotine Nasal Spray

Nicotine nasal spray is the least desirable formulation of NRT because of localized, intranasal side effects. A peppery sensation, sneezing, coughing, watery eyes, or runny nose may be experienced. The initial dose is two sprays once to twice per hour. The maximum number of doses is 5 per hour and 40 doses per day. The nasal spray may require a tapering down of the dose over 4 to 6 weeks before discontinuation. Since the dose is absorbed across the nasal mucosa, patients should avoid blowing their nose for 3 minutes after each dose.

TABLE 67-2	Nicotine Replacement Products[a]		
Dosage Form	**Doses**	**Instructions**	**Special Notes**
Patch[b,c]	21 mg, 14 mg, 7 mg (per 24 h)	21 mg daily × 6 wk[d] 14 mg daily × 2 wk 7 mg daily × 2 wk	24-h formulation
Gum[b]	2 mg, 4 mg	Wk 1-6: 1 piece every 1-2 h Wk 7-9: 1 piece every 2-4 h Wk 10-12: 1 piece every 4-8 h	Starting dose based on time to first cigarette after waking; under direct supervision of a health care provider—may use up to 24 pieces. <30 min: 4 mg >30 mg: 2 mg
Lozenge[b]	2 mg, 4 mg	Wk 1-6: 1 piece every 1-2 h Wk 7-9: 1 piece every 2-4 h Wk 10-12: 1 piece every 4-8 h	Starting dose based on time to first cigarette after waking; may use up to 20 lozenges <30 min: 4 mg >30 min: 2 mg
Nasal Inhaler[c]	0.5 mg (per spray)	Start 1-2 doses per h Max 5 sprays per h *or* 40 doses per day	Medication should be tapered for discontinuation over 4-6 wk
Oral Inhaler[c]	10 mg cartridge (4 mg available to absorb)	Start 6 cartridges per day May increase to 16 cartridges per day as needed	Cartridge is empty after 20 min of active puffing

[a]All forms of NRT are effective for smoking cessation. Use of NRT doubles the odds of quitting. Heart rate and blood pressure should be monitored periodically during nicotine replacement.
[b]Available over the counter.
[c]Available by prescription.
[d]If the patient smokes <10 cigarettes daily, then this is only a two-step process. Use step 2 daily for 6 wk and then step down to step 3 daily for 2 wk.

TABLE 67-3	Non-Nicotine Pharmacologic Agents Utilized for Smoking Cessation		
Medication	**Dosage Range**	**Duration**	**Comments/Monitoring**
Bupropion SR (Zyban)	Titrate up to 150 mg orally twice daily. May require reduced initial dose in elderly.	3-6 mo	Patients receiving bupropion and NRT should have blood pressure monitored. The extended-release tablet has an insoluble shell and may be visible in the stool. Substrate and inhibitor of CYP 450 (mostly minor and weak); exception, requires 2B6 for metabolism to active metabolite. Do not chew, crush, and divide extended-release tablets.
Varenicline (Chantix)	Titrate up to 1 mg orally twice daily. Reduce dose if creatinine clearance is less than 30 mL/min.	3-6 mo	Monitor renal function, especially in elderly patients. Nausea, headache, insomnia are dose-dependent side effects. Administer with food and full glass of water to minimize gastrointestinal upset. Should *not* be combined with nicotine replacement products due to the increased nausea.
Clonidine (Catapres)	Titrate to response; 0.15-0.75 mg per day. Consider dose reduction in elderly.	6-12 mo	Gradual withdrawal is needed (over 1 wk for oral), if medication needs to be stopped. Patient should be instructed about abrupt discontinuation (causes rapid increase in blood pressure and symptoms or sympathetic overactivity). Monitor blood pressure (standing, sitting/supine) mental status, and heart rate.
Nortriptyline (Aventyl, Pamelor)	Titrate up to 75-100 mg per day.	6-12 mo	Monitor blood pressure and pulse rate (ECG [electrocardiogram], cardiac monitoring) prior to and during initial therapy in elderly patients. Contraindicated in patients taking or received monoamine oxidase inhibitors in preceding 14 days.

Nicotine-Replacement Side Effects

Nicotine-replacement products have relatively few side effects. Nausea and light-headedness are possible symptoms of nicotine overdose that warrant a reduction of the nicotine dose. The most frequent side effect with the nicotine patch is skin irritation related to the adhesive or the medium containing nicotine and not to the nicotine itself. Approximately 50% of patients report skin irritation during the course of treatment with the patch. The patch site can be rotated to diminish this problem. Switching to a different brand of patch can alleviate the problem because different products use different adhesives or media. The gum can be used instead of the patch when the skin irritation is severe.

Non-nicotine Pharmacologic Agents

Bupropion and varenicline are the non-nicotine agents approved by Food and Drug Administration (FDA) to assist with tobacco cessation. Nortriptyline and clonidine are non-approved second-line medications for smoking cessation. Table 67-3 lists key components about non-nicotine pharmacologic agents for smoking cessation.

Bupropion

Bupropion is a weak inhibitor of dopamine, serotonin, and norepinephrine neuronal uptake. Since the pleasurable (and withdrawal) effects of nicotine are mediated by dopaminergic activity, bupropion attenuates the fluctuations between pleasure and dysphoria. Therefore, the physical adverse events of nicotine withdrawal are tolerable. Bupropion should be started 2 weeks before an attempt at smoking cessation because of a long time to reach steady state. The dose is 150 mg twice daily, starting with once-daily dosing for the first 3 days. Bupropion exhibits activity on dopamine, serotonin, and norepinephrine; therefore, the side effect profile includes high blood pressure, tachycardia, insomnia, weight loss, and headache. These effects are more pronounced in the first days of therapy if a dose titration is not utilized.

Bupropion is contraindicated in patients with a history of an eating disorder, seizures, and current or recent use of monoamine oxidase inhibitors (MAOI).

Varenicline

Varenicline is a mixed agonist and antagonist of CNS nicotinic receptors. Varenicline mildly stimulates the nicotinic receptors responsible for pleasure (or avoiding withdrawal), but also blocks the same receptors from receiving excessive stimulus. The dose for varenicline is titrated over 7 days before the planned quit date; start 0.5 mg daily for days 1 through 3 and increase to 0.5 mg twice daily for days 4 through 7. Administer the target dose of 1 mg twice daily on day 8. The treatment dose is adjusted for patients with a creatinine clearance less than 30 mL/min (0.5 mg twice daily) and patients on hemodialysis (target 0.5 mg daily). The most frequent varenicline side effects are nausea (worse if continue to smoke), insomnia, abnormal dreaming, and headache. Additionally, FDA has cautioned practitioners about suicidal ideations, erratic and aggressive behavior in patients using varenicline. Monitoring for behavioral changes and psychiatric symptoms should occur. The treatment should be discontinued and provider notified immediately with noted changes.

Clonidine

Clonidine is a second-line off-label medication for the treatment of tobacco dependence. Clonidine doses vary from 0.15 to 0.75 mg per day orally and 0.1 to 0.2 mg per day transdermally. There is a high incidence of dose-dependent side effects, especially dry mouth and sedation. Additionally, abrupt discontinuation may result in nervousness, agitation, headache, and tremor accompanied or followed by a rapid rise in blood pressure.

Nortriptyline

Nortriptyline is a second-line off-label medication for the treatment of tobacco dependence. Therapy is initiated 10 to 28 days prior to the planned quit date to allow for the medication to reach steady state. Nortriptyline side effects include sedation, dry mouth, blurred vision, urinary retention, light-headedness, and tremor.

SPECIAL CONSIDERATIONS

Tobacco cessation treatment is limited in patients that have contraindications or cannot tolerate NRT, bupropion, or varenicline. Examples include uncontrolled hypertension, unstable angina, cardiac arrhythmias, or pregnancy. NRT carries a pregnancy category D rating with FDA. Agents such as varenicline and bupropion are category C; varenicline lacks data in pregnant women and bupropion has mixed results.

Electronic nicotine delivery devices such as electronic cigarettes (e-cigarettes) are battery-powered devices that deliver nicotine, flavorings (eg, fruit, mint, and chocolate), and other chemicals via an inhaled aerosol. E-cigarettes that are marketed without a therapeutic claim by the product manufacturer are currently not regulated by FDA. One area of concern is the potential of e-cigarettes to cause acute nicotine toxicity. The most common adverse health effects in e-cigarette exposure calls are vomiting, nausea, and eye irritation. Clinicians should be aware that e-cigarettes have the potential to cause acute adverse health effects and represent an emerging public health concern.

CASE Application

1. JT is a 47-year-old man who is interested in quitting smoking. He has smoked 1.5 packs per day for the last 17 years. He successfully quit cold turkey in the past that lasted for approximately 16 months, but went back to smoking after starting a new job. Based on the various components of nicotine dependence, which reason most likely caused JT to return to smoking?

   a. Psychological dependence
   b. Physiologic dependence
   c. He did not use a pharmacologic aid to quit smoking.
   d. Most persons will relapse within 24 months of a quit attempt.

Questions 2 and 3 are related to the same patient.

2. HN has decided that she would like to quit smoking, but is not comfortable quitting without supportive NRT. She decides that the gum will be her best choice because it is easily concealable among friends, family, and coworkers. She has smoked 1 to 1.5 packs per day for the last 13 years. What is the appropriate starting dose for the nicotine polacrilex gum for HN?

   a. 4-mg piece of gum; not to exceed 24 doses in 24 hours
   b. 4-mg piece of gum; not to exceed 20 doses in 24 hours
   c. 2-mg piece of gum; not to exceed 24 pieces in 24 hours
   d. Not enough information provided to determine the correct dosage strength for this patient

3. Upon further consultation with HN, she indicates that she smokes within the 10 minutes after waking, when should HN reduce to the next dosage step/phase?

   a. She should not reduce the dosage formulation, but rather spread out the frequency of using the gum product.
   b. 8 weeks
   c. 6 weeks
   d. 4 weeks

4. IO is 31 years old and starting a new job in a dental clinic. She wishes to quit smoking before she starts her new job because the clinic does not allow employees to smoke during their shift. However, she would also like to quit to preserve her lung health. She smokes approximately 15 cigarettes daily and has her first one in the car on the way to work (about 95 minutes after waking). She wishes to use the lozenges for her quit attempt. What product would you suggest that IO use?

   a. Nicotrol 4 mg
   b. Nicotrol 2 mg
   c. Commit 4 mg
   d. Commit 2 mg

5. Which condition can be made worse using nicotine polacrilex gum?

   a. TMJ disorder
   b. Gingival hyperplasia
   c. Oropharyngeal candidiasis
   d. Episodic epistaxis

6. JE is a 72-year-old man smoking one pack per day for the last 40 years smoking history. He has never attempted to quit smoking, but feels he must try after being hospitalized for pneumonia for 3 days. While he was in the hospital he was given a nicotine patch to wear and change daily until discharge. Upon discharge, he was not given the nicotine patch, but wants to continue using it to abstain from smoking. What dose of the patch should JE start?

   a. 21 mg/d patch
   b. 14 mg/d patch
   c. 7 mg/d patch
   d. He does not smoke enough to warrant NRT with a patch.

7. JE has been without a cigarette for 3 days with the help of the nicotine patch. On the fourth day, JE is under a great deal of stress and needs to go outside for a cigarette. Since he is still wearing the nicotine replacement patch, what adverse events will he most likely experience?

   a. Excess fatigue
   b. Lower extremity cramping
   c. Nausea, vomiting, and headache
   d. Tinnitus

8. What would be a better choice for JE to use for break-through cravings while he is being treated with the nicotine patch?

   a. Nicorette gum
   b. Chantix 1 mg twice daily
   c. Zyban 150 mg twice daily
   d. He should not combine therapies for smoke tobacco cessation.

Questions 9 through 11 are related to the same case.

9. OH is a 41-year-old woman with multiple psychiatric medical conditions. She started smoking approximately 5 years ago and has slowly increased her daily ciga-rette consumption to 2 packs per day. She started using Nicoderm CQ 21-mg patches, but has experienced various abnormal dreams, causing her to lose sleep over the last 3 nights. She will not continue using the patches if the dreams continue. What alternative(s) may OH trial to help combat this side effects?

   a. Nicoderm CQ 14 mg/d patch
   b. Habitrol 21 mg/d patch
   c. Habitrol 14 mg/d patch
   d. Remove the Nicoderm CQ 21-mg patch prior to bed.

10. OH decides not to use the nicotine patches and switches to the Commit nicotine lozenge. Which of the following administration scenarios alters the pharmacokinetics of the lozenge? Select all that apply.

    a. In the morning, immediately after waking
    b. In the afternoon, during her scheduled work break
    c. In the evening, after her dinner and coffee
    d. Before bedtime, watching the evening news

11. OH's provider also decides to use a prescription, non-nicotine, smoking cessation aid because she feels that using lozenges as needed will not be sufficient. Which of the following medications would be discouraged/contraindicated?

    a. Varenicline
    b. Bupropion
    c. Nortriptyline
    d. Clonidine

12. Which disease should be screened before starting vareni-cline? Select all that apply.

    a. Hypertension
    b. Diabetes
    c. Chronic obstructive lung disease
    d. Renal insufficiency
    e. Past medical history for mental health disease

13. TY is a 40-year-old obese man with a medical history significant for hypertension and dyslipidemia. He also smokes cigarettes and has smoked 1.5 packs per day for the last 16 years. His most recent blood pressure was 161/94 mm Hg, which is consistent with his previous

three readings. His physician is convinced that if TY were to lose weight and quit smoking, many of his medical issues would be easier to manage. TY requests assistance to quit smoking. Which of the following medi-cations would be the best choice for TY?

   a. Bupropion
   b. Nicotine polacrilex gum
   c. Nicotine patch
   d. Varenicline

14. Insomnia and anxiety are common adverse events with bupropion, which of the following counseling points should be discussed with VX to minimize the side effects?

    a. Do not take the second dose after 5 o' clock in the evening.
    b. If the patient develops insomnia, omit the second dose of the day.
    c. Insomnia is a temporary adverse event and will resolve approximately 7 days after increasing the dose to twice daily.
    d. The insomnia and anxiety are most likely due to nicotine withdrawal and will resolve approximately 7 to 10 days after quitting smoking.

15. Combination therapy is ideal for many patients attempt-ing to quit smoking, which of the following combina-tions is/are appropriate? Select all that apply.

    a. Bupropion and nicotine polacrilex gum
    b. Nicotine patches and nicotine polacrilex gum
    c. Varenicline and nicotine polacrilex gum
    d. Nortriptyline and nicotine polacrilex gum

16. LK is a 62-year-old woman with osteoporosis, chronic allergic rhinitis, and a 50-pack-year history of smoking cig-arettes. At a recent trip to the dentist, she was told that due to poor oral hygiene and tooth decay, she needs her teeth removed and fitted for dentures. He also recommends that she quit smoking during this time period as it most likely contributed to her current predicament. Which agent listed below would be the best agent for LK to choose?

    a. Nicotine polacrilex gum
    b. Nicotine lozenge
    c. Nicotine nasal inhaler
    d. Nicotine transdermal patch

17. AI is a 28-year-old woman with a past medical history significant for polycystic ovarian syndrome (PCOS), hypertriglyceridemia, epilepsy, hyperthyroidism, and tobacco abuse for the last 9 years. Which of her medical conditions is considered a precaution for using bupro-pion therapy?

    a. PCOS
    b. Hypertriglyceridemia
    c. Epilepsy
    d. Hyperthyroidism

18. What is the brand name of clonidine?

    a. Chantix
    b. Pamelor
    c. Aventyl
    d. Catapres

19. Which of the following formulations is/are NRT available? Select all that apply.

    a. Patch
    b. Nasal inhaler
    c. Oral inhaler
    d. Lozenge

20. RI is a 54-year-old man on oral therapy for smoking cessation. He has been attempting to quit smoking for several years with no success. He is currently receiving second-line therapy for smoking cessation. RI feels the current therapy is helping; however, he is having dry mouth, sedation, and blurred vision. Additionally, he has been having difficulty in urinating. He went to his urologist because of the urination problem (he has a past medical history of benign prostatic hypertrophy); however, the urologist said his prostate specific antigen is within the reference range and was not causing his difficulty in urinating. RI presents to your pharmacy seeking guidance on his current symptoms. Which of the following medications could be contributing to RI's symptoms? Select all that apply.

    a. Nicoderm
    b. Aventyl
    c. Seroquel
    d. Pamelor
    e. Chantix

TAKEAWAY POINTS »

- Nicotine dependence displays psychological and physiologic components.
- Tobacco use and cessation should be continually addressed to maximize chances of cessation.
- Physical withdrawal symptoms are temporary and can be overcome with pharmacologic assistance. Psychological component remains indefinitely. A treatment plan should include medication(s) in conjunction with behavior modification.
- The nicotine patch is the only long-acting nicotine replacement formulation. It is a good initial choice (with or without bupropion) for tobacco cessation and can be combined with any of the other immediate release preparations.
- Nicotine gum is an appropriate agent to help cravings, but should be avoided in patients with dental hardware and TMJ disorder. It should be chewed and then placed in the mouth and *not* continuously chewed.

- Nicotine lozenges are an appropriate agent to help cravings, without the issues of dental hardware or TMJ. Like nicotine gum, this product is less effective when used within less than 15 minutes after eating or drinking an acidic product such as coffee or juices.
- The nicotine oral inhaler is an ideal option for persons who need to fulfill the hand-to-mouth motion associated with smoking a cigarette.
- Bupropion is a non-nicotine option for smoking cessation. Bupropion should be avoided in patients with a history of seizure and/or eating disorders.
- Varenicline should *not* be combined with nicotine replacement products due to the increased risk of nausea. The FDA has cautioned practitioners about suicidal ideations, erratic and aggressive behavior in patients using varenicline.

BIBLIOGRAPHY

Doering PL, Li R. Substance-related disorders II: alcohol, nicotine, and caffeine. In: DiPiro JT, Talbert RL, Yee GC, Matzke GR, Wells BG, Posey L, eds. *Pharmacotherapy: A Pathophysiologic Approach.* 9th ed. New York, NY: McGraw-Hill; 2014:chap 49.

Fiore MC, Bailey WC. Treating tobacco use and dependence. Clinical Practice Guidelines. Rockville, MD: United States Department of Health and Human Services, Public Health Service; June 2000 (updated May 2008).

Lüscher C. Drugs of abuse. In: Katzung BG, Masters SB, Trevor AJ, eds. *Basic & Clinical Pharmacology.* 12th ed. New York, NY: McGraw-Hill; 2012:chap 32.

O'Brien CP. Drug addiction. In: Brunton LL, Chabner BA, Knollmann BC, eds. *Goodman & Gilman's The Pharmacological Basis of Therapeutics.* 12th ed. New York, NY: McGraw-Hill; 2011:chap 24.

Perera S, Bullen C. Nicotine replacement therapy for smoking cessation. *Cochrane Collaboration.* 2009;4:1-63.

KEY ABBREVIATIONS

CNS = central nervous system
FDA = Food and Drug Administration
NRT = nicotine replacement therapy

PCOS = polycystic ovarian syndrome
TMJ = temporomandibular joint

68

Ocular Pharmacology

Karen H. McGee

FOUNDATION OVERVIEW

The eye is a specialized sensory organ that is relatively secluded from systemic access by the blood-retinal, blood-aqueous, and blood-vitreous barriers; as a consequence, the eye exhibits unique pharmacodynamic and pharmacokinetic properties.

Drug-Delivery Strategies

A number of delivery systems have been developed for treating ocular diseases. Most ophthalmic drugs are delivered in solutions, but for compounds with limited solubility, a suspension form facilitates delivery. Properties of varying ocular routes of administration are outlined in Table 68-1. Several formulations prolong the time a drug remains on the surface of the eye. These include gels, ointments, solid inserts, soft contact lenses, and collagen shields. Ophthalmic gels (eg, pilocarpine 4% gel) release drugs by diffusion following erosion of soluble polymers. The polymers used include cellulosic ethers, polyvinyl alcohol, carbopol, polyacrylamide, polymethylvinyl ether–maleic anhydride, poloxamer 407, and pluronic acid. Ointments usually contain mineral oil and a petrolatum base and are helpful in delivering antibiotics, cycloplegic drugs, or miotic agents. Solid inserts, such as the ganciclovir intravitreal implant, provide a *zero-order* rate of delivery by steady-state diffusion, whereby drug is released at a constant rate over a period of time rather than as a bolus. This surgical implant has been used to deliver anti-cytomegalovirus (CMV) medication in proximity to the retinal infection. The intent is to deliver a sustained dose of medication over several months with reduced spikes in drug delivery independent of patient compliance.

Pharmacokinetics

Pharmacokinetic principles based on studies of systemically administered drugs do not fully apply to all ophthalmic drugs. Although similar principles of absorption, distribution, metabolism, and excretion determine the fate of drug disposition in the eye, alternative routes of drug administration, in addition to oral and intravenous routes, introduce other variables in compartmental analysis.

Absorption

After topical instillation of a drug, the rate and extent of absorption are determined by the time the drug remains in the cul-de-sac and precorneal tear film, elimination by nasolacrimal drainage, drug binding to tear proteins, drug metabolism by tear and tissue proteins, and diffusion across the cornea and conjunctiva. A drug's residence time may be prolonged by changing its formulation. Residence time also may be extended by blocking the outlet of tears from the eye by closing the tear drainage ducts. Nasolacrimal drainage contributes to systemic absorption of topically administered ophthalmic medications. Absorption from the nasal mucosa avoids first-pass metabolism by the liver, and consequently, significant systemic side effects may be caused by topical medications, especially when used chronically.

Distribution

Topically administered drugs may undergo systemic distribution primarily by nasal mucosal absorption and possibly by local ocular distribution by transcorneal/transconjunctival absorption. Following transcorneal absorption, the aqueous humor accumulates the drug, which then is distributed to intraocular structures as well as potentially to the systemic circulation via the trabecular meshwork pathway.

Metabolism

Enzymatic biotransformation of ocular drugs may be significant because a variety of enzymes (esterases, oxidoreductases, and lysosomal enzymes) are found in the eye. The esterases have been of particular interest because of the development of prodrugs for enhanced corneal permeability (eg, dipivefrin hydrochloride is a prodrug for epinephrine, and latanoprost is a prodrug for prostaglandin $F_{2\alpha}$); both drugs are used for glaucoma management. Topically applied ocular drugs are eliminated by the liver and kidney after systemic absorption, but enzymatic transformation of systemically administered drugs also is important in ophthalmology.

Toxicology

All ophthalmic medications are potentially absorbed into the systemic circulation, so undesirable systemic side effects may occur. Most ophthalmic drugs are delivered locally to the eye, and the potential local toxic effects are due to hypersensitivity reactions or to direct toxic effects on the cornea, conjunctiva, periocular skin, and nasal mucosa. Eyedrops and contact lens

TABLE 68-1	**Characteristics of Ocualar Routes of Drug Administration**		
Route	**Absorption Pattern**	**Special Utility**	**Limitations and Precautions**
Topical	Prompt, depending on formulation	Convenient, economical, relatively safe	Compliance, corneal and conjunctival toxicity, nasal mucosal toxicity, systemic side effects from nasolacrimal absorption
Subconjunctival, sub-Tenon's, and retrobulbar injections	Prompt or sustained, depending on formulation	Anterior segment infections, posterior uveitis, cystoid macular edema	Local toxicity, tissue injury, globe perforation, optic nerve trauma, central retinal artery and/or vein occlusion, direct retinal drug toxicity with inadvertent globe perforation, ocular muscle trauma, prolonged drug effect
Intraocular (intracameral) injections	Prompt	Anterior segment surgery, infections	Corneal toxicity, intraocular toxicity, relatively short duration of action
Intravitreal injection or device	Absorption circumvented, immediate local effect, potential sustained effect	Endophthalmitis, retinitis, age-related macular degeneration	Retinal toxicity

Reproduced with permission from Brunton LL, Chabner BA, Knollmann BC: *Goodman & Gilman's The Pharmacological Basis of Therapeutics,* 12th ed. New York, NY: McGraw-Hill; 2011.

solutions commonly contain preservatives such as benzalkonium chloride for antimicrobial properties; however, benzalkonium chloride may cause an ulcerative keratopathy.

INFECTIOUS DISEASES OF THE EYE

Infectious diseases of the skin, eyelids, conjunctivae, and lacrimal excretory system are encountered regularly in clinical practice and a number of anti-infectives are formulated for topical ocular use. Appropriate selection of anti-infective and route of administration is dependent on the patient's symptoms, the clinical examination, and the culture/sensitivity results.

Antibacterial Agents

Indications for the use of topical antibiotics in ophthalmology are hordeolum, blepharitis, conjunctivitis, and keratitis. Table 68-2 summarizes topical antibiotics used in ophthalmology. Infectious processes of the lids include *hordeolum* and *blepharitis.*

- A hordeolum (stye) is an infection at the eyelid margins. The typical offending bacterium is *Staphylococcus aureus* and the treatment consists of warm compresses and topical antibiotic gel, drops, or ointment.

- Blepharitis is a common bilateral inflammatory process of the eyelids characterized by irritation and burning caused by *Staphylococcus* species. Local hygiene is the mainstay of therapy; topical antibiotics frequently are used, usually in gel, drop, or ointment form, particularly when the disease is accompanied by conjunctivitis and keratitis.

Conjunctivitis is an inflammatory process of the conjunctiva that varies in severity from mild hyperemia to severe purulent discharge. The more common causes of conjunctivitis include viruses, allergies, environmental irritants, contact lenses, and chemicals. The less common causes include other infectious pathogens, immune-mediated reactions, associated systemic diseases, and tumors of the conjunctiva or eyelid. The more commonly reported infectious agents are adenovirus and herpes simplex virus, followed by other viral (eg, enterovirus, coxsackie virus, measles virus, varicella zoster virus) and bacterial sources (eg, *Neisseria* species, *Streptococcus pneumoniae, Haemophilus* species, *S. aureus,* and chlamydial species). Fungi and parasites are rare causes of conjunctivitis. Effective management is based on selection of an appropriate antibiotic for suspected bacterial pathogens. Unless an unusual causative organism is suspected, bacterial conjunctivitis is treated empirically with a broad-spectrum topical antibiotic without obtaining a culture.

Keratitis (corneal inflammation) occurs at any level of the cornea (eg, epithelium, subepithelium, stroma, endothelium) and due to noninfectious or infectious causes. The mild, small, more peripheral infections usually are not cultured, and the eyes are treated with broad-spectrum topical antibiotics. In more severe, central, or larger infections, corneal scrapings for smears, cultures, and sensitivities are performed, and the patient is immediately started on intensive hourly, around-the-clock topical antibiotic therapy. The goal of treatment is to eradicate the infection and reduce the amount of corneal scarring and the chance of corneal perforation and severe decreased vision or blindness. The initial medication selection and dosage are adjusted according to the clinical response and culture and sensitivity results.

Antiviral Agents

The primary indications for the use of antiviral drugs in ophthalmology are viral keratitis and retinitis. There currently are no antiviral agents for the treatment of viral conjunctivitis caused by adenoviruses, which usually has a self-limited course and typically is treated by symptomatic relief of irritation. Table 68-3 summarizes antiviral drugs used in ophthalmology.

Viral keratitis is an infection of the cornea that involves the epithelium or stroma and is caused by herpes simplex type I and varicella zoster viruses. Less common viral etiologies include herpes simplex type II and CMV. Topical antiviral agents are indicated for the treatment of epithelial disease due

TABLE 68-2   Topical Antibacterial Agents for Ophthalmic Use

Generic Name (Trade Name)	Formulation[a]	Toxicity	Indications for Use
Azithromycin (azasite)	1% solution	H	Conjunctivitis
Bacitracin	500 units/g ointment	H	Conjunctivitis, blepharitis, keratitis, keratoconjunctivitis, corneal ulcers, blepharoconjunctivitis, meibomianitis, dacryocystitis
Besifloxacin (besivance)	0.6% suspension		Conjunctivitis
Chloramphenicol	1% ointment	H, BD	Conjunctivitis, keratitis
Ciprofloxacin hydrochloride (ciloxan, others)	0.3% solution; 0.3% ointment	H, D-RCD	Conjunctivitis, keratitis, keratoconjunctivitis, corneal ulcers, blepharitis, blepharoconjunctivitis, meibomianitis, dacryocystitis
Erythromycin (ilotycin, others)	0.5% ointment	H	Superficial ocular infections involving the conjunctiva or cornea; prophylaxis of ophthalmia neonatorum
Gatifloxacin (zymar)	0.3% solution	H	Conjunctivitis
Gentamicin sulfate (garamycin, genoptic, gent-ak, gentacidin, others)	0.3% solution; 0.3% ointment	H	Conjunctivitis, blepharitis, keratitis, keratoconjunctivitis, corneal ulcers, blepharoconjunctivitis, meibomianitis, dacryocystitis
Levofloxacin (quixin, iquix)	0.5% solution	H	Conjunctivitis
Levofloxacin (iquix)	1.5% solution	H	Corneal ulcers
Moxifloxacin (vigamox)	0.5% solution	H	Conjunctivitis
Ofloxacin (ocuflox, others)	0.3% solution	H	Conjunctivitis, corneal ulcers
Sulfacetamide sodium (bleph-10, cetamide, 30% solution; isopto cetamide, others)	1%, 10%, 15%, and 10% ointment	H, BD	Conjunctivitis, other superficial ocular infections
Polymyxin B combinations[b]	Various solutions and ointments		Conjunctivitis, blepharitis, keratitis
Tobramycin sulfate[c] (tobrex, aktob, defy, others)	0.3% solution; 0.3% ointment	H	External infections of the eye and its adnexa

[a]For specific information on dosing, formulation, and trade names, refer to the *Physicians' Desk Reference for Ophthalmic Medicines*, which is published annually.
[b]Polymyxin B is formulated for delivery to the eye in combination with bacitracin, neomycin, gramicidin, oxytetracycline, or trimethoprim.
[c]Tobramycin is formulated for delivery to the eye in combination with dexamethasone or loteprednol etabonate.
Abbreviations: H, hypersensitivity; BD, blood dyscrasia; D-RCD, drug-related corneal deposits.
Reproduced with permission from Brunton LL, Chabner BA, Knollmann BC: *Goodman & Gilman's The Pharmacological Basis of Therapeutics,* 12th ed. New York, NY: McGraw-Hill; 2011.

TABLE 68-3   Antiviral Agents for Ophthalmic Use

Generic Name (Trade Name)	Route of Administration	Ocular Toxicity	Indications for Use
Trifluridine (viroptic, others)	Topical (1% solution)	PK, H	Herpes simplex keratitis and keratoconjunctivitis
Acyclovir (zovirax)	Oral, intravenous (200-mg capsules, 400- and 800-mg tablets)		Herpes zoster ophthalmicus[a] Herpes simplex iridocyclitis
Valacyclovir (valtrex)	Oral (500- and 1000-mg tablets)		Herpes simplex keratitis[a] Herpes zoster ophthalmicus[a]
Famciclovir (famvir)	Oral (125-, 250-, and 500-mg tablets)		Herpes simplex keratitis[a] Herpes zoster ophthalmicus[a]
Foscarnet (foscavir)	Intravenous Intravitreal[a]		Cytomegalovirus retinitis
Ganciclovir (cytovene) (vitrasert)	Intravenous, oral Intravitreal implant		Cytomegalovirus retinitis
Valganciclovir (valcyte)	Oral		Cytomegalovirus retinitis
Cidofovir (vistide)	Intravenous		Cytomegalovirus retinitis

Abbreviations: H, hypersensitivity; PK, pharmacokinetic.
Reproduced with permission from Brunton LL, Chabner BA, Knollmann BC: *Goodman & Gilman's The Pharmacological Basis of Therapeutics,* 12th ed. New York, NY: McGraw-Hill; 2011.

TABLE 68-4	**Antifungal Agents for Ophthalmic Use**	
Drug Class/Agent	**Method of Administration**	**Indications for use**
Polyenes		
Amphotericin B[a]	0.1-0.5% (typically 0.15%) topical solution	Yeast and fungal keratitis and endophthalmitis
	0.8-1 mg subconjunctival	Yeast and fungal endophthalmitis
	5-mcg intravitreal injection	Yeast and fungal endophthalmitis
	Intravenous	Yeast and fungal endophthalmitis
Natamycin	5% topical suspension	Yeast and fungal blepharitis, conjunctivitis, keratitis
Imidazoles		
Fluconazole[a]	Oral, intravenous	Yeast keratitis and endophthalmitis
Itraconazole[a]	Oral	Yeast and fungal keratitis and endophthalmitis
Ketoconazole[a]	Oral	Yeast keratitis and endophthalmitis
Miconazole[a]	1% topical solution	Yeast and fungal keratitis
	5-10 mg subconjunctival	Yeast and fungal endophthalmitis
	10-mcg intravitreal injection	Yeast and fungal endophthalmitis

[a]Off-label use. Only natamycin (natacyn) is commercially available and labeled for ophthalmic use. All other antifungal drugs are not labeled for ophthalmic use and must be formulated for the given method of administration. For further dosing information, refer to the *Physicians' Desk Reference for Ophthalmic Medicines*.

Reproduced with permission from Brunton LL, Chabner BA, Knollmann BC: *Goodman & Gilman's The Pharmacological Basis of Therapeutics,* 12th ed. New York, NY: McGraw-Hill; 2011.

to herpes simplex infection. When treating viral keratitis topically, there is a very narrow margin between the therapeutic topical antiviral activity and the toxic effect on the cornea; hence, patients must be followed very closely.

Viral retinitis may be caused by herpes simplex virus, CMV, adenovirus, and varicella zoster virus. Treatment usually involves long-term parenteral administration of antiviral drugs. Intravitreal administration of ganciclovir is an effective alternative to the systemic route. Acute retinal necrosis and progressive outer retinal necrosis, most often caused by varicella zoster virus, can be treated by various combinations of oral, intravenous, intravitreal injection of, and intravitreal implantation of antiviral medications.

Antifungal Agents

The only currently available topical ophthalmic antifungal preparation is natamycin. Other antifungal agents may be compounded for topical, subconjunctival, or intravitreal routes of administration (Table 68-4). Ophthalmic indications for antifungal medications include fungal keratitis, scleritis, endophthalmitis, mucormycosis, and canaliculitis. Risk factors for fungal keratitis include trauma, chronic ocular surface disease, contact lens wear, and immunosuppression (including topical steroid use).

AUTONOMIC AGENTS OF THE EYE

Autonomic drugs are used extensively for diagnostic and surgical purposes and for the treatment of glaucoma. Glaucoma is a progressive eye disease classified as primary open angle glaucoma (POAG) and angle closure glaucoma. POAG is the most common type and will be the focus of this chapter. Angle closure glaucoma is a medical emergency as it may result in a sudden loss or blurring of vision, significantly elevated eye pressures, nausea, and vomiting. Both types of glaucoma may result in optic nerve damage and permanent blindness if not treated. Glaucoma asymptomatic in the majority of patients; therefore, it is important to counsel patients about routine eye examinations and glaucoma screenings. Risk factors associated with glaucoma include age more than 40 years, African American or Asian race, diabetes, hypertension, elevated intraocular pressure, myopia, and family history in a first-degree relative. Treatment is aimed at reduction in intraocular pressure via eye drops and surgery. The pharmacist's role in the care of patients with glaucoma includes disease and medication counseling, review of eye drop administration technique, eye drop adherence evaluations and recommendations for routine eye examinations.

Patients with glaucoma are asymptomatic until visual field destruction occurs. Visual field loss occurs in 8% to 20% of patients despite appropriate management. Eighty percent of patients without treatment will develop bilateral blindness. Patients with glaucoma may be involved in a motor vehicle accident because they have blind spots related to peripheral vision field defects. Elderly patients with long standing glaucoma often experience declining vision, headaches and eye pain. Patients may continue to use eye drops even after blindness to decrease the incidence of eye pain. Glaucoma is distinguished from other eye diseases that affect the optic nerve by performing a dilated eye examination. Ophthalmologists may note during examination that the rim of the optic nerve is thinning. This thinning is caused by loss of retinal nerve cells. Optic nerve thinning results in an enlarged cup-to-disc ratio, which is a hallmark visual finding. In glaucoma, increased pressures cause pathological cupping of the optic disc. As glaucoma advances, the cup enlarges to cover most of the disc.

TABLE 68-5 Drug-Induced Glaucoma

Medications Associated with Worsening Glaucoma

Corticosteroids
Anticholinergic medications
Antihistamines
Vasodilators
Cimetidine
Benzodiazepines
Topical sympathomimetics
Heterocyclic antidepressants
Phenothiazines
Theophylline
Selective serotonin reuptake inhibitors
Venlafaxine
Topiramate

The angle formed by the iris and cornea is measured to define the type of glaucoma present. The most common glaucoma type, POAG, is diagnosed when the angle is not obstructed.

Glaucoma can also be caused or worsened by certain classes of medications. Table 68-5 summarizes medications known to worsen glaucoma.

TREATMENT

The goals of glaucoma treatment are to preserve vision and decrease intraocular pressure. Medications are used first-line to decrease the intraocular pressure and administered topically using eye drops. Advantages of eye drops include quick absorption, increased efficacy, and decreased side effects. Oral medications are a second-line and surgery is also an option. Medications with different mechanisms of action are used to accomplish treatment goals (Table 68-6). For example:

- Prostaglandin analogs increase uveoscleral outflow;
- β-Blockers decrease aqueous humor production and improve outflow;
- Carbonic anhydrase inhibitors decrease aqueous humor production by inhibiting the enzyme carbonic anhydrase.

The two most effective classes are the prostaglandin analogs and the β-blockers. Each class has unique side effects and the incidence of side effects can be decreased by eye drop administration techniques. In most instances, minor eye irritations caused by eye drops improve over time.

Patients should be instructed to wash their hands prior to eye drop administration and avoid touching the tip of the medication bottle to the eye or any other surface to avoid contamination and eye infections (Table 68-7). Brinzolamide (Azopt®), betaxolol (Betoptic-S®), timolol and dorzolamide combination product (Cozopt®) and timolol gel forming solution (Timoptic XE®) are suspensions and should be shaken before use.

TABLE 68-6 Medications for Glaucoma

Category Generic and Brand Name	Usual Dose	Decrease IOP for the Class (%)	Mechanism for Category	Side Effects for Category (Local and Systemic)
β-Blockers				
Timolol, Timoptic 0.25%, 0.5%	1 drop twice daily	18%-34%	↓ Aqueous humor production	Burning, dry eyes, systemic β-blockade
Timoptic XE 0.25%, 0.5%	1 drop once daily			
Betaxolol, Betoptic 0.5, Betoptic S 0.25%	1 drop twice daily		Only β-1 agent selective agent	
Carteolol, Cartrol 1%	1 drop twice daily			
Levobunolol, Betagan 0.5%	1 drop twice daily			
Metipranolol, Optipranolol 0.3%	1 drop twice daily			
Prostaglandin Analogs				
Latanoprost, Xalatan 0.005%	1 drop every night	25%-36%	↑ Uveoscleral outflow	Iris pigmented, hyperpigment, hypertrichosis, itching, hyperemia
Travoprost, Travatan Z 0.004%	1 drop every night			
Bimatoprost, Lumigan 0.03%	1 drop every night			
Lantanoprostone Bunod, Vyzulta 0.025%	1 drop every night	14%-23%		
Tafluprost, Zioptan 0.0015%	1 drop every night			
α₂ Agonist				
Brimonidine, Alphagan P 0.15%, 0.1%	1 drop 2-3 times daily	15%-16%	↓ Aqueous humor production	Allergic, lid edema, itching
Apraclonidine, Iopidine 0.5%	1 drop 2-3 times daily			

TABLE 68-6 | **Medications for Glaucoma** *(Continued)*

Category Generic and Brand Name	Usual Dose	Decrease IOP for the Class (%)	Mechanism for Category	Side Effects for Category (Local and Systemic)
Sympathomimetics				
Dipivefrin, Propine 0.1%	1 drop twice daily	Not available	↑ Outflow of aqueous humor	Tearing, burning, brow ache, headache, tachycardia
Parasympathomimetics				
Pilocarpine, Pilocar 1%, 2%, 4%	1 drop 2-4 times a day Pilocar HS gel	20%-30%	↑ Outflow of aqueous humor	Brow ache, headache, myosis, blurred vision, edema
Carbachol, Carboptic 1.5%, 3%	1 drop hs 1 drop 2-4 times a day	Not available		
Carbonic Anhydrase Inhibitor[a]				
Brinzolamide, Azopt 1%	1 drop 2-3 times day	10%-26%	↓ Aqueous humor production	Stinging, bitter taste, acidosis, contains sulfa
Dorzolamide, Trusopt 2%	1 drop 2-3 times day			
Acetazolamide, Diamox 125 mg, 250 mg (sequels), 500 mg	1 tablet 2-4 times day			Systemic acidosis
Methazolamide, Neptazane 25 mg, 50 mg	1 tablet 2-3 times day			Systemic
Combination Agents				
Timolol/dorzolamide, Cosopt 0.5% and 2%	1 drop twice day	29%	See individual agents	See individual agents
Timolol/brimonidine Combigan 0.5% and 0.2%	1 drop twice day		See individual agents	See individual agents
Brinzolamide 1% and brimonidine 0.2%, Simbrinza	1 drop thrice daily		See individual agents	See individual agents

[a]Carbonic anhydrase inhibitors contain a sulfa moiety. Patients allergic to sulfa should not receive a carbonic anhydrase inhibitor.

β-Blockers

β-Blockers are effective options for POAG and considered first line of therapy. However, they are not the most commonly prescribed option because side effects may limit their tolerability. Stinging, dry eyes, blurred vision, and blepharitis are common local side effects. Systemic side effects are also common and include decreased blood pressure, decreased heart rate and bronchospasm. Systemic side effects are problematic for patients with diabetes, congestive heart failure, heart block, or severe chronic obstructive pulmonary disease. Nasolacrimal occlusion (NLO) helps decrease the frequency of side effects.

TABLE 68-7 | **Eye Drop Administration Technique With Nasolacrimal Occlusion**

1. Wash hands thoroughly.
2. Pull down lower eyelid to form a pocket with your forefinger.
3. Hold medicine bottle with forefinger and thumb of opposite hand.
4. Brace fingers against the side of the nose, place bottle close to eye.
5. Tilt the head back and administer the correct number of drops.
6. Immediately press finger gently against the inside corner of the eye (nasolacrimal occlusion).
7. Hold pressure to inside corner of eye for 1 to 3 min.
8. May also close the eye to increase medication absorption.

Prostaglandin Analogs

Prostaglandin analogs are the most commonly prescribed therapy for POAG. They are effective in lowering IOP and have a favorable side effect profile. Prostaglandin analogs have a diurnal IOP-lowering effect (effective at lowering IOP at night during sleep when IOP readings are the highest). Common side effects include hyperpigmentation of the iris and hypertrichosis of the eyelashes.

α₂ Agonist

α₂ Agonists decrease intraocular pressure by decreasing the production of aqueous humor and lower IOP by 15%. The unique use of α₂ agonists is after cataract or laser surgery. Side effects include lid edema, foreign body sensation, itching, and hyperemia. Systemic side effects include dizziness, fatigue, and dry mouth. NLO helps decrease the incidence of systemic side effects.

Sympathomimetics and Parasympathomimetics

Sympathomimetics and parasympathomimetics are used last line due to local and systemic side effects. Side effects include tearing, blurred vision, brow-ache, and hyperemia. Systemic side effects include headache, increased blood pressure, tachycardia, tremor, and anxiety.

Carbonic Anhydrase Inhibitors

Carbonic anhydrase inhibitors inhibit secretion of sodium and bicarbonate by enzyme inhibition. Local side effects include stinging, blurred vision, and conjunctivitis. Systemic side effects acidosis, nausea, weight loss, diaphoresis, and myopia. Oral therapy is a last-line option when eye drops are not effective or when eye drop technique is difficult (patients with mental disabilities).

Combination Therapy

Combination therapies such as Cosopt®, Combigan®, and Simbrinza® improve compliance and decrease eye drop burden. The combinations are more effective than the individual agents alone. Side effects are a culmination of the two individual agents.

CASE Application

KM is a 44-year-old African American female with decreased peripheral vision and a blind spot on the left side. She was in a motor vehicle accident because she did not see the car in the left lane. She complains of brow ache and headaches that have become worse over the past 2 weeks. Intraocular pressure measures 28 in the right eye and 26 in the left eye. She is on a fixed income and buying medications is often difficult. She works odd jobs with varying shifts. Blood pressure was 140/95.

Diagnosis: POAG, Hypertension, and Insomnia

Medications: Amlodipine 5 mg daily, Pilocarpine 2% both eyes four times daily, Tylenol PM® 2 at bedtime.

Allergies: Sulfa. Blue eyes turned brown on Xalatan® and she refused treatment.

1. Which of the following are true about KM? Select all that apply.

    a. She has at least three risk factors for glaucoma
    b. Pilocar® is first-line therapy for POAG
    c. She could have drug-induced glaucoma
    d. Diphenhydramine may worsen glaucoma
    e. Amlodipine may worsen glaucoma

2. Which of the following could affect KM's glaucoma therapy? Select all that apply.

    a. Titration of the blood pressure medication can affect intraocular pressures
    b. Adherence may be an issue
    c. Pilocarpine causes systemic side effects and NLO education could help
    d. Acetaminophen may increase intraocular pressure

3. Which glaucoma medication is contraindicated for KM?

    a. Timolol
    b. Iopidine
    c. Brimonidine

    d. Dorzolamide
    e. Tafluprost

4. Which medication may be causing KM to have brow aches?

    a. Amlodipine
    b. Acetaminophen
    c. Diphenhydramine
    d. Pilocarpine
    e. Latanoprost

5. Rank the following pharmacist recommendations by order of importance for KM's glaucoma therapy? Start with the most important. All options must be used.

Unordered Response	Ordered Response
Assess Refill histories every 3-6 months and provide adherence education as needed	
Discontinue Pilocarpine and start timolol XE if intraocular pressures remain high	
Review eye drop technique and educate about nasolacrimal occlusion	
Discontinue Tylenol PM	

6. Which class of medications is associated with darker, thicker, and longer eye lashes? Select all that apply.

    a. Prostaglandin analogs
    b. Carbonic anhydrase inhibitors
    c. α-Blockers
    d. Sympathomimetics
    e. β-Blockers

7. Which of the following medications can cause drug-induced glaucoma? Select all that apply.

    a. Corticosteroids
    b. Antihistamines
    c. Cimetidine
    d. Benazepril
    e. Aspirin

8. Which of the following are true regarding counseling about Nasolacrimal Occlusion? Select all that apply.

    a. Medication effectiveness
    b. Decrease side effects
    c. Increase systemic absorption of eye drops
    d. Increase the need for multiple eye drops
    e. Increase the cost of therapy

9. Rank the medication categories from highest to lowest ability to lower intraocular pressure (potency). All options must be used.

Unordered Response	Ordered Response
Brinzolamide	
Timolol	
Latanoprost	
Brimonidine	

10. Select the brand name for Latanoprost.

    a. Lumigan
    b. Xalatan
    c. Zioptan
    d. Alphagan

11. Rank the following β-adrenergic blocking agents in order of percent strength. Start with the lowest percent strength.

Unordered Response	Ordered Response
Metipranolol	
Carteolol	
Betaxolol	

12. Which of the following topical β-blockers utilized for the treatment of glaucoma are nonselective β-blockers? Select all that apply.

    a. Timolol
    b. Metipranolol
    c. Carbachol
    d. Levobunolol

13. Which of the following products contains timolol? Select all that apply.

    a. Combigan
    b. Timoptic
    c. Azopt
    d. Xalatan

14. Place the following topical antibiotics in order based upon formulation strength. Start with the lowest percent strength.

Unordered Response	Ordered Response
Azithromycin	
Moxifloxacin	
Ofloxacin	

15. Which of the following are topical fluoroquinolones used for the treatment of conjunctivitis? Select all that apply.

    a. Quixin
    b. Vigamox
    c. Ocuflox
    d. Ciloxan

16. Which of the following aminoglycoside antibiotics are formulated in a solution and ointment for ophthalmic use? Select all that apply.

    a. Tobramycin
    b. Azithromycin
    c. Gentamicin
    d. Erythromycin

17. Which of the following antiviral agents is commercially available as a topical solution for ophthalmic use?

    a. Trifluridine
    b. Valacyclovir
    c. Famciclovir
    d. Foscarnet

18. Rank the following antiviral medications based upon their lowest commercially available mg tablet dose. Start with the lowest mg.

Unordered Response	Ordered Response
Acyclovir	
Famciclovir	
Valacyclovir	

19. Which of the following antiviral agents is available in parenteral and oral formulations?

    a. Valganciclovir
    b. Ganciclovir
    c. Valacyclovir
    d. Acyclovir

20. Which of the following antifungals agents is commercially available as a 5% topical suspension? Select all that apply.

    a. Amphotericin b
    b. Natamycin
    c. Fluconazole
    d. Itraconazole

TAKEAWAY POINTS »

- A number of delivery systems have been developed for treating ocular diseases. Most ophthalmic drugs are delivered in solutions, but for compounds with limited solubility, a suspension form facilitates delivery.
- Indications for the use of topical antibiotics in ophthalmology are hordeolum, blepharitis, conjunctivitis, and keratitis.
- The primary indications for the use of antiviral drugs in ophthalmology are viral keratitis and retinitis.

- The only currently available topical ophthalmic antifungal preparation is natamycin. Other antifungal agents may be compounded for topical, subconjunctival, or intravitreal routes of administration.
- Autonomic drugs are used extensively for diagnostic and surgical purposes and for the treatment of glaucoma.
- Glaucoma is a progressive eye disease and early detection and treatment of glaucoma are important for preservation of vision.

- The two major types of glaucoma are POAG and angle closure glaucoma. POAG is the most common type.
- Topical medications are the first choice for treatment of POAG.
- Prostaglandin analogs and β-blockers are first-line medication choices.
- Drug of choice is based on concomitant disease states and medication side effects.
- Carbonic anhydrase inhibitors contain a sulfa moiety. Patients allergic to sulfa should not receive a carbonic anhydrase inhibitor.

- $α_2$ agonist, sympathomimetics and parasympathomimetics cause significant side effects and are last line in the treatment of glaucoma.
- Teaching eye drop administration technique and utilizing nasolacrimal occlusion improves medication efficacy and decreases the risk of systemic absorption and side effects.

BIBLIOGRAPHY

Fiscella RG, Lesar TS, Edward DP. Glaucoma. In: DiPiro JT, Talbert RL, Yee GC, Matzke GR, Wells BG, Posey L, eds. *Pharmacotherapy: A Pathophysiologic Approach.* 10th ed. New York, NY: McGraw-Hill; 2017:chap 94.

Henderer JD, Rapuano CJ. Ocular pharmacology. In: Brunton LL, Chabner BA, Knollmann BC, eds. *Goodman & Gilman's The Pharmacological Basis of Therapeutics.* 12th ed. New York, NY: McGraw-Hill; 2011:chap 64.

Horton JC. Disorders of the eye. In: Longo DL, Fauci AS, Kasper DL, Hauser SL, Jameson J, Loscalzo J, eds. *Harrison's Principles of Internal Medicine.* 18th ed. New York, NY: McGraw-Hill; 2012:chap 28.

Katzung BG. Special aspects of geriatric pharmacology. In: Katzung BG, Masters SB, Trevor AJ, eds. *Basic & Clinical Pharmacology.* 12th ed. New York, NY: McGraw-Hill; 2012:chap 60.

Robertson D, Biaggioni I. Adrenoceptor antagonist drugs. In: Katzung BG, Masters SB, Trevor AJ, eds. *Basic & Clinical Pharmacology.* 12th ed. New York, NY: McGraw-Hill; 2012:chap 10.

KEY ABBREVIATIONS

CMV = cytomegalovirus
NLO = Nasolacrimal occlusion

POAG = primary open angle glaucoma

69

Pregnancy and Lactation: Therapeutic Considerations

Renee Rose and Karen Whalen

FOUNDATION OVERVIEW

Drug use in pregnancy requires special considerations since medications have the potential to affect the developing fetus. In addition, pregnancy alters pharmacokinetic parameters of some medications, resulting in a need for dosage adjustment. Drug regimens for management of acute and chronic disorders in pregnancy should be tailored to optimize the health of the mother while minimizing risk to the fetus. After delivery, measures should be taken to minimize drug exposure to the breastfeeding infant. Pharmacists can play a key role in maximizing the safe and effective use of medications during pregnancy and lactation.

PRECONCEPTION CARE

Preconception care should be discussed with all women of childbearing age. The goal of preconception care is to minimize poor pregnancy, fetal/infant and maternal outcomes. Elements of preconception care include supplementation, dietary considerations, immunizations, and optimization of control of chronic diseases.

Vitamin and Mineral Supplementation

Folic acid deficiency is a major cause of neural tubal defects (NTDs), and adequate intake of folic acid can reduce the incidence of NTDs by 50% to 70%. Women of childbearing age should be advised to take a multivitamin (MVI) with 400 mcg of folic acid daily. During pregnancy, the recommended intake increases to 600 mcg. Higher doses (4-5 mg daily) are required for women with an increased risk of delivering a child with NTDs (eg, women taking antiepileptic medications). Initiation of supplementation should be at least 1 month before conception and continue throughout the first trimester.

Multivitamins offer additional benefit in meeting calcium (1000-1300 mg) and iron requirements. Calcium is important for bone health for the mother and fetus, and may reduce the risk of pre-eclampsia. Additional calcium supplementation with calcium carbonate or citrate may be needed if MVI and dietary intake is insufficient. The Center for Disease Control (CDC) recommends supplementation with 27 mg/d of elemental iron to support the increased demands of pregnancy.

Dietary Considerations

Caffeine consumption may increase risk of miscarriage and low birth weight. Low to moderate amounts of caffeine (<200 mg/d) appear to be safe. Seafood contains long-chain omega-3 polyunsaturated fatty acids and mercury. Fatty acids are beneficial to the central nervous system, but mercury can lead to birth defects. It is recommended to limit intake to 12 ounces of seafood per week with lower mercury content. Alcohol consumption may adversely affect fertility, contribute to complications during pregnancy, and cause fetal alcohol syndrome (physical, behavioral, and cognitive abnormalities) in infants. No level of alcohol consumption is considered safe during pregnancy.

Immunizations

Ideally, immunizations should be up-to-date before conception. Inactivated vaccines are safe during pregnancy and live vaccines (eg, varicella, measles, mumps, rubella [MMR]) should be avoided due to a theoretical risk of transmission to the fetus. Influenza is associated with high morbidity and mortality, and all pregnant women or women likely to become pregnant should receive the inactivated influenza vaccine. The CDC also recommends Tdap (tetanus, diphtheria, acellular pertussis vaccine) with each pregnancy, ideally given at 27 to 36-weeks gestation. The CDC does not recommend human papillomavirus (HPV) vaccine during pregnancy. If a woman becomes pregnant during the HPV vaccine series, the series should be delayed until after delivery. Please refer to the CDC recommendations (https://www.cdc.gov/vaccines/pregnancy/hcp/guidelines.html) for further information on immunizations during pregnancy.

TERATOGENIC EFFECTS OF DRUGS

Developmental toxicity may occur when an exposure coincides with a critical period of fetal development. The most critical time of fetal development is in the first 8 weeks of pregnancy. The goal of drug use during pregnancy is to treat conditions as necessary, while minimizing the risk to the fetus and maximizing medication safety.

Historically, risk of drug therapy to the fetus was denoted with the Food and Drug Administration (FDA) pregnancy risk

TABLE 69-1	**Previously Used FDA Pregnancy Categories**	
	Pregnancy Category	**Example Drugs**
A	Adequate and well-controlled studies have failed to demonstrate a risk to the fetus in the first trimester of pregnancy (and there is no evidence of risk in later trimesters).	Folic acid Levothyroxine Iron salts (eg, ferrous sulfate) Pyridoxine (vitamin B6)
B	Animal reproduction studies have failed to demonstrate a risk to the fetus and there are no adequate and well-controlled studies in pregnant women OR animal reproduction studies have shown an adverse effect, but adequate and well-controlled studies in pregnant women have failed to demonstrate a risk to the fetus.	Budesonide Enoxaparin H$_2$-receptor antagonists PPIs (except omeprazole)
C	Animal reproduction studies have shown an adverse effect on the fetus and there are no adequate and well-controlled studies in humans OR there are no animal reproduction studies and no adequate and well-controlled studies in humans. However, potential benefits may warrant use of the drug in pregnant women despite potential risks.	Albuterol Heparin Omeprazole Sertraline
D	There is positive evidence of human fetal risk based on adverse reaction data from investigational or marketing experience or studies in humans. However, potential benefits may warrant use of the drug in pregnant women despite potential risks.	ACE inhibitors Angiotensin receptor blockers Paroxetine Valproic acid
X	Studies in animals or humans have demonstrated fetal abnormalities and/or there is positive evidence of human fetal risk based on adverse reaction data from investigational or marketing experience. The risks involved in use of the drug in pregnant women clearly outweigh potential benefits.	Isotretinoin Misoprostol Statins Warfarin

Abbreviations: ACE, angiotensin-converting enzyme; PPI, proton pump inhibitor.

category using a letter rating of A, B, C, D, or X (Table 69-1). The letter categories had several limitations, did not provide detailed information, and sometimes created confusion about the relative risk of drugs. As such, the FDA implemented the Pregnancy and Lactation Labeling Rule (PLLR), which phases out pregnancy risk categories in favor of more comprehensive information. The PLLR requires removal of the letter risk categories from all prescription drug and biological product labeling. For prescription drugs approved on or after June 30, 2001, the pregnancy subsection of the label must include a risk summary (probability of adverse outcomes), clinical considerations (information to help with prescribing decisions), and data (summary of human and animal data). Over-the-counter products are not affected by the PLLR.

Drug exposures can be minimized by avoidance of drugs with known teratogenicity (Table 69-2), use of monotherapy for the shortest duration, and selection of drugs with a long history of safety. In addition, use of drugs with high molecular weight, strong ionization, high protein binding, and high water solubility limits entry to the placenta through passive diffusion. Several resources are available to access information pertaining to drug use during pregnancy. An example of a comprehensive resource is *Drugs in Pregnancy and Lactation: A Reference Guide to Fetal and Neonatal Risk* (also known as Briggs).

PHARMACOKINETIC CHANGES IN PREGNANCY

Pregnancy-induced physiological changes can influence pharmacokinetic parameters of drugs. Although gastric motility and gastric acid secretion are reduced in pregnancy, absorption of most medications does not appear to be significantly altered. Plasma volume is increased by about 50% during pregnancy, and this may result in an increased apparent volume of distribution (V_d) and lower maximum concentration (C_{max}) for some drugs (particularly those agents that are distributed mainly to water compartments).

Albumin concentrations decrease during the second trimester, resulting in decreased protein binding. For most drugs, the concentration of free (unbound) drug remains relatively unchanged, since unbound drug is more readily cleared by the liver and kidney. However, for low extraction drugs that are highly protein-bound and mainly eliminated by the liver (eg, phenytoin), an increase in the free (active) fraction of drug may occur. Therefore, monitoring total plasma concentrations of these drugs can be misleading, as the total concentration reflects both free and bound drug. Free drug levels should be obtained when possible.

Effects on hepatic metabolism are variable in pregnancy. The activity of the cytochrome P450 (CYP) isoenzymes CYP3A4, CYP2C9, and CYP2D6, as well as select uridine diphosphate glucuronosyltransferase (UGT) isoenzymes is increased, whereas the activity of CYP1A2 and CYP2C19 isoenzymes is diminished. Increased dosages may be needed for drugs metabolized via pathways with increased activity. Conversely, dosage reductions of drugs metabolized via pathways with reduced activity may be warranted to prevent adverse effects.

Renal blood flow and glomerular filtration are increased during pregnancy, potentially leading to lower plasma concentrations of drugs that are mainly excreted unchanged in the urine (eg, certain β-lactam antibiotics, digoxin). Therefore, medications that are predominantly renally excreted as unchanged drug may require an increase in dosage to maintain therapeutic concentrations.

TABLE 69-2 Medications With Proven Teratogenic Effects in Humans

Drug or Drug Class	Teratogenic Effects	Critical Period[a]
Alkylating agents	Malformations of many different organs	Organogenesis
Amiodarone	Transitory hypothyroidism (17%, goiter in some cases) or transitory hyperthyroidism	From 12th wk after LMP
Androgens (danazol, testosterone)	Masculinization of genital organs in female fetus	From 9th wk after LMP
Angiotensin-converting enzyme inhibitors Angiotensin II receptor antagonists	Renal failure, anuria, **oligohydramnios**, pulmonary hypoplasia, intrauterine growth restriction, limbs contracture, skull hypoplasia Contraindicated after first trimester	After the first trimester
Anticonvulsants (first generation) ■ Carbamazepine ■ Phenytoin ■ Phenobarbital ■ Valproic acid, divalproex	NTDs (carbamazepine and valproic acid); oral cleft, skeletal, urogenital, craniofacial, digital, and cardiac malformations; microcephalia Major malformations: 5%-10% depending on the agent used (10%-15% for valproic acid). Valproic acid: abnormal neurologic development	Organogenesis for structural anomalies Valproic acid: whole pregnancy for neurologic impairment
Corticosteroids (systemic)	Oral cleft (risk of 3-4/1000 vs 1/1000 in general population)	Organogenesis (most critical period for palate formation between 8 and 11 wk after LMP)
Diethylstilbestrol	Girls: cervical or vaginal adenocarcinoma, incidence about 1/1000 exposures. Structural genital anomalies (eg, of cervix, vagina) Boys: genital anomalies, spermatogenesis anomalies	First and second trimesters
Fluconazole high doses	Skeletal and craniofacial malformations, cleft palate, cardiac anomaly (with chronic dose > 400 mg/d; not reported with 150-mg single dose)	Not defined, but cases are reported where exposure was for most parts of pregnancy
Iodine (supraphysiologic dosage)	Hypothyroidism, goiter	From 12th wk after LMP
Isotretinoin, acitretin, and high dose of vitamin A (>10,000 IU/d)	Spontaneous abortion, CNS, skull, eyes and ears malformations, micrognathia, oral cleft, cardiac malformations, thymus anomalies, mental retardation: estimated at 25%-30% (may be higher for neurologic development impairment) Contraindicated throughout pregnancy Isotretinoin: discontinue 1 mo before pregnancy, prescribed under a special program called iPLEDGE Acitretin: discontinue 3 y before pregnancy	Organogenesis (risk of teratogenic effect after organogenesis not excluded)
Lithium	Cardiac malformations: risk of 0.9%-6.8% (higher risks from small studies) (compare to a baseline risk of ~1%) Includes **Ebstein anomaly**: risk estimated at 0.05%-0.1%	Cardiac organogenesis (5-10 wk after LMP)
Methimazole/ propylthiouracil	Methimazole: aplasia cutis, choanal atresia, esophageal atresia, minor facial anomalies, growth delay; risk probably low Methimazole/propylthiouracil: fetal hypothyroidism in 1%-5% of newborns, goiter	Organogenesis Second and third trimesters
Methotrexate, aminopterine	Spontaneous abortion, CNS and cranial malformations (large fontanelles, hydrocephalia, incomplete cranial ossification, craniosynostosis), oral cleft, ear, skeletal and limb malformations, mental retardation Do not use in pregnancy; stop 1-3 mo before pregnancy	Organogenesis (between 6 and 8 wk after LMP for structural anomalies but some exceptions reported)
Misoprostol	**Moebius syndrome** ± limb anomalies ± CNS anomalies Abortion, preterm birth	Organogenesis Throughout pregnancy for abortion/preterm birth
Mycophenolate mofetil, mycophenolic acid	Anomalies including ear anomalies (with or without ear canal), oral cleft, micrognathia; ophthalmic, cardiac and digital anomalies (risk of structural anomalies estimated from 20%-25%); spontaneous abortion (30%-50%)	Uncertain, probably organogenesis
Nonsteroidal anti-inflammatory drugs	In utero closure of **ductus arteriosus** (constriction is rare before 27 wk, 50%-70% at 32 wk (GA) and neonatal pulmonary hypertension Renal toxicity possible after prolonged use from second half of second trimester	Third trimester
Penicillamine	**Cutis laxa** Joints and CNS anomalies Risk probably low	Not defined

(Continued)

TABLE 69-2	Medications With Proven Teratogenic Effects in Humans *(Continued)*	
Drug or Drug Class	**Teratogenic Effects**	**Critical Period**[a]
Tetracyclines	Teeth discoloration	From 16 wk after LMP
Thalidomide	Limb anomalies (amelia, phocomelia) Cardiac, urogenital, gastrointestinal, and ear malformations Risk of 20%-50% Prescribed under a special program called STEPS (System for Thalidomide Education and Prescribing Safety)	34-50 d after LMP
Trimethoprim	Cardiac and urogenital malformations, neural tube defects, oral cleft; overall risk probably <6%	Organogenesis
Warfarin/acenocoumarol	Before 6 wk: no higher risk of anomaly Taken between 6 and 12 wk: nasal hypoplasia, epiphysis dysplasia, vertebral malformations, rarely ophthalmic anomalies, scoliosis, hearing loss; overall risk estimated between 6% and 10%. After 12 wk after LMP: more rarely, heterogeneous CNS anomalies	Between wk 6 and 12 after LMP

[a] Stages of pregnancy in this table are calculated after last menstrual period (gestational age) and not after conception to be more clinically useful.
Abbreviations: CNS, central nervous system; LMP, last menstrual period; NTD, neural tube defect.
Data from Chisholm-Burns MA, Schwinghammer TL, Barbara G. Wells BG, et al: *Pharmacotherapy Principles & Practice, 4th ed.* New York, NY: McGraw-Hill; 2016.

DRUG THERAPY FOR CONDITIONS IN PREGNANCY

Drug therapy is often required for optimal management of acute and chronic disorders in pregnancy. Gastrointestinal complaints such as heartburn, nausea and vomiting, and constipation are common during pregnancy. In addition, pregnancy may be complicated by the development of disorders, such as gestational diabetes, gestational hypertension, or occasionally, venous thromboembolism. Management of chronic conditions should be optimized prior to pregnancy, and medications switched, if needed, to those that present less risk to the fetus. Table 69-3 summarizes pharmacotherapy for common disorders in pregnancy.

Gestational Diabetes

Gestational diabetes mellitus (GDM) is glucose intolerance first diagnosed in pregnancy. Patients with risk factors for GDM (previous GDM, obesity, known glucose intolerance) should be screened for undiagnosed type 2 diabetes early in pregnancy, and all patients without known diabetes should be screened for GDM at 24 to 28 weeks of gestation. Adequate glucose control is important to prevent complications of GDM such as macrosomia and shoulder dystocia. Thus, glucose goals for GDM are more stringent than for other types of diabetes. Diet is the cornerstone of therapy for GDM, along with frequent self-monitoring of glucose. If drug therapy is needed, insulin is the preferred therapy. Metformin and glyburide are alternatives.

Gestational Hypertension

Gestational hypertension is defined as a blood pressure (BP) of greater than or equal to 140/90 mm Hg observed for the first time after 20 weeks of gestation. Severe gestational hypertension is BP greater than or equal to 160/110 mm Hg. Pregnant women may also develop pre-eclampsia (BP ≥140/90 mm Hg with proteinuria or other signs of end-organ dysfunction) which may progress to eclampsia (pre-eclampsia with seizures), a medical emergency. For women with BP less than 160/110 mm Hg, antihypertensive therapy is not recommended. Hydralazine, labetalol, and long-acting calcium-channel blockers are commonly used in the management of severe gestational hypertension.

Group B *Streptococcus*

Intrapartum transmission of group B *Streptococcus* from the mother to the infant can result in neonatal sepsis or death. Therefore, all pregnant women should have vaginal and rectal swabs to screen for colonization with group B *Streptococcus* between 35 and 37 weeks of gestation. Women with a positive screening test should receive intrapartum treatment with penicillin G (preferred) or ampicillin. Likewise, women with unknown screening results and a temperature of more than 100.4°F, membrane rupture of more than 18 hours, or those who are less than 37-weeks gestation should also receive intrapartum therapy. Cefazolin, clindamycin, and vancomycin are alternatives for penicillin-allergic patients. Vancomycin should be reserved for isolates resistant to other drugs.

Chronic Disorders in Pregnancy

If possible, management of chronic disorders such as asthma, epilepsy, hypothyroidism, diabetes, and hypertension should be optimized prior to conception. Suboptimal management of chronic health disorders may lead to complications of pregnancy, such as preterm labor, pre-eclampsia, intrauterine growth retardation, and miscarriage. For asthma management, albuterol is the preferred short-acting β_2-agonist, and should be recommended for all pregnant patients. For those with persistent asthma, budesonide is the inhaled corticosteroid of choice during pregnancy. Many antiepileptic drugs have been associated with congenital malformations; however, the risk of uncontrolled epilepsy is greater to the fetus than the risk associated with drug use in pregnancy. In general,

TABLE 69-3 Pharmacotherapy for Common Disorders in Pregnancy

Condition	Preferred Treatment	Comments

Asthma	Short-acting inhaled β₂-agonist
	  Albuterol (ProAir HFA, Proventil HFA, Ventolin HFA)
	Inhaled corticosteroid
	  Budesonide (Pulmicort)
		Long-acting β₂-agonists are also safe (similar safety to short-acting)
		Other inhaled corticosteroids may be used if used prior to pregnancy

Constipation	Bulk-forming laxatives
	  Polycarbophil (Fibercon)
	  Psyllium (Metamucil)
	Osmotic laxative
	  Polyethylene glycol (MiraLax)
		Drugs should be used if inadequate response to increased fiber and fluids
		Stool softener (docusate) may be used
		Stimulant laxatives (bisacodyl, senna) may be used short-term
		Avoid mineral oil and castor oil

Diabetes	Insulin therapy	Drug therapy should be used if not controlled with diet Glyburide, metformin are alternatives
Epilepsy	No preferred agent Optimize seizure control prior to pregnancy with monotherapy if possible	If monotherapy is not feasible, use as few drugs as possible Avoid valproic acid and carbamazepine High-dose folic acid (4-5 mg daily) should be used to reduce NTDs

Group B *Streptococcus*	Penicillin G
	Mild penicillin allergy
	  Cefazolin
	Severe penicillin allergy
	  Clindamycin
		Administer therapy IV from time of membrane rupture through delivery
		Ampicillin is an alternative to pen G
		Vancomycin can be used for isolates resistant to clindamycin

Heartburn	Antacids (preferred therapy)
	  Calcium- or magnesium-containing (various)
	H₂-receptor antagonist
	  Ranitidine (Zantac)
	Proton pump inhibitors (various)
		Lifestyle modifications (eg, smaller meals) should be tried before drugs
		Avoid aluminum-containing antacids and sodium bicarbonate
		Ranitidine may be used if no relief with antacids
		Proton pump inhibitors should be reserved for severe symptoms

Hypertension	Calcium-channel blockers Nifedipine extended-release (Adalat CC, Procardia XL) Labetalol (Trandate) Methyldopa	Avoid ACE inhibitors, ARBs, renin inhibitors (aliskiren), and mineralocorticoid receptor antagonists IV labetalol or hydralazine may be used for severe hypertension Patients with preeclampsia should receive IV magnesium sulfate to prevent occurrence of eclampsia
Hyperthyroidism	Methimazole (Tapazole) Propylthiouracil (PTU)	PTU is preferred in the first trimester After the first trimester, patients may be switched to methimazole to avoid risk of hepatotoxicity with PTU Avoid radioactive iodine
Hypothyroidism	Levothyroxine (Synthroid, Levothroid, Levoxyl)	For patients with hypothyroidism prior to pregnancy, dosing requirements may increase during pregnancy
Nausea/vomiting	Doxylamine/pyridoxine (Diclegis [delayed-release], Bonjesta [extended-release]; individual components also available separately)	Diphenhydramine, metoclopramide, phenothiazines, ginger are alternatives Ondansetron may be used for hyperemesis gravidarum
Urinary tract infection	Cephalexin (Keflex) Nitrofurantoin (Macrobid)	Nitrofurantoin should be avoided in late pregnancy (38-42 wk gestation) due to risk of hemolytic anemia in the neonate; do not use in first trimester if alternatives for treatment exist Avoid fluoroquinolones or TMP/SMX

Venous thromboembolism	Low-molecular-weight heparin
	  Dalteparin (Fragmin)
	  Enoxaparin (Lovenox)
		Unfractionated heparin is an alternative
		Avoid warfarin
		Women requiring anticoagulation for prosthetic heart valves may consider use of warfarin after the first trimester
		Avoid apixaban, dabigatran, rivaroxaban

Abbreviations: ACE, angiotensin-converting enzyme; ARB, angiotensin-receptor blocker; IV, intravenous; NTD, neural tube defect; TMP/SMX, trimethoprim/sulfamethoxazole.

monotherapy should be utilized to manage seizures whenever possible. Valproic acid and carbamazepine should be avoided, as they have been associated with a higher incidence of teratogenic effects, as well as developmental disorders in children exposed to the drug in utero. Hypothyroidism is of concern during pregnancy, as undertreatment may result in impaired neurological development in the fetus. Levothyroxine should be instituted to maintain a euthyroid state.

DRUG USE IN LACTATION

Exclusive breastfeeding is recommended whenever possible for the first 6 months of life. Most medications are compatible with breastfeeding and discouraging breastfeeding while taking medications should not be done without careful consideration. Table 69-4 reviews contraindicated drugs or drugs of concern during lactation. Most adverse effects occur in

TABLE 69-4	Drugs of Concern During Breast-Feeding
Drug or Class	**Comments**
Drugs that can decrease the breast milk production	
Clomiphene	Has been used to suppress lactation
Ergot derivatives (bromocriptine, cabergoline, ergotamine)	Have been used to suppress lactation
Estrogens	Hormonal contraceptives with ethinyle stradiol should be delayed for 4-6 wk following delivery
Pseudoephedrine	Do not use in women with low milk production; a few doses will probably not have significant effect
Drugs for which use during breast-feeding may expose the neonate to a significant quantity and may necessitate a strict follow-up	
β-Blocking agents (acebutolol, atenolol, sotalol)	Neonatal β-blockade reported Concern for acebutolol, atenolol, and sotalol, but other β-blocking agents such as metoprolol, propranolol, and labetalol are safe
Amiodarone	May accumulate because of long half-life; possible neonatal thyroid and cardiovascular toxicity
Antineoplastics	Neonatal myelosuppression possible
Chloramphenicol	Severe side effects reported when used to treat babies (blood dyscrasia, grey baby syndrome)
Ergotamine	Symptoms of ergotism (vomiting and diarrhea) reported
Illicit drugs	Unknown contents and effects
Lamotrigine	A breast-fed infant could have blood concentrations between 10% and 50% of maternal blood concentrations (can be in therapeutic range for babies). More than 100 breast-fed babies followed with rare side effects reported including apnea attributed to excessive sedation ($n = 1$), hepatotoxicity ($n = 1$) and a few cases of nonsevere or unrelated rashes. Monitor for CNS side effects (sedation, hypotonia, weight gain, and poor sucking) and rash
Lithium	Up to 50% of maternal serum levels have been measured in infants; cases of infant toxicity (lethargy, cyanosis, electrocardiogram anomalies, hypothyroidism, tremors) have been reported. Monitor infant serum lithium, creatinine, urea, and TSH levels every 4-12 wk and other side effects (jittery, feeding problems, signs of dehydration)
Phenobarbital/primidone	Drowsiness and reduced weight gain reported. Up to 25% of a pediatric dose can be ingested via breast milk. Monitor for CNS side effects (sedation, hypotonia, weight gain, and poor sucking)
Radioactive iodine-131	No breast-feeding for days to weeks to achieve nonsignificant radiation levels (long radioactive half-life). Monitor radioactive levels in milk before allowing breast-feeding
Tetracyclines	Chronic use may lead to dental staining or decreased epiphyseal bone growth

Data from Ferreira E, Martin E, Morin C: *Grossesse et allaitement: guide thérapeutique.* 2nd ed. Montreal: Éditions du CHU Ste-Justine, 2013; Briggs GG, Freeman RK, Yaffe SJ: *Drugs in pregnancy and lactation: a reference guide to fetal and neonatal risk.* 9th ed. Philadelphia, PA: Lippincott Williams & Wilkins, 2011; Hale TW, Rowe HE: *Medications and Mother's Milk,* 16th ed. Amarillo, TX: Hale Publishing, 2014.

breastfeeding infants younger than 2 months old. Drugs with high molecular weight, a pH less than 7.2, high protein binding, and high water solubility are less likely to transfer into breast milk through passive diffusion. Relative infant dose (RID) is a method used to estimate the risk associated with passage of drugs into the breast milk. RID is calculated by comparing the dosage (mg/kg/d) the infant receives through breast milk with the maternal dosage (mg/kg/d). An RID of less than 10% is considered acceptable, while an RID above 25% is considered unacceptable.

Passage of drugs between breast milk and plasma occurs in both directions. This continual movement rarely results in equilibrium and pumping and discarding milk does not speed up the elimination. Strategies to reduce drug exposure to the infant include: withhold the drug (often over-the-counter drugs), delay therapy, choose an alternative drug, use an alternate route of administration, avoid nursing at times of peak drug concentration, take medication before the infant's longest sleep period, use once-daily dosing whenever possible or use an alternate feeding for one to two feedings after the dose. Less desirable alternatives involve temporarily withholding breastfeeding or discontinuation of breastfeeding. An online comprehensive resource for information on drugs in lactation is LactMed.

Drugs may also affect milk by decreasing or increasing supply. Galactagogues are substances that increase milk supply. Metoclopramide is the most common. Galactagogues do not replace good lactation practices. If more frequent nursing fails to improve supply, the patient should be referred for further evaluation. Drugs that decrease milk supply include alcohol, anticholinergics, diuretics, dopaminergic agents, estrogens, and decongestants. If contraception is needed, progestin-only contraception is preferred for mothers who are breastfeeding, since it does not diminish milk production like estrogen-containing products. Pseudoephedrine decreases milk supply, and oral phenylephrine may have a similar effect. Topical nasal decongestants with oxymetazoline are preferred.

CASE Application

The following case pertains to questions 1 through 3.

SB is a 30-year-old woman who wants to start vitamins before she becomes pregnant. She wants to try to become pregnant sometime this year. She takes acetaminophen for headaches, her vaccines are current, and she consumes about 600 mg of caffeine per day.

1. Which component of a multivitamin is most important for SB to decrease the risk of NTDs?

   a. Calcium
   b. Iron
   c. Vitamin D
   d. Folic acid

2. If SB does become pregnant, which vaccines are safe to administer during pregnancy?

   a. Varicella and MMR
   b. Influenza (inactivated) and Tdap
   c. Tdap and HPV
   d. Influenza (inactivated) and MMR

3. Which statement is correct concerning SB's caffeine consumption?

   a. No change is necessary
   b. Caffeine is a known teratogen and she should avoid any consumption
   c. She should limit caffeine consumption to <200 mg daily
   d. She may safely consume caffeine up to 1000 mg daily

4. JW comes to the clinic today for a follow-up on her epilepsy. She would like to become pregnant within the next 12 months. Her current medications include prenatal vitamin, valproic acid, budesonide, albuterol, and acetaminophen. Which of her medications is of most concern in pregnancy?

   a. Valproic acid
   b. Acetaminophen
   c. Budesonide
   d. Prenatal vitamin

5. Which of the following medications may be dispensed to a pregnant patient? Select all that apply.

   a. Cephalexin
   b. Enoxaparin
   c. Isotretinoin
   d. Levothyroxine

6. Which of the following are strategies for minimizing teratogenicity of drug exposure during pregnancy? Select all that apply.

   a. Use monotherapy for the shortest duration
   b. Use a medication with a long history of safety
   c. Choose a drug with a high molecular weight
   d. Choose a drug with weak ionization

7. Which of the following is a pharmacokinetic parameter that should be considered when calculating an appropriate dosing regimen for a pregnant patient?

   a. Decreased renal clearance
   b. Increased absorption
   c. Increased plasma volume
   d. Increased protein binding

8. A patient who is 28-weeks gestation is prescribed cefuroxime for an upper respiratory tract infection. Cefuroxime is largely excreted unchanged in the urine. Which is correct regarding the use of cefuroxime in this patient?

   a. A reduction in dosage may be needed to adequately treat the infection.
   b. Antibiotics such as cefuroxime should be avoided in pregnancy.
   c. The maximum concentration (C_{max}) of cefuroxime may be increased.
   d. The volume of distribution of cefuroxime may be increased.

9. Which best summarizes changes in hepatic metabolism that occur during pregnancy?

   a. Decreased activity of cytochrome P450 isoenzymes
   b. Increased activity of cytochrome P450 isoenzymes
   c. No change in activity of cytochrome P450 isoenzymes
   d. Variable effects on activity of cytochrome P450 isoenzymes

10. A 36-year-old woman has gestational diabetes that is inadequately controlled with diet. Which medication would be best to initiate?

    a. Canagliflozin
    b. Glipizide
    c. Insulin
    d. Pioglitazone

11. Which of the following is appropriate for the management of gestational hypertension? Select all that apply.

    a. Captopril
    b. Labetalol
    c. Losartan
    d. Methyldopa

12. A 27-year-old woman who is 36-weeks gestation has a positive screening test for colonization with Group B *Streptococcus*. She displays no acute symptoms and has no known drug allergies. Which of the following therapies is most appropriate during labor and delivery?

    a. Intravenous cefazolin
    b. Intravenous penicillin G
    c. Oral ampicillin
    d. No therapy is warranted since she is afebrile

13. A patient who is 24-weeks gestation is suffering from occasional mild heartburn. Which of the following is the most appropriate therapy?

    a. Antacid containing calcium carbonate
    b. Famotidine
    c. Omeprazole sodium bicarbonate
    d. Pantoprazole

14. A 32-year-old who is 30-weeks gestation requires treatment for a urinary tract infection. She has no known drug allergies. Assuming that the infecting organism

is sensitive to the following antibiotics, which is an appropriate choice? Select all that apply.

a. Cephalexin
b. Ciprofloxacin
c. Nitrofurantoin
d. Sulfamethoxazole/trimethoprim

15. Which describes appropriate pharmacotherapy of a chronic medical condition in pregnancy?

a. Diabetes—exenatide
b. Dyslipidemia—rosuvastatin
c. Hypothyroidism—levothyroxine
d. Venous thromboembolism—warfarin

16. EH is a 27-year-old woman who is breastfeeding her 6-week-old infant every 4 hours without difficulty. Her current medications include multivitamin. She is suffering from a cold and would like to take a decongestant. Which of the following recommendations is best?

a. Phenylephrine 15 mg po q6h
b. Pseudoephedrine 30 mg po q6h
c. Oxymetazoline 2 sprays each nostril q12h for 3 days
d. No decongestant is safe for use while breastfeeding

17. Which of the following references would be an appropriate comprehensive resource for drug information in a patient that is breastfeeding? Select all that apply.

a. Clinical Pharmacology
b. Drugs in Pregnancy and Lactation: A Reference Guide to Fetal and Neonatal Risk
c. LactMed
d. Up to Date

18. PB is a 32-year-old woman presenting with a decrease in milk production. She has been breastfeeding her daughter for 4 months. Her medications include prenatal vitamin, ibuprofen, and calcium carbonate. She also recently started drospirenone/ethinyl estradiol for contraception. Which of the following medications is likely affecting her milk supply?

a. Calcium carbonate
b. Drospirenone/ethinyl estradiol
c. Ibuprofen
d. Prenatal vitamin

19. Which of the following medications is a galactagogue?

a. Metoprolol
b. Diphenhydramine
c. Metoclopramide
d. Warfarin

20. Which of the following are strategies for minimizing drug exposure to the breastfeeding infant? Select all that apply.

a. Choose an alternate route of administration
b. Choose an alternate drug
c. Take medication before the infant's longest sleep period
d. Prescribe low doses of medication more frequently

21. Which of the following is the brand name for the prescription product extended-release doxylamine/pyridoxine?

a. Bonjesta
b. Diclegis
c. Fragmin
d. Unisom

TAKEAWAY POINTS »

- Most women who are planning to become pregnant should take a daily multivitamin with 400 mcg of folic acid. Folic acid should be started at least 1 month prior to conception.
- All pregnant women should receive the inactivated influenza vaccine.
- Although developmental toxicity may occur at any time during pregnancy, the most critical time of development is in the first 8 weeks of pregnancy.
- Teratogenic effects from drug exposure can be minimized by avoidance of drugs with known teratogenicity, use of monotherapy for the shortest duration, selection of drugs with a long history of safety, and use of drugs less likely to cross the placenta through passive diffusion.
- The Pregnancy and Lactation Labeling Rule requires removal of the FDA pregnancy risk categories and inclusion of more comprehensive labeling information,

such as the fetal risk summary, clinical considerations, and human and animal data in pregnancy.
- Pharmacokinetic changes that may occur during pregnancy include an increased volume of distribution, reduced protein binding, and increased renal clearance. Effects on hepatic metabolism in pregnancy are variable, with some cytochrome P450 isoenzymes showing enhanced activity, and others showing less activity.
- Pregnant women often require drug therapy for gastrointestinal complaints, infections, and disorders of pregnancy such as gestational diabetes and gestational hypertension. Selection of drug therapy should be aimed at successful treatment of the disorder while minimizing risk to the fetus.
- Management of chronic conditions should be optimized prior to conception using medications with the least likelihood of causing harm to the fetus.

- Suboptimal management of chronic health disorders may lead to complications of pregnancy, such as preterm labor, preeclampsia, intrauterine growth retardation, and miscarriage.
- Most adverse effects associated with breastfeeding occur in infants younger than 2 months old.
- Most medications are compatible with breastfeeding. Strategies can be utilized to decrease infant exposure to medications during breastfeeding and to minimize the effect of drug therapy on supply of breast milk.
- Strategies to minimize drug exposure to the infant during breastfeeding include: withhold the drug, delay therapy, choose an alternative drug, use an alternate route of administration, avoid nursing at times of peak drug concentration, take medication before the infant's longest sleep period, use once-daily dosing whenever possible, or use an alternate feeding for one to two feedings after the dose.
- *Drugs in Pregnancy and Lactation: A Reference Guide to Fetal and Neonatal Risk* ("Briggs") is a comprehensive drug information resource for drug use in pregnancy and lactation. LactMed is a comprehensive database for drug use in lactation.

BIBLIOGRAPHY

American College of Obstetricians and Gynecologists, Task Force on Hypertension in Pregnancy. Hypertension in pregnancy. Report of the American College of Obstetricians and Gynecologists' Task Force on Hypertension in Pregnancy. *Obstet Gynecol.* 2013;122:1122.

Anderson GD. Pregnancy-induced changes in pharmacokinetics. *Clin Pharmacokinet.* 2005;44:989-1008.

Briggs GG. Developmental toxicity and drugs. In: Briggs GG, Nageotte M, eds. *Diseases Complications and Drug Therapy in Obstetrics: A Guide for Clinicians.* Maryland: American Society of Health-System Pharmacists, Inc.; 2009:chap 2.

Briggs GG. Drug use and lactation. In: Briggs GG, Nageotte M, eds. *Diseases Complications and Drug Therapy in Obstetrics: A Guide for Clinicians.* Maryland: American Society of Health-System Pharmacists, Inc.; 2009:chap 3.

Centers for Disease Control: Guidelines for Vaccinating Pregnant Women. https://www.cdc.gov/vaccines/pregnancy/hcp/guidelines.html. Accessed February 21, 2017.

Ferreira E, Rey E, Morin C, Theriault K. Pregnancy and lactation: therapeutic considerations. In: Chisholm-Burns MA, Schwinghammer TL, Wells BG, Malone PM, Kolesar JM, DiPiro JT, eds. *Pharmacotherapy Principles and Practice.* 4th ed. New York, NY: McGraw-Hill; 2016:chap 47.

LactMed: Drugs and lactation database. https://toxnet.nlm.nih.gov/newtoxnet/lactmed.htm. Accessed February 21, 2017.

National Institutes of Health. Folate Dietary Supplement Fact Sheet. https://ods.od.nih.gov/factsheets/Folate-HealthProfessional/. Accessed February 26, 2017.

US Food and Drug Administration. Pregnancy and lactation labeling final rule. https://www.fda.gov/BiologicsBloodVaccines/GuidanceComplianceRegulatoryInformation/ActsRulesRegulations/ucm445102.htm. Accessed February 21, 2017.

Ward KE. Pregnancy and lactation: therapeutic considerations. In: DiPiro JT, Talbert RL, Yee GC, Matzke GR, Wells BG, Posey L, eds. *Pharmacotherapy: A Pathophysiologic Approach.* 10th ed. New York, NY: McGraw-Hill; 2017:chap 78.

KEY ABBREVIATIONS

BP = blood pressure
CDC = Center for Disease Control
CYP = cytochrome P450
FDA = Food and Drug Administration
GDM = gestational diabetes mellitus
HPV = Human papillomavirus
MMR = measles, mumps, rubella

NTD = neural tubal defect
PLLR = Pregnancy and Lactation Labeling Rule
PPI = proton pump inhibitor
RID = relative infant dose
Tdap = tetanus, diphtheria, acellular pertussis vaccine
UGT = uridine diphosphate glucuronosyltransferase

70

Pharmacoeconomics

S. Scott Sutton

FOUNDATION OVERVIEW

Pharmacoeconomics is the description and analysis of the costs of drug therapy to health care systems and society. Pharmacoeconomic studies identify, measure, and compare the costs and consequences of pharmaceutical products and services. Decision-makers use these methods to evaluate and compare the total costs of treatment options and the outcomes associated with these options. To show this graphically, think of two sides of an equation: (1) the inputs (costs) used to obtain and use the drug and (2) the health-related outcomes (Figure 70-1). The center of the equation, the drug product, is symbolized by R_x. If only the left-hand side of the equation is measured without regard for outcomes, this is a cost analysis. If only the right-hand side of the equation is measured without regard to costs, this is a clinical or outcome study. A pharmacoeconomic analysis measures both sides of the equation. Outcomes research is defined as an attempt to identify, measure, and evaluate the end results of health care services. It may include not only clinical and economic consequences, but also outcomes, such as patient health status and satisfaction with their health care. Pharmacoeconomics is a type of outcomes research, but not all outcomes research is pharmacoeconomic research.

Models of Pharmacoeconomic Analysis

The four types of pharmacoeconomic analyses measure costs or inputs in dollars and assess the outcomes associated with these costs (Table 70-1). Pharmacoeconomic analyses are categorized by the method used to assess outcomes and include:

1. *Cost-minimization analysis* (CMA): outcomes are assumed to be equivalent;
2. *Cost-benefit analysis* (CBA): outcomes are measured in dollars;
3. *Cost-effectiveness analysis* (CEA): the costs are measured in natural units (eg, cures, years of life, blood pressure); and
4. *Cost-utility analysis* (CUA): outcomes take into account patient preferences (or utilities).

Assessment of Costs

The assessment of costs is the left-hand side of the equation in Figure 70-1. Costs are calculated to estimate the resources that are used in the production of an outcome. Pharmacoeconomic studies categorize costs into four types.

1. Direct medical costs are the medically-related inputs used *directly* in providing the treatment. Examples of direct medical costs include costs associated with pharmaceutical products, physician visits, emergency room visits, and hospitalizations.
2. Direct nonmedical costs are not medical in nature, but are directly associated with treatment. Examples include the cost of traveling to and from the physician's office or hospital, babysitting for the children of a patient, and food and lodging required for patients and their families during out-of-town treatment.
3. Indirect costs result from the loss of productivity due to illness or death. Please note that the **accounting** term *indirect costs*, which is used to assign overhead, is different from the **economic** term, which refers to a loss of productivity of the patient or the patient's family due to illness.
4. Intangible costs include the costs of pain, suffering, anxiety, or fatigue that occur because of an illness or the treatment of an illness. It is difficult to measure or assign values to intangible costs.

Treatment of an illness may include all four types of costs. For example, the cost of surgery would include the direct medical costs of the surgery (medication, room charges, laboratory tests, and physician services), direct nonmedical costs (travel and lodging for the preoperative day), indirect costs (cost due to the patient missing work during the surgery and recuperative period), and intangible costs (due to pain and anxiety). Most studies only report the direct medical costs. This may be appropriate depending on the objective of the study or the perspective of the study. For example, if the objective is to measure the costs to the hospital for two surgical procedures that differ in direct medical costs (eg, using a high-dose versus a low-dose of a new medication in cardiac bypass surgery), but that are expected to have similar nonmedical, indirect, and intangible costs, measuring all four types of costs may not be warranted.

In order to determine what costs are important to measure, the perspective of the study must be determined. Perspective is a pharmacoeconomic term that describes whose costs are relevant based on the purpose of the study. Economic theory suggests that the most appropriate perspective is that of society. Societal costs would include costs to the insurance company,

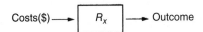

FIGURE 70-1 Pharmacoeconomic studies description. Reproduced with permission from Malone PM, Kier KL, Stanovich JE: *Drug Information: A Guide for Pharmacists*, 4th ed. New York, NY: McGraw-Hill; 2012.

costs to the patient, and indirect costs due to the loss of productivity. Although this may be the most appropriate perspective according to economic theory, it is rarely seen in the pharmacoeconomic literature. The most common perspectives used in pharmacoeconomic studies are the perspective of the institution or the perspective of the payer. The payer perspective may include the costs to the third-party plan, the patient, or a combination of the patient copay and the third-party plan costs.

Timing Adjustments for Costs

When costs are estimated from information collected for more than a year before the study or for more than a year into the future, adjustment of costs is needed. If retrospective data are used to assess resources used over a number of years, these costs should be adjusted to the present year. For example, if the objective of the study is to estimate the difference in the costs of antibiotic A versus B in the treatment of a specific type of infection, information on the past utilization of these two antibiotics might be collected from a review of medical records. If the retrospective review of these medical records dates back for more than a year, it may be necessary to adjust the cost of both medications by calculating the number of units (doses) used per case and multiplying this number by the current unit cost for each medication.

If costs are estimated based on dollars spent or saved in future years, another type of adjustment, called discounting, is needed. There is a time value associated with money. Most people (and businesses) prefer to receive money today, rather than at a later time. Therefore, a dollar received today is worth more than a dollar received next year (the time value of money). Discount rate, a term from finance, approximates the cost of capital by taking into account the projected inflation rate and the interest rates of borrowed money and then estimates the time value of money. From this parameter, the present value (PV) of future expenditures and savings can be calculated. The discount factor is equal to $1/(1 + r)^n$, where r is the discount rate and n is the year in which the cost or savings occur. For example, if the costs of a new pharmaceutical care program are $5000 per year for the next 3 years, and the discount rate is 5%, the PV of these costs is $14,297 ($5000 year one + $5000/1.05 year two + $5000/[1.05] year three) (note that discounting does not start until year two). The most common discount rates currently seen in the literature are 3% to 5%, the approximate cost of borrowing money today.

Assessment of Outcomes

The assessment of outcomes is the right-hand side of the equation in Figure 70-1. There are four ways to measure outcomes (CMA, CBA, CEA, and CUA) and each is associated with a different type of pharmacoeconomic analysis.

Cost-Minimization Analysis

A CMA measures cost in dollars and outcomes are assumed to be equivalent. An example is the measurement and comparison of costs for therapeutically equivalent products (eg, glipizide and glyburide). The outcomes (eg, efficacy, incidence of adverse drug interactions) are expected to be equal, but the costs are not. Some researchers contend that a CMA is not a true pharmacoeconomic study, because costs are measured, but outcomes are not. Others say that the strength of a CMA depends on the evidence that the outcomes are the same. This evidence can be based on previous studies, publications, or expert opinion. The advantage of this type of study is that it is simple compared to the other types of analyses because outcomes need not be measured. The disadvantage of this type of analysis is that it can only be used when outcomes are assumed to be identical.

Examples

A hospital needs to decide if it should add a new intravenous antibiotic to the formulary, which is therapeutically equivalent to the current antibiotic used in the institution and has the same side effect profile. The advantage of the new antibiotic is that it only has to be administered once per day versus three times a day for the comparison antibiotic. Because the outcomes are expected to be nearly identical, and the objective is to assess the costs to the hospital (eg, the hospital perspective), only direct medical costs need to be estimated and compared. The direct medical costs include the daily costs of each medication, the pharmacy personnel time used in the preparation of each dose, and the nursing personnel time used in the administration of each dose. Even if the cost of the new medication is a little higher than the cost of the current antibiotic, the lower cost of preparing and administering the new drug (once a day vs three times per day) may offset this difference. Direct nonmedical, indirect, and intangible costs are

Methodology	Cost Measurement Unit	Outcome Measurement Unit
TABLE 70-1	**Types of Pharmacoeconomic Analysis**	
Cost-minimization analysis (CMA)	Dollars	Assumed to be equivalent in comparable groups analysis
Cost-benefit analysis (CBA)	Dollars	Dollars
Cost-effectiveness analysis (CEA)	Dollars	Natural units (life years gained, mm Hg blood analysis (CEA) pressure, mmol/L blood glucose)
Cost-utility analysis (CUA)	Dollars	Quality-adjusted life year (QALY) or other utilities

Reproduced with permission from Malone PM, Kier KL, Stanovich JE: *Drug Information: A Guide for Pharmacists*, 4th ed. New York, NY: McGraw-Hill; 2012.

not expected to differ between these two alternatives and they need not be included if the perspective is that of the hospital, so these costs are not included in the comparison.

Aminoglycosides may be dosed once daily (consolidated dosing) or via traditional dosing every 8 hours. A CMA was conducted to compare the dosing methods. The drug acquisition cost was $43.70 for every 8 hours dosing and $55.39 for the single dose administration. The costs of Minibags ($29.32), preparation ($13.81), and administration ($67.63) were $110.76 for the three-times daily administration versus $42.23 (Minibags $10.90, preparation $6.20, and administration $25.13) for the single daily dose. With essentially equivalent clinical outcomes, the once-daily administration of the aminoglycoside minimized hospital costs ($97.62 vs $154.46). Note: the analysis did not include laboratory drug level measurements.

Cost-Benefit Analysis

A CBA measures inputs and outcomes in monetary terms. One advantage to using a CBA is that alternatives with different outcomes can be compared, because each outcome is converted to the same unit (dollars). For example, the costs (inputs) of providing a pharmacokinetic service versus a diabetes clinic can be compared with the cost savings (outcomes) associated with each service, even though different types of outcomes are expected for each alternative. CBAs are performed to determine how institutions can best spend their resources to produce monetary benefits. For example, a study conducted at a Medical Center looked at costs and savings associated with the addition of a pharmacist to its medical teams. Discounting of both the costs of the treatment or services and the benefits or cost savings is needed if they extend for more than a year. Comparing costs and benefits (outcomes in monetary terms) is accomplished by either of the two methods. One method divides the estimated benefits by the estimated costs to produce a benefit-to-cost ratio. If this ratio is more than 1.0, the choice is cost beneficial. The other method is to subtract the costs from the benefits to produce a net benefit calculation. If this difference is positive, the choice is cost beneficial.

Another more complex use of CBA consists of measuring clinical outcomes (eg, avoidance of death, reduction of blood pressure, and reduction of pain) and placing a dollar value on these clinical outcomes. This type of CBA is not often seen in the pharmacy literature. This use of the method offers the advantage that alternatives with different types of outcomes can be assessed, but a disadvantage is that it is difficult to put a monetary value on pain, suffering, and human life. There are two common methods that economists use to estimate a value for these types of consequences, the human capital (HC) approach and the willingness-to-pay (WTP) approach. The HC approach assumes that the values of health benefits are equal to the economic productivity that they permit. The cost of disease is the cost of the lost productivity due to the disease. A person's expected income before taxes and/or an inputted value for nonmarket activities (eg, housework and child care) is used as an estimate of the value of any health benefits for that person. The HC approach was used when calculating the costs and benefits of administering a meningococcal vaccine to college students. The value of the future productivity of a college student was estimated at $1 million in this study. There are disadvantages to using this method. People's earnings may not reflect their true value to society, and this method lacks a solid literature of research to back this notion. The WTP method estimates the value of health benefits by estimating how much people would pay to reduce their chance of an adverse health outcome. For example, if a group of people is willing to pay, on average, $100 to reduce their chance of dying from 1:1000 to 1:2000, theoretically a life would be worth $200,000 ($100/[0.001−0.0005]). Problems with this method include the issue that what people say they are willing to pay may not correspond to what they actually would pay, and it is debatable if people can meaningfully answer questions about a 0.0005 reduction in outcomes.

Example

An independent pharmacy owner is considering the provision of a new clinical pharmacy service. The objective of the analysis is to estimate the costs and monetary benefits of two possible services over the next 3 years. Clinical Service A would cost $50,000 in start-up and operating costs during the first year, and $20,000 in years two and three. Clinical Service A would provide an added revenue of $40,000 each of the 3 years. Clinical Service B would cost $40,000 in start-up and operating costs the first year and $30,000 for years two and three. Clinical Service B would provide added revenue of $45,000 for each of the 3 years. Table 70-2 illustrates the comparison of

TABLE 70-2 **CBA Example**

	Year 1 Dollars (No Discounting in Year 1)	Year 2 Dollars (Discounted Dollars)	Year 3 Dollars (Discounted Dollars)	Total Dollars (Discounted Dollars)	Benefit-to-Cost Ratio Dollars (Discounted Dollars)	Net Benefit Dollars (Discounted Dollars)
Costs of A	$50,000 ($50,000)	$20,000 ($19,048)	$20,000 ($18,140)	$90,000 ($87,188)	$120,000/$90,000 = 1.33:1 ($114,376/87,188 = 1.31:1)	$120,000 − $90,000 = $30,000 ($114,376 − 87,188 = 27,188)
Benefits of A	$40,000 ($40,000)	$40,000 ($38,095)	$40,000 ($36,281)	$120,000 ($114,376)		
Costs of B	$40,000 ($40,000)	$30,000 ($28,571)	$30,000 ($27,211)	$100,000 ($95,782)	$135,000/100,000 = 1.35:1 ($128,673/95,782 = 1.34:1)	$135,000 − 100,000 = 35,000 ($128,673 − 95,782 = 32,891)
Benefits of B	$45,000 ($45,000)	$45,000 ($42,857)	$45,000 ($40,816)	$135,000 ($128,673)		

both options using the perspective of the independent pharmacy with no discounting and when a discount rate of 5% is used. Although both services are estimated to be cost beneficial, Clinical Service B has both a higher benefit-to-cost ratio and a higher net benefit when compared to Clinical Service A.

Cost-Effectiveness Analysis

This is the most common type of pharmacoeconomic analysis and it measures costs in dollars and outcomes in natural health units (eg, cures, lives saved, or blood pressure). An advantage of using a CEA is that health units are common outcomes practitioners can readily understand and these outcomes do not need to be converted to monetary values. On the other hand, the alternatives used in the comparison must have outcomes that are measured in the same units, such as lives saved with each of two treatments. If more than one natural unit outcome is important when conducting the comparison, a cost-effectiveness ratio (CER) should be calculated for each type of outcome. Outcomes cannot be collapsed into one unit measure in CEAs as they can with CBAs (outcome = dollars) or CUAs (outcome = quality-adjusted life years [QALYs]). Because CEA is the most common type of pharmacoeconomic study in the pharmacy literature, many examples are available.

- An analysis of two medical treatments for gastroesophageal reflux disease (GERD) was conducted using both healed ulcers confirmed by endoscopy and symptom-free days as the outcomes measured.

- An analysis of two antidiabetic medications was conducted by comparing the percentage of patients achieving glycemic control as the outcome measure.

A cost-effectiveness grid (Table 70-3) can be used to illustrate the definition of cost-effectiveness. In order to determine if a therapy or service is cost-effective, both the costs and effectiveness must be considered. Think of comparing a new drug with the current standard treatment. If the new treatment is (1) both more effective and less costly (cell G), (2) more effective at the same price (cell H), or (3) has the same effectiveness at a lower price (cell D), the new therapy is considered cost-effective. On the other hand, if the new drug is (1) less effective and more costly (cell C), (2) has the same effectiveness but costs more (cell F), or (3) has lower effectiveness for the same costs (cell B), then the new product is *not* cost-effective. There are three other possibilities: (1) that the new drug is more expensive and more effective (cell I) - a very common finding, (2) less expensive but less effective (cell A), or (3) has the

TABLE 70-4 | Listing of Costs and Outcomes

Alternative	Costs for 12 Months of Medication	Lowering of LDL in 12 Months (mg/dL)
Current preferred medication	$1000	25
New medication	$1500	30

Abbreviations: LDL, low-density lipoprotein.
Reproduced with permission from Malone PM, Kier KL, Stanovich JE: *Drug Information: A Guide for Pharmacists*, 4th ed. New York, NY: McGraw-Hill; 2012.

same price and the same effectiveness as the standard product (cell E). For the middle cell E, other factors may be considered to determine which medication might be best. For the other two cells, an incremental cost-effectiveness ratio (ICER) is calculated to determine the extra cost for each extra unit of outcome. It is left up to the readers to determine if they think the new product is cost-effective, based on a value judgment. The underlying subjectivity as to whether the added benefit is worth the added cost is a disadvantage of CEA.

Example

A Medical Center is reviewing a new cholesterol-lowering medication and voting to decide if they should add it to the preferred formulary. The new product has a greater effect on lowering cholesterol than the current preferred formulary agent; however, the new medication is also more expensive. Using the perspective of the Medical Center (eg, direct medical costs of the product to the Medical Center), the results will be presented in three ways in Tables 70-4 to 70-6 to illustrate the various ways that costs and effectiveness are presented in the literature. Table 70-4 presents the simple listing of the costs and benefits of the two alternatives. Sometimes for each alternative, the costs and various outcomes are listed but no ratios are conducted, this is termed a cost-consequence analysis (CCA).

The second method of presenting results includes calculating the average CER for each alternative. Table 70-5 shows the CER for the two alternatives. The CER is the ratio of resources used per unit of clinical benefit, and implies that this calculation has been made in relation to doing nothing or no treatment. In this case, the current medication costs $40 for every 1 mg/dL decrease in LDL while the new medication under consideration costs $50 for the same decrease. In clinical practice, the question is *infrequently* "Should we treat the patient or not?" or "What are the costs and outcomes of this intervention versus no intervention?" More often the question

TABLE 70-3 | Cost-Effectiveness Grid

Cost-Effectiveness	Lower Cost	Same Cost	Higher Cost
Lower effectiveness	A	B	C
Same effectiveness	D	E	F
Higher effectiveness	G	H	I

Reproduced with permission from Malone PM, Kier KL, Stanovich JE: *Drug Information: A Guide for Pharmacists*, 4th ed. New York, NY: McGraw-Hill; 2012.

TABLE 70-5 | Cost-Effectiveness Ratios

Alternative	Costs for 12 Months of Medication	Lowering of LDL in 12 Months	Average Cost per Reduction in LDL
Current preferred medication	$1000	25 mg/dL	$40 per mg/dL
New medication	$1500	30 mg/dL	$50 per mg/dL

Abbreviation: LDL, low-density lipoprotein.
Reproduced with permission from Malone PM, Kier KL, Stanovich JE: *Drug Information: A Guide for Pharmacists*, 4th ed. New York, NY: McGraw-Hill; 2012.

TABLE 70-6	Incremental Cost-Effectiveness Ratio		
Alternative	Costs for 12 Months of Medication	Lowering of LDL in 12 Months	Incremental Cost per Marginal Reduction in LDL
Current preferred medication	$1000	25 mg/dL	($1,500 − $1,000)/ (30 mg/dL − 25 mg/dL) = $100 per mg/dL
New medication	$1500	30 mg/dL	

Reproduced with permission from Malone PM, Kier KL, Stanovich JE: *Drug Information: A Guide for Pharmacists*, 4th ed. New York, NY: McGraw-Hill; 2012.

is "How does one treatment compare with another treatment in costs and outcomes?" To answer this more common question, an ICER is calculated. The ICER is the ratio of the *difference* in costs divided by the *difference* in outcomes. Most economists agree that an ICER (the extra cost for each added unit of benefit) is the more appropriate way to present CEA results. Table 70-5 shows the incremental cost-effectiveness (the extra cost of producing one extra unit) of the new medication compared to the current medication. For the new medication, it costs an *additional* $100 for every *additional* decrease in LDL of 1 mg/dL. The formulary committee would need to decide if this increase in cost is worth the increase in benefit (improved clinical outcome). In this example, the costs and benefits of the medications are estimated for only 1 year; discounting is not needed. If incremental calculations produce negative numbers, this indicates that one treatment is both more effective and less expensive, or dominant, compared to the other option. The magnitude of the negative ratio is difficult to interpret, so it is suggested that authors instead indicate which treatment is the dominant one. As mentioned before, when one of the alternatives is both more expensive and more effective than another, the ICER is used to determine the magnitude of added cost for each unit in health improvement. Clinicians must then wrestle with this type of information and it becomes a clinical call. Many economists argue that this uncertainty is why cost-effectiveness may not be the preferred method of pharmacoeconomic analysis.

Cost-Utility Analysis

A CUA takes patient preferences, also referred to as utilities, into account when measuring health consequences. The most common unit used in conducting CUAs is QALYs. A QALY is a health-utility measure combining quality and quantity of life, as determined by some valuations process. The advantage of using this method is that different types of health outcomes can be compared using one common unit (QALYs) without placing a monetary value on these health outcomes (like CBA). The disadvantage of this method is that it is difficult to determine an accurate QALY value. This is a relatively new type of outcome measure and is not understood or embraced by all providers and decision-makers. Therefore, this method is not commonly seen in the pharmacy literature. One reason researchers are working to establish methods for measuring QALYs is the belief that 1 year of life (a natural unit outcome that can be used in CEAs) in one health state should not be given the same weight as 1 year of life in another health state. For example, if two treatments both add 10 years of life, but one provides an added 10 years of being in a healthy state and

the other adds 10 years of being in a disabled health state, the outcomes of the two treatments should not be considered equal. Adjusting for the quality of those extra years is warranted. When calculating QALYs, 1 year of life in perfect health has a score of 1.0 QALY. If health-related quality of life (HR-QOL) is diminished by disease or treatment, 1 year of life in this state is less than 1.0 QALY. This unit allows comparisons of morbidity and mortality. By convention, perfect health is assigned 1.0 per year and death is assigned 0.0 per year, but how are scores between these two determined? Different techniques for determining scales of measurement for QALY are discussed below.

There are three common methods for determining QALY scores: rating scales (RS), standard gamble (SG), and time trade-off (TTO). A RS consists of a line on a page, somewhat like a thermometer, with perfect health at the top (100) and death at bottom (0). Different disease states are described to subjects, and they are asked to place the different disease states somewhere on the scale indicating preferences relative to all diseases described. As an example, if they place a disease state at 70 on the scale, the disease state is given a score of 0.7 QALYs.

The second method for determining patient preference (or utility) scores is the SG method. For this method, each subject is offered two alternatives. Alternative one is treatment with two possible outcomes: either the return to normal health or immediate death. Alternative two is the certain outcome of a chronic disease state for life. The probability (p) of dying is varied until the subject is indifferent between alternative one and alternative two. As an example, a person considers two options: a kidney transplant with a 20% probability of dying during the operation (alternative one) or dialysis for the rest of his life (alternative two). If this percent is his point of indifference (he would not have the operation if the chances of dying during the operation were any higher than 20%), the QALY is calculated as 1−p or 0.8 QALY.

The third technique for measuring health preferences is the TTO method. Again, the subject is offered two alternatives. Alternative one is a certain disease state for a specific length of time *t*, the life expectancy for a person with the disease, then death. Alternative two is being healthy for time *x*, which is less than *t*. Time *x* is varied until the respondent is indifferent between the two alternatives. The proportion of the number of years of life a person is willing to give up (*t* − *x*) to have her remaining years (*x*) of life in a healthy state is used to assess her QALY estimate. For example, a person with a life expectancy of 50 years is given two options: being blind for 50 years or being completely healthy (including being able to see) for 25 years. If the person is indifferent between these two options (she would rather be blind than give up any more years of life), the QALY for this disease state (blindness) would be 0.5.

As one might surmise, QALY measurement is not regarded as being as precise or scientific as natural health unit measurements (like blood pressure and cholesterol levels) used in CEAs. Some issues in the measurement of QALYs are debated in the literature. One issue concerns whose viewpoint is the most valid. An advantage of having patients with the disease of interest determine health state scores is that these patients may understand the effects of the disease better than the general population; whereas, some believe these patients would provide a biased view of their disease compared with other diseases they have not experienced. Some contend that health care professionals could provide good estimates because they understand various diseases and others argue that these professionals may not rate discomfort and disability as seriously as patients or the general population.

Another issue that has been addressed regarding patient preference or utility-score measures is the debate over which is the best measure. Utility scores calculated using one method may differ from those using another. Finally, utility measures have been criticized for not being sensitive to small, but clinically meaningful, changes in health status.

Example

An analysis assessed the costs and utilities associated with two chemotherapy regimens (vindesine and cisplatin [VP], and cyclophosphamide, doxorubicin, and cisplatin [CAP]) and compared the results with the costs and utilities of using best supportive care (BSC) in patients with non–small cell lung cancer. The perspective was that of the health care system or the payer. Using the TTO method, treatment utility scores were estimated by personnel of the oncology ward. Although the chemotherapy regimens provide a longer survival (VP = 214 days, CAP = 165 days) than BSC (112 days), the quality of life TTO score was higher for BSC (0.61) compared with the chemotherapy regimens (0.34). When survival time is multiplied by the TTO scores, the use of BSC results in an estimated 0.19 QALYs, which is similar to VP (0.19 QALYs), but higher than CAP (0.15 QALY). The costs to the health care system for the three options are about $5000 for BSC, $10,000 for VP, and $7000 for CAP (the authors reported median costs instead of average costs due to the abnormality of the cost data). Cost-utility ratios are calculated similarly to CERs, except that the outcome unit is QALYs. Therefore, the cost-utility ratio is about $26,000/QALY for BSC and about $44,000 to $52,000/QALY for the chemotherapy regimens. Because BSC is at least as effective, as measured by QALYs, and is less expensive than the other two options, a marginal (or incremental) cost-utility ratio does not need to be calculated. Marginal cost-utility ratios only need to be calculated to estimate the added cost for an added benefit, not when the added benefit comes at a lower cost.

Conducting a Pharmacoeconomic Analysis

Conducting a pharmacoeconomic analysis can be challenging. Resources (time, expertise, data, and money) are limited. Data used to construct a model may be impossible to obtain due to lack of computer automation. Comparative studies of drug treatments may not be available or poorly designed. Results of clinical trials may not apply at the institution performing the analysis due to lack of resources. Methods for conducting a pharmacoeconomic analysis have been described. All four types of analyses described (CMA, CBA, CEA, and CUA) should follow 10 general steps.

Step 1: Define the Problem

This step is self-explanatory. What is the question or objective that is the focus of the analysis? An example might be, "The objective of the analysis is to determine what medications for the treatment of urinary tract infections (UTIs) should be included on our formulary." Perhaps one of the drugs being evaluated is a new drug recently approved by the FDA. Should the new drug be added to the drug formulary? The important thing to remember with this step is to be specific.

Step 2: Determine the Study's Perspective

It is important to identify from whose perspective the analysis will be conducted. Is the analysis being conducted from the perspective of the patient or from that of the hospital, clinic, insurance company, or society? Depending on the perspective assigned to the analysis, different results and recommendations based on those results may be identified. If deciding on whether to add a new antibiotic to a formulary for treating UTIs, the perspective of the institution or payer would probably be used.

Step 3: Determine Specific Treatment Alternatives and Outcomes

In this step, all treatment alternatives to be compared in the analysis should be identified. This selection should include the best clinical options and/or the options that are used most often in that setting at the time of the study. If a new treatment option is being considered, comparing it with an outdated treatment or a treatment with low efficacy rates is a waste of time and money. This new treatment should be compared with the next-best alternative or the alternative it may replace. Keep in mind that alternatives may include drug treatments and nondrug treatments. For the UTI example, a new antibiotic would probably be compared with fluoroquinolones or sulfa drugs. Today's expensive new chemical entities are very unlikely to cost less than standard therapy, and because of this, newer drugs are sometimes compared to the most recent, more expensive drugs used as alternative therapy.

The outcomes of those alternatives should include all anticipated positive and negative consequences or events that can be measured. Remember, outcomes may be measured in a variety of ways: lives saved, emergency room visits, hospitalizations, adverse drug reactions, dollars saved, QALYs, and so forth. For the UTI example, cure rates would be the most important outcome.

Step 4: Select the Appropriate Pharmacoeconomic Method or Model

The pharmacoeconomic method selected will depend on how the outcomes are measured. Costs (inputs) for all four types of analyses are measured in dollars. When all outcomes for each alternative are expected to be the same, a CMA is used. If all outcomes for each alternative considered are measured in monetary units, a CBA is used. When outcomes of each treatment alternative are measured in the same nonmonetary units, a CEA is used. When patient preferences for alternative treatments are being considered, a CUA is used. For the UTI example, cure rates are a natural clinical unit measure, so a CEA would be conducted.

Step 5: Measure Inputs and Outcomes

All resources consumed by each alternative should be identified and measured in monetary value. The cost for each alternative should be listed and estimated. The types of costs that will be measured will depend on the perspective chosen in Step 2. When evaluating alternatives over a long period of time (eg, >1 year), the concept of discounting should be applied. For the UTI example, if the perspective is an acute care hospital, only inpatient costs of treatment are measured. If the perspective is that of the third-party payer, all direct medical costs for the treatment are included whether they are provided on an inpatient or outpatient basis.

Measuring outcomes can be relatively simple (eg, cure rates) or relatively difficult (eg, QALYs). Outcomes may be measured prospectively or retrospectively. Prospective measurements tend to be more accurate and complete, but may take considerably more time and resources than retrospective data retrieval. Prospectively it is possible to define exactly what data to capture, but because it is necessary to wait for the patients to complete therapy, these types of studies may take months to years to complete. A data set on the shelf (computer) can be available now, and may have all the data fields of interest. For the UTI example, cure rates attributed to the new product may be estimated from previous clinical trials, expert opinion, or measured prospectively in the population of interest.

Step 6: Identify the Resources Necessary to Conduct the Analysis

The availability of resources to conduct the study is an important consideration. Lack of access to important data can severely limit the validity of an analysis, as can the accuracy of the data itself. Data may be obtained from a variety of sources, including clinical trials, medical literature, medical records, prescription profiles, or computer databases. Before proceeding with the project, evaluate whether reliable sources of data are accessible or the data can be collected within the timeframe and budget allocated for the project.

Step 7: Establish the Probabilities for the Outcomes of the Treatment Alternatives

Probabilities for the outcomes identified in Step 3 should be determined. This may include the probability of treatment failures or success, or adverse reactions to a given treatment or alternative. Data for these can be obtained from the medical literature, clinical trials, medical records, expert opinion, prescription databases, as well as institutional databases. For the UTI example, probabilities of a cure rate for the new medication can be found in clinical trials or obtained from the FDA-approved labeling information. Probabilities of cure rates for the previous treatments (eg, sulfas) can also be found in clinical trials or by accessing medical records. If prospective data collection is conducted, the probabilities of all alternatives will be directly measured instead of estimated.

Step 8: Construct a Decision Tree

Decision analysis can be a very useful tool when conducting a pharmacoeconomic analysis. Constructing a decision tree creates a graphic display of the outcomes of each treatment alternative and the probability of their occurrence. Costs associated with each treatment alternative can be determined and the respective cost ratios derived. An example using a decision tree is provided in Figure 70-2.

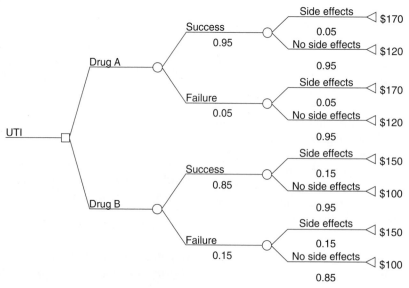

FIGURE 70-2   Decision tree for UTI example. Reproduced with permission from Malone PM, Kier KL, Stanovich JE: *Drug Information: A Guide for Pharmacists*, 4th ed. New York, NY: McGraw-Hill; 2012.

Step 9: Conduct a Sensitivity Analysis

Whenever estimates are used, there is a possibility that these estimates are not precise. These estimates may be referred to as assumptions. For example, if the researcher assumes that the discount rate is 5%, or assumes the efficacy rate found in clinical trials will be the same as the effectiveness rate in the general population, this is a best guess used to conduct the calculations. A sensitivity analysis allows one to determine how the results of an analysis would change when these best guesses or assumptions are varied over a relevant range of values. For example, if the researcher makes the assumption that the appropriate discount rate is 5%, this estimate should be varied from 0% to 10% to determine if the same alternative would still be chosen within this range. In order to vary many assumptions at one time, a probabilistic sensitivity analysis can be conducted that simulates many patients randomly being processed through the decision model using a range of estimates chosen for the analysis. This method will help determine the robustness of the analysis. Do small changes in probabilities produce significant differences in the outcomes of the treatment alternatives?

Step 10: Present the Results

The results of the analysis should be presented to the appropriate audience, such as P&T committees, medical staff, or third-party payers. The steps outlined in this section should be employed when presenting the results. State the problem, identify the perspective, and so on. It is imperative to acknowledge or clarify any assumptions. Although none of the models presented above are perfect, their utility may lead to better decision-making when faced with the difficult task of evaluating new drugs or technology for health care systems.

Decision Analysis

Decision analysis is a tool that can help visualize a pharmacoeconomic analysis. It is the application of an analytical method for systematically comparing different decision options. Decision analysis graphically displays choices and performs the calculations needed to compare these options. It assists with selecting the best or most cost-effective alternative. Decision analysis is a tool that has been utilized for years in many fields, but has been applied to medical decision-making more frequently in the last 10 years. This method of analysis assists in making decisions when the decision is complex and there is uncertainty about some of the information.

Discussions of the medical uses of decision analysis have been included in collections of pharmacoeconomic bibliographies, and in such specific topic areas as CEAs, CUAs, CBAs, CMAs, policies, formulary processes, pharmacy practices, and drug product development.

Steps in Decision Analysis

The six steps involved in performing a decision analysis are:

Step 1: Identify the Specific Decision

Clearly define the specific decision to be evaluated (what is the objective of the study?). Over what period of time will the analysis be conducted (eg, the episode of care, a year)? Will the perspective be that of the ill patient, the medical care plan, an institution/organization, or society? Specifying who will be responsible for the costs of the treatment will determine how costs are measured. For the UTI example, the decision was whether to add a new antibiotic to the formulary to treat UTIs. The perspective was that of the institution and the time period is 2 weeks.

Step 2: Specify Alternatives

Ideally, the two most effective treatments or alternatives should be compared. In pharmacotherapy evaluations, makers of innovative new products may compare or measure themselves against a standard (older or well-established) therapy. This is most often the case with new chemical entities. For pharmaceutical products, dosage and duration of therapy should be included. When analyzing costs and outcomes of pharmaceutical services, these services should be described in detail. For the UTI example, the use of the new medication (drug A) will be compared with that of a sulfa drug (drug B).

Step 3: Specify Possible Outcomes and Probabilities

Consequences and outcomes calculated in dollars yield a cost per outcome in natural medical units, such as mg/dL, which is a CEA. For each potential outcome, an estimated probability must be determined (eg, 95% probability of a cure or a 7% incidence of side effects). Table 70-7 shows the outcomes and probabilities for the UTI example. The probabilities represent the chances or likelihood of treatment success or side effects, and the costs associated with them.

Step 4: Draw the Decision Analysis Structure

Lines are drawn to joint decision points (branches or arms of a decision tree), represented either as choice nodes, chance nodes, or final outcomes. Nodes are places in the decision tree where decisions are allowed; a branching becomes possible at this point. There are three types of nodes: (1) a choice node is where a choice is allowed (as between two drugs or two treatments), (2) a chance node is a place where chance (natural occurrence) may influence the decision or outcome expressed as a probability, and (3) a terminal node is the final outcome of interest for that decision. Probabilities are assigned for each possible outcome, and the sum of the probabilities must add up to one. Most computer-aided software programs utilize a square box to represent a choice node, a circle to represent a chance node, and a triangle for a terminal branch or final

TABLE 70-7	Outcomes and Probabilities, UTI Example	
	Drug A	**Drug B**
Effectiveness probability	0.95	0.85
Side effect probability	0.05	0.15
Cost of medication	$120	$100
Cost of side effects	$50	$50

Reproduced with permission from Malone PM, Kier KL, Stanovich JE: *Drug Information: A Guide for Pharmacists*, 4th ed. New York, NY: McGraw-Hill; 2012.

TABLE 70-8	**Decision Analysis Calculations for Drug A**		
	Cost	**Probability**	**Probability × Cost ($)**
Outcome 1	$120 + $50 = $170	0.95 × 0.05 = 0.0475	8.08
Outcome 2	$120	0.95 × 0.95 = 0.9025	108.30
Outcome 3	$120 + $50 = $170	0.05 × 0.05 = 0.0025	0.42
Outcome 4	$120	0.05 × 0.95 = 0.0475	5.70
Total		1	122.5

Reproduced with permission from Malone PM, Kier KL, Stanovich JE: *Drug Information: A Guide for Pharmacists*, 4th ed. New York, NY: McGraw-Hill; 2012.

outcome. Figure 70-2 illustrates the decision tree for the UTI example.

Step 5: Perform Calculations

The first consideration should be the PV, or cost, of money. If the study is over a period of less than 1 year, actual costs are utilized in the calculations. If the study period is greater than 1 year, then costs should be discounted (converted to PV). For each branch of the tree, costs are totaled and multiplied by the probability of that arm of the tree. These numbers (costs × probabilities) calculated for each arm of the option are added for each alternative. Example calculations are given in Tables 70-8 to 70-10. The UTI example would be a cost-effectiveness type of study, so the difference in the cost for each arm would be divided by the difference in effectiveness for each arm to produce a marginal CER (see Table 70-10).

Step 6: Conduct a Sensitivity Analysis (Vary Cost Estimates)

Because these decision trees or models are constructed with best guesses, a sensitivity analysis is conducted. The highest and lowest estimates of costs and probabilities are inserted into the equations, to determine the best case and worse case answers. These estimates should be sufficiently varied to reflect all possible true variations in values. For the UTI example, the new drug (drug A) would be added to the formulary if the committee thought the added cost ($150) was worth the added benefit (one more successful treatment) (see Table 70-8). Some might not agree with the probability of the side effects of drug A; because the therapy is new, they may believe 5% may be an underestimate. If the estimate is increased to a 10% side effect rate for the new drug and the marginal CER is recalculated,

the recalculated ratio would be $175 per added treatment success. Again, the committee would have to decide if the added cost is worth the added benefit.

Example

A decision tree analysis was used to model the cost-effectiveness of enoxaparin compared to warfarin for the prevention of complications (deep vein thrombosis, venous thromboembolisms, and post thrombotic syndromes) due to hip replacement surgery. Data for this model were obtained through published literature and expert opinion. The model was created to assess both short-term (immediately after surgery) and long-term (followed until death or 100 years old) costs and consequences. The perspective was that of the payer, and a discount rate of 3% was used for the long-term analysis. For the short-term model, therapy with enoxaparin was more expensive (+ $133 per patient), but had a better outcome (+ 0.04 QALY per patient). For the long-term model, therapy with enoxaparin saved money (− $89 per patient) and had a better outcome (+ 0.16 QALY per patient), and was therefore the dominant choice. Both univariate and probabilistic sensitivity analyses were conducted and indicated that the results were robust.

Steps in Reviewing Published Literature

When evaluating the pharmacoeconomics literature for making a formulary decision, or selecting a best product for an institution, a systematic approach to evaluating the pharmacoeconomics literature can make the task easier. The steps for evaluating studies are similar to the steps for conducting studies, because the readers are determining if the proper steps

TABLE 70-9	**Decision Analysis Calculations for Drug B**		
	Cost	**Probability**	**Probability × Cost ($)**
Outcome 1	$100 + $50 = $150	0.85 × 0.15 = 0.1275	19.12
Outcome 2	$100	0.85 × 0.85 = 0.7225	72.25
Outcome 3	$100 + $50 = $150	0.15 × 0.15 = 0.0225	3.38
Outcome 4	$100	0.15 × 0.85 = 0.1275	12.75
Total		1	107.50

Reproduced with permission from Malone PM, Kier KL, Stanovich JE: *Drug Information: A Guide for Pharmacists*, 4th ed. New York, NY: McGraw-Hill; 2012.

TABLE 70-10	**Incremental Cost-Effectiveness Ratio**		
	Alternative Costs of Drug and Treating Side Effects ($)	Effectiveness in Treating UTI (%)	Incremental Cost per Treatment Success
Drug A	$122.50	95	($122.50 − $107.50)/(0.95 − 0.85) = $150
Drug B	$107.50	85	

Reproduced with permission from Malone PM, Kier KL, Stanovich JE: *Drug Information: A Guide for Pharmacists*, 4th ed. New York, NY: McGraw-Hill; 2012.

were followed when the researcher conducted the study. When evaluating a pharmacoeconomic study, at least the following 10 questions should be considered.

1. Was a well-defined question posed in an answerable form? The specific questions and hypotheses should be clearly stated at the beginning of the article.
2. Is the perspective of the study addressed? The perspective should be explicitly stated, not implied.
3. Were the appropriate alternatives considered? Head-to-head comparisons of the best alternatives provide more information than comparing a new product or service with an outdated or ineffective alternative.
4. Was a comprehensive description of the competing alternatives given? If products are compared, dosage and length of therapy should be included. If services are compared, explicit details of the services make the paper more useful. Could another researcher replicate the study based on the information given?
5. What type of analysis was conducted? The paper should address if a CMA, CEA, CBA, or CUA was conducted. Some studies may conduct more than one type of analysis (ie, a combination of a CEA and a CUA). Some studies, especially older published studies, incorrectly placed the terms *benefit* or *effectiveness analysis* in the title of the article, when many were actually CMA studies.
6. Were all the important and relevant costs and outcomes included? Check to see that all pertinent costs and consequences were mentioned. The clinician needs to evaluate his or her situation and compare it to his or her practice situation.
7. Was there justification for any important costs or consequences that were not included? Sometimes, the authors will admit that although certain costs or consequences are important, they were impractical (or impossible) to measure in their study. It is better that the authors state these limitations, than to ignore them.
8. Was discounting appropriate? If so, was it conducted? If the treatment cost or outcomes are extrapolated for more than 1 year, the time value of money must be incorporated into the cost estimates.
9. Are all assumptions stated? Were sensitivity analyses conducted for these assumptions? Many of the values used in pharmacoeconomic studies are based on assumptions. For example, authors may assume the side effect rate is 5%, or that compliance with a regimen will be 80%. These types of assumptions should be stated explicitly. For important assumptions, was the estimate varied within a reasonable range of values?

10. Was an unbiased summary of the results presented? Sometimes, the conclusions seem to overstate or exaggerate the data presented in the results section. Did the authors use unbiased reasonable estimates when determining the results? In general, are the study results believable?

CASE Application

1. Which of the following parameters is evaluated by a pharmacoeconomic analysis?
   a. Cost
   b. Outcomes
   c. Cost and outcomes
   d. Side effects
   e. Side effects and number needed to harm

2. What type of pharmacoeconomic analysis assumes the outcomes are equal?
   a. Epidemiologic study
   b. Retrospective study
   c. Cost-minimization
   d. Parametric analysis

3. A study is evaluating the cost associated with emergency room visits. What type of cost would emergency room visits represent? Select all that apply.
   a. Direct medical
   b. Direct nonmedical
   c. Indirect
   d. Intangible

4. A study is evaluating the cost associated with hotel and meal expenses for a patient traveling to see a subspecialist. What type of cost would hotel and meal expenses represent?
   a. Direct medical
   b. Direct nonmedical
   c. Indirect
   d. Intangible

5. A study is evaluating the cost associated with missing work due to an illness. What type of cost would missing work represent?
   a. Direct medical
   b. Direct nonmedical
   c. Indirect
   d. Intangible

6. A study is evaluating the cost associated with anxiety due to an illness. What type of cost would anxiety represent?

    a. Direct medical
    b. Direct nonmedical
    c. Indirect
    d. Intangible

7. A pharmacoeconomic analysis is to be conducted between simvastatin and atorvastatin. While these medications have different lowering of LDL (percentage points), they are considered equivalent in terms of decreasing primary cardiovascular mortality and safety per discussion with your attending physician. He wants you to conduct an analysis comparing the two agents. Which type of analysis would be utilized?

    a. CMA
    b. CBA
    c. CEA
    d. CUA

8. The pharmacy director at an academic medical center has been allotted on full time equivalent (FTE) to hire a clinical pharmacy specialist. He requested three FTEs in the area of cardiology, critical care, and infectious diseases. Now he has to decide which type of specialist he should hire. Instead of make a gut call, he has decided to include the economist faculty member from the College

of Pharmacy to assist. What type of analysis should be conducted to evaluate which position should be hired?

    a. CMA
    b. CBA
    c. CEA
    d. CUA

9. A medical center located in the Northeast part of the United States is dealing with resistant bacterial organisms at their institution. Specifically, they are overwhelmed with cases of extended spectrum β-lactamase gram-negative rods. The medical center director charges pharmacy service with comparing different types of treatment to optimize clinical cure outcomes. Which of the following types of pharmacoeconomic evaluations should be conducted?

    a. CMA
    b. CBA
    c. CEA
    d. CUA

10. Which of the following pharmacoeconomic models evaluated adjusted life years?

    a. CMA
    b. CBA
    c. CEA
    d. CUA

TAKEAWAY POINTS ❯❯

- Pharmacoeconomics is the description and analysis of the costs of drug therapy to health care systems and society. Pharmacoeconomic studies identify, measure, and compare the costs and consequences of pharmaceutical products and services.
- The four types of pharmacoeconomic analyses measure costs or inputs in dollars and assess the outcomes associated with these costs.
- CMA: Outcomes are assumed to be equivalent.
- CBA: Outcomes are measured in dollars.
- CEA: The costs are measured in natural units (eg, cures, years of life, blood pressure);

- CUA: Outcomes take into account patient preferences (or utilities).
- Pharmacoeconomic studies categorize costs into four types (direct medical costs, direct nonmedical costs, indirect costs, and intangible costs).
- Decision analysis is a tool that can help visualize a pharmacoeconomic analysis. It is the application of an analytical method for systematically comparing different decision options.

BIBLIOGRAPHY

Jolicoeur LM, Jones-Grizzle AJ, Boyer JG. Guidelines for performing a pharmacoeconomic analysis. *Am J Hosp Pharm.* 1992;49:1741-1747.

Mithani H, Brown G. The economic impact of once-daily versus conventional administration of gentamicin and tobramycin. *PharmacoEconom.* 1996;10(5):494-503.

Nadel HL. Formulary conversion from glipizide to glyburide: a cost-minimization analysis. *Hosp Pharm.* 1995;30(6):467-469, 472-474.

Shaw JW, Zachry WM. Application of probabilistic sensitivity analysis in decision analytic modeling. *Formulary (USA).* 2002;37:32-34, 37-40.

Wang Z, Salmon JW, Walton SM. Cost-effectiveness analysis and the formulary decision-making process. *J Manag Care Pharm.* 2004;10(10):48-59.

Wilson JP, Rascati KL. Pharmacoeconomics. In: Malone PM, Kier KL, Stanovich JE, eds. *Drug Information: A Guide for Pharmacists.* 4th ed. New York, NY: McGraw-Hill; 2012:chap 6.

KEY ABBREVIATIONS

BSC = best supportive care
CBA = cost-benefit analysis
CCA = cost-consequence analysis
CEA = cost-effectiveness analysis
CMA = cost-minimization analysis
CUA = cost-utility analysis
GERD = gastroesophageal reflux disease
HC = human capital

HR-QOL = health-related quality of life
PV = present value
QALYs = quality-adjusted life year
RS = rating scale
SG = standard gamble
TTO = time trade-off
UTI = urinary tract infection
WTP = willingness-to-pay

FOUNDATION OVERVIEW

Knowledge of statistics is essential to understand the biomedical science literature. The focus of this chapter is to describe concepts as they relate to evaluating medical literature, as opposed to mathematical calculation and programming of specific statistical tests.

Populations and Samples

A population refers to all objects of a similar type in the universe, while a sample is a fraction of the population chosen to be representative of the specific population of interest. Thus, samples are chosen to make generalizations about the population of interest. Researchers typically do not attempt to study the entire population as most often data cannot be collected for everyone within a population. This emphasizes why the sample must be chosen at random; that is, each member of the population must have an equal chance of being included in the sample. A random sample does not imply that the sample is drawn haphazardly or in an unplanned fashion. There are several approaches of selecting a random sample, with the most common method employing a random number table. A random number table contains all integers between one and infinity that have been selected without any trends or patterns (ie, completely random). Depending on the type of study design, a simple random sample may not be the best method for selecting a representative sample. On occasion, it may be necessary to separate the population into mutually exclusive groups called strata, where a specific factor (eg, patient race, gender) will be contained in separate strata to aid in analysis. In this case, the random sample is drawn within each stratum individually, termed a stratified random sample. Another method of randomly sampling a population is known as cluster sampling. Cluster sampling is appropriate when there are natural groupings within the population of interest. Another sampling method is known as systematic sampling. This method is used when information about the population is provided in list format, such as in the telephone book, election records, class lists, licensure records, and so forth. A form of systematic sampling is the equal-probability method where one individual is selected at random and every nth individual is then selected thereafter. Finally, it should be noted that researchers often use convenience sampling. A convenience sample selects participants based on the convenience of the researcher. That is, no attempt is made to select a random sample representative of the population. However, within the convenience sample, participants may be selected randomly. Obviously, there are significant weaknesses to this type of sampling, primarily, limited generalization (ie, external validity).

Variables and Data

A variable is a characteristic that is being observed or measured. Data are the measured values assigned to the variable for each individual member of the population. For example, a variable would be patient gender, while the data are whether the patient is male or female. There are three types of variables: dependent (DV), independent (IV), and confounding.

The DV is the response or outcome variable for a study, while an IV is a variable that is manipulated. A confounding variable is any variable that has an effect on the DV over and above the effect of the IV, but is not of specific research interest.

Scales of Measurement

There are four levels of measurement: nominal, ordinal, interval, and ratio scales. The scale of measurement is an important consideration when determining the appropriate statistical test to answer the research question and hypothesis. A nominal scale consists of categories that have no implied rank or order (male versus female; or absence versus presence). The patient can fit into only one category; that is, the data points are mutually exclusive. An ordinal scale has all of the characteristics of a nominal variable; however, the data are placed into rank-ordered categories. The distance between categories cannot be considered equal; that is, the data points can be ranked, but the distance between them may differ greatly (eg, New York Heart Association class I, II, III, and IV). Interval scales consist of ordered data points on a constant scale without a natural zero. Interval scales increase the information provided by an ordinal scale by allowing researchers to quantify a meaningful distance between two units (eg, temperature). Ratio scales differ from interval scales in that they have an absolute zero (eg, blood pressure). Although researchers should not confuse absolute and arbitrary zero points, this difference is nonessential as interval and ratio scales are analyzed by identical statistical procedures.

Continuous and Discrete Variables

Continuous variables consist of data measured on interval or ratio scales. Examples of continuous variables include age, body mass index (BMI) and uncategorized lab values (eg, a blood pressure of 160/95 as opposed to high blood pressure). Discrete variables consist of data measured on nominal or ordinal scales. Discrete variables are often termed nominal or categorical, or, if a variable is measured on a nominal scale with only two levels (eg, male versus female), it may be termed dichotomous.

Descriptive Statistics

There are two types of statistics: descriptive and inferential. Descriptive statistics present, organize, and summarize data in a very basic sense, while providing information regarding the appearance of the data and distributional assumptions. Descriptive statistics are often used to summarize study data numerically and/or graphically. Measures of central tendency (eg, mean, median, mode), variability, and shape are types of numerical representation, while histograms, boxplots, and scatterplots are common graphical representations. Inferential statistics (discussed later) test for differences or relationships, against random variation, within the study sample, allowing reliable findings to be generalized to the population of interest.

Measures of Central Tendency

Measures of central tendency are helpful in identifying the distribution of the data numerically. Common measures of central tendency are the mean, median, and mode. The appropriate measure of central tendency depends on the scale of measurement for the variable being studied.

- The mean is the most common and appropriate measure of central tendency for normally distributed data measured on an interval or ratio scale. It is best described as the average numerical value for data within a variable. The mean is calculated by summing all data for a variable and dividing by the total number of patients (total sample size or simply n).

- The median is most appropriate for data measured on an ordinal scale; however, it can also be presented for continuous variables to assist in describing the variable distribution. The median is the absolute middle value in the data (exactly at the 50th percentile); that is, half of the data points fall above and half below the median. It is important to note that outliers (ie, data points that are disconnected from the other data points) can significantly affect the mean, but not the median. Therefore, a comparison of the mean and median can give insight into whether outliers influenced the mean and overall distribution of the data points within a variable.

- The mode is the most appropriate measure of central tendency for nominal data. The mode is the most frequently occurring value or category within a variable. Further, a variable could have two, three, or more modes; thus, a variable with two modes is referred to as bimodal, with three modes, trimodal.

Measures of Variability

The most common measures of variability (or dispersion) are the range, interquartile range (IQR), variance, and standard deviation (SD). Measures of variability are useful in indicating the spread of data for a variable. These measures are also useful in association with measures of central tendency to assess how scattered the data are around the mean or median. The range can be used appropriately to describe data measured on an ordinal, interval, or ratio scale. The range is found by subtracting the minimum data point from the maximum data point. The IQR is another measure of dispersion used to describe data measured on ordinal, interval, or ratio scales. The IQR is a measure of variability directly related to the median. The IQR is the difference between the 75th and 25th percentile. Remember, the median is located at exactly the 50th percentile; therefore, the IQR presents the middle 50% of the data and always includes the median. This value is a stable measure of spread and is not as affected by extreme values (ie, outliers) in the data. The final two measures of variability described are the variance and SD. These measures are appropriate for normally distributed continuous variables measured on interval or ratio scales. The variance for a variable is the average squared deviation from the mean for all data points within a specific variable. The SD and variance are directly related, as the SD is the square root of the variance. Thus, if one value is known, the other can be calculated. SD is preferred over variance because it indicates the average deviation from the mean presented on the same scale as the original variable, unlike the variance, which is in square units. In comparing two groups with equal means, the SD can provide insight into the dispersion of scores around the mean, with larger values indicating greater variability. Finally, the coefficient of variation (CV) is a less commonly used measure that evaluates the dispersion of two or more variables measured on different scales. The CV is typically expressed as a percentage, with higher percentages indicating greater variation. It is calculated by dividing the SD by the mean and multiplying by 100. The higher the CV, the greater the dispersion.

Measures of Shape

Skewness and kurtosis are appropriate for variables measured on interval or ratio scales, and indicate asymmetry and peakedness, respectively. They are typically used by researchers to evaluate the distributional assumptions of a variable, but both measures are usually omitted in the biomedical literature. The distribution of the DV is incredibly important when determining the most appropriate statistical test to employ, as most parametric statistical tests require a normal distribution.

The mean, median, and mode of a normal distribution (discussed further) are identical; thus, skewness can be indicated when the mean is not directly in the middle of the distribution. Positive (or right) skewness occurs when the mode and median are less than the mean while negative (or left) skewness occurs when mode and median are greater than the mean. Kurtosis refers to the peakedness of the distribution of data points. A curve with a wide, flat top is referred to as platykurtic, while a narrow, peaked distribution is termed leptokurtic. A platykurtic curve often is an indicator of greater variability; that is, the data is spread over a larger range. In contrast, a leptokurtic distribution has less variability with a large percentage of data points close to the mean.

Graphical Representations

Graphical representations of data are incredibly useful, especially when sample sizes are large. They allow researchers to inspect visually the distribution of individual variables. There are typically three graphical representations presented in the literature—histograms, boxplots, and scatterplots. Note that graphical representations are typically used for continuous variables measured on ordinal, interval, or ratio scales. By contrast, nominal, dichotomous, or categorical variables are best presented as count data, typically as frequency and percentage.

A histogram presents data as frequency counts over some interval; that is, the *x*-axis presents the values of the data points, whether individual data points or intervals, while the *y*-axis presents the number of times the data point or interval occurs in the variable (ie, frequency). When data are plotted, it is easy to superimpose or visualize the normal distribution or bell curve to assess overall normality for the variable (ie, skewness and kurtosis) as well as outliers. A *boxplot* provides the reader with five descriptive statistics. The box in a boxplot is the IQR, which identifies the 25th to 75th percentiles of data. Within the box is a broad line depicting the median or 50th percentile. From both ends of the box extends a tail, or whisker, depicting the minimum and maximum data points. A scatterplot presents bivariate (ie, two variable) data for variables measured, typically, on continuous scales. That is, the *x*-axis contains the range of data for one variable, while the *y*-axis contains the range of data for the second variable. Scatterplots are useful in assessing association or correlation (discussed further), between two variables as well as assessing other assumptions of various statistical tests (eg, linearity, absence of outliers).

Common Probability Distributions

The distribution of the DV is of primary importance when determining which statistical test to employ. In the biomedical literature, a number of probability distributions are typically used to make inferences about the data and determine statistical significance. In the social, behavioral, and nursing sciences, the DV will often be continuous, requiring a normal distribution. In the biomedical literature, the DV could also be continuous, as well as categorical (eg, dead versus alive, disease present versus disease absent), which requires binomial or Poisson distributions.

The Normal Distribution

The normal distribution, also called Gaussian distribution, is one of the most important density curves. This distribution is the most commonly used distribution in statistics and one that occurs frequently in nature. It is very important to know

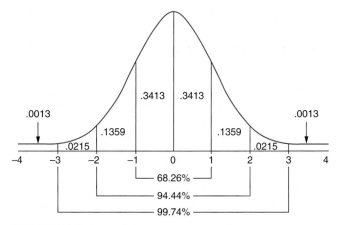

FIGURE 71-1 Bell curve. Reproduced with permission from Malone PM, Kier KL, Stanovich JE: *Drug Information: A Guide for Pharmacists*, 5th ed. New York, NY: McGraw-Hill; 2014.

whether a variable is distributed normally in the population, or whether the variable distribution approaches normal. A normal curve has several easily identifiable properties uncovered by analyzing the numerical measures of central tendency, variability, and shape (Figure 71-1). Specifically, this includes the following characteristics:

1. The primary shape is a bell-curve.
2. The mean, median, and mode are identical.
3. The curve is symmetric around the mean; that is, the distribution is symmetrical and reflects itself perfectly when folded in half.
4. Skewness and kurtosis are zero.
5. The area under a normal distribution is, by definition, 1.

The Binomial Distribution

Many discrete outcomes or events can be dichotomized into one of two mutually exclusive groups. The binomial distribution, also termed the Bernoulli distribution, is appropriate for this type of event or outcome (ie, DV), and calculates the exact probability of the event or outcome. Note the binomial distribution approximates the normal distribution when n is large and the probability of the outcome is 0.50 (ie, 50/50). The binomial distribution can only be used when an experiment assumes the four characteristics listed below:

1. The trial occurs a specified number of times (analogous to sample size, n).
2. Each trial has only two mutually exclusive outcomes (success or failure in a generic sense, x).
3. Each trial is independent, meaning that one outcome has no effect on the other.
4. The probability of success remains constant throughout the trial.

The binomial distribution counts the number of successes and failures during the study period. When all trials have been run, the probability of achieving exactly x successes (or failures) in n trials can be calculated. A classic example using the binomial distribution is flipping a coin. When the coin is flipped for a set number of trials, there are only two possible outcomes (ie, heads or tails); each trial is not affected by the last, and the probability of flipping heads or tails remains constant (ie, 0.50) throughout the trial. Say a coin is flipped ten times, of which it landed on heads six times. The binomial distribution allows for the calculation of the exact probability of achieving six heads in ten flips, which is 0.205. As mentioned above, if the coin was flipped 10,000 times, the binomial distribution would approximate the normal distribution.

In reality, however, the probability of an outcome is rarely 0.50. For example, often biomedical studies use all-cause mortality as the outcome variable. Most likely, the probability of suffering the event (ie, death) is much lower than staying alive. Regardless, at the end of the trial, patients experience only one mutually exclusive outcome—dead or alive. In this example, say the sample consists of 1000 patients, of which 154 die. The binomial distribution allows for the calculation of the exact probability of having 154 patients dying in a total sample of 1000 patients.

The Poisson Distribution

Similar to the binomial distribution, the Poisson distribution is a discrete probability distribution. However, the Poisson distribution typically involves count data or rates, allowing calculation of the mean probability of an event across time. The Poisson distribution can only be used when an experiment assumes the four characteristics listed below:

1. The probability of experiencing the event during a time interval is proportional to the length of the interval.
2. The probability of two events occurring during the time interval is low (ie, rare events).
3. The probability of experiencing the event across time intervals remains constant.
4. The probability of experiencing the event in one time interval is independent of all other intervals.

Epidemiological Statistics

The field of epidemiology investigates how diseases are distributed in the population and the various factors (or exposures) influencing this distribution. Pharmacoepidemiology is the study of the utilization and effects of drugs in large numbers of people; it provides an estimate of the probability of beneficial effects of a drug in a population and the probability of adverse effects. It can be called a bridge science spanning both clinical pharmacology and epidemiology.

Ratio, Proportions, and Rates

Ratios, proportions, and rates are frequent terms used interchangeably in the medical literature without regard for the actual mathematical definitions. A ratio expresses the relationship between two numbers. For example, consider the ratio of men to women diagnosed with rheumatoid arthritis (RA). If, in a sample consisting of only RA patients, 103 men and 57 women are diagnosed, the ratio of men to women is 103 to 57, or 103:57. Remember, that the order in which the ratio is presented is vitally important; that is, 103:57 is not the same as 57:103.

A proportion is a specific type of ratio indicating the probability or percentage of the total sample that experience an outcome or event without respect to time. Here, the numerator of the proportion (ie, patients with the disease) is included in the denominator (ie, all individuals at risk). For example, say 840 non-RA patients are added to the sample above for a total sample of 1000; thus, the proportion of patients with RA is 0.160 or 16.0% (ie, 160/1,000). Note that the probability of a specific proportion is assessed by the binomial distribution. A rate is a special form of proportion that includes a specific study period, typically used to assess the speed at which the event or outcome is developing. A rate is equal to the number events, in a specified time period, divided by the length of the time period. For example, say over a 1-year period, 50 cases of RA were diagnosed. Thus, the rate of new cases of RA within this sample is 50 per year.

Incidence and Prevalence

Incidence quantifies the occurrence of an event or outcome, for a specific study period, within a specific population. The incidence rate is calculated by dividing the number of new events by the total number of people capable of experiencing the event (ie, the population at risk). For example, consider the 50 new cases of RA that developed from the example above. The incidence rate is approximately 0.06 (ie, 50/840). Note the denominator did not include the 160 patients already diagnosed (ie, 1000 − 160 = 840) with RA because they were no longer considered at risk. Prevalence quantifies the number of patients who have already experienced the event or outcome at a specific time point. Prevalence is calculated by dividing the total number of patients experiencing the event by the total number of individuals in the population. For example, including all RA cases above (ie, 50 + 160 = 210), the prevalence of RA in this sample is 0.21.

Relative Risk and Odds Ratio

Relative risk is defined as the ratio (or probability) of the incidence of an event occurring in individuals exposed to a risk compared to the incidence of the event in those not exposed to the risk. Relative risk can be calculated directly from the cohort study design. This design is typically an observational design comparing the incidence of experiencing an event in exposed and unexposed individuals (ie, the cohort) over time. Upon study conclusion, a 2 × 2 contingency table (Table 71-1) is created containing frequency counts of events for the exposed and unexposed groups. This table provides all data necessary to calculate the incidence of the event for both exposed and unexposed individuals. Relative risk is calculated by dividing the proportion of individuals who suffered the event in the exposed group (ie, A/A+B) by the proportion of individuals who suffered the event in the unexposed group (ie, C/C+D). When calculated, relative risk provides a single number ranging from zero to infinity, and there are three interpretations resulting from this calculation.

1. If relative risk equals 1, the exposed and unexposed have equal risk, indicating no association between the event and exposure.

TABLE 71-1 | **2 × 2 Contingency Table**

	Event	No Event	
Exposed	A	B	A+B
Unexposed	C	D	C+D
	A+C	B+D	A+B+C+D

For Sensitivity, Specificity, and Predictive Values

	Disease Present	**Disease Not Present**	
Positive Test	TP	FP	TP + FP
Negative Test	FN	TN	TN + FN
	TP + FN	TP + FP	TP + FP + FN + TN

This 2x2 table helps in calculating sensitivity, specificity, and predictive values. Sensitivity is the true positive (TP) rate of the screening test. It is calculated by dividing true positives by all individuals who actually have the disease (TP/TP + FN). Specificity is the true negative (TN) rate of the screening test. It is calculated by dividing true negatives by all disease-free individuals (TN/TN + FP). Positive predictive values measures the accuracy of the screening test and is the proportion of individuals who test positive for the disease that actually have the disease. It is calculated by dividing true positives by all individuals with a positive test result (TP/TP + FP). Negative predictive value provides the proportion of individuals who test negative who are actually disease-free. It is calculated by dividing true negatives by all individuals with a negative test result (TN/TN + FN).

For Error Types

	Truth	
Decision	**Null Hypothesis is False**	**Null Hypothesis is True**
Reject Null Hypothesis	Correct decision (True Positive)	Type I error (False Positive)
Fail to Reject Null Hypothesis	Type II error (False Negative)	Correct decision (True Negative)

This 2 × 2 table helps in identifying the relationships between truth/false null hypothesis and the reject/fail to reject decision of the test. A Type I error occurs when the researcher indicates a statistically significant difference exists when, in fact, one actually does not (false positive). Thus, a Type I error can only occur when the null hypothesis is true. A Type II error occurs when the researcher fails to indicate a statistically significant difference when one actually exists (false negative).

2. If relative risk is greater than 1, the exposed group has greater risk than the unexposed group indicating a positive association with the risk factor.

3. If relative risk is less than 1, the exposed group has a lower risk than the unexposed group indicating a negative association or protective effect.

When relative risk cannot be calculated, researchers will present an odds ratio, which estimates relative risk. Odds are calculated by dividing the probability of experiencing an event by the probability of not experiencing an event. Thus, an odds ratio is a ratio of two odds; one for those exposed to the risk and the other for those not exposed to the risk. Odds ratios can be calculated for both cohort and case-control designs. A case-control study compares those who have experienced the event (ie, cases) and those who have not (ie, controls), and then assesses whether each individual was exposed to a risk. Thus, a case-control study is retrospective. A cohort study compares those exposed to a risk and those who were not exposed to a risk, and then assesses whether each individual will experience an event. In a cohort study, the odds ratio is calculated by dividing the odds of experiencing the event in the exposed group (ie, A/B) by the odds the unexposed group experienced the event (ie, C/D). In a case-control study, the odds ratio is calculated by dividing the odds that cases were exposed to the risk (ie, A/C) by the odds that the controls were exposed (ie, B/D).

Sensitivity, Specificity, and Predictive Values

Sensitivity, specificity, and predictive values (both positive and negative) measure the ability of a test to identify correctly those experiencing the event and those who did not. Four outcomes can result and are required for the calculation of sensitivity, specificity, and the predictive values:

1. True positives (TP) have the disease and have a positive test result.
2. False positives (FP) do not have the disease, but have a positive test result.
3. True negatives (TN) do not have the disease and have a negative test result.
4. False negatives (FN) have the disease, but have a negative test result.

Sensitivity is the probability that a diseased individual will have a positive test result. It is the TP rate of the test. It is calculated by dividing TPs by all individuals who actually have the disease (ie, TP/TP + FN). Specificity is the probability a disease-free individual will have a negative test result, and is the TN rate of the screening test. It is calculated by dividing TNs by all disease-free individuals (ie, TN/TN + FP). Positive and negative predictive values are calculated to measure the accuracy of the screening test. Both predictive values are directly related to disease prevalence; that is, the higher the prevalence, the higher the predictive value. Positive predictive value provides the proportion of individuals who test positive for the disease that actually have the disease. It is calculated by dividing TPs by all individuals with a positive test result (ie, TP/TP + FP). Negative predictive value provides the proportion of individuals who test negative who are actually disease-free. It is calculated by dividing TNs by all individuals with a negative test result (ie, TN/TN + FN).

Statistical Inference

Statistical analysis allows researchers to make rational decisions in the presence of random processes and variation. Inferential statistics provide the probability that a conclusion is true in the population, based on the analysis of sample data.

Sampling Distributions and the Central Limit Theorem

Statistical inference employs sample data to make conclusion about populations. Because good samples are chosen randomly, the means produced from these samples are also random. Thus, the mean may not be exactly representative of the population and varies from sample to sample. However, the law of large numbers states that as the size of the sample increases, the sample mean will move closer to the population mean. Further, as the number of samples increases, the mean of the sample means will begin to approximate the population mean. The central limit theorem states when equally sized samples are drawn from a non-normal distribution, the plotted mean values from each sample will approximate a normal distribution as long as the non-normality was not due to outliers. This distribution is termed the distribution of sampling means. As with any normal distribution, the SD of the distribution of sampling means can be calculated, termed the standard error of the mean (SEM). The SEM is equal to the SD divided by the square root of the sample size, and reflects variability within the sample means.

Hypothesis Testing

A hypothesis indicates a theory about the population regarding an outcome the researcher is interested in studying. Statistical analyses test two types of hypotheses, the null and alternative. The null hypothesis assumes no difference or association between the different study groups or variables, while the alternative hypothesis states there is a difference or association. When testing hypotheses, researchers often need to determine whether their hypothesis is directional; that is, using a one-sided (directional) or two-sided (nondirectional) hypothesis test. In the literature, it is generally more acceptable to use a two-sided test, even if the hypothesis is directional, as a two-sided test is considered stronger statistically and reduces the probability of committing a Type I error.

Error and Statistical Power

It is essential that researchers establish how much error they are willing to accept before the initiation of the study. A Type I error occurs when the researcher indicates a statistically significant difference exists when, in fact, one actually does not (ie, FP). Thus, a Type I error can only occur when the null hypothesis is true. A Type II error occurs when the researcher fails to indicate a statistically significant difference when one actually exists (ie, FN). Type I and Type II errors are interconnected; that is, as one type increases the other decreases. Researchers must consider these two errors carefully when designing studies. Statistical power was developed as a method allowing researchers to calculate the probability of finding a statistically significant result, when, in fact, one actually exists. Increasing statistical power reduces the probability of committing a Type II error; however, it can also increase the probability of committing a Type I error. Statistical power is influenced by four factors: alpha (the probability value at which the null hypothesis is rejected), effect size (the size of the treatment effect), error variance (the precision of the measurement instrument), and the sample size. Statistical power can be increased by increasing alpha (not advised), effect size, or sample size as well as deceasing error variance. Statistical power of at least 0.80 has been recommended. However, some researchers use 0.90 or higher in the biomedical sciences, indicating that an FN is more detrimental than an FP.

Statistical versus Clinical Significance

The next step in the research process is to employ a statistical test to assess whether a difference or relationship exists in the study sample. Primarily, the researcher is interested in determining whether to retain the null hypothesis or reject it in favor of the alternative hypothesis. Statistical tests produce probability values (ie, p values) which range from 0 to 1. The p value produced from a statistical test is the probability of committing a Type I error based on the assumption that the null hypothesis is true (ie, there is in reality no difference or relationship in the population and the actual observed difference or relationship is due to sampling error or random variation). If the p value is less than alpha, the difference or relationship is considered statistically significant.

Similar to p values, alpha ranges from 0 to 1; however, in most studies in the biomedical sciences use alpha set at 0.05. There may be occasions when alpha is set at 0.01 producing a more stringent statistical test (ie, less likely to find statistical significance); however, this is rare. Statistical significance can never prove a hypothesis, only support it. A more stringent statistical test (ie, alpha = 0.01 or 0.001) does not indicate in any way that a real treatment effect occurred. The set alpha level is a key contributor to the theoretical calculation of the true Type I error rate; that is, the level the researcher is willing to tolerate where a true null hypothesis may be falsely rejected. If a p value is less than the set alpha value, the researcher rejects the null hypothesis in favor of the alternative hypothesis, and the difference or relationship is considered statistically significant. If the *p* value is equal to or greater than alpha, the null hypothesis is retained, and the difference or relationship is not considered statistically significant.

Statistical significance can also be established by calculating a confidence interval (CI) around the estimated population parameters (eg, sample means) or test statistics. CIs account for sample size and variation; thus, a tighter CI indicates less variability in the data. A CI provides a range of scores likely to contain the unknown population parameter, and generally, a CI is reported using a 95% confidence level. However, similar to alpha, the confidence level is arbitrary, with some researchers using 99%. A 95% CI indicates that if repeated random sampling occurs within the population of interest under consistent conditions (eg, sample size), the true population parameter would be included in the interval 95% of the time. Thus, every value within the interval is considered a possible value of the population parameter. Remember from above that roughly 95% of scores in a normal distribution fall within two SDs of the mean (actually, within approximately 1.96 SDs), and, according to the central limit theorem, this same value is applicable to 95% of means in the sampling distribution of means. A 95% CI is calculated by multiplying 1.96 by the SEM and adding or subtracting this value from the estimated parameter to find the upper and lower confidence limits, respectively. Determining statistical significance using CIs around test statistics varies based on the statistical test. For most parametric tests of group differences and correlation (discussed further), a 95% CI around the test statistic containing zero is not considered statistically significant at an alpha of 0.05. That is, statistical significance for these types of analyses are essentially testing that the differences or relationship are different from zero. Thus, a 95% CI containing zero essentially indicates that it is plausible that the true population difference or relationship could be zero. Alternatively, the 95% CI for test statistics based on ratios (eg, logistic and Cox regression, discussed further) that contain 1 are not considered statistically significant at alpha equal to 0.05. Although this may seem different from above, it is actually very similar, and interpretation is identical. Statistical tests based on ratios produce odds or risks calculated by exponentiating the test statistic to create odds ratios. A 95% CI is calculated based on the exponentiated value. Because these values are exponentiated, converting these ratios back into the original unexponentiated metric requires calculating the natural log. Further, the natural log of 1 is zero. Thus, a 95% CI containing 1 for an odds ratio produced by logistic regression indicates that it is plausible that the true population parameter could in fact be zero (ie, the natural log of 1).

When evaluating the significance of the finding, keep in mind that statistical significance does not always indicate clinical significance. Statistical significance can be manipulated in several ways, most easily by increasing sample size drastically. This sample size increase may artificially reduce error variance, which in turn reduces the standard error on which the test statistic is based thereby increasing the probability of

statistical significance and the probability of committing a Type I error.

Experimental, Nonexperimental, and Quasi-Experimental Designs

The distinction between experimental, quasi-experimental, and nonexperimental research is important, both from a study design perspective and when evaluating literature. Although experimental designs are considered the gold standard by many, do not discount research conducted using quasi-experimental and nonexperimental designs, as long as the limitations are considered.

Experimental designs: In the biomedical sciences, experimental designs are referred to as a randomized control trial (RCT).

Nonexperimental designs: These studies are nonrandomized, retrospective, and correlational in nature. Nonexperimental designs have several advantages over RCTs, primarily, low cost, quicker timeline to publication, and a broader range of patients. The advantages of nonexperimental studies over RCTs have prompted their widespread use in the biomedical sciences.

Quasi-experimental designs: These studies appear experimental, but lack randomization.

Quasi-experimental designs are seldom used in biomedical studies, and are much more common in the social sciences.

The Design and Analysis of Clinical Trials

Parallel-Groups Design

The most common RCT is a parallel-groups design where the IV typically involves participants randomized into fixed levels of treatment (or arms), with each arm indicating a different treatment or comparison (eg, placebo, active control).

Crossover Design

The second most common RCT employs a crossover design, which has the primary purpose of having a participant serve as his or her own control. The primary advantage of this type of design is that it typically requires fewer participants in comparison to a parallel-groups design.

Adaptive Design

Adaptive designs implement changes (or adaptations) in the design or endpoint analyses based on the results of a predetermined (ie, prior to initiation of the study) set of interim analyses. Interim analyses can be based on blinded or unblinded data, with the resulting adaptation(s) aimed at establishing a more efficient, safer, and informative trial that is more likely to demonstrate treatment effects.

Intent-to-Treat and Per-Protocol Approaches

Two analytical approaches exist for clinical trials—intent-to-treat (ITT) and per-protocol (PP). The ITT approach is often employed in the presence of violations to protocol and patients being lost to follow-up, and is the approach most often used in the literature. ITT requires the analysis to include all participants in the arm to which they were randomized originally. That is, treatment effects are best evaluated by the planned treatment protocol rather than the actual treatment given. The PP approach evaluates only compliant participants with complete data. Although this analysis is straightforward analytically and allows researchers to evaluate a more accurate treatment effect, it has substantial limitations, primarily, reduced statistical power compared to an ITT approach, because participants with incomplete data are not considered in the analysis, and results in an inflated Type I error rate.

Analyzing Parallel-Groups Designs

When analyzing a parallel-groups design, the traditional approach is to conduct an endpoint analysis, which typically involves employing an independent samples t test (for two groups), one-way analysis of variance (ANOVA) (for more than two groups), or analysis of covariance (ANCOVA) (two or more groups, statistically controlling for a baseline measurement) using only the final measurement (ie, endpoint analysis).

Analyzing Crossover Designs

The purpose of the crossover design is to study treatment effects using the participant as his or her own control. A crossover design requires an initial test-for-order effect by assessing the interaction between order and the DV (ie, constipation symptoms) by means of a two-way mixed ANOVA. When testing for order effects, a statistically significant interaction indicates that the order in which the treatments were received influenced the treatment effect. If the interaction is nonsignificant (ie, no order effect), an endpoint analysis is typically evaluated via paired samples t test.

Analyzing Adaptive Designs

The statistical tests used on the study endpoint typically include an independent samples t test (ie, for comparing two groups), ANOVA (ie, for comparing more than two groups), or ANCOVA (ie, for statistically controlling baseline measurement).

Statistical Techniques

The decision of which statistical test to employ is based on several factors—research question, study design, DV and IV considerations, and assumption violations—all of which are interconnected.

Degrees of Freedom

Degrees of freedom (df) are a vital component of all statistical tests, as most probability distributions, and, thus, statistical significance, are based on them. Degrees of freedom are a useful indicator of adequate sample size in the presence of assumption violations.

Tests for Nominal and Categorical Data

Nonparametric Tests

Pearson's Chi Square Test Pearson's chi square test (or simply the chi square test) is one of the most common statistical tests used in the biomedical sciences. It is used to assess for significant differences between two or more mutually exclusive groups for two variables measured on nominal, dichotomous, or categorical scales.

Fisher's Exact Test Fisher's exact test is ubiquitous in the biomedical literature. The test can only be applied to 2×2 contingency tables; however, it is most useful when the sample size is small. Conceptually, Fisher's exact test is identical to the chi square test, in that, the two variables being compared must be discrete and have mutually exclusive categories.

Mantel-Haenszel Chi Square Test The Mantel-Haenszel chi square test (or Cochran-Mantel-Haenszel test or Mantel-Haenszel test) measures the association of three discrete variables, which usually consists of two dichotomous IVs and one categorical confounding variable or covariate.

Testing for Differences From the Population

Parametric Tests

One Sample Z Test The one sample z test is used to assess for a difference between the mean of the study sample and a known population mean.

One Sample T Test Only in rare cases is the population SD known; thus, test statistics often must be based on sample data (ie, SD and sample size). The one sample t test is used in situations where only the population mean is known, or can at least be estimated by very large amounts of data.

Nonparametric Tests

Binomial Test The binomial test is used when the DV is dichotomous (eg, inpatient or outpatient, male or female) and all of the possible data (or outcomes) fall into one, and only one, of the two categories. The binomial test uses the binomial distribution to test the exact probability of whether the sample proportion differs from the proportion expected by chance (ie, the expected population proportion).

Kolmogorov-Smirnov One Sample Test The Kolmogorov-Smirnov one sample test is a goodness-of-fit test used to determine the degree of agreement between the distribution of a researcher's sample data and a theoretical population distribution.

Testing for Between-Group Differences

Parametric Tests

Independent Samples T Test The independent samples t test (also referred to as Student's t test) is used to assess a statistically significant difference between the means of the two mutually exclusive (ie, independent) groups.

One-Way Analysis of Variance An ANOVA is an extension of the independent samples *t* test to situations where researchers want to assess for mean differences between three or more mutually exclusive groups.

Analysis of Covariance ANCOVA is an extension of ANOVA where main effects and interactions are assessed after statistically adjusting for one (or more) confounding variables called covariates. That is, ANCOVA adjusts all group means to create the situation as if all participants scored identically on the covariate.

Nonparametric Tests

Mann-Whitney Test The Mann-Whitney test is the nonparametric alternative to the independent samples *t* test and is one of the most powerful nonparametric tests. It is used when the distribution of a continuous DV is not normal or when the DV is measured on an ordinal scale. The Mann-Whitney test is based on ranked data. That is, instead of using the actual values of the DV, as an independent samples *t* test does, each participant's DV value is ranked with the highest value receiving the highest rank and the lowest value receiving the lowest rank. The ranks within each group are then summed, and the test assesses whether the difference in ranked sums between groups is statistically significant.

Kruskal-Wallis One-Way ANOVA by Ranks The Kruskal-Wallis one-way ANOVA by ranks (or simply, the Kruskal-Wallis test) is the nonparametric alternative to the one-way ANOVA. The test is an extension of the Mann-Whitney test to assess group differences between three or more mutually exclusive groups. The Kruskal-Wallis test is typically used when the distribution of a continuous DV is not normal or when the DV is measured on an ordinal scale.

Testing for Within-Group Differences

Parametric Tests

Paired Samples T Test The paired samples *t* test (also known as the matched *t* test or nested *t* test) is used when one group of participants is measured on the DV twice, or two groups of participants are matched on specific characteristics.

One-Way Repeated Measures ANOVA A one-way repeated measures ANOVA (or simply repeated measures ANOVA) is an extension of the paired samples *t* test to situations where the DV is measured three or more times. This can occur when the same participants are measured repeatedly or when three or more matched groups are measured once.

Nonparametric Tests

Wilcoxon Signed-Rank Test The Wilcoxon signed-rank test (or simply signed-rank test) is the nonparametric alternative to a paired samples *t* test. The test is used typically when the

distribution of the DV is not normal or when the DV is measured on an ordinal scale to assess for differences between two repeated measurements (or two matched groups).

Friedman Two-Way ANOVA by Ranks The Friedman two-way ANOVA by ranks test (or simply the Friedman test) is the nonparametric alternative to the one-way repeated measures ANOVA and is an extension of the signed-rank test to a situation with three or more repeated measurements. Similar to the other nonparametric tests, it is most often used when the distribution of the DV is not normal or the DV is measured on an ordinal scale. The Friedman test is based on ranked data, with higher scores receiving higher ranks, and is used to assess for statistically significant differences between repeated measurements.

The Sign Test The sign test is another nonparametric alternative to the paired samples *t* test. Similar to the signed-rank test, the sign test is used typically when the distribution of the DV is not normal or when the DV is measured on an ordinal scale.

The McNemar Test of Change The McNemar test of change (or simply the McNemar test) is an extension of the chi square and Fisher's exact test when participants are measured on two separate occasions and assesses the statistical significance of observed changes between the two repeated measurements.

The Cochran's Q Test The Cochran's Q test (or simply Cochran's Q) is an extension of the McNemar test to situations where participants are measured repeatedly on three or more separate occasions. Similar to the McNemar test, the DV must be measured repeatedly on a dichotomous scale.

Testing for Relationships or Associations

When exploring the association or relationship between two or more variables, two specific types of analyses are employed—correlation or regression. These analyses are applied to determine the magnitude and direction of an association or relationship. Correlation analysis indicates the corelationship of two variables (ie, how one variable changes in relationship to the other). It is critically important to note that correlation does not imply causation. Regression analysis is a type of correlational analysis used to predict the value of one variable from the value of another variable. In this type of analysis, researchers attempt to determine the amount of variance in the DV that is explained by the IV(s) or covariates. Note that regression analysis can also permit multiple IVs and/or covariates measured on any scale. This type of analysis is referred to as a multivariate or multivariable analysis.

Parametric Tests

Pearson's Product-Moment Correlation Pearson's product-moment correlation (or simply Pearson's correlation or Pearson's *r*) is one of the most commonly used correlation measures. It measures the direction and strength of a linear relationship between two variables measured on a continuous scale. Pearson's *r* ranges from −1 and +1, with *r* of 0 indicating no relationship. That is, as the correlation approaches −1 or 1, the relationship becomes stronger. A positive correlation (eg, 0.30 or 0.99) indicates that as the values of one variable increase so do the values of the other variable, while a negative correlation (eg, −0.50 or −0.80) indicates that as the values of one variable increase, the values of the other variable decrease.

Simple Linear Regression The magnitude of the correlation is directly related to the strength of the linear relationship. The pattern of this linear relationship is typically identified by the regression line. The regression line is a best fit line describing how a continuous response variable (DV) changes as the explanatory variable (IV) changes. The statistical test in simple linear regression is whether the slope of the regression line is statistically different from zero (ie, no slope or horizontal).

Multiple Linear Regression Multiple (sometimes called multivariate or multivariable) linear regression is an extension of simple linear regression for designs with one continuous DV and multiple IVs or covariates. Remember, an IV is defined as an explanatory variable of specific research interest, while a covariate is a nuisance variable that is significantly associated with the DV but not of specific research interest. That is, covariates are typically included because they are related to the DV or because previous research has indicated they are important. In multiple linear regression, IVs can be any combination of continuous or discrete variables (eg, height, gender, HbA1c). Further, this analysis is often a better option than simple linear regression because the inclusion of additional IVs often explains a higher percentage of variance in the DV, that is, higher *R* values.

Nonparametric Tests

Spearman Rank-Order Correlation Coefficient The Spearman rank-order correlation coefficient (r_s), also known as Spearman's rho (ρ), is the nonparametric alternative to Pearson's *r*. This correlation is used when the two variables being considered are not normally distributed, when the variables are measured on an ordinal scale, or when the relationship between the two variables is nonlinear. This correlation is based on rank-ordered data as opposed to the actual values.

Logistic Regression The interpretation of a logistic regression analysis is similar to linear regression; thus, a basic understanding of the interpretation of simple and multiple linear regressions is extremely useful. Logistic regression is used when the DV is measured on a discrete scale and the relationship between the DV and IV is nonlinear.

Survival Analysis Survival analysis (or failure analysis) consists of two of the most commonly used statistical techniques in the biomedical sciences—the Kaplan-Meier method and Cox regression. In general, survival analysis is concerned with time-to-event data; that is, the time to experience an outcome of interest. In survival analysis, participants who do not experience the outcome of interest (which for survival analysis is called the event) are considered to survive, while those who experience the event are considered to fail.

CASE Application

1. Which of the following is the outcome variable for a study? Select all that apply.

   a. DV
   b. IV
   c. Confounder
   d. Population

2. Which of the following represent scales of measurement? Select all that apply.

   a. Nominal
   b. Ordinal
   c. Interval
   d. Ratio scales

3. A pharmacy resident in South Carolina is charged with evaluating daptomycin as her research project for the year. She is evaluating all patients within 18 months and comparing them to vancomycin. The primary outcome is clinical response as defined by clearance of bacteremia within 5 days. Her data collection sheet has two boxes for the primary outcome (yes and no). What type of measurement scale is the resident collecting?

   a. Nominal
   b. Ordinal
   c. Interval
   d. Ratio scales

4. The pharmacy resident in question number 3 completed her study and demonstrated that vancomycin has a higher cure rate of bacteremia at 5 days as compared to daptomycin. She was concerned that she had introduced error into her study because of a low sample size (17 daptomycin patients and 34 vancomycin patients). Additionally, she was concerned that measuring the outcome as yes/no impacted the results. She is going to repeat the study and make two modifications: (1) she has recruited other pharmacy residents to participate to increase the sample size and (2) she has changed the primary outcome to days bacteremic. She will record the number of days until the patient has a negative blood culture. What type of measurement scale is the resident now collecting?

   a. Nominal
   b. Ordinal
   c. Interval
   d. Ratio scales

5. The pharmacy resident is also measuring the impact of obesity on the clinical outcomes. She is recording each

patient's weight, height, and BMI. What type of variables is she recording?

a. Continuous
b. Discrete
c. Categorical
d. Dichotomous

6. The resident is compiling the data of the repeat daptomycin study. A fellow resident collected the same variables she collected; however, instead of recording actual BMI, she categorized patients based on the World Health Organization's (WHO) classification of obesity. What type of variable is she recording by using the WHO system? Select all that apply.

a. Continuous
b. Discrete
c. Categorical
d. Dichotomous

7. Which of the following are measures of central tendency? Select all that apply.

a. Mean
b. Median
c. Mode
d. Average

8. Which of the following measures of central tendency is calculated by summing all data for a variable and dividing by the total number of patients? Select all that apply.

a. Mean
b. Median
c. Mode
d. 50th percentile

9. The pharmacy resident from question number 3 is writing her residency report about her study (the first study). She has to report measures of central tendency as appropriate. What measure of central tendency should she utilize for her primary outcome? Select all that apply.

a. Mean
b. Median
c. Mode
d. Average

10. The pharmacy resident has completed her study report and is not analyzing the second study. She has decided to utilize BMI as categorized by the WHO. What measure of central tendency should be utilized? Select all that apply.

a. Mean
b. Median
c. Mode
d. 50th percentile

11. Which of the following are measures of variability? Select all that apply.

a. SD
b. Range
c. IQR
d. Variance

12. Which of the following are measures of variability?

a. Mean
b. SD
c. Student paired t test
d. Nominal data

13. Which of the following terms describes variability around the median?

a. SD
b. IQR
c. Ordinal data
d. ANOVA

14. Which of the following statements identifies properties of a normal distribution (Gaussian distribution) regarding the central tendency, variability, and shape? Select all that apply.

a. Primary shape is a bell curve
b. Mean, median, and mode are identical
c. The distribution is symmetrical
d. Skewness and kurtosis are zero

15. What type of distribution is utilized for nominal data?

a. Gaussian
b. Binomial
c. Positive skew
d. Negative skew

16. A case-control study of 2300 participants looked at the association between acetaminophen and renal disease. The study included 537 cases. There were 224 cases and 130 controls taking acetaminophen. The 2×2 table has been filled in.

Acetaminophen	Renal Disease	No Renal Disease	
Exposed	224	130	354
Unexposed	313	1633	1946
	537	1763	2300

What is the odds ratio of this study?

a. OR = (224/354)/(313/1946) = 3.93
b. OR = (224/313)/(130/1633) = 8.99
c. OR = (224/2300) = 0.097

17. What is an example of a nonparametric test?

a. Student's t test
b. z test

c. ANOVA

d. Fisher's exact test

18. Which of the following statement(s) is true about statistical power? Select all that apply.

    a. Power increases when Type 1 error increases

    b. Power increases when sample size decreases

    c. Power increases when effect size increases

    d. Power is unaffected by error variance

19. Azithromycin was compared to amoxicillin and levofloxacin in a retrospective, observational pharmacoepidemiology study. The study used a national cohort of patients from an insurance claims database. The research question was: does azithromycin have a higher risk of all causes of death compared to a control antibiotic group? The hypothesis from the research group was that azithromycin will have a higher rate of all causes of death. The study produced the following study results:

Hazard Ratio (95% CIs) for Multiple Comparisons of All Causes of Death

Antibiotic	Amoxicillin
Azithromycin	1.48 (1.05-2.09)
Levofloxacin	2.49 (1.70-3.64)

Based upon the results of the study, select the statement that accurately describes the azithromycin and amoxicillin contrast.

    a. Amoxicillin has a 48% increased risk of death compared to azithromycin.

    b. Azithromycin has a 48% increased risk of death compared to amoxicillin.

    c. There is no statistical significance among the results of azithromycin compared to azithromycin.

    d. Levofloxacin has a 2.49-fold increased risk of death compared to amoxicillin.

20. Azithromycin was compared to amoxicillin and levofloxacin in a retrospective, observational pharmacoepidemiology study. The study used a national cohort of patients from an insurance claims database. The research question was: does azithromycin have a higher risk of arrhythmia compared to a control antibiotic group? The hypothesis from the research group was that azithromycin will have a higher rate of arrhythmia. The study produced the following study results:

Hazard Ratio (95% CIs) for Multiple Comparisons Arrhythmia

Antibiotic	Amoxicillin	Azithromycin	Levofloxacin
Amoxicillin	1	0.56 (0.38-0.83)	0.41 (0.26-0.64)
Azithromycin	1.77 (1.20-2.62)	1	0.73 (0.47-1.13)
Levofloxacin	2.43 (1.56-3.79)	1.37 (0.88-2.13)	1

Based upon the results of the study, select the statement that accurately describes the azithromycin and amoxicillin contrast(s).

21. Which of the following CIs indicates the results are statistically significant? Select all that apply.

Hazard Ratio (95% CIs) for Multiple Comparisons Arrhythmia

Antibiotic	Amoxicillin	Azithromycin	Levofloxacin
Amoxicillin	1	0.56 (0.38-0.83)	0.41 (0.26-0.64)
Azithromycin	1.77 (1.20-2.62)	1	0.73 (0.47-1.13)
Levofloxacin	2.43 (1.56-3.79)	1.37 (0.88-2.13)	1

    a. The amoxicillin to amoxicillin contrast

    b. The amoxicillin to levofloxacin contrast

    c. The levofloxacin to amoxicillin contrast

    d. The azithromycin to amoxicillin contrast

    e. The azithromycin to levofloxacin contrast

22. Which of the following definitions describes ITT?

    a. A design where the independent variable typically involves participants randomized into fixed levels of treatment (or arms), with each arm indicating a different treatment or comparison (eg, placebo, active control)

    b. A design which has the primary purpose of having a participant serve as his or her own control

    c. A design that implements changes (or adaptations) in the design or endpoint analyses based on the results of a predetermined (ie, prior to initiation of the study) set of interim analyses

    d. The analysis includes all participants in the arm to which they were randomized originally

    e. Evaluates only compliant participants with complete data

23. A study was evaluating the mortality of a new medication for acute coronary syndrome compared to the standard of care. The outcome of interest (mortality) was recorded as yes or no at the end of the 3-year study period. Patients were randomized to treatment groups and the results were reported as ITT. What would be the statistical test that can evaluate the outcome of interest?

    a. Pearson's chi square test

    b. Cochran-Mantel-Haenszel test

    c. Independent samples t test

    d. Student's t test

    e. Analysis of covariance

24. A study was evaluating the cholesterol values of a new medication for dyslipidemia compared to the standard of care. The outcome of interest (mean total cholesterol level) was recorded as a continuous variable (ie, ratio data).

The questions for #20's answer options (from the right column top):

    a. Amoxicillin has a 77% increased risk of arrhythmia compared to azithromycin.

    b. There is not statistical difference in arrhythmia risk between azithromycin and amoxicillin.

    c. Amoxicillin has a 56% lower risk of arrhythmia compared to azithromycin.

    d. Amoxicillin has a 44% lower risk of arrhythmia compared to azithromycin.

Patients were randomized to treatment groups and the results were reported as ITT. The total cholesterol values for the study represented a normal distribution. What would be the statistical test that can evaluate the outcome of interest?

a. Paired t test
b. ANOVA
c. T test
d. Mann-Whitney

25. A study was evaluating the mean blood pressure values of a new medication for hypertension compared to the

standard of care. The outcome of interest (mean blood pressure) was recorded as a continuous variable (ie, ratio data). Each patient served as their own control. The results were reported as ITT. The mean blood pressure values for the study had mean and median that were very different. What would be the statistical test that can evaluate the outcome of interest?

a. Paired t test
b. Wilcoxon signed-rank test
c. Kruskal-Wallis One-Way ANOVA
d. Fisher's exact test

TAKEAWAY POINTS »

- A population refers to all objects of a similar type in the universe, while a sample is a fraction of the population chosen to be representative of the specific population of interest. Thus, samples are chosen to make generalizations about the population of interest.

- A variable is a characteristic that is being observed or measured. Data are the measured values assigned to the variable for each individual member of the population. For example, a variable would be patient gender, while the data is whether the patient is male or female. There are three types of variables: dependent (DV), independent (IV), and confounding.

- There are four levels of measurement: nominal, ordinal, interval, and ratio scales. The scale of measurement is an important consideration when determining the appropriate statistical test to answer the research question and hypothesis.

- A nominal scale consists of categories that have no implied rank or order (male versus female; or absence versus presence).

- An ordinal scale has all of the characteristics of a nominal variable; however, the data are placed into rank-ordered categories.

- Interval scales consist of ordered data points on a constant scale without a natural zero.

- Ratio scales differ from interval scales in that they have an absolute zero.

- There are two types of statistics: descriptive and inferential.

- Descriptive statistics present, organize, and summarize data in a very basic sense, while providing information regarding the appearance of the data and distributional assumptions.

- Inferential statistics test for differences or relationships, against random variation, within the study sample, allowing reliable findings to be generalized to the population of interest.

- Measures of central tendency are helpful in identifying the distribution of the data numerically. Common measures of central tendency are the mean, median, and mode.

- Measures of variability (or dispersion) are the range, IQR, variance, and SD. Measures of variability are useful in indicating the spread of data for a variable. These measures are also useful in association with measures of central tendency to assess how scattered the data are around the mean or median.

- The field of epidemiology investigates how diseases are distributed in the population and the various factors (or exposures) influencing this distribution.

- Incidence quantifies the occurrence of an event or outcome, for a specific study period, within a specific population.

- Prevalence quantifies the number of patients who have already experienced the event or outcome at a specific time point.

- Relative risk is defined as the ratio (or probability) of the incidence of an event occurring in individuals exposed to a risk compared to the incidence of the event in those not exposed to the risk.

- Sensitivity, specificity, and predictive values (both positive and negative) measure the ability of a test to identify correctly those experiencing the event and those who did not.

- A hypothesis indicates a theory about the population regarding an outcome the researcher is interested in studying.

- A Type I error occurs when the researcher indicates a statistically significant difference exists when, in fact, one actually does not (ie, FP).

- A Type II error occurs when the researcher fails to indicate a statistically significant difference when one actually exists (ie, FN).

- Statistical power was developed as a method allowing researchers to calculate the probability of finding a statistically significant result, when, in fact, one actually exists.

- ITT requires the analysis to include all participants in the arm to which they were randomized originally.

BIBLIOGRAPHY

Bentley JP. Biostatistics and pharmacoepidemiology. In: Yang Y, West-Strum D, eds. *Understanding Pharmacoepidemiology.* New York, NY: McGraw-Hill; 2011:chap 5.

Dawson B, Trapp RG. Analyzing research questions about survival. In: Dawson B, Trapp RG, eds. *Basic & Clinical Biostatistics.* 4th ed. New York, NY: McGraw-Hill; 2004:chap 9.

Said Q. Other methodological issues. In: Yang Y, West-Strum D, eds. *Understanding Pharmacoepidemiology.* New York, NY: McGraw-Hill; 2011:chap 6.

Shargel L, Wu-Pong S, Yu AC. Appendix A: Statistics. In: Shargel L, Wu-Pong S, Yu AC, eds. *Applied Biopharmaceutics & Pharmacokinetics.* 6th ed. New York, NY: McGraw-Hill; 2012.

Walters RW, Kier KL. The application of statistical analysis in the biomedical sciences. In: Malone PM, Kier KL, Stanovich JE, eds. *Drug Information: A Guide for Pharmacists.* 4th ed. New York, NY: McGraw-Hill; 2012:chap 8.

KEY ABBREVIATIONS

ANCOVA = analysis of covariance
ANOVA = one-way analysis of variance
BMI = body mass index
CI = confidence interval
df = degrees of freedom
DV = dependent variable
FN = false negative
FP = false positive

IDV = independent variable
ITT = intent-to-treat
PP = per-protocol
RCT = randomized control trial
SEM = standard error of the mean
TN = true negative
TP = true positive
WHO = World Health Organization

72

Pharmacy Math I

Minou Khazan, Cynthia Phillips, Michaela Almgren, and S. Scott Sutton

FOUNDATION OVERVIEW

Units of Measure

Pharmaceutical calculations involve four different systems of measure: the International System of Units (SI), formerly known as the metric system, apothecaries', avoirdupois', and household. SI is an international decimalized system of measurement that recognizes the following units: gram, liter, and meter. SI is a decimal system, in the sense that all multiples and submultiples of the base units are factors of powers of ten of the unit. Examples of the SI system include:

Name	Prefix	Factor
Mega	M	10^6
Kilo	k	10^3
Deci	d	10^{-1}
Centi	c	10^{-2}
Milli	m	10^{-3}
Micro	μ	10^{-6}
Nano	n	10^{-9}
Pico	p	10^{-12}

The apothecaries' system is a traditional system of measurement using drams (liquids) and grains (solids) and is occasionally found in prescriptions. For example, a prescribed medicine being sold in four ounce (℥ iv) bottles or five grains (V gr.) of aspirin. The system consists of two basic units, grains for solids and minims for liquids. Examples of the apothecaries' system are listed in Table 72-1.

The avoirdupois system is a system of weights or mass commonly used in the United States for measuring body weight and in selling products. The avoirdupois ounce equals 437.5 grains. Sixteen ounces (7000 grains) corresponds to 1 pound (lb) (Table 72-2).

A common household unit of measure includes the teaspoon and tablespoon. A teaspoon is equivalent to 5 mL and a tablespoon is equivalent to 3 teaspoons. Other household liquid measurements are listed in Table 72-3.

Number Systems

Pharmaceutical calculations utilize two systems of numbers, Arabic and Roman. The Arabic system is more commonly used; however, the Roman system is occasionally utilized. The Roman numeral system uses letters to represent quantities and amounts. Common examples of Roman numerals include:

- ss = ½
- I = 1
- V = 5
- X = 10
- L = 50
- C = 100
- D = 500
- M = 1000

Roman numerals may be grouped together to express different quantities. To interpret these numbers, addition and subtraction may be needed. Key issues for Roman numerals include:

- When a numeral is repeated or a smaller numeral follows a larger one, the values are added together.
- ii = 2 (1 + 1 = 2)
- CXIII = 113 (100 + 10 + 1+ 1 + 1 = 113)
- When a smaller numeral comes before a larger numeral, subtract the smaller value.
- IV = 4 (5 – 1 = 4)
- IX = 9 (10 – 1 = 9)
- Numerals are never repeated more than three times in a sequence.
- III = 3
- IV = 4
- When a smaller numeral comes between two larger numerals, subtract the smaller numeral from the numeral following.
- XIV = 14 (10 + 5 – 1 = 14)
- XIX = 19 (10 + 10 – 1 = 19)

The Arabic system is a decimal system. The decimal point serves as the anchor. Each place to the left of the decimal signals a 10-fold increase and each place to the right signals a 10-fold decrease.

To access your complimentary online question exams, visit https://accesspharmacy.mhmedical.com/NAPLEX.aspx

TABLE 72-1	**Apothecaries' System of Measure**[a]			

Weight

- 20 grains = 1 scruple
- 60 grains = 3 scruples = 1 dram
- 480 grains = 24 scruples = 8 drams = 1 ounce
- 5760 grains = 288 scruples = 96 drams = 12 ounces = 1 pound

Pound (lb)	Ounce ($\mathfrak{Z}$)	Dram	Scruple	Grain
1	12	96	288	5760
	1	8	24	480
		1	3	60
			1	20

Volume

- 60 minims = 1 fluidram
- 480 minims = 8 fluidrams = 1 fl oz
- 7680 minims = 128 fluidrams = 16 fl oz = 1 pt
- 15360 minims = 256 fluidrams = 32 fl oz = 2 pt = 1 qt
- 61440 minims = 1024 fluidrams = 128 fl oz = 8 pt = 4 quarts = 1 gallon

Gallon (gal)	Quart (qt)	Pint (pt)	Fluidounce (f$\mathfrak{Z}$)	Fluidram	Minim
1	4	8	128	1024	61440
	1	2	32	256	15360
		1	16	128	7680
			1	8	480
				1	60

[a]Note: Apothecary and avoirdupois systems of measure have common terms—grain, pounds, and ounces. Pounds and ounces each have different values in each system. The grain, however, has the same value in both the avoirdupois and the apothecary systems.

Percentage and Ratio Strengths

Medications are administered as dosage forms that contain active and inactive ingredients; however, the amount of the active ingredient in a preparation needs to be expressed. A preparation may be a solution, but may also refer to a powder mixture, ointment, etc. There are several ways to do this and they include: (1) amount per individual dosage form (capsule, tablet); (2) concentration per dosing volume; (3) percent; (4) ratio strength; and (4) parts per million.

Percentage specifies the number of active parts per 100 parts (eg, the number of parts of solute in 100 total parts of solution). In pharmacy, this is expressed in three ways:

- Percent weight-in-weight: % (w/w) = grams of ingredient in 100 grams of product; assumed for mixtures of solids and semisolids

- Percent volume-in-volume: % (v/v) = milliliters of ingredient in 100 milliliters of product; assumed for solutions of liquids in liquids

- Percent weight-in-volume: % (w/v) = grams of ingredient in 100 milliliters of product; assumed for solutions, or suspensions of solids in liquids, or gases in liquids

Note: In performing calculations, percentages may be changed to a decimal fraction by eliminating the % sign and dividing the numerator by 100.

$$0.05\% = 0.05/100 \text{ or } 0.0005$$

In reverse, a concentration expressed as a decimal can be converted to a % by multiplying by 100.

$$0.50 \times 100 = 50\%$$

TABLE 72-2	**Avoirdupois System of Measure**[a]		

- 1 ounce	= 437.5 grains		
- 16 ounces	= 1 pound (lb)		
	= 256 drams		
	= 7000 grains		

Pound (lb)	Ounce (oz)	Grains (gr)
1	16	7000
	1	437.5

[a]Note: Apothecary and avoirdupois systems of measure have common terms—grain, pounds, and ounces. Pounds and ounces each have different values in each system. The grain, however, has the same value in both the avoirdupois and the apothecary systems.

TABLE 72-3	**Household System of Measure**

1 tablespoon (T) = 15 mL
1 teaspoon (tsp) = 5 mL
2 tablespoons = 1 fluid ounce (fl oz) = 1/8 cup
1 cup = 8 fl oz
1 pint = 16 fl oz = 2 cups
1 quart = 32 fl oz = 4 cups
1 gallon = 128 fl oz = 16 cups

Ratio and proportions are frequently encountered calculations in pharmacy. Ratio strength expresses concentration in terms of parts of active ingredient related to parts of the whole. When expressing a ratio strength, the numerator is preferably set as 1. It is written with a colon between the numbers. The expression 1:2 means there is 1 part in a total of 2 parts. A ratio of 1:100 means there is 1 part of a drug to 100 parts of a mixture or preparation.

Example: 5 ounces of drug A mixed with water to make 20 ounces of mixture is 5:20 or 1:4. The ratio may be written as 1:4 or as a fraction ¼.

A proportion is the expression of two ratios, which are equal. It is usually written in one of two ways: two equal fractions (a/b = c/d) or using a colon (a:b = c:d).

Parts per million is a special case of ratio strength used to express very dilute solution concentrations. Instead of fixing the numerator as 1, the denominator is fixed as 1,000,000. Parts per notation is used to denote relative proportions in measured quantities, particularly in low-value (high-ratio) proportions.

- ppm (parts per million) represents the number of parts of solute in 10^6 parts of solution

- ppb (parts per billion) represents the number of parts of solute in 10^9 parts of solution

- ppt (parts per trillion) represents the number of parts of solute in 10^{12} parts of solution

Preparations of Solutions—Dilution, Concentration, and Alligation

Dilution

Medications are often prepared by pharmaceutical manufacturers with adult usage as the primary intent. Pharmacists will encounter clinical situations in which patients are children or small in stature requiring the medication to be diluted.

Example: An aminoglycoside antibiotic injection is available as a 10 mg/mL preparation and the infant is to receive 4 mg. Volumes less than 1 mL are considered too small to measure accurately. Therefore, you must dilute the preparation. Prepare the dilution to a final concentration of 1 mg/mL. How much medication and how much diluent will you need if the aminoglycoside comes as 10 mg/mL in a 1 mL vial, and the entire contents of the vial are to be used?

$$\frac{1\ mg}{1\ mL} = \frac{10\ mg}{x\ mL} \quad x = 10\ mL \text{ (total volume of the preparation)}$$

- 10 mL – 1 mL (aminoglycoside) = 9 mL diluent Solution will then be 10 mg/10 mL (1 mg/mL).

$$\frac{1\ mg}{1\ mL} = \frac{4\ mg}{x\ mL} \quad x = 4\ mL \text{ (of solution will contain 4 mg of aminoglycoside)}$$

Concentration

A solution is a mixture of two or more substances. Solutions exist in three states: gas, liquid, or solid. A solution may exist in which the components are: (1) both liquids (a mixed drink); (2) a gas in a liquid (soda water); and (3) solid in a liquid (salt water). In a solution, the substance dissolved in the liquid is the solute and the liquid is the solvent. If both substances are liquids, the component with the least amount is the solute. Concentration may be defined as follows:

Concentration = Quantity of solute/Quantity of preparation

Examples:

- A 9% solution means there are 9 parts of the drug in 100 parts of solution.

- When the drug is a liquid, 1:50 means 1 mL of drug in 50 mL of solution.

- When the drug is a solid or in dry form, 1:50 means 1 g of drug in 50 mL of solution.

Powder Volume

A medication in a solid or dry form has a weight that is taken into account when preparing solutions or suspensions; however, when this solid or dry powder is added to the diluent, it also occupies a certain volume of space. When dealing with dry pharmaceuticals, this space is called powder volume. Powder volume is equivalent to the difference between the final volume and the volume of diluent added.

Example: QP is a cystic fibrosis patient prescribed a broad-spectrum antibiotic to treat a *Pseudomonas aeruginosa* infection. You are to reconstitute a dry powder that is 500 mg. The label states that you are to add 9.3 mL and the resultant solution will be 50 mg/mL. What is the powder volume?

$$\frac{500\ mg}{x\ mL} = \frac{50\ mg}{1\ mL} \quad x = 10\ mL$$

10 mL is the final volume. You added 9.3 mL, therefore the difference (10 mL – 9.3 mL = 0.7 mL) is the powder volume.

The same calculations may be made to determine powder volume for both dry powders intended for oral use and those intended for parenteral solution.

Alligation

The mixing of solutions or solids possessing different percentage strengths presents a calculation problem, which may be solved using an arithmetic method called alligation. In setting up an alligation formula, you must express the strength of each component as a percentage. Then you will determine how many parts of each different percent strength product you will need to create the final desired concentration of your product. Finally, you will be able to calculate the exact quantity of each beginning product you will need to create the final product. Alligation involves changing the percentages to parts and by using ratio and proportion, solving for the unknown amount of each initial product.

Example: Prepare 500 mL of dextrose 7.5% using dextrose 5% and dextrose 50%. How many milliliter of each solution will be needed?

Subtract the desired concentration from the larger starting concentration and subtract the lesser concentration from the desired concentration. Then add the difference from the first equation and the difference from the second equation to obtain the total parts of component.

Step 1:

$$\frac{45 \text{ parts}}{500 \text{ mL}} = \frac{2.5 \text{ parts}}{x \text{ mL D50W}} \quad x = 27.78 \text{ mL D50W}$$

Step 2:

$$\frac{45 \text{ parts}}{500 \text{ mL}} = \frac{42.5 \text{ parts}}{x \text{ mL D5W}} = 472.22 \text{ mL D5W}$$

Step 3: Check to see if the two volumes of the two ingredients are equal to the total required volume

$$472.22 \text{ mL} + 27.78 \text{ mL} = 500 \text{ mL}$$

Step 4: Another method to check your answer involves comparing the grams of dextrose of the three solutions. The grams of dextrose from the resultant 7.5% solution should equal the sum of the grams from the 50% and 5% solution.

(a) 500 mL total solution × 0.075 (7.5% solution was the desired final concentration) = 37.5 g of dextrose is the amount made in the solution. When we compare the grams of dextrose contributed by the D50W and the D5W, it should equal the 37.5 g.

(b) 27.78 mL × 0.50 (D50W) = 13.89 g of dextrose

(c) 472.22 mL × 0.05 (D5W) = 23.61 g of dextrose

(d) 13.89 g + 23.61 g = 37.5 g of dextrose

Other Units of Measure

Density and Specific Gravity

Density describes the relationship between the mass of a substance and the volume it occupies.

$$\text{Density} = \frac{\text{Mass}}{\text{Volume}}$$

Utilization of density allows conversion from a volume measure to a weight measure or vice versa and is usually expressed as grams per cubic centimeter or g/mL.

The specific gravity (sp gr) is a ratio of the weight of a material to the weight of the same volume of standard material. For liquids, the standard material is water, which has a density of 1 g/mL. Specific gravity is unit-less, because it is equal to the density divided by density of standard material; therefore, the units cancel out.

$$\text{Specific gravity} = \frac{\text{Weight of substance}}{\text{Weight of equal volume of water}}$$

Thus,

Weight of substance = Volume of substance × Specific gravity

or,

$$g = mL \times sp\ gr$$

Examples:

- Water is the standard material. It weighs 100 g/100 mL or a specific gravity of 1. Therefore, everything is compared to it.
- If the weight of 100 mL of a 50% solution of dextrose is 117 g, what is the specific gravity of the dextrose solution?
- 117 g (weight of the dextrose solution)/100 g (weight of a 100 mL of water) = 1.17 specific gravity
- If a liquid has a specific gravity of 0.75, what is the weight of 150 mL?
- g = mL × sp gr
- g = 150 × 0.75 = 112.5 g

Milliequivalents

A milliequivalent (mEq) describes the ability of an inorganic molecule to dissociate in a liquid and is a measurement of the chemical activity of an electrolyte based on its valence. The equivalent weight of an ion is the atomic weight of the ion divided by the absolute value of its valence. Thus, the equivalent weight of ferric ion, Fe^{3+} (atomic weight 55.9, valence 3) is 18.6. A milliequivalent is one-thousandth of an equivalent weight (eg, there are 1000 milliequivalent weights in 1 equivalent weight). For a molecule, the equivalent weight is obtained from the gram molecular weight (formula weight) divided by the total cation or the total anion charge.

Examples: Most electrolytes are measured by the milliequivalent method (the measure of the ion's combining power). The valence of an ion determines how many other ions it must combine with to form a stable compound. The valence is important, but not the positive or negative charge.

- Water (H_2O): Hydrogen has a valence of 1 and oxygen has a valance of 2. It takes two hydrogen ions to form a stable compound with 1 oxygen ion.
- Molecular weight, formula weight, and atomic weights are just numbers with no units attached.
- The atomic weight (with the unit of grams attached) and the valence determine the equivalent weight.
- Equivalent weight (in grams) = atomic weight/valence
- Sodium has an atomic weight of 22.99 and a valence of 1.
- 1 equivalent weight of sodium = 22.99/1 = 22.99 g or 23 g
- The milliequivalent (mEq) weight is one-thousandth the equivalent weight. The milliequivalent formula is similar to the equivalent weight formula; however, mEq weight is expressed in milligrams.
- Milliequivalent weight (in mg) = atomic weight/valence
- Sodium has an atomic weight of 22.99 and a valence of 1.
- 1 mEq weight of sodium = 22.99/1 valence = 22.99 mg or 23 mg
- The mEq weight may be used to convert between mg and mEq using the equation:
  - mg = mEq × molecular weight (atomic weight)/valence or
  - mEq = mg × valence/molecular weight (atomic weight)
- Sodium has an atomic weight of 23 and a valence of 1. How many mEq are present in 115 mg of sodium?

  - Using the equation above: $mEq = mg \times \dfrac{\text{Valence}}{\text{Atomic weight}}$
  - mEq = 115 × 1/23
  - mEq = 5, so 115 mg of Na is equivalent to 5 mEq of Na

- Or solving by proportion:

$$\frac{115 \text{ mg sodium}}{x \text{ mEq}} = \frac{23 \text{ mg sodium (atomic weight)}}{1 \text{ mEq}}$$

$$= 5 \text{ mEq in } 115 \text{ mg sodium}$$

Moles and Millimoles

A mole equals the molecular weight of a substance in grams. A millimole (mmol) equals the molecular weight or formula weight of a substance in milligrams. A one molar solution contains 1 g of molecular weight (1 GMW = 1 mole = weight in grams of Avogadro's number of particles) per liter of solution. The molarity expresses the number of moles per liter. The millimolarity (millimoles/liter) is 1/1000 times the molarity of a solution.

Examples: Magnesium has an atomic weight of 24. What is the weight of 1 millimole (mmol)?

$$1 \text{ mmol} = 24/1000 = 0.024 \text{ g or } 24 \text{ mg}$$

Milliosmoles

Osmotic concentration is a measure of the total number of particles in solution and is expressed in milliosmoles (mOsmol). Thus, the number of milliosmoles is based on the total number of cations and total number of anions. The milliosmolarity of a solution is the number of milliosmoles per liter of solution (mOsm/L):

$$\text{mOsmol/L} = \frac{\text{Weight of substance (g/L)} \times \text{number of species} \times 1000}{\text{Molecular weight (g)}}$$

Number of species = number of ionic species on complete dissociation (dextrose = 1; NaCl = 2, $MgCl_2$ = 3).

The total osmolarity of a solution is the sum of the osmolarities of the solute components of the solution. When calculating osmolarities in the absence of other information, assume that salts (eg, NaCl) dissociate completely. Be aware of the difference between osmolarity (milliosmoles of solute per liter of solution) and osmolality (milliosmoles of solute per kilogram of solvent).

Intravenous Fluid Rate of Flow

The prescriber must typically specify the flow rate of medication to be delivered via intravenous infusion. The flow rate is generally expressed as an amount of medication per unit of time (eg, milligrams per minute, milligrams per hour), as volume per unit of time (eg, milliliters per minute, liters per hour, drops per minute), or as an amount of medication per kg of patient body weight per unit of time (eg, mg/kg/min). The pharmacist needs to be able to make conversions between different units of flow rate, as well as determine flow rate when needed. Dimensional analysis is the best approach to these types of calculations.

Example: 1500 mg of ampicillin is added to 100 mL of D5W for IV infusion. The patient weighs 176 lb and the infusion will be given over 30 minutes. What should be the rate of infusion in drops per minute if the IV infusion set delivers 15 drops per mL?

$$\frac{100 \text{ mL}}{30 \text{ min}} \times \frac{15 \text{ drops}}{1 \text{ mL}} = 50 \text{ drops/min}$$

CASE Application

1. Identify the Roman numeral with a value of 50.
   a. X
   b. M
   c. I
   d. L

2. Identify the Arabic value of DCXXIV.
   a. 624
   b. 626
   c. 1024
   d. 1026

3. If 120 mL of a cough syrup contains 0.4 g of dextromethorphan, how many milligrams are contained in 1 teaspoonful?
   a. 0.016 mg
   b. 16 mg
   c. 160 mg
   d. 1.6 mg

4. Interferon injection contains 5 million U/mL. How many units are in 0.65 mL?
   a. 3,250 U
   b. 32,500 U
   c. 325,000 U
   d. 3,250,000 U

5. An inhalant solution contains 0.025% w/v of a drug in 5 mL. Calculate the number of milligrams in this solution.
   a. 0.125 mg
   b. 1.25 mg
   c. 12.5 mg
   d. 0.0125 mg

6. How many milligrams of a drug would be contained in a 10 mL container of a 0.65% w/v solution of a drug?
   a. 0.65 mg
   b. 6.5 mg
   c. 65 mg
   d. 650 mg

7. How many milliequivalents of potassium chloride are in 240 mL of a 10% solution of KCl? The gram molecular weight is 74.5 g (K 39 atomic weight; Cl 35.5 atomic weight).
   a. 24 mEq
   b. 0.0745 mEq

c. 2.4 mEq

d. 322 mEq

8. How many milliosmoles (mOsmol) of sodium chloride are there in 1 L of a 0.9% solution of normal saline solution? Molecular weight of NaCl = 58.5.

   a. 58.5 mOsmol

   b. 308 mOsmol

   c. 1 mOsmol

   d. 9000 mOsmol

9. What is the percentage concentration (w/v) of a 250 mL solution containing 100 mEq of ammonium chloride? Molecular weight of NH_4Cl is 53.5.

   a. 53.5%

   b. 5.35%

   c. 2.14%

   d. 21.4%

10. How many millimoles of HCl are contained in 130 mL of a 10% solution? Molecular weight = 36.5.

    a. 356 mmol

    b. 34 mmol

    c. 36.5 mmol

    d. 13 mmol

11. How many 60 mg tablets of codeine sulfate should be used to make this cough syrup?

    Rx :   Codeine SO_4 30 mg/teaspoon

    Cherry Syrup QS ad 150 mL

    Sig: 1 teaspoonful every 6 hours as needed for cough

    a. 7

    b. 15

    c. 20

    d. 24

12. How many milliliters of a 17% solution of benzalonium chloride is required to prepare 350 mL of a 1:750 w/v solution?

    a. 2.75 mL

    b. 0.275 mL

    c. 27.5 mL

    d. 275 mL

13. If 7 mL of a diluent is added to an injectable containing 0.5 g of a drug with a final volume of 7.3 mL, what is the final concentration of the parenteral solution in mg/mL?

    a. 6.85 mg/mL

    b. 0.069 mg/mL

    c. 685 mg/mL

    d. 68.5 mg/mL

14. A medication order of a drug calls for a dose of 0.6 mg/kg to be administered to a child weighing 31 lb. The drug is to be supplied from a solution containing 0.25 g in

50 mL bottles. How many milliliters of this solution are required to fill this order?

    a. 8.45 mL

    b. 0.00845 mL

    c. 1.69 mL

    d. 0.25 mL

15. A solution contains 2 mEq of KCl/mL. If a TPN order calls for the addition of 180 mg of K^+, how many milliliters of this solution should be used to provide the potassium required. Atomic weight of K = 39 and the atomic weight of Cl = 35.5.

    a. 343.85 mL

    b. 2.3 mL

    c. 39 mL

    d. 74.5 mL

16. A TPN solution contains 750 mL of D5W. If each gram of dextrose provides 3.4 kcal, how many kcal would the TPN solution provide?

    a. 127.5 kcal

    b. 37.5 kcal

    c. 34 kcal

    d. 75 kcal

17. Select the definition of specific gravity.

    a. Ratio of the weight of a material to the weight of the same volume of standard material.

    b. The mixing of solutions or solids possessing different percentage strengths.

    c. The expression of two ratios which are equal.

    d. Grams of ingredient in 100 g of product; assumed for mixtures of solids and semisolids.

18. Select the apothecary measure of volume.

    a. Grain

    b. Scruple

    c. Dram

    d. Minim

19. 480 minims equals:

    i. 8 fluidrams

    ii. 1 fl oz

    iii. 1 gallon

    a. i and ii

    b. i and iii

    c. ii and iii

    d. All of the above

20. 437.5 grains equal how many ounces?

    a. 1 oz

    b. 16 oz

    c. 30 oz

    d. 38 oz

21. What should be the flow rate of the medication in milliliters per hour if 100 mg of medication is added to 250 mL of NS and the desired rate of delivery is 5 mg/h?

TAKEAWAY POINTS »

- Pharmaceutical calculations involve four different systems of measure: metric, apothecaries, avoirdupois, and household.

- The International System of Units (SI), formerly called the metric system, is the most common system of measure in pharmacy and uses the following units: gram, liter, and meter. The metric system is decimal, in the sense that all multiples and submultiples of the base units are factors of powers of ten of the unit.

- The apothecaries' system is a traditional system of measurement occasionally found in prescriptions, for example: a prescribed medicine being sold in four ounce (℥ iv) bottles or five grains (V gr.) of aspirin. The system consists of two basic units, grains for solids, and minims for liquids.

- The avoirdupois system is a system of weights or mass. The avoirdupois ounce equals 437.5 grains. Sixteen ounces (7000 grains) correspond to 1 pound (lb).

- Common household units of measure include the teaspoon and tablespoon. A teaspoon is equivalent to 5 mL and a tablespoon is equivalent to three teaspoons.

- Pharmaceutical calculations utilize two systems of numbers: Arabic and Roman. The Arabic system is more commonly used; however, the Roman system is occasionally utilized.

- Medications are administered as dosage forms that contain active and inactive ingredients; however, the amount of the active ingredient needs to be expressed. There are several ways to do this and they include: (1) amount per individual dosage form (capsule, tablet); (2) concentration per dosing volume; (3) percentage; (4) ratio strength; and (5) parts per million.

- Percent weight-in-weight: %(w/w) = grams of ingredient in 100 g of product; assumed for mixtures of solids and semisolids.

- Percent volume-in-volume: %(v/v) = milliliters of ingredient in 100 milliliters of product; assumed for solutions of liquids in liquids.

- Percent weight-in-volume: %(w/v) = grams of ingredient in 100 mL of product; assumed for solutions or suspensions of solids in liquids, or gases in liquids.

- Medications are often prepared by pharmaceutical manufacturers with adult usage as the primary intent. Pharmacists will encounter clinical situations in which patients are children or small in stature requiring the medication to be diluted.

- A medication in a solid or dry form has a weight that is taken into account when preparing solutions; however, when this solid or dry powder is added to the solution, it also occupies a certain volume of space. When dealing with dry pharmaceuticals, this space is called powder volume. Powder volume is equivalent to the difference between the final volume and the volume of diluent added.

- Alligation is an arithmetic method of product preparation that involves using two initial products of differing percentage concentrations. Alligation involves changing the percentages to parts and by using ratio and proportion, solving for the unknown amount of each initial product.

- Density describes the relationship between the mass of a substance and the volume it occupies. Utilization of density allows conversion from a volume measure to a weight measure or vice versa.

- The specific gravity is a ratio of the weight of a material to the weight of the same volume of standard material. For liquids, the standard material is water, which has a density of 1 g/mL.

- A milliequivalent (mEq) is the measurement of the chemical activity of an electrolyte based on its valence and its ability to dissociate in a liquid. The equivalent weight of an ion is the atomic or formula weight of the ion divided by the absolute value of its valence.

- A one molar solution contains 1 g of molecular weight (1 GMW = 1 mole = weight in grams of Avogadro's number of particles) per liter of solution.

- Osmotic concentration is a measure of the total number of particles in solution and is expressed in milliosmoles (mOsmol).

BIBLIOGRAPHY

HC Ansel. *Pharmaceutical Calculations*. 13th ed. Philadelphia, PA: Lippincott Williams & Wilkins; 2010.

JL Zatz, M Teixeira. *Pharmaceutical Calculations*. 3rd ed. New York, NY: John Wiley and Sons, Inc.; 2005.

KEY ABBREVIATIONS

D5W = 5% dextrose solution
IV = intravenous

NS = Normal Saline
SI = International System of Units

73

Clinical Toxicology

Keith R. McCain and Howell R. Foster

FOUNDATION OVERVIEW

Clinical toxicology involves the assessment and management of disease caused by exposure to an agent(s) in which adverse effects may develop. All natural and synthetic xenobiotics are capable of causing toxicity in humans. It is paramount to recognize that all substances can be poisonous in a specific situation. As such, some agents are capable of severe consequence at microgram doses (botulinum toxin) while others are typically viewed as harmless, despite being lethal at extreme doses (water intoxication).

PREVENTION

Multiple avenues have been developed to reduce the incidents of unintentional poisoning. National Poison Prevention Week is designated by law (1961) as the third week in March and is used to increase public awareness of the incidents and dangers of poisoning. The Poison Prevention and Packaging Act (1970) (PPPA) requires some hazardous household products, as well as oral prescription medications and some over-the-counter medications, to utilize child-resistant containers. Additionally, the PPPA limits the quantity for packaging of some products. The Poison Control Center Enhancement and Awareness Act (2000) established a toll-free number (1-800-222-1222) to allow nationwide 24 hour access to PC consultation in the United States. Table 73-1 provides select tips that should be emphasized to the public to prevent poisoning emergencies.

GENERAL MANAGEMENT

General Approach to the Poisoned Patient

In the setting of known or suspected poisoning, patients commonly present with inadequate and unreliable histories. As such, the potential for rapid patient deterioration should be anticipated, and aggressive supportive care should be instituted early, with first consideration given to the "ABCs" (airway, breathing, circulation). In patients with concerning histories or abnormalities, interventions should also include administration of oxygen; establishment of intravenous access; obtaining a 12-lead electrocardiogram (EKG) and continuous cardiac monitoring; and determination of arterial blood gases (ABGs), blood glucose, and electrolyte values. Additionally, empiric administration of an intravenous "Coma Cocktail" consisting of 100 mg of thiamine, 25 to 50 g of dextrose, and 0.04 to 2 mg of naloxone should be considered early in the management of patients with altered mental status. Seizure and dysrhythmia potential should be considered, and potential need for treatment with a benzodiazepine (intravenous lorazepam or diazepam) and standard advanced cardiac life support (ACLS) measures anticipated. Upon stabilization, attention can be turned toward a more detailed physical examination, laboratory results, history of exposure, and potential decontamination measures.

Physical Examination

A thorough history and physical examination are essential in treating toxicologic emergencies. Close and ongoing evaluation of patient's vital signs and physical findings can provide invaluable information in determining appropriate supportive care, as well as aid in diagnosis. After the primary survey of the toxic patient and assuring that the ABCs have been addressed, a more detailed secondary survey should be performed. Recognition of a pattern or syndrome of symptoms may narrow the diagnosis to a particular class or group of offending agents. Several "toxidromes" have been developed and are described in Table 73-2. It is important to note that not all patients will be "classic" representations of the toxidrome. Some share overlapping characteristics. Health care providers must realize the limitations of toxidrome characteristics in conducting patient assessments.

Laboratory

In conjunction with history and physical examination, laboratory testing can provide important clues in treatment of the poisoned patient. While "toxicology" screens are commonly ordered in the setting of the poisoned patient, debate surrounds their utility. These tests are limited to a handful of agents, are associated with false-positive and negative results, do not prove impairment, and are infrequently associated with significant impact on overall patient management. More beneficial are the results from a basic metabolic panel, ABGs, EKG, and occasionally specific x-rays. Additionally, in all patients with suspected self-poisoning, an acetaminophen level, and

TABLE 73-1 | **Poison Prevention Tips**

1. Identify all potentially hazardous items in the home and workplace.
2. Keep all chemicals and medicines locked up and out of sight.
3. Do not transfer products from original containers.
4. Utilize and ensure proper use of child-resistant closures.
5. Do not store chemicals and medications with food items.
6. Read product labels prior to use.
7. Avoid taking medicine in front of children and never refer to medicine as candy.
8. Return products and medicine to proper storage immediately after use.
9. Do not take/administer medicine in the dark, and check the dose with every use.
10. Keep the Poison Center number (1-800-222-1222) readily available.

TABLE 73-2 | **Select Syndromes of Toxicity**

Toxidrome	**Symptoms**
Opiate	CNS depression, respiratory depression, miosis, decreased bowel motility
Cholinergic	Salivation, lacrimation, urination, defecation, GI distress, emesis, bronchorrhea, bradycardia
Anticholinergic	Delirium/hallucinations, urinary retention, decreased bowel motility, mydriasis, tachycardia, hyperthermia, flushed skin, dry mucous membranes
Sympathomimetic	Agitation, mydriasis, tachycardia, hyperthermia, diaphoresis, tremor, hypertension

possibly a salicylate level, should be determined. Serum levels of specific agents may prove useful and should be obtained depending on history or suspicion (ie, toxic alcohols, lithium, digoxin, heavy metals, etc). Other potentially useful determinations from laboratory data include evidence of an anion gap acidosis, osmolal gap, or oxygen saturation gap.

Decontamination

Dermal and ocular exposures should initially be managed with prompt and thorough irrigation of contaminated surfaces. Patients with inhalation exposure should be moved to fresh air. As 80% of exposures are associated with ingestion, the need and method of gastric decontamination following poisoning is a common decision associated with poisoning. There is extreme variance and controversy associated with the practice of gastric decontamination. Position papers have been developed by leading toxicology groups after evaluation of the available literature evidence with regard to gastric decontamination. These papers indicate there is limited evidence to support routine use of ipecac, gastric lavage, single dose—or multiple dose—activated charcoal, cathartics, or whole bowel irrigation. The decision for gastric decontamination should be made on an individual case basis with full understanding of the benefits and risks, as well as attention to the indications and contraindications for individual technique utilization. Table 73-3 outlines the variables and conditions that should be utilized in assessing if gastric emptying would be indicated. The indications and contraindications for orogastric lavage, and single dose-activated charcoal are detailed in Tables 73-4 and 73-5.

Antidotes

Supportive care is the mainstay of treatment in the majority of poisoned patients; however, there are instances in which antidotal therapy can be significant in reducing morbidity and mortality. Ideally antidotes would be highly effective in reversing or attenuating toxicity, readily available, associated

TABLE 73-3 | **Risk Assessment: When to Consider Gastric Emptying**

Gastric Emptying Is Usually Not Indicated If[a]	Gastric Emptying May Be Indicated If[b]
The xenobiotic has limited toxicity at any dose	There is reason to believe that, given the time of ingestion, a significant amount of the ingested xenobiotic is still present in the stomach
Although the xenobiotic ingested is potentially toxic, the dose ingested is less than that expected to produce significant illness	The ingested xenobiotic is known to produce serious toxicity, *or* the patient has obvious signs or symptoms of life-threatening toxicity
The ingested xenobiotic is well adsorbed by activated charcoal, and the amount ingested is not expected to exceed the adsorptive capacity of activated charcoal	The ingested xenobiotic is not adsorbed by activated charcoal, or activated charcoal is unavailable
Significant spontaneous emesis has occurred	Although the ingested xenobiotic is adsorbed by activated charcoal, the amount ingested exceeds the activated charcoal-to-xenobiotic ratio of 10:1 even when using a dose of activated charcoal that is twice the standard dose recommended
The patient presents many hours post-ingestion and has minimal signs or symptoms of poisoning	The patient has not had spontaneous emesis
The ingested xenobiotic has a highly efficient antidote (eg, acetaminophen and NAC)	No highly effective specific antidote exists or alternative therapies (eg, hemodialysis) pose a significant risk to the patient

[a]Patients who fulfill these criteria can be decontaminated safely with activated charcoal alone or may require no decontamination at all.
[b]Patients who fulfill these criteria should be considered candidates for gastric emptying *if* there are no contraindications. For individuals who meet some of these criteria but who are judged not to be candidates for gastric emptying, single- or multiple-dose activated charcoal and/or whole-bowel irrigation should be considered.
Reproduced with permission from Nelson L, Lewin N, Howland MA, et al: *Goldfrank's Toxicologic Emergencies*, 9th ed. New York, NY: McGraw-Hill; 2011.

TABLE 73-4	Indications and Contraindications to Orogastric Lavage
Indications	**Contraindications**
The patient meets criteria for gastric emptying (Table 73-3)	The patient does not meet criteria for gastric emptying (Table 73-3)
The benefits of gastric emptying outweigh the risks	The patient has lost or will likely lose his/her airway protective reflexes and has not been intubated. (After the patient has been intubated, orogastric lavage can be performed if otherwise indicated.)
	Ingestion of an alkaline caustic
	Ingestion of a foreign body (eg, a drug packet)
	Ingestion of a xenobiotic with a high aspiration potential (eg, a hydrocarbon) in the absence of endotracheal intubation
	The patient is at risk of hemorrhage or gastro-intestinal perforation because of underlying pathology, recent surgery, or other medical condition that could be further compromised by the use of orogastric lavage
	Ingestion of a xenobiotic in a form known to be too large to fit into the lumen of the lavage tube (eg, many modified-release preparations)

Reproduced with permission from Nelson L, Lewin N, Howland MA, et al: *Goldfrank's Toxicologic Emergencies*, 9th ed. New York, NY: McGraw-Hill; 2011.

with a low adverse effect profile, and inexpensive. Unfortunately, these characteristics are difficult to obtain as insufficient stocking of multiple antidotes have historically been an issue; several therapies have high acquisition cost; and antidotes often have adverse effect profiles that must be weighed against potential benefit. The most recent consensus guidelines recommend 24 antidotes that should be stocked by hospitals. Common antidotes and associated toxins are detailed in Table 73-6.

TREATMENT OF SELECT TOXINS

Acetaminophen

Excessive acute or chronic doses of acetaminophen can result in hepatic injury. Toxicity is due to production of the metabolite N-acetyl-p-benzoquinone imine (NAPQI), a potent electrophile by CYP2E1. Under therapeutic conditions, the small amount of NAPQI generated is detoxified by endogenous stores of glutathione. In excessive doses glutathione stores are depleted, allowing NAPQI to bind with hepatocytes leading to liver injury, which can range from mild transaminitis to fulminant failure. As toxicity is related to metabolite production, symptoms are delayed from time of ingestion and nausea and vomiting may be the only apparent symptoms in the first 24 hours following overdose. Acute ingestions of more than 10 g or 200 mg/kg (whichever is lower) warrant medical attention.

Chronic ingestions of doses more than 10 g or 200 mg/kg (whichever is less) over a 24-hour period, 6 g or 150 mg/kg (whichever is less) per 24-hour period for the prior 48 hours, or for children less than 6 years a dose of 100 mg/kg/24-hour period for the preceding 72 hour or longer period prompt need for medical evaluation. Patients potentially at increased risk of hepatic injury (alcoholism, concurrent therapy with CYP2E1 inducers, malnourished) should have medical evaluation at chronic doses more than 4 g or 100 mg/kg (whichever is less) per day. Medical evaluation should include determination of a serum APAP level and baseline liver function test. In acute overdose, the APAP level and known time post-ingestion can be plotted on the Rumack-Matthew nomogram to determine potential risk of hepatic injury and need for antidotal therapy with N-acetylcysteine (NAC, Acetadote, Mucomyst). NAC likely serves to maintain/restore glutathione stores or as an alternate substrate for NAPQI. For optimal liver protective effect, NAC should be administered within the first 8 hours of ingestion, as efficacy progressively diminishes further into the course of toxicity. NAC can be administered intravenously or orally; however, the dose and duration of treatment are different, with IV administration consisting of three different dose bags given over a 21-hour treatment period compared to the oral protocol that requires a loading dose followed by maintenance doses given every 4 hours for 72 hours. Besides patients with intractable vomiting or pregnant women for which intravenous administration is recommended, debate exists about

TABLE 73-5	Indications and Contraindications for Single-Dose Activated Charcoal Therapy Without Gastric Emptying
Indications	**Contraindications**
The patient does not meet criteria for gastric emptying (Table 73-3) or gastric emptying is likely to be harmful	Activated charcoal is known not to adsorb a clinically meaningful amount of the ingested xenobiotic
The patient has ingested a potentially toxic amount of a xenobiotic that is known to be adsorbed by activated charcoal	Airway protective reflexes are absent or expected to be lost and the patient is not intubated
The ingestion has occurred within a time frame amenable to adsorption by activated charcoal or clinical factors are present that suggest that not all of the xenobiotic has already been systemically absorbed	Gastrointestinal perforation is likely as in cases of caustic ingestions
	Therapy may increase the risk and severity of aspiration, such as in the presence of hydrocarbons with a high aspiration potential
	Endoscopy will be an essential diagnostic modality (caustics)

Reproduced with permission from Nelson L, Lewin N, Howland MA, et al: *Goldfrank's Toxicologic Emergencies*, 9th ed. New York, NY: McGraw-Hill; 2011.

TABLE 73-6 **Select Antidotes**

Antidote	Drug/Toxin	Comment
Acetylcysteine/NAC (IV = Acetadote, PO = Mucomyst or generic)	Acetaminophen	If IV route necessary and Acetadote unavailable, oral NAC can be given through appropriate filter IV Oral dose should be diluted to maximum 5% concentration
Crotalidae polyvalent immune Fab, ovine (CroFab)	North American crotaline snake (rattlesnakes, cottonmouth, copperheads)	Dosing is not weight based Reconstitution may take up to 1 h Potential for allergic reaction in patients with papaya or papain hypersensitivity
Antivenin (*Latrodectus mactans*)	Black widow spider	Horse serum-derived antitoxin, caution for immunogenic reactions and serum sickness
Antivenin (*Micrurus fulvius*)	Eastern/Texas coral snake	Product discontinued by manufacturer, some supply remains Horse serum-derived antitoxin
Atropine sulfate	Organophosphate and carbamate pesticides, nerve agents, drug/toxin-induced bradycardia	Cholinesterase inhibitor (CI) toxicity may require large doses Endpoint of therapy in CI toxicity is dry bronchial tree not mydriasis or tachycardia
Calcium chloride 10% Calcium gluconate 10%	Calcium channel blockers, hydrofluoric acid/fluoride	CaCl should be given through central IV due to vascular irritating properties For hydrofluoric acid burns, topical 2.5% calcium gluconate can be compounded from parenteral calcium gluconate and a water-based jelly.
Calcium disodium EDTA (Versenate)	Lead	Potential for medication error due to confusion with disodium EDTA
Calcium trisodium pentetate	Internal contamination with plutonium, americium, curium	Potential components of a radiological dispersal device ("dirty bomb")
Cyanide antidote kit or Cyanokit	Cyanide	Cyanide kit contains: amyl nitrite inhalant, parenteral sodium nitrite sodium thiosulfate Cyanokit contains: parenteral hydroxocobalamin and does not utilize induction of methemoglobinemia as any portion of its mechanism of action
Deferoxamine (Desferal)	Iron (acute)	Change in urine color is not always detected Use >24 h has been associated with acute respiratory distress syndrome (ARDS)
Digoxin immune Fab fragments (DigiFab, Digibind)	Digoxin/cardiac glycosides	Multiple methods of calculating dose, dependent on variables of specific case, consult prescribing information (1 vial binds ~0.5 mg of digoxin) Fab product will interfere with digoxin level measurements after administration Potential for allergic reaction in patients with papaya or papain hypersensitivity, previous digoxin immune Fab therapy, and ovine protein or latex allergy
Dimercaprol (BAL in Oil)	Arsenic, gold, mercury, lead	Must combine with calcium disodium EDTA for lead formulated with peanut oil
Ethanol	Methanol or ethylene glycol	Difficult to obtain, dose, and monitor levels; associated with multiple negative side effects if utilized
Fomepizole (Antizol)	Methanol or ethylene glycol	Requires dose increase on fifth dose
Flumazenil (Romazicon)	Benzodiazepines	Should utilize with caution if at all in the setting of acute overdose due to potential to precipitate withdrawal seizures or unmask coingestant toxicity Primary indication should be in the setting of iatrogenic oversedation Short duration of action
Glucagon	β-blockers, calcium channel blockers	Nausea and vomiting commo; caution in patients with decreased level of consciousness and unprotected airway
Methylene blue	Methemoglobinemia	Contraindicated in patients with G6PD deficiency as hemolysis may result
Naloxone (Narcan)	Opioids, opiates	Start with low dose to reduce potential to precipitate withdrawal Short duration of action
Octreotide (Sandostatin)	Oral sulfonylurea-induced hypoglycemia	Suppress sulfonylurea-induced insulin secretion Subcutaneous or IV administration, may require multiple doses over 24-48 h period
Physostigmine (Antilirium)	Anticholinergic syndrome, especially antimuscarinic delirium	Inhibits acetylcholinesterase, resulting in increased cholinergic tone; significant debate about appropriate use, especially in the setting of multidrug overdose or agents that may prolong QRS/QT intervals (tricyclics, neuroleptics) Side-effect potentials include seizures and SLUDGE syndrome
Potassium iodide	Thyroid radioiodine prophylaxis	Risk of associated cancer is most concerning in the very young (<18 years old with the exception of pregnant persons). Persons >40 years old have extremely small associated risk. Treatment is indicated in lactating mothers regardless of age
Pralidoxime/2-PAM (Protopam)	Organophosphate pesticides, nerve agents	Reactivates cholinesterase which have been inactivated by organophosphate pesticides and related compounds
Pyridoxine/Vitamin B$_6$	Isoniazid, hydrazines	Empiric 5 g dose requires #50 100 mg/mL 1 mL vials
Sodium bicarbonate	Agents producing wide QRS, urine, or serum alkalization	Multiple roles/mechanisms of action Attention to systemic pH, sodium, and potassium levels

which route of administration is preferred. The intravenous course is of shorter duration, requires fewer doses, and eliminates issues associated with nausea and vomiting, a common symptom of early toxicity; however, it has a higher acquisition cost and an increased incidence of adverse effect. Also, some concern exists in regard to the shorter duration of therapy in some scenarios. *The nomogram is not applicable to chronic poisoning and should not be utilized outside assessment of acute overdose.* There is less definitive standard for treatment following repeated supratherapeutic doses, but a conservative approach is to initiate NAC in patients with either signs or symptoms of hepatotoxicity, which are elevated AST values, or APAP level more than 10 mcg/mL. All other patients should be instructed to return to medical attention if symptoms develop.

Toxic Alcohols

Ethylene glycol and methanol are dangerous nonethanol alcohols. Small ingestions of either are capable of producing significant toxicity. Ethylene glycol is a common ingredient in antifreeze. Methanol can be found in windshield-washer fluid, canned fuel, paint removers, and deicer products. The toxicity of both is related to their metabolites. The initial metabolism of both occurs primarily via alcohol dehydrogenase, with ethylene glycol yielding glycolic and oxalic acids, and methanol yielding formic acid. These organic acid metabolites can result in profound metabolic acidosis with an elevated anion gap $([Na^+]) - ([Cl^-]+[HCO_3^-])$ and/or presence of an osmolal gap (measured serum osmolality – calculated osmolarity). Additionally, oxalic acid can complex with systemic calcium leading to calcium oxalate precipitates. These precipitates can result in renal and other organ dysfunction and hypocalcemia. Formic acid attacks the retinal and optic nerves and can result in visual impairment, including blindness. Prompt treatment to minimize formation of toxic metabolites is imperative. Ethanol and fomepizole (Antizol) are both inhibitors of alcohol dehydrogenase and effectively prevent formation of ethylene glycol and methanol metabolites. Fomepizole is preferred over alcohol as it does not cause inebriation or other additive toxicity, does not require blood monitoring, and has standardized dosing. Fomepizole is given as a 15 g/kg loading dose, then a 10 mg/kg maintenance dose every 12 hours for four doses, and then maintenance doses are increased to 15 mg/kg every 12 hours due to auto-induced metabolism. Hemodialysis may be a required concurrent therapy depending on patient disposition and serum glycol or methanol levels.

Benzodiazepines

Benzodiazepines (BZD) facilitate enhanced binding of gamma amino butyric acid (GABA) binding to the GABA$_A$ receptor, resulting in the hyperpolarization of post-synaptic neuron and causing central nervous system (CNS) inhibition. BZD are frequent agents involved in overdose. Symptoms of BZD toxicity include: CNS depression, ranging from ataxia, confusion, and drowsiness to coma; hypotension; and respiratory depression. BZD poisoning has low mortality when ingested alone, but in multidrug overdose with other CNS depressants, their additive

toxicity increases the risk of respiratory depression and mortality. Flumazenil (Romazicon) is an intravenous competitive antagonist of BZDs on the CNS and is classified as an antidote for BZD overdose; however, the utility of flumazenil in the overdose and nonspecific coma setting is associated with caveats and debate. Prior to utilization, thought should be given to the potential that it may precipitate a withdrawal syndrome such as seizures, or unmask coingestant toxicity. Flumazenil is given at an initial dose of 0.2 mg over 30 seconds with cautious titration to limit the risk of precipitating withdrawal or unmasking coingestant toxicity. An initial titration dose should be 0.3 mg. If necessary, further titration at 0.5 mg in 1 minute intervals to desired effect or until a cumulative dose of 3 to 5 mg have been administered are recommended. Doses more than this are not expected to be beneficial. Patients given flumazenil should be closely observed for resedation due to this drug's short half-life.

β-Adrenergic Antagonist

β-blockers competitively antagonize adrenergic β-receptors. Blockade of these receptors results in decreased intracellular phosphokinase A activation and, ultimately, a reduction in inotropy and chronotropy. The individual agents have significant inherent differences with regard to overall pharmacologic profiles. Potential differences within the class include cardioselectivity, intrinsic sympathomimetic activity, α-antagonism, membrane-stabilizing activity, and lipophilicity. β-Blocker receptor selectivity is lost in overdose, and effects not seen with standard therapeutic use can develop. Hypotension and bradycardia are the most common clinical findings associated with β-blocker toxicity. Other potential complications include: seizures, CNS depression, ventricular dysrhythmia, heart block, pulmonary edema, hypoperfusion, and bronchospasm. CNS depression, seizures, and dysrhythmia are particularly problematic with the more lipophilic agents (ie, propranolol). Classically, glucagon has been considered antidotal for β-blocker overdose. Stimulation of the glucagon receptor located on the β-receptor complex effectively bypasses the blockade of β-blocker antagonism, thus activating a shared G protein and increasing intracellular phosphokinase A activity. Glucagon should be given as a 3 to 5 mg IV bolus, additional boluses or a continuous infusion may be required due to short duration of effect. Nausea and vomiting should be anticipated from glucagon administration. Additionally, aggressive supportive care consisting of a combination of measures including fluid resuscitation, atropine, external pacing, vasopressor support, and high-dose insulin and dextrose therapy may be required.

Calcium Channel Antagonist

Calcium channel blockers reduce calcium flow through voltage-gated calcium channels. These channels are found in myocardial, smooth muscle, and pancreatic cells. Blockade of these channels results in reduction in intracellular calcium, leading to reduced actin-myosin interaction producing reduced vascular and myocardial contractility. Additionally a reduction in intracellular calcium causes a reduction in sinoatrial and atrioventricular nodal tone. At therapeutic doses, the dihydropyridines have peripheral action with vasodilatory effect. The nondihydropyridines (verapamil, diltiazem) express more direct cardiac effect. In overdose, these differences are lost. Common symptoms include hypotension, bradycardia, and conduction disturbances. Elevated blood glucose may be noted because of blockade of pancreatic islet cells, calcium channels, and a resultant decrease in insulin secretion. This metabolic impairment reduces carbohydrate supply to cardiac muscle and compounds myocardial dysfunction. Other potential symptoms include nausea and vomiting, CNS depression, hypoperfusion, and pulmonary edema. Initial therapies in the setting of calcium channel blocker toxicity should include intravenous fluids, atropine, and administration of calcium salts (10-20 mL 10% calcium gluconate via peripheral line or 5-10 mL 10% calcium chloride via central venous access). These methods commonly do not improve patient hemodynamics in moderate to severe poisoning and vasopressor support is required. If response remains inadequate glucagon and/or amrinone are additional treatment options. There is increasing support for early intervention using high-dose insulin and dextrose therapy (hyperinsulinemia-euglycemia therapy) in the setting of calcium channel blocker overdose. Insulin has positive inotropic activity and improves the carbohydrate delivery to cardiac myocytes. Current suggested dosing recommends a 1 Unit/kg bolus dose of regular insulin, followed by a 0.5 Unit/kg/h infusion adjusted to response. A dextrose infusion should be initiated at time of insulin bolus to maintain euglycemia, and close monitoring of glucose and potassium should be carried out throughout the therapy. Prior to initiating therapy, blood glucose and potassium levels should be checked, and if less than 200 mg/dL or less than 2.5 mEq/L respectively, supplementation should be provided. In many cases patients will require more than one of the above therapies to be initiated simultaneously.

Digoxin

Digoxin is a cardiac glycoside that inhibits the sodium/potassium ATPase pump. This effect increases inotropy and contractility as a result of increased intracellular calcium. Additionally, digoxin decreases heart rate via activity on both vagal and sympathetic tone. Digoxin has a narrow therapeutic window and a multitude of drug interactions (verapamil, carvedilol, spironolactone, alprazolam, macrolide antibiotics, etc). Comorbid conditions (renal dysfunction, reduced lean body mass) can help precipitate toxicity. Symptoms of toxicity vary between toxicities of acute or chronic nature. Early clinical symptoms of acute excess commonly include nausea, vomiting, confusion, lethargy, hyperkalemia, and a broad array of cardiovascular toxicity. Symptoms of chronic toxicity may be less obvious and may include nausea, vomiting, weight loss, confusion, drowsiness, and visual disturbances (chromatopsia and xanthopsia). A high degree of suspicion should be utilized in patients with potential for chronic digoxin poisoning. Excluding supraventricular tachydysrhythmia, digoxin toxicity can produce virtually every known dysrhythmia, with bidirectional ventricular tachycardia being a classic hallmark.

With exception of the administration of calcium salts to treat hyperkalemia and use of Class IA antidysrhythmics, both of which may increase mortality in the setting of suspected digoxin toxicity, standard supportive care measures should be utilized in the management of digoxin toxicity. More significant cardiac glycoside toxicity can be treated with digoxin-immune Fab. This antibody fragment antidote binds digoxin with higher affinity than the target pump, effectively blocking and reversing associated toxicities. Each vial of Fab fragment will bind approximately 0.5 mg of digoxin.

Antidotal treatment is indicated in any related life-threatening dysrhythmia, potassium levels more than 5 mEq/L due to acute toxicity, elevated digoxin concentration associated with dysrhythmia, significant gastrointestinal symptoms, altered mental status in patients chronically treated with digoxin, significant/refractory hemodynamic instability, acute ingestions of more than 10 mg in adults or more than 4 mg in children, a serum digoxin level of more than or equal to 15 ng/mL at any time post-ingestion, or a serum digoxin level more than or equal to 10 ng/mL 6 hours after ingestion. Determining appropriate antidote dose can be accomplished by the following methods:

1. Empirically, with recommended doses of 10 vials for acute overdose and 3 vials for chronic toxicity for all patient ages.
2. Based on a known dose ingested, as one vial of digoxin Fab fragments will complex 0.5 mg of digoxin.
3. Based on a steady-state serum level (must be drawn 4-6 hours post-ingestion to allow for complete distribution) and calculations listed in the product prescribing information.

Digoxin levels can rise dramatically following administration of digoxin immune Fab fragment as the levels indicate both bound and unbound drug. As such, total digoxin levels are not useful in guiding patient management after administration of Fab fragment antidote.

Tricyclic Antidepressants

Tricyclic antidepressants (TCAD) produce toxicity by multiple mechanisms: sodium channel antagonism, α-receptor antagonism, anticholinergic effects, and inhibition of norepinephrine and serotonin uptake. Moderate to severe toxicity can develop with doses of 10 to 20 mg/kg, with doses more than 20 mg/kg being potentially fatal. Clinical manifestations of toxicity can have abrupt onset and include CNS depression, respiratory depression, seizures, anticholinergic effects, conduction disturbances (particularly prolongation of the QRS interval), dysrhythmias, and profound hypotension. QRS duration more than 100 ms in the setting of TCAD poisoning is associated with a higher risk of seizure and durations more than 160 ms with malignant dysrhythmias. Hypotension is largely due to α-blockade, and direct-acting α agonists (norepinephrine or phenylephrine) are the vasopressors of choice. In addition to aggressive supportive care, serum alkalinization using sodium bicarbonate is utilized in TCAD poisoning with evidence of significant cardiovascular or neurologic toxicity with a goal of establishing a systemic pH of 7.5 to 7.55. In addition to providing higher levels of sodium in the setting of competitive sodium channel blockade, increased systemic pH is theorized to increase TCAD volume of distribution and enhance recovery time of blocked sodium channels. Alkalinization will potentially be of aid in correcting disturbances related to sodium channel blockade as well as treating metabolic acidosis associated with TCAD-induced seizure or hypotension. However, it will not address other mechanisms of TCAD toxicity, as such it is only a component of intervention.

Opioids

The hallmarks of opioid toxicity include miosis, CNS, and respiratory depression. Other potential complications include vomiting, hypoxia, decreased bowel motility, pulmonary edema, hypotension, bradycardia, seizures (meperidine and tramadol), dysrhythmia (methadone), and acidosis. The degree of interpatient tolerance can significantly affect the severity of symptoms observed related to dose. In addition to good ABCs, naloxone, an antagonist of opioid receptors, can reverse the CNS and respiratory depression related to opioid overdose. The lowest effective dose should be utilized initially (0.04-2 mg IV) with incremental titration (0.1 mg) to desired response in attempt to avoid opiate withdrawal syndrome. If no significant improvement in CNS/respiratory state has been achieved after administration of 10 mg of naloxone, other causes should be investigated. Duration of antagonism by naloxone may be shorter than opioid effect; as such patients should be monitored closely for resedation and may require continuous naloxone infusion. Toxicities of agents commonly formulated in combination with opioids should also be investigated (acetaminophen/aspirin).

Salicylates

Salicylates are ingredients in a number of prescription and over-the-counter products available in the United States. Toxicity is typically related to ingestion but can occur due to improper dermal use. Toxicity can result following acute overdose as well as chronic use either in supratherapeutic dose or in the setting of patients with decreased metabolism or renal function. In order to determine potential toxicity, individual agents must be converted to appropriate aspirin equivalents by multiplying the ingested dose by a corresponding individual salicylate aspirin equivalent factor (ie, aspirin = 1, methyl salicylate = 1.4, bismuth subsalicylate = 0.5, magnesium salicylate = 1.21, etc). Current guidelines recommend an emergency department evaluation for all symptomatic patients and ingestions more than 150 mg/kg or 6.5 g of aspirin equivalents in asymptomatic patients. Acute and chronic salicylate poisoning can result in gastrointestinal, CNS, and metabolic dysfunction. Potential symptoms include nausea and vomiting, tinnitus, tachypnea, diaphoresis, hypoglycemia, hyperthermia, altered mental status, seizures, CNS depression, a respiratory alkalosis (early), mixed respiratory alkalosis and metabolic acidosis (late), pulmonary edema,

and cerebral edema. Chronic toxicity is often not recognized early in diagnosis as the symptoms and salicylate blood levels may not be as pronounced or syndromic as acute toxicity. Delay in recognition of salicylism can prove lethal; therefore, salicylate toxicity should be investigated in all patients with unexplained altered mental status and metabolic disturbance. Interpretation of serum salicylate concentration is complex and requires consideration of more than just the serum concentration value. Salicylates have the potential for delayed or continual absorption due to formulation, pylorospasm, or concretion formation. For this reason serial levels are typically indicated in acute overdose. Decreasing levels do not always indicate resolving toxicity. While intuitively falling levels would seem to correspond with improving condition, in the setting of salicylate-induced acidemia the volume of distribution and tissue penetration into vital organs (especially the CNS) of salicylates increase resulting in more significant clinical toxicity. For these reasons, salicylate levels should never be the sole factor in assessing toxicity. Additionally, the Done nomogram is not considered appropriate for determination of salicylate toxicity and should not be utilized. There is no true antidote for salicylate poisoning. Treatment is aimed at decreasing absorption and enhancing elimination. Urinary alkalinization by administration of sodium bicarbonate with a goal of maintaining a urinary pH of 7.5 to 8 is an effective means of increasing renal elimination of salicylates as it increases retention of ionized salicylate in the urine. Hemodialysis effectively removes salicylate and is indicated in the salicylate-toxic patients with CNS dysfunction, renal failure, acute lung injury, severe acid-base or electrolyte disturbance, hepatic dysfunction with coagulopathy or salicylate levels more than 100 mg/dL regardless of symptoms.

SPECIAL POPULATIONS

Children, elderly, and the pregnant patient are groups in which special considerations may be required in the management of toxicity. Poisoning in toddlers are not attempts at self-harm and typically involve a small dose and single ingredient compared to exposures in older children and adults. However, due to their small size relative to dose, several medications or chemicals can be lethal in single tablet or mouthful ingestions. In elderly patients, drug toxicity may not be readily apparent or investigated as the cause of clinical symptoms. However, changes in hepatic or renal function may alter kinetics and elimination leading to increased serum levels. Additionally, older patients tend to take multiple pharmacologically active agents and have comorbid conditions that increase the risk of drug-drug interactions and additive clinical effects. In the pregnant patient as a general rule, treatment that is deemed necessary for the mother should not be held out of concern for the fetus. Of note in this population is the fact that intravenous acetylcysteine is recommended over oral acetylcysteine and that carbon monoxide is significantly more toxic to the fetal hemoglobin. Also, hyperbaric oxygen therapy is recommended at lower carboxyhemoglobin levels compared to nonpregnant patients.

Opioid Dependence

Opioid dependence has become an alarming epidemic over the past decade. Deaths due to opioid overdose have quadrupled since 1999. Up to 50% of opioid overdose deaths are due to prescription opioids, while the other half are due to recreational use of opioids. The most commonly abused prescription opioids include methadone, oxycodone, and hydrocodone, while heroin and nonpharmaceutical synthetic opioids account for illicit sources. Each day, 1000 individuals are treated in emergency departments (ED) for misuse of prescription opioids. There's a growing need to be prepared and alert to treat and manage patients with an opioid overdose. Pharmacists are starting to see an increasing need for action and education regarding patient care in overdose situations.

Naloxone (Narcan®, Evzio®) was originally approved in 1971 to treat opioid overdose. Naloxone can be administered intramuscularly, intravenously, subcutaneously, and as a nasal spray. Although several different formulations of naloxone currently exist, the intravenous form is preferred due to its quick onset of action. A continuous infusion of naloxone may be utilized for patients who have overdosed on long-acting opioids, such as methadone, or are requiring several bolus doses to maintain response. The auto injector (Evzio®) was FDA approved on April 3, 2014, and the nasal spray was approved on November 18, 2015. The nasal spray was granted fast-track, priority approval in order to aid in reducing the number of opioid overdose deaths in this nationwide epidemic.

Naloxone regulations for dispensing vary from state to state. Select states allow for standing orders written by physicians allowing the patient to receive naloxone without a traditional written prescription. Standing orders have expanded into outpatient practices, and 40 states have an authorized standing order for naloxone. The first naloxone Collaborative Drug Therapy Agreement was established in Washington in 2012. It allowed pharmacists to dispense naloxone to patients at high-risk of opioid overdose without a prescription from their physician. Under this agreement, pharmacists are required to document all patients to whom they dispense naloxone, in addition to attaching a training checklist with the patient's initials, acknowledging that they were trained in the appropriate administration techniques. In this structure, the pharmacist and physician perform regular quality assurance reviews together.

Patients should also be counseled on how to administer naloxone based on the dosage form that's dispensed. Administration varies greatly by dosage form. For example, Evzio® is dispensed with an auto-injector for training purposes and two true auto-injectors. The trainer has audible step-by-step instructions for injection. It's necessary to continue to monitor the breathing of the patient and administer another dose with the second auto-injector within 2 to 3 minutes if they don't wake up. The nasal spray should be administered when the patient is lying on their back. The nozzle should be placed inside either nostril while pressing the plunger to release the dose. After naloxone administration, the patient should be turned onto their side. Regardless of route of administration, naloxone counseling should include instructions to ALWAYS seek immediate medical attention following administration due to the short duration of naloxone action and risk of toxicity returning. Table 73-7 lists characteristics of opioids, opioid substitutes, and opioid antagonists.

TABLE 73-7	**Opioids, Opioid Substitutes, and Opioid Antagonists**			
Subclass, Drug	**Mechanism of Action**	**Effects**	**Clinical Applications**	**Pharmacokinetics, Toxicities**
Opioid Agonists				
• Morphine • Methadone • Fentanyl	Strong μ-receptor agonists • variable affinity for δ and κ receptors	Analgesia • relief of anxiety • sedation • slowed gastrointestinal transit	Severe pain • adjunct in anesthesia (fentanyl, morphine) • pulmonary edema (morphine only) • maintenance in rehabilitation programs (methadone only)	First-pass effect • duration 1-4 h except methadone, 4-6 h • *Toxicity*: Respiratory depression • severe constipation • addiction liability • convulsions
• *Hydromorphone, oxymorphone: Like morphine in efficacy, but higher potency* • *Meperidine: Strong agonist with anticholinergic effects* • *Oxycodone: Dose-dependent analgesia* • *Sufentanil, alfentanil, remifentanil: Like fentanyl but shorter durations of action*				
• Codeine • Hydrocodone	Less efficacious than morphine • can antagonize strong agonists	Like strong agonists • weaker effects	Mild-moderate pain • cough (codeine)	Like strong agonists, toxicity dependent on genetic variation of metabolism
Mixed Opioid Agonist Antagonists				
• Buprenorphine	Partial μ agonist • κ antagonist	Like strong agonists but can antagonize their effects • also reduces craving for alcohol	Moderate pain • some maintenance rehabilitation programs	Long duration of action 4-8 h • may precipitate abstinence syndrome
• Nalbuphine	κ Agonist • μ antagonist	Similar to buprenorphine	Moderate pain	Like buprenorphine

TABLE 73-7	Opioids, Opioid Substitutes, and Opioid Antagonists *(Continued)*			
Subclass, Drug	**Mechanism of Action**	**Effects**	**Clinical Applications**	**Pharmacokinetics, Toxicities**
Antitussives				
▪ Dextromethorphan	Poorly understood but strong and partial μ agonists are also effective antitussives	Reduces cough reflex • Dextromethorphan, levopropoxyphene not analgesic	Acute debilitating cough	30-60 min duration • *Toxicity*: Minimal when taken as directed
▪ *Codeine, levopropoxyphene: Similar to dextromethorphan*				
Opioid Antagonists				
▪ Naloxone	Antagonist at μ, δ, and κ receptors	Rapidly antagonizes all opioid effects	Opioid overdose	Duration 1-2 h (may have to be repeated when treating overdose) • *Toxicity*: Precipitates abstinence syndrome in dependent users
▪ *Naltrexone, nalmefene: Like naloxone but longer durations of action (10 h); naltrexone is used in maintenance programs and can block heroin effects for up to 48 h; naltrexone is also used for alcohol and nicotine dependence; when combined with bupropion, may be effective in weight-loss programs*				
▪ *Alvimopan, methylnaltrexone bromide: Potent μ antagonists with poor entry into the central nervous system; can be used to treat severe opioid-induced constipation without precipitating an abstinence syndrome*				
Other Analgesics Used in Moderate Pain				
Tapentadol	Moderate μ agonist, strong NET inhibitor	Analgesia	Moderate pain	Duration 4-6 h • *Toxicity*: Headache; nausea and vomiting; possible dependence
Tramadol	Mixed effects: weak μ agonist, moderate SERT inhibitor, weak NET inhibitor	Analgesia	Moderate pain • adjunct to opioids in chronic pain syndromes	Duration 4-6 h • *Toxicity*: Seizures • risk of serotonin syndrome

Abbreviations: NET, norepinephrine reuptake transporter; SERT, serotonin reuptake transporter.
Reproduced with permission from Katzung BG, Trevor AJ: *Basic & Clinical Pharmacology*, 13th ed. New York, NY: McGraw-Hill; 2015.

CASE Application

The following case pertains to questions 1 to 3.

1. RC is a 40-year-old, 170 lb man. He reports a toothache for which he has been taking four 500-mg acetaminophen tablets every 3 to 4 hours for the last 3 days without relief. Additionally, he complains of nausea and new onset of right upper quadrant pain. His last dose of acetaminophen was 2 hours prior to physical examination. Which of the following would be considered factors that would increase the risk of hepatotoxicity in RC? Select all that apply.

   a. Chronic alcohol use
   b. Concurrent isoniazid therapy
   c. Acquired immunodeficiency syndrome
   d. >40 years of age

2. Which of the following would be an appropriate measure in the evaluation/treatment of RC?

   a. Acetaminophen level should be plotted on the Rumack-Matthew nomogram to determine if antidote therapy is indicated.
   b. Antidote therapy should be initiated immediately.
   c. Acetaminophen level should be ordered to determine need for antidote therapy.
   d. Activated charcoal should be administered and acetaminophen level should be ordered to determine need for antidote therapy.

3. The decision is made to treat RC with the antidote for acetaminophen. Which of the following is a form of acetylcysteine that could be given intravenously as antidote therapy in acetaminophen poisoning? Select all that apply.

   a. Acetylcysteine solution 20%
   b. Acetadote injection
   c. Acetylcysteine solution 10%
   d. Acetylcysteine injection

4. MP is a 40-year-old, 107-lb woman brought to the emergency department by EMS after collapsing at a concert. On physical examination, MP is noted to be responsive only to painful stimuli, has a respiratory rate of 6, and constricted pupils. Which of the following agent(s) would be most likely associated with these physical findings?

   a. Methylphenidate
   b. Amitriptyline
   c. Donepezil
   d. Hydromorphone

5. ZW presents to the emergency department with a chief complaint of tinnitus and five episodes of emesis. She reports ingestion of #50 enteric coated aspirin tablets 90 minutes prior to arrival. On physical examination, her heart rate is 92 beats/min, blood pressure 115/80, respiratory rate is 32, and she is diaphoretic. If ZW's history

is accurate, arterial blood gases will most likely indicate which of the following acid-base derangements?

a. Metabolic acidosis
b. Respiratory alkalosis
c. Partially compensated metabolic acidosis
d. Partially compensated respiratory acidosis

6. How much aspirin equivalent is contained in 5 mL of the topical analgesic, oil of wintergreen (100% methyl salicylate)?

a. 140 mg
b. 500 mg
c. 1400 mg
d. 7 g

7. Which toxin antidote combination pairing is correct? Select all that apply.

a. Butorphanol and naloxone
b. Cyanide and hydroxocobalamin
c. Fomepizole and isopropyl alcohol
d. Pyridoxine and isoniazid
e. Deferoxamine and iron

The following case pertains to questions 8 and 9.

8. GL is a 58-year-old woman with history of congestive heart failure treated with digoxin. She presents to the emergency department with a history of ingesting #60 digoxin 0.25-mg tablets 6 hours ago. Her electrocardiogram revealed high-degree heart block with a ventricular rate of 40 to 50 beats/min, a potassium level of 5.8 mEq/L and a digoxin concentration of 12 ng/mL. Which of the following should GL's medical record be evaluated as a precaution, should digoxin immune Fab fragments' administration be necessary. Select all that apply.

a. Papaya or papain allergy
b. Patients treated previously with digoxin immune Fab fragments
c. Sheep protein allergy
d. Latex allergy

9. Digoxin immune Fab fragments in an appropriate dose for the given ingestion was initiated. Within 60 minutes, the patient's clinical status improved, but a repeat digoxin concentration 6 hours after Fab administration returned at 19 ng/mL. What is the best answer to explain the increase in GL's digoxin concentration?

a. Continued absorption of digoxin.
b. The time frame of ingestion was incorrect, and ingestion was closer to time of presentation.
c. Administration of digoxin immune Fab fragment has increased serum levels of total digoxin.
d. Endogenous digoxin-like immunoreactive substance.

10. The administration of which of the following agents would be indicated in the setting of tricyclic

antidepressant overdose associated with seizures or QRS interval more than 115 ms?

a. Sodium bicarbonate
b. Flumazenil
c. Physostigmine
d. Procainamide

11. Which vasopressor would be the best choice for hypotension due to tricyclic antidepressant toxicity that is refractory to fluid and sodium bicarbonate support?

a. Norepinephrine
b. Epinephrine
c. Dopamine
d. Dobutamine

12. Which of the following are differences between calcium gluconate and calcium chloride parenteral preparations?

a. The mechanism of action of calcium chloride is superior in calcium channel blocker poisoning.
b. The mechanism of action of calcium gluconate is superior in calcium channel blocker poisoning.
c. Calcium chloride provides three times more cation compared to calcium gluconate on an equal volume basis.
d. Calcium gluconate is more irritating when given intravenously than calcium chloride.

The following case pertains to questions 13 and 14.

13. RF, a 47-year-old, 205 lb man presents to the emergency department and states that he took an overdose of his "heart medication" 3 hours ago. He now feels lethargic and nauseated. His vitals reveal a heart rate of 45 beats/min and blood pressure of 85/40 mm Hg. The ED staff contacts the patient's pharmacy and is told the patient has prescriptions for atenolol, amlodipine, and digoxin. Which of the following agents should not be administered prior to return of digoxin serum concentration determination?

a. Atropine
b. Fluid bolus
c. Calcium salt
d. Glucagon

14. Administration of intravenous 0.9% saline, atropine, calcium chloride, dopamine, and norepinephrine does not result in adequate improvement in RF's clinical status, and the physician orders the initiation of hyperinsulinemia-euglycemia therapy. At an infusion rate of 0.5 Units/kg/h, how much regular insulin would be administered to RF in the first 30 minutes at this rate?

a. 23 Units
b. 47 Units
c. 51 Units
d. 103 Units

15. KR is a 39-year-old man brought to the emergency department by his wife. She states that he has been

vomiting for the last 2 hours and acting abnormal following an argument approximately 4 hours ago. Initial laboratory data results include: sodium of 144 mEq/L, potassium 3.8 mEq/L, bicarbonate 8 mEq/L, chloride 98 mEq/L, BUN 23 mg/dL, creatinine 0.7 mg/dL, glucose 93 mg/dL, calcium 9.6 mg/dL, and albumin 4 g/dL. Arterial blood gas values on room air were determined to be: pH 7.34, PCO_2 11 mm Hg, PO_2 93 mm Hg. What is the calculated anion gap for this patient?

  a. 23
  b. −49.8
  c. 147
  d. 38

16. Which opioid is associated with both proconvulsant activities in overdose?

  a. Meperidine
  b. Methadone
  c. Hydrocodone
  d. Heroin

17. ES is an 84 year-old, 200 lb man that presents to the emergency department after accidentally taking four of his metoprolol 200 mg tablets due to an error involving his weekly pill organizer. Which of the following is a first-line agent in the management of metoprolol toxicity associated with a high incidence of nausea and vomiting?

  a. Atropine
  b. Calcium gluconate
  c. Glucagon
  d. Milrinone

18. JD is a 39-year-old woman that presents to the emergency department at 3:00 pm and reports an acute ingestion of 10 g of acetaminophen 1 hour prior to arrival. On physical examination, she is emotional and upset but without other physical complaint. She reports a past medical history of depression treated with fluoxetine. What is the earliest time that an acetaminophen level can be drawn and plotted on the Rumack-Matthew nomogram to appropriately determine potential hepatotoxic risk and need for antidote administration for JD?

  a. Immediately on presentation to the emergency department
  b. 4:00 pm
  c. 6:00 pm
  d. 10:00 pm

19. ZM is a 44-year-old, 170 lb man who was found unresponsive in the middle of a city. He is noted to have a blood pressure of 115/60 mm Hg, a heart rate of 61 beats/min, and a respiratory rate of 6 breaths/min; his ECG reveals a normal sinus rhythm. He is afebrile, has no apparent trauma, and is noted to have an odor of alcohol on his breath. Prescription bottles for methadone and clonazepam were found in his shirt pocket. Which of these agents would be appropriate to administer with ZM's history? Select all that apply.

  a. Flumazenil
  b. Naloxone
  c. Thiamine
  d. Dextrose

20. Which of the following are requirements of The Poison Prevention and Packaging Act (PPPA) of 1970? Select all that apply.

  a. Limits the quantity of flavored "children's" aspirin tablets to #36, 81 mg tablets.
  b. With limited exceptions, requires pharmacists to dispense oral prescription drugs in child-resistant packaging unless the patient or prescribing practitioner requests non-child-resistant packaging.
  c. Allows manufactures of over-the-counter medications and certain household substances to package a single size, which does not comply with the PPPA if (1) it also supplies the substance in packages that do comply and (2) the packages of such substances bear conspicuous labeling that states "This package for households without young children."
  d. Requires child-resistant packaging for iron-containing over-the-counter and dietary supplements that contain a total of 250 mg or more of elemental iron per package.

TAKEAWAY POINTS »

- All substances can produce untoward and toxic effect in sufficient dose. Sufficient dose can be highly variable from patient to patient.
- All patients regardless of symptoms or expected toxicity should have medical evaluations following exposures that are attempts at self-harm.
- Urine drug screens are associated with a number of pitfalls, have limited utility, and rarely change treatment. Traditional laboratory tests generally provide better aid in diagnosis and treatment than "tox screens."

- There are significant limitations and little evidence to support routine utilization of gastric decontamination. Decisions to employ these techniques should thoroughly assess the risk-to-benefit ratio on an individual patient basis.
- There are limited circumstances and toxins in which antidotal therapy is available. As such, symptomatic and supportive care is the cornerstone in management of the poisoned patient.

- Acetaminophen overdose can produce hepatotoxicity to the point of fulminant failure. Acute doses more than 10 g or 200 mg/kg necessitate medical evaluation.
- Ethylene glycol and methanol can produce significant morbidity and mortality in very small dose. Toxicity can be prevented by inhibition of alcohol dehydrogenase by fomepizole or ethanol if given early in the course of poisoning prior to significant metabolite generation and resultant acidosis.
- Due to the potential for precipitating benzodiazepine withdrawal or unmasking of coingestant toxicity, flumazenil should not be routinely utilized in the treatment of benzodiazepine poisoning.
- Glucagon utilizes a mechanism of action that bypasses antagonized β-receptors in the setting of β-blocker toxicity.
- Calcium channel blockers can produce severe cardiovascular toxicity. High-dose insulin and dextrose therapy has increasingly been employed early in the course of toxicity.
- Digoxin inhibits the sodium-potassium ATPase pump resulting in increased intracellular calcium stores and increased extracellular potassium levels. Digoxin immune Fab fragments are extremely effective in reversing digoxin toxicity.
- TCAD can cause severe CNS depression and block sodium channels leading to prolonged QRS interval and significant dysrhythmia risk in 10 to 20 mg/kg dose.
- Opioid-toxic patients that respond to naloxone with improved level of consciousness or increased respiratory effort require close observation for resedation as the duration of action for naloxone may be as short as 45 minutes. Overdose of long-acting opiates may require a continuous naloxone infusion.
- Ion trapping with urinary alkalinization is an effective measure to increase salicylate elimination, but is not as effective as hemodialysis which should be utilized for more significant toxicity.
- Proper management of the poisoned patient necessitates sound understanding of the pathophysiology and pharmacology of poisoning and the risks and benefits associated with potential interventions. Consultation with a regional poison center (1-800-222-2222) provides free, 24-hour immediate expert advice.

BIBLIOGRAPHY

Chyka PA. Clinical toxicology. In: DiPiro JT, Talbert RL, Yee GC, Matzke GR, Wells BG, Posey L, eds. *Pharmacotherapy: A Pathophysiologic Approach.* 10th ed. New York, NY: McGraw-Hill; 2017.

Chyka PA, Erdman AR, Christianson G, et al. Salicylate poisoning: an evidence-based consensus guideline for out-of-hospital management. *Clin Toxicol.* 2007;45:95-131.

Dart RC, Borron SW, Caravati EM, et al. Expert consensus guidelines for stocking of antidotes in hospitals that provide emergency care. *Ann Emerg Med.* 2009;54(3):386-394.

Dart RC, Erdman AR, Olson KR, et al. Acetaminophen poisoning: an evidence-based consensus guideline for out-of-hospital management. *Clin Toxicol.* 2006;44:1-18.

Holstege CP, Dobmeier SG, Bechtel LK. Critical care toxicology. *Emerg Med Clin North Am.* 2008;26:715-739.

Marraffa JM, Cohen V, Howland MA. Antidotes for toxicological emergencies: a practical review. *Am J Health Syst Pharm.* 2012;69(3):199-212.

Nelsen LS, Lewin NA, Howland MA, et al. *Goldfrank's Toxicologic Emergencies.* 9th ed. New York, NY: McGraw-Hill Companies; 2011.

KEY ABBREVIATIONS

ABCs = airway, breathing, and circulation
ABG = arterial blood gases
ACLS = advanced cardiac life support
APAP = acetaminophen
AST = aspartate aminotransferase
BZD = benzodiazepine
CNS = central nervous system

EKG = electrocardiogram
GABA = gamma amino butyric acid
NAPQI = *N*-acetyl-p-benzoquinone imine
NAC = *N*-acetylcysteine
PC = poison center(s)
PPPA = Poison Prevention and Packaging Act

74

All Hazards Preparedness

Howell R. Foster and Keith R. McCain

FOUNDATION OVERVIEW

Paraphrasing the great scientist Louis Pasteur, "Luck favors the prepared!" When an event occurs, there will be a response, and that response will begin locally and radiate. While most events are small and local, some are incidences of national significance. The collapse of the I-35 bridge in Minneapolis in 2007 is a great example of local tragedy with a well-executed local response. According to Director of Pharmacy, University of Minnesota Medical Center, Scott Knoer, "All of the disaster training really pays off." "While this was a horrible tragedy for our city," reflected Knoer, "it was rewarding to see such a well-orchestrated response as our community pulled together."

It is the authors' opinion that, as health care professionals, it is pharmacists' ethical duty to assist during a disaster. Hospital pharmacists most likely have the easiest role to define because their participation in the hospital disaster plan should be clear. During a disaster, their service should be to their home institution. Pharmacists not associated with a health care facility will have to make their desire to volunteer known at the local or state level. Contacting your state's department of health, pharmacy association, or department of emergency management would all be good places to start.

Organization at the local or state level will vary, but virtually all plans will be based on the National Incident Management System (NIMS). NIMS provides a systematic, proactive approach to guide departments and agencies at all levels of government, nongovernmental organizations, and the private sector. The guide allows agencies to work seamlessly to prevent, protect against, respond to, recover from, and mitigate the effects of incidents, regardless of cause, size, location, or complexity, in order to reduce the loss of life and property and harm to the environment. Preparedness is achieved and maintained through a continuous cycle of planning, organizing, training, equipping, exercising, evaluating, and taking corrective action.

The Strategic National Stockpile (SNS) Program provides pharmaceuticals and medical supplies to the public free of charge in the event of a disaster. The governor of the afflicted state must ask for the SNS. If the request is granted, the material will be on site within 12 hours, hence they are often referred to as 12-Hour Push Packs. It is the requesting states' responsibility to manage the housing, dissemination, and administration of the material once it is received. However, this response time is inadequate for a nerve agent event, as treatment must be accomplished in less than 12 hours. The CHEMPACK container system is responsible for allowing storage of nerve agent antidote by various local and state agencies.

The pharmaceuticals initially found in the SNS were based on Category A threat agents. Presently, the pharmaceuticals are targeted for biologicals (smallpox, anthrax, botulism, viral hemorrhagic fevers (VHFs), plague, and tularemia), chemical agents (nerve agents), radiologicals, and recently the pandemic influenza. Pediatric dosing cards have been developed for the majority of these threats and would be extremely useful in the field.

BIOLOGICAL CATEGORY A AGENTS

The biologicals are typically referred to as the Category A threat agents. In regards to anthrax, plague, and tularemia, active cases will require intravenous (IV) antibiotics. These IV regimens will vary depending on the available agents prior to SNS delivery. The focus in this section will be on oral postexposure antibiotic prophylaxis for these infections. The use of ciprofloxacin and doxycycline in the pediatric population is not a common occurrence. However, the risk of mortality is so great with an exposure to a Category A Agent that pediatric use of the antibiotics is warranted.

Anthrax Inhalation Exposure

Bacillus anthracis is an encapsulated, aerobic, gram-positive, spore-forming, rod-shaped bacterium. The bacterium is known to cause cutaneous, gastrointestinal, respiratory, and oropharyngeal infections. Ciprofloxacin or doxycycline is indicated as initial therapy for postexposure prophylaxis to prevent inhalational anthrax from inhaled spores. Presently, no evidence exists to support either agent over the other for prophylaxis; therefore, a patient's individual history will be the determining factor.

Postexposure Prophylaxis (Adults)

Ciprofloxacin (Cipro) 500 mg every 12 hours for 60 days. Dose adjustment will be required for patients with a creatinine clearance (CrCl) less than 50 mL/min.

or

Doxycycline (Doryx, Doxy, Monodox, Vibramycin, and Vibra-Tabs) 100 mg every 12 hours for 60 days.

Postexposure Prophylaxis (Children)

Ciprofloxacin (Cipro) 10 to 15 mg/kg every 12 hours for 60 days.[a]

or

Doxycycline[a] (Doryx, Doxy, Monodox, Vibramycin, and Vibra-Tabs)

More than 8 year old and more than or equal to 45 kg: 100 mg every 12 hours for 60 days.

More than 8 year old and less than 45 kg: 2.2 mg/kg every 12 hours for 60 days.

Less than or equal to 8 year old: 2.2 mg/kg every 12 hours for 60 days.

Plague

Yersinia pestis is a gram-negative, rod-shaped facultative anaerobe known to cause bubonic and pneumonic plague. These diseases, although caused by the same organism, are different; however, both carry a high mortality. The pneumonic form is the greatest concern as a biologic weapon. The bacteria are aerosolized, and, once inhaled, the incubation period is 2 to 3 days. Pneumonia then develops, and patients often display stridor, cyanosis, and dyspnea. Pneumonic patients are highly contagious. Although it occurs naturally, bubonic plague could cause a mass casualty outbreak as it is considered the cause of the "Black Death" during the Middle Ages. Patients develop fever, malaise, and painful adenopathy (buboes). Patients can progress to the pneumonic form. Due to *Yersinia's* pathogenesis and its ability to replicate at a high rate, mortality is nearly 50% with treatment and nearly 100% if untreated; therefore, antibiotic therapy should be started immediately, and it should not be delayed while awaiting laboratory results.

Tularemia

Francisella tularensis is a gram-negative rod facultative intracellular pathogen. Tularemia is a naturally occurring disease most commonly associated with tick bites; however, it could be weaponized as an aerosol. Naturally occurring tularemia usually presents with a local skin ulcer, fever, chills, headache, and regional lymphadenopathy; progression to the pneumonic form is rare. Aerosolized tularemia is a potent entity, with inoculums as low as 25 colony-forming units/mL being capable of causing debilitating or fatal disease. The pneumonic form carries the highest mortality. An outbreak of the pneumonic form of tularemia should be considered an intentional event until proven otherwise.

Plague and Tularemia Postexposure Prophylaxis

Postexposure Prophylaxis (Adults)

Ciprofloxacin (Cipro) 500 mg every 12 hours for 7 days. Dose adjustment will be required for patients with a CrCl less than 50 mL/min.

or

Doxycycline (Doryx, Doxy, Monodox, Vibramycin, and Vibra-Tabs) 100 mg every 12 hours for 7 days.

Postexposure Prophylaxis (Children)

Ciprofloxacin (Cipro) 10 to 15 mg/kg every 12 hours for 7 days.

or

Doxycycline (Doryx, Doxy, Monodox, Vibramycin, and Vibra-Tabs) less than or equal to 45 kg: 2.2 mg/kg every 12 hours for 7 days.

Botulism

Clostridium botulinum is an anaerobic, gram-positive, spore-forming rod that produces a potent neurotoxin. The spores are heat-resistant and can survive in foods that are incorrectly or minimally processed. Seven types (A, B, C, D, E, F, and G) of botulism are recognized, based on the antigenic specificity of the toxin produced by each strain. Types A, B, E, and F cause human botulism naturally; therefore, human cases of other types would be suggestive of an act of terrorism. Types C and D cause most cases of botulism in animals. Animals most commonly affected are wild fowl and poultry, cattle, horses, and some species of fish. Botulinum-infected patients with extensive muscle weakness, ptosis, dysphagia, great frequency of gastrointestinal effects, and urinary retention are at a greater risk of developing respiratory failure. Mechanical ventilation may be required. Botulism is not communicable. A bivalent antitoxin preparation exists containing types A and B, and a monovalent antitoxin preparation type E (suggestive of contaminated seafood) exists for the treatment of botulism caused by the aforementioned toxins. (The trivalent antitoxin [types A, B, and E] is no longer available.) The monovalent type E is given only when it is suspected. To obtain the antitoxin preparations, call the Centers for Disease Control (CDC) at 770-488-7100. An investigational heptavalent antitoxin has also been developed and is maintained by the US military.

VIRAL HEMORRHAGIC FEVERS

VHFs are caused by viruses of four distinct families: arenaviruses (Lassa fever), filoviruses (Ebola and Marburg), bunyaviruses (Rift Valley fever), and flaviviruses (Yellow fever and dengue). They require a host and are ribonucleic acid (RNA) viruses. Naturally, VHFs are restricted geographically by their host. Human cases or outbreaks of VHFs caused by these viruses occur sporadically since humans are not their natural hosts. However once infected, human to human transmission is possible with some of the viruses. There are no cures; however, ribavirin may be useful against arenaviruses and bunyaviruses. Treatment is otherwise symptomatic and supportive.

Smallpox

The orthopoxvirus variola (smallpox) causes an acute febrile illness with a corresponding rash that develops into small,

---

[a]If ciprofloxacin and doxycycline are contraindicated, then amoxicillin (Amoxil; Polymox; Trimox) 80 mg/kg/d in divided doses every 8 hours.

pus-filled blisters. Mortality rates are as high as 30%. Survivors are often severely scarred and ocular involvement may lead to blindness in some. Prolonged face-to-face contact is generally required for transmission. A person is considered infectious to others from the onset of fever until the last pox scab sloughs off.

On the first day of a documented outbreak, the SNS will distribute smallpox vaccine to anyone who has been exposed. Over the next 5 to 6 days, the CDC will oversee the vaccination of the rest of the country as needed.

NERVE AGENTS

Organophosphate Compounds

These compounds are divided into the militarized agents GA (tabun), GB (sarin), GD (soman), and VX and the nonmilitarized or agricultural agents parathion, malathion, diazinon, and many other derivatives. The latter are considered less potent, but with a large dose, they can be formidable substances.

Organophosphates (OPs) are toxic by all routes of exposure. Regardless of the route of exposure, signs and symptoms are cholinergic in nature and will be muscarinic or nicotinic. Salivation, lacrimation, urination, defecation, gastrointestinal symptoms, and emesis form the acronym SLUDGE to assist in remembering the basic signs and symptoms. Pinpoint pupils, chest tightness, shortness of breath, excessive sweating, muscle twitching, confusion, seizures, paralysis, coma, respiratory paralysis, and death may also occur. With the more potent military agents, the incapacitating effects can occur within 1 minute and fatal effects can occur within 1 to 10 minutes. Fatigue, irritability, nervousness, and memory defects may persist for as long as 6 weeks after recovery from an exposure episode.

As a result of the rapid onset of severe signs and symptoms, nerve agents are stored and shipped differently than other treatments found in the SNS. As previously stated, they are stored under CHEMPACK. CHEMPACK is a voluntary program of the SNS operated by the CDC for the benefit of the US civilian population. Its mission is to provide state and local governments a sustainable nerve agent antidote cache. The CHEMPACK only contains materials for a nerve agent exposure and does not contain any other materials.

In the event of an OP poisoning, three agents need to be readily available (atropine, pralidoxime, and diazepam). Atropine will be used to counter the muscarinic effects commonly seen. However, it has little affinity for nicotinic receptors and will not reverse respiratory paralysis, fasciculation, or general muscle weakness. Pralidoxime will be used to reverse the binding of the OP to the acetylcholinesterase as long as aging has not occurred. Aging is the process by which the OP covalently binds the acetylcholinesterase rending it useless. Aging can occur in less than 12 hours with some of the militarized OPs; this is the principal reason for the CHEMPACK. Diazepam will be used to prevent or treat seizures.

Atropine

Adult: 2 to 6 mg (0.02-0.04 mg/kg) repeated every 2 to 30 minutes.

Pediatric: 0.05 to 0.1 mg/kg bolus every 2 to 30 minutes.

Pralidoxime (Protopam)

Adult: 1 to 2 g in 100 mL of 0.9% NS, IV, over 15 to 30 minutes followed by a continuous infusion of 500 mg/h. The infusion should be continued until symptoms have resolved for at least 24 hours.

Pediatric: 20 to 40 mg/kg in 100 mL of 0.9% normal saline (NS) over 30 minutes up to a maximum of 1 g followed by a continuous infusion of 10 to 20 mg/kg/h. The infusion should be continued until symptoms have resolved for at least 24 hours.

Central nervous system (CNS) damage from OP poisoning is currently thought to be due to seizure activity rather than a direct toxic effect. Prevention and treatment of seizures with diazepam is an important aspect of patient management. Seizures are more common in pediatric poisoning with cholinesterase inhibitors.

Diazepam (Dizac; Valium)

Adult: 5 to 10 mg, IV, every 5 to 10 minutes (one, 10-mg auto-injector, every 10 minutes × three doses maximum)

Pediatric: 0.2 mg/kg, IV, every 5 to 10 minutes.

RADIOLOGICS

Radioactive materials cannot be seen, tasted, felt, or smelled. It takes special equipment to detect them. Because of the unknown, they make an ideal weapon of terror. While a dirty bomb has been the focus of media reports in recent years, the biggest threat to life is most likely from the incendiary device used in the explosion and not the radiation itself. An atomic bomb is very different from a dirty bomb and the detonation of an atomic weapon would have very grave consequences. The following are recommendations for individuals near the blast area of a dirty bomb.

Dirty Bomb

If You Are Outside and Close to the Incident

- Cover your nose and mouth with a cloth to reduce the risk of breathing in radioactive dust or smoke.
- Don't touch objects thrown off by an explosion—they might be radioactive.
- Quickly go into a building where the walls and windows have not been broken. This area will shield you from radiation that might be outside.
- Once you are inside, take off your outer layer of clothing and seal it in a plastic bag if available. Put the cloth you used to cover your mouth in the bag, too. Removing outer clothes may get rid of up to 90% of radioactive dust.
- Put the plastic bag where others will not touch it and keep it until authorities tell you what to do with it.
- Shower or wash with soap and water. Be sure to wash your hair. Washing will remove any remaining dust.
- Tune to the local radio or television news for more instructions.

If You Are Inside and Close to the Incident

- If the walls and windows of the building are not broken, stay in the building and do not leave.

- To keep radioactive dust or powder from getting inside, shut all windows, outside doors, and fireplace dampers. Turn off fans and heating and air-conditioning systems that bring in air from the outside. It is not necessary to put duct tape or plastic around doors or windows.

- If the walls and windows of the building are broken, go to an interior room and do not leave. If the building has been heavily damaged, quickly go into a building where the walls and windows have not been broken. If you must go outside, be sure to cover your nose and mouth with a cloth. Once you are inside, take off your outer layer of clothing and seal it in a plastic bag if available. Store the bag where others will not touch it.

- Shower or wash with soap and water, removing any remaining dust. Be sure to wash your hair.

- Tune to local radio or television news for more instructions.

Treatment for many patients postexposure to radioactive materials will be symptomatic and supportive. However, if an individual has been exposed to I131, or Cs137, there may be an antidote.

Potassium Iodide KI is used for I131 acute exposures. Children are significantly more susceptible to the thyroid effects of I131. KI has to be given rapidly to be of benefit. Up to 90% of I131 uptake can be blocked in the first 2 hours postexposure. By 4 hours postexposure, only 50% of I131 is blocked. Maintenance doses may be given daily for 7 to 14 days to prevent recycling of I131 into the thyroid. Adults 40 years of age or older have low risk of thyroid damage and KI therapy is not warranted. If you live within 50 miles of a nuclear facility that produces or is capable of releasing I131, you should work with your medical association, local or state public health department, emergency response organizations, and elected representatives to ensure that a stockpile of KI is available and a distribution plan is in place.

Prussian Blue Prussian blue traps radioactive cesium in the intestines preventing reabsorption. The bound Cs is then excreted. Prussian blue reduces the T½ of Cs137 from about 110 days to about 30 days. Because Prussian blue reduces the time that radioactive Cs137 stays in the body, it helps limit the amount of time the body is exposed to radiation.

Nuclear Attack Under the National Response Plan and the Nuclear/Radiological Annex, HHS has the major role in protecting people's health by monitoring, assessing, and following up on people's health. Ensuring the safety of workers by assessing the amount of time they can safely work in an area contaminated with radioactive materials and providing them protective equipment such as respiratory devices and monitoring devices. Maintaining and ensuring the safety of the area's food and water supply will be paramount. Medical and

public health advice will be disseminated and the deployment of the SNS will occur if necessary.

PANDEMIC FLU

An influenza pandemic is a global disease outbreak that occurs when a new influenza A virus emerges for which there is little or no immunity in the human population. Since immunity is low, the virus can spread quickly. Pharmacist should be aware of http://www.flu.gov/. It is a comprehensive and up-to-date site for influenza information for both the public and healthcare professionals.

Antiviral drugs are stockpiled by HHS as part of the SNS. The US influenza antiviral drug stockpile includes supplies of both of the neuraminidase inhibitor agents, oseltamivir and zanamivir. These medications are to be used in the event that a novel influenza A subtype virus. Pandemic preparedness is a shared responsibility of all levels of government, businesses, families, and individuals.

CASE Application

1. Preparedness is achieved and maintained by which of the following? Select all that apply.

   a. Planning
   b. Organizing
   c. Training
   d. Exercising

2. Virtually all disaster plans are based on what national system?

   a. National Planning System (NPS)
   b. National Incidence Management System (NIMS)
   c. Federal Incidence Bureau System (FIBS)
   d. Strategic National Planning System (SNPS)

3. The SNS provides what during an incidence of national significance?

   a. Highly trained medical personal from around the country to disseminate supplies
   b. Pharmaceuticals only to the state
   c. Active military medical personnel to support the public
   d. Pharmaceuticals and medical supplies to the state in need

4. Which government official must request the SNS?

   a. President of the United States
   b. Director of Health and Human Services
   c. Governor
   d. Speaker of the House

5. The CHEMPACK Program stores nerve agent antidotes with participating local or state entities. What are the antidotes provided by this program? Select all that apply.

   a. Atropine
   b. Pyridoxine

c. Pralidoxime

d. Diazepam

6. Which of the following is considered a Category A threat agent? Select all that apply.

   a. Smallpox
   b. Novel H1N1
   c. Anthrax
   d. Botulism

7. Which agent is found in the SNS and is indicated for postexposure prophylaxis to inhaled *B. anthracis*?

   a. Dapsone
   b. Daptomycin
   c. Doxycycline
   d. Dicloxacillin

8. Antibiotic therapy for postexposure prophylaxis to inhaled *B. anthracis* should last for how many days?

   a. 30
   b. 40
   c. 60
   d. 90

9. An 18-year-old patient has been diagnosed with a pneumonic form of *Y. pestis*. What is the best course of action for the individual(s) exposed to the patient?

   a. Start ciprofloxacin 500 mg every 12 hours once symptoms appear.
   b. Start doxycycline 100 mg every 12 hours for 7 days in all individuals exposed during the patient's clinical course.
   c. Await the patient's culture and sensitivity results and start the most appropriate antibiotic as prophylaxis in the exposed individuals.
   d. Prophylaxis is not beneficial.

10. A pharmacist working in local retail pharmacy receives a call during a bioterrorism drill from an emergency department physician. He states they have a confirmed case of pneumonic tularemia. The patient states a former coworker threatened everyone in the workplace. Upon questioning from the police, it was determined the coworker had released *F. tularensis* into the air ducts of his former workplace approximately 3 days prior. There are six individuals in that area and he has written them each a prescription for ciprofloxacin 500 mg every 12 hours for 7 days as prophylaxis. However, the air duct system is shared with a daycare and eight children have been potentially exposed. All of the children are <30 kg. The physician asks for an antibiotic recommendation. Which of the following is the best treatment recommendation for all of the children?

    a. Doxycycline 50 mg every 12 hours for 7 days
    b. Doxycycline 2.2 mg/kg every 12 hours for 7 days
    c. Ciprofloxacin 500 mg once daily for 7 days
    d. Ciprofloxacin 25 mg/kg every 12 hours for 7 days

11. Which of the following botulism types can be treated with an antitoxin obtained from the CDC? Select all that apply.

    a. Type A
    b. Type B
    c. Type C
    d. Type E

12. Twelve patients with type G botulism have been diagnosed in the United States in the past 24 hours. All had recently flown through Toronto Pearson International Airport in the last 72 hours from various destinations. All are experiencing a rapid descending paralysis. What is the most likely reason for the outbreak?

    a. Contaminated seafood at an airport vendor
    b. Deliberate release of toxin within the airport
    c. Person to person contamination
    d. Serendipity

13. What is presently the best course of treatment for Ebola?

    a. Fluid replacement, ventilation, and additional supportive care as needed
    b. High dose ribavirin
    c. Cryotherapy to drop the core temperature to <95°F
    d. A cocktail of acyclovir, protease inhibitor, and interferon

14. A person with smallpox is no longer considered infectious when what event occurs?

    a. Defervescence
    b. The last pustule scabs over
    c. Sloughing of the last pustule scab
    d. When the rash turns to pustules

15. Which of the following signs and symptoms are considered clinically significant control with atropine in a postexposure OP patient?

    a. Miosis, salivation, and muscle twitching
    b. Mydriasis, dry mucous membranes, flushing, and tachycardia
    c. Tachycardia, bronchorrhea, and salivation
    d. Decreased bronchial secretions and increased ease of ventilation

16. An adult patient with sarin poisoning has been decontaminated and is now in the triage area. He has small pupils, sweating, and copious salivation and nasal secretions. He begins having a seizure almost immediately after being brought to the triage area. Which is the best course of treatment?

    a. Administer diazepam 10 mg, followed by a 2 mg bolus of atropine, and then pralidoxime 2 g in 100 cc of NS infused over 30 minutes.
    b. A 2 mg bolus of atropine and repeat as needed, then pralidoxime 2 g in 100 cc of NS infused over 30 minutes. If the seizure activity has not abated post pralidoxime, then give 5 mg of diazepam.

c. Administer 10 mg of diazepam for the seizure then no additional therapy as the other signs and symptoms are not concerning.

d. Administer 5 g of pralidoxime via *intravenous pyelography* (IVP) since it will replenish gamma-aminobutyric acid (GABA), then give atropine 2 g prn until bronchorrhea decreases.

17. A 3-year-old child and her 65-year-old grandmother were riding in car that was involved in a three-vehicle accident at 3 am. They have only minor injuries, but one of the other vehicles was carrying I131 for use as an imaging agent. The I131 container was not properly stored or sealed and it entered the side window of the vehicle with the child and grandmother. Many of the compounded I131 capsules were ruptured and dispersed throughout the car. They are 20 minutes postaccident and no one is answering the phone at the nuclear pharmacy; there is no paperwork with the I131 product and the delivery driver is unconscious. Which is the best advice for the grandmother and child?

a. Treat both with KI.

b. Treat the grandmother with KI and leave the child untreated.

c. Treat the child with KI and leave the grandmother untreated.

d. Treat both with Prussian blue.

18. The first case of novel H1N1 was reported in the United States in late March-early April 2009. By the end of June, reported cases topped 1 million US residents. The logical reason for rapid dissemination of the disease is most likely which of the following?

a. The seasonal flu vaccine weakened the immune system.

b. The wet spring months are better for viral survival.

c. The population lacks immunity.

d. Antivirals are infective.

19. Select the brand name for doxycycline.

a. Vibramycin

b. Zosyn

c. Zovirax

d. Valtrex

20. Select the brand name for ciprofloxacin.

a. Levaquin

b. Cipro

c. Avelox

d. Flagyl

TAKEAWAY POINTS »

- Organization at the local or state level will vary, but virtually all plans will be based on the NIMS. NIMS provides a systematic, proactive approach to guide departments and agencies at all levels of government, nongovernmental organizations, and the private sector.

- The SNS Program provides pharmaceuticals and medical supplies to the public free of charge in the event of a disaster.

- *Bacillus anthracis* is an encapsulated, aerobic, gram-positive, spore-forming, rod-shaped bacterium. The bacterium is known to cause cutaneous, gastrointestinal, respiratory, and oropharyngeal infections. Ciprofloxacin or doxycycline is indicated as initial therapy for postexposure prophylaxis to prevent inhalational anthrax from inhaled spores.

- *Yersinia pestis* is a gram-negative, rod-shaped facultative anaerobe that is known to cause bubonic and pneumonic plague. Treatment or prophylaxis on *Yersinia* consists of ciprofloxacin or doxycycline.

- *Francisella tularensis* is a gram-negative, rod-shaped facultative intracellular pathogen. Tularemia is a naturally occurring disease most commonly associated with tick bites; however, it could be weaponized as an aerosol. Treatment or prophylaxis on tularemia consists of ciprofloxacin or doxycycline.

- *Clostridium botulinum* is an anaerobic, gram-positive, spore-forming rod that produces a potent neurotoxin.

- VHFs are caused by viruses of four distinct families: arenaviruses (Lassa fever), filoviruses (Ebola and Marburg), bunyaviruses (Rift Valley fever), and flaviviruses (Yellow fever and dengue). There are no cures; however, ribavirin may be useful against arenaviruses and bunyaviruses. Treatment is otherwise symptomatic and supportive.

- The orthopoxvirus variola (smallpox) causes an acute febrile illness with a corresponding rash that develops into small, pus-filled blister. On the first day of a documented outbreak, the SNS will distribute smallpox vaccine to anyone who has been exposed. Then over the next 5 to 6 days the CDC will oversee the vaccination of the rest of the country as needed.

- In the event of an OP poisoning, three agents need to be readily available (atropine, pralidoxime, and diazepam).

BIBLIOGRAPHY

http://www.fema.gov/. Accessed June 12, 2018.

https://www.fema.gov/preparedness-checklists-toolkits. Accessed June 12, 2018.

http://emergency.cdc.gov/agent. Accessed June 12, 2018.

http://www.cdc.gov/DiseasesConditions/. Accessed June 12, 2018.

http://emergency.cdc.gov/radiation. Accessed June 12, 2018.

http://www.flu.gov/. Accessed June 12, 2018.

Suchard JR. Biological weapons. In: Hoffman RS, Howland M, Lewin NA, Nelson LS, Goldfrank LR, eds. *Goldfrank's Toxicologic Emergencies.* 10th ed. New York, NY: McGraw-Hill; 2015.

Terriff CM, Costanigro LT, McKeirnan KC, Hoeben BJ. Clinical management of potential bioterrorism-related conditions. In: DiPiro JT, Talbert RL, Yee GC, Matzke GR, Wells BG, Posey L, eds. *Pharmacotherapy: A athophysiologic Approach.* 10th ed. New York, NY: McGraw-Hill; 2017.

KEY ABBREVIATIONS

CDC = *Centers for Disease Control* and Prevention
CNS = central nervous system
CrCl = creatinine clearance
GABA = gamma-aminobutyric acid
IV = intravenous
IVP = intravenous pyelography
KI = potassium iodide

MRSA = methicillin-resistant *Staphylococcus aureus*
NIMS = National Incident Management System
NS = normal saline
RNA = ribonucleic acid
VHF = viral hemorrhagic fever
VRE = vancomycin resistant Enterococcus

75

Herbal and Nonherbal Dietary Supplements

Cydney E. McQueen and Andrea J. Potter

FOUNDATION OVERVIEW

Many patients regularly use or occasionally try supplements, either along with prescription and over-the-counter (OTC) therapies, or in place of some therapies. Because pharmacists must educate and advise patients on drug therapies, it is essential to have a basic understanding of dietary supplements (DS) in order to assist in avoiding harm, whether from drug interactions, use of a contraindicated supplement, or a poor quality product. Pharmacists do not control access to these products, but can provide essential advice and recommendations.

Although some dispensing software systems include a few DS and check for interactions, there are thousands of botanical and nonbotanical DS. Every pharmacy should have one or more comprehensive resources available to be able to look up information when necessary. However, all pharmacists should be familiar with the most commonly used DS and those that present possible risks of greatest severity. Additionally, familiarity with the key points for investigating safety and making recommendations when encountering previously unknown supplements is essential.

KEY POINTS FOR INVESTIGATING UNFAMILIAR SUPPLEMENTS

The following questions assume that the pharmacist has fully gathered pertinent information about a patient's medical history, current drug regimen, and reason for considering use of a DS.

1. **Does the supplement work?**

   What clinical trial data are available to support effectiveness? When this is minimal, the type and severity of the patient's disease state is a large factor in weighing risks and benefits, that is, what is risk of harm if the patient tries the supplement for a while and it is not effective? Risk is minimal with a self-limiting condition such as a cold but far greater for uncontrolled diabetes or hypertension. When the evidence to support effectiveness is stronger, it may be appropriate to use the supplement. For example, a trial period of 4 weeks in a patient with mild hypertension could be appropriate, but not with severe hypertension.

2. **Is the supplement safe?**

   Often, this information is not well-understood because of a lack of long-term clinical trials, and therefore must be extrapolated from the mechanism of action, small animal studies, or case reports. Both in mass media and in medical literature, safety issues are sometimes underemphasized and sometimes overemphasized. The possible risks to the particular patient should be realistically balanced with the possible benefits.

   Patient education rule for all supplements: stop all use 10 to 14 days before any scheduled surgical procedures to avoid possible drug and anesthesia interactions or increased bleeding risks.

3. **How does the supplement work?**

   This information is important for cautions and limitations in use. If well-researched, the mechanism of action may be available in general resources, but sometimes must be extrapolated from very limited in vitro or animal studies. For example, if animal studies have shown increased vasodilation, then it is reasonable to recommend caution, or to not use at all, when decreased blood pressure could be problematic, either due to a disease state or an additive effect with an antihypertensive medication.

4. **Are there quality considerations specific to this supplement?**

   To ensure patients are taking good quality supplements (ie, contain what is stated on the label without additional contaminants), it recommend that they only buy supplements that participate in a quality seal program. The Dietary Supplement Verification Program from the United States Pharmacopeia (USP) is probably the most recognizable and available. Alternatively, products that have been tested by third-party laboratories such as ConsumerLab.com could be recommended.

   When specific problems with quality are present, more patient education is needed. For example, butterbur extracts can be quite effective for seasonal allergy symptoms, but products must be free of unsaturated pyrrolizidine alkaloids (UPA), which are hepatotoxic. An issue more central to effectiveness, rather than safety, is ensuring the product purchased is of the appropriate standardization,

To access your complimentary online question exams, visit https://accesspharmacy.mhmedical.com/NAPLEX.aspx

if a botanical extract (eg, feverfew extract standardized to 0.2%-0.35% parthenolide) or a salt form for some nonbotanicals (eg, glucosamine sulfate, not hydrochloride).

5. **Does the patient have appropriate expectations of what this supplement might be able to do?**

   Generally, supplements are going to provide lesser effects than prescription drug treatments; onset of full benefit is often slower as well. The information-gathering process must include the patient's goals for therapy. For example, a postmenopausal woman experiencing 10 to 12 severe hot flashes every week who wants to reduce the frequency and severity by 30% to 50% may be very satisfied with black cohosh therapy, while a woman with 8 severe hot flashes per week who wants to reduce the number to zero is likely to be dissatisfied with results.

6. **A patient is going to use a product, despite your negative recommendation—what education is needed?**

   The goal is the same as with a recommended supplement—minimize any potential harm and maximize any potential benefits. Points of education are very similar to prescription drugs—dosing regimen, length of time to use/try, side effects/adverse effects, and drug or disease state interactions. Self-monitoring is very important, especially when a patient is using a supplement against recommendations. Instructions should be very specific, for example, say, "watch out for easy bruising," rather than "this might increase your bleeding risk."

DIETARY SUPPLEMENTS TO KNOW

Black Cohosh (*Actaea racemose or Cimicifuga racemosa*)

Primary Use: Postmenopausal symptoms such as hot flushes.

Mode of Action (MOA): Affects vasovagal and thermoregulatory system for hot flush suppression; may or may not have some minimal estrogen-modulator effects.

Evidence: Generally good effects in most trials, some with contradictory results, especially those using lower doses.

Dosage and Product Considerations: 20 mg extract standardized to contain 1 mg 27-deoxyacetin (or 2.5% triterpene glycosides) bid, which may be increased to 40 mg of extract bid if sufficient benefit is not seen. Most studies with positive results have used the German Remifemin® brand extract, which is available in the United States from enzymatic therapy.

Side Effects and Monitoring: Well-tolerated by most, with mild gastrointestinal (GI) effects most common, and allergic reactions and rashes possible. Rare reports of hypotension, bradycardia, and hepatic issues are controversial, but monitoring of liver function is advised for now. Regular well-woman gynecological exams should continue.

Contraindications and Interactions: Do not use in liver disease or bradycardia, or with hepatotoxic agents or estrogenic/

antiestrogenic agents; may have additive effects with antihypertensive agents. May inhibit CYP450 2D6; use with caution.

Key Knowledge: May take up to 8 weeks for full onset of effects. Treatment is not likely to reduce hot flush frequency and severity to the same extent as hormone therapy. It is not known to have beneficial effects on bone health in postmenopausal women.

Chondroitin Sulfate

Primary Use: Osteoarthritis (OA)

MOA: Chondroitin is a glycosaminoglycan that has slight anti-inflammation action, stimulates chondrocytes to produce cartilage, serves as a sulfur source for generation of molecular bonds within cartilage, and inhibits leukocyte elastase, an enzyme responsible for degradation of cartilage.

Evidence: There is far less evidence for chondroitin used alone than in combination with glucosamine. Although some trials of monotherapy for long periods in knee OA did demonstrate increased mobility, decreased pain, and fewer joint erosions, and hand OA trials resulted in less pain and stiffness, systemic analyses of later trials did not demonstrate a consistent clinically significant benefit for chondroitin.

Dosage and Product Considerations: Whether alone or in combination with glucosamine, the dose is 1200 mg/d in one or divided doses. Chondroitin is usually produced from cattle trachea; because this does not normally contain neural matter, there is little to no risk of bovine spongiform encephalopathy; however, microbial contamination is a possibility. Only high-quality products should be used—those participating in a quality seal program or tested by a third-party laboratory.

Side Effects and Monitoring: Generally well-tolerated. Headache and GI symptoms are most commonly reported; taking with food and dividing doses may alleviate these side effects.

Contraindications and Interactions: Case reports exist of increased international normalized ratio (INR) and bleeding when used with warfarin; use with any anticoagulant/antiplatelet agents should be avoided or closely monitored.

Key Knowledge: Due to the mechanism of action, chondroitin must be used for several months before any benefits can be expected to be observed; trial periods should be at least 6 months before any decision regarding efficacy is made. Chondroitin is an expensive product and cheap versions are very likely to not contain chondroitin in labeled amounts. In general, combination use with glucosamine is preferred over monotherapy (see glucosamine section).

Echinacea (*Echinacea purpurea, E. pallida, E. angustifolia*)

Primary Use: Treatment and/or prevention of colds/upper respiratory infections.

MOA: Multiple activities involved in immune system function: increased phagocytosis by macrophages, lymphocytic and natural killer cell activity, and cytokine (interferon, interleukins) secretion. Mild anti-inflammatory effects may exist via cyclooxygenase and 5-lipooxygenase inhibition. Antiviral action on certain respiratory illness viruses has been reported. Very recent information links some of the beneficial activities to bacteria living within the plants, rather than echinacea itself.

Evidence: Clinical trial evidence is extremely contradictory. Comparisons and meta-analyses can be difficult because of the variety of products—different species, plant parts, types of extracts, and methods of measuring outcomes. Results of a meta-analysis concluded that when echinacea was use for prevention after an initial illness, it resulted in about a third fewer recurrent infections than placebo. For treatment, current evidence supports a small reduction in "sick days" and a more than 50% reduction in development of colds in subjects exposed to cold viruses.

Dosage and Product Considerations: Data does not support one type of echinacea product or dose. Products with the most clinical evidence for benefits are not always available in the United States. Extracts are preferable to whole plant or root products and should be standardized to alkamide, chicoric acid, or echinoside content. For prevention, manufacturers' directions may be followed, while an increased dosing regimen of three to four times daily may be used for treatment. Treatment must begin at the very first onset of symptoms for best efficacy.

Side Effects and Monitoring: Generally well tolerated. Mild GI symptoms and headache are most common. Allergic reactions of varying severities, including anaphylaxis, are reported.

Contraindications and Interactions: Severe allergy to Asteracea/Compositae plants (chrysanthemums, ragweed) and patients with autoimmune diseases. Drug interactions are primarily minimal, although concomitant use with CYP1A2 substrates should be avoided or closely monitored. Avoid use with immunosuppressants. A prospective trial demonstrated no fetal harm from echinacea use in the first trimester; however, the limited information available, one trial and two retrospective reviews, prevents a recommendation of use during pregnancy; any use during pregnancy should be discussed with the primary healthcare provider.

Key Knowledge: Start standardized echinacea extracts at the very first sign of a cold or upper respiratory infection. To minimize risk of any adverse events, use for prevention should be limited to times when there is known exposure to an ill person. Only products participating in a quality seal program or that have been tested by a third-party laboratory should be recommended.

Evening Primrose Oil (EPO, *Oenothera biennis*)

Primary Use: Varying uses: atopic dermatitis, cyclic mastalgia, fibromyalgia and chronic fatigue syndrome, and asthma.

MOA: Evening primrose seeds contain oil with omega-6 fatty acids (primarily linoleic and gamma-linolenic acids).

In general, anti-inflammatory effects are achieved by influencing the balance of anti-inflammatory and pro-inflammatory cytokines through the production cascades. The gamma-linolenic component inhibits the pro-inflammatory effects of arachidonic acid's production of leukotrienes.

Evidence: Multiple clinical trials have resulted in a confusing and conflicting evidence picture. Despite some positive results noted in atopic dermatitis trials, a meta-analysis concluded oral EPO had no benefit; one trial with topical 10% EPO cream noted improvement over placebo. Half of the clinical trials for cyclic mastalgia demonstrated a reduction in breast pain, while an equal number of studies found no difference from placebo; the most recent high-quality trial found a small but significant decrease in pain compared to placebo. EPO has not been tested in fibromyalgia; a controlled study in patients with chronic fatigue syndrome found no improvements compared to placebo. Although trials in asthma have noted improvements in markers of inflammation, no differences from placebo in clinical symptoms were demonstrated.

Dosage and Product Considerations: Most studies have used EPO products containing at least 9% gamma-linolenic acid. For atopic dermatitis, dosage is 3 to 4 g/d for adults and 0.5 to 3 g/d for children; topical 10% EPO cream is generally used twice daily. Dosages for cyclic mastalgia, fibromyalgia, and chronic fatigue syndrome are 3 to 6 g/d.

Side Effects and Monitoring: Generally well-tolerated. Increased bleeding time is possible.

Contraindications and Interactions: Metabolic drug interactions are primarily theoretical and minor. Use with anticoagulants and antiplatelet agents should be avoided or occur only with low doses and careful monitoring. One report of seizure occurred in a patient taking several botanical therapies; use in seizure disorders or with anticonvulsant agents is best avoided. It should not be used in pregnancy, especially in the last trimester, due to potential for delivery complications and adverse effects on the newborn.

Key Knowledge: EPO is a supplement with great theoretical potential that has not been demonstrated in clinical trials. Because EPO has a good safety profile, patients who wish to try do not need to be discouraged unless there is a strict contraindication. Education should include the limited benefits likely in most individuals.

Fish Oil

Primary Use: Reduction of elevated triglycerides, hyperlipidemia, and cardiovascular risk reduction.

MOA: A source of the omega-3 fatty acids (O3FA), docosahexaenoic acid (DHA) and eicosapentaenoic acid (EPA). Resolvins and protectins from O3FA decrease inflammation of arterial plaque; cholesterol absorption is decreased and enzymes responsible for low-density lipoprotein production are inhibited, improving lipid profiles, especially triglycerides.

The increased DHA and EPA levels variously influence production of multiple cytokines having anti-inflammatory effects.

Evidence: Evidence for reduction of elevated triglycerides strongly supports use in mild-moderate hypertriglyceridemia (−9 to −26%). Effects on low-density lipoprotein (LDL) and total cholesterol levels are far smaller (0 to −11%) and little to no effects are generally seen for high-density lipoprotein (HDL). Though earlier studies supported a role in reducing cardiovascular risk, this has not always been borne out in later research; eating more fish may have more benefits than use of supplements.

Dosage and Product Considerations: To normalize dietary intake, 1 g/d. For triglyceride reduction, 2 to 4 g/d. Concerns over mercury and heavy metal contamination in fish generally do not extend to fish oil, because oil is expressed from fish skin, while contaminants are concentrated in the fish flesh. Use of a high-quality product is recommended: products either participating in the USP Dietary Supplement Verification program or tested by a third-party laboratory. Note: Although labeled amounts of DHA and EPA will not equal the total amount of fish oil per capsule, these amounts should consist of a fairly high percentage of the total in a high-quality product.

Side Effects and Monitoring: Generally well-tolerated; "fish burp" is the most common adverse effect, alleviated or minimized by use of enteric-coated capsules and/or by freezing the capsules. Reported side effects do include fishy halitosis, heartburn, nausea, and loose stools.

Contraindications and Interactions: Because of possible antiplatelet effects, doses greater than 3 g/d should be used very cautiously in patients on anticoagulants or antiplatelet agents. Administration of orlistat and fish oil should be separated by 2 to 3 hours. Monitor blood pressure in patients on antihypertensives, due to possible slight additive effects.

Key Knowledge: Patients should be educated that, though, fish oil can be a beneficial addition to decrease lipids, particularly triglycerides, benefits for overall cardiovascular risk reduction are likely to be much smaller.

Garlic (*Allium sativum*)

Primary Use: Hypertension and hyperlipidemia.

MOA: Though garlic contains multiple active components, the primary marker compound is allicin, produced from alliin when the enzyme alliinase is released upon damage to cells of the garlic bulb. Alliin and S-allylcysteine have antioxidant properties (preventing oxidation of lipids) and exhibit antiplatelet and antimicrobial effects. Antihypertensive effects are partly due to increased hydrogen sulfide, which dilates vasculature.

Evidence: In hypertension, decreases in systolic blood pressure average ~8 to 9 mm Hg and diastolic 4 to 6 mm Hg. A recent meta-analysis found reductions in total cholesterol of

15 to 20 mg/dL when used for extended periods of time; LDL decreases were smaller.

Dosage and Product Considerations: Aged garlic extracts with a minimum of 1.2 mg of S-allylcysteine daily or powdered garlic providing 3 to 5 mg of allicin daily; aged extracts may be more effective. Use of raw garlic and garlic oils are not supported.

Side Effects and Monitoring: Halitosis is the most common side effect. GI effects including heartburn and reflux are more prevalent with therapy initiation or with high doses. Garlic does affect platelet function; garlic must be stopped 10 to 14 days before any elective surgeries or dental procedures—reports of excessive bleeding are common.

Contraindications and Interactions: Supplement amounts should be avoided or used under close monitoring in patients on antithrombotics/anticoagulants. Garlic can enter breast milk, affecting taste and altering nursing time. Very limited and contradictory information is available for use in pregnancy; garlic does cross the placental barrier, so use is best avoided. Contradictory information indicates that garlic may induce some CYP450 enzymes to varying extent (2D6 and 3A4); use with saquinavir and isoniazid should be avoided while effects of other drugs during concomitant use should be closely monitored.

Key Knowledge: Effect sizes for reductions of both blood pressure and lipid levels are small, so garlic is only appropriate for mild hyperlipidemia and hypertension, and in patients who are making additional lifestyle changes to reduce their risks. However, due to the mild safety profile, patients with more severe disease wishing to use garlic do not have to be discouraged unless a specific contraindication exists.

Glucosamine Sulfate and Glucosamine Hydrochloride

Primary Use: Osteoarthritis.

MOA: Like chondroitin, glucosamine stimulates chondrocytes to synthesize cartilage while functioning as a source of building blocks, but also stimulates the product of synovial fluid. It reduces both inflammatory cytokines and matrix metalloproteinase, an enzyme involved in cartilage degradation. There are differences in salt forms; glucosamine sulfate reduces bone resorption to a greater extent than glucosamine hydrochloride.

Evidence: Clinical trial results vary widely with the type of glucosamine used. Glucosamine hydrochloride monotherapy is not supported. Both glucosamine sulfate monotherapy and glucosamine and chondroitin combination therapy do have sufficient clinical evidence to support use to decrease pain, increase mobility, and slow joint deterioration. A recent large comparison of glucosamine hydrochloride plus chondroitin sulfate to celecoxib found similar results at 6 months, though pain relief was achieved far more quickly with celecoxib. A crystalline glucosamine sulfate used in Europe has been demonstrated to reduce the need for knee joint replacement; European and International arthritis organizations have included the crystalline form in treatment guidelines as a first-line therapy.

Dosage and Product Considerations: There are significant differences between glucosamine sulfate and glucosamine hydrochloride. If monotherapy is used, then only glucosamine sulfate is recommended, 1500 mg/daily in one or divided doses. If utilized in combination with chondroitin, then either glucosamine sulfate or glucosamine hydrochloride is appropriate, at the same 1500 mg daily dose. A crystalline form of glucosamine made by Rotta Laboratories was used in many of the clinical trials with successful results; it is possible that other forms of glucosamine may not be as effective due to absorption differences.

Side Effects and Monitoring: GI symptoms are most commonly reported; splitting doses and taking with food can assuage discomfort.

Contraindications and Interactions: Glucosamine is commonly produced from the chitin of shellfish; although products are highly processed, and the likelihood of any remaining allergenic proteins is very low, patients with severe allergic reactions to shellfish should not use glucosamine. Although not demonstrated in clinical trials, there have been multiple case reports of increased INR in patients on warfarin who began glucosamine; this combination should be avoided.

Key Knowledge: Because of the mechanism of action, full benefits will not be evident for several months; patients trying glucosamine for OA, either monotherapy or with chondroitin, should use for a minimum of 6 months before assessing efficacy. Monotherapy should utilize only glucosamine sulfate, while glucosamine hydrochloride is acceptable for combination therapy with chondroitin.

Kava (*Piper methysticum*)

Primary Use: Anxiety disorders or occasional insomnia. Beverage preparations are used for ceremonial purposes and for social relaxation in much of Micronesia.

MOA: Enhances dopamine, inhibits noradrenaline, and increases expression of GABA receptors in the brain, preferentially in the limbic area of the brain.

Evidence: Although not all trials demonstrated benefit, evidence supports a clinically significant anxiolytic effect. A meta-analysis comparison of a commercially available European kava extract reported an odds ratio of efficacy compared to placebo of 3.3 (95% CI, 2.09-5.22) even though multiple differences in the Hamilton Anxiety (HAM-A) subscores were not significantly different. Although kava is often recommended for sleep, only two studies have assessed this use; one demonstrated benefit.

Dosage and Product Considerations: Varies dependent upon the product; the most tested extract is WS1490, standardized to 70% kavalactones, 50 to 100 mg three times daily

for anxiety. Because of significant concerns about toxicity and possible contamination of extracts, it is imperative that only products participating in a quality seal program or tested by a third-party laboratory be utilized by patients.

Side Effects and Monitoring: Hepatotoxicity. Liver effects were not reported in any medical literature until the late 1990s when kava became very popular and both production and use vastly expanded; cases of liver failure and death have occurred. Adverse events may have been a result of use of other plant parts, contamination by other plants, or contamination with pesticides. A genetic risk exists: individuals who are poor CYP2D6 metabolizers are at much higher risk of adverse events. After further research into the realistic extent of risks, Canada, France, and Germany recently lifted sales restrictions instituted by multiple countries a few years prior. Until more is known about the true causes of the hepatotoxicity, kava should not be recommended by healthcare professionals and use should be actively discouraged. Frequent monitoring of liver function is essential in patients who choose to use kava despite a negative recommendation. Other side effects include headache, GI effects, extrapyramidal effects, drowsiness, dizziness, and difficulty with eye movements.

Contraindications and Interactions: Liver disease or alcohol use is an absolute contraindication.

Key Knowledge: Despite good evidence of efficacy for anxiety, kava cannot currently be recommended, especially in the United States; European nations that have lifted kava sales bans regulate the quality of botanical medicine production far more rigorously. Kava is impairing; patients should not drive or operate heavy machinery while under its influence.

Melatonin

Primary Use: Insomnia and jet lag.

MOA: Produced and secreted by the pituitary gland in response to darkness to aid in controlling circadian rhythm; blind individuals often need provision of exogenous melatonin on an ongoing basis. It also functions as a hormone, aiding in ovulation and triggering sexual maturation at puberty.

Evidence: Some inconsistencies in trials, but overall evidence supports a small benefit for sleep improvement in chronic insomnia; children and adults with developmental delays or cognitive impairments may benefit more, well as patients with sleep disturbance induced by β-blockers. Melatonin is not effective for sleep disturbances due to shift work.

Dosage and Product Considerations: "Natural" melatonin extracted from bovine pituitary glands should be avoided due to the small risk of contamination with bovine spongiform encephalitis.

For insomnia, 0.3 to 5 mg 30 to 60 minutes prior to bedtime; for jet lag, 2 to 5 mg in the evening (5-10 pm) of arrival day at the destination, followed by use at bedtime for 5 days.

Side Effects and Monitoring: Very well-tolerated; all side effects reported are rare: GI, headache, tachycardia or other rhythm changes, morning sleepiness, and changes in depression status (worsening or improving).

Contraindications and Interactions: Use in adolescents should *only* occur under direction and supervision of a primary care provider. Melatonin may have the potential to decrease adverse effects of some cancer chemotherapy or radiotherapy treatments, but may interfere with others. Because information on these interactions changes rapidly, patients should discuss use with their oncologists.

Key Knowledge: Melatonin does not generally create a "sleepy" feeling, but use over time allows sleep attempts to be more successful, so chronic insomnia patients will benefit more than those with occasional sleeplessness. May be more effective for jet lag on return flights than for destination flights and for eastward rather than westward travel.

Red Yeast Rice (*Monascus purpureus*)

Primary Use: Hyperlipidemia

MOA: The red-tinged yeast that grows on rice contains an analog of lovastatin called monacolin K, an HMG-co-reductase inhibitor. Additional mechanisms occur, including increased bile acid secretion.

Evidence: Multiple clinical trials support lipid-lowering effects of total cholesterol (−13 to −26%), LDL (−21 to −33%), and triglycerides (−13 to −34%). HDL levels are affected minimally, if at all. No trials evaluating cardiovascular risk reduction have been performed. Some clinical trial evidence indicates red yeast rice (RYR) may be used by patients who cannot tolerate statins.

Dosage and Product Considerations: 1.2 to 2.4 g/d given once or twice daily. A high-quality product must be used, due to the possibility of contamination with citrinin, a toxin that may form during the fermentation process.

Side Effects and Monitoring: Generally well-tolerated. Dizziness and GI effects such as bloating and gas occur. Rarely, muscle pain and rhabdomyolysis have been reported with higher doses. Monitor liver function after 3 to 4 weeks of use, then regularly.

Contraindications and Interactions: Absolutely contraindicated in pregnancy; women of reproductive potential should use birth control. RYR should not be used by patients who have experienced severe reactions to statins, with liver disease, or who use alcohol heavily (>2 drinks/day). Do not use with fibric acids, niacin, or cyclosporine (increased risk of myopathies). Monacolin K is a CYP3A4 substrate, so use with potent inhibitors or inducers could affect levels of that component.

Key Knowledge: Effective for mild-moderate hyperlipidemia, but may not decrease cardiovascular risk. Many of the cautions and monitoring are due to the monacolin K component, which essentially is lovastatin. Some patients who cannot tolerate statins may be able to use RYR successfully, but those who have had very severe reactions to statins should avoid.

St. John's Wort (*Hypericum perforatum*)

Primary Use: Depression. Also used for seasonal affective disorder, anxiety, and postmenopausal symptoms.

MOA: Hyperforin affects the intra- and extracellular sodium gradients in neural synapses to influence sodium pumps used for reuptake of serotonin, norepinephrine, dopamine, and other neurotransmitters; may also affect serotonin receptor binding. Hypericin antagonizes gamma-aminobutyric acid (GABA) and other receptors.

Evidence: Not effective in severe depression. The latest meta-analyses have concluded that St. John's wort (SJW) is likely to have a smaller effect size than previously thought and use should be limited to mild to moderate depression. There is little evidence to support other uses, although concomitant use with black cohosh may provide additional benefit for postmenopausal symptoms.

Dosage and Product Considerations: 900 to 1800 mg/d of extract standardized to 5% hyperforin or to 0.3% hypericin in two to three divided doses.

Side Effects and Monitoring: Phototoxicity; sunscreen should be used at all times. Serotonin syndrome has been reported. Most common effects are mild GI symptoms, dry mouth, and headache. Sleep disturbances such as vivid dreaming and insomnia are reported and may be minimized by morning administration.

Contraindications and Interactions: Mania and hypomania are reported; use in bipolar patients is best avoided. SJW is a potent CYP3A4 inducer, which severely limits usefulness in therapy, induces 2C9 and 1A2 to a lesser extent, and also increases p-glycoprotein transporter activity, to increase drug absorption. Avoid use with serotonergic agents to avoid increased risk of serotonin syndrome.

Key Knowledge: Depression is not a self-treatable disease; patients using SJW should be monitored by their primary care provider. Avoid use with oral contraceptives, antiretroviral agents, and immunosuppressive agents; use with any prescription drugs should be closely monitored.

Saw Palmetto (*Serenoa repens, AKA Serenoa serrulata or Sabul serrulata*)

Primary Use: Symptoms of benign prostatic hyperplasia (BPH).

MOA: Inhibits both subtypes of 5-α-reductase, competitively inhibits dihydrotestosterone receptor binding, and has anti-inflammatory activity. May have anti-estrogenic activity. Does not decrease prostate size.

Evidence: Multiple early trials found significant decreases in multiple symptoms such as urinary flow rates or micturition rates; later trials have had negative results or demonstrated a smaller magnitude of benefit; a systematic review did not demonstrate clinically important improvements.

Dosage and Product Considerations: 320 mg/d of extract standardized to 80% to 95% fatty acids and sterols given in one or two doses daily.

Side Effects and Monitoring: Well tolerated; most common side effects are mild GI and headache. Reports exist for both worsening and improving erectile dysfunction and libido. Increased bleeding time has been reported at least twice.

Contraindications and Interactions: Absolutely contraindicated in pregnancy and lactation due to hormonal effects; although most often used in men for prostate issues, saw palmetto is frequently found in combination supplements for women marketed to "increase bust size." Metabolic drug interactions are theoretical, but use with antiplatelet agents or anticoagulants is best avoided. Due to hormonal effects, use with estrogenic or antiestrogenic therapies should be avoided.

Key Knowledge: Most appropriate for mild BPH symptoms. Does not decrease prostate size, so benefit for obstructive symptoms may be less than for irritative symptoms. Patients wishing to use for urinary symptoms must have a diagnosis of

BPH and have ruled out prostate cancer, due to the possibility of masking worsening cancer symptoms.

RELIABLE DIETARY SUPPLEMENT INFORMATION RESOURCES

A few recommended resources are listed in Table 75-1. In addition, here are some key questions to keep in mind when searching for information:

- Never use resources created/published by manufacturers or promotion groups, as their end goals concern sales, not information. However, reference lists from these resources may be useful.
- What is the publication/creation date of the resource? Information changes rapidly.
- Are statements about efficacy and safety based on analysis of complete clinical trials or upon only abstracts or the writers' opinions? Understanding trial quality is an essential component of assessing the accuracy of trial results.
- Is the resource reputable? False "publications" are common on the Internet and can look quite real.
- Are the authors healthcare professionals or scientists (Table 75-2)? Supplement information produced by ghost-writers and media groups is common (Table 75-3).

TABLE 75-1	Recommended Resources—For Additional Information on Individual Dietary Supplements[a]		
Resource	**Website**	**Cost**	**Comments**
Natural Medicines	https://naturalmedicines.therapeuticresearch.com/	$159/y or $15/mo	Resource is a merger of the Natural Medicines Comprehensive Database and the former Natural Standard resource. Includes monographs on individual supplements, an interactions checker, and clinical evidence tables with discussions of DS trials
ConsumerLab	www.consumerlab.com	$39/y or $64/2 y	A third-party laboratory that tests DS and reports on quality
Lexi-Comp	www.lexi.com	Variable	Mobile app (individual subscription) or website (pharmacy or institutional subscription) with monographs on individual supplements
Health Information at NIH Office of Dietary Supplements	http://ods.od.nih.gov/Health_Information/Health_Information.aspx	FREE	Dietary Supplement facts sheets, the Dietary Supplement Label Database, and link to MedWatch for reporting adverse events
Memorial Sloan-Kettering Cancer Center Integrative Medicine Service	http://www.mskcc.org/mskcc/html/1979.cfm	FREE	Focused on use in cancer patients; more information on chemotherapy interactions
CARDS Database (Computer Access to Research on Dietary Supplements)	https://ods.od.nih.gov/Research/CARDS_Database.aspx	FREE	A searchable listing of federally funded research projects on DS

[a]Note: Though many print information resources have been published, information regarding DS safety and interactions changes so rapidly that print resources have limited usefulness.

TABLE 75-2	Recommended Resources—For Discussions of Safe Use of Dietary Supplements
Resource	**Comments**
Bryant PJ, McQueen CE, Van Dyke. Literature Evaluation II: Beyond the Basics. In: Malone PM, Kier KL, Stanovich JE, et al., eds. *Drug Information: A Guide for Pharmacists*. 5th ed. New York City, NY: McGraw-Hill; 2014.	*Discusses supplements and clinical decision-making using a disease state approach.*
Dennehy CE, Tsourounis C. Dietary supplements & herbal medicines. In: BG Katzung, Trevor AJ, eds. *Basic & Clinical Pharmacology*. 13th ed. New York City, NY: McGraw-Hill; 2015.	*Provides botanical and nonbotanical supplement information with an emphasis on mechanisms and pharmacologic effects.*
McQueen CE. Complementary and alternative therapies. In: Schwinghammer TL, Koehler JM. *Pharmacotherapy Casebook: A Patient-Focused Approach*. 10th ed. New York City, NY: McGraw-Hill; 2016	*Discusses supplements and clinical decision-making using a disease state approach.*
McQueen CE, Orr K. Natural medicines. In: Krinsky DL, ed. *Handbook of Nonprescription Drugs*. 18th ed. Washington, DC: American Pharmacists Association; 2014.	*Discusses dietary supplements for multiple conditions using a body system approach.*
Shapiro K. *Natural Products: A Case-Based Approach For Health Care Professionals*. Washington, DC: American Pharmacists Association; 2006.	*Thoroughly discusses issues that impact clinical decisions regarding therapeutic use of dietary supplements in multiple disease states.*

TABLE 75-3	Common Dietary Supplement-Drug Interactions		
Product	**Possible CYP450 Enzyme Effects**	**Comments/Other Major Interactions**	**Common Substrate Examples[a]**
Black cohosh	2D6 inhibitor	Avoid combination with hepatotoxic drugs due to possible association with hepatotoxic effects. May see additive effects with antihypertensive medications.	**1A2:** caffeine, clopidogrel, diazepam, estradiol, warfarin, olanzapine, ropinirole, propranolol
Chondroitin sulfate	N/A	Several reports of increased INR, bruising, and bleeding with warfarin and glucosamine/chondroitin combination.	**2C9:** celecoxib, ibuprofen, losartan, torsemide, warfarin
Echinacea	1A2 inhibitor 3A4 inhibitor/inducer	Theoretically, may decrease effectiveness of immunosuppressants. Conflicting evidence regarding CYP interactions.	**2C19:** warfarin, citalopram, diazepam, omeprazole, phenytoin **2D6:** amitriptyline, haloperidol, metoprolol, ondansetron, paroxetine, risperidone, tramadol, venlafaxine
Evening primrose oil	N/A	Use cautiously with concomitant anticoagulant/antiplatelet medications. Use cautiously in combination with phenothiazines due to possible increase in seizures.	**2E1:** acetaminophen, ethanol, theophylline **3A4:** CCBs, antifungals, glucocorticoids, fentanyl, lidocaine, protease inhibitors, contraceptives, cyclosporine, NNRTIs
Fish oil	N/A	High doses may have antiplatelet effects. Use cautiously with concomitant anticoagulant/antiplatelet medications. May see additive effects with antihypertensive medications.	**P-glycoprotein:** digoxin, chemotherapy agents, cyclosporine, NNRTIs
Garlic	3A4 inducer 2E1 inhibitor 2D6 inducer	Contradictory and theoretical evidence regarding clinical significance of CYP interactions. Only some garlic preparations may cause 3A4 interaction. Antiplatelet effects; use cautiously with anticoagulant/antiplatelet medications. Blood pressure lowering effects; additive effects with antihypertensive medications possible. Avoid combination with saquinavir and isoniazid.	
Glucosamine	N/A	Several reports of increased INR, bruising, and bleeding with warfarin and glucosamine/chondroitin combination.	
Kava	See comments	Preliminary and contradicting evidence regarding CYP (1A2, 2C9, 2C19, 2D6, and 3A4) and p-glycoprotein interactions with kava. Synergistic effects possible with CNS; use with caution. May cause additive toxicity when combined with hepatotoxic drugs. Contraindicated with liver disease.	

TABLE 75-3	**Common Dietary Supplement-Drug Interactions** *(Continued)*		
Product	**Possible CYP450 Enzyme Effects**	**Comments/Other Major Interactions**	**Common Substrate Examples[a]**
Melatonin	1A2 substrate	Concomitant use with other CYP1A2 substrates can alter metabolism of either agent; 1A2 inducers/inhibitors can alter melatonin metabolism. May increase frequency of seizures. Use cautiously in combination with anticonvulsants and seizure threshold lowering drugs.	
Red yeast rice	3A4 substrate	Contains a lovastatin analog; all lovastatin interactions apply. Concomitant use of inducers/inhibitors of 3A4 can alter the metabolism of red yeast rice. May cause additive toxicity when combined with hepatotoxic drugs. Increased risk of myopathies if combined with cyclosporine, "statins," niacin, and gemfibrozil.	
St. John's wort	1A2 inducer 2C9 inducer 2C19 inducer 3A4 potent inducer P-glycoprotein transporter	Concomitant use with some antidepressants, tramadol, and "triptans" can increase serotonin syndrome risk. Preliminary and contradictory evidence regarding CYP1A2, 2C9, and 2C19. These are induced to a lesser extent compared to CYP3A4. Should not be taken by women using hormonal contraception due to reduced contraceptive efficacy.	
Saw palmetto	N/A	May prolong bleeding time; use cautiously with concomitant anticoagulant/antiplatelet medications. May have antiestrogenic effects; avoid use with estrogens, antihormonal agents, and contraceptives.	

Abbreviations: CCB, calcium channel blocker; CYP cytochrome; INR, international normalized ratio; N/A, not applicable; NNRTI, non-nucleoside reverse transcriptase inhibitors.

[a]List is not all inclusive.

Lexi-Comp Natural Medicine Database [online database]. Hudson, OH, Lexi-Comp, Inc, 2017.

Lissoni P, Barni S, Mandalà M, Ardizzoia A, Paolorossi F, Vaghi M, *et al*. Decreased toxicity and increased efficacy of cancer chemotherapy using the pineal hormone melatonin in metastatic solid tumour patients with poor clinical status. *Eur J Cancer.* 35:1688-92, 1999.

McQueen CE, Orr K. Natural Products. In Handbook of Nonprescription Drugs: An Interactive Approach to Self-Care, 18th edition, edited by DL Krinskey, SP Ferreri, BA Hemstreet, et al. Washington, DC, American Pharmacists Association, 2015 pp. 953-993.

Therapeutic Research Center. Drug-Supplement Interactions. *Pharmacist's Letter.* http://pharmacistsletter.therapeuticresearch.com. Accessed July 17, 2017.

Therapeutic Research Center. P-glycoprotein Drug Interactions. *Pharmacist's Letter.* http://pharmacistsletter.therapeuticresearch.com. Accessed July 17, 2017.

CASE Application

1. Which product affects circadian rhythm and also functions as a hormone to aid in ovulation and sexual maturity?

   a. Saw palmetto
   b. St. John's wort
   c. Black cohosh
   d. Melatonin

2. Which product can be utilized for postmenopausal symptoms, primarily hot flushes?

   a. Saw palmetto
   b. Kava
   c. Black cohosh
   d. RYR

3. A 42-year-old woman visits your pharmacy with complaints of increased sensitivity to the sun after starting a new natural product. Which of the following is most likely to cause this side effect?

   a. Garlic
   b. Kava
   c. Echinacea
   d. Chondroitin
   e. St. John's wort

4. What should be taken into consideration when a patient starts a new natural supplement? Select all that apply.

   a. The cheapest product
   b. Quality considerations
   c. Efficacy of the product
   d. How the supplement works
   e. The natural product must be more effective than the alternative prescription medication

5. A 78-year-old man with a history of BPH, hypertension, and depression wants to try saw palmetto for his

BPH. Which of the following is/are true regarding saw palmetto? Select all that apply.

a. It is usually well tolerated but increased bleeding time has been reported.
b. Saw palmetto has been shown to decrease prostate size.
c. It is not safe to use in pregnancy.
d. Can have additive effects with blood pressure medications.
e. This patient should not utilize saw palmetto due to known interactions with antidepressants.

6. A 55-year-old man with a history of hypertension and BPH was recently informed he has high cholesterol. He wants to try a natural product first before taking a "statin." Which of the following could he try for hypercholesterolemia? Select all that apply.

a. RYR
b. Garlic
c. Kava
d. Glucosamine sulfate
e. Fish oil

7. A 24-year-old woman wants to start taking St. John's wort for depression. She has a history of insomnia, anxiety, and asthma. Which of the following is/are true regarding St. John's wort? Select all that apply.

a. St. John's wort is a potent CYP3A4 inducer.
b. Drowsiness is a side effect of this product so it may help her insomnia.
c. St. John's wort has drug-drug interactions with oral contraceptives, immunosuppressive agents, and serotonergic agents.
d. St. John's wort may help with lowering blood pressure.
e. St. John's wort use should be limited to mild to moderate depression, not severe.

8. A patient is being discharged from the hospital on warfarin. Before leaving the hospital, you look over his prescriptions and natural products. Which natural products could increase his risk of bleeding with concomitant warfarin use due to the supplement's antiplatelet/anticoagulant properties? Select all that apply.

a. Chondroitin and glucosamine sulfate
b. Evening primrose oil
c. Black cohosh
d. Garlic
e. High doses of fish oil

9. Which of the following statement(s) is/are true about garlic? Select all that apply.

a. Garlic does NOT have GI side effects.
b. Medicinal doses of garlic are safe in pregnancy.
c. This product may be utilized for the treatment of acne.

d. It is safe to use with prescription medications since it does not interact with any drugs.
e. Garlic may need to be avoided in patients with low blood pressure.

10. A 60-year-old man wants to start glucosamine and chondroitin. He has a history of depression, hyperlipidemia, and OA and he's allergic to PCN (rash). He currently takes citalopram, atorvastatin, and ibuprofen as needed. Which of the following statements is NOT true in regard to glucosamine and chondroitin?

a. The most common side effects include GI-related symptoms.
b. There are different forms of glucosamine available.
c. Glucosamine and chondroitin are contraindicated with atorvastatin.
d. The mechanisms of these products are related to synthesis of cartilage or prevention of cartilage degradation.

11. Which of the following is/are true regarding safety and side effects of fish oil? Select all that apply.

a. Common side effects may include belching, bad breath, and nausea.
b. Common interactions with fish oil include antivirals and antibiotics.
c. Keeping fish oil capsules in the freezer or taking enteric-coated capsules can decrease some side effects.
d. It is known that fish oil inhibits several CYP enzymes.

12. Which of the following is considered an appropriate dose in regard for the mentioned supplement?

a. 2 grams of fish oil by mouth daily
b. 400 mg of melatonin by mouth 30 minutes prior to HS
c. 40 mg by mouth daily in divided doses of RYR
d. 100 mcg by mouth bid of black cohosh
e. 10 mg glucosamine sulfate with 5 mg chondroitin sulfate by mouth tid

13. A 23-year-old woman comes to your pharmacy stating she was exposed to the flu less than 24 hours ago. She has been feeling fine overall except for a runny nose. She would like to take a natural product for possible flu prevention. Which product do you recommend for her?

a. Evening primrose oil
b. Saw palmetto
c. Kava
d. Echinacea

14. Which of the following side effect(s) is/are associated with oral evening primrose oil use?

a. Weight loss
b. Kidney stone formation

c. Hair loss

d. Overall, evening primrose oil is well tolerated with some GI side effects

15. A patient comes to your pharmacy with a medication list containing efavirenz, tenofovir, emtricitabine, melatonin, and amlodipine. Which of the following natural products should NOT be recommended for this patient, considering the MAJOR interactions between the herbal product and their prescriptions?

a. Saw palmetto

b. St. John's wort

c. Kava

d. Glucosamine and chondroitin

16. Which of the following should NOT be recommended in patients with chronic liver damage or liver failure?

a. Melatonin

b. Evening primrose oil

c. Fish oil

d. Black cohosh

17. Which education points are appropriate to relay to a patient who is considering starting kava? Select all that apply.

a. Kava should not currently be recommended to patients.

b. Keep your healthcare providers updated on all prescription, OTC, and herbal products you are taking.

c. Kava has evidence to support efficacy for anxiety.

d. It is essential to monitor kidney function while taking kava.

18. Which of the following is true in regards to melatonin therapy? Select all that apply.

a. This is an endogenous substance naturally produced by the body.

b. Melatonin can be utilized for jet lag.

c. Glomerular filtration rate (GFR) and creatinine clearance (CrCl) need to be monitored if used chronically.

d. Melatonin may decrease adverse effects associated with radiation or chemotherapy.

e. Melatonin interacts with anticoagulant/antiplatelet medications due to increased risk of bleeding with concomitant use.

19. A 70-year-old female patient of yours wants to take glucosamine sulfate and chondroitin for her OA. She has taken Tylenol® in the past but it has not totally relieved her pain. She currently takes metformin, glimepiride, lisinopril, low-dose aspirin (81 mg), and hydrochlorothiazide. She has a history of hypertension, diabetes, and chronic kidney disease. She is allergic to cephalexin. Which of the following statements is an appropriate assessment regarding utilization

of glucosamine/chondroitin for OA therapy in this patient?

a. This patient should NOT take glucosamine/chondroitin because of its drug-disease interaction with diabetes.

b. This patient doesn't need the combination of glucosamine/chondroitin; she could safely take glucosamine hydrochloride as monotherapy for her OA.

c. This patient should NOT add glucosamine/chondroitin due to the increased risk of renal toxicity from the supplement.

d. This patient could try glucosamine/chondroitin but needs to have her kidney function closely monitored to prevent progression of her chronic kidney disease (CKD).

e. This patient could try glucosamine/chondroitin but needs to monitor for bleeding due to the increased risk from concomitant low-dose aspirin.

20. Which of the following medications may interact with medicinal doses of garlic? Select all that apply.

a. Metoprolol

b. Oral contraceptives

c. Rilpivirine

d. Metformin

e. Fentanyl

21. A 35-year-old woman wants to start taking oral evening primrose oil for "breathing and wheezing" in addition to her other medications. Upon review of her medical history, you find she has seasonal asthma, history of deep vein thrombosis (DVT), and high blood pressure. Her current medications include Xarelto®, Proair® inhaler PRN, enalapril, and metoprolol. Which of the following statements is the BEST assessment regarding starting oral evening primrose oil therapy for this patient?

a. Evening primrose oil could be considered in this patient since limited adverse events have been reported and this is an overall well-tolerated supplement.

b. Evening primrose oil should NOT be considered for this patient due to the CYP interaction with Xarelto, increasing the metabolism and clearance of Xarelto.

c. Evening primrose oil should be cautiously considered in this patient due to the antihypertensive effects of the supplement.

d. Evening primrose oil should NOT be recommended for this patient since it has not shown to be efficacious for asthma and it increases her risk of adverse bleeding if combined with Xarelto.

22. A 43-year-old man with OA is interested in adding glucosamine/chondroitin to his medication/herbal product regimen to decrease pain and increase mobility since he maintain a very active lifestyle. He is interested in this route before trying a prescription product. He currently takes fluticasone nasal spray for seasonal allergies, propranolol for blood pressure and heart

rate, bupropion XL for mood, and valacyclovir for cold sores. He is severely allergic to shellfish (anaphylaxis), and carries an EpiPen. Which of the following statements is the BEST assessment regarding glucosamine/chondroitin for this patient?

a. Glucosamine/chondroitin should be safe for this patient to try from a safety/interactions standpoint.
b. Due to the patient's allergy, glucosamine/chondroitin could be started in this patient with proper education and monitoring.
c. Glucosamine/chondroitin should be NOT be started in this patient since glucosamine is usually produced from shellfish chitin.
d. Glucosamine/chondroitin should be NOT be started in this patient due to the MAJOR drug-disease interactions with depression and cold sores.
e. Glucosamine/chondroitin interacts with valacyclovir but since the patient only takes this PRN for cold sores, it would be safe to be taken together.

TAKEAWAY POINTS »

- All pharmacies should have access to one or more reliable information resources on DSs, and all pharmacists should be familiar with the supplements that pose the greatest risks when used.
- Safety, efficacy, patient education, and product quality assurance all need to be considered when evaluating DSs to ultimately maximize benefits and minimize risks associated with the therapy.
- Under the guidance of a healthcare provider, some supplements may appropriately be utilized to aid in treatment of mild to moderate chronic diseases, such

as hyperlipidemia, hypertriglyceridemia, hypertension, and OA, or symptoms of life stages, such as menopausal hot flushes.
- St. John's wort's place in therapy is greatly limited by its safety profile, including numerous CYP450 drug interactions.
- Though kava has demonstrated some possible benefit for sleep or anxiety, it should not currently be recommended by healthcare providers due to the risk of hepatotoxicity.

BIBLIOGRAPHY

Bamford JT, Ray S, Musekiwa A, van Gool C, Humphreys R, Ernst E. Oral evening primrose oil and borage oil for eczema. *Cochrane Database Syst Rev*. 2013;4:CD004416.

Bruyére O, Altman RD, Reginster JY. Efficacy and safety of glucosamine sulfate in the management of osteoarthritis: evidence from real-life setting trials and surveys. *Semin Arthritis Rheum*. 2016;45:S12-S17.

Brzezinski A, Vangel MG, Wurtman RJ, et al. Effect of exogenous melatonin on sleep: a meta-analysis. *Sleep Med Rev*. 2005;9:41-50.

Calamia V, Mateos J, Fernández-Puente P, et al. A pharmacoproteomic study confirms the synergistic effect of chondroitin sulfate and glucosamine. *Sci Rep*. 2014;4:5069.

Gerards MC, Terlou RJ, Yu H, et al. Traditional Chinese lipid-lowering agent red yeast rice results in significant LDL reduction but safety is uncertain – a systematic review and meta-analysis. *Atherosclerosis*. 2015;240:415-423.

Gregory PJ, ed. Natural Medicines Database: Supplement monographs. www.naturalmedicines.therapeuticresearch.com Stockton, CA: 2017.

Kasper S, Caraci F, Forti B, et al. Efficacy and tolerability of Hypericum extract for the treatment of mild to moderate depression. *Eur Neuropsychopharmacol*. 2010;20:747-765.

Leach MJ, Moore V. Black cohosh (Cimicifuga spp.) for menopausal symptoms. *Cochrane Database Syst Rev*. 2012;9:CD007244.

Lexi-Comp Natural Medicine Database [online database]. Hudson, OH, Lexi-Comp, Inc, 2017.

McQueen CE, Orr K. Natural products. In: Krinskey DL, Ferreri SP, Hemstreet BA, et al. *Handbook of Nonprescription Drugs:*

An Interactive Approach to Self-Care. 18th ed. Washington, DC: American Pharmacists Association; 2015:953-993.

Ried K, Toben C, Fakler P. Effect of garlic on serum lipids: an updated meta-analysis. *Nutr Rev*. 2013;71:282-299.

Rohner A, Ried K, Sobenin IA, et al. A systematic review and meta-analysis on the effects of garlic preparations on blood pressure in individuals with hypertension. *Am J Hyperten*. 2015;28:414-423.

Schapowal A, Klein P, Johnston SL. Echinacea reduces the risk of recurrent respiratory tract infections and complications: a meta-analysis of randomized controlled trials. *Adv Ther*. 2015;32:187-200.

Siriwardhana N, Kalupahana NS, Moustaid-Moussa N. Health benefits of n-3 polyunsaturated fatty acids: eicosapentaenoic acid and docosahexaenoic acid. *Adv Food Nutr Res*. 2012;65:211-222.

Supplement card. In: Lawrence KS, ed. *Sigler's Dietary Supplement Drug Cards*. 2nd ed. SFI Medical Publishing; 2010.

Tacklind J, Macdonald R, Rutks I, et al. *Serenoa repens* for benign prostatic hyperplasia. *Cochrane Database Syst Rev*. 2012;12:CD001423.

Todd DA, Gulledge TV, Britton ER, et al. Ethanolic *Echinacea purpurea* extract contain a mixture of cytokine suppressive and cytokine-inducing compounds, including some that originate from endophytic bacteria. *PLoS ONE*. 2015;10:e0124276.

Witte S, Loew D, Gaus W. Meta-analysis of the efficacy of the acetonic kava-kava extract WS1490 in patients with non-psychotic anxiety disorders. *Phytother Res*. 2005;19:183-188.

Zeng C, Wei J, Li H, et al. Effectiveness and safety of glucosamine, chondroitin, the two in combination, or celecoxib in the treatment of osteoarthritis of the knee. *Scientific Rep*. 2015;5:16827.

KEY ABBREVIATIONS

CKD = chronic kidney disease
CrCl = creatinine clearance
DHA = docosahexaenoic acid
DS = dietary supplement
DVT = deep vein thrombosis
EPA = eicosapentaenoic acid
EPO = evening primrose oil
FDA = Food and Drug Administration
GABA = gamma-aminobutyric acid
GFR = glomerular filtration rate
GI = gastrointestinal
HDL = high-density lipoprotein

HIV = human immunodeficiency virus
INR = international normalized ratio
LDL = low-density lipoprotein
MOA = mode of action
NNRTI = non-nucleoside reverse-transcriptase inhibitors
O3FA = omega-3 fatty acids
OTC = over-the-counter
RYR = red yeast rice
SJW = St. John's wort
UPA = unsaturated pyrrolizidine alkaloid
USP = United States Pharmacopeia

76

Sterile Compounding Regulations and Best Practices for Sterile Compounding per USP 797

Michaela M. Almgren

FOUNDATION OVERVIEW

General Sterile Compounding Regulations

Sterile and nonsterile compounding are key elements of the pharmacy profession. Compounding plays an important role in modern pharmacotherapy, as doses of the medications can be prepared specifically for a patient. The Food and Drug Administration (FDA) divides compounded products into two categories. When medications are prepared for a specific patient according to orders from a licensed prescriber, the medication is considered to be a part of 503A section[1] of the Food, Drug, and Cosmetic (FD&C) Act. Section 503B was added to the FD&C Act by the Drug Quality and Security Act in 2013, and it defines a new category of compounders labeled as "outsourcing facilities".[1] Products that are prepared under the section 503A of the FD&C Act are what most clinicians consider as "traditional compounds". Compounders prepare medications for specific patients as they receive the prescription, with some minor exceptions when a pharmacy maybe compounding a product for physician in-office use, or in anticipation of a prescription. The majority of hospitals and the mainstream of retail compounding pharmacies fall into this category. Outsourcing facilities are subject to much more stringent current Good Manufacturing Practice (cGMP) regulations and can compound and distribute preparations that are not patient specific.

Sterile compounding is a skill that is very unique to pharmacists, as it requires specialized equipment and environment, as well as additional training. The resulting preparations are sterile and can be used in parenteral or any other type of application that requires sterile preparations. The term sterile is not relative, as preparation either is or is not sterile. The finished product must not become contaminated by microorganisms or any other chemical or physical contaminants during the process of preparation, as patient harm may result from exposure to nonsterile preparation when used parenterally. Until the recent past there were few official documents providing guidance on best practices for sterile compounding, but many patients were harmed as an outcome of poor standards and practices, because none of those documents were enforceable by any agency. In 2004, United States Pharmacopeia (USP) published in its USP compendium Chapter 797, which became the first enforceable guideline in 2008.[3] USP is a not for profit, independent, scientific, nongovernmental organization composed of scientists and practitioners from different fields, who offer their expertise on a variety of advisory boards. They create, validate, research, and publish guidelines, standard analytical methods, procedures for quality testing, and monographs for drugs, dietary supplements, and natural herbal products which are published and updated quarterly. Chapters 1 to 999 of the USP compendium are enforceable by FDA. In their pharmacy practice acts, many states have included USP 797 in its entirety or with some modifications as standards of sterile compounding.

USP Chapter 797

- **Gowning and hand hygiene**

  Gowning and hand hygiene are extremely important when it comes to sterile compounding in order to prevent sterile product contamination. Strict handwashing practices and gowning must be observed. These activities should take place in an anteroom prior to entering the buffer room. When gowning, one needs to remember to always cover from the dirtiest parts of the body to the cleanest, thus the shoe covers are donned first followed by the hair cover and face mask. All hair, including facial hair, must be covered when entering the clean room, thus special facial hair covers must be also utilized if applicable. Nail picks must be utilized to remove contaminants from under the nails, and antimicrobial soap to wash hands all the way up to the elbows for a minimum of 30 seconds is required. After drying hands with lint-free disposable towels or using an electric hand dryer, a nonshedding gown must be donned. The gown must have cuffs and be enclosed at the neck. While a gown may be reused during a typical shift in a nonhazardous compounding environment, the rest of the gowning materials should be new when re-entering the buffer room. Prior to donning powder-free sterile gloves, waterless antiseptic cleaner must be used. Sterile gloves must be donned without contamination from touching any nonsterile surfaces. Gloves should also be sterilized multiple times during the compounding activities. You must apply sterile 70% isopropyl alcohol (IPA): (1) after donning the gloves, (2) after cleaning of the laminar airflow workbenches (LAFW) prior to compounding, (3) if you are suspecting contamination, (4) periodically during more complex preparations (eg, total parenteral nutrition [TPN]), and (5) if you leave the LAFW and then come back (even if for very short period of time) to resume compounding. Other important points to remember—outer personal garments such as jackets, sweatshirts, bandanas; visible jewelry such as watches, rings, bracelets; nail polish, artificial nails; and make up are not allowed in the clean room at any time.

- **Primary engineering controls (PECs)**

LAFW, often referred to as the PECs, also sometimes called hoods, are key equipment in sterile compounding. LAFWs are the actual equipment inside of which the sterile compounding takes place. The term **laminar** refers to the **unidirectional** air flow which is produced by the LAFWs, and the air is purified by a high efficiency particulate air (HEPA) filter which is more than 99.97% efficient in removing particles as small as 0.3 microns. The environment inside of the LAFW is classified as International Standards Organization (ISO) class 5, which refers to a high level of cleanliness. There are different types of LAFWs available. **Horizontal or vertical positive airflow pressure** workbenches are used for compounding of **nonhazardous medications**. Vertical **negative airflow pressure** biological safety cabinets (BSCs) are used for compounding of **hazardous medications**, as they offer additional protections for the compounders to shield them from exposure to the hazardous drugs. Compounding aseptic isolators (CAIs) or "glove boxes" are also a type of PEC, and are used to prepare nonhazardous sterile compounds. Compounding aseptic containment isolators (CACIs) are for compounding of hazardous medications. Important note on the proper use of CAIs and CACIs: you must follow all hand hygiene and gowning requirements while working in the isolators, and sterile gloves should be donned on top of your isolator gloves.

When cleaning the PECs, always start from the cleanest parts and finish with the dirtiest/most likely contaminated, which is the bottom working surface of the hood. Lint-free wipes moistened with sterile IPA should be used for cleaning any PECs, and the alcohol should remain on the surfaces for at least 30 seconds prior to use. Use a new wipe for each surface cleaned. Also, the motion of cleaning should be perpendicular to the airflow, using overlapping strokes from the inside of the LAFW (cleanest)

to the outside (dirtiest). For horizontal airflow LAFW, the correct order is: top (from side to side, from inside corners of the hood working toward the outside), hanging pole and hooks (using gripping motion), sides (top to bottom, from the inside toward outside), and then the deck/bottom (from side to side, start from inside, work to the outside), using one new clean wipe for each surface cleaned. Vertical airflow LAFW or BSC order is: IV pole, back of the hood (using horizontal wiping motion starting from top and working down), sides (side to side motion, from inside out), sash (if present, same as back), and then deck (start in the back, move side to side towards the front). Cleaning of the diffuser (the grate in front of the HEPA filter) is a somewhat controversial topic, as some sites prohibit any interaction with the diffuser unless heavily soiled, and some LAFW manufacturers recommend cleaning it only when the LAFW is down for certification due to possibility of filter contamination. But other sites, in particular outsourcing compounding facilities that use LAFWs for 503B type of compounding require diffuser cleaning as a part of the daily routine cleaning per their institutional SOPs. If the diffuser is to be included in daily cleaning activities, it should be cleaned as one of the initial areas to avoid any cross contamination. You should clean the LAFW or BSC prior to beginning any compounding activity at the beginning of each shift, at least every 30 minutes while compounding, in case of any spills or suspected contamination, and in between different preparations. LAFWs typically run continuously. However, if the LAFW is turned off for any reason, it must run at least 30 minutes once turned back on prior to use. BSC should also run continuously, but in any case of interruption, it should run at least 4 minutes prior to cleaning and use. All PECs must be certified and monitored for viable and nonviable particle levels prior to initial use, or if any repairs or maintenance were performed, and then re-certified at least semiannually.

- **Secondary engineering controls (SECs)**

SECs also play a vital role in keeping sterile compounds safe, as they provide limited access, and a safe and clean environment for the PECs. Per USP Chapter 797, SECs include "facilities physically designed and environmentally controlled to minimize airborne contamination from contacting critical sites".[4] The **ante area** is typically used for gowning and handwashing, and it is typically ISO class 7 or 8, depending on whether the buffer area that it connects to is a positive air pressure room (in which case the anteroom can be ISO 7 or 8) or negative air pressure room (when an anteroom ISO class 7 is required). The **buffer area** must always be ISO class 7 category, as it is the main area where LAFWs are housed, and it must provide (can also be in combination with PECs) a minimum of 30 air exchanges per hour through the HEPA filter. USP 797 also currently allows PECs to be placed in a segregated compounding area where preparation for low-risk level CSPs with 12-hour beyond use dates (BUDs) are prepared.

Low-Risk Level	Medium-Risk Level	High-Risk Level
Prepared in PECS, not more than three commmpercialy prepared products, no more than two entries into vial	Prepared in PECS, multiple injections, all sterile products and equipment used, more complex compounding	Either nonsterile environment, drug or equipment used in the compounding process, sterilization required
Room Temperature: 48 hours	Room Temperature: 30 hours	Room Temperature: 24 hours
Refrigerated: 14 days	Refrigerated: 9 days	Refrigerated: 3 days
Freezer: 45 days	Freezer: 45 days	Freezer: 45 days

FIGURE 76-1 BUD and risk levels.

SECs are also cleaned regularly. Floors and counters need to be wiped daily, while walls, ceilings and storage shelves, plus any items stored in the room must be wiped once every month. All items must be wiped and decontaminated prior to being placed into the buffer room. A disinfecting agent needs to be used for cleaning and mopping of SECs, and cleaning materials must be area specific. SECs must be monitored for both viable and nonviable particle levels to assure the safest compounding environment. This monitoring is usually needed when starting a new compounding facility, thereafter at least semiannually, in case of any repairs, or if monitoring detects problems. The facility must have SOPs listing corrective steps if any positive results are detected.

- **Risk levels and BUD assignment**

Commercially prepared products have expiration dates determined by stability studies required by the FDA and typically performed by drug manufacturers. Products that are prepared per 503A regulations have a BUD that is assigned by the pharmacist/compounder based on USP 797 guidelines. The BUD is assigned based on the risk level of the preparation as defined by USP Chapter 797. **Low-Risk CSP** is defined as a preparation compounded in proper LAFW/SECs and involving not more than three sterile medications, and not more than two entries into the containers.[4] Reconstitution of a lyophilized drug powder is an example of this risk level. If preparation of the low-risk compound takes place in a LAFW which is not placed inside of appropriate SECs, the BUD is 12 hours or less per USP 797. This is particularly useful in the preparation of single-dose diagnostic agents that are prepared on demand. **Medium-Risk CSPs** can be described

as anything more complex, as long as all medications are sterile from the manufacturer and the compounding takes place in the proper LAFW and SECs using sterile equipment. Compounding of a TPN is considered medium-risk preparation. **High-risk CSP** is anything that involves a nonsterile component—medication, bulk drug powder, equipment, or environment (with the exception of immediate risk level products)—and therefore requires sterilization prior to use. As the risk levels increase, BUD in room temperature/refrigerator decreases. **Immediate use products are** prepared outside of LAFW due to urgency of preparation (example—ED patient needs a dose of lifesaving medication STAT) and their BUD is 1 hour (Figure 76-1).

- **Personnel training requirement, aseptic technique, terminology**

Proper training of all personnel performing sterile compounding is crucial, as sterile technique is the single most important factor when it comes to the safety of the CSPs. USP Chapter 797 dedicates a long section to proper training and documentation requirements for compounding personnel. The personnel must be familiar with proper procedures and aseptic technique, and perform a number of assessments prior to preparing CSPs for patients. LAWF design has a direct influence on compounders' technique, as **first air**, which is the air coming directly from the HEPA filter in the PECs, must not be blocked at any time. All **critical sites** must be in contact with first air **at all times**. Critical sites are defined as areas that if touched will lead to contamination of the final product. Critical sites of the syringe are the ribs of the plunger and tip where the needle attaches.

The entire needle is considered a critical site; it should only be handled by its cover. Other examples of critical sites are the top of the vial through which the needle will enter, as well as the additive port of the IV bag. When entering the vial, put the needle against the top of the vial at a 45° angle and bevel up to avoid coring. Always remember to replace the volume removed from the vial with air to avoid negative pressure build up as well as to remove excess air from the vial into which you are injecting fluid equal to the volume injected to avoid positive pressure build up. Also, all items prior to being placed into any LAFW, BSC, CAI, or CACI should be wiped clean using nonshedding wipes saturated with sterile 70% IPA to further reduce the risk of contamination. Media fill testing is used to assess each compounder's ability to prepare sterile products without contamination. This test should be done at least annually and the procedure should mimic the most complex preparation for which the compounder is responsible. Personnel garbing and hand washing also needs to be assessed, and can be done by direct observation of the activities, as well as by using gloved fingertip sampling.

- **Hazardous drug handling**

Hazardous medications should only be prepared in BSC or CACI (vented to the outside) located in the proper negative air pressure SECs. It is important to protect the health of the compounder and reduce the chance of exposure. Gowning requirements are also slightly different for hazardous drug handling—a nonpervious gown with closure on the back is required, and double gloving is required using chemotherapy resistant ASTM rated gloves. Proper PPE should also be worn when unpacking and stocking hazardous agents, as evidence shows that various chemotherapeutic agents have been detected on the outside of sealed and unopened drug vials shipped from manufacturers. Strict labeling must be implemented with hazardous medications to reduce the potential for exposure. Closed system transfer devices (CSTDs) can be used in compounding but do not replace the use of PECs and SECs. Personnel preforming hazardous drug compounding should have further training on aseptic technique demonstrating negative pressure utilization and hazardous agent spill cleanup.

- **Other topics**

USP Chapter 797 also briefly discusses other relevant topics—here are the relevant highlights:

- Handling of radiopharmaceuticals requires properly shielded compounding equipment inside of ISO class 5PECs and ISO class 8 SECs.
- Allergen extracts are not subject to risk levels and BUD dating as long as proper handling technique, hand hygiene, and gowning requirements are met as listed in the Chapter 797.
- Proprietary systems such as ADD-Vantage® or Mini Bag Plus® do not need BUD; follow manufacturer's recommendations.

- **Calculations**

Prior to tackling applications and review questions, please review the following calculation topics:

- Dilutions
- Powder volume calculations
- Flow rate calculations

CASE Application

1. What is the proper order of gowning and hand hygiene when preparing to enter the clean room?

   a. Don on shoe covers, mask, hair cover, facial hair cover, gown, perform hand hygiene
   b. Don on hair cover, mask, facial hair cover, gown, shoe covers, perform hand hygiene
   c. Don on shoe covers, hair cover, mask, facial hair cover, perform hand hygiene, gown
   d. Perform hand hygiene, don on shoe covers, hair cover, face mask, facial hair cover, gown

2. When cleaning positive air pressure horizontal LAFW, the correct order of cleaning surfaces and the motion to clean is:

   a. Top using side to side motion from inside out, IV hanging pole using gripping motion, bottom using back to front motion going from one side to the other, sides using up, and down motion working from inside out.
   b. Bottom using side to side motion from inside out, top using side to side motion from inside out, IV hanging pole using gripping motion, sides using up, and down motion from inside out.
   c. Top using side to side motion from inside out, hanging pole using gripping motion, sides using top to bottom motion from inside out, bottom using side to side motion from inside out.
   d. Top using front to back motion from one side to the other, hanging pole using gripping motion, sides using side to side motion from top to bottom, bottom from side to side inside out.

3. When referring to laminar air flow in the LAFW, we are talking about:

   a. Horizontal flow of air coming from HEPA filter in the LAFW
   b. Vertical flow of air coming from the HEPA filter in the BSC
   c. Unidirectional flow of air coming from HEPA filter
   d. Turbulent flow of air produced by HEPA filter

4. Which of the statements regarding media fill testing is correct?

   a. It is used to assess personnel's ability to don on sterile gloves.
   b. It is used to test SECs performance.

c. It is used to test performance of the cleaning and sanitizing agents.

d. It is used for assessment of aseptic technique of compounding personnel.

5. A pharmacy technician prepared TPN (from sterile components only) for one patient inside of ISO class 5 LAFW that was inside of the ISO class 7 compliant buffer room. What is the appropriate BUD for this product?

a. 9 days if refrigerated

b. 48 hours if refrigerated

c. 14 days if refrigerated

d. 3 days if refrigerated

6. Adenosine injection was prepared as a STAT dose in the emergency room at bedside by withdrawing liquid from one vial into a syringe but without access to LAFW or buffer room. What would be the correct BUD for this preparation?

a. 24 hours refrigerated

b. 24 hours at room temperature

c. 1 hour at room temperature

d. Cannot determine BUD, insufficient amount of information provided

7. If turned off, for a minimum of how long should a BSC and horizontal positive air flow LAFW run prior to use?

a. The BSC should run for at least 4 minutes and the horizontal LAFW should run for at least 30 minutes.

b. The BSC should run for at least 30 minutes and the horizontal LAFW should run for at least 10 minutes.

c. The BSC should run for at least 30 minutes and the horizontal LAFW should run for at least 1 hour.

d. Both should run for at least 30 minutes.

8. When entering a vial with a needle, which is appropriate technique to use?

a. Enter the vial at a 90° angle, bevel down.

b. Enter the vial at a 90° angle, bevel up.

c. Enter the vial at a 45° angle, bevel down.

d. Enter the vial at a 45° angle, bevel up.

9. What is the appropriate BUD for a Minibag Plus® product assembled in the LAFW under proper conditions as a part of batch?

a. 45 days if frozen

b. BUD does not apply as with proprietary products expiration date is assigned based on manufacturer's recommendations.

c. 9 days in refrigerator

d. Unable to determine, as not sufficient amount of information is provided.

10. Which of the following is an example of a primary engineering control?

a. Buffer room

b. BSC

c. Anteroom

d. SEC

11. Which of the following statements discussing the term "critical site" are correct? Select all that apply.

a. Hub of the needle as well as the shaft are considered critical sites of the needle.

b. Critical sites should be exposed to first air at all times.

c. Critical sites must not be contaminated by microorganisms but it is acceptable to expose them to physical contaminants, if sterility is preserved.

d. If critical site is touched and contamination is suspected, it must be wiped with sterile 70% IPA to prevent contamination.

12. According to USP Chapter 797, minimum frequency of cleaning floors in the buffer room is:

a. Hourly

b. Daily

c. Weekly

d. Monthly

13. Which of the following statements is true regarding proper hand hygiene prior to entering buffer room?

a. Wash your arms from the wrists toward the finger tips making sure your gown stays dry.

b. Jewelry, such as rings, is allowed as long as it is properly cleaned with 70% IPA.

c. Wash your hands all the way up to your elbows with antimicrobial soap for 30 seconds.

d. You can use waterless sanitizer in place of thorough hand wash.

14. Which of the following PECs should NOT be used to prepare hazardous medications?

a. BSC

b. Compounding aseptic containment isolator

c. Horizontal positive LAFW

d. All of the above are appropriate to prepare hazardous medications.

15. Which of the following statements regarding hazardous drug compounding per USP 797 is correct? Select all that apply.

a. Personnel needs additional training when handling hazardous medications.

b. CSTDs can be used in place of PECs and SECS, as they provide sufficient amount of protection to the compounder.

c. Proper PPE must be worn when unpacking shipment of chemotherapeutic agents.

d. When gowning for hazardous drug compounding, one must use impervious gown to avoid/limit any exposure.

16. Label instructions on a pharmacy bulk package of 10 g of vancomycin HCl state that when 95 mL of SWFI are added to the powder, the resultant solution will have

concentration of 500 mg per 5 mL. How many milliliters of SWFI should the pharmacist add to the dry powder to prepare the concentration of 1000 mg per 5 mL?

17. Due to national drug shortage, you need to prepare 250 mL NS bags using 23.4% NaCl vial and sterile water. How many milliliters of 23.4% NaCl solution will you need to prepare 10 bags of 250 mL NS?

18. How many milliliters of injection containing 40 mg of gentamicin in each 1 mL should be used in filling a medication order calling for 85 mg of gentamicin to be administered IV in a 100 mL NS small volume parenteral IV bag?

19. A pharmacist received a medication order to add 50,000 units of heparin to 1 L of D5W for a 175 lb patient. The rate of infusion was prescribed as 5000 units/h. What is the dose of heparin received by the patient on a unit/kg/min basis?

20. A physician prescribed continuous heparin infusion of 18 units/kg/h for a patient with VTE. It is to be prepared in 250 mL IV NS and it is to run over next 6 hours for a patient who weighs 91 kg. How many mL of 10,000 units per 10 mL heparin do you need to add to the IV bag?

TAKEAWAY POINTS ❱❱

- USP Chapter 797 is the first set of enforceable guidelines providing guidance on best practices for sterile compounding.
- Proper hand hygiene and gowning are extremely important in prevention of CSP contamination.
- When gowning, one needs to remember to always cover from the dirtiest parts of the body to the cleanest.
- When cleaning LAFWs, start from the cleanest areas, with the bottom being the last area to clean to avoid contamination.
- The motion used to clean LAFWs must be perpendicular to the airflow.
- CSPs that are prepared per 503A regulations have a BUD that is assigned by the pharmacist/compounder based on the risk level of the preparation as defined by USP 797.
- Critical sites must be in contact with first air at all times.
- Compounder's sterile technique has the greatest impact on quality and safety of the CSP.

BIBLIOGRAPHY

https://www.fda.gov/downloads/Drugs/GuidanceCompliance RegulatoryInformation/Guidances/UCM496286.pdf. Accessed August 18, 2017.

https://www.fda.gov/downloads/Drugs/GuidanceCompliance RegulatoryInformation/Guidances/UCM469119.pdf. Accessed August 18, 2017.

https://www.usp.org/frequently-asked-questions/pharmaceutical-compounding-sterile-preparations. Accessed August 18, 2017.

USP Chapter<797> from USP 40–NF 35—published on November 1, 2017 in English, and becomes official December 1, 2017.

KEY ABBREVIATIONS

BSC = biological safety cabinet
BUD = beyond use date
CAI = compounding aseptic isolator
CACI = compounding aseptic containment isolator
CSPs = compounded sterile products
CSTDs = closed system transfer devices
D5W = 5% dextrose IV solution
FDA = Food and Drug Administration
HEPA = high efficiency particulate air
IPA = isopropyl alcohol
ISO = International Standards Organization

IV = intravenous
LAFW = laminar airflow workbench
NS = normal saline, 0.9% NaCl
PECs = primary engineering controls
PPE = personal protective equipment
RT = room temperature
SECs = secondary engineering controls
SOPs = standard operating procedures
SWFI = sterile water for injection
USP = United States Pharmacopeia

Pharmacy Math II

Minou Khazan and S. Scott Sutton

CALCULATIONS REVIEW PROBLEMS

1. Interpret the following codes taken from prescriptions:

   a. Propranolol HCl 10 mg po tid ac & hs
   b. 1 tsp q6h x 10d
   c. Flurazepam 30 mg at HS prn sleep
   d. Caps i tid pc

   Solution:

   a. 10 mg of propranolol HCl by mouth three times a day before meals and at bedtime
   b. Take 1 teaspoon (5 mL) every 6 hours for 10 days
   c. 30 mg of flurazepam at bedtime as needed for sleep
   d. Take 1 capsule three times a day after meals

2. An injection for dental anesthesia contains 4% (w/v) of prilocaine hydrochloride and 1:200,000 (w/v) of epinephrine. Express the concentration of prilocaine as a ratio strength and the concentration of epinephrine as a percentage.

   Solution:

   a. Prilocaine hydrochloride: $\dfrac{4}{100} = \dfrac{1}{25}$ so ratio is 1:25 w/v

   b. Epinephrine: $\dfrac{1}{200,000} = 0.000005 \rightarrow 0.000005$

   $\times\, 100\% = 0.0005\%$ w/v

3. Norgestrel and ethinyl estradiol tablets are available containing 0.25 mg of norgestrel and 75 mcg of ethinyl estradiol. If a manufacturer wants to make 15,000 tablets, how many grams of each ingredient would be needed?

   Solution:

   a. Norgestrel:

   $$\frac{0.25\ \text{mg}}{\text{tablet}} \times \frac{1\ \text{g}}{1000\ \text{mg}} \times 15,000\ \text{tablets} = 3.75\ \text{g}$$

   b. Ethinyl estradiol:

   $$\frac{75\ \text{mcg}}{\text{tablet}} \times \frac{1\ \text{g}}{10^6\ \text{mcg}} \times 15,000\ \text{tablets} = 1.125\ \text{g}$$

4. A prescription balance has a sensitivity requirement of 6 mg. Explain how you would weigh 20 mg of acetaminophen with an error not greater than 5%.

   Solution:

   Least weighable quantity: $\dfrac{100\% \times 6\ \text{mg}}{5\%} = 120\ \text{mg}$

   $$\frac{20\ \text{mg (APAP needed)}}{120\ \text{(APAP} - \text{diluent mix)}}$$

   $$= \frac{120\ \text{(total APAP weighed)}}{x\ \text{(total amount of APAP} - \text{diluent mix)}}\ \text{so } x = 720\ \text{mg}$$

   Weigh 120 mg of acetaminophen, dilute with 600 mg diluent to make 720 mg of mixture, and take 120 mg of mixture to contain 20 mg of acetaminophen needed.

5. A pharmacy technician attempts to weigh 350 mg of morphine sulfate on a balance of unknown accuracy. When the pharmacist checked the weight on a highly accurate balance, the actual weight is discovered to be 375 mg. Calculate the percentage error of the inaccurate balance.

   Solution:

   $$\frac{\text{Error} \times 100\%}{\text{Desired quantity}} = \frac{25 \times 100\%}{350\ \text{mg}} = 7.14\%$$

6. An injection contains 60 mcg of drug A, 0.05 mg of drug B, and 8.18 mg of drug C in each milliliter. Calculate the milligrams percent (w/v) of drug A and the percentage (w/v) of drug B in the injection.

Solution:

Drug A: $\dfrac{60 \text{ mcg}}{1 \text{ mL}} \times \dfrac{1 \text{ mg}}{1000 \text{ mcg}} \times 100 \text{ mL} = 6 \text{ mg\%}$

Drug B: $\dfrac{0.05 \text{ mg}}{1 \text{ mL}} \times \dfrac{1 \text{ g}}{1000 \text{ mg}} \times 100 \text{ mL} = 0.005\% \text{ w/v}$

7. What is the volume, in milliliters, of 3 lb of mineral oil with a specific gravity of 0.85?

Solution:

1 lb = 454 g

$\dfrac{1362 \text{ g}}{x} = 0.85$ so volume $= 1602.35 \text{ mL}$

8. A vial contains 10 g of a powdered drug for reconstitution prior to use in an IV infusion. The label states that when 18.5 mL of diluent are added, the concentration of the resulting solution is 500 mg/mL. A medication order calls for a drug concentration of 300 mg/mL. How many mL of diluent should be added to the vial?

Solution:

$\dfrac{10,000 \text{ mg}}{x} = \dfrac{500 \text{ mg}}{\text{mL}}$, x = 20 mL so powder volume = 1.5 mL

$\dfrac{300 \text{ mg}}{\text{mL}} = \dfrac{10,000 \text{ mg}}{x}$, x = 33.3 mL so 33.3 − 1.5 mL powder

$= 31.8 \text{ mL diluent added}$

9. How many grams of a 4% w/w hydrocortisone ointment must be mixed with a 0.5% w/w hydrocortisone ointment to achieve 30 g of an ointment with 2.5% strength?

Solution:

4   2   parts 4% ointment

    2.5

0.5   1.5   parts 0.5% ointment

$\rightarrow \dfrac{30 \text{ g}}{3.5 \text{ parts}} = \dfrac{x}{2 \text{ parts}}$

$\rightarrow 17.1 \text{ g 4\% ointment}$

10. A pharmacist added 6 g of salicylic acid to 30 g of an ointment containing 4% salicylic acid, what would be the final concentration of the resulting mixture?

Solution:

$30 \text{ g} \times \dfrac{4 \text{ g}}{100 \text{ g}} = 1.2 \text{ g salicylic acid} \rightarrow 1.2 \text{ g} + 6 \text{ g}$

$= 7.2 \text{ g} \rightarrow \dfrac{7.2 \text{ salicylic acid}}{36 \text{ g mixture}} = 20\%$

11. If 500 mL of a 35% w/v solution are diluted to 1.75 L, what would be the resulting percentage strength?

Solution:

$(500 \text{ mL})(35\%) = (1750 \text{ mL})(x) \rightarrow x = 10\% \text{ w/v}$

12. The phenytoin loading dose in children is 20 mg/kg infused at a rate of 0.5 mg/kg/min. Over how many minutes should the dose be administered to a 50-lb child?

Solution:

$\dfrac{20 \text{ mg}}{\text{kg}} \times 22.7 \text{ kg} = 454 \text{ mg} \rightarrow \dfrac{0.5 \text{ mg}}{\text{kg}} \times 22.7 \text{ kg}$

$= \dfrac{11.35 \text{ mg}}{\text{min}} \rightarrow 454 \text{ mg} \times \dfrac{\text{min}}{11.35 \text{ mg}} = 40 \text{ min}$

13. The following formula is for 60 sertraline hydrochloride capsules. Calculate the amount of sertraline HCl in grams required to prepare 500 sertraline capsules.

Sertraline HCl	450 mg
Silica gel	9 g
Calcium citrate	6 g

Solution:

$\dfrac{450 \text{ mg}}{60 \text{ caps}} = \dfrac{x}{500 \text{ caps}} \rightarrow x = 3750 \text{ mg} = 3.75 \text{ g}$

14. The typical dose of digoxin for congestive heart failure in dogs is 0.005 mg/kg. Calculate the dose for a dog weighing 65 lb.

Solution:

$65 \text{ lb} \times \dfrac{1 \text{ kg}}{2.2 \text{ lb}} \times \dfrac{0.005 \text{ mg}}{1 \text{ kg}} = 0.15 \text{ mg}$

15. The dose of a drug is 45 mg/kg/d. What would be the infusion rate in milliliters per hour of a 0.6% solution of the drug if administered to a patient weighing 140 lb?

Solution:

$$140 \text{ lb} \times \frac{1 \text{ kg}}{2.2 \text{ lb}} \times \frac{45 \text{ mg}}{\text{kg}} = 2{,}863.6 \frac{\text{mg}}{\text{day}}$$

$$\frac{2863.6 \text{ mg}}{\text{day}} \times \frac{1 \text{ g}}{1000 \text{ mg}} \times \frac{100 \text{ mL}}{0.6 \text{ g}} \times \frac{1 \text{ d}}{24 \text{ h}} = 19.88 \rightarrow 20 \text{ mL/h}$$

16. What is the concentration, in mg/mL, of a solution containing 25 mEq of NaCl per milliliter? (MW of NaCl = 58.5)

Solution:

$$\frac{25 \text{ mEq}}{1 \text{ mL}} \times \frac{58.5 \text{ mg}}{1 \text{ mEq}} = 1{,}462.5 \text{ mg/mL}$$

17. A physician orders a 1 g vial of a drug to be added to 500 mL of D5W. If the administration rate is 100 mL/h, how many milligrams of the drug will the patient receive per minute?

Solution:

$$\frac{1000 \text{ mg}}{500 \text{ mL}} \times \frac{100 \text{ mL}}{1 \text{ h}} \times \frac{1 \text{ h}}{60 \text{ min}} = 3.33 \text{ mg/min}$$

18. An ophthalmic solution contains the equivalent of 0.3% tobramycin base (MW 467.5). How many milligrams of tobramycin sulfate (MW 565.6) may be used to prepare each 10 mL of the solution?

Solution:

$$\frac{0.3 \text{ g}}{100 \text{ mL}} = \frac{0.03 \text{ g}}{10 \text{ mL}} \rightarrow \frac{0.03 \text{ g tobra base}}{467.5} = \frac{\text{x tobra sulfate}}{565.6} \rightarrow \text{x}$$

$$= 36 \text{ mg tobramycin sulfate}$$

19. Calculate the ideal body weight for a female patient weighing 150 lb and measuring 68 inches tall.

Solution:

$$\text{IBW} = 45.5 \text{ kg} + (2.3)(8) = 63.9 \text{ kg or } 140.58 \text{ lb}$$

20. The directions for a prescription for insulin glargine state the following: 27 u SubQ q pm. How many vials will the patient require for 1 month, if each bottle of insulin glargine contains 1000 units.?

Solution:

$$\frac{27 \text{ units}}{\text{day}} \times \frac{30 \text{ d}}{} \times \frac{1 \text{ bottle}}{1000 \text{ units}} = 0.81 \text{ bottles} \rightarrow 1 \text{ bottle}$$

21. Calculate the milliequivalents of potassium in 20 mL of a 5% w/v solution of potassium chloride (MW 74.5).

Solution:

$$\frac{5 \text{ g}}{100 \text{ mL}} = \frac{\text{x g}}{20 \text{ mL}} \rightarrow \frac{1 \text{ g}}{} \times \frac{1000 \text{ mg}}{1 \text{ g}} \times \frac{1 \text{ mEq}}{74.5 \text{ mg}}$$

$$\rightarrow 13.42 \text{ mEq of potassium}$$

22. A certain over-the-counter (OTC) antacid contains 800 mg of calcium carbonate ($CaCO_3$) per tablet. How many milliequivalents of calcium does each tablet contain? (AW of Ca = 40, AW of C = 12, AW of O = 16)

Solution:

Calcium: 40 × 1 = 40 Carbon: 12 × 1 = 12 Oxygen: 16 × 3 = 48

Formula MW = 40 + 12 + 48 = 100 mg for calcium carbonate

Calcium is a divalent ion. $1 \text{ mEq of } CaCO_3 = \frac{100}{2} = \frac{50 \text{ mg } CaCO_3}{}$

$$800 \text{ mg } CaCO_3 \times \frac{1 \text{ mEq } CaCO_3}{50 \text{ mg } CaCO_3} = 16 \text{ mEq of } CaCO_3 \text{ and}$$

calcium per tablet

23. A prescription calls for a benzalkonium chloride Solution 1:10,000 w/v to be compounded. Express the benzalkonium chloride concentration in mg/mL, mg%, and %.

Solution:

a. $$\frac{1 \text{ g}}{10{,}000 \text{ mL}} \rightarrow \frac{1000 \text{ mg}}{10{,}000 \text{ mL}} \rightarrow \frac{1000 \text{ mg}}{10{,}000 \text{ mL}} = \frac{\text{x mg}}{\text{mL}} \rightarrow \text{x}$$

$$= 0.1 \text{ mg/mL}$$

b. $$\frac{1000 \text{ mg}}{10{,}000 \text{ mL}} = \frac{\text{x}}{100} \rightarrow \text{x} = 10 \text{ mg\%}$$

c. $$10 \text{ mg x} \frac{1 \text{ g}}{1000 \text{ mg}} = 0.01 \text{ g} \rightarrow \frac{0.01 \text{ g}}{100 \text{ mL}} \text{x } 100 = 0.01\%$$

24. You are asked to compound 90 mL of a concentrated chlorhexidine gluconate solution, so that the patient may dilute 1 tablespoonful of the concentrated solution with 1 pint of water and produce a final solution with a concentration of 0.12% v/v to use as a mouth wash. How many mL of pure chlorhexidine gluconate liquid are needed to prepare the prescription order?

Solution:

$$(15 \text{ mL})(x) = (473 \text{ mL} + 15 \text{ mL})(0.12\%)$$

$$x = \frac{(488)(0.12)}{15} = 3.9\% \rightarrow \frac{3.9}{100 \text{ mL}} = \frac{x}{90} \rightarrow x$$

$$= 3.51 \text{ mL required}$$

25. If 50 mL of a 1:20 w/v solution is diluted to 500 mL, what is the % strength? Ratio strength?

Solution:

a. $\dfrac{1}{20} = \dfrac{x}{100} \rightarrow x = 5\% \rightarrow (50 \text{ mL})(5\%)$

$$= (500 \text{ mL})(x\%) \rightarrow x = 0.5\%$$

b. $\dfrac{0.5 \text{ g}}{100 \text{ mL}} = \dfrac{1}{x} \rightarrow 0.5(x) = 100 \rightarrow x$

$$= \frac{100}{0.5} = 200 \rightarrow \frac{1}{200} \rightarrow 1:200$$

CASE Application ANSWERS

CHAPTER 1 | Chronic Heart Failure

1. MM is a 58-year-old woman with cardiomyopathy (left ventricular ejection fraction [LVEF] 25%) following an acute MI. Immediately following her MI, she developed signs and symptoms of HF including shortness of breath (SOB) at rest. Which of the following best characterizes MM's current ACC/AHA HF stage and NYHA class?

   a. Stage A, NYHA class not applicable
   b. Stage B, NYHA class I
   c. Stage C, NYHA class II
   d. Stage C, NYHA class IV

Answer d is correct. MM meets the criteria for Stage C. Patients such as MM who are Stage C have developed signs and/or symptoms of HF. Additionally, MM has symptoms at rest; therefore, she is NYHA class IV.

Answers a, b, and c are incorrect. Answers a to c are incorrect because MM has symptoms at rest and is post-MI. Patients who are Stage A are at risk for developing left ventricular dysfunction and HF (eg, due to hypertension, coronary artery disease). Patients who are Stage B have developed structural heart disease but have not developed signs and symptoms of HF. The NYHA classification system categorizes patients as class I if they are relatively asymptomatic and physical activity is not limited by the HF disease process. Patients who are NYHA class II and III are symptomatic with minimal and moderate physical activity, respectively.

2. Which of the following therapies decreases HR via inhibition of the I_f current in the sinoatrial node?

   a. Metoprolol succinate
   b. Carvedilol
   c. Digoxin
   d. Ivabradine

Answer d is correct. Ivabradine inhibits I_f current in the sinoatrial node, leading to reductions in HR without affecting myocardial contractility.

Answers a and b are incorrect. Metoprolol succinate and carvedilol are β-blockers, and decrease HR by inhibiting the effects of adrenergic neurotransmitters (eg, epinephrine) on $β_1$ receptors in myocardial tissue. Consequently, transient reductions in myocardial contractility may also occur.

Answer c is incorrect. Although a precise mechanism of action for digoxin has not been well-elucidated, it is thought to lower HR via parasympathetic (ie, vagal) activation.

3. Which of the following laboratory values may be helpful in differentiating HF from other disease states that cause similar symptoms?

   a. Serum sodium
   b. Serum creatinine
   c. BNP
   d. Norepinephrine

Answer c is correct. Increased BNP occurs in the setting of left ventricular stretch secondary to fluid overload. It may be helpful in differentiating HF from other disease states that cause similar symptoms (eg, pneumonia).

Answer a is incorrect. Reduced serum sodium (hyponatremia) may occur in HF and is a predictor of poor outcomes. Sodium levels may be affected by numerous conditions and therefore cannot distinguish between HF and other disease states.

Answer b is incorrect. Increased serum creatinine or worsening renal function is a common objective measure of low output. Serum creatinine may be affected by numerous conditions and therefore cannot distinguish between HF and other disease states.

Answer d is incorrect. In response to a decline in cardiac output, numerous compensatory mechanisms are activated to maintain adequate CO, including activation of the SNS with increased norepinephrine. Other disease states may also cause elevated norepinephrine levels.

4. KW is a 53-year-old man with HF (NYHA class I) receiving furosemide 40 mg twice daily, lisinopril 10 mg daily, metoprolol succinate 50 mg daily, digoxin 0.125 mg daily, and spironolactone 25 mg daily. During a routine clinic visit today, pertinent findings include: BP 120/80 mm Hg, HR 70 beats/min, RR 14, K^+ 5.1 mmol/L, BUN 35 mg/dL, and creatinine 1.2 mg/dL (baseline). Which of the following is the most appropriate change to optimize KW's medical regimen? Select all that apply.

   a. Increase ACE inhibitor dose
   b. Increase β-blocker dose
   c. Add ivabradine
   d. Increase spironolactone dose

Answer b is correct. For HF management, ACE inhibitor and β-blocker therapy should be titrated to target doses associated with improved outcomes in clinical trials. This patient has adequate blood pressure to increase either therapy. In addition, HR is adequate to further titrate β-blocker therapy. Uptitration of β-blocker therapy is the safest medication change for this patient.

Answer a is incorrect.   ACE inhibitors are associated with dose-related hyperkalemia and this patient already has borderline high serum potassium.

Answer c is incorrect.   Although the patient's HR is ≥70 beats/min, β-blocker therapy is not yet at target dose and the patient does not have any evidence of intolerance that might preclude dose uptitration. Because β-blockers improve mortality (whereas ivabradine primarily reduces hospitalizations), ivabradine should be reserved for patients who remain symptomatic with a HR ≥70 beats/min despite maximally tolerated β-blocker therapy.

Answer d is incorrect.   Aldosterone antagonists such as spironolactone are associated with hyperkalemia. Thus, the spironolactone dose should not be increased and may even need to be reduced to 12.5 mg daily if hyperkalemia persists or worsens.

Questions 5 through 8 pertain to the following case.

JC is a 64-year-old African American man with HFrEF presenting with a 2-week history of SOB which limits his normal daily activities and increased lower extremity edema. His weight has recently increased by 10 lb. His physical examination is notable for BP 148/72 mm Hg, HR 68 beats/min, RR 24, rales, and 3+ lower extremity edema. Pertinent laboratory values include: sodium 138 mmol/L, potassium 5.4 mmol/L, BUN 35 mg/dL, creatinine 0.9 mg/dL, and digoxin 2.1 ng/mL. Past medical history is significant for HTN, gout, and chronic obstructive pulmonary disease (COPD). Current medications include lisinopril 20 mg daily, diltiazem CD 120 mg daily, digoxin 0.250 mg daily, and salmeterol/fluticasone 250/50 two puffs bid. JC recently began taking naproxen 220 mg tid for gout pain.

5. In addition to counseling on salt and fluid restriction, which of the following pharmacologic options is most appropriate for managing JC's fluid overload?

    a. Initiate hydrochlorothiazide 50 mg daily.
    b. Initiate furosemide 40 mg twice daily.
    c. Initiate metolazone 2.5 mg daily.
    d. Initiate spironolactone 25 mg daily.

Answer b is correct.   Loop diuretics, such as furosemide, are the treatment of choice for managing volume overload in HF patients.

Answers a and c are incorrect.   Thiazide diuretics such as hydrochlorothiazide and metolazone are not effective diuretics as monotherapy; however, these therapies may be added if patients are not responding adequately to loop diuretic dose escalation.

Answer d is incorrect.   Spironolactone has been shown to be effective in reducing mortality when added to standard HF therapy in moderate to severe (NYHA class II-IV) patients. The low doses (eg, 12.5-25 mg/d) used to manage HF do not result in clinically significant diuresis.

6. Within the following 24 hours, JC experiences a brisk diuresis with considerable improvement in HF signs and symptoms. What additional medication changes should be considered?

    a. Continue current regimen and initiate hydrochlorothiazide 50 mg daily.
    b. Continue current regimen and initiate spironolactone 25 mg daily.
    c. Discontinue lisinopril and initiate combination hydralazine 25 mg and ISDN 20 mg three times daily.
    d. Discontinue over-the-counter naproxen and initiate colchicine 0.6 mg bid until gout pain resolves.

Answer d is correct.   Medications that may exacerbate fluid retention should be avoided in HF patients. The NSAID that JC is taking for gout pain should be discontinued and colchicine initiated as a safe alternative. While colchicine should not affect the patient's HF status, it is associated with other toxicities that warrant patient education.

Answer a is incorrect.   Addition of hydrochlorothiazide would not be indicated unless JC demonstrated resistance to loop diuretic therapy.

Answer b is incorrect.   Spironolactone should not be considered unless JC continues to have symptomatic HF (NYHA class II-IV) despite receiving β-blocker therapy. In addition, current hyperkalemia would also preclude use of this agent.

Answer c is incorrect.   Combination hydralazine and ISDN should only be used in lieu of ACE inhibitor therapy, if JC exhibits intolerable renal dysfunction or hyperkalemia with ACE inhibitor. In addition, combination hydralazine and ISDN may be added to ACE inhibitor in African American patients with NYHA class III to IV symptoms despite standard HF therapy.

---

7. Once optimal fluid status has been achieved, which of the following represents the best option to manage JC's HTN?

    a. Initiate amlodipine 5 mg daily.
    b. Initiate carvedilol 3.125 mg twice daily.
    c. Initiate hydrochlorothiazide 25 mg daily.
    d. Initiate prazosin 2 mg daily.

Answer b is correct.   In addition to assisting with managing JC's HTN, carvedilol is one of the three β-blockers shown to reduce mortality in HF patients. Importantly, although the blood pressure-lowering effects of carvedilol may be helpful at initiation of therapy, they tend to dissipate with time.

Answer a is incorrect.   Amlodipine has not been shown to reduce mortality and would not be considered until HF medications that reduce blood pressure and mortality have been initiated.

Answer c is incorrect.   Although hydrochlorothiazide would be helpful for the treatment of hypertension in the absence of HF, other HF therapies with antihypertensive effects should be optimized first. Additionally, the addition of hydrochlorothiazide to loop diuretic therapy may elicit excess diuresis.

Answer d is incorrect. Prazosin may be useful for managing benign prostatic hypertrophy (BPH); however, it has been shown to worsen outcomes in HF patients.

8. What additional medication change should be considered to optimize JC's medical regimen? Select all that apply.

   a. Discontinue diltiazem.
   b. Reduce digoxin to 0.125 mg daily.
   c. Initiate spironolactone 25 mg daily.
   d. Initiate candesartan 4 mg daily.
   e. Initiate ivabradine 5 mg twice daily.

Answers a and b are correct. Diltiazem should be discontinued, as it exerts negative inotropic effects and may provoke an HF decompensation. While digoxin does not reduce mortality in HF, it has been shown to reduce hospitalization and improve symptoms. The goal serum digoxin concentration is <1 ng/mL and serum digoxin concentrations >1 ng/mL may negatively impact JC's mortality. JC's digoxin dose should be reduced to 0.125 mcg daily in an attempt to lower his serum digoxin concentration <1 ng/mL.

Answer c is incorrect. Adding spironolactone is not indicated unless JC remains symptomatic (NYHA class II-IV) despite standard HF therapy. In addition, current hyperkalemia precludes initiation of this potassium-sparing therapy.

Answer d is incorrect. Candesartan is also likely to worsen JC's current hyperkalemia and should be avoided at this time. The benefit of adding an ARB to standard HF therapy is not as clinically meaningful as adding an aldosterone antagonist. In addition, therapy with an ARB, aldosterone antagonist, and ACE inhibitor therapy is discouraged due to the risk of hyperkalemia. In fact, such "triple therapy" is given a class III recommendation (harm > benefit) in the ACC/AHA guidelines.

Answer e is incorrect. Ivabradine is indicated in patients with normal sinus rhythm and HR greater than 70 beats/min. JC's HR is less than 70 beats/min. Furthermore, it should only be considered in patients whose HR remains greater than 70 beats/min despite receiving maximally tolerated β-blocker which is not yet the case for JC.

Questions 9 and 10 pertain to the following case.

RJ is a 61-year-old woman with a history of ischemic cardiomyopathy who presents to clinic with symptoms consistent with NYHA class IV HF. Past medical history includes hyperlipidemia, diabetes mellitus, MI, and hypothyroidism. RJ complains of progressive weight gain (~6 lb increase since visit 3 months ago), SOB at rest, 2 pillow orthopnea, and occasional paroxysmal nocturnal dyspnea (PND). Her physical examination is positive for 1+ pitting edema in her ankles and minimal jugular vein distention (JVD). Vital signs include BP 105/70 mm Hg and HR 91 beats/min. Laboratory results include: potassium 3.6 mmol/L, BUN 39 mg/dL, and creatinine 1.4 mg/dL (baseline creatinine 1.2-1.6 mg/dL). RJ's current medications are levothyroxine 0.05 mg daily, furosemide 40 mg twice daily,

lisinopril 20 mg daily, atorvastatin 40 mg daily, aspirin 81 mg daily, insulin glargine 46 units at bedtime, and insulin as part 6 units before meals.

9. Which of the following is the best treatment option to manage RJ's hypokalemia and fluid overload? Select all that apply.

   a. Continue furosemide 40 mg twice daily.
   b. Increase furosemide to 80 mg twice daily.
   c. Initiate spironolactone 25 mg once daily.
   d. Initiate hydrochlorothiazide 25 mg daily.

Answers b and c are correct. Increasing the furosemide dose alone is inappropriate as it will worsen RJ's low serum potassium. While the addition of a potassium supplement could be considered, the addition of spironolactone along with the increased diuretic dose would provide additional mortality benefit as well as potassium retention. When added to standard HF therapy in patients with NYHA class II to IV HF symptoms, spironolactone has been shown to reduce mortality. Spironolactone alone at the low doses used to reduce mortality in HF does not commonly result in clinically meaningful diuresis. It is important to recognize that spironolactone alone may be insufficient to maintain adequate serum potassium levels and close monitoring is indicated.

Answer a is incorrect. The patient is already receiving this dose of furosemide and has not experienced a weight change. Therefore, continuation of current dose/interval would not be appropriate.

Answer d is incorrect. Thiazide diuretics are not utilized for fluid management of HF unless the patient is refractory to a loop diuretic (at which point one may be added for the purposes of sequential nephron blockade).

10. Which of the following represents the next best option to manage RJ's HF?

   a. Initiate metoprolol succinate 25 mg daily immediately.
   b. Initiate metoprolol succinate 25 mg daily once euvolemia is achieved.
   c. Initiate metoprolol tartrate 12.5 mg bid immediately.
   d. Initiate digoxin 0.25 mg daily.

Answer b is correct. Given the mortality benefit associated with β-blockers in HF, this medication should be part of the patient's medical regimen. However, β-blockers should only be initiated once euvolemia is obtained.

Answer a is incorrect. β-Blockers should only be initiated once euvolemia is obtained.

Answer c is incorrect. Metoprolol tartrate is not used in the management of HFrEF. The succinate form of metoprolol is utilized in HF management.

Answer d is incorrect. Digoxin is indicated for symptomatic patients despite standard HF therapy (ACE inhibitor and β-blocker). In addition, a lower digoxin dose should be initiated in an elderly patient to achieve a serum digoxin concentration less than 1 ng/mL.

11. Which of the following are absolute contraindications to the use of β-blockers? Select all that apply.

    a. Asthma with active bronchospasm
    b. Diabetes
    c. Chronic obstructive pulmonary disease
    d. Peripheral vascular disease
    e. Complete heart block

Answer a is correct. There are very few *absolute* contraindications to β-blocker therapy: asthma with active bronchospasm and symptomatic hypotension or bradycardia. Relative contraindications to β-blocker therapy include: diabetes with recurrent hypoglycemia, asthma without active bronchospasm, HR <55 beats/min, second- or third-degree heart block, and systolic blood pressure <80 mm Hg.

Answer e is correct. Complete heart block is an absolute contraindication to β-blocker therapy.

Answers b, c, and d are incorrect. Given that benefit exceeds risk in most HFrEF patients, β-blockers should not be avoided in diabetes mellitus (Answer b), chronic obstructive pulmonary disease (Answer c), asthma without active bronchospasm, and peripheral vascular disease (Answer d).

Questions 12 and 13 pertain to the following case.

SD is a 54-year-old man with NYHA class III HF due to non-ischemic cardiomyopathy. His past medical history is notable for moderate asthma since childhood and HTN. Current medications include salmeterol, one inhalation twice daily; fluticasone 88 mcg, inhaled twice daily; furosemide 80 mg twice daily; enalapril 20 mg twice daily; and spironolactone 25 mg daily.

12. Which of the following β-blockers is the best option to treat SD's HF and minimize aggravating his asthma?

    a. Carvedilol
    b. Metoprolol succinate
    c. Propranolol
    d. Atenolol

Answer b is correct. Only three β-blockers have been demonstrated to reduce mortality in HF: carvedilol, metoprolol succinate, and bisoprolol. Metoprolol succinate is the correct answer because it has proven mortality benefit in HFrEF and it is a cardio-selective β-blocker. While metoprolol is β-1 selective, it is important to recognize that β-receptor selectivity may decrease as the dose is up-titrated.

Answer a is incorrect. Carvedilol is a nonselective β-blocker and may aggravate underlying lung disease.

Answers c and d are incorrect. Propranolol (Answer c) and atenolol (Answers d) have not been studied in HF.

Additionally, propranolol is a nonselective β-blocker and could aggravate underlying lung disease.

13. Which of the following medication changes may provide further mortality benefit for SD once stabilized on β-blocker therapy?

    a. Addition of digoxin 0.125 mg daily.
    b. Substitution of sacubitril/valsartan 49 mg/51 mg for enalapril 20 mg twice daily.
    c. Addition of valsartan 160 mg twice daily.
    d. Addition of amlodipine 5 mg daily.

Answer b is correct. The combination of sacubitril and valsartan demonstrated a significant mortality benefit over ACE inhibitors in patients with symptomatic HF despite receiving optimal HF therapy with β-blockers and ACE inhibitors.

Answer a is incorrect. Digoxin improves symptoms and reduces hospitalization, but does not confer a mortality benefit.

Answer c is incorrect. Valsartan reduces HF exacerbations in combination with background ACE inhibitor therapy, but not all-cause mortality when added to an ACE inhibitor.

Answer d is incorrect. Amlodipine has neutral effects on mortality in HF patients.

14. Which of the following is appropriate rationale for switching an ACE inhibitor to an ARB? Select all that apply.

    a. Hypotension
    b. Renal dysfunction
    c. Hyperkalemia
    d. Cough
    e. Angioedema

Answers d and e are correct. An ARB may be considered for patients who have cough (Answer d) or angioedema with an ACE inhibitor. These side effects are attributed to the elevation in bradykinin caused by ACE inhibitors, which is less likely with an ARB. It is important to exert extreme caution if an ARB is initiated following ACE inhibitor-induced angioedema, as cross-sensitivity has been reported.

Answers a, b, and c are incorrect. Hypotension (Answer a), renal dysfunction (Answer b), and hyperkalemia (Answer c) are likely to reoccur with an ARB if a patient experienced these side effects with an ACE inhibitor. Although ACE inhibitors and ARBs have different mechanisms of action, their overall function is to inhibit the effects of angiotensin II. Blocking the hormone angiotensin II is responsible for these adverse effects.

15. IH is a 44-year-old African American man presenting with dizziness and orthostatic hypotension. His laboratory values reveal the following: potassium 5.8 mmol/L, BUN 60 mg/dL

(baseline 18), and serum creatinine 2.0 mg/dL (baseline 0.9). IH's medications include furosemide 80 mg twice daily, ramipril 5 mg twice daily, and metoprolol XL 50 mg daily. Which of the following immediate medication adjustments are appropriate? Select all that apply.

a. Temporarily hold furosemide.
b. Temporarily hold metoprolol XL.
c. Temporarily hold ramipril.
d. Continue current regimen with no changes.
e. Increase metoprolol XL to 100 mg daily.

Answers a and c are correct.   IH's vital signs and laboratory values suggest dehydration with orthostatic hypotension and an elevated BUN/serum creatinine ratio; therefore, temporarily holding furosemide (Answer a) is indicated until IH becomes euvolemic. Additionally, the patient is experiencing hyperkalemia secondary to renal dysfunction; therefore, temporarily holding ramipril (Answer c) is an optimal response.

Answer b is incorrect.   Temporarily holding metoprolol XL or downtitration of dose should be considered, if recent initiation or uptitration results in fluid retention or worsening HF (neither of which is the case in this patient).

Answer d is incorrect.   To continue the current regimen with no changes would be inappropriate given patient's vital signs and laboratory values.

Answer e is incorrect.   The patient is already hypotensive so increasing the metoprolol dose would be inappropriate.

---

16. Which of the following β-blocker regimens would represent target therapy for most HF patients?

    a. Toprol XL 150 mg once daily
    b. Coreg 25 mg twice daily
    c. Tenormin 100 mg once daily
    d. Zebeta 2.5 mg once daily

Answer b is correct.   Three β-blockers have been shown to reduce mortality in HF patients. In these studies, target doses of these therapies included: Toprol XL (metoprolol succinate) 200 mg once daily, Coreg (carvedilol) 25 mg twice daily, and Zebeta (bisoprolol) 10 mg once daily.

Answer a is incorrect.   Toprol XL (metoprolol succinate) 150 mg once daily is the mean dose achieved in the HF study demonstrating a mortality benefit; however, the target dose in this study was 200 mg once daily. The mortality benefit of β-blocker is dose-related, and thus, reaching target dose as tolerated is important.

Answer c is incorrect.   Tenormin (atenolol) has not been studied in a randomized controlled trial of HF patients, and thus should not be considered.

Answer d is incorrect.   Zebeta (bisoprolol) 2.5 mg once daily is an appropriate starting dose to consider in HF patients. The target dose is 10 mg once daily.

---

17. Which of the following are important to consider when initiating combination hydralazine and ISDN in an African American patient with HF? Select all that apply.

    a. Initiate hydralazine 37.5 mg and ISDN 20 mg one tablet three times daily.
    b. Discontinue background ACE inhibitor therapy.
    c. Utilize a nitrate-free interval.
    d. Lower doses may be used in patients who develop a headache with therapy.
    e. Discontinue background β-blocker therapy.

Answers a and d are correct.   In African American patients with HF, hydralazine 37.5 mg and ISDN 20 mg tid are the appropriate starting doses, and hydralazine 75 mg and ISDN 40 mg tid are the appropriate target doses. Headache is a common adverse effect that usually responds to temporary dose-reduction.

Answer b is incorrect.   In African American patients with HF, the hydralazine/isosorbide combination therapy should be initiated in addition to background ACE inhibitor therapy.

Answer c is incorrect.   A nitrate-free interval is not required in patients taking concomitant hydralazine.

Answer e is incorrect.   Patients are not required to discontinue β-blocker therapy when initiating ISDN with hydralazine.

---

18. Patients should be counseled to monitor for which of the following when initiating β-blocker therapy?

    a. Tachycardia
    b. Dehydration
    c. Fatigue
    d. Hypokalemia

Answer c is correct.   When initiating β-blocker therapy, it is important that patients monitor for worsening HF, including fatigue and fluid retention. Worsening HF may occur as a result of the acute negative inotropic effects of therapy.

Answer a is incorrect.   Bradycardia rather than tachycardia is a common side effect of β-blocker.

Answer b is incorrect.   An increase in volume may be associated with β-blocker initiation or uptitration (fluid retention). Dehydration is not associated with β-blockers.

Answer d is incorrect.   Hyperkalemia occurs with many HF therapies including ACE inhibitors, ARBs, and ARAs. Hypokalemia is a common side effect of loop or thiazide diuretic therapy.

19. In which HF patients should aldosterone antagonists be avoided? Select all that apply.

    a. Serum potassium <3.5 mmol/L
    b. Creatinine clearance <30 mL/min
    c. Concomitant sacubitril/valsartan therapy
    d. NYHA class III to IV despite standard HF therapy
    e. Serum potassium >5 mmol/L

Answers b and e are correct. Aldosterone antagonists (ARA) can cause hyperkalemia and renal dysfunction and thus should be avoided in patients with a serum potassium >5 mmol/L (Answer e). Patients with creatinine clearance <30 mL/min (Answer b) are at higher risk of hyperkalemia and thus is a contraindication to ARA therapy.

Answer a is incorrect. ARAs can safely prescribed in a patient with a serum potassium <3.5 mmol/L.

Answer c is incorrect. Therapy with an ARA may be initiated with concomitant sacubitril/valsartan as long as hyperkalemia is not present.

Answer d is incorrect. ARA therapy is recommended in patients who are NYHA class III to IV despite standard HF therapy. ARAs are also beneficial in NYHA class II HF.

20. Select the brand name of torsemide.

    a. Lasix
    b. Bumex
    c. Toprol XL
    d. Demadex

Answer d is correct. The brand name of torsemide is Demadex.

Answer a is incorrect. The brand name of furosemide is Lasix.

Answer b is incorrect. The brand name of bumetanide is Bumex.

Answer c is incorrect. The brand name of metoprolol succinate is Toprol XL.

CHAPTER 2 | **Acute Decompensated Heart Failure**

Questions 1 through 3 pertain to the following case.

RF is a 62-year-old man with nonischemic cardiomyopathy (LVEF 30%-35%) presenting to the emergency department (ED) with an acute HF exacerbation. His vital signs include BP 155/90 mm Hg, heart rate (HR) 85 beats/min, RR 20, and O_2 sat 94% on 4 L/min of oxygen by nasal cannula (NC). Physical examination reveals jugular venous distension (JVD), regular rate and rhythm (RRR), crackles bilaterally at bases, and 2+ bilateral lower extremity edema. He admits to a 12-lb weight gain in the past 2 weeks since his carvedilol dose was increased and reports strict adherence to both dietary

restrictions and medications. In the ED, he has already received furosemide 80 mg IV ×1 dose with minimal response in urine output. Pertinent laboratory results include potassium 3.9 mmol/L, BNP 1550 pg/mL, BUN 37 mg/dL, and SCr 1.3 mg/dL (baseline). RF's home medications include lisinopril 10 mg daily, carvedilol 25 mg twice daily, digoxin 0.125 mg/d, and furosemide 80 mg orally twice daily.

1. Based on the BNP lab, RF is experiencing which one of the following?

    a. Active myocardial ischemia
    b. Shortness of breath due to a non-cardiac etiology
    c. Significant volume overload and ventricular wall stretch
    d. Renal insufficiency

Answer c is correct. Brain natriuretic peptide (BNP) is released and elevated in the setting of significant volume overload causing stretch of the ventricular wall.

Answer a is incorrect. Common laboratory tests for assessing active myocardial ischemia include creatinine kinase, creatinine kinase-myocardial fraction, and troponin.

Answer b is incorrect. BNP may be used to rule out other etiologies of shortness of breath due to a noncardiac etiology, in which cases the BNP level will be normal. RF's shortness of breath (SOB) is due to a heart failure exacerbation with pulmonary edema from cardiac failure, which would be a cardiac etiology.

Answer d is incorrect. While BNP may be altered in the setting of renal insufficiency, it is not to the same degree as the level of elevations which occurs in the setting of fluid overload.

2. Which of the following interventions is best for RF on arrival to the intensive care unit (ICU)?

    a. Dobutamine 2.5 mcg/kg/min infusion
    b. Milrinone 0.375 mcg/kg/min infusion
    c. Metolazone 10 mg po now and then daily
    d. Furosemide 120 mg IV twice daily

Answer d is correct. RF is clearly experiencing fluid overload secondary to acute decompensated heart failure (ADHF). RF has failed an initial dose of IV furosemide but the dose was small. Therefore, it is appropriate to try a higher dose of IV furosemide such as 120 mg IV twice daily.

Answers a and b are incorrect. Currently, RF is *not* exhibiting any signs or symptoms of low cardiac output that would necessitate administration of an inotropic agent such as dobutamine (Answer a) or milrinone (Answer b).

Answer c is incorrect. Metolazone is a thiazide-type diuretic, which acts synergistically with loop diuretics for refractory fluid overload. At this time, RF is not refractory to higher furosemide doses.

3. Select the appropriate management of RF's β-blocker based upon his history and clinical presentation?

   a. Continue carvedilol 25 mg twice daily.
   b. Increase carvedilol to 50 mg twice daily.
   c. Decrease carvedilol to 12.5 mg twice daily.
   d. Discontinue carvedilol.

Answer c is correct. RF experienced fluid accumulation in association with recent up-titration of his β-blocker dose. Therefore, a decrease to carvedilol 12.5 mg twice daily is indicated in this situation.

Answer a is incorrect. RF experienced fluid accumulation in association with recent up-titration of his β-blocker dose. Thus, continuation of this same dose, carvedilol 25 mg twice daily, is inappropriate at this time.

Answer b is incorrect. An increase to carvedilol 50 mg twice daily would be warranted *if* JP was tolerating the current dose with no fluid accumulation or worsening HF.

Answer d is incorrect. Discontinuing carvedilol should occur only in the setting of cardiogenic shock.

4. Which of the following should be closely monitored during initial intravenous diuretic administration?

   a. Hypokalemia
   b. Hypernatremia
   c. Hypertension
   d. Hypouricemia

Answer a is correct. Hypokalemia is a common side effect of loop and thiazide diuretics. Diuretics can cause potassium (K^+) imbalances in extracellular fluid. Changes in the K^+ concentration in the extracelluar fluid will affect the membrane potential of cells. Changes in the membrane potential may cause problems with electrical activity in the heart, nervous system, and muscles.

Answer b is incorrect. Aggressive diuretic administration may result in hyponatremia rather than hypernatremia. Hyponatremia is a predictor of poor outcome in HF patients.

Answer c is incorrect. Diuretic administration may cause hypotension rather than hypertension, especially if over diuresis occurs.

Answer d is incorrect. Hyperuricemia rather than hypouricemia may occur with diuretic use.

Questions 5 through 7 pertain to the following case.

BG is a 72-year-old woman complaining of being "extremely tired all the time." Her exercise tolerance is significantly less than it was 2 months ago; she now has to rest during daily activities. This has come on gradually. She has a history of hypertensive cardiomyopathy (LVEF 25%-30% by ECHO 1 year ago). She is strictly adherent with both diet restrictions and medications. Vital signs include BP 92/63 mm Hg, HR 105 beats/min with symptomatic orthostasis upon standing, and RR 14. BG does complain of recent dizziness; however, she denies palpitations and her electrocardiogram (ECG) is normal. On physical examination, her lungs are clear and she has no jugular venous distention, ascites, or lower extremity edema. Laboratory analysis reveals sodium 129 mmol/L, potassium 4.2 mmol/L, BUN 65 mg/dL, and SCr 2.1 mg/dL (baseline BUN/SCr 32/0.9). BG has been stable on the following oral regimen for several months: valsartan 80 mg twice daily, metoprolol XL 50 mg/d, furosemide 40 mg twice daily, amiodarone 200 mg/d, and digoxin 0.125 mg/d.

5. Which one of the following clinical categories best describes BG?

   a. Warm and dry
   b. Warm and wet
   c. Cold and dry
   d. Cold and wet

Answer c is correct. Being cold and dry best describes BG's current status. Administration of fluid would assist with correcting her volume depletion. In addition, it may or may not correct her low output.

Answer a is incorrect. BG is complaining of fatigue which is a common symptom of low cardiac output (ie, cold); therefore, she is not warm and dry (Answer a). BG's worsening renal function may be associated with low output.

Answers b and d are incorrect. BF is not experiencing any signs of pulmonary or peripheral edema (ie, not "wet") based upon physical examination and thus she is not warm and wet (Answer b) or cold and wet (Answer d). In fact, the presence of orthostasis and a BUN/SCr ratio >20 suggests volume depletion.

6. Which one of the following is the optimal initial intervention for BG?

   a. Change furosemide to 80 mg intravenously twice daily.
   b. Hold furosemide and begin cautious hydration with IV fluids.
   c. Hold metoprolol and begin dobutamine at 2 mcg/kg/min.
   d. Increase metoprolol XL to 100 mg/d.

Answer b is correct. At a minimum, her diuretic dose should be held and administration of IV fluids would be reasonable, especially given worsening renal function.

Answer a is incorrect. Since BG is volume depleted, a decision to change furosemide to the more aggressive intravenous route is incorrect.

Answer c is incorrect. Since recent up-titration of β-blocker has not occurred and symptomatic hypotension or cardiogenic shock is not present, the β-blocker should be continued at the current dose. Additionally, inotropic therapy

(Answer c) would not be indicated until BG's low volume status and filling pressures are corrected.

Answer d is incorrect. β-Blocker up-titration would not be indicated until low output has been corrected.

---

7. After your intervention, BG feels much better. Her vital signs today include BP 132/76 mm Hg, HR 78 beats/min, and RR 14, and her orthostasis has resolved. An echocardiogram (performed today) reveals LVEF of 15% to 20% with increasing ventricular dilation. Her relevant laboratory values are sodium 129 mmol/L, potassium 5.1 mmol/L, BUN 40 mg/dL, and SCr 1.2 mg/dL.

    Which one of the following most likely explains BG's change in EF?

    a. Acute arrhythmia
    b. Dietary nonadherence
    c. Renal insufficiency
    d. Progression of heart failure

Answer d is correct. BG's SCr did not return to baseline suggesting that some level of HF progression may exist (Answer d). Also, the presence of hyponatremia also suggests worsening HF.

Answer a is incorrect. BG's ECG was normal and thus acute arrhythmia is likely not the cause of her decompensation.

Answer b is incorrect. The patient reports strict compliance with her medications and diet (Answer b).

Answer c is incorrect. While renal insufficiency did occur in the setting of volume overload, the elevated BUN/SCr ratio improved. Unfortunately, BG's SCr did not return to baseline suggesting that some level of HF progression may exist (Answer d). Also, the presence of hyponatremia also suggests worsening HF.

Questions 8 through 12 pertain to the following case.

JF is a 57-year-old woman who presents to the hospital with ADHF. Vital signs include BP 105/67 mm Hg, HR 83 beats/min, and RR 21. Physical examination reveals 12 cm JVD elevated, +S_3, bilateral rales on auscultation, abdominal ascites, and 4+ bilateral edema extending to her thighs. Chest radiograph reveals pulmonary edema and pleural effusions. Hemodynamic measurements obtained by PAC include PCWP 29 mm Hg, CI 1.7 L/min/m², and SVR 700. Her laboratory values are all normal, except sodium 132 mmol/L, BUN 49 mg/dL, and SCr 2.1 mg/dL (baseline BUN/SCr 32 and 0.9). Her drugs on admission include enalapril 10 mg twice daily, carvedilol 12.5 mg twice daily, bumetanide 2 mg twice daily, hydralazine 50 mg three times daily, isosorbide dinitrate 40 mg three times daily, and aspirin 81 mg/d.

8. Which of the following is a reasonable choice for diuretic therapy in JF?

    a. JF should not receive diuretic therapy because she is volume-depleted.
    b. Intravenous loop diuretic therapy should be given to provide a net fluid loss of 500 to 2000 mL/d.

    c. Metolazone should be considered a first-line option because of JF's impaired renal function.
    d. Nesiritide therapy should be used as a replacement for diuretic therapy because JF is volume overloaded.

Answer b is correct. Loop diuretics are the mainstay of initial therapy for fluid overload and 500 to 2000 mL/d net fluid loss is appropriate. Loop diuretics rapidly reduce ventricular filling pressures and decrease PCWP by blocking sodium and chloride reabsorption in the Loop of Henle leading to fluid excretion.

Answer a is incorrect. Avoiding diuretic administration in JF is not an option as she is volume overloaded.

Answer c is incorrect. Loop diuretics are the diuretic of choice in patients with renal insufficiency; therefore, metolazone should only be considered in the setting of refractory volume overload, and should be added to background loop diuretic therapy.

Answer d is incorrect. JF's low BP and SVR preclude nesiritide administration since this agent is a potent vasodilator. Also, the cost of nesiritide prohibits it from being used first line for diuresis.

---

9. Which of the following best describes what PCWP represents in JF? Select all that apply.

    a. Fluid status
    b. Inotropy
    c. Afterload
    d. Chronotropy

Answer a is correct. Pulmonary capillary wedge pressure (PCWP) is a marker of intravascular fluid status and ventricular filling pressures. Normal, healthy individuals have a PCWP of 10 mm Hg, but those with HF may require a PCWP of 15 to 18 to optimize cardiac output. Patients with a PCWP >18 mm Hg are generally considered "wet" as a consequence of fluid overload; whereas those with a PCWP of 15 to 18 mm Hg are considered "dry" (euvolemic).

Answer b is incorrect. Inotropy or the force of myocardial contraction is reflected in cardiac output (CO) and cardiac index (CI).

Answer c is incorrect. The term preload rather than afterload (Answer c) represents the pressure stretching the ventricle of the heart and also reflects fluid status.

Answer d is incorrect. Chronotropy reflects the time or rate of the heart.

---

10. What is the desired PCWP for JF? Select all that apply.

    a. Less than 2.2 L/min/m²
    b. Greater than 2.2 L/min/m²
    c. Between 6 and 12 mm Hg
    d. Between 15 and 18 mm Hg

Answer d is correct. For patients with left ventricular dysfunction, the optimal PCWP is 15 to 18 mm Hg as maintaining mildly elevated filling pressures is essential to optimizing the Starling curve and assuring optimal cardiac output.

Answers a and b are incorrect. These numbers represent cardiac index. A cardiac index of greater than 2.2 L/min/m² is necessary to maintain adequate tissue perfusion.

Answer c is incorrect. For patients with normal cardiac function, the desired PCWP is between 6 and 12 mm Hg. Most patients with heart failure will require higher than normal ventricular filling pressures in order to maximize cardiac output.

11. Once JF has undergone successful diuresis and returned to her euvolemic weight, her CI and SVR do not change substantially. Her vital signs and oral HF medications remain unchanged with the exception of her diuretic dose. Her renal function has improved to baseline. Which of the following therapies are now appropriate to manage JF's ADHF?

    a. Nitroprusside
    b. Nesiritide
    c. Dopamine
    d. Milrinone

Answer d is correct. Milrinone is an inotrope that works through phosphodiesterase inhibition. A possible side effect of milrinone therapy is hypotension, so loading doses are often omitted and low doses should be initiated with slow titration.

Answers a and b are incorrect. Nitroprusside (Answer a) and Nesiritide (Answer b) are potent vasodilators and JF's current BP and SVR preclude their safe use. In the setting of low blood pressure and worsening renal function, current guidelines recommend inotropic therapy.

Answer c is incorrect. Current literature does not support the routine use of dopamine in the management of ADHF as it has been associated with no benefit and possible harm (eg, tachycardia).

12. Discharge for JF is planned with outpatient inotropic therapy based on your recommendations. According to the American College of Cardiology/American Heart Association (ACC/AHA) HF performance measures, which one of the following should be completed prior to JF's discharge?

    a. BNP measurement
    b. Written documentation of her EF
    c. Care of her IV access site
    d. Advance directives

Answer b is correct. Measurement of BNP (Answer a), intravenous access site care (Answer c), and advance directives (Answer d) are all important to address prior to discharging a patient for ADHF. However, written documentation of EF (Answer b) is one of several performance

measures recommended by ACC/AHA to be obtained prior to discharge for ADHF. Prescribing of an ACE inhibitor or ARB as well as a β-blocker in HF with reduced ejection fraction (HFrEF) is also a current performance measure. In JF's case, if she is unable to tolerate these guideline-recommended medications (ie, due to hypotension or other adverse effects), intolerance should be documented in the medical record.

13. Which of the following should be assured prior to administering intravenous inotropes and vasodilators?

    a. Adequate filling pressures with a PCWP 6 to 12 mm Hg
    b. Adequate filling pressures with a PCWP >15 mm Hg
    c. Adequate filling pressure with an SVR >1200 dyne/s/cm⁵
    d. Adequate filling pressure with an SVR >1500 dyne/s/cm⁵

Answer b is correct. Adequate filling pressures as reflected by a PCWP 15 to 18 mm Hg (Answer b) should be assured prior to safely administering IV inotropes or vasodilators.

Answer a is incorrect. While a PCWP 6 to 12 mm Hg would suggest adequate filling pressures in a patient with normal cardiac function, patients with HFrEF require a higher filling pressure to optimize cardiac output (starling curve).

Answers c and d are incorrect. An SVR measurement (Answers c and d) reflects vascular tone or afterload and not filling pressure.

14. Which of the following would be an absolute contraindication to intravenous vasodilators?

    a. Heart rate >90 beats/min
    b. Heart rate >110 beats/min
    c. Systolic blood pressure <90 mm Hg
    d. Systolic blood pressure <110 mm Hg

Answer c is correct. Intravenous vasodilators are considered for persistent ADHF despite aggressive treatment with diuretics *in the absence* of low blood pressure (SBP <90 mm Hg). A systolic blood pressure <90 mm Hg is an absolute contraindication to intravenous vasodilators.

Answers a and b are incorrect. Vasodilators do not affect heart rate unless extreme hypotension occurs. In this setting, a reflex tachycardia would occur, thus a heart rate >90 beats/min (Answer a) or 110 beats/min (Answer b) would not be a contraindication to therapy.

Answer d is incorrect. A systolic blood pressure <100 mm Hg is a relative contraindication to therapy, but not 110 mm Hg.

15. Which of the following are adverse effects of dobutamine? Select all that apply.

    a. Hyponatremia
    b. Renal dysfunction

   c. Hypokalemia
   d. Arrhythmia
   e. Thrombocytopenia

Answers c and d are correct. Hypokalemia has been reported with dobutamine and is likely associated with direct stimulation of β-receptors. Arrhythmia is a known adverse effect of inotropes. Intravenous inotropic agents promote increased myocardial contractility via elevation of myocyte calcium concentrations, a mechanism that is known to promote the development of cardiac arrhythmias.

Answers a, b, and e are incorrect. Inotropic therapy improves cardiac output and will potentially improve hyponatremia (Answer a) and renal dysfunction (Answer b) in patients with ADHF. Thrombocytopenia (Answer c) is a rare adverse effect of milrinone, not dobutamine.

---

16. Which of the following is referred to as an "inodilator," having both inotropic and vasodilatory properties?

   a. Milrinone
   b. Dobutamine
   c. Nesiritide
   d. Nitroprusside

Answer a is correct. Milrinone decreases the breakdown of cyclic adenosine monophosphate (cAMP) in cardiac tissue, resulting in an increase in cardiac contractility and output. By increasing cAMP in vascular smooth muscle, systemic and pulmonary vascular resistance are reduced, thus milrinone is often referred to as an "inodilator" (inotrope and vasodilator).

Answer b is incorrect. Dobutamine is an inotrope. While dobutamine stimulates β-2 receptors in the periphery causing mild vasodilation, it also stimulates alpha receptors, which counteracts with mild vasoconstriction. Therefore, the decrease in SVR that occurs with dobutamine is a reflexive response to the increase in cardiac output.

Answers c and d are incorrect. Nesiritide (Answer c) and nitroprusside (Answer d) are potent arterial and venous vasodilators. These agents dilate the arterial vessels (decrease in SVR) and cause a reflex increase in cardiac output.

---

17. JT is an 81-year-old man (70 kg) admitted for ADHF refractory to outpatient titration of oral diuretics, including torsemide and metolazone. He is now receiving intravenous furosemide 20 mg/h and chlorothiazide 500 mg intravenously twice daily. While JT's vital signs and renal function appear stable (BP 127/65 mm Hg, HR 90 beats/min, SCr 1.2 mg/dL), his urine output is unchanged despite over 24 hours of the above regimen. Additionally, review of continuous telemetry demonstrates multiple 10-beat runs of ventricular tachycardia. Which of the following is an appropriate next step in therapy?

   a. Initiate milrinone 0.1 mcg/kg/min
   b. Initiate dobutamine 2.5 mcg/kg/min

   c. Initiate nesiritide 0.01 mcg/kg/min
   d. Increase furosemide to 60 mg/h

Answer c is correct. Nesiritide is a recombinant BNP molecule that promotes natriuresis, venodilation, and arterial vasodilation. When administered as a continuous infusion, nesiritide decreases PCWP, decreases SVR (indirectly increasing CO), and assists in diuresis when coadministered with loop diuretics. Appropriate pharmacotherapy options for diuretic resistance include a drug with an alternative mechanism of action such as a thiazide-type diuretic or nesiritide. JT has already received therapy with chlorothiazide. MJ's systolic blood pressure is >100 mm Hg, making nesiritide a safe option.

Answers a and b are incorrect. JT is demonstrating refractory fluid overload. While the inotropic agents, milrinone (Answer a) and dobutamine (Answer b), can be considered in this setting, ventricular tachycardia precludes use of these proarrhythmic agents.

Answer d is incorrect. JT is already receiving a rather high dose of continuous furosemide and further uptitration of the furosemide dose is not expected to enhance diuresis.

---

18. Which of the following is associated with the use of IV nitroglycerin alone for ADHF?

   a. Natriuresis
   b. Increased risk of ventricular arrhythmias
   c. Accumulation of toxic metabolites in hepatic or renal impairment
   d. Primarily venous dilation at lower doses (ie, <100 mcg/min)

Answer d is correct. At lower doses, nitroglycerin produces primarily venodilation; doses in excess of 100 mcg/min are typically required to produce both venous and arterial dilation. At higher doses (>100 mcg/min), nitroglycerin also dilates the arterial vasculature, decreasing afterload and SVR and increasing CO.

Answer a is incorrect. Although IV nitroglycerin can enhance diuresis when added to a loop diuretic, this occurs indirectly via vasodilation and mobilization of fluid from the extravascular space.

Answer b is incorrect. While ventricular arrhythmias are common with IV inotropes, this is uncommon with IV nitroglycerin.

Answer c is incorrect. Nitroprusside forms toxic byproducts that may accumulate in patient's hepatic or renal impairment, but this is not true of nitroglycerin.

---

19. Place the following diuretics in order of potency. Start with the least potent agent. Select all that are in the correct order.

   a. Torsemide, furosemide, bumetanide
   b. Furosemide, torsemide, bumetanide

c. Bumetanide, furosemide, torsemide

d. Lasix, demadex, bumex

e. Bumex, lasix, demadex

Answers b and d are correct. The relative equivalent potency of loop diuretics are furosemide (Lasix) 40 mg = torsemide (Demadex) 20 mg = bumetanide (Bumex) 0.5-1 mg.

20. Select the intravenous agent(s) utilized for ADHF that has a neutral effect on heart rate (no change when utilized at recommended doses). Select all that apply.

a. Loop diuretics

b. Nitroprusside

c. Nesiritide

d. Dobutamine

e. Milrinone

Answers a and c are correct. Loop diuretics and nesiritide have a neutral effect on heart rate. Additionally, nitroglycerin is expected to have a neutral or minimal effect on heart rate.

Answers b, d, and e are incorrect. Nitroprusside, dobutamine, and milrinone are expected to have a significant increase in heart rate. Nitroprusside's effect on heart rate is indirect through reducing blood pressure resulting in reflex tachycardia, whereas dobutamine and milrinone have a direct effect on heart rate through their positive chronotropic properties.

CHAPTER **3 | Hypertension**

1. According to the 2017 guidelines for hypertension. What is the BP goal for a 58-year-old African American male with diabetes and chronic kidney disease?

a. <130/80 mm Hg

b. <140/90 mm Hg

c. <150/90 mm Hg

d. <160/100 mm Hg

Answer a is correct. All patients with hypertension and cardiovascular disease or other comorbid conditions such as CKD and diabetes should have a goal blood pressure of <130/80 mm Hg.

Answers b, c, d are incorrect. For adults with confirmed hypertension and known stable CVD or ≥10% 10-year ASCVD risk, a BP target of <130/80 mm Hg is recommended. BP should be categorized as normal, elevated, or stages 1 or 2 hypertension to prevent and treat high BP. Normal BP is defined as <120/<80 mm Hg; elevated BP 120-129/<80 mm Hg; hypertension stage 1 is 130-139 or 80-89 mm Hg, and hypertension stage 2 is ≥140 or ≥90 mm Hg. Prior to labeling a person with hypertension, it is important to use an average based on ≥2 readings obtained on ≥2 occasions to estimate the individual's level of BP.

2. Which of the following recommendations for lifestyle modification is correct?

a. A minimum weight loss of 15 lb

b. Sodium restriction of 4 g or less per day

c. Reduce alcohol intake to no more than two drinks a day for a woman, one for a man

d. Exercise for at least 30 minutes most days of the week

e. Adopt an eating plan low in potassium and carbohydrates

Answer d is correct. Thirty minutes per day is the minimum recommendation for physical activity in most patient populations. Regular physical activity can lower BP by 2 to 9 mm Hg. It is important to make sure that all patients have been clinically cleared to engage in physical activity by their primary care provider, cardiologist, or other responsible provider.

Answer a is incorrect. Although many patients may require a weight loss of 15 lb or more, the recommendation is to maintain normal body weight, which is a BMI of 18.5 to 24.9 kg/m². Maintaining normal body weight can lower BP by 5 to 20 mm Hg/10 kg weight loss.

Answer b is incorrect. The recommendation is no more than 2.4 g of sodium per day. Restriction of sodium can decrease BP by 2 to 8 mm Hg.

Answer c is incorrect. Alcohol should be no more than one drink per day for a woman and two drinks per day for a man. A drink is considered to be a 12 ounces of beer, a 5 ounces glass of wine, or 1.5 ounces of 80-proof whiskey. Moderating the intake of alcohol can lower BP by 2 to 4 mm Hg.

Answer e is incorrect. The DASH plan is low in sodium and fat (saturated and total) and high in potassium, fruits, and vegetables, and low-fat dairy products. Adopting the DASH eating plan can lower BP by 8 to 14 mm Hg.

3. JD is a 55-year-old African American woman with newly diagnosed hypertension. Her average BP is 164/91 mm Hg. Which of the following is the best recommendation for JD?

a. Begin hydrochlorothiazide and return to clinic in 3 months.

b. Begin metoprolol and prescribe monitoring blood pressure at home.

c. Begin two medications since most patients with stage 2 hypertension will not reach goal with one agent alone.

d. Prescribe lifestyle modifications first, and return to clinic in 1 month to determine if pharmacotherapy is warranted.

e. Begin clonidine patch since a once weekly patch increases patient compliance.

Answer c is correct. Since JD has been classified with Stage 2 hypertension at the time of diagnosis, dual therapy would be recommended for this patient. With JD being

African American, it would be recommended to make sure that at least one of the medications initiated is a thiazide and/or a DHP CCB.

Answer a is incorrect. Although JD will most likely require two medications as she has stage 2 hypertension, it is equally logical to begin one and add the other at follow-up to determine efficacy of the first agent. However, follow-up should be monthly until the patient is at goal.

Answer b is incorrect. At home BP monitoring should be prescribed and implemented for any hypertensive patient who is willing and able. However, metoprolol is not the best initial choice for this patient. Results are more inconsistent with β-blockers than other medication classes for the treatment of hypertension, and JD does not have any concomitant conditions that would warrant starting with a β-blocker (post-MI, heart failure).

Answer d is incorrect. Lifestyle modifications are essential to the treatment and management of hypertension. They should always be prescribed. However, JD definitely requires medications with a BP of 167/92 mm Hg as she will most likely not reach goal with lifestyle modifications alone and in the meantime possess significant cardiovascular risk with an elevated BP at this level.

Answer e is incorrect. Although transdermal systems are good options for patients with compliance problems, clonidine and other centrally acting agents are reserved as last-line options for patients who do not respond to first-line agents. RAAS agents, CCBs, and BBs should be tried before centrally acting medications.

---

4. TM was started on a new medication for her blood pressure. About a week later she noticed a persistent cough. Which of the following medications could be the cause?

   a. Maxzide
   b. Bystolic
   c. Vasotec
   d. Aldactone
   e. Catapres

Answer c is correct. Vasotec is enalapril, an ACEI. ACEIs inhibit the breakdown of bradykinin, a vasodilator that is in high concentrations in the lungs. Increased levels of bradykinin by ACEI are hypothesized to cause the side effect of a nagging, unproductive cough. The cough occurs in 5% to 35% of patients and resolves in 1 to 4 weeks, though in some it has been reported to last up to 3 months.

Answer a is incorrect. Maxide is triamterene and hydrochlorothiazde, a combination of two diuretics. Cough is not an expected side effect. Both may cause electrolyte abnormalities, glucose and lipid intolerance, and sexual dysfunction.

Answer b is incorrect. Bystolic is nebivolol, a BB. Cough is not an expected side effect. BBs cause glucose and lipid disturbances, fatigue, bradycardia, exercise intolerance, and sexual dysfunction.

Answer d is incorrect. Aldactone is sprinolactone, an aldosterone antagonist (potassium-sparing diuretic) and not readily known to cause cough. The most common side effect to spironolactone is gynecomastia.

Answer e is incorrect. Catapres is clonidine, which does not cause a cough as a side effect. The most common adverse reaction is orthostatic hypotension.

---

5. You have identified the cause of the cough. At the next visit, TM wants to change the medication as she cannot tolerate the cough. Unfortunately, she missed her follow-up and returns to you in 6 months. In between appointments she was admitted to the hospital and diagnosed with type 2 diabetes. Which of the following recommendations is best for TM assuming no insurance or cost issues?

   a. Switch to Lopressor
   b. Switch to Atacand
   c. Switch to Altace
   d. Switch to Cardizem
   e. Continue her current medication as this side effect usually resolves in a couple of months.

Answer b is correct. Due to the new diagnosis of diabetes in addition to her hypertension, TM should be on an RAAS agent, either an ACEI or an ARB (Atacand = candesartan). RAAS agents are proven to slow the progression of target organ damage in patients with diabetes and should be used unless contraindicated. Since cough was the reason for discontinuing the ACEI, switching to an ARB is the best option to control TM's hypertension. ARBs do not cause the breakdown of bradykinin and therefore do not induce a nagging cough.

Answer a is incorrect. Although a BB (Lopressor = metoprolol) is an alternative option for the treatment of hypertension, other medications should be utilized in this patient. In addition, TM's diabetes may be worsened due to glucose intolerance caused by BBs. However, this would not be a reason to avoid BB in the case of compelling indications (myocardial infarction or heart failure) or if nothing else is a viable option to reach BP goal.

Answer c is incorrect. Altace is another ACEI (ramipril). Switching to another medication of the same class may not provide relief of the cough. Not all ACEI-cough occur with every challenged ACEI, therefore it could be an alternative option if she was not able to trial an ARB due to cost or insurance issues.

Answer d is incorrect. Although CCBs are viable hypertensive agents (Cardizem = diltiazem), TM has diabetes and if not contraindicated requires the addition of a RAAS agent (eg, ARB).

Answer e is incorrect. Since it is 6 months post initiation of the medication, the chances of TM's cough going away are limited. Important to note is that the cough is nonproductive and essentially benign. If a patient is not bothered by the cough, the ACEI does not necessarily have to be discontinued.

---

6. FS is a 50-year-old woman diagnosed with osteoporosis and hypertension. Which of the following antihypertensives is likely to help the FS's osteoporosis in addition to lowering her BP?

    a. Demadex
    b. Microzide
    c. Capoten
    d. Toprol XL

Answer b is correct. Microzide (HCTZ) is a thiazide diuretic, the preferred initial therapy for the treatment of hypertension. Unlike loop diuretics, thiazide diuretics decrease the excretion of calcium, and added benefit in a patient with concomitant osteoporosis.

Answer a is incorrect. Demadex (torsemide) is a loop diuretic. These agents are generally not used as monotherapy for hypertension. In addition, these agents increase the excretion of calcium, rendering this agent least appropriate for a patient with osteoporosis.

Answer c is incorrect. Capoten (captopril) is an ACEI. Although ACEI is viable first-line options for the treatment of hypertension, there are no compelling indications to use this agent over HCTZ.

Answer d is incorrect. Toprol XL (metoprolol) is a BB. This class of medication is not currently recommended as first-line agents for the treatment of hypertension in the absence of compelling comorbid conditions.

---

7. Which of the following statements is true regarding lifestyle modifications (LSM)? Select all that apply.

    a. LSM decreases the risk for cardiovascular disease.
    b. LSM decreases the risk for renal disease.
    c. LSM decreases morbidity.
    d. LSM is critical for the prevention of hypertension but not the treatment.

Answers a, b, and c are correct. All forms of cardiovascular disease, renal disease, and stroke are decreased. Additionally, both morbidity and mortality are decreased through lifestyle modifications.

Answer d is incorrect. Hypertension represents a major public health challenge. Lifestyle modifications are essential to the *management and prevention* of hypertension. These modifications simply represent a healthy lifestyle and should be adopted by all regardless of health status.

---

8. A patient presents to the emergency department with signs and symptoms of hyperkalemia. Electrolyte testing reveals serum potassium of 6.7 mmol/L. Which agents could cause or exacerbate the electrolyte abnormality? Select all that apply.

    a. Bumex
    b. Mavik
    c. Dyrenium
    d. Aldactone
    e. Cozaar

Answer b is correct. Mavik (trandolapril) is an ACEI. This class causes an increase in serum potassium.

Answer c is correct. Dyrenium (triamterene) is a potassium-sparing diuretic which can increase the concentration of serum potassium.

Answer d is correct. Aldactone (spironolactone) is an aldosterone antagonist. Blocking aldosterone increases the concentration of serum potassium.

Answer e is correct. Cozaar (losartan) is an ARB. Like ACEI, these agents also increase the serum concentration of potassium.

Answer a is incorrect. Bumex (bumetanide) is a loop diuretic. Loop diuretics profoundly increase the excretion of potassium, lowering the serum concentration.

---

9. Which of the following is *true* regarding the use of combination treatment with an ACEI and an ARB for the treatment of hypertension?

    a. The combination significantly reduces the risk of cardiovascular events.
    b. The combination increases the risk of hyperkalemia.
    c. The combination is more effective for controlling blood pressure than monotherapy.
    d. This combination is recommended because it does not reduce cardiovascular events in this setting.

Answer b is correct. If this combination is to be used, prudent electrolyte (potassium) monitoring is required. However, there is also an increased risk for syncope, renal dysfunction, and hypotension.

Answer a is incorrect. Although additional blood pressure lowering *may* be achieved with the combination, it is at the expense of increased syncope, hypotension, renal dysfunction, and hyperkalemia.

Answer c is incorrect. This statement is false—the combination does not significantly lower BP compared with monotherapy.

Answer d is incorrect. An ACEI does not inhibit all forms of angiotensin production. It would theoretically make sense to test the effect of additional blockade by adding an ARB, which blocks angiotensin at the receptor directly. However, until more evidence demonstrates an increase in benefit to risk ratio, this combination is not currently recommended.

---

10. DL is a 35-year-old man recently diagnosed with type 2 diabetes, hypertension, hyperlipidemia, and sexual dysfunction induced by diabetic neuropathy. Which of the following

two-drug regimens is most appropriate to initiate in DL for antihypertensive therapy?

    a. Amlodipine + lisinopril
    b. Short-acting nifedipine + trandolapril
    c. Doxazosin + HCTZ
    d. Pindolol + losartan
    e. HCTZ + lisinopril

Answer a is correct. A RAAS agent, such as an ACEI or an ARB, is indicated for renal protection in the diabetes population. Therefore, lisinopril is an appropriate first-line option for the treatment of hypertension in this patient. A CCB such as amlodipine is appropriate, given that calcium channel blockers have equal antihypertensive efficacy (compared to an ACEI or a diuretic) and have neutral effects on glucose homeostasis and on the lipid profile. This regimen is also least likely to worsen sexual function.

Answer b is incorrect. Although an ACEI (trandolapril) is a good choice, short-acting CCBs should be avoided because of an increase in side effects from the immediate release formulations (flushing, headache).

Answer c is incorrect. The alpha-1 blocker doxazosin would be a viable option in patients with concomitant BPH; however, it is less effective in lowering blood pressure and not a first-line agent. HCTZ, normally the agent of choice, would not be appropriate in this patient since diuretics have negative effects on the lipid and glucose profile. In addition, other agents are available (CCBs). Diabetes and hyperlipidemia are not absolute contraindications for diuretics but if they can be avoided they should be.

Answer d is incorrect. Losartan is a viable option since patients with diabetes should be on an ACEI or an ARB. However, pindolol is not the best option since BBs are not first-line and they often cause sexual dysfunction. BBs with ISA, such as pindolol, have neutral effects on the lipid profile but can still worsen glucose homeostasis. In addition, BBs can mask signs and symptoms of hypoglycemia (except for sweating).

Answer e is incorrect. This would be a good first-line regimen, except HCTZ can worsen glucose intolerance and the lipid profile, whereas CCBs have neutral effects. Since a CCB like amlodipine is not contraindicated in this patient, it is a better choice than HCTZ.

---

11. ER is a 72-year-old man who presents to clinic. He is currently on lisinopril 40 mg daily, HCTZ 25 mg daily, and Amlodipine 10 mg daily. His blood pressure in clinic supports his elevated home readings, providing an average BP of 162/89 mm Hg. He is open to going adding therapy in addition to altering his diet with reduced sodium intake (however, in discussion his diet seemed appropriate). You have agreed to start spironolactone 25 mg daily. What side effects do you educate the patient about regarding the addition of spirlonlactone?

    a. retrograde ejaculation
    b. rebound hypertension if immediate discontinuation occurs

    c. hypokalemia
    d. gynecomastia

Answer d is correct. Due to spironolactone's affinity toward progesterone and androgen receptors, gynecomastia is a common side effect and the patient should be informed of this.

Answers a is incorrect. In retrograde ejaculation, the muscle that shuts the bladder does not function normally. This allows all or part of the semen to travel backward (retrograde) into the bladder at the time of ejaculation. Medications that may cause retrograde ejaculation include drugs to treat:

Prostate enlargement—tamsulosin (Flomax) or terazosin (Cardura)

Depression—especially selective serotonin reuptake inhibitors (SSRIs) such as fluoxetine (Prozac), sertraline (Zoloft) and several others

Psychosis—such as chlorpromazine (Thorazine), thioridazine (Mellaril) and risperidone (Risperdal)

Answer b is incorrect. Rebound hypertension associated with immediate discontinuation is related to clonidine.

Answer c is incorrect. Sprionolactone is associated with hyperkalemia. Medications that faciliate fluid loss are associated with hypokalemia and include thiazide and loop diuretics.

---

12. Which of the following is correct regarding the pathophysiology of hypertension?

    a. Most patients with hypertension have an identifiable secondary cause such as hyperaldosteronism.
    b. Cardiac output and peripheral vascular resistance are the two key factors that determine blood pressure.
    c. Stroke volume and heart rate are the two key factors that determine blood pressure.
    d. In the elderly, cardiac output rises, increasing the risk of hypertension, especially diastolic hypertension.

Answer b is correct. The stroke volume multiplied by the heart rate is the cardiac output.

Answer a is incorrect. 90% of patients have essential hypertension.

Answer c is incorrect. Stroke volume and heart rate are the parameters that determine cardiac output. Blood pressure is determined by cardiac output and peripheral vascular resistance.

Answer d is incorrect. Isolated systolic hypertension accounts for more than two-thirds of hypertensive cases in the elderly population. As individuals age, their risk of developing systolic hypertension increases while diastolic hypertension tends to stabilize or decrease.

---

13. AC is a 46-year-old white man with a medical history significant for type 2 diabetes obesity, and new-onset hypertension. His current HA1c is 7.2%. He was started on lisinopril 10 mg daily 6 weeks ago and the dose was increased after 2 weeks to 20 mg daily. It has been 4 weeks since any alterations in therapy and in clinic his BP is 146/94 mm Hg and his heart rate is 67 beats/min. Which of the following is the most appropriate recommendation for AC?

    a. Continue current regimen.
    b. Discontinue lisinopril and start diltiazem.
    c. Discontinue lisinopril and start HCTZ.
    d. Add atenolol.
    e. Add amlodipine.

Answer e is correct. The CCB, amlodipine, is the best option due to limited side effects and its ability to work on peripheral vascular resistance without the risk of electrolyte abnormalities and limited glucose abnormalities caused by particular blood pressure agents.

Answer a is incorrect. The patient's blood pressure is not at goal and requires intervention. BP reductions are required to decrease morbidity and mortality associated with hypertension.

Answers b and c are incorrect. ACEI therapy is warranted in hypertensive patients with diabetes and should be continued unless the patient has contraindications to ACEI therapy (this patient does not have any contraindications).

Answer d is incorrect. BB therapy is controversial in the management of hypertension, except when the patient has a compelling indication (myocardial infarction and heart failure).

---

14. TJ is a 64-year-old man with long-standing hypertension. He has recently been diagnosed with chronic kidney disease and his estimated glomerular filtration rate (eGFR) is 24 mL/min. He is currently taking ramipril 10 mg daily. His blood pressure is 148/86 mm Hg, heart rate is 58 beats/min, and electrolytes notable for a potassium of 5.1 mEq/L. Upon physical examination, the patient is noted to have slight peripheral edema; however, ECHO was without evidence of systolic heart failure (ejection fraction estimated at 60%) however noted left ventricular dysfunction. Which of the following would be the most appropriate recommendation at this time?

    a. Continue current therapy and monitor BP regularly.
    b. Add HCTZ 12.5 mg daily.
    c. Add furosemide 20 mg daily.
    d. Start verapamil ER to 360 mg daily.
    e. Add spironolactone 25 mg daily.

Answer c is correct. Loop diuretics such as furosemide may be used in hypertensive patients with reduced CrCl.

Loop diuretics are filtered and secreted, so when a patient loses kidney filtration ability (CrCl <30 mL/min), the loop diuretics may still be effective (thiazide diuretics would most likely not be effective in this setting because they are only filtered). The patient is also noted to have peripheral edema and due to the great excretion of Na/H_2O by this agent it would be better than a thiazide or potassium-sparing diuretic.

Answer a is incorrect. The patient's blood pressure is not at goal and requires intervention.

Answer b is incorrect. HCTZ is unlikely to be effective because the patient has kidney dysfunction (CrCl <30 mL/min) and it has minimal water excretion effects due to its side of action.

Answer d is incorrect. TJ does not have any compelling indication to start an NDHP CCB and with the possibility of LVD the negative chronotropic effects could be detrimental and increase risk for HF diagnosis.

Answer e is incorrect. Spironolactone use in the setting of renal dysfunction would increase the risk of hyperkalemia. The patient's potassium level is already on the high end of the normal range.

---

15. RH is a 47-year-old white woman who has been seen by her family physician twice in the last 2 weeks, and her BP (measured properly) was similar at both visits, averaging 138/88 mm Hg. RH has no significant medical history or risk factors for cardiovascular disease; she is relatively active and likes to exercise. Which of the following would be the most appropriate recommendation for RH?

    a. She should be seen again by her physician within 3 months to see if she has hypertension, but in the meantime work with recommended lifestyle modifications listed within this chapter.
    b. She should be counseled to undertake an intensive weight reduction program, with follow-up in 2 years.
    c. Initiate treatment with ramipril.
    d. Initiate treatment with atenolol.
    e. Initiate treatment with clonidine.

Answer a is correct. RH has prehypertension and at this point guidelines do not recommend starting drug therapy; however, it would be recommended to take preventative actions and provide education as often as possible to delay the diagnosis of hypertension and other chronic disease states.

Answer b is incorrect. A prehypertensive patient should be followed up more routinely. While weight loss is recommended, telling a patient in 2 years for follow-up is negligence.

Answers c, d, and e are incorrect. At this time drug therapy is not warranted.

16. In a patient with risk factors for hyperkalemia and history of hyperkalemia, which of the following agents would be acceptable treatment to avoid hyperkalemia risk?

    a. Amiloride
    b. Amlodipine
    c. Enalapril
    d. Spironolactone
    e. Valsartan

Answer b is correct. CCBs (such as amlodipine) are not associated with hyperkalemia.

Answer a is incorrect. Amiloride is a potassium-sparing diuretic (similar to triamterene).

Answer c is incorrect. ACEI (such as enalapril) are associated with hyperkalemia because of their effects on aldosterone.

Answer d is incorrect. Spironolactone is a potassium-sparing diuretic (aldosterone antagonist).

Answer e is incorrect. ARBs (such as valsartan) are associated with hyperkalemia because of their effects on aldosterone.

---

17. Which of the following agents is likely to increase blood glucose? Select all that apply.

    a. Chlorthalidone
    b. Furosemide
    c. Hydrochlorothiazide
    d. Lisinopril
    e. Propranolol

Answers a, b, c, and e are correct. These are all associated with blood glucose effects.

Answer d is incorrect. ACEI (such as lisinopril) are not associated with hyperglycemia. ACEI are beneficial in diabetic patients.

---

18. FS is a 56-year-old man with diabetes mellitus and newly diagnosed hypertension. His mean blood pressure in clinic today after three proper measurements is 158/101 mm Hg. He is not currently on treatment. Which of the following drug regimens would be the most appropriate to treat FS?

    a. Chlorthalidone
    b. Quinapril
    c. Benazepril + amlodipine
    d. Benazepril + losartan
    e. Atenolol + HCTZ

Answer c is correct. Because the patient has diabetes, ACEI therapy should be part of the combination regimen. The addition of a CCB has been shown to be beneficial in this setting.

Answer a is incorrect. While chlorthalidone is an effective hypertensive medication, ACEI are preferred in a hypertensive patient with diabetes.

Answer b is incorrect. ACEI therapy is warranted in this patient; however, since this patient is more than 20 mm Hg away from BP goal, combination therapy should be used.

Answer d is incorrect. While this patient should be given an ACEI, combination therapy with an angiotensin-receptor blocker is not warranted in hypertension or to patients with diabetes (PER THE ON-TARGET TRIAL).

Answer e is incorrect. Because the patient has a history of diabetes, the combination regimen needs to include an ACEI.

---

19. What diagnostic classification is an average blood pressure of 158/104 mm Hg on June 1st and an average blood pressure of 150/110 mm Hg on June 4th (both blood pressure averages were taken on two separate clinic dates as the patient refused to go to the emergency department)?

    a. Normal
    b. Elevated
    c. Stage 1 hypertension
    d. Stage 2 hypertension

Answer d is correct. Stage 2 is systolic BP greater than or equal to 160 mm Hg, and diastolic BP is greater than or equal to 100 mm Hg. While the systolic BP appears to be stage 1, the diastolic BP is stage 2. Classification is driven by which one is the highest stage.

Answer a is incorrect. Normal BP would be less than 120/80 mm Hg.

Answer b is incorrect. Prehypertension is systolic BP 120-139 mm Hg and diastolic BP 80-89 mm Hg.

Answer c is incorrect. Stage 1 is systolic BP 140-159 mm Hg and diastolic BP 90-99 mm Hg.

---

20. Which of the following requires monitoring in a patient on HCTZ? Select all that apply.

    a. Renal function
    b. Hepatic function
    c. Electrolytes
    d. Uric acid
    e. Blood glucose

Answers a, c, d, and e are correct. These are all effects of HCTZ and should be monitored or followed.

Answer b is incorrect. HCTZ is not associated with liver effects and therefore hepatic function does not need to be monitored.

---

21. Which of the following should be considered in patients with resistant hypertension? Select all that apply.

    a. Volume overload is a common cause.
    b. Spironolactone might be effective.
    c. Minoxidil might be effective.
    d. A loop diuretic might be necessary.

Answer a is correct. Patients with volume overload may have resistant hypertension.

Answer b is correct. Spironolactone may be used in the treatment of resistant hypertension.

Answer c is correct. Minoxidil is a direct-acting vasodilator that may be used in the treatment of resistant hypertension, but probably is not your first agent when thinking about resistant hypertension due to side effects.

Answer d is correct. Diuretic therapy might be necessary in resistant hypertension.

---

22. Which of the following blood pressure classifications would include lifestyle modifications as a recommended intervention? Select all that apply.

    a. Blood pressure 130/84
    b. Elevated
    c. Stage 1 hypertension
    d. Stage 2 hypertension
    e. Blood pressure 149/92

Answer a is correct. A blood pressure of 130/84 mm Hg is considered prehypertension. Lifestyle recommendations are recommended in all classifications. All patients with prehypertension and hypertension should be prescribed lifestyle modifications. However, lifestyle modifications should never be used as a replacement for antihypertensive drug therapy for patients with hypertension who are not at goal BP, especially in those with additional CV risk factors or hypertension-associated complications. Aside from lowering BP in patients with known hypertension, strict adherence with lifestyle modification can decrease the progression to hypertension in patients with prehypertension BP values. A sensible dietary program is one that is designed to reduce weight gradually (for overweight and obese patients) and one that restricts sodium intake with only moderate alcohol consumption if one consumes alcohol. The rationale for dietary intervention in hypertension can be explained to patients as follows:

1. Weight loss, as little as 5% to 10% of your body weight, can decrease BP significantly in overweight or obese patients.

2. Diets rich in fruits and vegetables and low in saturated fat have been shown to lower BP in patients with hypertension.

3. Most people experience some BP lowering with sodium restriction.

The Dietary Approaches to Stop Hypertension (DASH) eating plan is a diet that is rich in fruits, vegetables, and low-fat dairy products with a reduced content of saturated and total fat. It is recommended as a reasonable and feasible diet that has proven to lower BP. Intake of sodium should be minimized as much as possible, ideally to 1.5 g/d, although an interim goal of less than 2.3 g/d may be reasonable considering the difficulty in achieving these low intakes. Patients should be aware of the multiple sources of dietary sodium (eg, processed foods,

soups, and table salt) so that they may follow these recommendations. Potassium intake should be encouraged through fruits and vegetables with high content (ideally 4.7 g/d) in those with normal kidney function or without impaired potassium excretion. Excessive alcohol use can either cause or worsen hypertension. Patients with hypertension who drink alcoholic beverages should restrict their daily intake.

Answers b, c, and d are correct. Lifestyle recommendations are recommended in all types of classifications.

Answer e is correct. A blood pressure of 140/92 mm Hg is considered stage 1 hypertension. Lifestyle recommendations are recommended in all classifications.

---

23. Place the lifestyle modifications of weight reduction, moderation of alcohol consumption, and physical activity in order of the decrease in expected/approximate systolic blood pressure reduction. Start with the lowest expected decrease in SBP.

    a. Moderation of alcohol consumption, physical activity, weight reduction
    b. Weight reduction, physical activity, moderation of alcohol consumption
    c. Physical activity, moderation of alcohol consumption, weight reduction

---

Answer a is correct. Moderation of alcohol consumption has an approximate range of a 2 to 4 mm Hg decrease in SBP. Physical activity has an approximate range of 4 to 9 mm Hg decrease in SBP. Weight reduction has an approximate range of 5 to 20 mm Hg per 10 kg decrease in SBP.

Answers b and c are incorrect. Those answers are not the correct ordered response of blood pressure reduction starting with the lowest expected decrease in SBP.

---

24. Which of the following lifestyle recommendation would have the potential to decrease the SBP the greatest in a 58-year-old patient with chronic kidney disease, diabetes, atrial fibrillation, and hypertension. The patient currently has stage 2 hypertension and is not receiving pharmacologic therapy.

    a. Physical activity
    b. Moderation of alcohol consumption
    c. Adopting the DASH eating plan
    d. Initiating an ACEI + chlorthalidone

Answer c is correct. The DASH diet is a recommendation to consume fruits, vegetables, and low-fat dairy products with a reduced content of saturated and total fat. The diet has an approximate decrease in SBP of 8 to 14 mm Hg.

Answer a is incorrect. Physical activity consisting of regular aerobic exercise such as brisk walking at least 30 min/d for most days of the week has an approximate SBP decrease of 4 to 9 mm Hg.

Answer b is incorrect. Moderation of alcohol consumption is limiting consumption to no more than two drinks (eg, 24 oz beer, 10 oz wine, or 3 oz 80-proof whiskey) per day in most men, and to no more than one drink per day in women and lighter weight persons. This lifestyle modification has an approximate SBP decrease of 2 to 4 mm Hg.

Answer d is incorrect. The patient has stage 2 hypertension and stage 2 recommendations often include a two drug regimen. However, the question specifically asked for lifestyle modifications. Additionally, since the patient has chronic kidney disease, the use of the thiazide diuretic chlorthalidone may not be the best option for select stages of CKD (eg, CrCl <30 mL/min).

CHAPTER **4 | Acute Coronary Syndromes**

Questions 1 to 3 refer to the following patient case.

LC is a 76-year-old woman who presents to ED via EMS to a large academic medical center (with a coronary catheterization laboratory) complaining of sudden onset of diaphoresis and nausea. She states, "About 5 hours ago my chest started hurting and I just don't feel well." LC's weight is 65 kg.

Past medical history: CAD and arthritis

Family history: Father died of acute myocardial infarction at 76 years of age and mother passed away at age 70 from pneumonia

Social history: Does not drink alcohol; smokes 1 pack of cigarettes per week

Medications: ASA 81 mg orally once daily, atorvastatin 40 mg orally at bedtime, conjugated estrogens 0.625 mg orally daily, and celecoxib 200 mg orally daily

Laboratory data: Serum creatinine (SCr) = 1.9 mg/dL, total cholesterol 250 mg/dL, triglycerides 150 mg/dL, high-density lipoprotein (HDL) 40 mg/dL, LDL 130 mg/dL, troponin I = 5.7 ng/mL

Electrocardiogram: ST-segment elevation

1. Which one of the following is the preferred approach to reperfuse this patient?

   a. Chew ASA 81 mg, clopidogrel 75 mg, UFH for 48 hours
   b. Reteplase 10 units IV for two doses 30 minutes apart and UFH for 48 hours
   c. Chew ASA 325 mg, administer ticagrelor 180 mg orally once, abciximab 16.25 mcg IV bolus and percutaneous intervention with coronary stent placement
   d. Streptokinase 1,500,000 units IV over 30 minutes, ASA 81 mg, clopidogrel 300 mg

---

Answer c is correct. LC is experiencing a STEMI that requires emergent reperfusion and has presented to a hospital with cardiac catheterization capabilities. The patient should be loaded (higher doses) with antiplatelets, and started on abciximab since he will be going to catheterization emergently.

Answer a is incorrect. LC is experiencing a STEMI and the goal for these patients is always primarily reperfusion. ASA, clopidogrel, and UFH will prevent further platelet aggregation and thrombus formation but they do not dissolve current clots.

Answer b is incorrect. A regimen including reteplase is a possibility for LC's treatment since reperfusion can occur either with fibrinolytic or PCI. However, if the facility has PCI capabilities, the patient should receive PCI as it is more effective than thrombolysis.

Answer d is incorrect. This is a possibility for treatment since this patient is a STEMI and will need reperfusion either with fibrinolytic or PTCA. However, streptokinase is not a common or highly recommended fibrinolytic due to its lack of specificity and capability of allergic reactions. Newer second generation fibrinolytics are preferred. Also, if the facility has PCI capabilities, the patient should receive PCI as it is more effective than thrombolysis.

---

2. The physicians are debating on whether LC should receive early oral β-blockers after receiving ASA, ticagrelor, oxygen, nitrates, and morphine. Which of the following vital signs for TS would be conducive for early β-blocker use?

   a. Heart rate 110 beats/min; SBP 85 mm Hg
   b. Heart rate 50 beats/min; SBP 120 mm Hg
   c. Heart rate 120 beats/min; SBP 120 mm Hg
   d. Heart rate 120 beats/min; SBP 120 mm Hg with rales and rhonchi on physical examination

---

Answer c is correct. These vitals show tachycardia and normal systolic so this patient would be a candidate for β-blockade.

Answer a is incorrect. Oral β-blocker therapy should be initiated in the first 24 hours for patients who do not have any signs of HF, evidence of a low-output state (hypotension or cardiogenic shock) or contraindications to β-blockade (bradycardia or active asthma). These vitals show hypotension, a sign of low-output state.

Answer b is incorrect. These vitals show a heart rate of 50 beats/min. A normal heart rate is around 70 beats per min and so this represents bradycardia. β-Blocker therapies are not recommended for patients with bradycardia.

Answer d is incorrect. This patient is hemodynamically stable but has signs of reactive airway disease or HF with the rales and rhonchi.

---

3. Which one of the following statements would you suggest to the attending physician prior to patient discharge regarding her home medication regimen? Select all that apply.

   a. Discontinue conjugated estrogens
   b. Continue ASA
   c. Discontinue celecoxib
   d. Start a β-blocker
   e. Start prasugrel

Answer a is correct. Conjugated estrogens should be discontinued prior to discharge. Estrogen therapy was once thought to decrease cardiovascular events; however, the Women's Health Initiative study revealed increased incidence of breast cancer, heart attacks, and strokes in women receiving HRT. Based on these findings, it is now recommended that women take prescribed HRT treatment at the lowest feasible dose, for the shortest possible time. ACS guidelines also recommend discontinuation of therapy post-MI.

Answer b is correct. This patient has extensive CAD and should remain on an ASA, at least 75 mg daily.

Answer c is correct. Patients routinely taking NSAIDs (except for ASA), both nonselective as well as COX-2 selective agents, have an increased risk of cardiovascular mortality compared to those not receiving these therapies. Upon presentation with STEMI, these agents should be discontinued to prevent adverse effects including re-infarction, hypertension, HF, and myocardial rupture associated with their use.

Answer d is correct. β-Blocker initiation should be recommended before discharge, if the patient is stable.

Answer e is incorrect. Because patient is 75 years old, the use of prasugrel is not ideal in this patient. Prasugrel has a black box warning regarding increased bleeding and recommends against use in patients ≥75 years old, less than 60 kg, and with history of ischemic stroke or TIA (absolute contraindication).

4. A patient experiencing chest pain for a few hours decides to take an SL tablet of NTG. The first tablet provides no pain relief, so EMS is contacted. The patient continued to take the NTG every 5 minutes. The third tablet she took provided relief. How do oral nitrates decrease chest pain?

   a. Vasoconstriction of venous vasculature
   b. Vasoconstriction of arterial vasculature
   c. Vasodilation of venous vasculature
   d. Decreased cardiac output

Answer c is correct. Nitrates cause venous vasodilation as well as peripheral vasodilation at higher doses. This decreases the pressure going into the heart (preload) and decreases the pressure the heart has to push against in the arteries (afterload). This decreases the workload on heart. Nitrates also facilitate collateral flow in coronary arteries.

Answer a is incorrect. Nitrates cause vasodilation of venous vasculature, not constriction.

Answer b is incorrect. Nitrates cause vasodilation of the venous vasculature, not arterial.

Answer d is incorrect. Nitrates increase cardiac output by decreasing the work load on the heart and improving coronary perfusion.

5. What is the mechanism of ticagrelor's benefit in a STEMI patient that has already received ASA, oxygen, nitrates, and morphine?

   a. Ticagrelor improves myocardial oxygen supply.
   b. Ticagrelor opens up the infarct-related artery.
   c. Ticagrelor reduces myocardial oxygen demand.
   d. Ticagrelor prevents myocardial reinfarction.

Answer d is correct. Ticagrelor along with ASA will prevent the infarct from expanding further as well as prevent future myocardial infarctions and reinfarction (thrombosis) after reperfusion with thrombolytics or PCI.

Answer a is incorrect. Ticagrelor cannot dissolve platelets that are already in a platelet clot covered by thrombin; therefore, it will not improve myocardial oxygen supply by the removal of the clot. It also does not cause vasodilation or improve blood supply to heart.

Answer b is incorrect. Antiplatelets cannot disable platelets that are already in a platelet clot covered by thrombin. A fibrinolytic is needed to break up a fibrin-bound clot.

Answer c is incorrect. Ticagrelor will not decrease heart rate or afterload that would decrease myocardial oxygen demand.

Questions 6 to 8 refer to the following patient case.

SK is a 68-year-old man who presents to his local physician's office after eating lunch at a local fast food restaurant. He complains of chest pain with radiation to his jaw. His physician has him chew ASA 325 mg and calls 911. He is transported to the local hospital where electrocardiogram shows ST-segment elevation.

Past medical history: Hypertension, CAD, chronic obstructive pulmonary disease (COPD), stage IV chronic kidney disease, cerebrovascular accident 2 months ago

Family history: Mother died of a stroke at 85 years and father passed away at 75 years in a car accident.

Social history: Smokes 1.5 packs of cigarette per day for 50 years; no alcohol history

Medications: Hydrochlorothiazide 25 mg orally daily, metoprolol tartrate 25 mg orally bid, tiotropium 18 mcg inhaled once daily, albuterol inhaler 1 puff every 6 hours as needed, fluticasone/salmeterol 250/50 mcg inhaled bid

Vital signs: Blood pressure 185/90 mm Hg, heart rate 98 beats/min, respiratory rate 22, O_2 saturation 88%, weight 100 kg

Laboratory data: Unavailable

Allergies: Heparin

6. SK presents at a hospital that does not have a cardiac catheterization laboratory; therefore, they have 30 minutes to verify his candidacy for fibrinolytic therapy. Which of the following is a contraindication (relative or absolute) to SK receiving a fibrinolytic? Select all that apply.

   a. SK already received ASA and clopidogrel.
   b. SK's blood pressure is 185/90 mm Hg.
   c. SK had a recent cerebrovascular accident.
   d. SK has an allergy to heparin.
   e. SK has a respiratory rate of 22

Answer b is correct. Severe uncontrolled hypertension on presentation is classified as SBP >180 mm Hg, and is a relative contraindication. Remember that even if SK's BP was >180 mm Hg it should be treated prior to fibrinolysis, but does not preclude treatment.

Answer c is correct. Ischemic stroke in the last 3 months is a contraindication to fibrinolysis. The possibility of having an intracranial hemorrhage in SK outweighs the benefits of administering fibrinolytic therapy.

Answer a is incorrect. Patients that receive fibrinolytic therapy should also receive antiplatelet therapy with ASA and a thienopyridine.

Answer d is incorrect. Anticoagulation is required with thrombolysis but heparinoids are not the only anticoagulant option.

Answer e is incorrect. Respiratory rate is not a contraindication to fibrinolytic therapy.

7. Given SK's contraindication to fibrinolytic therapy, he was life-flighted to a hospital with 24 hour cardiac catheterization capabilities. The plan is for emergent PCI on arrival. Rank the anticoagulants in the order of shortest half-life to longest half-life.

Unordered Options	Ordered Response
Heparin	
Enoxaparin	
Fondaparinux	
Bivalirudin	

Answer. Bivalirudin 25 to 57 minutes → Heparin 1.5 hours → Enoxaparin 4.5 to 7 hours → Fondaparinux 17 to 21 hours

8. Which anticoagulant is the treatment of choice in a STEMI patient that is also dialysis dependent?

a. Enoxaparin
b. Dalteparin
c. Fondaparinux
d. Heparin

Answer d is correct. Heparin is not renally eliminated.

Answer a is incorrect. Enoxaparin is renally eliminated and does not have data for treatment in hemodialysis patients.

Answer b is incorrect. Dalteparin does not have dosing data for hemodialysis patients and is renally eliminated.

Answer c is incorrect. Fondaparinux is contraindicated, if the creatinine clearance is less than 30 mL/min.

9. What laboratory value may be used to monitor the level of anticoagulation achieved with UFH?

a. International normalized ratio (INR)
b. Prothrombin time (PT)
c. Anti-Xa level
d. aPTT

Answer d is correct. aPTTs are used to monitor UFH anticoagulation. When treating ACS, the goal aPTT is 1.5 to 2 times a patient's baseline (approximately 50-70 seconds).

Answer a is incorrect. INR is used to monitor vitamin K antagonism therapy (warfarin).

Answer b is incorrect. PT is the unstandardized laboratory value associated with INR. Therefore, it is also used to monitor warfarin therapy.

Answer c is correct. Anti-Xa levels can be monitored when patients are on LMWH. There are also an increasing number of institutions using anti-Xa levels to monitor UFH.

10. Which of the following antiplatelet/anticoagulant regimens would be recommended for treatment of an NSTEMI patient with a heparin allergy? The patient is going to receive PCI later in the day.

a. Bivalirudin
b. Eptifibatide and LMWH
c. Abciximab and UFH
d. Fondaparinux

Answer a is correct. In patients with UA and NSTEMI, bivalirudin may be started prior to PCI (if PCI is planned). It is a direct thrombin inhibitor and does not require concomitant use with heparin or GPI.

Answer b is incorrect. Eptifibatide therapy is appropriate, but administration with LMWH is not appropriate in this patient due to heparin allergy.

Answer c is incorrect. Abciximab may be used in this patient since it is indicated when PCI is planned. However it is not necessary to start it early. Also, this patient has a heparin allergy and should not receive heparin.

Answer d is incorrect. Fondaparinux would be safe to use in patients with heparin allergies; however, it is not recommended when PCI is planned.

11. Which of the following agents is indicated in the setting of NSTEMI? Select all that apply.

a. Eptifibatide
b. UFH
c. ASA
d. Reteplase
e. Clopidogrel

Answer a is correct. Eptifibatide can be used as an adjunct for PCI in NSTEMI and for the medical management of ACS.

Answer b is correct. UFH is indicated in PCI as well as the medical management of NSTEMI.

Answer c is correct. ASA should be given to all patients experiencing ACS unless significant contraindication.

Answer e is correct. Clopidogrel plus ASA has been found to have added benefit over ASA alone in treatment of NSTEMI.

Answer d is incorrect. Fibrinolytics are not indicated in the treatment of NSTEMI or UA. They break fibrin clots, also known as "red clots," that occur with complete occlusion of coronary arteries, which occur with STEMI only.

12. Once the acute phase of myocardial infarction has passed, which of the following therapies is most likely to slow the development of HF?

    a. Clopidogrel
    b. Atenolol
    c. Ramipril
    d. Amiodarone

Answer c is correct. ACEI, like ramipril, have been shown to prevent ventricular remodeling. This is the main pathophysiologic change that results in HF following myocardial infarction.

Answer a is incorrect. Clopidogrel prevents recurrent ischemic events and provides an important reduction in morbidity post-MI, however does not alter progression of left ventricular dysfunction.

Answer b is incorrect. Atenolol prevents recurrent ischemic events and provides mortality benefits post-MI, however does not alter progression of left ventricular dysfunction.

Answer d is incorrect. Amiodarone treats atrial and ventricular arrhythmias, which occur with increased frequency following ACS. However, it does not affect HF progression.

13. PR is an 82-year-old woman who is status post drug-eluting stent placement following presentations with a STEMI. She has a past medical history significant for hypertension, dyslipidemia, and hypothyroidism. She has no known drug allergies. Which of the following is the best choice of long-term antiplatelet therapy?

    a. ASA 325 mg orally daily
    b. ASA 325 mg plus Ticagrelor 90 mg orally twice daily
    c. Ticagrelor 180 mg orally twice daily
    d. ASA 81 mg plus clopidogrel 75 mg orally daily

Answer d is correct. This regimen of low-dose ASA and a thienopyridine represents the best option in this patient. ASA plus clopidogrel should be continued for at least a year following drug-eluting stent placement.

Answer a is incorrect. Following treatment with drug-eluting coronary artery stents, DAPT is indicated (ASA plus thienopyridine).

Answer b is incorrect. Although use of low-dose ASA is appropriate, Ticagrelor is only approved to be given with 75-100 mg/d of ASA.

Answer c is incorrect. Following treatment with coronary artery stents, DAPT is indicated (ASA plus thienopyridine). The dose for ticagrelor is 90 mg orally twice daily.

14. A patient with recent NSTEMI with an LDL of 150 mg/dL, total cholesterol (TC) of 192 mg/dL, triglycerides (TG) of 140 mg/dL, and HDL of 47 mg/dL and needs to be on a statin. Rank the following statins in order of lowest to highest potency.

Unordered Options	Ordered Responses
Pravastatin 20 mg po daily	
Simvastatin 20 mg po daily	
Atorvastatin 20 mg po daily	
Rosuvastatin 20 mg po daily	

Answer. Pravastatin → simvastatin → atorvastatin → rosuvastatin

Pravastatin would lower this patient's LDL by approximately 30%.

Simvastatin would lower this patient's LDL by approximately 38%.

Numerous trials have evaluated the use of atorvastatin post-MI. This is the medication of choice to prevent future ischemic events albeit in higher doses (40 mg or 80 mg). It would also reduce this patients LDL by approximately 41%.

Rosuvastatin is the most potent statin and would decrease LDL by approximately 55%.

15. Which of the following therapies requires routine monitoring of serum creatinine and potassium?

    a. Carvedilol
    b. Spironolactone
    c. Atenolol
    d. Pravastatin

Answer b is correct. Initiation of spironolactone should only occur in patients with SCr <2.5 and K <5.0. Dose reductions are used in patients with SCr 1.5 to 2.5 as well. This medication requires frequent monitoring of both laboratory values during initiation and occasionally thereafter.

Answer a is incorrect. Carvedilol is not renally eliminated nor does it have much effect on serum potassium levels.

Answer c is incorrect. Atenolol is renally eliminated. Therefore, it would be appropriate to monitor SCr occasionally. However, effect on potassium is minimal and does not require routine monitoring.

Answer d is incorrect. Pravastatin requires monitoring of hepatic function tests and lipid levels only.

16. Which of the following is an appropriate fibrinolytic dosing regimen for a 78-kg person with STEMI?

    a. Streptase 1 million units intravenously over 20 minutes
    b. Reteplase or rPA 10 units IV bolus twice 30 minutes apart
    c. Tenecteplase or TNK 80 mg IV bolus once
    d. Alteplase 100 mg IV over 2 hours

Answer b is correct. Reteplase or rPA is given as two 10 units boluses 30 minutes apart.

Answer a is incorrect. Streptokinase, SK, or streptase is rarely used, and the dose is 1.5 million units over 60 minutes.

Answer c is incorrect. TNK or tenecteplase is given as a single weight-based bolus. This patient's weight would require a bolus of 40 mg, not 80 mg.

Answer d is incorrect.   This dose of alteplase (tPA) is for treatment of pulmonary embolism. When given for STEMI, it is administered in three phases 15 mg IV bolus followed by 0.75 mg/kg IV over 30 minutes (max 50 mg) followed by 0.5 mg/kg (max 35 mg) over 60 minutes.

---

17. KE presents with chest pain, nausea, vomiting, and diaphoresis. He is diagnosed with an NSTEMI. Current blood pressure is 92/56 mm Hg and HR is 105 beats/min. Which of these medications should be given to this patient?

    a. ASA EC 325 mg orally once
    b. ASA 81 mg two tablets chewed once
    c. NTG IV drip at 20 mcg/min
    d. IV metoprolol 5 mg IV once

Answer b is correct.   ASA 162 to 325 mg should be chewed upon presentation with ACS.

Answer a is incorrect.   Enteric-coated ASA products by design have delayed absorption. In the setting of ACS, it is important to have rapid absorption of ASA.

Answer c is incorrect.   This patient is currently hypotensive; the risks of giving NTG do not outweigh the benefits.

Answer d is incorrect.   This patient does have an elevated heart rate; however, IV β-blockers should be avoided in patients demonstrating signs of reduced cardiac output, like hypotension.

---

18. PR is a 62-year-old woman who presents to the ED with an NSTEMI. She has no significant past medical history. Pertinent data include: blood pressure 125/79 mm Hg, heart rate 75 beats/min, SCr 1.2 mg/dL, platelet count 142 k/uL, weight 94 kg. She has allergies to penicillin, sulfa, and ASA. Which of the following regimens are okay to give PR while she waits for her PCI? Select all that apply.

    a. ASA 324 mg once, then 81 mg daily
    b. Clopidogrel 300 mg once, then 75 mg daily
    c. ASA 162 mg once, then 81 mg daily plus clopidogrel 600 mg once, then 75 mg daily
    d. Prasugrel 60 mg once then 10 mg daily

Answer b is correct.   Clopidogrel alone may be used in patients with ASA allergies.

Answer d is correct.   Prasugrel would be a reasonable option in this patient given her ASA allergy.

Answer a is incorrect.   PR has an ASA allergy. Although desensitization protocols exist, this is not the time to attempt this; so ASA products should be avoided.

Answer c is incorrect.   As with answer a, ASA should be avoided in this patient secondary to ASA allergy.

---

19. Which of the following β-blockers are available in both oral and IV formulations? Select all that apply.

    a. Atenolol
    b. Esmolol
    c. Metoprolol
    d. Carvedilol
    e. Labetalol

Answer a is correct.   Atenolol is available in both an IV solution and oral tablets.

Answer c is correct.   Metoprolol is available in both an IV solution and oral tablets (sustained and immediate release).

Answer e is correct.   Labetalol is available in IV solution and oral tablets.

Answer b is incorrect.   Esmolol is only available intravenously.

Answer d is incorrect.   Carvedilol is only available orally (immediate and controlled release).

---

20. Secondary prevention of an ACS in a patient with resulting HF (EF 35%) should include which of the following therapies assuming normal blood pressure? Select all that apply.

    a. HMG-CoA reductase inhibitors
    b. ASA
    c. Calcium channel blockers
    d. Fenofibrates
    e. ACE-I

Answer a is correct.   Statins are indicated for all patients post-ACS unless contraindicated. They reduced major adverse cardiovascular endpoints. If patients have been intolerant to one statin, another should be tried before moving to another class of cholesterol lowering medication.

Answer b is correct.   ASA should also be used in all patients without contraindications.

Answer e is correct.   Because this patient's ACS resulted in systolic dysfunction, an ACE inhibitor would be recommended as long as the patient's blood pressure could tolerate it.

Answer c is incorrect.   Calcium channel blockers, specifically dihydropyridine calcium channel blockers may be used as third line treatment for hypertension in patients with a history of ACS. Both β-blockers and ACEI should be utilized first.

Answer d is incorrect.   Fenofibrates may be added to statins for treatment of hypertriglyceridemia; however, they are not required for secondary prevention.

CHAPTER **5** | Dyslipidemia

1. CX is a 62-year-old patient that presents to your pharmacy seeking guidance on an appropriate diet to reduce heart disease risk in a patient with high cholesterol. Which of the following lifestyle changes should be recommended to patients with dyslipidemia?

    a. Increase intake of animal products and low carbohydrate vegetables, and limit grains and fruit

b. Reduce trans fat and limit saturated fat to <10% of calories
c. Engage in regular physical activity
d. Eat one serving per week of fatty fish

Answer c is correct. Increased activity is important for all patients without physical restrictions. AHA/ACC lifestyle management guidelines endorse three to four sessions a week of moderate to vigorous intensity physical activity with an average duration of 40 minutes per session.

Answers a, b, and d are incorrect. The AHA/ACC lifestyle management guidelines advise eating a diet rich in vegetables, fruits, and whole grains, including low-fat dairy products, fish, poultry, legumes, and nuts, with limited intake of saturated fat, trans fat, sweets, sugar-sweetened beverages, and red meats. Dietary adaptations are available for vegetarians or vegans. Although trans fat should be reduced or preferably eliminated, the favored saturated fat intake is also just 5% to 6% of calories. The AHA recommends consuming at least two servings of fish per week for the general population and approximately 1 g of EPA + DHA daily (preferably from oily fish) for those with documented CHD.

---

2. RR is a 56-year-old Asian man with an LDL-C of 180 mg/dL, HDL-C 28 mg/dL, and TG 140 mg/dL. His fasting glucose is 96 mg/dL, waist circumference 41 inches, and BP 128/82 mm Hg. Medications include hydrochlorothiazide and gemfibrozil. Which of the following indicates a risk for metabolic syndrome? Select all that apply.

a. HDL-C
b. TG
c. Fasting glucose
d. Waist circumference
e. BP

Answer a is correct. HDL-C <40 mg/dL in men and <50 mg/dL in women is defined as a potential risk factor. ATP III guidelines classify a patient with *three* such risk factors as having metabolic syndrome.

Answer b is correct. Although ATP III only defines TG ≥150 mg/dL as a potential risk factor, the diagnostic criteria were recently expanded to include drug treatment of elevated TG.

Answer d is correct. ATP III defines abdominal obesity (waist circumference >40 inches in men, >35 in women) as a risk factor. For Asian Americans, newer diagnostic criteria recommend using a lower waist of >35 in men and >31 in women.

Answer e is correct. Although ATP III only defines BP ≥130/85 mm Hg as a potential risk factor, diagnostic criteria were later expanded to include drug treatment of hypertension.

Answer c is incorrect. Although ATP III considers fasting glucose ≥110 mg/dL as a potential risk factor, the definition was lowered to ≥100 mg/dL based upon the ADA's revised

definition of impaired fasting glucose. RR's fasting glucose is currently <100 mg/dL, so glucose is not a risk factor at this time.

---

3. MM is a 54-year-old woman with a past medical history of unstable angina, hypertension, and diabetes. She smokes two packs of cigarettes daily. Her LDL-C is 120 mg/dL, HDL-C 48 mg/dL, and TG 220 mg/dL. Which of the following therapy is recommended?

a. Simvastatin 80 mg daily
b. Atorvastatin 80 mg daily
c. Pravastatin 20 mg daily
d. Lovastatin 40 mg daily

Answer b is correct. Because MM has clinical ASCVD, the ACC/AHA expert panel recommends high-intensity statin, lowering LDL-C ≥50% (ie, atorvastatin 40 mg and 80 mg or rosuvastatin 20 mg and 40 mg daily). The 80 mg atorvastatin and 20 mg rosuvastatin doses are preferred and best supported by randomized clinical trials.

Answer a is incorrect. Patients should not be started on or titrated to simvastatin 80 mg due to increased risk of rhabdomyolysis.

Answer c is incorrect. Pravastatin 20 mg is a low-intensity statin therapy, lowering LDL-C <30%.

Answer d is incorrect. Lovastatin 40 mg is a moderate-intensity therapy, lowering LDL-C 30 to <50%.

---

4. CE is a 72-year-old man with no clinical ASCVD, no diabetes, and a 10-year ASCVD risk of 12%. Which of the following is recommended for this patient?

a. Simvastatin 10 mg daily
b. Fluvastatin 40 mg daily
c. Pitavastatin 1 mg daily
d. Rosuvastatin 10 mg daily

Answer d is correct. Rosuvastatin 10 mg is a moderate-intensity therapy, lowering LDL-C 30 to <50%. The guidelines recommend moderate- or high-intensity statin for this individual who is classified in group four.

Answers a, b, and c are incorrect. These doses represent low-intensity therapy, lowering LDL-C <30%.

---

5. KW is a 53-year-old Asian woman with an LDL-C of 210 mg/dL, HDL-C 56 mg/dL, and TG 182 mg/dL. Her PMH is notable for hypertension with a recent BP of 118/70 mm Hg on lisinopril monotherapy. She is a nonsmoker. Her father died of a myocardial infarction at 58 years of age. Her physician elects to use rosuvastatin and requests a dosing recommendation. Although a high-intensity statin is preferred for most patients with LDL-C >190 mg/dL, what is the most appropriate starting dose for KW considering genetic factors?

a. 5 mg daily
b. 10 mg daily

c. 20 mg daily
d. 40 mg daily

Answer a is correct. Asian patients have a twofold increase in median exposure to rosuvastatin compared to Caucasians. The recommended starting dose is 5 mg in these patients.

Answers b, c, and d are incorrect. The starting doses are too high for an Asian patient. The 40-mg dose in Answer d is reserved for patients not responding to and tolerating the 20-mg dose. Even higher doses of 80 mg were associated with proteinuria in clinical trials and are not advised.

---

6. MJ has a history of subtherapeutic anticoagulation on warfarin (due to poor adherence) until the administration time was changed from evening to morning. The patient also frequently skips meals and takes antacids for reflux. Which of the following statins is optimal for this patient?

   a. Pravastatin
   b. Atorvastatin
   c. Lovastatin
   d. Rosuvastatin

Answer b is correct. Atorvastatin has a longer half-life and can be dosed at any time of day. Atorvastatin is also unlikely to interact with warfarin.

Answer a is incorrect. Pravastatin has a short half-life and should be dosed at bedtime since cholesterol synthesis is maximal between midnight and 2:00 AM Fluvastatin is another statin that should be dosed at bedtime.

Answer c is incorrect. Lovastatin should be dosed in the evening with food for optimal efficacy, while other statins may be given with or without food. Both lovastatin and simvastatin can increase the effects of warfarin through CYP-3A4 inhibition.

Answer d is incorrect. Rosuvastatin has the longest half-life and can be given at any time of day. However, rosuvastatin should also be dosed at least 2 hours apart from antacids due to reduced absorption. In addition, it may cause a pronounced prothrombin increase in patients on warfarin due to CYP-3A4 and possibly CYP-2C9 inhibition. Fluvastatin is another statin that potently inhibits CYP-2C9, potentially increasing warfarin effects.

---

7. CE is a 74-year-old man with a PMH of CHD, stroke, and hypothyroidism. He currently takes aspirin, levothyroxine, and simvastatin and has now been prescribed cholestyramine. What will you discuss with the patient?

   a. Take on an empty stomach once daily.
   b. Mix each dose with at least 12 ounces of juice or soda.
   c. Sip slowly to reduce side effects.
   d. Take other medications at least 1 to 2 hours before or 4 to 6 hours after taking cholestyramine.

Answer d is correct. Cholestyramine and colestipol can bind a wide array of medications, including digoxin,

warfarin, levothyroxine, phenytoin, niacin, oral contraceptives, ezetimibe, fibrates, statins, and aspirin. Interacting medications should be given 1 to 2 hours before or 4 to 6 hours after these resins. Colesevelam has the lowest likelihood of interactions, but the manufacturer still recommends either closely monitoring or separating medications with a narrow therapeutic index by 4 hours.

Answer a is incorrect. BAS should be taken with or just after meals in two to three divided doses daily, with the exception of colesevelam (625 mg, six tablets per day), which may be dosed all at once if tolerated.

Answer b is incorrect. Cholestyramine (and colestipol) powder should be mixed with 2 to 6 ounces of water, a noncarbonated beverage such as orange, apple, or grape juice, or a high moisture content pulpy fruit (eg, applesauce).

Answer c is incorrect. Powdered resins may cause teeth discoloration, erosion, and decay and must be swallowed quickly.

---

8. Select the brand name for fenofibrate. Select all that apply.

   a. Fenoglide®
   b. Tricor®
   c. Triglide®
   d. Lipofen®
   e. Lopid®

Answers a, b, c, and d are correct. All are brand names for fenofibrate. Generic fenofibrate is also available.

Answer e is incorrect. Lopid® is brand name for gemfibrozil.

---

9. What medication or combination is safest to use for a patient with advanced hepatic disease?

   a. Colesevelam
   b. Ezetimibe/simvastatin
   c. Niacin
   d. Gemfibrozil

Answer a is correct. BAS are not contraindicated in hepatic disease, although these patients may be more susceptible to GI side effects. No dose adjustment is necessary for drugs in this class.

Answer b is incorrect. Statins are contraindicated in patients with active hepatic disease. Although there is newer evidence of safety in patients with nonalcoholic fatty liver disease and hepatitis B and C, this patient has advanced unspecified disease. Ezetimibe is also not recommended in patients with moderate or severe hepatic impairment.

Answer c is incorrect. Niacin is contraindicated in patients with active hepatic disease.

Answer d is incorrect. Fibrates are contraindicated in patients with hepatic dysfunction.

10. JM is a 64-year-old woman with a PMH of pancreatitis (when TG 2200 mg/dL), uncontrolled gout, severe psoriasis, recurrent infections requiring hospitalization, and lovastatin-associated myopathy. Her current medications include rosuvastatin, prednisone, and allopurinol. Colchicine was also added a few days ago for a gout exacerbation. She reports an anaphylactic reaction after eating seafood in college. Her LDL-C is 96 mg/dL, HDL-C 42 mg/dL, and TG 640 mg/dL. Which of the following is the safest addition to her therapy?

    a. Niacin
    b. Colesevelam
    c. Fish oil
    d. Fenofibrate

Answer d is correct. Fenofibrate does not appear to interfere with statin metabolism and has a rhabdomyolysis rate significantly lower than that of gemfibrozil when combined with statins. Gemfibrozil is a potent inhibitor of several components of statin metabolism, inhibiting glucuronidation, OATP1B1-mediated uptake of statin acids, and biliary excretion. New guidelines also advise against use of gemfibrozil with statins.

Answer a is incorrect. Theoretically, the niacin-statin combination may have greater risk of myopathy over statin monotherapy, although confirming evidence is weak. Niacin should be primarily avoided in this patient with uncontrolled gout since it may increase uric acid.

Answer b is incorrect. BAS can increase TG and are contraindicated in patients with TG >500 mg/dL or history of pancreatitis caused by elevated TG.

Answer c is incorrect. Fish oil is best avoided considering her severe allergic reaction to seafood. EPA and DHA in doses >3 g/d may also suppress T- and B-cell function and lead to more infections in combination with prednisone.

11. Select the brand name for lovastatin.

    a. Lescol®
    b. Crestor®
    c. Mevacor®
    d. Zocor®

Answer c is correct. Mevacor® is the brand name for lovastatin.

Answer a is incorrect. Lescol® is the brand name for fluvastatin.

Answer b is incorrect. Crestor® is the brand name for rosuvastatin.

Answer d is incorrect. Zocor® is the brand name for simvastatin.

12. Which of the following statin(s) should be temporarily discontinued for a patient starting a short course of clarithromycin? Select all that apply.

    a. Simvastatin
    b. Pravastatin
    c. Lovastatin
    d. Atorvastatin
    e. Rosuvastatin

Answer a is correct. Simvastatin is metabolized by the CYP-3A4 isoenzyme and should not be coadministered with clarithromycin.

Answer c is correct. Lovastatin is metabolized by the CYP-3A4 isoenzyme and should not be coadministered with clarithromycin. Both lovastatin and simvastatin should never be given with itraconazole, ketoconazole, telithromycin, clarithromycin, erythromycin, protease inhibitors, and nefazodone. Patients especially taking higher doses of simvastatin and lovastatin should also avoid grapefruit juice in quantities over 1 quart per day, which has been associated with rhabdomyolysis.

Answer b is incorrect. Pravastatin does not require dose adjustment. It is metabolized through non-CYP enzymes.

Answer d is incorrect. Although atorvastatin is metabolized by CYP-3A4 to a small extent, there are no specific recommendations for therapy adjustment with clarithromycin.

Answer e is incorrect. Rosuvastatin does not interact with clarithromycin.

13. Which of the following statin doses may be dispensed to a patient also taking gemfibrozil? Select all that apply.

    a. Rosuvastatin 20 mg
    b. Simvastatin 20 mg
    c. Lovastatin 40 mg
    d. Fluvastatin 40 mg

Answer d is correct. There is no dose limit for fluvastatin in combination with gemfibrozil. Studies suggest that fluvastatin is the only statin that may be safely combined with gemfibrozil, although caution is still advised.

Answer a is incorrect. Although rosuvastatin has few drug interactions since 90% is eliminated unchanged, doses should not exceed 5 mg for patients on cyclosporine and 10 mg for those on gemfibrozil, ritonavir, lopinavir, and oral contraceptives.

Answer b is incorrect. Simvastatin doses should not exceed 10 mg for patients on gemfibrozil, danazol, and cyclosporine and 20 mg for those on amiodarone and verapamil.

Answer c is incorrect. Lovastatin doses should not exceed 20 mg for patients on gemfibrozil, fenofibrate, cyclosporine, and niacin (≥1 g/d) and 40 mg for those on amiodarone and verapamil.

14. LR is a 54-year-old woman with elevated TG who wants to substitute over-the-counter (OTC) fish oil instead of omega-3-acid ethyl esters (Lovaza®) to save money. Her physician approves this change. She mentions past gastrointestinal problems with dietary fish. What should you advise the patient regarding a

product with 180 mg of EPA and 120 mg of DHA per capsule? Select all that apply.

a. Change to the more concentrated cod liver oil
b. Six capsules a day will equal the dose of the prescription product
c. Take with meals to improve tolerability
d. Eleven capsules a day will equal the dose of the prescription product
e. Have your mercury levels tested periodically

Answer c is correct. Fish oil tolerability may be improved by dosing with meals, spacing doses apart, using enteric-coated products, and freezing capsules (however, the manufacturer recommends against freezing Lovaza®).

Answer d is correct. Lovaza® contains 840 mg of EPA and DHA per 1000-mg capsule and is dosed four capsules once daily or two capsules bid with meals. Since at least 11 capsules a day of this fish oil would provide an equivalent therapeutic dose, a higher potency product should be considered.

Answer a is incorrect. Cod liver oil can cause toxicity with long-term use or large doses due to vitamin A content.

Answer b is incorrect. Since OTC fish oil capsules usually contain only 30% to 50% of EPA and DHA per 1000- to 1200-mg capsule, an even larger number of capsules would be needed to lower TG.

Answer e is incorrect. The majority of OTC products have no detectable levels of mercury and other toxins.

---

15. Select a patient risk factor for development of myopathy on statin therapy. Select all that apply.

a. Larger body size
b. Hyperthyroidism
c. Female sex
d. Vitamin D deficiency
e. Young age

Answer c is correct. Women have greater risk.

Answer d is correct. Vitamin D deficiency has been found to predispose patients to statin-induced myopathy, and many patients demonstrate resolution of symptoms after replacement.

Answer a is incorrect. Small body frame and frailty are risk factors.

Answer b is incorrect. Hypothyroidism is a risk factor, and thyroid-stimulating hormone should be screened at baseline or checked in patients who develop symptoms.

Answer e is incorrect. Advanced age is a risk factor. Other risk factors are alcoholism, major surgery, trauma, strenuous physical activity, multisystem disease, history or family history of myopathy with lipid-lowering therapy, history of CK elevation, hypomagnesemia, Asian ancestry, higher statin dose, and the presence of concomitant interacting drugs.

---

16. What lipid-lowering medication(s) should be adjusted in a patient with renal impairment?

a. Atorvastatin
b. Gemfibrozil
c. Ezetimibe
d. Cholestyramine
e. Niacin

Answer b is correct. Fibrates require renal adjustment in patients with mild to moderate renal impairment. Fibrates are also contraindicated in patients with severe renal impairment, defined by manufacturers as <30 mL/min for fenofibrate and <10 mL/min for gemfibrozil.

Answer a is incorrect. Atorvastatin and fluvastatin (≤40 mg) are confirmed to be safe in this population. Atorvastatin has even been shown safe in patients with diabetes on dialysis. Although statins at currently approved doses are not considered nephrotoxic, all other drugs in this class should be given at lower doses to reduce myopathy risk.

Answer c is incorrect. Ezetimibe does not require adjustment.

Answer d is incorrect. Cholestyramine and other BAS do not require adjustment.

Answer e is incorrect. There are no specific renal adjustments for niacin, although niacin should be used with caution in this population.

---

17. A patient on simvastatin complains of muscle pain, weakness, and cramps since running a marathon this past weekend. His CK is 1760 U/L today (normal range, 50-160) and 280 U/L when checked 3 months ago. His Cr is 1.0 mg/dL. How should you manage this patient?

a. Continue therapy and closely monitor the CK.
b. Stop simvastatin until symptoms and CK improve, then try another statin.
d. Add coenzyme Q10.
e. Change simvastatin to ezetimibe.

Answer b is correct. If symptoms are caused by statin therapy, they usually resolve within a few weeks after discontinuation. Many patients can tolerate another statin without problems, but start low and gradually increase the dose as tolerated. No studies have directly compared incidence of myopathy but there are likely differences. For example, fluvastatin was associated with lower incidence of muscle-related symptoms in a large observational trial. There have also been no documented cases of fatal rhabdomyolysis associated with fluvastatin. Less lipophilic statins with fewer drug interactions (ie, pravastatin and rosuvastatin) theoretically may have reduced risk. Retrospective studies and case reports also suggest benefit from altered dosing regimens of atorvastatin and rosuvastatin (ie, one to three times a week).

Answer a is incorrect. Statins should be stopped for intolerable muscle complaints, progressively increasing CK, and/or moderate CK elevations (>10 times ULN). If symptoms are tolerable, the National Lipid Panel Muscle Safety Expert Panel recommends continuing therapy for CK elevations <10 times ULN with closer CK monitoring. Milder CK elevations less than five times the ULN with tolerable symptoms may be followed every 3 to 6 months.

Answer c is incorrect. Statins block the synthesis of coenzyme Q10, and a small trial found a significant 40% reduction in pain severity when 100 mg/d was added to therapy. Coenzyme Q10 can be considered for patients with no benefit from other approaches, but it has a variable response and insufficient evidence.

Answer d is incorrect. Although he may tolerate ezetimibe better, this option should be reserved for patients who fail other strategies.

---

18. JT is a 62-year-old woman with low HDL-C who was prescribed niacin. She did not fill her prescription because of the expense and instead took five 100-mg immediate-release crystalline niacin tablets at bedtime. She complains of flushing and dizziness after the first dose that almost caused her to fall. What is the best recommendation to improve overall tolerability?

    a. Change to a "no-flush" formulation and take 81 mg of aspirin 30 to 60 minutes before each dose.
    b. Start with 100 mg bid after breakfast and supper.
    c. Take with food and a hot liquid.
    d. Change to sustained-release OTC formulation.

Answer b is correct. Niacin should be slowly titrated to reduce flushing. A common starting dose for immediate-release niacin is 100 mg two to three times a day or 250 mg two times a day after meals.

Answer a is incorrect. "No-flush" niacin products are ineffective for cholesterol lowering. A higher aspirin dose of 325 mg is also most commonly used to prevent flushing.

Answer c is incorrect. Although dosing with food can improve tolerability, concomitant hot liquids, alcohol, and spicy foods can worsen symptoms.

Answer d is incorrect. Although this product may reduce flushing, hepatic toxicity may occur more frequently with sustained-release formulations (with the exception of prescription extended-release niacin).

---

19. LE is a 33-year-old woman currently attempting to become pregnant. Her physician decides that benefits of dyslipidemia treatment outweigh fetal risks. Her LDL-C is 240 mg/dL, HDL-C 64 mg/dL, and TG 132 mg/dL. Her PMH includes recent cholelithiasis. What is the most appropriate medication for LE?

    a. Rosuvastatin
    b. Niacin
    c. Colesevelam
    d. Gemfibrozil
    e. Omega-3-acid ethyl esters

Answer c is correct. Cholesterol and cholesterol derivatives are critical for normal fetal development. Because BAS are not systemically absorbed, they are considered the treatment of choice for women of childbearing age who are lactating or pregnant, or could become pregnant. Colesevelam is pregnancy category B and also not expected to be excreted in breast milk. Clofibrate and cholestyramine are pregnancy category C.

Answer a is incorrect. Statins are pregnancy category X and should only be given to women of childbearing age, if they are highly unlikely to conceive.

Answer b is incorrect. Niacin is pregnancy category C and insufficiently studied in pregnancy.

Answer d is incorrect. Gemfibrozil is pregnancy category C, not indicated since TG are controlled, and contraindicated in patients with gallstones.

Answer e is incorrect. Omega-3-acid ethyl esters (Lovaza®) is pregnancy category C, not indicated since TG are controlled, and may actually increase LDL-C further.

---

20. CL is a 10-year-old boy with familial hyperlipidemia (FH). His physician wishes to use drug therapy since lifestyle changes have failed. His LDL-C is 320 mg/dL. Which of the following medications would you recommend?

    a. Atorvastatin
    b. Colesevelam
    c. Ezetimibe
    d. Niacin
    e. Fenofibrate

Answer a is correct. Atorvastatin is approved for treatment of FH in children 10 years of age and older. Pravastatin and simvastatin are also approved for treatment of FH in children 8 and 10 years of age and older, respectively.

Answers b, c, and d are incorrect. Colesevelam is dangerous in this population due to its large tablet size. Cholestyramine is approved for treating hypercholesterolemia in children but has poor adherence. Although ezetimibe appears effective and tolerable in children ages 10 to 17 years, it is not FDA-approved in this population. It also causes only a modest LDL-C reduction compared to atorvastatin. Niacin and the fibrates have not been adequately studied in this population and are not recommended.

CHAPTER **6 | Stroke**

1. A 38-year-old white man with a past medical history. (PMH) significant for hypertension, diabetes, and chronic alcoholism comes to your clinic for routine follow-up. His social history is significant for alcohol and tobacco abuse. He currently drinks one case of beer per night and smokes two packs per day. Pertinent laboratory findings are as follows: total cholesterol (TC) 182 mg/dL, TG 218 mg/dL, low density lipoprotein

(LDL) 96 mg/dL, high density lipoprotein (HDL) 52 mg/dL, glucose 146 mg/dL. Current blood pressure is 158/94 mm Hg and heart rate (HR) is 92 beats/min. He is 69 in tall and weighs 232 lb.

Which of the following are risk factors for ischemic stroke in this patient? Select ALL that apply.

a. Hypertension
b. Tobacco abuse
c. Diabetes
d. African-American race
e. Age

Answers a is correct. Hypertension is the single most important modifiable risk factor for ischemic stroke. Most estimates for hypertension indicate a relative risk of stroke of approximately 4 when hypertension is defined as systolic blood pressure ≥160 mm Hg and/or diastolic blood pressure ≥95 mm Hg.

Answer b is correct. Cigarette smoking increases risk of ischemic stroke nearly two times. In both the Framingham Study and the Nurses' Health Study, cessation of smoking led to a prompt reduction in stroke risk—major risk was reduced within 2 to 4 years.

Answer c is correct. Persons with diabetes have an increased susceptibility to atherosclerosis and an increased prevalence of atherogenic risk factors, notably hypertension, obesity, and abnormal blood lipids. Case-control studies of stroke patients and prospective epidemiological studies have confirmed an independent effect of diabetes with a relative risk of ischemic stroke in persons with diabetes from 1.8 to 3.0.

Answer d is correct. Stroke incidence and mortality rates vary widely between racial groups. Blacks are more than twice as likely to die of stroke as whites are. Between the ages of 45 and 55, mortality rates are four to five times greater for African-Americans than for whites; the difference decreases with increasing age.

Answer e is incorrect. This patient is 38 years of age. Younger age groups (25-44 years) are at lower risk. However, age is the single most important risk factor for stroke. For each successive 10 years after age 55, the stroke rate more than doubles in both men and women.

---

2. Which of the following statements accurately describes the acute presentation of ischemic stroke?

a. Acute infarction of the central nervous system tissue, one-sided weakness, systolic blood pressure >200 mm Hg
b. Neurologic dysfunction without infarction, one-sided weakness, visual impairment
c. Acute infarction of the central nervous system tissue, one-sided weakness, visual impairment
d. Neurologic dysfunction without infarction, one-sided weakness, blood glucose >200 mg/dL

Answer c is correct. Acute ischemic stroke is caused by a local thrombus formation leading to acute infarction. Visual impairment, weakness on one side of the body, and inability to speak are all other common symptoms of acute stroke.

Answer a is incorrect. Patients do commonly present with one-sided weakness; however, they may or may not present with elevated blood pressure. Further, there is not an upper limit of systolic blood pressure that is indicative of acute ischemic stroke.

Answer b is incorrect. Stroke is defined as infarction of the central nervous system tissue. Neurological dysfunction without acute infarction is a TIA. Patients do commonly present with one-sided weakness and visual impairment. They may also present with the inability to speak.

Answer d is incorrect. Stroke is defined as infarction of the central nervous system tissue. Neurological dysfunction without acute infarction is a TIA. Patients do commonly present with one-sided weakness, and, while diabetes is a risk factor for having an ischemic stroke, there is not a correlation with elevated blood glucose levels and acute stroke.

---

3. JS is a 78-year-old white woman with a PMH significant for atrial fibrillation, systolic heart failure with an ejection fraction of 35%, and hypertension. She presents to the emergency department with symptoms of right-sided paralysis. She is not able to communicate, but her family member states that the symptoms began approximately 5 hours ago. MRI of the brain confirms the patient has had an ischemic stroke. At home she takes metoprolol 100 mg po bid, lisinopril 40 mg po daily, and furosemide 20 mg po daily. Which of the following medications would be the most appropriate for secondary stroke prevention in JS?

a. Ticlopidine
b. Clopidogrel
c. Warfarin
d. Extended-release dipyridamole plus aspirin

Answer c is correct. Oral anticoagulant therapy is the most effective treatment option for the secondary prevention of stroke in patients with a cardioembolic source (atrial fibrillation). All patients with atrial fibrillation should be on antithrombotic therapy with warfarin, dabigatran, apixaban, rivaroxaban, or aspirin for primary stroke prevention. The decision to use one over the other is made based on a patients risk for having a stroke.

Answers a, b, and d are incorrect. Aspirin, clopidogrel, and extended-release dipyridamole plus aspirin are all appropriate options of secondary prevention of ischemic stroke, if the patient does not have a cardioembolic source.

---

4. HB is a 54-year-old African American man who presents to the emergency department with symptoms of left-sided paralysis and visual impairment. He has a PMH significant for hypertension, dyslipidemia, and benign prostatic hyperplasia. MRI of the brain confirms the patient has had an ischemic stroke.

Which of the following medications would be the most appropriate for secondary stroke prevention in HB?

a. Ticlopidine
b. Dipyridamole
c. Aspirin
d. Clopidogrel plus aspirin

Answer c is correct. Aspirin is the most well-studied antiplatelet agent used in the secondary prevention of stroke. Currently, aspirin, clopidogrel, and extended-release dipyridamole plus aspirin are all appropriate antiplatelet options for initial therapy.

Answer a is incorrect. Ticlopidine is not currently recommended by the American Heart Association Stroke Council due to its significant side-effect profile. It can cause severe gastrointestinal side effects and there have been reports of neutropenia, agranulocytosis, aplastic anemia, and thrombotic thrombocytopenic purpura.

Answer b is incorrect. Dipyridamole should not be used as monotherapy in the secondary prevention of ischemic stroke. The combination of extended-release dipyridamole plus aspirin is an acceptable antiplatelet option for initial therapy.

Answer d is incorrect. The American Heart Association Stroke Council currently does not recommend the combination of clopidogrel with aspirin as there is an increased risk of hemorrhage when used together.

---

5. Which of the following is a common side effect of extended-release dipyridamole plus aspirin?

a. Agranulocytosis
b. Visual disturbances
c. Pancreatitis
d. Headache

Answer d is correct. The incidence of headache in patients taking extended-release dipyridamole plus aspirin approaches 40% and is the most common reason for discontinuation.

Answer a is incorrect. Extended-release dipyridamole plus aspirin has not been shown to cause agranulocytosis. Anemia has been reported in approximately 1% of patients. Agranulocytosis is a side effect of ticlopidine.

Answer b is incorrect. Extended-release dipyridamole plus aspirin has not been shown to cause visual disturbances.

Answer c is incorrect. Extended-release dipyridamole plus aspirin has not been shown to cause pancreatitis. It has been shown to cause abdominal pain, indigestion, and diarrhea with incidences approaching 20%.

---

6. A 63-year-old African American man with a PMH significant for dyslipidemia presented to the emergency department several days ago with symptoms of an acute stroke. The physician you are working with wants your recommendations on what to

send this patient home on for blood pressure control. Current vitals are as follows: BP 138/88 mm Hg, HR 86 beats/min What do you recommend?

a. β-Blocker
b. Nondihydropyridine calcium channel blocker
c. Angiotensin-converting enzyme inhibitor plus a diuretic
d. No blood pressure medication. The patient's blood pressure is at goal.

Answer c is correct. Currently the American Heart Association Stroke Council recommends the use of diuretics or the combination of diuretics plus an angiotensin-converting enzyme inhibitor.

Answer a is incorrect. There is no data to support the use of a β-blocker postischemic stroke, and this patient does not have any compelling indications that warrant β-blocker use. Currently the American Heart Association Stroke Council recommends the use of diuretics or the combination of diuretics plus an angiotensin-converting enzyme inhibitor.

Answer b is incorrect. There is no data to support the use of a calcium channel blocker, both nondihydropyridine and dihydropyridine, postischemic stroke. Currently the American Heart Association Stroke Council recommends the use of diuretics or the combination of diuretics plus an angiotensin-converting enzyme inhibitor.

Answer d is incorrect. Per the American Heart Association Stroke Council, antihypertensive treatment is recommended for all patients with a history of ischemic stroke regardless of whether or not the patient has a history of hypertension.

---

7. What is the brand name of extended-release dipyridamole 200 mg plus aspirin 25 mg?

a. Angiomax
b. Aggrastat
c. Aggrenox
d. Abraxane

Answer c is correct. The generic name for Aggrenox is extended-release dipyridamole 200 mg plus aspirin 25 mg. The dose used in the secondary prevention of stroke is one capsule po bid.

Answer a is incorrect. The generic name for Angiomax is bivalirudin. Bivalirudin is a direct thrombin inhibitor.

Answer b is incorrect. The generic name for Aggrastat is tirofiban. Tirofiban is a glycoprotein IIb/IIIa inhibitor.

Answer d is incorrect. The generic name for Abraxane is paclitaxel. Paclitaxel is an antineoplastic agent.

---

8. A 49-year-old white man with a PMH significant only for osteoarthritis was diagnosed with an ischemic stroke due to an atherosclerotic process several days ago. The patient drinks one to two beers per day and denies smoking. Family history is

unremarkable. His current lipid panel is as follows: TC 168 mg/dL, TG 88 mg/dL, HDL 44 mg/dL, LDL 116 mg/dL. Vitals: BP 136/84 mm Hg, HR 78 beats/min. The physician you are working with wants to know if this patient needs to be placed on statin therapy. What do you recommend?

a. This patient's only major risk factor for coronary heart disease is his age. He does not need to be placed on statin therapy.

b. This patient's only major risk factors for coronary heart disease are his age and history of previous ischemic stroke. He does not need to be placed on statin therapy.

c. This patient's only major risk factors for coronary heart disease are his age and history of previous ischemic stroke. He does not need to be placed on statin therapy, but therapeutic lifestyle recommendation should be initiated.

d. Statin therapy is recommended for all patients with an atherosclerotic ischemic stroke. He should be put on statin therapy.

Answer d is correct. All patients with atherosclerotic, ischemic stroke should receive statin therapy to reduce the risk of recurrent events.

Answers a, b, and c are incorrect. If this patient had not had an atherosclerotic ischemic stroke, then he would need to have his 10-year risk assessed because he is between the ages of 40 and 75 years of age with an LDL between 70 and 189 mg/dL. If his 10-year risk was ≥7.5%, he would need statin therapy.

9. Which of the following medications inhibit platelet activity? Select all that apply.

a. Clopidogrel
b. Aspirin
c. Dipyridamole
d. Warfarin
e. Ticlopidine

Answers a, b, c, and e are correct. Aspirin causes irreversible inhibition of platelet cyclooxygenase ultimately leading to a reduction in platelet aggregation. Clopidogrel and ticlopidine work through selective, irreversible inhibition of adenosine diphosphate–induced platelet aggregation. Dipyridamole is an inhibitor of phosphodiesterase.

Answers d is incorrect. Warfarin is an anticoagulant that inhibits vitamin K dependent clotting factors.

10. Which of the following is an appropriate way to counsel patients on taking extended-release dipyridamole plus aspirin therapy?

a. Extended-release dipyridamole 200 mg plus aspirin 25 mg po daily

b. Extended-release dipyridamole 25 mg plus aspirin 200 mg po daily

c. Extended-release dipyridamole 200 mg plus aspirin 25 mg po bid

d. Extended-release dipyridamole 25 mg plus aspirin 200 mg po bid

Answer c is correct. Aggrenox is supplied as a capsule containing extended-release dipyridamole 200 mg plus aspirin 25 mg. This capsule is given twice daily.

Answers a, b, and d are incorrect.

11. CS is a 61-year-old white woman who has a PMH significant for hypertension and diabetes mellitus. She presented to the emergency department yesterday with signs and symptoms of an ischemic stroke. CT of the brain confirmed this diagnosis. Which of the following medications would be the most appropriate for secondary stroke prevention in CS?

a. Extended-release dipyridamole 200 mg plus aspirin 25 mg two capsules po bid

b. Aspirin 81 mg po daily

c. Clopidogrel 75 mg po bid

d. Warfarin 5 mg po daily

Answer b is correct. Aspirin is an acceptable antiplatelet option for initial therapy. The dosing range varies from 50 to 325 mg/d.

Answer a is incorrect. Aggrenox is supplied as a capsule containing extended-release dipyridamole 200 mg plus aspirin 25 mg. This capsule is given twice daily, not two capsules twice daily.

Answer c is incorrect. Clopidogrel is an acceptable antiplatelet option for initial therapy; however, the dose is 75 mg once daily.

Answer d is incorrect. Warfarin should only be used when there is a cardioembolic source such as atrial fibrillation.

12. Which of the following describes the mechanism of action of clopidogrel?

a. Irreversible inhibition of adenosine diphosphate–induced platelet aggregation

b. Irreversible inhibition of platelet cyclooxygenase

c. Reversible inhibition of adenosine diphosphate–induced platelet aggregation

d. Reversible inhibition of platelet cyclooxygenase

Answer a is correct. Clopidogrel works via irreversible inhibition of adenosine diphosphate–induced platelet aggregation.

Answer b is incorrect. Aspirin works via irreversible inhibition of platelet cyclooxygenase.

Answer c and d are incorrect. Clopidogrel works via inhibition of adenosine diphosphate–induced platelet aggregation and aspirin works via inhibition of platelet cyclooxygenase; however, both of the medications cause irreversible inhibition, not reversible.

13. Which of the following medications works by binding to fibrin and subsequently converting plasminogen to plasmin?

a. Plavix
b. Aggrenox

c. Argatroban
d. Activase

Answer d is correct. Activase is the brand name for rtPA. rtPA is a fibrinolytic agent used to dissolve clots associated with acute ischemic stroke.

Answer a is incorrect. Plavix is the brand name for clopidogrel. It works by irreversibly inhibiting adenosine diphosphate–induced platelet aggregation.

Answer b is incorrect. Aggrenox is the brand name for the combination of extended-release dipyridamole plus aspirin. Dipyridamole inhibits phosphodiesterase, and aspirin irreversibly inhibits cyclooxygenase.

Answer c is incorrect. Argatroban is a direct thrombin inhibitor.

14. Which of the following is the correct dose of aspirin for use during an acute stroke? Select all that apply.

   a. Aspirin 81 mg within 24 hours
   b. Aspirin 81 mg within 48 hours
   c. Aspirin 325 mg within 24 hours
   d. Aspirin 325 mg within 48 hours
   e. Aspirin 162 mg within 24 hours

Answers c and d are correct. All answers include the correct timeframe of aspirin use (within 24-48 hours of acute stroke); however, the only dose approved dose for the treatment of acute stroke is aspirin 325 mg.

Answers a, b, and e are incorrect.

15. A 68-year-old man with a PMH significant for diabetes mellitus, DVT 5 years ago, and GI bleed 2 weeks ago presents with right-sided weakness and right facial droop that began 2 hours ago. CT of the head confirms ischemic stroke. Home medications include: warfarin 5 mg po daily, pantoprazole 40 mg po daily, and metformin 1000 mg po bid. Pertinent laboratory values on admission include INR 1.4, hemoglobin 14, hematocrit 41, platelets 175,000, and glucose 200 mg/dL. Blood pressure on admission is 160/90 mm Hg. Which of the following is a relative exclusion criterion for this patient to receive rtPA?

   a. Elevated INR
   b. Low platelets
   c. Recent GI bleed
   d. Elevated blood pressure on admission

Answer c is correct. Gastrointestinal bleeds within the previous 3 weeks qualify as relative exclusion criteria for rtPA use.

Answer a is incorrect. Patients taking warfarin who have a current INR of ≤1.7 may be considered for rtPA, if it is given within the 3-hour window from symptom onset.

Answer b is incorrect. Patients may be considered for rtPA if platelets are >100,000.

Answer d is incorrect. In order to receive rtPA, blood pressure must remain <185/110 mm Hg.

16. A 72-year-old woman (68 in, 111 kg) is admitted for acute ischemic stroke confirmed by CT of the head. She presents within 1.5 hours of symptom onset and meets all criteria to receive rtPA. The physician asks you what the appropriate dose is for this patient and how to administer it. Your response is:

   a. Give 10 mg over 1 minute and then 90 mg over an hour
   b. Give 9 mg over 1 minute and then 81 mg over an hour
   c. Give 10 mg over 10 minutes and then 90 mg over an hour
   d. Give 9 mg over 10 minutes and then 81 mg over an hour

Answer b is correct. Because our patient is over 100 kg, the maximum rtPA dose is 90 mg. Ten percent (9 mg) is given as an IV bolus over 1 minute, and the remainder of the dose (81 mg) is given over an hour.

Answer a is incorrect. The maximum rtPA dose is 90 mg in patients over 100 kg.

Answer c is incorrect. The maximum total rtPA dose is 90 mg in patients over 100 kg. Also, the bolus dose should be given over 1 minute, not 10 minutes.

Answer d is incorrect. The dosing is correct, including the percentages given as bolus and infusion; however, the bolus dose should be administered over 1 minute, not 10 minutes.

17. Current guidelines recommend the use of rtPA up to 4.5 hours after symptom onset in many patients. Patients who are candidates to receive rtPA in this extended time window include: Select all that apply.

   a. Age younger than 80 years
   b. Patients taking oral anticoagulants regardless of INR
   c. Score of less than 25 on the National Institutes of Health Stroke Scale (NIHSS)
   d. History of both previous stroke and diabetes together
   e. History of intracranial hemorrhage

Answer a is correct. Patients age 80 and younger may receive rtPA out to 4.5 hours. Age greater than 80 is a relative exclusion criterion for receiving rtPA 3 to 4.5 hours after symptom onset, but these patients may still undergo consideration of rtPA, if symptom onset is within 3 hours.

Answer c is correct. Patients with a score of greater than (not less than) 25 on the NIHSS are excluded from consideration of the 4.5 hour window. On the NIHSS, higher scores correlate with greater severity of stroke.

Answer b is incorrect. Oral anticoagulant use (regardless of INR) is a relative exclusion criteria for rtPA use in the 3 to 4.5 hour window. Patients taking warfarin may receive rtPA, if given less than 3 hours from symptom onset as long as INR is ≤1.7.

Answer d is incorrect. History of both previous stroke and diabetes is a relative exclusion criterion for receiving rtPA 3 to 4.5 hours after symptom onset. These patients may still undergo consideration of rtPA, if symptom onset is within 3 hours.

Answer e is incorrect. Patients with a history of intracranial hemorrhage may not receive rtPA no matter what the time window is.

---

18. An 81-year-old man with a PMH significant for diabetes, hypertension, and ischemic stroke 3 years ago presents with slurred speech and left-sided weakness that began 3.5 hours ago. NIH stroke score is calculated to be 15. Home medications include lisinopril 40 mg po daily and glipizide 5 mg po bid. Laboratory values are within normal limits and blood pressure is 150/84 mm Hg. The patient weighs 80 kg. Which of the following may be used as initial treatment for ischemic stroke in this patient?

    a. rtPA 72 mg (10% IV bolus over 1 minute and the remainder over 1 hour)
    b. Aspirin 325 mg po
    c. Aspirin 162 mg po
    d. Lovenox 1 mg/kg SQ q12h

Answer b is correct. He should initially receive aspirin at a dose of 325 mg within 24 to 48 hours.

Answer a is incorrect. This patient does not qualify for rtPA. He presented within the extended 4.5-hour time frame but is excluded from consideration due to age >80 *and* PMH significant for both a history of diabetes and a stroke.

Answer c is incorrect. The initial aspirin dose in acute stroke is 325 mg within 24 to 48 hours.

Answer d is incorrect. Lovenox is not beneficial in the treatment of acute stroke and should not be used.

---

19. Which of the following may be used to treat elevated blood pressure in acute stroke patients who have concomitant renal dysfunction? Select all that apply.

    a. Labetalol
    b. Nicardipine
    c. Sodium nitroprusside
    d. Perindopril
    e. Indapamide

Answers a and b are correct. Both labetalol and nicardipine may be initiated in patients with renal dysfunction and they both are the preferred medications to use for blood pressure lowering in acute stroke.

Answer c is incorrect. Sodium nitroprusside's metabolite accumulates in renal insufficiency and can lead to cyanide toxicity.

Answer d is incorrect. Perindopril is not indicated for blood pressure treatment in the acute stroke setting; however, ACE inhibitors may be used for blood pressure control starting after the initial 24 hours.

Answer e is incorrect. Indapamide is not indicated for blood pressure treatment in the acute stroke setting; however, thiazide-like diuretics may be used for blood pressure control starting after the initial 24 hours.

---

20. A 62-year-old woman is admitted 2 hours after onset of acute stroke symptoms including blurred vision, slurred speech, and right facial droop. CT of the head confirms ischemic stroke. Past medical history is nonsignificant, and the patient takes no medications at home. All laboratory values are within normal limits. Blood pressure is 200/110 mm Hg. Patient meets all other inclusion criteria for rtPA use. Which of the following is the best option for blood pressure control in this patient?

    a. No treatment should be given since the systolic blood pressure is <220 mm Hg and the diastolic blood pressure is <120 mm Hg.
    b. Since the patient meets all other inclusion criteria for rtPA, labetalol should be given to lower blood pressure to <185/110 mm Hg so that the patient can receive rtPA.
    c. Since the patient meets all other inclusion criteria for rtPA, nicardipine infusion should be initiated to lower blood pressure to <140/90 mm Hg.
    d. Since the patient meets all other inclusion criteria for rtPA, sodium nitroprusside should be initiated to lower the blood pressure by 15% within the first day.

Answer b is correct. Assuming this patient meets all inclusion criteria for rtPA use, then it is prudent to lower blood pressure to below 185/110 mm Hg. Labetalol is an appropriate first-line option.

Answer a is incorrect. Normally antihypertensive treatment is not necessary until blood pressure rises above 220/120 mm Hg. However, if blood pressure lowering would result in patient becoming an rtPA candidate, then it is prudent to lower blood pressure to below 185/110 mm Hg.

Answer c is incorrect. Blood pressure should not be dropped to 140/90 mm Hg. Lower blood pressures in the acute setting can cause neurological deterioration. A reasonable goal is to lower the blood pressure by 15% within the first 24 hours. The goal is to lower the blood pressure to <185/110 mm Hg when a patient is a candidate for rtPA.

Answer d is incorrect. Sodium nitroprusside is typically reserved for situations when blood pressure remains elevated despite adequate use of both labetalol and nicardipine. The goal is to lower the blood pressure to <185/110 mm Hg when a patient is a candidate for rtPA.

---

21. TP is a 62-year-old patient presenting at 8 pm to the emergency department. The patient has symptoms of weakness to the left side and inability to speak. A CT scan was ordered and revealed an ischemic stroke. The time is now 10:30 pm and the physician wants to treat the patient with rtPA. Which of the following would be exclusion criteria that would prevent TP from receiving rtPA? Select all that apply.

    a. Platelets <100,000 mm³
    b. Oral anticoagulation *and* INR >1.7 or PT >15 seconds

c. Active internal bleeding

d. Blood pressure of 156/92 mm Hg

Answers a, b, and c are correct. Exclusion criteria for rtPA include:

- Symptom onset >4.5 h
- Significant head trauma or prior stroke in previous 3 months
- Symptoms suggest subarachnoid hemorrhage
- Arterial puncture at a noncompressible site within the preious 7 days
- History of previous intracranial hemorrhage
- Intracranial neoplasm, arteriovenous malformation, or aneurysm
- Recent intracranial or intraspinal surgery
- Elevated blood pressure (systolic >185 or diastolic > 110 mm Hg)
- Active internal bleeding
- Acute bleeding diathesis
- Platelets <100,000 mm³
- Heparin therapy within previous 48 h *and* aPTT above upper limit of normal
- Oral anticoagulation *and* INR >1.7 or PT >15 seconds
- Current use of direct thrombin inhibitors or direct factor Xa inhibitors with elevated sensitivity lab tests
- Blood glucose <50 mg/dL
- CT with multilobar infarction

Answer d is incorrect. Exclusion criteria for rtPA related to blood pressure is systolic >185 or diastolic >110 mm Hg.

CHAPTER **7** | Anticoagulation/Venous Thromboembolism

1. A 59-year-old man with past medical history significant for diabetes, hypertension, hyperlipidemia, seizure disorder, and depression presents to the anticoagulation clinic for management of his warfarin. His current medication list includes metformin, lisinopril, cholestyramine, phenytoin, levetiracetam, and mirtazapine. His physician asks you which of his current medications could interact with his warfarin. Select all that apply

a. Metformin

b. Cholestyramine

c. Phenytoin

d. Levetiracetam

e. Mirtazapine

Answers b and c are correct. Phenytoin is a CYP 2C9 inducer and can result in a decreased INR. Cholestyramine can decrease the absorption of warfarin, resulting in a decreased INR.

Answers a, d, and e, are incorrect. They do not pose major interactions with warfarin.

2. KP is 72-year-old woman who presents to the emergency department and reports hematuria for the past 2 days. The patient's INR is 7.2 and KP reports she may have accidentally taken old 10 mg warfarin tablets instead of her currently prescribed 5 mg tablets for the past week. Which agent is the most appropriate reversal agent to be used in the case of warfarin overdose?

a. Phenprocoumon

b. Protamine sulfate

c. Vitamin K

d. Idarucizumab

Answer c is correct. Vitamin K reverses the anticoagulant effects of vitamin K antagonists (VKAs) such as warfarin. VKAs reduce thrombus formation by inhibiting the activation of the vitamin K-dependent clotting factors II, VII, IX, and X. The anticoagulant effect of VKAs is a fine balance between the amount of vitamin K available to activate the clotting factors and ultimately produce thrombin. Ingestion of additional Vitamin K upsets this equilibrium and reverses the anticoagulant effects.

Answer a is incorrect. Phenprocoumon is a vitamin K antagonist available in countries outside the United States. The addition of this agent would have an additive effect to warfarin and increase the severity of the adverse effects.

Answer b is incorrect. Protamine sulfate is the agent of choice for the reversal of unfractionated heparin (UFH) overdose. The recommended dose for reversal of UFH effects is 1 mg of protamine per 100 U of heparin.

Answer d is incorrect. Idarucizumab reverses the anticoagulant effects of dabigatran for emergent surgery, urgent procedures, or in the instance of life-threatening or uncontrolled bleeding. The manufacturer recommended dose is 5 g (2 vials, each contains 2.5 g) administered intravenously as two consecutive infusions or bolus injection by injecting both vials consecutively one after another via syringe.

3. Which adverse reaction(s) may be associated with vitamin K antagonist use? Select all that apply.

a. Melena

b. Cardiac arrhythmias (QT prolongation)

c. Bleeding

d. Purple toe syndrome

e. Anemia

Answer a is correct. Melena is the medical term used for the passing of black, tarry stools. It is a potential sign of an upper gastrointestinal bleed and/or supratherapeutic level of vitamin K antagonist.

Answer c is correct. Bleeding is the most common adverse reaction associated with any of the anticoagulant agents.

Answer d is correct. Purple toe syndrome is rare but potentially serious adverse reaction usually associated with warfarin use.

Answer e is correct. Anemia may be a sign of potential bleeding which is a common adverse reaction with warfarin use.

Answer b is incorrect. Vitamin K antagonists may be used to prevent clot formation in atrial fibrillation. However, they do not impact the rate or rhythm of the heart.

---

4. JC is a 36-year-old pregnant woman with an active DVT. She takes no other medications and has no significant past medical history. Which agent is the best choice for the initial treatment of her DVT?

    a. Enoxaparin
    b. Aspirin
    c. Warfarin
    d. Dabigatran

Answer a is correct. UFH or LMWH are the agents of choice for anticoagulation during pregnancy. LMWHs are the agents of choice for outpatient use due to less monitoring and subcutaneous route of administration. UFH requires close monitoring and is generally given intravenously.

Answer b is incorrect. Aspirin is an antiplatelet medication. Antiplatelet and anticoagulant therapies may often be confused since they both may be used for the prevention of stroke and thrombus formation in certain situations. However, they differ in their mechanisms of action and are not interchangeable.

Answer c is incorrect. Warfarin has a pregnancy category of X and is considered teratogenic.

Answer d is incorrect. Dabigatran has a pregnancy category of C and very little data in pregnancy so would not be a first-line agent.

---

5. A 55-year-old woman is diagnosed with a new DVT. She weighs 80 kg and her SCr is 1.0 and CrCl is 89 mL/min. Her past medical history includes type 2 diabetes and hypertension. Which is an appropriate initial treatment recommendation?

    a. Xarelto® 20 mg once daily with the evening meal
    b. Eliquis® 10 mg bid for 7 days then 5 mg bid
    c. Lovenox® 120 mg bid
    d. Pradaxa® 150 mg bid

Answer b is correct. For treatment of DVT or PE, apixaban must be dosed at 10 mg bid for 7 days, then continued with 5 mg bid.

Answer a is incorrect. The appropriate dose for DVT/PE treatment with rivaroxaban is 15 mg bid for 21 days followed by 20 mg once daily with the evening meal.

Answer c is incorrect. The appropriate dose of enoxaparin for DVT/PE treatment is 1 mg/kg bid or 1.5 mg/kg once daily. The appropriate dose for this patient who is 80 kg would be 80 mg bid or 120 mg once daily.

Answer d is incorrect. If considering the use of dabigatran for DVT/PE treatment, parenteral anticoagulation must be used for the first 5-10 days prior to dabigatran use.

---

6. Which drug can be used safely in a Heparin-induced thrombocytopenia (HIT) patient with a creatinine clearance of 25 mL/min?

    a. Enoxaparin
    b. Dalteparin
    c. Fondaparinux
    d. Argatroban

Answer d is correct. Argatroban, a direct thrombin inhibitor, should be used to prevent and treat thrombosis associated with HIT. It is metabolized in the liver and therefore, safe to use in patients with renal insufficiency.

Answers a and b are incorrect. Enoxaparin and dalteparin are LMWHs and should not be used in patients who have developed heparin-induced thrombocytopenia. Although LMWH have a lower incidence of HIT, they still interact with platelets and could worsen HIT.

Answer c is incorrect. Fondaparinux is contraindicated in patients with creatinine clearance less than 30 mL/min.

---

7. Which agent has a delayed onset of anticoagulant effect?

    a. Arixtra®
    b. Coumadin®
    c. Fragmin®
    d. Lovenox®

Answer b is correct. The anticoagulant effect of warfarin is dependent on the depletion of vitamin K-dependent clotting factors, II, VII, IX, and X. Factor II, thrombin, is largely responsible for warfarin's anticoagulant effect, and it also has the longest half-life.

Answers a, c, and d are incorrect. These anticoagulants have a rapid onset of anticoagulant effect.

Questions 8 and 9 refer to the following case.

A 64-year-old woman (70 kg) followed in your anticoagulation clinic presents for routine monitoring of her warfarin. Her past medical history is significant for recurrent DVT, hypertension, and osteoarthritis. She currently takes warfarin 5 mg daily, lisinopril 10 mg daily, and acetaminophen 1000 mg four times daily as needed. Her current laboratory values are INR 2.0, SCr 1.1 mg/dL, K^+ 4.5 meq/L, and TSH 10.5 μIU/mL. The primary care provider plans to initiate levothyroxine today due to her symptoms of hypothyroidism.

8. Initiation of levothyroxine for this patient's hypothyroidism is most likely going to result in which effect?

    a. Decreased INR
    b. Increased INR
    c. Increased TSH
    d. Increased SCr

Answer b is correct. Hypothyroid patients metabolize vitamin K dependent clotting factors more slowly compared to patients who are euthyroid. Once levothyroxine is initiated and the patient progresses toward a euthyroid state, clotting factors are metabolized more rapidly and could result in an increased INR if the warfarin dose remains the same. Careful monitoring is warranted.

Answer a is incorrect. The INR would be expected to increase.

Answer c is incorrect. Initiation of levothyroxine should result in a decrease in TSH.

Answer d is incorrect. Levothyroxine does not affect serum creatinine.

9. The patient returns to clinic and her primary care provider has decided to transition the patient from warfarin to a direct oral anticoagulant (DOAC) today. Her INR is 2.7. Which DOAC can be safely initiated today?

    a. Xarelto®
    b. Eliquis®
    c. Pradaxa®
    d. Savaysa®

Answer a is correct. It is recommended that when a patient's INR value is less than 3, warfarin can be stopped and Xarelto® (rivaroxaban) can be safely initiated.

Answers b, c, and d are incorrect. When transitioning from warfarin to other oral anticoagulants, it is important to determine how to safely do that. Switching from warfarin to Savaysa® (edoxaban) would require the INR to be less than 2.5. Switching from warfarin to Eliquis® (apixaban) or Pradaxa® (dabigatran) would require INR to be less than 2.

10. Select all of the factors that could result in a supratherapeutic INR.

    a. Binge alcohol use
    b. Diarrhea
    c. Missed doses
    d. Increased dietary vitamin K
    e. Initiation of azole antifungal agents

Answers a, b, and e are correct. Binge alcohol use can increase anticoagulation by decreasing the metabolism of warfarin. In contrast, chronic alcohol use can result in a subtherapeutic INR due to increased metabolism of warfarin. Diarrhea can result in malabsorption, specifically reducing absorption of dietary vitamin K and can result in an

increased INR. Initiation of medications affecting the CYP 450 group, especially CYP2C9, can increase or decrease the INR depending upon if they are inhibitors or inducers. Azole antifungals are inhibitors of CYP2C9 and can result in decreased warfarin metabolism and increased INR.

Answers c and d are incorrect. Extra doses not missed doses would be expected to increase the INR. Also less vitamin K intake would increase the INR, not more vitamin K intake.

11. A 57-year-old woman (65 kg, BMI 28) was just admitted to the hospital for treatment of a pulmonary embolism. An order was written for heparin IV bolus 80 units/kg followed by a continuous infusion of 18 units/kg/h. What are respective heparin bolus dose and continuous infusion rate for this patient?

    a. 5000 units IV bolus; 1200 units/h infusion
    b. 4000 units IV bolus; 800 units/h infusion
    c. 6000 units IV bolus; 1150 units/h infusion
    d. 4000 units IV bolus; 1150 units/h infusion

Answer a is correct. Heparin is dosed based on actual body weight. For the initial bolus dose, 65 kg × 80 units/kg = 5200 units. The dose is rounded to 5000 units for ease of administration. Heparin is prepared as a 5000 units syringe. Alternatively, it would be difficult to draw up a dose to the nearest 100 units dose. For the continuous infusion, 65 kg × 18 units/kg/h = 1170 units/kg/h. In this case, the dose is rounded to the nearest 100 units because most IV pumps could not be programmed to the nearest 50 units dose.

Answer b is incorrect. Actual body weight and not ideal body weight is used in calculating the dose.

Answer c is incorrect. The bolus dose is rounded too high. The IV pump would be unable to program the continuous IV infusion dose.

Answer d is incorrect. The bolus dose is based on actual body weight. The continuous infusion rate should be rounded to the nearest 100 units for purposes of programming the IV pump and accuracy of dosing.

12. Select the appropriate routes of administration for unfractionated heparin. Select all that apply.

    a. Intravenous
    b. Subcutaneous
    c. Intramuscular
    d. Oral
    e. Intrathecal

Answers a and b are correct. Heparin may be administered IV and SC only.

Answers c, d, and e are incorrect. Intramuscular administration of heparin may cause hematoma and should be avoided. Heparin is not available orally and is not indicated for intrathecal use.

Questions 13 and 14 pertain to the following patient case.

JT is a 62-year-old woman with a history of atrial fibrillation, coronary heart disease, hypertension, and diabetes mellitus. Her current medications include warfarin 5 mg daily, amlodipine 5 mg daily, clopidogrel 75 mg daily, lisinopril 10 mg daily, metformin XR 1000 mg daily, and ibuprofen 600 mg three times daily.

13. Which of her medications increases the risk of bleeding with warfarin? Select all that apply.

    a. Clopidogrel
    b. Amlodipine
    c. Metformin
    d. Ibuprofen
    e. Lisinopril

Answers a and d are correct. Clopidogrel, an antiplatelet agent, can increase bleeding risk when used alone and this risk is increased when it is used concomitantly with warfarin. Ibuprofen is a non-steroidal anti-inflammatory drug that increases the risk of gastric ulcer and gastrointestinal bleed when administered concurrently with warfarin.

Answers b, c, and e are incorrect. Amlodipine, metformin, and lisinopril do not increase the risk of bleeding with warfarin.

14. JT presents to her PCP with polyuria and pain on urination and is diagnosed with a urinary tract infection. Which antibiotic would be expected to have the least effect on her warfarin therapy?

    a. Sulfamethoxazole-trimethoprim
    b. Nitrofurantoin
    c. Ciprofloxacin
    d. Fluconazole

Answer b is correct. Nitrofurantoin can be used safely in patients receiving warfarin therapy without interaction.

Answers a, c, and d are incorrect. These antibiotics have been known to interact with warfarin. Sulfamethoxazole-trimethoprim, ciprofloxacin, and fluconazole can increase the INR.

15. A patient returns to the anticoagulation clinic for routine monitoring of her INR, which is below the goal range of 2 to 3 today. The patient stated she has recently started a multivitamin. Which ingredient in the patient's multivitamin is likely to have contributed to a decrease in the INR?

    a. Zinc
    b. Riboflavin
    c. Phytonadione
    d. Selenium

Answer c is correct. Multivitamin supplements containing vitamin K (phytonadione) can interact with warfarin and cause a decrease in the INR.

Answers a, b, and d are incorrect. None of these components in the multivitamin have an effect on warfarin metabolism.

16. A middle-aged woman presents a new prescription for her husband to your pharmacy for enoxaparin (Lovenox®) 240 mg subcutaneously once daily for 7 days for deep venous thrombosis. The patient's weight is 150 kg. What is the most appropriate action for dispensing the medication?

    a. Dispense 21 80-mg syringes with instructions to inject three 80-mg syringes daily.
    b. Repackage the 240-mg dose in one syringe and dispense seven 220-mg syringes.
    c. Call the prescriber and recommend changing the dose to 150 mg twice daily.
    d. Call the prescriber and recommend changing the dose to 200 mg daily.

Answer c is correct. Enoxaparin has not been adequately studied in doses more than 150 mg. Because this patient is at the upper end of the studied weight, he will be unable to use the 1.5 mg/kg once daily dose and must use the 1 mg/kg bid dosing instead.

Answer a is incorrect. It would be difficult and painful for the patient to inject three syringes to make one dose.

Answer b is incorrect. Sterile products cannot be repackaged and dispensed to patients.

Answer d is incorrect. The dose of 200 mg exceeds the maximum number of milligrams that may be given in one dose.

17. An 87-year-old man presents to the anticoagulation clinic for follow-up after recent initiation of warfarin for treatment of a PE. You ask the patient what dose he is currently taking but the patient cannot remember. You then ask him what color tablets the patient has and how many he takes per day. The patient responds that he takes 1 blue tablet every day. Based upon this information, what is the patient's current warfarin dose?

    a. 2.5 mg daily
    b. 4 mg daily
    c. 5 mg daily
    d. 7.5 mg daily

Answer b is correct. All manufacturers of warfarin produce each tablet strength in the same color to provide an easier way to determine a patient's dose if they forget the numerical strength. The table below describes the available warfarin tablet strengths and corresponding tablet color.

Answers a, c and d are incorrect. These tablet strengths are green, peach, and yellow in color, respectively.

Tablet Strength	Tablet Color
1	Pink
2	Lavender
2.5	Green
3	Tan
4	Blue
5	Peach

6	Teal
7.5	Yellow
10	White

18. A patient comes to your pharmacy asking for Boost® dietary supplement. In your discussion, she tells you that she is also taking warfarin for recurrent DVT. Which of the following is a likely consequence of starting this dietary supplement in someone who is receiving chronic warfarin therapy?

    a. Increased risk of bleeding
    b. Increase in the INR
    c. Decrease in the INR
    d. Decrease in warfarin dose

Answer c is correct. Boost® dietary supplement contains vitamin K which can interact with warfarin and make it more difficult for the patient to be appropriately anticoagulated.

Answers a, b, and d are incorrect. These are all consequences for a patient who is taking an interacting medication with warfarin that increases the INR.

Questions 19 to 21 correspond to the following patient case.

TS is a 46-year-old man who was admitted to your hospital with an acute DVT. The patient has no other significant medical history and this is the first episode of DVT in this patient. Warfarin was initiated 2 days ago and a therapeutic INR has not yet been achieved. The patient is being discharged today with discharge prescriptions for warfarin and Lovenox.

19. What counseling information should be provided to TS upon discharge from the hospital? Select all that apply.

    a. Rotate injection site to minimize bruising and pain.
    b. Inject at least 2 inches from your belly button and out toward your sides.
    c. Prior to injection, gently press the plunger to remove the air bubble from the syringe.
    d. Avoid rubbing site of injection after administration to minimize risk of bruising.
    e. Store unused syringes in the refrigerator until just before use.

Answers a, b, and d are correct. These statements are accurate.

Answer c is incorrect. This is a false statement. Attempting to remove the air bubble from the syringe may result in loss of medication.

Answer e is incorrect. Lovenox® syringes should be stored at room temperature.

20. TS presents to the anticoagulation clinic for his initial visit, what counseling information is appropriate for educating TS about taking chronic warfarin therapy? Select all that apply.

    a. All herbal therapies are safe in combination with warfarin therapy.
    b. Report any missed warfarin doses to your physician or clinic.

    c. Over-the-counter analgesics are safe in combination with warfarin therapy.
    d. Avoid wide fluctuations in the consumption of foods high in vitamin K content.
    e. Alcohol consumption does not affect warfarin therapy.

Answers b and d are correct. Lack of adherence to therapy is a major cause of subtherapeutic INRs in patients receiving warfarin therapy. A decrease in the INR may be seen even after only one missed warfarin dose. For this reason, it is important that patients report any missed doses to their physician or anticoagulation-monitoring service. Patients should be educated to maintain a consistent intake of vitamin K-containing foods. Many of these foods are a recommended part of our diets and should not be avoided indefinitely. Additionally, small changes in vitamin K intake have a greater impact on warfarin therapy and INR values in patients who consistently receive minimal vitamin K in their diets.

Answer a is incorrect. Many herbal therapies can interact with warfarin and patients should check with their physician or anticoagulation-monitoring service before starting any new herbal therapies.

Answer c is incorrect. Many OTC analgesics, such as NSAIDs, can increase the risk of bleeding when used concomitantly with warfarin. When used in high doses, acetaminophen may also interact with warfarin by increasing the INR value.

Answer e is incorrect. Alcohol use can interfere with warfarin therapy. Chronic excessive alcohol use can result in a decrease in the INR. An acute alcohol binge can cause an increase in the INR due to an inhibition of hepatic microsomal enzymes.

21. Which agent would be the best pain management option for TS to utilize while on chronic warfarin therapy?

    a. Celebrex®
    b. Excedrin®
    c. Aspirin
    d. Acetaminophen

Answer d is correct. Although use of high doses of acetaminophen over several days can cause an interaction with warfarin therapy, as needed, doses less than 1500 mg daily is a safe option. Acetaminophen is the recommended over-the-counter agent for the management of mild-moderate pain with chronic warfarin therapy.

Answer a is incorrect. Celebrex® is the brand name for celecoxib, a COX-2 inhibitor. COX-2 inhibitors increase bleeding risk in warfarin patients due to their potential to cause gastrointestinal ulceration.

Answer b is incorrect. Excedrin® contains aspirin. Aspirin reduces platelet aggregation and increases risk for bleeding.

Answer c is incorrect. Aspirin reduces platelet aggregation and increases risk for bleeding.

22. In which procedure should Lovenox® use be avoided?

    a. Computed tomography (CT) scan
    b. Magnetic resonance imaging (MRI) scan
    c. Epidural anesthesia
    d. Liver biopsy

Answer c is correct. LMWHs should be avoided in patients undergoing epidural anesthesia due to the potential of developing a spinal hematoma, which can result in long-term or permanent paralysis.

Answers a and b are incorrect. These procedures are noninvasive and pose no added bleeding risk in patients receiving LMWHs.

Answer d is incorrect. There is no contraindication to the use of LMWHs in patients undergoing liver biopsy.

23. The effects of which anticoagulant(s) can be reversed by idarucizumab? Select all that apply.

    a. Rivaroxaban
    b. Dabigatran etexilate mesylate
    c. Warfarin
    d. Apixaban
    e. Heparin

Answer b is correct. The effects of dabigatran can be reversed by idarucizumab (Praxbind).

Answers a and d are incorrect. Apixaban and rivaroxaban can be reversed by andexanet alpha (Andexxa).

Answer c is incorrect. Warfarin can be reversed by utilizing vitamin K, fresh frozen plasma (FFP), or prothrombin complex concentrate (PCC).

Answer e is incorrect. Heparin can be reversed by utilizing protamine.

24. Dose adjustment or avoidance may be necessary in a patient with renal dysfunction for which of the following agents? Select all that apply.

    a. Argatroban
    b. Warfarin
    c. Dabigatran etexilate
    d. Rivaroxaban
    e. Enoxaparin sodium

Answers c, d, and e are correct. Each of these agents has a recommended dose modification or contraindication due to renal insufficiency.

Answers a and b are incorrect. Argatroban and warfarin have no specific dose adjustment due to renal insufficiency.

25. A 62-year-old female patient presents with acute PE and is initially managed with enoxaparin sodium. The patient has a past medical history significant only for hypertension. The patient has no history of renal or hepatic dysfunction. Which of the following would be appropriate for continued treatment? Select all that apply.

    a. Warfarin
    b. Dabigatran etexilate
    c. Apixaban
    d. Aspirin
    e. Rivaroxaban

Answers a, b, c, and e are correct. Dabigatran etexilate, warfarin, apixaban, and rivaroxaban are approved for treatment of PE.

Answer d is incorrect. Aspirin is not an oral anticoagulant and would not be appropriate for treatment of PE.

26. Rank the following anticoagulants in order from shortest to longest half-life. (ALL options must be used.)

Unordered Options	Ordered Response
Enoxaparin	
Warfarin	
Heparin	
Fondaparinux	
Rivaroxaban	

Answer.

Unordered Options	Ordered Response
Enoxaparin	Heparin
Warfarin	Enoxaparin
Heparin	Rivaroxaban
Fondaparinux	Fondaparinux
Rivaroxaban	Warfarin

27. A 76-year-old woman with atrial fibrillation, hypertension, and diabetes mellitus presents to the clinic with complaints of indigestion, bloating, and nausea. Her current medications include dabigatran 150 mg bid, lisinopril 20 mg daily, chlorthalidone 25 mg daily, metformin 1000 mg bid, and glipizide 10 mg bid. Which medication is the likely cause?

    a. Dabigatran
    b. Lisinopril
    c. Chlorthalidone
    d. Glipizide

Answer a is correct. One of the most common adverse effects associated with dabigatran is dyspepsia.

Answers b, c, and d are incorrect. None of the drugs commonly cause dyspepsia.

28. A patient tells you she has recently started a new diet that has given her more energy and an optimistic outlook on life. You

see from her medication list she is currently taking warfarin. You ask her about her new diet and she tells you she eats protein smoothies for breakfast (bananas, strawberries, spinach, kale, protein powder), onion broth soup for lunch, and baked chicken, collard greens, and an apple at dinner. What foods in her new diet can affect her INR? Select all that apply.

a. Strawberries
b. Spinach
c. Kale
d. Chicken
e. Protein powder

Answers b and c, are correct. These are foods rich in vitamin K. Foods rich in vitamin K could lead to a decrease in the INR.

Answers a, d, and e are incorrect. They are not rich in vitamin K and therefore, do not affect her INR.

29. A 42-year-old male patient presents with new onset non-valvular atrial fibrillation. The patient's past medical history is significant for simple partial seizures, hypertension, and type 2 diabetes. Current medications include Tegretol-XR® 400 mg bid, Januvia® 100 mg daily, metformin 500 mg bid, and lisinopril 20 mg daily. The patient's physician would like to initiate rivaroxaban for treatment of atrial fibrillation. Which medication the patient is currently receiving presents the most significant interaction with rivaroxaban?

a. Lisinopril
b. Januvia®
c. Tegretol-XR®
d. Metformin

Answer c is correct. Carbamazepine is a strong CYP-3A4 and P-gp inducer and may reduce the efficacy of rivaroxaban.

Answers a, b, and d are incorrect. Lisinopril, Januvia®, and metformin are not strong CYP-3A4 and P-gp inhibitors or inducers and would not be expected to interact with rivaroxaban.

30. A 45-year-old man on lifelong therapy with warfarin for recurrent DVT has been prescribed metronidazole for *Clostridium difficile* infection. Addition of metronidazole to this patient's warfarin will likely have what effect on the INR and by what mechanism?

a. Increase INR due to CYP2C9 inhibition
b. Decrease INR due to CYP2D6 inhibition
c. Increase INR due to CYP1A2 inhibition
d. Decrease INR due to CYP3A4 inhibition

Answer a is correct. Metronidazole and azole antifungals are inhibitors of CYP2C9. The more potent warfarin isomer, S-warfarin, is primarily metabolized by CYP2C9. Inhibition of this enzymes leads to increased concentrations of warfarin and increased INR.

Answers b, c, and d are incorrect. The primary inhibitor effect of metronidazole is not related to CYP2D6, CYP1A2, or CYP3A4.

CHAPTER 8 | Peripheral Arterial Disease

1. A 42-year-old smoker with hypertension, diabetes, hypercholesterolemia, and PAD complains of pain in his calves when he walks two to three blocks. What therapy might offer him the greatest benefit in symptom reduction and in overall mortality?

a. Limb revascularization procedure
b. Cilostazol
c. Smoking cessation
d. Pravastatin

Answer c is correct. Tobacco cessation is the most important intervention to improve cardiovascular morbidity and mortality in high-risk patients and to improve claudication symptoms.

Answer a is incorrect. A limb revascularization procedure is indicated with an acute arterial occlusion that threatens limb viability.

Answer b is incorrect. Cilostazol may help with claudication symptoms but will not affect cardiovascular mortality.

Answer d is incorrect. Pravastatin will not help with claudication symptoms.

2. Which of the following are contraindications to the use of aspirin? Select all that apply.

a. Asthma
b. Hypersensitivity to NSAIDS
c. Nasal polyps
d. 30-year-old man with influenza

Answer a is correct. Asthma is a contraindication to the use of aspirin.

Answer b is correct. Hypersensitivity to NSAIDS is a contraindication to the use of aspirin.

Answer c is correct. Nasal polyps is a contraindication to the use of aspirin.

Answer d is incorrect. Aspirin is contraindicated in adolescents less than 16 years of age with chickenpox, influenza, or flu-like symptoms.

3. Which of the following is recommended as an alternative antiplatelet therapy for patients with PAD who do not tolerate aspirin?

a. Pentoxifylline 400 mg twice daily
b. Clopidogrel 225 mg daily
c. Clopidogrel 75 mg daily
d. Pentoxifylline 400 mg three times daily

Answer c is correct. The recommended dosage of clopidogrel in the treatment of PAD is 75 mg daily orally.

Answer b is incorrect. The recommended dosage of clopidogrel in the treatment of PAD is 75 mg daily orally.

Answers a and d are incorrect. The use of pentoxifylline in the treatment of PAD is for symptoms of claudication, not to reduce cardiovascular risk. It is not a replacement for aspirin in patients who do not tolerate aspirin and no longer recommended for claudication symptom relief due to lack of efficacy.

---

4. Which of the following pharmacologic interventions may achieve a reduction in cardiovascular events for a patient with established peripheral arterial disease? Select all that apply.

   a. Aspirin
   b. Clopidogrel
   c. Statin therapy
   d. Pentoxifylline

Answer a is correct. Aspirin achieves a reduction in cardiovascular events. Aspirin carries non-FDA labeled indications (Evidence Class IIb, Category B) for peripheral arterial disease and the medical literature strongly supports the use of low and medium-dose aspirin (75 to 325 mg daily).

Answer b is correct. Clopidogrel achieves a reduction in vascular events. Clopidogrel (Plavix) is recommended as an alternative antiplatelet therapy for patients who do not tolerate aspirin. Clopidogrel carries an FDA-labeled indication (Evidence Class IIb, Category A) for the treatment of PAD.

Answer c is correct. Statins achieve a reduction in cardiovascular events and are recommended by the American Heart Association/American College of Cardiologists for all patients with PAD.

Answer d is incorrect. Pentoxifylline does not achieve a reduction in vascular events and is not recommended by the American Heart Association/American College of Cardiologists for the treatment of PAD. Recent studies have demonstrated no benefit over placebo with walking distance improvements in several trials.

---

5. Which of the following antiplatelet agents is not generally used in the treatment of PAD and should be monitored with periodic complete blood count testing related to potential hematologic complications that include agranulocytosis and aplastic anemia?

   a. Aspirin
   b. Simvastatin
   c. Ticlopidine
   d. Dipyridamole plus aspirin

Answer c is correct. Ticlopidine has a black box warning for potential life-threatening hematologic reactions, including neutropenia, agranulocytosis, thrombotic thrombocytopenic

purpura (TTP), and aplastic anemia. Routine monitoring is required for ticlopidine. Monitor for signs and symptoms of neutropenia and thrombocytopenia. Discontinue therapy if the absolute neutrophil count falls less than 1200/mm³ or if the platelet count falls less than 80,000/mm³.

Answer a is incorrect. Aspirin does not require periodic monitoring of the complete blood count.

Answer b is incorrect. Simvastatin does not require periodic monitoring of the complete blood count.

Answer d is incorrect. Dipyridamole plus aspirin does not require monitoring of the complete blood count.

---

6. Which of the following patients would have a contraindication for receiving cilostazol as treatment for peripheral arterial disease?

   a. A 49-year-old woman with hypertension
   b. A 60-year-old man with a history of benign prostatic hypertrophy
   c. A 48-year-old man with congestive heart failure
   d. A 52-year-old woman with hypothyroidism

Answer c is correct. Cilostazol is contraindicated in all degrees of heart failure.

Answer a is incorrect. Although cilostazol can cause edema, having hypertension is not an absolute contraindication to cilostazol.

Answer b is incorrect. Benign prostatic hyperplasia (BPH) is not a contraindication to the use of cilostazol.

Answer d is incorrect. Hypothyroidism is not a contraindication to cilostazol.

---

7. A 58-year-old male patient with heart failure, erectile dysfunction, and CAD with stable angina underwent testing for PAD after having findings suggestive of PAD on physical examination at his last primary care office visit. Which of the following diagnostic tests is most appropriate to confirm a PAD diagnosis in this patient?

   a. Fecal occult blood test
   b. Toe-brachial index
   c. Cardiac catheterization
   d. Ankle-brachial index

Answer d is correct. Resting ankle-brachial index is the preferred test to confirm diagnosis of PAD in patients who have findings suggestive of PAD upon examination or who are high risk of PAD.

Answer a is incorrect. Fecal occult blood test is used to screen for colorectal cancer or to test for blood in stool samples.

Answer b is incorrect. Toe-brachial index is only recommended as an alternative to ankle-brachial index as a PAD diagnostic test.

Answer c is incorrect. Cardiac catheterization can diagnose atherosclerotic arterial disease in the heart vasculature, not in the lower extremities.

---

8. The 58-year-old male patient with heart failure and CAD was diagnosed with PAD after recent testing. Current medications: carvedilol 25 mg po bid, lisinopril 40 mg po daily, aspirin 81 mg po daily. The patient describes his lower extremity pain as cramping up and down the backs of his legs, worse during busy times at the restaurant and resolves with rest. Which of the following therapies would be the best treatment for his leg symptoms?

    a. Cilostazol 100 mg po twice daily
    b. Structured walking exercise therapy
    c. Pentoxifylline 400 mg po three times daily
    d. Clopidogrel 75 mg po daily

Answer b is correct. Structured walking exercise therapy should be recommended as first-line therapy for claudication. Structured exercise therapy results in improved functional status and quality of life and decreases leg symptoms.

Answer a is incorrect. Cilostazol is contraindicated in patients with heart failure.

Answer c is incorrect. Pentoxifylline is not recommended for PAD due to lack of efficacy in improving walking symptoms compared to placebo.

Answer d is incorrect. Clopidogrel is an antiplatelet therapy option for reducing cardiovascular risk in patients with PAD; however, this patient is currently taking aspirin for this purpose. Clopidogrel is not used for symptom management of PAD.

---

9. Select the treatment goal(s) for PAD in patients with intermittent claudication. Select all that apply.

    a. Increase maximal walking distance
    b. Increase duration of walking
    c. Increase amount of pain-free walking
    d. Decrease preload
    e. Decrease afterload

Answer a is correct. Increasing maximal walking distance is a treatment goal for patients with PAD.

Answer b is correct. Increasing duration of walking is a treatment goal for patients with PAD.

Answer c is correct. Increasing amount of pain-free walking is a treatment goal for patients with PAD.

Answers d and e are incorrect. Decreasing preload (venous vasodilation) and afterload (arterial vasodilation) are not utilized in the management of PAD. Preload and afterload reducers (eg, BiDil, ACE inhibitors) are utilized in the management of heart failure and other cardiovascular diseases.

---

10. Select the risk factors (comorbidities) that should be controlled in a patient with PAD. Select all that apply.

    a. Blood pressure
    b. Cholesterol
    c. Blood glucose
    d. International normalized ratio (INR)

Answers a, b, and c are correct. Risk factor reduction and controlling underlying causes, such as diabetes mellitus, hypertension, and hyperlipidemia, should be included in the overall treatment strategy for PAD. Improving control of comorbid conditions can result in improvement in overall quality of life and reduction in cardiovascular morbidity and mortality.

Answer d is incorrect. The INR is not monitored during the management of PAD. **This is used to manage Coumadin therapy.**

---

11. Select the primary pharmacologic management for PAD.

    a. Anticoagulants
    b. Antiplatelet agents
    c. Antihypertensive agents
    d. Sympatholytic agents

Answer b is correct. Primary pharmacologic interventions for PAD involve antiplatelet drug therapies. Antiplatelet therapy is indicated to reduce the risk of myocardial infarction, stroke, or vascular death in individuals with atherosclerotic lower extremity PAD. Aspirin, clopidogrel, cilostazol, and pentoxifylline are commonly prescribed antiplatelet agents for the treatment of PAD.

Answer a is incorrect. Anticoagulants (eg, warfarin, heparin) are not first-line agents in the management of PAD.

Answer c is incorrect. Antihypertensives are not utilized in the management of PAD; however, control of blood pressure is a key factor to decreasing complications. Improving control of comorbid conditions (eg, hypertension, hyperlipidemia, and diabetes) can result in improvement in overall quality of life and reduction in cardiovascular complications and death.

Answer d is incorrect. Sympatholytics (eg, β blockers) are not utilized in the management of PAD due to lack of long-term data showing efficacy and safety in the management of PAD.

---

12. A 28-year-old mother with no significant medical history asks her pharmacist if she can start taking low-dose aspirin herself and also thinks it is a good idea to keep a bottle in the house in case anyone in her family gets a headache or has some mild pain. Which of the following counseling points should be discussed with the patient? Select all that apply.

    a. Low-dose aspirin is perfectly fine to have around the house. Many people find it works well for mild pains and headache and it is safe for anyone over the age of 12.

b. You should discuss this with your physician. Some of the common side effects include indigestion and nausea and some of the serious side effects include bleeding, ringing in the ears, and peptic ulcer disease.

c. Should you decide to become pregnant while you are taking aspirin, let your doctor know right away because aspirin may not be safe while pregnant, especially during the third trimester.

d. Do not give aspirin to anyone who has asthma or breathing problems without discussing with their physician because aspirin may cause bronchospasm.

Answer b is correct. These are common side effects and serious adverse effects.

Answer c is correct. Aspirin is not recommended in pregnancy, especially during the third trimester.

Answer d is correct. Aspirin can cause bronchospasm (especially in the triad of asthma, allergic rhinitis with nasal polyps).

Answer a is incorrect. Aspirin should be avoided in anyone under the age of 16 due to the risk of Reye syndrome. Low-dose aspirin has limited efficacy when used for pain disorders.

13. Select the dose(s) of aspirin utilized in the management of PAD. Select all that apply.

a. 81 mg
b. 162 mg
c. 50 mg
d. 325 mg

Answers a, b, and d are correct. Aspirin may be dosed 75 to 325 mg for management of PAD. *Note:* Side effects associated with aspirin may be encountered with low dose (81 mg) aspirin.

Answer c is incorrect. Aspirin 50 mg is used as an antiplatelet agent when combined with dipyridamole (Aggrenox).

14. Clopidogrel works by which of the following mechanisms?

a. Selectively and irreversibly inhibits ADP-induced platelet aggregation.
b. Reversibly inhibits platelet aggregation.
c. Reduces blood viscosity by inhibiting phosphodiesterase.
d. Suppresses cyclic adenosine monophosphate (cAMP) degradation, which produces vasodilation.

Answer a is correct. Clopidogrel requires in vivo biotransformation to an active metabolite. The clopidogrel active metabolite inhibits platelet aggregation by selectively and irreversibly inhibiting the binding of adenosine diphosphate (ADP) to its platelet receptor and the subsequent activation of ADP-mediated glycoprotein GPIIb/IIIa complex. Since this action is irreversible, the remainder of the platelet life span is affected.

Answer b is incorrect. Clopidogrel irreversibly inhibits platelets.

Answer c is incorrect. This is the mechanism of action of pentoxifylline.

Answer d is incorrect. This is the mechanism of dipyridamole.

15. Which of the following medications is contraindicated in patients with hypersensitivity to xanthines?

a. Aspirin
b. Plavix
c. Trental
d. Pletal

Answer c is correct. Trental (pentoxifylline) is contraindicated in patients with hypersensitivity to xanthines.

Answer a is incorrect. Aspirin is not contraindicated in patients with hypersensitivity to xanthines.

Answer b is incorrect. Plavix (clopidogrel) is not contraindicated in patients with hypersensitivity to xanthines.

Answer d is incorrect. Pletal (cilostazol) is not contraindicated in patients with hypersensitivity to xanthines.

16. Which of the following medications require dosage reduction when administered with strong CYP3A4 inhibitors?

a. Aspirin
b. Cilostazol
c. Pentoxifylline
d. Clopidogrel

Answer b is correct. Cilostazol dose should be reduced to 50 mg twice daily when given with strong CYP3A4 inhibitors such as diltiazem, erythromycin, itraconazole, and ketoconazole.

Answer a is incorrect. Aspirin is not a CYP3A4 substrate.

Answer c is incorrect. Pentoxifylline is not a CYP3A4 substrate.

Answer d is incorrect. Clopidogrel is a minor CYP3A4 substrate. There is no clinically significant drug interaction between clopidogrel and CYP3A4 inhibitors.

17. Which of the following immunizations is recommended for patients with PAD?

a. Pneumococcal PPSV-23
b. Pneumococcal PCV-13
c. Annual influenza vaccine
d. Zoster vaccine

Answer c is correct. Influenza vaccination is recommended for all patients with PAD because they are at a high risk of cardiovascular morbidity and mortality. There is clinical evidence that the seasonal influenza vaccine was associated with a significant reduction in 1-year cardiovascular death rates among patients with established cardiovascular disease.

Answers a and b are incorrect. Current guidelines do not identify PAD as a compelling indication for pneumococcal vaccinations, although pneumococcal vaccines are recommended for patients with cardiac conditions.

Answer d is incorrect. Current guidelines do not identify PAD as a compelling indication for zoster vaccination.

---

18. Which of the following symptoms suggest limb-threatening ischemia and should prompt immediate referral for further evaluation? Select all that apply.

    a. Toenail dystrophy
    b. Gangrene
    c. Paralysis
    d. Severe lower extremity pain at rest

Answers b, c, and d are correct. Gangrene, paralysis, ischemic rest pain, and non-healing wounds suggest the affected limb is threatened and the patient should be referred for immediate medical evaluation.

Answer a is incorrect. Toenail dystrophy can be a symptom of PAD, but is not generally a life-threatening or limb-threatening condition.

---

19. Which of the following treatments are recommended as standard therapy for all patients with PAD? Select all that apply.

    a. Aspirin or clopidogrel
    b. Cilostazol
    c. Statin
    d. Ticlopidine
    e. Pentoxifylline

Answers a and c are correct. Antiplatelet therapy with asprin or clopidogrel and statin are recommended for all patients with PAD by the American Heart Association/American College of Cardiology.

Answer b is incorrect. Cilostazol is recommended as pharmacotherapy only for patients with PAD and claudication.

Answer d is incorrect. Ticlopidine is not recommended as a standard treatment for any patients with PAD due to the risk of harm related to hematologic adverse effects.

Answer e is incorrect. Pentoxifylline is not recommended for PAD due to lack of efficacy in improving walking symptoms as compared to placebo.

---

20. A 66-year-old female patient with PAD and exertional pain in her lower extremities is currently taking cilostazol, aspirin, atorvastatin, and lisinopril. Which of the following is the most

common adverse effect of taking cilostazol and aspirin in combination?

    a. Heart failure hospitalizations
    b. Subtherapeutic effects of cilostazol
    c. Skeletal muscle soreness
    d. Increased bleeding risk

Answer d is correct. Cilostazol and aspirin are both antiplatelet agents. The risk of bleeding is greater when multiple antiplatelet agents are taken in combination.

Answer a is incorrect. Combination cilostazol and aspirin are not known to increase heart failure risk. Cilostazol is contraindicated in patients with heart failure because of increased risk of death.

Answer b is incorrect. Aspirin does not reduce the effectiveness of cilostazol. Cilostazol levels are increased when taken in combination with strong CYP3A4 inhibitors. Atorvastatin does have CYP3A4 effects, but is not a strong inhibitor.

Answer c is incorrect. Skeletal muscle soreness is not an effect of taking cilostazol and aspirin in combination or as monotherapy. Muscle soreness is a potential adverse effect of atorvastatin.

CHAPTER **9 | Arrhythmias**

1. The onset of AF is associated with which patient characteristics? Select all that apply.

    a. Hepatitis
    b. Increasing age
    c. Female sex
    d. Cardiovascular disease

Answer b is correct. AF is associated with increasing age.

Answer d is correct. AF is associated with the presence of cardiovascular disease.

Answer a is incorrect. AF is not associated with hepatitis.

Answer c is incorrect. AF is more common in the male sex.

---

2. A 68-year-old woman weighing 60 kg presents to the emergency room in AF and is hemodynamically unstable. It is decided to proceed with DCC. Which of the following would be appropriate anticoagulation therapy to administer prior to DCC? Select all that apply.

    a. Enoxaparin 60 mg
    b. Unfractionated heparin 4800 unit bolus followed by 1100 units/h by continuous infusion
    c. Enoxaparin 40 mg
    d. Enoxaparin 30 mg

Answer a is correct. The appropriate dose of enoxaparin prior to DCC is the full treatment dose of 1 mg/kg.

Answer b is correct. The appropriate dose of unfractionated heparin prior to DCC is the full VTE treatment dose of 80 units/kg IV bolus followed by 18 units/kg/h IV continuous infusion. The exact calculation for the infusion dosing is 1080 units, but this needs to be rounded to the nearest 100 unit increment.

Answer c is incorrect. The appropriate dose of enoxaparin prior to DCC is the full treatment dose of 1 mg/kg.

Answer d is incorrect. The appropriate dose of enoxaparin prior to DCC is the full treatment dose of 1 mg/kg.

---

3. Which of the following is/are available in oral and IV preparations? Select all that apply.

   a. Diltiazem
   b. Dofetilide
   c. Dronedarone
   d. Amiodarone

Answer a is correct. Diltiazem is available in both oral and IV preparations.

Answer d is correct. Amiodarone is available in both oral and IV preparations.

Answer b is incorrect. Dofetilide is only available as an oral formulation.

Answer c is incorrect. Dronedarone is only available as an oral formulation.

---

4. A patient with an HR of 53 beats/min is complaining of SOB, light-headedness, and has a blood pressure (BP) of 80/58 mm Hg. Transcutaneous pacing is being prepared. What is the first drug and dose that should be administered?

   a. Epinephrine 1 mg IV
   b. Atropine 0.5 mg IV
   c. Atropine 1 mg IV
   d. Dopamine 1-5 mcg/kg/min IV

This patient is in sinus bradycardia with an HR of 53 beats/min. The patient is considered unstable due to SOB, light-headedness, and hypotension (BP 80/58 mm Hg). Therefore, intervention is warranted.

Answer b is correct. Atropine 0.5 mg IV is the first drug and dose that should be administered while transcutaneous pacing is being prepared.

Answer a is incorrect. Epinephrine is an appropriate drug to administer for bradycardia, but in the form of an infusion after atropine has failed.

Answer c is incorrect. The dose is too high. Atropine 0.5 mg is the correct dose for symptomatic bradycardia and may be repeated up to 3 mg total.

Answer d is incorrect. Dopamine is an appropriate drug to administer for bradycardia. However, it should be tried after atropine has failed and the correct dose range is dopamine 2 to 10 mcg/kg/min.

---

5. You respond with the code team to a patient that is in cardiac arrest. High-quality chest compressions are being given. The patient is intubated and an IV has been started. ECG reveals that the patient is in asystole. The first IV drug and dose to administer is:

   a. Amiodarone 300 mg IV
   b. Epinephrine 1 mg IV
   c. Dopamine 1 to 5 mcg/kg/min
   d. Lidocaine 1 to 1.5 mg/kg IV

Answer b is correct. Epinephrine 1 mg IV is the initial drug and dose to be administered for asystole.

Answer a is incorrect. Class III antiarrhythmics have no role in asystole.

Answer c is incorrect. Dopamine has no role in asystole.

Answer d is incorrect. Class Ib antiarrhythmics have no role in asystole.

---

6. Which of the following antiarrhythmic drugs is *likely* to cause TdP? Select all that apply.

   a. Quinidine
   b. Sotalol
   c. Lidocaine
   d. Dofetilide

Answer a is correct. Class Ia antiarrhythmics prolong the QT interval and can cause TdP.

Answer b is correct. Sotalol, a Class III antiarrhythmic can prolong the QT interval and cause TdP.

Answer d is correct. Dofetilide, a Class III antiarrhythmic can prolong the QT interval and cause TdP.

Answer c is incorrect. Lidocaine, a Class Ib antiarrhythmic has a low potential of causing TdP.

---

7. A nonresponsive patient in ventricular fibrillation has received multiple appropriate defibrillations and epinephrine 1 mg IV twice. Which antiarrhythmic drug can be used next?

   a. Cordarone
   b. Isoptin
   c. Brevibloc
   d. Quinidex

Answer a is correct. Once the primary CAB algorithm for VF/pulseless VT has been followed, drugs should be administered followed by shocks in between. Since the patient has already received the first drug of choice, epinephrine, antiarrhythmic therapy should be initiated. Amiodarone 300 mg IV is a good choice.

Answer b is incorrect. Non-DHP calcium channel blockers have no role in the treatment of VF.

Answer c is incorrect. β-Blockers have no role in the treatment of VF.

Answer d is incorrect. Quinidex (Quinidine), a Class Ia antiarrhythmic, has no role in the treatment of VF.

---

8. A 79-year-old man weighing 80 kg presents to your hospital emergency room with newly discovered AF with rapid ventricular response and is symptomatic with little rate control achieved after initiation of a diltiazem drip. It is decided by the attending physician to proceed with electrical cardioversion. The patient's wife reports that he underwent a cardiac workup the day before for routine knee replacement surgery. The ECG from that workup is retrieved and shows normal sinus rhythm. What is the next appropriate step in this patient's care?

    a. Proceed with synchronized direct cardioversion after receiving enoxaparin 80 mg.
    b. Anticoagulate with warfarin for 3 weeks, target INR 2.0 to 3.0, then cardioversion.
    c. Obtain transesophageal ECHO to rule out thrombus then cardioversion.
    d. Proceed with synchronized direct current cardioversion without anticoagulation.

The first goal of managing a patient presenting with AF is rate control. This has been attempted with the diltiazem drip. However, the patient is still very symptomatic. Because of the symptoms, immediate cardioversion should be considered.

Answer a is correct. Because the patient has been in AF for less than 48 hours, it is appropriate to proceed with immediate cardioversion as long as the patient is anticoagulated with full VTE treatment dose heparin, full treatment dose enoxaparin, a therapeutic INR on warfarin, or currently on maintenance therapy with one of the new oral anticoagulants (NOAC).

Answer b is incorrect. Because the patient is still symptomatic despite rate control, an attempt should be made to cardiovert now.

Answer c is incorrect. Because we know that the patient's AF has been occurring for less than 48 hours, it is appropriate to proceed with cardioversion without the TEE.

Answer d is incorrect. Patients receiving DCC should be cardioverted only after receiving full dose anticoagulation.

---

9. A 65-year-old patient presents with AF and HF. Which of the following is the best choice for pharmacologic cardioversion of AF in this patient?

    a. Flecainide
    b. Sotalol
    c. Dofetilide
    d. Dronedarone

Answer c is correct. Dofetilide, a Class III antiarrhythmic is a safe drug to use in patients with structural heart disease and LV dysfunction. Amiodarone is the other antiarrhythmic that is safe in this patient population.

Answers a, b, and d are all incorrect. Flecainide, sotalol, and dronedarone are not safe for use in patients with structural heart disease.

---

10. Amiodarone requires substantial safety monitoring during long-term therapy due to its numerous side effects. Which of the following is required to be routinely performed in a patient on long-term amiodarone therapy?

    a. Hepatic function panel
    b. Renal function panel
    c. Erythrocyte sedimentation rate
    d. B-type natriuretic peptide (BNP) levels

Answer a is correct. Amiodarone can cause elevations in liver function test (LFT) and may require dose adjustment in patients with liver impairment. Hepatic function panels should be monitored routinely.

Answer b is incorrect. Amiodarone is not appreciably eliminated by the kidneys.

Answer c is incorrect. Amiodarone is not known to affect sedimentation rates.

Answer d is incorrect. Amiodarone does not affect BNP levels, which is considered a measurement of HF status and response to ventricular stretch.

---

11. Dofetilide is indicated in which of the following?

    a. A patient initiated in an outpatient setting
    b. A patient with creatinine clearance (CrCl) <20 mL/min
    c. A baseline QTc 510 millisecond
    d. A patient with LV hypertrophy

Answer d is correct. Dofetilide is safer in patients with structural heart disease and ventricular hypertrophy.

Answer a is incorrect. Dofetilide must be initiated in an inpatient setting under telemetry.

Answer b is incorrect. Dofetilide is contraindicated in patients with a CrCl <20 mL/min.

Answer c is incorrect. Dofetilide is contraindicated in patients with a QTc >440 millisecond (or 500 millisecond with a ventricular conduction abnormality).

---

12. Which antiarrhythmic drug is safer to use for maintenance of sinus rhythm in a patient with AF, HF, and an ejection fraction of 15%?

    a. Sotalol
    b. Flecainide
    c. Amiodarone
    d. Procainamide

Answer c is correct.   Amiodarone is safe for use in patients with HF and impaired ventricular output.

Answer a is incorrect.   Sotalol, a Class III antiarrhythmic, while used often for AF and ventricular arrhythmias, is not safe for use in patients with LV dysfunction and HF.

Answer b is incorrect.   Flecainide, a Class Ic antiarrhythmic, while used often for AF, is not safe for patients with impaired LV function.

Answer d is incorrect.   Procainamide, a Class Ia antiarrhythmic is not safe for this patient. Class Ia agents are not typically recommended for atrial arrhythmias any longer.

---

13. RT is a 65-year-old woman who presents with PSVT with a regular rhythm. RT is experiencing mild symptoms and was given unilateral carotid sinus massage with no success. If the patient has a narrow QRS interval, what medication(s) is(are) first-line agent(s) to treat this patient? Select all that apply.

    a. Adenosine
    b. Verapamil
    c. Procainamide
    d. Amiodarone

Answer a is correct.   Adenosine is indicated for the treatment of patients with PSVT with a narrow QRS interval and a regular rhythm.

Answer b is correct.   Verapamil is indicated for the treatment of patients with PSVT with a narrow QRS interval and a regular rhythm.

Answer c is incorrect.   Procainamide is used for the treatment of patients with PSVT and an irregular rhythm.

Answer d is incorrect.   Amiodarone is used for patients with PSVT with a wide QRS interval.

---

14. Which antiarrhythmic drug has the potential for causing taste disturbances?

    a. Norpace
    b. Mexitil
    c. Betapace
    d. Rythmol

Answer d is correct.   Rythmol (propafenone) can illicit taste disturbances.

Answer a is incorrect.   Norpace (disopyramide) has not been shown to produce taste disturbances.

Answer b is incorrect.   Mexitil (mexiletine) has not been shown to produce taste disturbances.

Answer c is incorrect.   Betapace (sotalol) has not been shown to produce taste disturbances.

---

15. KG is a 55-year-old man who presents with recurrent complaints of SOB and describes feeling like his heart is racing. An ECG is performed and it is determined that he is in AF with a ventricular rate of 160 beats/min. An evaluation of his LV function concluded that his ejection fraction is 35%. While the patient was still in the examination room, he reports that his symptoms have subsided and a repeat ECG was completed and it was found that the patient was in normal sinus rhythm. What medication should be prescribed to KG to control his rate?

    a. Flecainide
    b. Amiodarone
    c. Diltiazem
    d. Verapamil

Answer b is correct.   If a patient presenting with AF is stable, the initial focus of therapy is rate control. In patients with decreased LV function (EF ≤40%), digoxin or amiodarone are the recommended treatments for rate control.

Answer a is incorrect.   Flecainide is contraindicated in patients with structural heart disease and low EF.

Answer c is incorrect.   Diltiazem or other calcium channel blockers are used in AF rate control if the patient has no comorbid conditions. In addition, diltiazem is contraindicated in patients with LV dysfunction.

Answer d is incorrect.   Verapamil or other calcium channel blockers are used in AF rate control if the patient has no comorbid conditions. In addition, verapamil is contraindicated in patients with LV dysfunction.

---

16. Potential side effect(s) of dronedarone is (are): (select all that apply)

    a. Gingival hyperplasia
    b. Increased serum creatinine
    c. QT prolongation
    d. Hypothyroidism

Answer b is correct.   Increased serum creatinine is a potential side effect of dronedarone.

Answer c is correct.   QT prolongation is a potential side effect of dronedarone.

Answer a is incorrect.   Gingival hyperplasia is a side effect of nifedipine.

Answer d is incorrect.   Hypothyroidism is a potential side effect of amiodarone.

---

17. CB is a 56-year-old woman who presents with palpitations, dyspnea, and presyncope. An ECG is performed and PVCs are found. CB has a past medical history of hypertension, hyperlipidemia, and postmyocardial infarction 2 years ago. What is the treatment of choice for CB?

    a. Flecainide
    b. Propafenone
    c. Metoprolol succinate
    d. Amiodarone

Answer c is correct.   β-Blockers, such as metoprolol, are indicated for treatment of symptomatic patients with PVCs.

Answer a is incorrect.   Class Ic antiarrhythmic agents, such as flecainide, should be avoided in patients with premature ventricular contractions (PVCs) due to the increased risk of mortality postmyocardial infarction.

Answer b is incorrect.   Class Ic antiarrhythmic agents, such as propafenone, should be avoided in patients with PVCs due to the increased risk of mortality postmyocardial infarction.

Answer d is incorrect.   Amiodarone is not indicated for the treatment of PVCs.

---

18. What is the initial step in therapy for a stable patient presenting with monomorphic VT?

    a. Epinephrine
    b. Adenosine
    c. Lidocaine
    d. Immediate DCC

Answer b is correct.   The initial treatment for a stable patient with monomorphic VT is adenosine.

Answer a is incorrect.   Epinephrine is utilized in the treatment of VF or pulseless VT. Following CPR and DCC, epinephrine 1 mg IV is given every 3 to 5 minutes with no maximum dose.

Answer c is incorrect.   Lidocaine is given during the treatment of VF or pulseless VT. Following CPR, DCC, and epinephrine therapy, lidocaine 1 to 1.5 mg/kg IV can be given and repeated at a dose of 0.5 mg to 0.75 mg/kg IV every 5 to 10 minutes (maximum cumulative dose of 3 mg/kg).

Answer d is incorrect.   Immediate DCC is utilized if the patient is unstable.

---

19. Which of the following medications given during the treatment of VF or pulseless VT has no dose maximum?

    a. Vasopressin
    b. Epinephrine
    c. Lidocaine
    d. Amiodarone

Answer b is correct.   During the treatment of VF or pulseless VT, epinephrine is given 1 mg IV every 3 to 5 minutes with no maximum dose.

Answer a is incorrect.   Vasopressin no longer has a role for VF or pulseless VT.

Answer c is incorrect.   During the treatment of VF or pulseless VT, lidocaine has a maximum cumulative dose of 3 mg/kg.

Answer d is incorrect.   During the treatment of VF or pulseless VT, amiodarone can be given as a single dose of 300 mg IV, followed by a dose of 150 mg IV only.

---

20. JL is a 47-year-old man with new onset AF and seasonal allergies. After cardioversion and 4 weeks of anticoagulation, which of the following would be appropriate therapy to prevent thromboembolic complications in JL long-term?

    a. No therapy necessary
    b. Warfarin with a target INR 2.5
    c. Aspirin 325 mg daily
    d. Rivaroxaban 20 mg once daily

Answer a is correct.   Patient, JL's, CHA_2DS_2-VASc score is 0; therefore, it is appropriate to not use any antithrombotic therapy.

Answer b is incorrect.   Warfarin therapy is reserved for use in patients with a CHA_2DS_2-VASc score of 1 or more.

Answer c is incorrect.   Aspirin therapy is appropriate for use in patients with a CHA_2DS_2-VASc score of 1.

Answer d is incorrect.   Rivaroxaban therapy is reserved for use in patients with a CHA_2DS_2-VASc score of 1 or more.

---

21. Which of the following medications slows depolarization through sodium channel blockade?

    a. Brevibloc
    b. Tambocor
    c. Tiazac
    d. Covert

Answer b is correct.   Tambocor (flecainide) slows depolarization through sodium channel blockade.

Answer a is incorrect.   Brevibloc (esmolol) slows AV nodal conduction through β-blockade.

Answer c is incorrect.   Tiazac (diltiazem) slows AV nodal conduction through calcium channel blockade.

Answer d is incorrect.   Covert (ibutilide) slows repolarization through potassium channel blockade.

---

22. TG is an 85-year-old woman who is currently hospitalized for pneumonia. Her current medications include levofloxacin, albuterol via nebulization, zolpidem, and acetaminophen. On the second day of her hospitalization, her ECG reveals that she is experiencing polymorphic VT. If TG remains stable, what would be the first step of treatment?

    a. Immediate DCC
    b. Epinephrine 1 mg IV
    c. Discontinue levofloxacin
    d. Amiodarone 150 mg over 10 minutes

Answer c is correct.   If a patient is experiencing polymorphic VT (TdP) and is stable, the first step is to discontinue any agents that may be causing the arrhythmia. In this case, levofloxacin has the potential for causing polymorphic VT and should be discontinued.

Answer a is incorrect.   Immediate DCC is indicated for unstable patients with polymorphic VT.

Answer b is incorrect. Epinephrine 1 mg IV is utilized in the treatment of VF or pulseless VT.

Answer d is incorrect. Amiodarone 150 mg is utilized in the treatment of monomorphic VT.

23. Place the following Class I antiarrhythmics in order based upon classification. Start with Class Ia.

Unordered Response	Ordered Response
Lidocaine	Procainamide (Ia)
Procainamide	Lidocaine (Ib)
Flecainide	Flecainide (Ic)

24. Place the following antiarrhythmics in order based upon classification. Start with Class I.

Unordered Response	Ordered Response
Esmolol	Mexiletine Ib
Sotalol	Esmolol II
Verapamil	Sotalol III
Mexiletine	Verapamil IV

CHAPTER 10 | Oncology Overview and Supportive Care

1. Which of the following is the correct route of administration for vincristine administration?

   a. Intramuscular
   b. Intrathecal
   c. Intravenous
   d. Subcutaneous

Answer c is correct. Vincristine may be administered intravenously by short (10-15 minute) infusion, slow IV push (1-2 minutes), or 24 hour continuous infusion.

Answer a is incorrect. Vincristine is a vesicant and should not be administered intramuscularly due to causing severe tissue damage.

Answer b is incorrect. Vincristine and the other vinca alkaloids are fatal if administered intrathecally.

Answer d is incorrect. Vincristine is a vesicant and should not be administered subcutaneously due to causing severe tissue damage.

2. Select the supportive care medication that is associated with fluid retention.

   a. Darbepoetin
   b. Peg-filgrastim
   c. Amifostine
   d. Oprelvekin

Answer d is correct. Oprelvekin may cause fluid retention; therefore, use caution in heart failure and hypertension patients. Other significant cardiovascular events associated with oprelvekin include arrhythmia, pulmonary edema, and cardiac arrest.

Answer a is incorrect. Darbepoetin is not associated with causing fluid retention. It has been associated with worsening outcomes in patients with cancer and should only be used in patients who have cancer that is considered to be incurable.

Answer b is incorrect. Peg-filgrastim is not associated with causing fluid retention. The most common side effected attributed to CSFs, such as peg-filgrastim, is bone pain.

Answer c is incorrect. Amifostine is not associated with causing fluid retention. The most notable side effects from amifostine are hypotension and nausea/vomiting.

Use the following scenario to answer questions 3 to 8.

WF is a 70-year-old man with a recent diagnosis of stage IV colorectal cancer with the primary tumor in the sigmoid colon and multiple metastases found in his liver. The oncologist indicated that cure is not a realistic goal of treatment for WF because of his advanced disease. He is scheduled to begin chemotherapy with the regimen FOLFOXIRI, which contains 5-fluorouracil, leucovorin, oxaliplatin, and irinotecan. In addition, the patient is to receive bevacizumab.

3. What is the term for chemotherapy that is being used with the intention of prolonging life and improving quality of life but not of curing the patient?

   a. Curative intent
   b. Stabilization intent
   c. Palliative intent
   d. Hospice intent

Answer c is correct. When a patient has cancer that is considered incurable, such as many cancers that are metastatic or cancers that have relapsed the goal of treatment is to prolong the patient's life and to improve their quality of life.

Answer a in incorrect. In certain situations, it is highly unlikely that a cancer can be cured. Such situations include when a cancer has relapsed (returned after a prior therapy) or certain cancers that are metastatic. In these situations, the cancer is not treated with curative intent.

Answer b is incorrect. Stabilization intent is not a term that is used to describe intent of therapy. SD is used to describe response to therapy where the cancer has not decreased or increased in size by a significant amount.

Answer d is incorrect. Hospice intent is not a term that is used to describe intent of therapy. Hospice is frequently employed when patients have exhausted their treatment options. Chemotherapy is seldom used in patients on hospice.

4. Which of the medications that WF is to receive as part of his treatment regimen is not chemotherapy?

   a. 5-Fluorouracil
   b. Leucovorin
   c. Oxaliplatin
   d. Irinotecan

Answer b is correct. In this regimen, leucovorin is a drug that is being used to enhance the cytotoxicity of 5-fluorouracil. It achieves this by stabilizing the binding of 5-fluorouracil to its target site.

Answer a is incorrect. 5-fluorouracil is a chemotherapy agent that is classified as an antimetabolite.

Answer c is incorrect. Oxaliplatin is a chemotherapy agent that is classified as an alkylating agent and is also classified as a heavy metal or platinum analogue.

Answer d is incorrect. Irinotecan is a chemotherapy agent that is classified as a topoisomerase I inhibitor.

5. Which of the medication(s) in WF's treatment regimen is a cell cycle specific drug? Select all that apply.

   a. 5-Fluorouracil
   b. Oxaliplatin
   c. Irinotecan
   d. Bevacizumab

Answers a and c are correct. 5-fluorouracil is classified as an antimetabolite and acts on cells in S phase of the cell cycles. Irinotecan is classified as a topoisomerase I inhibitor and acts on cells in the S phase.

Answer b is incorrect. Oxaliplatin is an alkylating agent that is also classified as a heavy metal or platinum analogue. It is cell cycle nonspecific.

Answer d is incorrect. Bevacizumab is an MAB that binds to vascular endothelial growth factor. It is cell cycle nonspecific.

6. Shortly after receiving his first dose of chemotherapy, WF begins to experience numbness and painful tingling that is exacerbated by cold. Which of the medications in his treatment regimen is most likely causing these new symptoms?

   a. 5-Fluorouracil
   b. Leucovorin
   c. Oxaliplatin
   d. Irinotecan

Answer c is correct. Platinum agents (oxaliplatin, carboplatin, cisplatin) are known to cause neuralgias. Oxaliplatin is unique in the neuralgias it causes are typically associated with cold. This could include cold air in the environment as well as cold food or drink.

Answer a is incorrect. 5-fluorouracil is not associated with causing neuropathy.

Answer b is incorrect. Leucovorin is not associated with causing neuropathy.

Answer d is incorrect. Irinotecan is not associated with causing neuropathy.

7. Approximately 8 weeks after the beginning of his chemotherapy, WF begins complaining about feeling more tired and weak lately. He also mentions that he becomes short of breath after even moderate physical activity. Blood tests showed a hemoglobin level of 8.6 g/dL. Which of the following is correct regarding WF's anemia?

   a. He should begin treatment with erythropoietin to treat chemotherapy-induced anemia.
   b. He should receive a blood transfusion to treat severe anemia from blood loss.
   c. He should begin treatment with darbepoetin once his hemoglobin level fall below 8 g/dL.
   d. He is not a candidate for treatment with an erythropoiesis stimulating agent since his cancer is being treated with curative intent.

Answer a is correct. Anemia is a common complication from chemotherapy. Typically, treatment with an erythropoiesis stimulating agent (erythropoietin or darbepoetin) will be considered in these patients. Due to concerns over safety, including evidence that shows these drugs can worsen cancer outcomes, the erythropoietin stimulating agents should only be used in patients who are receiving chemotherapy for palliative intent. That is to say, the cancer is considered to be incurable.

Answer b is incorrect. The patient is experiencing mild to moderate symptoms of anemia and blood transfusion is not typically used in this situation. Most clinician will consider transfusion when hemoglobin falls below 7 g/dL or if patient is experiencing severe symptoms such as hypotension or shortness of breath at rest.

Answer c is incorrect. There is no need to wait for the hemoglobin to fall below 8 g/dL prior to initiation of darbepoetin.

Answer d is incorrect. As stated in the case scenario, WF's cancer is considered to be incurable. This indicates that his cancer treatment is being used with palliative intent.

8. After the completions for 4 cycles of his chemotherapy, WF undergoes imaging scans to determine the cancer's response to therapy. The imaging tests reveal that the patient's total tumor burden has decreased by approximately 65%. Which of the following best describes WF's response to his treatment?

   a. Progressive disease
   b. Stable disease
   c. Partial response
   d. Complete response

Answer c is correct. A PR occurs when the tumor decreases in size by at least 50%.

Answer a is incorrect. PD in the term for cancer that grows despite treatment.

Answer b is incorrect. SD indicates that the cancer has not grown and may have decreased in size by up to 50%.

Answer d is incorrect. CR describes the complete absence of any known cancer cells following treatment. Patients who achieve a CR are described as being in remission.

---

9. Rank the following MABs in order for lowest immunogenicity to highest immunogenicity.

Unordered options	Ordered response
Ibritumomab	Denosumab
Rituximab	Bevacizumab
Pertuzumab	Rituximab
Denosumab	Ibritumomab

For MABs, the immunogenicity can be predicted based on the nomenclature. The syllable immediately preceding the "-mab" indicates the degree of foreign protein. "-mo" refers to mouse, and is most immunogenic, "-xi" is chimeric, a mix of foreign and human protein, "-zu-" is humanized, mostly human protein, and "-u-" is fully human and least immunogenic.

---

10. A patient is newly initiated on erlotinib for the treatment of nonsmall cell lung cancer. Which of the following medications may pose a drug/drug interaction with his new medication?

    a. Phenytoin
    b. Pregabalin
    c. Heparin
    d. Sulfamethoxazole/trimethoprim

Answer a is correct. Many kinase inhibitors, including erlotinib have multiple drug interactions through the CYP450 system. Erlotinib is an inhibitor and substrate of 3A4 and is thus sensitive to other substrates of the enzyme as well as inducers and inhibitors of the enzyme, such as amiodarone.

Answer b is incorrect. Erlotinib has drug/drug interactions with many anticonvulsants due to activity related to CYP450 3A4. Pregabalin does not affect this enzyme system.

Answer c is incorrect. Heparin does not have drug/drug interaction with erlotinib. However, erlotinib can cause myelosuppression, including thrombocytopenia, and should be used with caution in patients receiving medications that can increase risk of bleeding.

Answer d is incorrect. There are no known drug interactions between sulfamethoxazole/trimethoprim and erlotinib.

Use the following scenario to answer questions 11 to 15.

YM is a 62-year-old woman with a recent diagnosis of stage III diffuse large B-cell lymphoma. Her disease is characterized by multiple areas of involvement including the spleen, pelvic lymph nodes, and mediastinal lymph nodes. She is scheduled to begin chemotherapy with the regimen EPOCH-R, which includes etoposide, prednisone, vincristine, cyclophosphamide, doxorubicin, and rituximab.

11. Oncovin is the brand name of which of the medications in YM's treatment regimen?

    a. Etoposide
    b. Vincristine
    c. Doxorubicin
    d. Rituximab

Answer b is correct. Oncovin is the brand name of vincristine. In many chemotherapy regimens, including EPOCH, it is represented by the letter O.

Answer a is incorrect. The brand name of etoposide is VePesid. It is also available under other brand names such as Toposar. It is sometimes referred to as VP-16.

Answer c is incorrect. The original brand name of doxorubicin is Adriamycin. In some chemotherapy regimens, such as ABVD for Hodgkin's lymphoma, it is represented by the letter A. It is also represented by the letter H, like in EPOCH, due to another name for doxorubicin, hydroxydaunorubicin.

Answer d is incorrect. Rituxan is the brand name of rituximab.

---

12. The medical team asks the pharmacists if YM needs to receive any medications to prevent allergic reactions from her treatment regimen. Which of the medications in her treatment regimen is most likely to cause an infusion reaction and could benefit from premedication with acetaminophen and diphenhydramine?

    a. Cyclophosphamide
    b. Vincristine
    c. Doxorubicin
    d. Rituximab

Answer d is correct. Rituximab is a chimeric MAB ("-xi-") indicating that it has a substantial amount of nonhuman protein. Because of this, patients receiving rituximab are at risk of developing a reaction during the infusion. Patients typically receive acetaminophen and diphenhydramine to lessen the risk of infusion reactions from rituximab.

Answer a is incorrect. Cyclophosphamide is not associated with infusion reactions.

Answer b is incorrect. Vincristine is not associated with infusion reactions. The primary concern with infusion of vincristine is risk of extravasation since it is a vesicant.

Answer c is incorrect. Doxorubicin is not associated with infusion reactions. The primary concern with infusion of doxorubicin is risk of extravasation since it is a vesicant.

13. The EPOCH-R regimen that YM is receiving is considered to be a high risk of developing febrile neutropenia. Which of the following is a medication that could be used to help YM's white blood cell count recover faster and decrease her risk of developing febrile neutropenia? Select all that apply.

    a. Peg-filgrastim
    b. Oprelvekin
    c. Sargramostim
    d. Darbepoetin

Answers a and c are correct. Because this patient is at high risk for developing febrile neutropenia preventative medication is warranted. The CSFs (filgrastim, sargramostim, and peg-filgrastim) have been shown to decrease the risk of febrile neutropenia in patients receiving myelosuppressive chemotherapy. They are recommended to use if the risk of developing febrile neutropenia is at least 20%. The agents decrease the duration and severity of neutropenia following chemotherapy, thus decreasing the risk of infection.

Answer b is incorrect. Oprelvekin is a drug that is used to decrease the risk of thrombocytopenia following chemotherapy.

Answer d is incorrect. Darbepoetin is used in the treatment of chemotherapy-induced anemia in patients who are receiving chemotherapy for the treatment of incurable cancer.

14. Approximately 4 hours after the infusion of the first cycle of chemotherapy, YM begins experience severe nausea and has episodes of vomiting. Which of the medications in her treatment regimen is the most likely to be causing her nausea and vomiting?

    a. Etoposide
    b. Prednisone
    c. Cyclophosphamide
    d. Vincristine

Answer c is correct. Cyclophosphamide is an alkylating agent and is considered to be a noncell cycle specific chemotherapy. Like all alkylating agents, CINV is a concern. At doses typically used in the treatment of cancer, cyclophosphamide is moderately emetogenic (risk of nausea/vomiting is 30%-90%). However, when you use high doses (greater than 1000 mg/m^2) or in combination with an anthracycline such as doxorubicin, it is highly emetogenic (≥90% risk of nausea/vomiting)

Answer a is incorrect. Etoposide is a topoisomerase II inhibitor and is considered to be cell cycle specific chemotherapy. It has a low emetogenic potential.

Answer b is incorrect. Prednisone is a corticosteroid. The oral use of prednisone could be associated with some nausea and vomiting and taking it with food should be considered. Corticosteroids like prednisone, and especially dexamethasone, are frequently used to prevent chemotherapy-induced nausea/vomiting.

Answer d is incorrect. Vincristine is a vinca alkaloid and is considered to be cell cycle specific. It is considered to be minimally emetogenic.

15. On her second cycle, during the infusion of the doxorubicin YM begins experiencing extreme pain at the injection site. The nurse observes new onset redness and swelling around the infusion site and is concerned that extravasation has occurred. Which of the following agents is the most appropriate to treat this extravasation injury?

    a. Hyaluronidase
    b. Dexrazoxane
    c. Sodium thiosulfate
    d. Silver sulfadiazine

Answer b is correct. Dexrazoxane is indicated for the treatment of extravasation injury from anthracyclines. It works by inhibiting the production of free radicals. It should be administered as soon as extravasation is detected and repeated for 3 total days of therapy.

Answer a is incorrect. Hyaluronidase is incorrect. Hyaluronidase breaks down hyaluronic acid, allowing an extravasated drug to dissipate, decrease the concentration of the drug at the site of extravasation. Before dexrazoxane was known to be beneficial for anthracycline extravasation, hyaluronidase was commonly used.

Answer c is incorrect. Sodium thiosulfate is used in the treatment of extravasation of alkylating agents. It binds to the active sites on the alkylating agents, thus neutralizing them.

Answer d is incorrect. Silver sulfadiazine is a topical preparation that is used in the treatment of skin burns. It does not have a role in the treatment of chemotherapy extravasation.

16. Select the chemoprotectant that supplies a free thiol that binds to acrolein preventing a major antineoplastic adverse reaction.

    a. Mesna
    b. Leucovorin
    c. Dexrazoxane
    d. Hydroxyurea

Answer a is correct. Mesna is oxidized to dimesna which in turn is reduced in the kidney back to mesna, supplying a free thiol group which binds to and inactivates acrolein, the urotoxic metabolite of ifosfamide and cyclophosphamide.

Answer b is incorrect. Leucovorin is used as a rescue agent to decrease toxicity from methotrexate. It is also used to enhance the toxicity of 5-fluorouracil.

Answer c is incorrect. Dexrazoxane is utilized to decrease the risk of cardiac toxicity from anthracyclines. It is also administered to prevent tissue damage following extravasation of an anthracycline.

Answer d is incorrect. Hydroxyurea is a miscellaneous chemotherapy agent. It is used to acutely lower white blood cell counts in patients with leukocytosis. It is also used to decrease the frequency of painful crises in patients with sickle cell disease.

Use the following scenario to answer questions 17 to 21.

JH is a 56-year-old woman who was recently diagnosed with stage IIIa adenocarcinoma of the lung. She has an extensive smoking history, smoking one and a half packs of cigarettes per day for 30 years. Her oncologist indicated that the cancer is too large to operate on and she will receive chemotherapy first to shrink the tumor, followed later by surgery. She is to receive chemotherapy with cisplatin and pemetrexed.

17. Prior to her diagnosis of lung cancer, would JH have been an appropriate candidate for lung cancer screening?

    a. Yes, she would have been a good candidate for lung cancer screening.
    b. No, she would not have been a good candidate for lung cancer screening because she is too old.
    c. No, she would not have been a good candidate for lung cancer because she smoked too much.
    d. No, she would not have been a good candidate for lung cancer screening because she does not have chronic obstructive pulmonary disease (COPD).

Answer a is correct.   Screening for lung cancer is recommended for people between the ages of 55 and 80 years who have at least a 30-pack year history and have been an active smoker at some point in the last 15 years. The screening test that is used is a helical CT scan.

Answer b is incorrect.   The patient's current age is 56, she is within the recommended 55 to 80 years range for lung cancer screening.

Answer c is incorrect.   Her smoking history is more than 30-pack years. She has smoked 1.5 packs per day for 30 years, giving her a 45-pack year history.

Answer d is incorrect.   Presence or absence of comorbid conditions, including COPD are not considered when recommended screening for lung cancer.

18. What is the term that best describes the timing of JH's chemotherapy in relation to her surgery?

    a. Adjuvant
    b. Adjunct
    c. Neoadjuvant
    d. Neoadjunct

Answer c is correct.   When a cancer is so large that it is difficult to operate on, chemotherapy is frequently given first to shrink the tumor. This is referred to as "neoadjuvant" therapy.

Answer a is incorrect.   Adjuvant chemotherapy is given after surgery.

Answer b is incorrect.   Adjunct is not a term used to describe chemotherapy timing.

Answer d is incorrect.   Neoadjunct is not a term used to describe chemotherapy timing.

19. Which of the following organ toxicities is most likely to occur as a result of the patient receiving cisplatin?

    a. Hepatotoxicity
    b. Nephrotoxicity
    c. Pulmonary toxicity
    d. Cardiotoxicity

Answer b is correct.   The dose limiting toxicity of cisplatin is nephrotoxicity. Cisplatin is eliminated renally and can cause direct damage to the kidneys. This can result in increased serum creatinine and electrolyte disturbance such as hypokalemia. Cisplatin is typically administered with aggressive hydration to promote the elimination of cisplatin and decrease nephrotoxicity.

Answer a is incorrect.   Cisplatin is not known to cause hepatotoxicity.

Answer c is incorrect.   Cisplatin is not known to cause pulmonary toxicity.

Answer d is incorrect.   Cisplatin is not known to cause cardiotoxicity.

20. Which of the following medications should the patient receive to decrease toxicity from pemetrexed? Select all that apply.

    a. Folic acid
    b. Cyanocobalamin
    c. Thiamine
    d. Dexamethasone

Answers a, b, and d are correct.   Dexamethasone is given to patients receiving pemetrexed to prevent the development of rash. Cyanocobalamin (vitamin B12) is administered intramuscularly once a month and folic acid is given orally every day to decrease the severity of myelosuppression and other toxicities from pemetrexed.

Answer c is incorrect.   Thiamine does not prevent toxicity from pemetrexed.

21. Two year after her initial lung cancer diagnosis, JH has achieved a complete remission and has been cancer free for over a year following the completion of all her therapy. She is interested in early detection of other types of cancer. Which of the following types of cancer should JH be screened for? Select all that apply.

    a. Breast cancer
    b. Colorectal cancer
    c. Melanoma
    d. Uterine cancer

Answers a and b are correct.   The patient's current age is 58. Screening for breast cancer is recommended to start at ages 40 to 45 years of age and continue as long as a patient's life expectancy is at least 10 years. Given that her cancer is currently in remission, there is no reason to think her life expectancy is shortened. Screening for colorectal cancer is recommended to commence at age 50.

Answer c is incorrect. Routine screening for the early detection of melanoma is not recommended for the general population.

Answer d is incorrect. Routine screening for the early detection of uterine cancer is not recommended for the general population. Screening for cervical cancer may be appropriate for JH at this time.

Use the following scenario to answer questions 22 to 26.

HM is a 51-year-old postmenopausal female with a recent diagnosis of stage II ductal carcinoma of the breast. Pathology reports revealed her tumor is estrogen/progesterone receptor positive and HER2 negative. She undergoes a bilateral mastectomy and is scheduled to begin chemotherapy with the regimen AC → T. This regimen contains doxorubicin and cyclophosphamide followed by paclitaxel.

22. Which of the following toxicities may occur as the result of administration of paclitaxel in HM?

    a. Ototoxicity
    b. Nephrotoxicity
    c. Cerebellar toxicity
    d. Peripheral neuropathy

Answer d is correct. Paclitaxel, like all microtubule causing drugs is known to cause peripheral neuropathy.

Answer a is incorrect. Paclitaxel is not known to cause ototoxicity. An example of a chemotherapy agent that causes ototoxicity is cisplatin.

Answer b is incorrect. Paclitaxel is not known to cause nephrotoxicity. An example of a chemotherapy agent that causes nephrotoxicity is cisplatin.

Answer c is incorrect. Paclitaxel is not known to cause cerebellar toxicity. An example of a chemotherapy agent that causes cerebellar toxicity is cytarabine.

---

23. Which of the following is a long-term toxicity that may occur in HM as a result of the administration of doxorubicin?

    a. Cardiotoxicity
    b. Nephrotoxicity
    c. Colitis
    d. Pulmonary toxicity

Answer a is correct. Anthracyclines are well known to cause a delayed cardiotoxicity directly linked to the cumulative dose of the drug. This late onset cardiotoxicity manifests as heart failure.

Answer b is incorrect. Doxorubicin is not known to cause nephrotoxicity. An example of a chemotherapy known to cause nephrotoxicity is cisplatin.

Answer c is incorrect. Doxorubicin is not known to cause colitis. An example of an anticancer medication known to cause colitis is ipilimumab.

Answer d is incorrect. Doxorubicin is not known to cause pulmonary toxicity. An example of a chemotherapy known to cause pulmonary toxicity is bleomycin.

---

24. After the completion of her chemotherapy, the oncologist plans to initiate hormonal therapy. Which of the following hormonal therapies is an appropriate choice to treat HM's breast cancer?

    a. Degarelix
    b. Bicalutamide
    c. Letrozole
    d. Raloxifene

Answer c is correct. Aromatase inhibitors such as letrozole are indicated for the treatment of hormone receptor positive breast cancer. They are typically initiated after the completion of chemotherapy. Aromatase inhibitors can only be used in postmenopausal women while tamoxifen is preferred in premenopausal women.

Answer a is incorrect. Degarelix is a liutenizing-hormone releasing hormone (LHRH) antagonist indicated for the treatment of prostate cancer.

Answer b is incorrect. Bicalutamide is an antiandrogen indicated for the treatment of prostate cancer.

Answer d is incorrect. Raloxifene is a select estrogen receptor modulator. It was originally indicated for the treatment of osteoporosis in postmenopausal women. It has shown efficacy in the prevention of breast cancer and is also approved for this indication. It has not been studied in the treatment of women who have already developed breast cancer.

---

25. HM is concerned about her daughter developing breast cancer and is asking about early detection recommendations for her. Her daughter is 29. Which of the following is the most appropriate breast cancer screening recommendation for HM's 29-year-old daughter?

    a. Breast cancer screening is not recommended for the general population.
    b. She should begin screening for breast cancer now.
    c. She should begin screening for breast cancer when she turns 50 years old.
    d. She should begin screening for breast cancer when she turns 55 years old.

Answer c is correct. Multiple organizations including the American Cancer Society (ACS) and the United States Preventative Services Task Force (USPSTF) recommend screening for breast cancer. There is disagreement between ACS (age 40-45) and USPSTF (age 50) at what age screening should begin.

Answer a is incorrect. Multiple organizations including the ACS and the USPSTF recommend screening for breast cancer.

Answer b is incorrect. She is currently not old enough to benefit from screening for breast cancer.

Answer d is incorrect. Both ACS (age 40-45) and USPSTF (age 50) recommend beginning screening for breast cancer prior to age 55.

---

26. Three years after the completion of her chemotherapy, HM presents to her primary care provider with abdominal pain and increased yellowing of the skin. Laboratory evaluation showed increased bilirubin and markedly elevated liver function tests. Imaging scans showed breast cancer recurrence with widespread metastases to the liver. Which of the following chemotherapy agents used in the treatment of relapsed breast cancer should be used with caution in HM due to her liver disease?

    a. Eribulin
    b. Docetaxel
    c. Gemcitabine
    d. Ixabepilone

Answers a, b, and d are correct. Each of these agents is eliminated hepatically and should be used in caution with patients who have cancer that has spread to the liver, especially if there are signs of liver damage such as increased bilirubin or liver function tests. Dose adjustments are recommended depending on the level of hepatic impairment.

Answer c is incorrect. Gemcitabine is eliminated renally and does not require any special considerations in patients with liver metastases or otherwise compromised hepatic function.

CHAPTER **11 | Immune System**

1. The immune system is designed to attack and destroy foreign antigens and should be able to differentiate self from nonself. Failure to differentiate self from nonself may lead to which of the following? Select all that apply.

    a. Addison disease
    b. Rheumatoid arthritis (RA)
    c. Systemic lupus erythematosus (SLE)
    d. Multiple sclerosis (MS)

Failure to differentiate self from nonself may lead to an autoimmune disease. An autoimmune disease is a condition that occurs when the immune system mistakenly attacks and destroys healthy body tissue.

Answer a is correct. Addison disease is an autoimmune disease. Addison disease is a disorder that results when your body produces insufficient amount of certain hormones produced by your adrenal glands. The gradual destruction of the adrenal cortex, the outer layer of the adrenal glands, by the body's immune system causes up to 80% of Addison cases. In autoimmune disorders, the immune system makes antibodies that attack the body's own tissues or organs and slowly destroy them. Adrenal insufficiency occurs when at least 90% of the adrenal cortex has been destroyed. As a result, often both cortisol and aldosterone are lacking.

Answer b is correct. RA is a chronic disease that leads to inflammation of the joints and surrounding tissues. The cause of RA is unknown, but is considered to be an autoimmune disease. The disease usually begins gradually with fatigue, loss of appetite, morning stiffness, widespread muscle aches, and weakness. Eventually, joint pain appears. When the joint is not used for a while, it can become warm, tender, and stiff. When the lining of the joint becomes inflamed, it gives off more fluid and the joint becomes swollen. Joint pain is often felt on both sides of the body and may affect the fingers, wrists, elbows, shoulders, hips, knees, ankles, toes, and neck. Additional symptoms include: anemia, eye burning, hand and feet deformities, limited range of motion, low-grade fever, lung inflammation (pleurisy), nodules under the skin (sign of severe disease), numbness/tingling, and paleness. Joint destruction may occur within 1 to 2 years after the appearance of the disease.

Answer c is correct. SLE is a chronic, inflammatory autoimmune disorder. SLE may affect the skin, joints, kidneys, and other organs. Symptoms vary from person to person, and may come and go. The condition may affect one organ or body system at first. Others may become involved later. Almost all people with SLE have joint pain and most develop arthritis. Frequently affected joints are the fingers, hands, wrists, and knees. Inflammation of various parts of the heart may occur as pericarditis, endocarditis, or myocarditis. Chest pain and arrhythmias may result from these conditions. General symptoms include arthritis, fatigue, fever, general discomfort (malaise), muscle aches, nausea and vomiting, pleural effusions, pleurisy, seizures, sensitivity to sunlight, and skin rash. (A butterfly rash over the cheeks and bridge of the nose, affects about half of those with SLE. The rash gets worse when in sunlight.)

Answer d is correct. MS is a potentially debilitating disease in which your body's immune system eats away at the protective sheath (myelin) that covers your nerves. Damage to myelin causes interference in the communication between your brain, spinal cord, and other areas of your body. This condition may result in deterioration of the nerves themselves, a process that's not reversible.

---

2. Select the nonspecific functional division of the immune system.

    a. Innate
    b. Adaptive

c. Granulocytes

d. Lymphocytes

Answer a is correct. The innate immune system is the nonspecific functional division of the immune system. There are two functional divisions, innate (nonspecific) and adaptive (specific).

Answer b is incorrect. While the adaptive immune system is a functional division of the immune system, it is the specific division.

Answer c is incorrect. Granulocytes are WBCs that make up part of the innate (nonspecific) immune system.

Answer d is incorrect. Lymphocytes are WBCs that make up part of the adaptive (specific) immune system.

---

3. The difference between the innate and adaptive immune system is described by which of the following? Select all that apply.

a. Specificity
b. Memory
c. Strength
d. Size

Answer a is correct. The adaptive immune exhibits specificity compared to the innate division. The adaptive immune response can evolve with each subsequent infection, whereas the innate immune response stays the same with each infection.

Answer b is correct. The adaptive immune exhibits memory compared to the innate division. The adaptive immune response can evolve with each subsequent infection, whereas the innate immune response stays the same with each infection.

Answer c is incorrect. Both the adaptive and innate immune divisions display a significant amount of strength to fight off pathogens. While we are describing the innate and adaptive systems separately, they work collectively to attack and destroy foreign antigens/pathogens.

Answer d is incorrect. Size is not a factor in the action of the WBCs. Size is measured when describing red blood cells. The size of the red blood cell is measured via the mean corpuscular volume (MCV).

---

4. Physical and chemical defenses compose the innate immune system and consist of which of the following? Select all that apply.

a. Skin
b. Lymphocytes
c. Granulocytes
d. Normal urine flow

Answers a and d are correct. The skin and coughing are examples of physical defenses of the innate immune system.

Other examples of physical innate immunity are: pH of the stomach, coughing, cilia lining the epithelium, normal bacterial flora of the throat, and gastrointestinal tract.

Answer c is correct. Granulocytes are part of the chemical defense of the innate immune system. Cells that make up the granulocytes are: neutrophils, basophils, eosinophils, and monocytes.

Answer b is incorrect. Lymphocytes are part of the adaptive immune system.

---

5. Examples of physical defense innate immunity include which of the following? Select all that apply.

a. Skin
b. Stomach pH
c. Normal flora of gastrointestinal tract
d. Coughing

Answer a is correct. The skin is an example of physical innate immunity.

Answer b is correct. The pH of the stomach is an example of physical innate immunity.

Answer c is correct. The normal flora of the gastrointestinal tract is an example of physical innate immunity.

Answer d is correct. Coughing is an example of physical innate immunity.

---

6. Select the medication that may cause SJS and in turn alter the skin, leading to an easy portal of entry for bacterial pathogens. Select all that apply.

a. Carbamazepine
b. Lamotrigine
c. Loratadine
d. Levothyroxine

SJS is a *rare*, serious disorder in which the skin and mucous membranes react severely to a medication or infection.

Answer a is correct. Carbamazepine has been associated with causing SJS.

Answer b is correct. Lamotrigine has been associated with causing SJS. Lamotrigine has a black box warning stating: severe and potentially life-threatening skin rashes requiring hospitalization have been reported; risk may be increased by coadministration with valproic acid, higher than recommended starting doses, and rapid dose titration. The majority of the cases occur in the first 8 weeks; however, isolated cases may occur after prolonged treatment. Discontinue at first sign of rash unless rash is clearly not drug related.

Answer c is incorrect. Loratadine has not been associated with SJS.

Answer d is incorrect. Levothyroxine is not expected to cause SJS.

---

7. Select the agent(s) that may cause pneumonia by altering the pH of the stomach. Select all that apply.

   a. Omeprazole
   b. Ranitidine
   c. Ceftriaxone
   d. Sucralfate

Medications with the ability to alter the pH of the stomach may change the gastrointestinal bacterial flora and increase risk of infections. Antisecretory agents such as proton pump inhibitors have been associated with the development of bacterial infections. Given the frequency with which antisecretory agents are utilized, this is a rare adverse reaction (although causal relationship has not been established). Gram-negative nosocomial pneumonia may result from retrograde colonization of the pharynx from the stomach, and this may be more likely when the gastric pH is relatively high.

Answer a is correct. Omeprazole and other proton pump inhibitors may cause infections by altering the normal bacterial flora.

Answer b is correct. Ranitidine and other H_2 antagonists may cause infections by altering the normal bacterial flora.

Answer c is incorrect. Ceftriaxone does not have any effect on the pH of the stomach.

Answer d is incorrect. Sucralfate provides a protective coating within the stomach to minimize contact with acid. Sucralfate would not be expected to have an effect on the pH.

---

8. Select the medication that may alter the normal flora of the gastrointestinal tract leading to infection. Select all that apply.

   a. Lansoprazole
   b. Clindamycin
   c. Pantoprazole
   d. Levofloxacin

Answer a is correct. Lansoprazole may alter the normal flora of the gastrointestinal tract leading to an infection. Medications with the ability to alter the pH of the stomach may change the gastrointestinal bacterial flora and increase risk of infections. Antisecretory agents such as proton pump inhibitors have been associated with the development of bacterial infections.

Answer b is correct. Clindamycin and other anti-infectives that alter gastrointestinal flora leave the patient at an increased risk of infection (*Clostridium difficile* infection).

Answer c is correct. Pantoprazole may alter the normal flora of the gastrointestinal tract leading to an infection. Medications with the ability to alter the pH of the stomach may change the gastrointestinal bacterial flora and increase

risk of infections. Antisecretory agents such as proton pump inhibitors have been associated with the development of bacterial infections.

Answer d is correct. Levofloxacin and other anti-infectives that alter gastrointestinal flora leave the patient at an increased risk of infection (*C. difficile* infection).

---

9. Select the chemical cell(s) of the innate immune system. Select all that apply.

   a. Neutrophils
   b. Eosinophils
   c. Basophils
   d. Granulocytes

Answer a is correct. Neutrophils are chemical cells of the innate immune system. Neutrophils may also be known as segs, mature neutrophils, polymorphonuclear cells, and PMNs. Bands or stabs are immature neutrophils.

Answer b is correct. Eosinophils are chemical cells of the innate immune system.

Answer c is correct. Basophils are chemical cells of the innate immune system.

Answer d is correct. Granulocytes are chemical cells of the innate immune system. Granulocytes are composed of neutrophils, basophils, eosinophils, and monocytes. Sometimes the term granulocyte is used incorrectly. Clinicians often use the term granulocytes to refer to neutrophils. This is done because neutrophils make up 80% to 90% of the granulocytes.

---

10. Innate cells may be evaluated clinically by ordering which laboratory test? Select all that apply.

   a. CRP
   b. Chemokines
   c. Complete blood cell count
   d. CD4 count

Answer a is correct. CRP is an innate cell and has become very useful clinically. CRP is a plasma protein that can increase up to 1000 times its baseline concentration. Clinical evidence found that CRP is also released in response to inflammatory markers present within atherosclerotic plaques and leads to cardiovascular disease. Cholesterol medications (HMG-CoA reductase inhibitors/statins) decrease CRP levels and rosuvastatin was found to decrease cardiovascular disease in patients with elevated CRP levels.

Answer c is correct. The innate cells are one of the most widely monitored clinical laboratory tests. Innate cells may be evaluated by ordering a CBC. When a CBC is ordered, part of the laboratory test reports a tally of the total WBCs in a given volume of blood plus the relative percentages of each cell type contributes to the total. A CBC also reports lymphocytes, part of the adaptive immune system.

Answer b is incorrect.   Chemokines are not part of the innate immune system, but rather play an essential role in linking the innate and adaptive immune response by orchestrating traffic. The chemokine system consists of a group of small polypeptides and their receptors. Chemokines possess four cysteines. Based upon the positions of the cysteines, chemokines fall into one of two categories: (1) CC group or (2) CXC group. Maraviroc selectively and reversibly binds to the chemokine receptor (CCR5) co-receptors located on CD4 cells. A CCR5 assay must be ordered before a patient can be prescribed maraviroc for HIV. Not all HIV patients will have the CCR5 chemokine on their CD4 cell.

Answer d is incorrect.   A CD4 count is a T-lymphocyte that is part of the adaptive system.

---

11. Select the innate cell that represents the majority of granulocytes and serves as the primary defense against bacterial infections.

    a. Lymphocytes
    b. Neutrophils
    c. Monocytes
    d. Eosinophils
    e. Basophils

Answer b is correct.   Neutrophils represent the majority of granulocytes (80%-90%) and leukocytes (40%-70%) and serve as the primary defense against bacterial infections. Neutrophils, also termed as segs or polymorphonuclear cells, migrate from the bloodstream into infected or inflamed tissue. In this migration process known as chemotaxis, neutrophils reach the desired site and recognize, adhere to, and phagocytose pathogens. During phagocytosis, the pathogen is internalized within the phagocyte. The neutrophil releases its granular contents which lead to destruction of the engulfed pathogen.

Answer a is incorrect.   Lymphocytes are not part of the granulocyte cells; they are key cells for the adaptive immune system and consist of B lymphocytes (humoral) and T lymphocytes (cell-mediated). T lymphocytes are tailored to defend against infections that are intracellular (viral infections), whereas B lymphocytes secrete antibodies that neutralize pathogens prior to their entry into host cells.

Answer c is incorrect.   Monocytes account for 1% to 10% of circulating granulocytes and leukocytes, remove dead/damaged tissues, destroy cancer cells, and regulate against foreign substances.

Answer d is incorrect.   Eosinophils account for less than 7% of circulating granulocytes and leukocytes and are present in the intestinal mucosa and lungs, two locations where foreign proteins enter the body. Eosinophils can phagocytize, kill, and digest bacteria and yeast. Elevations of eosinophil counts are highly suggestive of parasitic infections, or may be associated with allergies and asthma.

Answer e is incorrect.   Basophils are the least common granulocyte, accounting for 0.1% to 0.3% of granulocytes. Signs and symptoms of allergic responses are linked to basophil and mast cell products. Basophils may be associated with immediate hypersensitivity and delayed hypersensitivity reactions, and increase in chronic inflammation and leukemia.

---

12. Select the innate cell that is immature.

    a. Basophil
    b. Eosinophil
    c. Band
    d. Neutrophil
    e. Macrophage

Answer c is correct.   The neutrophil (mature and immature) releases its granular content, which leads to destruction of the engulfed pathogen. The less mature form of a neutrophil is a band. During an acute infection, there is an increase in the percentage of neutrophils as they are released from the bone marrow. Less mature band forms may also be released. These immature neutrophils are still considered active. The appearance of band cells is called a shift to the left.

Answer a is incorrect.   Basophils are mature cells.

Answer b is incorrect.   Eosinophils are mature cells.

Answer d is incorrect.   Neutrophils are mature cells.

Answer e is incorrect.   Macrophages are mature cells.

---

13. Select the cell that is part of cell-mediated immunity.

    a. B lymphocyte
    b. Neutrophil
    c. Macrophage
    d. T lymphocyte
    e. Complement

Answer d is correct.   T lymphocytes compose the cell-mediated part of the adaptive functional division and are tailored to defend against infections that are intracellular (viral infections).

Answer a is incorrect.   B lymphocytes compose the humoral part of the adaptive immune system and secrete antibodies that neutralize pathogens prior to their entry into host cells. B cells, once activated by T cells or antigen presenting cells, become a plasma cell that will produce one of five immunoglobulin types: IgA, IgD, IgE, IgG, or IgM.

Answer b is incorrect.   Neutrophils are key cells of the innate chemical immunity that fight off bacterial infections.

Answer c is incorrect.   Macrophages are the main scavenger cells of the immune system. In addition to attacking foreign cells, they are involved in the destruction of old erythrocytes, denatured plasma proteins, and plasma lipids.

Answer e is incorrect. The complement system is a mediator of innate immunity. The complement system consists of multiple proteins that play a key role in immune defense. The complement system serves as an adjunct or "complement" to humoral immunity.

---

14. B and T lymphocytes may be distinguished from each other by the presence of lineage specific membrane markers termed:

   a. CD
   b. Complement
   c. CRP
   d. Chemokines
   e. CCR5 coreceptor

Answer a is correct. Morphologic differentiation of lymphocytes is difficult and visual inspection of a blood smear cannot distinguish between T and B cells. Fortunately, lymphocytes can be distinguished by the presence of lineage-specific membrane markers, termed CD. Mature T cells are CD4 or CD8 and B cells are CD20. Identification of the subtype of lymphocyte is not a routine clinical hematology test; lymphocytes are reported as a total lymphocyte count on the CBC. An exception is the reporting/monitoring of CD4 cells for patients with HIV.

Answer b is incorrect. The complement system is a mediator of innate immunity. The complement system consists of multiple proteins that play a key role in immune defense. The complement system serves as an adjunct or "complement" to humoral immunity.

Answer c is incorrect. CRP is an acute phase reactant produced by the liver during early stages of infection or inflammation. Acute phase reactants or proteins increase in response to inflammatory stimuli such as tissue injury or infection. Recent clinical evidence found that CRP is also released in response to inflammatory markers present within atherosclerotic plaques and leads to cardiovascular disease. Cholesterol medications (HMG-CoA reductase inhibitors/statins) decrease CRP levels and rosuvastatin was found to decrease cardiovascular disease in patients with elevated CRP levels.

Answer d is incorrect. Chemokines play an essential role in linking the innate and adaptive immune response by orchestrating traffic. The chemokine system consists of a group of small polypeptides and their receptors. Chemokines possess four cysteines. Based upon the positions of the cysteines, almost all chemokines fall into one of two categories: (1) CC group or (2) CXC group.

Answer e is incorrect. CCR5 is a chemokine receptor located on CD4 cells. Maraviroc blocks CCR5 and this CCR5 antagonism prevents interaction between the human CCR5 co-receptor and the gp120 subunit of the viral envelope glycoprotein, thereby inhibiting gp120 conformational change required for fusion of CCR5 HIV with the CD4 cell and subsequent entry.

---

15. A neutrophil count greater than 12,000 cells/mm^3 is termed which of the following?

   a. Neutrophilia
   b. Bandemia
   c. Lymphocytosis
   d. Agranulocytosis

Answer a is correct. Neutrophilia is an elevated neutrophil count. A normal neutrophil count is 2.3 to 7.7×10^3 cells/mm^3. Rarely do you hear clinicians say the term neutrophilia. The term leukocytosis will most likely be used since neutrophils are the predominant WBC. The term leukocytosis could be caused by any of the five WBCs.

Answer b is incorrect. A bandemia is an increase in immature neutrophils and is termed a shift to the left. A normal band count is 0 to 10×10^3 cells/mm^3. However, it is possible with a neutrophil count of 12,000 cells/mm^3 that a bandemia may also be present.

Answer c is incorrect. Lymphocytosis is an increase in lymphocytes. A normal lymphocyte count is 1.6 to 2.4×10^3 cells/mm^3.

Answer d is incorrect. Agranulocytosis means a failure of the bone marrow to make enough WBCs (neutrophils).

---

16. Select the cause(s) of neutrophilia. Select all that apply.

   a. Acute bacterial infections
   b. G-CSF
   c. Glucocorticoids
   d. Lithium

Answer a is correct. Acute bacterial infections can increase neutrophils. Neutrophils are the predominate cell that fights bacterial infections.

Answer b is correct. The actions of cytokine medications such as G-CSF and GM-CSF may intensify neutrophil activity. G-CSF (filgrastim [Neupogen]) is a G-CSF used to stimulate granulocyte production in chemotherapy induced neutropenia and severe chronic neutropenia. GM-CSF (sargramostim [Leukine]) is a GM-CSF used in AML, bone marrow transplant, and stem cell transplant to shorten time to neutrophil recovery and reduce infections.

Answer c is correct. Glucocorticoids may cause neutrophilia and different glucocorticoids seem to have different effects. Neutrophils are primarily located intravascularly; they do not normally reside extravascularly in the tissues. The total blood granulocyte pool is composed of two equal parts, the circulating pool and the noncirculating pool). Cells in the noncirculating pool are adherent to the vascular endothelium in areas of decreased blood flow. After administration of a glucocorticoid, noncirculating cells are released into the circulating pool, making a neutrophilia. The WBC count returns to normal within 24 hours.

Answer d is correct. Lithium is also associated with a release of noncirculating cells (demargination).

---

17. Select the drug-induced cause of a neutrophil count less than 1500 cells/mm³. Select all that apply.

    a. Zidovudine
    b. β-lactam antibiotics
    c. Angiotensin-converting enzyme (ACE) inhibitors
    d. Ticlopidine

Answer a is correct. Zidovudine may cause neutropenia.

Answer b is correct. β-lactam antibiotics may cause neutropenia, although this occurs rarely.

Answer c is correct. ACE inhibitors, particularly captopril, may cause neutropenia, although this is a rare occurrence.

Answer d is correct. Ticlopidine may cause neutropenia.

---

18. Select the cause(s) of an eosinophil count greater than 350 cells/mm³. Select all that apply.

    a. Asthma
    b. Parasitic infections
    c. Antibiotics (allergic reaction)
    d. Lymphoma

Answer a is correct. Asthma may cause an eosinophilia.

Answer b is correct. Parasitic infections may cause an eosinophilia.

Answer c is correct. Allergic reactions to antibiotics may cause an eosinophilia.

Answer d is incorrect. Lymphomas would not have an effect on the eosinophil count.

---

19. HIV is most likely to cause which of the following?

    a. Neutrophilia
    b. Eosinophilia
    c. Monocytosis
    d. Lymphocytosis
    e. Lymphopenia

Answer e is correct. Lymphopenia may be caused by HIV since HIV disease attacks and destroys T lymphocytes (CD4 cells). Lymphopenia may also be caused by: radiation exposure, lymphoma, aplastic anemia, and glucocorticoids. Glucocorticoids may cause leukocytosis as well, by demargination (increasing noncirculating WBCs). However, administration of glucocorticoids may also decrease WBC counts.

Answer a is incorrect. HIV may cause neutropenia, but it is not the predominant cell line affected by HIV.

Answer b is incorrect. Eosinophilia may be caused by allergic disorders, asthma, parasitic infections, leukemia, and antibiotics (allergic reaction).

Answer c is incorrect. Monocytosis may be caused by tuberculosis, endocarditis, protozoal infection, and leukemia.

Answer d is incorrect. Lymphocytosis may be caused by mononucleosis, viral infections, pertussis, tuberculosis, syphilis, and lymphoma.

---

20. A patient that is found to have a granulocyte count less than 500 cells/mm³ would be classified as which of the following?

    a. Lymphopenia
    b. Basophilia
    c. Agranulocytosis
    d. Eosinophilia

Answer c is correct. Agranulocytosis is defined as a severe form of neutropenia with a total granulocyte count <500/mm³.

Answer a is incorrect. Lymphopenia is a decreased lymphocyte count.

Answer b is incorrect. Basophilia is an increased basophil count. Because basophils represent a small portion of the granulocytes, a basophilia would be unlikely to have an effect on the total granulocyte count.

Answer d is incorrect. Eosinophilia is an increased eosinophil count. Because eosinophils represent a small portion of the granulocytes, an eosinophilia or eosinopenia would be unlikely to have an effect on the total granulocyte count.

---

21. Which of the following functions is performed by neutrophils?

    a. Antigen presentation to T lymphocytes
    b. Engulfing pathogens
    c. Lysing virally infected cells
    d. Secreting antibody

Answer b is correct. The major role of neutrophils is to engulf and destroy the infectious pathogen.

Answer a is incorrect. Because only APCs (eg, macrophages and dendritic cells) present antigen to T-lymphocytes (specifically helper T lymphocytes).

Answer c is incorrect. Only CD8(+) cytotoxic T lymphocytes have the machinery to lyse cells that are infected with viruses.

Answer d is incorrect. B lymphocytes become activated to plasma cells which secrete antibody or immunoglobulin.

---

22. Which of the following cell types can present peptide fragments from an engulfed pathogen in association with MHC class II to T lymphocytes?

    a. Neutrophils
    b. Basophils
    c. Dendritic cell
    d. Eosinophils

Answer c is correct. Dendritic cells are a potent APC.

Answer a is incorrect. Neutrophils simply engulf and destroy the pathogen. They cannot present antigen to T lymphocytes.

Answer b is incorrect. Basophils play a role in allergic reactions, like other granulocytes, they cannot present antigen.

Answer d is incorrect. Eosinophils play an important role in parasitic infections and allergic disorders. Like other granulocytes, they cannot present antigen to T lymphocytes.

---

23. Which of the following cell types plays a critical role in parasitic infections?

    a. Basophil
    b. Macrophage
    c. Plasma cell
    d. Eosinophil

Answer d is correct. Eosinophils play a major role in parasitic infections.

Answer a is incorrect. Basophils play a major role in allergic reactions.

Answer b is incorrect. Macrophages also engulf pathogens and present fragments of the pathogen to T lymphocytes. They do not play a major role in parasitic infections.

Answer c is incorrect. Plasma cells are activated B lymphocytes that secrete antibody.

CHAPTER **12 | Anemia**

1. JM is a 43-year-old man with metastatic small-cell lung cancer that is currently receiving chemotherapy. He was recently diagnosed with chemotherapy-induced anemia with a hemoglobin level of 7.7 g/dL and was initiated on erythropoietin therapy. Two weeks after initiating erythropoietin, his hemoglobin level is 9.5 g/dL. Which of the following represents the most appropriate course of action for JMs erythropoietin?

   a. Continue erythropoietin at the same dose
   b. Decrease the dose of erythropoietin by 25%
   c. Increase the dose of erythropoietin by 50%
   d. Discontinue the erythropoietin

Answer b is correct. This patient had >1 g/dL increase in hemoglobin 2 weeks after initiating therapy with an ESA. The appropriate course of action is a 25% dose reduction.

Answer a is incorrect. This patient has had too rapid of an increase in hemoglobin and needs to have the dose reduced.

Answer c is incorrect. This is the recommendation for dose adjustment in patients who have an inadequate increase in hemoglobin after initiation of ESA therapy.

Answer d is incorrect. The patient has benefitted from the erythropoietin therapy and continuing therapy at a lower dose is the most appropriate course of action.

The following case pertains to questions 2 and 3:

MG is a 62-year-old woman with a prior medical history of CKD, hypertension, and stage II colon cancer. Her social history is significant for a long standing history of alcoholism. She underwent surgical resection of her primary cancer 6 months ago and is currently undergoing chemotherapy with the intent to cure her cancer. Routine laboratory monitoring revealed the patient has a hemoglobin level of 8.8 g/dL.

2. MG's nephrologist wants to start him on an ESA. Which of the following is true regarding the use of ESAs in MG?

   a. Darbepoetin can be used in MG at a dose of 500 mcg every 3 weeks
   b. Epoetin can be used in MG at a dose of 40,000 units every week
   c. Darbepoetin can be used in MG at a dose of 0.45 mcg/kg every week
   d. ESAs should not be used in MG

Answer d is correct. MG has active cancer that is being treated with curative intent. The risk evaluation mitigation strategy for ESAs clearly indicates that these agents should not be used in patients in this setting, regardless of the cause of anemia. The reason for this contraindication is that clinical trial evidence has shown an increased risk of tumor progression in patients receiving ESAs.

Answer a is incorrect. ESAs are contraindicated as stated above. The dose provided in answer a is an appropriate dose for chemotherapy-induced anemia. If ESA therapy was appropriate in this patient, determining the optimal dose would be difficult since his anemia is multifactorial (chemotherapy and CKD).

Answer b is incorrect. This is the appropriate dose for the treatment of chemotherapy-induced anemia. However, ESA therapy is contraindicated in this patient.

Answer c is incorrect. This is the appropriate dose for the treatment of anemia from CKD. However, ESA therapy is contraindicated in this patient.

---

3. Due to her social history, MG should be evaluated for his anemia being complicated by deficiency in:

   a. Vitamin B_{12}
   b. Iron
   c. Vitamin D
   d. Thiamine

Answer a is correct. MG has a long standing history of chronic alcoholism. Vitamin B_{12} deficiency is a frequent complication that is seen in this patient population. It is important to assess his vitamin B_{12} status because deficiency could lead to neurological complications in addition to anemia.

Answer b is incorrect. Iron deficiency is not correlated to alcoholism. Although if this patient were to start ESA therapy, an assessment of iron status would be warranted.

Answer c is incorrect. Vitamin D deficiency is not associated with anemia.

Answer d is incorrect. Thiamine deficiency commonly occurs in patients with chronic alcoholism; however, it is not associated with anemia.

---

4. Most flour in the United States is fortified with which of the following?

   a. Folic acid
   b. Potassium
   c. Vitamin B_{12}
   d. Vitamin C

Answer a is correct. In the United States, flour is fortified with multiple vitamins. Relevant to anemia, flour is fortified with folic acid and iron. The goal is to increase the average daily intake of these key nutrients and prevent conditions that may result from their deficiency.

Answer b is incorrect. Potassium is not added to flour.

Answer c is incorrect. Currently flour is not fortified with vitamin B12. There is a growing movement worldwide to add vitamin B_{12} to flour to help prevent neurologic complications of vitamin B_{12} deficiency.

Answer d is incorrect. Vitamin C is not added to flour.

---

5. SL is a 57-year-old man who is admitted to the hospital for pneumonia. During his clinical and laboratory evaluation, he was found to have a microcytic anemia. Which of the following additional diagnostic tests would be most useful in determining if SL has anemia as a result of iron deficiency?

   a. Ferritin
   b. Red cell distribution width
   c. Transferrin saturation
   d. Reticulocyte count

Answer c is correct. There are multiple indices that can be useful in assessing iron stores, including ferritin and transferrin saturation. Ferritin is an acute phase reactant and is elevated in patients with an acute illness, such as pneumonia. Transferrin saturation is not affected by acute illness and is a more reliable indicator of iron stores in this situation.

Answer a is incorrect. Ferritin is an acute phase reactant and is falsely elevated in acute illnesses. This can lead to clinicians falsely concluding the patient is not deficient in iron.

Answer b is incorrect. The red cell distribution width measures the variability in sizes of RBCs. It is a tool that is especially useful when multiple causes of anemia are suspected.

Answer d is incorrect. In the assessment of anemia, the reticulocyte count is a good measure of bone marrow response. In the setting of anemia, the reticulocyte count should be elevated as the marrow works to produce more RBCs. If the reticulocyte count is not elevated, it could indicate there is difficulty with production of new RBCs. It will not help determine iron status.

---

6. Which of the following iron preparations requires a prescription?

   a. Ferrous fumarate
   b. Polysaccharide-iron complex
   c. Ferrous sulfate
   d. Ferrous gluconate

Answer b is correct. Polysaccharide-iron complex is a prescription only medication. The original brand name product is Niferex.

Answer a is incorrect. Ferrous fumarate is available without a prescription under the brand name Feostat (among others).

Answer c is incorrect. Ferrous sulfate is available without a prescription under the brand name Feosol (among others).

Answer d is incorrect. Ferrous gluconate is available without a prescription under the brand name Fergon (among others).

The following case pertains to questions 7 through 9:

DE is a 49-year-old woman with a diagnosis of breast cancer that is currently being treated with chemotherapy. Her prior medical history is significant for allergic rhinitis and chronic heartburn. Her home medications include cetirizine, pantoprazole, and transdermal norelgestromin/ethinyl estradiol. The patient was recently diagnosed with chemotherapy-induced anemia with a hemoglobin level of 8.8 g/dL. She was prescribed darbepoetin to treat her anemia.

7. DE may require supplementation with which of the following agents to optimize the effectiveness of darbepoetin?

   a. Folic acid
   b. Iron
   c. Vitamin B_{12}
   d. Thiamine

Answer b is correct. Patients receiving ESA therapy may develop a functional iron deficiency and require iron supplementation. Clinical trials have also shown that empiric iron supplementation without assessment of iron stores increases the hemoglobin response from erythropoietin.

Answer a is incorrect. Typical dietary intake of folic acid is sufficient to compensate for increased use in the setting of increased RBC in response to anemia.

Answer c is incorrect. Typical dietary intake of vitamin B_{12} is sufficient to compensate for increased use in the setting of increased RBC in response to anemia.

Answer d is incorrect. Thiamine is not essential in the production of RBCs.

---

8. Six weeks after initiating darbepoetin, DEs hemoglobin level is 9.6 g/dL. Which of the following represents the most appropriate course of action for DEs darbepoetin?

    a. Continue darbepoetin at the same dose
    b. Decrease the dose of darbepoetin by 25%
    c. Increase the dose of darbepoetin by 50%
    d. Discontinue the darbepoetin

Answer c is correct. This patient has had an inadequate increase in hemoglobin (<1 g/dL in 4-6 weeks) and a dose increase is warranted. The recommended dose increase in ESA nonresponders is 25%.

Answer a is incorrect. The patient has not had an adequate response to his ESA therapy so a dose increase is indicated.

Answer b is incorrect. The dose of ESAs is decreased in patients whose hemoglobin exceeds the goal level or who have too rapid of a rise in hemoglobin level.

Answer d is incorrect. The patient has not had an adequate response in hemoglobin since initiating ESA therapy. Six weeks of therapy is not long enough

---

9. Four months after the patient began treatment with darbepoetin, she began experiencing edema and warmth of her left lower extremity. She was diagnosed with a deep vein thrombosis (DVT). Which of her medications contributed to her increased risk of DVT? Select all that apply.

    a. Cetirizine
    b. Darbepoetin
    c. Pantoprazole
    d. Norelgestromin/ethinyl estradiol

Answers b and d are correct. One of the primary safety concerns of ESAs is development of DVT. This class of agents should be used with caution in patients receiving other medications that increase risk of DVT such as hormonal contraceptives (like norelgestromin/ethinyl estradiol).

Answer a is incorrect. There is no correlation between cetirizine and increased risk of DVT.

Answer c is incorrect. There is no correlation between pantoprazole and increased risk of DVT.

10. Vitamin B_{12} supplementation is available by which of the following routes? Select all that apply.

    a. Oral
    b. Transdermal
    c. Injectable
    d. Intranasal

Answers a, c, and d are correct. Vitamin B_{12} supplementation is available in many forms, including an injectable forms that are administered intramuscularly or intravenously, various oral formulation, sublingual formulations, and an intranasal formulation.

Answer b is incorrect. While there are many products available to purchase claiming to be vitamin B_{12} patches, these products are not approved by the FDA and are not recommended.

---

11. Rank the following oral iron salts in order from highest percentage of elemental iron to lowest percentage of elemental iron.

Unordered options	Ordered response
Ferrous fumarate	Ferrous fumarate
Ferrous gluconate	Ferrous sulfate anhydrous
Ferrous sulfate anhydrous	Ferrous sulfate
Ferrous sulfate	Ferrous gluconate

The correct order from highest to lowest percentage of elemental iron is ferrous fumarate (33% elemental iron), ferrous sulfate anhydrous (30%-32% elemental iron), ferrous sulfate (20% elemental iron), and ferrous gluconate (12% elemental iron).

The following case pertains to questions 12 and 13:

JS is an 18-year-old woman who presents to urgent care with a chief complaint of increasing fatigue that has gotten progressively worse over the last 2 months. Physical examination is notable for diffuse pallor and tachycardia. Her prior medical history is significant only for occasional reflux disease that she manages with OTC omeprazole and calcium carbonate. She also notes she has a history of heavy menstrual blood flow. Laboratory examination reveals a hemoglobin level of 9.4 g/dL and a mean corpuscular volume (MCV) of 73 fL.

12. Based on the information provided, JS most likely has anemia as a result in deficiency of:

    a. Iron
    b. Vitamin B_{12}
    c. Folic acid
    d. Erythropoietin

Answer a is correct. Based on the patient's MCV, she has microcytic anemia. Iron deficiency is the most common cause of iron-deficiency anemia. Additionally, patients with a history of heavy menstrual blood flow can develop iron deficiency as a result of having increased iron needs for the production of new blood.

Answer b is incorrect. Vitamin B_{12} deficiency results in macrocytic anemia.

Answer c is incorrect. Folic acid deficiency results in macrocytic anemia.

Answer d is incorrect. Anemia resulting from deficiency in erythropoietin (such as anemia of CKD) is typically normocytic. Anemia in this population may present with a slight elevation in MCV as a result of increased reticulocytes in the blood stream.

---

13. The decision is made to treat JS's anemia with medication instead of blood transfusion. Which of the following medications used in the treatment of anemia may have a drug interaction with JS's current medications?

    a. Ferrous sulfate
    b. Cyanocobalamin
    c. Folic acid
    d. Epoetin

Answer a is correct. Optimal absorption of iron occurs in an acidic environment. Use of agents that increase gastric pH (such as omeprazole and calcium carbonate) can decrease iron's bioavailability. Additionally, calcium carbonate can bind to iron, also decreasing its bioavailability.

Answer b is incorrect. There are no drug interactions between cyanocobalamin and JS's medications.

Answer c is incorrect. There are no drug interactions between folic acid and JS's medications.

Answer d is incorrect. There are no drug interactions between epoetin and JS's medications.

The following case pertains to questions 14 and 15:

LJ is a 38-year-old woman who recently underwent gastric resection for the management of extreme obesity that was complicated by hypertension and type 2 diabetes. Twelve weeks after her surgery, she is complaining of fatigue and become short of breath when climbing steps. Laboratory evaluation revealed a hemoglobin level of 10.2 g/dL and an MCV of 120 fL.

14. LJs anemia is best described as:

    a. Normocytic
    b. Macrocytic
    c. Hypochromic
    d. Normochromic

Answer b is correct. The patient's MCV is above the normal range (80-100 fL). This indicates that the RBCs are larger than normal and is termed macrocytic.

Answer a is incorrect. Normocytic describes RBC sizes that result in an MCV in the normal range.

Answer c is incorrect. Hypochromic refers to the appearance of RBCs. Hypochromic anemias tend to be microcytic

as well (MCV <80). An example of a hypochromic anemia is iron-deficiency anemia.

Answer d is incorrect. Normochromic refers to anemia that is normal in color appearance. Normochromic anemias tend to be normocytic as well. An example of normochromic anemia is aplastic anemia.

---

15. Which of the following deficiencies is most likely responsible for LJs anemia?

    a. Erythropoietin
    b. Iron
    c. Vitamin B_{12}
    d. Folic acid

Answer c is correct. Patients who undergo gastric resection have a decrease in intrinsic factor, a protein necessary for optimal vitamin B_{12} absorption. Vitamin B_{12} deficiency is common in this patient population when empiric supplementation is not utilized. Additionally, her MCV indicates a macrocytic anemia, which is consistent with vitamin B_{12} deficiency.

Answer a is incorrect. Erythropoietin deficiency typically occurs in patients with CKD and results in normocytic anemia.

Answer b is incorrect. It is possible that patients who undergo weight loss surgery to develop iron deficiency as a result of decreased iron intake, however iron-deficiency anemia is microcytic.

Answer d is incorrect. Folic acid deficiency is not associated with gastric resection.

---

16. JR is a 37-year-old female patient who was previously diagnosed with iron-deficiency anemia. She has been taking oral iron supplementation as directed for 16 weeks without achieving her goal hemoglobin of 12 g/dL. Her most recent hemoglobin level was 9.8 g/dL. The decision has been made to administer IV iron dextran. She is 5' 4" tall and weighs 150 lb. What is the correct dose of iron dextran for CR?

    a. 19.5 mL
    b. 21.1 mL
    c. 24.4 mL
    d. 29.2 mL

Answer a is correct. Dose of iron dextran, in milliliters can be calculated by using this equation: Dose (mL) = 0.0442 (Desired Hb - Observed Hb) × LBW + (0.26 × LBW) her dose calculates at 27 mL. The variable used are: desired hemoglobin 12 g/dL, observed hemoglobin 9.8 g/dL, LBW (lean body weight) 54.7 kg. LBW is calculated for a male as 45.5 + 2.3 (Ht-60) where Ht is measured in inches.

Answer b is incorrect. This is the value that is calculated if you use the LBW formula for a male patient.

Answer c is incorrect. This is the value if you calculated the dose using actual body weight instead of LBW.

Answer d is incorrect. This is the value if you calculated the dose using 16 g/dL as your target hemoglobin.

17. Which of the following types of deficiencies typically results in a macrocytic anemia? Select all that apply.

 a. Erythropoietin
 b. Iron
 c. Vitamin B_{12}
 d. Folic acid

Answers c and d are correct. Deficiencies in vitamin B_{12} and folic acid arrest RBC production early in the development process. Reticulocytes decrease in size as they progress towards maturation. Without vitamin B_{12} and folic acid, the cells fail to develop properly and are larger in size than a normal RBC (macrocytic).

Answer a is incorrect. Deficiency in erythropoietin does not affect RBC size. The maturation process is not affected. Low levels of erythropoietin decrease the stimulus to produce new RBCs. The resulting anemia is typically normocytic.

Answer b is incorrect. Iron is a component of hemoglobin and is incorporated into the RBC late in the development process. In a setting of iron deficiency, there is less fully functional hemoglobin to be incorporated into the cells, resulting in cells that are smaller than normal (microcytic).

18. Venofer is the brand name for which of the following iron preparations?

 a. Iron sucrose
 b. Ferumoxytol
 c. Ferric sodium gluconate
 d. Polysaccharide-iron complex

Answer a is correct. Venofer is an injectable formulation of iron sucrose.

Answer b is incorrect. Feraheme is an injectable formulation of ferumoxytol.

Answer c is incorrect. Ferrlecit is an injectable formulation of ferric sodium gluconate.

Answer d is incorrect. Niferex is a brand name of oral polysaccharide-iron complex.

19. Deficiency in which of the following can result in severe neurologic complications?

 a. Erythropoietin
 b. Iron
 c. Vitamin B_{12}
 d. Folic acid

Answer c is correct. Deficiency in vitamin B_{12} can cause severe neurologic complications such as paraesthesia, ataxia,

and psychotic symptoms. B_{12} deficiency frequently goes undetected until profound deficiency has occurred. Because of the risk of neurological complications, it is essential to assess B_{12} in patients with macrocytic anemia, even when folic acid deficiency has already been identified.

Answer a is incorrect. Deficiency in erythropoietin is a common complication of CKD, particularly in advanced stages. Erythropoietin deficiency will result in an underproductive bone marrow that can lead to anemia.

Answer b is incorrect. Iron deficiency is known to impact immune system function in addition to causing anemia but it is not associated with neurologic consequences.

Answer d is incorrect. In addition to macrocytic anemia, folic acid deficiency is associated with neural tube defects in developing fetuses. However, there are not known neurologic complications to folic acid deficiency in the individual patient.

20. GC is a 72-year-old man with stage 4 CKD, not receiving dialysis. He was recently diagnosed with anemia. He is currently not receiving any medications to treat his anemia. Assessment of iron stores revealed the patient to be iron deficient. Which of the following is an IV iron preparation that is indicated for CF? Select all that apply.

 a. Iron dextran
 b. Iron sucrose
 c. Sodium ferric gluconate
 d. Ferumoxytol

Answers b and d are correct. Iron sucrose and ferumoxytol are both indicated to treat iron deficiency in adult patients with anemia secondary to CKD. These agents are indicated regardless of use of ESAs or hemodialysis.

Answer a is incorrect. Iron dextran is indicated for the treatment of iron-deficiency anemia when oral iron is not unsatisfactory or not possible.

Answer c is incorrect. Sodium ferric gluconate is only indicated to treat iron deficiency in patients with CKD requiring hemodialysis and receiving ESA therapy.

CHAPTER 13 | Lung Cancer

1. What is the brand name of crizotinib?

 a. Xalkori
 b. Opdivo
 c. Cyramza
 d. Iressa

Answer a is correct. The brand name of crizotinib is Xalkori.

Answer b is incorrect. Opdivo is the brand name of nivolumab.

Answer c is incorrect. Cyramza is the brand name of ramucirumab.

Answer d is incorrect. Iressa is the brand name of gefitinib.

2. A 59-year-old man with recently diagnosed limited-stage small-cell lung cancer comes to clinic for treatment. Which of the following would be the most appropriate treatment for him?

 a. Cisplatin plus vinorelbine
 b. Surgery followed by adjuvant cisplatin plus etoposide
 c. Carboplatin, paclitaxel, and bevacizumab
 d. Cisplatin and etoposide along with concurrent thoracic radiation therapy

Answer d is correct. For limited stage small-cell lung cancer (SCLC) to maximize survival, one should utilize concurrent thoracic radiation therapy and cisplatin plus etoposide.

Answer a is incorrect. Cisplatin and vinorelbine is a potential adjuvant treatment for squamous NSCLC.

Answer b is incorrect. Surgery is not recommended for the treatment of SCLC.

Answer c is incorrect. Carboplatin, paclitaxel, and bevacizumab are the regimens used for the treatment of advanced non-squamous NSCLC.

3. A 60-year-old woman comes into your pharmacy to pick up her usual prescription for her maintenance medications. She asks you about taking vitamin supplements to decrease her risk of lung cancer. Her social history is significant for smoking a pack of cigarettes a day for 25 years, but she stopped 3 years ago. Based upon this information, you should recommend which of the following?

 a. β-Carotene
 b. Vitamin E plus β-carotene
 c. β-Carotene plus retinyl palmitate
 d. No supplement is recommended

Answer d is correct. To date, randomized trials of chemopreventive agents (eg, vitamin E, β-carotene, and retinyl palmitate) have not demonstrated a benefit in preventing lung cancer in patients at high risk for developing lung cancer. In two randomized clinical trials, β-carotene has been associated with an increased risk of lung cancer and mortality in patients at high risk for developing lung cancer.

Answer a is incorrect. In two randomized clinical trials, β-carotene has been associated with an increased risk of lung cancer and mortality in patients at high risk for developing lung cancer.

Answer b is incorrect. In two randomized clinical trials, β-carotene has been associated with an increased risk of lung cancer and mortality in patients at high risk for developing

lung cancer. Additionally, vitamin E (tocopherol) offers no benefit in lowering the risk of developing lung cancer.

Answer c is incorrect. In two randomized clinical trials, β-carotene has been associated with an increased risk of lung cancer and mortality in patients at high risk for developing lung cancer. Additionally, retinyl palmitate offers no benefit in lowering the risk of developing lung cancer.

4. A 62-year-old woman who quit smoking 15 years ago comes to clinic asking, "Should I undergo screening for lung cancer?" Her past medical history is significant for hypertension and chronic obstructive pulmonary disease. Her social history is significant for a 31-pack year history of smoking and drinks a beer or two a day. Which of the following represent appropriate lung cancer screening recommendations for this patient?

 a. Annual chest MRI
 b. Annual chest x-ray
 c. Annual sputum cytology
 d. Annual helical CT scan

Answer d is correct. The NLST showed that in patients aged 55 to 74 with at least a 30 pack year smoking history annual low-dose helical CT scan decreases lung cancer related mortality by 20% compared to annual chest x-ray. Guidelines have been adopted based on these findings.

Answer a is incorrect. MRI of the chest has not been demonstrated to be an effective screening tool for the early detection of lung cancer.

Answer b is incorrect. Randomized trials have not demonstrated that chest x-rays either every 6 months or annually reduce mortality associated with lung cancer.

Answer c is incorrect. Randomized trials have not demonstrated that sputum cytology reduce the mortality associated with lung cancer.

Use the following scenario to answer questions 5 to 8.

SM is a 52-year-old man with a new diagnosis of metastatic adenocarcinoma of the lung. Complete pathologic review revealed the following profile: ALK negative, EGFR negative, BRAF V600E negative. The oncologist has recommended to start chemotherapy with carboplatin/pemetrexed.

5. The carboplatin for SM should be dosed based on:

 a. Body surface area
 b. Target area under the curve
 c. Ideal body weight
 d. Actual body weight

Answer b is correct. Carboplatin doses are based on target area under the curve (AUC). The dose is calculated using the Calvert formula: Dose = Target AUC × (GFR + 25), where GFR is glomerular filtration rate.

Answer a is incorrect.   Most chemotherapy is dosed based on area under the curve however carboplatin is not.

Answer c is incorrect.   Ideal body weight is seldom used as a dosing parameter for chemotherapy.

Answer d is incorrect.   Actual body weight is used as a dosing parameter for some chemotherapy agents; however, body surface area is most commonly used. For carboplatin, target AUC is the correct dosing parameter.

---

6. Which of the following monoclonal antibodies could be added to SM's chemotherapy regimen to help improve efficacy?

    a. Necitumumab
    b. Atezolizumab
    c. Cetuximab
    d. Pembrolizumab

Answer d is correct.   Pembrolizumab has been shown to improve the efficacy of combination chemotherapy in the treatment of metastatic, non-squamous NSCLC. It has specifically been studied in combination with carboplatin and pemetrexed.

Answer a is incorrect.   Necitumumab has been shown to improve the efficacy of the cisplatin/gemcitabine in the treatment of squamous cell NSCLC. In clinical trials it was ineffective in the treatment of non-squamous NSCLC and had increased risk of side effects.

Answer b is incorrect.   Like pembrolizumab, atezolizumab targets the programmed cell death 1 pathway. It has not been shown to be effective as first-line chemotherapy in NSCLC and it has not been studied in combination with chemotherapy.

Answer c is incorrect.   Like necitumumab, cetuximab is a monoclonal antibody that inhibits EGFR. It has been studied in various lung cancer scenarios and has provided only slight benefit with increased toxicities. It is not recommended for the treatment of NSCLC in patients such as the one provided in the question.

---

7. Which of the following should the patient receive to lessen the severity of side effects from pemetrexed? Select all that apply.

    a. Dexamethasone
    b. Vitamin B_{12}
    c. Pyridoxine
    d. Folic acid

Answer a is correct.   Dexamethasone is given the day before, the day of, and the day after pemetrexed to decrease the incidence of severe rash from pemetrexed.

Answer b is correct.   Monthly administration of vitamin B_{12} is recommended for patients receiving pemetrexed to decrease the severity of the myelosuppressive effects of pemetrexed.

Answer d is correct.   Daily administration of folic acid is recommended for patients receiving pemetrexed to decrease the severity of the myelosuppressive effects of pemetrexed.

Answer c is incorrect.   Vitamin B_6 (pyridoxine) is sometimes used to lessen neurological toxicities from some chemotherapy agents, such as cytarabine. It has no role for the prevention of pemetrexed toxicity.

---

8. SM continued on his prior treatment for 14 months with stable disease. Unfortunately his lung cancer has now progressed and he is to begin a new lung cancer treatment. Which of the following would be most appropriate for him at this time?

    a. Cisplatin/gemcitabine
    b. Docetaxel/ramucirumab
    c. Carboplatin/paclitaxel
    d. Paclitaxel/erlotinib

Answer b is correct.   Recurrent/relapsed NSCLC that is negative for all biomarkers (EGFR, ALK, BRAF V600E) is treated with single agent chemotherapy, such as docetaxel. Clinical trial evidence has shown the addition of ramucirumab to docetaxel in this setting improved median overall survival. Ramucirumab may be used in all types of NSCLC.

Answer a is incorrect.   Cisplatin/gemcitabine is a combination chemotherapy regimen that is most often used in the initial treatment of squamous cell NSCLC.

Answer c is incorrect.   Carboplatin/paclitaxel is a commonly used combination chemotherapy regimen; however, single agent chemotherapy is most appropriate for the patient since his disease has progressed after initial therapy.

Answer d is incorrect.   This combination is not used in the treatment of NSCLC.

---

9. Rank the following chemotherapy agents used in the treatment of lung cancer in order of their emetogenicity, from least emetogenic to most emetogenic.

Unordered options	Ordered response
Cisplatin	Bevacizumab
Bevacizumab	Docetaxel
Docetaxel	Carboplatin
Carboplatin	Cisplatin

The correct ordered response from least emetogenic to most emetogenic is bevacizumab (minimal emetogenicity), docetaxel (low emetogenicity), carboplatin (moderate emetogenicity), cisplatin (high emetogenicity).

10. A 68-year-old man with recently diagnosed adenocarcinoma of the lung is found to have stage IV disease (liver metastases). He tests negative for ALK and EGFR mutations. At home, he is bedridden due to severe chronic obstructive pulmonary disease that requires home oxygen. His social history is significant for

an 80-pack year history. Which of the following chemotherapy regimens would be rational?

a. Best supportive care
b. Crizotinib
c. Carboplatin, pemetrexed, and pembrolizumab
d. Cisplatin plus gemcitabine and necitumumab

Answer a is correct. The patient has a performance status of 4 due to COPD. Treatment of NSCLC in patients with a poor performance status (PS) has not been shown to improve survival. The Eastern Cooperative Oncology Group (ECOG) PS (Table 13-3) delineation ranges from fully active to confinement to bed. Generally, patients with a PS of 3 and 4 are not treated, but offered best supportive care.

Answer b is incorrect. Crizotinib is indicated in NSCLC that is ALK positive. The evidence suggesting no benefit to treatment of lung cancer for severely ill and debilitated patients was evaluating the benefit of chemotherapy. It is unknown if patients who have specific pathologic features, like ALK positivity would benefit from treatment. The patient in this scenario is ALK negative, making crizotinib inappropriate regardless of performance status.

Answer c is incorrect. If the patient was a good performance status and able to handle aggressive therapy, the combination of carboplatin, pemetrexed, and pebrolizumab would be a valid option.

Answer d is incorrect. The combination of cisplatin, gemcitabine, and necitumumab is used in the treatment of squamous NSCLC. This patient has adenocarcinoma (non-squamous) NSCLC.

11. What is the best treatment option for a 61-year-old man who is chemotherapy naïve and was recently diagnosed with extensive-stage small-cell lung cancer?

a. Carboplatin, pemetrexed, plus pembrolizumab
b. Cisplatin plus gemcitabine
c. Carboplatin plus paclitaxel
d. Cisplatin plus etoposide

Answer d is correct. For extensive-stage SCLC to maximize survival, one should utilize cisplatin plus etoposide regimen.

Answer a is incorrect. Carboplatin, pemetrexed, and pembrolizumab can be used together for the treatment of metastatic non-squamous NSCLC.

Answer b is incorrect. Cisplatin and gemcitabine are the regimens typically used in squamous NSCLC.

Answer c is incorrect. Carboplatin and paclitaxel are the regimens utilized in NSCLC not in SCLC.

Use the following scenario to answer questions 12 to 14.

MK is a 62-year-old woman with a recent diagnosis of stage II squamous NSCLC. Complete pathological evaluation showed ALK positive, EGFR negative, BRAF V600E negative. She has a prior medical history of hypertension, type 2 diabetes, stage 3b chronic kidney disease (last estimated glomerular filtration rate 35 mL/min), and gastroesophageal reflux disease. She underwent surgery and is ready to receive chemotherapy.

12. Which of the following therapies is most appropriate for MK at this time?

a. Carboplatin and pemetrexed
b. Carboplatin, pemetrexed, and bevacizumab
c. Cisplatin and etoposide
d. Cisplatin, etoposide, and bevacizumab

Answer c is correct. The patient is due to start adjuvant chemotherapy for the treatment of early stage squamous NSCLC. The combination of cisplatin and etoposide is one of the combination regimens that is recommended in this situation.

Answer a is incorrect. Pemetrexed containing recommends are not recommended for the treatment of squamous NSCLC.

Answer b is incorrect. In addition to pemetrexed being inappropriate, bevacizumab is also not recommended in this situation. Bevacizumab is only used in the treatment of non-squamous NSCLC and is only approved for use in patients with metastatic disease.

Answer d is incorrect. Bevacizumab is only used in the treatment of non-squamous NSCLC and is only approved for use in patients with metastatic disease.

13. Which of the problems in the patient's prior medical history is most likely to be worsened by her receiving platinum-based chemotherapy?

a. Hypertension
b. Type 2 diabetes
c. Chronic kidney disease
d. Gastroesophageal reflux disease

Answer c is correct. Cisplatin and carboplatin are both associated with nephrotoxicity, with cisplatin having the most nephrotoxic potential. To decrease the risk of nephrotoxicity patients should be encouraged to stay hydrated to maintain renal perfusion and promote the elimination of the platinum chemotherapy agent.

Answer a is incorrect. The platinum chemotherapy agents are not typically associated with hypertension.

Answer b is incorrect. The platinum chemotherapy agents themselves do not have effect on blood sugar. It is worth noting that patients receiving cisplatin or carboplatin will receive dexamethasone to prevent nausea and vomiting. In patients with diabetes the dexamethasone could affect glycemic control.

Answer d is incorrect. While both platinum agents are associated with significant nausea/vomiting, reflux disease is not a known side effect of these drugs.

---

14. Four years after completing chemotherapy, MK presents to her primary care physician with new onset coughing with hemoptysis. Complete evaluation revealed the patient's lung cancer has relapsed, now with multiple tumors in the original lung as well as several suspicious tumors in the liver. The pathologic evaluation reveals the same genetic features as her original tumor. Which of the following is the most appropriate treatment for MK at this time?

    a. Docetaxel and ramucirumab
    b. Atezolizumab
    c. Crizotinib
    d. Erlotinib

Answer c is correct. The patient is positive for ALK. Since her initial regimen was used in the adjuvant setting for the treatment of early stage lung cancer chemotherapy was initially used. Now, in the relapsed setting, targeted therapy is preferred when possible. Since the patient is positive for ALK, therapy targeting this kinase can be used. Crizotinib is the preferred initial anti-ALK drug.

Answer a is incorrect. Since her tumor is ALK positive she should receive targeted therapy prior to receiving any further chemotherapy. Typically patients who are ALK positive will receive multiple ALK targeted drugs before receiving chemotherapy for relapsed disease.

Answer b is incorrect. Since her tumor is ALK positive she should receive therapy targeted at this mutation prior to other targeted therapies like the PD-1/PDL-1 inhibitors. Typically patients who are ALK positive will receive multiple ALK targeted drugs before attempting other therapies for relapsed disease.

Answer d is incorrect. This patient has ALK positive, EGFR negative lung cancer, targeted EGFR kinase inhibitors such as erlotinib would not be recommended until the patient has failed ALK-targeted medications.

---

15. Which of the following patients with small-cell lung cancer should receive prophylactic cranial irradiation?

    a. Patients with limited-stage SCLC who achieve a complete response to their initial therapy.
    b. Patients with extensive-stage SCLC who do not respond to their initial therapy.
    c. All patients with limited-stage SCLC.
    d. All patients with extensive-stage SCLC.

Answer a is correct. Whether limited or extensive stage, patients with SCLC who achieve a complete response to their chemotherapy regimen should receive prophylactic cranial irradiation (PCI). In this situation, PCI decreases the incidence of brain metastases and improves overall survival.

Answer b is incorrect. Prophylactic cranial irradiation is only recommended in SCLC, whether limited or extensive stage, if the patient achieves a complete response to their chemotherapy regimen.

Answer c is incorrect. Prophylactic cranial irradiation is only recommended in SCLC, whether limited or extensive stage, if the patient achieves a complete response to their chemotherapy regimen.

Answer d is incorrect. Prophylactic cranial irradiation is only recommended in SCLC, whether limited or extensive stage, if the patient achieves a complete response to their chemotherapy regimen.

---

16. A 64-year-old man with a performance status of 1 returns to clinic with relapsed SCLC, new bone and liver metastases. He completed his previous chemotherapy of carboplatin and etoposide 5 months ago and reports no other medical problems. He and his wife request further treatment if it is reasonable. Based upon this information, which of the following treatments would be rational?

    a. Topotecan
    b. Osimertinib
    c. Pembrolizumab
    d. Best supportive care

Answer a is correct. Topotecan demonstrates activity in patients with relapsed SCLC and has a FDA-approved indication for this patient population.

Answer b is incorrect. Osimertinib is utilized for NSCLC not SCLC.

Answer c is incorrect. Pembrolizumab is utilized for NSCLC not SCLC.

Answer d is incorrect. Because his SCLC relapsed more than 3 months since completing first-line therapy, his performance status is a one, and he requests therapy, it is rational to give him second-line therapy by offering a clinical trial, topotecan, gemcitabine, or taxanes.

---

17. HM is a 54-year-old man with a recent diagnosis of metastatic squamous NSCLC. He is scheduled to receive chemotherapy with cisplatin and gemcitabine. Which monoclonal antibody should be added to HM's chemotherapy to improve the efficacy of his chemotherapy?

    a. Bevacizumab
    b. Necitumumab
    c. Pembrolizumab
    d. Ramucirumab

Answer b is correct. In clinical trials necitumumab added to cisplatin/gemcitabine in the treatment of metastatic squamous NSCLC was shown to improve median overall survival.

Answer a is incorrect. Bevacizumab has shown benefit when added to carboplatin/paclitaxel in the treatment of non-squamous NSCLC. Bevacizumab should not be used in the treatment of squamous NSCLC due to increased risk of bleeding.

Answer c is incorrect. Pembrolizumab has shown to improve the efficacy of carboplatin/pemetrexed for the treatment of non-squamous NSCLC. It has not been shown to improve the efficacy of chemotherapy for squamous NSCLC. Pembrolizumab is approved as a monotherapy for the treatment of metastatic NSCLC, regardless of histology.

Answer d is incorrect. Ramucirumab has been shown to improve the efficacy of docetaxel when used in the treatment of relapsed NSCLC. This patient is receiving his first chemotherapy regimen and ramucirumab-containing therapy would not be appropriate at this time.

18. Which of the following kinase inhibitors should be used in the treatment of metastatic NSCLC that tests positive for the BRAF V600E mutation? Choose all that apply.

    a. Afatinib
    b. Trametinib
    c. Ceritinib
    d. Dabrafenib

Answers b and d are correct. Dabrafenib targets the BRAF kinase resulting from the V600E mutation. Trametinib targets the MEK enzymes, which are downstream signals of the BRAF pathway. They have been shown to have strong activity in NSCLC that is positive for BRAF V600E.

Answer a is incorrect. Afatinib is a kinase inhibitor active in NSCLC that is positive for activating mutations in EGFR. It can be used as an initial EGFR targeting therapy.

Answer c is incorrect. Ceritinib is a kinase inhibitor active in NSCLC that is positive for ALK. It is used in patients who have failed prior crizotinib therapy.

19. Which of the following chemotherapy agents should be added to carboplatin for the adjuvant treatment of stage III adenocarcinoma of the lung?

    a. Pemetrexed
    b. Etoposide
    c. Vinorelbine
    d. Cisplatin

Answer a is correct. The combination of carboplatin or cisplatin with pemetrexed is one of the most commonly used regimens for the adjuvant treatment of non-squamous NSCLC.

Answer b is incorrect. Etoposide is added to cisplatin for the adjuvant treatment of squamous NSCLC.

Answer c is incorrect. Vinorelbine can be added to cisplatin for the adjuvant treatment of squamous NSCLC.

Answer d is incorrect. Cisplatin and carboplatin have the same mechanism of action and a very similar toxicity profile.

It is never appropriate to combine platinum agents in the treatment of any cancer.

20. Rank the following histologies of lung cancer in order of prevalence, from least prevalent to most prevalent.

Unordered Options	Ordered Response
Small-cell carcinoma	Large cell carcinoma
Adenocarcinoma	Small cell carcinoma
Large-cell carcinoma	Squamous cell carcinoma
Squamous cell carcinoma	Adenocarcinoma

The correct ordered resposne from least prevalent to most prevalent is large cell carcinoma (<10% of lung cancers), small cell carcinoma (15%), squamous cell carcinoma (30%), and adenocarcinoma (50%).

CHAPTER 14 | Prostate Cancer

1. A 62-year-old man with a recent diagnosis of prostate cancer presents to oncologist. His oncologist tells him that his prostate cancer has a Gleason score of 3 + 3 or 6. A prostate cancer with a Gleason score of 6 is considered:

    a. Not differentiated
    b. Poorly differentiated
    c. Differentiated
    d. Moderately differentiated
    e. Well differentiated

Answer d is correct. Prostate cancer can be graded systematically according to the histologic appearance of the malignant cell and then grouped into well, moderately, or poorly differentiated grades. Gland architecture is examined and then rated on a scale of 1 (well differentiated) to 5 (poorly differentiated). Two different specimens are examined, and the score for each specimen is added. Poorly differentiated tumors grow rapidly (poor prognosis), while well-differentiated tumors grow slowly (better prognosis). A Gleason score of 5 to 6 is considered moderately differentiated.

Answer a is incorrect. The term "not differentiated" is not used in the Gleason scoring system.

Answer b is incorrect. A Gleason score of 7 to 10 is considered poorly differentiated.

Answer c is incorrect. The term "differentiated" is not used alone in the Gleason scoring system.

Answer e is incorrect. Well differentiated is equal to a Gleason score of 2 to 4.

2. HH is a 72-year-old African American man with a family history of prostate cancer who presents to his primary care physician for his annual examination. He has a past medical history of hypertension, diabetes, and heart failure. He asks about

prostate cancer screening. According to the AUA, which of the following is the most appropriate course of action? Select all that apply.

a. Observation because he is not eligible for prostate cancer screening due to his age being >70.
b. Patient should be screened with a DRE and a PSA level.
c. Observation because he is not eligible for prostate cancer screening due to his family history.
d. Patient should be screened with a DRE alone.
e. Observation because his life expectancy is less than 10 to 15 years.

Answers a and e are correct. The AUA does not recommend routine screening for any man with a life expectancy less than 10-15 years, men under 40, men between 40 and 54 years at average risk, or men over the age of 70. Shared decision making is recommended for men age 55-69 years who are considering screening based on patients' values and preferences.

Answer b is incorrect. Neither DRE nor PSA is sensitive or specific enough to be used alone as a screening test. Therefore, if screening is recommended, the combination of a DRE plus PSA determination is a better method in detecting prostate cancer than DRE alone.

Answer c is incorrect. AUA does not take into effect family history when considering prostate cancer screening and therefore this patient would not be eligible based on this reason. He is not eligible because he is over the age of 70 and has a life expectancy of less than 10-15 years due to his past medical history.

Answer d is incorrect. DRE as a single screening method, has poor compliance, and has had little effect on preventing metastatic prostate cancer. Therefore, prostate screening with a DRE alone is currently not recommended.

3. JJ is a 52-year-old man with a history of BPH. His most recent DRE was normal, but last PSA was 5.1 ng/mL. JJ is concerned about getting prostate cancer and wants to discuss preventative therapy. Which of the following is true pertaining to the use of 5-α reductase inhibitors for prostate cancer prevention?

a. 5-α reductase inhibitors are approved for prostate cancer prevention.
b. 5-α reductase inhibitors increase libido.
c. 5-α reductase inhibitors decrease prostate cancer, but increase the Gleason score in patients who develop cancer.
d. 5-α reductase inhibitors increase the risk of prostate cancer.
e. 5-α reductase inhibitors can increase the PSA level.

Answer c is correct. Studies reveal 5-α reductase inhibitors reduce the rate of prostate cancer, but may increase the cancer grade (Gleason grade 7-10) in those who develop prostate cancer.

Answer a is incorrect. 5-α reductase inhibitors are not approved for prostate cancer prevention.

Answer b is incorrect. 5-α reductase inhibitors can decrease libido not increase.

Answer d is incorrect. Studies reveal 5-α reductase inhibitors reduce the rate of prostate cancer, not increase. 5-α reductase inhibitors are not approved for prevention of prostate cancer.

Answer e is incorrect. 5-α reductase inhibitors falsely lower the PSA in patients and this needs to be accounted for when measuring the PSA

4. Which of the following agents is considered a GnRH antagonist?

a. Goserelin
b. Degarelix
c. Leuprolide
d. Triptorelin
e. Sipuleucel-T

Answer b is correct. Degarelix is a GnRH antagonist that binds to GnRH receptors on cells in the pituitary gland, reducing the production of testosterone to castrate levels.

Answer a is incorrect. Goserelin is an LH-RH agonist.

Answer c is incorrect. Leuprolide is an LH-RH agonist.

Answer d is incorrect. Triptorelin is an LH-RH agonist.

Answer e is incorrect. Sipuleucel-T is an autologous immunologic agent.

5. BD is a 59-year-old man with hypertension and dyslipidemia. He reports to the ER in status epilepticus. Which medication is the most likely cause?

a. Bicalutamide
b. Flutamide
c. Nilutamide
d. Enzalutamide
e. Abiraterone

Answer d is correct. Enzalutamide may cause seizures and would require immediate treatment.

Answer a is incorrect. Bicalutamide may cause gynecomastia, hot flashes, diarrhea, liver function abnormalities, and breast tenderness.

Answer b is incorrect. Flutamide may cause gynecomastia, hot flashes, diarrhea, liver function abnormalities, breast tenderness, and methemoglobinemia.

Answer c is incorrect. Nilutamide may cause gynecomastia, hot flashes, diarrhea, liver function abnormalities, breast tenderness, and visual disturbances.

Answer d is incorrect. Abiraterone may cause diarrhea, edema, hypokalemia, hypophosphatemia, liver function abnormalities, and hypertriglyceridemia.

6. What is the trade name of abiraterone?

    a. Xtandi
    b. Nilandron
    c. Avodart
    d. Casodex
    e. Zytiga

Answer e is correct. The trade name for abiraterone is Zytiga.

Answer a is incorrect. Xtandi is the trade name for enzalutamide.

Answer b is incorrect. Nilandron is the trade name for nilutamide.

Answer c is incorrect. Avodart is the trade name for dutasteride.

Answer d is incorrect. Casodex is the trade name for bicalutamide.

7. MN is a newly diagnosed prostate cancer patient being treated with androgen deprivation. Which of the following are appropriate counseling points for a new patient starting on an LH-RH agonist? Select all that apply.

    a. Patient may experience side effects such as a loss in libido, hot flushes, and impotence.
    b. ADT is associated with osteoporosis and therefore the patient should take a calcium/vitamin D supplement.
    c. Patient may experience worsening symptoms during the first week related to "tumor flare."
    d. Patient may experience nausea/vomiting, alopecia, and weight loss.

Answers a, b, and c are correct. MN may experience side effects such as loss in libido, hot flushes, and impotence from androgen ablation. MN should take calcium/vitamin D supplementation because the androgen deprivation therapy is associated with osteoporosis. MN may experience worsening of symptoms during the first week because of a tumor flare.

Answer d is incorrect. Patient will not likely experience nausea/vomiting, alopecia, and weight loss. These symptoms are most likely associated with chemotherapy.

8. SL is a 69-year-old man who was recently diagnosed with prostate cancer and is initiated on a hormone agent for the first time for androgen deprivation. The pharmacist tells the patient he should not experience tumor flare with this new medication. Which of the following agents was this patient initiated on?

    a. Leuprolide
    b. Goserelin
    c. Triptorelin
    d. Degarelix
    e. Enzalutamide

Answer d is correct. Degarelix is a GnRH antagonist and therefore tumor flare is not expected with this agent due to its mechanism of action.

Answer a is incorrect. Leuprolide is an LH-RH agonist and therefore a disease flare-up during the first week may be expected.

Answer b is incorrect. Goserelin is an LH-RH agonist and therefore a disease flare-up during the first week may be expected.

Answer c is incorrect. Triptorelin is an LH-RH agonist and therefore a disease flare-up during the first week may be expected.

Answer e is incorrect. Enzalutamide is not an LH-RH or a GnRH agent, and therefore tumor flare is not an expected side effect. Additionally, this agent is only approved for use in castrate resistant prostate cancer, which this patient does not have.

9. CC is a 56-year-old man with metastatic castrate resistant prostate cancer. He has several other comorbid diseases including chronic heart failure (CHF), diabetes, and hypertension. Which of the following chemotherapy or systemic agents is the most appropriate for this patient? Select all that apply.

    a. Abiraterone
    b. Enzalutamide
    c. Cabazitaxel
    d. Docetaxel + prednisone

Answers a, b, and d are correct. Abiraterone, enzalutamide, and docetaxel and prednisone are all approved for first-line therapy in patients with castrate resistant prostate cancer.

Answer c is incorrect. Cabazitaxel is only approved in metastatic castrate resistant prostate cancer patients who have previously failed docetaxel.

10. BB is a 69-year-old man with metastatic prostate cancer who is receiving chemotherapy and denosumab. Which of the following side effects may potentially occur while on denosumab?

    a. Hypocalcemia
    b. Osteonecrosis of the jaw
    c. Loss of libido
    d. Hypokalemia
    e. Renal failure

Answer a is correct. Hypocalcemia may occur with denosumab. Patients should be on a calcium and vitamin D supplement while on denosumab.

Answer b is incorrect. Zoledronic acid may cause osteonecrosis of the jaw. Baseline dental assessment should be made prior to initiation.

Answer c is incorrect. While chemotherapy may cause some loss of libido in additional to some hormone agents, denosumab has not been associated with this side effect.

Answer d is incorrect. Abiraterone has been associated with hypokalemia, not denosumab.

Answer e is incorrect. Zoledronic acid may cause some renal dysfunction or renal failure while receiving treatment. Baseline monitoring of SCr is recommended. Denosumab is not renally eliminated and therefore does not have to be adjusted for renal dysfunction.

---

11. Which of the following side effects is associated with docetaxel use? Select all that apply.

    a. Myelosuppression
    b. Gynecomastia
    c. Alopecia
    d. Cardiotoxicity
    e. Blue/Green secretions

Answers a and c are correct. Docetaxel may cause myelosuppression, alopecia, mucositis, or neuropathy.

Answer b is incorrect. Antiandrogens are associated with gynecomastia.

Answer d is incorrect. Antiandrogens are not associated with a rash.

Answer e is incorrect. Mitoxantrone is associated with blue/green secretions.

---

12. Which of the following antiandrogens is associated with interstitial pneumonitis?

    a. Flutamide
    b. Bicalutamide
    c. Nilutamide
    d. Enzalutamide
    e. Abiraterone

Answer c is correct. Nilutamide has been associated with interstitial pneumonitis.

Answer a is incorrect. Flutamide is not associated with interstitial pneumonitis.

Answer b is incorrect. Bicalutamide is not associated with interstitial pneumonitis.

Answer d is incorrect. Enzalutamide is not associated with interstitial pneumonitis.

Answer e is incorrect. Abiraterone is not an antiandrogen and is not associated with interstitial pneumonitis.

---

13. Which of the following patients with prostate cancer can be managed with observation alone?

    a. Patient with a Gleason score of 3 and PSA of 5 ng/mL
    b. Patient with a Gleason score of 8 and PSA of 40 ng/mL
    c. Patient with a Gleason score of 2 and PSA of 15 ng/mL
    d. Patient with a Gleason score of 5 and PSA of 20 ng/mL
    e. Patient with a Gleason score of 6 and a PSA of 100 ng/mL

Answer a is correct. Asymptomatic patients with a low risk of recurrence, a Gleason score of 2 through 6, and a PSA of less than 10 ng/mL (10 mcg/L) may be managed by observation, radiation (external beam or brachytherapy), or radical prostatectomy.

Answer b is incorrect. The treatment of patients at high risk of recurrence (Gleason score ranging from 8-10, and a PSA value greater than 20 ng/mL, 20 mcg/L) should be treated with androgen ablation for 2 to 3 years combined with radiation therapy.

Answer c is incorrect. Individuals with moderate disease or a Gleason score of 7, and a PSA ranging from 10 to 20 ng/mL (10-20 mcg/L) are considered at intermediate risk for prostate cancer recurrence.

Answer d is incorrect. Individuals with moderate disease or a Gleason score of 7, and a PSA ranging from 10 to 20 ng/mL (10-20 mcg/L) are considered at intermediate risk for prostate cancer recurrence.

Answer e is incorrect. The treatment of patients at high risk of recurrence (Gleason score ranging from 8-10, and a PSA value greater than 20 ng/mL, 20 mcg/L) should be treated with androgen ablation for 2 to 3 years combined with radiation therapy.

---

14. A 61-year-old is seeing his primary care physician for an annual physical today. As part of the shared-decision making, the physician reviews the data pertaining to prostate cancer screening. Which of the following is true?

    a. DRE is highly specific and highly sensitive for detecting prostate cancer and should be used alone for diagnosis.
    b. PSA is highly specific and highly sensitive for detecting prostate cancer and should be used alone for diagnosis.
    c. DRE and PSA are highly specific and highly sensitive for detecting prostate cancer and should be used in combination for diagnosis.
    d. Neither DRE nor PSA are highly specific or highly sensitive when used alone for detecting prostate cancer. Therefore, these agents should be used in combination for diagnosis.
    e. DRE is highly specific and PSA is low is sensitivity and therefore it doesn't matter if these screening methods are used separately or in combination.

Answer d is correct. Neither DRE nor PSA are highly specific or highly sensitive when used alone for detecting prostate cancer. However, because of the lack of specificity and sensitivity when used alone, these tests should be used in combination for diagnosis.

Answer a is incorrect. DRE is not highly specific or highly sensitive when used alone for detection of prostate cancer.

Answer b is incorrect. PSA is not highly specific or highly sensitive when used alone for detection of prostate cancer.

Answer c is incorrect. DRE and PSA are neither highly specific nor highly sensitive for detecting prostate cancer. However, because of the lack of specificity and sensitivity when used alone, these tests should be used in combination for diagnosis.

Answer e is incorrect. DRE and PSA are neither highly specific nor highly sensitive for detecting prostate cancer. However, because of the lack of specificity and sensitivity when used alone, these tests should be used in combination for diagnosis.

15. Which of the following agents has an adherence concern due to the dosing concern?

    a. Flutamide
    b. Bicalutamide
    c. Nilutamide
    d. Enzalutamide
    e. Abiraterone

Answer a is correct. Flutamide is dose three times daily and therefore adherence is a concern.

Answer b is incorrect. Bicalutamide is a once-daily drug and therefore adherence is less of a concern.

Answer c is incorrect. Nilutamide is a once-daily drug and therefore adherence is less of a concern.

Answer d is incorrect. Enzalutamide is a once-daily drug and therefore adherence is less of a concern.

Answer e is incorrect. Abiraterone is a once-daily drug and therefore adherence is less of a concern.

16. Which of the following agents should be utilized in patients with castrate resistant prostate cancer with bone pain for assistance with pain reduction?

    a. Flutamide
    b. Bicalutamide
    c. Docetaxel
    d. Radium-223
    e. Sipuleucel-T

Answer d is correct. Radium-223 is approved for patients with metastatic prostate cancer with bone metastases. In the approval studies, this agent was found to reduce the pain associated with bone metastases.

Answer a is incorrect. Flutamide has not been shown to reduce pain in patients with bone metastases in clinical trials.

Answer b is incorrect. Bicalutamide has not been shown to reduce pain in patients with bone metastases in clinical trials.

Answer c is incorrect. Although Docetaxel may ultimately reduce bone pain, this was not an outcome on the landmark studies.

Answer e is incorrect. Sipuleucel-T is approved for patients with minimally symptomatic disease, and therefore less severe pain.

17. MN is seeing his oncologist today and receives a prescription for both leuprolide and flutamide. The use of an antiandrogen and an LH-RH agonist together is called:

    a. Concurrent chemoprevention
    b. Concurrent chemoradiotherapy
    c. CAB
    d. Castrate resistant prostate cancer
    e. Concurrent chemotherapy

Answer c is correct. CAB is the use of an antiandrogen and LH-RH agonists concurrently.

Answer a is incorrect. Chemoprevention is a term that defines agents used to prevent cancer.

Answer b is incorrect. Concurrent chemoradiotherapy is the use of chemotherapy and radiation concurrently.

Answer d is incorrect. Castrate or hormone resistant prostate cancer describes a patient with an increasing PSA while receiving hormonal therapy.

Answer e is incorrect. Concurrent chemotherapy is utilizing two chemotherapy agents together at the same time.

18. Which of the following agents should only be utilized as second-line therapy for metastatic castrate resistant prostate cancer? Select all that apply.

    a. Docetaxel plus prednisone
    b. Abiraterone plus prednisone
    c. Enzalutamide plus prednisone
    d. Mitoxantrone plus prednisone
    e. Cabazitaxel plus prednisone

Answers d and e are correct. Mitoxantrone plus prednisone has not demonstrated a survival improvement after failure of docetaxel, but remains a palliative therapeutic option, specifically in men who are not candidates for cabazitaxel or radium-223 therapy. Cabazitaxel is only approved as second line therapy.

Answer a is incorrect. Docetaxel may be utilized in the first or subsequent lines of therapy.

Answer b is incorrect. Abiraterone is approved for use in first-line therapy but may be utilized in second or subsequent lines of therapy.

Answer c is incorrect. Enzalutamide should not be administered with prednisone. Enzalutamide may be utilized in first or subsequent lines of therapy.

19. Which of the following hormonal therapies is administered via depot? Select all that apply.

    a. Lupron
    b. Zoladex
    c. Trelstar
    d. Viadur
    e. Firmagon

Answers a, c, and e are correct.   Lupron, Trelstar, and Firmagon are all depot formulations. Zoladex and Viadur are implants. Firmagon is administered SQ, but it forms a depot once administered.

Answer b is incorrect.   Zoladex, or Goserelin, is an implant.

Answer d is incorrect.   Viadur, or Leuprolide, is an implant.

20. GS is a 58-year-old man who was diagnosed with prostate cancer several years ago. He was recently referred to oncology as his disease was deemed castrate resistant. The physician recommends docetaxel with prednisone for GS every 3 weeks. Which of the following premedication regimens would you recommend?

    a. Diphenhydramine and ranitidine
    b. Loperamide
    c. Allopurinol
    d. Calcium and magnesium
    e. Mesna

Answer a is correct.   Due to hypersensitivity reactions, diphenhydramine and ranitidine are recommended for prevention.

Answer b is incorrect.   Loperamide may be utilized to prevent diarrhea in other chemotherapy regimens, but is not necessary with docetaxel.

Answer c is incorrect.   Hyperuricemia is not common therefore allopurinol is not recommended.

Answer d is incorrect.   Calcium and magnesium may sometimes be administered with agents utilized for colon cancer, but not recommended for use with docetaxel.

Answer e is incorrect.   Docetaxel does not cause hemorrhagic cystitis and therefore would not be appropriate to initiate Mesna prior to therapy.

CHAPTER 15 | Leukemias

For questions 1 to 7 use patient DC vignette.

1. DC is a 59-year-old Caucasian man who reports to his primary care physician complaining of 2-week history of fatigue and fever. A CBC with differential reveals an elevated WBC (25,000 U/L) and profound thrombocytopenia (platelets 30,000 U/L). His peripheral blood has 20% blasts. A bone marrow biopsy was performed and DC was diagnosed with acute myeloid leukemia (AML-M4). Molecular testing revealed—FLT3 negative, NPML1 negative, C-KIT negative. Initial induction therapy should consist of the following:

    a. Mitoxantrone
    b. Cytarabine + idarubicin
    c. Cytarabine + imatinib
    d. Asparaginase

Answer b is correct.   The most active agents in AML are anthracyclines and the antimetabolite cytarabine. Cytarabine in combination with idarubicin is often referred to as "7+3" regimen (cytarabine 100 mg/m² days 1-7, idarubicin 12 mg/m² days 1-3). Accounting for age, other comorbidities, and patient's ejection fraction, this combination should be recommended for initial induction therapy.

Answer a is incorrect.   Mitoxantrone is recommended in adult AML, however, is usually not given as monotherapy for induction. For patients less than 60 years old, they should receive standard dose cytarabine + (daunorubicin or idarubicin) per National Comprehensive Cancer Network (NCCN) guidelines.

Answer c is incorrect.   Imatinib is not recommended in AML induction. Imatinib is recommended in CML, GIST tumors, and Ph+ ALL.

Answer d is incorrect.   Asparaginase in not recommended in the treatment of adult AML. Asparaginase is recommended in pediatric and adult ALL regimens.

2. Physician asks you about tumor lysis syndrome (TLS) prevention and management for patient DC. Which of the following suggestions should include? Select all that apply.

    a. Initiating allopurinol
    b. Treating electrolyte disturbances
    c. Aggressive hydration
    d. Minimize hydration

Answer a is correct.   Allopurinol is indicated in preventing and managing TLS. Allopurinol acts as a competitive inhibitor of xanthine oxidase, thereby blocking the conversion of the purine metabolites to uric acid.

Answer b is correct.   Electrolyte disturbances commonly seen in TLS include hyperuricemia, hyperkalemia, hyperphosphatemia, and hypocalcemia. Agents such as sodium polystyrene sulfonate (Kayexalate) for hyperkalemia or oral phosphate binders, such as calcium acetate (PhosLo) or sevelamer (Renagel), may be warranted in some clinical situations.

Answer c is correct.   Hydration enhances urine flow and promotes the excretion of uric acid and phosphate by improving intravascular volume, renal blood flow, and glomerular filtration. The use of sodium bicarbonate in IV fluids to alkalinize the urine is often performed to protect kidney function.

Answer d is incorrect.   Hydration is recommended.

3. TLS is characterized by the following:

    a. Hypocalcemia, hypouricemia, hyperkalemia
    b. Hyperphosphatemia, hyperkalemia, hyperuricemia
    c. Hypercalcemia, hyperkalemia, hypomagnesium
    d. Hypokalemia, hyperphosphatemia, hypouricemia

Answer b is correct. Electrolyte disturbances commonly seen in TLS include hyperuricemia, hyperkalemia, hyperphosphatemia, and hypocalcemia.

Answer a is incorrect. Hyperuricemia is commonly seen in TLS. Uric acid levels are often more than 7.5 mg/dL, which may require drug therapy such as rasburicase.

Answer c is incorrect. Alterations in serum magnesium levels are not associated with TLS.

Answer d is incorrect. Serum potassium and uric acid levels are often increased in TLS.

---

4. Following induction therapy, DC achieves a complete remission. Next month he arrives at your institution to receive high-dose cytarabine (HDAC) for consolidation therapy. You receive the following order—

    Cytarabine 3000 mg/m² IV q12h days 1, 3, and 5

    Patient characteristics: Height 6'0", Weight 165 lb

    Which of the following represents a correct dosing strategy for patient DC?

    a. Cytarabine 5850 mg IV days 1, 3, and 5
    b. Cytarabine 5850 mg IV q12h days 1, 3, and 5
    c. Cytarabine 5550 gm IV days 1, 3, and 5
    d. Cytarabine 5550 mg IV q12h days 1, 3, and 5

Answer b is correct. DC's calculated BSA is 1.95 m² since height is 182.88 cm and weight is 75 kg. This answer represents correct dosing and strategy.

Answer a is incorrect. DC should receive cytarabine twice daily given every 12 hours.

Answer c is incorrect. This dose would represent a major dosing error. Note units of gm not mg.

Answer d is incorrect. DC's calculated BSA is 1.95 m² since height is 182.88 cm and weight is 75 kg. This answer represents a dosing strategy for a BSA of 1.85 m².

---

5. Which type of biological safety cabinet (BSC) should the cytarabine be prepared in?

    a. Vertical flow, class I
    b. Vertical flow, class II
    c. Horizontal flow, class II
    d. Horizontal flow, class I

Answer b is correct. A vertical flow class II BSC, HEPA filtered air (ISO class 5) is required for personnel in handling hazardous agents. For reference—ASHP Guidelines on Handling Hazardous Drugs. *Am J Health-Syst Pharm.* 2006;63:1172-93.

Answer a is incorrect. When asepsis is not required a Class I BSC can be used. However, USP Chapter <797> Pharmaceutical Compounding: Sterile Preparations details the procedures and requirements for sterile compounding preparations for hospitals.

Answer c is incorrect. See answer B for rationale.

Answer d is incorrect. See answer B for rationale.

---

6. What toxicities should DC be counseled on prior to receiving high-dose cytarabine?

    a. Infusion-related reactions, paralytic ileus, cardiotoxicity
    b. Cerebellar toxicity, peripheral neuropathy, infusion-related reactions
    c. Nausea, peripheral neuropathy, ocular toxicity
    d. Cerebellar toxicity, nausea, ocular toxicity

Answer d is correct. Cytarabine is associated with cerebellar, nausea, and ocular toxicity particularly in the high-dose (g/m²) setting. Cerebellar toxicity is characterized by nystagmus, slurred speech, and ataxia. HDAC is listed as a moderate emetogenic risk (30%-90% frequency of emesis) agent by NCCN guidelines. Ocular toxicity manifests itself by conjunctivitis; this can be prevented with the use of prophylactic dexamethasone eye drops.

Answer a is incorrect. Cytarabine is not associated with infusion related reactions, paralytic ileus, or cardiotoxicity.

Answer b is incorrect. Cytarabine is not associated with peripheral neuropathy or infusion related reactions.

Answer c is incorrect. Cytarabine is not associated with peripheral neuropathy.

---

7. A newly diagnosed patient with acute promyelocytic leukemia (APL) begins treatment with tretinoin 40 mg orally twice daily. Within 48 hours of the initiation, the patient develops fever, dyspnea, and respiratory distress. Which of the following should be immediately initiated to treat apparent differentiation syndrome (DS)?

    a. Dexamethasone
    b. Acetaminophen
    c. Diphenhydramine
    d. Epinephrine

Answer a is correct. Dexamethasone 10 mg IV every 12 hours is recommended for 3 days or until resolution of symptoms, immediately starting at onset of symptoms of DS. Steroids have shown a mortality benefit.

Answer b is incorrect. Acetaminophen is not recommended in the management of DS.

Answer c is incorrect. Diphenhydramine is not recommended in the management of DS.

Answer d is incorrect. Epinephrine is used for anaphylactic reactions, not applicable in this clinical setting.

For questions 8 to 10 use patient AB vignette.

8. AB is a 60-year-old African American man newly diagnosed with acute lymphoblastic leukemia (ALL). His physician has recommended part A hyper-CVAD regimen (cyclophosphamide, vincristine, doxorubicin, and dexamethasone). Which of the following is a correct dose for doxorubicin?

   Patient specifics: Height 5'8", Weight 180 lb

   Notable labs: SrCr 1 mg/dL, Total bilirubin 2.5 mg/dL

   Dosing recommendations: CrCl <50 mL/min: No dosage adjustment necessary; Serum bilirubin 1.2-3 mg/dL: Administer 50% of dose; Serum bilirubin 3.1-5 mg/dL: Administer 25% of dose.

   Regimen

   Cyclophosphamide 300 mg/m² IV q12h days 1-3

   Mesna 600 mg/m² CIVI days 1-3

   Vincristine 2 mg IV day 4 and 11

   Doxorubicin 50 mg/m² IV over 24 hours day 4

   Dexamethasone 40 mg po days 1-4 and days 11-14

   a. 50 mg doxorubicin IV over 24 hours
   b. 100 mg doxorubicin IV over 24 hours
   c. 75 mg doxorubicin IV over 24 hours
   d. 100 mg doxorubicin IV push

Answer a is correct. Given patient characteristics (height 172.72 cm, weight 81.8 kg, BSA 1.98 m²) patient would normally receive doxorubicin 100 mg dose. However, MJ has elevated serum bilirubin which should lead to a 50% dose reduction.

Answer b is incorrect. This answer does not represent the dose adjustment that is recommended.

Answer c is incorrect. This answer does not reflect an accurate dose due to miscalculations of BSA.

Answer d is incorrect. This answer does not represent the dose adjustment that is recommended. Some institutions give this doxorubicin over 15 minutes, but reference listed above states doxorubicin should be administered over 24 hours.

9. Why is AB receiving mesna given continuously with cyclophosphamide on days 1-3?

   a. Prevention of renal toxicity associated with cyclophosphamide
   b. Chemotherapy induced nausea and vomiting prevention
   c. Neutropenic fever prophylaxis
   d. Reduce incidence of cyclophosphamide-induced hemorrhagic cystitis

Answer d is correct. Mesna binds to and inactivates the toxic oxazaphosphorine metabolite (acrolein) in the urine to prevent hemorrhagic cystitis.

Answer a is incorrect. Mesna does not prevent renal toxicity associated with aklyating agents.

Answer b is incorrect. Mesna does not improve CINV symptoms.

Answer c is incorrect. Mesna does increase granulocyte or macrophage colony stimulating factor production.

10. AB is to receive CNS prophylaxis. Which of the following can be safely administered intrathecally (IT)? Select all that apply.

    a. Cytarabine
    b. Methotrexate
    c. Vincristine
    d. Vinblastine

Answer a is correct. Intrathecal cytarabine is recommended in ALL patients due to CNS involvement.

Answer b is correct. Intrathecal methotrexate is recommended in ALL patients due to CNS involvement.

Answers c and d are incorrect. Vincristine and vinblastine should never be given intrathecally; this may cause severe neurologic toxicity and/or death.

11. You are an oncology pharmacist counseling a parent and their child undergoing treatment for pediatric ALL. Patient will be treated with a Children's Oncology Group (COG) protocol. All of the following adverse events should be discussed with them regarding asparaginase? Select all that apply.

    a. Hyperglycemia
    b. Risk of allergic reactions
    c. Potential for bleeding
    d. Alopecia

Answer a is correct. Hyperglycemia/glucose intolerance has been reported in ~10% of patients which receive asparaginase.

Answer b is correct. Hypersensitivity reactions are a major concern with patients which receive asparaginase. A test dose is recommended with first dose of therapy. Practitioners are instructed to have epinephrine, diphenhydramine, and hydrocortisone available at bedside due to risk.

Answer c is correct. Thrombosis, fatal bleeding, consumption coagulopathy, and intracranial hemorrhage have all been reported.

Answer d is incorrect. Asparaginase is not associated with alopecia.

For questions 12 to 15 use patient TC vignette.

12. TC is a 62-year-old man recently diagnosed with Stage 3 CLL. TC has been recently complaining of painful lymphadenopathies as well as easy bruising. His physician has chosen to begin rituximab for 6 cycles. Which of the following adverse events should be discussed with the patient prior to first cycle infusion? Select all that apply.

    a. Hepatitis B reactivation
    b. Infusion-related reactions
    c. Tumor lysis syndrome
    d. Flu-like symptoms

Answer a is correct. Hepatitis B reactivation has been reported in patients treated with rituximab in combination with chemotherapy. As a result, it is recommended that hepatitis B testing be performed prior to the initiation of rituximab.

Answer b is correct. Infusion related reactions are common and can be severe. Reactions include bronchospasms, hypoxia, hypotension, and in more severe cases pulmonary infiltrates. Infusion related reactions are a Black Box warning.

Answer c is correct. TLS has occurred within first 24 hours of rituximab dose. This is listed as a Black Box warning.

Answer d is correct. Adverse events associated with rituximab include infusion related reactions, tumor lysis syndrome, flu-like symptoms, skin rash, and cytopenias. Hepatitis B reactivation has been reported in patients treated with rituximab in combination with chemotherapy.

13. Which of the following is true regarding the monoclonal antibody rituximab (Rituxan®)?

    a. Humanized, targets CD33+ myeloid cells
    b. Chimeric, targets CD20+ B cells
    c. Humanized, targets CD52+ lymphocytes
    d. Chimeric, targets CD33+ myeloid cells

Answer b is correct. Monoclonal antibody nomenclature includes that (-xi-) in name represents a chimeric monoclonal antibody. Rituximab binds specifically to CD20, a hydrophobic protein, located on pre-B and mature B lymphocytes. The Fab domain of rituximab binds to the CD20 antigen and the Fc domain recruits the immune system to mediate cell lysis.

Answer a is incorrect. Rituximab is not a humanized monoclonal antibody or targets CD33+ myeloid cells

Answer c is incorrect. Rituximab is not a humanized monoclonal antibody or targets CD33+ myeloid cells. An example of this would be alemtuzumab (Campath®), which is used in CLL treatment.

Answer d is incorrect. See above for rationale.

14. Patient TC relapses following rituximab therapy and now their oncologist is contemplating an oral therapy option such as ibrutinib, idelalisib, or ventoclax. TC has been experiencing diarrhea episodes from irritable bowel syndrome. Which of the following novel oral therapies should not be recommended for patient TC?

    a. Ibrutinib
    b. Idelalisib
    c. Ventoclax
    d. None of the above

Answer b is correct. Idelalisib has FDA Black Box warnings for diarrhea or colitis as well as fatal/serious intestinal perforations. With these warning, idelalisib should be avoided in patient TC.

Answer a is incorrect. Ibrutinib is an effective option for CLL and does not have any contraindications for TC.

Answer c is incorrect. Ventoclax is an effective option for relapsed CLL and does not have any contraindications for TC.

Answer d is incorrect. See above for rationale for answer b.

15. For CLL patients such as TC, which of the following agents should be recommended for patients who present with recurrent infections? Select all that apply.

    a. Annual influenza vaccine
    b. Monthly intravenous immunoglobulin (when serum IgG <400 mg/dL)
    c. Pneumococcal vaccine every 5 years
    d. Annual pneumococcal vaccine

Answer a is correct. Annual influenza vaccine is recommended. In patients who have received rituximab, B-cell recovery occurs by approximately 9 months. Prior to B-cell recovery, patients generally do not respond to influenza vaccine and if given should not be considered vaccinated per NCCN guidelines.

Answer b is correct. Due to hypogammaglobulinemia, which occurs in most CLL patients, select patients should receive monthly IVIG infusions.

Answer c is correct. Per NCCN guidelines, patients should receive a pneumococcal vaccine every 5 years.

Answer d is incorrect. Pneumococcal vaccine is administered every 5 years.

For questions 16 to 19, please refer to patient DD vignette.

16. DD is a 55-year-old woman who has been in excellent health until 2 weeks ago. Since that time she has complained about fatigue, night sweats, and early satiety. She presented to her PCP where labs revealed the following—WBC 62,000 mm³, platelets 190,000 mm³, and hemoglobulin 12.3 g/dL.

    She was referred to an oncologist where a bone marrow biopsy was performed.

    Cytogenetics: + translocation (9;22)

    Diagnosis: chronic myelogenous leukemia (CML)

    Which of the following is an approved first-line treatment for CML?

    a. Allogeneic stem cell transplant
    b. Interferon-α + cytarabine
    c. Imatinib (Gleevec)
    d. Sunitinib (Sutent)

Answer c is correct. for the above mentioned reason. Imatinib is recommended as first-line therapy for CML at 400 mg/d in chronic phase CML.

Answer a is incorrect. Patients will receive oral tyrosine kinase inhibitors (imatinib, dasatinib, or nilotinib) prior to stem cell transplant.

Answer b is incorrect. Imatinib was shown to provide better response rates than interferon-α + cytarabine in a clinical trial. This combination regimen is no longer recommended for first-line therapy.

Answer d is incorrect. Sunitinib is FDA approved for renal cell carcinoma and gastrointestinal stromal tumors (GIST).

---

17. It is established that DD has chronic phase (CP-CML). Which of the following BCR-ABL inhibitors are FDA labeled for the treatment of CP-CML?

    a. Imatinib only
    b. Imatinib and dasatinib only
    c. Imatinib, dasatinib, and nilotinib
    d. Imatinib, dasatinib, nilotinib, and erlotinib

Answer c is correct. Imatinib, dasatinib, and nilotinib are all approved in the treatment of CP-CML.

Answer a is incorrect. Imatinib is approved in CP-CML; however, other second generation BCR-ABL inhibitors have been approved since the impressive IRIS study with imatinib.

Answer b is incorrect. Both imatinib and dasatinib have FDA approved indications in CP-CML, but the Phase III ENESTnd demonstrated effectiveness of nilotinib in this clinical study.

Answer d is incorrect. The presence of erlotinib in this answer makes this incorrect. Erlotinib has an FDA labeled indication in non-small lung cancer as well as pancreatic cancer.

---

18. Select the brand name for nilotinib.

    a. Tasigna
    b. Sprycel
    c. Gleevec
    d. Nexavar

Answer a is correct. Tasigna is the brand name for nilotinib.

Answer b is incorrect. Sprycel is the brand name for dasatinib.

Answer c is incorrect. Gleevec is the brand name for imatinib.

Answer d is incorrect. Nexavar is the brand name for sorafenib.

---

19. Which of the following adverse events associated with dasatinib should be discussed with DD? Select all that apply.

    a. Pleural effusion
    b. Bruising
    c. Alopecia
    d. Fatigue

Answer a is correct. Fluid retention is an adverse event associated with dasatinib. Eighteen percent (all grade toxicity) of patients receiving dasatinib at 100 mg/d reported pleural effusions.

Answers b and d are correct. Treatment with dasatinib is associated with severe (grade 3 or 4) neutropenia, anemia (fatigue), and thrombocytopenia (bruising). CBCs should be performed weekly for the first 2 months and then monthly thereafter, or as clinically indicated.

Answer c is incorrect. Alopecia is not a common adverse event associated with dasatinib.

---

20. QTc monitoring is warranted with which BCR-ABL inhibitor?

    a. Imatinib
    b. Dasatinib
    c. Nilotinib
    d. Bosutinib

Answer c is correct. Nilotinib prolongs the QT interval. It is recommended that patients should have corrected hypokalemia or hypomagnesemia prior to initiation. Sudden deaths have been reported. Recommend ECGs at baseline, 7 days following initiation, and periodically thereafter.

Answer a is incorrect. Imatinib is not associated with QTc prolongation.

Answer b is incorrect. Dasatinib should be used with caution in patients with history of QTc prolongation. Currently it is not recommended to routinely monitor QTc. In 865 patients in Phase 2 studies, only 1% of patients experienced a QTcF more than 500 ms.

Answer d is incorrect. In a single-arm phase I/II study, only 0.2% experienced QTcF interval more than 500 ms.

CHAPTER **16 | Breast Cancer**

1. Select the agent that is administered via intramuscular injection for the treatment of metastatic ER positive breast cancer.

    a. Anastrozole
    b. Avastin
    c. Herceptin
    d. Faslodex

Answer d is correct. Faslodex is administered by IM injection to women with ER+ metastatic breast cancer.

Answer a in incorrect. Anastrozole is administered orally to patients with ER+ metastatic breast cancer.

Answer b is incorrect. Avastin is administered intravenously to patients with breast cancer.

Answer c is incorrect. Herceptin is administered intravenously to patients with breast cancer characterized by an overexpression of HER-2.

---

2. Which of the following conditions would be a contraindication to administration of tamoxifen for the prevention of breast cancer in a "high-risk" premenopausal patient?

   a. History of deep venous thrombosis
   b. First-degree relative with ER negative breast cancer
   c. History of diabetes mellitus
   d. History of seizures

Answer a is correct. Tamoxifen is associated with an increased risk for developing thromboembolic events. Administration of tamoxifen to prevent breast cancer is contraindicated in patients with a history of deep venous thrombosis or pulmonary emboli.

Answer b is incorrect. The ER status of first degree relatives is not a contraindication to prescribing tamoxifen to reduce the risk for developing breast cancer.

Answer c is incorrect. Diabetes mellitus is not a contraindication to prescribing tamoxifen to reduce the risk for developing breast cancer.

Answer d is incorrect. A history of seizures is not a contraindication to prescribing tamoxifen to reduce the risk for developing breast cancer.

---

3. A premenopausal woman with ER negative, node positive breast cancer is starting doxorubicin and cyclophosphamide adjuvant treatment. What would you recommend to determine the severity of the most common toxicity associated with this treatment regimen?

   a. An electrocardiogram
   b. A complete blood count including platelets 1 week after administration of the chemotherapy
   c. Serum bilirubin and aspartate transaminase
   d. Urinalysis

Answer b is correct. Myelosuppression (neutropenia, thrombocytopenia) is the most common treatment related adverse effect associated with this adjuvant treatment regimen. Nearly 100% of patients receiving this treatment regimen will experience myelosuppression.

Answer a is incorrect. Although doxorubicin has been associated with cardiomyopathy that increases in incidence with cumulative doses exceeding 400 mg/m^2, it is not the most common toxicity associated with this treatment regimen. The incidence of cardiomyopathy in patients administered cumulative doses exceeding 400 mg/m^2 is in the range of 5%.

Answer c is incorrect. Although these drugs may cause elevations of serum bilirubin and aspartate transaminase, it occurs less frequently than myelosuppression.

Answer d is incorrect. Although urinalysis could be useful in detecting hematuria caused by cyclophosphamide, this adverse effect (hemorrhagic cystitis) occurs infrequently with this adjuvant chemotherapy regimen.

---

4. Select the toxicity that has been associated with the administration of both trastuzumab and bevacizumab.

   a. Myelosuppression
   b. Gastrointestinal (GI) perforation
   c. Alopecia
   d. Infusion reactions

Answer d is correct. Trastuzumab and bevacizumab are monoclonal antibodies administered by intravenous infusion. Infusion reactions (the onset of chills, fever, changes in blood pressure within 1 hour of administration) have been reported to occur with both agents.

Answer a is incorrect. Trastuzumab and bevacizumab are monoclonal antibodies that are rarely associated with myelosuppression.

Answer b is incorrect. Although GI perforation is a proven bevacizumab toxicity, it is not associated with trastuzumab.

Answer c is incorrect. Monoclonal antibodies are not associated with hair loss.

---

5. Which of the following medications are recommended to be administered prior to an infusion of paclitaxel in order to prevent infusion reactions? Select all that apply.

   a. Dexamethasone
   b. Ranitidine
   c. Meperidine
   d. Diphenhydramine
   e. Acetaminophen

Answers a, b, and d are correct. Pretreatment with a glucocorticoid, an H_2 antagonist, and an H_1 antagonist is recommended to prevent or lessen the severity of hypersensitivity reactions occurring with paclitaxel administration.

Answers c and e are incorrect. Meperidine and acetaminophen are not included in the recommended pretreatment regimen to prevent or lessen the severity of hypersensitivity reactions occurring with paclitaxel administration.

---

6. A patient taking capecitabine for metastatic breast cancer describes to you the development of tenderness on her hands and feet, making it difficult for her to be on her feet. Select the most appropriate recommendation for this patient.

   a. Her symptoms describe the onset of a known side effect of capecitabine. You recommend she call her physician and describe the onset of these symptoms before taking any more doses of capecitabine.

b. Her symptoms are classic for individuals with vitamin B6 deficiency. You recommend she schedule an appointment with her physician to discuss these symptoms.

c. Her symptoms are commonly caused by capecitabine. You reassure her that there is nothing to worry about and recommend she avoid standing as much as possible while she completes the last week of capecitabine.

d. Her symptoms are commonly caused by capecitabine. You recommend the symptoms are self-limiting and easily managed by spraying her hands and feet with benzocaine first-aid spray four times daily.

Answer a is correct. The hand-foot syndrome is a known toxicity of capecitabine and will likely worsen if she continues taking the drug. The patient's physician should be informed and evaluate the benefits/risks of continuing therapy.

Answer b is incorrect. The symptoms are consistent with the onset of capecitabine induced hand-foot syndrome and require evaluation by the patient's physician.

Answer c is incorrect. The symptoms often become progressively worse. The patient's physician should be informed and evaluate the benefits/risks of continuing therapy.

Answer d is incorrect. The symptoms often become progressively worse. There is no clinical trial data supporting the efficacy of using a topical anesthetic to manage the symptoms while the capecitabine is continued. The patient's physician should be informed and evaluate the benefits/risks of continuing therapy.

7. A patient presents her prescription for capecitabine to you. Review of her medication profile documents she is also taking 5 mg of warfarin daily for atrial fibrillation and metformin for type II diabetes mellitus. Select the appropriate assessment of potential drug interactions for this patient.

a. Capecitabine has been shown to increase metabolism of warfarin and result in subtherapeutic INRs. More frequent monitoring of this patient's INRs is recommended.

b. Capecitabine has been shown to decrease metabolism of warfarin and result in elevated INRs and bleeding. More frequent monitoring of this patient's INRs is recommended.

c. Capecitabine has been shown to decrease metabolism of metformin and result in hypoglycemia. The importance of scheduled blood glucose monitoring and possible need for holding metformin doses needs to be discussed with this patient.

d. Capecitabine has been shown to increase metabolism of metformin and result in hyperglycemia. The importance of daily blood glucose monitoring and possible need for increasing metformin doses needs to be discussed with this patient.

e. Metformin has been shown to decrease metabolism of capecitabine and result in the increased severity of capecitabine induced-myelosuppression. A 25% reduction in the dose of capecitabine is indicated.

Answer b is correct. Case reports document significant elevation of INR values and bleeding when capecitabine was given to patients on a stable dose of warfarin. Capecitabine is responsible for elevated warfarin activity by inhibition of the CYP2C9 isoenzyme.

Answer a is incorrect. Capecitabine has been shown to decrease metabolism of warfarin.

Answer c is incorrect. Capecitabine has not been shown to alter metformin metabolism.

Answer d is incorrect. Capecitabine has not been shown to alter metformin metabolism.

Answer e is incorrect. Metformin has not been shown to alter capecitabine metabolism.

8. A patient presents a new prescription to you for tamoxifen. Her doctor said he was prescribing it as adjuvant treatment for breast cancer following her surgery last month. You review her medication profile and document that she is also taking metoprolol, hydrochlorothiazide, and fluoxetine. Select the appropriate assessment of potential drug interactions for this patient.

a. There are no clinically significant drug interactions to alter her medication regimen.

b. You explain that a number of selective serotonin reuptake inhibitors (SSRIs) including fluoxetine decrease the effectiveness of tamoxifen by interfering with its metabolism to an active metabolite. You will call the patient's physician to consider alternative antidepressant options.

c. You explain that hydrochlorothiazide has been documented to decrease the effectiveness of tamoxifen by interfering with its metabolism to an active metabolite. You will call the patient's physician to consider alternative diuretic.

d. You explain that metoprolol has been documented to decrease the effectiveness of tamoxifen by interfering with its metabolism to an active metabolite. You will call the patient's physician to consider alternative β-blocker.

Answer b is correct. SSRIs that are strong inhibitors of CYP2D6 have been documented to decrease the effectiveness of tamoxifen by decreasing the metabolism of tamoxifen to its potent metabolite endoxifen. It would be appropriate to notify the patient's physician and discuss alternative antidepressant options.

Answer a is incorrect. There is a potentially clinically significant drug interaction between tamoxifen and Prozac (fluoxetine).

Answer c is incorrect. Hydrochlorothiazide has not been shown to interfere with the activation of tamoxifen.

Answer d is incorrect. Metoprolol has not been shown to interfere with the activation of tamoxifen.

9. Select the endocrine therapy associated with an increased incidence of endometrial cancer.

a. Letrozole
b. Raloxifene
c. Toremifene

d. Fulvestrant

e. Tamoxifen

Answer e is correct. In the Breast Cancer Prevention Trial, the difference in the incidence of uterine cancer was statistically significant; tamoxifen 36 cases in 6,576 patients versus placebo 5 cases in 6,599 patients (risk ratio 2.53 with 95% confidence interval 1.35-4.97).

Answer a is incorrect. Letrozole and the other AIs have not been proven to increase the risk for uterine cancer.

Answer b is incorrect. Raloxifene is a SERM that has less estrogenic effects on the uterus. It has not been associated with an increased risk for uterine cancer.

Answer c is incorrect. Toremifene is a SERM but has not been associated with an increased risk for uterine cancer.

Answer d is incorrect. Fulvestrant is a pure estrogen antagonist that has not been associated with an increased risk for uterine cancer.

---

10. Which of following conditions would be a contraindication for prescribing an AI?

    a. The development of arthralgias and myalgias

    b. A patient with a history of thromboembolic events

    c. A premenopausal patient

    d. A postmenopausal patient with a history of thromboembolic events

    e. There are no contraindications for the administration of AIs

---

Answer c is correct. The administration of AIs to premenopausal women with breast cancer is contraindicated because they are ineffective in depleting estrogen production in women with functioning ovaries.

Answer a is incorrect. Arthralgias and myalgias are documented adverse effects of the AIs. If a patient develops these toxicities, a trial of an alternative AI is indicated.

Answer b is incorrect. A patient with a history of thromboembolic events is not a contraindication for administration of AIs.

Answer d is incorrect. The administration of AIs are not contraindicated for postmenopausal patients with a history of thromboembolic events.

Answer e is incorrect. The administration of AIs is contraindicated in premenopausal women and in women with a known hypersensitivity to these agents or any of their excipients.

---

11. Which of the following statements are true regarding palbociclib? Select all that apply.

    a. It is a signal transduction inhibitor that inhibits CDK 4 and 6.

    b. It is a signal transduction inhibitor that inhibits intracellular tyrosine kinase activity at EGFR-1 and EGFR-2.

    c. It is approved for treatment of ER positive and HER-2 negative metastatic breast cancer, in combination with letrozole as initial endocrine therapy for postmenopausal women.

    d. It is approved in combination with fulvestrant for metastatic disease, following progression on endocrine therapy.

    e. It is approved as monotherapy for patients with metastatic disease.

Answers a, c, and d are correct.

Answers b and e are incorrect. Palbociclib does not target tyrosine kinase. Palbociclib is only approved as combination therapy for patients with metastatic breast cancer.

---

12. Select the brand name for letrozole.

    a. Arimidex

    b. Nolvadex

    c. Avastin

    d. Evista

    e. Femara

Answer e is correct. Femara is the trade name for letrozole.

Answer a is incorrect. Arimidex is the trade name for anastrozole.

Answer b is incorrect. Nolvadex is the trade name for tamoxifen.

Answer c is incorrect. Avastin is the trade name for bevacizumab.

Answer d is incorrect. Evista is the trade name for raloxifene.

---

13. Select the taxane effective in treating advanced breast cancer that is formulated as an albumin nanoparticle product.

    a. Abraxane

    b. Taxol

    c. Jevtana

    d. Taxotere

Answer a is correct. Abraxane is the trade name for paclitaxel that is formulated as a nanoparticle suspension.

Answer b is incorrect. Taxol is the trade name for paclitaxel that is formulated in a Cremaphor solvent.

Answer c is incorrect. Jevtana is the trade name for cabazitaxel, which is indicated for the treatment of prostate cancer.

Answer d is incorrect. Taxotere is the trade name for docetaxel a non-nanoparticle taxane formulation.

---

14. A 69-year-old woman is taking anastrozole for ER positive/ PR positive, HER-2 negative stage IV breast cancer. Upon returning for her third refill she tells you that she has noticed increased stiffness and joint pain in knees. She started taking

ibuprofen 400 mg four times daily and at bedtime without much benefit for the past week. Your recommendation is to:

a. Increase the ibuprofen dosage to 800 mg four times daily and at bedtime.
b. The symptoms of joint and muscle pain are likely caused by anastrozole. You offer to call her physician to discuss switching to letrozole or exemestane.
c. The symptoms are consistent with a hypersensitivity reaction to anastrozole. You recommend she take some diphenhydramine and go to the emergency room for evaluation.
d. The symptoms have not been associated with anastrozole; she is likely developing rheumatoid arthritis.

Answer b is correct. AIs are known to cause joint and muscle pain. Switching to an alternative AI is a reasonable option as reports support other AIs may be better tolerated.

Answer a is incorrect. The recommended maximum dose of ibuprofen is 3200 mg daily. Switching to an alternative AI would be the preferred option.

Answer c is incorrect. These symptoms are not consistent with a hypersensitivity reaction.

Answer d is incorrect. The symptoms are likely caused by anastrozole rather than symptoms consistent with the development of rheumatoid arthritis.

15. MK is a 63-year-old woman with newly diagnosed metastatic breast cancer scheduled to receive her first dose of trastuzumab. She is 5' 6" tall and weighs 175 lb. You receive the following order: trastuzumab 440 mg IV infusion over 1.5 hours. Select the appropriate assessment to discuss with the prescriber.

a. Trastuzumab causes significant nausea and vomiting warranting premedication with a serotonin antagonist antiemetic. It would be best to call the prescriber and suggest administration of an antiemetic.
b. Trastuzumab can safely be administered as an IV bolus injection. It would be appropriate to call the prescriber and suggest the order be changed to be administered as an IV bolus injection.
c. Trastuzumab has been shown effective as an adjuvant treatment but not treatment of metastatic disease. It would be appropriate to call the prescriber and clarify the indication for trastuzumab for this patient.
d. The recommended initial dose of trastuzumab is 4 mg/kg (320 mg total for this patient). It would be appropriate to call the prescriber and clarify dosage for this patient.
e. Trastuzumab ordered appropriately for this patient. No clarification is indicated.

Answer d is correct. The standard initial dose for this patient would be 4 mg/kg or 320 mg for this patient. It would be appropriate to clarify this patient's dose.

Answer a is incorrect. Trastuzumab is not associated with nausea and vomiting that requires pretreatment antiemetic therapy.

Answer b is incorrect. Trastuzumab should not be administered as an IV bolus injection.

Answer c is incorrect. Trastuzumab has been shown effective as treatment for both micrometastatic and metastatic breast cancer characterized by overexpression of HER-2.

Answer e is incorrect. Clarification of the dose ordered for this patient is warranted.

16. JK is a 48-year-old woman scheduled to receive her first 175 mg/m^2 dose of paclitaxel for metastatic breast cancer. She is 5'3" tall and weighs 127 lb. Using the Mosteller formula (BSA (m^2) = $\sqrt{\text{Ht [cm]} \times \text{Wt [kg]}/3600}$) what dose of paclitaxel would you prepare?

a. 2780 mg
b. 278 mg
c. 412 mg
d. 4120 mg

Answer b is correct. The patient's BSA is 1.6 m^2 - (175 mg/m^2 × 1.6 m^2 = 278 mg)

Answer a is incorrect. A dose of 2780 mg represents a 10-fold over dose that could result by misplacing a decimal point during calculations.

Answer c is incorrect. This dose would have resulted by failing to convert the patient's weight to kg when calculating the BSA.

Answer d is incorrect. This dose would have resulted by failing to convert the patient's weight to kg when calculating the BSA and misplacing a decimal point when performing calculations.

17. You receive the following order for a patient with stage IV breast cancer. Albumin-bound paclitaxel 470 mg administer as an IV infusion at a rate of 10 mg/min. You verify that an appropriate dose is 260 mg/m^2 administered over 30 minutes. The patient has a BSA of 1.81 m^2. Is this dose and infusion rate ordered correctly?

a. Yes, the order is correct.
b. No, the order is incorrect because the dose and the infusion rate are miscalculated.
c. No, the order is incorrect because the dose is correct, but the infusion rate should be 15 mg/min.
d. No, the order is incorrect because the infusion rate is correct but the dose is miscalculated.

Answer c is correct. The correct dose is 470 mg but the correct infusion is 15 mg/min.

Answer a is incorrect. The correct dose is 470 mg but the infusion rate should be 15 mg/min.

Answer b is incorrect. Only the infusion rate is miscalculated.

Answer d is incorrect. The correct dose is ordered but the infusion rate is not correct.

18. A 65-year-old patient brings in her tamoxifen prescription for a refill. Upon reviewing her medication profile, you discover that she began taking tamoxifen 20 mg daily in June 2000 for the prevention of breast cancer and she has been having it refilled regularly since then. What if anything should you discuss with the patient's physician?

    a. The recommended duration of tamoxifen when prescribed to decrease the risk of breast cancer is 10 years. There is no need to clarify this patient's tamoxifen regimen.
    b. The merits of increasing the dose to 40 mg daily based on results of a recent study documenting superior efficacy of a 40 mg daily dose.
    c. Switching this patient to an AI based on recent studies that have documented improvement in efficacy and tolerability with AIs.
    d. The merits of decreasing the dose to 10 mg daily based on results of a recent study documenting equal efficacy but superior tolerability of a 20 mg daily dose.
    e. The recommended duration of tamoxifen when prescribed to decrease the risk of breast cancer is 5 years.

Answer e is correct. Results from the National Surgical Adjuvant Breast Project (NSABP) Breast Cancer Prevention Trial established that the risks associated with continuing tamoxifen beyond 5 years (increased incidence of uterine cancer, deep venous thrombosis) exceeded the benefits.

Answer a is incorrect. Results from the NSABP Breast Cancer Prevention Trial established that the risks associated with continuing tamoxifen beyond 5 years (increased incidence of uterine cancer, deep venous thrombosis) exceeded the benefits.

Answer b is incorrect. The dose of tamoxifen established as effective in the prevention of breast cancer is 20 mg daily.

Answer c is incorrect. Results from the NSABP Breast Cancer Prevention Trial established that the risks associated with continuing tamoxifen beyond 5 years (increased incidence of uterine cancer, deep venous thrombosis) exceeded the benefits.

Answer d is incorrect. The dose of tamoxifen established as effective in the prevention of breast cancer is 20 mg daily.

19. This patient asks you if you could recommend a dietary supplement that has been proven effective in decreasing the risk of breast cancer.

    a. You explain that vitamin A 100 IU daily has been proven effective to decrease the risk of breast cancer.
    b. You explain that vitamin D 200 mg daily has been proven effective to decrease the risk of breast cancer.
    c. You explain that vitamin C 500 IU daily has been proven effective to decrease the risk of breast cancer.
    d. You explain that there are not any dietary supplements that have been proven effective in lowering the risk of breast cancer.
    e. You explain that vitamin E 100 IU daily has been proven effective to decrease the risk of breast cancer.

Answer d is correct. No dietary supplement has been proven effective in reducing the risk of breast cancer.

Answer a is incorrect. Vitamin A has not been proven effective in reducing the risk of breast cancer.

Answer b is incorrect. Vitamin D has not been proven effective in reducing the risk of breast cancer.

Answer c is incorrect. Vitamin C has not been proven effective in reducing the risk of breast cancer.

Answer e is incorrect. Vitamin E has not been proven effective in reducing the risk of breast cancer.

20. Which of the following organizations publishes on their website evidence-based clinical practice guidelines for cancers that affect over 90% of patients with cancer?

    a. The American Cancer Society
    b. The Eastern Cooperative Oncology Group
    c. NCCN
    d. The National Cancer Institute
    e. The American Society of Health-System Pharmacy

Answer c is correct. The NCCN Clinical Practice Guidelines are evidence-based guidelines for the treatment of cancers that affect over 90% of cancer patients. The guidelines can be accessed at the following link: http://www.nccn.org/professionals/physician_gls/f_guidelines.asp.

Answer a is incorrect. The American Cancer Society website is not a source for evidence-based clinical practice guidelines for cancers that affect over 90% of cancer patients.

Answer b is incorrect. The Eastern Cooperative Oncology Group website is not a source for evidence-based clinical practice guidelines for cancers that affect over 90% of cancer patients.

Answer d is incorrect. The National Cancer Institute website is not a source for evidence-based clinical practice guidelines for cancers that affect over 90% of patients with cancer.

Answer e is incorrect. American Society of Health-System Pharmacy website is not a source for evidence-based clinical practice guidelines for cancers that affect over 90% of cancer patients.

21. Which of the following antineoplastic agents are likely to cause arthralgias and myalgias? Select all that apply.

    a. Docetaxel, ixabepilone, letrozole, exemestane
    b. Paclitaxel, ixabepilone, anastrozole
    c. Anastrozole, exemestane
    d. Letrozole, anastrozole, exemestane

Answers a, b, c, and d are correct. Arthralgias and myalgias are commonly experienced by patients taking agents belonging to the taxane, AI, and epothilone classes.

22. Which of the following antineoplastic agents are vesicants? Select all that apply.

    a. 5-Fluorouracil
    b. Fulvestrant
    c. Doxorubicin
    d. Methotrexate
    e. Epirubicin

Answer c is correct. Extravasation of doxorubicin can cause tissue necrosis. The administration of doxorubicin and other anthracycline antitumor antibiotics should only be performed by trained personnel.

Answer e is correct. Extravasation of epirubicin can cause tissue necrosis. It should only be administered by trained personnel.

Answer a is incorrect. Extravasation of 5-fluorouracil does not cause tissue necrosis.

Answer b is incorrect. Fulvestrant is not a vesicant. It is administered as an IM injection.

Answer d is incorrect. Extravasation of methotrexate does not cause tissue necrosis.

23. Which of the following antineoplastic agents would be effective as adjuvant therapy for postmenopausal patients with breast cancer that is ER negative and does not overexpress HER-2? Select all that apply.

    a. Cyclophosphamide
    b. Epirubicin
    c. Doxorubicin
    d. Letrozole

Answer a is correct. Cyclophosphamide is effective in treating ER negative, HER-2 negative breast cancer.

Answer b is correct. Epirubicin is effective in treating ER negative, HER-2 negative breast cancer.

Answer c is correct. Doxorubicin is effective in treating ER negative, HER-2 negative breast cancer.

Answer d is incorrect. Letrozole would not be effective in treating breast cancer that is ER negative.

24. The goal of neoadjuvant chemotherapy is to:

    a. Eradicate micrometastatic disease following localized modalities such as surgery or radiation or both.
    b. Attempt to shrink large tumors and make them more amenable to subsequent surgical resection.
    c. Reduce the symptoms of the cancer without affecting the underlying tumor.
    d. Rapidly treat and reduce tumor volume for a cure without other treatment modalities.

Answer b is correct. Neoadjuvant therapy administered prior to surgery has been proven effective in decreasing tumor size, facilitating subsequent resection, and resulting in improved postsurgical outcomes.

Answer a is incorrect. While neoadjuvant therapy may eradicate micrometastatic disease, it is administered before, not following surgery and/or radiation.

Answer c is incorrect. It is administered to decrease the size of the tumor, not reduce symptoms.

Answer d is incorrect. Neoadjuvant therapy is always followed by surgery and/or radiation.

CHAPTER **17** | **Solid Organ Transplantation**

1. JP is a kidney transplant patient whose biopsy showed cellular rejection. Select the statement that most accurately describes mechanism of JP's rejection.

    a. An orchestrated immune response that involves alloantigen presentation via APCs that then leads to alloreactive T lymphocytes.
    b. A cytotoxic immune response mediated via preformed antibodies against antigens present on vascular endothelium.
    c. A slow process of graft fibrosis and arteriopathy, which results in graft dysfunction.
    d. A process which inhibits the entire process of immune activation, including antigen presentation by APCs, the release of cytokines such as IL-1, IL-2, IL-6, and TNF α, and subsequently lymphocyte proliferation.

Answer a is correct. This is a description of ACR. ACR requires the production of alloreactive T cells via T cell binding at the T cell receptors on APCs, with subsequent cytokine release and immune activation.

Answer b is incorrect. Antibody-mediated rejection typically occurs hours to days after transplant if donor-specific antibodies are present at the time of transplant. This type of rejection most frequently results from mismatched blood types and positive cross matches, and the incidence has decreased with the advent of screening.

Answer c is incorrect. This is a description of chronic rejection. The etiology of chronic rejection is not known and there is no treatment for this condition. However, ACR has been shown to be a primary risk factor for the development of chronic rejection, thus prevention is a key modifier.

Answer d is incorrect. This is a description of the ubiquitous immunosuppressive action that steroids have on immune response.

2. SK is a 16-year-old boy who is waiting for kidney transplantation. He states that he has been doing research on the Internet and heard that ACR is a major complication of kidney

transplantation. What can a pharmacist counsel him regarding the time frame for risk of ACR after transplant?

a. The risk is greatest during the first hours to days after transplantation
b. The risk is greatest during the first several months after transplantation
c. The risk increases with increased time from transplant
d. The risk is the same regardless of time after transplant

Answer b is correct. The time period of greatest risk for ACR is during the first 6 months after transplantation, with risk dropping precipitously after 1 year.

Answer a is incorrect. This time period describes the time of greatest risk for antibody mediated rejection.

Answer c is incorrect. The further out from transplant a patient is, the less likely they are to have an episode of ACR. However, as time passes from date of transplant, a patient is at increased risk for chronic rejection, especially if they have a history of multiple episodes of ACR.

Answer d is incorrect. The risk for ACR varies with time, with risk decreasing with time from transplant.

3. SK received kidney transplantation from his brother today. Which "triple drug regimen" describes the most commonly used maintenance immunosuppression?

a. Cyclosporine, prednisone, and basiliximab
b. Cyclosporine, tacrolimus, and prednisone
c. Tacrolimus, mycophenolate mofetil, and rabbit ATG
d. Tacrolimus, mycophenolate mofetil, and prednisone

Answer d is correct. This regimen contains a calcineurin inhibitor (tacrolimus), an antiproliferative agent (mycophenolate mofetil), and a corticosteroid (prednisone), with three distinct mechanisms of action.

Answer a is incorrect. This regimen contains a calcineurin inhibitor (cyclosporine), a corticosteroid (prednisone), and an IL-2 receptor antagonist (basiliximab). Basiliximab is an induction agent and does not make up the maintenance regimen. This regimen should include an antiproliferative agent such as mycophenolate or azathioprine.

Answer b is incorrect. This regimen contains two calcineurin inhibitors (cyclosporine and tacrolimus) and a corticosteroid. The "triple drug regimen" is designed to optimize therapy, without excessive toxicity. A patient should never take two calcineurin inhibitors simultaneously, as their risk for serious side effects, such as nephrotoxicity, neurotoxicity, and electrolyte disturbances, are greatly increased without much added benefit. The three drugs in the triple drug regimen should have different mechanisms of action, thus allowing decreased doses of each and therefore decreased incidence of dose-dependent side effects.

Answer c is incorrect. This regimen contains a calcineurin inhibitor, an antiproliferative agent (mycophenolate mofetil),

and an ATG. Although rabbit ATG is commonly employed in kidney transplant recipients, it is used as an induction agent or treatment for rejection.

4. GH presents to your pharmacy with a prescription for clarithromycin. He says that his primary care physician prescribed this medication to treat community-acquired pneumonia. You review GH's medication profile and you see that he received a renal transplant 2 years ago and his immunosuppressive regimen includes tacrolimus, mycophenolate mofetil, and prednisone. Which of the following would be most appropriate as your next course of action?

a. Dispense clarithromycin and counsel on avoiding grapefruit juice.
b. Contact the prescriber about the interactions between clarithromycin and tacrolimus as clarithromycin will inhibit the metabolism of tacrolimus resulting in supratherapeutic levels and toxicity.
c. Contact the prescriber about the interactions between clarithromycin and mycophenolate mofetil as clarithromycin will inhibit the metabolism of mycophenolate mofetil resulting in supratherapeutic levels and toxicity.
d. Recommend an alternative as clarithromycin is not an appropriate therapy for community-acquired pneumonia in an immunosuppressed host.

Answer a is incorrect. Avoiding grapefruit juice is a good counseling point for a patient taking clarithromycin or tacrolimus (CYP 3A substrates). However, answer B is more critical than A to avoid tacrolimus toxicity.

Answer b is correct. Clarithromycin is an inhibitor of CYP 3A, and therefore will inhibit the metabolism of tacrolimus resulting in supratherapeutic concentrations and potential toxicity.

Answer c is incorrect. Mycophenolate mofetil is metabolized to its active metabolite, MPA which then undergoes enterohepatic recirculation until it is eventually cleared via hepatic glucuronidation. Clarithromycin will not significantly affect mycophenolate clearance.

Answer d is incorrect. General immunosuppressed state is not a contraindication for the use of clarithromycin, as long as the organisms isolated or suspected is susceptible to this agent.

5. AJ is a lung transplant recipient who is found to have *Aspergillus* on routine bronchoscopy. AJ's transplant physician wants to begin treatment with the antifungal voriconazole. The patient is currently taking prednisone, cyclosporine, azathioprine, clotrimazole, rabeprazole, cotrimoxazole, valganciclovir, and inhaled amphotericin. Which of the following medications will interact with voriconazole?

a. Prednisone
b. Azathioprine
c. Cyclosporine
d. Valganciclovir

Answer c is correct. Voriconazole is a potent inhibitor of CYP 3A and P-glycoprotein. Cyclosporine is extensively metabolized via CYP 3A and also a substrate of P-glycoprotein. Voriconazole will significantly increase cyclosporine levels, and it is recommended to decrease cyclosporine dosing empirically by more than 50% to avoid toxic cyclosporine blood concentrations.

Answer a is incorrect. Voriconazole is a potent inhibitor of CYP 3A and P-glycoprotein. Prednisone is not suspected to interact, as it is not involved with either of these mechanisms.

Answer b is incorrect. Voriconazole is a potent inhibitor of CYP 3A and P-glycoprotein. Azathioprine is not suspected to interact, as it is metabolized to its inactive metabolite via xanthine oxidase.

Answer d is incorrect. Voriconazole is a potent inhibitor of CYP 3A and P-glycoprotein. Following oral administration, valganciclovir is hydrolyzed to ganciclovir, which is then excreted renally. Therefore, no interaction is suspected between these agents.

---

6. PW is a transplant patient taking a stable dose of cyclosporine and rosuvastatin was recently added. Which counseling information should a pharmacist provide to PW? Select all that apply.

   a. Avoid grapefruit and grapefruit juice.
   b. Report unexplained muscle pain, muscle weakness, or dark urine.
   c. Cyclosporine dose should be decreased within days after starting rosuvastatin.
   d. Inform the prescriber of rosuvastatin that PW is taking cyclosporine.

Answer a is correct. Grapefruit (and juice) increased both blood levels of cyclosporine and rosuvastatin and thereby their side effects. Patients taking cyclosporine or rosuvastatin should avoid grapefruit and grapefruit juice.

Answer b is correct. Cyclosporine can increase rosuvastatin exposure sevenfold, resulting in increased risk for myopathy and rhabdomyolysis. Patients taking cyclosporine and rosuvastatin together should be monitored for symptoms of statin-induced myopathy.

Answer d is correct. Due to the increased risk of myopathy, rosuvastatin dose should be limited to 5 mg po daily when used with cyclosporine. The prescriber should be informed about PW's concomitant drug and monitor him closely for statin-induced myopathy.

Answer c is incorrect. Rosuvastatin does not inhibit CYP 3A or P-glycoprotein and thus increased cyclosporine concentrations are not expected. However, an interaction like this is expected with such agents as diltiazem, voriconazole, and clarithromycin.

The following case pertains to Questions 7 through 11.

CJ is a 24-year-old female patient who received kidney transplantation 3 months ago. She fills her prescription for tacrolimus, mycophenolate sodium, and prednisone at your pharmacy.

7. Which of the following represents two adverse effects specific to tacrolimus that CJ may experience?

   a. Diarrhea and leukopenia
   b. Alopecia and hyperglycemia
   c. Hypertriglyceridemia and nephrotoxicity
   d. Hirsutism and gingival hyperplasia

Answer b is correct. Alopecia and hyperglycemia are adverse effects specific to tacrolimus. Hyperglycemia is further exacerbated by the concomitant use of corticosteroids and can lead to post-transplant diabetes mellitus.

Answer a is incorrect. Diarrhea and leukopenia are adverse effects specific to mycophenolate products. Diarrhea can be associated with tacrolimus, but leukopenia is not common with tacrolimus.

Answer c is incorrect. Both cyclosporine and tacrolimus can cause nephrotoxicity, but hypertriglyceridemia is more frequently associated with mTOR inhibitors such as sirolimus and everolimus.

Answer d is incorrect. Hirsutism and gingival hyperplasia are adverse effects specific to cyclosporine. It is important to counsel patients who are initiating cyclosporine on the importance of good oral hygiene.

---

8. Which of the following represents two adverse effects specific to corticosteroids that CJ may experience?

   a. Diarrhea and leukopenia
   b. Alopecia and hyperglycemia
   c. Water retention and osteoporosis
   d. Hirsutism and nephrotoxicity

Answer c is correct. Water retention and osteoporosis both are adverse effects specific to corticosteroids. Water retention leads to wait gain and hypertension. It is important to ensure adequate calcium intake and screening for bone mineral density in patients taking corticosteroids chronically.

Answer a is incorrect. Diarrhea and leukopenia are adverse effects specific to mycophenolate products. Gastrointestinal adverse effects of corticosteroids include indigestion and ulcers, but diarrhea is not particularly associated with corticosteroids. Corticosteroids cause leukocytosis.

Answer b is incorrect. Alopecia and hyperglycemia are adverse effects specific to tacrolimus. Corticosteroids can cause hirsutism. Hyperglycemia is further exacerbated by the concomitant use of corticosteroids and can lead to post-transplant diabetes mellitus.

Answer d is incorrect. Hirsutism and nephrotoxicity are adverse effects specific to cyclosporine. Corticosteroids can cause hirsutism, but nephrotoxicity is not associated with corticosteroids.

9. Which of the following should be included in patient counseling about mycophenolate sodium for CJ? Select all that apply.

   a. Educate CJ regarding higher risks of miscarriage and birth defects.
   b. Counsel CJ regarding pregnancy planning.
   c. Ensure the use of acceptable contraception during the first 6 weeks of starting mycophenolate.
   d. Perform pregnancy tests only before starting mycophenolate.

Answers a and b are correct.

Answer c is incorrect. Female patients of reproductive potential must use acceptable contraception during entire treatment with mycophenolate and for 6 weeks after stopping mycophenolate.

Answer d is incorrect. Pregnancy tests should be performed immediately before initiation of mycophenolate, 8 to 10 days later, and at routine follow-up visits.

10. CJ approaches the counter at your pharmacy and would like you to suggest an over-the-counter (OTC) remedy for her mild headache. What would you suggest for her headache?

    a. That she should proceed immediately to a local emergency room as this might be a symptom of severe tacrolimus toxicity.
    b. That she may take OTC acetaminophen, and alert the transplant physician if the headache does not resolve.
    c. That she may take OTC naproxen, and alert the transplant physician if the headache does not resolve.
    d. That she may take OTC ibuprofen, and alert the transplant physician if the headache dose not resolve.

Answer a is incorrect. While neurotoxicity such as headaches and tremors are associated with supratherapeutic calcineurin inhibitor concentrations, headache is a common side effect, especially a few hours after the dose is administered, as this is the time when drug levels in the body are highest. Because her headache is only mild, the most reasonable suggestion would be to try the OTC analgesic acetaminophen, and if the headache does not dissipate, to contact the transplant physician. If the headache was severe, immediate medical attention would be warranted.

Answer b is correct. Transplant patients that are taking calcineurin inhibitors should avoid taking NSAIDs because NSAIDs cause inhibition of renal prostaglandin production and can increase the risk for nephrotoxicity induced by calcineurin inhibitors. Therefore, acetaminophen is the preferred OTC analgesic agent.

Answers c and d are incorrect. Naproxen and ibuprofen are NSAIDs; therefore, they are not recommended in

combination with her tacrolimus due to the pharmacodynamic interaction which can lead to increased nephrotoxicity.

11. CJ presents to the hospital with symptoms concerning for a bowel obstruction. She is receiving mycophenolate sodium 720 mg po bid. The physician wants to convert the patient from oral mycophenolate sodium to IV due to po intolerance resulting from her bowel obstruction. Which of the following would result in comparable plasma concentrations of MPA?

    a. Mycophenolate sodium 720 mg IV bid
    b. Mycophenolate sodium 1000 mg IV bid
    c. Mycophenolate mofetil 720 mg IV bid
    d. Mycophenolate mofetil 1000 mg IV bid

Answer d is correct. CellCept, or mycophenolate mofetil, is available in an oral and intravenous formulation. When converting a patient from PO Myfortic (mycophenolate sodium) to intravenous therapy, IV mycophenolate mofetil (CellCept) can be used at a therapeutically equivalent dose. 720 mg of Myfortic is equivalent to 1000 mg of CellCept.

Answers a and b are incorrect. Myfortic, or mycophenolate sodium, is an enteric-coated delayed-release oral formulation and it is not available intravenously.

Answer c is incorrect. The dosing conversion between mycophenolate sodium and mycophenolate mofetil (CellCept) is not 1:1, but rather 720 mg of mycophenolate sodium is equivalent to 1000 mg of mycophenolate mofetil.

12. Which of the following agents would be most appropriate to prevent a gout flare in a transplant patient who is currently receiving tacrolimus, azathioprine, and prednisone?

    a. Indomethacin
    b. Allopurinol
    c. Diclofenac
    d. Probenecid

Answer d is correct. Probenecid is indicated for the prevention of gouty attacks, and is not expected to interact with any medication in this patient's immunosuppressive regimen as it is excreted renally. However, if this patient had renal insufficiency with a CrCl less than 50 mL/min, this agent should be avoided.

Answer a is incorrect. Indomethacin is an NSAID. NSAIDs are not recommended in combination with calcineurin inhibitors like tacrolimus due to increased potential for nephrotoxicity via decrease in renal prostaglandin production.

Answer b is incorrect. Allopurinol inhibits xanthine oxidase and is typically the drug of choice to prevent gouty attacks. The metabolite of azathioprine (6-mercaptopurine) is inactivated via xanthine oxidase. If allopurinol is administered concomitantly with azathioprine, the other metabolic pathway that produces 6-thioguanine nucleotides can be enhanced, leading to severe pancytopenia. Allopurinol should be avoided in patients who are currently receiving azathioprine.

Answer c is incorrect. Diclofenac is an NSAID. NSAIDs are not recommended in combination with calcineurin inhibitors like tacrolimus due to increased potential for nephrotoxicity via decrease in renal prostaglandins.

---

13. You are counseling HD who is being discharged today. He received a living related renal transplant 3 days ago, and his postoperative course has been uncomplicated except for mild hypertension. When reconciling his home medications, you notice that the medical team has not restarted his home diltiazem. What is the most appropriate action to control his blood pressure at this point?

    a. Notify the patient's medical team and request a discharge prescription for amlodipine.
    b. Notify the patient's medical team and instruct the patient to resume his home regimen of diltiazem after discharge.
    c. Notify the patient's medical team and request a discharge prescription for verapamil.
    d. Notify the patient's medical team and request addition of diltiazem at discharge.

Answer a is correct. Many patients will experience higher postoperative blood pressures following solid organ transplant due to high doses of steroids and calcineurin inhibitors. Patients with pre-existing hypertension may have a more difficult time maintaining blood pressure control, while patients who receive renal transplants may experience resolution of their hypertension with resolution of their kidney disease. While the nondihydropyridine calcium channel blockers, such as diltiazem and verapamil may be appropriate choices for some patients prior to transplant, they may complicate management of calcineurin inhibitors post operatively, due to their interaction mediated via CYP 3A and P-glycoprotein. Dihydropyridine calcium channel blockers, such as nifedipine and amlodipine, have less potential for clinically significant pharmacokinetic interactions with calcineurin inhibitors.

Answers b, c, and d are incorrect. The nondihydropyridine calcium channel blockers (diltiazem and verapamil) inhibit CYP3A and P-glycoprotein, resulting in elevated concentrations and toxicity of calcineurin inhibitors. These agents can be used safely, with close monitoring of trough levels of calcineurin inhibitors, but reinitiation of these agents at discharge is not appropriate.

---

14. Which of the following statement is correct about sirolimus?

    a. Sirolimus is not metabolized via cytochrome P450 enzymes, thus decreasing the propensity for drug interactions.
    b. Sirolimus is less nephrotoxic than calcineurin inhibitors.
    c. Sirolimus is available in many different formulations, thereby facilitating ease of dosing.
    d. Sirolimus does not require therapeutic drug monitoring.

Answer b is correct. Sirolimus has decreased risk for nephrotoxicity compared to calcineurin inhibitors, therefore, it is commonly used in calcineurin inhibitor-sparing regimens to protect patients from calcineurin inhibitor-induced renal insufficiency.

Answer a is incorrect. CYP 3A is the major metabolic pathway for sirolimus. Like cyclosporine and tacrolimus, sirolimus is affected by inducers and inhibitors of CYP 3A.

Answer c is incorrect. Sirolimus is only available orally and there is no IV formulation. Furthermore, the tablet is triangular, disallowing splitting to create unavailable tablet strengths.

Answer d is incorrect. Therapeutic drug monitoring was deemed unnecessary during clinical trials, as sirolimus was used primarily as an adjunctive agent, in the place of an antiproliferative agent. However, the risk of drug interactions and variability in pharmacokinetics warrant monitoring of sirolimus concentrations.

---

15. What is the drug target for the immunosuppressive agent MPA?

    a. mTOR
    b. Cyclophilin
    c. FKBP-12
    d. IMPDH

Answer d is correct. IMPDH is an enzyme required for the de novo synthesis of purines, and is inhibited by MPA the active metabolite of the mycophenolate derivatives. This is the mechanism that allows these agents to selectively inhibit lymphocyte proliferation, as these cells are unable to utilize salvage pathways of purine synthesis.

Answer a is incorrect. Sirolimus is a selective immunosuppressant that exerts its affect via inhibition of the mTOR. Blockade of mTOR results in inhibition of lymphocyte proliferation via cell cycle arrest in the G1 to S phase.

Answer b is incorrect. Cyclophilin is the binding target of cyclosporine that facilitates inhibition of calcineurin, a phosphatase enzyme that is responsible for the dephosphorylation of NFAT, which is a required transcription factor in the process of cytokine production. This inhibition in turn suppresses T cell activation, and thus cellular immune response.

Answer c is incorrect. FKBP-12 is the binding target of tacrolimus that facilitates inhibition of calcineurin which results in the same outcome as inhibition by cyclosporine, although the intercellular mediators are different.

---

16. Which of the following is generally considered as a narrow therapeutic ratio drug?

    a. Cyclosporine
    b. Prednisone
    c. Mycophenolate mofetil
    d. Mycophenolate sodium

Answer a is correct. Cyclosporine is generally considered to have a narrow therapeutic ratio as the blood concentration ranges to effectively prevent rejection overlap with that of nephrotoxic potential, and cyclosporine concentration monitoring is required.

The FDA does not formally designate the narrow therapeutic ratio drugs. According to 21 CFR 320.33(c), narrow therapeutic ratio is defined as follows:

1. There is less than a twofold difference in median lethal dose (LD50) and median effective dose (ED50) values or there is less than a twofold difference in the minimum toxic concentrations and minimum effective concentrations in the blood, and

2. safe and effective use of the drug products require careful titration and patient monitoring.

Answers b, c and d are incorrect. Prednisone and mycophenolate derivatives do not meet the FDA criteria for narrow therapeutic ratio drugs and serum concentrations are not typically monitored.

---

17. DD is a liver transplant patient who presents with elevated liver function tests. She admits to not taking her immunosuppressive regimen for the past week as she was out of town and forgot her medications. The medical team wants to treat her for ACR. Which of the following would treat ACR most effectively?

    a. Basiliximab
    b. Rabbit ATG
    c. Belatacept
    d. Rituximab

Answer b is correct. ATGs deplete T cells and can be used for both induction regimens as well as treatment of ACR.

Answer a is incorrect. While basiliximab (IL-2 receptor antagonist) can be used in induction regimens, it is not indicated for the treatment of ACR.

Answer c is incorrect. Belatacept (costimulation blocker) can be used as part of maintenance regimen in kidney transplant patients. Belatacept is not indicated for the treatment of ACR or for use in liver transplant patients.

Answer d is incorrect. Rituximab is a monoclonal antibody directed against CD20 on B cells. Rituximab currently has no role in the treatment of ACR, as this type of rejection is largely mediated by T cells.

---

18. Which of the following should be confirmed before administering belatacept in a kidney transplant patient? Select all that apply.

    a. Positive cytomegalovirus serostatus
    b. Positive EBV serostatus
    c. Normal renal and liver function
    d. Absence of any new or worsening neurological abnormalities

---

Answer b is correct. Belatacept was associated with the increased risk of PTLD predominantly involving the central nervous system. It is contraindicated in patients who are EBV seronegative or with unknown EBV serostatus.

Answer d is correct. Before each dose of belatacept, patients should be assessed for signs and symptoms of PTLD and progressive multifocal leukoencephalopathy. If the patient reports any new or worsening problems such as a new or sudden change in thinking, memory, speech, mood, behavior, vision, balance, strength, fever, night sweats, persistent tiredness, weight loss, or swollen glands, belatacept should not be administered and the patient should be referred to appropriate medical management.

Answer a is incorrect. Although positive EBV serostatus is required to receive belatacept, cytomegalovirus status is not pertinent.

Answer c is incorrect. Belatacept dose is determined based on actual body weight and does not need to be adjusted for renal or hepatic dysfunction.

---

19. During interdisciplinary rounds, the medical resident states that TK has a low white blood cell (WBC) count. TK received a combined kidney pancreas transplant for juvenile onset diabetes mellitus 2 months ago and presented 2 days ago with hyperglycemia and elevated amylase and lipase. ACR of the pancreas transplant was confirmed on a subsequent biopsy. Her rejection episode is being treated with rabbit ATG. Her home immunosuppressive regimen consists of tacrolimus, mycophenolate mofetil, and prednisone. She is receiving antiviral prophylaxis with valganciclovir, antibacterial prophylaxis with trimethoprim-sulfamethoxazole, and antifungal prophylaxis with nystatin. Which of the following approach is most appropriate for this patient's new onset leukopenia?

    a. Suggest the physician to hold her prednisone until her WBC count normalizes.
    b. Suggest the physician to hold her mycophenolate mofetil until her WBC count normalizes.
    c. Suggest the physician to hold her current therapy, but to closely monitor her WBC count.
    d. Suggest the physician to hold her valganciclovir until her WBC count normalizes.

Answer c is correct. This patient's leukopenia is likely caused by rabbit ATG infusion. WBC count along with the rest of hematology labs should be monitored closely. If there is a significant decrease in her WBC or platelet counts, a reduction of or withholding the dose of rabbit ATG may be warranted.

Answer a is incorrect. Prednisone usually causes leukocytosis and not leukopenia.

Answer b is incorrect. While mycophenolate mofetil can cause leukopenia, the likely agent inducing this patient's leukopenia is rabbit ATG. It is important to review the patient's medication administration record in this case to see if her blood sample was drawn during the infusion of rabbit ATG, as this will produce a significant leukopenia. However, even if the blood draw occurred after the infusion, the leukopenia is likely due to this agent, and the antiproliferative agent need not be held. This is especially true in light of her current presentation with ACR.

Answer d is incorrect.   While valganciclovir can cause leukopenia, the likely agent inducing this patient's leukopenia is rabbit ATG. During an episode of rejection, patients are treated with immunosuppressive intensification, and therefore are at increased risk for reactivation of latent viral infections. Therefore, care must be taken to not inaccurately hold a patient's antiviral prophylaxis, but thoroughly investigate the cause of leukopenia and act on the most likely cause.

20. Which of the following medications require a REMS by FDA? Select all that apply.

    a. Mycophenolate mofetil
    b. Mycophenolate sodium generic products
    c. Belatacept
    d. Tacrolimus

Answers a, b, and c are correct.   REMS is required for all products containing mycophenolate mofetil or mycophenolate sodium including generic products given their risk for teratogenicity. REMS is also required for belatacept given its risk for PTLD and progressive multifocal leukoencephalopathy in patients whose EBV status is negative.

Answer d is incorrect.

21. Which of the following vaccines will need to be administered prior to transplant as they are relatively contraindicated post-transplant? Select all that apply.

    a. Pneumococcal polysaccharide
    b. Varicella
    c. MMR
    d. Meningococcal conjugate

Answer b is correct.   Varicella must be administered prior to transplant for anyone who has never been exposed to chicken pox virus and who has not been vaccinated. Some experts recommend a minimum of 4 weeks between live vaccine administration and transplantation. Live vaccines are generally not contraindicated after transplant.

Answer c is correct.   MMR must be administered prior to transplant for anyone who has never been exposed to chicken pox virus and who has not been vaccinated. Some experts recommend a minimum of 4 weeks between live vaccine administration and transplantation. Live vaccines are generally not contraindicated after transplant.

Answer a is incorrect.   Pneumococcal polysaccharide vaccine may be given after transplant as it is an inactivated vaccine. Some experts recommend to wait at least 3 months after transplant prior to administering nonlive vaccines as

response to vaccines is diminished early after transplant due to the potent immunosuppression given immediately after transplant.

Answer d is incorrect.   Meningococcal conjugate may be given after transplant as it is an inactivated vaccine. Some experts recommend to wait at least 3 months after transplant prior to administering nonlive vaccines as response to vaccines is diminished early after transplant due to the potent immunosuppression given immediately after transplant.

CHAPTER 18 | Skin and Melanoma

1. AE is a 28-year-old woman in clinic today for routine annual check-up with her general practitioner. AE's older brother was recently treated for basal cell carcinoma. Which of the following are risk factor(s) associated with melanoma AE should be educated about?

    a. Presence of multiple dysplastic nevi
    b. Presence of genetic factors
    c. Individuals with fair skin type who sunburns easily
    d. Individuals who are immunosuppressed

Answer a is correct.   Presence of multiple dysplastic nevi is a risk factor associated with melanoma.

Answer b is correct.   Presence of inherited genetic factors (ie, xeroderma pigmentosum, familial atypical multiple mole syndrome, and hereditary dysplastic nevus syndrome) are risk factors associated with melanoma.

Answer c is correct.   Individuals with fair skin type who sunburns easily are more likely to develop melanoma.

Answer d is correct.   Individuals who are immunosuppressed are more likely to develop melanoma.

2. Which of the following statement(s) is (are) true regarding the subtypes of melanoma? Select all that apply.

    a. Superficial spreading melanomas are the most common type of melanomas with lesions usually arising from preexisting nevus.
    b. Nodular melanomas are slow-growing lesions that develop and spread in a vertical growth phase pattern.
    c. Lentigo maligna melanomas are more commonly reported in children, with lesions less likely to metastasize.
    d. Uveal melanomas are rare lower extremity malignancies arising from pigmented epithelium of the choroids, with lesions more likely to metastasize to liver.

Answer a is correct.   Superficial spreading melanoma is the most common type of melanoma, making up about 70% of all cases of melanoma, and is more common in women than men. The lesions usually arise from a preexisting nevus, with initial presentation appears as flat which later develops as irregular and asymmetrical.

Answer b is correct. Nodular melanoma is the second most common type of melanoma, making up about 15% to 30% of all cases of melanoma, and is more common in men than women. Unlike superficial spreading melanoma, nodular melanoma has a more aggressive and rapid growth pattern, with lesions develop and spread in a vertical growth phase pattern. The lesions are usually dark blue-black and uniform in color, and are most commonly located on the head, neck, and trunk.

Answer c is correct. Lentigo maligna melanoma comprise a smaller percentage of all cases of melanoma and commonly occurs in older age group, typically located on the face of elderly Caucasians. Compared to the other subtypes of melanoma, lentigo maligna melanoma does not usually metastasize.

Answer d is correct. Uveal melanoma is an ocular melanoma which arises from the pigmented epithelium of the choroids. Although incidence of uveal melanoma is rare, it is the most common intraocular lesions reported in adults, with metastases most frequently occurring in the liver.

3. FB is a 25-year-old woman presented to dermatology clinic for her initial check-up after noticing multiple lesions and dark spot on her skin after 1 month of tanning session. Which of the following is not a part of the ABCDE rule used to identify and evaluate a suspicious lesion? Select all that apply.

   a. Asymmetry
   b. Border irregularity
   c. Color of lesions
   d. Depths of the lesions
   e. Evolving or changing characteristics of a lesion

Answer a is correct. *A* is asymmetry where one half of the mole does not match the other half.

Answer b is correct. *B* is border irregularity where the edges of the mole are often irregular, blurred, ragged, or notched.

Answer c is correct. *C* is color where the color of the mole is not uniform, it may appears with different shades of tan or blue-black, and sometimes mixed with colors of red, purple, and white.

Answer e is correct. *E* is evolving or changing characteristics of a lesion.

Answer d is incorrect. *D* is diameter where lesions are often >6 mm in diameter, although melanoma can sometimes present with lesions of <6 mm in diameter (ACS).

4. TS is a 35-year-old man in dermatology clinic today for follow-up visit on a suspicious lesion that was identified last week. Which is the best method in confirming the diagnosis?

   a. Obtain a complete clinical examination, and medical history of patient and family members.

   b. Obtain complete laboratory studies with hematology, electrolytes, liver function test, and lactate dehydrogenase (LDH).
   c. Consider full-thickness excisional biopsy with 1 to 3 mm margin of normal-appearing skin.
   d. Consider ordering a chest x-ray and a computerized tomography (CT) scan for confirming diagnosis.

Answer c is correct. Excisional biopsy of the suspicious lesions is the only way to confirm the diagnosis of melanoma. A full-thickness excisional biopsy with 1 to 3 mm margin of normal-appearing skin is the preferred method of choice as it removes the entire lesion.

Answer a is incorrect. A complete clinical examination, and medical history of patient and family members is done to identify and assess potential risk factors, but not enough to confirm the diagnosis of melanoma.

Answer b is incorrect. Laboratory studies including hematology, electrolytes, liver function test, and/or LDH are done to identify and assess the clinical status of patient, NOT to confirm the diagnosis of melanoma.

Answer d is incorrect. Diagnostic tests such as chest x-ray, CT scan, magnetic resonance imaging (MRI), positron emission tomography (PET) scan, and/or bone scan are used to identify and assess for possible local regional lymph nodes involvement or metastases, and are NOT used to confirm the diagnosis of melanoma.

5. According to the ACS, what is the latest recommendation for the prevention and screening of melanoma? Select all that apply.

   a. Wear proper protective clothing to cover as much exposed skin as possible (ie, sun glasses, hat with wide brim, long sleeve clothing, etc.).
   b. Use sunscreen lotion with an SPF of at least 15 or higher.
   c. Avoid direct sun exposure between 10 AM to 4 PM when ultraviolet rays are the most intense.
   d. Avoid the use of tanning beds or sunlamps to minimize exposure to ultraviolet radiation.

Answer a is correct. Protect your skin from sun exposure by wearing clothing. Long-sleeved shirts, long skirts, or long pants offer the most protection. Dark colors clothing offers more protection than light colors clothing.

Answer b is correct. Use sunscreen and lip balms with at least an SPF factor of 15 or higher on areas where skin are exposed to the sun. Best to apply sunscreen about 20 to 30 minutes prior to sun exposure, and reapplied at least every 2 hours or more frequently if you sweat or swim for maximum benefits.

Answer c is correct. Avoid direct sun exposure between 10 AM to 4 PM when the ultraviolet radiations are the most intense. Practice sun safety if you have to be outdoors by wearing protective clothing and use sunscreen.

Answer d is correct. Avoid the use of tanning beds or sunlamps to minimize exposure to ultraviolet radiation. There are more evidence on the potential hazardous of the ultraviolet radiation they deliver and the increase risk of melanoma.

---

6. Which of the following molecular targeted marker is relevant for the treatment of metastatic melanoma?

    a. EGFR (+) mutation
    b. Kras wild-type
    c. BRAF V600 (+) mutation
    d. VEGF (+) mutation
    e. ALK (+) mutation

Answer c is correct.   Both BRAF V600E or V600K mutation status have been identified as useful molecular marker for treatment selection in patients with metastatic or unresectable melanoma.

Answer a is incorrect.   EGFR mutation status has not been identified as molecular marker for treatment selection in patients with metastatic or unresectable melanoma.

Answer b is incorrect.   Kras wild-type has not been identified as molecular marker for treatment selection in patients with metastatic or unresectable melanoma.

Answer d is incorrect.   VEGF mutation status has not been identified as molecular marker for treatment selection in patients with metastatic or unresectable melanoma.

Answer e is incorrect.   ALK mutation status has not been identified as molecular marker for treatment selection in patients with metastatic or unresectable melanoma.

---

7. TN is a 54-year-old man with newly diagnosed stage IV metastatic melanoma. TN has good PS with no comorbid conditions, thought to be perfect candidate for immunotherapy. Which of the following immunotherapy would be treatment of choice for TN?

    a. Interferon alfa-2b
    b. Dacarbazine
    c. Carmustine
    d. IL-2
    e. Paclitaxel

Answer d is correct.   High-dose IL-2 is an immunotherapy that is FDA approved in treatment of metastatic melanoma in selected patients with good PS.

Answer a is incorrect.   High dose interferon-alfa 2b is an immunotherapy agent that is FDA approved for use in the adjuvant setting for treatment of melanoma in patients who are free of disease (nonmetastatic) but at high risk for systemic recurrence within 56 days of surgery.

Answer b is incorrect.   Dacarbazine is a chemotherapy agent with FDA approval as single agent for treatment of metastatic melanoma.

Answer c is incorrect.   Carmustine is a chemotherapy agent used in combination with other chemotherapeutic agents in the Dartmouth regimen for the treatment of Stage IV metastatic melanoma.

Answer e is incorrect.   Paclitaxel is a chemotherapy agent that has been used in treatment of metastatic melanoma; however, response rate are relatively lower (6%-18%) compared to single agent Dacarbazine.

---

8. Which of the following oral chemotherapeutic agent has been used in the treatment of unresectable melanoma?

    a. Capecitabine
    b. Lapatinib
    c. Erlotinib
    d. Procarbazine
    e. Vemurafenib

Answer e is correct.   Vemurafenib (Zelboraf™) is a BRAF kinase inhibitor FDA approved for treatment of metastatic or unresectable melanoma with BRAF V600E mutation (+) disease.

Answer a is incorrect.   Capecitabine (Xeloda™) is FDA approved for metastatic colorectal and breast cancer, and as adjuvant for Stage III colon cancer.

Answer b is incorrect.   Lapatinib (Tykerb™) is FDA approved for advanced or metastatic breast cancer in combination with Capecitabine.

Answer c is incorrect.   Erlotinib (Tarceva™) is FDA approved for advanced or metastatic nonsmall cell lung and pancreatic cancer.

Answer d is incorrect.   Procarbazine (Matulane™) is FDA approved for Hodgkin disease as part of the MOPP chemotherapy regimen which contains chemotherapy with *Mechlorethamine*, *Oncovin*™, *Procarbazine*, and *Prednisone*.

---

9. KT is a 45-year-old woman with newly diagnosed stage III melanoma; KT tumor was surgically resected 3 months ago but was found to have (+) lymph node 4/10 involvement. KT is in clinic today to discuss adjuvant treatment. Which of the following is the best treatment option for KT?

    a. Ipilimumab
    b. IL-2
    c. Interferon-alpha 2b
    d. Procarbazine
    e. Trametinib

Answer a is correct.   Ipilimumab (Yervoy) is a monoclonal antibody that targets the CTLA-4 receptor resulting in an immune response directed against melanoma. Ipilimumab is FDA approved for adjuvant treatment of resected melanoma and metastatic or unresectable melanoma.

Answer b is incorrect.   High-dose IL-2 is an immunotherapy that is FDA approved in treatment of metastatic melanoma in selected patients with good PS.

Answer c is incorrect.   High dose interferon-alfa 2b is an immunotherapy agent that is FDA approved for use in the adjuvant setting for treatment of melanoma in patients who are free of disease (nonmetastatic) but at high risk for systemic recurrence within 56 days of surgery.

Answer d is incorrect. Procarbazine is a chemotherapy agent FDA approved for used in combination with other chemotherapeutic agents in MOPP regimen for the treatment of Hodgkin lymphoma.

Answer e is incorrect. Trametinib (Mekinist) is an MEK inhibitor with FDA approval for treatment of metastatic or unresectable melanoma with BRAF V600E or V600K mutations. Trametinib is a selective and reversible MEK inhibitor with activity downstream to BRAF.

---

10. DS is a 35-year-old man with stage IV unresectable melanoma who is in dermatology clinic for follow-up visit and assessment for his second treatment with ipilimumab. What side effect(s) would you monitor in DS prior to treatment?

    a. Immune-mediated constipation
    b. Immune-mediated enterocolitis
    c. Capillary leak syndrome
    d. Myelosuppression
    e. Immune-mediated depression

Answer b is correct. Enterocolitis (eg, diarrhea) was reported as the most common adverse reaction observed with ipilimumab. Median onset occurs about 6 to 7 weeks after initiation of treatment. Moderate cases of noninfectious enterocolitis (diarrhea ≤ six stools) can be treated with antidiarrheals. For severe cases of diarrhea, high-dose corticosteroids (eg, methylprednisolone 1-2 mg/kg/d) should be given intravenously until symptoms subsided, then continue steroids taper over ≥1 month to avoid exacerbation of symptoms. Treatment should be withheld for moderate and severe enterocolitis.

Answer a is incorrect. Constipation is not an immune-mediated side effect associated with Ipilimumab.

Answer c is incorrect. Capillary leak syndrome is not an immune-mediated side effect associated with ipilimumab.

Answer d is incorrect. Myelosuppression is not an immune-mediated side effect associated with ipilimumab.

Answer e is incorrect. Depression is not an immune-mediated side effect associated with ipilimumab.

---

11. CD is a 28-year-old woman who is to start immunotherapy treatment with high-dose interferon-alfa 2b. Select the side effect(s) associated with interferon. Select all that apply.

    a. Flu-like symptoms requiring premedication with antipyretic
    b. Fatigue
    c. Depression
    d. Somnolence and confusion

Answer a is correct. Majority of patients (>80%) develop flu-like symptoms with fever, chills, headache, myalgias, and arthralgias. Symptoms usually occur few hours after

treatment and can last up to 24 hours and can be dose-limiting for some patients. Incidence of symptoms is lower with subsequent injections. Premedication with an antipyretic (ie, acetaminophen or indomethacin) is recommended to minimize risk and severity of fever and chills.

Answer b is correct. Fatigue (8%-96%) has been reported as dose-limiting side effects commonly associated with high dose interferon-alfa 2b. Caution if use in patients (>65 years of age) as these patients are at increased risk of developing fatigue and neurological toxicities secondary to high dose interferon-alfa 2b.

Answer c is correct. Depression (3%-40%) has been reported as side effect commonly associated with high dose interferon-alfa 2b. Caution if use in patients with history of depression and/or other psychological disorders, or in patients (>65 years of age) as these patients are at increased risk of developing neurological toxicities secondary to high dose interferon-alfa 2b.

Answer d is correct. Somnolence (<33%) and confusion (<12%) have been reported as side effects commonly associated with high dose interferon-alfa 2b. Caution if use in patients (>65 years of age) as these patients are at increased risk of developing neurological toxicities secondary to high dose interferon-alfa 2b.

---

12. HM is a 52-year-old man with newly diagnosed BRAF V600E mutation (+) unresectable melanoma. HM has untreated CNS involvement, with poor PS. Which of the following treatment option is appropriate for HM?

    a. IL-2
    b. Temozolomide
    c. Vemurafenib
    d. Dacarbazine
    e. Ipilimumab

Answer c is correct. Vemurafenib (Zelboraf) is a BRAF kinase inhibitor FDA approved for treatment of metastatic or unresectable melanoma with BRAF V600E mutation (+) disease. The use of vemurafenib is considered first-line treatment in newly diagnosed patient with unresectable melanoma with BRAF V600E mutation (+) disease, untreated brain involvement, and with poor PS.

Answer a is incorrect. High-dose IL-2 has been used in treatment of metastatic melanoma in selected patients with good PS and no CNS involvement as treatment with IL-2 is associated with many severe side effects requiring continuous monitoring.

Answer b is incorrect. Temozolomide (Temodar) is an oral alkylating agent with off-labeled indication in treatment of metastatic or unresectable melanoma. Myelosuppression (eg, leukopenia and thrombocytopenia) is the dose-limiting toxicity associated with temozolomide. The use of chemotherapy is considered fourth-line treatment in newly diagnosed patient with unresectable melanoma with BRAF

V600E mutation (+) disease, untreated brain involvement, and with poor PS.

Answer d is incorrect. Dacarbazine (DTIC) is an alkylating agent FDA approved for treatment of metastatic melanoma as single or combination therapy. As with other chemotherapy agent, the use of dacarbazine is associated with many side effects (eg. myelosuppression, high emetogenic potential, flu-like symptoms, and phlebitis). The use of chemotherapy is considered fourth-line treatment in newly diagnosed patient with unresectable melanoma with BRAF V600E mutation (+) disease, untreated brain involvement, and with poor PS.

Answer e is incorrect. Ipilimumab (Yervoy) is an immunotherapy used in treatment of metastatic or unresectable melanoma in patients with good or poor PS who is not candidate for IL-2 as treatment with ipilimumab is associated with immune-mediated adverse events requiring continuous monitoring prior to treatment. The use of ipilimumab is considered third-line treatment in newly diagnosed patient with unresectable melanoma with BRAF V600E mutation (+) disease, untreated brain involvement, and with poor PS.

---

13. LG is a 40-year-old woman in dermatology clinic today to discuss vemurafenib treatment with her oncologist. Which of the following are side effect(s) associated with vemurafenib in the treatment of unresectable melanoma? Select all that apply.

    a. Arthralgia
    b. Cutaneous squamous cell carcinoma
    c. QTc prolongation
    d. Photosensitivity

Answer a is correct. Arthralgia is the most common noncutaneous adverse effect observed with vemurafenib.

Answer b is correct. Cutaneous squamous cell carcinoma is a side effect observed with vemurafenib. Median onset of presentation is about 6 to 8 weeks into treatment, can be managed with surgical excision without discontinuing treatment. Keratoacanthomas and melanoma have also been reported. Incidence is reported to be higher in patients ≥65 years of age, chronic sun exposure, and history of skin cancer.

Answer c is correct. QTc prolongation has been observed with vemurafenib. Consider withholding treatment if QTc >500 msec. Monitor and adjust electrolytes particularly potassium and magnesium. Monitor EKG at baseline, repeat in 2 weeks following initiation of treatment, and monthly to every 3 months based on clinical assessment.

Answer d is correct. Dermatologic with photosensitivity reaction has been observed with vemurafenib. Case reports of SJS have also been observed requiring treatment discontinuation.

---

14. Which of the follow is the only FDA-approved combination tyrosine kinase oral chemotherapy regimen approved for the treatment of unresectable or metastatic V600E or V600K mutated melanoma?

    a. Ipilimumab + Dacarbazine
    b. IL-2 + Temozolomide
    c. Interferon-alpha 2b + Temozolomide
    d. Vemurafenib + Dabrafenib
    e. Dabrafenib + Trametinib

Answer e is correct. Combination use of trametinib and dabrafenib has recently obtained FDA accelerated approved for use in the treatment of metastatic or unresectable melanoma as the combination therapy allows for greater inhibition of the MAPK pathway and improved outcome in patients with BRAF V600 mutation (+) disease.

Answer a is incorrect. Ipilimumab is an intravenous immunotherapy agent and Dacarbazine is an intravenous chemotherapy agent.

Answer b is incorrect. IL-2 is an intravenous immunotherapy agent and Temozolomide is an oral alkylating chemotherapy agent.

Answer c is incorrect. Interferon-alpha 2b is an intravenous immunotherapy agent and Temozolomide is an oral alkylating chemotherapy agent.

Answer d is incorrect. Both vemurafenib and dabrafenib are tyrosine kinase oral chemotherapy regimen approved for the treatment of unresectable or metastatic V600E or V600K mutated melanoma; however, its approval is for single agent usage and not for combination use.

---

15. PF is a 42-year-old man with newly resected stage III melanoma who is in dermatology clinic today to discuss adjuvant treatment option. Which of the following is the correct FDA-approved dosing of interferon-alfa 2b when used as single agent for adjuvant treatment of melanoma?

    a. 375 mg/m^2 IVPB on days 1 and 15 with cycle repeat every 28 days
    b. 20 million IU/m^2 IVPB five times weekly for 4 weeks, then 10 million IU/m^2 subcutaneously three times weekly for 48 weeks
    c. 250 mg/m^2 IVPB on days 1 to 5 with cycle repeat every 21 days
    d. 600,000 IU/kg IVPB every 8 hours for a maximum of 14 doses; repeat after 9 days for a total of 28 doses per course
    e. 150 mg/m^2 po daily for 5 days with cycle repeat every 28 days

---

Answer b is correct. The FDA approved dosing of Interferon-alfa 2b when use as single agent for treatment of melanoma is 20 million IU/m^2 IVPB five times weekly for 4 weeks, then 10 million IU/m^2 subcutaneously three times weekly for 48 weeks

Answer a is incorrect. Incorrect dosing of Interferon-alpha 2b when use as single agent for treatment of melanoma.

Answer c is incorrect. Incorrect dosing of Interferon-alpha 2b when use as single agent for treatment of melanoma.

Answer d is incorrect. Incorrect dosing of Interferon-alpha 2b when use as single agent for treatment of melanoma.

Answer e is incorrect. Incorrect dosing of Interferon-alpha 2b when use as single agent for treatment of melanoma.

16. WK is a 36-year-old man with newly diagnosed unresectable BRAF V600E (+) melanoma. He is in excellent health with no comorbid conditions. WK is being admitted to oncology unit to start treatment with IL-2. Which of the following is the correct FDA-approved dosing of IL-2 when used as single agent for treatment of unresectable melanoma?

    a. 375 mg/m^2 IVPB on days 1 and 15 with cycle repeat every 28 days
    b. 20 million IU/m^2 IVPB five times weekly for 4 weeks, then 10 million IU/m^2 subcutaneously three times weekly for 48 weeks
    c. 250 mg/m^2 IVPB on days 1 to 5 with cycle repeat every 21 days
    d. 600,000 IU/kg IVPB every 8 hours for a maximum of 14 doses; repeat after 9 days for a total of 28 doses per course
    e. 150 mg/m^2 po daily for 5 days with cycle repeat every 28 days

Answer d is correct. The FDA approved dosing of IL-2 when use as single agent for treatment of melanoma is 600,000 IU/kg IVPB every 8 hours for a maximum of 14 doses; repeat after 9 days for a total of 28 doses per course. Retreat if needed in 7 weeks after previous course.

Answer a is incorrect. Incorrect dosing of IL-2 when use as single agent for treatment of melanoma.

Answer b is incorrect. Incorrect dosing of IL-2 when use as single agent for treatment of melanoma.

Answer c is incorrect. Incorrect dosing of IL-2 when use as single agent for treatment of melanoma.

Answer e is incorrect. Incorrect dosing of IL-2 when use as single agent for treatment of melanoma.

17. GK is a 62-year-old man who has just completed his adjuvant treatment for advanced stage III melanoma. Which of the following is (are) appropriate follow-up care recommendations for patients with melanoma? Select all that apply.

    a. Annual skin examination and surveillance by a dermatologist for all patients with melanoma regardless of stage of lesions.
    b. Educate patients to perform monthly self-examination of their skin and lymph nodes.
    c. Educate patients about skin cancer prevention including sun protection and proper use of sunscreen with at least SPF of 15 or higher.
    d. None of the above is appropriate follow-up care recommendations for patients with melanoma.

Answer a is correct. Life-time annual skin examination and surveillance by a dermatologist for all patients with melanoma regardless to stage of lesions, and including those with

stage 0, in-situ melanoma is recommended by the NCCN clinical practice guidelines for melanoma.

Answer b is correct. The NCCN clinical practice guidelines for melanoma recommend clinicians to consider educating patients to perform monthly self-examination of their skin and lymph nodes. Any suspicious lesions should be follow-up with health care professional for further work-up and evaluation.

Answer c is correct. Patients and their family should be educated on skin cancer prevention including sun protection measures and the proper use of sunscreen with at least SPF of 15 or higher.

Answer d is incorrect. All of the above are appropriate follow-up care recommendations for patients with melanoma.

18. RC is a 47-year-old man with stage IV unresectable melanoma who is in the hospital for his treatment with high-dose IL-2. Select the side effect associated with IL-2 that can lead to hypotension and reduced organ perfusion.

    a. Capillary leak syndrome
    b. Myelosuppression
    c. Anemia
    d. Hepatotoxicity
    e. Delirium

Answer a is correct. Vascular or capillary leak syndrome is a dose-limiting toxicity commonly reported with IL2. It can be observed immediately after initiation of therapy; clinical presentations may include weight gain, ascites, peripheral edema, arrhythmias and/or tachycardia, hypotension, oliguria and renal insufficiency, pleural effusions, and pulmonary congestion.

Answer b is incorrect. Myelosuppression with neutropenia, anemia, and thrombocytopenia have been reported with IL2, but does not usually lead to hypotension and reduced organ perfusion. Monitor patients closely for any infectious process.

Answer c is incorrect. Anemia has been reported with IL2, but does not usually lead to hypotension and reduced organ perfusion.

Answer d is incorrect. Hepatotoxicity has been reported with IL2, but does not usually lead to hypotension and reduced organ perfusion.

Answer e is incorrect. Deliriums have been observed with IL2 and generally resolve when therapy is discontinued, but does not usually lead to hypotension and reduced organ perfusion.

19. AC is a 35-year-old woman with newly diagnosed stage IV metastatic melanoma who presents to clinic for treatment with Nivolumab. Which of the following is the correct FDA-approved dosing for Nivolumab monotherapy?

    a. 240 mg IVPB every 2 weeks
    b. 240 mg IVPB every 3 weeks

c. 200 mg IVPB every 2 weeks
d. 1 mg/kg IVPB every 2 weeks
e. 1 mg/kg IVPB every 3 weeks

Answer a is correct. The FDA-approved fixed dosing of Nivolumab when used as monotherapy for metastatic or unresectable melanoma is 240 mg IVPB over 60 minutes every 2 weeks until disease progression or unacceptable toxicity.

Answer b is incorrect. Incorrect dosing frequency of Nivolumab when use as monotherapy for treatment of metastatic or unresectable melanoma.

Answer c is incorrect. Incorrect dosing of Nivolumab when use as monotherapy for treatment of metastatic or unresectable melanoma.

Answer d is incorrect. Incorrect dosing of Nivolumab when use as monotherapy for treatment of metastatic or unresectable melanoma.

Answer e is incorrect. Incorrect dosing of Nivolumab when use as monotherapy for treatment of metastatic or unresectable melanoma.

20. GS is a 52-year-old man who has developed severe immune-mediated colitis after receiving 12 cycles of pembrolizumab. He was started on prednisone 2 mg/kg/d, but has not improved after 1 week of treatment. Which of the following is the most appropriate treatment option for GS now?

a. Prednisone 4 mg/kg/d
b. Infliximab 5 mg/kg IVPB
c. Tacrolimus 0.06 mg/kg po twice daily
d. Loperamide 2 mg po every 2 hours
e. Atropine 0.4 mg IV

Answer b is correct. Based on a growing number of case reports, the immunosuppressant infliximab can provide rapid improvement in patients with serious or steroid-refractory immune-mediated colitis. It works by binding to human tumor necrosis factor alpha (TNFα), whose biological activities include the induction of proinflammatory cytokines, enhancement of leukocyte migration, activation of neutrophils and eosinophils, and the induction of acute phase reactants and tissue degrading enzymes. Many cases reported only one dose of infliximab was needed to dramatically improve symptoms. Infliximab should not be used in cases of perforation or sepsis. In addition, it should not be used for immune-mediated hepatitis as it confers its own risk of hepatotoxicity.

Answer a is incorrect. Patient has been on high-dose corticosteroid treatment for 1 week, now considered to be steroid-refractory, will need to switch to a different immunosuppressant for optimal outcome.

Answer c is incorrect. Tacrolimus has been used in attempts to manage high-grade immune-mediated hepatitis.

Answer d is incorrect. Loperamide is not effective in managing immune-mediated colitis.

Answer e is incorrect. Atropine is not effective in managing immune-mediated colitis.

21. DK is a 45-year-old woman with stage IV unresectable melanoma who presents to clinic today for her third cycle of Pembrolizumab. She has tolerated the previous 2 cycles of treatment very well, except for some mild nausea. Which of the following is the most appropriate supportive care to add to DK's treatment today?

a. Acetaminophen 650 mg po
b. Hydrocortisone 100 mg IV
c. Dexamethasone 10 mg IV
d. Diphenhydramine 25 mg po
e. Ondansetron 8 mg IV

Answer e is correct. Serotonin receptor antagonists can be used as antiemetic prophylaxis.

Answer a is incorrect. Acetaminophen is used as premedication for infusion-related reactions.

Answer b is incorrect. Steroids should be avoided during immunotherapy treatment unless it is for a life-threatening hypersensitivity or anaphylactic reaction or severe immune-mediated adverse effects.

Answer c is incorrect. Steroids should be avoided during immunotherapy treatment unless it is for a life-threatening hypersensitivity or anaphylactic reaction or severe immune-mediated adverse effects.

Answer d is incorrect. Diphenhydramine is used as premedication for infusion-related reactions, not nausea.

CHAPTER 19 | Colorectal Cancer

Use the following scenario to answer questions 1 through 3:

GC is a 58-year-old man with a recent diagnosis of stage IV colon cancer. His prior medical history is significant for hypertension (on lisinopril and hydrochlorothiazide [HCTZ]), deep vein thrombosis (on warfarin), and atrial fibrillation (on amiodarone). The oncologist informs the patient the plan is for him to receive neoadjuvant chemotherapy followed by surgery. The oncologist informs GC that he will receive the chemotherapy regimen XELOX (capecitabine and oxaliplatin).

XELOX:

Capecitabine 1000 mg/m^2 orally twice daily for 14 days

Oxaliplatin 130 mg/m^2 IV on day 1

Repeat cycle every 3 weeks

1. GC presents to your pharmacy with a prescription for capecitabine. Which of his home medications has a significant drug interaction with his capecitabine?

a. Lisinopril
b. HCTZ

c. Warfarin

d. Cetirizine

Answer c is correct. Capecitabine has a black boxed warning for increased risk of bleeding in patients receiving warfarin therapy. This is thought to be due to an increase in S-warfarin. R-warfarin levels are not affected. Consideration should be given to switching anticoagulants in patients who are to receive warfarin. In patients receiving concomitant capecitabine and warfarin, strict monitoring of prothrombin time (PT)/international normalized ratio (INR) is recommended.

Answer a is incorrect. Lisinopril does not interact with capecitabine.

Answer b is incorrect. Theoretically, HCTZ may increase risk of myelosuppression in patients receiving chemotherapy. However, this is not considered to be a clinically significant drug interaction and concomitant use of HCTZ and capecitabine is not contraindicated.

Answer d is incorrect. Cetirizine does not interact with capecitabine.

---

2. Which of the following points should the pharmacist council GC on regarding his capecitabine?

   a. Take tablets with food.
   b. If he has trouble swallowing the tablets, crush them and mix in applesauce.
   c. Avoid eating grapefruit or drinking grapefruit juice while taking capecitabine.
   d. Avoid drinking cold liquids while taking capecitabine.

Answer a is correct. Capecitabine should be taken with food.

Answer b is incorrect. Capecitabine is a chemotherapeutic agent, as such it should never be crushed or otherwise adulterated except by professionals trained in safe handling of cytotoxic drugs using appropriate equipment and safety procedures.

Answer c is incorrect. There is no drug-food interaction with grapefruit products.

Answer d is incorrect. This is a counseling point related to cold-intolerance related to oxaliplatin, not capecitabine.

---

3. How many 500 mg capecitabine tablets are required to fill GC's capecitabine prescription for 1 cycle of XELOX? GC's BSA is 2.0 m².

   a. 28 tablets
   b. 56 tablets
   c. 112 tablets
   d. 168 tablets

Answer c is correct. The patient's dose would be 2000 mg twice daily for 14 days. It will take 4 tablets to make 2000 mg.

Four tablets, twice daily for 14 days requires 112 tablets. One cycle consists of 14 days of capecitabine therapy followed by an off week.

Answer a is incorrect. This is the answer if the patient only had to take 1 tablet twice daily for 14 days.

Answer b is incorrect. This is the answer if the patient took 4 tablets once per day for 14 days.

Answer d is incorrect. This is the answer if the patient took 4 tablets, twice daily for 3 weeks.

---

4. PL is a 67-year-old man with a history of diabetes and alcoholism. PL presents to the clinic for his seventh cycle of oxaliplatin. He is currently taking capecitabine at home. PL's complete blood count (CBC) with differential is within normal limits. Before preparing the oxaliplatin for infusion, which parameters would determine if he requires a dose reduction or for this dose to be held? Select all that apply.

   a. Total bilirubin
   b. Renal function estimated by creatinine clearance
   c. Assessment of neurotoxicity side effects
   d. Liver function estimated by aspartate transaminase (AST), alanine transaminase (ALT)

Answers b and c are correct. Oxaliplatin is primarily renally excreted like other platinum chemotherapy agents. There are creatinine clearance specific recommendations in the FDA approved labeling, but caution is recommended for severe renal dysfunction. The labeling does have dose modification guidelines based on grade 2 persistent neurosensory events and recommends consideration to discontinue therapy for grade 3 events. Dose modifications are also recommended for severe GI toxicities and myelosuppression.

Answers a and d are incorrect. Hepatic metabolism is not a major pathway of oxaliplatin clearance and should not affect the dose. However, severe impairment should prompt you to carefully monitor capecitabine toxicities due to reduced clearance.

---

5. PY is a 62-year-old woman diagnosed with stage IV colon cancer with a primary tumor in the sigmoid colon that has spread to the liver. The patient has undergone surgery 2 weeks ago to remove the solitary tumor in the liver and is ready to begin drug therapy including combination chemotherapy (FOLFOX) and a monoclonal antibody. The patient tested negative for KRAS, NRAS, BRAF, MSI, and MMR. What is the most appropriate monoclonal antibody for PY to receive with FOLFOX?

   a. Bevacizumab
   b. Nivolumab
   c. Cetuximab
   d. Ramucirumab

Answer c is correct. The patient has a tumor on the left side of the colon (sigmoid colon) and no mutations that confer resistance to EGFR antibodies (negative for KRAS/NRAS/BRAF) and is likely to respond to cetuximab or panitumumab.

Answer a is incorrect. Bevacizumab is a vascular endothelial growth factor (VEGF) inhibitor and can prolong wound healing times. It is recommended that patients wait at least 4 weeks after a surgical procedure to receive bevacizumab. If there was not another viable option, chemotherapy could be started then bevacizumab added later. However, in this case cetuximab is an acceptable alternative to bevacizumab.

Answer b is incorrect. The PD-1 inhibitors, nivolumab and pembrolizumab, are only indicated in MSI-H or dMMR positive tumors that have failed multiple therapies. PY does not meet these criteria.

Answer d is incorrect. Like bevacizumab, ramucirumab is a VEGF inhibitor and should not be used soon after surgery. Additionally, it is only indicated as a second-line agent in combination with FOLFIRI. This patient is receiving initial chemotherapy with FOLFOX.

6. Which of the following monoclonal antibodies used in the treatment of CRC is associated with causing hypomagnesemia? Select all that apply.

    a. Panitumumab
    b. Bevacizumab
    c. Cetuximab
    d. Nivolumab

Answers a and c are correct. Magnesium wasting appears to be a class effect for monoclonal antibodies that target EGFR. Both panitumumab and cetuximab have been shown to cause hypomagnesemia. Patients receiving either of these agents should have their magnesium levels monitored regularly. Potassium should also be monitored as hypomagnesemia can lead to hypokalemia.

Answers b is incorrect. Bevacizumab is not known to have effect on magnesium levels.

Answer d is incorrect. Nivolumab is not known to have effect on magnesium levels.

7. During a routine colonoscopy, KG was diagnosed with stage I colon cancer but is otherwise healthy. He is experiencing no symptoms and has no complications from his cancer so far. His oncologist will likely recommend which therapy?

    a. Surgery
    b. Radiation
    c. Neoadjuvant chemotherapy
    d. Adjuvant chemotherapy

Answer a is correct. Surgical removal for cure is the primary therapy for early stage colon cancers.

Answer b is incorrect. Radiation is not commonly used for colon cancer. It is sometimes used if patients are not surgical candidates, if the tumor is very large, or as local therapy to control local recurrences. These treatment strategies are not applicable for this patient.

Answer c is incorrect. Neoadjuvant chemotherapy would only be necessary to turn an unresectable cancer into one that can be surgically removed.

Answer d is incorrect. Adjuvant chemotherapy is recommended for stage III disease or stage II disease with high-risk features.

8. Which of the following medications is part of the CRC regimen FOLFIRI?

    a. Fludarabine
    b. Lomustine
    c. Oxaliplatin
    d. Irinotecan

Answer d is correct. FOLFIRI contains fluorouracil, leucovorin, and irinotecan.

Answer a is incorrect. Fludarabine is a purine derivative used in the treatment of follicular lymphoma and chronic lymphocytic leukemia.

Answer b is incorrect. Lomustine is an alkylating agent that is used in the treatment of malignant brain tumors.

Answer c is incorrect. While oxaliplatin is used in the treatment of CRC, it is not part of this regimen. The most common oxaliplatin-containing regimens include FOLFOX, XELOX, and CapeOx.

9. Which of the following targeted therapies can delay wound healing and should not be used until at least 4 weeks after a surgical procedure. Select all that apply.

    a. Cetuximab
    b. Ramucirumab
    c. Bevacizumab
    d. Pembrolizumab

Answers b and c are correct. Both ramucirumab and bevacizumab are VEGF inhibitors that can delay wound healing. It is recommended they not be given until at least 4 weeks after a surgical procedure.

Answer a is incorrect. EGFR targeting antibodies such as cetuximab have no effect on wound healing.

Answer d is incorrect. PD-1 inhibiting antibodies such as pembrolizumab have no effect on wound healing.

10. GW is a 58-year-old man with metastatic colon cancer on irinotecan plus cetuximab therapy. When he arrives to the infusion center, he is complaining of new "pimples" appearing all over his chest and face. The oncology nurse asks you to counsel him on managing this new finding. Your counseling points would include which of the following? Select all that apply.

    a. Reassure him that this side effect actually may be predictive of a positive tumor response to this regimen.
    b. Warn him to use sunscreen since direct sunlight can exacerbate his condition.

c. Recommend him to ask his doctor about isotretinoin, give him the FDA approved med guide, and explain about the iPLEDGE program to reduce birth defects.

d. Recommend him to ask his doctor about initiating a tetracycline such as doxycycline or minocycline.

Answer a is correct. This is a valid counseling point. Although response is correlated with rash, severe rash may still require dose modifications or delays of cetuximab.

Answer b is correct. This is a valid counseling point. Recommend sun precautions such as hats and clothing or adequate sun block.

Answer d is correct. This is a valid counseling point. Tetracyclines have been shown to be useful in treating EGFR rash to reduce its severity, albeit with little clinical evidence.

Answer c is incorrect. This is not an appropriate counseling point. Although rash caused by EGFR agents have been described in the literature as acneiform, typical acne treatments like retinoids will have no efficacy and may even exacerbate the rash.

---

11. Which of the following may increase a person's risk of CRC? Select all that apply.

a. Family history of CRC
b. Hormone replacement therapy (HRT)
c. Obesity
d. HNPCC

Answer a is correct. Family history of CRC and family history of adenomatous polyps are known risk factors for the development of CRC.

Answer c is correct. Obesity is a known risk factor for developing CRC.

Answer d is correct. HNPCC is a genetic syndrome characterized by an increased risk of CRC, typically occurring earlier in life than in patients without this disease. HNPCC is an inherited disorder that leads to defects in DNA mismatch repair and predisposes a person to a number of different cancers including colorectal, endometrium, ovarian, stomach, among others.

Answer b is incorrect. HRT lowers risk of CRC. However, due to other risks associated with HRT, including increased risk of other types of cancers, HRT is not recommended for prophylaxis.

---

12. KY is a 74-year-old man with a diagnosis of relapsed metastatic rectal cancer. His tumor is positive for KRAS mutation. The patient has undergone extensive prior therapies including fluorouracil/leucovorin, XELOX with bevacizumab, and FOLFIRI with ramucirumab. The patient wishes to receive further therapy; however, he is not interested in having to come to the clinic to receive intravenous medications. Which of the following medications is most appropriate for KY at this time?

a. Capecitabine
b. Trifluridine/tipiracil
c. Regorafenib
d. Ziv-aflibercept

Answer b is correct. The trifluridine/tipiracil is an oral drug approved for the treatment of metastatic CRC in patients who have failed multiple therapies. It is an oral medication that differs significantly from his prior regimens.

Answer a is incorrect. KY has received three fluorouracil-based regimens, including one regimen that contains capecitabine (XELOX). He is unlikely to respond to fluorouracil-based therapy.

Answer c is incorrect. The patient has already received two prior VEGF inhibitors (bevacizumab and ramucirumab). Regorafenib has not been studied in this situation and is unlikely to be effective in this patient.

Answer d is incorrect. The patient has already received two prior VEGF inhibitors (bevacizumab and ramucirumab). Ziv-aflibercept has not been study in this situation and is unlikely to be effective in this patient. Additionally, ziv-aflibercept is only indicated in combination with chemotherapy. This is an intravenous agent, which is not desired by the patient at this time.

---

13. SL is 53 years old with advanced CRC that has progressed despite multiple prior chemotherapy regimens. Pathologic review of her tumor reveals she is positive for mutation in KRAS, negative for mutation in BRAF, and positive for deficiency in mismatch repair (dMMR). Which of the following medications is most likely to benefit SL at this time? Select all that apply.

a. Cetuximab
b. Nivolumab
c. Pembrolizumab
d. Trastuzumab

Answers b and c are correct. The PD-1 inhibitors, pembrolizumab and nivolumab, are indicated for the treatment of relapsed cancers that are MSI-H or have dMMR. Pembrolizumab has this indication for all solid tumors, while nivolumab has this indication specifically for CRC.

Answer a is incorrect. Because this patient has mutation in KRAS, medications such as cetuximab that act on the EFGR will be ineffective for this patient.

Answer d is incorrect. Trastuzumab is a medication that is used in cancers that are positive for the HER-2 receptor, such as some types of breast cancer.

---

14. According to national guidelines, what is the recommended age to begin screening for CRC in a person with average risk?

a. No later than 21 years old
b. 40 years old
c. 45 years old
d. 50 years old

Answer d is correct. The frequency of screening tests depends on the method of screening.

Answer a is incorrect. Average risk women should receive Pap tests beginning 3 years after first vaginal intercourse, but no later than 21 years old.

Answer b is incorrect. Average risk women should receive annual mammograms starting at age 40.

Answer c is incorrect. High-risk men, such as African Americans, should be offered prostate cancer screening at age 45 per the American Cancer Society with careful consultation about the risks and benefits of screening. Of note, other organizations such as the National Comprehensive Cancer Network recommends a baseline evaluation and consultation begin at age 40.

---

15. Which of the following chemotherapy agents is safe to use in patients with dihydropyridine dehydrogenase (DPD) deficiency? Select all that apply.

    a. Fluorouracil
    b. Trifluridine/tipiracil
    c. Capecitabine
    d. Irinotecan

Answers b and d are correct. Neither trifluridine/tipiracil nor irinotecan are metabolized by DPD, thus they are unaffected by DPD deficiency. It is worth noting that irinotecan metabolism is delayed in patients with certain polymorphisms in the UGT1A1 enzyme, such as UGT1A1*28. This leads to decreased irinotecan clearance and potentially life-threating side effects.

Answer a is incorrect. Fluorouracil is metabolized by DPD in the liver. Undetected DPD deficiency can lead to increased fluorouracil toxicity including severe myelosuppression, diarrhea, and even death.

Answer c is incorrect. Capecitabine is metabolized to fluorouracil. After conversion to fluorouracil, DPD is responsible for ultimate metabolism. Patients with DPD deficiency would be at increased risk of side effects while on capecitabine.

Use the following scenario to answer questions 16 through 18:

JM is a 63-year-old woman with a recent diagnosis of stage IV CRC with widespread metastatic disease. She has a prior medical history of hypertension, type 2 diabetes, peripheral neuropathy, and inflammatory bowel disease. She is scheduled to begin chemotherapy with FOLFOX and bevacizumab.

FOLFOX and Bevacizumab:

Fluorouracil 400 mg/m^2 bolus then 600 mg/m^2 continuous infusion day 1 and 2

Leucovorin 200 mg/m^2 intravenous infusion day 1 and 2

Oxaliplatin 85 mg/m^2 intravenous infusion day 1

Bevacizumab 10 mg/kg intravenous infusion day 1

Repeat every 2 weeks

16. Which of the medications JM is scheduled to receive does not have anticancer activity when used by itself?

    a. Fluorouracil
    b. Leucovorin
    c. Oxaliplatin
    d. Bevacizumab

Answer b is correct. Leucovorin is not a chemotherapeutic agent. It is used in patients with CRC who are receiving fluorouracil to enhance the binding of the fluorouracil to the target site. It enhances the antitumor activity of the fluorouracil as well as potentially increasing side effects. In oncology, leucovorin is also used as a rescue agent to decrease side effects from methotrexate therapy.

Answer a is incorrect. Fluorouracil is a chemotherapy agent that is classified as an antimetabolite. It has activity against many cancers including gastrointestinal cancers and breast cancer.

Answer c is incorrect. Oxaliplatin is a chemotherapy agent that is classified as a platinum agents.

Answer d is incorrect. Bevacizumab is a targeted therapy that binds to circulating VEGF. It has activity against many cancers.

---

17. Which of the conditions from JM's prior medical history may be exacerbated by her receiving bevacizumab?

    a. Hypertension
    b. Diabetes
    c. Peripheral neuropathy
    d. Inflammatory bowel disease

Answer a is correct. Bevacizumab is known to cause hypertension in patients and its prescribing information includes warning and precaution regarding bevacizumab-induced hypertension. Patients receiving bevacizumab should have their blood pressure monitored regularly, especially in the setting of preexisting hypertension.

Answer b is incorrect. Bevacizumab has no known effect on blood sugars.

Answer c is incorrect. Bevacizumab is not known to cause, or worsen neuropathy.

Answer d is incorrect. Bevacizumab is not known to cause, or worsen inflammatory bowel disease.

18. Avastin is the brand name of which medication that JM is receiving for her CRC?

    a. Fluorouracil
    b. Leucovorin
    c. Oxaliplatin
    d. Bevacizumab

Answer d is correct. The brand name of bevacizumab is Avastin.

Answer a is incorrect. Fluorouracil is available under various brand names. The original brand name was Adrucil.

Answer b is incorrect. Leucovorin is available under numerous brand names.

Answer c is incorrect. The brand name of oxaliplatin is Eloxatin.

19. Which of the following statements about CRC is *correct*? Select all that apply.

    a. FOLFOX with bevacizumab can be used as a first-line therapy.
    b. FOLFIRI with bevacizumab can be used as a first-line therapy.
    c. Surgery and other local therapies are almost never a valid option.
    d. Colon cancer tends to first spread to the liver.

Answer a is correct. FOLFOX with bevacizumab is a commonly used regimen in patients with metastatic or relapsed disease.

Answer b is correct. Although the FDA-approved labeling for bevacizumab is for combination with IFL, FOLFIRI is generally recommended instead due to improved tolerability.

Answer d is correct. The liver is typically the first site of metastasis in patient with CRC. This is thought to be related to portal blood flow. The lungs are the second most common site of metastases.

Answer c is incorrect. Surgery is an important part of therapy and is performed in most patients with stages I, II, or III disease. In patients with stage IV disease, surgery is still a therapeutic option if the number of metastases is limited. RT, another localized therapy, is used in many patients with rectal cancer.

20. JL is a 55-year-old African American man concerned about CRC screening. He inquires about screening recommendations for someone his age. Which of the following screening tests is most appropriate for JL?

    a. FSIG
    b. Digital rectal examination
    c. CEA blood test
    d. Colonoscopy

Answer d is correct. The advantages of colonoscopy are that the full colon is visualized and any abnormal polyps can be removed for a biopsy. The disadvantages include the invasiveness, cost, and need for sedation.

Answer a is incorrect. FSIG only images the lower part of the colon and requires a follow-up full colonoscopy if any abnormalities are found.

Answer b is incorrect. However, JL should get a digital rectal examination and prostate-specific antigen (PSA) blood test to detect prostate cancer if he has not gotten one this year.

Answer c is incorrect. CEA may be elevated in other malignant and benign conditions and is not considered a valid screening method for CRC. The level may be helpful to determine extend of disease already diagnosed by other means, evaluate treatment response, and for recurrence surveillance.

CHAPTER 20 | Antimicrobial Principles

1. Select the antimicrobial that may cause collateral damage by selecting for a nontargeted organism (ie, *Clostridium difficile*) leading to a colitis infection. Select all that apply.

    a. Clindamycin
    b. Levofloxacin
    c. Ciprofloxacin
    d. Ceftriaxone

Clostridium difficile, also known as *C. difficile*, is a species of gram-positive bacteria of the genus *Clostridium*. Clostridia are anaerobic, spore-forming rods (bacillus). *C. difficile* is the most serious cause of antibiotic-associated diarrhea (AAD) and can lead to pseudomembranous colitis, a severe infection of the colon, often resulting from eradication of the normal gut flora by antibiotics. The *C. difficile* bacteria, which naturally reside in the body, become overpopulated. The overpopulation is harmful because the bacterium releases toxins that can cause bloating, constipation, and diarrhea with abdominal pain, which may become severe. Discontinuation of causative antibiotic treatment is often curative. In more serious cases, oral administration of metronidazole or vancomycin is the treatment of choice. Relapses of *C. difficile* AAD have been reported in up to 20% of cases.

Answer a is correct. Clindamycin may cause/select for a *C. difficile* infection.

Answer b is correct. Levofloxacin may cause/select for a *C. difficile* infection.

Answer c is correct. Ciprofloxacin may cause/select for a *C. difficile* infection.

Answer d is correct. Ceftriaxone may cause/select for a *C. difficile* infection.

2. Select the correct dose of cefepime (Maxipime) for a patient with normal renal function and empirically treated for an infection (at this time the site or source of infection have not been identified). Select all that apply.

   a. 1 g IV every 12 hours
   b. 2 g IV every 12 hours
   c. 2 g IV every 8 hours
   d. 4.5 g every 6 hours

Answer a is correct. Cefepime 1 g every 12 hours may be utilized for patients with community-acquired pneumonia and UTIs.

Answer b is correct. Cefepime 2 g every 12 hours may be utilized for patients with intra-abdominal infections, skin and skin structure infections, and UTIs.

Answer c is correct. Cefepime 2 g every 8 hours may be utilized for patients with febrile neutropenia and suspected resistant pathogens (ie, *Pseudomonas aeruginosa infections*)

All of the above doses of cefepime may be utilized, depending upon the site of infection and the potential for bacterial resistance. High doses of cefepime are often utilized empirically, especially when the site or source of infection has not been identified, as is the situation with our current case application question. Since this patient has been diagnosed with an infection and cefepime is going to be utilized, high doses would likely be the best option until the site or source has been identified. Once the site and/or source have been identified, the dose or anti-infective may be required to be changed. Also, if a patient were suspected to have a multidrug resistant organism, other methods of dosing may be utilized (eg, *extended infusion* β-lactam therapy). Please note this case application question was about dosing of anti-infectives, not selection of anti-infectives, with cefepime serving as an example.

Answer d is incorrect. 4.5 g every 6 hours is the dose/ interval for piperacillin/tazobactam.

3. Select the antimicrobial PK property that impacts the dose and/or interval. Select all that apply.

   a. Bioavailability
   b. Volume of distribution
   c. Metabolism
   d. Elimination

Answer a is correct. Bioavailability (absorption) is a key PK property in describing antimicrobial properties.

Answer b is correct. Volume of distribution (V_d) is a key PK property in describing antimicrobial properties. V_d may change during therapy and is an important factor to monitor. Patients that may have altered V_d include: ascites, edema, pregnant, burn, obese, thin, loss of extremities (ie, above the knee amputation), and dehydrated patients.

Answer c is correct. Metabolism is a key PK property in describing antimicrobial properties. Understanding drug interactions and its impact on the antimicrobial concentration are important factors in determining anti-infective dose and/or interval.

Answer d is correct. Elimination is a key PK property in describing antimicrobial properties. Understanding renal and/or hepatic function are important factors in determining anti-infective dose and/or interval. Renally eliminated anti-infectives are usually dose-based upon results from the approximation of the glomerular filtration rate (GFR) via calculation of the creatinine clearance (Cockroft-Gault or modification of diet in renal disease [MDRD] equations). Anti-infectives eliminated via the hepatic system may be dosed upon a Child-Pugh score, although recommendations for dosing anti-infectives in patients with liver dysfunction are not as formalized as guidelines for patients with renal dysfunction.

4. Select the factor that may affect the bioavailability of an oral anti-infective.

   a. A medication that is a substrate of the CYP-450 system
   b. Dosage formulation of the anti-infective
   c. A patient that has peripheral vascular disease
   d. A patient that has renal dysfunction

Answer b is correct. The dosage formulation of the anti-infective may have significant effects on the bioavailability. A classic example is vancomycin. Vancomycin is available as oral and parenteral formulations. Oral vancomycin is not absorbed and reserved for treatment of *C. difficile* infections (AAD). Intravenous vancomycin has a bioavailability of 100% (F = 1) and is used for treatment of systemic gram-positive infections (ie, methicillin resistant *Staphylococcus aureus*). Parenteral formulations of an anti-infective may also have various degrees of bioavailability. Examples include a potential difference in bioavailability of β-lactams when administered via IV versus intramuscular routes.

Answer a is incorrect. Anti-infective CYP-450 activity (substrates, inhibitors, inducers) will not affect the bioavailability. P-450 activity will affect the metabolism and elimination, but not absorption. Anti-infectives administered orally that are circulated through the liver may be affected by the first-pass effect. The first-pass effect will eliminate some of the anti-infective and would indirectly affect the amount of medication able to be absorbed. The first-pass effect is a phenomenon of drug metabolism whereby the concentration of a drug is reduced before it reaches the systemic circulation. It is the fraction of lost drug during the process of absorption which is generally related to the liver and gut wall. Notable drugs that experience a significant first-pass effect are imipramine, propranolol, and lidocaine.

Answer c is incorrect. A patient with peripheral vascular disease would not be expected to have different bioavailability. However, comorbidities (like peripheral vascular disease) may impact other PK properties of anti-infectives like distribution and elimination.

Answer d is incorrect. Renal dysfunction would not have an impact on bioavailability. Renal dysfunction would affect the elimination of the anti-infective.

---

5. Select the factor that would usually necessitate a patient to be given IV anti-infectives.

    a. Fever of 101.9°F
    b. Severe cough
    c. G6PD deficiency
    d. Blood pressure of 91/52 mm Hg with signs of hypoperfusion (baseline blood pressure for patient is 129/86 mm Hg)

Answer d is correct. Patients manifesting systemic signs of infection such as hypotension and hypoperfusion should receive IV anti-infectives.

Answer a is incorrect. Hyper- or hypothermia would not necessitate a patient to be given IV anti-infectives. Patients diagnosed with sepsis (overwhelming infection) would be recommended to receive IV anti-infectives. Septic patients will most likely present with hyper- or hypothermia, but they must have other signs and symptoms to be classified as sepsis. Fever is one of the factors that is utilized in the recommendation of switching from IV to oral anti-infectives. The factors that are involved in streamlining patients from IV to oral anti-infectives are: (1) display of clinical improvement, (2) lack of fever for 8 to 24 hours, (3) decreased WBC count, and (4) functioning gastrointestinal tract.

Answer b is incorrect. Cough would not impact the decision to utilize IV or oral anti-infectives.

Answer c is incorrect. G6PD deficiency would not impact the decision to recommend oral or IV anti-infectives. Patients should not receive certain anti-infectives if they have G6PD deficiency because they may develop hemolysis, but it would not impact oral/IV decision. Anti-infectives that may lead to hemolysis in G6PD deficient patients are sulfonamides and dapsone.

---

6. Select the oral anti-infective(s) that displays good bioavailability. Select all that apply.

    a. Fluconazole
    b. Linezolid
    c. Levofloxacin
    d. Vancomycin

Answer a is correct. Oral fluconazole displays good bioavailability (>90%). Other azole antifungals (itraconazole and ketoconazole) have critical bioavailability concerns. They must be administered and absorbed in an acidic gastrointestinal pH. Major drug interactions with ketoconazole and itraconazole are acid suppressing agents (H2 blockers and proton pump inhibitors).

Answer b is correct. Oral linezolid displays good bioavailability (rapid and extensive).

Answer c is correct. Oral levofloxacin displays good bioavailability (rapid and complete).

Answer d is incorrect. Oral vancomycin displays poor bioavailability.

---

7. Select the infection that requires excellent tissue penetration (distribution). Select all that apply.

    a. Meningitis
    b. Acute cystitis
    c. Bronchitis
    d. Cellulitis

Answer a is correct. Meningitis infections require anti-infective distribution within the CSF. Anti-infectives that do not reach significant concentrations in the CSF should be avoided or instilled directly. Anti-infectives with moderate to good penetration within the CSF will still require higher doses. For example, the dose/interval for IV ceftriaxone in meningitis is 2 g every 12 hours, compared to 1 g every 24 hours for community-acquired pneumonia.

Answer b is correct. Acute cystitis infections require the anti-infective to be renally eliminated to be able to reach the site of infection.

Answers c and d are incorrect. Bronchitis and cellulitis infections do not require specific distribution properties of the anti-infectives.

Sites of infections that require specific distribution properties of the anti-infectives include CSF, urine, synovial fluid, and peritoneal fluid. Apart from these areas, more attention should be paid to clinical efficacy, antimicrobial spectrum, adverse effects, and cost than to comparative data on penetration.

Please note that this case application question focuses on selection of anti-infectives based upon the PK property distribution. This question *did not* focus on selection of oral or parenteral administration of an anti-infective. There are *infectious disease states* that *may* require parenteral administration. These disease states are considered sequestered infections and include: meningitis, osteomyelitis, endocarditis, and pneumonia.

---

8. Select the anti-infective that exhibits the pharmacodynamic property of concentration dependent activity.

    a. Ceftriaxone
    b. Amoxicillin
    c. Ciprofloxacin
    d. Meropenem

Answer c is correct. Ciprofloxacin exhibits the pharmacodynamic property of concentration-dependent activity. Other anti-infectives that exhibit concentration-dependent activity include: aminoglycosides, metronidazole, and other fluoroquinolones. Concentration dependent activity is maximized when the peak concentration (C_{max}) to MIC ratio is greater than or equal to 10:1 for aminoglycosides. Quinolone pharmacodynamic properties are maximized according to the area under the curve (AUC) to MIC ratio. For gram-positive bacteria, the ideal AUC:MIC ratio is greater than or equal to 30:1. For gram-negative bacteria, the ideal AUC:MIC ratio is greater than or equal to 125:1.

Answer a is incorrect.   Ceftriaxone and other cephalosporins exhibit the pharmacodynamic property of time-dependent activity.

Answer b is incorrect.   Amoxicillin and other penicillins exhibit the pharmacodynamic property of time-dependent activity.

Answer d is incorrect.   Meropenem and other carbapenems exhibit the pharmacodynamic property of time-dependent activity.

---

9. Select the anti-infective that exhibits the pharmacodynamic property of time-dependent activity.

    a. Levofloxacin
    b. Doripenem
    c. Amikacin
    d. Metronidazole

Answer b is correct.   Doripenem (other carbapenems, penicillins, cephalosporins) exhibit time-dependent activity. The pharmacodynamic property of time-dependent activity is maximized when the free concentration (nonprotein bound) exceeds the MIC for a certain period of time. For the cell wall agents to exhibit ***bactericidal*** time-dependent activity, the following parameters must be met:

- Carbapenems require that the concentration be above the MIC for 40% of the dosing interval.

- Cephalosporins require that the concentration be above the MIC for 60% to 70% of the dosing interval.

- Penicillins require that the concentration be above the MIC for 50% of the dosing interval.

    For the cell wall agents to exhibit ***bacteriostatic*** time-dependent activity, the following parameters must be met:

- Carbapenems require that the concentration be above the MIC for 20% of the dosing interval.

- Cephalosporins require that the concentration be above the MIC for 35% to 40% of the dosing interval.

- Penicillins require that the concentration be above the MIC for 30% of the dosing interval.

    The best pharmacodynamic property for the glycopeptide vancomycin is debatable. Traditionally, vancomycin was considered to display time-dependent activity; however, more recently the AUC:MIC ratio was found to be the best predictor of successful outcomes. Pharmacodynamic properties of vancomycin are maximized then the AUC:MIC ratio

is greater than or equal to 400:1. A vancomycin *trough* of 15 to 20 mcg/mL would achieve an AUC:MIC ratio greater than 400:1, as long as the MIC was less than or equal to 1 mcg/mL.

Answer a is incorrect.   Levofloxacin (and other quinolones) exhibit the pharmacodynamic property of concentration-dependent activity.

Answer c is incorrect.   Amikacin and other aminoglycosides exhibit the pharmacodynamic property of concentration-dependent activity.

Answer d is incorrect.   Metronidazole exhibits the pharmacodynamic property of concentration-dependent activity. *Note:* Please be able to differentiate between metronid*azole* and the azole antifungals (flucon*azole*, voricon*azole*, itracon*azole*, and ketocon*azole*). Metronidazole (Flagyl) is an antibiotic used to treat anaerobic infections (ie, *Bacteroides fragilis*) and AAD caused by *C. difficile*. The azole antifungals are used to treat fungal infections (yeast or mold). There are also major differences in side effects and drug interactions between these agents with similar ending names. Metronidazole may cause a disulfiram reaction when administered with alcohol. The azole antifungals have significant drug interactions (CYP-450) and may cause hepatitis.

---

10. A patient with a health care-associated pneumonia infection is found to have a multidrug resistant organism (this was found by the culture and susceptibility and the pathogen *P. aeruginosa* exhibits high MIC to all antibiotics). Since the pathogen exhibits high-level resistance, modifications to the dose or interval will be required to achieve successful outcomes. Currently, the patient is receiving the β-lactam piperacillin/tazobactam 4.5 g intravenously every 6 hours infused over 30 minutes. Select the factor that may be done to piperacillin/tazobactam that could optimize the pharmacodynamic property.

    a. Increase the infusion time
    b. Increase the dose
    c. Add combination therapy with another β-lactam
    d. Decrease the dose to 3.375 g

Answer a is correct.   β-lactam antimicrobials are often administered intravenously as 30-minute infusions. An example is piperacillin/tazobactam (Zosyn) 4.5 g intravenously every 6 hours infused over 30 minutes. In efforts to optimize the time-dependent activity of β-lactams, extending the infusion interval is being clinically utilized (piperacillin/tazobactam 3.375 g intravenously every 8 hours infused over 4 hours). Extending the infusion interval allows for the concentration to remain above the MIC for longer periods of time (time-dependent activity).

Answer b is incorrect.   Increasing the dose would optimize the pharmacodynamic property for concentration-dependent agents, not time-dependent agents.

Answer c is incorrect.   A common subject of debate involves the utilization of combination anti-infective therapy.

Proponents state that double coverage may be synergistic, prevent the emergence of resistance, and improve outcomes. However, there are few clinical examples in the literature to support these assertions. Double antimicrobial coverage may be beneficial for selected infections associated with high bacterial loads or for initial empirical coverage of critically ill patients in whom antimicrobial-resistant organisms are suspected. Monotherapy usually is satisfactory once antimicrobial susceptibilities are known. In the case application question above, the combination of the two anti-infectives would not be ideal because they are of the same mechanism of action (β-lactams). When the clinical situation calls for combination therapy, utilization of drugs with different mechanisms of action is preferred.

Answer d is incorrect. Decreasing the dose would not assist in optimizing the PK/PD property of piperacillin/tazobactam. *Note:* Some providers may decrease the dose when they increase the infusion time.

---

11. CNS side effects (seizures and mental status changes) are associated with β-lactam and quinolone anti-infectives. A risk factor for development of the CNS reactions is:

    a. Duration of therapy
    b. Infusion interval
    c. Bioavailability
    d. Renal dysfunction

Answer d is correct. Antibiotic-associated CNS toxicities may be common effects for penicillin, cephalosporin, carbapenem, and quinolone anti-infectives, especially if the dose or interval is not adjusted for renal dysfunction.

Answer a is incorrect. Duration of therapy would not be a factor in CNS side effects of β-lactams or quinolones, unless the patient was accumulating (not eliminating) the anti-infective.

Answer b is incorrect. The infusion interval would not impact the CNS side effect.

Answer c is incorrect. Bioavailability would not impact the CNS side effect.

---

12. Select the anti-infective that is associated with the adverse effects of nephrotoxicity and ototoxicity.

    a. Amoxicillin/clavulanate
    b. Cefpodoxime
    c. Moxifloxacin
    d. Gentamicin

Answer d is correct. The aminoglycoside gentamicin (Garamycin) is associated with nephrotoxicity and ototoxicity.

Answer a is incorrect. The penicillin β-lactam amoxicillin/clavulanate (Augmentin) is not associated with nephrotoxicity and ototoxicity.

Answer b is incorrect. The cephalosporin β-lactam cefpodoxime (Vantin) is not associated with nephrotoxicity and ototoxicity.

Answer c is incorrect. The fluoroquinolone moxifloxacin (Avelox) is not associated with nephrotoxicity and ototoxicity.

---

13. Select the anti-infective(s) that is associated with the adverse reaction of AAD (*C. difficile*). Select all that apply.

    a. Augmentin
    b. Levaquin
    c. Cleocin
    d. Vancocin

Answer a is correct. Amoxicillin/clavulanate (Augmentin) and other β-lactams are associated with the adverse reaction of AAD (*C. difficile*). Please note that anti-infectives may also cause gastrointestinal disturbances leading to diarrhea that is different than *C. difficile* infections. Augmentin has a high rate of diarrhea from gastrointestinal disturbance as well. Just because a patient develops diarrhea on anti-infectives, it does not mean it is caused by *C. difficile*.

Answer b is correct. Levofloxacin (Levaquin) and other fluoroquinolones are associated with the adverse reaction of AAD (*C. difficile*).

Answer c is correct. Clindamycin (Cleocin) is associated with the adverse reaction of AAD (*C. difficile*). Clindamycin has the highest incidence of *C. diff* infections.

Answer d is incorrect. Vancomycin (Vancocin) is not associated with the adverse reaction of AAD (*C. difficile*). Oral vancomycin is used to treat *C. diff* infections.

---

14. JG is a patient with an immediate allergic reaction to ticarcillin/clavulanate (Timentin). Select the antimicrobial that JG may take in relation to his allergy.

    a. Piperacillin/tazobactam
    b. Amoxicillin/clavulanate
    c. Cephalexin
    d. Aztreonam

Answer d is correct. Aztreonam (Azactam) is a monobactam antimicrobial. The place in therapy for aztreonam is for patients with a hypersensitivity reaction to penicillins.

Answer a is incorrect. JG has an immediate allergic reaction to penicillin (Timentin) and, therefore, cannot take penicillin antimicrobials.

Answer b is incorrect. JG has an immediate allergic reaction to penicillin (Timentin) and, therefore, cannot take penicillin antimicrobials.

Answer c is incorrect. JG has an immediate allergic reaction to penicillin (Timentin) and, therefore, cannot take select cephalosporin antimicrobials.

15. Select the host factor(s) that may impact antimicrobial therapy. Select all that apply.

   a. Age
   b. Pregnancy
   c. Metabolic abnormalities
   d. Organ dysfunction

Answer a is correct. Age is an important factor in determining causative pathogens for certain infections (ie, meningitis) and PK factors (renal dysfunction).

Answer b is correct. Antimicrobial agents must be used with caution in pregnant and nursing women. Some agents are known or likely to be teratogenic (eg, metronidazole), and others pose potential threats to the fetus or infant (eg, quinolones, tetracyclines, and sulfonamides). PK variables also are altered during pregnancy. Both the clearance and volume of distribution are increased during pregnancy. As a result, increased dosages and/or more frequent administration of certain drugs may be required to achieve adequate concentrations.

Answer c is correct. Inherited or acquired metabolic abnormalities influence infectious diseases therapy. Patients with peripheral vascular disease may not absorb drugs given by intramuscular injection. Other examples include: patients who are phenotypically slow acetylators of isoniazid are at greater risk for peripheral neuropathy; patients with G6PD deficiency can develop hemolysis when exposed to sulfonamides and dapsone.

Answer d is correct. Patients with renal or hepatic dysfunction will accumulate certain drugs unless the dosage is adjusted.

16. Select the risk factor(s) for the acquisition of exogenous pathogens. Select all that apply.

   a. Nursing home admission
   b. Pregnancy
   c. Recent antimicrobial use
   d. Hospital admission for 7 days

Answers a and d are correct. Nursing home and hospital admission may expose the patient to different types of bacteria and change the patient's normal flora. This change in normal flora may necessitate a change in empiric treatment of infections.

Answer c is correct. Patients with a history of recent antimicrobial use may have altered normal flora (acquisition of exogenous pathogen).

Answer b is incorrect. Pregnancy would not change the normal (endogenous) flora. Pregnancy may change PK parameters such as volume of distribution.

17. Select the potential cause of a fever. Select all that apply.

   a. Infection
   b. Piperacillin

   c. Trauma
   d. Cancer

Answer a is correct. Infections may cause a fever. However, patients with infections may also present with hypothermia (eg, patients with overwhelming infection, sepsis). Elderly patients may be afebrile, as well as patients with localized infection (eg, uncomplicated UTIs).

Answer b is correct. Medications may cause a fever. Examples of mediations that have been associated with a drug fever are: anticonvulsants, minocycline, penicillins, cephalosporins, allopurinol, and heparin.

Answer c is correct. Trauma may cause a fever.

Answer d is correct. Malignancy may cause a fever

18. Select the information that is revealed by a gram stain.

   a. MIC
   b. Genre and species of the bacteria
   c. Morphologic characteristics of the bacteria
   d. Antibiotic susceptibility

Answer c is correct. A gram stain is performed to identify if bacteria are present and to determine morphologic characteristics of bacteria (such as gram-positive or negative; shape—cocci or bacilli).

Answers a and d are incorrect. MIC and antibiotic susceptibility are revealed by the culture and susceptibility test.

Answer b is incorrect. The genre and species of the bacteria are revealed by the culture and susceptibility test.

19. Select the pathogen(s) that is classified as an atypical organism.

   a. *Escherichia coli*
   b. *Klebsiella pneumoniae*
   c. *Mycoplasma pneumoniae*
   d. *Streptococcus pneumoniae*

Answer c is correct. *M. pneumoniae* is an aerobic gram-negative bacteria, but it retains the gram stain poorly and thus cannot be reliably seen on routine gram stain, and therefore referred to as an atypical pathogen. Other atypical organisms are *Legionella pneumophila* and *Chlamydia pneumoniae*.

Answer a is incorrect. *E. coli* is an aerobic lactose-positive fermenting gram-negative rod. *E. coli* belongs to the Enterobacteriaceae (Enteric) family.

Answer b is incorrect. *Klebsiella* species are aerobic lactose-positive fermenting gram-negative rods. *Klebsiella* species belong to the Enterobacteriaceae (Enteric) family.

Answer d is incorrect. *S. pneumoniae* is an aerobic gram-positive organism.

20. Select the pathogen that represents an exogenous bacteria flora (ie, acquired from the hospital). Characteristics of this pathogen are nonlactose fermenting gram-negative bacilli.

    a. *Neisseria meningitidis*
    b. *Enterobacter cloacae*
    c. *Streptococcus pneumoniae*
    d. *Pseudomonas aeruginosa*

Answer d is correct. *P. aeruginosa* is a nonlactose fermenting gram-negative bacilli. Other nonlactose fermenting gram-negative bacilli include *Proteus, Serratia, Morganella, Stenotrophomonas,* and *Acinetobacter.*

Answer a is incorrect. *N. meningitidis* is a gram-negative cocci.

Answer b is incorrect. *E. cloacae* is a lactose-fermenting gram-negative bacilli.

Answer c is incorrect. *S. pneumoniae* is a gram-positive cocci (diplococcic).

21. Select the penicillin antimicrobial that is broad spectrum and has coverage against nonlactose negative (oxidase-positive) gram-negative bacilli.

    a. Amoxicillin
    b. Nafcillin
    c. Cefepime
    d. Doripenem
    e. Piperacillin/tazobactam

Answer e is correct. Piperacillin/tazobactam is a broad-spectrum penicillin antimicrobial that has activity against the nonlactose negative (oxidase-positive) gram-negative bacilli (*P. aeruginosa*).

Answer a is incorrect. Amoxicillin is a narrow-spectrum antimicrobial and it does not have activity against the nonlactose negative (oxidase-positive) gram-negative bacilli (*P. aeruginosa*).

Answer b is incorrect. Nafcillin is a narrow-spectrum gram-positive antimicrobial and it does not have activity against the nonlactose negative (oxidase-positive) gram-negative bacilli (*P. aeruginosa*) or any gram negative.

Answer c is incorrect. Cefepime is broad-spectrum and it does have coverage against nonlactose negative (oxidase-positive) gram-negative bacilli (*P. aeruginosa*); however, it is a cephalosporin.

Answer d is incorrect. Doripenem is broad-spectrum and it does have coverage against nonlactose negative (oxidase-positive) gram-negative bacilli (*P. aeruginosa*); however, it is a carbapenem.

22. Select the pathogen(s) that is part of the normal (endogenous) flora of the large intestine. Select all that apply.

    a. *Escherichia coli*
    b. Viridans streptococci
    c. *Neisseria meningitidis*
    d. *Enterococcus* species

Answers a and d are correct. *E. coli* and *Enterococcus* species reside within the normal flora of the large intestine. Other organisms that reside with the large intestine include: Enterobacteriaceae, *Enterococcus* species, and anaerobes. *E. coli* also resides in the small intestine.

Answer b is incorrect. Viridans *streptococci* reside within the normal flora of the mouth and are a potential cause of endocarditis.

Answer c is incorrect. *N. meningitidis* reside within the normal flora of the upper respiratory tract and may cause meningitis.

23. Select the best answer that represents part of the normal (endogenous) flora of the lower respiratory tract.

    a. Enterobacteriaceae
    b. *Streptococcus pneumoniae*
    c. *Enterococcus* species
    d. Normally sterile

Answer d is correct. The lower respiratory tract is normally sterile. Other areas that are normally sterile include the CSF and urine.

Answer a is incorrect. Enterobacteriaceae reside as part of the normal flora in the small and large intestines.

Answer b is incorrect. *S. pneumoniae* reside as part of the normal flora in the upper respiratory tract.

Answer c is incorrect. *Enterococcus* species reside as part of the normal flora in the small and large intestines.

24. Select the drug interaction(s) with aminoglycosides. Select all that apply.

    a. Amphotericin B
    b. Vancomycin
    c. Furosemide
    d. Cisplatin

Answer a is correct. Amphotericin B has a drug interaction with the aminoglycosides. The mechanism/effect is additive adverse effects (nephrotoxicity).

Answer b is correct. Vancomycin has a drug interaction with the aminoglycosides. The mechanism/effect is additive adverse effects (nephrotoxicity).

Answer c is correct. Furosemide has a drug interaction with the aminoglycosides. The mechanism/effect is additive adverse effects (ototoxicity).

Answer d is correct. Cisplatin has a drug interaction with the aminoglycosides. The mechanism/effect is additive adverse effects (nephrotoxicity and ototoxicity).

Other drug interactions with the aminoglycoside antimicrobials are neuromuscular blocking agents, cyclosporine, nonsteroidal anti-inflammatory drugs, and radio contrast. The clinical management for the aminoglycoside drug interactions is to monitor aminoglycoside serum drug concentrations and renal function (except when combined with neuromuscular blocking agents, it is best to avoid utilization of aminoglycosides and neuromuscular blocking agents).

25. RL is a patient with a past medical history of iron deficiency anemia. He is being treated with ferrous sulfate. Select the antimicrobial(s) that would have a decreased bioavailability when combined with ferrous sulfate. Select all that apply.

    a. Moxifloxacin
    b. Tetracycline
    c. Azithromycin
    d. Doxycycline

Answer a is correct. Moxifloxacin (and other fluoroquinolones) have decreased absorption when combined with multivalent cations (antacids, iron, sucralfate, zinc, vitamins, dairy, and citric acid). The clinical management for this interaction is to separate administration of the two agents by at least 2 hours.

Answers b and d are correct. Tetracycline and doxycycline have decreased absorption when combined with iron, antacids, calcium, and sucralfate. The clinical management for this interaction is to separate administration of the two agents by at least 2 hours.

Answer c is incorrect. Azithromycin and the macrolide antimicrobials are not affected by concurrent administration of multivalent cations.

CHAPTER 21 | **Lower Respiratory Tract Infections**

1. Select the infection(s) that is/are an LRTI. Select all that apply.

    a. Pneumonia
    b. Sinusitis
    c. Bronchitis
    d. Otitis

Answer a is correct. Pneumonia is an LRTI. There are different classifications of pneumonia, including community-acquired, aspiration, and hospital-acquired.

Answer c is correct. Bronchitis is an example of LRTI. Bronchitis has two subsets: acute bronchitis and chronic bronchitis. Acute bronchitis is usually a self-limiting viral infection.

Answers b and d are incorrect. Sinusitis is an upper respiratory tract infection. Other examples of upper respiratory tract infections include otitis media and pharyngitis.

2. AS is a 54-year-old man with fever, cough, and shortness of breath. He has been diagnosed with an LRTI. Select bacterial pathogen(s) that is a common cause of LRTI. Select all that apply.

    a. *Haemophilus influenzae*
    b. *Moraxella catarrhalis*
    c. Influenza
    d. *Streptococcus pneumoniae*

Answers a and b are correct. *H. influenzae* is a Gram-negative coccobacillus and *M. catarrhalis* is a Gram-negative diplococcus—they are a common bacterial causes of LRTIs.

Answer d is correct. *S. pneumoniae*, or pneumococcus, is a Gram-positive organism that is a common bacterial cause of LRTIs.

Answer c is incorrect. Influenza is a viral pathogen that is a common cause of LRTIs. Be able to recognize and differentiate the difference between *H. influenzae* (*H. flu*) and influenza. Both are causes of LRTIs; however, one is a bacteria and the other a virus.

3. QW is a patient admitted to a rehabilitation hospital to improve strength after cardiac surgery. He does not want to develop an infection (especially pneumonia) because it hurts when he coughs. He questions how he can prevent the development of pneumonia. Which of the following may prevent pneumonia? Select all that apply.

    a. Infection control/prevention measures
    b. *Streptococcus pneumoniae* vaccine
    c. Influenza vaccine
    d. Levofloxacin

Answer a is correct. Infection control/prevention measures may prevent pneumonia cases. Examples of infection prevention measures are: respiratory hygiene measures (use of hand hygiene and masks or tissues for patients with cough), hospitalized patients should be kept in a semirecumbent position, and enteral nutrition is preferred over parenteral.

Answer b is correct. Pneumococcal vaccine prevents pneumonia and is recommended in the following groups: all people ≥65 years of age, people ≥2 years old with chronic conditions, smokers, immunocompromised patients, and people without spleens.

Answer c is correct. Annual influenza vaccine is recommended for everyone over the age of 6 months. Since a serious possible consequence of influenza infection is bacterial pneumonia, it helps prevent this superinfection by preventing the primary influenza infection. When influenza does occur in vaccinated patients, it is generally less severe than in the unvaccinated population.

Answer d is incorrect. Levofloxacin or other antibiotics are not administered to prevent pneumonia infections.

4. A pharmacy student is on his pediatric acute care clerkship and is charged with developing a list of antibiotics that may be used to treat pediatric pneumonia. Select anti-infectives that may be used to treat pediatric CAP. Select all that apply.

    a. Levofloxacin
    b. Doxycycline
    c. Ceftriaxone
    d. Azithromycin

Answers c and d are correct. Ceftriaxone may be used to treat pediatric infections, including pneumonia. Other antimicrobials utilized in the treatment of pediatric pneumonia include outpatient—high-dose amoxicillin, amoxicillin-clavulanate, intramuscular ceftriaxone, azithromycin, and clarithromycin; inpatient—IV cefuroxime, cefotaxime, ceftriaxone, and ampicillin-sulbactam.

Answer a is incorrect. Levofloxacin and other fluoroquinolones should not be used to treat pediatric infections. Although the systemic use of fluoroquinolones in children is only Food and Drug Administration (FDA) indicated for the treatment of complicated urinary tract infections, plague, and postexposure treatment of inhalation anthrax, use of fluoroquinolones in pediatric patients is increasing. Current recommendations by the American Academy of Pediatrics note that systemic use of these agents in children should be restricted to infections caused by multidrug resistant (MDR) pathogens with no safe or effective alternative.

Answer b is incorrect. Doxycycline is incorrect. Doxycycline and tetracyclines may cause tissue hyperpigmentation, enamel hypoplasia, or permanent tooth discoloration; use of tetracyclines should be avoided during tooth development (children <8 years of age) unless other drugs are not likely to be effective or are contraindicated.

5. AQ is a 44-year-old female patient with a past medical history of hypertension (HTN) and dyslipidemia. Medications include lisinopril and simvastatin. AQ has developed pneumonia and would like to take an oral agent that will not interact with her medications. Which of the following antibiotics used in the treatment of CAP is a strong inhibitor of the CYP-450 3A4 hepatic enzyme and would have a drug interaction with her medications?

    a. Azithromycin
    b. Clarithromycin
    c. Amoxicillin
    d. Cefpodoxime

Answer b is correct. Clarithromycin is utilized for treatment of CAP, inhibits protein synthesis, and is a strong inhibitor of the CYP-450 3A4 hepatic enzyme. Therefore, drug interactions with the macrolide antimicrobial may be common. Medications that are substrates of the CYP-450 3A4 hepatic enzyme will have their metabolism/clearance decreased. Common examples of substrates of the CYP-450 3A4 hepatic enzyme are the azole antifungals, calcium channel blockers (verapamil and diltiazem), and

hydroxymethylglutaryl-coenzyme A (HMG-CoA) reductase inhibitors, and many others.

Answer a is incorrect. The azalide azithromycin is utilized for CAP and inhibits protein synthesis; however, it is a weak inhibitor of the CYP-450 3A4 hepatic enzyme. Drug interactions are a major difference between the macrolides (erythromycin and clarithromycin) and the azalide azithromycin.

Answer c is incorrect. Amoxicillin may be used as part of a treatment regimen for CAP; however, amoxicillin *does not* inhibit the CYP-450 system.

Answer d is incorrect. Cefpodoxime may be used as part of a treatment regimen for CAP; however, cefpodoxime *does not* inhibit the CYP-450 system.

6. KC is a 33-year-old pregnant woman with a bacterial LRTI. Select the antimicrobial that is preferred in LRTIs in pregnant patients. Select all that apply.

    a. Clarithromycin
    b. Azithromycin
    c. Doxycycline
    d. Cefuroxime

Answer b is correct. Azithromycin is pregnancy category B. Adverse events were not observed in animal studies; therefore, azithromycin is classified as pregnancy category B. Although no adverse reports in human or animal fetuses have been documented, information in pregnant women is limited.

Answer d is correct. Cefuroxime is pregnancy category B. Adverse events were not observed in animal studies; therefore, cefuroxime is classified as pregnancy category B. Most cell wall antimicrobials are pregnancy category B (exception imipenem). Recommendation: If you are not familiar with pregnancy category of antimicrobials, focus on the agents that you cannot use. For example, cell wall antimicrobials are often utilized; whereas, protein synthesis and DNA gyrase inhibitors are often contraindicated.

Answer a is incorrect. Clarithromycin is pregnancy category C. Although no teratogenic effects have been reported in humans, adverse fetal effects have been documented in animal studies; therefore, clarithromycin is classified as pregnancy category C. Clarithromycin should not be used in pregnant women unless there are no alternative therapies.

Answer c is incorrect. Doxycycline is pregnancy category D. Because use during pregnancy may cause fetal harm, doxycycline is classified as pregnancy category D. Exposure to tetracyclines during the second or third trimester may cause permanent discoloration of the teeth.

7. Which of the following antibiotics has the same oral and IV dose?

    a. Doxycycline
    b. Amoxicillin/clavulanate
    c. Piperacillin/tazobactam

d. Ceftriaxone

e. Ciprofloxacin

Answer a is correct. Doxycycline is available in oral and parenteral formulations. The pneumonia dose of doxycycline for oral and IV utilization is 100 mg every 12 hours.

Answer b is incorrect. Amoxicillin/clavulanate is available in an oral formulation only. Amoxicillin/clavulanate is available in immediate and extended release formulations. The immediate release dose of amoxicillin/clavulanate is 500 mg every 8 hours or 875 mg every 12 hours; the dose for the extended release preparation is 2000 mg every 12 hours.

Answer c is incorrect. Piperacillin/tazobactam is available in a parenteral formulation only. The pneumonia dose of piperacillin/tazobactam is 3.375 g every 4 to 6 hours or 4.5 g every 6 hours.

Answer d is incorrect. Ceftriaxone is available in a parenteral formulation only. The pneumonia dose of ceftriaxone is 1 to 2 g daily.

Answer e is incorrect. Ciprofloxacin is available in oral and parenteral formulations; however, the dose is different based upon the formulation utilized. The oral dose for ciprofloxacin is 500 to 750 mg every 12 hours. The IV dose is 400 mg every 8 to 12 hours. *Note*: Fluoroquinolones are often referred to as medications that have excellent bioavailability. The majority of fluoroquinolones have complete absorption; however, the bioavailability of ciprofloxacin is 50% to 85%, hence the difference in the oral and IV dose of ciprofloxacin. Levofloxacin and moxifloxacin have higher bioavailability and equivalent oral and IV doses.

8. Select the antimicrobial(s) that is associated with the adverse effect of photosensitivity. Select all that apply.

a. Doxycycline

b. Ciprofloxacin

c. Cefepime

d. Sulfamethoxazole/trimethoprim

Answers a, b, and d are correct. Tetracyclines, fluoroquinolones, and sulfamethoxazole/trimethoprim are associated with photosensitivity.

Answer c is incorrect. Cephalosporin antimicrobials are not associated with photosensitivity.

9. Select the antimicrobials that are associated with a *C. difficile* infection. Select all that apply.

a. Ciprofloxacin

b. Clindamycin

c. Cefotaxime

d. Cephalexin

Answer a is correct. Fluoroquinolones may lead to *C. difficile* infections.

Answer b is correct. Clindamycin may lead to *C. difficile* infections.

Answers c and d are correct. Cephalosporins may lead to *C. difficile* infections.

All antimicrobials can lead to *C. difficile* infections, even those that are indicated to treat it. *C. difficile* overgrowth occurs when normal flora is disturbed by antibiotics or other drugs (eg, chemotherapy agents). *C. difficile* infections are treated by metronidazole, oral vancomycin, or fidaxomicin.

10. ZT is a patient with an LRTI. She has a past medical history for HTN and reflux. Medications include amlodipine and pantoprazole. She has an allergy to Unasyn (delayed/rash). Select the antimicrobial(s) that a patient with a delayed allergic hypersensitivity reaction to Unasyn may receive. Select all that apply.

a. Ceftriaxone

b. Moxifloxacin

c. Piperacillin/tazobactam

d. Oral vancomycin

Note: Unsayn = ampicillin/sulbactam a penicillin antibiotic.

Answer a is correct. Ceftriaxone and cephalosporin antimicrobials may be utilized in patients with delayed hypersensitivity (rash) reactions to penicillin. There is a low chance of cross reaction (but monitoring/counseling is needed).

Answer b is correct. Moxifloxacin and fluoroquinolone antimicrobials are chemically unrelated to β-lactams and may be utilized in patients with *delayed* (rash) or *immediate* (anaphylaxis) hypersensitivity reactions to penicillin or any other β-lactam. Though patients with a history of hypersensitivity to any one drug are more likely to react to a second drug than patients with no allergy history, the reactions are idiosyncratic.

Answer c is incorrect. Like ampicillin, piperacillin is a penicillin antimicrobial and cannot be used in patients with an allergic reaction to penicillin.

Answer d is incorrect. While oral vancomycin may be administered to a patient with an allergy to ampicillin/sulbactam, oral vancomycin is not utilized in the management of LRTIs.

11. Select the penicillin antimicrobial that is combined with a β-lactamase inhibitor. Select all that apply.

a. Zosyn

b. Unasyn

c. Augmentin

d. Primaxin

Note: Clavulanate, sulbactam, tazobactam, and avibactam are β-lactamase inhibitors that have little intrinsic antibacterial activity but inhibit the activity of a number of plasmid-mediated β-lactamases. They generally do not inhibit chromosomally mediated β-lactamases. Combination of these agents with ampicillin, amoxicillin, ticarcillin, piperacillin, ceftolozane, and ceftazidime results in antibiotics with an enhanced spectrum of activity against many, but not all, organisms containing plasmid-mediated β-lactamases.

Answer a is correct. Zosyn is piperacillin/tazobactam. Tazobactam is a β-lactamase inhibitor.

Answer b is correct. Unasyn is ampicillin/sulbactam. Sulbactam is a β-lactamase inhibitor.

Answer c is correct. Augmentin is amoxicillin/clavulanate. Clavulanate is a β-lactamase inhibitor.

Answer d is incorrect. Primaxin is imipenem/cilastatin. Imipenem is a carbapenem antibiotic. Imipenem is partially inactivated by an enzyme in the kidney and this can reduce its effectiveness. Cilastatin blocks the action of this enzyme, thereby increasing the activity of the imipenem. Cilastatin does not have antibacterial effects.

---

12. Select the β-lactam antimicrobial that requires dose or interval modifications in patients with significant renal dysfunction. Select all that apply.

    a. Amoxicillin
    b. Azithromycin
    c. Ceftriaxone
    d. Moxifloxacin
    e. Cefepime

Answer a is correct. The β-lactam amoxicillin and other *penicillin* antimicrobials used for the treatment of pneumonia are required to have dose and/or interval modifications in patients with renal dysfunction.

Answer e is correct. The fourth generation cephalosporin cefepime is a β-lactam that requires dose or interval changes in patients with renal dysfunction.

Answer b is incorrect. Azithromycin does not require dose or interval changes in patients with renal dysfunction (azithromycin undergoes hepatic metabolism/elimination) and it is not a β-lactam. Azithromycin is an azalide antimicrobial, which is a type of macrolide.

Answer c is incorrect. The β-lactam ceftriaxone undergoes dual elimination. Even though ceftriaxone has renal excretion, it does not require dose/interval changes in patients with renal dysfunction.

Answer d is incorrect. While moxifloxacin does not require dose or interval reductions in patients with renal dysfunction (moxifloxacin undergoes hepatic metabolism and renal and feces elimination), it is not a β-lactam. Moxifloxacin is a fluoroquinolone antimicrobial. All other fluoroquinolones (levofloxacin, ciprofloxacin, gemifloxacin) require dose or interval modifications in patients with renal dysfunction.

---

13. Select the side effect(s) associated with fluoroquinolone antimicrobials. Select all that apply.

    a. Hypoglycemia
    b. *Clostridium difficile* infection

c. Confusion in the elderly
d. QTc prolongation

Answer a is correct. Fluoroquinolones can cause glucose problems. Fluoroquinolones have been associated with hypo- and hyperglycemia. Gatifloxacin (Tequin) was a fluoroquinolone pulled from the market because of this effect. While fluoroquinolones may have a different incidence of causing glucose homeostasis issues, it is a class wide effect.

Answer b is correct. Fluoroquinolones can cause *C. difficile* infections.

Answer c is correct. Fluoroquinolones can cause central nervous system side effects, such as confusion.

Answer d is correct. Fluoroquinolones can prolong the QTc interval, especially when combined with Class 1a or III antiarrhythmics. The QTc prolongation caused solely by the fluoroquinolones is usually not clinically significant. Combination with other agents that prolong the QTc interval may lead to clinically significant events.

Use the patient case scenario to answer questions 14 and 15.

KP is a 78-year-old man who was admitted to the hospital 6 days ago for a COPD exacerbation. Today KP is complaining of shortness of breath and cough. A chest X-ray reveals a left lower lobe infiltrate. His vitals today are: Tmax 100.9, blood pressure (BP) 132/80, heart rate (HR) 97, respiratory rate (RR) 20.

Labs

143 | 102 | 19   Glucose 140   WBC 15   H/H 12.7/39   Plt 220K
4.2 | 30 | 1.0

KP is diagnosed with pneumonia.

14. What type of pneumonia does KP have?

    a. CAP
    b. Influenza pneumonia
    c. Aspiration pneumonia
    d. Hospital-acquired pneumonia

Answer d is correct. The patient has been in the hospital >48 hours; he is at risk for hospital acquired pathogens.

Answer a is incorrect. With a length of stay (>48 hours) in a health care facility, he is at risk for hospital-acquired pathogens.

Answer b is incorrect. Although influenza can cause pneumonia, we have no information in this case that the patient has the flu.

Answer c is incorrect. There is no evidence that KP aspirated, such as a witnessed aspiration or a seizure.

---

15. Based on the above patient case, what MDR pathogen may be causing his pneumonia? Select all that apply.

    a. *Pseudomonas aeruginosa*
    b. *Klebsiella pneumoniae*

c. *Acinetobacter* species

d. Methicillin-resistant *Staphylococcus aureus*

Answer a is correct. *P. aeruginosa* is an example of an MDR organism. Very few antimicrobials have clinical activity against *Pseudomonas* species. Examples include piperacillin/tazobactam (Zosyn), cefepime (Maxipime), ceftazidime (Fortaz), imipenem (Primaxin), meropenem (Merrem), doripenem (Doribax), the aminoglycosides (gentamicin, tobramycin, and amikacin), and the antipseudomonal quinolones (ciprofloxacin and levofloxacin).

Answer b is correct. *K. pneumoniae* is an example of an MDR organism. It often produces an extended-spectrum β-lactamase (ESBL) that leads to resistance to many types of drugs, and these organisms frequently express resistance to many non-β-lactams. Treatment of ESBL enteric Gram-negative rods (GNRs) like *K. pneumoniae* is often with carbapenems (ertapenem, imipenem, meropenem, doripenem).

Answer c is correct. Acinetobacter species is an example of an MDR organism.

Answer d is correct. MRSA is an example of an MDR organism. Antimicrobials used to treat MRSA infections include vancomycin, linezolid, tigecycline, and daptomycin. *Note*: While daptomycin is utilized to treat MRSA infections, it *cannot* be used to treat *MRSA pneumonia* since it is inactivated by pulmonary surfactant in human lungs.

Use the patient case scenario to answer questions 16 and 17.

AL is a 67-year-old WM in the emergency room with a 3-day history of subjective fever, productive cough, chills, and increasing shortness of breath, to the point where he now has difficulty walking up the stairs in his home.

History of previous illness (HPI): 2 weeks ago AL was diagnosed with bronchitis and a Z-Pak was prescribed by his primary care physician. He states that he "hasn't felt completely better since."

Past medical history (PMH):

Diabetes mellitus (DM), type II

Hx of venous thromboembolism (VTE) (deep vein thrombosis [DVT] 5 years ago)

HTN

Past cerebrovascular accident (CVA)

Allergies: Unknown

Meds (home):

Metformin XL 1 g po daily

Glipizide 5 mg po daily

Lisinopril 10 mg po daily

Warfarin 5 mg po MWF

Warfarin 7.5 mg po TThSS

ASA 81 mg 1 po daily

Physical examination:

Ht 5′ 9″, Wt 170 lb, T=101°F, BP 110/72, HR 100, RR 21, Pulse Ox 95% Room Air

Gen: WDWN WM in obvious distress

Cardiac: RRR, no murmurs, rubs or gallops

Lungs: Decreased bilateral breath sounds

Ext: normal

Labs:

$\dfrac{143 \mid 102 \mid 19}{4.2 \mid 30 \mid 1.0}$ Glucose 180   WBC 14.2   H/H 13/38   Plt 180 K

Sputum and blood cultures are sent, and a chest radiograph shows a right lower lobe (RLL) infiltrate, suggestive of pneumonia. AL is admitted to the internal medicine service.

16. What pathogen is the likely cause of the pneumonia this patient is presenting with?

a. *Streptococcus pneumoniae*

b. *Mycoplasma pneumoniae*

c. MRSA

d. *Acinetobacter baumannii*

Answer a is correct. *S. pneumoniae* is a Gram-positive coccus that is a common bacterial cause of LRTIs. It is frequently resistant to macrolides and azalides such as the azithromycin that he received.

Answer b is incorrect. *M. pneumoniae* is an aerobic Gram-negative atypical pathogen. It commonly causes CAP, but it rarely causes disease that is severe enough to lead to hospitalization. Azithromycin is reliably active against it also and likely would have worked.

Answer c is incorrect. CA-MRSA rarely causes CAP; however, when it is the cause, the pneumonia is very severe and can be rapidly fatal.

Answer d is incorrect. *A. baumannii* is a highly drug-resistant GNR that causes disease primarily in hospitalized patients. It often causes second infections in patients who have already received antibiotics for an initial infection.

---

17. What empiric antibiotic regimen would you start on AL?

a. Azithromycin + ceftriaxone

b. Clarithromycin + ceftriaxone

c. Azithromycin + ceftriaxone + vancomycin

d. Vancomycin + piperacillin/tazobactam

Answer a is correct. Even though AL received azithromycin previously, he failed monotherapy. A likely cause of his treatment failure was macrolide resistance to *S. pneumoniae*, which carries a 30% to 40% failure rate. Coverage of *S. pneumoniae* will be required as it a common cause of this CAP. On this admission, he should be treated with ceftriaxone due to the possibility of macrolide resistance and continue with azithromycin for atypical bacterial coverage.

Answer b is incorrect. Though clarithromycin is a macrolide and can be used in this scenario it also more likely to interact with his medications (particularly warfarin) since it is a potent CYP3A4 inhibitor.

Answer c is incorrect.   Based on AL's clinical presentation, it is unlikely that MRSA is the cause of AL's pneumonia. If he were admitted to the intensive care unit (ICU) with severe respiratory problems, vancomycin or linezolid should be given for the possibility of this pathogen.

Answer d is incorrect.   Vancomycin and piperacillin/tazobactam is indicated in late-onset hospital-acquired pneumonia.

Use the patient case scenario to answer questions 18 through 22.

ZX is a 29-year-old man with no significant past medical history who was in a serious motor vehicle collision 3 weeks ago, and has been in the ICU sedated and on a ventilator since. Recently he has been spiking fevers up to 103.2°F, producing purulent sputum, and he has a WBC that has been trending upward. A chest x-ray is performed and shows an RLL infiltrate. The team diagnoses him with pneumonia, collects a deep sputum sample and blood cultures, and wishes to begin therapy.

Chem 7 = normal   CBC = elevated WBC and bands   Tmax = 103.2°F

18. Based on the above case which bacterial organisms should be covered? Select all that apply.

    a. *Streptococcus pneumoniae*
    b. *Pseudomonas aeruginosa*
    c. MRSA
    d. *Klebsiella pneumoniae*

Answer a is correct.   ZX has been in the hospital for a prolonged stay; therefore, the risk of MDR organisms increases. However, *S. pneumoniae* should still be covered.

Answers b and d are correct.   ZX will need antibiotic coverage against multiple drug-resistant organisms due to his prolonged hospital stay. In addition to *P. aeruginosa* and MRSA, *K. pneumoniae, A. baumannii,* and other resistant GNRs could cause infection in ZX.

Answer c is correct.   ZX has been admitted for well over 5 days and is at risk for MRSA.

---

19. ZX is allergic to penicillin (type I/anaphylaxis). Based on this, what antibiotic regimen would be most appropriate for him?

    a. Cefepime + tobramycin + vancomycin
    b. Azithromycin + ceftriaxone
    c. Levofloxacin + gentamicin + vancomycin
    d. Gentamicin + vancomycin

Answer c is correct.   Given the patient's allergy to penicillin this answer would be the best choice to cover for MDR organisms. The antipseudomonal fluoroquinolone and gentamicin provide double coverage for GNRs, and the vancomycin covers MRSA.

Answer a is incorrect.   In this scenario, given the history of anaphylaxis with penicillins it would be contraindicated to give a cephalosporin such as cefepime, even if the risk of cross-reactivity is rather low. Tobramycin and vancomycin would be reasonable choices.

Answer b is incorrect.   This is a CAP regimen that is inappropriate for ventilator associated pneumonia because it will not cover for MDR organisms. Ceftriaxone, a cephalosporin, should also be avoided in patients with a history of anaphylaxis to penicillin.

Answer d is incorrect.   This regimen is missing double GNR coverage, which is recommended for hospital-acquired pneumonia with MDR risk factors.

---

20. ZX is placed on a regimen of linezolid, tobramycin, and ciprofloxacin. What are potential adverse effects associated with the drugs in this regimen? Select all that apply.

    a. Ototoxicity
    b. Nephrotoxicity
    c. QTc prolongation
    d. Thrombocytopenia

Answers a, b, c, and d are correct.   Aminoglycosides can cause ototoxicity and nephrotoxicity especially when the trough is elevated. Vancomycin can additionally cause nephrotoxicity. Fluoroquinolones can increase the risk for QTc prolongation especially when the patient is on concomitant QTc prolonging agents. Linezolid has been associated with thrombocytopenia, particularly in courses of 2 weeks or more.

---

21. A sputum Gram stain shows few epithelial cells, many WBCs, and moderate gram-negative rods. Two days later, the following data are known:

    Sputum: *K. pneumoniae*

    Susceptible to: ampicillin/sulbactam, piperacillin/tazobactam, imipenem, cefepime, levofloxacin, gentamicin, tobramycin, amikacin

    Resistant to: ampicillin, piperacillin

    Blood cultures (2/2): No growth

    Chem 7 normal   CBC normal   Tmax = 37.8°C

    Based on the susceptibility report, what should his therapy be now?

    a. Continue current therapy
    b. Stop current therapy, start Levaquin
    c. Stop current therapy, start Rocephin
    d. Stop current therapy, start Unasyn

Answer b is correct.   Given the susceptibility to levofloxacin (Levaquin), it is appropriate to continue this antimicrobial and discontinue the gentamicin and vancomycin.

Answer a incorrect.   Now that susceptibility reports have confirmed the organism, it is appropriate to narrow the spectrum of activity.

Answer c is incorrect. Rocephin is the brand for ceftriaxone, a cephalosporin. Patient has a penicillin allergy resulting in anaphylaxis and, therefore, should avoid a cephalosporin despite the true cross reactivity being fairly low (3%-5%).

Answer d is incorrect. Unasyn is the brand for ampicillin/sulbactam and, therefore, patient has an allergy to the penicillin component and cannot receive this antimicrobial.

---

22. How many days in total should ZX receive antibiotics?

    a. 3 days
    b. 5 days
    c. 7 days
    d. 14 to 21 days

Answer c is correct. 7 or 8 days is the recommendation duration of therapy for most patients with hospital-acquired pneumonia. ZX has also responded clinically.

Answer a is incorrect. Duration is too short for pneumonia. This is the recommended duration for uncomplicated cystitis.

Answer b is incorrect. Duration is too short for pneumonia.

Answer d is incorrect. Duration is excessive for pneumonia, unless the patient had not responded to initial therapy.

CHAPTER **22** | **Upper Respiratory Tract Infections**

1. Select the upper respiratory tract condition that is defined as the presence of fluid in the middle ear without symptoms of acute illness.

    a. OME
    b. Sinusitis
    c. Pharyngitis
    d. Laryngitis
    e. Rhinitis

Answer a is correct. OME is the presence of fluid in the middle ear without symptoms of acute illness. It is important to differentiate between OME and AOM because antimicrobials are only useful for AOM. AOM is a symptomatic middle ear infection that occurs rapidly with effusion.

Answer b is incorrect. Sinusitis is an inflammation and/or infection of the paranasal sinus mucosa.

Answer c is incorrect. Pharyngitis is an acute throat infection caused by viruses or bacteria.

Answer d is incorrect. Laryngitis is a common and acute inflammation of the larynx that is usually caused by acute vocal strain, irritation of the mucosal surface of the larynx, or an URTI.

Answer e is incorrect. Rhinitis is the presence of any one of the following: sneezing, nasal congestion, rhinorrhea, or nasal itching.

---

2. JH is a 4-year-old patient that is brought to his pediatrician with a 36-hour history of rhinorrhea, nasal congestion, cough, and mild otalgia. He does not have any concurrent purulent conjunctivitis. His current temperature is 38°C (100.4°F). He has no known drug allergies and no known past medical conditions. He has not received amoxicillin in the previous 30 days. He is 36 lb. Which of the following would be the most appropriate option for JH?

    a. Acetaminophen 10 mg/kg po qid prn
    b. Amoxicillin 30 mg/kg po tid
    c. Pseudoephedrine HCl 15 mg po qid
    d. Diphenhydramine 6.25 mg po qid
    e. Levofloxacin 10 mg/kg po bid

Answer a is correct. The most appropriate option for JH currently would be to watch and wait and provide adequate pain control. The patient is >2 years old; he had ear pain for <48 hours, and only has mild ear pain. Antimicrobials are not indicated at this time. The signs of rhinorrhea, nasal congestion and cough would also be consistent with viral etiology.

Answer b is incorrect. Antimicrobials are not indicated at this time.

Answer c is incorrect. There is limited literature to support efficacy in using decongestions for AOM. The potential risks outweigh the potential benefits and should not be recommended.

Answer d is incorrect. There is limited literature to support efficacy in using antihistamines for AOM. The potential risks outweigh the potential benefits and should not be recommended.

Answer e is incorrect. Again, JH does not currently require treatment and levofloxacin would not be a preferred option for AOM.

Questions 3 and 4 pertain to the following case:

JM is a 6-year-old patient that presents to his pediatrician with a 5 days history of otalgia and otorrhea. Upon otoscopic review, his pediatrician notices moderate bulging of his tympanic membrane. His temperature is 38.5°C (101.3°F). He has a history of penicillin allergy, and his reaction was itchy legs. He does not have concurrent purulent conjunctivitis and he has not received amoxicillin in the previous 30 days. He is 44 lb.

3. Which of the following would be the most appropriate treatment option for JM?

    a. Amoxicillin 600 mg po tid
    b. Amoxicillin 1375 mg po tid
    c. Cefdinir 300 mg po bid
    d. Cefdinir 140 mg po bid
    e. Levofloxacin 600 mg po bid

Answer d is correct. Although the JM had a mild skin reaction with penicillin, the "cross-reactivity" between penicillins and cephalosporins is low. The benefit gained in using the narrowest spectrum antimicrobial outweighs the risk of exposing both the patient and society to unnecessary broad-spectrum antimicrobials and subsequently increasing the risk for developing microbial resistance. Furthermore, due to the differences in the chemical structures, cefdinir, cefuroxime, cefpodoxime, and ceftriaxone are unlikely to be associated in cross-reactivity with penicillin.

Answer a is incorrect. JM has a penicillin allergy; amoxicillin is an aminopenicillin and may cause him to have a mild skin reaction.

Answer b is incorrect. JM has a penicillin allergy, and this dose is too high for him.

Answer c is incorrect. This is a twofold overdose. The appropriate dose is 14 mg/kg/d in one to two divided doses. This would equate to 7 mg/kg/dose. The patient is 20 kg.

Answer e is incorrect. This would be an example of an unnecessary broad-spectrum antimicrobial.

---

4. Which of the following pathogens might be the cause of JM's AOM. Select all that apply.

    a. *Streptococcus pneumoniae*
    b. *Moraxella catarrhalis*
    c. *Haemophilus influenzae*
    d. Influenza virus
    e. Adenovirus

Answer a is correct. *S. pneumoniae* is an aerobic, Gram-positive diplococcus that is one of the three most prevalent bacterial pathogens for AOM.

Answer b is correct. *M. catarrhalis* is a Gram-negative diplococcus that is again one of the three most prevalent bacterial pathogens for AOM.

Answer c is correct. *H. influenzae* is a small aerobic, Gram-negative coccobacillus that is mainly found in the respiratory tract and is the last of the three most prevalent bacterial pathogens for AOM.

Answer d is correct. As you may recall, viruses are actually the most common cause of URTIs and play a predominant role in OM. One of the most common viral causes is influenza virus.

Answer e is correct. The most common viruses to cause AOM include RSV, influenza virus, rhinovirus, and adenovirus.

---

5. When considering treatment failure and mechanisms of bacterial resistance, which of the following might be present in any one of the three most common bacterial pathogens for AOM? Select all that apply.

    a. Reduction in antimicrobial drug accumulation due to the upregulation of bacterial efflux pumps

b. Inability of the antimicrobial to bind to the targeted bacteria due to bacterial alterations of their PBPs
    c. Enzymatic inactivation of the antimicrobial via bacterial production of β-lactamase
    d. Reduction in antimicrobial drug accumulation due to decreased bacterial membrane permeability
    e. Enzymatic inactivation of the antimicrobial via bacterial production of penicillinase

---

Answer a is correct. *H. influenzae* is known to have intrinsic efflux resistance mechanisms which can limit the activity of macrolides (azithromycin and clarithromycin).

Answer b is correct. This is the most common mechanism of resistance for *S. pneumoniae*. It is also the reason that bacterial resistance cannot be easily overcome with the addition of a β-lactamase inhibitor.

Answer c is correct. This the most common mechanism of resistance in *M. catarrhalis* and is also widely present in *H. influenzae*.

Answer d is correct. This is a potential mechanism of resistance for both *M. catarrhalis* and *H. influenzae*; it is an additional mechanism of resistance for *M. catarrhalis* to the aminopenicillins.

Answer e is correct. Penicillinase is a specific type of β-lactamase which again can be commonly found in both *M. catarrhalis* and *H. influenzae*.

Questions 6 through 8 pertain to the following case:

JS is a 16-year-old patient with purulent nasal discharge, headache, cough and congestion, bad breath, and anosmia (loss of smell) for the past 2 days. He has a temperature of 38.3°C (100.9°F). He has no known drug allergies. He has no known past medical history; however, he did receive 5 days of an unknown antibiotic to treat a skin and soft tissue infection about 20 days ago. He is 140 lb.

6. Which of the following treatment options should be recommended?

    a. Acetaminophen 325 mg po q4h prn
    b. Amoxicillin 875 po tid
    c. Pseudoephedrine HCl 60 mg po qid
    d. Amoxicillin/clavulanate 875 mg po bid
    e. Amoxicillin/clavulanate 2 g XR po bid

Answer a is correct. The most appropriate option for JS currently would be to provide adequate pain control. The most likely cause of sinusitis is viral and antimicrobials are overprescribed. Viral infections typically are self-limiting and will resolve within 7 to 10 days.

Answer b is incorrect. Considering his current symptoms are not severe and the timing of his symptomatology, antimicrobials are not indicated.

Answer c is incorrect. There is currently no literature to support efficacy in using decongestions for sinusitis. Therefore, the potential risks outweigh the potential benefits and, hence, should not be recommended.

Answer d is incorrect. The most likely cause of sinusitis is viral and antimicrobials are overprescribed. Viral infections typically are self-limiting and will resolve within 7 to 10 days.

Answer e is incorrect. Antimicrobials are not indicated.

---

7. After providing JS with an appropriate treatment option, 4 to 5 days after his initial presentation, he started to feel much better. On day 5, he even decided to go outside and ride his scooter with his friends. However, the next morning he woke up with chills, nausea, headache, and increased nasal discharge. He had a temperature of 38.3°C (100.9°F). Which of the following is the most appropriate recommendation?

    a. Acetaminophen 325 mg po q4h prn
    b. Amoxicillin 875 mg po tid
    c. Levofloxacin 500 mg po daily
    d. Amoxicillin/clavulanate 875 mg po bid
    e. Amoxicillin/clavulanate 2 g XR po bid

Answer e is correct. The patient is at risk for drug resistant *S. pneumoniae* and, therefore, would need a higher dose to overcome potential resistance.

Answer a is incorrect. Although it would be appropriate to give JS acetaminophen analgesia and thermoregulation, this answer is not the most appropriate. At this time, JS needs antimicrobial therapy. When a viral respiratory infection occurs, patients can be at risk for developing a secondary bacterial infection. This phenomenon is sometimes referred to as "double-sickening" and can be easily identified following a viral URTI (lasting 5-6 days) that was initially improving followed by a new onset of worsening symptoms, that is fever, headache, or increase in nasal discharge.

Answer b is incorrect. Amoxicillin is no longer recommended empirically due to the increasing prevalence of β-lactamase producing respiratory pathogens (*H. influenzae* and *M. catarrhalis*).

Answer c is incorrect. The patient does not have a history of hives/anaphylaxis to penicillin.

Answer d is incorrect. The patient has received an antibiotic within the previous 30 days and, therefore, is at risk for drug resistant *S. pneumoniae* which will not be overcome with a β-lactamase inhibitor.

---

8. Which of the following are common side effects that JS could experience while taking this recommended treatment? Select all that apply.

    a. Hepatotoxicity
    b. Diarrhea
    c. Prolonged QT interval
    d. Tendon rupture
    e. Candidiasis

Answer b is correct. Amoxicillin/clavulanate (and most antibiotics in general) are known to cause diarrhea. One way

to keep diarrhea to a minimum is by dosing the amoxicillin to clavulanate at 14:1 ratio.

Answer e is correct. Oral candidiasis can occur following exposure to antimicrobials and is particularly common for amoxicillin/clavulanate. This is due to the fact that amoxicillin/clavulanate eliminates most of the bacteria located within the normal oral flora; this leads to the overgrowth of the yeast (*Candida spp.*) which can also reside in the normal oral flora.

Answer a is incorrect. If hepatotoxicity was a common side effect for any of the treatment options listed in the above question, they would not be commonly used (if at all). Hepatotoxicity is, however, a rare side effect for amoxicillin/clavulanate, acetaminophen, and levofloxacin.

Answer c is incorrect. Levofloxacin is known to prolong the QTc interval; the clinical significance of this side effect is most apparent when the patient is elderly, receiving concurrent QTc prolonging medications, or having electrolyte disturbances and/or underlying cardiac conditions.

Answer d is incorrect. Levofloxacin has a rare side effect of tendonitis/tendon rupture. This risk is increased when the patient is elderly, participates in strenuous activity, has underlining tendon disorders, renal failure, organ transplantation, and/or is taking corticosteroids.

Questions 9 through 11 pertain to the following case:

TM is a 17-year-old patient who initially presented to the ED with a fever of ≥40°C/104°F, severe headache, purulent nasal discharge, and facial pain for the last four consecutive days. He is 143 lb, has no known drug allergies, and no significant past medical history. He was originally worked up for meningitis and received the following medications:

1. Vancomycin 30 mg/kg IV over 2 hours (placed in 500 mL of normal saline [NS])
2. Ceftriaxone 2 g IV over 30 minutes (placed in 50 mL of D5W [5% dextrose in water])
3. Dexamethasone 10 mg IV over 5 minutes (10 mg/1 mL)

Unfortunately, after his lumbar puncture TM got increasingly nauseous which prompted an intern to give an additional:

4. Piperacillin/tazobactam 4.5 g IV over 4 hours (placed in 100 mL of D5W)

Fortunately, after his lumbar puncture returned grossly negative and consulting with an otolaryngologist, TM was diagnosed with severe acute sinusitis and was ultimately given:

5. Ampicillin/sulbactam 3 g IV over 30 minutes q6h (placed in 100 mL of NS)

9. Calculate each IV dose in "mg/min" that TM received and then order the medications from highest to lowest "mg/min" given.

Unordered Options	Ordered Response
Vancomycin 30 mg/kg IV over 2 h	Ampicillin/sulbactam
Ceftriaxone 2 g IV over 30 min	Ceftriaxone
Dexamethasone 10 mg IV over 5 min	Piperacillin/tazobactam

| Piperacillin/tazobactam 4.5 g IV over 4 h | Vancomycin |
| Ampicillin/sulbactam 3 g IV over 30 min | Dexamethasone |

1. **Ampicillin/sulbactam = 100 mg/min**

   3 g/30 min = 6 g/h; 6 g/h = 6000 mg/h; 6000 mg/h = 100 mg/min

2. **Ceftriaxone = 66.7 mg/min**

   2 g/30 min = 4 g/h; 4 g/h = 4000 mg/h; 4000 mg/h = 66.67 mg/min

3. **Piperacillin/tazobactam = 18.8 mg/min**

   4.5 g/4 h = 1.125 g/h; 1.125 g/h = 1125 mg/h; 1125 mg/h = 18.75 mg/min

4. **Vancomycin = 16.7 mg/min**

   TM = 143 lb; 143 lb = 65 kg; 30 mg/kg = 1950 mg (rounded to 2 g for ease of dosing)

   2000 mg over 2 hours = 1000 mg/h; 1000 mg/h = 16.67 mg/min

5. **Dexamethasone = 2 mg/min**

   10 mg/5 min = 2 mg/min

10. Which of the following vaccines may have prevented TMs sinusitis? Select all that may apply.

    a. Comvax
    b. Prevnar 13
    c. Fluzone
    d. Ipol
    e. Twinrix

Answer a is correct. Comvax is a combination vaccination against *H. influenzae*/Hepatitis B.

Answer b is correct. Prevnar 13 is a pneumococcal vaccine providing immunologic protection against 13 strains of *S. pneumoniae*.

Answer c is correct. Fluzone is a vaccine against the influenza virus which is a very common cause of URTIs. Viral respiratory infections can predispose patients to secondary bacterial infections or "double-sickening."

Answer d is incorrect. Ipol is an inactivated poliovirus.

Answer e is incorrect. Twinrix is a vaccination against Hepatitis A and B.

11. Calculate each drip rate in "mL/min" that TM received and then order the medications from fastest to slowest drip rate.

Unordered Options	Ordered Response
Vancomycin 30 mg/kg IV over 2 h	Vancomycin
Ceftriaxone 2 g IV over 30 min	Ampicillin/sulbactam
Dexamethasone 10 mg IV over 5 min	Ceftriaxone

| Piperacillin/tazobactam 4.5 g IV over 4 h | Piperacillin/ tazobactam |
| Ampicillin/sulbactam 3 g IV over 30 min | Dexamethasone |

1. **Vancomycin = 4.2 mL/min**

   500 mL over 2 hours = 250 mL/h; 250 mL/h = 4.17 mL/min

2. **Ampicillin/sulbactam = 3.3 mL/min**

   100 mL over 30 minutes = 200 mL/h; 200 mL/h = 3.33 mL/min

3. **Ceftriaxone = 1.7 mL/min**

   50 mL over 30 minutes = 100 mL/h; 100 mL/h = 1.67 mL/min

4. **Piperacillin/tazobactam = 0.4 mL/min**

   100 mL over 4 hours = 25 mL/h; 25 mL/h = 0.42 mL/min

5. **Dexamethasone = 0.2 mL/min**

   1 mL over 5 minutes = 0.2 mL/min

Questions 12 and 13 pertain to the following case:

ES is a 12-year-old patient who was brought to her pediatrician with complaints of sore throat, odynophagia, and vomiting for 24 hours. She has a temperature of 38.5°C (101.3°F). Upon physical examination, she is noted to have enlarged cervical lymph nodes and red uvula.

12. In an ideal situation, which of the following would occur first?

    a. Give penicillin 250 mg po tid
    b. Give saline nasal spray each nostril qid
    c. Obtain a rapid antigen detection test or throat culture
    d. Give a diphenhydramine 25 mg po qid
    e. Give Comvax

Answer c is correct. A throat culture is a cost effective method to obtain accurate microbiologic data; however, results often take 48 hours to complete. Similarly, a rapid antigen detection test is a time effective method to obtain microbiologic data; however, it is costly and in certain patient populations, negative results should be confirmed with a throat culture.

Answer a is incorrect. Viruses are the most common cause of pharyngitis and there is limited ability to easily distinguish viral and bacterial pathogens. Additional diagnostics should be performed first.

Answer b is incorrect. In the treatment of sinusitis, saline nasal sprays are sometimes used to moisturize the nasal canal and inhibit crusting of secretions along with promoting ciliary function. However, there are no controlled studies that support efficacy of this practice.

Answer d is incorrect. There is currently no literature to support efficacy in using antihistamines for laryngitis and, therefore, the potential risks outweigh the potential benefits and should not be recommended.

Answer e is incorrect. Comvax is a combination vaccination against *H. influenzae* and Hepatitis B. *H. influenzae* is not a predominant pathogen for pharyngitis; also, typically a complete immune response does not occur until 2 weeks after the receipt of a vaccination.

13. Given that ES has bacterial pharyngitis, what are the goals of therapy? Select all that apply.

    a. Eradicate infection
    b. Prevent infectious complications
    c. Shorten the disease course
    d. Reduce infectivity and spread to others
    e. Reduce sore throat and odynophagia

Answer a is correct.   Eradication of infection is the goal of antimicrobial therapy.

Answer b is correct.   Particularly with *S. pyogenes*, antimicrobial treatment can prevent uncommon infectious complications such as peritonsillar abscess.

Answer c is correct.   Antimicrobials can often shorten the duration of the disease course.

Answer d is correct.   Rapid eradication of bacteria can minimize the risk of a prolonged duration of infection, and can minimize the ability to spread the infection to other individuals.

Answer e is correct.   Reducing pain and discomfort is a goal of therapy.

14. Historically, which of the following rare sequelae might be prevented with full treatment of "strep throat"? Select all that apply.

    a. Peritonsillar abscess
    b. Cervical lymphadenitis
    c. Rheumatic fever
    d. Poststreptococcal glomerulonephritis
    e. Appendicitis

Answer a is correct.   Peritonsillar abscesses are often polymicrobial. However, *Streptococcus pyogenes* or GAS is a predominant pathogen.

Answer b is correct.   Second to viral etiology, cervical lymphadenitis is usually caused by *S. aureus* or *group A streptococcus*.

Answer c is correct.   Streptococcal pharyngitis has been associated with the development of rheumatic fever.

Answer d is incorrect.   Antimicrobial therapy is not effective at preventing poststreptococcal glomerulonephritis.

Answer e is incorrect.   *S. pyogenes* is not associated with appendicitis.

Questions 15 and 16 pertain to the following case:

MM is a 15-year-old patient that was recently diagnosed with acute bacterial sinusitis. She has a complicated past medical history including venous thromboembolism (left leg) 2/2 severe systemic

lupus erythematosus/antiphospholipid antibody syndrome, lupus nephritis, seizures, and depression. At age 13, she has had an anaphylactic reaction to amoxicillin resulting in an intensive care unit (ICU) admission, requiring intubation and mechanical ventilation; she has no other known drug allergies. She is 115 lb. Her current medications include:

1. Prednisone 15 mg po daily
2. Ibuprofen 400 mg po tid
3. Warfarin 5 mg po daily
4. Sertraline 50 mg po daily
5. Flintstones + iron multivitamin po daily

15. A concerned otolaryngologist would like to treat MM's sinusitis with levofloxacin 500 mg po daily to avoid any potential risk of anaphylaxis. Which of the following medications could potentially interact with levofloxacin 500 mg po daily? Select all that apply.

    a. Prednisone
    b. Ibuprofen
    c. Warfarin
    d. Sertraline
    e. Flintstones + iron

Answer a is correct.   Levofloxacin can enhance the toxic effect of systemic prednisone. This includes risk of tendon-related side effects.

Answer b is correct.   Ibuprofen can increase the serum concentration of levofloxacin which may enhance the neuro-excitatory effects of levofloxacin and, therefore, increase the risk of seizures. This interaction has increased significance for MM given her history of seizures. Furthermore, we are uncertain of her renal function, which may be compromised given her lupus nephritis, which would put her at additional risk for toxicity.

Answer c is correct.   Levofloxacin may increase the international normalized ratio (INR)/enhance the anticoagulant effects of warfarin.

Answer d is correct.   The risk of QTc-prolongation is enhanced when multiple QTc-prolonging agents are being used concurrently; both sertraline and levofloxacin can prolong the QTc interval.

Answer e is correct.   Multivalent cations (iron, magnesium, aluminum, or zinc) can chelate oral levofloxacin and, therefore, decrease efficacy. This interaction is particularly relevant because MM is being prescribed PO levofloxacin. This reaction can be reduced by administering oral levofloxacin at least 2 hours before, or 6 hours after, the dose of her Flintstone + iron vitamins.

16. While receiving levofloxacin, which of the following might MM be at risk for given her past medical history and current medication history? Select all that apply.

    a. Tendinitis
    b. Bleeding/bruising

c. Clotting
d. QTc prolongation
e. Seizures

Answer a is correct. Given MM's past medical history (lupus) and current medications (prednisone, ibuprofen, levofloxacin), MM might be at risk for tendonitis.

Answer b is correct. Given the drug-drug interaction between levofloxacin and warfarin, MM's INR can increase, putting her at risk for bleeding. INR should be monitored and warfarin doses should be reduced accordingly.

Answer d is correct. Given the drug-drug interaction between levofloxacin and sertraline, MM has a slightly higher risk of QTc-prolongation due to additive effects.

Answer e is correct. Given MM's past medical history (seizures, lupus nephritis) and current medication interactions (ibuprofen, levofloxacin), MM might be at risk for seizures.

Answer c is incorrect. While receiving levofloxacin, the INR can increase. However, it is important to continue monitoring the INR after levofloxacin has been discontinued, as the INR may decrease upon discontinuation (putting MM at risk for clots). This is especially true if the warfarin dose had been reduced while taking levofloxacin.

---

17. Select the parenteral cephalosporin that is often administered intramuscularly for AOM.

    a. Clarithromycin
    b. Amoxicillin/clavulanate
    c. Trimethoprim-sulfamethoxazole
    d. Clindamycin
    e. Ceftriaxone

Answer e is correct. Ceftriaxone is a third generation cephalosporin that is available only as a parenteral formulation. Ceftriaxone is used intramuscularly.

Answer a is incorrect. Clarithromycin is used for treatment of OM; however, it is a macrolide and only available orally.

Answer b is incorrect. Amoxicillin/clavulanate is used for the treatment of OM; however, it is a penicillin and only available orally.

Answer c is incorrect. Trimethoprim-sulfamethoxazole is not recommended for the empiric treatment of OM; furthermore, it is a sulfonamide antibiotic. Trimethoprim-sulfamethoxazole is available in oral and parenteral formulations.

Answer d is incorrect. Clindamycin is used for the treatment of OM (used for PRSP—it does not have coverage against Gram-negative bacteria); however, it is a lincosamide antibiotic. Clindamycin is available in oral and parenteral formulations; however, only the oral formulation is utilized for OM.

18. Correctly assign the following antimicrobials that can be used (either alone or in combination) for the treatment of sinusitis with their assigned mechanisms of actions: cefixime, clavulanate, clindamycin, doxycycline, levofloxacin

Unordered Options	Ordered Response
Inhibits protein synthesis by primarily binding to the 30S ribosomal subunit	Doxycycline
Inhibits DNA-gyrase, promoting the breakage of DNA strands	Levofloxacin
Binds and inhibits β-lactamase production	Clavulanate
Inhibits protein synthesis by reversibly binding to the 50S ribosomal subunit	Clindamycin
Inhibits bacterial cell wall synthesis by binding to penicillin-binding proteins	Cefixime

1. **Doxycycline:** Inhibits protein synthesis by primarily binding to 30S ribosomal subunits
2. **Levofloxacin:** Inhibits DNA-gyrase, promoting the breakage of DNA strands
3. **Clavulanate:** Binds and inhibits β-lactamase production
4. **Clindamycin:** Inhibits protein synthesis by reversibly binding to 50S ribosomal subunit
5. **Cefixime:** Inhibits bacterial cell wall synthesis by binding to penicillin binding proteins

---

19. Correctly rank the following antimicrobials based on their respective half-lives in order from shortest to longest. (Hint, consider appropriate dosing intervals and available dosage formulations.)

Unordered Options	Ordered Response
Amoxicillin/clavulanate	Amoxicillin/clavulanate
Cefixime	Clindamycin
Clindamycin	Cefixime
Doxycycline	Levofloxacin
Levofloxacin	Doxycycline

1. **Amoxicillin/clavulanate:** Has a half-life of 1.3 hours (dosed tid)
2. **Clindamycin:** Has a half-life of 2.4 hours (dosed tid)
3. **Cefixime:** Has a half-life of 3.1 hours (dosed bid)
4. **Levofloxacin:** Has a half-life of 7 hours (dosed daily)
5. **Doxycycline:** Has a half-life of ~12 hours (dosed one to two times daily); half-life varies with different formulations

---

20. DV is a 26-year-old patient with chronic/recurrent sinus infections. Which of the following are most likely to occur? Select all that apply.

    a. Sinus infections three to four times yearly
    b. Excellent symptomatic response to steam/vapor
    c. Symptomatic cure with nasal decongestions
    d. Chronic unproductive cough
    e. Frequent headaches

Answer a is correct. Chronic/recurrent infections occur three to four times a year.

Answer d is correct. Chronic/recurrent infections are often associated with a nonproductive cough.

Answer e is correct. Chronic/recurrent infections are often associated with headaches.

Answer b is incorrect. Chronic/recurrent infections are unresponsive to steam.

Answer c is incorrect. Chronic/recurrent infections are unresponsive to decongestions. The potential risk outweighs potential benefit.

CHAPTER **23 | Urinary Tract Infections**

Questions 1 through 3 are related to the same case.

1. GB is a 28-year-old woman with a chief complaint of dysuria. Symptoms started 3 days ago. The physician orders a urinalysis and a urine culture. What is the most likely bacterial cause of the UTI?

   a. *Acinetobacter baumannii (A. baumannii)*
   b. *Escherichia coli (E. coli)*
   c. *Pseudomonas aeruginosa (P. aeruginosa)*
   d. *Staphylococcus saprophyticus (S. saprophyticus)*

Answer b is correct. The majority of UTIs are caused by gram-negative bacteria, of which *E. coli* is the most common pathogen. Table 23-1 lists the bacterial causes of UTIs and *E. coli* is the most common organism of uncomplicated and complicated UTIs. However, empiric therapy with *E. coli* will often cover/treat other organisms listed within Table 23-1. The exception would be Pseudomonas, select bacter organisms (eg, Citrobacter), and Enterococci.

Answer a is incorrect. *A. baumannii* is a nosocomial organism and a cause of catheter-associated UTIs.

Answer c is incorrect. *P. aeruginosa* is a nosocomial organism and causes <20% of UTIs.

Answer d is incorrect. *S. saprophyticus* only causes 5% to 10% of uncomplicated UTIs. It is the most common gram-positive bacteria causing uncomplicated UTIs.

---

2. What is appropriate empiric therapy for GB? Patient has normal renal function and no medication allergies. Medications include metoprolol and omeprazole.

   a. Cefdinir
   b. Linezolid
   c. Amoxicillin
   d. TMP-SMX

Answer d is correct. TMP-SMX is appropriate empiric therapy for GB. If the local *E. coli* resistance rate for TMP-SMX is high, ciprofloxacin would be an appropriate choice.

Answer a is incorrect. Cefdinir is an oral third-generation cephalosporin commonly used for acute otitis media in pediatrics. It is not indicated for treatment of UTIs. Although cefdinir is not indicated for treatment of UTIs, you may see an oral cephalosporin utilized. Bacteria are becoming increasingly more resistant and management is driven by in vitro results of a culture and susceptibility report. There are often times when an *E. coli* UTI is resistant to TMP-SMX and quinolones; therefore, alternative therapy may be utilized (even if it is not indicated).

Answer b is incorrect. Linezolid is an antibiotic that covers gram-positive bacteria exclusively. It is primarily used to treat methicillin-resistant *S. aureus* (MRSA) and vancomycin-resistant enterococci (VRE). Both MRSA and VRE can cause UTIs, but GB does not need to be empirically covered with linezolid.

Answer c is incorrect. *E. coli* resistance rate to amoxicillin is high (37% and higher in select regions). Therefore, aminopenicillins (eg, amoxicillin) would not be ideal for empiric therapy. Because *E. coli* and other fermenting gram-negative rods (eg, *Klebsiella*) produce β-lactamase, the addition of clavulanate to amoxicillin (Augmentin) may be utilized in the treatment of *E. coli* UTIs.

---

3. What is the appropriate duration of therapy for GB?

   a. 1 day
   b. 3 days
   c. 7 days
   d. 14 days

Answer b is correct. The Infectious Disease Society of America (IDSA) recommends 3-day therapy for treatment of uncomplicated lower tract infections in women.

Answer a is incorrect. Multiple reviews have concluded that 3 days of therapy is better than 1 day of therapy. The IDSA recommends 3-day therapy for treatment of uncomplicated lower tract infections in women.

Answer c is incorrect. Seven days is recommended in pregnant women or women with a history of UTIs caused by antibiotic-resistant bacteria or >7 days of symptoms.

Answer d is incorrect. Fourteen days is the recommended duration of therapy for men and those with pyelonephritis.

---

4. Who should be screened for asymptomatic bacteriuria?

   a. College students
   b. Men
   c. Patients with indwelling catheters
   d. Pregnant women

Answer d is correct. The IDSA recommends pregnant women should be screened for bacteriuria by urine culture at least once during early pregnancy (12-16 weeks gestation) or at their first prenatal visit. All positive urine cultures, including asymptomatic bacteriuria, should be treated in pregnant women.

Answer a is incorrect. College students do not need to be screened for asymptomatic bacteriuria.

Answer b is incorrect. Men do not need to be screened for asymptomatic bacteriuria.

Answer c is incorrect. Patients with indwelling catheters do not need to be screened for asymptomatic bacteriuria. Patients with chronic catheters universally have asymptomatic bacteriuria.

5. Which of the following patient groups are considered to have complicated UTIs? Select all that apply.

   a. Children
   b. Men
   c. Pregnant women
   d. Catheter-associated

Answers a, b, c, and d are correct. UTIs in men, pregnant women, children, and patients who are hospitalized or in health care-associated settings are considered complicated. These infections are more likely to be caused by resistant organisms.

Questions 6 through 10 are related to the same case.

6. NK is a 62-year-old man presenting to urgent care today with dysuria, increased urinating frequency, and flank pain. His past medical history includes hyperlipidemia and migraines. He is allergic to penicillin and sulfa drugs. The patient has a high fever and severe nausea and vomiting. What is the probable diagnosis?

   a. Benign prostatic hyperplasia (BPH)
   b. Cystitis
   c. Prostate cancer
   d. Pyelonephritis

Answer d is correct. NK has classic symptoms of pyelonephritis. Pyelonephritis is characterized as cystitis symptoms plus systemic symptoms such as fever, flank pain, nausea, and vomiting.

Answer a is incorrect. BPH produces lower urinary tract symptoms, but is not commonly associated with fever or flank pain.

Answer b is incorrect. Cystitis does not cause flank pain.

Answer c is incorrect. Prostate cancer does not present with fever or flank pain.

7. What is the most appropriate therapy for NK?

   a. Amoxicillin 500 mg po tid
   b. Ciprofloxacin 500 mg po bid
   c. Ciprofloxacin 400 mg IV twice daily
   d. TMP-SMX 1 double strength (DS) tablet po bid

Answer c is correct. Ciprofloxacin is the appropriate therapy because NK is allergic to penicillin and sulfa drugs.

Answer a is incorrect. NK is allergic to penicillin so amoxicillin would be an inappropriate choice. Additionally, amoxicillin would not be utilized as empiric therapy.

Answer b is incorrect. Oral therapy would most likely not be utilized at this time because of the severe N&V. Once the N&V have resided, a transition to oral therapy will be utilized.

Answer d is incorrect. NK is allergic to sulfa drugs, and TMP-SMX includes a sulfa component. If the patient did not have an allergy, sulfa antibiotics can be utilized in uncomplicated pyelonephritis. An uncomplicated pyelonephritis would be a mild case where a patient could be treated as an outpatient with oral antibiotics.

8. What is the most appropriate duration of therapy for NK?

   a. 7 days
   b. 3 days
   c. 14 days
   d. 1 day

Answer c is correct. Fourteen days is the appropriate duration of therapy for complicated pyelonephritis. In some circumstances, levofloxacin (not ciprofloxacin) is approved for a 5-day course for uncomplicated pyelonephritis.

Answer a is incorrect. Seven days may be utilized for a patient with uncomplicated pyelonephritis (eg, mild symptoms).

Answer b is incorrect. Three days is the recommendation for a patient with acute uncomplicated cystitis.

Answer d is incorrect. One day of therapy is not recommended for any type of UTI.

9. NK completes prescribed therapy and feels better. Two weeks later, he returns to the emergency department (ED) with general malaise, a temperature of 101.7°F, pelvic pain, dysuria, and increased urination. The basic metabolic panel was within the references ranges for each laboratory. Additionally, the complete blood count laboratory values were also within the reference rages. The prostate specific antigen (PSA) was 12 ng/mL (reference less than 4.0 ng/mL), the erythrocyte sedimentation rate was 10 mm/h (reference range less than 15 mm/h) and the C-reactive protein (CRP) was 11 mg/dL (reference range less than 3.0 mg/dL). What is the probable diagnosis?

   a. Acute bacterial prostatitis
   b. Benign prostatic hyperplasia
   c. Cystitis
   d. Epididymitis

Answer a is correct. NK's initial therapy resolved his pyelonephritis. The prostate is a common site of bacteria persistence. Two weeks later, he displays symptoms of acute bacterial prostatitis which is supported by the PSA and CRP labs. CRP measures general levels of inflammation in your body. PSA is a protein produced by prostate gland cells. Elevated levels may indicate prostate cancer, but PSA levels can also be affected by other things, such as enlarged prostate or a UTI. High levels of CRP are caused by infections and many long-term diseases. But a CRP test cannot show where the inflammation is located or what is causing it. Other tests are needed to find the cause and location of the inflammation.

Answer b is incorrect. BPH does not present with these symptoms. Patients with BPH have a urinary stream that may be weak, or stop and start. In some cases, BPH can lead to infection, bladder stones, and reduced kidney function.

Answer c is incorrect. Cystitis does not typically produce a fever.

Answer d is incorrect. Epididymitis is an inflammation of the epididymis, a tube near the testicles that stores and carries sperm. Epididymitis in adults is most often caused by gonorrhea or chlamydia, while epididymitis in children is likely caused by direct trauma or a UTI. Epididymitis causes unilateral testicular pain and swelling.

10. NK is admitted to the hospital. Blood and urine cultures are collected. He is started on ceftriaxone 1 g IV daily. On day 3, blood cultures are negative, and the urine culture is positive for *E. coli*. The isolate is resistant to amoxicillin. On day 4, NK is ready for discharge. What is the most appropriate outpatient therapy for NK?

    a. Ciprofloxacin 500 mg po bid for 3 days
    b. Ciprofloxacin 500 mg po bid for 14 days
    c. Ciprofloxacin 500 mg po bid for 28 days
    d. Nitrofurantoin 100 mg po bid for 28 days

Answer c is correct. Acute bacterial prostatitis is treated for 4 weeks to reduce the risk of developing chronic prostatitis. Treatment of bacterial prostatitis is hampered by the lack of an active antibiotic transport mechanism and the relatively poor penetration of most antibiotics into infected prostate tissue and fluids. Most antibiotics are weak acids or bases that convert in biological fluids, which inhibits their crossing prostatic epithelium. Fluoroquinolones have emerged as preferred antibiotics for treating bacterial prostatitis; however, concern with these agents is the growing problem of fluoroquinolone resistance. TMP-SMX may also be used for the treatment of acute bacterial prostatitis but would not be appropriate for NK due to his allergy to sulfa drugs.

Answer a is incorrect. Short-course therapy (3 days) is not recommended in prostatitis.

Answer b is incorrect. Fourteen days is the appropriate duration of treatment for men with a UTI.

Answer d is incorrect. Nitrofurantoin is indicated for uncomplicated UTIs only and not for bacterial prostatitis.

11. What is the most common gram-positive cause of a UTI?

    a. *Streptococcus aureus*
    b. *Staphylococcus epidermidis*
    c. *Staphylococcus saprophyticus*
    d. *Streptococcus pneumoniae*

Answer c is correct. *S. saprophyticus* is the most common gram-positive bacteria causing UTIs (5%-10%). *S. saprophyticus* may be treated with TMP-SMX, amoxicillin/clavulanate, cephalosporins, and quinolones.

Answer a is incorrect. *S. aureus* may cause UTI; however, it is not a common cause. *S. aureus* (including MRSA) may cause catheter-associated UTIs.

Answer b is incorrect. *S. epidermidis* is an infrequent cause of UTIs. Please note that *S. epidermidis* is often reported as coagulase-negative Staphylococci. *S. saprophyticus* is also a coagulase-negative Staph species.

Answer d is incorrect. *Streptococcus pneumoniae* (pneumococcus) is an infrequent cause of UTIs. Pneumococcus is a common cause of respiratory tract infections.

12. Which antibiotic is most appropriate for prophylaxis of recurrent UTIs?

    a. Amoxicillin/clavulanic acid
    b. Levofloxacin
    c. Moxifloxacin
    d. Nitrofurantoin

Answer d in correct. Nitrofurantoin and TMP-SMX are recommended for the prophylaxis of UTIs in select patients.

Answer a is incorrect. Amoxicillin/clavulanic acid is used for the treatment of UTIs and in rare cases prophylaxis only when allergies to other agents are present or resistance patterns dictate use. It would not be a first-line agent for prophylaxis.

Answer b is incorrect. Levofloxacin is used for the treatment of UTIs.

Answer c is incorrect. Moxifloxacin is metabolized in the liver via glucuronide and sulfate conjugation with little renal excretion, and it is not indicated for the treatment of UTIs. Ciprofloxacin and levofloxacin are the two fluoroquinolones indicated for UTIs.

13. Select the correct statement regarding nitrofurantoin.

    a. Does not have a renal dosing recommendations/requirements
    b. Appropriate throughout pregnancy
    c. Is not indicated for the treatment of pyelonephritis
    d. Is an antifungal

Answer c is correct. Nitrofurantoin is an antibiotic indicated specifically for uncomplicated UTIs.

Answer a is incorrect. Nitrofurantoin is contraindicated in patients with a creatinine clearance less than 40 mL/min.

Answer b is incorrect. Nitrofurantoin is contraindicated in pregnant patients at term (38-42 weeks gestation) and during labor and delivery due to the risk of hemolytic anemia via immature erythrocyte enzyme systems.

Answer d is incorrect. Nitrofurantoin (FURADANTIN, MACROBID, others) is a synthetic nitrofuran that is used for the prevention and treatment of bacterial infections of the urinary tract. Nitrofurantoin is absorbed rapidly and completely from the GI tract. The macrocrystalline form of the drug is absorbed and excreted more slowly. Antibacterial concentrations are not achieved in plasma following ingestion of recommended doses because the drug is eliminated rapidly; therefore, the primary role is treatment of cystitis.

Questions 14 through 16 are related to the same case.

14. LA is 30-year-old pregnant woman. She is 16 weeks pregnant and reports dysuria at her appointment today. Urinalysis and urine culture are conducted, and she is started on TMP-SMX 1 DS tablet po bid. What is the appropriate duration of therapy?

    a. 3 days
    b. 7 days
    c. 14 days
    d. 28 days

Answer b is correct. Initial therapy for pregnant women should be 7 days, and a follow-up urine culture 1 to 2 weeks post therapy and then monthly until birth is recommended.

Answer a is incorrect. Three days of therapy at standard doses is effective treatment for uncomplicated lower UTIs in women.

Answer c is incorrect. Fourteen days is the recommended duration of therapy for pyelonephritis.

Answer d is incorrect. Twenty-eight days is the recommended duration of therapy for prostatitis.

15. Three days later, the clinic calls LA to tell her the culture results are back and she needs to change therapy. The culture was positive for *E. coli*, and it is resistant to TMP-SMX only. What would be the new appropriate therapy for LA?

    a. Amoxicillin 500 mg po tid for 3 days
    b. Ciprofloxacin 500 mg po bid for 7 days
    c. Nitrofurantoin 100 mg po bid for 7 days
    d. TMP-SMX 2 DS tablets po bid for 7 days

Answer c is correct. Initial therapy for pregnant women should be 7 days, and a follow-up urine culture 1 to 2 weeks post therapy and then monthly until birth is recommended. Nitrofurantoin is contraindicated in pregnant patients at term (38-42 weeks gestation) and during labor and delivery. LA is only 16 weeks pregnant; so she can take nitrofurantoin.

Answer a is incorrect. Three days of therapy at standard doses is effective treatment for uncomplicated lower UTIs in women.

Answer b is incorrect. Pregnant women should avoid fluoroquinolones due to the risk of arthropathies and the potential to inhibit cartilage and bone development in the newborn.

Answer d is incorrect. The isolate is resistant to TMP-SMX. Increasing the dose will not overcome the resistance.

16. Does LA need a follow-up culture? If so, when?

    a. No follow-up culture is needed
    b. Yes, in 2 days
    c. Yes, a day after the therapy is complete
    d. Yes, 7 to 14 days after the therapy is complete

Answer d is correct. Pregnant women are recommended to have a follow-up urine culture 1 to 2 weeks post therapy and then monthly until birth is recommended.

Answers a, b, and c are incorrect. A follow-up culture will be needed after the therapy is complete.

17. Which antibiotic is appropriate for UTI treatment in pregnant women who are not near-term? Select all that apply.

    a. Amoxicillin/clavulanic acid
    b. Doxycycline
    c. Nitrofurantoin
    d. TMP-SMX

Answers a, c, and d are correct. Sulfonamides, amoxicillin, amoxicillin/clavulanic acid, cephalexin, and nitrofurantoin may be given to pregnant women and are effective in 70% to 80% of patients. TMP-SMX should be avoided near term due to risk of kernicterus but may be used in other times during pregnancy.

Answer b is incorrect. Tetracyclines should be avoided during pregnancy. An agent with low adverse effect potential and which is safe for mother and child should be selected.

18. Patients with chronic indwelling catheters usually have asymptomatic bacteriuria. What should be done if the patient becomes symptomatic? Select all that apply.

    a. Remove the catheter; insert new sterile catheter before treatment
    b. Remove the catheter; insert new sterile catheter after treatment
    c. Start antibiotic therapy
    d. Leave the same catheter in place

Answers a and c are correct. Asymptomatic bacteriuria is universal in patients with chronic indwelling catheters (≥30 days). Antimicrobial therapy for asymptomatic bacteriuria will not prevent bacteriuria or symptomatic infection, but will aid in the emergence of resistance. However, symptomatic patients must have their catheter removed, be recatheterized, and then treated to prevent the development of pyelonephritis or bacteremia.

Answers b and d are incorrect. A new catheter should be placed prior to treatment.

---

19. What is the brand name for TMP-SMX? Select all that apply.

    a. Bactrim
    b. Macrobid
    c. Septra
    d. Trimprex

Answers a and c are correct. Bactrim and Septra are both brand names for TMP-SMX.

Answer b is incorrect. Macrobid is the brand name for nitrofurantoin.

Answer d is incorrect. Trimprex is the brand name for trimethoprim.

---

20. Short-course therapy (3 days) is appropriate for which patient group.

    a. Women with a history of UTIs caused by antibiotic-resistant bacteria
    b. Men
    c. Women with >7 days of symptoms
    d. Women with uncomplicated cystitis

Answer d is correct. The IDSA recommends 3-day therapy for treatment of uncomplicated lower tract infections in women.

Answer a is incorrect. Short-course therapy (3 days) is not recommended in women with a history of UTIs caused by antibiotic-resistant bacteria. These patients should receive 7 to 14 days of therapy.

Answer b is incorrect. Short-course therapy (3 days) is not recommended in men.

Answer c is incorrect. Short-course therapy (3 days) is not recommended in women with >7 days of symptoms. These patients should receive 7 to 14 days of therapy.

---

21. TC is a 19-year-old woman diagnosed with acute cystitis. She is allergic to sulfa drugs. What is an appropriate empiric regimen for her? Select all that apply.

    a. Ciprofloxacin 250 mg po bid for 3 days
    b. Trimethoprim 100 mg po bid for 3 days
    c. Sulfamethoxazole/trimethoprim 1 DS tablet twice daily for 3 days
    d. Moxifloxacin 400 mg daily for 3 days

Answers a and b are correct. Both ciprofloxacin and trimethoprim are appropriate for TC. TC is allergic to sulfa drugs so trimethoprim is okay. Please note that trimethoprim is usually used in combination with a sulfonamide in Bactrim/Septra. Patients allergic to sulfonamides may not take

Bactrim/Septra, but could take trimethoprim. It is possible to still be allergic to trimethoprim (unrelated to sulfa allergy).

Answers c and d are incorrect. Patient is allergic to sulfa; therefore, cannot take sulfamethoxazole. Moxifloxacin is hepatically metabolized and is not indicated for UTI management.

---

22. YI is a 26-year-old patient being treated with TMP-SMX for a UTI. The current dose is 1 DS tablet twice daily. What gram-negative organisms would TMP-SMX treat that are potentially causes of a complicated UTI? Select all that apply.

    a. *Staphylococcus saprophyticus*
    b. *Escherichia coli*
    c. *Klebsiella pneumoniae*
    d. *Pseudomonas aeruginosa*
    e. *Proteus mirabilis*

Answer b is correct. *E. coli* is a gram negative organism that is the most common bacterial cause of UTIs. TMP-SMX has activity against *E. coli* and is a good appropriate treatment for select UTIs (eg, cystitis).

Answer c is correct. *Klebsiella pneumoniae* is a gram negative organism and is a potential bacterial etiology of UTIs. TMP-SMX has activity against *Klebsiella pneumoniae* and is a good appropriate treatment for select UTIs (eg, cystitis).

Answer e is correct. *Proteus mirabilis* is a gram negative organism and is a potential bacterial etiology of UTIs. TMP-SMX has activity against *Proteus mirabilis* and is a good appropriate treatment for select UTIs (eg, cystitis).

Answer a is incorrect. Although TMP-SMX has activity against *S. saprophyticus* and is a good appropriate treatment for select UTIs (eg, cystitis); it is a gram-positive organism and the question asked for gram-negative organisms.

Answer d is incorrect. TMP-SMX does not have clinical activity against *P. aeruginosa*; therefore, TMP-SMX would not be an appropriate antibiotic to empirically treat complicated UTIs where Pseudomonas is a potential pathogen.

---

23. Place the following antibiotics in order of dosing frequency. Start with the antibiotic that should be dosed most frequently in a patient with an estimated glomerular filtration of 100 mL/min (calculated by the Cockcroft-Gault equation).

Unordered Response	Ordered Response
Macrodantin 50 mg	Macrodantin 50 mg four times per day
Levaquin 500 mg	Septra 160/800 mg twice daily
Septra 160/800 mg	Levaquin 500 mg daily

---

24. Select the antibiotic that is available as a 3-gram single dose for management of adult acute uncomplicated cystitis?

    a. Nitrofurantoin
    b. Ciprofloxacin

c. Amoxicillin/clavulanate
d. Fosfomycin

Answer d is correct. For uncomplicated UTIs, a single oral dose of fosfomycin tromethamine 5.61 g (equivalent to 3 g of fosfomycin) dissolved in liquid is used. A longer treatment course is probably necessary for infections at other sites (eg, prostate). Fosfomycin is a novel class of antibacterial with a chemical structure unrelated to other known antibiotics. It is a bactericidal drug that disrupts cell wall synthesis by inhibiting phosphoenolpyruvate synthetase and thus interferes with the production of peptidoglycan. It is available as a powder formulation of fosfomycin tromethamine, which can be dissolved in liquid and taken orally. Oral bioavailability of the fosfomycin tromethamine salt is low (about 40%), and consequently, serum levels are low relative to the minimum inhibitory concentrations (MICs). For this reason, the drug is used to treat uncomplicated lower UTIs, not pyelonephritis. Fosfomycin is used mainly for uncomplicated UTIs caused by *E. coli* or *E. faecalis*. However, because it has a broad spectrum of activity, fosfomycin is sometimes used to treat infections with multidrug-resistant organisms at other anatomic sites.

Answer a is incorrect. Nitrofurantoin is typically dosed as: (1) regular release: 50 to 100 mg orally four times a day for 1 week or for at least 3 days after urine sterility is obtained or (2) dual release: 100 mg orally twice a day for 7 days.

Answer b is incorrect. Ciprofloxacin dose is (1) Acute uncomplicated: Immediate-release, 250 mg po q12hr for 3 days; extended-release, 500 mg po q24hr for 3 days; (2) Mild/moderate: 250 mg po q12hr or 200 mg IV q12hr for 7 to 14 days; (3) Severe/complicated: 500 mg po q12hr or 400 mg IV q12hr for 7 to 14 days. Reminder: Reserve fluoroquinolones for patients who do not have other available treatment options for uncomplicated UTIs.

Answer c is incorrect. Amoxicillin/clavulanate dose is: 250 mg orally every 8 hours or 500 mg orally every 8 to 12 hours for 3 to 7 days. For more severe infections, 500 mg orally every 8 hours or 875 mg orally every 12 hours may be administered.

CHAPTER **24 | Skin and Soft Tissue Infections**

1. Which organism(s) is(are) the most common cause of SSTIs? Select all that apply.

   a. *Streptococcus pyogenes*
   b. *Staphylococcus aureus*
   c. *Pasteurella multicida*
   d. *Enterobacter cloacae*

Answer a is correct. Acute bacterial SSTIs are predominantly caused by Gram-positive organisms, particularly those that are present on skin. *S. pyogenes*, a Gram-positive

bacteria, is a normal human skin colonizing organism which in the right circumstances can cause infection.

Answer b is correct. *S. aureus* is another Gram-positive bacteria that can colonize certain parts of the human body and is among the most implicated cause of SSTIs.

Answer c is incorrect. *P. multicida* is only a common cause of infections from dog and cat bites.

Answer d is incorrect. *E. cloacae*, a Gram-negative bacteria, may cause SSTIs. However, it is not a common pathogen and usually implicated in patients with predisposing comorbidities (eg, diabetics) and those with already damaged tissue.

2. TR is a 29-year-old pregnant patient with a diagnosis of cellulitis. TR has no drug allergies and is not on any other medications. Select the most appropriate antibiotic that may be used to treat TR's infection.

   a. Cefazolin
   b. Doxycycline
   c. Imipenem-cilastatin
   d. Levofloxacin

Answer a is correct. Cefazolin is pregnancy category B and is generally considered safe for use during pregnancy. In addition, cefazolin is active against MSSA and GAS, the two most common causes of cellulitis.

Answer b is incorrect. Doxycycline is classified as pregnancy category D due to harmful risks to the fetus. Doxycycline crosses the placenta to cause discoloration of teeth and may also deposit into long bone to inhibit growth. Other adverse effects have been described as well.

Answer c is incorrect. Imipenem-cilastatin belongs to pregnancy category C, denoting observations of adverse effects in animal studies.

Answer d is incorrect. Levofloxacin belongs to pregnancy category C, denoting observations of adverse effects in animal studies.

The following patient case pertains to questions 3 through 5.

3. AB, a 30-year-old man who does not have any significant previous medical history nor drug allergies, was admitted to the hospital with an abscess and associated cellulitis. After appropriate drainage of the abscess, AB was initiated on intravenous vancomycin therapy. The culture from the incision and drainage grew caMRSA. AB's clinical status improved with 2 days of vancomycin therapy and thus will be discharged home with an oral antibiotic to finish his therapy. Which of the following antibiotic(s) is(are) appropriate step-down options for AB? Select all that apply.

   a. Cephalexin
   b. Minocycline
   c. Tigecycline
   d. TMP-SMX

Answer b is correct. Minocycline is an oral antibiotic active against caMRSA used for the treatment of SSTIs.

Answer d is correct. TMP-SMX is an oral antibiotic active against caMRSA and can be used for the treatment of SSTIs.

Answer a is incorrect. As the culture was positive for caMRSA, any step-down therapy chosen should have activity against it. Cephalexin is not active against caMRSA.

Answer c is incorrect. Tigecycline, while active against caMRSA, is only available as a parenteral formulation.

---

4. Doxycycline is chosen as the step-down therapy for AB's cellulitis. What pertinent counseling point(s) should be provided to AB regarding this medication? Select all that apply.

   a. Doxycycline may cause your teeth to turn brown.
   b. Avoid direct sunlight for prolonged periods and wear sunscreen.
   c. Doxycycline may turn your urine and tears into an orange-red color.
   d. Avoid taking this medication with antacids.

Answer b is correct. Doxycycline, as with all tetracyclines, can cause photosensitivity.

Answer d is correct. Divalent and trivalent cations (eg, iron, calcium, and magnesium) bind to doxycycline and other tetracyclines, reducing the amount of antibiotic absorption. Patients should avoid taking these two medications concurrently.

Answer a is incorrect. Tetracyclines may cause irreversible brown staining of teeth in young children (therefore is contraindicated in children ≤8 except in exceptional cases). As AB is 30 years old, this is not pertinent to him.

Answer c is incorrect. Doxycycline does not cause color change in bodily fluids. Other antibiotics, such as metronidazole and rifampin, cause bodily fluids to turn orange.

---

5. During discharge counseling, AB expresses concern that he may spread his infection to others. What are some measures he can take to minimize this risk? Select all that apply.

   a. Wash linens with cold water.
   b. Keep wound covered with a clean and dry dressing until it has healed.
   c. Avoid sharing personal hygiene products with others.
   d. As the infection is being treated with antibiotics, there are no precautions needed.

Answer b is correct. In order to prevent spread of infection, the wound should be covered until healed.

Answer c is correct. Sharing personal hygiene products such as razors may spread infection to others.

Answer a is incorrect. Linens should be washed using hot (not cold) water.

Answer d is incorrect. Even during treatment with effective antibiotics, it is possible to spread it to others.

---

6. RD is an 18-year-old woman who presents to a clinic with cellulitis. The local antibiogram reveals that <1% of *S. aureus* that were isolated last year were methicillin resistant. The treating physician would like to prescribe an oral antibiotic regimen that covers both *S. aureus* and GAS. Which of the following regimens is the most appropriate for monotherapy?

   a. Amoxicillin
   b. Cephalexin
   c. Ciprofloxacin
   d. Trimethoprim-sulfamethoxazole

Answer b is correct. Cephalexin is a first-line antibiotic regimen for cellulitis. It is active against both methicillin-sensitive *S. aureus* and GAS. As the local prevalence of MRSA is low and the patient does not have specific history to suggest so, RD does not need a MRSA-active treatment.

Answer a is incorrect. Amoxicillin is active against GAS, but is inactivated by penicillinases that most *S. aureus* strains produce.

Answer c is incorrect. Ciprofloxacin has very unreliable activity against Gram-positive organisms such as *S. aureus* and GAS.

Answer d is incorrect. While TMP-SMX has excellent activity against *S. aureus* (including caMRSA, which is not needed for this patient), it lacks activity against GAS. Therefore, another agent would need to be added to adequately cover both *S. aureus* and GAS.

---

7. What is the brand name of linezolid?

   a. Teflaro
   b. Tygacil
   c. Zosyn
   d. Zyvox

Answer d is correct. Zyvox is the brand name of linezolid.

Answer a is incorrect. Teflaro is the brand name of ceftaroline.

Answer b is incorrect. Tygacil is the brand name of tigecycline.

Answer c is incorrect. Zosyn is the brand name of piperacillin-tazobactam.

---

8. OT is a 45-year-old man with diabetes who was diagnosed with a mild foot infection. Since he has a history of chronic renal insufficiency, the provider would like to use an antibiotic that does not have to be adjusted for renal dysfunction. To treat his diabetic foot infection, select the antibiotic(s) that does(do) not require adjustment for renal dysfunction.

   a. Cefazolin
   b. Linezolid

c. Nafcillin
d. Vancomycin

Answer b is correct. Linezolid is metabolized through oxidation and is mostly excreted through nonrenal routes. It does not require adjustment for renal insufficiency.

Answer c is correct. Nafcillin undergoes hepatic metabolism and is primarily eliminated in the feces. Adjustment of dose or interval is only required in patients with both renal and hepatic insufficiency.

Answer a is incorrect. The major route of elimination for cefazolin is through the kidneys; therefore, cefazolin requires renal dose adjustment.

Answer d is incorrect. The major route of elimination of vancomycin is through the kidneys; therefore, vancomycin requires dose adjustment for renal dysfunction.

9. Select the antibiotic that may cause an adverse reaction during or soon after infusion characterized by itching, warmth, flushing, and rash (among other symptoms), especially if infused at a rate faster than recommended.

    a. Ampicillin
    b. Cefazolin
    c. Daptomycin
    d. Vancomycin

Answer d is correct. Vancomycin, if infused too quickly may cause Redman syndrome. Redman syndrome is caused by a nonimmune release of histamine and is characterized by itching, warmth, flushing, and rash (typically on face and upper torso). In some cases, angioedema, tachycardia, and hypotension may also occur. It typically occurs during, or soon after administration of vancomycin and resolves within a few hours after the infusion. For most patients, extending the infusion of vancomycin and/or pretreating with an antihistamine resolves future episodes of Redman syndrome.

Answer a is incorrect. Ampicillin may cause a hypersensitivity reaction similar to what is described in the question, but it is not infusion related.

Answer b is incorrect. Daptomycin is not associated with an infusion-related reaction as described.

Answer d is incorrect. Cefazolin is not associated with an infusion-related reaction as described.

The following patient case pertains to questions 10 and 11.

10. BC is a 40-year-old woman, who has hypertension and drug allergies to penicillins (angioedema, hives) and sulfa drugs (rash), presents to urgent care with a dry and intensely red lesion about 5 cm by 5 cm in size, with well-demarcated and raised borders on her right lower extremity. She describes having pain and burning sensation. What is the most likely type of SSTI that BC is experiencing?

    a. Cellulitis
    b. Folliculitis

c. Impetigo
d. Erysipelas

Answer d is correct. The clinical presentation is most consistent with erysipelas, an SSTI that affects the epidermis and lymphatics.

Answer a is incorrect. Cellulitis typically presents with flat, diffuse borders.

Answer b is incorrect. Folliculitis is an SSTI that is associated with hair follicles and is much smaller in size than described.

Answer c is incorrect. Impetigo is characterized by multiple small lesions and often pruritic.

11. What is the most appropriate oral antibiotic for BC's SSTI?

    a. Amoxicillin
    b. Cefuroxime
    c. Clindamycin
    d. Vancomycin

Answer c is correct. Clindamycin, an antibiotic available in an oral formulation, is active against GAS, which is the most common cause of erysipelas. It is a rational alternative for treating erysipelas in patients who have serious penicillin allergies.

Answer a is incorrect. While amoxicillin is active against GAS, the most common cause of erysipelas, BC has a serious allergy to penicillins.

Answer b is incorrect. While cefuroxime is active against GAS, the most common cause of erysipelas, BC's serious allergy to penicillins limits the use of cephalosporins.

Answer d is incorrect. While vancomycin does come in oral form, the oral form is not systemically absorbed through the gastrointestinal tract and is limited to the treatment of *Clostridium difficile* infections.

12. Among the following, select the β-lactam(s) that have activity against penicillinase-producing *S. aureus*. Select all that apply.

    a. Ampicillin
    b. Cefazolin
    c. Dicloxacillin
    d. Doxycycline

Answer b is correct. Cefazolin is a first-generation cephalosporin with activity against penicillinase-producing *S. aureus*.

Answer c is correct. Dicloxacillin is a penicillin antibiotic resistant to hydrolysis by penicillinases that are produced by *S. aureus*.

Answer a is incorrect. Ampicillin is hydrolyzed by the penicillinases that are produced by *S. aureus* and, therefore, lacks activity against *S. aureus*.

Answer d is incorrect.   Doxycycline is not a β-lactam antibiotic.

13. GT is a 60-year-old man who was initiated on vancomycin and piperacillin-tazobactam for a rapidly progressing cellulitis in the emergency department. Upon arrival to the critical care unit, GT was determined to have necrotizing fasciitis. What, if anything, should be adjusted to the patient's antibiotic regimen?

    a. Add clindamycin.
    b. Change piperacillin-tazobactam to cefepime.
    c. Discontinue piperacillin-tazobactam.
    d. The current regimen is optimal, with no changes necessary.

Answer a is correct.   Clindamycin should be added to halt toxin production (by inhibiting protein synthesis) to minimize further damage to the tissues. It also provides additional activity for infections with high bacterial inoculum like necrotizing fasciitis.

Answer b is incorrect.   By switching from piperacillin-tazobactam to cefepime, the regimen loses anaerobic coverage. Anaerobes are the predominant organisms that cause type I necrotizing fasciitis.

Answer c is incorrect.   In type I necrotizing fasciitis, anaerobes and, to a lesser extent, Gram-negative bacteria are the etiologic pathogens. As such, it is important for the empiric regimen to contain antibiotics that are active against these pathogens.

Answer d is incorrect.   Because of the serious nature of necrotizing fasciitis with its significant morbidity and mortality, it is important to promptly minimize the damage caused by the infection. As such, clindamycin should be added to stop toxin production.

14. What is the generic name of Omnicef?

    a. Cefdinir
    b. Cefpodoxime
    c. Cefuroxime
    d. Cephalexin

Answer a is correct.   Cefdinir is the generic name of Omnicef.

Answer b is incorrect.   Cefpodoxime is the generic name of Vantin.

Answer c is incorrect.   Cefuroxime is the generic name of Ceftin and Zinacef.

Answer d is incorrect.   Cephalexin is the generic name of Keflex.

The following patient case pertains to questions 15 and 16.

15. HW is a 7-year-old girl who was bitten on the forearm by a dog. While the wound was superficial, it now shows signs of infection. The wound was thoroughly irrigated and cleaned. The patient does not have any allergies. What are the most common organisms that may cause the infection? Select all that apply.

    a. *Pasteurella multocida*
    b. *Escherichia coli*
    c. *Eikenella corrodens*
    d. Streptococci

Answer a is correct.   Bite infections are typically caused by organisms present in the biting animal's mouth and, to a lesser extent, the victim's skin. *P. multocida* is a normal flora in the mouths of dogs and cats that is implicated in bite infections.

Answer d is correct.   Streptococci are present in both mouths of dogs and on the human skin.

Answer b is incorrect.   *E. coli* is a Gram-negative organism that is not typically present in dog mouths or the skin of healthy humans.

Answer c is incorrect.   *E. corrodens* causes infections after human bites, but not dog bites.

16. What is the most appropriate antibiotic monotherapy for HW's dog bite wound infection?

    a. Augmentin
    b. Avelox
    c. Cleocin
    d. Doxycycline

Answer a is correct.   Augmentin (amoxicillin/clavulanic acid) is active against the typical organisms responsible for dog bite infections and is the drug of choice for those who do not have contraindications.

Answer b is incorrect.   While Avelox (moxifloxacin) is active against the typical organisms responsible for dog bite infections, fluoroquinolones are generally not recommended in children due to increased risk of severe adverse effects.

Answer c is incorrect.   Cleocin (clindamycin) is not active against *Pasteurella*, one of the major pathogens isolated from dog bite infections. If clindamycin is prescribed, it should be combined with another agent that is active against *Pasteurella*.

Answer d is incorrect.   While doxycycline is an alternative for dog bite infections in penicillin-allergic patients, tetracyclines are not recommended for children 8 years old and younger due to risk of permanent discoloration of teeth.

The following patient case pertains to questions 17 and 18.

17. PT is a 58-year-old woman with diabetes who will be started on Zosyn and an MRSA-active antibiotic for her diabetic foot infection with osteomyelitis. The patient's other medications include simvastatin, metoprolol, fenofibrate, escitalopram, and metformin. The team is concerned with potential drug

interactions and wants to avoid medications that interact with the patient's chronic medications. Which of the following medications is the most appropriate for MRSA coverage?

a. Daptomycin
b. Linezolid
c. Moxifloxacin
d. Vancomycin

Answer d is correct. There are no significant drug interactions with vancomycin and the patient's current medications.

Answer a is incorrect. Daptomycin, when used concurrently with simvastatin and fenofibrate, may increase the risk of myopathy. If there are no other options, simvastatin and fenofibrate may be temporarily discontinued, during daptomycin therapy, if deemed safe for the patient.

Answer b is incorrect. Linezolid used in concurrently with an SSRI may increase risk of serotonin syndrome. It is a relative contraindication and should be avoided unless there are no alternatives. Alternatively, SSRIs may be temporarily discontinued, during linezolid therapy, if deemed safe for the patient.

Answer c is incorrect. Fluoroquinolones, including moxifloxacin, are usually not active against MRSA, especially haMRSA.

18. Which of the following is a reasonable duration of antimicrobial therapy for PT's infection?

a. 1 week
b. 2 weeks
c. 3 weeks
d. 6 weeks

Answer d is correct. The typical duration of therapy for osteomyelitis is 4 to 6 weeks.

Answer a is incorrect. This is shorter than the typical treatment duration for osteomyelitis.

Answer b is incorrect. This is shorter than the typical treatment duration for osteomyelitis.

Answer c is incorrect. This is shorter than the typical treatment duration for osteomyelitis.

19. ZD is a 50-year-old man (83.3 kg) who was admitted into the hospital for cellulitis and was empirically initiated on vancomycin 15 mg/kg every 12 hours. Because of an adverse reaction he suffered when he previously received vancomycin, the medical team would like to infuse vancomycin at a rate of 500 mg/h. The pharmacy policy for final concentration of reconstituted vancomycin is at 5 mg/mL. What is the correct rate of infusion (mL/h) for his vancomycin and how long will it take to infuse each dose?

a. 50 mL/h for 5 hours
b. 100 mL/h for 2.5 hours
c. 125 mL/h for 2 hours
d. 200 mL/h for 2.5 hours

Answer b is correct. 100 mL/h would deliver 500 mg of vancomycin per hour. Infusion over 2.5 hours should reach the prescribed dose of 1250 mg.

Answer a is incorrect. 83.3 kg × 15 = 1250 mg (vancomycin dose)

1250 mg/5 mg/mL = 250 mL solution bag (the only volume that meets the 5 mg/mL criteria). 50 mL/hr would deliver only 250 mg of vancomycin per hour, lower than the desired 500 mg/h.

Answer c is incorrect. 125 mL/h would deliver 625 mg of vancomycin per hour, higher than the desired 500 mg/h.

Answer d is incorrect. 200 mL/h would deliver 1000 mg of vancomycin per hour, higher than the desired 500 mg/h.

20. TY is a 29-year-old woman with a mild penicillin allergy who is being treated with an intravenous antibiotic in the hospital for a severe lymphangitis. The patient is not receiving any other medications. One week into therapy, TY's creatine phosphokinase (CPK) elevated to six times above the normal level and she complains of muscle aches. Which antimicrobial agent is TY most likely receiving and contributing to this lab abnormality and symptom?

a. Cefuroxime
b. Daptomycin
c. Linezolid
d. Vancomycin

Answer b is correct. Daptomycin is associated CPK elevation and myopathy.

Answer a is incorrect. Cefuroxime is not associated with CPK elevation and myopathy.

Answer c is incorrect. Linezolid is not associated with CPK elevation and myopathy.

Answer d is incorrect. Vancomycin is not associated with CPK elevation and myopathy.

21. DM is a 51-year-old man with uncontrolled diabetes, 20-year 1 pack/d smoking history who just finished treatment for his first episode of a mild diabetic foot infection. He is interested in learning preventive strategies to reduce his chances of another infection. Which counseling point is appropriate for DM? Select all that apply.

a. Obtain periodic foot exams.
b. Work toward improving his control of diabetes.
c. Work toward smoking cessation.
d. Walk in open-toed shoes or barefoot as much as possible to keep feet dry.

Answer a is correct. It is important for diabetic patients to have periodic foot exams to ensure that their feet are in good condition and to screen for potential problems (such as worsening neuropathy through the monofilament test).

Answer b is correct. Improving control of his diabetes will reduce the progression of neuropathy, vasculopathy, and other diabetic complications which contribute to risk of foot infections.

Answer c is correct. Smoking is an independent risk factor for peripheral vascular disease, which contributes to poor blood supply to extremities and poor wound healing, and thereby increases risk of diabetic foot infections.

Answer d is incorrect. Well-fitting, closed footwear are recommended for diabetic patients to protect the feet from accidental trauma.

CHAPTER 25 | **Central Nervous System Infections**

1. A 13-day-old former 35-week gestational age baby presents to the emergency room with a temperature of 102°F. The mother reports that the baby has been feeding less, is constipated, and is very irritable. Which of the following is a common symptom of meningitis in a neonate? Select all that apply.

   a. Temperature of 102°F
   b. Decreased feeding
   c. Constipation
   d. Irritable appearance

Answer a is correct. Fever is a common symptom of meningitis in a neonate.

Answer b is correct. Decreased feeding is a common symptom of meningitis in a neonate.

Answer d is correct. Irritability is a common symptom of meningitis in a neonate.

Answer c is incorrect. Constipation is not a common symptom of meningitis in a neonate.

---

2. The emergency physician is unable to obtain CSF after multiple attempts. Based on clinical findings, the team believes that the 13-day-old former 35-week gestational age baby may have meningitis. What is the best empiric therapy to begin in this baby before sending her to a pediatric hospital?

   a. Ampicillin and gentamicin
   b. Ceftriaxone and gentamicin
   c. Vancomycin and cefotaxime
   d. Ampicillin and ceftriaxone

Answer a is correct. Ampicillin provides appropriate empiric coverage for *L. monocytogenes* and *S. agalactiae* (may cover some aerobic Gram-negative bacilli as well). Gentamicin provides appropriate empiric coverage against aerobic Gram-negative bacilli (and some synergy with ampicillin against Gram-positives, like *L. monocytogenes*). Ampicillin and cefotaxime would also be an appropriate regimen.

Answer b is incorrect. While gentamicin is appropriate, this regimen is missing first-line empiric coverage for

L. monocytogenes (ie, ampicillin). Also, ceftriaxone is not a first-line agent for bacterial meningitis in neonates (≤28 days) due to risk of adverse events, for example, biliary sludging, kernicterus, and potentially life-threatening precipitation with calcium-containing products.

Answer c is incorrect. While cefotaxime is appropriate, this regimen is missing empiric coverage for *L. monocytogenes* (ie, ampicillin). Also, vancomycin is broader empiric Gram-positive coverage than is generally needed for neonates.

Answer d is incorrect. While ampicillin is appropriate, cefotaxime is the preferred third-generation cephalosporin in neonates. Ceftriaxone is not a first-line agent for bacterial meningitis in neonates (≤28 days) due to risk of adverse events, for example, biliary sludging, kernicterus, and precipitation potentially life-threatening with calcium-containing products.

---

3. When the 13-day-old former 35-week gestational age baby is examined at the pediatric hospital, she is also noted to have some lesions. The team has just sent cultures of the lesions as well as HSV PCR of the CSF. Which of the following is an appropriate pharmacologic approach in this patient?

   a. Wait for the cultures and PCR results to come back, then modify therapy if needed.
   b. Change antibiotic therapy to ceftriaxone and vancomycin.
   c. Add IV acyclovir to the current antibiotic regimen.
   d. Add oral voriconazole therapy to the current antibiotic regimen.

Answer c is correct. IV acyclovir should be added as soon as possible as empiric therapy for HSV encephalitis while awaiting the results of diagnostic studies. The earlier the treatment is started, the lower the risk of death or serious sequelae.

Answer a is incorrect. Culture and PCR results may take hours to days to return. Such a delay in therapy against HSV would increase the risk of death or serious sequelae in an infected patient.

Answer b is incorrect. This change in antibiotics to ceftriaxone and vancomycin would offer no antiviral coverage against HSV. Also, ceftriaxone and vancomycin would be inappropriate empiric therapy for bacterial meningitis in a neonate (see Question 2).

Answer d is incorrect. This addition of antifungal therapy with voriconazole would offer no antiviral coverage against HSV. In addition, antimicrobial therapy for CNS infections is generally given the IV route (vs oral) in order to ensure adequate CNS penetration.

---

4. If a neonate is begun on acyclovir for HSV-associated encephalitis, which of the following should be routinely monitored? Select all that apply.

   a. Serum creatinine
   b. WBC count

c. Urine output
d. International normalized ratio (INR)

Answer a is correct. Serum creatinine should be monitored as a marker of renal function because acyclovir may cause nephrotoxicity secondary to precipitation in the renal tubules (particular at high doses used to treat encephalitis).

Answer b is correct. WBC count should be monitored as a marker of bone marrow function because acyclovir may cause bone marrow suppression, resulting in a decrease in WBCs or other blood cell lines.

Answer c is correct. Urine output should also be monitored as a marker of renal function because acyclovir may cause nephrotoxicity secondary to precipitation in the renal tubules (particular at high doses used to treat encephalitis).

Answer d is incorrect. The INR is not generally used to monitor for toxicity secondary to acyclovir therapy.

5. What is the brand name for ceftriaxone?

a. Ceftin
b. Keflex
c. Maxipime
d. Rocephin

Answer d is correct. Rocephin is the brand name for ceftriaxone.

Answer a is incorrect. Ceftin is the brand name for cefuroxime.

Answer b is incorrect. Keflex is the brand name for cephalexin.

Answer c is incorrect. Maxipime is the brand name for cefepime.

6. Which of the following patients are recommended to receive a vaccine against *Streptococcus pneumoniae*? Select all that apply.

a. Healthy infants
b. A 40 year old with chronic obstructive pulmonary disease (COPD)
c. A healthy 55 year old
d. A 35-year-old asplenic patient

Answer a is correct. Healthy infants should receive the pneumococcal vaccination as part of their routine pediatric vaccination schedule beginning at 2 months of age (minimum age for dose 1 is 6 weeks).

Answer b is correct. This patient is between 19 and 64 years old, but has COPD which is a risk factor for pneumococcal disease. The patient should therefore be vaccinated.

Answer d is correct. This patient is between 19 and 64 years old, but has anatomic asplenia which is a risk factor

for pneumococcal disease. The patient should therefore be vaccinated.

Answer c is incorrect. Adults age 19 to 64 only require pneumococcal vaccination if they are at risk for pneumococcal disease. These include patients with any chronic disease (eg, cardiovascular, respiratory, diabetes mellitus, alcoholism, cirrhosis, CSF leak, or cochlear implants) or immunocompromising conditions (eg, medication-induced, functional, or anatomic asplenia).

7. A 66-year-old woman with coronary artery disease, peripheral artery disease, diabetes, and hypertension is transferred from a nursing home to the hospital secondary to fever and altered mental status. A lumbar puncture was performed and CSF was sent for fluid analysis and culture. Which of the following findings are consistent with bacterial meningitis in this patient? Select all that apply.

a. CSF WBC 5000 cells/mm^3
b. CSF WBC with 70% lymphocytes
c. CSF glucose of 23 mg/dL
d. CSF protein of 250 mg/dL

Answer a is correct. Elevated CSF WBC of 1000-10,000 cells/mm^3 is consistent with bacterial meningitis.

Answer c is correct. Low CSF glucose of <40 mg/dL (likely with a CSF:serum glucose ratio of ≤0.4) is consistent with bacterial meningitis.

Answer d is correct. Elevated CSF protein of >100 mg/dL is consistent with bacterial meningitis.

Answer b is incorrect. In bacterial meningitis, the WBC differential is typically shifted to a predominance of neutrophils (>80%). A lymphocytic predominance can be seen with viral meningitis or other CNS infections.

8. The physician decides to start the patient on vancomycin, ampicillin, and ceftriaxone, but the patient has a history of difficult IV access. Which of the following is an appropriate plan for treatment of this patient's bacterial meningitis?

a. Attempt immediate IV line placement and administer antibiotics IV for the duration of therapy.
b. Administer antibiotics orally for the duration of therapy.
c. Administer antibiotics intramuscularly for the duration of therapy.
d. Immediately insert an external ventricular drain into the brain and administer antibiotics intraventricularly for the duration of therapy.

Answer a is correct. IV therapy is the preferred route for antimicrobial treatment of CNS infections in order to ensure optimal CNS penetration (including allowing for administration of high-dose regimens).

Answer b is incorrect. Oral administration is not the preferred route for treatment of bacterial meningitis.

Also, alternative antibiotics would have to be used for oral administration.

Answer c is incorrect. Intramuscular administration is not the preferred route for treatment of bacterial meningitis. Also, an alternative to vancomycin would have to be used for intramuscular administration.

Answer d is incorrect. Intraventricular administration may be considered as adjunctive therapy is some patients (eg, CNS shunt infections), yet IV remains the preferred route of administration for treatment of bacterial meningitis to ensure optimal drug penetration into the CNS. Also, placement of an external ventricular drain is a more invasive procedure that may cause more delay than IV line placement.

---

9. Nephrotoxicity is one of the common side effects for which of the following IV antimicrobial agents? Select all that apply.

   a. Acyclovir
   b. Ceftriaxone
   c. Gentamicin
   d. Vancomycin

Answer a is correct. Nephrotoxicity is one of the common side effects of acyclovir.

Answer c is correct. Nephrotoxicity is one of the common side effects of gentamicin.

Answer d is correct. Nephrotoxicity is one of the common side effects of vancomycin, especially with troughs greater than 15 mcg/mL or combined with gentamicin.

Answer b is incorrect. Nephrotoxicity is not one of the common side effects of ceftriaxone.

---

10. A 12-year-old boy presents to his pediatrician for a routine follow-up visit. The patient denies having any complaints. Physical examination, vital signs, and laboratory values are all within normal limits. Which of the following vaccinations should the patient receive today as part of routine care for a healthy adolescent?

    a. MCV4
    b. MPSV4
    c. PCV13
    d. PPSV23

Answer a is correct. MCV4 is the specific formulation of the meningococcal vaccine recommended as a routine vaccination for adolescents aged 11 to 12 years, with a booster dose at age 16 years. MCV4 is also recommended for children aged 9 months to 10 years, if risk factors for meningococcal disease are present, such as persistent complement deficiencies, anatomic or functional asplenia (eg, sickle cell disease), presence during an outbreak caused by a vaccine serogroup, or travel to the African meningitis belt or to the Hajj.

Answer b is incorrect. MPSV4 is not a formulation of meningococcal vaccine generally recommended for adolescents. It is preferred for vaccine-naïve patients ≥56 years of age who are at risk for meningococcal disease.

Answer c is incorrect. PCV13 is the specific formulation of the pneumococcal vaccine recommended as a routine vaccination for children, not adolescents. Children should receive a series of PCV13 beginning at age 2 months (minimum age 6 weeks). PCV13 may also be given as vaccination for patients in other age groups, including adolescents, if risk factors for pneumococcal disease are present. These may include chronic disease (eg, cardiovascular, respiratory, diabetes mellitus, alcoholism, cirrhosis, CSF leak, or cochlear implants) or an immunocompromised state (eg, medication-induced, asplenia).

Answer d is incorrect. PPSV23 is the specific formulation recommended as a routine vaccination for adults aged ≥65 years, not adolescents. PPSV23 may also be given to patients aged ≥2 years who are at risk for pneumococcal disease.

---

11. A 22-year-old man (94 kg) with no significant past medical history presents to your hospital with fever, severe headache, photophobia, and neck pain. The physician does a lumbar puncture and sends the CSF collections to the laboratory. Based upon clinical diagnosis, the patient is suspected to have bacterial meningitis. Which of the following are likely pathogens associated with bacterial meningitis in this patient?

    a. *Streptococcus pneumoniae* and *Haemophilus influenzae*
    b. *Neisseria meningitidis* and *Listeria monocytogenes*
    c. *L. monocytogenes* and *Streptococcus agalactiae* (group B)
    d. *S. pneumoniae* and *N. meningitidis*

Answer d is correct. *N. meningitidis* and *S. pneumoniae* are the most likely causative pathogens of bacterial meningitis in adult patients <50 years of age.

Answer a is incorrect. While *S. pneumoniae* is correct, *H. influenzae* is not a likely pathogen in adult patients <50 years of age. *H. influenzae* is a likely pathogen for young infants aged 1 to 23 months.

Answer b is incorrect. While *N. meningitidis* is correct, *L. monocytogenes* is not a likely pathogen in adult patients <50 years of age. *L. monocytogenes* is a likely pathogen in neonates and adults >50 years old.

Answer c is incorrect. Neither *L. monocytogenes* nor *S. agalactiae* (group B) are likely pathogens in adult patients <50 years of age. *S. agalactiae* (group B) is a likely pathogen in neonates and young infants aged 1 to 23 months.

---

12. What is an appropriate empiric antibiotic therapy for this 22-year-old patient with suspected bacterial meningitis?

    a. Ceftriaxone
    b. Ceftriaxone and ampicillin
    c. Cefotaxime and vancomycin
    d. Ampicillin and gentamicin

Answer c is correct.   Cefotaxime provides appropriate empiric coverage for *N. meningitidis* and most *S. pneumoniae*. Vancomycin provides additional empiric coverage against multidrug-resistant *S. pneumoniae* (resistant to third-generation cephalosporins like cefotaxime).

Answer a is incorrect.   Ceftriaxone provides appropriate empiric coverage for *N. meningitidis* and most *S. pneumoniae*; yet, this therapy is missing empiric coverage against multi-drug-resistant *S. pneumoniae* (ie, vancomycin).

Answer b is incorrect.   Ceftriaxone provides appropriate empiric coverage for *N. meningitidis* and most *S. pneumoniae*. Ampicillin provides additional empiric coverage for *L. monocytogenes*, which is unnecessary for a young adult patient. This therapy is also missing empiric coverage against multidrug resistant *S. pneumoniae* (ie, vancomycin).

Answer d is incorrect.   Ampicillin and gentamicin are inadequate empiric coverage for *S. pneumoniae* and *N. meningitidis*. This regimen would instead be preferred in neonates given appropriate empiric coverage for *S. agalactiae*, aerobic Gram-negative bacilli, and *L. monocytogenes*.

13. The physician orders vancomycin 1500 mg IV Q12h for this 22-year-old man (among other antimicrobials). In order to minimize the risk of infusion-related reactions, for example, Red Man Syndrome, the drug will be administered at a concentration of 5 mg/mL and rate of 10 mg/min. What is the resulting infusion rate and duration for each vancomycin dose?

    a. 120 mL/h over 150 minutes
    b. 300 mL/h over 90 minutes
    c. 120 mL/h over 90 minutes
    d. 300 mL/h over 150 minutes

Answer a is correct.   1500 mg/(5 mg/mL) = 300 mL total volume. 1500 mg/(10 mg/min) = 150 min infusion time. 150 min/(60 min/h) = 2.5 h infusion time. 300 mL/2.5 h = 120 mL/h.

Answer b is incorrect.   This would represent 1500 mg in 450 mL, concentration of 3.3 mg/mL, rate of 16.7 mg/min.

Answer c is incorrect.   This would represent 1500 mg in 180 mL, concentration of 8.3 mg/mL, rate of 16.7 mg/min.

Answer d is incorrect.   This would represent 1500 mg in 450 mL, concentration of 3.3 mg/mL, rate of 10 mg/min.

14. The 22-year-old male patient received antibiotics prior to CSF collection. CSF, blood, sputum, and urine specimens were sent for Gram stain and culture. Which of the following is correct regarding diagnosis of bacterial meningitis?

    a. The likelihood of a bacteria being identified from CSF Gram stain and/or culture is unchanged, despite the patient receiving antibiotics prior to CSF collection.

    b. CSF Gram stain and culture are not reliable for diagnosis of bacterial meningitis.
    c. There is no role for blood cultures in the diagnosis of bacterial meningitis.
    d. A bacteria will be identified in majority of CSF cultures in bacterial meningitis cases.

Answer d is correct.   Bacterial identification is possible in 60% to 90% of CSF Gram stains and 70% to 85% of CSF cultures.

Answer a is incorrect.   The likelihood of identifying bacteria by either Gram stain or culture significantly decreases if antibiotics are administered prior to CSF collection. However, best practice is not to withhold antibiotics while awaiting diagnostic testing, for example lumbar puncture, if it will result in a significant delay (30-60 min) in antibiotic administration to the patient.

Answer b is incorrect.   CSF Gram stain and culture are the most important tools for diagnosis of bacterial meningitis.

Answer c is incorrect.   Blood cultures may play an important role in diagnosis of bacterial meningitis. For instance, they may aid in bacterial identification if CSF culture is negative or they may assist in evaluating the source, extent, and/or prognosis of the infection.

15. The CSF culture is growing *N. meningitidis*. Close contacts of this patient needing chemoprophylaxis for meningococcal disease are identified. Which of the following are therapeutic options for chemoprophylaxis? Select all that apply.

    a. Ceftriaxone
    b. Vancomycin
    c. Ciprofloxacin
    d. Rifampin

Answer a is correct.   Ceftriaxone as a single intramuscular dose is a recommended option for chemoprophylaxis against meningococcal disease.

Answer c is correct.   Ciprofloxacin as a single oral dose is a recommended option for chemoprophylaxis against meningococcal disease.

Answer d is correct.   Rifampin as a 2-day oral regimen (given po q12h) is an option for chemoprophylaxis against meningococcal disease.

Answer b is incorrect.   Vancomycin is not a recommended option for chemoprophylaxis against meningococcal disease.

16. A 4-year-old girl with no significant past medical history is admitted for suspected bacterial meningitis and started on empiric therapy with ceftriaxone and vancomycin. What is the purpose of adding vancomycin to this empiric regimen for bacterial meningitis?

    a. To provide coverage against resistant *L. monocytogenes*
    b. To provide coverage against resistant *N. meningitidis*

c. To provide coverage against resistant *S. pneumoniae*
d. Vancomycin is not needed in a 4 year old with bacterial meningitis because *S. aureus* is unlikely

Answer c is correct. While third-generation cephalosporins, for example ceftriaxone, provide adequate coverage against most isolates of *S. pneumoniae*, some resistance has been reported. Vancomycin is added to provide empiric coverage against these resistant strains of *S. pneumoniae*.

Answer a is incorrect. *L. monocytogenes* is not a likely pathogen for bacterial meningitis in patients aged >1 month to 50 years. If the patient was a neonate or >50 years old, then empiric coverage for *L. monocytogenes* would be appropriate and ampicillin (not vancomycin) would be added to the regimen for this specific pathogen.

Answer b is incorrect. Ceftriaxone alone is sufficient empiric coverage for *N. meningitidis*.

Answer d is incorrect. *S. aureus* is not a likely pathogen for bacterial meningitis in otherwise healthy patients. Instead, vancomycin is used to provide empiric coverage against resistant *S. pneumoniae*.

17. The 4-year-old patient is diagnosed with bacterial meningitis secondary to *N. meningitidis*. This case is identified as being part of an outbreak in the patient's day care center. Which meningococcal vaccine is recommended for use in control of an outbreak caused by a vaccine-preventable serogroup of *N. meningitidis* (ie, A, C, Y, and W135)? Select all that apply.

a. Hib-MenCY
b. MCV4
c. MPSV4
d. MCV4, followed by administration of MPSV4

Answer a is correct. Hib-MenCY is a recommended option for use in controlling outbreaks secondary to serogroups C and Y in the age group for which it is licensed (6 weeks to 18 months).

Answer b is correct. MCV4 is a recommended option for use in controlling outbreaks secondary to serogroups A, C, Y, and W135. It is the preferred formulation in the age group for which it is licensed (9 months to 55 years).

Answer c is incorrect. MPSV4 is not currently recommended for use in controlling outbreaks of meningococcal disease.

Answer d is incorrect. MPSV4 is not currently recommended for use in controlling outbreaks of meningococcal disease. There is no recommendation suggesting the need for administration of MPSV4 following administration of MCV4 for this indication.

18. In which of the following groups has dexamethasone demonstrated a mortality benefit?

a. A 2 week old with *S. agalactiae* (group B) meningitis
b. A 17 year old with *N. meningitidis* meningitis

c. A 35 year old with *S. pneumoniae* meningitis
d. It has not demonstrated clear benefit for any type of bacterial meningitis

Answer c is correct. One randomized controlled trial and two subsequent meta-analyses have shown a mortality benefit of administering adjunctive corticosteroids in adult patients with *S. pneumoniae* meningitis.

Answer a is incorrect. There is a lack of data demonstrating a mortality benefit of adjunctive corticosteroids in *S. agalactiae* (group B) meningitis.

Answer b is incorrect. There is a lack of data demonstrating a mortality benefit of adjunctive corticosteroids in *N. meningitidis* meningitis.

Answer d is incorrect. A mortality benefit has been shown for adults with *S. pneumoniae* meningitis.

19. A 70-year-old man presents with fever, nausea, vomiting, severe headache, and extreme photophobia. CSF results: WBC 2500 cells/mm^3, 87% neutrophils, glucose 37 mg/dL, and protein 240 mg/dL. What type of CNS infection is considered based upon the information provided?

a. Bacterial meningitis
b. Aseptic meningitis
c. Viral encephalitis
d. HSV Encephalitis

Answer a is correct. Elevated WBC (1000-10,000 cells/mm^3), predominance of neutrophils (80%-90%), and elevated CSF protein (>100 mg/dL) as well as low CSF glucose (<40 mg/dL, and a likely CSF:serum glucose ratio of ≤0.4) are all consistent with bacterial meningitis.

Answer b is incorrect. Aseptic meningitis (commonly viral meningitis) would likely demonstrate lower CSF WBC, neutrophils, and protein than seen in this case, as well as a normal CSF glucose.

Answer c is incorrect. Viral encephalitis results in similar CSF changes as viral meningitis. It would likely demonstrate lower CSF WBC, neutrophils, and protein than seen in this case, as well as a normal CSF glucose.

Answer d is incorrect. Bacterial meningitis alone is the most likely CNS infection in this patient. A concurrent viral infection cannot be completely excluded based on the information provided, yet mixed bacterial/viral CNS infections would also likely have more mixed CSF findings.

20. Which of the following is consistent with the recommended antibacterial therapy for a 70-year-old patient with bacterial meningitis?

a. Vancomycin and ceftriaxone
b. Vancomycin, ceftriaxone, and ampicillin
c. Ampicillin and ceftriaxone
d. Ceftriaxone

Answer b is correct. Ceftriaxone provides appropriate empiric coverage for *N. meningitidis*, aerobic Gram-negative bacilli, and most *S. pneumoniae*. Vancomycin provides additional empiric coverage for multidrug-resistant *S. pneumoniae*. Ampicillin provides additional empiric coverage for *L. monocytogenes*.

Answer a is incorrect. Empiric coverage for *L. monocytogenes* with ampicillin is missing.

Answer c is incorrect. Empiric coverage for multidrug-resistant *S. pneumoniae* with vancomycin is missing.

Answer d is incorrect. Empiric coverage for *L. monocytogenes* with ampicillin is missing and empiric coverage for multidrug-resistant *S. pneumoniae* with vancomycin is missing.

21. The 70-year-old patient also has a significant past medical history of hypertension, diabetes, and stroke. What is the *optimal* order of events for delivery of care for this patient (assuming no delays in any of these procedures)?

Unordered Response	Ordered Response
Dexamethasone	Lumbar puncture for CSF culture
Lumbar puncture for CSF culture	Dexamethasone
Restart chronic home medications	Antibiotic therapy
Antibiotic therapy	Restart chronic home medications

CSF culture is the most important diagnostic tool and chances of bacterial identification decrease significantly if antibiotics are given beforehand. Lumbar puncture should be done first, as long as it does not result in significant delay in delivery of antibiotic therapy. Dexamethasone should be given before or with the first dose of antibiotics (not after). Management of CNS infections is a medical emergency. Reinitiating chronic home medications should occur as soon as possible following delivery of the more emergent care for suspected bacterial meningitis.

CHAPTER 26 | Sepsis Syndromes

1. Select the definition that describes a patient with septic shock.
   a. GH has the presence of bacteria within the blood.
   b. HH has a systemic inflammatory response to a clinical insult.
   c. JA has an infection associated with organ dysfunction.
   d. KS has an infection with persistent hypotension despite fluid resuscitation.

Answer d is correct. Adult patients with septic shock can be identified using the clinical criteria of hypotension requiring use of vasopressors to maintain mean blood pressure of 65 mm Hg or greater and having a serum lactate level greater than 2 mmol/L persisting after adequate fluid resuscitation.

Answer a is incorrect. Bacteremia (or fungemia) is the presence of viable bacteria (or fungi) within the bloodstream.

Answer b is incorrect. Systemic inflammatory responses to a variety of clinical insults can be either infectious or non-infectious.

Answer c is incorrect. This fits more with the definition of sepsis as outlined in the 2016 guideline update.

2. ZB is a patient with sepsis in the intensive care unit. ZB is currently receiving piperacillin/tazobactam, tobramycin, and vancomycin to treat his infection. The source of his infection is currently unknown. What type of organism(s) may cause septic shock? Select all that apply.
   a. Gram-positive bacteria
   b. Gram-negative bacteria
   c. Fungal species
   d. Viruses

Answer a is correct. Gram-positive and gram-negative bacteria, fungal species, and viruses cause sepsis. Gram-positive infections account for 30% to 50% of sepsis and septic shock cases. Additionally, multidrug resistant bacteria are responsible for approximately 25% of sepsis cases, are difficult to treat, and increase mortality.

Answer b is correct. Gram-negative bacteria sepsis cases represent 25% of cases and multidrug resistant bacteria are common.

Answer c is correct. The rate of fungal sepsis has increased 200% in recent years. This patient is not currently receiving fungal treatment. If the patient was not responding to the initial treatment a thorough evaluation of fungal risk factors should occur and empiric antifungal therapy should be considered.

Answer d is correct. Viral infections represent 4% of sepsis cases and could include viruses such as influenza and herpes simplex. An evaluation for risk factors and patient history should occur to guide consideration for empiric antiviral therapy.

3. Which of the following components make up the qSOFA score? Select all that apply.
   a. Respiratory rate ≥22
   b. Altered mentation
   c. Systolic blood pressure ≤100 mm Hg
   d. Diastolic blood pressure ≤60 mm Hg
   e. Heart rate ≥100 beats per minute

Answers a, b, and c are correct. Each of these components are criteria for calculating a qSOFA score which stands for Quick Sequential (Sepsis-Related) Organ Failure Assessment. If a patient has any two of these criteria, further investigation of infection and organ dysfunction should occur promptly with initiation or escalation of therapy.

Answers d and e are incorrect. While these criteria are important in evaluating and managing septic patients, they are not a part of the qSOFA score.

---

4. Which of the following may reduce or prevent morbidity and mortality associated with sepsis? Select all that apply.

   a. Preventing organ failures
   b. Early fluid resuscitation
   c. Acquisition of microbiologic cultures
   d. Administration of narrow spectrum anti-infectives

Answers a and b are correct. Reducing sepsis-related morbidity and mortality requires multiple interventions including preventing organ failure, early fluid resuscitation, and treating (and eliminating) infections.

Answer a – organ failure: The three most frequent organ dysfunctions are respiratory, circulatory, and renal. Septic shock is associated with several complications, including disseminated intravascular coagulation, acute respiratory distress syndrome, and multiple organ failure.

Answer b – early fluid resuscitation: Septic patients may have enormous fluid requirements as a result of peripheral vasodilation and capillary leakage. Fluids alone will reverse hypotension and restore hemodynamic stability in approximately 50% of septic hypotensive patients. Rapid fluid resuscitation improves the 28-day survival rate in patients with sepsis-induced hypoperfusion. The goal of fluid therapy is to maximize cardiac output by increasing the left ventricular preload, which will ultimately restore tissue perfusion. Fluid administration should be titrated based on a constellation of static and dynamic indices of fluid responsiveness, which may include central venous pressure, passive leg raise, and stroke volume variation, in conjunction with clinical endpoints, such as blood pressure, heart rate, and urine output. Increased serum lactate, a by-product of cellular anaerobic metabolism, should normalize as tissue perfusion improves. When fluid resuscitation alone provides inadequate arterial pressure and organ perfusion, vasopressors and inotropic agents should be initiated.

Answer c is incorrect. Microbiologic cultures (as clinically appropriate) should be obtained before anti-infective therapy as long as there is not a significant delay in obtaining (microbiologic cultures should be obtained within 45 minutes; do not withhold antibiotics if it takes longer than 45 minutes to obtain cultures). However, microbiologic cultures do not prevent morbidity and mortality. Administration of effective intravenous anti-infectives should be initiated within the first hour to improve morbidity and mortality.

Answer d is incorrect. Anti-infective therapy should be targeted against all likely pathogens and could include one or more drugs.

---

5. XJ is a 33-year-old woman (weight 70 kg) who presents with sepsis (hypotension and decreased urine output). Past medical history is significant for diabetes, hypertension, hypothyroidism, and gastroesophageal reflux. Medications include metformin, lisinopril, levothyroxine, and omeprazole. Select the appropriate initial regimen for fluid resuscitation in XJ.

   a. 5% dextrose 500 mL
   b. 5% albumin 1000 mL
   c. 0.9% sodium chloride 2000 mL
   d. 0.45% sodium chloride 2000 mL

Answer c is correct. It is appropriate to use 0.9% sodium chloride (normal saline) 1000 mL for fluid resuscitation in sepsis. Infusion of 1 L of 0.9% sodium chloride (isotonic saline) adds 275 mL to the plasma volume and 825 mL to the interstitial volume. Note that the total volume expansion (1100 mL) is slightly greater than the infused volume. This is the result of a fluid shift from the intracellular to extracellular space, which occurs because isotonic saline is actually hypertonic to the extracellular fluids.

Answer a is incorrect. Five percent dextrose is not an appropriate resuscitation fluid because only 8% of the administered volume stays intravascular. 5% glucose (dextrose) is widely used as a maintenance fluid (a substitute for patients unable to drink water) or to correct a free water deficit when oral fluids cannot be given. It has no place in the restoration of circulating volume because it is rapidly distributed throughout the entire body water compartment of about 40 liters.

Answer b is incorrect. Colloids, like albumin, can be used for fluid resuscitation in sepsis, especially in patients who cannot tolerate high volumes of fluid; however, only 300 to 500 mL should be used. They also should generally not be used for initial resuscitation but reserved for patients requiring large fluid volumes.

Answer d is incorrect. Sodium chloride 0.45% (1/2 normal saline) is not an appropriate fluid for resuscitation, because it provides only half of the intravascular volume that normal saline provides.

---

6. AA is a patient with hypotension secondary to sepsis. Past medical history is significant for heart failure with active fluid overload, hypertension, diabetes, previous myocardial infarction, and dyslipidemia. Medications include lisinopril, spironolactone, glipizide, metoprolol succinate, atorvastatin, and a baby aspirin. Labs were within normal limits except for a SCr of 1.9 mg/dL, glucose 180 mg/dL, and potassium of 5.6 mEq/L Select the appropriate colloid therapy for fluid resuscitation in this patient.

   a. 5% albumin 500 mL
   b. 5% dextrose 500 mL
   c. 0.45% sodium chloride with 5% dextrose 500 mL
   d. 0.45% sodium chloride 500 mL

Answer a is correct. Five percent albumin is a colloid resuscitation fluid used for patients at risk for fluid overload. Colloids are large molecules that do not pass across diffusional barriers as readily as crystalloids. The plasma expansion with albumin is nearly twice that produced by an equivalent volume of isotonic saline (500 mL vs 275 mL, respectively). In theory, colloid fluids infused into the vascular space should have a greater tendency to stay put and enhance the plasma volume than do crystalloid fluids. However, clinical superiority over crystalloid resuscitation has not been established and therefore isotonic crystalloids remain first-line resuscitation agents. In this case, no isotonic crystalloid answer is given and therefore answer a is correct.

Answer b is incorrect. Five percent dextrose is a crystalloid fluid and has no place in the restoration of circulating volume because it is rapidly distributed throughout the entire body water component of about 40 liters.

Answer c is incorrect. Sodium chloride 0.45% is a hypotonic crystalloid fluid and is inappropriate for fluid resuscitation. Five percent dextrose is a crystalloid fluid and has no place in the restoration of circulating volume because it is rapidly distributed throughout the entire body water component of about 40 liters.

Answer d is incorrect. Sodium chloride 0.45% is a hypotonic crystalloid fluid and is inappropriate for fluid resuscitation.

7. KT is a 65-year-old man with a history of end-stage renal disease on hemodialysis admitted with sepsis likely secondary to an infected dialysis catheter. KT was diagnosed 30 minutes ago and has not yet received intervention. Which of the following represents the best order of events to manage KT?

a. Vasopressors, fluids, microbiologic cultures, antimicrobial therapy
b. Vasopressors, antimicrobial therapy, microbiologic cultures, fluids
c. Fluids, microbiologic cultures, antimicrobial therapy, insulin for glucose >180 mg/dL
d. Fluids, antimicrobial therapy, microbiologic cultures, insulin for glucose >180 mg/dL

Answer c is correct. In patients with sepsis syndromes, early fluid resuscitation should be administered first. Microbiologic cultures should be collected prior to antimicrobial therapy, unless waiting for cultures might cause a significant delay in antibiotic administration (>45 minutes). A protocolized approach to insulin therapy is recommended for patients with sepsis when two consecutive blood glucose levels are >180 mg/dL.

Answer a is incorrect. In patients with sepsis syndromes, priority is placed on fluid resuscitation and antimicrobial therapy. Vasopressors are utilized for hypotension that does not respond to initial fluid resuscitation.

Answer b is incorrect. Priority should be placed on fluid resuscitation and antimicrobial therapy. Vasopressors are utilized for hypotension that does not respond to initial fluid resuscitation.

Answer d is incorrect. Microbiologic cultures should be obtained prior to administration of antimicrobial therapy to help ensure their accuracy.

8. TP is a 63-year-old male patient with a past medical history of hypertension, diabetes, chronic obstructive pulmonary disease, and dyslipidemia. Medications include amlodipine, metformin, tiotropium, albuterol as needed, and pravastatin. TP is diagnosed with sepsis. Pertinent labs include a pH of 7.25, white blood cell count of 13,500 cells/mm³, glucose of 170 mg/dL, serum creatinine of 2.3 mg/dL, and blood pressure of 85/43 mm Hg. What therapy should be administered within 1 hour of the recognition of sepsis?

a. Broad-spectrum antimicrobial therapy
b. Corticosteroids
c. Sodium bicarbonate
d. Vasopressor therapy

Answer a is correct. Administration of broad-spectrum antimicrobial(s) therapy within the first hour of recognition improves mortality in septic shock. Obtaining vascular access and starting aggressive fluid resuscitation are the first priorities when managing patients with septic shock. Prompt administration of anti-infective agent(s) is also a priority. Each hour delay in achieving administration of effective antibiotics is associated with an increase in mortality.

Answer b is incorrect. Optimal timing of corticosteroids in sepsis is not well-defined, but it most likely would not be within first hour. Additionally, adrenal insufficiency is no longer routinely assessed because hydrocortisone should NOT be used to treat sepsis IF fluid resuscitation or vasopressor therapy is able to restore hemodynamic stability. Fluid resuscitation and vasopressors (if needed) would be initiated prior to hydrocortisone therapy. Therefore, in cases where fluid resuscitation and vasopressor therapy do not achieve hemodynamic goals, intravenous hydrocortisone at a dose of 200 mg per day in divided daily doses may be used.

Answer c is incorrect. The sepsis guidelines recommend against using sodium bicarbonate for improving hemodynamics or reducing vasopressor requirements in patients with hypoperfusion-induced lactic acidosis with a pH > 7.15. Effects of bicarbonate on patients with a pH < 7.15 are not currently known.

Answer d is incorrect. There is no specific timing of vasopressor therapy in sepsis. It should be administered in patients with persistent hypotension following aggressive fluid resuscitation.

9. SL is a 32-year-old man with sepsis secondary to an intra-abdominal abscess. He has no significant past medical history and currently has been fluid resuscitated with an MAP of 70 mm Hg. What is the best treatment plan for SL?

a. Cefoxitin 2 g IV every 6 hours and transfer to the intensive care unit

b. Cefoxitin 2 g IV every 6 hours and surgical drainage of the abscess
c. Amoxicillin/clavulanic acid 875 mg/125 mg po every 12 hours and transfer to the intensive care unit
d. Amoxicillin/clavulanic acid 875 mg/125 mg po every 12 hours and surgical drainage of the abscess

Answer b is correct.   Intravenous antimicrobial therapy with cefoxitin is appropriate because it provides coverage of enteric gram-negatives and anaerobes likely to be present in an intra-abdominal abscess. In addition, treatment of abscesses should include surgical drainage (referred to as source control within sepsis guidelines), as antimicrobial therapy alone is unlikely to be curative. The principles of source control include rapid diagnosis of the specific infection site and identification of a focus of infection amenable to source control measures (eg, drainage of an abscess, debridement of necrotic tissue, removal of infected device).

Answer a is incorrect.   Intravenous antimicrobial therapy with cefoxitin is appropriate because it provides coverage of enteric gram-negatives and anaerobes likely to be present in an intra-abdominal abscess. However, definitive management and treatment of abscesses must include surgical drainage (source control). The patient's hemodynamic status is stable after fluid resuscitation so escalation of care to an intensive care unit is not necessary.

Answer c is incorrect.   Oral antimicrobial therapy initially is inappropriate in a patient with sepsis and hypotension. In addition, abscesses require surgical drainage.

Answer d is incorrect.   Although surgical drainage of the abscess is warranted, initial oral therapy is inappropriate in a patient with sepsis.

10. XC is a 41-year-old patient admitted to the intensive care unit for septic shock. Appropriate therapy was initiated within the desired times. The critical care attending asks the pharmacy student during rounds how long antimicrobial therapy should be continued for XC. Select the duration of antimicrobial therapy in most patients with septic shock.

a. 1 to 3 days
b. 3 to 5 days
c. 7 to 10 days
d. 24 to 28 days

Answer c is correct.   Although not specifically studied, guidelines recommend 7 to 10 days of antimicrobial therapy in sepsis syndromes. Longer courses of therapy may be appropriate in patients demonstrating a slow clinical response, undrainable source of infection, or bacteremia with *Staphylococcus aureus*.

Answer a is incorrect.   One to three days of therapy is too short for sepsis.

Answer b is incorrect.   A duration of therapy of 3 to 5 days is too short for sepsis; however, the 3 to 5 day time interval is discussed within the sepsis guidelines. Empiric combination therapy should not be administered for more than 3 to 5 days. De-escalation therapy should be employed based upon results of culture and susceptibility reports.

Answer d is incorrect.   Sepsis is a severe life-threatening infection; however, most patients do not benefit from an extended duration of therapy.

11. UC is a patient in the medical intensive care unit with a diagnosis of septic shock. During rounds the pulmonary critical care attending questions the pharmacy student about the utilization of corticosteroids. Which corticosteroid should be used to treat patients with septic shock refractory to aggressive fluid resuscitation and vasopressor therapy?

a. Prednisone
b. Hydrocortisone
c. Methylprednisolone
d. Dexamethasone

Answer b is correct.   Hydrocortisone therapy has been studied and is recommended in patients with septic shock refractory to aggressive fluid resuscitation and vasopressors. NOTE: hydrocortisone should not be used as a treatment of adult septic shock patients that respond to fluid resuscitation or vasopressor therapy.

Answer a is incorrect.   Prednisone has not been studied in patients with septic shock.

Answer c is incorrect.   Methylprednisolone has not been studied in patients with septic shock.

Answer d is incorrect.   Dexamethasone was *previously* used in sepsis prior to the return of cortisol levels when adrenal insufficiency is suspected. NOTE: The ACTH stimulation test should *not* be used to identify patients who should receive corticosteroid therapy. The use of dexamethasone and the ACTH stimulation test are *old recommendations*. Current recommendations are for hydrocortisone in hypotensive patients that did not respond to fluid resuscitation and vasopressor therapy (no ACTH stimulation test needed).

12. What is the brand name for hydrocortisone?

a. Deltasone
b. Sterapred
c. Solu-Medrol
d. Solu-Cortef

Answer d is correct.   Solu-Cortef is the brand name for hydrocortisone.

Answer a is incorrect.   Deltasone is the brand name for prednisone.

Answer b is incorrect.   Sterapred is the brand name for prednisone.

Answer c is incorrect. Solu-Medrol is the brand name for methylprednisolone.

The Following Case Pertains to Questions 13 and 14.

13. LA is a patient in the medical intensive care unit with sepsis. Past medical history includes hypertension, myocardial infarction 3 years ago, dyslipidemia, and gastroesophageal reflux. Medications include lisinopril, metoprolol, atorvastatin, aspirin and omeprazole. Labs include: white blood cell count of 12,000 cells/mm³, serum creatinine 1.8 mg/dL, and blood glucose 190 mg/dL. What is the goal blood glucose for patients with sepsis?

    a. 80 to 110 mg/dL
    b. ≤120 mg/dL
    c. ≤150 mg/dL
    d. 140 to 180 mg/dL

Answer d is correct. A protocolized approach to blood glucose management in ICU patients with sepsis is recommended when two consecutive blood glucose levels are greater than 180 mg/dL. The target upper blood glucose level is less than or equal to 180 mg/dL. Additionally, blood glucose values should be monitored every 1 to 2 hours until the glucose and insulin infusion rates are stable. At that time monitoring should be every 4 hours. Glucose levels obtained with point of care testing of capillary blood should be interpreted with caution, because it may not accurately estimate arterial blood or plasma glucose values.

Answer a is incorrect. The range for normal blood glucose is 80 to 100 mg/dL (normal host, non-septic patient).

Answer b is incorrect. Less than 120 mg/dL is not the range for blood glucose in patients with sepsis.

Answer c is incorrect. Previous sepsis guidelines recommended a target blood glucose in patients with sepsis of less than 150 mg/dL.

14. Select the most appropriate regimen for glycemic control in LA. Select all that apply.

    a. Metformin 1000 mg po bid
    b. Sitagliptin 100 mg po daily
    c. Insulin glargine 50 units qhs
    d. Regular insulin infusion

Answer d is correct. Insulin infusion is appropriate for a patient with sepsis because it is rapidly titrated and can accommodate the rapid changes in blood glucose seen in patients with sepsis.

Answer a is incorrect. Oral antihyperglycemic therapy is inappropriate in a patient with sepsis. Additionally, the patient has a contraindication to metformin therapy (Serum creatinine is 1.8 mg/dL).

Answer b is incorrect. Oral antihyperglycemic therapy is inappropriate in a patient with sepsis.

Answer c is incorrect. Insulin glargine is a long-acting insulin. Patients with sepsis need insulin therapy that can be rapidly titrated.

15. VB is admitted to the medical intensive care unit with sepsis and acute respiratory failure requiring mechanical ventilation. She is currently receiving crystalloid resuscitation, doripenem and amikacin. The critical care attending requests pharmacy to handle the nutrition recommendations for VB as it has been nearly a week prior to admission that VB has had any nutritional intake. Which of the following nutrition regimens is (are) most appropriate in a patient with sepsis secondary to pneumonia with a functioning GI tract?

    a. Continuous tube feeding via a nasoduodenal tube
    b. Parenteral nutrition via a central IV catheter
    c. Parenteral nutrition via a peripheral IV catheter
    d. Intravenous glucose

Answer a is correct. Parenteral nutrition increases a patient's risk for infection and should be avoided unless a patient cannot be fed via the enteral route. Continuous tube feeding into the small intestine will avoid this risk and this location in the gut will decrease the risk for aspiration.

Answer b is incorrect. Parenteral nutrition increases a patient's risk for infection and should be avoided unless a patient cannot be fed via the enteral route. In a patient with pneumonia, the patient's gastrointestinal tract is unlikely to be affected and is an appropriate route for feeding.

Answer c is incorrect. Parenteral nutrition increases a patient's infection risk. In addition, parenteral nutrition is not typically given via a peripheral line.

Answer d is incorrect. Within the first 48 hours after a diagnosis of sepsis or septic shock, oral or enteral (if necessary) feedings should be administered rather than complete fasting or intravenous glucose.

16. Which of the following is a risk factor for stress-induced gastrointestinal bleeding? Select all that apply.

    a. Mechanical ventilation ≥48 hours
    b. Coagulopathy
    c. Warfarin therapy (Therapeutic INR)
    d. Hypertension

Answer a is correct. Mechanical ventilation induces physiologic stress and is a risk factor for stress-induced GI bleeding when used more than or equal to 48 hours.

Answer b is correct. Coagulopathy for any reason increases a patient's risk for GI bleeding.

Answer c is correct. Warfarin therapy induces a pharmacologic coagulopathy and increases a patient's risk for GI bleeding.

Answer d is incorrect. Patients with sepsis have hypotension. Hypertension does NOT appear to be a risk factor for the development of a stress ulcer.

---

17. RE is a patient with sepsis from an *Escherichia coli* urinary tract infection. RE is receiving ertapenem for management of the infection. Select the medication that may be used for RE for stress-ulcer prophylaxis. RE does not have any risk factors for the development of a stress ulcer. Select all that apply.

    a. Proton pump inhibitor
    b. H$_2$ blocker
    c. Sucralfate
    d. Prophylaxis is not recommended

Answer d is correct. Stress ulcer prophylaxis is not recommended in patients without risk factors. Risk factors (coagulopathy, mechanical ventilation for 48 hours, hypotension) are often present in patients with sepsis or septic shock. However, RE does not exhibit any risk factors.

Answers a and b are incorrect. Proton pump inhibitors and H$_2$ blockers are recommended for the prophylaxis of stress ulcers to patients with sepsis or septic shock who have bleeding risk factors. Additionally, the benefit of prevention of upper GI bleeding must be weighed against the potential effect of increased stomach pH on a greater incidence of VAP and *Clostridium difficile* infection. Additionally, if prophylaxis is used, patients should be periodically evaluated for the continued need for prophylaxis.

Answer c is incorrect. Suppression of acid production is the recommended treatment modality for stress ulcer prophylaxis. Therefore, sucralfate (barrier protection) is not recommended.

---

18. QP is a 68-year-old man diagnosed with sepsis. Past medical history includes heart failure (ejection fraction 25%), diabetes, and dyslipidemia. Patient was initially hospitalized for a heart failure exacerbation (20 lb of fluid overload). Select the initial fluid resuscitation for QP.

    a. Dextrose
    b. Albumin
    c. Hydroxyethyl starch
    d. 0.45% normal saline

Answer b is correct. Albumin is recommended for fluid resuscitation of sepsis and septic shock when patients require substantial amounts of crystalloids. Given the patients past medical history of heart failure and his current exacerbation, administration of albumin would be recommended.

Answer a is incorrect. Dextrose is a crystalloid fluid and has no place in the restoration of circulating volume because it is rapidly distributed throughout the entire body water component of about 40 liters.

Answer c is incorrect. The sepsis guidelines recommend against the use of hydroxyethyl starch for fluid resuscitation in sepsis and septic shock.

Answer d is incorrect. Sodium chloride 0.45% (1/2 normal saline) is not an appropriate fluid for resuscitation, because it provides only half of the intravascular volume that normal saline provides.

---

19. CX is an adult patient in septic shock. Crystalloid fluid resuscitation at 40 mL/kg did not improve hemodynamics. Further assessment of CX's clinical variables indicate that he is not fluid responsive. Select the agent to increase CX's blood pressure.

    a. Normal saline
    b. Norepinephrine
    c. Dopamine
    d. Phenylephrine

Answer b is correct. Norepinephrine is recommended as the vasopressor of choice by the sepsis guidelines. Norepinephrine increases MAP by its vasoconstriction effects, with little change in heart rate and less increase in stroke volume as compared to dopamine. Norepinephrine is more potent than dopamine and may be more effective at reversing hypotension in patient with septic shock.

Answer a is incorrect. Adult patients with septic shock can be identified using the clinical criteria of hypotension requiring use of vasopressors to maintain mean blood pressure of 65 mm Hg or greater and having a serum lactate level greater than 2 mmol/L persisting after adequate fluid resuscitation. Therefore, a vasopressor should be utilized in the hemodynamic management for septic shock patients. Therefore, a vasopressor should be utilized in the hemodynamic management for septic shock patients who are not fluid responsive.

Answer c is incorrect. Dopamine is an alternative vasopressor to norepinephrine only in select patients. Dopamine increases MAP and cardiac output, primarily due to an increase in stroke volume and heart rate. Dopamine may be useful in patients with compromised systolic function but causes more tachycardia and may be more arrhythmogenic than norepinephrine.

Answer d is incorrect. Phenylephrine is not recommended in the treatment of septic shock except in select situations; such as when norepinephrine has been associated with serious arrhythmias; when cardiac output is known to be high and blood pressure persistently low; when salvage therapy including combined inotrope/vasopressor drugs and low dose vasopressin have failed to achieve MAP goal, or in patients with active coronary ischemia in order to decrease the risk of worsening the ischemia as compared to norepinephrine or dopamine.

20. ER is a patient in septic shock currently receiving vasopressor therapy and broad spectrum anti-infective therapy. ER has continued signs of hypoperfusion (although he has achieved adequate intravascular volume and MAP). ER is currently receiving a low dose of norepinephrine. What inotropic agent should be utilized to manage his continued hypoperfusion?

    a. Vasopressin
    b. Dopamine
    c. Dobutamine
    d. Phenylephrine

Answer c is correct. A trial of dobutamine (up to 20 mcg/kg/min) may be administered or added to vasopressor therapy (if in use) if a patient exhibits ongoing signs of hypoperfusion, despite achieving adequate intravascular volume and adequate MAP. Additionally, a dobutamine trial may be used in the presence of myocardial dysfunction as suggested by elevated cardiac filling pressures and low cardiac output.

Answer a is incorrect. Vasopressin is a vasopressor that can be added to norepinephrine with the intent of either raising MAP or decreasing norepinephrine dosage.

Answer b is incorrect. Dopamine is an alternative vasopressor to norepinephrine only in select patients. Dopamine increases MAP and cardiac output, primarily due to an increase in stroke volume and heart rate. Dopamine may be useful in patients with compromised systolic function but causes more tachycardia and may be more arrhythmogenic than norepinephrine.

Answer d is incorrect. Phenylephrine is not recommended in the treatment of septic shock except in select situations such as the following: to decrease the risk of serious arrhythmias compared to norepinephrine or dopamine; when cardiac output is known to be high and blood pressure persistently low; and as salvage therapy when combined inotrope/vasopressor drugs and low dose vasopressin have failed to achieve MAP goal.

21. KJ is an 87-kg male receiving a norepinephrine infusion (4 mg/250 mL) at 2 mcg/kg/min for management of his septic shock. At what rate (mL/h) should the infusion be administered?

    a. 652.5 mL/h
    b. 652,500 mL/h
    c. 7.5 mL/h
    d. 10.9 mL/h

Answer a is correct. Infusion concentration = 4 mg/250 mL = 0.016 mg/mL = 16 mcg/mL

2 mcg/kg/min × 87 kg = 174 mcg/min × 60 min/1 h = 10,440 mcg/h

10,440 mcg/x mL = 16 mcg/1 mL

x= 652.5 mL

In clinical practice, often when rates of this magnitude are needed the pharmacy can compound bags with much higher concentrations so that nursing does not have to change the bag so often.

Answer b is incorrect. The incorrect concentration (0.016 mcg/mL) was used in the calculations.

Answer c is incorrect. Weight was not included in the calculation.

Answer d is incorrect. This is the rate calculated in mL/min.

22. JZ is a 48-year-old man admitted to the hospital with sepsis. He receives initial therapy with fluid resuscitation and antibiotic therapy but remains hypotensive. The physician decides to initiate therapy with a norepinephrine continuous infusion and phones the pharmacy for dosing recommendations. What reference(s) would be appropriate to find information on appropriate dosing? Select all that apply.

    a. *Drug Information Handbook*
    b. *Micromedex*
    c. PubMed
    d. *Drug Facts and Comparisons*
    e. Lexi-Comp

Answer a is correct. *Drug Information Handbook* is a tertiary reference that contains dosing information.

Answer b is correct. *Micromedex* is a tertiary reference that contains dosing information.

Answer d is correct. *Drug Facts and Comparisons* is a tertiary reference that contains dosing information.

Answer e is correct. Lexi-Comp is an appropriate tertiary reference that contains dosing information.

Answer c is incorrect. PubMed is a secondary reference that compiles primary literature. While dosing information can be found, specifics related to sepsis and dosing can be difficult to locate.

23. BD is a 44-year-old man with severe alcoholism who is intubated due to hypoxia from community-acquired pneumonia complicated by sepsis. Which of the following sedation regimens if given via continuous infusion may induce a metabolic acidosis?

    a. Ativan
    b. Precedex
    c. Valium
    d. Versed

Answer a is correct. Ativan contains propylene glycol in its diluent which can result in an osmolar gap metabolic acidosis when given in high doses as a continuous infusion. High doses of benzodiazepines are often given in alcoholic patients in alcohol withdrawal in order to prevent symptoms such as delirium tremens.

Answer b is incorrect. Precedex does not induce a metabolic acidosis. The two major side effects of Precedex are hypotension and bradycardia, especially with loading doses.

Answer c is incorrect. Valium is rarely given as a continuous infusion and does not cause a metabolic acidosis.

Answer d is incorrect. Versed does not cause a metabolic acidosis.

---

24. Which of the following is the generic name of Precedex?
    a. Dexamethasone
    b. Dexmedetomidine
    c. Dextroamphetamine
    d. Dextromethorphan

Answer b is correct. Precedex is the brand name for dexmedetomidine.

Answer a is incorrect. Decadron is the brand name of dexamethasone.

Answer c is incorrect. Dexedrine or Dextrostat are brand names of dextroamphetamine.

Answer d is incorrect. There are many brand names for dextromethorphan such as Delsym.

---

25. LL is an 80-year-old woman who was admitted to the ICU with presumed sepsis due to a urinary tract infection. Upon review of the medical record, you note that the patient has several allergies including heparin (history of heparin-induced thrombocytopenia 1 month ago) and also penicillin (anaphylaxis). Which of the following is recommended in LL to prevent the occurrence of venous thromboembolism?
    a. Unfractionated heparin 5000 units SQ every 8 hours
    b. Enoxaparin 40 mg SQ every 24 hours
    c. Rivaroxaban 20 mg po daily with food
    d. Mechanical prophylaxis only (eg, graduated compression stockings or intermittent compression devices)

Answer d is correct. In patients who have a contraindication to heparin use (eg, thrombocytopenia, severe coagulopathy, active bleeding, recent intracerebral hemorrhage, or heparin allergy) the guidelines recommend mechanical prophylaxis only.

Answer a is incorrect. Although unfractionated heparin and low-molecular weight heparins are recommended for DVT prophylaxis, this patient has a recent history of heparin-induced thrombocytopenia. Chemical prophylaxis should be avoided.

Answer b is incorrect. Although unfractionated heparin and low-molecular weight heparins are recommended for DVT prophylaxis, this patient has a recent history of heparin-induced thrombocytopenia. Chemical prophylaxis should be avoided.

Answer c is incorrect. Rivaroxaban is approved for the prevention of venous thromboembolism in patients undergoing orthopedic surgery, for stroke prevention in non-valvular

atrial fibrillation and treatment of DVT or pulmonary embolism. The 20-mg dose is used for either atrial fibrillation or venous thromboembolism treatment.

---

26. Which of the following best describes the hemodynamic properties of norepinephrine?
    a. Minimal α- and β-adrenergic agonist effects
    b. Potent α-adrenergic activity with less potent β-adrenergic agonist properties
    c. Potent β-adrenergic agonist effects and minimal α-adrenergic effects
    d. Potent α- and β-adrenergic agonist properties

Answer b is correct. Norepinephrine is an endogenous catecholamine with potent α_1 and less potent β_1 adrenergic activity which primarily is utilized to increase systemic vascular resistance and blood pressure. Compared to dopamine, norepinephrine is more potent in terms of vasopressor activity and is less arrhythmogenic.

Answer a is incorrect. Minimal α- and β-adrenergic effects would likely correspond to low dose dopamine. At a low range, dopamine demonstrates agonist activity at dopaminergic receptors. Higher doses must be achieved in order to stimulate β and α receptors.

Answer c is incorrect. Dobutamine is a synthetic sympathomimetic amine with potent β-adrenergic agonist activity and minor α-adrenergic effects. Therefore, hemodynamic effects include an increase in cardiac output through an increase in heart rate and contractility.

Answer d is incorrect. Epinephrine is an endogenous catecholamine with potent α- and β-adrenergic activity.

CHAPTER 27 | **Human Immunodeficiency Virus**

1. YP is a patient recently diagnosed with HIV. The patient presents to your pharmacy to fill a prescription for Triumeq. During the counseling session, YP ask the pharmacist, when is a person living with HIV classified as having AIDS? Select all that apply.
    a. Diagnosis of *Pneumocystis jiroveci* pneumonia
    b. CD4 count of 350 μL
    c. HIV viral load of >100,000 copies/mL
    d. CD4 count of 150 μL
    e. CD4% of 10%

Answer a is correct. *P. jiroveci* (formerly known as *P. carinii*) pneumonia is considered an AIDS defining condition, so an HIV patient with this diagnosis would be considered to have progressed to AIDS. Other AIDS defining conditions include esophageal candidiasis, Kaposi's sarcoma, and *Mycobacterium avium* complex.

Answers d and e are correct. A CD4 count of ≤200 μL, CD4% of <14%, or development of an AIDS defining condition indicates an AIDS diagnosis.

Answer b is incorrect. A CD4 count of ≤200 μL or development of an AIDS defining condition indicates an AIDS diagnosis.

Answer c is incorrect. An AIDS classification is independent of viral load.

---

2. LF is a 31-year-old male patient recently diagnosed with HIV. He presents to the HIV clinic for the first time and is eager to start treatment, what is your most appropriate course of action? Select all that apply.

   a. Begin therapy with TFV, emtricitabine, and efavirenz
   b. Counsel the patient regarding HIV, transmission, prevention of transmission to others, answer his questions, and schedule another follow-up visit
   c. Obtain baseline viral load and CD4
   d. Begin therapy with emtricitabine, lamivudine, darunavir/ritonavir
   e. Obtain genotype

Answer b is correct. Newly diagnosed HIV patients need extensive counseling regarding the disease, how to prevent transmission and need their questions answered. Follow-up visits are necessary to review labs and evaluate the patients understanding of the disease. Follow-up appointments can be used to assess if patients are candidates for therapy, because if they miss follow-up appointments, they are likely not be adherent to HIV therapy.

Answer c is correct. Baseline labs are required to determine if opportunistic infection prophylaxis is indicated and to have a baseline CD4 and viral load to measure treatment effectiveness (if antiretrovirals are started).

Answer e is correct. When antiretroviral treatment is started, a minimum of three agents is required. Three active agents are associated with increased viral suppression and CD4+ cell count. Therefore, naïve and treatment experienced patients should have therapy guided by a genotype or phenotype resistance profile.

Answers a and d are incorrect. Patients diagnosed with HIV are not immediately started on drug therapy. Baseline labs need to be obtained to determine if therapy is indicated and the patient's likelihood of compliance needs to be assessed. If a patient is not going to be compliant/adherent, it is best to hold therapy until patient is ready to commit. Answer a is a regimen that can be utilized as cART, when it is time to start therapy. Additionally, this regimen is available as a single tablet therapy (Atripla). Answer d is a regimen that CANNOT be utilized as cART. Although NRTIs are utilized together, there are select NRTIs that are contraindicated (emtricitabine and lamivudine; stavudine and zidovudine). Foundation pharmacologic principles for combination therapy include using medications with a different mechanism of action (this is for most disease states, not just HIV). Although HIV therapy often utilizes at least two NRTIs concurrently, they actually have a different mechanism of action; however, we have to use NRTIs with different DNA base pairs. Recall the primary nucleobases are cytosine (DNA and RNA), guanine (DNA and RNA), adenine (DNA and RNA), thymine (DNA) and uracil (RNA), abbreviated as C, G, A, T, and U, respectively. If you review the names for the NRTIs, you will see which ones can and cannot be used together. For example zidovudine (AZT) and stavudine (D4T) are the same base pairs. Additionally, lamivudine (3TC) and emtricitabine (FTC) are the same base pairs and cannot be utilized together.

---

3. Select the signs and symptoms of primary HIV infection (acute infection) in an adult patient. Select all that apply.

   a. Mononucleosis-like illness (fever, sore-throat, fatigue, weight loss)
   b. GI-upset (nausea, vomiting, diarrhea)
   c. Lymphadenopathy
   d. Night sweats

Answers a, b, c, and d are correct. Mononucleosis-like illness (fever, sore-throat, fatigue, weight loss), gastrointestinal (GI) upset (nausea, vomiting, diarrhea), lymphadenopathy, and night sweats are all signs and symptoms of primary HIV infection in adult patients. Symptoms are typically self-limiting, resolving often without intervention. Pediatric patients that acquire infection perinatally typically do not have symptoms.

---

4. Which of the following statements about HIV prevention is TRUE?

   a. Condoms are 100% effective in preventing HIV transmission.
   b. All pregnant women should be screened for HIV.
   c. Only pregnant women who engage in high-risk behaviors should be screened for HIV.
   d. IV drug abusers can reuse/share syringe hubs as long as a new needle is used.

Answer b is correct. Pregnant women should be screened for HIV. Patients that are positive should be initiated on ART to decrease her viral load and decrease the chance of transmitting the infection to the infant.

Answer a is incorrect. Abstinence is the only 100% effective way to prevent sexual transmission of HIV. While condoms may reduce transmission rates, they are not 100% effective.

Answer c is incorrect. All pregnant women should be screened for HIV; however, nonpregnant persons engaging in high risk behaviors should be routinely screened for HIV.

Answer d is incorrect. Sharing of any drug paraphernalia can cause HIV transmission (not just needles).

5. A patient presents to the hospital with a 2-week history of a mono-like illness. Basic metabolic and complete blood count tests are within normal limits and an ELISA test is negative (nonreactive). The patient reports being sexually active with multiple partners. Which of the following counseling points should be discussed with the patient? Select all that apply.

    a. Inform her she most likely had viral sinusitis.
    b. Inform her that she does not have HIV.
    c. Inform her that she will need to complete a follow-up ELISA in 1 month to evaluate for HIV.
    d. Provide counseling on HIV and STD prevention.

Answers c and d are correct. The patient should have a follow-up ELISA screen in 1 month since. After the acute syndrome, HIV antibody production takes 2 to 4 weeks and up to 6 months, so this patient may have a false negative ELISA. However, given her high risk behavior it is important that she be counseled about HIV and STD prevention.

Answer a is incorrect. An ELISA is not utilized to evaluate patients for a viral sinusitis.

Answer b is incorrect. After the acute syndrome, HIV antibody production takes 3 to 4 weeks and up to 6 months, so this patient may have a false negative ELISA.

6. In a patient receiving zidovudine therapy, which of the following could you expect to be elevated on laboratory evaluation?

    a. Blood urea nitrogen (BUN)
    b. Mean corpuscular volume (MCV)
    c. SCr
    d. Potassium

Answer b is correct. MCV is a marker of RBC size and utilized in the diagnosis of anemia. An elevated MCV is common with zidovudine therapy as a result of macrocytic anemia. This can be used as an indirect marker of patient adherence to therapy.

Answers a and c are incorrect. Zidovudine is not expected to affect BUN levels or SCr creatinine levels. However, the NRTI TFV does affect renal filtration and monitoring of BUN and SCr is required.

Answer d is incorrect. Zidovudine is not expected to impact potassium concentrations.

7. A treatment experienced patient receiving atazanavir therapy should avoid the addition of which of the following medications?

    a. Omeprazole
    b. Metronidazole
    c. Pravastatin
    d. Metoprolol

Answer a is correct. Atazanavir requires an acidic environment for optimal absorption. In treatment experienced patients, combination therapy with proton pump inhibitors is contraindicated. In treatment naïve patients, doses of omeprazole 20 mg equivalence or less, may be used *with caution*. The risk versus benefit should be weighed when combining these agents.

Answer b is incorrect. There is no known or anticipated drug interaction between metronidazole and atazanavir therapy.

Answer c is incorrect. There is no known or anticipated drug interaction between pravastatin and atazanavir therapy. Pravastatin (3-hydroxy-3-methylglutaryl-coenzyme [HMG-CoA] reductase inhibitors, also known as statins) does not undergo metabolism through the CYP450 enzyme system.

Answer d is incorrect. There is no known or anticipated drug interaction between metoprolol and atazanavir therapy.

8. Which of the following treatment regimens would be considered appropriate in a treatment naïve patient?

    a. Maraviroc + Efavirenz + Nevirapine
    b. Raltegravir + ABC + Indinavir + Ritonavir
    c. TFV + Zidovudine + ABC
    d. Lamviudine + Zidovudine + Lopinavir + Ritonavir

Answer d is correct. This regimen includes two NRTIs (lamivudine and zidovudine) plus a preferred boosted PI (lopinavir). The two NRTIs are different base pairs; therefore, they may be used concurrently as part of the antiretroviral regimen. The most commonly utilized NRTIs combinations include lamivudine plus abacavir OR emtricitabine plus tenofovir. The vast majority of patients receiving protease inhibitor therapy will be receiving the pharmacokinetic enhancer ritonavir. Lopinavir/ritonavir are coformulated (Kaletra). Recall that ritonavir is a PI, but it is not being utilized as a PI. Ritonavir is being used for drug interaction properties to decrease the metabolism of lopinavir, so patients do not have to take the medication as often. This is done in efforts to improve patient adherence.

Answer a is incorrect. Two NNRTIs (efavirenz and nevirapine) should not be used in combination. Additionally, there are no two NRTI backbones in this regimen and Maraviroc is utilized in treatment experienced patients.

Answer b is incorrect. There is only one NRTI (ABC) in this treatment regimen, whereas two are optimal for a complete NRTI backbone. Although indinavir plus ritonavir could be used, indinavir is not a preferred PI.

Answer c is incorrect. The triple combination of NRTI therapy is not preferred due to high failure rates.

9. In a patient with a history of acute or chronic pancreatitis, which of the following medications should be avoided?

    a. Didanosine
    b. Darunavir
    c. TFV
    d. Enfuvirtide

Answer a is correct. Didanosine is a known cause of drug-induced pancreatitis and should be avoided in patients with a history of pancreatitis. In cases of unavoidable use, risk versus benefit should be carefully weighed.

Answer b is incorrect. Darunavir is not associated with drug-induced pancreatitis.

Answer c is incorrect. TFV is not associated with drug-induced pancreatitis. Adverse effects from TFV are most commonly linked to renal impairment.

Answer d is incorrect. Enfuvirtide is not associated with drug-induced pancreatitis. Adverse effects from enfuvirtide are most commonly injection site reactions.

---

10. Which of the following properties are true regarding efavirenz? Select all that apply.

    a. Should be taken with a high fat meal
    b. Is a common cause of vivid dreams and hallucinations
    c. Is the NNRTI of choice in pregnancy
    d. Lacks significant drug interactions
    e. Teratogenic in nonhuman primates and potentially teratogenic in first trimester of pregnancy

Answer b is correct. Central nervous system adverse events of efavirenz include hallucinations, vivid dreams, and altered mental status. Dosing at bedtime on an empty stomach is preferred and may help with daytime symptoms.

Answer e is correct. Regarding embryo-fetal toxicity, the Food and Drug Administration (FDA) advises women to avoid becoming pregnant while taking efavirenz and healthcare providers to avoid administration in the first trimester of pregnancy as fetal harm may occur. However, efavirenz should be continued in pregnant women receiving a virologically suppressive EFV-based regimen, because ARV drug changes during pregnancy may be associated with loss of viral control and increased risk of perinatal transmission.

Answer a is incorrect. Taking efavirenz with a high-fat meal will result in significant increases in peak drug concentrations (Cmax). These increased concentrations may increase side effects, notably CNS-related adverse events. Therefore, efavirenz should be taken on an empty stomach.

Answer c is incorrect. Efavirenz is pregnancy category D, specifically during the first trimester. Careful risk versus benefit should be weighed if using this drug at any point during pregnancy, or in young females intending on becoming pregnant.

Answer d is incorrect. Efavirenz is associated with significant drug interactions. Efavirenz is a substrate, inhibitor, and inducer of the cytochrome P450 system.

---

11. Which of the following antiretrovirals is/are available in a parenteral form? Select all that apply.

    a. Zidovudine
    b. Etravirine
    c. Dolutegravir
    d. Rilpivirine
    e. Enfuvirtide

Answer a is correct. Zidovudine is available in the IV form (10 mg/mL IV solution).

Answer e is correct. Enfuvirtide is available in a parenteral (subcutaneous) form (90 mg/mL syringes).

Answer b is incorrect. Etravirine is only available as an oral capsule.

Answer c is incorrect. Dolutegravir is only available as oral tablet.

Answer d is incorrect. Rilpivirine is only available as an oral tablet.

---

12. Which of the following patients would be at highest risk for developing hepatotoxicity secondary to nevirapine therapy?

    a. 31-year-old woman with a CD4+ = 91 cells/mm^3
    b. 21-year-old man with CD4+ = 270 cells/mm^3
    c. 50-year-old man with CD4+ = 260 cells/mm^3
    d. 25-year-old woman with CD4+ = 265 cells/mm^3

Answer d is correct. Her CD4+ count is >250 cells/mm^3 putting this patient into a high risk category. Nevirapine is associated with severe hepatic dysfunction, especially in women with CD4+ counts >250 cells/mm^3 and men >400 cells/mm^3.

Answer a is incorrect. Females with CD4+ counts >250 cells/mm^3 are at an increased risk. Her CD4 count is below this threshold.

Answer b is incorrect. Males with CD4+ counts >400 cells/mm^3 are at an increased risk. His CD4+ count is below this threshold.

Answer c is incorrect. His CD4+ count is below the 400 cells/mm^3 threshold. Also, age has not been directly linked with increased risk of hepatotoxicity.

---

13. Which of the following combinations of antiretrovirals should be avoided because of contraindications?

    a. Rilpivirine and TFV
    b. Efavirenz and nevirapine
    c. Lamivudine and zidovudine
    d. Fosamprenavir and ritonavir

Answer b is correct. Efavirenz and nevirapine are NNRTIs. Dual NNRTI therapy is contraindicated.

Answer a is incorrect. Rilpivirine is an NNRTI and TFV is an NRTI. These drugs are commonly used together and are coformulated as part of Complera.

Answer c is incorrect. Lamivudine and zidovudine are both NRTIs and are coformulated together in Combivir. There are no contraindications to this combination.

Answer d is incorrect. Fosamprenavir and ritonavir are both PIs. Ritonavir is used in combination with fosamprenavir as a boosting agent, through its inhibition of CYP3A4 enzyme system.

---

14. Which of the following regarding Truvada® PrEP is true?

    a. Should only be given to HIV-positive patients.
    b. Should be administered under direct medical supervision in an emergency situation.
    c. Should be taken daily in high-risk patients to prevent acquisition of HIV.
    d. A negative HIV screening test is required monthly prior to prescribing.

Answer c is correct. PrEP should be taken daily on a continuous basis in HIV-negative individuals (eg, serodiscordant heterosexuals, IV drug users) to prevent acquisition.

Answer a is incorrect. PrEP is indicated in patients that are HIV negative to prevent acquisition.

Answer b is incorrect. PrEP should be taken daily on a continuous basis to prevent acquisition.

Answer d is incorrect. A maximum of 90-day prescriptions should be provided at one time. Prior to the next prescription, confirmation of a negative HIV test is required.

---

15. Dosing of *maraviroc* should be increased to 600 mg twice daily when combined with which of the following medications?

    a. Ketoconazole
    b. Clarithromycin
    c. Rifampin
    d. Warfarin

Answer c is correct. Rifampin is a potent *inducer* of CYP 3A and 2C. When a 3A4 inducer is combined with maraviroc, the dose should be increased to 600 mg twice daily.

Answer a is incorrect. Ketoconazole is a potent *inhibitor* of CYP 3A. When a 3A4 inhibitor is combined with maraviroc, the dose should be decreased to 150 mg twice daily.

Answer b is incorrect. Clarithromycin is a potent *inhibitor* of CYP 3A. When a 3A4 inhibitor is combined with maraviroc, the dose should be decreased to 150 mg twice daily.

Answer d is incorrect. Warfarin is a *substrate* of primarily CYP 3A and 2C. There would be no dose adjustment of maraviroc when the two are combined.

---

16. Which of the following is true regarding PEP?

    a. PEP should be administered within 1 week of HIV exposure.
    b. A two-drug regimen of TFV plus zidovudine is preferred for PEP.
    c. A three-drug regimen of TFV, emtricitabine, and raltegravir is preferred for PEP.
    d. Nevirapine should be included in PEP regimen when possible.

Answer c is correct. The three-drug regimen of Truvada® (TFV plus emtricitabine) plus raltegravir is preferred. Treatment should be started within 72 hours of exposure, but delayed treatment *may* still provide a benefit, particularly in high-risk exposure settings, and should be continued for 4 weeks. PEP consists of the NRTI backbone TFV plus emtricitabine plus twice daily raltegravir. PI-based regimens may be utilized as alternatives.

Answer a is incorrect. PEP should be administered as soon as possible after potential exposure and within 72 hours.

Answer b is incorrect. A three-drug regimen is preferred for PEP.

Answer d is incorrect. Nevirapine should be avoided due to increased risk of hepatotoxicity in patients with higher baseline CD4+ cell counts.

---

17. Which of the following is true regarding Stribild® therapy?

    a. This medication should be taken on an empty stomach at bedtime.
    b. This medication will commonly increase SCr value.
    c. This medication should only be used in patients with an eGFR <60 mL/min.
    d. This medication will commonly increase indirect bilirubin.

Answer b is correct. The cobicistat boosting agent commonly increases SCr without impacting renal function. The increase in SCr will affect the calculated estimated glomerular filtration (eGFR), but will not affect the actual glomerular filtration.

Answer a is incorrect. Stribild® should be taken with a meal to maximize bioavailability.

Answer c is incorrect. Stribild® should not be used in patients with CrCl <70mL/min because the individual agents requiring varied dose adjustments in renal dysfunction.

Answer d is incorrect. Stribild® has not been commonly associated with increases in indirect bilirubin. The PI atazanavir is commonly associated with this lab abnormality.

---

18. Which of the following laboratory tests should be evaluated on a patient prior to starting ABC therapy?

    a. MCV
    b. Hemoglobin
    c. SCr
    d. HLA-B*5701

Answer d is correct. The abacavir hypersensitivity reaction (ABC HSR) is a multiorgan clinical syndrome typically seen within the initial 6 weeks of ABC treatment. This reaction has been reported in 5% to 8% of patients participating in clinical trials when using clinical criteria for the diagnosis and it is the major reason for early discontinuation of ABC. Discontinuing ABC usually promptly reverses HSR, whereas subsequent rechallenge can cause a rapid, severe, and even life-threatening recurrence Several groups have reported a highly significant association between ABC HSR and the presence of the major histocompatibility complex (MHC) class I allele HLA-B*5701. Recommendations include:

1. Screening for HLA-B*5701 before starting patients on an ABC-containing regimen to reduce the risk of HSR.
2. HLA-B*5701-positive patients should not be prescribed ABC.
3. The positive status should be recorded as an ABC allergy in the patient's medical record.
4. When HLA-B*5701 screening is not readily available, it is reasonable to initiate ABC with appropriate clinical counseling and monitoring for any signs of HSR.

Answers a, b, and c are incorrect. ABC is not expected to impact or be affected by MCV, hemoglobin, or SCr.

19. Which of the following medications has hepatitis B virus (HBV) activity and if stopped in a patient with HBV, may cause a hepatitis flare? Select all that apply.

   a. Emtricitabine
   b. Nevirapine
   c. Lamivudine
   d. TFV
   e. ABC

Answers a, c, and d are correct. Emtricitabine, lamivudine, and TFV have HBV activity. In a coinfected patient with HIV and HBV, if a patient stops the medication a flare of the HBV could occur.

Answers b and e are incorrect. Nevirapine and ABC do not have HBV activity.

20. Which of the following HIV medications is associated with increased bilirubin?

   a. Acyclovir
   b. Atazanavir
   c. ABC
   d. TFV

Answer b is correct. Atazanavir therapy (similar to indinavir) causes an increase in unconjugated (indirect) and total serum bilirubin that can manifest as jaundice in up to 10% of patients. The jaundice, however, is not indicative of hepatic injury. These elevations are due to the inhibition of UDP (Uridine 5'-diphospho) glucuronyl transferase, the hepatic enzyme responsible for conjugation of bilirubin. The hyperbilirubinemia is usually mild, the increases averaging 0.3 to 0.5 mg/dL.

Answers a is incorrect. Acyclovir is an antiviral medication; however, it is not utilized for HIV management nor is it associated with increased bilirubin.

Answers c and d are incorrect. ABC and TFV are commonly used HIV medications belonging to the nucleoside reverse transcriptase inhibitor class. However, they are not associated with increased bilirubin.

21. Based upon the development of central nervous system side effects, which of the following NNRTIs would you expect to have the highest concentration distributed into the CNS? Select all that apply.

   a. Viramune
   b. Sustiva
   c. Atripla
   d. Stribild

Answers b and c are correct. Efavirenz is associated with central nervous system side effects and include hallucinations and vivid dreams. The brand name of efavirenz is Sustiva; however, efavirenz is also part of the STR Atripla.

Answer a is incorrect. Nevirapine (Viramune) is an NNRTI, but is not associated with significant CNS side effects. The main side effects of nevirapine are rash and hepatotoxicity.

Answer d is incorrect. Stribild does not contain an NNRTI and is not associated with significant CNS side effects.

22. Place the following NNRTIs in order based upon initial starting dose. Start with the lowest mg NNRTI.

Unordered Response	Ordered Response
Nevirapine	Rilpivirine (25 mg daily)
Efavirenz	Nevirapine (200 mg daily; then bid)
Rilpivirine	Etravirine (200 mg twice daily)
Etravirine	Efavirenz (600 mg daily)

23. Which of the following medication regimen(s) contain efavirenz?

   a. Triumeq
   b. Atripla
   c. Genvoya
   d. Complera
   e. Odefsey

Answer b is correct. Efavirenz, emtricitabine, TFV—tdf (Atripla)

Answer a is incorrect. ABC, dolutegravir, lamivudine (Triumeq)

Answer c is incorrect. Elvitegravir, cobicistat, emtricitabine, TFV—taf (Genvoya)

Answer d is incorrect. Emtricitabine, rilpivirine, TFV—tdf (Complera)

Answer e is incorrect. Emtricitabine, rilpivirine, TFV—taf (Odefsey)

24. Which of the following medication(s) contain TFV? Select all that apply.

    a. Stribild
    b. Triumeq
    c. Genvoya
    d. Prezcobix
    e. Descovy

Answer a is correct. Elvitegravir, cobicistat, emtricitabine, TFV—tdf (Stribild)

Answer c is correct. Elvitegravir, cobicistat, emtricitabine, TFV—taf (Genvoya)

Answer e is correct. Emtricitabine, TFV—taf (Descovy)

Answer b is incorrect. ABC, dolutegravir, lamivudine (Triumeq)

Answer d is incorrect. Darunavir, cobicistat (Prezcobix)

25. Which of the following medication(s) contact TFV alafenamide (taf)? Select all that apply.

    a. Evotaz
    b. Kaletra
    c. Truvada
    d. Odefsey
    e. Genvoya

Answer d is correct. Emtricitabine, rilpivirine, TFV—taf (Odefsey)

Answer e is correct. Elvitegravir, cobicistat, emtricitabine, TFV—taf (Genvoya)

Answer a is incorrect. Atazanavir, cobicistat (Evotaz)

Answer b is incorrect. Lopinavir, ritonavir (Kaletra)

Answer c is incorrect. Emtricitabine, TFV—tdf (Truvada)

26. Which of the following antiretrovirals are STRs?

    a. Epzicom
    b. Sustiva
    c. Triumeq
    d. Complera
    e. Atripla

Answer c is correct. ABC, dolutegravir, lamivudine (Triumeq)

Answer d is correct. Emtricitabine, rilpivirine, TFV—tdf (Complera)

Answer e is correct. Efavirenz, emtricitabine, TFV—tdf (Atripla)

Answer a is incorrect. ABC, lamivudine (Epzicom)

Answer b is incorrect. Efavirez (Sustiva)

27. A patient presents to your pharmacy with severe muscle weakness. The patient has a past medical history of hypertension and HIV. Medications include lisinopril, TFV alafenamide, emtricitabine, and raltegravir. The patient was referred to you to evaluate the medications and see if the symptom is associated with one of his medications. Which of the following medications may be causing the patients symptom of muscle weakness?

    a. Emtricitabine
    b. TFV alafenamide
    c. Simvastatin
    d. Raltegravir
    e. Daptomycin

Answer d is correct. *Myopathy* refers to a clinical disorder of the skeletal muscles. Abnormalities of muscle cell structure and metabolism lead to various patterns of weakness and dysfunction. In some cases, the pathology extends to involve cardiac muscle fibers, resulting in a hypertrophic or dilated cardiomyopathy. Treatment with the HIV integrase inhibitor raltegravir (*Isentress*) is associated with an increased risk of skeletomuscular side effects. Toxicities included muscle pain and muscle weakness and wasting. Case reports have associated raltegravir with rhabdomyolysis—the breakdown of skeletal muscle fiber. Elevations in creatinine kinase levels have also been observed in people treated with raltegravir. However, in most instances, these side effects were mild and in the case of muscle wasting/weakness disappeared with the cessation of raltegravir therapy.

Answer a is incorrect. Emtricitabine is not associated with muscle weakness/myopathy.

Answer b is incorrect. TFV (TDF or TAF) is not associated with muscle weakness/myopathy.

Answer c is incorrect. Simvastatin is associated with muscle weakness/myopathy; however, the patient is not receiving this medication.

Answer e is incorrect. Daptomycin is associated with muscle weakness/myopathy; however, the patient is not receiving this medication.

CHAPTER **28 | Opportunistic Infections**

1. Pyrimethamine has been shown to cause bone marrow suppression. Which agent can be given in conjunction with pyrimethamine to lessen the suppressive effects?

    a. Vitamin B_{12}
    b. Levofloxacin
    c. Dapsone
    d. Leucovorin

Answer d is correct. Leucovorin has similar functionality when used with methotrexate.

Answer a is incorrect. Vitamin B_{12} will not have an effect on the bone marrow suppression of pyrimethamine.

Answer b is incorrect. Levofloxacin, a fluoroquinolone, has not been shown to decrease bone marrow suppression.

Answer c is incorrect. Dapsone prevents bacterial folic acid synthesis but has not been demonstrated to be helpful in bone marrow suppression.

---

2. Treatment for PCP during pregnancy has been associated with hemolytic anemia in G6PD deficient states. Select the medication that may be implicated in this condition. Select all that apply.

   a. Azithromycin
   b. Primaquine
   c. Dapsone
   d. Atovaquone

Answers b and c are correct. Primaquine and dapsone can cause mild maternal hemolysis that ultimately precipitates hemolytic anemia in G6PD deficient states.

Answers a and d are incorrect. Azithromycin and Atovaquone have not been shown to be associated with hemolytic anemia in G6PD deficient states.

---

3. What is the brand name for moxifloxacin?

   a. Avelox
   b. Septra
   c. Mepron
   d. Aczone

Answer a is correct. Avelox is the brand name of moxifloxacin.

Answer b is incorrect. Septra is the brand name of sulfamethoxazole and trimethoprim.

Answer c is incorrect. Mepron is the brand name of atovaquone.

Answer d is incorrect. Aczone is the brand name of dapsone.

---

4. JK is a patient at a local clinic with a recent diagnosis of AIDS. His past medical history includes hypertension, dyslipidemia, and depression. Medications include losartan, atorvastatin, and escitalopram. Labs include: CD_4 count of 120 cells/mm³, serum and potassium 4.8 mEq/L (increased from 3.5 mEq/L). Which agent is recommended as a preferred therapy for PCP prophylaxis?

   a. Clindamycin
   b. TMP-SMX
   c. Amikacin
   d. Levofloxacin

Answer b is correct. TMP-SMX is the preferred therapy for PCP prophylaxis despite its potassium retaining capabilities.

Answer a is incorrect. Clindamycin, a lincosamide, is an alternative therapy for PCP prophylaxis.

Answer c is incorrect. Amikacin, an aminoglycoside, is not preferred therapy for PCP prophylaxis.

Answer d is incorrect. Levofloxacin, a fluoroquinolone, is not considered preferred therapy for PCP prophylaxis.

---

5. RA is a nonpregnant female with a past medical history of AIDS (diagnosed 5 years ago). Due to denial of her status, she refused treatment. RA presents to the clinic today with a CD_4 count of 80 cells/mm³. Which of the following primary prophylaxis medications should be recommended for RA? Select all that apply.

   a. MAC
   b. TE
   c. PCP
   d. No prophylaxis is recommended for RA

Answers b and c are correct. Prophylaxis is warranted in TE and PCP when the CD_4 count falls below 100 cells/mm³ and 200 cells/mm³, respectively.

Answer a is incorrect. Prophylaxis is warranted in MAC when the CD_4 count falls below 50 cells/mm³.

Answer d is incorrect. Prophylaxis is desired in AIDS patients with CD_4 counts below 200 cells/mm³.

---

6. LZ is a 52-year-old patient admitted to the hospital with complications of AIDS. The nurse informs the pharmacy resident that he is being treated for a PJP infection. She is unclear of the duration of therapy and asks the pharmacy resident for clarification. Select the approximate duration of antimicrobial therapy in most patients with PJP infection.

   a. 7 days
   b. 10 days
   c. 14 days
   d. 21 days

Answer d is correct. The recommended duration of therapy for treatment of PJP is ≥21 days.

Answer a is incorrect. Seven days is below the recommended duration of therapy for treatment of PJP.

Answer b is incorrect. Ten days is below the recommended duration of therapy for treatment of PJP.

Answer c is incorrect. Fourteen days is below the recommended duration of therapy for treatment of PJP.

---

7. The diagnostic criterion for which of the following opportunistic infections is seropositive for immunoglobulin G (IgG)?

   a. Candidiasis
   b. Toxoplasmosis

c. MAC
d. PJP

Answer b is correct. Diagnosis of Toxoplasmosis can be made by seropositivity for IgG.

Answer a is incorrect. Diagnosis of TB can be made by an induration greater than 5 mm upon exposure to purified protein derivative (PPD).

Answer c is incorrect. Diagnosis of MAC can be made by a positive acid fast bacilli (AFB) culture from a blood specimen.

Answer d is incorrect. Diagnosis of PJP can be made by polymerase chain reaction (PCR) procedures.

8. Which of the agents listed below is available in an aerosolized preparation used in the primary prophylaxis of PJP?

   a. Dapsone
   b. Leucovorin
   c. Trimethoprim
   d. Pentamidine

Answer d is correct. Pentamidine is administered in aerosolized and intravenous preparations.

Answer a is incorrect. Dapsone is administered in tablet and topical gel preparations.

Answer b is incorrect. Leucovorin is administered in tablet (outpatient setting) and intravenous (inpatient setting) preparations.

Answer c is incorrect. Trimethoprim is administered in tablet and oral solution preparations.

9. Which of the agents listed below are utilized for primary prophylaxis in both PJP and toxoplasmosis? Select all that apply.

   a. Atovaquone
   b. Dapsone
   c. Leucovorin
   d. Pentamidine

Answers a, b, and c are correct. Atovaquone, dapsone, and leucovorin are indicated in prophylactic measures for PJP and TE.

Answer d is incorrect. Pentamidine is indicated in primary prophylaxis of PJP but not TE.

10. Which of the agents listed below can be given once weekly in primary prophylaxis for MAC?

    a. Azithromycin
    b. Aztreonam
    c. Clindamycin
    d. Cefazolin

Answer a is correct. Azithromycin, a macrolide, has a long half-life which often results in administration once weekly.

Answer b is incorrect. Aztreonam, a monobactam, is not indicated for primary prophylaxis of MAC.

Answer c is incorrect. Clindamycin, a lincosamide, is not indicated for primary prophylaxis of MAC.

Answer d is incorrect. Cefazolin, a first generation cephalosporin, is not indicated in primary prophylaxis for MAC.

11. What is the generic name for Biaxin?

    a. Clindamycin
    b. Sulfamethoxazole-Trimethoprim
    c. Clarithromycin
    d. Vancomycin

Answer c is correct. Clarithromycin is the generic name for Biaxin.

Answer a is incorrect. Clindamycin is the generic name for Cleocin.

Answer b is incorrect. Sulfamethoxazole-Trimethoprim is the generic name for Bactrim or Septra.

Answer d is incorrect. Vancomycin is the generic name for Vancocin.

12. IT is a male patient with a past medical history of HIV. CD_4 count is 115 cells/mm³ and HIV RNA is currently undetectable (3 months ago he was started on tenofovir (TDF)/emtricitabine/rilpivirine). He presents to the clinic today with pain upon swallowing and white patches in his mouth. He is diagnosed with oropharyngeal candidiasis (first episode). Which of the following medications may be used for an initial episode of oropharyngeal candidiasis and is available as a troche?

    a. Fluconazole
    b. Clotrimazole
    c. Itraconazole
    d. Posaconazole
    e. Voriconazole

Answer b is correct. Clotrimazole is effective for initial episodes of oropharyngeal candidiasis and is available in a troche formulation.

Answers a, c, d, and e are incorrect. While these azoles are effective in the management of thrush, they are not available in troche formulations.

13. GY is an HIV patient with a past medical history of HIV (CD4 150). Medications include tenofovir (TDF)/emtricitabine and lopinavir/ritonavir, TMP/SMZ (PJP prophylaxis), Amiodarone (history of atrial fibrillation), and clarithromycin (started 3 days for a respiratory tract infection—day 3 of 10 day treatment course). He presents to the clinic with complaints of thrush. This is his third case of thrush this year. Which of the

following medications may be utilized for the management of GY's esophageal candidiasis and would have a potential drug interaction with his medications? Select all that apply.

a. Fluconazole
b. Clotrimazole
c. Itraconazole
d. Voriconazole

Answers a, c, and d are correct. Fluconazole, Itraconazole, and Voriconazole may be utilized in the management of esophageal candidiasis (fluconazole is utilized most often). Additionally, they have drug interactions via cytochrome P450 activity. Therefore, interactions with amiodarone, clarithromycin, and lopinavir/ritonavir could occur. Clinical evaluation of risk/benefit should be conducted for each medication.

Answer b is incorrect. Clotrimazole should not be used for esophageal candidiasis. Additionally, clotrimazole lacks drug interaction potential mediated via the CYP450 system.

14. Select the brand name for amphotericin B products. Select all that apply.

a. Amphocin
b. Fungizone
c. Ambisome
d. Ancobon

Answers a, b, and c are correct. Amphocin and fungizone are brand names for amphotericin B deoxycholate. Ambisome is the brand name for liposomal Amphotericin B.

Answer d is incorrect. Ancobon is the brand name for flucytosine.

15. RT is a patient with HIV on the following medications: simvastatin, pantoprazole, TMP/SMZ, and as needed ibuprofen. Because his CD$_4$ count has decreased, he is to be placed on MAC primary prophylaxis. Which of the following medications may be utilized for MAC prophylaxis in RT?

a. Azithromycin
b. Clarithromycin
c. Clindamycin
d. Clotrimazole

Answer a is correct. Azithromycin may be utilized as MAC primary prophylaxis.

Answer b is incorrect. Clarithromycin may be utilized as MAC primary prophylaxis; however, clarithromycin should not be administered to a patient receiving simvastatin because of a drug interaction potential and increased risk of rhabdomyolysis.

Answers c and d are incorrect. Clindamycin and clotrimazole are not utilized in MAC prophylaxis.

16. Which of the following medications is available in a powder for nebulization formulation?

a. Dapsone
b. Pentamidine
c. Clindamycin
d. Primaquine

Answer b is correct. Pentamidine is available in 300 mg powder for injection and 300 mg powder for nebulization.

Answer a is incorrect. Dapsone is available in 25 and100 mg tablets.

Answer c is incorrect. Clindamycin is available in 300, 600, 900 mg premixed IV; 150 mg/mL IV solution; and 150, 300 mg capsules.

Answer d is incorrect. Primaquine is available in 26.3 mg (15 mg base) tablets.

17. What is the brand name of posaconazole?

a. Diflucan
b. Vfend
c. Sporanox
d. Noxafil

Answer d is correct. Noxafil is the brand name for posaconazole.

Answer a is incorrect. Diflucan is the brand name for fluconazole.

Answer b is incorrect. Vfend is the brand name for voriconazole.

Answer c is incorrect. Sporanox is the brand name for itraconazole.

18. Place the following echinocandins in order based upon day 1 initial dose for esophageal candidiasis. Start with the lowest mg dose.

Unordered Response	Ordered Response
Micafungin	Caspofungin
Anidulafungin	Anidulafungin
Caspofungin	Micafungin

19. Which of the following azole antifungal medication is associated with hallucinations? Select all that apply.

a. Voriconazole
b. Metronidazole
c. Clotrimazole
d. Fluconazole

Answer a is correct. Voriconazole is associated with central nervous system side effects including hallucination and visual changes.

Answers b, c, and d are incorrect. Metronidazole is not an azole antifungal and is not associated with hallucinations. Clotrimazole and fluconazole are not associated with hallucinations.

---

20. Which of the following medications is associated with optic neuritis?

    a. Clarithromycin
    b. Itraconazole
    c. Ethambutol
    d. Amphotericin

Answer c is correct. Ethambutol is associated with optic neuritis. Optic neuropathies are disorders of the optic nerve involving degeneration of the nerve. Optic neuropathy should not be confused with optic neuritis. Both can lead to vision problems; optic neuritis involves inflammation of the optic nerve while optic neuropathy refers to damage from any cause. Optic neuritis is one of the many causes of optic neuropathy. Ethambutol is contraindicated in patients with a history of optic neuritis unless clinical judgment warrants its use. Baseline and periodic eye examinations should be conducted; the prescribing information for ethambutol recommends monthly examinations for patients taking more than 15 mg/kg/d. Some have suggested that annual testing may be appropriate for those patients taking less than 15 mg/kg/d, with more frequent monitoring for those at high risk of developing optic neuropathy. This would include patients over 60 years or under 16 years; those with renal disease, alcoholism, or peripheral neuropathy; those taking more than 15 mg/kg/d; or treatment for longer than 6 months. Patients exhibiting symptoms of optic neuropathy should be evaluated, and the drug should be discontinued.

Answers a, b, and d are incorrect. They are not associated with optic neuritis.

CHAPTER **29** | Invasive Fungal
                  Infections

1. TI is a 44-year-old patient with an aspergillosis infection. She is to receive treatment with amphotericin B. Which one of the following adjunctive measures is used to lessen the occurrence of nephrotoxicity associated with amphotericin B?

    a. Test dose of amphotericin B
    b. Diphenhydramine premedication
    c. Normal saline boluses
    d. Furosemide

Answer c is correct. Although not proven via large scale controlled trials, data from animal and small human studies suggest a decrease in nephrotoxicity. Patients will often receive a 500 mL IV bolus of normal saline solution before starting the amphotericin B infusion. Saline doses are also often administered after the dose of amphotericin B.

Answer a is incorrect. This may help to identify patients who might develop an infusion-related adverse effect (fevers, chills, rigors, or hypotension) or anaphylaxis. Most experts do not advocate this anymore due to the poor predictive value. However, during initial dosing, the drug should be administered under close monitoring.

Answer b is incorrect. This is believed to reduce the occurrence of infusion-related adverse effects (fevers, chills, and rigors). Other medications that might be used to treat/prevent the infusion-related reactions include acetaminophen, nonsteroidal anti-inflammatory medications, and hydrocortisone. If the patient continues with severe rigors despite the premedication, meperidine may be used.

Answer d is incorrect. Use of furosemide can often contribute to renal insufficiency in patients receiving amphotericin B.

---

2. PT is a 33-year-old HIV patient. He has a high viral load and low CD4. He has been nonadherent with medication and provider appointments. PT is admitted to the medical center for a change in mental status. He is undergoing a complete work-up to identify the cause. An India Ink stain is reported as positive. Which one of the following organisms is likely to manifest a positive India ink stain on a CSF sample?

    a. *Candida albicans*
    b. *Candida glabrata*
    c. *Aspergillosis fumigatus*
    d. *Candida neoformans*

Answer d is correct. The India ink stain adheres to the capsule around *C. neoformans.*

Answers a, b, and c are incorrect. *Cryptococcus* is evaluated via an India ink stain. The other organisms do not respond to the India ink stain.

---

3. When preparing an IV formulation of amphotericin B deoxycholate, the lyophilized amphotericin B powder must first be reconstituted with sterile water. What type of IV fluid must the reconstituted amphotericin B be placed in for IV administration?

    a. 0.9% sodium chloride
    b. 5% dextrose in water
    c. Lactated Ringer's solution
    d. Any of the above solutions

Answer b is correct. This solution will maintain the micellular distribution that is required for IV amphotericin B deoxycholate.

Answer a is incorrect. This solution will not maintain the micellular distribution.

Answer c is incorrect. This solution will not maintain the micellular distribution.

Answer d is incorrect. Only 5% dextrose in water should be used.

---

4. Which of the following agents is recommended as therapy for invasive aspergillosis? Select all that apply.

   a. Amphotericin B
   b. Fluconazole
   c. Voriconazole
   d. Liposomal amphotericin B
   e. Terbinafine

Answer a is correct. Amphotericin B is a drug of choice for *Aspergillus* species.

Answer c is correct. Voriconazole is a drug of choice for *Aspergillus* species.

Answer d is correct. Lipid formulations of amphotericin B are a drug of choice for *Aspergillus* species.

Answer b is incorrect. Fluconazole lacks activity against molds like *Aspergillus*.

Answer e is incorrect. Terbinafine is used for topical infections.

---

5. IT is receiving initial therapy for *Cryptococcus*. His provider has been monitoring for toxicity and identified that IT has a low granulocyte count (previously within normal limits). Which of the following antifungal agents is associated with bone marrow suppression?

   a. Fluconazole
   b. Amphotericin B
   c. Voriconazole
   d. Flucytosine

Answer d is correct. 5-FC is known to cause blood dyscrasias. Bone marrow toxicity (as well as hepatic) is dose-related; monitor levels closely and adjust dose accordingly.

Answers a and c are incorrect. The azoles have not been identified as a common cause of blood dyscrasias. *Note:* Be careful about using drug information resources when looking up or studying adverse reactions. Azole antifungals have hematologic side effects listed, but they are extremely rare.

Answer b is incorrect. Amphotericin B may cause a normocytic-normochromic anemia. The drug has been rarely associated with neutropenia.

---

6. Lipid-based or liposomal amphotericin B formulations have what advantage over conventional amphotericin B (deoxycholate)?

   a. Less expensive than conventional amphotericin B
   b. Decreased mortality
   c. Decreased rates of nephrotoxicity
   d. More efficacious than conventional amphotericin B

Answer c is correct. Changes in serum creatinine are less pronounced with lipid-based formulations.

Answer a is incorrect. Liposomal formulations are considerably more expensive.

Answer b is incorrect. This has not been shown in well-designed trials.

Answer d is incorrect. This has not been shown in well-designed trials.

---

7. Which antifungal preparation carries a relative contraindication against use in patients with severe renal insufficiency (due to risk of renal complications from a carrier molecule)?

   a. IV posaconazole
   b. IV voriconazole
   c. Oral itraconazole
   d. IV caspofungin
   e. Oral voriconazole

Answers a and b are correct. IV voriconazole uses a cyclodextrin carrier molecule. Related cyclodextrins have been associated with nephrotoxicity in some animal studies.

Answer c is incorrect. Oral itraconazole solution uses a cyclodextrin carrier molecule, but it does not enter the systemic circulation.

Answers d and e are incorrect. No carrier molecule is contained in these formulations.

---

8. A patient with a histoplasmosis infection is to be discharged from the hospital and started on oral itraconazole capsules. Which one of the following statements would you tell the patient about his medication to maximize the oral absorption?

   a. Take with food and avoid concomitant use of antacids
   b. Take on an empty stomach
   c. Food will not affect the oral absorption
   d. Do not take this with cola

Answer a is correct. For optimal dissolution and absorption of itraconazole capsules an acidic pH is desired.

Answer b is incorrect. Itraconazole should be taken with food.

Answer c is incorrect. Studies have shown that food can significantly improve oral absorption.

Answer d is incorrect. Administration with cola has been one way to provide some acidic fluid to increase dissolution and absorption.

---

9. A patient is to receive home infusion therapy with amphotericin B. What laboratory values should be monitored? Select all that apply.

   a. Serum creatinine
   b. Serum potassium

c. Serum magnesium
d. Serum creatine phosphokinase (CPK)

Answer a is correct. Amphotericin B is nephrotoxic.

Answer b is correct. Due to nephrotoxicity the kidney loses ability to maintain potassium.

Answer c is correct. Due to nephrotoxicity the kidney loses ability to maintain magnesium.

Answer d is correct. Muscle weakness is a clinical sign of hypokalemia.

10. Which of the following antifungal agents has been shown to cause visual acuity side effects? Select all that apply.

a. Amphotericin B
b. Flucytosine
c. Fluconazole
d. Voriconazole
e. Caspofungin

Answer d is correct. About 30% of patients in clinical trials reported some degree of reversible changes in visual acuity with voriconazole.

Answers a, b, c, and e are incorrect. as they have not been associated with visual disturbances.

11. A 54-year-old man with leukemia developed neutropenia 10 days ago after a chemotherapy course. His absolute neutrophil count (ANC) is 200, and he has been febrile for 7 days despite empiric bacterial therapy with imipenem and vancomycin. He was ordered amphotericin B 5 days ago. His CrCl has diminished to <30 mL/min. Which one of the following antifungal agents would be an option for a febrile neutropenic patient with renal insufficiency? The provider would like a broad-spectrum antifungal that covers yeasts and molds and an agent that does not affect the kidneys as much as conventional amphotericin B.

a. Liposomal amphotericin B
b. Fluconazole
c. Posaconazole
d. Ketoconazole

Answer a is correct. Although liposomal amphotericin B can still contribute to continued renal failure, it affects renal function less. This agent is a broad-spectrum antifungal (yeasts and molds).

Answer b is incorrect. This agent is not advised due to narrow spectrum of activity and fungistatic killing rate.

Answer c is incorrect. This agent is primarily used in the prophylaxis of invasive fungal infections, not treatment. Furthermore, the cyclodextrin carrier is relatively contraindicated with his current CrCl.

Answer d is incorrect. This drug is only available in an oral formulation with poor absorption. There is limited data on using this drug in this indication.

12. A 58-year-old febrile woman in the surgical intensive care unit has one out of two blood culture bottles growing yeast and is hemodynamically stable. A urine sample collected 2 days ago is growing *C. glabrata*. What is the best empiric decision for this patient?

a. Start fluconazole 400-800 mg daily
b. Wait for a susceptibility report and then start with a sensitive antifungal agent
c. The one out of two blood bottles and the urine culture do not require therapy
d. Initiate caspofungin 70 mg × 1 dose, then 50 mg daily

Answer a is correct. This option could be used, but many *C. glabrata* strains may require higher doses of fluconazole based on in vitro susceptibilities (S-DD). Therefore, doses of 400-800 mg would be appropriate. Therapy or dose could be changed after susceptibilities become known.

Answer b is incorrect. Generally antifungal therapy is initiated and changed if needed based on the susceptibility results or clinical situation.

Answer c is incorrect. All positive blood cultures growing yeast should receive treatment.

Answer d is incorrect. While caspofungin would be active against *C. glabrata*, caspofungin undergoes extensive hepatic metabolism and would not be the best agent for a urinary source.

13. Genetic variability in cytochrome P-450 CYP 2C19 has been linked to significant interpatient pharmacokinetic differences for which antifungal agent?

a. Fluconazole
b. Voriconazole
c. Micafungin
d. Flucytosine

Answer b is correct. Studies indicated that CYP 2C19 is significantly involved in the metabolism of voriconazole. This enzyme exhibits genetic polymorphism. About 3% to 5% of Caucasians and 12% to 23% of Asians are expected to be poor metabolizers.

Answer a is incorrect. Fluconazole is not a significant substrate for CYP 2C19.

Answer c is incorrect. Micafungin is not a CYP-450 substrate.

Answer d is incorrect. Flucytosine is not a CYP-450 substrate.

14. A 55-year-old man is to be treated for invasive aspergillosis. He weighs 100 kg. What amphotericin B formulation dose(s) would be appropriate for this patient? Select all that apply.

    a. Amphotericin B deoxycholate 80 mg
    b. Amphotericin B deoxycholate 400 mg
    c. Liposomal Amphotericin B 400 mg
    d. Liposomal Amphotericin B 80 mg
    e. Liposomal Amphotericin B 800 mg

Answer a is correct. The recommended dose of amphotericin B deoxycholate is 0.5 to 1.5 mg/kg.

Answer c is correct. The recommended dose for liposomal amphotericin B is 3 to 5 mg/kg

Answer b is incorrect. This dose would be too high.

Answer d is incorrect. This dose would be too low.

Answer e is incorrect. This dose would be too high.

15. The fungal cell wall component (1, 3) β-D-glucan is not a key structure in *C. neoformans* and therefore explains the poor activity of what class of antifungal agents for *Cryptococcus*?

    a. Triazoles
    b. Amphotericin B
    c. Echinocandins
    d. 5-FC

Answer c is correct. Echinocandins inhibit (1, 3) β-D-glucan synthase enzyme that makes (1, 3) β-D-glucan fibrils. They lack activity for cryptococcal infections.

Answer a is incorrect. Triazoles inhibit 14-α-demethylase. They are usually effective for cryptococcal infections.

Answer b is incorrect. Amphotericin B binds to ergosterol. It usually is effective for cryptococcal infections.

Answer d is incorrect. 5-FC causes defective fungal protein synthesis. It can be effective for cryptococcal infections.

16. What drug interaction would be exhibited by adding fluconazole to a person's medication regimen that includes warfarin (stabilized at an INR of 2.5)?

    a. Fluconazole and warfarin concentrations would both be reduced
    b. An increase in INR would be expected
    c. Warfarin cytochrome P-450 metabolism would be induced
    d. An interaction would not be expected

Answer b is correct. Fluconazole can interact with warfarin primarily through CYP 2C9 and some CYP 3A4 inhibition, increasing warfarin concentrations and therefore the patient's INR.

Answer a is incorrect. The major interaction causes an increase in warfarin concentrations.

Answer c is incorrect. The interaction is through metabolic inhibition.

Answer d is incorrect. This interaction is well reported.

17. BK is a 40-year-old HIV-positive patient. He develops CSF culture-positive cryptococcal meningitis. He has no hepatic or renal insufficiency and his complete blood count is within normal limits. Select the preferred antifungal regimen for a patient with cryptococcal meningitis.

    a. Amphotericin B deoxycholate + flucytosine
    b. Amphotericin B deoxycholate
    c. Liposomal amphotericin B
    d. Fluconazole

Answer a is correct. This is regarded as the first-line regimen. Flucytosine has excellent CSF penetration. Historically, it was used as monotherapy, but resistance quickly developed. It is now used as adjunctive therapy with amphotericin B to avoid failure due to resistance and to optimized killing due to synergistic killing of both agents.

Answer b is incorrect. This would be a second-line alternative. Amphotericin B alone may not be as good during the initial part of the treatment. Amphotericin B does not penetrate the CSF as well as flucytosine.

Answer c is incorrect. This would be a second-line alternative. Liposomal amphotericin B alone may not be as good during the initial part of the treatment. Amphotericin B does not penetrate the CSF as well as flucytosine.

Answer d is incorrect. This would be a second-line alternative. Fluconazole is not fungicidal enough to use for induction therapy. It is however used as antifungal consolidation after about 2 weeks of amphotericin B deoxycholate + flucytosine and as a chronic suppression therapy in HIV patients.

18. Which antifungal agent is only available as a parenteral formulation? Select all that apply.

    a. Amphotericin B lipid-complex
    b. Voriconazole
    c. Posaconazole
    d. Fluconazole

Answer a is correct. This is available as IV only.

Answer b is incorrect. This is available as oral and IV.

Answer c is incorrect. This is available as oral suspension and IV.

Answer d is incorrect. This is available as oral and IV.

19. Which antifungal agent has the greatest 24-hour urinary excretion percentage?

    a. Amphotericin B deoxycholate
    b. Fluconazole
    c. Voriconazole
    d. Caspofungin

Answer b is correct. About 80% of a fluconazole dose is eliminated unchanged in the urine.

Answer a is incorrect. Urinary elimination of amphotericin B happens over a prolonged duration in small amounts.

Answer c is incorrect. Less than 2% of a dose of voriconazole appears in the urine.

Answer d is incorrect. Less than 2% of a dose of caspofungin appears in the urine.

Note: Most antifungals undergo hepatic metabolism and small amounts of active medication undergo renal elimination. The exceptions are fluconazole and flucytosine.

---

20. At the end of initial treatment (amphotericin and flucytosine) for cryptococcal meningitis (CSF-sterilized) in an HIV-positive patient, what is generally recommended in terms of cryptococcal infection? Select all that apply.

    a. Once weekly doses of azithromycin
    b. Four weeks of fluconazole oral therapy
    c. Indefinite low-dose suppressive fluconazole therapy
    d. No further antifungal therapy is needed
    e. Once weekly doses of fluconazole for 4 weeks

Answer b is correct. Longer fluconazole therapy may be needed in some cases where CSF is still positive or was slow to sterilize. Higher doses may be used.

Answer c is correct. HIV-positive patients will receive indefinite therapy after the patient displays clinical cure and a negative CSF. Dose is 200 mg.

Answer a is incorrect. This is used to prevent *Mycobacterium* avium-intracellulare complex (MAC).

Answer d is incorrect. HIV-positive patients will receive indefinite therapy after the patient displays clinical cure and a negative CSF.

Answer e is incorrect. Daily dosing of fluconazole would be warranted in these infections.

---

21. What is the generic name for Cresemba?

    a. Itraconazole
    b. Isavuconazole
    c. Posaconazole
    d. Ketoconazole

Answer b is correct. Cresemba is the FDA approved name for isavuconazole.

Answer a is incorrect. Itraconazole is Sporanox.

Answer c is incorrect. Posaconazole is Noxafil.

Answer d is incorrect. Ketoconazole is Nizoral.

CHAPTER **30 | Tuberculosis**

1. JK is a 32-year-old HIV-negative patient presenting to your clinic. He receives a Mantoux skin test that returns positive 2 days later. He was born in the United States and works as a prison guard. He injects heroin on a regular basis. His chest x-ray comes back normal, he has no symptoms of tuberculosis, and his smear culture is negative. What type of drug therapy would be appropriate for this patient?

    a. Isoniazid 300 mg daily × 9 months
    b. Rifampin 100 mg daily × 4 months
    c. No drug therapy needed
    d. Isoniazid 300 mg and rifampin 600 mg × 6 months
    e. Isoniazid, rifampin, ethambutol, and pyrazinamide

Answer a is correct. The patient does not have any symptoms or indications of active TB disease; so he needs treatment for latent TB infection. This is the correct first-line regimen for treatment of latent TB infection.

Answer b is incorrect. Rifampin is a second-line treatment for latent TB infection. It can be used in patients with intolerance to isoniazid or in areas where isoniazid-resistant strains of TB are prevalent. The dose of rifampin is also too low.

Answer c is incorrect. Treating latent TB infection significantly reduces his risk of converting to active disease. He works in a high-risk setting prison where if he were to get active disease it could be spread more easily as well.

Answer d is incorrect. Latent TB infection typically only requires monotherapy.

Answer e is incorrect. Latent TB infection typically only requires monotherapy. This four drug regimen is used in treating active TB disease.

---

2. BCG vaccine should be routinely given to which patient in the United States?

    a. A 10-year-old child
    b. A 2-month-old infant
    c. A 65-year-old man
    d. A 6-month-old infant
    e. BCG vaccine is not routinely recommended in the United States.

Answer e is correct. BCG vaccination should *not* be routinely given to any specific age group in the United States.

Answers a, b, c, and d are incorrect. BCG vaccination should *not* be routinely given to any specific age group in the United States.

---

3. RL is a 37-year-old man who presents to your pharmacy with a prescription for rifampin. His other medications include: acetaminophen 1000 mg four times daily, phenytoin 100 mg twice daily, warfarin 3 mg daily, and omeprazole 20 mg once daily.

Which of the following is important to counsel RL on his new medication? Select all that apply.

a. This medication can cause your body secretions to be an orange-red color.
b. You should limit your acetaminophen use as much as possible during therapy with this medication.
c. This medication can cause you to need a decrease in your warfarin dose.
d. This medication may cause gastrointestinal upset.
e. This medication can cause your phenytoin concentrations to go down.

Answer a is correct. Rifampin does cause secretions to turn an orange-red color.

Answer b is correct. Rifampin can be hepatotoxic and patients should limit their use of other medications that can increase risk of hepatotoxicity. This includes acetaminophen.

Answer d is correct. Rifampin has the potential to cause gastrointestinal upset.

Answer e is correct. Rifampin can induce the metabolism of phenytoin which would decrease the concentration of phenytoin.

Answer c is incorrect. Rifampin induces cytochrome P-450 enzymes that increase the metabolism of warfarin. Thus you would likely need an increase in your warfarin dose.

4. RS is a 25-year-old Hispanic woman who is recently diagnosed with active tuberculosis. Her physician asks what drug regimen you would recommend to treat her disease. She does not have any contraindications to any of the tuberculosis medications. You do not have susceptibility testing back yet.

a. INH, RIF, PZA × 8 weeks, then INH, RIF ×18 weeks
b. INH × 9 months
c. INH, RIF × 9 months
d. INH, RIF, EMB, FQ × 8 weeks, then INH, RIF × 18 weeks
e. INH, RIF, EMB, PZA × 8 weeks, then INH, RIF × 18 weeks

Answer e is correct. This is the correct first-line initial four-drug regimen and two-drug continuation phase regimen in adults. Drug susceptibility could ultimately influence your drug choices in the future.

Answer a is incorrect. Ethambutol is also part of the initial 8-week regimen in adults.

Answer b is incorrect. This is the treatment for latent TB infection. This patient has active disease.

Answer c is incorrect. There are typically two phases of treatment in active TB disease, an initial 8 weeks and then a continuation phase of approximately 18 weeks. Ethambutol and pyrazinamide are part of the initial 8-week treatment in active TB treatment in adults unless the patient is pregnant. If the patient is pregnant the pyrazinamide is not given.

Answer d is incorrect. Fluoroquinolones are not first-line agents in active TB treatment.

5. Which of the following is true regarding acid-fast bacteria?

a. They cause the majority of bacterial infectious diseases in the United States.
b. *Mycobacterium tuberculosis* is the only type of acid-fast bacteria.
c. Cultures of acid-fast bacteria grow faster than other bacteria.
d. They retain their stained color even with acid-alcohol washes.

Answer d is correct. Acid-fast bacteria keep their stain color despite acid-alcohol washes. *Mycobacterium tuberculosis* is acid fast.

Answer a is incorrect. Acid-fast bacilli cause a small subset of bacterial illnesses in the United States.

Answer b is incorrect. There are other acid-fast bacteria. Examples include: *Mycobacterium bovis* and *Mycobacterium leprae.*

Answer c is incorrect. Mycobacterium tuberculosis is an acid-fast bacteria and it grows in culture at a slow rate.

6. Select the primary method for transmission of tuberculosis.

a. Inhalation
b. Exposure to blood and/or bodily fluids
c. Exposure to dead birds
d. Hospitalization

Answer a is correct. Inhalation of respiratory droplets is the primary mechanism for contracting tuberculosis infection.

Answer b is incorrect. Tuberculosis is not transmitted this way. Viral infections such as HIV and hepatitis B/C can be transmitted this way.

Answer c is incorrect. Tuberculosis is not transmitted through animals to humans.

Answer d is incorrect. Suspected tuberculosis patients in the hospital are typically in isolation. It is possible to be exposed to TB in the hospital, but it is not the primary method for contracting TB.

7. What time period is the risk highest for conversion to active disease in those patients with latent tuberculosis infection?

a. 10 years after exposure
b. 8 years after exposure
c. 6 years after exposure
d. 4 years after exposure
e. 2 years after exposure

Answer e is correct. Risk of converting from latent TB infection to active disease is highest in the first 2 years. Drug therapy for latent TB reduces this risk significantly.

Answers a, b, c, and d are incorrect. Risk of converting from latent TB infection to active disease is highest in the first 2 years. Drug therapy for latent TB reduces this risk significantly.

8. Which of the following is a sign/symptom of pulmonary tuberculosis? Select all that apply.

    a. Weight loss
    b. Productive cough
    c. Headache
    d. Fever
    e. Night sweats

Answers a, b, d, and e are correct. These are common signs/symptoms of pulmonary TB.

Answer c is incorrect. Headache is not typical with TB infection.

---

9. How long after a Mantoux skin test for TB infection is placed should it be read?

    a. 12 hours
    b. 24 hours
    c. 48 hours
    d. 96 hours
    e. 120 hours

Answer c is correct. Mantoux skin tests should be read within 48 to 72 hours of administering them.

Answers a, b, d, and e are incorrect. This time period is too soon/long to read a skin test.

---

10. Which patient group should get drug-susceptibility testing?

    a. All latent tuberculosis patients
    b. Latent tuberculosis patients over age 35
    c. All active tuberculosis disease patients
    d. Active tuberculosis patients over age 35
    e. Foreign-born cases of latent and active tuberculosis

Answer c is correct. Drug-susceptibility testing should be initially done in all patients with active disease to determine proper drug therapy to control spread of drug-resistant strains.

Answer a is incorrect. Latent TB patients do not need drug-susceptibility testing.

Answer b is incorrect. Latent TB patients do not need drug-susceptibility testing regardless of age.

Answer d is incorrect. All active TB patients should receive susceptibility regardless of age.

Answer e is incorrect. A patient being born in a foreign country does not typically affect decisions to do drug-susceptibility testing.

---

11. TF is a 10-year-old girl recently diagnosed with active tuberculosis. Her other medications include: methylphenidate 10 mg twice daily. She is HIV negative. Which medication should not be included in her regimen for active TB?

    a. Isoniazid
    b. Rifampin

    c. Pyrazinamide
    d. Ethambutol

Answer d is correct. Ethambutol is not typically included in a child's regimen because of the potential inability to adequately assess visual acuity. Changes in visual acuity and color vision need to be assessed during ethambutol therapy due to the drug having the potential to cause retrobulbar neuritis.

Answers a, b, and c are incorrect. These are first-line regimens in children with active TB disease.

---

12. The addition of which of the following drugs necessitates follow-up liver function tests in a patient being treated for latent TB infection treated with isoniazid?

    a. Naproxen
    b. Multivitamin
    c. Sertraline
    d. Acetaminophen
    e. Lisinopril

Answer d is correct. Acetaminophen can increase the risk of isoniazid-induced hepatotoxicity. If patients are placed on scheduled acetaminophen you need to closely monitor for hepatotoxicity including liver enzymes. You may want to recommend an alternative pain regimen while on isoniazid.

Answer a is incorrect. Naproxen does not commonly cause changes in isoniazid metabolism and is not known to commonly cause hepatotoxicity or elevate liver enzymes.

Answer b is incorrect. Multivitamins do not commonly cause changes in isoniazid metabolism and are not known to commonly cause hepatotoxicity or elevate liver enzymes.

Answer c is incorrect. Sertraline does not commonly cause changes in isoniazid metabolism and is not known to commonly cause hepatotoxicity or elevate liver enzymes.

Answer e is incorrect. Lisinopril does not commonly cause changes in isoniazid metabolism and is not known to commonly cause hepatotoxicity or elevate liver enzymes.

---

13. What is the preferred regimen for treating latent tuberculosis infection in adults?

    a. Isoniazid 300 mg daily × 6 months
    b. Isoniazid 300 mg daily × 9 months
    c. Rifampin 600 mg daily × 6 months
    d. Rifampin 600 mg daily × 9 months

Answer b is correct. Isoniazid is the preferred drug and 9 months is the preferred time period. It is been found to be superior to 6 months.

Answer a is incorrect. Isoniazid is the preferred drug and can be used for 6 months in certain cases; however, this is not the preferred time period of treatment.

Answer c is incorrect. Rifampin is second-line regimen in latent TB treatment if the patient is intolerant to isoniazid or if isoniazid resistance is high in the area. Rifampin is also typically given for 4 months.

Answer d is incorrect. Rifampin is second-line regimen in latent TB treatment if the patient is intolerant to isoniazid or if isoniazid resistance is high in the area. Rifampin is also typically given for 4 months.

---

14. RS is a 45-year-female who was placed on isoniazid for latent tuberculosis. Medications include: metformin 1000 mg twice daily, glipizide 10 mg twice daily, lisinopril 20 mg daily, and atorvastatin 40 mg daily. She presents to your pharmacy to purchase some vitamin B6 (pyridoxine) as recommended by her doctor. Which adverse effect of isoniazid does pyridoxine reduce?

    a. Hepatotoxicity
    b. Peripheral neuropathy
    c. Gastrointestinal upset
    d. Rash

Answer b is correct. Isoniazid promotes excretion of pyridoxine. This pyridoxine deficiency can cause neuropathy so one can supplement with pyridoxine to prevent peripheral neuropathies from isoniazid.

Answer a is incorrect. There are no protective drugs to give against isoniazid hepatotoxicity.

Answer c is incorrect. Gastrointestinal upset can be alleviated potentially by taking the isoniazid with food.

Answer d is incorrect. There are no protective drugs to give to prevent rash.

---

15. Which rifamycin is the least potent in terms of CYP450 induction?

    a. Rifampin
    b. Rifabutin
    c. Rifapentine
    d. Rocephin

Answer b is correct. Rifabutin is the least potent cytochrome P-450 inducer and has the least amount of drug interactions.

Answer a is incorrect. Rifampin is the strongest cytochrome P-450 inducer and has the most drug interactions.

Answer c is incorrect. Rifapentine has less drug interactions than rifampin; however, rifabutin is thought to have the least and recommended in most HIV-positive patients on antiretroviral regimens.

Answer d is incorrect. Rocephin is a cephalosporin antibiotic.

16. ZK is a 56-year-old woman who has been on treatment for active TB for the past month. Her regimen includes: isoniazid, rifampin, ethambutol, and pyrazinamide. She reports to her doctor for routine monitoring. She reports no adverse effects. Which of the following tests should be done?

    a. Creatinine
    b. Foot examination
    c. Snellen visual chart examination
    d. Complete blood count
    e. Triglycerides

Answer c is correct. Ethambutol can cause retrobulbar neuritis which causes changes in visual acuity and red-green color blindness. Visual acuity can be checked with the Snellen visual chart examination and should be done as baseline and throughout treatment.

Answer a is incorrect. None of the medications require creatinine monitoring.

Answer b is incorrect. While some medications in the regimen may cause peripheral neuropathies, routine foot examinations are not required for monitoring.

Answer d is incorrect. None of the medications require routine monitoring of CBC.

Answer e is incorrect. None of the medication requires routine monitoring of triglycerides.

---

17. Which of the following is a contraindication to pyrazinamide therapy? Select all that apply.

    a. Acute gout attacks
    b. Chronic obstructive pulmonary disease
    c. Rheumatoid arthritis
    d. Asthma

Answer a is correct. Pyrazinamide can cause hyperuricemia which puts patients at higher risk for developing acute gout attacks.

Answer b is incorrect. Pyrazinamide does not exacerbate chronic obstructive pulmonary disease or shortness of breath.

Answer c is incorrect. Pyrazinamide does not typically exacerbate rheumatoid arthritis.

Answer d is incorrect. Pyrazinamide does not exacerbate asthma or shortness of breath.

---

18. Place the following patient groups in order of lowest reaction to highest reaction size (that defines a positive PPD reaction).

Unordered Response	Ordered Response
No risk factor	HIV 5 mm
HIV	Injection drug user ≥ 10 mm
Injection drug user	No risk factor ≥ 15 mm

19. Place the following latent TB treatments in order based upon duration of therapy. Start with the shortest duration.

Unordered Response	Ordered Response
Rifampin	Isoniazid + Rifapentine
Isoniazid + Rifapentine	Rifampin
Isoniazid	Isoniazid

20. Which of the following medications would be expected to interact with INH? Select all that apply.

    a. Carbamazepine
    b. Warfarin
    c. Phenytoin
    d. Theophylline

Answers a, b, c, and d are correct. Carbamazepine, warfarin, phenytoin, and theophylline are expected to interact with INH via the CYP450 system.

CHAPTER 31 | **Sexually Transmitted Diseases**

1. AS is a 27-year-old patient with a new diagnosis of a chlamydia infection. The patient is concerned about the infection, the treatment, and complications from the infection. Complications of chlamydia genital infection include which of the following?

    a. Granulomatous and cardiovascular diseases
    b. Vesicular lesions on the external genitalia
    c. PID and infertility
    d. General paresis, dementia, and sensory ataxia

Answer c is correct. Without appropriate and timely treatment for chlamydia, complications such as PID, ectopic pregnancy, premature delivery, and infertility can result.

Answer a is incorrect. Granulomatous and cardiovascular diseases are manifestations of tertiary syphilis and represent some of the long-term complications of syphilis.

Answer b is incorrect. Vesicular lesions on the external genitalia are manifestations of genital herpes infection.

Answer d is incorrect. General paresis, dementia, and sensory ataxia are clinical manifestations of late neurosyphilis, a form of tertiary syphilis.

2. TD is 27-year-old man who presents to a local STD clinic with complaints of painful urination and urethral discharge over the past 4 days. He is sexually active, reporting one partner within the past 30 days. He has no known drug allergies. A diagnosis of chlamydia is made. Select the most appropriate therapy for TD.

    a. Doxycycline
    b. Azithromycin + cefixime
    c. Ceftizoxime
    d. Acyclovir + ofloxacin

Answer a is correct. Doxycycline is a recommended agent for the treatment of chlamydia.

Answer b is incorrect. While azithromycin is a recommended agent for the treatment of chlamydia, cefixime is not necessary to be added. Cefixime in combination with azithromycin is an alternative regimen for the treatment of gonorrhea.

Answer c is incorrect. Ceftizoxime is not a recommended therapy for chlamydia, although it is an alternative agent for gonorrhea treatment.

Answer d is incorrect. Acyclovir is an antiviral agent and would not be effective against a chlamydia bacterial infection. Although ofloxacin is an alternative agent for chlamydia treatment, this combination is inappropriate.

3. Which of the following is a contraindication to doxycycline therapy? Select all that apply.

    a. Age less than 8 years
    b. Concomitant use of QTc interval-prolonging drugs
    c. Diabetes mellitus
    d. Documented penicillin allergy

Answer a is correct. The calcium-binding effects of tetracyclines cause permanent darkening of teeth in children and effects on developing bone. For this reason, tetracyclines are contraindicated in pregnancy and children under the age of eight.

Answer b is incorrect. This statement refers to fluoroquinolone and macrolide antibiotics, both of which can prolong the QTc interval.

Answer c is incorrect. Diabetes mellitus is not a contraindication to tetracycline therapy. However, fluoroquinolones have the potential to cause dysglycemia (hypo- or hyperglycemia), and this adverse effect has been most commonly reported in patients with underlying diabetes mellitus.

Answer d is incorrect. Tetracyclines are not contraindicated in penicillin allergy. Tetracyclines represent an alternative antibiotic class option for patients with susceptible infections and penicillin allergy.

4. JM is a 23-year-old woman who is 28 weeks pregnant. She presents to her primary care physician (PCP) with symptoms of dysuria and unusual vaginal discharge. A diagnosis of chlamydia is made. JM has no medication allergies. Select appropriate therapy for JM.

    a. Doxycycline
    b. Amoxicillin
    c. Cefixime
    d. Levofloxacin

Answer b is correct. Amoxicillin is recommended for the treatment of chlamydia in pregnancy and is classified in pregnancy category B.

Answer a is incorrect. While tetracyclines are effective agents against chlamydia genital infection, they are contraindicated in pregnancy.

Answer c is incorrect. Although cephalosporins are safe to use in pregnancy (pregnancy category B), they are not recommended agents for the treatment of chlamydia.

Answer d is incorrect. Fluoroquinolones have not adequately been studied in pregnancy, and their use is generally discouraged.

---

5. Which of the following represents an adverse effect associated with fluoroquinolone use? Select all that apply.

    a. Permanent tooth darkening
    b. Esophageal ulceration
    c. Dysglycemia
    d. Jarisch-Herxheimer reaction

Answer c is correct. Fluoroquinolones have the potential to cause dysglycemia (hypo- or hyperglycemia), and this adverse effect has been most commonly reported in patients with underlying diabetes mellitus.

Answer a is incorrect. Permanent tooth darkening is associated with tetracycline use in children younger than 8 years of age.

Answer b is incorrect. Esophageal ulceration can occur with tetracycline antibiotics. For this reason, patients are recommended to take them with an adequate amount of fluid and to remain upright after the dose.

Answer d is incorrect. The Jarisch-Herxheimer reaction is an acute febrile reaction that can occur within hours of initiation of therapy for syphilis.

---

6. Which of the following is true regarding gonococcal urethritis and/or cervicitis?

    a. Gonorrhea infections are treated with oral vancomycin.
    b. Men are typically asymptomatic or have minor symptoms.
    c. Increased transmission of HIV infection is associated with gonococcal infection.
    d. Antibiotic susceptibility data can be obtained using nonculture diagnostic tests for gonorrhea.

Answer c is correct. In both men and women, gonorrhea can cause increased susceptibility to and transmission of HIV infection.

Answer a is incorrect. Oral vancomycin is utilized to treat *Clostridium difficile* infection.

Answer b is incorrect. Women with gonorrhea are usually asymptomatic or have only minor symptoms. In men, symptoms of gonorrhea include dysuria and purulent urethral discharge. Because of the early presentation and discomfort associated with symptoms in men, treatment is often sought early enough to prevent complications.

Answer d is incorrect. Nonculture diagnostic tests cannot provide antibiotic susceptibility results, which may be necessary in cases of infection that persists after treatment.

---

7. IT is a patient that reports to her primary care provider for evaluation of a vaginal discharge, dysuria, and vaginal bleeding. The provider orders several labs and cultures. A Gram stain reveals gram-negative diplococci. The presence of gram-negative diplococci on Gram stain is suggestive of which organism?

    a. *Treponema pallidum*
    b. *Chlamydia trachomatis*
    c. HSV-2
    d. *Neisseria gonorrhoeae*

Answer d is correct. *N. gonorrhoeae* is a Gram-negative diplococcus.

Answer a is incorrect. *T. pallidum* is a spiral-shaped organism that is invisible on light microscopy.

Answer b is incorrect. *C. trachomatis* is an obligate intracellular pathogen.

Answer c is incorrect. Herpes is a viral organism.

---

8. AF is a 19-year-old college student who is considering becoming sexually active. During her annual Pap smear, she asks her gynecologist for information on STD and pregnancy prevention. Which of the following statements is true regarding STD prevention? Select all that apply.

    a. Vaccines are currently available for chlamydia, gonorrhea, and syphilis.
    b. Diaphragm use is a reliable method of STD prevention.
    c. Hormonal contraception is effective in preventing pregnancy and STDs.
    d. Condom use reduces the acquisition and transmission of STDs.

Answer d is correct. Condom use and STD/HIV counseling have been shown to be effective in reducing the acquisition and transmission of STDs.

Answer a is incorrect. Vaccines *are not* currently available for chlamydia, gonorrhea, and syphilis.

Answer b is incorrect. Diaphragm use *is not* a reliable method of STD prevention.

Answer c is incorrect. Hormonal contraception *is not* an effective method of preventing STDs.

---

9. Select the mechanism of action for cephalosporin antibiotics.

    a. Bind to the 30S bacterial ribosomal subunit, ultimately inhibiting bacterial protein synthesis
    b. Bind and inactivate a family of enzymes required for bacterial cell wall synthesis, causing cell death
    c. Bind and stabilize DNA complexes with topoisomerase II and topoisomerase IV enzymes, causing DNA-strand breakage and cell death

d. Bind to the 23S component of the 50S ribosomal subunit, inhibiting RNA-dependent protein synthesis

Answer b is correct. Cephalosporins bind and inactivate a family of enzymes, called penicillin-binding proteins, which are required for bacterial cell wall synthesis. This action causes cell death and is bactericidal.

Answer a is incorrect. Tetracyclines bind to the 30S bacterial ribosomal subunit, ultimately inhibiting bacterial protein synthesis.

Answer c is incorrect. Fluoroquinolones bind and stabilize DNA complexes with topoisomerase II and topoisomerase IV enzymes, causing DNA-strand breakage and cell death.

Answer d is incorrect. Macrolides bind to the 23S component of the 50S ribosomal subunit, inhibiting RNA-dependent protein synthesis.

---

10. SA is a 33-year-old man with no known drug allergies who presents to the local STD clinic with complaints of extreme pain on urination and urethral discharge for 2 days. A diagnosis of gonococcal urethritis is made. Select the most appropriate therapy for SA.

   a. Ceftriaxone + azithromycin
   b. Benzathine penicillin
   c. Azithromycin
   d. Levofloxacin + azithromycin

Answer a is correct. The CDC recommends combination therapy AND does not recommend cefixime first line due to the emergence of resistance. Parenteral cephalosporins (intramuscular) in combination with azithromycin or doxycycline is recommended.

Answer b is incorrect. Benzathine penicillin is a recommended agent for the treatment of syphilis.

Answer c is incorrect. Azithromycin is a recommended agent for the treatment of chlamydia.

Answer d is incorrect. Fluoroquinolones are no longer recommended for the treatment of gonorrhea in the United States due to increasing rates of fluoroquinolone-resistant *N. gonorrhoeae*.

---

11. TE is a 33-year-old patient with genital herpes. Which of the following describes a current goal of therapy for genital herpes infection? Select all that apply.

   a. Disease eradication
   b. Viral suppression
   c. Transmission prevention
   d. Decrease recurrence frequency

Answer b is correct. Viral suppression is a goal of therapy for genital herpes.

Answer c is correct. Prevention of disease transmission is a goal of therapy for genital herpes.

Answer d is correct. Decreasing the frequency of recurrence (outbreaks) is a goal of therapy for genital herpes.

Answer a is incorrect. Since genital herpes cannot currently be eradicated, this is not a goal of therapy.

---

12. Which of the following is true regarding genital herpes infection?

   a. Genital herpes is an acute, self-limiting disease.
   b. Genital lesions are typically vesicular in nature and accompanied by pain, itching, and burning.
   c. The rate of recurrence increases over time in most patients.
   d. Transmission risk in a mother with recurrent disease but no visible lesions is high.

Answer b is correct. Clinical manifestations of genital herpes include the development of papular and vesicular lesions on the external genitalia which are accompanied by pain, itching, and burning. Involvement may also include perianal, buttock, and thigh areas.

Answer a is incorrect. Genital herpes is a chronic, lifelong viral infection.

Answer c is incorrect. The rate of genital herpes recurrence generally decreases over time.

Answer d is incorrect. The risk of transmission in a mother with recurrent disease but no visible lesions is thought to be low.

---

13. EV is a 29-year-old pregnant patient with a past medical history of genital HSV herpes. Which of the following is true regarding genital herpes infection and pregnancy?

   a. The risk of herpes transmission is lowest in mothers who have the initial outbreak at the time of delivery.
   b. Acyclovir, famciclovir, and valacyclovir are classified in pregnancy category D.
   c. Use of antiviral therapy late in pregnancy decreases herpes transmission to the neonate.
   d. Herpes disease in the neonate commonly manifests as a scalp abscess or ophthalmic infection.

Answer c is correct. Herpes transmission from an infected mother can cause symptomatic disease in the neonate. Use of antiviral therapy late in pregnancy decreases herpes recurrences near term as well as transmission to the neonate.

Answer a is incorrect. The risk of herpes transmission is highest in mothers who have the initial outbreak at the time of delivery.

Answer b is incorrect. Acyclovir, famciclovir, and valacyclovir are classified in pregnancy category B.

Answer d is incorrect. Gonococcal disease in the neonate commonly manifests as a scalp abscess or ophthalmic infection.

14. HF is a 29-year-old woman who was diagnosed with genital herpes 6 years ago. She reports approximately one to two recurrences each year since diagnosis. Recently she has experienced an increase in outbreaks, having three in a 6-month period. The decision is made to start HF on daily suppressive therapy. Select the most appropriate therapy for HF.

    a. Valacyclovir po
    b. Erythromycin ointment
    c. Tetracycline po
    d. Acyclovir ointment

Answer a is correct. Valacyclovir is a prodrug of acyclovir that has increased oral bioavailability. It is a recommended agent for daily suppressive therapy.

Answer b is incorrect. Erythromycin is an antibacterial agent and would be ineffective against the herpes virus.

Answer c is incorrect. Tetracycline is an antibacterial agent and would be ineffective against the herpes virus.

Answer d is incorrect. Use of topical antiviral therapy (eg, acyclovir ointment) is discouraged due to limited clinical benefit.

15. Which of the following is true regarding the stages of syphilis infection?

    a. The characteristic lesion of primary syphilis is a diffuse rash, usually affecting the palms and soles.
    b. Manifestations of latent syphilis include regional lymphadenopathy and meningitis.
    c. Tertiary syphilis is highly transmissible.
    d. Neurosyphilis can present at any stage of syphilis.

Answer d is correct. CNS involvement can present at any stage of syphilis. Early neurosyphilis occurs within first few years of infection and usually coexists with primary or secondary syphilis. Late neurosyphilis occurs years to decades after the initial infection and represents a tertiary manifestation of syphilis.

Answer a is incorrect. The characteristic lesion of primary syphilis is the chancre (ulcer). The chancre is usually painless and appears at the site of *T. pallidum* entrance into the body approximately 3 weeks after transmission.

Answer b is incorrect. Latent syphilis refers to patients with a positive serologic diagnosis for syphilis, but no clinical symptoms. This stage occurs after secondary syphilis symptoms have subsided and there are two possible outcomes: progression to tertiary syphilis or clinical cure.

Answer c is incorrect. Tertiary syphilis encompasses the long-term complications of syphilitic disease such as granulomatous disease (also called gummatous syphilis) and cardiovascular syphilis. Tertiary syphilis is now uncommon due to antibiotic treatment and is not transmissible.

16. Which of the following is true regarding the diagnosis of syphilis?

    a. The diagnosis of syphilis is made through direct techniques such as culture.
    b. Serologic testing is the standard method of detecting primary, secondary, latent, and tertiary syphilis in the United States.
    c. The VDRL-CSF is the standard serologic test for secondary syphilis.
    d. Nontreponemal serologic testing alone is sufficient for a definitive diagnosis of syphilis.

Answer b is correct. Serologic testing, including treponemal and nontreponemal tests, provides a presumptive diagnosis and is the standard method of detecting primary, secondary, latent, and tertiary syphilis in the United States.

Answer a is incorrect. *T. pallidum* cannot be cultured, so indirect diagnostic techniques must be used.

Answer c is incorrect. The VDRL-CSF is the standard serologic test for neurosyphilis, not secondary syphilis.

Answer d is incorrect. Nontreponemal tests, such as the VDRL and RPR, are used for initial syphilis screening. Nontreponemal tests should be confirmed by treponemal-specific tests (such as the *T. pallidum* particle agglutination or fluorescent treponemal antibody absorption test) due to the rate of false-positive results.

17. Select the brand name for benzathine penicillin.

    a. Bicillin C-R
    b. Wycillin
    c. Bicillin L-A
    d. Pen-VK

Answer c is correct. Bicillin L-A is the brand name for benzathine penicillin.

Answer a is incorrect. Bicillin C-R is the brand name for a procaine-benzathine penicillin mix.

Answer b is incorrect. Wycillin is the brand name for procaine penicillin.

Answer d is incorrect. Pen-VK is the brand name for oral penicillin V potassium.

18. TP is a 26-year-old woman who is 31 weeks pregnant. She visits her obstetrician-gynecologist because of a sore throat, generalized weakness, and a rash on her palms and soles for the past week. Testing is performed and a diagnosis of secondary syphilis is made. The treating physician requests pharmacist consultation because the patient is allergic to penicillin. Select the most appropriate therapy for TP.

    a. Doxycycline
    b. Cefoxitin + probenecid
    c. Levofloxacin
    d. Desensitization + benzathine penicillin G

Answer d is correct.   Penicillin regimens, appropriate for the stage of disease, are recommended for the treatment of syphilis in pregnant women. No proven alternatives to penicillin exist for the treatment of syphilis during pregnancy. It is recommended that pregnant patients with a penicillin allergy undergo desensitization and subsequent treatment with penicillin.

Answer a is incorrect.   While doxycycline is an appropriate choice for the treatment of secondary syphilis in the setting of penicillin allergy, tetracyclines are contraindicated in pregnancy.

Answer b is incorrect.   Cefoxitin plus probenecid is not a recommended antibiotic combination for the treatment of syphilis.

Answer c is incorrect.   Levofloxacin is not a recommended agent for the treatment of syphilis. Furthermore, fluoroquinolones have not adequately been studied in pregnancy and their use is generally discouraged.

19. The Jarisch-Herxheimer reaction is an acute febrile reaction associated with therapy for which STD?

    a. Genital herpes
    b. Gonorrhea
    c. Chlamydia
    d. Syphilis

Answer d is correct.   The Jarisch-Herxheimer reaction is an acute febrile reaction that may occur within hours of initiation of therapy for syphilis. It is most common in patients with early syphilis and usually subsides within a 24-hour period. Complications of the Jarisch-Herxheimer reaction include induction of early labor and fetal distress in pregnant women.

Answer a is incorrect.   The Jarisch-Herxheimer reaction is not associated with genital herpes.

Answer b is incorrect.   The Jarisch-Herxheimer reaction is not associated with gonorrhea.

Answer c is incorrect.   The Jarisch-Herxheimer reaction is not associated with chlamydia.

20. Which of the following is true regarding the treatment of STDs in special populations?

    a. The treatment of STDs in pregnancy can decrease pregnancy complications and prevent disease transmission to the child.
    b. Children diagnosed with congenital or acquired STDs should not be treated until they reach 2 years of age due to antimicrobial toxicities.
    c. In general, adolescent patients require lower doses of recommended antimicrobials for the treatment of STDs.
    d. Management of genital herpes in patients with HIV infection is the same as the management in patient who are HIV negative.

Answer a is correct.   The treatment of STDs in pregnancy can decrease pregnancy complications and prevent disease transmission to the child.

Answer b is incorrect.   Children, including neonates and infants, who are diagnosed with congenital or acquired STDs should be treated according to guideline recommendations.

Answer c is incorrect.   In general, pharmacologic treatment for STDs in adolescent patients is the same as in adults.

Answer d is incorrect.   Because severe or prolonged herpes episodes may occur in immunocompromised patients, doses for patients with HIV infection are typically higher and/or treatment durations longer than in patients who are HIV negative.

CHAPTER **32 | Influenza**

1. Select the statement that accurately describes a patient with influenza.

    a. MP has a bacterial illness caused by *Haemophilus influenzae*.
    b. BA has a viral illness caused by respiratory syncytial virus (RSV).
    c. JJ has a viral illness caused by rhinovirus.
    d. FJ has a viral illness caused by influenza A and B.

Answer d is correct.   Influenza A and B are the two types of influenza viruses that cause epidemic human disease. There are two subtypes of influenza A based upon surface antigens (hemagglutinin [H] and neuraminidase [N]). Influenza B is separated into two genetic lineages (Yamagata and Victoria), but not categorized by subtypes. Since 1977, influenza A subtype H1N1, influenza A subtype H3N2, and influenza B have been circulating globally.

Answer a is incorrect.   Influenza is a viral illness—not a bacterial illness. It is easy to confuse influenza viral infections with *H. influenzae* bacterial infections. Even though the species name of *Haemophilus* is *influenzae*, it is a bacterial pathogen. *H. influenzae* is a common cause of respiratory tract infections.

Answer b is incorrect.   RSV is a respiratory virus that infects the lungs and breathing passages. RSV is not influenza, although RSV is a viral infection. RSV is the most common cause of bronchiolitis (inflammation of the small airways in the lung) and pneumonia in children under 1 year of age in the United States. Most healthy people recover from RSV infection in 1 to 2 weeks. However, infection can be severe in some people, such as certain infants, young children, and older adults.

Answer c is incorrect.   Rhinoviruses are the most common viral infective agents in humans, and a causative agent of the common cold.

2. ZC is a 35-year-old woman. She does not have a significant past medical history and is currently taking a multivitamin and calcium supplementation. She has a 3-year-old child. Based upon the information provided, provide influenza vaccination recommendations.

   a. ZC is 35 years old and influenza only affects the elderly and young children. Vaccination not recommended.
   b. ZC does not have comorbidities that place her at risk for influenza complications. Vaccination not recommended.
   c. ZC has a child that is at risk for influenza complications. Vaccination recommended for ZC.
   d. ZC has a child that is at risk for influenza complications. Vaccination recommended for ZC and her 3-year-old child.

Answer d is correct.   Both ZC and the 3-year-old child should be recommended to receive influenza vaccination, barring any contraindication. Counseling and discussion with patient would reveal if mother or child had contraindication to receiving influenza vaccination.

Answer a is incorrect.   Influenza can cause illness in any person, regardless of age. Children and elderly individuals are often at risk for influenza complications. ZC is at low risk for influenza complications because of her age and lack of comorbidities; however, influenza vaccination is recommended for providers of children because children are at high risk for influenza complications.

Answer b is incorrect.   Because of ZC's age and lack of comorbidities, she is at low risk for influenza complications. However, influenza vaccination is recommended for providers of children, because children are at high risk for influenza complications.

Answer c is incorrect.   Because the child is at risk for influenza and influenza complications, it is important to vaccinate the mother and child.

The following case should be used for questions 3 and 4:

A 33-year-old woman who runs a daycare for children 6 months of age to 5 years of age calls your pharmacy for information pertaining to the transmission of influenza.

3. What primary method of transmission for seasonal influenza should she be most concerned with?

   a. Inhalation
   b. Exposure to blood
   c. Exposure to dead birds
   d. Exposure to body fluids

Answer a is correct.   Inhalation of respiratory droplets is the primacy mechanism for contracting the influenza illness.

Answers b and d are incorrect.   Influenza is not transmitted via these routes. Other viral infections such as human immunodeficiency virus (HIV) may be transmitted via blood and/or bodily fluids.

Answer c is incorrect.   Exposure to dead birds has been associated with the West Nile virus and bird flu. The bird flu consists of different antigens than the traditional (seasonal) flu. Bird flu is H5N1 and traditional flu is H1N1 or H3N2.

4. What other information should be provided to this caller to help reduce the transmission of seasonal influenza? Select all that apply.

   a. Influenza vaccination is strongly encouraged given the caller's place of work.
   b. Cover your nose and mouth with a tissue when you cough or sneeze.
   c. Wash your hands often with soap and water.
   d. Stay at home when worker or child has a fever.

Answer a is correct.   Seasonal influenza vaccination is strongly encouraged for the caller and her staff since they are taking care of persons who are at a higher risk of influenza infection and influenza related complications (ie, children 6 months to 59 months). The parents of these children should also be encouraged to seek vaccinations for the children and themselves as well.

Answers b and c are correct.   The CDC recommends covering your nose and mouth with a tissue when you cough or sneeze and washing your hands often with soap and water to prevent transmission of seasonal influenza.

Answer d is correct.   If you are sick with flu-like illness, CDC recommends that you stay home for at least 24 hours after your fever is gone except to get medical care or for other necessities. (Your fever should be gone without the use of a fever-reducing medicine.) Keep away from others as much as possible to keep from making others sick.

5. DB is a 40-year-old man with a history of hypertension. DB has not been feeling well for the past 2 days and decides to go to his doctor. Based on his symptoms, DB's doctor diagnoses him with influenza. What could be some of DB's symptoms that led to his diagnosis? Select all that apply.

   a. Rapid onset of fever
   b. Myalgia
   c. Headache
   d. Nonproductive cough

Answers a, b, c, and d are correct.   Classic signs and symptoms of influenza include rapid onset of fever, myalgia, headache, malaise, nonproductive cough, sore throat, and rhinitis. Nausea, vomiting, and otitis media are commonly reported in children. Signs and symptoms resolve in 3 to 7 days; however, cough and malaise may persist for more than 2 weeks.

6. BC is a 28-month-old child with no significant past medical history. BC has not had a wheezing episode in the last 12 months. Select the best statement as it relates to influenza vaccination.

   a. BC should be vaccinated with IIV.
   b. BC should be vaccinated with LAIV.

c. BC should be vaccinated with RIV or ccIIV₃.

d. BC should be administered oseltamivir for prophylaxis.

Answer a is correct.   All children greater than 6 months of age should receive vaccination. Children greater than 2 years of age without a history of asthma or wheezing episode within past 12 months may receive IIV or LAIV. Children 6 months to 2 years should only receive IIV.

Answer b is incorrect.   All children greater than 6 months of age should receive vaccination. LAIV, or the nasal spray vaccine, is not recommended for use during the 2017-2018 season because of concerns about its effectiveness. For subsequent influenza seasons, please refer to the CDC recommendations.

Answer c is incorrect.   ccIIV3 is an IIV, but only persons age 18 years and older should receive this vaccine. RIV should only be given to people who are 18 to 49 years of age.

Answer d is incorrect.   Antiviral drugs used for prophylaxis should be considered adjuncts and not a replacement for annual vaccination with TIV or LAIV.

7. Select the agent that is administered via intramuscular injection for influenza prevention or postexposure prophylaxis.

a. IIV

b. LAIV

c. Zanamivir

d. Amantadine

Answer a is correct.   IIV should be administered via intramuscular injection.

Answer b is incorrect.   LAIV is administered intranasally (mist). Also, LAIV is not used as postexposure prophylaxis.

Answer c is incorrect.   Zanamivir is administered via oral inhalation.

Answer d is incorrect.   Amantadine is administered orally. Also, because of increased levels of adamantane resistance, amantadine and rimantadine are not used in the United States for postexposure prophylaxis or treatment, unless combined with other antiviral agents.

8. XW is a 28-year-old pregnant patient. She is currently receiving amoxicillin for a urinary tract infection caused by *Escherichia coli*. She comes to your pharmacy wanting an influenza vaccination. She hates shots and prefers not to receive any injection. During last year's influenza season, she received treatment with oseltamivir. What is the appropriate agent for influenza vaccination for XW? Select all that apply.

a. LAIV

b. IIV

c. RIV

d. Oseltamivir

Answer b is correct.   IIV may be administered to pregnant patients. Vaccination is recommended regardless of the stage of pregnancy.

Answer c is correct.   RIV may be administered to pregnant patients. Vaccination is recommended regardless of the stage of pregnancy.

Answer a is incorrect.   LAIV should not be used in pregnant patients at this time. LAIV is indicated for healthy, nonpregnant patients 2 years of age to 49 years of age. However, LAIV, or the nasal spray vaccine, is **not** recommended for use during the 2017-2018 season because of concerns about its effectiveness. For subsequent influenza seasons, please refer to the CDC recommendations.

Answer d is incorrect.   Oseltamivir should not replace TIV or LAIV as prevention of influenza unless the patient has a contraindication to receiving either TIV or LAIV (egg allergy). Also, there are insufficient human data to determine the risk to a pregnant woman or developing fetus.

9. Which of the following condition(s) would be a contraindication for receiving LAIV? Select all that apply.

a. Diabetes mellitus

b. Development of GBS within 6 weeks of receiving previous influenza vaccine

c. Egg allergy

d. Recently received amantadine (within 48 hours)

Note: LAIV, or the nasal spray vaccine, is *not* recommended for use during the 2017-2018 season because of concerns about its effectiveness. For subsequent influenza seasons, please refer to the CDC recommendations.

Answer a is correct.   Diabetes is currently a contraindication for receiving LAIV. Currently, LAIV is indicated for healthy patients from the age of 2 to 49 years. Patients with a significant past medical history (diabetes, chronic obstructive pulmonary disease [COPD], asthma, atrial fibrillation, coronary heart disease, etc.) will not be candidates for LAIV. The only past medical history that does not exclude patients from receiving LAIV is hypertension.

Answer b is correct.   Development of GBS within 6 weeks of receiving an influenza vaccine (this includes LAIV, IIV, and RIV) is contraindication for receiving influenza vaccine.

Answer c is correct.   Influenza vaccine (IIV and LAIV) are made from eggs and should not be utilized in patients with an egg allergy. RIV could be used in this instance if the person is 18 to 49 years of age.

Answer d is correct.   Antiviral agents (such as amantadine) have the potential to inhibit the replication of live vaccine virus, and could interfere with the effectiveness of the vaccine. Therefore, LAIV should not be administered within 2 weeks before or 48 hours after administration of amantadine. IIV or RIV may be administered at any time relative to amantadine.

10. Which of the following condition(s) would be a contraindication for receiving IIV?

    a. Diabetes mellitus
    b. Egg allergy
    c. Recently received amantadine (within 48 hours)
    d. Concerned about development of autism from thimerosal in IIV

Answer b is correct. Patients with an egg allergy should not receive IIV. Patients with an egg allergy cannot receive LAIV either. RIV could be used in this instance if the person is 18 to 49 years of age.

Answer a is incorrect. Diabetic patients can and should receive influenza vaccination with IIV unless they have a contraindication.

Answer c is incorrect. IIV may be administered within 48 hours of adamantanes (rimantadine and amantadine). LAIV should not be administered within this time frame because the adamantanes could inhibit viral replication and interfere with the effectiveness of LAIV.

Answer d is incorrect. There is no association with influenza vaccines and the development of autism or from thimerosal in the vaccines. Thimerosal is used as a preservative in the influenza vaccines and the amount of thimerosal has been reduced or eliminated from the vaccine (except from multidose vials).

11. Adamantanes have activity against which influenza types?

    a. Influenza A
    b. Influenza B
    c. Influenza C
    d. *Haemophilus influenzae*

Answer a is correct. Adamantanes (rimantadine and amantadine) have activity against influenza A; however, over the past few influenza seasons, resistance to the adamantanes has significantly increased.

Answer b is incorrect. Adamantanes do not have activity against influenza B.

Answer c is incorrect. Influenza C is not a common cause in influenza infections.

Answer d is incorrect. *H. influenzae* is a Gram-negative bacterial organism that causes upper respiratory tract infections.

12. Select the brand name for zanamivir.

    a. Relenza
    b. Tamiflu
    c. Symmetrel
    d. Fluzone

Answer a is correct. Relenza is the brand name for zanamivir.

Answer b is incorrect. Tamiflu is the brand name for oseltamivir.

Answer c is incorrect. Symmetrel is the brand name for amantadine.

Answer d is incorrect. Fluzone is the brand name for IIV. IIV has several different brand names because there are different manufacturers. Of note Flublok is the brand name for RIV.

13. Select the anti-influenza agent that is formulated as a Rotadisk inhaler.

    a. Rimantadine
    b. Amantadine
    c. Oseltamivir
    d. Zanamivir

Answer d is correct. Zanamivir is formulated as a Rotadisk inhaler (5 mg/blister).

Answer a is incorrect. Rimantadine is formulated as a tablet (100 mg).

Answer b is incorrect. Amantadine is formulated as syrup (50 mg/mL), tablet (100 mg), and capsule (100 mg).

Answer c is incorrect. Oseltamivir is formulated as a capsule (30 mg, 45 mg, 75 mg) and powder for oral suspension (6 mg/mL)

14. YQ is a 59-year-old man with a past medical history significant for COPD, diabetes mellitus, hypertension, and hyperlipidemia. YQ wanted to receive influenza vaccination, but the United States has a short supply of IIV and RIV. YQ's physician recommended postexposure prophylaxis if he is exposed to influenza. If YQ is exposed to influenza, which agent should be used as postexposure prophylaxis?

    a. Amantadine
    b. Rimantadine
    c. Oseltamivir
    d. Zanamivir

Answer c is correct. Oseltamivir may be used as postexposure prophylaxis, but only when influenza vaccines cannot be used. Since this patient cannot obtain the vaccine because of a short supply, postexposure prophylaxis with oseltamivir would be appropriate.

Answer a is incorrect. Amantadine should not be used for postexposure prophylaxis because it does not have activity against influenza B and because of an increase in adamantanes resistance to influenza A.

Answer b is incorrect. Rimantadine should not be used for postexposure prophylaxis because it does not have activity against influenza B and because of an increase in adamantanes resistance to influenza A.

Answer d is incorrect. Zanamivir may cause bronchospasm in patient's COPD or asthma. Therefore, this agent is not ideal for patient YQ.

15. A 24-year-old woman with a history of asthma presents to your pharmacy to ask a question about influenza prevention and symptom resolution. She was diagnosed with influenza B. She still has cough and malaise. What should you discuss with the patient? Select all that apply.

    a. Influenza symptoms will disappear within 48 hours. If you are still having symptoms, see your provider.
    b. Influenza symptoms typically last 3 to 7 days. Cough and malaise may last up to 2 weeks. If your symptoms have increased/worsened, you may need to see your provider.
    c. As long as a patient does not have a fever, there is no need to worry. Cough and malaise symptoms will go away.
    d. Influenza vaccination on an annual basis is strongly encouraged given the patient's history of asthma.

Answer b is correct.   Influenza symptoms typically last 3 to 7 days, while cough and malaise may persist for longer.

Answer d is correct.   Emphasis should be placed upon vaccinating certain groups at higher risk of influenza infection and influenza related complications. This patient has a history of asthma (one of the high risk groups) and should be encourage to receive the influenza vaccine annually.

Answer a is incorrect.   Influenza symptoms may (and often do) last longer than 48 hours.

Answer c is incorrect.   Influenza complications can lead to high morbidity and mortality. Just because a patient lacks a fever does not mean they will not develop influenza complications.

16. SW is a 32-year-old woman who is in her third trimester of pregnancy. Her doctor suggested that she be vaccinated with the seasonal influenza vaccine since she is at a higher risk of having influenza and influenza-related complications due to pregnancy. She comes to your pharmacy for the vaccination and inquires about side effects. Select the most common adverse reaction of IIV.

    a. Injection site soreness
    b. Birth defects
    c. GBS
    d. Autism

Answer a is correct.   Injection site soreness is a common adverse reaction from administration of IIV since it is administered as an intramuscular injection.

Answer b is incorrect.   There is no conclusive documentation that IIV causes birth defects. IIV should be administered to pregnant patients.

Answer c is incorrect.   IIV has not been associated with the development of GBS. If a patient developed GBS within 6 weeks after an influenza vaccine, they should not receive the vaccine again.

Answer d is incorrect.   IIV has not been associated with the development of autism.

17. Which of the following patient(s) should receive influenza vaccination? Select all that apply.

    a. CH who is 8-year-old boy with a history of cystic fibrosis
    b. GS who is a healthy 10-month-old baby girl
    c. KL who is a 48-year-old man with diabetes
    d. RC who is a healthy 65-year-old woman

Answer a is correct.   Chronic pulmonary patients are at a higher risk of having influenza and influenza related complications. He should receive influenza vaccination with IIV. He would not be a candidate for LAIV because he has cystic fibrosis or RIV because of his age. LAIV, or the nasal spray vaccine, is **not** recommended for use during the 2017-2018 season because of concerns about its effectiveness. For subsequent influenza seasons, please refer to the CDC recommendations.

Answer b is correct.   Children 6 to 59 months of age are at a higher risk of having influenza and influenza related complications. She should receive influenza vaccination with IIV. She would not be a candidate for LAIV or RIV because of her age. LAIV, or the nasal spray vaccine, is **not** recommended for use during the 2017-2018 season because of concerns about its effectiveness. For subsequent influenza seasons, please refer to the CDC recommendations.

Answer c is correct.   Diabetic patients are at a higher risk of having influenza and influenza related complications. He should receive influenza vaccination with IIV or RIV. He would not be a candidate for LAIV because he has diabetes. LAIV, or the nasal spray vaccine, is **not** recommended for use during the 2017-2018 season because of concerns about its effectiveness. For subsequent influenza seasons, please refer to the CDC recommendations.

Answer d is correct.   All persons aged 50 years and greater are at a higher risk of having influenza and influenza related complications. She should receive influenza vaccination with IIV. She would not be a candidate for LAIV or RIV since she is more than 49 years of age. LAIV, or the nasal spray vaccine, is **not** recommended for use during the 2017-2018 season because of concerns about its effectiveness. For subsequent influenza seasons, please refer to the CDC recommendations.

18. LWS is a 28-year-old man returning home from a military tour of duty from overseas. LWS is an OEF (operation enduring freedom) veteran. He received IIV 7 days ago. Today he presents with symptoms of influenza. Select the reason LWS could develop influenza symptoms, even if he received the appropriate vaccine.

    a. IIV is a dead virus and can cause influenza.
    b. LWS was not a candidate for influenza vaccination; therefore, he should not have received IIV.
    c. LWS does not have influenza. He has the common cold.
    d. Influenza vaccines are not 100% effective.

Answer d is correct. Influenza vaccines are not 100% effective. Therefore, even if you received the influenza vaccine, it is possible that you could develop influenza.

Answer a is incorrect. IIV is a dead virus and cannot replicate. There is currently no documentation that IIV can cause influenza.

Answer b is incorrect. LWS was a candidate for influenza vaccine. Any person wishing to not develop influenza is a candidate for influenza vaccine.

Answer c is incorrect. The symptoms of the common cold and influenza can overlap. There is not enough information given to be able to differentiate the common cold versus influenza.

19. Select the surface antigens that categorize influenza A. Select all that apply.
    a. Hemagglutinin
    b. Thimerosal
    c. Neuraminidase
    d. GBS

Answer a is correct. Hemagglutinin is a surface antigen for influenza A (ie, H3N2).

Answer c is correct. Neuraminidase is a surface antigen for influenza A (ie, H1N1).

Answer b is incorrect. Thimerosal is a preservative that is used in multidose vials of IIV. Thimerosal is not in LAIV, RIV, or prefilled syringes containing IIV.

Answer d is incorrect. Guillain-Barré syndrome is a disorder where the immune system attacks the peripheral nervous system.

20. TK is a 32-year-old HIV-positive patient. He does not want to develop influenza and would like to be vaccinated since he is immunocompromised. He has a severe egg allergy (wheezing). Select the appropriate vaccination for TK.
    a. LAIV
    b. RIV
    c. IIV
    d. Immunocompromised patients should not be vaccinated

Answer b is correct. RIV may be used in immunocompromised patients, including HIV. He has a history of egg allergies so IIV would not be preferred in this instance.

Answer a is incorrect. LAIV is indicated for healthy, nonpregnant patients aged 2 to 49 years. Since TK has HIV, he is not a candidate for LAIV. LAIV, or the nasal spray vaccine, is **not** recommended for use during the 2017-2018 season because of concerns about its effectiveness. For subsequent influenza seasons, please refer to the CDC recommendations.

Answer c is incorrect. IIV may be used in immunocompromised patients, including HIV. He has a history of egg allergies so IIV would not be preferred in this instance.

Answer d is incorrect. Immunocompromised patients should be vaccinated with IIV or RIV, unless there is a contraindication.

21. You are working in an outpatient clinic and a 27-year-old man comes in with a 2-day history of myalgia, headache, malaise, nonproductive cough, sore throat, and rhinitis. He also has a fever that started this morning. The doctor at the clinic diagnoses him with influenza after a positive rapid antigen test and wants to prescribe oseltamivir therapy for 5 days to the patient. The doctor asks you for a dose. What reference(s) would you consult to find this information?
    a. PubMed
    b. *Drug Information Handbook*
    c. Index Medicus
    d. *Martindale: The Complete Drug Reference*

Answer b is correct. *Drug Information Handbook* is a tertiary reference that contains dosing information.

Answer a is incorrect. PubMed is a secondary reference that compiles primary literature. Dosing information could be found, but specifics related to oseltamivir and dosing may not be retrievable in a timely fashion.

Answer c is incorrect. Index Medicus is a secondary reference that indexes bibliographic information of medical science journals. Dosing information could eventually be found, but specifics related to oseltamivir and dosing may not be retrievable in a timely fashion.

Answer d is incorrect. *Martindale: The Complete Drug Reference* is a tertiary reference that lists medications used throughout the world in monograph form. It is most useful for identifying foreign proprietary names of medications.

CHAPTER **33** | Estimating Renal Function

Questions 1 through 3 apply to the following case.

BG is a 50-year-old African American woman who is 63 in tall and weighs 130 lb. Her current SCr is 1.6 mg/dL.

1. What is BG's IBW?
    a. 125 lb
    b. 115 lb
    c. 135 lb
    d. 165 lb

Answer b is correct. IBW (women) = 45.5 + 2.3 (3 in over 5 ft) = 52.4 kg × 2.2 lb/1 kg = 115 lb

2. What is BG's CrCl as estimated by the Cockcroft-Gault equation?

   a. 41 mL/min
   b. 35 mL/min
   c. 50 mL/min
   d. 58 mL/min

Answer b is correct. CrCl = [(140 − 50) × 52.4 kg /72 × 1.6 mg/dL] × 0.85 = ~35 mL/min

3. What is BG's GFR as estimated by the MDRD equation?

   a. 25 mL/min
   b. 35 mL/min
   c. 45 mL/min
   d. 55 mL/min

Answer b is correct. GFR = $186 × 1.6^{-1.154} × 50^{-0.203} × 0.742 = $ ~36 mL/min

Questions 4 through 6 apply to the following case.

GS is a 79-year-old African American man who is 71 in tall and weighs 190 lb. His current SCr is 1.2 mg/dL.

4. What is GS's IBW?

   a. 145 lb
   b. 156 lb
   c. 166 lb
   d. 254 lb

Answer c is correct. IBW (man) = 50 + 2.3 (11 in over 5 ft) = 75.3 kg × 2.2 lb/1 kg = 166 lb

5. What is GS's CrCl as estimated by the Cockcroft-Gault equation?

   a. 69 mL/min
   b. 45 mL/min
   c. 81 mL/min
   d. 53 mL/min

Answer d is correct. CrCl = (140 − 79) × 75.3 kg /72 × 1.2 mg/dL = ~53 mL/min

6. What is GS's GFR as estimated by the MDRD equation?

   a. 45 mL/min
   b. 55 mL/min
   c. 65 mL/min
   d. 75 mL/min

Answer d is correct. GFR = $186 × 1.2^{-1.154} × 79^{-0.203} × 1.210 = $ ~75 mL/min

7. JK is a 4-year-old girl who is 42 in tall and weighs 50 lb. Her current SCr is 0.6 mg/dL. What is JK's estimated GFR based on the Schwartz equation?

   a. ~30 mL/min
   b. ~60 mL/min

   c. ~80 mL/min
   d. ~100 mL/min

Answer d is correct. 42 in × 2.54 cm/in × 0.55/0.6 mg/dL = ~100 mL/min

8. LO is a 6-month-old infant who is 25 in long and weighs 15 lb. His current SCr is 0.4 mg/dL. What is LO's estimated GFR based on the Schwartz equation?

   a. 60 mL/min
   b. 70 mL/min
   c. 80 mL/min
   d. 90 mL/min

Answer b is correct. 25 in × 2.54 cm/in × 0.45/0.4 mg/dL = ~70 mL/min

9. Which of the following factors independent from GFR affect SCr? Select all that apply.

   a. Age
   b. Diet
   c. Gender
   d. Race

Answers a, b, c, and d are correct. Age, diet, gender, and race all can affect SCr in patients.

10. Which of the following patients would be most likely to have a baseline SCr of <0.8 mg/dL?

    a. A 25-year-old man in very good health
    b. A 36-year-old man adhering to the Atkins diet
    c. A 92-year-old woman who is wheelchair bound
    d. A bodybuilder taking creatine supplements

Answer c is correct. This patient likely has very little muscle mass, which will contribute to a below normal SCr.

Answer a is incorrect. This patient is most likely to have a SCr in the normal range of 0.8 to 1.2.

Answer b is incorrect. Since the Atkins diet is extremely high in protein, this patient will likely have a SCr in the high end of the normal range or slightly above the normal range. Excessive protein intake can increase SCr.

Answer d is incorrect. This patient will likely have a higher than normal SCr due to the addition of creatine supplements to the diet.

11. Which of the following is considered the gold standard for measurement of GFR?

    a. Cockcroft-Gault equation
    b. MDRD equation
    c. 24-Hour urine creatinine
    d. Inulin clearance

Answer d is correct. Inulin clearance method is considered the gold standard for measurement of GFR. It is rarely done in clinical practice due to cost and complexity issues.

Answer a is incorrect. The Cockcroft-Gault equation is the most commonly used method to estimate CrCl but does not *measure* GFR.

Answer b is incorrect. The MDRD equation estimates but does not measure GFR.

Answer c is incorrect. Twenty-four hour urine creatinine analysis has shown to be no more accurate than the Cockcroft-Gault and MDRD equations and does not measure GFR.

---

12. Which of the following factors are important to consider when dosing a medication based on renal function? Select all that apply.

    a. The extent to which the drug is renally eliminated
    b. SCr
    c. The manufacturer-recommended dosing guidelines for the agent
    d. Aspartate aminotransferase (AST)

Answers a, b, and c are correct. All of these factors are important to consider when dosing a medication based on renal function.

Answer d is incorrect. AST is a clinical biochemistry assay designed to give information about the liver. Liver transaminases (eg, AST) are useful biomarkers of liver injury.

---

13. GU is a 50-year-old man who is admitted with SCr of 1.1 mg/dL. Twenty-four hours later, his SCr is 2.2 mg/dL. GU is on several medications that need to be dose-adjusted for renal function. What is the most appropriate course of action?

    a. Calculate GU's GFR using the MDRD equation and dose adjust based on the result.
    b. Calculate GU's CrCl using the Cockcroft-Gault equation and dose-adjust based on the result.
    c. Discontinue all of GU's medications until his renal function improves.
    d. Assess each of GU's medications and use clinical judgment to determine the best course of action, balancing the risk of treatment failure with drug toxicity.

Answer d is correct. Each medication should be assessed to determine the most appropriate course of action based on the patient's condition and the combined risks of drug toxicity and treatment failure.

Answer a is incorrect. The MDRD equation may overestimate GFR in this patient who is in acute renal failure. This could lead to overdosing and potential toxicities.

Answer b is incorrect. The Cockcroft-Gault equation may also overestimate renal function in a patient with acute renal failure.

Answer c is incorrect. It would be inappropriate to simply discontinue necessary medications.

---

14. LN is an 88-year-old man who weighs 70 kg and is 71 in tall. His current SCr is 0.6 mg/dL. What is his CrCl as estimated by the Cockcroft-Gault equation?

    a. 101 mL/min
    b. 51 mL/min
    c. 92 mL/min
    d. 46 mL/min

Answer b is correct. LN has a SCr <1.0 mg/dL, so we should round up to 1.0 mg/dL when using the Cockcroft-Gault equation. CrCl = (140 − 88) × 70 kg/72 × 1.0 = 51 mL/min.

---

15. FW is a 33-year-old woman with a SCr of 1.3 mg/dL. She is 64 in tall and weighs 118 lb. She has no past medical history. Which of the following methods is the most appropriate way to estimate her renal function? Select all that apply.

    a. Schwartz equation
    b. MDRD equation
    c. Cockcroft-Gault equation
    d. Jelliffe equation

Answers b and c are correct. The MDRD may be used to estimate the renal function in this patient. The Cockcroft-Gault equation may be used to estimate the renal function in this patient. Both the MDRD and Cockcroft-Gault equations would be appropriate methods to estimate this patient's renal function. The vast majority of medications use Cockcroft-Gault for determining dosing based on renal function.

Answer a is incorrect. The Schwartz equation is used for pediatric patients.

Answer d is incorrect. The Jelliffe equation is used to estimate GFR in patient with changing SCr values. Clinical judgment must be used to adjust medication dosages in patients with rapidly changing renal function as even the Jelliffe equation has limited supporting data for these patient scenarios.

Questions 16 through 18 apply to the following case.

DA is a 32-year-old African American woman who is 67 in tall and weighs 88 lb. Her current SCr is 0.8 mg/dL.

16. What is DA's IBW?

    a. 135 lb
    b. 125 lb
    c. 145 lb
    d. 85 lb

Answer a is correct. IBW (women) = 45.5 + 2.3 (7 in over 5 ft) = 61.6 kg × 2.2 lb/1 kg = 135 lb

17. What is DA's CrCl as estimated by the Cockcroft-Gault equation?

    a. 98 mL/min
    b. 115 mL/min
    c. 64 mL/min
    d. 75 mL/min

Answer c is correct. Since DA's actual body weight is less than her IBW, actual body weight should be used. CrCl = $[(140 - 32) \times 40 \text{ kg}/72 \times 0.8] \times 0.85 = {\sim}60$ to 65 mL/min

18. What is DA's GFR as estimated by the MDRD equation?

    a. 54 mL/min
    b. 66 mL/min
    c. 75 mL/min
    d. 88 mL/min

Answer d is correct. GFR = $186 \times 0.8^{-1.154} \times 32^{-0.203} \times 0.742 = {\sim}88$ mL/min

19. Select the normal SCr for an adult patient.

    a. 0.3 mg/dL
    b. 0.7 mg/dL
    c. 1.7 mg/dL
    d. 2.0 mg/dL

Answer b is correct. The normal range for SCr is from 0.6 to 1.2 mg/dL; however, just because this serum creatinine value lies within a normal range does not mean that the patient has effective kidney filtration. Other factors would have to be evaluated to estimate GFR, such as age, weight, sex, race (for the MDRD), muscle mass, and urine output.

Answer a is incorrect. The normal range for SCr is from 0.6 to 1.2 mg/dL; however, this can vary between assays. A SCr value of 0.3 mg/dL may indicate low muscle mass.

Answer c is incorrect. A SCr of 1.7 mg/dL lies outside the normal range for SCr.

Answer d is incorrect. A SCr of 2.0 mg/dL lies outside the normal range of SCr.

20. Select the weight that should be used to calculate the CrCl via the Cockcroft-Gault method.

    a. IBW
    b. Actual body weight
    c. Adjusted body weight
    d. No weight should be used

Answer a is correct. IBW should be used to calculate CrCl. However, the Cockcroft-Gault equation is a population mathematical model used to estimate kidney filtration within an individual patient. Patient extremes may introduce variability and the mathematical model will lose accuracy. For example, the Cockcroft-Gault method was not validated on using extreme patient populations; therefore, obese patients may have an inaccurate estimation of GFR compared to non-obese patients. The IBW should be used in obese patients for purposes of estimating CrCl.

Answer b is incorrect. Actual body weight is not used in calculating the CrCl *unless* the actual body weight is less than the calculated IBW. However, refer to package insert of select medications for specific recommendations as this is a general rule.

Answer c is incorrect. Adjusted body weight takes into account the patients lean body mass and a percentage of the total body weight. Adjusted body weight = IBW + 0.4 (actual body weight – IBW). This equation may be used for calculation of volume of distribution for certain drugs that are heavily distributed into tissues for obese patients. Adjusted body weight would not be used for estimation of GFR.

Answer d is incorrect. The IBW should be used for calculation of CrCl, unless the actual body weight is less than the IBW.

CHAPTER **34 | Acute Kidney Injury**

1. AH is a 72-year-old woman who presents to the emergency room complaining of severe nausea and vomiting for 3 days. On admission, her SCr is 2.5 mg/dL (her baseline is 1.1 mg/dL). She has not been able to eat or drink for 3 days and has lost 2.5 kg. Her medications on admission include: hydrochlorothiazide 25 mg po every day, lisinopril 10 mg po every day. Which of the following statements is *true* regarding AH at this time? Select all that apply.

    a. Nausea and vomiting may have caused a decrease in her EABV leading to prerenal AKI.
    b. AH should not receive radiocontrast media unless absolutely necessary until her kidneys recover.
    c. Hydrochlorothiazide may have caused vasoconstriction of the afferent arteriole leading to prerenal AKI.
    d. Lisinopril should be discontinued until AH's kidney function returns near her baseline.
    e. AH's weight loss suggests fluid volume depletion.

Answer a is correct. Nausea and vomiting can lead to decreased fluid volume and a decrease in EABV. A decrease in EABV will result in decreased perfusion to the kidneys and may result in prerenal AKI.

Answer b is correct. Radiocontrast media can cause ATN, and given that this patient already has AKI, the administration of any known nephrotoxins should be avoided if possible. If the use of radiocontrast media is necessary, AH should be adequately hydrated prior to the administration.

Answer d is correct. Lisinopril is an ACE-I and acts to vasodilate the efferent arteriole. This action, in combination with the volume depletion AH is experiencing may have contributed to the prerenal AKI. While ACE-I may be beneficial in slowing progression of CKD, further decreasing the intraglomerular pressure during any type of AKI may potentiate or prolong the damage to the kidney.

Answer e is correct. AH's sudden weight loss is likely due to acute water loss. Volume depletion, in combination with the other risk factors likely caused AH's prerenal AKI.

Answer c is incorrect. Hydrochlorothiazide is a thiazide-type diuretic. It acts in the distal tubule to block sodium reabsorption and thereby enhances sodium and water excretion. While this agent may have contributed to AH's AKI by this mechanism, it does not constrict the afferent arteriole.

---

2. Which of the following findings is consistent with the diagnosis of prerenal AKI?

   a. Specific gravity 1.029, FENa 0.85%, uOsmol 550 mOsm/kg
   b. Specific gravity 1.013, FENa 1.75%, uOsmol 350 mOsm/L
   c. Specific gravity 1.009, FENa 2.04%, uOsmol 213 mOsm/L
   d. UA: 1+ protein, 10 to 15 RBC, 10 to 15 WBC

Answer a is correct. A high specific gravity, low FENa, and high uOsmol is indicative of a prerenal AKI, a state in which the kidneys will avidly reabsorb sodium and water in an attempt to increase the perfusion to the kidneys and increase the intraglomerular pressure.

Answer b is incorrect. The specific gravity suggests normal urine density. The FENa is within the normal range of 1% to 2%. The uOsmol is also normal. These urine findings are not suggestive of any specific kidney damage.

Answer c is incorrect. In this situation the specific gravity is low, suggesting more dilute urine. The FENa is possibly a little elevated, suggesting excess sodium loss. The uOsmol is a bit low. These findings are the opposite of what might be seen in a prerenal AKI.

Answer d is incorrect. The protein and cellular matter in this UA are suggestive of some type of intrinsic AKI. Typically, in prerenal AKI there will not be any particulate matter in the urine.

---

3. A patient in the intensive care unit develops AKI. You review the medications the patient has been taking to evaluate for drug-induced AKI. Which of the following agents would be *most likely* to cause AIN?

   a. Labetalol
   b. Diltiazem
   c. Nafcillin
   d. Propofol

Answer c is correct. AIN is a hypersensitivity reaction and is most commonly associated with nafcillin and penicillin derivatives.

Answer a is incorrect. Labetalol is a nonselective β_1 and β_2 antagonist as well as an α-1 antagonist. Although it is possible to mount an allergic response to any foreign substance, labetalol is not a common cause of AIN. This agent would more

likely contribute to a prerenal AKI through its ability to lower blood pressure and decrease renal perfusion.

Answer b is incorrect. Diltiazem is a nondihydropyridine calcium channel antagonist. Although it is possible to mount an allergic response to any foreign substance, diltiazem is not a common cause of AIN. This agent would more likely contribute to a prerenal AKI as it can lower blood pressure and heart rate which could decrease cardiac output and therefore decrease renal perfusion.

Answer d is incorrect. Propofol is a sedative agent commonly used in the critical care setting. Although it is not a common cause of an allergic reaction (AIN), it may contribute to prerenal AKI due to a decrease in blood pressure and therefore renal perfusion. Patients with sulfite allergies can sometimes have general allergic reactions to propofol.

---

4. Which of the following statements is *true* regarding the use of diuretics in patients with oliguric AKI?

   a. Diuretics increase urine output and reverse kidney damage.
   b. Diuretics can be used in very high doses with little concern for toxicity.
   c. Thiazides and potassium-sparing diuretics are the preferred agents in AKI.
   d. Diuretics may improve urine output and help manage fluid and electrolyte abnormalities.

Answer d is correct. While studies have shown that nonoliguric patients have better outcomes than oliguric/anuric patients, there is no evidence that demonstrates that enhancing urine production through diuretic use confers these better outcomes. Diuretics may be helpful in controlling fluid overload and electrolyte abnormalities (particularly hyperkalemia).

Answer a is incorrect. Diuretics remove fluid, predominantly from the intravascular space. For this reason, they may actually worsen AKI and must be used with extreme caution.

Answer b is incorrect. High doses of diuretics can have serious consequences such as ototoxicity. While higher doses may be necessary to overcome diuretic resistance in AKI, careful monitoring should be employed.

Answer c is incorrect. While thiazide-type diuretics may be used in combination with loop diuretics to enhance urine production, they are not generally effective in cases of decreased kidney function. Potassium-sparing diuretics are generally contraindicated, especially if the patient is anuric/oliguric as hyperkalemia may occur rapidly and is potentially life threatening.

---

5. Which of the following agents can cause constriction of the *afferent* arteriole? Select all that apply.

   a. Ibuprofen
   b. Tacrolimus
   c. Captopril
   d. Rocephin
   e. Cyclosporine

Answers a, b, and e are correct. Vasodilatory prostaglandins such as PGE2 and PGI maintain the tone in the afferent arteriole. Nonsteroidal anti-inflammatory agents act by inhibiting cyclooxygenase and thereby prevent the production of prostaglandins. Thus, NSAIDs may lead to constriction of the afferent arteriole and a decrease in intraglomerular pressure. Calcineurin inhibitors like cyclosporine may also cause afferent arteriole constriction.

Answer c is incorrect. ACE-Is decrease/prevent the production of angiotensin II. Angiotensin II acts to vasoconstrict the efferent arteriole and maintain tone and pressure. A decrease in angiotensin II leads to vasodilation of the efferent arteriole and a subsequent decrease in intraglomerular pressure.

Answer d is incorrect. Cephalosporin antibiotics are not associated with afferent arteriole constriction.

---

6. Which of the following combinations would be effective to enhance urine production in a patient who has oliguric AKI secondary to ATN?

    a. Furosemide and ethacrynic acid
    b. Triamterene and hydrochlorothiazide
    c. Bumetanide and spironolactone
    d. Furosemide and metolazone

Answer d is correct. The combination of a loop-type (furosemide) and a thiazide diuretic (metolazone) synergistically enhances urine production. By preventing the reabsorption in the loop of Henle, more sodium remains in the tubular lumen and is delivered to the distal tubule. Blocking sodium channels in the distal tubule (thiazides) promotes the excretion of the sodium and water (now from both the loop of Henle and the distal tubule).

Answer a is incorrect. Both furosemide and ethacrynic acid are loop-type diuretics. They share the same mechanism of action, inhibiting sodium reabsorption in the loop of Henle. The use of two agents with the same mechanism of action would not be expected to produce synergistic effects.

Answer b is incorrect. Triamterene is a potassium-sparing diuretic and would be relatively contraindicated in oliguria/anuria. Hydrochlorothiazide works in the distal tubule. In oliguria, the delivery of sodium to the distal tubule is decreased and therefore the efficacy of hydrochlorothiazide would also be decreased.

Answer c is incorrect. While bumetanide is a loop-type diuretic that would be useful in oliguric ATN, spironolactone would be relatively contraindicated. Spironolactone is aldosterone antagonist and would therefore increase the elimination of sodium (and water) but enhance the reabsorption of potassium.

7. A patient with ATN with anuria has a serum potassium concentration of 6.8 mEq/L with associated electrocardiogram changes of peaked T waves. Which intervention should be initiated first?

    a. Regular insulin 10 units and 25 g of dextrose 50% IV push over 2 to 5 minutes
    b. Sodium bicarbonate 8.4% 50 mEq IV push over 2 to 5 minutes
    c. Calcium gluconate 1 g IV push over 2 to 5 minutes
    d. Sodium polystyrene sulfonate 15 g po

Answer c is correct. This patient has signs of cardiotoxicity secondary to hyperkalemia. The most important first step is to antagonize the effect of potassium on the myocardial cells. One gram of calcium (either chloride or gluconate) should be given immediately if any EKG abnormalities are noted.

Answer a is incorrect. Insulin stimulates the cellular uptake of potassium, decreasing the extracellular concentration. This is an appropriate step to manage hyperkalemia, though not the first step in this patient.

Answer b is incorrect. Administering sodium bicarbonate causes the efflux of H^+ from within in the cell in exchange for K^+. While this might be an appropriate strategy to manage hyperkalemia (especially if the patient had a metabolic acidosis), it is not the first step in this patient.

Answer d is incorrect. Sodium polystyrene sulfonate is an appropriate adjunctive agent to promote elimination of potassium from the body in the feces. It acts to exchange sodium for potassium ions in the gastrointestinal tract. It does not work immediately and would not be the first step.

---

8. Which of the following regimens would be the most appropriate prophylaxis option for contrast-induced nephropathy in a high-risk patient?

    a. Acetadote 150 mg/kg IV for 6 hours preprocedure
    b. Sodium chloride 0.9% IV infusion 6 hours before and 8 hours after
    c. Theophylline 200 mg po every 12 hours, two doses before, two doses after
    d. Dopamine 0.5 mcg/kg/min IV infusion 6 hours before and 6 hours after

---

Answer b is correct. Adequate hydration is important to protect the tubules of the kidneys. The IV solution of choice should be an isotonic crystalloid so that it remains in the intravascular space.

Answer a is incorrect. The recommended practice is to hydrate the patient prior to the administration of contrast media. While N-acetylcysteine (Acetadote) is an agent that has shown some benefit and is relatively safe, it would be used in conjunction with hydration, not alone. Additionally, this dose is the loading dose for the indication of acetaminophen toxicity, not prophylaxis of ATN.

Answer c is incorrect. There are conflicting data on the effectiveness of theophylline in reducing the incidence of contrast-induced nephropathy and its use is not supported by current guidelines. The primary prevention that is recommended is IV hydration.

Answer d is incorrect. The use of dopamine as well as fenoldopam has been shown to be deleterious in patients with AKI and ineffective as a prophylactic agent for ATN. The use of these agents is not recommended.

---

9. Which of the following circumstances can lead to ATN? Select all that apply.

    a. Administration of a direct nephrotoxin
    b. Prolonged hypotension
    c. Prolonged prerenal AKI
    d. Metronidazole
    e. Colistin

Answer a is correct. One mechanism of damage leading to ATN is direct toxicity. Substances that can bind to tubular cells and cause cellular damage include aminoglycosides, radiocontrast agents, myoglobin, and cisplatin.

Answer b is correct. There are two basic mechanisms that can cause ATN. Prolonged hypotension, decreases in renal perfusion, and decreases in intraglomerular pressure will lead to ischemia and necrosis in the tubular cells.

Answer c is correct. As in Answer b, any sustained episode of hypotension or hypoperfusion can lead to apoptosis of tubular cells and ATN.

Answer e is correct. Polymyxin E (Colistin) is a direct nephrotoxin and can cause ATN.

Answer d is incorrect. Metronidazole (Flagyl) is not a direct nephrotoxic medication and is not associated with ATN.

---

10. Which of the following statements is *true* regarding drug dosing in AKI?

    a. All patients should be dosed for a CrCl <10 mL/min.
    b. Pharmacokinetic parameters do not usually change so dose adjustment is not needed.
    c. Although elimination may be decreased, the volume of distribution should remain unchanged in AKI.
    d. The estimation of kidney function should include urine output.

Answer d is correct. It is difficult to quantify renal function and results from current equations and formulas should be interpreted with care. The patient's renal function should be evaluated with regard to the urine output and other clinical information. All of the available information should be used to obtain a more accurate assessment of the patient's renal function and status.

Answer a is incorrect. While it is difficult to quantify renal function during an episode of AKI, many patients will retain at least some kidney function. Assuming that there is no clearance, dosing conservatively may lead to subtherapeutic concentrations and inefficacy.

Answer b is incorrect. Many of the pharmacokinetic parameters (absorption, distribution, metabolism, and excretion) may be altered during AKI. While all of the changes are difficult to quantify, they must be considered and professional judgment must be exercised when determining drug dosing.

Answer c is incorrect. While decreases in elimination are easier to observe, changes in protein binding are common as metabolic byproducts, drugs and drug metabolites, and other substances accumulate in the body and compete for plasma protein binding sites. For example, patients with AKI in critical illness may experience increases in volume of distribution.

---

11. Which of the following UA findings would be *indicative* of acute GN?

    a. Protein
    b. Muddy brown casts
    c. pH 8.0
    d. Eosinophils

Answer a is correct. Proteins are large molecule substances that should not be able to cross the barriers in the glomerulus to be excreted in the urine. The presence of proteinuria is most indicative of glomerular nephritis.

Answer b is incorrect. Muddy brown casts are the cellular components of necrotic tubular epithelial cells. This is the hallmark finding of ATN.

Answer c is incorrect. The pH of the urine may have little to do with the pathophysiology of AKI. A high pH may predispose crystal formation of alkaline substances. This information would be more useful in the evaluation of postobstructive nephropathy.

Answer d is incorrect. The presence of eosinophils in the urine is unusual and would be more indicative of a hypersensitivity reaction (AIN).

---

12. Which of the following statements appropriately defines urine volume?

    a. Anuria is defined as <50 mL of urine per day.
    b. Oliguria is defined as <50 mL of urine per day.
    c. Polyuria is defined as <50 mL of urine per day.
    d. Anuria is defined as no urea in the urine.

Answer a is correct. Anuria, the absence of urine, is defined as urine output of <50 mL/d. Quantifying urine output is very important as it provides information about the GFR, the prognosis of the patient (worse outcomes) as well as anticipating needs for RRT as fluid, electrolyte, and acid–base balance will be severely compromised.

Answer b is incorrect. Oliguria, "little urine" is defined as urine output 50-400 mL/d. The judicious use of diuretics may enhance urine production to convert oliguria to nonoliguria (>400 mL/d). Patients who are nonoliguric have better outcomes.

Answer c is incorrect. Polyuria means a great deal of urine, generally any amount greater than normal output (~ 1.5-2 L/d). Polyuria maybe caused by aggressive diuresis or in the recovery phase of ATN as the glomerulus regains the ability to filter but the tubules have not yet regained the ability to properly reabsorb water, sodium, and other solutes.

Answer d is incorrect. The suffix "uria" refers to urine. While the urine may not contain a great deal of urea, the body is still producing urea and other nitrogenous wastes.

13. Place the acronym "AEIOU" in the correct order as it relates to the indications for RRT.

    a. A, *a*cid–base imbalance; E, *E*KG changes; I, *i*nflammation; O, *o*btundation; U, *u*remia
    b. A, *a*cute distress; e, *e*lectrolyte disturbance; I, *i*nflammation; O, *o*vert proteinuria; U, *u*remia
    c. A, *a*cid–base imbalance; E, *e*lectrolyte disturbance; I, *i*ngestion/intoxication; O, fluid *o*verload; U, *u*remia
    d. A, *a*cid–base imbalance; E, *E*KG abnormality; I, *i*ngestion/intoxication; O, *o*liguria; U, *u*remia

Answer c is correct. Remembering the acronym AEIOU can aid in the clinical evaluation of patients with AKI who may require emergent dialysis and other care.

Answer a is incorrect. While EKG changes may occur as a result of severe kidney insufficiency, the "E" stands for *e*lectrolytes. In fact, the most common (and potentially life-threatening) electrolyte disturbance in AKI is hyperkalemia. Increased serum potassium concentrations can lead to EKG changes, specifically peaked T waves, prolonged QRS waves, and even ventricular fibrillation. Additionally, the "I" is for *i*ngestion or *i*ntoxication, not inflammation. Inflammation is a common finding in patients with AKI and other comorbidities; unfortunately, renal replacement therapy will not help it. While obtundation is a parameter that should be carefully monitored, the "O" in the acronym stands for fluid *o*verload. The "U" is for *u*remic syndrome. For explanations I and O please also see Answers b and d.

Answer b is incorrect. The "A" stands for *a*cid–base disturbances. Metabolic acidosis is the most common finding in AKI. The "I" stands for *i*ngestion or *i*ntoxication. Renal replacement therapies may be able to remove toxic substances from the body. The "O" does not stand for overt proteinuria, but refers to fluid *o*verload. See Answer d.

Answer d is incorrect. The "O" stands for fluid *o*verload. While many patients with AKI may be oliguric (upon presentation or afterward), fluid accumulation secondary to decreased urine production can result in life-threatening

pulmonary edema. Auscultation of the lungs should be part of the physical examination to assess rales.

14. CB is a 24-year-old man brought to the hospital by his roommate. He states that he has been having diarrhea and vomiting for 3 days. He reports a 3 kg weight loss and cannot keep down anything, even water. In the emergency department his BP is 96/46 mm Hg, HR 120 beats/min, temp is 102.6°F, weight is 65 kg. On examination, his mucous membranes are dry and he has no peripheral edema. He does not recall the last time that he urinated but thinks it may have been yesterday. Which of the following findings would you expect from his serum and urine laboratory analysis?

    a. SpGr 1.035, 0 protein, dark yellow urine, no casts, FENa <1%
    b. SpGr 1.035, 0 protein, hazy-red urine, granular casts, FENa >2%
    c. SpGr 1.016, 2+ protein, light-yellow urine, many WBC and RBCs
    d. SpGr 1.005, 0 protein, hazy-red urine, granular casts, FENa >1%

Answer a is correct. The high SpGr, dark color, decreased FENa (<1%), and the absence of cellular matter and protein are all consistent with a prerenal AKI secondary to circumstances such as dehydration.

Answer b is incorrect. The FENa >2% suggests that the tubules are not reabsorbing as much sodium as possible. In a volume-depleted state (prerenal), the tubules should reabsorb as much water as possible and excrete as little as possible. In this situation, the FENa should be very low, <1%.

Answer c is incorrect. Dehydration causes a prerenal AKI. There is no intrinsic damage to the nephrons, so there should not be any cellular matter or protein in the urine (a bland sediment).

Answer d is incorrect. This is very dilute urine (SpGr 1.003). The FENa is inconsistent with prerenal AKI as is hazy-red appearance and presence of casts.

15. Which of the following statements best describes the BUN to SCr ratio?

    a. In situations of dehydration, the BUN:SCr ratio will be <10:1.
    b. In situations of dehydration, the BUN:SCr ratio will be >15:1.
    c. In situations of volume overload, the BUN:SCr ratio will be <10:1.
    d. In situations of volume overload, the BUN:SCr ratio will be >15:1.

Answer b is correct. Generally, the BUN:SCr ratio is approximately 10:1 to 15:1. In states of water conservation, the increased water reabsorption in the proximal tubule leads to increased reabsorption of urea back into systemic circulation and therefore an increase in BUN:SCr ratio.

Answer a is incorrect. Dehydration will cause the proximal tubule to reabsorb more sodium and water to compensate for the decreased EABV. Urea (BUN) is passively reabsorbed in the proximal tubule and the diffusion is increased with the increase in water reabsorption. This process leads to a disproportionately higher BUN than SCr concentration in states of dehydration.

Answer c is incorrect. While an elevated BUN:SCr ratio is helpful in assessing dehydration or a prerenal AKI, a low BUN:SCr ratio is not specific or sensitive for other disorders.

Answer d is incorrect. As noted in Answer b, an elevated BUN:SCr ratio is indicative of a dehydrated, prerenal AKI. It is important to remember that there are factors that may elevate the BUN that are not associated with a decline in renal function. Such factors include upper gastrointestinal bleeding or therapy with corticosteroids.

16. MT is a 38-year-old man brought to the ED after being found at the bottom of the stairs to his apartment. Apparently, while he was intoxicated, MT fell down the stairs, and remained unresponsive for approximately 6 to 12 hours. In the ED, he was diagnosed with rhabdomyolysis. Which of the following statements best describes rhabdomyolysis?

    a. Rhabdomyolysis may cause AIN.
    b. Rhabdomyolysis may cause ATN.
    c. Rhabdomyolysis may cause eosinophilia and eosinophiluria.
    d. MT should undergo RRT for his rhabdomyolysis.

Answer b is correct. Rhabdomyolysis is the breakdown of muscle tissue. Myoglobin is released during muscle breakdown and is directly toxic to tubular cells. Muddy brown casts are the remnants of the tubular cells that are often visualized upon urine microscopy.

Answer a is incorrect. AIN is a hypersensitivity reaction (allergic reaction) causing inflammation and damage to the interstitium. This is unrelated to rhabdomyolysis.

Answer c is incorrect. Increased eosinophil count in the serum and the presence of eosinophils in the urine would be more indicative of either a parasitic infection or an allergic reaction, including AIN.

Answer d is incorrect. MT has no indications (AEIOU) for RRT. While renal replacement therapy may be useful to remove certain toxins, it is not routinely used for ethanol intoxication.

17. Hyperkalemia may result from AKI and can lead to which one of the following life-threatening complications?

    a. Seizures
    b. Arrhythmias
    c. Hypertension
    d. Acidosis

Answer b is correct. Hyperkalemia can lead to EKG changes such as peaked T waves, prolonged QRS waves, and eventually ventricular fibrillation.

Answer a is incorrect. Patients with AKI may experience acid–base abnormalities or other electrolyte abnormalities that increase risk for seizures.

Answer c is incorrect. Hypertension is not indicative of acute hyperkalemia, and patients with AKI may be normotensive, hypotensive, or hypertensive.

Answer d is incorrect. Metabolic acidosis can worsen hyperkalemia by causing a shift of potassium from the intracellular to extracellular space. Hyperkalemia, however, does not cause an acidosis.

18. TB is a 62-year-old woman with a history of CKD and heart failure. Her baseline SCr is 1.8 mg/dL with a corresponding CrCl of approximately 50 mL/min. Today she is brought by ambulance to the emergency room with dyspnea at rest (currently has an oxygen saturation of 100% on 2 L room air of oxygen) and lower extremity edema all the way up to her thighs. Laboratory analysis shows a SCr of 3.6 mg/dL and she does not recall urinating at all in the past 24 hours. Which of the following best describes TB's kidney injury?

    a. Her CrCl is essentially zero as she is not making urine.
    b. Her CrCl is approximately 25 mL/min.
    c. Her CrCl is still approximately 50 mL/min.
    d. Acute hemodialysis is indicated.

Answer a is correct. Clearance is defined as the volume of solvent cleared of solute per unit time. If the patient is not urinating, her clearance is essentially zero.

Answer b is incorrect. This answer seems appropriate given that TB's SCr doubled. Doubling of the SCr would "seem" to cause the CrCl to decrease by one-half, from 50 mL/min to 25 mL/min. However, the SCr is the amount of creatinine in the serum at the time. If the patient stops urinating the GFR is zero, but the SCr will not reflect this change until more SCr is made and accumulates in the serum. SCr values lag behind kidney dysfunction.

Answer c is incorrect. TB's CrCl on presentation was approximately 50 mL/min. Now that she is not urinating and her SCr has started to increase, this value is no longer valid. This baseline value would be a good reference point and goal to achieve during her recovery from AKI.

Answer d is incorrect. While the patient has essentially a CrCl of 0 (Answer a), there is no acute indication for hemodialysis (AEIOU).

19. CG is a 58-year-old woman with a history of stage 4 ovarian cancer. She has metastases in her colon, abdominal cavity, liver, and bone. Recently, she has undergone chemotherapy and radiation as palliative treatment. Today she is admitted due to

1-week history of fatigue, malaise, nausea, vomiting, and she notes that she has not urinated for days. Upon examination, the doctor notes that her bladder is palpable and distended. Which of the following tests would be best to confirm a postrenal obstruction in this patient? Select all that apply.

   a. MRI with contrast media
   b. CT abdomen with contrast media
   c. KUB
   d. Renal ultrasound
   e. MRI of the bladder without contrast

Answer c is correct. A KUB is an abdominal X-ray of the kidneys, ureters, and bladder and is an effective tool in identifying bone and structural abnormalities, as well as identifying masses, perforations, or obstruction. Other causes of postrenal obstruction, including kidney stones, may also be identified.

Answer d is correct. A renal ultrasound is a noninvasive procedure that can be done at the bedside. This study is particularly well suited to detect hydronephrosis.

Answer a is incorrect. A different, less expensive, or time-consuming test would evaluate the bladder as effectively and contrast media could potentially worsen or further AKI.

Answer b is incorrect. As with Answer a, a CT scan would not evaluate the presence of hydronephrosis as effectively, and contrast media is relatively contraindicated in this patient.

Answer e is incorrect. Again, an MRI is an expensive diagnostic test that is not always available. An ultrasound is the easiest, least invasive procedure to determine hydronephrosis.

20. Which of the following agents may be used to treat AIN?

   a. Prednisone
   b. Furosemide
   c. Lisinopril
   d. Ibuprofen

Answer a is correct. Although the data are minimal, corticosteroids can be used to treat the immune reaction and inflammation that causes the damage to the interstitium. The decision to use steroids should be made on a case-by-case basis.

Answer b is incorrect. While furosemide can be used to enhance urine production and manage fluid balance, it does not treat the underlying pathophysiology of AIN.

Answer c is incorrect. Lisinopril has no role in the treatment of AIN. Additionally, the use of ACE-I or ARB during an episode of AKI is relatively contraindicated. By vasodilating the efferent arteriole, these agents may decrease the intraglomerular pressure, thwarting filtration.

Answer d is incorrect. While ibuprofen is an anti-inflammatory agent, the effects of inhibiting vasodilatory prostaglandins in the afferent arteriole may cause a worsening of kidney function in the setting of AKI.

CHAPTER **35** | Chronic Kidney Disease/ End-Stage Renal Disease

The following case should be used for questions 1 through 6 below.

A 79-year-old African American woman with HTN and diabetes presents to her primary care physician for a routine visit. Her spot urine albumin:urine creatinine ratio is 200 mg/g and GFR is estimated at 50 to 55 mL/min/1.73 m^2. The patient reports that she does not drink alcohol. She is a smoker but is willing to quit. She participates in an aerobics and strength training class for 30 minutes every day and enjoys a low-sodium diet. Pt denies medication allergies. Medications include lisinopril, metformin, aspirin, and nicotine replacement therapy.

1. Which of the following are risk factors for development of CKD as related to this patient? Select all that apply.

   a. HTN
   b. DM
   c. Smoking
   d. Diet and exercise

Answer a is correct. HTN and diabetes are the most common causes of CKD that lead to kidney failure.

Answer b is correct. Diabetes and HTN are the most common causes of CKD that lead to kidney failure.

Answer c is correct. Cigarette smoking is associated with abnormal albuminuria and progression of CKD.

Answer d is incorrect. The main nonpharmacologic interventions in patients with CKD include diet therapy (dietary sodium limited to 2,300 mg/d to help control blood pressure) and exercise (20-30 minutes of physical activity every day).

2. Based on this patient's ACR, she would be classified as having what category of albuminuria?

   a. A1 (normal to mildly increased)
   b. A2 (moderately increased)
   c. A3 (severely increased)
   d. Classification cannot be determined

Answer b is correct. The ACR detects elevated urinary protein (albuminuria) and is a marker of kidney damage. ACR 30 to 300 mg/g is categorized as A2 (moderately increased).

Answer a is incorrect. ACR less than 30 mg/g is categorized as A1 (normal to mildly increased).

Answer c is incorrect. ACR greater than 300 mg/g (or nephrotic syndrome) is categorized as A3 (severely increased).

Answer d is incorrect. ACR, the first method of preference to detect elevated urinary protein (albuminuria), is a marker of kidney damage and can be categorized accordingly.

---

3. Based on this patient's GFR, she would be categorized as having what stage of CKD?

   a. Stage 1
   b. Stage 2
   c. Stage 3a
   d. Stage 3b
   e. Stage 4

Answer c is correct. Staging is important in that it identifies patients at higher risk of worsening clinical manifestations and complications secondary to CKD. CKD is staged based on GFR. Renal function worsens from Stage 1 (greater than 90 mL/min/1.73 m^2) to Stage 5 (less than 15 mL/min/1.73 m^2). GFR 45 to 59 mL/min/1.73 m^2 is categorized as Stage 3a.

Answer a is incorrect. GFR greater than 90 mL/min/1.73 m^2 is categorized as Stage 1.

Answer b is incorrect. GFR 60 to 89 mL/min/1.73 m^2 is categorized as Stage 2.

Answer d is incorrect. GFR 30 to 44 mL/min/1.73 m^2 is categorized as Stage 3b.

Answer e is incorrect. GFR 15 to 29 mL/min/1.73 m^2 is categorized as Stage 4.

---

4. Due to a change in formulary medications, the patient will have to be switched to an alternative antihypertensive. Which of the following agents is classified as first-line therapy for patients with HTN in the setting of CKD and will inhibit the RAAS to slow the progression of proteinuria? Select ALL that apply.

   a. Benazepril
   b. Mavik
   c. Losartan
   d. Amlodipine
   e. Toprol XL

Answer a is correct. HTN is a risk factor for progression of kidney disease by accelerating proteinuria and activation of the RAAS. When tolerated, ACE inhibitors or ARBs are considered first-line therapy for blood pressure control and to reduce albuminuria. Benazepril (Lotensin) is an ACE inhibitor.

Answer b is correct. Trandolapril (Mavik) is an ACE inhibitor.

Answer c is correct. Losartan (Cozaar) is an ARB.

Answer d is incorrect. Amlodipine (Norvasc) is a dihydropyridine Ca channel blocker and may cause peripheral edema (fluid retention may be a manifestation of kidney disease).

Answer e is incorrect. Metoprolol (Toprol XL) is a β-blocker.

---

5. In general, common patient counseling pearls that should be shared regarding the use of an ACE inhibitor include which of the following? Select all that apply.

   a. ACE inhibitors are safe to use during pregnancy.
   b. Monitoring of potassium levels is necessary while taking an ACE inhibitor.
   c. A common side effect associated with ACE inhibitor use includes dry cough.
   d. Per the KDIGO guidelines, the ideal blood pressure in patients with diabetes, HTN, and CKD is less than 140/90 mm Hg (with a lower goal of less than 130/80 mm Hg, if the patient has proteinuria).

Answer b is correct. ACE inhibitors may cause hyperkalemia in patients with CKD or in those receiving a potassium-sparing diuretic, aldosterone antagonist, angiotensin receptor blocker, or direct renin inhibitor.

Answer c is correct. A common side effect associated with ACE inhibitors is a dry cough (3%-4%). This may warrant a switch to an ARB.

Answer d is correct. In patients with diabetes, HTN, and CKD the blood pressure goals are: systolic blood pressure should be treated to <140 mm Hg and diastolic blood pressure should be treated to <90 mm Hg. Lower goal systolic blood pressure <130 mm Hg and/or diastolic blood pressure <80 mm Hg may be appropriate for some, such as younger patients or patients with diabetes and urine albumin excretion >30 mg/24 h, if attained without undue treatment burden.

Answer a is incorrect. ACE inhibitors are teratogenic and should not be used in pregnancy.

---

6. Which of the following medications may provide CV protection by inhibiting platelet aggregation in the setting of CKD?

   a. Lisinopril
   b. Metformin
   c. Aspirin
   d. Amlodipine

Answer c is correct. Patients with CKD are at increased risk of CV mortality. Consideration for low dose aspirin 81 mg by mouth daily may minimize bleeding risk while providing heart protection through inhibition of platelet aggregation.

Answer a is incorrect. While lisinopril may assist with blood pressure control which may decrease CV mortality, it works through the RAAS.

Answer b is incorrect.   Metformin, an antidiabetic agent, is a medication of concern in patients with CKD as it may increase likelihood of lactic acidosis and is best avoided.

Answer d is incorrect.   Amlodipine (Norvasc) is a dihydropyridine Ca channel blocker and may cause peripheral edema (fluid retention may be a manifestation of kidney disease).

The following case should be used for questions 7 through 17 below.

A 44-year-old man with comorbid diabetes, HTN, and peripheral neuropathy was recently diagnosed with ESRD requiring hemodialysis on Monday-Wednesday-Friday. You receive a pharmacy consult for medication therapy management for this complicated patient. The patient states that he does not like taking medications with meals and experienced two episodes of hypoglycemia in the last month. He denies medication or food allergies and does not recall his recent immunizations.

Height 5'11" Weight 90 kg

Vitals: BP 160/89 (baseline BP prior to hemodialysis 145/80); heart rate, 72; respiratory rate, 18; temperature, 98.6

Pertinent labs:

Hgb	9.2
Hematocrit	30
T$_{sat}$	18
Serum ferritin	69
Retic count	1.01
Albumin	2.9
Phos	7.5
Ca^{2+}	7.8
iPTH	420
HbA1c	10.5

Current Medications

EC aspirin 81 mg po daily

Insulin glargine 30 units subcutaneous (SubQ) QHS

Regular insulin 10 units SubQ QAC

Metoprolol tartrate 25 mg po bid

Losartan 50 mg po daily

Iron dextran 100 mg IV QHD to be initiated today (was receiving oral ferrous sulfate)

Epoetin alfa 4000 units IV QHD

Amitriptyline 50 mg po QHS

Calcium carbonate 500 mg po tid

7. Which of the following would be the most appropriate vitamin supplement to recommend for this patient?

    a. Prenatal vitamin 1 tab po daily
    b. Vitamin A 4000 units po daily
    c. Multivitamin with iron 1 tab po daily
    d. Vitamin B complex-folic acid-vitamin C 1 tab po daily

Answer d is correct.   Supplementation of water soluble vitamins (B complex, folic acid, vitamin C) commonly provided as a "renal vitamin" may be necessary in patients requiring hemodialysis. Water soluble vitamins are typically removed via the process of hemodialysis.

Answer a is incorrect.   This is a male patient with CKD. Prenatal vitamins contain B complex (water soluble) and vitamins A, E (fat soluble). Fat soluble should be avoided in patients with renal disease. In addition, prenatal vitamins are typically given to pregnant women.

Answer b is incorrect.   Fat soluble vitamins (A, E) should be avoided in patients with renal disease.

Answer c is incorrect.   Multivitamins may contain fat and water soluble vitamins; however, the water soluble vitamins may not be at the adequate concentrations required in a patient with CKD and the fat soluble vitamins may accumulate. While patients with CKD are often anemic, the low dose iron in a daily multivitamin tablet will likely not achieve goal elemental iron amounts (200 mg/d) to prevent or treat anemia.

---

8. Assuming the patient does not have any contraindications, which of the following preventive health measures does the patient qualify for? Select all that apply.

    a. Influenzae vaccine
    b. PCV13
    c. PCV23
    d. Hepatitis B series (standard dose)
    e. Hepatitis B series (twice the standard dose)

Answer a is correct.   Patients with CKD/ESRD should be screened appropriately for administration of influenza, pneumococcal, and hepatitis B immunizations.

Answer b is correct.   Patients with CKD/ESRD are at a higher risk of developing pneumococcal disease and should receive both the PCV13 and PCV23 vaccines with the PCV23 given at least 8 weeks after PCV13 regardless of age.

Answer c is correct.   Patients with CKD/ESRD are at a higher risk of developing pneumococcal disease and should receive both the PCV13 and PCV23 vaccines with the PCV23 given at least 8 weeks after PCV13 regardless of age.

Answer e is correct.   All patients who are currently or potentially could receive hemodialysis should receive hepatitis B vaccine due to possible exposure to blood. Studies have shown that patients with ESRD have a decreased immune response to the vaccine so it is recommended that CKD patients receive the vaccine course as early as possible. Once the patient is receiving dialysis or becomes uremic, the patient should receive the vaccine at twice the standard dose (40 mcg doses in a four-dose schedule).

Answer d is incorrect.   All patients who are currently or potentially could receive hemodialysis should receive hepatitis B vaccine due to possible exposure to blood. Studies have shown that patients with ESRD have a decreased immune response to the vaccine so it is recommended that CKD patients receive the vaccine course as early as possible. Once the patient is receiving dialysis or becomes uremic, the patient should receive the vaccine at twice the standard dose (40 mcg doses in a four-dose schedule).

---

9. The patient expresses frustration with taking medications around mealtimes. Which medication is most effective when taken with meals and may require motivational interviewing to change the patient's mindset?

    a. EC aspirin
    b. Calcium carbonate
    c. Iron dextran
    d. Epoetin alfa

Answer b is correct. Patients with CKD are prone to developing mineral and bone disorders (CKD–MBD). Irregularities in Ca intake coupled with Phos abnormalities may lead to bone disease. When limiting dietary Phos intake is ineffective at lowering these levels, pharmacotherapy with a phosphate binder such as calcium carbonate may be necessary. As Phos is found in highest concentrations in food, it is important to counsel the patient on taking calcium carbonate with meals in order to bind up the most Phos and also refer the patient to a nutritionist.

Answer a is incorrect. EC aspirin may be administered with food or a full glass of water to minimize GI distress (not for therapeutic effect).

Answer c is incorrect. IV iron dextran may be given without regard to meals and is typically given by the health care provider during hemodialysis sessions.

Answer d is incorrect. IV epoetin alfa may be given without regard to meals and is typically given by the health care provider during hemodialysis sessions.

---

10. The nephrologist is considering starting cinacalcet for this patient to help regulate PTH and treat mineral and bone disorders common in patients with chronic kidney disease (CKD–MBD). Select the best recommendation to the provider in regards to initiation of cinacalcet.

    a. It is safe to start cinacalcet but it is best to administer with food.
    b. The starting dose of cinacalcet is 180 mg by mouth daily with aggressive titration to goal PTH and serum Ca levels.
    c. Cinacalcet is typically well-tolerated with low incidence of GI irritation and minimal drug-drug interactions.
    d. It is unsafe to start cinacalcet as the patient has hypocalcemia that may be worsened by this calcimimetic.

Answer d is correct. Cinacalcet hydrochloride (Sensipar) is the only calcimimetic agent approved for treatment of secondary hyperparathyroidism in patients with CKD on dialysis. Cinacalcet increases the sensitivity of the parathyroid gland to extracellular Ca, subsequently reducing PTH secretion and decreasing serum Ca. The most frequent adverse events associated with cinacalcet are nausea/vomiting and hypocalcemia (do not initiate if the serum Ca is less than 8.4 mg/dL). This patient's Ca level is 7.8 and corrects for low albumin to approximately 8 mg/dL.

Answer a is incorrect. Calcitriol may be administered without regard to food.

Answer b is incorrect. The typical starting dose is 30 mg by mouth daily with titration every 2 to 4 weeks to a maximum dose of 180 mg once daily until the desired PTH values are achieved and to maintain goal serum Ca. Slow titration helps to minimize nausea/vomiting.

Answer c is incorrect. The most frequent adverse events associated with cinacalcet are nausea/vomiting and hypocalcemia (do not initiate if the serum Ca is less than 8.4 mg/dL). Cinacalcet is known to interaction with other medications utilizing the cytochrome P450 CYP3A4 pathway.

---

11. Of the following brand name medications that may be used for the treatment of hyperphosphatemia in patients with CKD, which contain a non-Ca based or iron-based binder? Select all that apply.

    a. Auryxia
    b. Tums
    c. Renvela
    d. Fosrenol
    e. AlternaGel

Answer a is correct. Pharmacologic therapy aimed at regulating parathyroid levels (and ultimately Ca and Phos) include Ca-based, non-Ca based, and iron-based phosphate binders. Ca-based include calcium carbonate (Tums, Os-Cal, Caltrate), calcium acetate (PhosLo, Phoslyra). Non-Ca based include sevelamer (Renvela, Renagel), lanthanum carbonate (Fosrenol), and aluminum hydroxide (AlternaGel). Iron-based include ferric citrate (Auryxia) and sucroferric oxyhydroxide (Velphoro).

Answer c is correct. Non-Ca based include sevelamer (Renvela, Renagel), lanthanum carbonate (Fosrenol), and aluminum hydroxide (AlternaGel).

Answer d is correct. Non-Ca based include sevelamer (Renvela, Renagel), lanthanum carbonate (Fosrenol), and aluminum hydroxide (AlternaGel).

Answer e is correct. Non-Ca based include sevelamer (Renvela, Renagel), lanthanum carbonate (Fosrenol), and aluminum hydroxide (AlternaGel).

Answer b is incorrect. Ca-based include calcium carbonate (Tums, Os-Cal, Caltrate) and calcium acetate (PhosLo, Phoslyra).

12. This patient is receiving pharmacotherapy for the treatment of mineral and bone disorders that are common in patients with chronic kidney disease (CKD–MBD). Starting with reduced renal function, identify the sequence of pathophysiological events that can result in this complication.

    a. Increased PTH production resulting in increased bone breakdown
    b. Elevations of Phos concentrations in the blood as the result of reduced renal function
    c. Reduction in intestinal absorption of Ca and reduced serum Ca levels
    d. Reduction in plasma levels of vitamin D due to decreased activation by the kidney

Answers d, c, b, and a are correct. The sequence of events that lead to the development of mineral and bone disorders that are common in patients with chronic kidney disease (CKD–MBD) are: Patients with CKD/ESRD have reduced plasma levels of vitamin D resulting in reduced intestinal absorption of Ca and also decreased Phos elimination leading to hyperphosphatemia and hypocalcemia. To compensate for the low Ca, the body increases production of PTH which alters Ca and Phos concentrations in the kidney and bone. This process results in secondary hyperparathyroidism, more commonly referred to as CKD–MBD. Clinical symptoms manifest as itchy skin, bone pain/fractures, neuropathies, and heart problems.

13. This patient is receiving pharmacotherapy to manage anemia of CKD. In patients with anemia where endogenous stores of erythropoietin are adequate, the body is able to compensate for hypoxic states. Identify the correct sequence of this normal compensatory mechanism.

    a. Erythropoietin acts on E-progenitor cells in the bone marrow to produce new red blood cells
    b. Kidney decreases erythropoietin production
    c. Kidney senses increased tissue oxygenation
    d. Kidney senses hypoxia and increases endogenous erythropoietin production

Answers d, a, c, and b are correct. In anemic patients where endogenous stores of erythropoietin are adequate, the body is able to compensate for hypoxic states by: kidney senses hypoxia and increases endogenous erythropoietin production, erythropoietin acts on E-progenitor cells in the bone marrow to produce new red blood cells, kidney senses increased tissue oxygenation, and kidney decreases erythropoietin production. As an individual's stage of CKD progresses and approximates a GFR <60 mL/min/1.73 m^2, anemia develops. Anemia of CKD occurs in approximately 90% of patients receiving dialytic therapy. Symptoms of anemia include fatigue, weakness, angina, and shortness of breath. Anemia in patients with CKD/ESRD is usually the result of decreased production of erythropoietin in the kidneys but can be multifactorial including blood loss, iron deficiency, folate and B12 deficiency, and aluminum toxicity. Treatment of anemia in patients with CKD requires effective use of exogenous ESAs, guided by appropriate monitoring of blood indices including Hgb. ESAs induce erythropoiesis by stimulating the division and differentiation of committed erythroid progenitor cells and the release of reticulocytes from bone marrow into the bloodstream.

14. The patient is receiving IV epoetin alfa (Procrit) with each hemodialysis session for anemia of CKD. Identify the correct statement regarding the use of ESAs for the treatment of anemia of CKD. Select all that apply.

    a. ESAs have a boxed warning that highlights increased risk of CV events (death, heart attacks, stroke, venous thromboembolism, thrombosis of vascular access).
    b. Prior to ESAs initiation and during treatment with ESAs, evaluation of and maintenance of iron stores is necessary.
    c. Common side effects with ESAs include elevated blood pressure, nausea/vomiting, diarrhea, headache, muscle pain, swelling, or rash.
    d. In general, a target Hgb value of less than 11.5 g/dL when on ESAs allows for individualized patient dosing and monitoring for safety and efficacy.

Answer a is correct. Various ESAs therapy including rHuEPO (ie, epoetin alfa or Procrit®, Epogen®), NESP (ie, darbepoetin alfa or Aranesp®), and methoxy polyethylene glycol-epoetin beta (Mircera®) are used for the management of patients with anemia secondary to renal disease. It is important to note that, in patients with CKD, ESAs carry a blackbox warning for increased mortality, serious CV events, thromboembolic events, and stroke when administered ESAs to target an Hgb level of greater than 11 g/dL.

Answer b is correct. Hgb formation is dependent on both effective erythropoiesis and adequate iron stores. Anemia of CKD is common and typically responds to exogenous ESAs therapy when concomitant iron therapy is used to maintain adequate iron stores.

Answer c is correct. Common side effects with ESAs include elevated blood pressure, nausea/vomiting, diarrhea, headache, muscle pain, swelling, or rash.

Answer d is correct. Safety and efficacy can be monitored when doses are individualized for the patient to maintain target Hgb values between 9 and 11.5 g/dL.

15. This patient was previously receiving oral ferrous sulfate with initiation of IV iron dextran at the current visit. Which of the following statements is accurate regarding common patient counseling tips for patients with CKD receiving oral iron replacement products? Select all that apply.

    a. Oral ferrous sulfate contains approximately 65 mg elemental iron per 325 mg tablet.
    b. Oral iron replacement products may cause constipation, darkening of stools, nausea/vomiting, and stomach cramps.
    c. Absorption of ferrous gluconate is best when given with a concomitant proton pump inhibitor like lansoprazole.

d. It is important to keep oral iron replacement products out of children's reach and in child-resistant containers as severe toxicity may occur if inadvertently ingested.

Answer a is correct. Each oral iron replacement product contains a different amount of elemental iron. Oral ferrous sulfate comes in several different formulations and the 325 mg tablet contains approximately 65 mg elemental iron per tablet.

Answer b is correct. Oral iron replacement products are known for causing GI irritation including constipation, darkening of stools, epigastric pain, nausea/vomiting, and stomach cramps.

Answer d is correct. Iron is a leading cause of fatal poisoning in children. Store out of children's reach and in child-resistant containers.

Answer c is incorrect. Acid-suppressing therapies such as histamine-2-antagonists and proton pump inhibitors may decrease the absorption of oral iron salts.

16. This patient will be initiated on IV iron dextran today. Which of the following IV iron products require monitoring of the patient for 30 to 60 minutes following an infusion to ensure tolerance? Select all that apply.

    a. INFed
    b. Venofer
    c. Sodium ferric gluconate
    d. Ferric carboxymaltose

Answer a is correct. Common side effects associated with all parenteral iron products (dextran or nondextran containing) include hypotension, peripheral edema, headache, nausea, and muscle cramps. Although rare (<1%), anaphylactic/anaphylactoid reactions including serious or life-threatening responses have been reported. Cardiopulmonary resuscitation equipment and personnel should be available during initial administration until tolerance has been demonstrated. INFed is the brand name of iron dextran.

Answer b is correct. Cardiopulmonary resuscitation equipment and personnel should be available during initial administration until tolerance has been demonstrated. Venofer is the brand name of iron sucrose.

Answer c is correct. Cardiopulmonary resuscitation equipment and personnel should be available during initial administration until tolerance has been demonstrated. Sodium ferric gluconate's corresponding brand name is Ferrlecit.

Answer d is correct. Cardiopulmonary resuscitation equipment and personnel should be available during initial administration until tolerance has been demonstrated. Ferric carboxymaltose's corresponding brand name is Injectafer.

17. In this patient with ESRD (hemodialysis) and insulin-requiring diabetes, HTN, and peripheral neuropathy, select the most appropriate hemoglobin A1c (HbA1c) goal (in percentage)?

    a. Less than 6
    b. Less than 6.5
    c. Less than 7
    d. Less than 8

Answer d is correct. Optimal glucose control for patients with diabetes prior to the development of kidney disease may delay its occurrence. However, once kidney disease is present, tight glucose control has not been shown to be more beneficial than less control in the progression of kidney disease. Less stringent HbA1c goal (<8%) may be appropriate in patients with a history of severe hypoglycemia, limited life expectancy, advanced micro/macrovascular complications or comorbidities, or in difficult to reach goal patients despite adequate therapy. In patients with end stage renal disease (microvascular complication), insulin requirements are reduced due to changes in insulin clearance and metabolism. Some resources suggest to administer insulin at 50% of normal dose and monitor glucose closely to minimize hypoglycemia (this patient has history of hypoglycemia).

Answer a is incorrect. HbA1c values between 5.7% and 6.4% are classified as prediabetes.

Answer b is incorrect. HbA1c goal should be individualized, with <6.5% if achieved without significant hypoglycemia or adverse effects in younger, long-life expectancy, and no CV disease patients.

Answer c is incorrect. HbA1c goal for nonpregnant adults in general is <7%.

18. Which of the following medications are best to avoid in patients with Stage 4 or Stage 5 CKD? Select ALL that apply.

    a. Ibuprofen
    b. Phenazopyridine
    c. Glucophage
    d. Doxycycline
    e. Macrobid

Answer a is correct. Stage 4 CKD is defined as a GFR 15 to 29 mL/min/1.73 m^2 or severely decreased renal function. Stage 5 is GFR less than 15 mL/min/1.73 m^2 or kidney failure. Pharmacists may suggest appropriate timing of medication administration (typically after IHD on dialysis days) or medication prescribing alterations (lower daily dose or supplemental dosing after IHD, increased administration interval such as every other day or a combination of change in dosing and interval) to facilitate adequate drug concentrations while minimizing toxicities. In addition, avoidance of some medications may be recommended. Ibuprofen (Motrin) is not recommended if GFR <30 mL/minute/1.73 m^2.

Answer b is correct. Pharmacists may recommend avoidance of some medications in the setting of CKD and

ESRD due to safety and efficacy concerns. Phenazopyridine (Pyridium) use is contraindicated in renal impairment. In order for this azo dye to exert local anesthetic and analgesic action on the urinary tract mucosa, it must be able to reach the kidney (decreased efficacy with renal impairment).

Answer c is correct. Pharmacists may recommend avoidance of some medications in the setting of CKD and ESRD due to safety and efficacy concerns. Metformin (Glucophage) use is contraindicated if GFR <30 mL/minute/1.73 m². Use cautiously in patients at risk for lactic acidosis such as in renal impairment.

Answer e is correct. Pharmacists may recommend avoidance of some medications in the setting of CKD and ESRD due to safety and efficacy concerns. Nitrofurantoin (Macrobid) use is contraindicated if CrCl <60 mL/minute (per manufacturer's labeling). Urinary nitrofurantoin concentrations are variable in patients with impaired renal function and there is increased risk of hemolytic anemia and pulmonary fibrosis.

Answer d is incorrect. Pharmacists may recommend avoidance of some medications in the setting of CKD and ESRD due to safety and efficacy concerns. Doxycycline (Vibramycin) does not require renal dose adjustment and is poorly dialyzed (0%-5%); no supplemental dose or dosage adjustment is necessary, including patients on IHD, PD, or CRRT. Thus, it is safe to use in renal impairment.

19. In the setting of CKD, some medications require careful assessment. By ordering the answers, select which adverse event is appropriately matched with each medication and its metabolite.

Medication	Metabolite	Adverse Drug Event
Allopurinol	Oxypurinol	
Glipizide	Norglipizide	
Meperidine	Normeperidine	

   a. Hypoglycemia
   b. Kidney stone
   c. Seizure

Answers b, a, and c are correct. Pharmacists may suggest appropriate timing of medication administration (typically after IHD on dialysis days) or medication prescribing alterations (lower daily dose or supplemental dosing after IHD, increased administration interval such as every other day, or a combination of change in dosing and interval) to facilitate adequate drug concentrations while minimizing toxicities. In addition, avoidance of some medications may be recommended due to accumulation of the active drug or active metabolites. Oxypurinol is a metabolite of allopurinol and may cause kidney stones. Norglipizide is a metabolite of glipizide and may cause hypoglycemia. Normeperidine is a metabolite of meperidine and may cause seizures.

The following case should be used for question 20 below.

20. A 67-year-old man with community acquired pneumonia and CKD due to diabetic nephropathy is admitted to the hospital for failure of standard outpatient treatment with oral levofloxacin. The patient will be initiated on piperacillin/tazobactam (Zosyn).

Patient specific information: NKDA, Height 5'11", Weight 80 kg

Renal function trends:

Baseline serum creatinine (SCr) = 1.5; Yesterday SCr = 2.0; Today SCr = 2.3

Baseline urine output (UOP) 2000 mL/24 h; Yesterday UOP 1000 mL/24 h; Today UOP 300 mL/24 h

As the hospital pharmacist assigned the renal dosing queue, which of the following parameters may be considered when making a renal dose adjustment recommendation? Select all that apply.

   a. Piperacillin/tazobactam-induced adverse effects if drug accumulates in renal insufficiency
   b. Renal function trends as determined by SCr and UOP (improving or declining)
   c. Clinical status of the patient (mild infection or severe infection)
   d. Availability of alternative drug that does not require renal dose adjustment

Answer a is correct. In the setting of CKD, the pharmacist may suggest medication dose adjustment based on several parameters including side effects or toxicity if the medication accumulates.

Answer b is correct. In the setting of CKD, the pharmacist may suggest medication dose adjustment based on several parameters including renal function trends as determined by SCr and UOP. If the renal function is improving, more aggressive therapy may be suggested. If the renal function is declining, a more conservative approach may be necessary.

Answer c is correct. In the setting of CKD, the pharmacist may suggest medication dose adjustment based on several parameters including clinical status of the patient. If mild infection, a conservative approach may be appropriate. If severe infection, more aggressive therapy may be warranted.

Answer d is correct. In the setting of CKD, the pharmacist may suggest medication dose adjustment based on several parameters including availability of alternative drugs that do not require renal dose adjustment but will provide similiar efficacy and ensure safety.

CHAPTER 36 | Acid–Base Disorders

Questions 1 and 2 pertain to the following case.

A 35-year-old woman is in the intensive care unit, intubated after a recent abdominal surgery. While in the operating room, she received more than 8 L of fluid and blood products, but has been aggressively diuresed since that time. In the past 3 days she has generated 6 L of urine output, her BUN and Cr have *increased* to

35 mg/dL and 1.4 mg/dL, respectively (baseline of 10 mg/dL and 0.7 mg/dL), and her blood pressure has decreased to 100/60 mm Hg. This morning, her ABG shows the following: pH 7.50, P_aCO_2 48 mm Hg, and HCO_3 37 mEq/L.

1. Which of the primary acid–base disturbances is present in this patient?

   a. Metabolic acidosis
   b. Metabolic alkalosis
   c. Respiratory acidosis
   d. Respiratory alkalosis

Answer b is correct. The pH is elevated, indicating alkalosis, and the bicarbonate more than 28, indicating metabolic alkalosis.

Answers a and c are incorrect. The pH is alkalemic; therefore, acidosis can be excluded.

Answer d is incorrect. The P_aCO_2 >40 mm Hg which would be inappropriate for a respiratory alkalosis. The patient has a metabolic alkalosis secondary to over-diuresis which has led to volume contraction.

2. Has the patient appropriately compensated for the primary disorder?

   a. Yes, the P_aCO_2 is elevated, indicating appropriate compensation.
   b. Yes, the HCO_3 is elevated, indicating appropriate compensation.
   c. No, the HCO_3 is low, indicating the patient has not yet been compensated.
   d. No, the P_aCO_2 is low, indicating the patient has not yet been compensated.

Answer a is correct. In metabolic alkalosis we would expect the P_aCO_2 to be elevated as compensation to hold on to acid.

Answers b and c are incorrect. The patient does not have a primary respiratory problem.

Answer d is incorrect. The P_aCO_2 is low therefore this is incorrect. Furthermore, the patient does not have a metabolic acidosis. Therefore the best answer is a.

3. Which of the following acid–base disturbances would *most likely* be exhibited in a person with GOLD 3 (severe) chronic obstructive pulmonary disease (COPD)? Select all that apply.

   a. Respiratory alkalosis
   b. Respiratory acidosis
   c. Respiratory acidosis compensation
   d. Metabolic alkalosis compensation
   e. Metabolic acidosis compensation

Answers b and d are correct. In patients with restrictive airway diseases, such as COPD, there is an inability to properly ventilate CO_2. This will result in a buildup of P_aCO_2 in the lungs, leading to respiratory acidosis. As a compensatory response to the chronically elevated P_aCO_2 levels, the kidneys will retain bicarbonate to attempt to normalize pH, creating a metabolic alkalosis.

Answers a, c, and e are incorrect.

4. Which of the following acid–base disturbances would you expect to see in the early stages of an acute asthma exacerbation?

   a. Respiratory acidosis
   b. Respiratory alkalosis
   c. Metabolic acidosis
   d. Metabolic alkalosis

Answer b is correct. In acute asthma exacerbations, the bronchioles have become inflamed, resulting in airflow obstruction. This obstruction causes patients with acute exacerbations to breathe more rapidly in an effort to oxygenate their tissues more. Therefore, an increased respiratory rate causes CO_2 to be exhaled, resulting in low P_aCO_2 levels—respiratory alkalosis.

Answer a is incorrect. Respiratory acidosis occurs only in late stage acute asthma exacerbations that are untreated.

Answers c and d are incorrect. This is a primary respiratory process.

5. A patient presents to the emergency department unconscious, after ingesting a bottle of temazepam. What acid–base disturbance would you expect to see?

   a. Increased anion gap metabolic acidosis
   b. Respiratory alkalosis
   c. Normal gap metabolic acidosis
   d. Respiratory acidosis

Answer d is correct. Benzodiazepine overdose results in suppression of the respiratory center of the brain. This, therefore, leads to decreased exhalation of CO_2 and increased levels of P_aCO_2. Thus, the patient who overdoses on benzodiazepines will have a respiratory acidosis.

Answer a is incorrect. This could occur if the patient was given too high a dose of intravenous lorazepam due to the excipient in the formulation, propylene glycol.

Answers b and c are incorrect. B is incorrect because benzodiazepine overdose results in suppression of the respiratory center of the brain, leading to decreased exhalation of CO_2. This leads to increased P_aCO_2, which would cause a respiratory acidosis, not alkalosis. Answer c is incorrect because ingestion of a benzodiazepine causes a primary respiratory acidosis.

Questions 6 to 8 pertain to the following case.
A 62-year-old woman has been hospitalized in the ICU for several weeks. She has had a complicated hospital course with sepsis

secondary to pneumonia, requiring prolonged courses of antibiotics. Over the past few days, she began spiking fevers and is having a lot of diarrhea. Her stool was positive for *C. difficile* by polymerase chain reaction. Laboratory values include: Na⁺ 140 mEq/L, Cl⁻ 110 mEq/L, HCO₃⁻ 17 mEq/L, albumin 4.1 g/dL, pH 7.32, and P$_a$CO₂ 33 mm Hg.

6. Place the following answers in the correct order to assess the acid–base disorder:

   a. Calculate the anion gap
   b. Assess the patient
   c. Assess P$_a$CO₂ and HCO₃⁻
   d. Assess the pH to determine if acidotic or alkalotic

Answer: b, d, c, a. The first step in assessing any acid–base disorder is assessing the patient. Then, you look at the pH to determine if the patient is acidemic or alkalemic. Once that is determined, assess P$_a$CO₂ and HCO₃⁻ to determine the primary cause. Once that is done and you determine that this is a metabolic acidosis, calculate the anion gap to determine if the cause is due to unmeasured anions, or if it is a normal gap.

7. What is the *most likely primary* acid–base disturbance?

   a. Increased anion gap metabolic acidosis
   b. Normal anion gap metabolic acidosis
   c. Metabolic alkalosis
   d. Respiratory acidosis

Answer b is correct. The patient is experiencing diarrhea from an infection with *C. difficile*. This leads us to believe there is a metabolic process occurring. Looking at the pH, we note the patient to be acidemic. We should examine the HCO₃⁻ next, because we believe this to be a primary metabolic disorder, based upon patient presentation, and discover it to be low (metabolic acidosis). When we discover this, it is recommended to next check the anion gap, and it is (140−110−17) 13. The patient's expected anion gap is 12.3 (3 × albumin of 4.1); therefore, the anion gap is *not* elevated, nor is there anything in the history to point toward an increased anion gap (KILU). Answers a, c, and d would then be incorrect.

8. Has the patient appropriately compensated for the primary disorder?

   a. No, the P$_a$CO₂ is elevated, indicating the patient has not yet been compensated.
   b. Yes, the HCO₃ is elevated, indicating appropriate compensation.
   c. No, the HCO₃ is low, indicating the patient has not yet been compensated.
   d. Yes, the P$_a$CO₂ is low, indicating appropriate compensation.

Answer d is correct. For a primary metabolic acidosis, the lungs compensate by "blowing off" excess acid (P$_a$CO₂).

Therefore, one should expect to see such a patient exhibit an increased respiratory rate and, on blood gas, a decreased P$_a$CO₂. In this case the P$_a$CO₂ is in fact low (<40 mm Hg); therefore, answer d is the best choice.

Answers a and b are incorrect. The P$_a$CO₂ is low and the HCO₃ is low.

Answer c is incorrect. The primary disturbance is a metabolic acidosis; therefore, compensation has to occur through the respiratory (P$_a$CO₂) route and the patient has appropriately compensated with a low P$_a$CO₂.

Questions 9 and 10 pertain to the following case.

A 17-year-old girl with no known medical history is brought to the emergency department (ED) in a difficult-to-arouse state. Her parents report she was been complaining of a vague abdominal pain earlier in the morning, and then began vomiting and urinating frequently in the hours before admission. Urine and blood were positive for ketones. The following laboratory values were taken: Na⁺ 145 mEq/L, K⁺ 4.7 mEq/L, Cl⁻ 105 mEq/L, HCO₃⁻ 8 mEq/L, glucose 625 mg/dL, pH 7.22, and P$_a$CO₂ 22 mm Hg.

9. What is the *most likely primary* acid–base disturbance?

   a. Increased anion gap metabolic acidosis
   b. Normal anion gap metabolic acidosis
   c. Metabolic alkalosis
   d. Respiratory alkalosis

Answer a is correct. The patient is vomiting, urinating frequently, and is difficult to arouse. There is no reason to suspect any pulmonary processes based upon the information given, so a primary metabolic disorder is likely. Looking at the pH, we determine the patient to be acidemic. The P$_a$CO₂ is low, while the HCO₃ is also low, indicating a metabolic acidosis. When we discover this, it is recommended to next check the anion gap, and it is (145−105−8) 32. Without an albumin, we estimate the patient's normal anion gap to be 12, thus the anion gap is elevated. This is a classic case of diabetic ketoacidosis where a patient has been exhibiting symptoms of hyperglycemia that eventually lead to her near comatose state. Because the cells are starved of energy (no glucose is being utilized due to a lack of insulin), ketone bodies (unmeasured anions) are produced from the breakdown of free fatty acids for energy. Therefore, an increase in the anion gap will be exhibited in DKA.

Answer b is incorrect. The patient has an anion gap of approximately 32.

Answers c and d are incorrect. The patient is acidemic.

---

10. Has the patient appropriately compensated for the primary disorder?

   a. Yes, the P$_a$CO₂ is elevated, indicating appropriate compensation.
   b. Yes, the HCO₃ is elevated, indicating appropriate compensation.

c. Yes, the P_aCO_2 is low, indicating appropriate compensation.
d. Yes, the HCO_3 is low, indicating appropriate compensation.

Answer c is correct. In this case of metabolic acidosis, the most appropriate compensation would be for the lungs to exhale excess acid. By doing this, one would expect to see a low P_aCO_2, and therefore a respiratory alkalosis. As we can see this to be the case, the P_aCO_2 is 22 mm Hg (lower than 40 mm Hg), thus a respiratory alkalosis is taking place.

Answer a is incorrect. The P_aCO_2 is actually decreased.

Answers b and d are incorrect. This is a primary metabolic problem; therefore, the primary disorder, not compensatory disorder, will be a problem of bicarbonate.

Questions 11 and 12 pertain to the following case.

A 22-year-old man with no medical history is admitted after being "found down" at a party after drinking a lot of alcohol over a 20-minute time period. Upon arrival to the emergency department, he was neurologically unresponsive and had the following laboratory values: pH 7.15, P_aO_2 55, P_aCO_2 60 mm Hg, HCO_3^- 25 mEq/L, Na^+ 132 mEq/L, Cl^- 95 mEq/L, and albumin 4.2 g/dL. Urine drug screen is positive for benzodiazepines.

11. What is the *primary* acid–base disturbance?

    a. Increased anion gap metabolic acidosis
    b. Normal anion gap metabolic acidosis
    c. Metabolic alkalosis
    d. Respiratory acidosis

Answer d is correct. In this case of acute intoxication of alcohol and benzodiazepines, we would expect a primary respiratory disorder, due to the combination causing respiratory depression.

Answers a, b, and c are incorrect. The pH is low indicating acidemia and the P_aCO_2 is elevated, indicating respiratory acidosis. None of the other answers therefore are correct.

---

12. Has the patient appropriately compensated for the primary acid–base disorder?

    a. Yes, the P_aCO_2 is elevated, indicating appropriate compensation.
    b. Yes, the P_aCO_2 is low, indicating appropriate compensation.
    c. Yes, the HCO_3 is elevated, indicating appropriate compensation.
    d. Unsure, it is too soon after the acute respiratory event to assess metabolic compensation at this time.

Answer d is correct. Because the range in normal bicarbonate is wide (22-28 mEq/L), and because it is unknown where the patient's bicarbonate level was prior to this episode, we cannot say whether or not the patient is appropriately compensated, as the bicarbonate is within the expected range.

Answers a and b are incorrect. The compensation for a primary respiratory acidosis would involve HCO_3 not P_aCO_2.

Answer c is incorrect. Compensation has not had time to occur.

Questions 13 and 14 pertain to the following case.

A 45-year-old woman with previous peptic ulcer disease was admitted with persistent vomiting. She looked dehydrated, with dry mucus membranes and skin tenting. Her blood results were Na^+ 142 mEq/L, K^+ 2.6 mEq/L, Cl^- 88 mEq/L, pH 7.52, P_aCO_2 51 mm Hg, and HCO_3^- 42 mEq/L.

13. What is the primary acid–base disorder?

    a. Increased anion gap metabolic acidosis
    b. Normal anion gap metabolic acidosis
    c. Metabolic alkalosis
    d. Respiratory acidosis

Answer c is correct. Given the patient's presentation of persistent vomiting, we would expect to see a primary metabolic disorder due to loss of hydrogen ions from the upper GI tract.

Answers a and b are incorrect. Looking at the HCO_3, we see it is markedly elevated, indicating a metabolic alkalosis.

Answers d is incorrect. There is no information given to suspect a respiratory disorder, so answer d can be excluded.

---

14. Has the patient appropriately compensated for the primary acid–base disorder?

    a. Yes, the P_aCO_2 is elevated, indicating appropriate compensation.
    b. Yes, the P_aCO_2 is low, indicating appropriate compensation.
    c. Yes, the HCO_3^- is elevated, indicating appropriate compensation.
    d. Yes, the HCO_3^- is low, indicating appropriate compensation.

Answer a is correct. Knowing there is a primary metabolic disorder, we can exclude answers c and d immediately. Because the pH is elevated secondary to metabolic alkalosis, the most appropriate respiratory compensation would be for the lungs to hold on to acid (P_aCO_2) resulting in a respiratory acidosis, which is the case here with a P_aCO_2 of 51 mm Hg.

Answer b is incorrect. The P_aCO_2 is 51 mm Hg, which is elevated, not low.

Answers c and d are incorrect. The patient has a primary metabolic disorder so the lungs would have to compensate through P_aCO_2.

Questions 15 and 16 pertain to the following case.

A 55-year-old man was admitted to the hospital with a 3-day history of persistent vomiting. The following laboratory values are taken: pH 7.40, P_aCO_2 40 mm Hg, HCO_3 24 mEq/L, Na 149 mEq/L, Cl 100 mEq/L, BUN 110 mg/dL, and Cr 8.7 mg/dL.

15. What would you *expect* the pH, P_aCO_2, and HCO_3 to be in a patient who has persistent vomiting ($\uparrow$, $\downarrow$, or N)?

    a. pH $\uparrow$; P_aCO_2 $\downarrow$; HCO_3 $\uparrow$
    b. pH $\downarrow$; P_aCO_2 $\downarrow$; HCO_3 $\downarrow$
    c. pH $\uparrow$; P_aCO_2 N; HCO_3 $\uparrow$
    d. pH $\downarrow$; P_aCO_2 N; HCO_3 $\downarrow$

Answer c is correct. In a patient with persistent vomiting, one would expect to see metabolic alkalosis, with or without respiratory compensation. Therefore, the pH should be elevated, the HCO_3 should be elevated (because of a loss of hydrogen ions from the upper GI tract), and the P_aCO_2 should be normal or elevated (depending on the duration of metabolic alkalosis).

Answer a is incorrect. P_aCO_2 should be normal or elevated (depending on the duration of metabolic alkalosis).

Answers b and d are incorrect. The patient should be alkalemic not acidemic.

16. What acid–base disturbance would you expect in this patient who has acute-on-chronic kidney failure?

    a. Increased anion gap metabolic acidosis
    b. Normal anion gap metabolic acidosis
    c. Metabolic alkalosis
    d. Respiratory acidosis

Answer a is correct. Patients with renal failure and uremia will exhibit an increased anion gap metabolic acidosis (recall: KILU, where "U" stands for uremia).

Answers b, c, and d are incorrect.

17. A 55-year-old woman with a history of severe chronic obstructive pulmonary disease is admitted after several days of worsening shortness of breath. Recently, she was discharged from the hospital with a similar episode and was doing fine until 3 days before admission, when she developed a productive cough, requiring an increase in her home O_2, and more frequent albuterol/ipratropium use. What would you *expect* the pH, P_aCO_2, and HCO_3 to be in this patient ($\uparrow$, $\downarrow$, N)?

    a. pH $\uparrow$; P_aCO_2 $\downarrow$; HCO_3 $\uparrow$
    b. pH $\downarrow$; P_aCO_2 $\uparrow$; HCO_3 $\uparrow$
    c. pH $\uparrow$; P_aCO_2 N; HCO_3 $\uparrow$
    d. pH $\downarrow$; P_aCO_2 N; HCO_3 $\downarrow$

Answer b is correct. In a patient with chronic obstructive pulmonary disease, one would expect to see a primary respiratory process, with metabolic compensation. Because COPD is a restrictive airway disease, patients have difficulty "blowing off" or ventilating P_aCO_2. Therefore, you should see an increase in P_aCO_2 which will result in a decrease in the pH (respiratory acidosis). As compensation for this chronic process, patients with COPD hold onto bicarbonate to try and normalize the pH; therefore you will see a metabolic

alkalosis. Chronically, patients with COPD will have a normal pH because the increase in P_aCO_2 is compensated for by a chronic metabolic alkalosis. However, acutely, as in this case, the increase in the P_aCO_2 that occurs will result in an acute respiratory acidosis.

Answers a, c, and d are incorrect. See above explanation.

18. What acid–base disturbance might you see in a person from New Orleans, LA (1 ft. below sea level) who just flew to Denver, CO and is hiking up Pike's Peak (over 14,000 ft. above sea level)?

    a. Increased anion gap metabolic acidosis
    b. Normal anion gap metabolic acidosis
    c. Metabolic alkalosis
    d. Respiratory alkalosis

Answer d is correct. Hiking in high altitude areas results in a state of hypoxemia. This low level of oxygen will cause a person's respiratory system to increase ventilation in an effort to oxygenate tissues. Therefore, you would expect to see a respiratory alkalosis.

Answers a, b, and c are incorrect.

19. Which of the following antifungals may cause a normal anion gap metabolic acidosis?

    a. Flucytosine
    b. Amphotericin B
    c. Caspofungin
    d. Voriconazole

Answer b is correct. Amphotericin B can cause a normal anion gap metabolic acidosis through hydrogen ion retention and potassium excretion.

Answers a, c, and d are incorrect. These agents are not associated with normal anion gap metabolic acidosis.

20. Which of the following analgesics is associated with a respiratory alkalosis especially with toxic doses?

    a. Acetaminophen
    b. Aspirin
    c. Hydrocodone
    d. Fentanyl

Answer b is correct. Aspirin which is a salicylate is well known for inducing a respiratory alkalosis early in toxic concentrations with a metabolic acidosis as a late finding if untreated. Hemodialysis is indicated for patients who do not respond to other supportive measures as aspirin can be dialyzed.

Answer a is incorrect. Acetaminophen's primary toxicity is hepatotoxicity in excessive doses.

Answers c and d are incorrect. Toxic levels of hydrocodone or fentanyl would induce a respiratory acidosis due to respiratory depression and subsequent hypoventilation.

---

21. Excessive use of bumetanide may lead to what acid–base disorder?

    a. Metabolic acidosis
    b. Metabolic alkalosis
    c. Respiratory acidosis
    d. Respiratory alkalosis

Answer b is correct. Bumetanide is a loop diuretic similar to furosemide. Overdiuresis results in volume depletion with decreased kidney perfusion. The kidneys attempt to absorb more sodium in the proximal tubule, a place where it is reabsorbed with bicarbonate, in order to increase blood pressure and perfusion. The end result is an increase in the serum bicarbonate with a metabolic alkalosis. Therefore, answers a, c, and d are incorrect.

CHAPTER 37 | Enteral Nutrition

1. Which of the following statements is <u>NOT</u> true regarding enteral nutrition?

   a. Enteral nutrition should be used only if parenteral nutrition is contraindicated in the patient.
   b. Enteral nutrition is associated with less glucose intolerance compared to parenteral nutrition.
   c. Enteral nutrition is associated with lower rates of infection compared to parenteral nutrition.
   d. Enteral nutrition can be used even if the patient is eating by mouth.

Answer a is correct. This statement is not true. In general, enteral nutrition is preferred over parenteral nutrition if the patient's GI system is functional.

Answer b is incorrect. This statement is true as enteral nutrition is associated with significantly less metabolic complications compared to parenteral nutrition.

Answer c is incorrect. This statement is true as parenteral nutrition is associated with a higher risk of infection compared to enteral nutrition.

Answer d is incorrect. This statement is true as enteral nutrition can be used as a supplement to food when oral intake is insufficient.

---

2. While administering medications via nasogastric tubes:

   a. The medication must be compatible with basic fluids.
   b. Tablets must be fully crushed and mixed with 15 to 30 mL of water.
   c. The tube must be flushed with 250 mL of water before and after medication administration.
   d. Capsule beads should be crushed and mixed with 15 to 30 mL of water.

Answer b is correct. Tablets that are able to be crushed must be ground into a very fine powder and mixed with water prior to administration.

Answer a is incorrect. The tip of a nasogastric tube terminates in the gastrum of the stomach which is acidic. There is no requirement for compatibility with basic medium.

Answer c is incorrect. Nasogastric tubes should be flushed with 30 mL before and after medication administration.

Answer d is incorrect. Capsule beads should not be crushed. For those capsules that can be opened, the beads should be given intact and flushed with 30 mL water before and after administration.

---

3. JK is a 28 yo admitted with seizures secondary to alcohol withdrawal. The medical team starts JK on oral phenytoin regimen of 100 mg three times daily and also initiates the patient on continuous tube feedings since his oral food intake is inadequate at this time to provide optimal nutrition. All of the following counseling points are appropriate to give the medical team EXCEPT:

   a. The patient's phenytoin should always be converted to IV when on continuous tube feedings.
   b. Tube feedings should be held 1-2 hours before and after the patient's phenytoin dose.
   c. It is important that the nurse adjust the patient's tube feeding rate to adjust for the time held for phenytoin administration.
   d. Tube feedings lead to reduced bioavailability of phenytoin.

Answer a is correct. The patient's phenytoin does not necessarily have to be converted to IV when patients are on enteral nutrition, but can be considered if the patient is unable to reach therapeutic serum concentrations on oral therapy.

Answer b is incorrect. This statement is appropriate as holding tube feedings before and after phenytoin administration should be done to prevent the interaction of reduced bioavailability of phenytoin due to enteral nutrition.

Answer c is incorrect. This statement is true. Since tube feedings are held before and after the phenytoin dose, it is important to appropriate adjust the patient's tube feeding rate to adjust for the time held to ensure the patient is still meeting their caloric and dietary requirements.

Answer d is incorrect. This statement is appropriate and correct.

---

4. When administering drugs via enteral feeding tube:

   a. Liquid medications are always preferable to solid dosage forms.
   b. As long as tablets are crushed very finely they will retain their pharmacokinetic properties.

c. All drugs that a patient receives should be given simultaneously to minimize feeding interruptions.
d. Liquid medications may interact with nutritional formula.

Answer d is correct. As stated above, some liquid medications have physical incompatibilities with enteral nutrition products which may thicken the products or form a gel.

Answer a is incorrect. Liquid medications are *not* always preferable. Gastrointestinal intolerance is a common adverse effect of some liquid medications, especially those that contain sorbitol, and some may be physically incompatible with enteral nutrition.

Answer b is incorrect. Many tablets cannot be crushed at all, and crushing often changes the pharmacokinetic properties of the tablet.

Answer c is incorrect. Even in patients taking medications by mouth, there may be incompatibilities. These same restrictions apply when administering medications per tube.

5. Which of the following statements is correct?

a. Modular formulas contain a balanced mixture of carbohydrates and lipids.
b. Calorically dense formulas provide nutrition targeted to a specific disease state.
c. Elemental formulas contain intact proteins and polysaccharides.
d. Standard formulas contain intact proteins.

Answer d is correct. Standard formulas contain intact proteins and are meant for patients who can fully digest proteins and do not require hydrolyzed proteins.

Answer a is incorrect. Modular formulas contain a single nutrient entity that is used to supplement traditional formulas; therefore, targeting specific patient needs.

Answer b is incorrect. Calorically dense formulas are complete nutrition sources and contain a balanced mix of nutrients.

Answer c is incorrect. Elemental formulas contain hydrolyzed proteins (peptides and amino acids) which are easier to digest than intact proteins.

6. Aspiration risks during enteral nutrition feedings are increased by which of the following?

a. Feeding in an elevated or upright position
b. High gastric residual prior to feeding
c. Continuous feeding regimens
d. High-protein modular feeding

Answer b is correct. Initiating enteral feeds when the gastric residual is high increases the risk for aspiration.

Answer a is incorrect. An elevated or upright position is preferable to a supine position if a risk of aspiration exists.

Answer c is incorrect. Continuous feeding regimens are protective against aspiration.

Answer d is incorrect. High-protein modular feeding does not have an effect on aspiration risk.

7. Which of the following statements is true regarding aspiration pneumonia?

a. Is usually viral
b. Is usually preceded by a bacterial infection
c. Is a chemical pneumonitis initially
d. Is decreased by H_2 antagonists

Answer c is correct. Aspiration pneumonia initially causes a chemical pneumonitis.

Answer a is incorrect. Aspiration pneumonia is initially a chemical pneumonitis and in most cases sterile. When it occurs it usually is bacterial in nature.

Answer b is incorrect. Aspiration pneumonitis is caused by aspirating the stomach contents into the lung. In some cases true infection or aspiration pneumonia develops.

Answer d is incorrect. H_2 blockers do not appear to have an effect on susceptibility to aspiration pneumonia, but by lowering the acid content of the stomach they allow bacteria to remain in the gut. So if a patient does develop aspiration pneumonia, it is more likely to be complicated by bacterial growth if the patient is taking an H_2 antagonists (or PPI).

8. Which of the following factors is most important for initial selection of an enteral formulation?

a. Formula osmolality
b. Cost of formulation
c. Location of tube
d. Nutritional needs

Answer d is correct. Nutritional needs of the patient should be the guiding factor in all decisions about enteral nutrition. While osmolality, cost, and tube location are certainly important, attaining optimal nutrition status is the overall goal.

Answer a is incorrect. Osmolality, while important because it may influence tolerability, is not usually the primary concern when making the initial product selection.

Answer b is incorrect. Again, while important, cost is not the overriding factor in product selection.

Answer c is incorrect. Tube location is dictated by patient's disease state, and while it may have some influence on the decision of which formula to select, it is not the primary consideration.

9. Enteral nutrition may be contraindicated or cautioned against use in which of the following situations?

a. Gastrointestinal bleeding
b. Gastric cancer
c. Short bowel syndrome
d. Colostomy

Answer a is correct. Enteral feeding is relatively contra-indicated in gastrointestinal bleeding as it may potentiate bleeding. In some cases, once the cause of the GI bleeding has been determined and treated, it may be acceptable, and even preferred to restart the feeding.

Answer b is incorrect. Gastric cancer is a common reason to initiate enteral nutrition. Patients with gastric cancer often have obstruction or gastric pain associated with their disease, and enteral feeds beyond the point of obstruction are beneficial.

Answer c is incorrect. As with answer b, short bowel syndrome is a common reason to initiate enteral feeding. Those with short bowel syndrome do not absorb nutrients well, so close attention to nutrient content is warranted.

Answer d is incorrect. The colon is beyond the point that most nutrients are absorbed, and as such, colostomies do not interfere with enteral feeds any more than oral feeding.

10. MJ is a hospitalized man who weighs 78 kg and has a BMI of 24 kg/m². What is his calculated daily fluid requirement?

a. 2160 mL
b. 2660 mL
c. 3160 mL
d. 3660 mL

Answer b is correct. The average adult requires 1500 mL for the first 20 kg of body weight and 20 mL/kg of body weight over 20 kg. Therefore, the calculations for daily fluid requirement for a 78-kg adult are: 1500 mL + [(78 kg − 20 kg) × 20 mL) = 2660 mL.

Answers a, c, and d are incorrect.

11. Which of the following daily calorie counts would be most appropriate for MJ (from Question 10)?

a. 1500 kcal
b. 2000 kcal
c. 2500 kcal
d. 3000 kcal

Answer c is correct. Adult patients on bedrest require an average of 30 to 35 kcal/kg of body weight per day. The calculations for calorie intake are from 78 kg × 30 to 78 kg × 35 kcal/d = 2340 to 2730 kcal.

Answer a is incorrect. This regimen does not supply enough calories for a 78-kg man (19 kcal/kg/d).

Answer b is incorrect. This regimen does not supply enough calories for a 78-kg man (25 kcal/kg/d).

Answer d is incorrect. This regimen supplies too many calories for a 78-kg man (38 kcal/kg/d).

12. Which of the following is a common complication of enteral nutrition therapy?

a. Weight loss
b. Diarrhea
c. Weight gain
d. Hypoglycemia

Answer b is correct. Diarrhea is a common complication of enteral nutrition and may be caused by malabsorption, infection, or high osmolar concentration of formula or drugs.

Answer a is incorrect. Weight loss is not a common complication of enteral nutrition therapy. If unintentional weight loss is thought to be caused by enteral nutrition, a reassessment of the feeding regimen needs to be performed.

Answer c is incorrect. Weight gain is not a common complication of enteral nutrition and like weight loss can be managed through appropriate nutrition management.

Answer d is incorrect. Hypoglycemia is not a common complication of enteral feeding unless feedings are held in diabetic patients receiving insulin.

13. Fluid retention associated with enteral nutrition is a problem that is commonly encountered in which of the following disease states?

a. Heart failure
b. Respiratory distress
c. Hyperthyroidism
d. Diabetic ketoacidosis

Answer a is correct. Heart failure will likely cause increased fluid retention.

Answer b is incorrect. Respiratory distress is not a cause of fluid retention, increased respiratory rate will actually increase fluid losses because expired air has higher water content than inspired air.

Answer c is incorrect. Hyperthyroidism is not a common cause of fluid retention.

Answer d is incorrect. Patients with diabetic ketoacidosis often are volume depleted upon presentation due to their hyperglycemic polyuria.

14. ED is a 62-year-old woman with type 2 diabetes and end-stage renal disease who requires enteral nutrition. She was recently placed on hemodialysis therapy 3 times/wk. Please select the most appropriate nutrition combination.

a. Low protein, high carbohydrate
b. Low protein, low carbohydrate
c. Moderate protein, low carbohydrate
d. High protein, high carbohydrate

Answer c is correct. A moderate protein diet in a hemodialysis patient decreases the risk of protein malnutrition; there is no risk of further renal deterioration. A low-carbohydrate diet may prove beneficial for patient with diabetes.

Answer a is incorrect. A low-protein diet in hemodialysis may lead to protein malnutrition due to increased protein loss. A high carbohydrate diet is likely to lead to loss of glycemic control.

Answer b is incorrect. A low-protein diet in hemodialysis may lead to protein malnutrition due to increased protein loss. A low carbohydrate diet may prove beneficial for patient with diabetes.

Answer d is incorrect. High-protein diets have not been proved to be beneficial in preventing protein malnutrition. A high-carbohydrate diet is likely to lead to loss of glycemic control.

15. Patients with hepatic encephalopathy may benefit from nutritional formulations containing:

    a. High branched chain amino acids (BCAA), low aromatic amino acids (AAA)
    b. Low branched chain amino acids, high aromatic amino acids
    c. High protein, low amino acids
    d. Protein and amino acid content does not affect hepatic encephalopathy

Answer a is correct. Patients with hepatic encephalopathy tend to have low levels of BCAA and high levels of AAA.

Answer b is incorrect. Supplementing already high AAA may worsen hepatic encephalopathy.

Answer c is incorrect. High-protein diets may worsen hepatic encephalopathy through elevated blood ammonia levels because the impaired liver cannot synthesize the excess nitrogen into urea for disposal.

Answer d is incorrect. See answer c for explanation of protein content and hepatic encephalopathy.

16. TR is a 72-year-old man with diabetes and COPD. He is currently hospitalized and on a ventilator for community-acquired pneumonia. Which of the following regimens would be most appropriate dietary therapy?

    a. 50% carbohydrate, 30% fat, 20% protein
    b. 65% carbohydrate, 30% fat, 35% protein
    c. 35% carbohydrate, 25% fat, 40% protein
    d. 35% carbohydrate, 50% fat, 15% protein

Answer d is correct. The low carbohydrate diet has been supplemented by a higher fat content. This will help decrease the CO_2 load while providing adequate calories.

Answer a is incorrect. Patients with pulmonary disease should be given a low carbohydrate diet to decrease CO_2

production as well as to decrease the risk of hyperglycemia in a diabetic patient.

Answer b is incorrect. See answer a above.

Answer c is incorrect. The carbohydrate load is appropriate, but the caloric deficit should be replaced with fat.

17. TR (from Question 16) has been in your facility on the ventilator for 4 days and the resident asks how the risk of aspiration can be decreased. Which of the following methods is an appropriate intervention for this patient?

    a. Elevating head of the bed during and after feedings
    b. Initiating intermittent bolus feedings rather than continuous feedings
    c. Placing gastric tube and stopping proton-pump inhibitor use
    d. Placing gastric tube instead of duodenal tube

Answer a is correct. Elevating the head of the bed is an appropriate method to decrease the risk of aspiration.

Answer b is incorrect. Use of continuous feeds decreases the risk of aspiration compared to intermittent bolus feeds.

Answer c is incorrect. Gastric tube placement actually increases the risk of aspiration compared to duodenal placement; proton-pump inhibitor use is appropriate in this patient for stress ulcer prophylaxis since he has been intubated for more than 48 hours.

Answer d is incorrect. Duodenal tube placement decreases the risk of aspiration when compared to gastric tube placement.

18. Which of the following statements applies to fiber in enteral formulations?

    a. Decreases tolerability in most patients
    b. May increase diarrhea
    c. May increase constipation
    d. May contribute to GI obstruction

Answer d is correct. Fiber-containing products may increase the risk of GI obstruction in those already at risk.

Answer a is incorrect. Fiber increases the tolerability of enteral feedings for most patients.

Answer b is incorrect. Fiber-containing formulas are often given to decrease the incidence of diarrhea.

Answer c is incorrect. Fiber-containing formulas are often given to decrease the incidence of constipation.

19. Which of the following tubes are correctly matched to their preferred use or tube type?

    a. Nasogastric tube, long-term use
    b. Orogastric tube, small bore
    c. Percutaneous gastric tube, short-term use
    d. Nasojejunal tube, large bore

Answer b is correct. Orogastric tubes should be small bore to increase patient comfort and tolerability.

Answer a is incorrect. Nasogastric tubes should not be used long term as they are not well tolerated.

Answer c is incorrect. Percutaneous placement is typically reserved for long-term feeding access.

Answer d is incorrect. Small-bore tubes are preferred for both oral and nasal tube placement to decrease the risk of physical irritation from the tube and increase tolerability.

---

20. Which of the following patient groups have increased metabolic needs? Select all that apply.
    a. Type 1 diabetics
    b. Trauma patients
    c. Burn patients
    d. Critically ill patients

Answer b is correct. Trauma patients do have increased metabolic needs; recovering from trauma is a catabolic process that increases baseline energy needs.

Answer c is correct. Burn patients are in a highly catabolic state and have greatly increased metabolic rates.

Answer d is correct. Critical illness induces a catabolic state and energy needs are increased over baseline.

Answer a is incorrect. Patients with type 1 diabetes do not have increased metabolic/caloric needs over those of a non-diabetic patient.

CHAPTER **38 | Parenteral Nutrition**

1. LC is a 48-year-old man who underwent small bowel resection for a volvulus (gut twisting) that caused bowel necrosis. He is receiving PN and has required a nasogastric tube for suction. He develops metabolic alkalosis. Which of the following is the most appropriate adjustment to LC's PN solution?
   a. Add sodium bicarbonate
   b. Decrease acetate and increase chloride
   c. Increase acetate and decrease chloride
   d. Increase sodium and potassium

Answer b is correct. Acetate in PN solutions tends to have an alkalinizing effect (because of its conversion to bicarbonate in the liver), whereas chloride has an acidifying effect. Therefore, decreasing acetate and increasing chloride should help to improve a metabolic alkalosis.

Answer a is incorrect. Sodium bicarbonate is generally not added to PN solutions due to compatibility issues. When a source of base is desired to be added to a PN solution, acetate is usually utilized. Acetate is converted to bicarbonate in the liver. Adding sodium bicarbonate to a PN solution

would tend to worsen a metabolic alkalosis rather than to improve this condition.

Answer c is incorrect. As explained above for Answer b, increasing acetate and decreasing chloride in a PN solution might be helpful in correcting a metabolic acidosis, but it would be expected to worsen a metabolic alkalosis and would therefore be inappropriate for a patient with metabolic alkalosis.

Answer d is incorrect. Not enough information is given to determine whether increasing sodium in the PN is appropriate for this patient, and these changes would not directly affect acid-base balance. Fluid overload can be a problem in some PN patients, and excess sodium in the PN could exacerbate this problem. The amount of the potassium in the PN should not generally affect acid-base balance.

---

2. Which of the following statements is true regarding macrosubstrates found in PN solutions? Select all that apply.
   a. Dextrose and amino acids can be mixed together by the manufacturer, heat sterilized, and then shipped to hospitals.
   b. Glycerin and amino acids can be mixed together by the manufacturer, heat sterilized, and then shipped to hospitals.
   c. Clinimix is a two compartment PN solution containing dextrose and amino acid that is available in the United States.
   d. Kabiven is a three compartment PN solution containing dextrose, amino acid, and lipid that is available in the United States.
   e. Glycerin and dextrose can be mixed together by the manufacturer, heat sterilized, and then shipped to hospitals.

Answer b is correct. Because glycerin does not contain a carbonyl group, the Maillard reaction does not occur when combinations of glycerin and amino acids are heat sterilized. The commercially available product called ProcalAmine contains these components in a premixed formulation.

Answer c is correct. Clinimix and Clinimix E are premixed or ready-to-use PN solutions available in the United States supplied in two compartment bags, with each compartment containing either amino acid or dextrose. A septum between the two chambers is broken immediately before use and the two solutions are mixed together.

Answer d is correct. Kabiven and Perikabiven are premixed or ready-to-use PN solutions available in the United States supplied in three compartment bags, with each compartment containing either dextrose, amino acid, or lipid. Septa between the three chambers are broken immediately before use and the three solutions are mixed together.

Answer a is incorrect. When heated, carbonyl groups on dextrose will react with amino groups on amino acids in what is called the Maillard or browning reaction. Therefore, dextrose and amino acid combinations are not available premixed by the manufacturer.

Answer e is incorrect. You would not use dextrose and glycerin together in a PN solution.

3. A patient is receiving ProcalAmine postoperatively at 100 mL/h. ProcalAmine contains 3% final concentration of glycerin (4.3 kcal/g) and 3% final concentration of amino acid. How many total calories and how much protein are provided per day by this solution?

   a. 598 kcal and 72 g amino acid
   b. 533 kcal and 72 g amino acid
   c. 720 kcal and 60 g amino acid
   d. 747 kcal and 60 g amino acid

Answer a is correct.   Calculation of kcal and amino acid is as follows:

   100 mL/h × 24 h/d = 2400 mL/d

   Glycerin provides 4.3 kcal/g

   3 g glycerin/100 mL = x g glycerin/2400 mL; x = 72 g

   72 g × 4.3 kcal/g = 310 kcal

   Amino acid provides 4 kcal/g

   3 g amino acid/100 mL = x g amino acid/2400 mL; x = 72 g

   72 g × 4 kcal/g = 288 kcal

   310 kcal + 288 kcal = 598 kcal

Answers b, c, and d are incorrect.   Note that IV dextrose supplies 3.4 kcal/g and oral carbohydrate supplies 4 kcal/g. Although ProcalAmine may be appropriate as a PPN solution, the amount of kcal and protein that it provides is limited by low concentrations.

4. A 51-year-old patient has hepatic encephalopathy that is refractory to standard medical therapy including lactulose. He is intolerant of enteral feedings and is being considered for PN. When compared to a standard amino acid formulation, which of the following amino acid profiles best describes a specialty formulation designed for patients such as this?

   a. Higher in branched chain amino acids, same level of aromatic amino acids
   b. Higher in branched chain amino acids, lower in aromatic amino acids
   c. Higher in essential amino acids, lower in nonessential amino acids
   d. Fortified with dipeptides containing glutamine

Answer b is correct.   Aromatic amino acids tend to accumulate in hepatic failure, whereas branched chain amino acids in the blood are decreased. According to the false neurotransmitter theory, aromatic amino acids compete for transport across the blood–brain barrier with branched chain amino acids and are converted to false neurotransmitters such as octopamine, leading to hepatic encephalopathy. Feeding of a parenteral amino acid formula fortified with branched chain amino acids and with lesser amounts of aromatic amino acid formulas can help normalize amino acid levels in the blood. Such formulas have been shown to help patients "wake up" from hepatic encephalopathy, but data demonstrating improved outcomes in terms of mortality with

use of these products are limited. They should be reserved for use in hepatic encephalopathy patients who have failed standard medical therapy.

Answer a is incorrect.   Products containing more branched chain amino acids but the same amount of aromatic amino acids as in standard products have been marketed as Aminosyn-HBC or FreAmine HBC for use in highly stressed patients. Branched chain amino acids are preferentially broken down during stress and are thus fortified in these products. These products are not frequently utilized, largely because of expense and stability concerns limiting their concentration and therefore the amount that can be delivered to a patient in a reasonable fluid load.

Answer c is incorrect.   Specialty products for use in renal failure contain higher amounts of essential amino acids and lower amounts of nonessential amino acids compared to standard amino acid formulations. This allows for recycling of some endogenous urea nitrogen for synthesis of nonessential amino acids. Although some data support lowering of blood urea nitrogen in patients with renal failure receiving these products, data on improved clinical outcomes are limited.

Answer d is incorrect.   Amino acid products available in the United States do not contain glutamine due to stability issues. Some products available in other parts of the world do provide dipeptides containing glutamine; the dipeptides overcome the stability issues with glutamine. Glutamine is often depleted during stress and is the preferred fuel source for small intestinal cells.

5. MF is a 68-year-old woman with cancer cachexia. She has lost 10% of her body weight since her diagnosis with colon cancer about 6 months ago. Her cancer treatments are causing severe nausea and vomiting. The physician wants to start PN. The dietitian expresses concern regarding refeeding syndrome. Which electrolyte abnormalities are characteristic of this syndrome? Select all that apply.

   a. Hypomagnesemia
   b. Hypercalcemia
   c. Hypokalemia
   d. Hypophosphatemia
   e. Hypernatremia

Refeeding syndrome occurs in the setting of chronic malnutrition when a patient is refed with aggressive amounts of dextrose. Although more likely to occur with parenteral feeding, it has also been reported with enteral and oral feedings. In extreme cases, it can be associated with pulmonary and cardiac failure and central nervous system involvement and can be life threatening.

Answer a is correct.   Although hypophosphatemia is the hallmark electrolyte abnormality of refeeding syndrome, hypokalemia and hypomagnesemia may also occur as outlined under answer d below.

Answer c is correct. Although hypophosphatemia is the hallmark electrolyte abnormality of refeeding syndrome, hypokalemia and hypomagnesemia may also occur as outlined under answer d below.

Answer d is correct. With carbohydrate refeeding, phosphorus, magnesium, and potassium, which are primarily intracellular electrolytes, are forced intracellularly by the action of insulin. This leads to lower levels of these electrolytes in the extracellular space, including the blood, where levels are routinely measured. Therefore, hypophosphatemia, hypomagnesemia, and hypokalemia are expected with refeeding. Hypophosphatemia is the hallmark electrolyte abnormality. Phosphorus is important in diaphragm function and in energy metabolism as a component of adenosine triphosphate (ATP). Thus hypophosphatemia can contribute to respiratory failure in severe refeeding syndrome.

Answer b is incorrect. Although hypercalcemia is common in patients with cancer, it is not the hallmark of refeeding syndrome.

Answer e is incorrect. Hypernatremia is not a complication of refeeding syndrome but can be a complication of PN therapy if the formula is concentrated.

---

6. A national shortage of IV multivitamin products leads a hospital to ration this product in patients receiving PN. Which vitamins would be most crucial to supplement as individual entities to a hospitalized patient receiving PN for a few weeks in the setting of an IV multivitamin shortage? Select all that apply.

    a. Pantothenic acid
    b. Biotin
    c. Folic acid
    d. Thiamine
    e. Phytonadione

Nationwide shortages of IV multivitamin products have occurred intermittently during the past several decades. In settings of shortages, patients may be given oral multivitamins if they are able to absorb them. Remaining IV multivitamin product may need to be rationed; instead of daily administration, a regimen of 2 or 3 times per week may be implemented. Some of the vitamins found in the IV multivitamin products are not available as individual IV entities. On the other hand, some vitamins are available as individual entities and should be added on a daily basis in a shortage situation. Three vitamins of particular importance available as individual IV entities are thiamine, folic acid, and pyridoxine.

Answer c is correct. Folic acid deficiency is associated with megaloblastic anemia which has been reported in patients receiving folate-free PN for 4 to 5 weeks.

Answer d is correct. The classic deficiency disease of thiamine is beriberi. Wet beriberi, characterized by a congestive heart failure picture, has been described in patients receiving PN for 3 to 4 weeks without thiamine.

Answer a is incorrect. Pantothenic acid deficiency should not be a problem over the short term. It is not available as an individual commercially available IV product.

Answer b is incorrect. Although biotin is considered an essential nutrient, it is not likely to become deficient during short-term PN in a hospitalized patient. It is not available as an individual commercially available IV product.

Answer e is incorrect. Phytonadione (Vitamin K) should not be a problem in the short term.

---

7. Which of the following increases the solubility of calcium and phosphate in a PN solution? Select all that apply.

    a. Increased temperature
    b. Decreased pH
    c. Use of calcium gluconate instead of calcium chloride
    d. Increased amino acid concentration in the PN
    e. Decreased acidity

Solubility of calcium and phosphate in PN solutions is important because precipitation of these substances has led to patient harm. Precipitates large enough to cause adverse events are not always visible to the human eye, although visual checking of PN solutions is still a vital part of quality assurance. Furthermore, TNA are opaque and therefore precipitates in these admixtures are typically undetectable by visual checks. Final filtering of PN solutions is vital for prevention of infusion of large particulates into the patient.

Answer b is correct. Decreases in pH increase the solubility of calcium and phosphate.

Answer c is correct. Calcium gluconate is the preferred form of calcium for addition to PN in the United States. Calcium gluconate is more soluble than calcium chloride.

Answer d is correct. Increasing the amino acid concentration of the PN tends to decrease the pH of the solution, thus increasing the solubility of calcium and phosphate. The low amino acid concentration of neonatal PN solutions, together with high requirements for calcium and phosphate in neonates, leads to challenges relating to calcium and phosphate solubility in PN solutions for this population.

Answer a is incorrect. Although solubility of many substances increases with increased temperatures, the opposite is true for calcium and phosphate.

Answer e is incorrect. Increased acidity increases calcium and phosphate solubility in PN solution.

---

8. A hospital is transitioning from use of dextrose/amino acid solutions plus piggybacked lipid for PN to a system utilizing TNA. The former practice was to use 0.22 μm filters for dextrose/amino acid solutions and to use 1.2 μm filters for piggybacked lipid emulsion. Which one of the following

best describes proper use of final filters with the new TNA system?

a. A switch from use of 0.22 μm filters to use of 1.2 μm filters is appropriate.

b. A switch from use of 0.22 μm filters to use of 5 μm filters is appropriate.

c. No switch in filtration practices is necessary; use of 0.22 μm filters may continue.

d. Switching from the current 0.22 μm filters to no filters is most appropriate.

Answer a is correct.   It is recommended that dextrose/amino acid solutions be filtered through a 0.22 μm final filter. Such filters remove both particulates and microbes. Lipid emulsions and TNA cannot be passed through a 0.22 μm filter, because particles within these emulsions typically range up to about 0.5 μm in size and would thus be disrupted or deformed by passage through the smaller filter. Lipid emulsions administered via piggyback should be passed through a 1.2 μm filter.

Answer b is incorrect.   Although 5 μm filters are also available, it is recommended that TNA be passed through a 1.2 μm filter.

Answer c is incorrect.   TNA should not be administered through a 0.22 μm filter as outlined under answer a.

Answer d is incorrect.   It is very important to administer TNA through a filter. Adverse outcomes have been reported when this step was omitted. Infusion of particles greater in size than about 0.5 μm can cause lung damage.

---

9. PS is a 28-year-old man receiving PN because of intolerance to enteral feeding following multiple trauma. He is receiving 150 g of protein each day. A 24-hour urine collection for urea nitrogen (UUN) yields a value of 20 g. What is the estimated nitrogen balance in grams per day for this patient?

a. +4
b. 0
c. −30
d. −120

Answer b is correct.   To calculate the number of grams of nitrogen from the number of grams of protein, divide by 6.25 or multiply by 0.16. Thus, the amount of nitrogen going into the patient is 150/6.25 = 24 g. Applying the correction factor given above for nonurinary urea nitrogen losses, the nitrogen balance is calculated as follows:

Nitrogen balance = nitrogen in - (nitrogen out + 4), or

Nitrogen balance = 24 - (20 + 4) = 0

Thus the patient is estimated to be in neutral nitrogen balance. The goal is to have patients in positive nitrogen balance; therefore, increasing the protein and/or kcal of the PN may be appropriate in this situation to achieve a positive balance. Achievement of a positive nitrogen balance is frequently unrealistic in patients undergoing high stress.

Answer a is incorrect.   It does not take into account nonurinary urea nitrogen losses. A correction factor of 4 g/d is generally allowed for such losses.

Answers c and d are incorrect.   Negative numbers of this magnitude would not be expected in the setting of PN feeding.

---

10. TL is a 41-year-old mechanically ventilated woman receiving propofol for sedation. The drug is provided as 10 mg/mL propofol and is being delivered at 100 mg/h. Propofol is commercially provided in a 10% lipid emulsion vehicle. How many calories per day is TL receiving via the propofol infusion?

a. 22
b. 43
c. 216
d. 264

Propofol is commonly used as a sedative in mechanically ventilated critically ill patients. The rate of administration for this use frequently provides significant lipid kcal and should be taken into account when calculating kcal and lipid administration. In patients receiving PN concomitantly, IV lipid emulsion may need to be held or the rate of administration cut while the patient is receiving propofol.

Answer d is correct.   Calculation is as follows:

Propofol being infused at 100 mg/h/10 mg/mL = 10 mL/h
10 mL/h × 24 h/d = 240 mL/d

240 mL/d × 1.1 kcal/mL = 264 kcal

Answers a, b, and c are incorrect.   See above for correct calculation.

---

11. Which of the following statements is true regarding TNA?

a. A cracked TNA may be safely administered to a patient, but a creamed TNA is unsafe for administration.

b. A creamed TNA may be safely administered to a patient, but a cracked TNA is unsafe for administration.

c. Neither a creamed nor a cracked TNA may be safely administered to a patient.

d. Both creamed and cracked TNA may be safely administered to a patient.

TNAs are inherently less stable than dextrose/amino acid solutions. The so-called zeta potential is a negative charge on the surface of lipid globules. This zeta potential prevents clumping of lipid globules. If this negative surface charge is neutralized by cations, coalescence of lipid globules may occur. Trivalent cations are the worst culprits for neutralizing the negative surface charge, followed by divalent cations; monovalent cations have a lesser effect. TNA stability is decreased with decreasing pH due to increases in hydrogen ion concentration.

A creamed TNA is one in which lipid globules have separated out of the emulsion, but gentle inversion of the container results in the globules redispersing, and the original homogeneous appearance of the admixture reappears. On the other hand, in a cracked TNA, lipid globules have coalesced and separated out of the emulsion, and gentle inversion cannot result in reappearance of the original homogeneous condition of the admixture.

Answer b is correct. A creamed TNA may be safely administered after redispersion, whereas a cracked TNA cannot be restored to its original condition and therefore should be discarded.

Answer a is incorrect. A cracked TNA may not be safely administered to a patient, whereas a creamed TNA may be administered after the separated fat globules have been redispersed.

Answer c is incorrect. Creamed TNA may be safely administered to patients after redispersion to their original condition.

Answer d is incorrect. Cracked TNA cannot be rehomogenized.

---

12. A 19-year-old patient is involved in a serious motor vehicle accident. He is admitted to the ICU and is initiated on tube feeding. However, on day 8 of hospitalization, he remains in the ICU and is not tolerating tube feeding. A TNA is ordered. Which of the following additives to the TNA would be expected to remain stable for at least 24 hours and also not adversely affect stability of the TNA? Select all that apply.

    a. Famotidine
    b. Regular insulin
    c. Iron dextran
    d. Manganese
    e. Glargine insulin

Answer a is correct. All parenteral H_2 antagonists are stable for at least 24 hours in PN solutions. These are added to PN solutions, either dextrose/amino acids or TNA, for continuous infusion in some hospitals.

Answer b is correct. Regular insulin is commonly added to PN solutions. Although insulin may be adsorbed to glass, tubing, and other surfaces, it does not significantly affect stability of a TNA.

Answer d is correct. Although manganese is a divalent cation, it is commonly added to PN solutions (including TNA) in small amounts as part of a multitrace element package.

Answer c is incorrect. As a multivalent cation, iron dextran has the capacity to neutralize the zeta potential on fat globules, thus destabilizing a TNA. If parenteral iron is required in a patient receiving a TNA, it can either be administered outside the PN, or it can be administered via a dextrose/amino acid solution on days when the lipid is omitted from the formulation.

Answer e is incorrect. Only regular insulin may be added to PN formulas.

---

13. AM is to receive cycled PN over 16 h/d at home. The PN is to be infused at half the goal rate for the first and last hours of the 16-hour cycle. If the final concentration of amino acid in the solution is 5%, what goal rate of PN (in mL/h) will supply about 80 g of protein per day?

    a. 62
    b. 77
    c. 92
    d. 107

Answer d is correct. Calculation is as follows:

5 g/100 mL = 80 g/x mL; x = 1600 mL

14 Y + 2(1/2 Y) = 1600 mL; 15 Y = 1600 mL; Y = 107 mL; ½ Y = 53.5 mL

Therefore, infuse 107 mL/h × 14 h + 53.5 mL/h × 2 h = 1605 mL/d.

Answers a, b, and c are incorrect.

---

14. A 71-year-old woman is in the intensive care receiving PN following surgical repair of a fistula. Which of the following most closely reflects the current recommendation for the optimal goal blood glucose range for this critically ill PN patient?

    a. 80 to 110 mg/dL
    b. 90 to 130 mg/dL
    c. 140 to 180 mg/dL
    d. 180 to 240 mg/dL

Answer c is correct. The 2013 American Society for Parenteral and Enteral Nutrition (ASPEN) guidelines for nutrition support in adult patients with hyperglycemia call for keeping blood sugar between 140 and 180 mg/dL in most patients. The 2009 American Diabetes Association and American Association of Clinical Endocrinologists joint guidelines for control of diabetes in the hospital setting call for goal blood glucose less than 140 mg/dL fasting and less than 180 mg/dL for random blood glucose checks.

Answer a is incorrect. Although at one time it was recommended to try to maintain euglycemia in critically ill patients, particularly surgical patients, concerns regarding hypoglycemia and increased morbidity in groups of patients in whom intensive insulin protocols were utilized in the Normoglycemia in Intensive Care Evaluation–Survival Using Glucose Algorithm Regulation (NICE-SUGAR) Study have led authoritative bodies to recommend less intensive blood sugar control in most patients. Cardiac surgery patients are an exception to this rule in many institutions; goal ranges in these patients are frequently set lower than goal ranges for other patient populations.

Answer b is incorrect. For the reasons outlined for Answer a above.

Answer d is incorrect. Maintenance of blood glucose in the 180 to 240 mg/dL range could lead to increased risk of infection and other complications in both critically ill and other hospitalized general medical-surgical patients.

15. LF is a 56-year-old man who is receiving PN following a bowel resection for mesenteric ischemia. He is receiving a dextrose/amino acid solution with final concentrations of 15% dextrose and 5% amino acid. This solution is being administered at 75 mL/h continuously over 24 hours. He is also receiving 200 mL of 20% lipid each day. Renal function is normal. LF weighs 60 kg, which is near his ideal body weight of 62 kg. Which of the following best describes the amount of kcal, protein, and dextrose that LF is receiving?

   a. Calories are excessive, but the amounts of protein and dextrose are within recommended ranges.
   b. The amounts of dextrose and protein are lower than recommended ranges as is the amount of calories.
   c. Protein is below the recommended range, but calories and dextrose are adequate.
   d. The number of calories, as well as the amounts of protein and dextrose, are within recommended ranges.

LF is currently receiving the following:

Dextrose/amino acid solution: 75 mL/h × 24 h/d = 1800 mL/d

Dextrose: 15 g/100 mL = x g/1800 mL; x = 270 g/d; 270 g/60 kg = 4.5 g/kg/d; 270 g × 3.4 kcal/g = 918 kcal/d

Amino acid: 5 g/100 mL = x g/1800 mL; x = 90 g; 90 g/60 kg = 1.5 g/kg/d; 90 g × 4 kcal/g = 360 kcal/d

Lipid: 200 mL/d × 2 kcal/mL = 400 kcal/d

Total kcal/d = 918 + 360 + 400 = 1678 kcal/d; 1678 kcal/60 kg = 28 kcal/kg/d

Typical recommendations for calories are to provide about 20 to 35 kcal/kg/d to patients who are not overweight or obese. These patients typically should receive 1.2 to 2 g protein/kg/d and no more than 7 g dextrose/kg/d. Lipid is typically recommended at <2.5 g/kg/d; some authorities recommend limiting lipid to 1 or 2 g/kg/d, especially in immunocompromised patients.

Answer d is correct. At 28 kcal/kg/d, calories are being administered within the recommended range of 20 to 35 kcal/kg/d. At 1.5 g/kg/d, protein is being administered within the recommended range of 1.2 to 2 g/kg/d. At 4.5 g/kg/d, dextrose is being administered at the recommended range of <7 g/kg/d; generally at least 100 g/d of dextrose should be provided to fuel dextrose-obligate organs such as the brain.

Answer a is incorrect. Calories being administered are not excessive.

Answer b is incorrect. The amounts of dextrose, protein, and calories being administered are within recommended ranges and are not too low.

Answer c is incorrect. Protein being administered is within the recommended range.

16. Which of the following vitamins commonly included in PN solutions could interfere with warfarin anticoagulation?

   a. Vitamin A
   b. Vitamin K
   c. Riboflavin
   d. Vitamin B_6

Answer b is correct. Warfarin acts by inhibiting the synthesis of vitamin K-dependent clotting factors II, VII, IX, and X and the anticoagulant proteins C and S. Vitamin K can actually be given in the setting of overcoagulation to reverse the effects of warfarin. Although it could be argued that patients receiving oral medications such as warfarin are not good candidates for PN, the combination of oral warfarin and PN is sometimes encountered. Most of the parenteral multivitamin preparations now commercially available contain 150 mcg of vitamin K to be administered as a daily dose.

Answers a, c, and d are incorrect. Vitamin A, riboflavin, and vitamin B_6 do not significantly interfere with the anticoagulant effect of warfarin.

17. Which of the following trace elements are commonly included in PN solutions? Select all that apply.

   a. Iron
   b. Zinc
   c. Manganese
   d. Copper
   e. Chloride

Answers b, c, and d are correct. Zinc, manganese, copper, and chromium are the four most common trace elements supplied in PN solutions. Selenium is also commonly included.

Answer a is incorrect. Iron is not added routinely to PN, although iron dextran may be added occasionally to dextrose/amino acid solutions, especially in long-term patients. Iron dextran is incompatible with TNA.

Answer e is incorrect. While chloride is almost always included in PN, it is not as a trace element but as a standard electrolyte.

18. YN is a 38-year-old man with short bowel syndrome who receives home PN. What is the most common PN-related reason that patients on home PN require hospitalization?

   a. Metabolic bone disease
   b. Catheter-related sepsis
   c. Trace element deficiency
   d. Hyperglycemia

Answer b is correct. Catheter-related sepsis is a common adverse event in patients on home PN that often, although not always, results in hospitalization. Because placement of a central venous catheter is an invasive procedure, and suitable venous sites for placement of such catheters are limited, efforts are made if possible to salvage infected catheters rather than removing and replacing them. Treatments include infusion of systemic antibiotics and placement of antibiotic lock solutions within the catheter. Catheter-related sepsis is most commonly caused by gram-positive bacteria but can also be caused by gram-negative bacteria and fungi. Fungal infections almost universally require catheter removal and replacement.

Answer a is incorrect. Although metabolic bone disease is a common problem in long-term home PN patients, it is not the most common cause of hospitalization in this population. The etiology of metabolic bone disease in long-term PN is not well elucidated.

Answer c is incorrect. Trace element deficiencies do occur during long-term home PN, although they can be difficult to definitively diagnose. When a trace element deficiency is suspected, higher amounts of that trace element are generally provided by the PN; this does not usually require hospitalization.

Answer d is incorrect. Hyperglycemia is a potential adverse event during PN, either short term or long term. It is prudent to stabilize blood glucose prior to initial discharge from the hospital on home PN. One setting in which hyperglycemia may develop in a patient on home PN is in the setting of infection such as catheter-related sepsis. In this situation, it is typically the signs and symptoms of infection such as fever, chills, and rigors, rather than hyperglycemia that bring the patient to the hospital.

19. HS is a 61-year-old critically ill, morbidly obese woman (BMI 42 kg/m²) with severe acute pancreatitis in whom EN has failed. On day 7 of hospitalization, PN is initiated. HS weighs 150 kg; ideal body weight is 82 kg. The PN regimen consists of 1800 kcal/d and 180 g protein per day. The patient's renal and liver functions are not severely compromised. What is the most appropriate assessment of this PN regimen?

    a. Appropriate calories and protein
    b. Appropriate calories; too much protein
    c. Appropriate protein; too many calories
    d. Too little protein; too many calories

Answer a is correct. According to the 2016 ASPEN nutrition support guidelines for the hospitalized adult patient with obesity, hypocaloric high protein feedings are appropriate for patients without severe renal or hepatic dysfunction. HS's regimen provides 12 kcal/kg actual body weight per day. Protein is being provided at 2.2 g/kg/d based on ideal body weight and 1.2 g/kg/d based on actual body weight. These are within the ranges set forth by the ASPEN obesity guidelines.

Answer b is incorrect. HM's regimen does not contain too much protein.

Answer c is incorrect. HM's regimen does not contain too many calories.

Answer d is incorrect. HM's regimen does not contain too little protein or too many calories.

20. Order the following components of a typical PN solution from highest to lowest volume contribution.

Unordered Options	Ordered Response
Electrolytes	
Amino acids	
Vitamins	
Water	

Correct ordered response. Water, amino acids, electrolytes, vitamins

Water is the largest volume component of a PN solution; the dextrose and amino acid components of a PN solution are in a water base. Even for TNAs containing lipid, water will be the largest volume component. Amino acids will typically comprise a large volume of a PN solution. Electrolytes will comprise a much smaller volume; a typical volume for a PN solution containing standard amounts of electrolytes would be about 20 mL of electrolyte per liter of PN. Vitamins are typically added at 10 mL/d.

21. A TNA is compounded using 1000 mL of dextrose 10%, 1000 mL of amino acid 8.5%, and 250 mL of 20% lipid emulsion. Which one of the following is true regarding stability of this TNA?

    a. Should be stable.
    b. Could be unstable because of low concentrations of dextrose and amino acids.
    c. Could be unstable because of low concentrations of amino acids and fat.
    d. Could be unstable because of high concentrations of dextrose and fat.

Answer b is correct. The final concentration of dextrose is less than 10% and the final concentration of amino acid is less than 4%.

Final concentrations in this TNA are as follows:

1000 mL dextrose × 10 g/100 mL = 100 g dextrose; 100 g/2250 mL final volume = 4.4%

1000 mL amino acid × 8.5 g/100 mL = 85 g amino acid; 85 g/2250 mL = 3.7%

250 mL lipid × 20 g/100 mL = 50 g lipid; 50 g/2250 mL = 2.2%

Answer a is incorrect. Minimum final concentrations of amino acid of 4%, dextrose 10%, and fat 2% are recommended for maximal TNA stability. The dextrose and amino acid concentrations of this TNA are too low.

Answer c is incorrect. The final concentration of amino acid is less than 4%, but the final concentration of fat is greater than 2%.

Answer d is incorrect. Limits on TNA stability are described in terms of minimum final concentrations, not maximum.

22. A peripheral PN solution has final concentrations of 4.25% amino acid and 5% dextrose; no fat is included in this admixture. What is the approximate osmolarity of this

solution (without electrolytes and other additives), and is that osmolarity appropriate for peripheral administration?

   a. 675; appropriate
   b. 675; inappropriate
   c. 1025; appropriate
   d. 1025; inappropriate

To estimate osmolarity of a PN solution, use 100 mOsm/L for each 1% final concentration of amino acid, and add 50 mOsm/L for each 1% final concentration of dextrose. Therefore, the solution in this question has an approximate osmolarity of 425 + 250 = 675. An osmolarity of less than 900 mOsm/L is considered acceptable for peripheral administration in adults. Lipid has an osmolarity of 280 to 340 mOsm/L, contributing to a lower osmolarity of TNA compared to dextrose/amino acid alone. Electrolytes and other additives typically add about 100 to 150 mOsm/L to these solutions.

Answer a is correct. The approximate osmolarity is 675 mOsm/L as outlined above. Since this osmolarity is less than 900 mOsm/L, this is appropriate for peripheral administration.

Answers b, c, and d are incorrect.

---

23. UN is a 34-year-old man admitted to the ICU following a motor vehicle accident in which he suffers major trauma. He was well nourished prior to the accident, and although his injuries are significant, it is anticipated that he is not at high nutritional risk. Enteral feedings (tube feedings) are started on day 2 of admission, but on day 4 they are discontinued due to intolerance. What is the best approach at this time?

   a. Start PN with dextrose, amino acids, and soybean oil fat emulsion as soon as possible.
   b. Start PN with dextrose and amino acids as soon as possible; hold soybean oil fat emulsion for now.
   c. Keep trying to reinitiate enteral feedings and wait on starting PN until about day 8 of admission if the tube feedings are still not successful.
   d. Because the patient was previously well nourished, hold both PN and enteral feedings until about day 14 of the hospitalization.

Answer c is correct. ASPEN intensive care guidelines promote holding PN for the first 7 days of an intensive care admission in patients who were well nourished prior to admission and are not at high nutritional risk. These guidelines also promote early initiation of enteral feedings if these can be safely administered.

Answer a is incorrect. ASPEN intensive care guidelines promote holding PN for the first 7 days of an intensive care admission in patients who were well nourished prior to admission and are not at high nutritional risk. These guidelines recommend holding soybean oil for the first 7 days of an intensive care admission regardless of the patient's nutritional status and nutritional risk.

Answer b is incorrect. ASPEN intensive care guidelines promote holding PN for the first 7 days of an intensive care admission in patients who were well nourished prior to admission and are not at high nutritional risk.

Answer d is incorrect. Fourteen days without nutrition would be longer than recommended for intensive care patients.

CHAPTER 39 | Electrolyte Disorders

1. A 72-year-old man is admitted for a low serum sodium level at a routine check-up. The patient states he feels fine. Past medical history includes chronic obstructive pulmonary disease, depression, gout, and hypertension. Current medications are albuterol, allopurinol, lisinopril, and sertraline. Physical examination is unremarkable. Pertinent laboratory values include a serum sodium of 123 mEq/L, urine sodium of 90 mEq/L, and a urine osmolarity of 585 mOsm/L. The patient is diagnosed with SIADH. Which of the following represents appropriate treatment to correct this patient's sodium abnormality?

   a. 3% Saline infusion
   b. Demeclocycline
   c. Stopping the offending agent and fluid restriction
   d. Normal saline infusion

Answer c is correct. In addition to stopping the offending agent, fluid restriction is the mainstay of therapy for acute management of SIADH. The negative water balance can correct serum sodium.

Answer a is incorrect. Hypertonic saline is not indicated in asymptomatic patients. It should be reserved for patients with life-threatening symptoms, such as seizures or coma.

Answer b is incorrect. Agents that interfere with ADH activity in the collecting duct are not typically used when the causative agent can be removed. The cause in this patient is most likely sertraline. Demeclocycline and vasopressin receptor agents may be useful in patients with chronic SIADH who are unresponsive to or cannot tolerate water restriction.

Answer d is incorrect. Infusion of normal saline in a patient with SIADH is inappropriate. Since the patient's renal handling of sodium is intact with an increased absorption of free water, serum sodium can actually fall with a normal saline infusion.

---

2. Choose the statement that best describes SIADH based on the underlying disorder and common cause.

   a. Hypervolemic hypotonic hypernatremia and hydrochlorothiazide
   b. Hypervolemic hypotonic hypernatremia and cirrhosis
   c. Euvolemic hypotonic hyponatremia and lithium
   d. Euvolemic hypotonic hyponatremia and sertraline

Answer d is correct. SIADH is classified as a euvolemic hypotonic hyponatremia and commonly caused by selective serotonin reuptake inhibitors.

Answer a is incorrect. Thiazide diuretics are commonly associated with hypovolemic hyponatremia, but do not cause SIADH. Antidiuretic hormone stimulation with thiazide therapy is an appropriate response to the modest hypovolemia caused by thiazides.

Answer b is incorrect. Cirrhosis is most commonly associated with hyponatremia and not hypernatremia or SIADH.

Answer c is incorrect. Lithium is a common cause of nephrogenic diabetes insipidus (hypernatremia). Lithium antagonizes adenyl cyclase and cyclic adenosine monophosphate (cAMP), and inhibits the opening of aquaporin channels in the renal tubules. This leads to a loss of free water causing hypernatremia when water losses are not replaced. SIADH is classified as a euvolemic hypotonic hyponatremia.

---

3. A 68-year-old woman is brought to the hospital because of progressive drowsiness and syncope. She complains of diarrhea for the past 3 days. She is lethargic but has no focal neurologic deficits. Past medical history is significant for lung cancer, depression, hypertension, gastroesophageal reflux disease (GERD), and osteoarthritis. Medications include acetaminophen, hydrochlorothiazide, fluoxetine, ranitidine, and magnesium oxide. Physical examination reveals a blood pressure of 96/56 mm Hg, pulse of 110 beats/min, dry mucous membranes, and reduced skin turgor. Laboratory value is significant for serum sodium of 125 mEq/L. The most appropriate treatment to correct this patient's sodium abnormality includes which of the following?

   a. 3% Saline infusion
   b. Demeclocycline
   c. Fluid restriction of <1000 mL/d
   d. Normal saline infusion

Answer d is correct. Patients with hypovolemic hyponatremia require volume replacement and correction of serum sodium with isotonic saline infusion. Serum sodium should not be corrected faster than 10 to 12 mEq/L in 24 hours or 18 mEq/L in 48 hours.

Answer a is incorrect. Hypertonic saline is not indicated in patients with mild symptoms. It should be reserved for patients with life-threatening symptoms, such as seizures or coma.

Answer b is incorrect. Demeclocycline is used in chronic SIADH and is not indicated for hypovolemic hyponatremia.

Answer c is incorrect. Fluid restriction is used in isovolemic hyponatremia and is not indicated for hypovolemic hyponatremia.

---

4. A 54-year-old man is admitted to the hospital from the outpatient clinic with abdominal swelling, weight gain, and abnormal laboratory values. Medical history is significant for cirrhosis and hepatitis C. Medications include furosemide and propranolol. His physical examination is significant for distended abdomen with shifting dullness. Significant laboratory values include serum sodium of 124 mEq/L, INR of 1.9, and albumin of 2.1. The most appropriate treatment to correct this patient's sodium abnormality includes:

   a. 3% Saline with IV furosemide
   b. Fluid restriction

   c. Normal saline infusion
   d. Sodium restriction and diuretics

Answer d is correct. The cornerstone of therapy for hyponatremia associated with edema is dietary sodium restriction and diuretic therapy.

Answer a is incorrect. Hypertonic saline is not indicated in patients without severe CNS symptoms.

Answer b is incorrect. Fluid restriction can be helpful in symptomatic hypervolemic hyponatremia. This patient, however, does not have CNS symptoms.

Answer c is incorrect. Normal saline would be inappropriate in a cirrhotic patient without evidence of volume depletion.

---

5. An 82-year-old man was brought to the emergency department by his daughter for worsening confusion and diarrhea. The daughter reports he has had poor oral intake over the last week. Medical history is significant for hypertension, ischemic stroke, reflux, and chronic constipation. Medications include aspirin, lactulose, lisinopril, omeprazole, and simvastatin. His physical examination is significant for orthostatic hypotension, tachycardia, and dry mucous membranes. Significant laboratory values include serum sodium of 162 mEq/L, blood urea nitrogen (BUN) of 66, and serum creatinine of 2.5. Appropriate initial treatment for this patient would include:

   a. 0.45% Saline infusion
   b. 5% Dextrose infusion
   c. Desmopressin
   d. Normal saline infusion

Answer d is correct. This patient is showing signs of hemodynamic instability (orthostatic hypotension, tachycardia) and should first receive isotonic saline until volume status is restored. After volume repletion, hypotonic fluids would be appropriate to correct serum sodium.

Answer a is incorrect. While hypotonic fluids will help correct this patient's serum sodium, patients with hemodynamic instability (orthostatic hypotension, tachycardia) should first receive normal saline until euvolemia is restored. Free water, from 0.45% saline or 5% dextrose, distributes throughout the intracellular fluid (ICF) and ECF. Normal saline is the appropriate initial choice. Since it is confined to the ECF, it will restore intravascular volume more efficiently than hypotonic fluids.

Answer b is incorrect. See explanation for Answer a.

Answer c is incorrect. Desmopressin is indicated in patients with central diabetes insipidus.

---

6. A 39-year-old man presents to the emergency department with abnormal laboratory values from a local psychiatric hospital. He is 4 days post neurosurgical repair of intraventricular hemorrhage secondary to bilateral self-enucleation. He is currently constrained to the hospital bed and hallucinating. Medical

history includes hypertension and schizophrenia. Medications include haloperidol, fluphenazine, and benztropine. Physical examination is normal. Pertinent laboratory values include sodium of 158 mEq/L and a urine osmolarity of 76 mOsm/kg. Urine output was 6500 mL over the last 24 hours. The patient is admitted for the treatment of central diabetes insipidus. The most appropriate treatment to correct this patient's sodium abnormality includes:

a. Desmopressin
b. Free water orally
c. Hydrochlorothiazide
d. Normal saline infusion

Answer a is correct. Patients with central diabetes insipidus require exogenous ADH.

Answer b is incorrect. Oral replacement of water would be difficult in a restrained, hallucinating patient. Free water should be given in the form of intravenous hypotonic fluids when oral replacement is not possible.

Answer c is incorrect. Hydrochlorothiazide can be useful in nephrogenic diabetes insipidus. This patient requires exogenous ADH replacement.

Answer d is incorrect. Normal saline is not appropriate in hypernatremic patients without signs of volume depletion.

7. What is the drug of choice for lithium-induced diabetes insipidus when lithium must be continued?

a. Amiloride
b. Desmopressin
c. Hydrochlorothiazide
d. Indomethacin

Answer a is correct. Amiloride closes sodium channels in the luminal membrane of the collecting tubule cells. This is the site where lithium enters cells and interferes with the actions of ADH.

Answer b is incorrect. Patient's with nephrogenic diabetes insipidus have a defect in the vasopressin-2 receptor and have an impaired response to ADH. Desmopressin is generally not effective in nephrogenic diabetes insipidus, but may provoke a partial response at high doses.

Answer c is incorrect. Hydrochlorothiazide is useful in the treatment of other forms of nephrogenic diabetes insipidus.

Answer d is incorrect. Indomethacin is useful as adjunctive therapy in the treatment of other forms of nephrogenic diabetes insipidus.

8. Which of the following are potential side effect(s) of potassium replacement (all dosage forms)? Select all that apply.

a. Irritation of the vein
b. Constipation
c. Nausea/vomiting

d. Cardiac arrhythmias
e. Dyspepsia

Answer a is correct. Intravenous administration of potassium may cause vein irritation and phlebitis. Intravenous potassium should be diluted and infused at a slower rate when given through a peripheral vein.

Answer c is correct. Nausea, vomiting, abdominal pain, diarrhea, and indigestion are common side effects of potassium chloride preparations, but all potassium salt formulations have been associated with adverse GI effects. In particular, liquid forms of potassium often have a strong, bitter smell and taste which may result in nausea and vomiting. Microencapsulated formulations are less likely to cause this effect. Administering large doses of potassium replacement orally may also increase the risk of GI upset.

Answer d is correct. Cardiac arrhythmias may result when the rate of potassium administration is too high. ECG monitoring is recommended when the rate of potassium administration exceeds 10 mEq/h.

Answer e is correct. Dyspepsia is a common adverse effect of oral potassium replacement. Administering large doses of potassium orally increases the likelihood of this effect. It is also recommended to take many formulations of potassium replacement with food and/or a full glass of water to prevent GI irritation.

Answer b is incorrect. Constipation is not commonly associated with potassium replacement. Adverse GI effects related to potassium replacement generally involve nausea and/or vomiting, dyspepsia, and diarrhea.

9. A 66-year-old man is seen for annual follow-up. He has a history of hypertension, type 2 diabetes, coronary artery disease, and heart failure (EF 30%). Current medications include spironolactone 25 mg daily, lisinopril 20 mg daily, metoprolol succinate XL 100 mg once daily, furosemide 40 mg daily, simvastatin 40 mg daily, metformin 500 mg twice daily, and aspirin 81 mg daily. Laboratory values reveal Na 141, K 6, BUN 11, serum creatinine (SCr) 1.1, Phos 3.5, and Mg 2.2. Patient has no complaints at this time. What is the most likely cause of this patient's potassium disorder?

a. Spironolactone
b. Metoprolol
c. Albuterol
d. Furosemide

Answer a is correct. Spironolactone is a potassium-sparing diuretic. The development of hyperkalemia with spironolactone and other drugs, which decrease the activity of aldosterone, is well described. Serum potassium concentration should be monitored periodically after administration or dose titration of these types of drugs.

Answer b is incorrect. β-Blockers may cause a slight rise in serum potassium levels. However, total body potassium is not affected during treatment with these drugs. Isolated case reports of hyperkalemia with β-blocking agents in patients experiencing acute acid–base disorders can be found; however, these reports are rare.

Answer c is incorrect. Albuterol in large doses is more likely to cause hypokalemia and may be used to manage hyperkalemia.

Answer d is incorrect. Furosemide is not associated with hyperkalemia. Conversely, this and other loop and thiazide diuretics are commonly associated with the development of hypokalemia through increased renal elimination of potassium.

---

10. Which hyperkalemia treatment results in the permanent removal of potassium from the body?

    a. Insulin and dextrose
    b. Calcium gluconate
    c. Kayexalate
    d. Nebulized albuterol

Answer c is correct. Sodium polystyrene sulfonate (Kayexalate) is a cation exchange resin which works by exchanging sodium for potassium as it passes through the intestine or colon. The bound potassium ions are then excreted with normal GI transit, effectively removing potassium from the body and reducing total body potassium.

Answer a is incorrect. Insulin decreases the serum potassium concentration through stimulation of the Na^+-K^+-ATPase pump. This results in the shift of potassium ions from the serum intracellularly. Dextrose is usually administered concurrently to prevent the development of hypoglycemia from insulin administration. Additionally, dextrose stimulates the secretion of endogenous insulin.

Answer b is incorrect. The intent of calcium administration in the treatment of hyperkalemia is not to affect the serum potassium concentration. Rather, it slows conduction and stabilizes the cardiac membrane potential to prevent development of cardiac arrhythmias, which may result from excessive serum potassium concentrations.

Answer d is incorrect. β-agonists result in reduction in serum potassium concentration via two separate mechanisms. β-agonists, including albuterol, stimulate the Na^+-K^+-ATPase pump to move potassium intracellularly. Additionally, these agents increase the release of insulin through stimulation of pancreatic β-cells.

---

11. Which statement best describes a mechanism of potassium homeostasis? Select all that apply.

    a. Insulin increases the intracellular uptake of potassium.
    b. Aldosterone increases potassium excretion.
    c. Calcitonin increases the tubular reabsorption of potassium.
    d. Increasing the plasma pH decreases the uptake of potassium into the cells.

    e. β-Receptor stimulation increases movement of potassium extracellularly.

Answer a is correct. Insulin increases the intracellular uptake of potassium through stimulation the Na^+-K^+-ATPase pump to move potassium intracellularly.

Answer b is correct. Aldosterone promotes urinary excretion of potassium in the distal tubule and collecting duct as it increases reabsorption of sodium and water.

Answer c is incorrect. Calcitonin increases the urinary excretion of sodium, chloride, magnesium, calcium, phosphate, and potassium by limiting tubular reabsorption.

Answer d is incorrect. Increasing the plasma pH increases the uptake of potassium inside cells as extracellular potassium is exchanged for intracellular hydrogen ions. This is the therapeutic effect desired when sodium bicarbonate is administered in the treatment of hyperkalemia.

Answer e is incorrect. Stimulation of β-receptors increases the intracellular uptake of potassium through stimulation of the Na^+-K^+-ATPase pump.

---

12. A 48-year-old man presents to the ambulatory clinic with complaints of palpitations over the past few days. Current medications are ramipril 10 mg daily, aspirin 325 mg daily, and omeprazole 20 mg daily. Vitals are blood pressure 152/90 mm Hg, pulse 90, temp 98.6°F, and respiratory rate 14 breaths/min. Laboratory values reveal Na 141, K 5.9, Cl 101, HCO_3 25, BUN 12, SCr 1.1, and glucose (Glu) 115. ECG showed peaked T waves. Which is the most appropriate initial management for this patient's potassium disorder?

    a. PO SPS
    b. Calcium chloride
    c. Sodium bicarbonate
    d. Albuterol

Answer b is correct. IV calcium should be administered initially because the patient has symptomatic ECG changes from hyperkalemia. Stabilization of the cardiac membrane potential should be addressed immediately, but quickly followed with measures to alleviate the burden of the serum potassium concentration. This can be accomplished rapidly by stimulating the shift of potassium ions intracellularly. IV sodium bicarbonate, nebulized albuterol, and IV insulin and dextrose will all stimulate transcellular potassium shifting. The best choice for this patient is likely IV insulin and dextrose. Sodium bicarbonate is especially useful for patients with concomitant metabolic acidosis which this patient lacks, and high doses of albuterol may exacerbate this patient's hypertension and tachycardia. It is important to remember that the effect of transcellular shift is transient, so additional therapy which enhances the elimination of potassium from the body should be administered early in the course of therapy. SPS is commonly employed, but it will take several hours to see the therapeutic effect.

Answer a is incorrect. Oral SPS should be administered early in the course of therapy for this patient, but the effect will not be seen for several hours. Because the patient is symptomatic from the hyperkalemia, IV calcium should be given initially to provide cardiovascular protection.

Answer c is incorrect. Because the patient is symptomatic from the hyperkalemia, IV calcium should be given initially to provide cardiovascular protection. IV sodium bicarbonate is effective in causing intracellular shifting of potassium ions and is especially useful in patients with concomitant metabolic acidosis.

Answer d is incorrect. Because the patient is symptomatic from the hyperkalemia, IV calcium should be given initially to provide cardiovascular protection. Nebulized albuterol is effective in causing intracellular shifting of potassium ions but may exacerbate concomitant hypertension and/or tachycardia.

13. Which of the following is an expected symptom of significant (>10 meq/L) hypermagnesemia? Select all that apply.

    a. Hypotension
    b. Flushing
    c. Coma
    d. ECG changes
    e. Diarrhea

Answer a is correct. Hypotension is a common symptom of hypermagnesemia. It typically appears as the magnesium concentration exceeds 3 mEq/L.

Answer b is correct. Flushing is a common symptom of hypermagnesemia. Flushing results from cutaneous vasodilation.

Answer c is correct. Coma can result from hypermagnesemia. It does not usually appear until the serum magnesium concentration is around 10 mEq/L.

Answer d is correct. ECG changes associated with hypermagnesemia typically begin with QT interval prolongation but can progress to heart block and asystole especially in levels 10 meq/L and higher.

Answer e is incorrect. Diarrhea is not commonly associated with hypermagnesemia. Diarrhea is a common adverse effect of oral magnesium *replacement* for hypomagnesemia. Additionally, diarrhea is a common cause of hypomagnesemia.

14. Which commonly causes hypomagnesemia? Select all that apply.

    a. Amphotericin B
    b. Amiloride
    c. Lithium
    d. Ethacrynic acid
    e. Amoxicillin

Answer a is correct. Magnesium and potassium wasting are commonly associated with amphotericin B therapy and usually require replacement.

Answer d is correct. Ethacrynic acid, a loop diuretic, is associated with both hypokalemia and hypomagnesemia.

Answer b is incorrect. Hypomagnesemia is not commonly associated with amiloride treatment.

Answer c is incorrect. Hypomagnesemia is not commonly associated with lithium treatment.

Answer e is incorrect. Hypomagnesemia is not commonly associated with amoxicillin treatment.

15. Loop diuretics are commonly associated with which of the following effects? Select all that apply.

    a. Hypokalemia
    b. Hypocalcemia
    c. Hypermagnesemia
    d. Hypomagnesemia
    e. Hyperkalemia

Answer a is correct. Hypokalemia commonly occurs with loop diuretic administration due to decreased renal reabsorption. Monitoring of potassium concentration is required.

Answer b is correct. Hypocalcemia is not unexpected with loop diuretic administration and may be used to treat hypercalcemia. Monitoring of calcium is recommended.

Answer d is correct. Hypomagnesemia is not unexpected with loop diuretic administration due to decreased renal reabsorption. Monitoring of magnesium is recommended.

Answer c is incorrect. Loop diuretics cause renal wasting of potassium, calcium, and magnesium. This would result in hypomagnesemia as opposed to hypermagnesemia.

Answer e is incorrect. See answer a.

16. Which statement accurately describes hormonal regulation of calcium and phosphate homeostasis?

    a. Vitamin D reduces calcium and phosphate serum levels.
    b. Calcitonin decreases serum calcium levels.
    c. PTH decreases calcium levels and increases phosphate levels.
    d. Vitamin D causes renal wasting of potassium, calcium, and magnesium.

Answer b is correct. Calcitonin decreases calcium mobilization from the bone and increases renal excretion of calcium.

Answer a is incorrect. Vitamin D increases calcium and phosphate levels by increasing intestinal absorption and renal reabsorption.

Answer c is incorrect. PTH increases calcium levels and decreases phosphate levels.

Answer d is incorrect. Loop diuretics (not vitamin D) cause renal wasting of potassium, calcium, and magnesium.

---

17. A 55-year-old woman with a past medical history of multiple myeloma is admitted to the hospital with nausea, abdominal pain, and severe constipation. Current laboratory values are Na 140, K 4.2, Cl 103, CO_2 24, BUN 13, SCr 0.9, Glu 123, Mg 2.2, Ca 11.5, Phos 4, and albumin 1.3. She is currently receiving normal saline and furosemide 20 mg IV q4h with adequate urine output. Select the best treatment to prevent recurrence of her calcium disorder.

    a. Intranasal calcitonin
    b. IV potassium phosphate
    c. Sevelamer
    d. IV pamidronate 90 mg

Answer d is correct. The patient has hypercalcemia with a corrected calcium of 12.2. Pamidronate is a bisphosphonate. These are the drugs of choice for treatment and prevention of malignancy-induced hypercalcemia. Bisphosphonates inhibit osteoclast activity and decrease bone resorption and osteolysis.

Answer a is incorrect. Intranasal calcitonin is used to acutely manage hypercalcemia in patients who would not tolerate IV fluids and furosemide. Bisphosphonate therapy is the preferred treatment for malignancy-induced hypercalcemia.

Answer b is incorrect. This patient's potassium and phosphate are within normal limits, and she does not need to receive IV replacement of phosphate or potassium.

Answer c is incorrect. Sevelamer is a phosphate binder used to manage hyperphosphatemia. It is most commonly used in patients with CKD.

---

18. Which adverse effect may be associated with pamidronate therapy?

    a. Constipation
    b. Tachycardia
    c. Osteonecrosis of the jaw
    d. Increased blood sugar

Answer c is correct. Intravenous administration of bisphosphonate therapy has been associated with acute renal failure, and esophagitis has occurred after oral administration. Recently, numerous case reports have described a new complication: osteonecrosis of the jaw.

Answer a is incorrect. Bisphosphonate therapy is used to treat malignancy-induced hypercalcemia, which may commonly be associated with constipation.

Answer b is incorrect. Bisphosphonate therapy is not commonly associated with tachycardia.

Answer d is incorrect. Pamidronate is not expected to affect glucose levels.

19. A patient with hyperparathyroidism is admitted to the medical intensive care unit with pneumonia and respiratory distress requiring mechanical ventilation. Current laboratory values are Na 144, K 3.4, Cl 105, CO_2 24, BUN 16, SCr 0.9, Glu 130, Mg 1.9, Ca 9, Phos 0.8, and albumin 4. Select the best medication to manage this patient's phosphate disorder.

    a. IV sodium phosphate
    b. IV potassium phosphate
    c. IV calcium chloride
    d. PO Neutra-Phos

Answer b is correct. The patient has significant hypophosphatemia with a phosphate level less than 1. This patient's phosphate is severely low and may by contributing to the respiratory distress, which warrants intravenous phosphate administration. Additionally, the patient is hypokalemic; therefore, the patient should receive intravenous potassium phosphate. The dose should be infused over 4 to 6 hours to prevent precipitate formation.

Answer a is incorrect. Patient has a normal sodium level and should not receive sodium phosphate.

Answer c is incorrect. This patient's calcium is within normal limits and the patient is not displaying signs and symptoms of hypocalcemia.

Answer d is incorrect. This patient has severe hypophosphatemia with respiratory distress; therefore, the patient should receive intravenous phosphate replacement.

---

20. A 70-year-old man on hemodialysis with Stage 5 CKD presents to the nephrology clinic for routine follow-up. Past medical history includes end-stage renal disease (ESRD), hypertension, and type II diabetes. Current medications include amlodipine 10 mg daily, lisinopril 20 mg daily, glipizide 10 mg daily, and aspirin 325 mg daily. Current laboratory values are BUN 60, SCr 4.5, Ca 9, Phos 8, and albumin 2. Which is the best initial management of this patient's phosphate disorder?

    a. Calcium acetate
    b. Sevelamer
    c. Discontinuation of lisinopril
    d. Calcium carbonate

Answer b is correct. The patient has hyperphosphatemia. Sevelamer (Renagel) is the best initial management for this patient because his corrected calcium is 10.6 and his calcium-phosphate product is 84.8 mg/dL. This would increase his risk of soft tissue calcifications. Sevelamer is a noncalcium-, nonaluminum-containing phosphate binder that reduces phosphate absorption in the GI tract and does not further increase calcium levels.

Answers a and d are incorrect. This patient's corrected calcium is 10.6 (corrected calcium = measured calcium + [0.8 (4 - measured albumin)]), and his calcium-phosphate product is 84.8 mg/dL. This would increase his risk of soft tissue calcifications; therefore, he should receive a noncalcium-containing phosphate binder. It will minimize phosphate absorption in the GI tract and not further increase calcium levels.

Answer c is incorrect.   Lisinopril is an ACE-I that is associated with hyperkalemia, not calcium or phosphate disorders.

---

21. Which of the following represents an appropriate counseling point for patients prescribed a phosphate binder?

    a. Take with meals to reduce phosphate absorption
    b. Take with meals to increase phosphate absorption
    c. Take with meals to reduce GI side effects
    d. Take between meals to reduce food–drug interactions

Answer a is correct.   Phosphate binders are to be given with meals to minimize the absorption of dietary phosphate.

Answers b, c, and d are incorrect.   Phosphate binders are taken with meals to reduce not increase phosphate absorption.

---

22. Which electrolyte abnormalities commonly occur in patients with CKD? Select all that apply.

    a. Hyperkalemia
    b. Hyperphosphatemia
    c. Hypomagnesemia
    d. Hypercalcemia
    e. Hypernatremia

Answer a is correct.   CKD is associated with hyperkalemia.

Answer b is correct.   CKD is commonly associated with hyperphosphatemia.

Answer c is incorrect.   CKD is not associated commonly with hypomagnesemia but more common hypermagnesemia.

Answer d is incorrect.   CKD is associated more often with hypocalcemia not hypercalcemia due to decreased activation of vitamin D thus limiting GI absorption.

Answer e is incorrect.   Hypernatremia is not a common finding with CKD patients who are often volume overloaded, resulting in hyponatremia more commonly.

---

23. Which drug/disease state is matched with the correct drug-induced electrolyte disorder?

    a. Lisinopril and hyperkalemia
    b. Fluoxetine and hypernatremia
    c. Alcoholism and hypermagnesemia
    d. Diabetes insipidus and hyponatremia

Answer a is correct.   Lisinopril is an ACE-I and most commonly associated with the development of hyperkalemia.

Answer b is incorrect.   Fluoxetine is an SSRI; SSRIs are associated with the development of a euvolemic hypotonic hyponatremia not hypernatremia.

Answer c is incorrect.   Chronic alcoholism is commonly associated with low magnesium levels due to poor dietary intake.

Answer d is incorrect.   Diabetes insipidus causes an increase in sodium and therefore hypernatremia.

---

24. Place the following electrolytes in order based upon their normal serum concentration. Start with the lowest concentration.

Unordered Response	Ordered Response
Sodium	Magnesium
Potassium	Potassium
Magnesium	Sodium

---

25. Place the following NaCl solution in order based upon the chloride concentration. Start with the lowest.

Unordered Response	Ordered Response
0.9% NaCl	0.45% NaCl
3% NaCl	0.9% NaCl
0.45% NaCl	3% NaCl

---

26. Place the following calcium products in order based upon their Meq calcium concentration. Start with the lowest.

Unordered Response	Ordered Response
Acetate 250 mg	Gluconate 90 mg
Gluconate 90 mg	Acetate 250 mg
Carbonate 400 mg	Carbonate 400 mg

CHAPTER 40 | **Liver Cirrhosis and Complications**

DT is a 42-year-old man with a 20-year history of alcohol abuse who presents with altered mental status, anorexia, mild weight loss over the past 3 months, recent abdominal swelling, and general malaise. Current medications include rosuvastatin, niacin, acetaminophen, and diazepam. Upon examination he was found to have palmar erythema and splenomegaly and his labs were significant for mildly elevated AST, ALT, bilirubin, and blood glucose. He is diagnosed with hepatic cirrhosis.

1. Which of the following is the most likely cause of DT's cirrhosis?

    a. Rosuvastatin
    b. Ethanol
    c. Acetaminophen
    d. Niacin

Answer b is correct.   Alcoholism and hepatitis C are the most common causes of cirrhosis in the western world.

Answer a is incorrect.   Statins can cause liver damage, but it would be more likely to be associated with significant AST and ALT elevations and less likely to be the cause of this patient's cirrhosis, given the patient's history of alcohol abuse.

Answer c is incorrect.   Acetaminophen can also cause acute hepatotoxicity but the pattern of injury is similar to acute hepatitis, not cirrhosis.

Answer d is incorrect.   Nicotinic acid (Niacin) can also cause acute hepatotoxicity but the pattern of injury is similar to acute hepatitis, not cirrhosis.

2. An arterial ammonia level is drawn for DT with the following results:125 mcg/dL (Normal: 15-60 mcg/dL)

   This laboratory abnormality is most closely associated with which of the symptoms reported by DT?

   a. Abdominal swelling
   b. Altered mental status
   c. Jaundice
   d. Palmar erythema

Answer b is correct.   Elevated venous and arterial ammonia levels are associated with hepatic encephalopathy which can cause altered mental status.

Answer a is incorrect.   Significant abdominal swelling is associated with ascites, a complication of cirrhosis.

Answer c is incorrect.   Jaundice is associated with liver damage and cirrhosis; however, it is not associated with an increased ammonia level.

Answer d is incorrect.   Palmar erythema is a symptom of cirrhosis; however, it is not associated with an increased ammonia level.

3. A consultation with DT should include recommendations to prevent the exacerbation or progression of his cirrhosis and complications. Select the counseling points that should be discussed by the pharmacist. Select **ALL** that apply.

   a. Limit alcohol intake
   b. Limit protein intake
   c. Limit total caloric intake
   d. Limit sodium intake
   e. Limit fluid intake

Answer a is correct.   Alcoholism is a common cause of cirrhosis. Continued abuse of alcohol can worsen cirrhosis and cirrhosis complications. Additionally, alcohol will exacerbate ascites (a complication DT currently has abdominal swelling).

Answer b is correct.   Reduction in protein reduces the level of ammonia in the blood. Increased blood ammonia levels can cause hepatic encephalopathy, a cirrhosis complication.

Answer d is correct.   Sodium restriction is a key management principle for ascites.

Answer c is incorrect.   Muscle wasting, anorexia, and weight loss are seen in cirrhosis. Proper nutrition including appropriate caloric intake is recommended. There is no indication for limiting total caloric intake in DT as described in the case.

Answer e is incorrect.   Restriction of fluid intake is not a principle measure in the management of cirrhosis or cirrhosis complications.

4. Your patient is a 52-year-old woman who presents with the following liver function test results:

   AST: 200 U/L (Normal: 8-20 U/L)

   ALT: 520 U/L (Normal: 5-40 U/L)

   Your patient's liver function test results are most likely associated with which of the following?

   a. Acute acetaminophen toxicity
   b. Cirrhosis
   c. Chronic hepatitis C infection
   d. Nonalcoholic fatty liver disease

Answer a is correct.   Patients with marked increase in AST and ALT typically have acute liver injury, such as that which would occur after acute ingestion of toxic amounts of acetaminophen.

Answers b, c, and d are incorrect.   Cirrhosis, chronic hepatitis C infection, and nonalcoholic fatty liver disease may cause elevations in AST and ALT, but typically not to the same degree as acute insults. Additionally, AST and ALT may test within the normal range in patients with cirrhosis or another chronic liver disease.

Utilize the following case to answer the next four questions.

KD is a 65-year-old man who has been diagnosed with cirrhosis for the past 2 years. KD presents with mild ascites, esophageal and gastric varices with no bleeding, and no apparent encephalopathy. Pertinent laboratory values are: total bilirubin 2.5 mg/dL (normal: 0.3-1.2 mg/dL), albumin 2.9 g/dL (normal: 3.2-4.6 g/dL), prothrombin time 19.5 seconds (normal:12.5-15.2 seconds).

5. KD is currently having difficulty with overactive bladder and his physician is considering starting him on darifenacin. Based on the patient's Child-Pugh score and the following information from darifenacin's dosing information, what dose will you recommend for KD.

No Liver Disease	Mild Hepatic Insufficiency	Moderate Hepatic Insufficiency	Severe Hepatic Insufficiency
15 mg daily	15 mg daily	7.5 mg daily	No clinical experience

   a. KD has grade A cirrhosis and should be started on 15 mg daily.
   b. KD has grade B cirrhosis and should be started on 7.5 mg daily.

c. KD has grade C cirrhosis and should be started on 7.5 mg daily.

d. KD has grade A cirrhosis and should not be given darifenacin.

KD's Child-Pugh score is calculated as follows:

Bilirubin 2.5 (0.3-1.2 mg/dL) = 2 points

Albumin 2.9 (3.2-4.6 g/dL) = 2 points

Mild ascites = 2 points

No encephalopathy = 1 point

Prothrombin time 19.5 (12.5-15.2 seconds) = 2 points

Child-Pugh score = 9 points = Grade B moderate liver dysfunction

---

Answer c is correct. KD has grade B liver disease; therefore should receive 7.5 mg daily as his initial dose.

Answer a is incorrect. KD has grade B liver disease.

Answer b is incorrect. KD has grade B liver disease.

Answer d is incorrect. KD has grade B liver disease.

---

6. Which of the following drugs would be expected to have a decreased therapeutic effect in KD due to pharmacodynamic changes associated with chronic liver disease?

a. Hydromorphone
b. Propranolol
c. Alprazolam
d. Zolpidem

Answer b is correct. Certain diuretics (furosemide, triamterene, torsemide, and bumetanide) as well as non-selective β-blockers such as propranolol have been found to exert a decreased therapeutic effect due to pharmacodynamic changes that occur in cirrhosis.

Answer a is incorrect. Hydromorphone (an opioid analgesic) would be expected to have an increased therapeutic effect in cirrhosis.

Answer c is incorrect. Anxiolytics such as the benzodiazepine alprazolam would be expected to exert an increased effect in a patient with cirrhosis (and also increases the patient's risk of developing hepatic encephalopathy; in fact, benzodiazepines should be avoided in patients at risk for hepatic encephalopathy).

Answer d is incorrect. Zolpidem, a sedative, would be more likely to have an increased effect in a patient with cirrhosis rather than a decreased effect.

---

7. Which of the following statements is true for KD regarding volume of distribution and half-life of drugs highly protein bound to albumin in the blood?

a. Albumin is increased in chronic liver disease leading to increased protein binding, increased volume of distribution, and potentially decreased half-life.

b. Albumin is decreased in chronic liver disease leading to decreased protein binding, increased volume of distribution, and potentially increased half-life.

c. Albumin is decreased in chronic liver disease leading to decreased protein binding, decreased volume of distribution, and potentially decreased half-life.

d. No changes in albumin concentrations, volume of distribution, or half-life normally occur in chronic liver disease.

Answer b is correct. Albumin is decreased in chronic liver disease which leads to decreased binding of drugs bound to albumin in the blood. This increases those drugs' volumes of distribution and potentially increases their half-live.

Answer a is incorrect. Albumin is not increased in liver disease. It is potentially decreased in chronic liver disease.

Answer c is incorrect. Albumin concentrations are usually decreased in severe chronic liver disease.

Answer d is incorrect. Albumin is decreased in chronic liver disease which leads to decreased binding of drugs bound to albumin in the blood. This increases those drugs' volumes of distribution and potentially increases their half-live.

---

8. Which of the following is true about the oral bioavailability of high hepatic ratio drugs in KD if portal-systemic shunting has occurred?

a. Oral bioavailability will be unchanged and no initial dosage adjustment should be considered.

b. Oral bioavailability will be decreased and initial dosage should be increased.

c. Oral bioavailability will be increased but no dosage adjustment need be considered.

d. Oral bioavailability will be increased and initial dosage should be decreased.

Answer d is correct. Oral bioavailability of a high hepatic ratio drug would be expected to be increased if portal-systemic shunting is present. Hepatic elimination of high hepatic extraction ratio drugs is dependent upon blood flow. Blood flow in portal systemic shunting is altered so that blood flows directly from the portal vein into systemic circulation bypassing the liver. If the drug is normally cleared to a large extent by first-pass effect, this could change drastically the serum concentration that would be achieved after the initial dose.

Answer a is incorrect. In this situation, oral bioavailability would be expected to be increased.

Answer b is incorrect. Oral bioavailability would be expected to be increased, not decreased.

Answer c is incorrect. Due to the possibility for significantly higher serum concentrations following initial dosing, consideration should be given to lowering the initial dose given to the patient.

9. Hepatic drug elimination is dependent upon which of the following?

   a. Blood flow, drug binding in blood, and hepatic extraction ratio
   b. Blood flow, drug binding in blood, and bioavailability
   c. Drug binding in blood, bioavailability, and hepatic extraction ratio
   d. Blood flow, drug binding in blood, hepatic intrinsic clearance

___

Answer d is correct. Hepatic drug elimination is dependent upon blood flow, protein binding of the drug in the blood, and hepatic intrinsic clearance.

Answer a is incorrect. Hepatic drug elimination is dependent upon blood flow, protein binding of the drug in the blood, and hepatic intrinsic clearance. Hepatic extraction ratio is not one of the primary determinants of hepatic drug elimination.

Answer b is incorrect. Hepatic drug elimination is dependent upon blood flow, protein binding of the drug in the blood, and hepatic intrinsic clearance. Bioavailability is not one of the primary determinants of hepatic drug elimination.

Answer c is incorrect. Hepatic drug elimination is dependent upon protein binding of the drug in the blood but is not dependent upon bioavailability or hepatic extraction ratio.

___

10. Patients who have cirrhosis and edema may have an increased volume of distribution for hydrophilic drugs. In this situation, what adjustments should be made to the loading doses if a rapid drug effect is required?

    a. Loading doses should be eliminated in these patients
    b. Loading doses should be increased
    c. Loading doses should be decreased
    d. Hydrophilic drugs are contraindicated in patients with cirrhosis

___

Answer b is correct. Loading doses of hydrophilic drugs may need to be increased in patients with cirrhosis and edema.

Answer a is incorrect. Loading doses of hydrophilic drugs may need to be increased in patients with cirrhosis and edema.

Answer c is incorrect. Loading doses of hydrophilic drugs may need to be increased in patients with cirrhosis and edema.

Answer d is incorrect. Hydrophilic drugs are not contraindicated but loading doses may need to be increased in patients with cirrhosis and edema.

___

11. Dosage adjustment of low hepatic extraction ratio/low plasma protein bound drugs should be aimed at maintaining which of the following?

    a. Normal unbound plasma concentrations
    b. Normal bound plasma concentrations
    c. Normal total (bound plus unbound) plasma concentrations
    d. No dosage adjustments need be considered

___

Answer c is correct. Dosage adjustment for a low hepatic extraction ratio/low plasma protein bound drug should be aimed at maintaining normal total plasma concentrations. Low hepatic extraction ratio drugs are affected most by changes in protein binding and hepatic intrinsic clearance. Since this drug is not highly protein bound, a change in the amount of drug that is protein bound is unlikely to significantly change the amount of drug free to act in the body in this situation. Therefore, bound versus unbound concentration is less important. Total plasma concentration should be the target of dosage adjustments in this case.

Answer a is incorrect. Dosage adjustment for a low hepatic extraction ratio/low plasma protein bound drug should be aimed at maintaining normal total plasma concentrations.

Answer b is incorrect. Dosage adjustment for a low hepatic extraction ratio/low plasma protein bound drug should be aimed at maintaining normal total plasma concentrations.

Answer d is incorrect. Dosage adjustment for a low hepatic extraction ratio/low plasma protein bound drug should be aimed at maintaining normal total plasma concentrations.

___

12. Which of the following statements is true?

    a. In liver disease, phase II conjugation metabolism is affected to a greater extent than phase I oxidative reactions.
    b. In liver disease, phase I oxidative metabolism is affected to a greater extent than phase II conjugation reactions.
    c. Chronic liver disease is associated with uniform reductions in metabolism via the different cytochrome P450 pathways.
    d. Serum creatinine is an accurate reflection of renal function in chronic liver disease.

___

Answer b is correct. Phase I oxidative reactions (which typically involve the cytochrome P450 enzymatic pathways) are affected to a greater extent in cirrhosis than phase II reactions such as glucuronidation. This is because the cytochrome P450 enzymes are dependent upon oxygen to act. In cirrhosis, there is a relative lack of oxygen due to shunting, sinusoidal capillarization, and reduced liver perfusion. In severe cirrhosis, glucuronidation may be affected.

Answer a is incorrect. Phase I oxidative reactions are affected to a greater extent in cirrhosis than phase II conjugation reactions.

Answer c is incorrect. Chronic liver disease is associated with non-uniform reductions in metabolism via the cytochrome P450 system. For example, in early-stage liver disease, drug metabolism through the cytochrome P450 2C19 enzyme can be expected to be reduced while the cytochrome P450 1A2, 2D6, and 2E1 enzyme pathways retain normal or near normal activity. As liver disease progresses, the activity levels of the different cytochrome P450 enzyme pathways change.

Answer d is incorrect.   Serum creatinine is not considered a reliable predictor of renal function in chronic liver disease. This is because of the reduced muscle mass and impaired metabolism of creatine to creatinine that accompany severe liver disease.

---

13. Your patient has just been diagnosed with cirrhosis and undergoes an endoscopy. Several large esophageal varices are noted and his hepatologist decides that he should be started on drug therapy to prevent variceal bleeding. Which of the following describes appropriate therapy for primary prevention of variceal bleeding in this patient?

    a. No primary prevention therapy needed; only patients who have experienced an episode of variceal bleeding in the past should receive prophylaxis therapy.
    b. Norfloxacin 400 mg po bid.
    c. Sulcralfate 1 g po four times daily.
    d. Propranolol 20 mg po bid.

Answer d is correct.   Propranolol 20 mg po bid is an appropriate drug and dosing schedule for primary prevention of variceal bleeding in portal hypertension. Non-selective β-blockers reduce portal pressure by diminishing portal venous inflow via two mechanisms: a decrease in cardiac output through β_1 receptor antagonism and a decrease in splanchnic blood flow through β_2 receptor antagonism. Propranolol should be titrated to the maximum tolerated dose. Possible side effects of non-selective β-blocker therapy include fatigue, shortness of breath, inability to recognize hypoglycemia in patients with diabetes, depression, and erectile dysfunction.

Answer a is incorrect.   Patients found to have varices should receive primary prophylaxis therapy in an effort to prevent variceal hemorrhage.

Answer b is incorrect.   Norfloxacin is an antibiotic that is indicated in the treatment of variceal bleeding. Prophylactic antibiotic therapy is indicated for variceal bleeding.

Answer c is incorrect.   Sucralfate, an aluminum complex, has no indication for the primary prophylaxis of variceal bleeding in portal hypertension, but is used to manage duodenal ulcer.

---

14. The physician decides to treat your patient's ascites with oral diuretic therapy and starts him on 100 mg spironolactone and 40 mg furosemide every day. After 5 days the patient is re-evaluated and the physician decides to increase the spironolactone to 150 mg/d and a further adjustment to 200 mg/d occurs after an additional 3 days. What is the appropriate dose of oral furosemide that should be given with this dose of spironolactone?

    a. Furosemide 100 mg/d
    b. Furosemide 40 mg/d
    c. Furosemide 60 mg/d
    d. Furosemide 80 mg/d

Answer d is correct.   The starting ratio for spironolactone and furosemide combination therapy is 100:40. Also with alcohol avoidance and sodium restriction, diuretic therapy is one of the mainstays of ascites management. This ratio helps to maximize fluid loss while maintaining electrolyte (particularly serum potassium) balance within normal range. Spironolactone may be increased to 400 mg po daily and furosemide may be increased to 160 mg po daily in 3 to 5 day increments as needed and as tolerated with proper electrolyte monitoring. When the dose of Spironolactone is increased to 150, this represents a 50% increase in dosage (100 mg × 1.5 = 150 mg). The dose of furosemide must also be increased by 50% in order to maintain the ratio of 100:40. The correct dose of furosemide will be 60 mg (40 mg × 1.5 = 60 mg) at 5 days. After an additional 3 days the dosage of spironolactone is increased by another 50 mg to a total of 100% of the initial dose. The correct dose of furosemide is now 80 mg (40 mg × 2 = 80 mg)

Answers a, b, and c are incorrect.   When the dose of spironolactone is increased to 200, this represents a 100% increase in dosage (100 mg × 2 = 200 mg). The dose of furosemide must also be increased by 100% in order to maintain the ratio of 100:40. The correct dose of furosemide will be 80 mg (40 mg × 2 = 80 mg).

---

15. A 65-year-old man with a 20-year history of heavy alcohol use, cirrhosis, and portal hypertension presents for emergent care after experiencing hematemesis and is diagnosed with acute esophageal variceal bleeding. Which of the following is appropriate therapy for this patient at this time?

    a. Nadolol 40 mg po daily plus norfloxacin 400 mg po bid
    b. Octreotide 50 mcg IV bolus, then 50 mcg/h infusion plus norfloxacin 400 mg po bid
    c. Octreotide 50 mcg IV bolus, then 50 mcg/h infusion plus pantoprazole 40 mg IV daily
    d. Octreotide 50 mcg IV bolus then 50 mcg/h infusion plus propranolol 20 mg po bid

---

Answer b is correct.   Octreotide decreases splanchnic arterial blood flow as well as portal inflow and is therefore useful in the management of acute variceal hemorrhage. Octreotide has a short half-life and therefore must be given as IV infusion. Short-term antibiotic therapy is recommended in a patient with acute variceal hemorrhage because patients with variceal hemorrhage are at risk of infection and sepsis due to aspiration and translocation of the gastrointestinal bacterial flora. Norfloxacin po 400 mg bid for 7 days is appropriate.

Answer a is incorrect.   Non selective β-blockers are indicated for the prophylaxis of variceal bleeding, not the treatment for active bleeding.

Answer c is incorrect.   Octreotide is appropriate, but pantoprazole is not (IV proton pump inhibitor therapy may be appropriate for a gastric bleed related to peptic ulcer disease, it is not appropriate for variceal bleeding).

Answer d is incorrect. Antibiotic prophylaxis should be provided. Antibiotic prophylaxis in cases of acute variceal hemorrhage has been found to decrease re-bleeding rates and increase rates of short-term survival. Octreotide is the vaso-active drug that is indicated for active variceal bleeding.

---

16. Octreotide is ordered to be infused at a rate of 50 mcg/h and the pharmacy prepares 1 mg of Octreotide in 1 L of normal saline. What amount of the preparation will need to be infused per hour in order to attain the prescribed rate?

    a. 10 mL/h
    b. 25 mL/h
    c. 50 mL/h
    d. 250 mL/h

Answer c is correct. 1 mg = 1000 mcg; 1000 mcg in 1 L of solution is equivalent to 1 mcg/mL (1000 mcg /1000 mL = 1 mcg/mL). In order to achieve a rate of 50 mcg/h you multiply the concentration of 1 mcg/mL × 50 = 50 mcg/50 mL; therefore, you will need to infuse 50 mL per hour.

Answers a, b, and d are incorrect.

Use the following questions to answer the next three questions.

AB is a 65-year-old woman with a history of cirrhosis who was just admitted with severe ascites and undergoes paracentesis. AB's poly-morphonuclear count is found to be 300 cells/mm³ and she is diag-nosed with spontaneous bacterial peritonitis.

17. Which of the following antibiotics is available in IV formula-tion and is appropriate empiric therapy for AB's spontaneous bacterial peritonitis?

    a. Vancomycin
    b. Cephalexin
    c. Tigecycline
    d. Cefotaxime

Answer d is correct. The ideal antibiotic choice in this case would be cefotaxime 2 g IV every 8 hours. Ofloxacin po 400 mg twice daily may be substituted for cefotaxime in patients *without* prior exposure to quinolones, vomiting, shock, grade II or higher encephalopathy, or serum creatinine greater than 3 mg/dL.

Answer a is incorrect. Vancomycin is not the ideal antibi-otic choice in this case as it would not adequately cover two of the likely pathogens often involved in spontaneous bacte-rial peritonitis, *Escherichia coli* and *Klebsiella pneumoniae* Vancomycin is dosed via IV administration, however.

Answer b is incorrect. Cephalexin is not the ideal antibiotic choice in this case as it is a first-generation cepha-losporin. Also, cephalexin is not available in IV formulation. A third-generation cephalosporin is preferable for empiric treatment of spontaneous bacterial peritonitis.

Answer c is incorrect. Tigecycline may be a viable option in this case as it would likely cover all three of the

likely pathogens in spontaneous bacterial peritonitis, *E. coli, K. pneumoniae,* and *Streptococcus pneumoniae.* However, the most recent guideline statement supported by the American Association for the Study of Liver Diseases recommends the third-generation cephalosporin, cefotaxime, as empiric therapy for cases of likely spontaneous bacterial peritonitis. Tigecycline is administered via the IV route, however.

---

18. Which of the following resources would be appropriate to use to determine compatibility for an IV solution for AB's antibiotic? Select **ALL** that apply.

    a. King Guide
    b. Red Book
    c. Orange Book
    d. Trissel's
    e. Sanford Guide

Answer a is correct. The King Guide contains compatibility information for drugs related to concomitant Y-site administration, administration in a single syringe, and admixture administration. Information about compatible IV solution options is also available.

Answer d is correct. Trissel's contains compatibility information for drugs related to concomitant Y-site admin-istration, administration in a single syringe, and admixture administration. Information about compatible IV solution options is also available.

Answer b is incorrect. Red Book contains information primarily about drug pricing.

Answer c is incorrect. Orange Book contains information about drug product equivalency.

Answer e is incorrect. Sanford Guide contains informa-tion about antimicrobial therapy.

---

19. The treatment for AB is effective and she recovers from her spontaneous bacterial peritonitis but develops symptoms of hepatic encephalopathy. Place the following drug options for hepatic encephalopathy in proper order from first line, to second line, to third line.

    a. Neomycin, lactulose, rifaximin
    b. Lactulose, rifaximin, neomycin
    c. Rifaximin, lactulose, neomycin
    d. Lactulose, neomycin, rifaximin

Answer b is correct. Lactulose is considered first-line therapy for hepatic encephalopathy. Rifaximin is considered second line for patients who cannot tolerate lactulose or may be used in conjunction with lactulose for patients who have an inadequate response to lactulose alone. Neomycin is considered third line.

Answer a is incorrect. Neomycin would be considered no earlier than third line.

Answer c is incorrect. Lactulose remains the first-line drug.

Answer d is incorrect.   Neomycin would be considered no earlier than third line.

---

20. Your patient presents with a prescription for Flagyl® which his physician has chosen in the management of his hepatic encephalopathy. The script indicates substitution permitted. Which of the following generic agents would be an appropriate substitution for Flagyl®?

    a. Neomycin
    b. Rifaximin
    c. Metronidazole
    d. Cefotaxime

Answer c is correct.   Flagyl® is the brand name for metronidazole.

Answer a is incorrect.   Neo-Fradin® is the brand name for neomycin.

Answer b is incorrect.   Xifaxan® is the brand name for rifaximin.

Answer d is incorrect.   Claforan® is the brand name for cefotaxime.

---

21. PA is a 42-year-old woman who is at risk for developing cirrhosis. Identify the correct sequence of events that can result in the development of cirrhosis.

    a. Shunting of hepatic blood supply
    b. Distortion of hepatic vasculature
    c. Hepatic cell injury
    d. Replacement of injured tissue by scar tissue

Answers c, d, b, and a are the correct sequence.   The sequence of events that lead to the development of cirrhosis are hepatic cell injury followed by the replacement of injured tissue by scar tissue. This scar tissue results in a distortion of hepatic tissue which leads to a shunting of the hepatic blood supply.

---

22. Which of the following decreases splanchnic blood flow through mechanisms other than β-adrenergic antagonism?

    a. Inderal®
    b. Corgard®
    c. Sandostatin®
    d. Xifaxan®

Answer c is correct.   Sandostatin®, octreotide, is not a β-adrenergic antagonist, rather mimics the effects of somatostatin and causes, among other effects, a decrease in splanchnic blood flow.

Answer a is incorrect.   Inderal®, propranolol, is a β-adrenergic antagonist.

Answer b is incorrect.   Corgard®, nadolol, is a β-adrenergic antagonist.

Answer d is incorrect.   Xifaxan®, rifaximin, is not a β-adrenergic antagonist, and has no effect on splanchnic blood flow.

---

23. Which of the following medications is useful in the prevention of esophageal variceal bleeding? Select **ALL** that apply.

    a. Sandostatin®
    b. Pravastatin
    c. Corgard®
    d. Calan®
    e. Carvedilol

Answer c is correct.   Corgard® is the brand name for nadolol, a non-selective β-adrenergic antagonist, which decreases portal venous inflow by decreasing cardiac output (β1) and decreasing splanchnic blood flow (β2).

Answer e is correct.   Carvedilol, a non-selective β-adrenergic antagonist/α-1 antagonist, which decreased portal venous inflow by decreasing cardiac output (β1) and decreasing splanchnic blood flow (β2).

Answer a is incorrect.   Sandostatin® is the brand name for octreotide which decreases splanchnic blood flow and is indicated in the treatment, not prevention, of esophageal varices.

Answer b is incorrect.   Pravastatin is an inhibitor of HMG CoA Reductase and has no effect on esophageal varices.

Answer d is incorrect.   Calan® is the brand name for verapamil, a calcium channel blocker. Although calcium channel blockers are useful to reduce blood pressure, they are not utilized in the prophylaxis or treatment of esophageal varices.

---

24. KR is a 45-year-old man who has been diagnosed with chronic hepatitis C. Which of the following would indicate that KR is developing or has developed cirrhosis? Select **ALL** that apply.

    a. Gynecomastia
    b. Hypogonadism
    c. Aplastic anemia
    d. Type 2 diabetes
    e. Thrombocytopenia

Answer a is correct.   Gynecomastia is a symptom that is associated with cirrhosis.

Answer b is correct.   Hypogonadism is a symptom that is associated with cirrhosis.

Answer d is correct.   Type 2 diabetes is a symptom that is associated with cirrhosis.

Answer e is correct.   Thrombocytopenia is a symptom that is associated with cirrhosis.

Answer c is incorrect.   Aplastic anemia is not a symptom that is associated with cirrhosis.

Answer d is incorrect. Mesalamine is not available in the United States in an injectable formulation.

CHAPTER 41 | Inflammatory Bowel Disease

1. A 67-year-old man, RJ, presents with complaints of 2 months of 2 to 3 loose bloody stools per day without accompanying fever or weight loss. His gastroenterologist performs a colonoscopy to determine the extent and severity of his suspected IBD. RJ is found to have UC, which is confined to the rectum. Select all of the characteristics that are features of UC but not of CD.

    a. Disease distribution limited to the colon
    b. Inflammation interspersed with healthy tissue
    c. Inflammation affecting only the mucosal layer
    d. Inflammation penetrating below the mucosal layer

Answer a is correct. Ulcerative colitis (UC) is confined to the colon, whereas Crohn disease (CD) may affect any area within the gastrointestinal (GI) tract.

Answer b is incorrect. UC is associated with continuous lesions whereas CD in characterized by areas of inflammation or lesions interspersed with healthy tissue, or skip lesions.

Answer c is correct. Inflammation affecting only the mucosal layer of the GI tract is indicative of UC.

Answer d is incorrect. Crohn disease is associated with much deeper intestinal inflammation compared to UC. The inflammation often penetrates into the submucosal and muscular layers of the intestinal tract.

2. Which drug formulation of mesalamine is most effective as initial therapy for RJ's UC confined to the rectum?

    a. Suppository
    b. Enema
    c. Tablet
    d. Intravenous injection

Answer a is correct. Ulcerative proctitis is a subset of UC in which inflammation is localized to the rectum. Mesalamine is a first-line agent for mild to moderate proctitis. The suppository formulation delivers mesalamine directly to the site of action and treats up to 20 cm of the rectal area, thus it is the preferred formulation for treatment of proctitis.

Answer b is incorrect. While the enema form of mesalamine would treat proctitis, it delivers the drug up to the splenic flexure. This would result in unnecessary coverage of this area of the GI tract and would be more appropriate for a patient with distal or left-sided disease.

Answer c is incorrect. While the tablet form of mesalamine would treat proctitis, it delivers the drug either throughout the small and large intestine or just throughout the colon, depending on the formulation. This would result in unnecessary coverage of this area of the GI tract and would be more appropriate for a patient with extensive disease.

3. Three years later, RJ's UC has advanced to moderately severe disease. After a course of steroids, his gastroenterologist wants to start him on azathioprine. Which enzyme should be tested to determine RJ's ability to metabolize azathioprine?

    a. Rasburicase
    b. Dihydrofolate reductase
    c. Thiopurine methyltransferase
    d. Hyaluronidase

Answer c is correct. Thiopurine methyltransferase is an enzyme that is partially responsible for the metabolism of azathioprine. Genetic polymorphisms of this enzyme may result in reduced enzyme activity. This may predispose patients to higher blood levels of azathioprine and increase the potential for toxicity. Patients should have their thiopurine methyltransferase activity level measured prior to initiating therapy with azathioprine.

Answer a is incorrect. Rasburicase is not an enzyme, but rather a drug used in the treatment of tumor lysis syndrome.

Answer b is incorrect. Dihydrofolate reductase is an enzyme that is involved in the metabolism of methotrexate and does not affect azathioprine.

Answer d is incorrect. Hyaluronidase is a substance, which increases the permeability of connective tissue. It is often used in surgical procedures to increase drug absorption.

4. A 33-year-old African American woman is newly diagnosed with moderate extensive UC. She reports a drug allergy to sulfonamide-containing medications, which manifests as a rash. Which product would be most appropriate as initial therapy for this patient?

    a. Canasa
    b. Colazal
    c. Entocort
    d. Azulfidine

Answer b is correct. Colazal is balsalazide, which contains mesalamine linked to an inert carrier molecule. This formulation delivers mesalamine to the colon. Since this patient has extensive disease, this would be a favorable formulation. Balsalazide also lacks a sulfa moiety and can be used safely in patients with an allergy to sulfonamide-containing drugs.

Answer a is incorrect. Mesalamine is an appropriate agent for this patient. However, Canasa is the suppository formulation of mesalamine. This patient has extensive disease, which indicates that the majority of the colon is affected. The suppository formulation would deliver mesalamine only to the rectal area and not to the colon where it is needed.

Answer c is incorrect. Entocort is budesonide, which is a corticosteroid that is used for patients with CD who have disease located in the ileum and ascending colon.

Answer d is incorrect. Azulfidine is sulfasalazine. This would be an appropriate first-line agent for extensive UC; however, the patient has a sulfa allergy, which precludes the use of sulfasalazine.

---

5. Which of the following products is available only as an intravenous solution for injection?

    a. Flagyl
    b. Purinethol
    c. Colazal
    d. Remicade

Answer d is correct. Infliximab is available only as an injection for intravenous use.

Answer a is incorrect. Metronidazole is available as both oral tablets and as an injection.

Answer b is incorrect. Mercaptopurine is available only as a tablet.

Answer c is incorrect. Balsalazide is available only as a tablet.

---

6. A 56-year-old man, QC, has a history of CD and is maintained in remission with daily oral mesalamine 800 mg daily and oral prednisone 30 mg daily. He is interested in trying weekly subcutaneous injections of methotrexate with a goal of discontinuing his prednisone therapy. Which monitoring parameters should be assessed prior to intiating and periodically during methotrexate therapy? (Please choose all that apply)

    a. Liver transaminases
    b. Chest radiography
    c. Complete blood count
    d. Serum potassium

Answer a is correct. Methotrexate is associated with hepatotoxicity. Liver function tests, specifically liver transaminases, should be monitored in patients receiving methotrexate.

Answer b is correct. Methotrexate is associated with the development of pneumonitis. Chest radiography and pulmonary function tests should be assessed at baseline and periodically during methotrexate therapy.

Answer c is correct. Methotrexate is a folate antagonist that can cause bone marrow suppression. A complete blood count should be routinely monitored in patients receiving methotrexate.

Answer d is incorrect. Methotrexate is not commonly associated with alterations in serum potassium concentrations except in the instance of severe nephrotoxicity caused by methotrexate.

7. Eight months later, JJ presents to the gastroenterologist's office again. He complains that his symptoms are not controlled on methotrexate therapy. His physician is considering initiating JJ on infliximab. Which of the following conditions is considered a contraindication to receiving a TNF-α antagonist?

    a. Asthma
    b. Migraine headache
    c. Previous myocardial infarction
    d. Sepsis

Answer d is correct. Since TNF-α antagonists are associated with development of severe infections, patients should not have a preexisting severe infection when initiating therapy. Sepsis is a condition associated with severe infections and would be a contraindication to therapy.

Answer a is incorrect. Asthma or COPD are not considered contraindications to therapy.

Answer b is incorrect. Migraine headache is not considered a contraindication to therapy. Neurologic disorders, such as optic neuritis or demyelinating diseases, would be potential contraindications.

Answer c is incorrect. Previous myocardial infarction is not considered a contraindication to therapy; however, the presence of advanced heart failure would be a cardiac condition that is considered a contraindication.

---

8. A 49-year-old woman has been receiving maximal doses of Delzicol for treatment of UC, but continues to have daily moderate symptoms including urgency, abdominal pain, and rectal bleeding. Which therapy would be best for treatment of her symptoms at this time?

    a. Trexall
    b. Remicade
    c. Entocort EC
    d. Apriso

Answer b is correct. Remicade (infliximab) is indicated in patients with moderate to severe symptoms who are unresponsive to other therapies, such as aminosalicylates or corticosteroids. Infliximab works faster than azathioprine and would be a better choice for this patient based on the fact that she is experiencing moderate symptoms on a daily basis.

Answer a is incorrect. Methotrexate is used more in the setting of CD and, like azathioprine, has a delayed onset of action, taking at least 3 to 4 months to work. This patient needs more rapid control of her symptoms.

Answer c is incorrect. Entocort EC (budesonide) is a corticosteroid that is only indicated for patients with CD, who have involvement of the terminal ileum or ascending colon.

Answer d is incorrect. Apriso is a once daily formulation of mesalamine. Since this patient is already failing maximal doses of mesalamine, switching to another mesalamine product would provide minimal benefit.

---

9. A 38-year-old female patient with CD is prescribed Humira for treatment of severe symptoms. Which counseling point is best to provide to this patient prior to starting this therapy?

    a. Correct number of tablets to take on a daily basis
    b. The next dose should be given in 8 weeks
    c. Proper injection technique
    d. Monitor for development of diarrhea

Answer c is correct. Since Humira is administered by subcutaneous injection and is available as a single-dose syringe or a pen device, that patient should be instructed on how to use the formulation and administer the injection properly. The manufacturer medication guide has detailed instructions, which can be used to educate patients on this process.

Answer a is incorrect. Humira is an injectable product, and is not available in an oral tablet formulation.

Answer b is incorrect. Following the initial dose, the next two doses occur at 2 weeks intervals, followed then by an every other week dose schedule.

Answer d is incorrect. Humira is not commonly associated with development of diarrhea.

10. A 53-year-old man with CD for 25 years is experiencing draining, non-healing fistulas. He is interested in beginning therapy with infliximab. Which of the following are important to discuss with this patient prior to starting infliximab therapy? (Please choose all that apply)

    a. Rule out tuberculosis prior to infliximab therapy
    b. Infliximab may be self-administered subcutaneously
    c. Premedication with acetaminophen and diphenhydramine prevents infusion reactions
    d. Administration of a test dose is required before the initial injection

Answer a is correct. Infliximab may predispose patients to infections. Patients must be evaluated for latent tuberculosis prior to initiating therapy.

Answer c is correct. Infliximab is associated with a flu-like infusion reaction. This adverse effect may be prevented by premidicating patients with acetaminophen and diphenhydramine prior to each infusion.

Answer b is incorrect. Infliximab is administered as an intravenous solution, whereas other available TNF-α agents (certolizumab, adalimumab, and golimumab) are administered subcutaneously.

Answer d is incorrect. A test dose is not required or recommended with infliximab therapy.

11. A 27-year-old man presents with an 8-week history of new-onset cramping abdominal pain together with 2 to 3 bloody stools per day. He is diagnosed with left-sided UC.

Which one of the following is the most appropriate initial therapy?

    a. Sulfasalazine orally 1 g 4 times per day
    b. Mesalamine enema rectally 4 g every night
    c. Hydrocortisone enema rectally 100 mg every night
    d. 6-Mercaptopurine (6-MP) orally 75 mg/d

Answer b is correct. An aminosalycilate would be appropriate initial therapy for a patient with mild to moderate UC. Topical therapy with an enema would treat from the rectum up to the splenic flexure, which is the portion of the colon affected in left sided UC. Therefore, a mesalamine enema formulation would be the most appropriate initial therapy for this patient.

Answer a is incorrect. While oral aminosalycilate therapy is an option, use of topical therapy first provides good efficacy while minimizing systemic drug exposure and adverse effects.

Answer c is incorrect. Topical corticosteroid therapy is effective for the induction of remission in mild to moderate left-sided UC; however, they are reserved for patients who are not successfully treated with aminosalycilate therapy.

Answer d is incorrect. 6-Mercaptopurine is effective for the maintenance of remission of UC. Because it may take several months to experience the full effect of this agent, it is not appropriate for use in the induction of remission.

12. A 38-year-old male patient is newly diagnosed with mild to moderate CD confined to the ileum and ascending colon. What is the best recommendation for this patient?

    a. Mesalamine enema 1 g PR at bedtime
    b. Prednisone 40 mg daily orally
    c. Certolizumab pegol 400 mg subcutaneously
    d. Budesonide 9 mg daily orally

Answer d is correct. Oral budesonide is effective for the induction of remission of mild to moderate disease affecting the ileum or ascending colon. Budesonide undergoes first pass metabolism, which limits systemic exposure and adverse effects.

Answer a is incorrect. Topical mesalamine enema would only be effective for left-sided disease that is distal to the splenic flexure. It would not be effective for disease the affects the ileum and ascending colon.

Answer b is incorrect. Systemic corticosteroid therapy is reserved for the induction of remission in moderate to severe CD.

Answer c is incorrect. TNF-α antagonists are reserved for the induction of remission for patients with moderate to severe CD who are unresponsive to corticosteroid therapy. It would not be appropriate to initiate a TNF-α antagonist for a patient with mild to moderate disease who is treatment-naïve.

13. Order the following formulations of mesalamine from least to most area of exposure within the GI tract:

Unordered Options	Ordered Response
Asacol	
Rowasa	
Pentasa	
Canasa	

Correct Response:

Unordered Options	Ordered Response
Asacol	Canasa (Suppository – rectum only)
Rowasa	Rowasa (Enema – rectum, descending colon)
Pentasa	Asacol (Entire colon)
Canasa	Pentasa (Colon + small intestine)

14. A 42-year-old patient presents to his community pharmacy with a prescription for Entocort. What is the generic drug name for Entocort EC?

   a. Methylprednisolone
   b. Prednisone
   c. Hydrocortisone
   d. Budesonide

Answer d is correct. Budesonide is the correct generic name for Entocort.

Answer a is incorrect. Methylprednisolone is available as tablets (Medrol) or injectable products (Solu-Medrol, Depo-Medrol).

Answer b is incorrect. Prednisone is available generically and is typically not referred to by brand name.

Answer c is incorrect. Hydrocortisone is available as a suppository (Proctocort), foam (Cortifoam), tablet (Cortef, Hydrocortone), and injectable product (Solu-Cortef).

15. A patient receiving Tysabri for CD develops mental status changes after 24 weeks of therapy. This may indicate development of which adverse effect of Tysabri?

   a. Progressive multifocal leukoencephalopathy
   b. Central pontine myelinolysis
   c. Cerebrovascular accident
   d. Multi-infarct dementia

Answer a is correct. Tysabri (natalizumab) is associated with development of progressive multifocal leukoencephalopathy as a potential adverse neurologic effect. For this reason, prescribers must enroll in the manufacturer's prescribing program in order to prescribe this agent. Patients should also be closely monitored for signs or symptoms of neurologic changes while receiving therapy.

Answer b is incorrect. Central pontine myelinolysis is an adverse neurologic event associated with nerve demyelination, often due to rapid correction of hyponatremia.

Answer c is incorrect. Tysabri (natalizumab) is not commonly associated with development of cerebrovascular accident as a potential adverse neurologic effect.

Answer d is incorrect. Multi-infarct dementia is a neurologic disorder associated with having multiple strokes over time, many of which are clinically silent. This is not a condition associated with natalizumab use.

16. A 41-year-old woman with UC affecting most of her colon (pancolitis) has been taking balsalazide 6.75 g/d for 2 years and prednisone 40 mg/d for 1 year. When the dose of prednisone is reduced to less than 40 mg, the patient develops fever, abdominal pain, and five or six bloody bowel movements a day. Which modification to this patient's drug regimen is the most appropriate at this time?

   a. Initiate therapy with methotrexate 25 mg intramuscularly once weekly.
   b. Initiate infliximab 5 mg/kg intravenous infusion.
   c. Change balsalazide to sulfasalazine orally 6 g/d.
   d. Add mesalamine suppository 1000 mg rectally once daily.

Answer b is correct. This patient's UC is steroid dependent. Infliximab therapy may result in steroid-sparing effects and allow for reduction of the steroid dose or discontinuation of the steroid.

Answer a is incorrect. Methotrexate is effective for the maintenance of remission of CD and would not be appropriate to use for this patient's UC.

Answer c is incorrect. Balsalazide and sulfasalazine are both aminosalicylates with similar effectiveness, so switching to sulfasalazine would not improve this patient's symptoms.

Answer d is incorrect. This patient is already receiving an oral mesalamine formulation for her pancolitis. A mesalamine suppository would be appropriate if the patient was experiencing ulcerative proctitis, but it would not be likely to reduce the patient's with moderate to severe CD has been dependence on her steroid therapy.

17. A 34-year-old woman presents to the emergency department with a 2-day history of cramping abdominal pain, fever, fatigue, and 10 to 12 bloody stools a day. She has had CD for 5 years; typically, she is maintained on mesalamine (Pentasa) 250 mg 4 capsules two times/day. On admission, her vital signs include temperature 101°F, heart rate 110 beats/min, respiratory rate 18 breaths/min, and blood pressure 118/68 mm Hg. Which therapeutic choice is best?

   a. Administer cyclosporine 4 mg/h by continuous infusion.
   b. Increase the dose of mesalamine (Pentasa) to 4 g/d.
   c. Obtain a surgery consult for immediate colectomy.
   d. Administer hydrocortisone 100 mg intravenously every 8 hours.

Answer d is correct. Intravenous systemic corticosteroid therapy is the most appropriate initial approach to inducing remission in a patient with severe CD.

Answer a is incorrect. Cyclosporine continuous intravenous infusion is reserved for induction of remission in severe CD that is unresponsive to intravenous corticosteroid therapy.

Answer b is incorrect. This patient is experiencing a severe episode of CD. Mesalamine is appropriate for the induction of remission of mild to moderate CD and will not be effective in this situation.

Answer c is incorrect. Colectomy may be considered after drug therapy has failed, or in emergent situations. It would not be appropriate initial therapy for this patient presenting to the hospital.

---

18. A 58-year-old male patient is receiving long-term therapy with metronidazole for the prevention of pouchitis following ileal pouch-anal anastomosis. This patient should be monitored for the development of which adverse effect?

    a. Anemia
    b. Peripheral neuropathy
    c. Hepatitis
    d. Pulmonary fibrosis

Answer b is correct. Metronidazole may cause peripheral neuropathy when administered in high doses over extended periods of time. Long-term use should be avoided, if possible. Patients should be monitored for signs of peripheral neuropathy if long-term use is necessitated.

Answer a is incorrect. Metronidazole is not commonly associated with development of anemia.

Answer c is incorrect. While metronidazole is metabolized hepatically, development of hepatitis is not commonly associated with metronidazole use.

Answer d is incorrect. Pulmonary fibrosis is associated with methotrexate use and is not commonly associated with metronidazole.

---

19. A 56-year-old woman with a history of UC presents to the emergency department with 1 day of abdominal pain, which she rates as 10 out of 10. The pain worsens when she eats and improves slightly when she lies down. She denies alcohol, tobacco, and illicit drug use. Her laboratory findings include a serum lipase level of 3,794 U/L (normal 0-160 U/L). She states that she started taking a new medication to control her UC but cannot recall the name of it. Which drug is most likely causing this adverse effect?

    a. Methotrexate
    b. Adalimumab
    c. Azathioprine
    d. Natalizumab

Answer c is correct. Azathioprine is commonly associated with development of pancreatitis. This adverse effect often occurs within the first 4 to 6 weeks of therapy. Patients should

be monitored for signs or symptoms that may be consistent with pancreatitis.

Answer a is incorrect. Methotrexate is associated with development of hepatic, pulmonary, renal, and bone marrow toxicity; however, it is not commonly associated with development of pancreatitis.

Answer b is incorrect. Adalimumab is associated with development of infections, heart failure, and neurologic complications among others, but is not commonly associated with development of pancreatitis.

Answer d is incorrect. Adalimumab is associated with development of infusion-related reactions, neurologic complications, and development of infection, but is not commonly associated with development of pancreatitis.

---

20. A 26-year-old woman has been able to maintain remission of her UC for the past year with the use of oral mesalamine, oral azathioprine, and intravenous infliximab therapy. This patient is not up to date with her vaccines. Which of the following vaccines are recommended for this patient? (Please choose all that apply.)

    a. Injectable influenza vaccine
    b. Human papilloma virus (HPV)
    c. Measles, mumps, rubella (MMR)
    d. Tetanus, diphtheria, pertussis (Tdap)

Answer a is correct. The injectable inactivated viral influenza vaccine is not a live vaccine and would therefore be appropriate to administer on an annual basis for this patient. A previously available intranasal influenza vaccine was a live attenuated viral vaccine. Because this patient is receiving multiple immunosuppressive treatments, live vaccines are contraindicated.

Answer b is correct. Human papilloma vaccine is an inactivated viral vaccine. Three doses are recommended for administration to patients younger than 26 years old, and would be appropriate for this patient.

Answer d is correct. Tdap is an inactivated viral vaccine that is recommended for use in immunosuppressed patients and should be administered to this patient.

Answer c is incorrect. The measles, mumps, rubella (MMR) vaccines is a live attenuated viral vaccine, making it contraindicated in patients who are immunosuppressed.

---

21. A 38-year-old man with moderate to severe CD has been experiencing numerous relapses on his current medication regimen. He is taking azathioprine and infliximab for maintenance therapy. What changes would be best to make to his maintenance regimen?

    a. Stop infliximab and initiate intravenous cyclosporine
    b. Stop infliximab and azathioprine and initiate dexamethasone
    c. Stop infliximab and azathioprine and initiate vedolizumab
    d. Continue azathioprine and infliximab and begin natalizumab

Answer c is correct. Vedolizumab is an anti-integrin antibody that may be used in patients who fail immunomodulator and TNF-α antagonist therapies. It is now preferred over natalizumab due to the reduced risk of PML.

Answer a is incorrect. Cyclosporine is only used in severe UC exacerbations to delay time to colectomy and is not appropriate as a maintenance therapy.

Answer b is incorrect. Dexamethasone is a systemic corticosteroid. Corticosteroids are useful for the induction of remission of CD. Due to their limited long-term efficacy and risk of adverse effects, systemic corticosteroids are not recommended for maintenance therapy.

Answer d is incorrect. The anti-integrins, vedolizumab and natalizumab, should not be used in combination with TNF-α antagonists. In addition, natalizumab is not preferred prior to vedolizumab due to the risk for PML.

---

22. A 58-year-old woman, AK, with a history of severe UC presents to the emergency department with profuse, bloody diarrhea. She is hypotensive and tachycardic on admission, and is initiated on intravenous fluids. The decision is made to start the patient on glucocorticoid therapy. Rank the following steroids in order of glucocorticoid potency from least potent (1) to most potent (4).

Unordered Options	Ordered Response
Prednisone	
Dexamethasone	
Hydrocortisone	
Methylprednisolone	

Correct response.

Unordered Options	Ordered Response
Prednisone	2
Dexamethasone	4
Hydrocortisone	1
Methylprednisolone	3

23. AK is initiated on intravenous methylprednisolone for her UC exacerbation; however, she continues to decompensate and the surgery team is considering colectomy. Which medication can you recommend to potentially eliminate the need for surgical intervention?

a. Intraveous natalizumab
b. Oral methotrexate
c. Intraveous cyclosporine
d. Intraveous infliximab

Answer c is correct. Intraveous cyclosporine infusion has been used in cases of refractory ulcerative colitis exacerbation to delay the time to colectomy and potentially eliminate the need for procedure.

Answer a is incorrect. Intravenous natalizumab is used as a maintenance therapy for chronic treatment and has no role in the setting of an acute UC exacerbation.

Answer b is incorrect. Oral methotrexate is an immunomodulator, which may limit the need for long-term steroids in IBD, and mainly CD, patients. It is not useful in emergent situations and would not be effective in delaying the need for surgical intervention.

Answer d is incorrect. Intravenous infliximab is a TNF-α antagonist, which is used as a long-term maintenance medication. Although it is available in IV formulation and has steroid-sparing effects, it is unlikely to prevent the need for colectomy in this situation.

CHAPTER 42 | Nausea and Vomiting

Questions 1 to 6 pertain to the following case.

MR is a 42-year-old woman diagnosed with stage 2 breast cancer. Past medical history is significant for heavy alcohol use. She is single and has no children. She presents to clinic today to begin treatment with doxorubicin and cyclophosphamide.

1. Which of the following are risk factors MR has for developing nausea and vomiting? Select all that apply.

a. Heavy alcohol use
b. Female gender
c. Age
d. No children

Answer b is correct. Female patients tend to have more nausea and vomiting than male patients.

Answer c is correct. Patients younger than 50 years of age are more susceptible to nausea and vomiting.

Answer a is incorrect. Patients with a history of long-term heavy alcohol consumption have a lower risk of nausea and vomiting.

Answer d is incorrect. Having no children is a risk for developing breast cancer, but not for nausea and vomiting.

---

2. Select which antiemetic combination will give MR optimal prevention of acute and delayed CINV?

a. Aprepitant, prochlorperazine, and dexamethasone
b. Fosaprepitant, dolasetron, and prochlorperazine
c. Netupitant/palonosetron and haloperidol
d. Rolapitant, palonosetron, and dexamethasone

Answer d is correct. The doxorubicin and cyclophosphamide regimen is categorized as a highly emetic regimen. Rolapitant is FDA-approved to be given in combination with a corticosteroid (dexamethasone) and 5-HT3 receptor antagonist (palonosetron) to prevent acute and delayed CINV with highly emetic regimens.

Answer a is incorrect. Aprepitant is FDA-approved in combination with a corticosteroid (dexamethasone) and 5-HT3 receptor antagonist to prevent acute and delayed CINV with highly emetic regimens. This combination lacks the 5-HT3 receptor antagonist.

Answer b is incorrect. Fosaprepitant is FDA-approved in combination with a corticosteroid and 5-HT3 receptor antagonist (dolasetron) to prevent acute and delayed CINV with highly emetic regimens. This combination lacks the corticosteroid.

Answer c is incorrect. Netupitant/palonosetron (NEPA) is FDA-approved in combination with a corticosteroid to prevent acute and delayed CINV with highly emetic regimens. This combination lacks the corticosteroid.

3. You note that MR is appropriately treated for acute CINV, but not delayed CINV. Her day 1 regimen includes ondansetron, dexamethasone, and fosaprepitant 150 mg IV prior to chemotherapy. What is the best regimen to prevent delayed CINV for MR?

   a. Dexamethasone 8 mg po daily on days 2 through 4
   b. Dexamethasone 8 mg po daily on day 2 and 8 mg bid on days 3 and 4
   c. Ondansetron 8 mg po bid and dexamethasone 8 mg po daily on day 2 and 8 mg bid on days 3 and 4
   d. No treatment is needed as MR is not at risk for delayed nausea and vomiting

Answer b is correct. Only dexamethasone should be continued when fosaprepitant 150 mg IV is used prior to chemotherapy. The recommended dose is 8 mg daily on day 2 and 8 mg bid on days 3 and 4.

Answer a is incorrect. When fosaprepitant 150 mg IV is used prior to chemotherapy, the recommended dose of dexamethasone is 8 mg daily on day 2 and 8 mg bid on days 3 and 4.

Answer c is incorrect. Ondansetron has not been shown to be more effective than dexamethasone alone for delayed nausea and vomiting and should not be used for initial treatment.

Answer d is incorrect. The cyclophosphamide and doxorubicin combination can cause significant delayed CINV and prophylaxis is needed.

4. MR tolerated cycle 2 well, but had significant nausea and vomiting with cycle 3 requiring hospitalization. When MR arrives to the clinic for cycle 4, she immediately feels nauseous. This is an example of what kind of CINV?

   a. Acute
   b. Anticipatory
   c. Breakthrough
   d. Delayed

Answer b is correct. Anticipatory CINV is a conditioned response caused by poor CINV control. The patient was hospitalized after her last cycle of chemotherapy for uncontrolled CINV.

Answer a is incorrect. Acute CINV occurs within 24 hours after chemotherapy administration, and the patient has not received her chemotherapy yet today.

Answer c is incorrect. Breakthrough CINV occurs despite adequate antiemetic prophylaxis prior to chemotherapy administration and the patient has not received chemotherapy since her last cycle.

Answer d is incorrect. Delayed CINV occur >24 hours after chemotherapy administration and the patient has not received chemotherapy since her last cycle.

5. What is the best treatment for the type of CINV that MR is experiencing?

   a. Dexamethasone
   b. Dronabinol
   c. Lorazepam
   d. Palonosetron

Answer c is correct. Lorazepam and other benzodiazepines are useful in the treatment and prevention of anticipatory CINV.

Answer a is incorrect. Dexamethasone is used for the prevention of acute and delayed CINV.

Answer b is incorrect. Dronabinol is generally used for refractory CINV.

Answer d is incorrect. Palonosetron is used for the prevention of acute and delayed CINV.

6. MR is ready to go home from the clinic and would like a prescription for something in case she gets sick at home. What would be the most appropriate antiemetic for MR?

   a. Aprepitant
   b. Droperidol
   c. Ondansetron
   d. Prochlorperazine

Answer d is correct. Dopamine antagonists such as prochlorperazine are effective for the treatment of breakthrough CINV.

Answer a is incorrect. Aprepitant is used to prevent acute and delayed CINV and should not be prescribed for breakthrough CINV.

Answer b is incorrect. Droperidol is available only in an injectable form, so it would not be a good option for use at home for breakthrough CINV.

Answer c is incorrect. Ondansetron should not be prescribed for breakthrough CINV when a 5-HT3 receptor antagonist is used as part of the regimen used to prevent acute CINV.

---

7. Which of the following statements is correct concerning delayed CINV?

   a. Is easier to prevent than acute nausea and vomiting
   b. Occurs ≥24 hours following drug administration
   c. Occurs more commonly with etoposide and docetaxel
   d. No 5-HT3 receptor antagonist has been shown to be more effective in the prevention of delayed CINV

Answer b is correct. Delayed CINV is nausea and vomiting that occurs ≥24 hours following the administration of chemotherapy.

Answer a is incorrect. Delayed CINV is more difficult to prevent than acute CINV. Most of the clinical studies have focused on acute nausea and vomiting, thus we have well-defined guidelines for acute CINV. Fortunately, drug therapy is improving with many of the new drugs such as aprepitant and palonosetron being helpful in the prevention of delayed nausea and vomiting.

Answer c is incorrect. Etoposide and docetaxel are two low emetic chemotherapy agents that are general not associated with delayed CINV.

Answer d is incorrect. Palonosetron has been shown to be more effective in preventing delayed CINV than any of the other 5-HT3 receptor antagonists.

---

8. Which neurotransmitter(s) are involved in CINV? Select all that apply

   a. Dopamine
   b. Neurokinin-1
   c. Norepinephrine
   d. Serotonin

Answer a is correct. The neurotransmitter dopamine plays an important role in CINV. Dopamine antagonists such as promethazine are routinely prescribed in the prevention/treatment of CINV.

Answer b is correct. The neurotransmitter neurokinin-1 (substance P) plays an important role in CINV. Neurokinin-1 receptor antagonists such as aprepitant are prescribed in the prevention of CINV.

Answer d is correct. The neurotransmitter serotonin plays an important role in CINV. Serotonin (5-HT3) antagonists such as ondansetron are routinely prescribed in the prevention of CINV.

Answer c is incorrect. The neurotransmitter norepinephrine has not been shown to play a role in CINV. Thus, there are no drugs used in the treatment of CINV that inhibit norepinephrine.

Questions 9 and 10 pertain to the following case.

9. MB is a 42-year-old woman undergoing a laparoscopic cholecystectomy. She has a history of PONV and motion sickness and denies alcohol or tobacco use. Which drug(s) should be administered at induction or at the end of surgery for the prevention of PONV? Select all that apply.

   a. Dexamethasone
   b. Ondansetron
   c. Aprepitant
   d. Scopolamine

Answer a is correct. Because the patient has 3 of the 4 risk factors (female, history of motion sickness and is a non-smoker) used to stratify risk, she should receive at least 2 medications to prevent PONV. The laparoscopic cholecystectomy may add an additional risk and justify a 3-drug regimen. Dexamethasone should be administered at induction and is appropriate to include as part of the antiemetic regimen.

Answer b is correct. Because the patient has 3 of the 4 risk factors (female, history of motion sickness and is a non-smoker) used to stratify risk, she should receive at least 2 medications to prevent PONV. The laparoscopic cholecystectomy may add an additional risk and justify a 3-drug regimen. Ondansetron should be administered at the end of surgery and is appropriate to include as part of the antiemetic regimen.

Answer c is correct. Because the patient has 3 of the 4 risk factors (female, history of motion sickness and is a non-smoker) used to stratify risk, she should receive at least 2 medications to prevent PONV. The laparoscopic cholecystectomy may add an additional risk and justify a 3-drug regimen. Aprepitant should be administered at induction and is appropriate to include as part of the antiemetic regimen.

Answer d is incorrect. Transdermal scopolamine has been shown to control for up to 24 hours but must be applied the night before or at least 2 to 4 hours before anesthesia because of the 2- to 4-hour delay in onset of effect so it would not be appropriate to use at induction or at the end of surgery. If the scopolamine patch were applied at least 2 hours prior to surgery, it would be a viable choice as part of SG's regimen.

---

10. You receive a call from the physician who cannot remember the correct dose of aprepitant for the prevention of PONV and when it should be administered. What is your response?

    a. 40 mg orally within 3 hours of induction
    b. 80 mg orally within 3 hours of induction
    c. 40 mg IV at the end of surgery
    d. 150 mg IV at the end of surgery

Answer a is correct. The recommended dose of aprepitant for prevention of PONV is 40 mg orally administered within 3 hours prior to surgery.

Answer b is incorrect. While the timing is appropriate, 80 mg is not an approved dose for PONV.

Answer c is incorrect. While the dose is correct, the approved route is oral, and the timing should be within 3 hours of induction.

Answer d is incorrect. Aprepitant 150 mg IV is the approved dose to be given on day 1 of chemotherapy, not for PONV.

---

11. RL is a 72-year-old man being treated for non-small cell lung cancer. He is scheduled to receive carboplatin and etoposide today. You receive the following antiemetic orders: ondansetron 32 mg IV and dexamethasone 12 mg IV 30 minutes before chemotherapy. What is your assessment of the regimen for prophylaxis of acute CINV? Select all that apply.

    a. Aprepitant 125 mg IV prior to chemotherapy should be added to the regimen.
    b. Ondansetron should be decreased to 16 mg po prior to chemotherapy.
    c. Rolapitant 180 mg po should be added to the regimen prior to chemotherapy and the dexamethasone dose should be increased to 20 mg po prior to chemotherapy.
    d. Ondansetron must be changed to palonosetron and the dexamethasone dose should be increased to 20 mg.

Answer b is correct. Ondansetron 32 mg IV is no longer recommended because of increased risk of QT prolongation. The dose range is 8 to 16 mg IV, with 16 mg being the maximum single dose recommended for IV ondansetron. Because there is no indication that the patient cannot take po, it would be preferred that ondansetron be changed to po.

Answer c is correct. Because carboplatin is known to cause delayed nausea and vomiting, adding rolapitant would be appropriate for prevention of both acute and delayed nausea and vomiting. Rolapitant does not affect CYP3A4 metabolism, so the dexamethasone dose should be increased to 20 mg po prior to chemotherapy as the oral route is preferred.

Answer a is incorrect. Because carboplatin is known to cause delayed nausea and vomiting, adding aprepitant would be appropriate for prevention of both acute and delayed nausea and vomiting. The appropriate aprepitant dose for day 1 though is 150 mg IV before chemotherapy.

Answer d is incorrect. When an NK-1 receptor antagonist is not used, palonosetron is a reasonable option, but until more information is available, a specific 5-HT3 receptor antagonist is not preferred. Since Rolapitant is appropriate in this patient, any of the 5-HT3 receptor antagonists are appropriate in this patient.

---

12. Which statement concerning 5-HT3 receptor antagonist therapy for CINV is correct?

    a. Dolasetron has similar efficacy to ondansetron when used at equipotent doses.
    b. Granisetron is the only 5-HT3 receptor antagonist approved for prevention of delayed CINV with HEC.
    c. Palonosetron is superior to prochlorperazine for the treatment of breakthrough CINV.
    d. The IV route of administration of ondansetron is superior to oral administration.

Answer a is correct. Studies show that when 5-HT3 receptor antagonists are given at equipotent doses they have similar efficacy in the prevention of acute CINV.

Answer b is incorrect. Granisetron has not been shown to improve delayed CINV. Palonosetron is the only 5-HT3 receptor antagonist that has been show to improve delayed CINV when given without an NK-1 receptor antagonist in moderately emetic chemotherapy.

Answer c in incorrect. Dopamine antagonists such as prochlorperazine should be used in the treatment of breakthrough CINV. Superiority of the 5-HT3 receptor antagonists has not been shown.

Answer d is incorrect. The IV route of administration of 5-HT3 receptor antagonists is equal to the oral route in regards to efficacy.

Questions 13 and 14 pertain to the following case.

RN is a 64-year-old man who will be coming to clinic to receive a 3-day chemotherapy regimen that includes cisplatin on all 3 days. He has no history of alcohol use and is otherwise healthy.

13. The oncologist contacts you and asks for your antiemetic regimen recommendations to prevent acute and delayed CINV for RN. Which regimen(s) is/are appropriate? Select all that apply.

    a. Dolasetron 100 mg po prior to chemotherapy each day and fosaprepitant 150 mg IV on day 1 before chemotherapy. Dexamethasone 12 mg po given daily prior to chemotherapy each day and then dexamethasone 8 mg po bid on days 4 through 6 alone after chemotherapy.
    b. Granisetron transdermal patch applied 24 hours before chemotherapy, dexamethasone 12 mg po and aprepitant 125 mg po on day 1 before chemotherapy, then aprepitant 80 mg po daily on days 2 and 3 and dexamethasone 8 mg po daily on days 2 through 6.
    c. Ondansetron 32 mg IV and dexamethasone 20 mg IV daily before chemotherapy. Aprepitant 125 mg po on day 1 and 80 mg po on days 2 and 3.
    d. Palonosetron 0.25 mg IV, dexamethasone 12 mg IV and fosaprepitant 150 mg IV on day 1 before chemotherapy, then dexamethasone 8 mg po daily on day 2 and dexamethasone 8 mg po bid on days 3 through 6.

Answer a is correct. For a 3-day chemotherapy regimen the recommendation is to give a 5-HT3 receptor antagonist and dexamethasone prior to each dose of chemotherapy, and to give an NK-1 receptor antagonist on day 1 only unless oral aprepitant is used. Dexamethasone should be given for 2 to 3 days after then end of chemotherapy.

Answer b is correct. Granisetron transdermal patch is indicated for multi-day chemotherapy and can be worn for up to 7 days, depending on the chemotherapy regimen. It should be left in place for 24 hours after the last chemotherapy dose. Dexamethasone should be given for 2 to 3 days after the end of chemotherapy.

Answer d is correct.   Palonosetron, because of its longer half-life, should provide anti-emetic coverage throughout the 3-day regimen and is only needed on day 1.

Answer c is incorrect.   Ondansetron 32 mg IV is no longer recommended because of the increased risk of QT prolongation and the dexamethasone dose should be reduced to 12 mg on day 1 because of the increased levels seen when given with aprepitant. Dexamethasone 8 mg on days 2 and 3 should be added as well.

---

14. RN is sent home with prescriptions for lorazepam and prochlorperazine. He calls 3 days later to say that the lorazepam and prochlorperazine are not working. The nurse tells RN to take the prochlorperazine q6h scheduled and calls in a prescription for ondansetron as needed. He calls back the next day to say he is not getting any relief. What agent is commonly used for refractory nausea and vomiting?

    a. Droperidol
    b. Olanzapine
    c. Palonosetron
    d. Promethazine

Answer b is correct.   While the treatment of refractory nausea and vomiting is many times trial and error, olanzapine has shown efficacy in refractory CINV.

Answer a is incorrect.   Droperidol is only available as an injection and would not be a good choice to administer to a patient at home.

Answer c is incorrect.   The patient has already received ondansetron. Giving him a drug with the same mechanism of action will probably not be helpful.

Answer d is incorrect.   Promethazine is a phenothiazine and RN did not respond to prochlorperazine. RN probably would not benefit from additional phenothiazine treatment.

---

15. Which antiemetic(s) should be avoided in patients with the potential for a prolonged QT-interval? Select all that apply.

    a. Aprepitant 150 mg IV
    b. Palonosetron 0.25 mg IV
    c. Droperidol 1.25 mg IV
    d. Ondansetron 24 mg IV

Answer c is correct.   QT-interval prolongation may occur with recommended doses of droperidol. Droperidol now has a black box warning alerting practitioners of the serious potential for QT-interval prolongation.

Answer d is correct.   Because of the risk of QT-interval prolongation the maximum ondansetron single IV dose

recommended is 16 mg. Using a lower dose of 8 mg IV dose would be safer but the patient would need to be monitored closely.

Answer a is incorrect.   QT-interval prolongation is not a concern with aprepitant.

Answer b is incorrect.   Palonosetron is the only 5-HT3 receptor antagonist that has shown to cause infrequent QT prolongation, and this would be a good choice for those patients at risk.

---

16. VP is a 47-year-old woman and is admitted for abdominal pain. She denies alcohol or tobacco use but does have issues with motion sickness. CT scan shows an inflamed gall bladder, and the patient is scheduled for a cholecystectomy. With the information you have, what is VP's risk of developing PONV?

    a. Low
    b. Moderate
    c. High
    d. Very high

Answer c is correct.   Risk factors used to assess risk include female sex, nonsmokers, history of PONV or motion sickness, and postoperative opioid use. With the information you have, she would have a high risk of developing PONV because she has 3 identified risk factors. Her age and the surgery type also increase her risk of developing PONV.

Answer a is incorrect.   Low risk is defined as 0-1 risk factors for developing PONV. VP has ≥3 risk factors that increase her risk of developing PONV.

Answer b is incorrect.   Moderate risk is defined as 2 risk factors for developing PONV. VP has ≥3 risk factors that increase her risk of developing PONV.

Answer d is incorrect.   There is not a risk level defined as very high.

Questions 17 and 18 pertain to the following case.

JS is a 64-year-old woman who presents to the clinic for cycle 1 of single-agent gemcitabine for pancreatic cancer. She has no history of nausea and vomiting with pregnancy or motion and no heavy alcohol use.

17. Categorize this patient's risk for CINV based on the chemotherapy agent to be given.

    a. Minimal risk
    b. Low risk
    c. Moderate Risk
    d. High risk

Answer b is correct.   Gemcitabine is classified as low risk.

Answer a is incorrect.   Gemcitabine is classified as low risk.

Answer c is incorrect.   Gemcitabine is classified as low risk.

Answer d is incorrect. Gemcitabine is classified as low risk.

---

18. Based on the emetic risk classification of gemcitabine, what medication(s) should JS receive for prevention of acute nausea and vomiting?

    a. Ondansetron, aprepitant, and dexamethasone
    b. Dexamethasone
    c. Lorazepam
    d. Olanzapine

Answer b is correct. For low emetic risk chemotherapy, the recommended prophylaxis is dexamethasone or a dopamine receptor antagonist.

Answer a is incorrect. The 3-drug regimen is appropriate for highly emetic chemotherapy, but since gemcitabine is classified and a low risk of causing nausea and vomiting, this is inappropriate.

Answer c is incorrect. Benzodiazepines are recommended for anticipatory CINV, and as an adjunct to recommended antiemetic therapy, but should not be used alone for prevention of CINV.

Answer d is incorrect. Olanzapine is reserved for highly emetic chemotherapy or for patients who are refractory to traditional antiemetic therapy.

---

19. Which antiemetic should be diluted when given intravenously to minimize extravasation potential?

    a. Droperidol
    b. Fosaprepitant
    c. Palonosetron
    d. Promethazine

Answer d is correct. Promethazine can cause serious tissue damage when extravasation occurs. Several organizations recommend diluting promethazine prior to injection to minimize the extravasation potential.

Answer a is incorrect. Extravasation is not a major concern with droperidol.

Answer b is incorrect. Extravasation is not a major concern with fosaprepitant.

Answer c is incorrect. Extravasation is not a major concern with palonosetron.

---

20. A 34-year-old woman is admitted for a total abdominal hysterectomy and bilateral oophorectomy. The nurse calls and tells you she is asked to write antiemetic orders for ondansetron to prevent PONV but she can't remember the dose. What do you tell her?

    a. Ondansetron 16 mg IV given at the beginning of surgery
    b. Ondansetron 32 mg IV given in postoperative recovery
    c. Ondansetron 8 mg IV given 2 hours before surgery
    d. Ondansetron 4 mg IV given at the end of surgery

Answer d is correct. The appropriate dose of ondansetron to prevent PONV is 4 mg IV given at the end of surgery.

Answer a is incorrect. Ondansetron 16 mg IV is a dose used to prevent CINV and 5-HT3 receptor antagonists should be given at the end of surgery to prevent PONV.

Answer b is incorrect. Ondansetron 32 mg IV is a dose that was previously used to prevent CINV but is no longer recommended due to QT prolongation risk and 5-HT3 receptor antagonists should be given at the end of surgery to prevent PONV.

Answer c is incorrect. Ondansetron 8 mg IV is a dose used to prevent CINV and 5-HT3 receptor antagonists should be given at the end of surgery.

---

21. Rank the 5-HT3 receptor antagonists in order of mg per dose. Start with the lowest mg.

Unordered Response	Ordered Response
Rolapitant	Aprepitant
Netupitant (as part of NEPA)	Fosaprepitant
Fosaprepitant	Rolapitant
Aprepitant	Netupitant (as part of NEPA)

CHAPTER **43** | **Upper Gastrointestinal Disorders**

1. Patients with NSAID-induced ulcers are more likely to have which of the following? Select all that apply.

    a. Superficial ulcer depth
    b. A duodenal ulcer
    c. Stress related mucosal bleeding
    d. Damage to the gastric mucosa
    e. More severe GI bleeding involving a single vessel

Answer d is correct. NSAID-induced ulcers typically develop in the gastric mucosa.

Answer e is correct. NSAID-induced ulcers are often deeper and have more severe GI bleeding involving a single blood vessel.

Answer a is incorrect. Superficial ulcer depth is common with *H. pylori* induced ulcers.

Answer b is incorrect. Ulcers caused by *H. pylori* are more common in the duodenum than the stomach.

Answer c is incorrect. Stress related mucosal bleeding is associated with a major stressful event (mechanical ventilation, trauma, burns, surgery, organ failure, or sepsis).

2. You are asked for pharmacotherapy recommendations for a 59-year-old man with a documented NSAID-induced ulcer who is *H. pylori* negative. He needs to continue taking an NSAID for severe osteoarthritis. Which is the preferred medication for treating an NSAID-induced ulcer?

   a. Lansoprazole
   b. Misoprostol
   c. Ranitidine
   d. Sucralfate

Answer a is correct.   A PPI is the agent of choice if the NSAID must be continued in the presence of ulcer disease. If a patient tests positive for *H. pylori*, treatment is recommended.

Answer b is incorrect.   Misoprostol is indicated in the *prevention* of NSAID-induced gastric ulcers.

Answer c is incorrect.   H2RA antagonists have been shown to prevent only duodenal ulcers and, therefore, should not be recommended for prophylaxis of gastric ulcers.

Answer d is incorrect.   Sucralfate has not been shown to be effective in preventing or treating NSAID-related ulcers.

3. A 43-year-old woman with epigastric pain was just diagnosed with a duodenal ulcer. A urea breath test confirmed *H. pylori*. The patient denies any allergies to medications, and recently completed a course of azithromycin for community-acquired pneumonia. In addition to PPI, which of the following is/are recommended as primary initial therapy for *H. pylori*? Select all that apply.

   a. Amoxicillin + levofloxacin for 14 days
   b. Metronidazole + clarithromycin for 7 days
   c. Amoxicillin + clarithromycin for 14 days
   d. Metronidazole + bismuth + tetracycline for 14 days
   e. Levofloxacin + nitazoxanide + doxycycline for 10 days

Answer a is correct.   Levofloxacin-based triple therapy is a suggested option for initial therapy of *H. pylori* infection.

Answer d is correct.   The regimen of PPI, bismuth, metronidazole, and tetracycline (bismuth quadruple therapy) is a recommended therapy. Bismuth quadruple therapy is particularly attractive in patients with prior macrolide exposure or in cases of penicillin allergy.

Answer e is correct.   The regimen of PPI, levofloxacin, nitazoxanide, and doxycycline is considered a first-line regimen for *H. pylori* eradication.

Answer b is incorrect.   Clarithromycin triple therapy is a recommended therapy in regions where *H. pylori* resistance is known to be <15% and in patients with no prior macrolide exposure. Additionally, the treatment duration should be extended to 14 days.

Answer c is incorrect.   Clarithromycin triple therapy is a recommended therapy in regions where *H. pylori* resistance

is known to be <15% and in patients with no prior macrolide exposure.

4. Which of the following is a nonendoscopic test used to diagnose active *H. pylori* PUD?

   a. Urea breath test
   b. Mucosal biopsy
   c. Culture
   d. Antibody detection

Answer a is correct.   Urea breath test and fecal antigen are reliable for identifying active *H. pylori* before treatment. The urea breath test is the most commonly utilized test for diagnosis of *H. pylori*.

Answer b is incorrect.   Mucosal biopsy is an endoscopic test that can be used to diagnose *H. pylori*.

Answer c is incorrect.   Culture is an endoscopic test that can be used to diagnose *H. pylori*.

Answer d is incorrect.   Antibody detection is a nonendoscopic test, but is unable to distinguish between active or cured infection.

5. A patient calls the pharmacy to complain about her tongue turning black after starting a new regimen for PUD. Which medication is causing the side effect?

   a. Amoxicillin
   b. Metronidazole
   c. Bismuth subsalicylate
   d. Clarithromycin

Answer c is correct.   Bismuth may cause nausea and a dark tongue and/or stool.

Answer a is incorrect.   Amoxicillin may cause headache, diarrhea, or GI upset.

Answer b is incorrect.   Metronidazole can cause metallic taste, dyspepsia, peripheral neuropathy, and a disulfiram-like reaction with alcohol.

Answer d is incorrect.   Clarithromycin may cause GI upset, diarrhea, QTc prolongation, or altered taste (bitter or metallic).

6. A patient was treated initially with PPI, amoxicillin, and clarithromycin for 10 days but failed to eradicate *H. pylori*. Which regimen(s) would you recommended for salvage therapy? Select all that apply.

   a. PPI + amoxicillin for 10 days
   b. PPI + tetracycline + metronidazole + bismuth for 14 days
   c. PPI + metronidazole + clarithromycin for 14 days
   d. PPI + nitazoxanide + levofloxacin + doxycycline for 10 days
   e. PPI + amoxicillin + clarithromycin for 14 days

Answer b is correct. Bismuth quadruple therapy is commonly used as the second course or salvage therapy. Salvage therapy should avoid antibiotics that were previously utilized for treatment of *H. pylori*.

Answer d is correct. Levofloxacin-based therapies have been used as salvage therapy. This regimen is referred to as LOAD (see Table 43-4). Nitazoxanide is a nitroimidazole antibiotic related to metronidazole. In situations where it is unavailable or too costly, metronidazole could be substituted.

Answer a is incorrect. All regimens for the treatment of *H. pylori* should contain two antibiotics.

Answer c is incorrect. Clarithromycin was used in the initial treatment regimen; therefore, it should be avoided in the salvage regimen. In the United States, clarithromycin resistance is believed to exceed 15% to 20%.

Answer e is incorrect. This is the same regimen that was used initially. In the United States, clarithromycin resistance is believed to exceed 15% to 20%. Extending the treatment duration would not be expected to overcome any underlying antimicrobial resistance.

---

7. What is the recommended duration of treatment for *H. pylori* if clarithromycin-based triple therapy is initially used?

   a. 5 days
   b. 7 days
   c. 10 days
   d. 14 days

Answer d is correct. In the United States, 14 days is the recommended treatment duration for clarithromycin-based triple therapy due to increasing rates of resistance.

Answer a is incorrect. Five days of therapy is not recommended due to lower eradication rate when compared to 14-day therapy.

Answer b is incorrect. Seven days of therapy is not recommended due to lower eradication rate when compared to 14-day therapy.

Answer c is incorrect. Ten days of therapy is no longer recommended due to increasing resistance.

---

8. A 62-year-old woman with rheumatoid arthritis and atrial fibrillation (AF) requires chronic NSAID therapy. She controls her arthritis pain with high-dose nabumetone and takes warfarin for AF. Patient is considered as low CV risk. Which medication regimen(s) is/are recommended for prevention of NSAID ulcer complications? Select all that apply.

   a. Change to celecoxib plus PPI
   b. Add PPI to current NSAID
   c. Change to celecoxib
   d. No change is needed
   e. Change to indomethacin

Answer a is correct. COX-2 plus either misoprostol or PPI is recommended for patients at high risk for GI toxicity and low CV risk.

Answer b is correct. Patients at high risk of GI toxicity may be treated with NSAID plus PPI. Nabumetone is considered a nonselective NSAID with low risk of GI toxicity.

Answer c is incorrect. In patients at high-risk of GI toxicity, celecoxib alone is not preferred over celecoxib plus PPI.

Answer d is incorrect. In patients with multiple risk factors of NSAID, GI toxicity should be treated with COX-2 inhibitor or an NSAID plus either misoprostol or PPI.

Answer e is incorrect. Indomethacin has low COX-2 selectivity and moderate-high GI risk. Compared to current NSAID, this regimen would increase GI risk.

---

9. A patient heard on television that indomethacin can cause ulcers. She calls the pharmacy to find out if there is a better alternative to treat her arthritis. She prefers an NSAID with a similar treatment effect but a lower risk of GI toxicity. The patient is aged 55 and does not have any other significant medical problems. What recommendation would be most appropriate?

   a. Sulindac
   b. Etodolac
   c. Piroxicam
   d. Naproxen

Answer b is correct. Etodolac is an NSAID with high COX-2 selectivity and low risk of GI toxicity.

Answer a is incorrect. Sulindac is an NSAID with moderate COX-2 selectivity and moderate risk of GI toxicity.

Answer c is incorrect. Piroxicam is an NSAID with moderate COX-2 selectivity and high risk of GI toxicity.

Answer d is incorrect. Naproxen is an NSAID with low COX-2 selectivity and moderate risk of GI toxicity. It is similar to indomethacin, but with a slightly improved CV risk profile.

---

10. A 55-year-old woman with prior PUD, hyperlipidemia, MI (2 years ago), and hypertension (HTN) requires chronic NSAID therapy for hip pain. Medications include atorvastatin 20 mg once daily, *acetylsalicylic acid* (ASA) 81 mg once daily, and metoprolol 100 mg bid. What would you recommended for treatment of her hip pain +/- ulcer prevention?

   a. Celecoxib 100 mg daily
   b. Naproxen
   c. Celecoxib 100 mg daily plus omeprazole 20 mg daily
   d. Naproxen plus ranitidine

Answer c is correct. Although some of the gastroprotective effect is lost with COX-2 inhibitors in patients taking low-dose aspirin despite the addition of a PPI, it represents the best choice in this patient. The daily dose of COX-2 inhibitors should be limited due to increased risk of CV events, and this patient has a history of CV disease.

Answer a is incorrect. The gastroprotective effect is lost with COX-2 inhibitors in patients taking low-dose aspirin. The daily dose of celecoxib is considered low-dose; however, this patient is considered at high-risk of GI toxicity due to prior PUD and need for aspirin and NSAID. Guidelines recommend the addition of PPI or misoprostol for these patients.

Answer b is incorrect. Naproxen is a preferred NSAID in patients with CV disease, but for high-risk (due to prior PUD) patients on low-dose aspirin the addition of PPI or misoprostol is recommended.

Answer d is incorrect. The patient is at high risk for NSAID-induced GI toxicity due to prior PUD and high CV risk due to prior MI. Naproxen is a preferred NSAID in patients with CV disease; however, guidelines recommend the addition of PPI or misoprostol. Ranitidine is an H2RA and is not sufficient to prevent NSAID ulcers.

---

11. Which of the following describes the clinical presentation of duodenal ulcers?

    a. Pain may be accompanied by coughing up blood.
    b. Pain is worse at night or between meals.
    c. Pain is worse with food.
    d. Pain is caused by damage from NSAIDs.

Answer b is correct. Pain due to a duodenal ulcer may be worse on an empty stomach.

Answer a is incorrect. Coughing up blood is associated with the complications of PUD such as perforation or a GI bleed.

Answer c is incorrect. Gastric ulcer pain may be worse with eating.

Answer d is incorrect. Gastric ulcers are associated with NSAID use.

---

12. Which of the following requires a negative pregnancy test prior to starting therapy?

    a. Celecoxib
    b. Misoprostol
    c. PPIs
    d. Amoxicillin

Answer b is correct. Female patients should have a negative pregnancy test within 2 weeks prior to starting therapy. Patients should start misoprostol on the second or third day of their next normal menstrual cycle. Misoprostol is pregnancy category X.

Answer a is incorrect. Celecoxib does not require a pregnancy test prior to starting therapy. Celecoxib is

pregnancy category C prior to 30 weeks gestation and category D at 30 or more weeks gestation.

Answer c is incorrect. PPIs do not require a pregnancy test prior to starting therapy. PPIs are either pregnancy category B or C.

Answer d is incorrect. Amoxicillin does not require a pregnancy test prior to starting therapy. Amoxicillin is pregnancy category B.

---

13. A patient is admitted to the intensive care unit after a car accident. The patient has been on mechanical ventilation for 72 hours and has a head injury. Which of the following is recommended for this patient for stress ulcer prophylaxis?

    a. Ranitidine by mouth
    b. Intravenous pantoprazole
    c. Sucralfate by nasogastric tube
    d. Patient does not require stress ulcer prophylaxis

Answer b is correct. PPIs and H2RAs are preferred treatment options and IV would be the best route of administration.

Answer a is incorrect. H2RAs and PPIs are preferred treatment options, but they are not preferred by mouth since the patient is on mechanical ventilation. Nasogastric administration would make this an acceptable choice.

Answer c is incorrect. Sucralfate is not first line for high-risk patients on a ventilator.

Answer d is incorrect. The patient is considered at high risk for stress ulcers because mechanical ventilation has been used for more than 48 hours and head injury patients are at higher risk of SRMD.

---

14. Which of the following factors may worsen symptoms in GERD patients? Select all that apply.

    a. Alcohol consumption
    b. Caffeine consumption
    c. Obesity or recent weight gain
    d. Smoking
    e. Furosemide

Answer a is correct. Alcohol consumption may worsen GERD symptoms by increasing acid secretion, reducing LES tone and esophageal motility, and slowing gastric emptying.

Answer b is correct. Caffeine is believed to reduce LES pressure causing increased GERD symptoms.

Answer c is correct. Obesity is believed to cause GERD symptoms for several reasons including increased intra-abdominal pressure and increased output of bile and pancreatic enzymes. Additionally, obese patients have a higher incidence of hiatal hernia.

Answer d is correct. Smoking has been shown to prolong acid clearance and decrease LES pressure.

Answer e is incorrect.   Furosemide would not be expected to affect GERD symptoms. Anticholinergics, estrogen/progesterone, nicotine, nitrates, tetracyclines, and theophylline are medications that may decrease LES tone resulting in increased GERD symptoms.

15. A 45-year-old obese woman with HTN and diabetes presents with complaints of "severe" heartburn after meals and occasionally at night. She admits to smoking and occasional alcohol consumption. She consumes four to five caffeinated beverages daily. Medications include: hydrochlorothiazide (HCTZ) 12.5 mg daily and metformin 850 mg twice daily. Which of the following represents the best initial treatment option with the highest probability of symptom control?

    a. Ranitidine
    b. Metoclopramide
    c. Lansoprazole
    d. Sucralfate

Answer c is correct.   PPIs have the highest rate of symptom control and healing rates when esophagitis is present or suspected. All PPIs are considered equally effective.

Answer a is incorrect.   H2RAs are effective for many patients with mild to moderate GERD symptoms; however, this patient presents with severe reflux symptoms. Overall, PPIs are the most effective pharmacologic option for control of symptoms and healing of esophagitis.

Answer b is incorrect.   Due to significant risk of side effects and lack of benefit in clinical trials, metoclopramide is not considered as first-line therapy. It could be used as an adjunctive medication in patients with known GI motility disorders, but should always be used in conjunction with acid suppressive therapy.

Answer d is incorrect.   Sucralfate is not effective for patients with GERD and cannot be recommended.

16. A 65-year-old woman with osteoporosis, GERD, and HTN is taking alendronate 70 mg weekly, calcium carbonate 600 mg + vitamin D 400 units twice daily, omeprazole 20 mg daily, and enalapril 10 mg twice daily. Which of the following are possible consequences of this regimen? Select all that apply.

    a. Alendronate may worsen GERD symptoms.
    b. Enalapril may worsen GERD symptoms.
    c. Omeprazole may reduce calcium absorption.
    d. Omeprazole may decrease alendronate metabolism.
    e. Omeprazole may decrease absorption of vitamin D.

Answer a is correct.   Bisphosphonates can cause a myriad of GI symptoms including dyspepsia, reflux, and ulcer formation. These symptoms may be worsened in patients who do not remain in an upright position for at least 30 minutes after taking bisphosphonates such as alendronate.

Answer c is correct.   Calcium carbonate requires an acidic environment for adequate absorption. Acid suppressant

therapy, particularly potent PPIs, raise the pH reducing calcium absorption. Older patients taking omeprazole had an increased risk of fracture compared to equally matched patients. Calcium citrate may be recommended in these patients as it does not require an acidic environment for adequate absorption.

Answer b is incorrect.   Angiotensin-converting-enzyme (ACE)-inhibitors do not cause an increase in GERD symptoms or interact with medications commonly used for treatment.

Answer d is incorrect.   Omeprazole is not expected to interact with alendronate.

Answer e is incorrect.   Omeprazole is not expected to interact with vitamin D.

17. Which of the following is a typical sign or symptom of patients with GERD?

    a. Iron deficiency anemia
    b. Dysphagia
    c. Regurgitation
    d. Weight loss

Answer c is correct.   Regurgitation is a common symptom of uncomplicated GERD. Additional typical symptoms include heartburn, belching, and hypersalivation.

Answer a is incorrect.   The presence of iron deficiency in patients with GERD is a complicating factor. This may be an indication of GI bleeding; therefore, additional diagnostic testing (endoscopy and/or colonoscopy) would be indicated.

Answer b is incorrect.   Dysphagia, or difficulty swallowing, is a concerning alarm symptom because it may indicate stricture or malignancy.

Answer d is incorrect.   Unexplained weight loss is not a typical symptom of patients with GERD and warrants further investigation.

18. Which of the following acts by competitively inhibiting histamine at the H2 receptor of gastric parietal cells? Select all that apply.

    a. Omeprazole
    b. Rabeprazole
    c. Cimetidine
    d. Ranitidine
    e. Misoprostol

Answer c is correct.   Cimetidine is an H2RA.

Answer d is correct.   Ranitidine is an H2RA.

Answer a is incorrect.   Omeprazole is a proton pump inhibitor.

Answer b is incorrect.   Rabeprazole is a proton pump inhibitor.

Answer e is incorrect. Misoprostol is a prostaglandin analog.

19. A 50-year-old woman presented to her physician approximately 8 weeks ago with complaints of heartburn, regurgitation, and dysphagia which resulted in an endoscopy. At that time, her physician diagnosed GERD with erosive esophagitis and prescribed 2 months of lansoprazole 30 mg daily. Today at her follow-up visit, she reports improvement in her symptoms. What would you recommend as an initial trial of maintenance therapy for NJ?

    a. Famotidine 20 mg twice daily
    b. Lansoprazole 30 mg daily
    c. No further therapy required
    d. Sucralfate 1 g twice daily

Answer b is correct. Chronic maintenance therapy with PPI will be required by most patients with symptoms severe enough to warrant initial therapy. Patients may be continued on the previous dose as relapse of heartburn and other GERD symptoms is common; however, dosage reduction should be attempted at some point. Daily maintenance with a PPI with erosive esophagitis is recommended.

Answer a is incorrect. Chronic maintenance therapy with PPI will be required by most patients with symptoms severe enough to warrant initial therapy. Many patients may tolerate dosage reduction and maintain adequate symptom control. Daily maintenance with a PPI for erosive esophagitis is recommended over maintenance with H2RA.

Answer c is incorrect. GERD is a chronic condition requiring maintenance therapy. For most patients, continuous PPI therapy is recommended to maintain the healed mucosa, and discontinuing therapy results in recurrent heartburn or erosions.

Answer d is incorrect. Sucralfate is not as effective compared to a PPI for erosive esophagitis. In some cases, it may be added as an adjunct in the initial period after diagnosis, but it has no role in maintenance therapy.

20. Select the brand name for pantoprazole.

    a. Axid
    b. Aciphex
    c. Prevacid
    d. Protonix

Answer d is correct. Protonix is the brand name for pantoprazole.

Answer a is incorrect. Axid is the brand name for nizatidine.

Answer b is incorrect. Aciphex is the brand name for rabeprazole.

Answer c is incorrect. Prevacid is the brand name for lansoprazole

21. Which of the following would be appropriate health information to discuss with a patient presenting to your pharmacy with GERD symptoms? Select all that apply.

    a. Eating smaller meals more often
    b. Elevating the head of the bed 6 inches if nighttime symptoms are present
    c. Weight reduction for patients who are overweight
    d. Smoking cessation for those who smoke
    e. Avoid eating within 6 hours before bedtime

Answer a is correct. Eating smaller meals more often may be beneficial in reducing reflux symptoms.

Answer b is correct. Elevating the head of the bed may be a helpful nonpharmacologic strategy for patients who experience frequent nighttime GERD symptoms.

Answer c is correct. Patients who are overweight often have increased GERD symptoms. Losing weight has been shown to improve symptoms.

Answer d is correct. Cigarette smoking has been shown to reduce lower esophageal pressure and prolong acid clearance. The duration of smoking is also an important risk factor for GERD symptoms; smokers with more than 20-year history of tobacco use were more likely to have reflux symptoms when compared with those who smoked for less than 1 year.

Answer e is incorrect. Patients should avoid eating within 3 hours of bedtime.

22. Select the counseling points for a patient receiving omeprazole 40 mg daily.

    a. Take in the evening 30 minutes prior to going to bed.
    b. The capsule may be chewed or crushed.
    c. Administer with food.
    d. Delayed release capsule may be opened and added to 1 tablespoon of applesauce.

Answer d is correct. Delayed release capsules may be opened and contents added to 1 tablespoon of applesauce. It should be used immediately after adding to applesauce. The mixture should not be chewed or warmed.

Answer a is incorrect. PPIs should be taken in the morning 30 minutes prior to breakfast.

Answer b is incorrect. The capsule or tablet should be swallowed whole. Delayed release capsules may be opened and contents added to 1 tablespoon of applesauce. It should be used immediately after adding to applesauce. The mixture should not be chewed or warmed.

Answer c is incorrect. Omeprazole should be administered on an empty stomach 30 minutes prior to eating.

23. Order the following NSAIDs in order of risk of GI toxicity. Place in order starting with the lowest to highest risk: Salsalate, Piroxicam, Aspirin.

    a. Salsalate < Piroxicam < Aspirin
    b. Salsalate < Aspirin < Piroxicam
    c. Aspirin < Piroxicam < Salsalate
    d. Piroxicam < Aspirin < Salsalate

Answer b is correct. Salsalate has a low risk of GI toxicity; Aspirin has a moderate risk of GI toxicity; and piroxicam has a high risk of GI toxicity.

CHAPTER **44 | Viral Hepatitis**

1. Select the most common mode of transmission for the hepatitis A virus (HAV).

    a. Blood
    b. Fecal-oral route
    c. Perinatal exposure
    d. Semen

Answer b is correct. The fecal-oral route is the most common mode of transmission of HAV and often occurs through contact with contaminated food, poor hygienic practices, and in poorly developed countries.

Answer a is incorrect. Intravenous drug users can acquire HAV through exposure to HAV infected blood but this is not a common mode of transmission.

Answer c is incorrect. Perinatal transmission is not associated with HAV, but is infrequently associated with HBV and very rarely for HCV.

Answer d is incorrect. Transmission of viral hepatitis from semen is not associated with HAV, but is rarely associated with other viral hepatitis types.

2. Which of the following forms of viral hepatitis can be cured with drug therapy?

    a. Chronic hepatitis A
    b. Chronic hepatitis B
    c. Chronic hepatitis C
    d. Viral hepatitis can never be cured

Answer c is correct. Hepatitis C can be cured if a patient has no measurable HCV 6 months after completing treatment.

Answer a is incorrect. Hepatitis A is an acute infection and patients eventually clear the virus. HAV does not develop into a chronic form.

Answer b is incorrect. Chronic hepatitis B cannot be cured with drug therapy. The goals are to suppress the viral load and to prevent complications (eg, cirrhosis and hepatocellular carcinoma).

Answer d is incorrect. HCV can be cured.

3. Which of the following represent a rare side effect associated with Twinrix (hepatitis A/B vaccine)?

    a. Stevens-Johnson syndrome
    b. Neuroleptic syndrome
    c. Guillain-Barré syndrome
    d. Red-man syndrome

Answer c is correct. Guillain-Barré syndrome is a rare side effect associated with Twinrix.

Answer a is incorrect. Stevens-Johnson syndrome is not a reported side effect of Twinrix.

Answer b is incorrect. Neuroleptic syndrome is not a reported side effect of Twinrix.

Answer d is incorrect. Red-man syndrome is not a reported side effect of Twinrix.

4. Which of the following best represents the pregnancy category when ribavirin is added to a HCV regimen?

    a. B
    b. C
    c. D
    d. X

Answer d is correct. Peg-interferon monotherapy is pregnancy class C but when combined with ribavirin, the cotherapy is pregnancy class X. Ribavirin is extremely teratogenic during and up to 6 months after therapy. Female partners of ribavirin treated patients are at equal risk. Women and men of childbearing age should use two forms of contraception until 6 months following discontinuation of therapy. A Ribavirin Registry tracks pregnancies that have been exposed to ribavirin.

Answers a, b, and c are incorrect.

5. A 58-year-old man diagnosed with chronic hepatitis C (HCV) genotype 1a is to begin therapy with ledipasvir/sofosbuvir + ribavirin. Which of the following counseling topics is appropriate? Select all that apply.

    a. He should use two forms of birth control.
    b. His HCV treatment will last 48 weeks.
    c. He likely developed HCV from a contaminated food source.
    d. He should not share razors or toothbrushes with anyone.

Answer a is correct. Ribavirin has a black box warning about its teratogenic effects in both pregnant women taking ribavirin and in pregnant women whose partner is taking ribavirin and up to 6 months following completion of ribavirin therapy. Two forms of birth control are recommended even in patients who believe they are infertile or have low fertility. A Ribavirin Registry exists for women who became pregnant while they or their partner took ribavirin.

Answer d is correct. HCV is transmitted via contaminated blood. Patients are advised not to share razors, toothbrushes, or other personal care products that may come in contact with HCV-infected blood.

Answer b is incorrect. Therapy with ledipasvir/sofosbuvir lasts 12 weeks in most patients. Some treatment-naive patients meeting certain criteria can be treated for 8 weeks.

Answer c is incorrect. HCV is transmitted via the bloodstream.

---

6. LO is a 28-year-old woman who found out her boyfriend has chronic hepatitis B (HBV). They are sexually active and plan to marry in 6 months. Which of the following is the best course of action? Select all that apply.

   a. Administer HBIG
   b. Begin the HBV vaccine series
   c. Initiate lamivudine
   d. Offer HBV screening

Answers a and b are correct. The CDC recommends initiating the HBV vaccine series and giving HBIG as postexposure prophylaxis for HBV in both individuals.

Answer d is correct. LO can be offered screening to determine if she has been exposed to HBV infection. This should be done before considering any treatment.

Answer c is incorrect. Neither of these alone represents the *best* option for postexposure prophylaxis to HBV.

---

7. Which of the following signs and symptoms may LO experience if she develops HBV? Select all that apply.

   a. Jaundice
   b. Nausea
   c. Elevated liver enzymes
   d. She may experience no physical symptoms

Answers a, b, c, and d are correct. Viral hepatitis may initially present with jaundice, nausea, and elevated liver enzymes. Some patients experience no physical symptoms.

---

8. MO is a 19-year-old Asian man diagnosed with chronic HBV acquired from perinatal exposure. He will begin therapy with entecavir today. Entecavir will likely

   a. Be combined with ribavirin
   b. Eradicate the HBV virus
   c. Develop resistance
   d. Cause minimal side effects

Answer d is correct. All of the nucleoside reverse transcriptase inhibitors are typically well tolerated with the most common adverse events being gastrointestinal in nature. This is in stark contrast to the only other drug available to treat chronic HBV (peg-interferon α-2a).

Answer a is incorrect. Ribavirin is not used in the treatment of chronic HBV. It is used to treat chronic HCV along with peg-interferon α-2a or 2b or interferon alfacon-1.

Answer b is incorrect. It is not possible to eradicate chronic HBV with the drugs currently on the market. The goal for therapy is to suppress the virus in order to prevent long-term complications of hepatocellular carcinoma or cirrhosis.

Answer c is incorrect. Entecavir has low viral resistance (<1% up to 4 years of use).

---

9. Rank the following HCV treatment regimens based on their likelihood of clinical cure (SVR) from lowest to highest cure rate. (ALL options must be used.)

Unordered Options	Ordered Response
Interferon α monotherapy	Interferon α monotherapy
Peg-interferon α-2b, ribavirin, and telaprevir	Peg-interferon α-2b and ribavirin
Peg-interferon α-2b and ribavirin	Peg-interferon α-2b, ribavirin, and telaprevir
Sofosbuvir/velpatasvir	Sofosbuvir/velpatasvir

---

10. Immune globulin (GamaSTAN) is indicated for postexposure prophylaxis for which of the following?

   a. Autoimmune hepatitis
   b. Hepatitis A virus
   c. Hepatitis B virus
   d. Hepatitis C virus

Answer b is correct. Immune globulin (GamaSTAN) is used to provide passive immunity in susceptible individuals under the following circumstances: Hepatitis A, Measles, Varicella, Rubella, and Immunoglobulin deficiency.

Answer a is incorrect. Autoimmune hepatitis is not acquired from people or the environment but is instead an autoimmune disease.

Answer c is incorrect. The only immune globulin formulated for HBV exposure is the hepatitis B immune globulin (HBIG).

Answer d is incorrect. There are no products in the market that provide passive immunity to HCV.

---

11. Which of the following drugs has the highest incidence of hemolytic anemia?

   a. Ribavirin
   b. Peg-interferon α-2a
   c. Lamivudine
   d. Tenofovir

Answer a is correct. The incidence of hemolytic anemia for ribavirin is 10% to 13%. The FDA requires a black box warning regarding this risk in the package insert.

Answers b, c, and d are incorrect. While peg-interferon α-2a, lamivudine, and tenofovir are associated with anemia, they do not cause hemolytic anemia.

---

12. DP is a 42-year-old woman who has developed chronic HBV from longstanding intravenous drug use. Her physician asks you to recommend an NRTI that has both high potency and low viral resistance. Rank the following HBV treatment regimens from best to worse choice. (ALL options must be used.)

Unordered Options	Ordered Response
Telbivudine	Lamivudine
Lamivudine	Telbivudine
Entecavir	Adefovir
Adefovir	Entecavir

---

13. A 54-year-old man with HCV genotype 2 infection, treatment-naive, and no cirrhosis presents for treatment initiation. Which of the following would be the best treatment option?

    a. Peg-interferon and ribavirin for 24 weeks
    b. Peg-interferon and ribavirin for 48 weeks
    c. Glecaprevir/pibretansvir for 8 weeks
    d. Sofosbuvir and ribavirin for 24 weeks

Answer c is correct. Treatment-naive, non-cirrhotic patients with genotype 2 infection can be treated with 8 weeks of glecaprevir/pibrentasvir. In clinical trials, this regimen cured HCV infection in 99% of genotype 2, treatment-naive patients.

Answers a and b are incorrect. Peg-interferon and ribavirin regimens are no longer recommended due to the availability of more effective treatments with fewer side effects.

Answer d is incorrect. Sofosbuvir and ribavirin for 24 weeks was a previously recommended regimen effective in approximately 90% of patients. However, it has been replaced in the guidelines to more effective regimens with fewer side effects.

---

14. RM is a man who has just learned he is coinfected with HIV/HCV. When should RM's chronic HCV be treated?

    a. Immediately.
    b. As soon as his HIV is well controlled with medication.
    c. Never. His HCV is not treatable.
    d. After he develops decompensated cirrhosis.

Answer b is correct. RM should wait until his HIV is well controlled with medications to increase his likelihood of response.

Answer a is incorrect. RM should wait until his HIV is well controlled with medications.

Answer c is incorrect. It is possible to treat his chronic HCV, and new regimens are as effective in HIV/HCV co-infection as with HCV mono-infection.

Answer d is incorrect. Patients who have more extensive liver disease are more difficult to cure of HCV. Whenever possible, treatment should be initiated early before further liver disease progression.

---

15. DA has been diagnosed with chronic HCV genotype 1. His past medical and social histories include a history of IV drug abuse, alcoholism, a wife (married 30 years) with chronic HCV, and a blood transfusion in 2002. During your patient counseling session, DA asks you how he most likely acquired HCV. You correctly tell him.

    a. Blood transfusion in 2002
    b. Sexually transmitted from his wife
    c. Intravenous drug abuse
    d. Alcoholism

Answer c is correct. Contact with blood contaminated with the HCV virus is the most common route of transmission with intravenous drug use being the number one method of transmission.

Answer a is incorrect. After 1992, blood banks began screening blood for HCV; his risk for acquiring HCV from his blood transfusion in 2002 is extremely low.

Answer b is incorrect. Transmission of HCV from one monogamous heterosexual partner to another is extremely low. In fact, it is not necessary for HCV patients to wear a condom to protect the partner *unless* they are on peg-interferon and ribavirin treatment, since the risk of spreading via sexual contact is very low.

Answer d is incorrect. Chronic alcohol use and untreated chronic HCV can both lead to cirrhosis but alcoholism does increase the susceptibility of acquiring HCV.

---

16. BR is a 47-year-old woman coinfected with HBV and HIV. The physician wants to prescribe a nucleoside reverse transcriptase inhibitor (NRTI) monotherapy to treat BR's chronic HBV. Which of the following NRTIs should you recommend?

    a. Lamivudine
    b. Entecavir
    c. Telbivudine
    d. Tenofovir

Answer c is correct. The only drug that does not result in HIV resistance is telbivudine. It is therefore the only NRTI that can be safely used as monotherapy in patients coinfected with HIV.

Answers a, b, and d are incorrect. because each drug is associated with the development of HIV resistance.

---

17. Which of the following drugs has been given a black box warning by the FDA for the risk of severe depression and suicidal risk?

    a. Ribavirin
    b. Peg-interferons

c. Nucleoside reverse transcriptase inhibitors
d. Hepatitis B immune globulin (HBIG)

Answer b is correct.   Peg-interferon as well as all forms of interferon is associated with severe depression and a risk of suicidal and homicidal thoughts. Patients should be educated and monitored for this risk.

Answers a, c, and d are incorrect.   Ribavirin, NRTIs, and HBIG are not associated with a high incidence of severe depression and suicidal risk.

18. Which of the following products should not be given concomitantly with live vaccines?

   a. Engerix-B
   b. Recombivax HB
   c. Twinrix
   d. GamaSTAN

Answer d is correct.   GamaSTAN is an immune globulin that stimulates the immune system. A live vaccine contains weakened live virus that can become virulent if given concomitantly with an immune globulin product.

Answers a, b, and c are incorrect.   The HAV, HBV, and HAV/HBV combination vaccines are safe to give with both live and inactivated vaccines.

19. MM, a 21-year-old woman, has been exposed to hepatitis C. Which of the following is the most appropriate course of action?

   a. Do nothing unless MM acquires hepatitis C.
   b. Administer immune globulin.
   c. Begin peg-interferon and ribavirin.
   d. Begin lamivudine.

Answer a is correct.   There is no postexposure prophylaxis available for HCV exposure (no vaccine and no immune globulin). Some patients will clear the virus on their own. If acute HCV develops, treatment is usually deferred for 3 to 6 months to see if this will occur before proceeding to antiviral treatment.

Answer b is incorrect.   There is no immune globulin for postexposure prophylaxis of HCV.

Answer c is incorrect.   Peg-interferon and ribavirin are no longer recommended for treatment of chronic infection. If the decision to treat acute infection is made, it would be with a newer oral regimen (see Tables 44-3 and 44-4).

Answer d is incorrect.   Lamivudine is a nucleotide reverse transcriptase inhibitor indicated for the treatment of chronic HBV. It has no action against HCV.

20. TO is a 42-year-old patient prescribed lamivudine for HBV. Which of the following products contain lamivudine and may be used for HBV in TO?

   a. Viread
   b. Combivir

   c. Epivir
   d. Emtriva

Answer c is correct.   Lamivudine (Epivir) may be used for the management of HBV. However, lamivudine is plagued with a high incidence of viral resistance and cross-resistance.

Answer a is incorrect.   Viread is tenofovir (although tenofovir can be used for HBV).

Answer b is incorrect.   Combivir is a combination product containing zidovudine and lamivudine. This product is used in combination with a non-nucleoside inhibitor, protease inhibitor, or integrase strand inhibitor to manage HIV. However, if a patient is coinfected with HIV and HBV—then combivir could be utilized. TO cannot receive Combivir because he is HBV only.

Answer d is incorrect.   Emtricitabine (Emtriva) is an NRTI similar to lamivudine.

CHAPTER 45 | **Chronic Obstructive Pulmonary Disease**

1. A patient presents with symptoms of shortness of breath, nonproductive cough, and the following spirometry results: prebronchodilator FEV_1: 69% predicted; postbronchodilator FEV_1: 70% predicted; FEV_1/FVC ratio: 0.64. How would you interpret these findings?

   a. This patient has COPD with reversible airway obstruction.
   b. This patient has COPD with irreversible airway obstruction.
   c. This patient has asthma with reversible airway obstruction.
   d. This patient does not have asthma since the airway obstruction is irreversible.
   e. This patient does not have COPD or asthma.

Answer b is correct.   This patient does have COPD, which is irreversible since the predicted FEV_1 did not change with administration of a bronchodilator.

Answer a is incorrect.   This patient does have COPD (an *irreversible* condition), and it is not reversible since the predicted FEV_1 did not change with administration of a bronchodilator.

Answer c is incorrect.   This patient does not have asthma, since airway obstruction in this patient was irreversible (demonstrated by the lack of change in FEV_1 post-bronchodilator).

Answer d is incorrect.   This patient does not have asthma, since airway obstruction is reversible.

Answer e is incorrect.   This patient does have COPD; patient has a FEV_1/FVC ratio less than 0.7.

2. AB is a 41-year-old white male with COPD confirmed by spirometry. His physician would like to test him for alpha

1 antitrypsin (AAT) deficiency. Which of the following characterizes this disease? Select ALL that apply.

a. Onset at an early age (<50 years)
b. Disease caused by environmental factors
c. Disease caused by genetic factors
d. Prominent in African American populations
e. Disease caused by oxidative stress

Answer a is correct. Alpha 1 antitrypsin deficiency presents at an *early* age (20-50 years).

Answer c is correct. Alpha 1 antitrypsin deficiency is a *genetic* disorder.

Answer b is incorrect. Alpha 1 antitrypsin deficiency is caused by *genetic* factors, not environmental.

Answer d is incorrect. Alpha 1 antitrypsin deficiency is prominent in those of Northern European descent.

Answer e is incorrect. Alpha 1 antitrypsin deficiency is a genetic disorder.

3. AF is a 59-year-old African American male who currently smokes and has recently been diagnosed with COPD. He currently is classified by the Global Initiative for Chronic Obstructive Lung Disease (GOLD) guidelines as patient group A. Which of the following would be recommended as the first-line treatment for AF?

a. Short-acting bronchodilator
b. Long-acting anticholinergic
c. Long-acting β-agonist
d. Inhaled corticosteroid
e. Oral theophylline

Answer a is correct. According to the GOLD guidelines, a short-acting bronchodilator PRN should be given to those in patient group A. An example of the short-acting bronchodilator would be albuterol or levalbuterol. These β$_2$-agonists are similar in mechanism and dosing. Along with the short-acting bronchodilator should be a spacer.

Note: All patients should utilize a spacer device or valved holding chamber when using a metered-dose inhaler; in addition, face masks should be used in children less than 4 years of age.

Answer b is incorrect. A long-acting anticholinergic (tiotropium) can be added in patient group B. Ipratropium (Atrovent) is a short-acting anticholinergic and is often used in the early stages of COPD. Ipratropium is often combined with albuterol and is coformulated with albuterol (Combivent).

Answer c is incorrect. A long-acting β-agonist (salmeterol or formoterol) can be added in patient group B.

Answer d is incorrect. Inhaled corticosteroids are recommended in patient group C. In symptomatic patients with severe COPD (FEV$_1$ <50% predicted) and frequent exacerbations, regular treatment with *inhaled* corticosteroids

decreases the number of exacerbations per year and improves health status; however, corticosteroid therapy does not slow the long-term decline in pulmonary function.

Answer e is incorrect. Theophylline is often the last agent prescribed in COPD patients (after the β$_2$-agonists, anticholinergic, and inhaled corticosteroid). Theophylline has a narrow-therapeutic index and requires close monitoring due to the pharmacokinetic considerations.

4. BD is a 59-year-old man with COPD, hypertension, and dyslipidemia. He reports to your pharmacy complaining of developing a tremor since starting one of his medications. Which medication is the most likely cause?

a. Ipratropium
b. Tiotropium
c. Fluticasone
d. Prednisone
e. Albuterol

Answer e is correct. Tremor is a common side effect of β-agonists. Other common effects include tachycardia and central nervous system stimulation/excitation.

Answer a is incorrect. Tremor is not a side effect of inhaled anticholinergics.

Answer b is incorrect. Tremor is not a side effect of inhaled anticholinergics.

Answer c is incorrect. Tremor is not a side effect of inhaled corticosteroids.

Answer d is incorrect. Tremor is not a side effect of oral corticosteroids.

5. ZH is a 59-year-old with COPD who was recently prescribed a fluticasone inhaler for COPD. He is concerned about the side effects of inhaled corticosteroids and you conduct inhaler counseling for him. Which of the following is the most likely side effect to be caused by inhaled corticosteroids?

a. Oral candidiasis
b. Glucose intolerance
c. Tachycardia
d. Immunosuppression
e. Weight gain

Answer a is correct. Inhaled corticosteroids can cause candidiasis of the mouth and/or throat.

Answer b is incorrect. Long-term systemic (not inhaled) corticosteroids can cause glucose intolerance.

Answer c is incorrect. Inhaled β$_2$-agonists can cause tachycardia.

Answer d is incorrect. Long-term systemic (not inhaled) corticosteroids can cause immunosuppression.

Answer e is incorrect. Long-term systemic (not inhaled) corticosteroids can cause weight gain.

6. Which of the following are advantages of using a spacer device with a metered-dose inhaler? Select all that apply.

   a. Decreased oropharyngeal deposition
   b. Enhanced lung delivery
   c. Less hand-lung coordination needed
   d. Reduced side effects from inhaled corticosteroids

Answers a, b, c, and d are correct. Spacer devices decrease oropharyngeal deposition, enhance lung delivery, require less hand-lung coordination, and reduce the side-effects from inhaled corticosteroids (thrush, hoarseness).

7. SS is a 68-year-old woman who smokes and has recently been diagnosed with COPD. In addition to a short-acting bronchodilator, what would you recommend for her treatment? Select all that apply.

   a. Smoking cessation
   b. Influenza vaccine yearly
   c. Pneumococcal vaccine
   d. Oxygen therapy

Answers a, b, and c are correct. Smoking cessation and influenza and pneumococcal vaccinations are recommended for all COPD patients, regardless of stage or symptoms

Answer d is incorrect. Oxygen therapy is added in late, very severe COPD.

8. The clinical presentation of COPD can include which of the following? Select all that apply.

   a. Dyspnea
   b. Chronic cough
   c. Sputum production
   d. Exposure to risk factors

Answers a, b, c, and d are correct. Dyspnea and chronic cough are common in the presentation of COPD. Sputum production is common especially in COPD patients with chronic bronchitis. The most common risk factor is smoking, followed by air pollution.

9. CP is a 65-year-old man with COPD, classified by the GOLD guidelines as patient group C. He is currently using albuterol inhaler PRN, salmeterol inhaler twice a day, and tiotropium inhaler once a day. His COPD is still uncontrolled with frequent symptoms and a recent exacerbation. What recommendations would you make to his medication regimen?

   a. Add theophylline once daily.
   b. Change salmeterol inhaler to fluticasone/salmeterol combination inhaler scheduled twice a day.
   c. Add an oral corticosteroid once daily.

   d. Change tiotropium inhaler to ipratropium inhaler scheduled four times a day.
   e. Do not make any changes.

Answer b is correct. Inhaled corticosteroids are recommended for patients in patient group C. In COPD patients with FEV_1 less than 60% predicted regular treatment with *inhaled* corticosteroids improves symptoms, lung function, quality of life, and decreases the number of exacerbations. Combination therapy with an inhaled corticosteroid and long-acting β agonist is more effective than either component alone. This combination also has been shown to be beneficial in addition to tiotropium.

Answer a incorrect. Theophylline is less effective and less well tolerated than other options.

Answer c is incorrect. Oral corticosteroids should only be used during exacerbation and should not be recommended for long-term treatment.

Answer d is incorrect. Ipratropium is much shorter acting and less effective than tiotropium and the dosing would be inconvenient for the patient.

Answer e is incorrect. The patient is uncontrolled so a medication change should be made.

10. PL is a 75-year-old man who has been experiencing increased dyspnea for the last month. He was diagnosed with COPD 3 years ago and has been taking albuterol metered-dose inhaler on an as needed (prn) basis. He has not had any exacerbations within the last year, and he has an mMRC score of 2. Which of the following is the best choice for changing his medication regimen?

   a. Add scheduled inhaled tiotropium and continue prn albuterol.
   b. Add scheduled inhaled fluticasone and continue prn albuterol.
   c. Add prn inhaled salmeterol and continue prn albuterol.
   d. Add scheduled oral theophylline and continue prn albuterol.
   e. No changes are necessary at this time.

Answer a is correct. The patient is in patient group B since he has had less than or equal to 1 exacerbation/year, and his mMRC is more than or equal to 2. The guidelines recommend adding regular treatment with one or more long-acting bronchodilators.

Answer b is incorrect. Inhaled corticosteroids are only recommended in patient group C.

Answer c is incorrect. Salmeterol could be added in patient group B as a long-acting bronchodilator, but it should be scheduled, not prn.

Answer d is incorrect. Theophylline can be considered patient group C.

Answer e is incorrect. The patient is symptomatic and in patient group B and therefore, needs additional medication.

11. Select the COPD medications that can be used concurrently in a maintenance regimen for a patient classified by the GOLD guidelines as patient group C.

    a. Levalbuterol and albuterol
    b. Albuterol and formoterol
    c. Formoterol and salmeterol
    d. Fluticasone and mometasone
    e. Theophylline and aminophylline

Answer b is correct. Albuterol is a short-acting β_2-agonist and formoterol is a long-acting β_2-agonist. Even though these medications have a similar mechanism of action (β_2-agonists), they can be used concurrently.

Answer a is incorrect. Levalbuterol and albuterol are both short-acting β_2-agonists. A rule of thumb for combination therapy is to use medications with a different mechanism of action.

Answer c is incorrect. Salmeterol and formoterol are long-acting β_2-agonists and because they work the same, would not be recommended for concurrent therapy. A rule of thumb for combination therapy is to use medications with a different mechanism of action.

Answer d is incorrect. Fluticasone and flunisolide are inhaled corticosteroids. Concurrent therapy with inhaled corticosteroids is not recommended (same mechanism of action).

Answer e is incorrect. The methylxanthines, theophylline, and aminophylline would not be used concurrently. Aminophylline is a salt formulation of theophylline. Aminophylline is the methylxanthine that is used intravenously and theophylline is the methylxanthine used orally.

12. Select the disease state or factor that can affect the clearance of theophylline. Select all that apply.

    a. Smoking history
    b. Hepatic cirrhosis
    c. Drug interactions (cytochrome P-450 inhibitors especially 1A2, 2E1, 3A4)
    d. Occasional alcohol use

Answer a is correct. Cigarette smokers have a theophylline clearance about 1.5 to 2 times that of nonsmokers. The effects of smoking (one pack of cigarettes per day) appear to last several months after the cigarettes have been discontinued. Therefore, patients admitted to the hospital with a recent history of smoking should be considered smokers throughout their hospitalization, even if they refrain from smoking during hospitalization.

Answer b is correct. Theophylline is eliminated hepatically. Therefore, hepatic damage will decrease theophylline clearance and leads to elevated levels.

Answer c is correct. Theophylline is a substrate of the cytochrome P-450 system (1A2—major; 2C9—minor; 2D6—minor; 2E1—major; 3A4—major). Therefore, medications that inhibit these CYP enzymes (especially the major pathways—1A2; 2E1; and 3A4) will decrease the elimination/metabolism of theophylline leading to increase in theophylline levels. Macrolide antibiotics (erythromycin and clarithromycin) decrease the clearance of theophylline by as much as 25% to 50%. Phenytoin and Phenobarbital increase the clearance of theophylline by as much as 30% to 50%. Cimetidine appears to reduce the clearance of theophylline by as much as 40%. Rifampin can increase theophylline clearance/metabolism by 20% to 25%. Unfortunately, the predictability of clearance changes secondary to the addition of these drugs is poor indicating that while some change may be expected, each patient will need to be evaluated individually. Please refer to a drug interaction reference to review the numerous agents that interact with theophylline.

Answer d is incorrect. Alcohol does not affect the clearance of theophylline.

13. Select the formulation of the corticosteroid that should be utilized in maintenance therapy for COPD.

    a. IV/injection (methylprednisolone)
    b. Oral (prednisone)
    c. Inhalation (fluticasone)
    d. Nasal (fluticasone)

Answer c is correct. Inhalation is the preferred formulation/dosage route for maintenance therapy with COPD. This method minimizes adverse reactions.

Answer a is incorrect. IV medications are not ideal for the maintenance therapy of any disease state. Also, because of the adverse reactions of systemic therapy with corticosteroids, maintenance therapy is not recommended with systemic corticosteroids. Methylprednisolone could be utilized for exacerbations of COPD.

Answer b is incorrect. Because of the numerous adverse reactions associated with systemic oral corticosteroids (prednisone), maintenance therapy is not recommended. Prednisone could be utilized for exacerbations of COPD.

Answer d is incorrect. Nasal preparations are used for allergic rhinitis.

14. BD is a 59-year-old Caucasian man with advanced COPD who has been hospitalized with an acute exacerbation. He has been receiving IV aminophylline. His current aminophylline level is 22 mcg/mL. What adverse events would be possible at this level? Select all that apply.

    a. Hypotension
    b. Arrhythmias
    c. Nausea and vomiting
    d. Seizures

Answer a is correct. Hypotension is a cardiac side effect of theophylline and usually occurs when patients have exceeded the concentration range of theophylline (>20 mcg/mL).

Answer b is correct. Arrhythmias are cardiac side effects of theophylline and usually occur when patients have exceeded the concentration range of theophylline (>20 mcg/mL).

Answer c is correct. Nausea and vomiting are gastrointestinal side effects of theophylline. Gastrointestinal side effects may occur when theophylline levels are within the therapeutic range (<20 mcg/mL) and they may also occur when levels are outside the therapeutic range (>20 mcg/mL). Gastrointestinal side effects outside the therapeutic range are often repetitive and persistent.

Answer d is correct. Seizures are the central nervous system side effect that most commonly occur when patients have supra-therapeutic theophylline levels. Other central nervous system side effects (occurring within therapeutic range) are: headache, hyperactivity (children), insomnia, and restlessness.

---

15. PW is a 49-year-old Caucasian female recently diagnosed with COPD. Her physician plans to start her on a short-acting bronchodilator. Which of the following would be appropriate for the treatment of COPD? Select all that apply.

    a. Albuterol inhalation (metered-dose inhaler—90 mcg/puff) as needed "rescue" (prn)
    b. Levalbuterol inhalation (metered-dose inhaler—90 mcg/puff) as needed "rescue" (prn)
    c. Albuterol oral 4 mg tid
    d. Ipratropium inhalation (metered-dose inhaler—17 mcg/puff) as needed "rescue" (prn)

Answer a is correct. A short-acting β-agonist PRN is recommended first line by the GOLD guidelines for those in patient group A.

Answer b is correct. A short-acting β-agonist PRN is recommended first line by the GOLD guidelines for those in patient group A. Levalbuterol may cause less side effects than albuterol, but is significantly more expensive.

Answer d is correct. A short-acting anticholinergic PRN is recommended first line by the GOLD guidelines for those in patient group A.

Answer c is incorrect. Systemic albuterol is not preferred for COPD treatment. Inhalation treatment is the preferred method for treatment of COPD.

---

16. AZ is a 67-year-old white male who is receiving 32 mg/h of aminophylline in the hospital. He is ready to be changed to oral theophylline. What would the daily dose of theophylline be that would equal 32 mg/h of aminophylline? Aminophylline's salt factor is 0.8.

    a. 614 mg
    b. 768 mg
    c. 300 mg
    d. 900 mg

Answer a is correct. 32 mg/h of aminophylline would equal a daily theophylline dose of 614 mg. 32 mg/h × 24 h = 768 mg of aminophylline in a daily dose. Multiply by the aminophylline salt factor (0.8) to get the daily dose of theophylline equal to 614.4.

Answers b, c, and d are incorrect. 768 mg is the daily dose of aminophylline.

---

17. Select the generic name of Symbicort.

    a. Fluticasone + salmeterol
    b. Albuterol + ipratropium
    c. Budesonide + formoterol
    d. Mometasone + formoterol

Answer c is correct. The brand name of budesonide + formoterol is Symbicort.

Answer a is incorrect. The brand name of fluticasone + salmeterol is Advair.

Answer b is incorrect. The brand name of albuterol + ipratropium is Combivent.

Answer d is incorrect. The brand name of mometasone + formoterol is Dulera

---

18. KT is a patient that presents to your clinic on Theo-24 (a sustained release/once a day theophylline product). She has experienced the dose-dumping effect when the agent is taken with a high-fat meal. She would like to be changed to another sustained release theophylline product that does not have the dose-dumping effect. Which of the following oral products can be used in replace of Theo-24? Select all that apply.

    a. Theo-Dur twice daily
    b. Slo-Bid twice daily
    c. Uniphyl once daily
    d. Aminophylline drip

Answer a is correct. Theo-Dur is a sustained-release formulation that does not appear to be associated with dose-dumping. Be cautious—just because a product is labeled as sustained release that does not mean it will be dosed once a day. Sometimes, sustained- or extended-release products will be dosed twice daily.

Answer b is correct. Slo-Bid is a sustained-release formulation that does not appear to be associated with dose-dumping. Be cautious—just because a product is labeled as sustained release that does not mean it will be dosed once a day. Sometimes, sustained- or extended-release products will be dosed twice daily.

Answer c is correct. Uniphyl is a sustained-release product that is taken once daily. While no dose-dumping was observed following ingestion of Uniphyl with a high-fat meal, a change in the rate of absorption was apparent. For this reason, clinicians often use the sustained released theophylline products that are dosed twice daily more often.

A large number of sustained-release dosage forms of theophylline have been marketed. These products are designed to release theophylline slowly so that patients who metabolize the drug rapidly (children and smokers) can maintain theophylline-plasma concentrations within the therapeutic range. Most of these drugs products are completely absorbed; however, there are major differences between these products with regard to duration of absorption. Some of the dosage forms are absorbed over 3 to 4 hours, while others are absorbed over 8 to 12 hours. Nevertheless, as the duration of absorption increases, the possibility of incomplete bioavailability increases because the duration of absorption begins to exceed the gastrointestinal transit time. Therefore, when switching theophylline products/dosage forms caution must be taken and pharmacokinetic considerations taken into account.

Answer d is incorrect. Aminophylline is the parenteral salt form of theophylline that is used to manage COPD exacerbations.

19. Select the COPD medication that is a phosphodiesterase inhibitor.

    a. Albuterol
    b. Salmeterol
    c. Ipratropium
    d. Fluticasone
    e. Roflumilast

Answer e is correct. Roflumilast is a phsopodiesterase-4 inhibitor approved for COPD.

Answer a is incorrect. Albuterol increases cAMP, thereby relaxing bronchial smooth muscle.

Answer b is incorrect. Salmeterol increases cAMP, thereby relaxing bronchial smooth muscle.

Answer c is incorrect. Ipratropium blocks the action of acetylcholine at the parasympathetic sites in bronchial smooth muscle causing bronchodilation.

Answer d is incorrect. Fluticasone is a corticosteroid and has anti-inflammatory properties.

20. AB is a 60-year-old woman recently discharged from the hospital following an exacerbation of her COPD. She was prescribed Advair, Spiriva, and Daliresp. She also has albuterol for prn use. She complains of nausea and weight loss when she is picking up her refills and wants to know if one of these medications could be responsible. Which of the medications is most likely to cause these effects?

    a. Advair (fluticasone/salmeterol)
    b. Daliresp (roflumilast)
    c. Spiriva (tiotropium)
    d. Proair (albuterol)

Answer b is correct. The most common adverse effects of roflumilast are gastrointestinal effects (nausea, diarrhea) and weight loss.

Answer a is incorrect. The most common adverse effects associated with ICS are thrush and hoarseness. The most common adverse effect of LABAs is anxiety.

Answer c is incorrect. The most common adverse effect associated with tiotropium is dry mouth.

Answer d is incorrect. The most common adverse effect associated with albuterol is anxiety and tremor.

CHAPTER 46 | Asthma

1. Select the statement(s) that most accurately characterizes asthma. Select all that apply.

    a. Airway inflammation
    b. Esophageal hyperresponsiveness
    c. Adrenal inflammation
    d. Bronchial hyperresponsiveness

Answer a is correct. The major characteristics of asthma are airway inflammation and bronchial hyperresponsiveness which cause variable degree of airflow obstruction.

Answer d is correct. The major characteristics of asthma are airway inflammation and bronchial hyperresponsiveness which cause variable degree of airflow obstruction.

Answer b is incorrect. Esophageal hyperresponsiveness due to acid reflux may be a precipitating factor for asthma that is not well controlled; however, is not a major characteristic.

Answer c is incorrect. Adrenal inflammation is not part of the pathophysiological process of asthma but suppression may occur when oral or high dose steroids are used.

2. Select the mechanism(s) for development of asthma. Select all that apply.

    a. Ectopy
    b. Activation of natural killer cells
    c. Atopy
    d. Exposure to environmental triggers

Answer c is correct. In the asthmatic response, a genetically predisposed or atopic individual is exposed to a specific reactive stimuli or trigger.

Answer d is correct. In the asthmatic response, a genetically predisposed or atopic individual is exposed to a specific reactive stimuli or trigger.

Answer a is incorrect.   Ectopy does not play a role in asthma development.

Answer b is incorrect.   Natural killer cells do not play a role in asthma development.

The following text pertains to questions 3 and 4.

JB is started on fluticasone 220 mcg MDI 2 puffs bid, albuterol MDI 2 puff q4-6 hour prn cough, montelukast 10 mg 1 tablet at bedtime and lortadine 10 mg daily. Patient returns 1 month later with dysphonia and was recently treated for thrush.

3. Which medication is most likely to cause the patients current side effects?

    a. Fluticasone
    b. Loratadine
    c. Montelukast
    d. Albuterol

Answer a is correct.   The most common side effects of low to medium dose-ICSs are thrush and dysphonia.

Answer b is incorrect.   Second generation antihistamine do not cause thrush or dysphonia.

Answer c is incorrect.   Leukotriene modifiers do not cause thrush or dysphonia.

Answer d is incorrect.   Short acting β-agonist do not cause thrush or dysphonia.

4. What intervention(s) can the pharmacist recommend to manage or prevent JB current side effects? Select all that apply.

    a. Rinse and spit with water after use
    b. Inhale medication quickly
    c. Use a spacer or holding chamber
    d. Rinse inhaler sleeve after use

Answer a is correct.   Rinsing and spitting with water decrease upper airway deposition of medication thus decreasing side effects.

Answer c is correct.   Spacer/holding chambers allow larger drug particle to fall out in the device verse the oral cavity thus decreasing potential side effects.

Answer b is incorrect.   Inhaling quickly will not minimize oral medication deposition and prevents the delivery of a therapeutic dose.

Answer d is incorrect.   Rinsing inhaler sleeve may help with delivery of medication. It will not minimize or prevent side effects.

5. AJ is a 5 year old who has been experiencing daytime rhinorrhea, nighttime cough that woke him two times this past week, enuresis two times in the past months, and has a history of

reflux. Which symptom is most likely to warrant a work up for asthma?

    a. Rhinorrhea
    b. Cough
    c. Reflux
    d. Enuresis

Answer b is correct.   Although wheezing is considered one of the classic symptoms of asthma, nighttime cough has been shown to be a common symptom requiring further work up for asthma.

Answer a is incorrect.   Rhinorrhea is upper airway symptom and may contribute to poor asthma control; however, it does not warrant a work up for asthma.

Answer c is incorrect.   Reflux may play a role in asthma that does not respond to treatment; however, it is not a symptom that leads to the work up for asthma.

Answer d is incorrect.   There has been no correlation between asthma and enuresis.

6. What is the preferred treatment for an 18-year-old man with off and on chest tightness that occurred 4 days this past week with no nocturnal awakening, $FEV_1/FVC = 83\%$, and $FEV_1 = 75\%$? Select all that apply.

    a. Scheduled low-dose ICS
    b. Scheduled medium-dose ICS
    c. Schedule low-dose ICS and LABA
    d. Short-acting β-agonist as needed

Answer b is correct.   Therapy is always recommended based on the most severe presenting sign or symptom. In the case, the FEV1/FVC and FEV1 is in the moderate persistent category. Preferred treatment is ICS + LABA or medium dose ICS.

Answer c is correct.   Therapy is always recommended based on the most severe presenting sign or symptom. In the case, the FEV1/FVC and FEV1 is in the moderate persistent category. Preferred treatment is ICS + LABA or medium dose ICS.

Answer d is correct.   All patient with asthma regardless of severity require as need short acting β-agonist for acute symptoms.

Answer a is incorrect.   Treatment of mild persistent asthma not moderate persistent asthma.

7. You are providing follow-up education for a 3-year-old child with asthma who in the last month is scheduling their AccuNeb 1.25 mg tid for symptoms. Parents indicate that he wakes up at least once a night due to cough.

What is/are the best treatment option(s) given the patients current asthma control? Select all that apply.

    a. Continue current treatment
    b. Step up one step

c. Step down one step
d. Oral steroid burst

Answer b is correct. Patient is using SABA several times per day with night awakening greater than one time per week which is indicative of very poorly controlled asthma requiring step up treatment.

Answer d is correct. An oral steroid burst will quickly suppress excessive lung inflammation due to very poorly controlled asthma.

Answer a is incorrect. Symptom presents and mediation used not consistent with well control.

Answer c is incorrect. Symptom presents and mediation used not consistent with well control.

8. CM is started on fluticasone/salmeterol DPI 100/50 mcg 1 puff bid. She returns for a follow-up visit with minimal improvement of symptoms and an FEV1 of 70% indicating not well-controlled asthma. After assessing environmental control and medication adherence, what additional factor should be addressed prior to stepping up her asthma therapy?

a. Inhaler technique assessment for slow deep inhale
b. Albuterol use in the last month
c. Adherence to morning and evening peak flows
d. Inhaler technique assessment for forceful deep inhale

Answer d is correct. Prior to stepping up therapy adherence, environment and inhaler technique are assessed and in this case when assessing DPI technique a forceful deep inhale should be observed to maximize medication deposition to the lungs.

Answer a is incorrect. Although assessment of inhaler technique is correct, DPIs require a forceful deep inhale.

Answer b is incorrect. Albuterol use is assessed initially in the assessment of control not after step-up therapy is being considered.

Answer c is incorrect. Peak flow are used to monitor disease and are used initially in the assessment of control, however, not after step up therapy is being considered.

9. Which medication(s) are available as an MDI and nebulization? Select all that apply.

a. Albuterol
b. Fluticasone
c. Levalbuterol
d. Budesonide

Answer a is correct. Albuterol is commercially available as a nebulizer and meter dose inhaler.

Answer c is correct. Levalbuterol is available as a meter dose inhaler and nebulization.

Answer b is incorrect. Fluticasone is available as a DPI and meter dose inhaler.

Answer d is incorrect. Budesonide is available as a DPI and nebulization.

10. Select the brand name for levalbuterol.

a. Serevent
b. Flovent
c. Xolair
d. Xopenex

Answer d is correct. Brand name of levalbuterol.

Answer a is incorrect. Brand name of salmeterol.

Answer b is incorrect. Brand name of fluticasone.

Answer c is incorrect. Brand name of omalizumab.

11. Rank the following corticosteroids as low, medium, or high potency for a 10 year old.

Unordered Options	Ordered Response
Beclomethasone MDI 80 mcg 2 puff bid	Medium = 320 mcg per day
Budesonide DPI 180 mcg 1 puff bid	Low = 320 mcg per day
Fluticasone MDI 110 mcg 2 puffs bid	High = 440 mcg per day
Mometasone 220 mcg 1 puff daily	Medium = 220 mcg per day

12. A 16-year-old African American patient is admitted to the hospital for an asthma exacerbation. The patient was prescribed the following medications: albuterol MDI 2 puffs prn wheezing, mometasone DPI 1 inhalation daily, fexofenadine 180 mg 1 tablet daily, and formoterol DPI 1 capsule bid. Which has demonstrated an increased risk of death when administered as monotherapy for daily control of asthma?

a. Albuterol
b. Mometasone
c. Fexofenadine
d. Formoterol

Answer d is correct. Formoterol is a long acting β-agonist. This class has a black box warning for increased risk of death if used as monotherapy for asthma.

Answer a is incorrect. Albuterol is used for relief of symptoms thus it is not recommended to be used as a controller medication.

Answer b is incorrect. Mometasone is an ICS and may be used as monotherapy to control asthma.

Answer c is incorrect. Fexofenadine is a second generation antihistamine used for allergies.

13. Despite adherence to combination high-dose ICS/LABA therapy, a patient remains symptomatic. What is a potential cause for this patient's lack of control?

    a. Polymorphism of the β-receptor (Arg/Arg or Arg/Gly combination)
    b. Over production of IgG as a result of immunotherapy
    c. Downregulation of muscarinic receptors (M3) on bronchial smooth muscle
    d. Inability of IgE to bind to Fc receptor on mast cells

Answer a is correct. Genetic variants of the β-receptor may contribute to suboptimal response to β-agonist medications.

Answer b is incorrect. The goal of immunotherapy is to stimulate a greater IgG response which in many instances improves asthma control.

Answer c is incorrect. Muscarinic receptor are stimulated by anticholinergic agent.

Answer d is incorrect. IgE inability to bind to the Fc receptor on mast cell, as when bound to Omalizumab, normally improves asthma control.

---

14. Using the diagram below, identify where omalizumab exerts its mechanism of action.

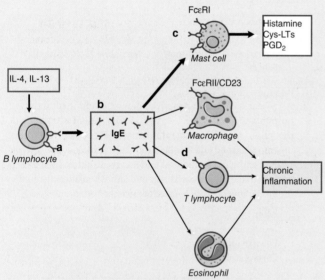

Reproduced with permission from Brunton LL, Hilal-Dandan R, Knollmann BC: *Goodman & Gilman's: The Pharmacological Basis of Therapeutics*, 13th ed. New York, NY: McGraw-Hill; 2018

Answer b is correct. Omalizumab binds to free circulating IgE preventing bind to mast cells.

Answer a is incorrect. Omalizumab has no binding affinity to lymphocytes.

Answer c is incorrect. Omalizumab has no binding affinity to mast cells.

Answer d is incorrect. Omalizumab has no binding affinity to lymphocytes.

15. What is the preferred treatment option for a 46-year-old man with the diagnosis of asthma? Current complaints are wheezing in morning that gets better as day progresses. One episode of cough in last month and has required three courses of oral steroids within the last year. Current FEV_1 = 55%.

    a. Medium-dose ICS
    b. Low-dose ICS and LABA
    c. Medium-dose ICS and LABA
    d. Theophylline

Answer c is correct. Patient is exhibiting severe persistent asthma which requires high dose step 4-6 combination therapy.

Answer a is incorrect. Patient is exhibiting severe persistent asthma which requires high dose step 4-6 combination therapy.

Answer b is incorrect. Patient is exhibiting severe persistent asthma which requires high dose step 4-6 combination therapy.

Answer d is incorrect. Patient is exhibiting severe persistent asthma which requires high dose step 4-6 combination therapy.

---

16. Select the brand name for ciclesonide.

    a. Ventolin
    b. Asmanex
    c. Pulmicort
    d. Alvesco

Answer d is correct. Alvesco is brand name of ciclesonide.

Answer a is incorrect. Ventolin is brand name of albuterol.

Answer b is incorrect. Asmanex is brand name of mometasone.

Answer c is incorrect. Pulmicort is brand name of budesonide.

---

17. What is the follow-up treatment recommendation for a 16-year-old girl currently on QVAR 80 mcg 2 puffs bid who is experiencing no limitation on activity and has not used her SABA in over 3 months?

    a. Step up therapy
    b. Step down therapy
    c. Continue current treatment
    d. Discontinue SABA

Answer b is correct. When a patient's is well controlled for at least 3 months, therapy is stepped down.

Answer a is incorrect. When a patient's is well controlled for at least three months, therapy is stepped down.

Answer c is incorrect. Patient who is well controlled would benefit from decrease in steroid dosing.

Answer d is incorrect. All persons with asthma regardless of severity require access to SABA.

---

18. Which vaccination(s) are specifically recommended for a 23-year-old person with asthma? Select all that apply.

    a. MMR
    b. Influenza
    c. Herpes Zoster
    d. PPSV

Answer b is correct. Patient with respiratory disease require annual influenza injections.

Answer d is correct. Patient with respiratory disease should have 1-2 doses in their lifetime.

Answer a is incorrect. Part of the childhood vaccination schedule.

Answer c is incorrect. Not appropriate given patient age and not specifically recommended for patient with respiratory disease.

---

19. You are counseling the parents of a 2-year-old child who will be released from the hospital with a new prescription for a medium-dose ICS. What side effect should you educate the parents about?

    a. Reduced glucose production leading to hypoglycemia
    b. Permanente growth suppression
    c. Intermitted expiratory wheezing
    d. Reduced growth over the first few years but not progressive

---

Answer d is correct. The Childhood Asthma Management Program (CAMP) trials demonstrated a reduction in growth within the first few years of inhaled steroid that is not regained in adulthood but no permeate growth suppression.

Answer a is incorrect. Medium dose ICSs do not effect glucose production, however, high dose and oral corticosteroids may increase glucose levels.

Answer b is incorrect. The CAMP trials demonstrated a reduction in growth within the first few years of inhaled steroid that is not regained in adulthood but no permeate growth suppression.

Answer c is incorrect. ICSs suppress inflammation which aids in minimization of bronchoconstriction and subsequent symptoms such as wheezing.

---

20. You are counseling a 25-year-old woman with asthma who is well controlled with Advair 250/50 mcg 1 puff bid and albuterol 2 puffs every 4 to 6 hours prn. She presents a prescription for prenatal vitamin from her initial obstetric appointment. What is the safest medication to recommend for *control* of her asthma?

    a. Albuterol 2 puffs qid
    b. Advair 250/50 1 puffs bid
    c. Alvesco 160 mcg 1 puff daily
    d. Pulmicort 90 mg 1 puff bid

Answer b is correct. In pregnancy when a patient is well controlled on a current regimen, continue treatment. If initiating controller therapy, budesonide is the only category B ICS.

Answer a is incorrect. Used for quick relief of symptom not for control.

Answer c is incorrect. In pregnancy when a patient is well controlled on a current regimen, continue treatment. If initiating controller therapy, budesonide is the only category B ICS.

Answer d is incorrect. In pregnancy when a patient is well controlled on a current regimen, continue treatment. If initiating controller therapy, budesonide is the only category B ICS.

CHAPTER 47 | Cystic Fibrosis

1. JN is a 2-year-old (8 kg) with repeat visits to her physician for pneumonia. There is a positive family history for CF. What test should be ordered in this patient to diagnose CF?

    a. Chest x-ray
    b. Sputum culture
    c. Sweat test
    d. DNA test

Answer c is correct. With repeat pneumonias and a positive family history for CF, this patient should receive a sweat test.

Answers a and b are incorrect. They are tests that would be ordered to diagnose pneumonia.

Answer d is incorrect. Most patients with CF can be diagnosed with the less expensive sweat test. If the sweat test is inconclusive then DNA testing can be used for diagnosis.

---

2. JN is diagnosed with CF and treatment for her pneumonia needs to be initiated. Which test should be ordered to guide the antibiotic selection?

    a. Sputum culture and sensitivity
    b. Chest x-ray
    c. Chest MRI
    d. Chest CAT scan

Answer a is correct. The sputum culture and sensitivity will identify the organism(s) in the lungs and will show the organism's sensitivity to antibiotics.

Answer b is incorrect. The chest x-ray and clinical symptoms are used to diagnose pneumonia in children. This test will not help guide antibiotic selection.

Answers c and d are incorrect. These tests are used to distinguish pathologic tissue, such as a tumor, from normal tissue in the body. These tests will not help guide antibiotic selection.

Questions 3 and 4 pertain to the same patient case.

3. TY is an 18-year-old patient with repeat visits for pneumonia. The patient has a past medical history for CF. Which organism would you empirically treat/target for in this patient with CF?

    a. *Burkholderia cepacia*
    b. *Pseudomonas aeruginosa*
    c. *Stenotrophomonas maltophilia*
    d. *Haemophilus influenzae*

Answer b is correct.   Empiric antibiotic therapy is usually aimed at *Pseudomonas aeruginosa* in CF patients. During the first decade of life of CF patients, *Staphylococcus aureus* and *Hemophilus influenzae* are the most common bacteria isolated from the sputum, but in the second and third decade of life, *Pseudomonas aeruginosa* is the prevalent bacteria.

Answers a and c are incorrect.   *Burkholderia cepacia* and *Stenotrophomonas maltophilia* are resistant organisms seen in CF patients later in life after exposure to many broad-spectrum antibiotics.

Answer d is incorrect.   This organism may be a copathogen but CF exacerbations are correlated with *Pseudomonas aeruginosa* density in the airways. Antibiotic treatment should be aimed at *Pseudomonas aeruginosa's* sensitivities.

4. Which combination of antibiotics would be appropriate to treat TY's pneumonia?

    a. Tobramycin and amoxicillin
    b. Tobramycin and ceftriaxone
    c. Tobraymcin and piperacillin/tazobactam
    d. Ciprofloxacin

Answer c is correct.   The treatment of *Pseudomonas aeruginosa* is double-antibiotic therapy with a synergistic combination of aminoglycoside and extended-spectrum penicillin.

Answer a is incorrect.   Oral therapy should not be initiated in a patient with CF and pneumonia. Amoxicillin is only available in an oral dosage form and does not have activity against *Pseudomonas aeruginosa*.

Answer b is incorrect.   Ceftriaxone would not have activity to treat the *Pseudomonas aeruginosa*.

Answer d is incorrect.   Ciprofloxacin is reserved for CF patients in the outpatient setting who need oral antipseudomonal therapy. Additionally, initial therapy is usually started with combination treatment.

5. CF patients are unique in respect to volume of distribution and clearance. What is expected to be needed for antibiotic doses of CF patients?

    a. CF patients may require a larger dose.
    b. CF patient may require a smaller dose.
    c. CF patients have a smaller volume of distribution.
    d. CF patients have a slower rate of clearance.

Answer a is correct.   CF patients are unique in respect to a larger volume of distribution and a faster rate of clearance. With a larger volume of distribution, patients may require larger antibiotic doses. Dosing intervals become shorter because drugs are eliminated faster. Critically ill patients may vary from their baseline function and require closer monitoring. However, as patients age, they tend to approach normal population parameters.

Answers b and c are incorrect.   With a larger volume of distribution, CF patients may require larger antibiotic doses.

Answer d is incorrect.   Dosing intervals become shorter because drugs are eliminated faster.

6. What general statement can you make regarding the initial dose of antibiotics in CF patients? Select all that apply.

    a. Higher antibiotic doses are needed in CF patients.
    b. The same doses are needed in CF patients as other patients with pneumonia.
    c. Doses vary with each patient and should be individualized.
    d. Lower antibiotic doses are needed in CF patients.

Answers a and c are correct.   CF patients are hypermetabolizers of hepatically and renally eliminated drugs. In general, higher antibiotic doses are needed for CF patients. All patients should have doses individualized based on patient specific parameters. In the CF population, those individualized doses will be higher than those in the general population.

Answer b is incorrect.   CF patients are hypermetabolizers of drugs and lower doses or usual doses would not be adequate for this population.

Answer d is incorrect.   CF patients are hypermetabolizers of hepatically and renally eliminated drugs; therefore, higher doses should be employed but via an individualized approach.

7. Give two reasons why double IV antibiotic therapy should be used to treat an acute pulmonary exacerbation caused by Pseudomonas aeruginosa.

    a. Antibiotic synergy and decreased bacterial resistance
    b. Antibiotic synergy and increased bacterial resistance
    c. Minimize side effects of the antibiotics because of using lower doses
    d. Narrower antibacterial coverage and antibiotic synergy

Answer a is correct.   The combination of an aminoglycoside and β-lactam antibiotic provides synergistic bacterial killing. The combination may also prevent resistance in the exposed bacteria.

Answer b is incorrect.   Antibiotic synergy will be achieved with double IV antibiotic therapy (assuming we select antibiotics with a different mechanism of action, for example, piperacillin and tobramycin). This double combination therapy will not increase bacterial resistance, hence it may prevent antibiotic resistance.

Answer c is incorrect. Side effects may be increased because of using multiple agents; additionally, higher doses are typically utilized.

Answer d is incorrect. Two antibiotics will not provide narrower antibiotic coverage.

8. What other therapy should be initiated along with antibiotics for an acute pulmonary exacerbation?

 a. Airway clearance (high-frequency chest wall oscillation)
 b. Pancreatic enzyme replacement therapy
 c. Vitamin replacement therapy
 d. Insulin replacement therapy

Answer a is correct. Three mainstays of pulmonary treatment in CF patients are antibiotics, anti-inflammatories, and chest physiotherapy.

Answers b and c are incorrect. These are used to treat the gastrointestinal disease in CF patients.

Answer d is incorrect. This is used in late-stage CF when cystic fibrosis related diabetes (CFRD) is present.

9. VC is a 3-year-old (36 months) patient with cystic fibrosis. VC is ready to be discharged from the Children's Hospital. She needs to be started on pancreatic enzyme replacement therapy. She eats three meals each day and has three snacks. How would you instruct VC's mother to administer her pancreatic enzyme replacement therapy?

 a. Administer the capsule whole with water.
 b. Administer the capsule whole with juice.
 c. Open the capsule and sprinkle over soft, non-alkaline food. Do not chew the beads.
 d. Open the capsule and sprinkle over soft, alkaline food. Do not chew the beads.

Answer c is correct. The beads can be sprinkled over soft food if swallowed whole and not chewed. Non-alkaline food should be used to support the enteric coating on the microspheres. Pancrelipase should be used as part of a high-calorie diet, appropriate for age and clinical status. Administer with meals or snacks and swallow whole with a generous amount of liquid. Do not crush or chew. Delayed-release capsules containing enteric-coated microspheres or microtablets may also be opened and the contents sprinkled on soft food with a low pH such as applesauce, gelatin, banana, sweet potato, baby food, or baby formula. Dairy products, such as milk, custard, and ice cream, may have a high pH and should be avoided.

Answers a, b, and d are incorrect. This would work in an older patient but **most** 3-year-old children will not be able to swallow a capsule. Water or juice would not breakdown the

enteric coating. Alkaline food should not be taken with the pancreatic enzymes.

10. How would you instruct VC's mother to monitor the effectiveness of her child's pancreatic enzyme replacement therapy?

 a. ↓ Steatorrhea, ↑ weight
 b. ↓ Steatorrhea, ↓ weight
 c. ↑ Steatorrhea, ↑ weight
 d. ↑ Steatorrhea, ↓ weight

Answer a is correct. When the pancreatic enzyme dose is correct, malabsorption will decrease and the mother will see a decrease in the fat in the stool (steatorrhea) and an increase in VC's weight.

Answer b is incorrect. The weight will increase as the malabsorption improves.

Answers c and d are incorrect. The pancreatic enzymes will improve the absorption of fat and steatorrhea will decrease.

11. What side effects would you instruct VC's mother to monitor with the pancreatic enzyme replacement therapy? Select all that apply.

 a. Soar mouth
 b. Sunburn
 c. Diaper rash
 d. Decreased appetite

Answers a and c are correct. If the microspheres are chewed the enzymes will breakdown the lining of the mouth. When too much enzyme is given, the excess comes through in the stool and produces a diaper rash on the skin.

Answer b is incorrect. Pancreatic enzymes do not produce sun sensitivity.

Answers d is incorrect. Pancreatic enzymes are not expected to decrease appetite.

12. PR is a child with cystic fibrosis. The doctors would like to administer a medicine shown to decrease the time between pulmonary infections. What would you recommend?

 a. Inhaled tobramycin
 b. Inhaled albuterol
 c. Inhaled DNAse
 d. Inhaled hypertonic saline

Answer c is correct. Inhaled DNAse has been shown to increase the time between CF exacerbations and hospitalizations.

Answer a is incorrect. Inhaled tobramycin has been shown to improve PFTs in CF patients.

Answer b is incorrect. Inhaled albuterol will improve gas exchange in a patient with an asthmatic component to their CF.

Answer d is incorrect. Inhaled hypertonic saline has been shown to slow the progression of damage in the lungs of CF patients.

---

13. If a mother has a child with CF, what is the likelihood of development of CF in other children she may have. Neither she nor her husband has been diagnosed with CF.

    a. 25%
    b. 50%
    c. 75%
    d. 100%

Answer a is correct. With recessive heterozygous (homozygous) transmission, two carriers must marry. They will have normal children (25%), asymptomatic carriers (50%), and CF children (25%).

Hh (asymptomatic carrier)	+	Hh (asymptomatic carrier)
	↓	
	↓	
1 HH (normal child) + 2 Hh (asymptomatic carriers) + 1 hh (CF child)		
25%	50%	25%

Answers b, c, and d are incorrect.

---

14. Which vitamins should be supplemented in patients with CF? Select all that apply.

    a. Vitamin B
    b. Vitamin C
    c. Vitamin D
    d. Vitamin K

Answers c and d are correct. People with cystic fibrosis have trouble absorbing fats, which means they have trouble absorbing vitamins that need fat to be absorbed—A, D, E and K. These fat-soluble vitamins are critical to normal growth and good nutrition.

Answers a and b are incorrect. People with CF also need to ensure that they get vitamins from the water-soluble group, which contains vitamin C and the B-complex vitamins.

---

15. Which anti-inflammatory therapy is recommended and safe for patients with CF?

    a. Azithromycin
    b. High-dose ibuprofen
    c. Inhaled corticosteroids
    d. Oral corticosteroids

Answer a is correct. Studies with macrolides have shown an inhibition of the neutrophil migration and a decrease in production of proinflammatory mediators. It is unclear at this point if the anti-inflammatory effects of macrolides are a combination of antimicrobial and/or immunomodulatory mechanisms of action.

Answers b, c, and d are incorrect. Steroids and non-steroidal anti-inflammatory drugs (NSAIDs) are not widely used because of long-term safety concerns. High-dose ibuprofen (20-30 mg/kg of body weight twice daily) has proven efficacious in a study where patients showed less decline in pulmonary function when compared with patients given placebo. Patients on high dose ibuprofen were able to maintain weight and had less hospital admissions. The benefits of this regimen exceed the risks of GI complications and nephrotoxicity. Despite these outcomes, less than 5% of CF patients in the United States are on this regimen.

CHAPTER **48 | Gout**

1. Which of the following is the generic name for Colcrys?

    a. Probenecid
    b. Colchicine
    c. Sulindac
    d. Febuxostat

Answer b is correct. Colchicine is the generic name for Colcrys.

Answer a is incorrect. Probenecid is the generic name for Benamid.

Answers c is incorrect. Sulindac is the generic name for Clinoril.

Answer d is incorrect. Febuxostat is the generic name for Uloric.

---

2. JJ is a patient who is receiving medication therapy management services from your pharmacy. Since he has a past medical history of gout, which of the following foods should you counsel him to avoid eating as it contains a high purine content?

    a. Liver
    b. Apple
    c. Popcorn
    d. Potatoes

Answer a is correct. Red meats, particularly organ meats, have high purine content and should be avoided in patients with gout.

Answers b, c, and d are incorrect. These foods have low purine content.

---

3. Which of the following is consistent with the typical clinical presentation of gout? Select all that apply.

    a. Commonly affects the great toe
    b. Bilateral joint involvement
    c. Rapid onset of symptoms
    d. Self-limiting pain and erythema

Answers a, c, and d are correct. Patients with gout frequently present with rapid onset of self-limiting pain and erythema, commonly involving the great toe.

Answer b is incorrect. Gout is typically a monoarthritis and is usually not characterized by bilateral joint involvement.

4. A 76-year-old woman with a 10-year history of gout presents to the clinic with painful MSU crystal deposits in her hand. Which of the following terms most accurately describes this complication of gout?

    a. Atheromas
    b. Podagra
    c. Tophi
    d. Uric acid nephrolithiasis

Answer c is correct. Tophi are painful MSU crystals which deposit in the skin and can cause tissue damage. These complications often occur in patients with long-standing hyperuricemia and chronic gout.

Answer a is incorrect. Atheroma is a lipid deposit within the arterial wall and is not related to gout.

Answer b is incorrect. Podagra is a term used to describe gout-related symptoms in the great toe.

Answer d is incorrect. Uric acid nephrolithiasis is a complication of gout characterized by MSU crystal deposits in the kidney which can contribute to renal failure.

5. A 60-year-old man presents to the pharmacy with a past medical history of hypertension and gout. After reviewing his medication profile, which of the following medications is most likely to cause elevated SUA levels?

    a. Hydrochlorothiazide
    b. Lisinopril
    c. Metoprolol
    d. Indomethacin

Answer a is correct. The antihypertensive hydrochlorothiazide can contribute to hyperuricemia, and if possible, it should be avoided in patients with gout.

Answers b and c are incorrect. These antihypertensive agents are not associated with elevated SUA levels and are good choices for many patients with gout.

Answer d is incorrect. This NSAID is used to treat pain and inflammation associated with gout, and it does not cause elevated SUA levels.

6. Which of the following is the brand name for allopurinol?

    a. Uloric
    b. Zyloprim
    c. Zebeta
    d. Benemid

Answer b is correct. Zyloprim is the brand name for allopurinol.

Answer a is incorrect. Uloric is the brand name for febuxostat.

Answer c is incorrect. Zebeta is the brand name of bisoprolol.

Answer d is incorrect. Benemid is the brand name of probenecid.

7. Which of the following is a *true* statement regarding allopurinol drug interactions?

    a. Use of allopurinol increases warfarin levels and increases theophylline levels.
    b. Use of allopurinol increases warfarin levels and decreases theophylline levels.
    c. Use of allopurinol decreases warfarin levels and decreases theophylline levels.
    d. Use of allopurinol decreases warfarin levels and increases theophylline levels.

Answer a is correct. Use of allopurinol may inhibit the metabolism of warfarin and theophylline, resulting in increased levels of each drug.

Answers b, c, and d are incorrect. Allopurinol may inhibit the metabolism of warfarin and theophylline, resulting in increased levels of each drug.

8. A resident physician approaches you about a patient admitted for an acute gout flare. He wants to start the patient on corticosteroid therapy. Which of the following would be important to communicate to the resident regarding monitoring parameters?

    a. Recommend to monitor serum creatinine for renal dysfunction.
    b. Recommend to monitor blood glucose levels.
    c. Recommend to monitor for diarrhea.
    d. Recommend to monitor for presence of skin rash.

Answer b is correct. It is important to monitor blood glucose levels in patients who are started on corticosteroid therapy—regardless if patients are diabetic or not, due to corticosteroid's ability to increase blood glucose levels.

Answer a is incorrect. Corticosteroids are a gout treatment option for patients who have renal insufficiency; corticosteroids do not cause renal impairment.

Answer c is incorrect. This would be an important monitoring parameter if the patient was started on colchicine.

Answer d is incorrect. It would be important to monitor for this possible side effect if the patient was started on allopurinol once the initial episode was under control.

9. A 63-year-old man presents to your clinic complaining of excruciating pain in his left big toe. After being diagnosed with

an acute gout flare, his physician wants to start him on therapy. His medical history is positive for hypertension, hyperlipidemia, peptic ulcer disease, and glaucoma. Which of the following is appropriate therapy for this patient?

a. Ibuprofen
b. Indomethacin
c. Allopurinol
d. Prednisone

Answer d is correct. This would be an option for patients who have contraindications to other acute gout therapy, such as NSAIDs with peptic ulcer disease.

Answers a and b are incorrect. They are both NSAIDs and should be avoided in patients with a history of peptic ulcer disease.

Answer c is incorrect. Allopurinol should not be initiated as treatment for an acute gout flare as this medication may worsen the flare by rapidly decreasing uric acid and causing mobilization of uric acid stores.

10. In a patient with a CrCl of less than 10 mL/min, which acute gout medication is most appropriate?

a. Prednisone
b. Ibuprofen
c. Nabumetone
d. Colchicine

Answer a is correct. Corticosteroids are the drugs of choice for acute gout in patients with renal insufficiency.

Answers b and c are incorrect. They are both NSAIDs and so should be avoided in patients with a history of renal dysfunction.

Answer d is incorrect. Colchicine should also be avoided in patients with renal insufficiency due to increased risk for toxicities.

11. A patient is picking up a new prescription for colchicine. Which of the following are the appropriate counseling points to discuss with the patient?

a. The patient should be counseled on GI side effects of nausea, vomiting, diarrhea, and abdominal pain.
b. The patient should be counseled on possibility of a rash.
c. The patient should be counseled on signs and symptoms of bleeding.
d. The patient should be counseled on close monitoring of blood glucose levels.

Answer a is correct. The major side effects which can limit the use of colchicine are gastrointestinal.

Answer b is incorrect. This would be a counseling point for allopurinol.

Answer c is incorrect. This would be a counseling point for NSAIDs.

Answer d is incorrect. This would be a counseling point for corticosteroids.

12. Which of the following statements accurately describes NSAIDs mechanism of action in the treatment of gout?

a. NSAIDs work by reducing phagocytosis and lactic acid production in joints, thereby reducing deposition of urate crystals.
b. NSAIDs work by blocking the conversion of xanthine to uric acid.
c. NSAIDs work by exerting anti-inflammatory, analgesic, and antipyretic effects by inhibiting the synthesis of prostaglandin.
d. NSAIDs work by inhibiting proximal renal tubule reabsorption of uric acid to decrease serum levels.

Answer c is correct. NSAIDs work by exerting anti-inflammatory, analgesic, and antipyretic effects by inhibiting the synthesis of prostaglandin.

Answers a, b, and d are incorrect. This is the mechanism of action of colchicine, allopurinol, and probenecid, respectively.

13. Which of the following statements is *true* regarding febuxostat?

a. Febuxostat is a good choice for patients with liver failure.
b. Febuxostat is the drug of choice for acute gout.
c. Febuxostat is an option for patients with renal insufficiency.
d. Febuxostat has no drug interactions.

Answer c is correct. Febuxostat is an option for patients with renal insufficiency (hepatically metabolized).

Answer a is incorrect. Febuxostat is metabolized through the liver and should not be used in liver failure.

Answer b is incorrect. Febuxostat is used as treatment in chronic gout.

Answer d is incorrect. Febuxostat does interact with drugs, including azathioprine, 6-mercaptopurine, and theophylline.

14. You are on the internal medicine rounding service and taking care of a patient who has developed an acute gouty flare. The resident physician on your team would like to start the patient on indomethacin. Which of the following is a *true* statement regarding the use of NSAIDs in the treatment of gout and as such, you would communicate the information to the resident physician?

a. Indomethacin is the NSAID of choice for treating gout.
b. Short-acting NSAIDs at equipotent, anti-inflammatory doses are the drugs of choice for acute gout in the absence of contraindications.
c. Intravenous administration of NSAID is the preferred route of administration for the treatment of gout.
d. NSAIDs are second-line treatment behind colchicine for the treatment of gout.

Answer b is correct. Short-acting NSAIDs at equipotent, anti-inflammatory doses are the drugs of choice for acute gout in the absence of contraindications.

Answer a is incorrect. Any NSAID used at anti-inflammatory doses can be efficacious for the treatment of gout.

Answer c is incorrect. Fast-acting oral administration is usually preferred.

Answer d is incorrect. Colchicine is usually second-line to NSAIDs for the treatment of gout due to adverse effect profile.

---

15. A 68-year-old man presents to the clinic with a history of three acute episodes of gout in the past year. He is classified as an overproducer of uric acid. He has severe liver impairment but no renal insufficiency. Which of the following medications is appropriate for chronic prophylaxis of gout?

    a. Allopurinol
    b. Febuxostat
    c. Probenecid
    d. Sulfinpyrazone

Answer a is correct. Allopurinol is used for chronic prophylaxis of gout in patients who are overproducers of uric acid.

Answer b is incorrect. Febuxostat should not be used in hepatic impairment.

Answers c and d are incorrect. These agents are used as underexcretors of uric acid, not overproducers.

---

16. What is the mechanism of action by which probenecid produces its effect?

    a. Inhibition of xanthine oxidase
    b. Blocks excretion of uric acid
    c. Blocks reuptake of uric acid at the proximal tubule
    d. Inhibits prostaglandin synthesis

Answer c is correct. Probenecid blocks reuptake of uric acid at the proximal tubule.

Answer a is incorrect. This is the mechanism of action of allopurinol and febuxostat.

Answer b is incorrect. Probenecid increases uric acid excretion.

Answer d is incorrect. This is the mechanism of action of NSAIDs.

Questions 17 and 18 relate to the following text.

A 75-year-old man is started on allopurinol for gout prevention. His baseline SUA level is 11.6 mg/dL. He is overweight (body mass index [BMI] 30 mg/m²) and drinks 1 to 2 cans of beer a day.

17. Which of the following statements describes allopurinol and its role in gout prevention?

    a. Allopurinol is most effective when initiated within 24 to 48 hours of an acute attack.
    b. The usual starting dose is 300 mg po daily.
    c. Treatment with allopurinol should be continued for 3 to 12 months.
    d. Serious side effects include myopathy and bone marrow suppression.

Answer c is correct. Treatment with allopurinol should be continued for 3 to 12 months.

Answer a is incorrect. Allopurinol should not be initiated during an acute attack.

Answer b is incorrect. The usual starting dose is 100 mg daily (for this age range).

Answer d is incorrect. These side effects are reported with colchicine.

---

18. Which of the following measures may be recommended in a patient with gout? Select all that apply.

    a. Weight loss
    b. Reduction of alcohol consumption
    c. Application of cold packs
    d. Application of heat

Answers a, b, and c are correct. Weight loss, reduction of alcohol, and application of cold packs are utilized in the management of gout.

Answer d is incorrect. The affected joints should be rested and treated with cold packs (application of heat should be avoided).

---

19. Select the target SUA level when treating gout.

    a. ≤6 mg/dL
    b. ≤7 mg/dL
    c. ≤8 mg/dL
    d. ≤9 mg/dL

Answer a is correct. The target SUA level should be ≤6 and patients typically require 3 to 12 months of continued therapy.

Answers b, c, and d are incorrect. Target SUA level should be ≤6 and patients typically require 3 to 12 months of continued therapy.

---

20. Place the following gout medication in order based upon their mg dose. Start with the lowest dose.

Unordered Response	Ordered Response
Methylprednisolone	Colchicine 1.2 mg
Colchicine	Methylprednisolone 10-40 mg
Naproxen	Indomethacin 50 mg
Indomethacin	Naproxen 250 mg

CHAPTER 49 | Osteoporosis

1. SD is a 55-year-old woman with no significant past medical history. However, she currently smokes one pack a day and drinks alcohol socially (2 beers every other week). She attends a health fair and learns her T-score is −1.5. Which statement represents the best course of action for the patient?

   a. SD has osteopenia and should be started on alendronate 70 mg po every week.
   b. SD should be advised to quit smoking and to have her BMD checked again in 6 months.
   c. SD should be started on teriparatide 20 mcg SQ daily to rebuild her bone mass to normal levels.
   d. SD should be started on calcium 1200 mg po daily and vitamin D 800 IU po daily.

Answer d is correct. SD is not currently taking calcium or vitamin D per World Health Organization (WHO) guidelines. Though this may or may not fully explain her low BMD score, it is the most logical starting point to minimize the risk of developing osteoporosis. She should be referred for further testing (ie, DXA).

Answer a is incorrect. It is unknown if SD does or does not have osteopenia based on the WHO guidelines, as a heel ultrasound cannot be used for diagnostic purposes. Therefore, it would be prudent to do a more thorough assessment before initiating a bisphosphonate at this point. Furthermore, if a bisphosphonate is ultimately deemed appropriate, the "prevention" dose of alendronate is 5 mg po daily or 35 mg po every week.

Answer b is incorrect. It should be recommended that SD go for a more thorough assessment and be advised to quit smoking, as active or previous smoking is a risk factor. However, repeating a BMD is generally not recommended more than every other year per the National Osteoporosis Foundation (NOF).

Answer c is incorrect. Teriparatide is recommended for patients with (severe) osteoporosis with high risk of fracture. SD should be referred for further assessment to determine her condition based on WHO guidelines.

2. JR is a 58-year-old white man who presents to the emergency department with a hip fracture after rolling out of his bed in his home. He is 5′ 8″ and weighs 133 lb. His medical history includes rheumatoid arthritis, currently treated with prednisone 10 mg daily (× 2 years), methotrexate 15 mg weekly (× 2 years) and folic acid 1 mg daily (× 2 years). Which statement represents the best course of action for the patient?

   a. JR should have a BMD checked immediately to determine if he has osteoporosis.
   b. JR is a candidate for zoledronic acid 5 mg intravenously (IV) with repeat dosing every other year.
   c. JR is a candidate for raloxifene 60 mg po daily.
   d. JR is a candidate for teriparatide 20 mcg SQ daily.

Answer d is correct. JR appears to have glucocorticoid-induced osteoporosis with a high risk of fracture (following his previous low-trauma fracture) and is a candidate for teriparatide.

Answer a is incorrect. Whether JR should have a BMD checked immediately is a matter of clinical debate, and hence, not the best answer. It may be useful to have a BMD as a baseline to track the effects of therapy moving forward. However, JR has suffered a low-trauma hip fracture in the presence of multiple osteoporosis risk factors (low BMI, rheumatoid arthritis, and prednisone). JR most likely has osteoporosis regardless of the BMD score at this point.

Answer b is incorrect. JR may be a candidate for a bisphosphonate, including zoledronic acid. However, zoledronic acid 5 mg IV with every other year dosing is for prevention and JR is a candidate for treatment .

Answer c is incorrect. Raloxifene is a SERM and is only indicated in women.

3. Select the antiresorptive agent that can be administered monthly for osteoporosis treatment. Select all that apply.

   a. Risedronate
   b. Raloxifene
   c. Zoledronic acid
   d. Alendronate
   e. Ibandronate

Answer a and e is correct. Risedronate is taken orally either daily, weekly, every 2 consecutive days, or monthly. Ibandronate is also available as an oral monthly formulation.

Answer b is incorrect. Raloxifene is taken orally daily for treatment.

Answer c is incorrect. Zoledronic acid is given IV annually for treatment.

Answer d is incorrect. Alendronate is taken orally daily or weekly for treatment.

4. RS is a 67-year-old Asian woman with a T-score −2.7. She is 5′ 6″ and 127 lb. She has a past medical history of deep vein thrombosis (DVT), 6 months ago. Her medical history includes hypertension, osteoarthritis, and diabetes. She currently takes furosemide, celecoxib, lisinopril, metformin, and aspirin. Which statement represents the best course of action for the patient?

   a. RS is a candidate for calcitonin 200 units intranasally daily.
   b. RS is a candidate for estrogen 0.625 mg po daily
   c. RS is a candidate for ibandronate 3 mg IV every 3 months.
   d. RS is a candidate for raloxifene 60 mg po daily.

Answer c is correct. RS is a candidate for osteoporosis treatment, including ibandronate IV, as bisphosphonates are first-line therapy. She has no contraindications to bisphosphonate therapy. She should also begin taking calcium 1200 mg po daily and vitamin D 800 to 1000 IU po daily.

Answer a is incorrect. Calcitonin is typically a last-line option for the treatment of osteoporosis.

Answer b is incorrect. Based on the WHO, it is no longer appropriate to initiate estrogen as first-line therapy for the treatment of osteoporosis. HRTs are also associated with venous thromboembolism and can lead to DVTs (particularly in this high-risk patient).

Answer d is incorrect. The SERM has been associated with venous thromboembolism and should be used with caution in a patient with a history of DVT.

---

5. Identify the contraindication for a bisphosphonate in the prevention and/or treatment of osteoporosis. Select all that apply.

    a. CrCl <30 mL/min
    b. Peanut allergy
    c. History of stroke
    d. History of Paget disease
    e. Hypocalcemia

Answer a and e is correct. Renal dysfunction described as a CrCl <30 mL/min is a contraindication to the oral and intravenous bisphosphonates. Hypocalcemia is also a contraindication to oral and intravenous bisphosphonates.

Answer b is incorrect. There is no known association between a peanut allergy and any sensitivity to bisphosphonates.

Answer c is incorrect. There is no known association between stroke and sensitivity to bisphosphonates.

Answer d is incorrect. Paget disease, which is essentially a disorder of abnormally high, erratic bone remodeling leading to deformities, pain, and fractures, is commonly treated with bisphosphonates.

---

6. Identify the correct statement regarding teriparatide for the treatment of osteoporosis.

    a. It may be associated with hypocalcemia.
    b. It is contraindicated in a patient with Paget disease.
    c. It is available as a monthly intramuscular injection.
    d. It should only be used for a maximum of 3 years.

Answer b is correct. Paget disease is associated with high, erratic bone turnover, which could be worsened by the anabolic effects of teriparatide.

Answer a is incorrect. Teriparatide increases overall bone remodeling with a preference toward osteoblastic function and may cause hypercalcemia and hypercalciuria.

Answer c is incorrect. Teriparatide is Food and Drug Administration (FDA) approved as a daily, subcutaneous injection.

Answer d is incorrect. Teriparatide should only be used for a maximum of 2 years, based on available data, due to the black boxed warning of osteosarcoma.

---

7. A patient visits the pharmacy counter regarding bisphosphonates. Which statement would be correct when educating the patient about this class of medications?

    a. Ibandronate oral should be taken with food to minimize GI side effects.
    b. Risedronate should be taken sitting down to minimize the risk of dizziness.
    c. A patient receiving zoledronic acid should avoid drinking high-mineral water.
    d. A patient taking alendronate should also routinely be taking calcium and vitamin D.

Answer d is correct. A patient taking alendronate, or any bisphosphonate, should routinely take calcium and vitamin D per WHO guidelines. One caveat for oral bisphosphonates, however, is to avoid taking supplements within 60 minutes of administration to avoid effecting bioavailability.

Answer a is incorrect. All oral bisphosphonates, including ibandronate, should be taken on an empty stomach, as food greatly diminishes absorption. For daily or weekly bisphosphonates, the patient should remain upright and avoid food for 30 minutes. For monthly bisphosphonates, the patient should remain upright and avoid food for 60 minutes. Oral bisphosphonates should be taken with 6 to 8 oz of water.

Answer b is incorrect. All oral bisphosphonates, including risedronate, should be taken first thing in the morning, with a full glass of water while the patient remains upright to avoid esophageal irritation. Teriparatide should be taken sitting down as it may cause orthostasis.

Answer c is incorrect. Zoledronic acid is given IV and will not be affected by water intake. Patients should avoid high-mineral water when taking oral bisphosphonates due to the decreased bioavailability.

---

8. KG is a 59-year-old postmenopausal woman who had her BMD checked (T-score = −2.3). Her past medical history is unremarkable and she only takes a multivitamin with additional calcium and vitamin D. Her family history is remarkable for a mother who had osteoporosis and died of breast cancer. Which statement indicates the most appropriate management for the patient? Select all that apply.

    a. KG has osteopenia but is taking appropriate calcium and vitamin D.
    b. KG may be a good candidate for risedronate 5 mg po daily.
    c. KG may be a good candidate for alendronate 70 mg po weekly.
    d. KG may be a good candidate for raloxifene 60 mg po daily.
    e. KG may be a good candidate for calcitonin 200 units intranasally daily.

Answers b and c are correct. Technically, KG could be a candidate for risedronate or alendronate based on her T-score and risk factors. However, daily oral bisphosphonates are rarely recommended first-line since there are weekly and monthly options (which help improve compliance).

Answer d is correct. Raloxifene is a good choice for two reasons: osteoporosis prevention (and arguably treatment based on risk factors) and prevention of breast cancer based on her potential risk. Her family history makes the SERM a logical option based on the information given.

Answer a is incorrect. Based on her T-score, KG is osteopenic, but may not be taking enough calcium and vitamin D. It would be prudent to consider checking a serum vitamin D, particularly in light of her family history of osteoporosis.

Answer e is incorrect. Calcitonin intranasally is indicated for treatment of osteoporosis (she is osteopenic, but may be a candidate for treatment based on risk factors). Calcitonin intranasally is rarely used first-line based on cost and the availability of other agents that seem to offer greater fracture reduction.

9. MF is a 63-year-old postmenopausal woman having a T-score of −2.9 (−2.8, 1 year ago) despite being on an oral bisphosphonate, calcium, and vitamin D. Which counseling point would be the most appropriate statement to the patient?

   a. Explain to her that at her age and being postmenopausal, such a small change in BMD is not surprising.
   b. Suggest she talk to her doctor about taking a different bisphosphonate.
   c. Recommend to her physician that raloxifene should be added to the current regimen.
   d. Counsel the patient to see how she is taking her medications and review her refill records to see if she is filling the bisphosphonate as expected.

Answer d is correct. Oral bisphosphonates can be difficult to take for some patients, and are often associated with poor compliance (and poor outcomes). One of the most important roles a pharmacist has is to educate patients, in hopes of improving issues like poor compliance. The pharmacist may determine that education can solve the problem or decide that consultation with the prescribing physician is needed to redesign the therapeutic plan.

Answer a is incorrect. MF needs to have her T-score addressed. It is well below -2.5, appears to be worsening, and merits further investigation with her and her physician.

Answer b is incorrect. Different bisphosphonates do have different potencies, as well as different routes of administration that may need to ultimately be considered. However, the two most common reasons patients see worsening BMDs while on therapy are noncompliance with their bisphosphonate and/or inadequate calcium and vitamin D intake. These factors should be examined prior to recommending a switch in treatment.

Answer c is incorrect. Adding or changing therapy may be warranted, but not until the cause of the inadequate response is examined.

10. SM is a 65-year-old postmenopausal woman with a T-score of −3.0. Her past medical history is notable for osteoarthritis. She currently takes naproxen, as well as calcium 1200 mg po and vitamin D 1000 IU po daily. Which statement is correct regarding potential recommendations options for the patient? Select all that apply.

   a. SM is on the appropriate doses of calcium and vitamin D according to WHO guidelines.
   b. SM is a candidate for risedronate 150 mg po every month, despite the fact she is on naproxen.
   c. SM should have her vitamin D level checked, despite the high dose of vitamin D she is currently taking.
   d. SM is a candidate for zoledronic acid 5 mg IV once a year, but normal renal function should be observed prior to receiving each dose.
   e. She should take a multivitamin to receive 2000 IU of vitamin D per day.

Answer a is correct. SM is on the appropriate doses of calcium and vitamin D according to WHO guidelines.

Answer b is correct. SM is a candidate for treatment doses of a bisphosphonate, including risedronate. The use of a nonsteroidal anti-inflammatory drug (NSAID), like naproxen, is not a contraindication to taking an oral bisphosphonate. However, the patient should be reminded to take the bisphosphonate separately from the NSAID and be made aware of the potential GI side effects of either medication.

Answer c is correct. Despite the fact that SM is on the recommended dose of vitamin D, she may still have low serum levels. It is important to remember that if her baseline levels were low, she may need a vitamin D loading dose to get her to goal.

Answer d is correct. SM is a candidate for treatment doses of a bisphosphonate, including zoledronic acid. Patients may only receive IV zoledronic acid if CrCl is ≥35mL/min.

Answer e is incorrect. SM does not need additional vitamin D, as she is receiving an adequate daily amount per WHO guidelines.

11. QW is a 43-year-old female patient with a past medical history of absence epilepsy, rheumatoid arthritis, reflux, depression, and hypertension. Medications include valproic acid, prednisone (7.5 mg daily for past year), omeprazole, sertraline, and furosemide. She presents to emergency care because of a broken bone. Which medication is the patient receiving that can increase her risk of osteoporosis and osteoporotic-related fracture? Select all that apply.

   a. Valproic acid
   b. Prednisone
   c. Omeprazole
   d. Sertraline
   e. Furosemide

Answers a, b, c, d, and e are correct. All of the medication QW is receiving may decrease BMD or increase fracture risk.

---

12. Identify the correct dosing regimen of vitamin D supplementation for a patient with vitamin D deficiency.

    a. 400 IU
    b. 800 IU
    c. 50,000 IU one time per week
    d. 50,000 IU one to two times per week

Answer d is correct. For vitamin D deficiency, ergocalciferol is warranted as 50,000 units one to two times per week for 8 to 12 weeks. Vitamin D levels can be repeated after this treatment duration to re-evaluate the level.

Answer a is incorrect. This dose is not sufficient for vitamin D deficiency.

Answer b is incorrect. This dose is not sufficient for vitamin D deficiency. It may be recommended as maintenance vitamin D supplementation, once vitamin D levels are replenished.

Answer c is incorrect. This dose is not adequate for vitamin D deficiency, but would be used if vitamin D levels were assessed as insufficient.

---

13. Identify the medication that affects osteoblast activity.

    a. Teriparatide
    b. Calcitonin
    c. Risedronate
    d. Raloxifene

Answer a is correct. Teriparatide is an anabolic medication for the treatment of osteoporosis. It is the only medication that targets osteoblast activity and function to build bone.

Answer b is incorrect. Calcitonin is an antiresorptive agent which suppresses osteoclast activity to slow the breakdown of bone.

Answer c is incorrect. Risedronate is an antiresorptive agent which suppresses osteoclast activity to slow the breakdown of bone.

Answer d is incorrect. Raloxifene is an antiresorptive agent which suppresses osteoclast activity to slow the breakdown of bone.

---

14. AP is a 45-year-old patient presenting to your pharmacy to pick up a prescription for Atelvia. Identify the appropriate educational point to discuss with the patient. Select all that apply.

    a. Administer first thing in the morning on an empty stomach.
    b. Take immediately following breakfast.
    c. Remain upright for at least 30 minutes following administration.
    d. Remain upright for at least 60 minutes following administration.
    e. Take with a full glass of mineral water (8 ounces).

Answers b and c are correct. Risedronate (Atelvia) is a delayed release formulation and unlike other bisphosphonates it is designed to be administered immediately following breakfast. As with other agents, you need to stay upright for at least 30 minutes.

Answer a is incorrect. This is true for most bisphosphonates including risedronate (Actonel).

Answer d is incorrect. Ibandronate (Boniva) requires patients to be upright for at least 60 minutes.

Answer e is incorrect. Bisphosphonates should be administered with 8 ounces of plain water (not mineral water).

---

15. A patient is taking calcium carbonate 1250 mg with breakfast and dinner due to inadequate intake from dietary sources. Calculate the daily amount of elemental calcium based on this supplement.

Answer. 1000 mg of elemental calcium (1250 mg × 2 doses = 2500 mg/d × 0.40 [40% elemental calcium] = 1000 mg/d).

---

16. Place the following bisphosphonates in order based upon their lowest treatment milligrams dose that it available. Start with the lowest dose.

Unordered Response	Ordered Response
Alendronate	Risedronate 5 mg
Risedronate	Alendronate 10 mg
Ibandronate	Ibandronate 150 mg

---

17. Identify the antiresorptive agent that would be contraindicated in a pregnant patient.

    a. Ibandronate
    b. Raloxifene
    c. Alendronate
    d. Risedronate

Answer b is correct. Raloxifene is a SERM and should not be used among patients who wish to become pregnant or who are pregnant. It is contraindicated in this patient population.

Answers a, c, and d are incorrect. Ibandronate, alendronate, and risedronate can be used in pregnancy as there are no studies to show fetal adverse events; however, the benefit of a bisphosphonate should outweigh the risk. Calcium levels should be monitored among a pregnant patient, if a bisphosphonate is prescribed.

18. AS is a 54-year-old female patient at risk for osteoporosis and would like assistance with calcium and vitamin D supplements. Identify the correct educational point to discuss with the patient. Select all that apply.

    a. Maintain adequate hydration.
    b. Maintain adequate fiber intake.
    c. Maintain adequate exercise.
    d. Take 1000 mg of elemental calcium.
    e. Take 400 IU of vitamin D.

Answers a, b, and c are correct.   Hydration, fiber, and exercise all important parameters for the disease state osteoporosis and calcium intake. Calcium can cause kidney stones and constipation.

Answer d is incorrect.   Women 51 to 70 years of age should take 1200 mg of elemental calcium.

Answer e is incorrect.   Women older than 51 years should take at least 800 IU of vitamin D.

19. An infusion of zoledronic acid (5 mg/100 mL) will be infused over 30 minutes. How many milliliters will be administered per minute?

Answer.   3.33 mL/min (100 mL/30 min = 3.33 mL/min).

20. Identify the medication that can affect osteoblast activity and function.

    a. Calcitonin
    b. Teriparatide
    c. Risedronate
    d. Raloxifene

Answer b is correct.   Teriparatide is the only anabolic agent for the treatment of osteoporosis. It targets osteoblast activity and function to build bone.

Answers a, c, and d are incorrect.   These medications are antiresorptive agents and focus on suppressing osteoclast activity.

21. Identify a common adverse event associated with Prolia.

    a. Dermatitis
    b. Orthostasis
    c. Hot flashes
    d. Acute phase reactions

Answer a is correct.   Cutaneous reactions, such as dermatitis, are common with Prolia (denosumab).

Answer b is incorrect.   Orthostasis is associated with teriparatide.

Answer c is incorrect.   Hot flashes are common with raloxifene.

Answer d is incorrect.   Acute phase reactions, such as fever or flu-like reactions, can occur with intravenous bisphosphonates.

22. A patient is taking calcium citrate 950 mg at breakfast and dinner due to inadequate intake from dietary sources. Calculate the amount of elemental calcium in each dose. Round to the nearest whole number.

Answer.   200 mg of elemental calcium (950 mg × 1 dose = 950 mg × 0.21 [21% elemental calcium] = 199.5 mg/dose, rounded to 200 mg/dose).

23. Identify the agents that have been associated with osteonecrosis of the jaw. Select all that apply.

    a. Teriparatide
    b. Raloxifene
    c. Alendronate
    d. Zoledronic acid
    e. Denosumab

Answers c, d, and e are correct.   These medications have been associated with a rare, but serious adverse event known as osteonecrosis of the jaw. Patients should be instructed on this adverse events and the importance of proper dental hygiene.

Answers a and b are incorrect.   These specific medications have not been associated with osteonecrosis of the jaw.

24. RS is a 65-year-old man with a FRAX risk score of 13.5% for a major osteoporotic fracture and 1.5% for a hip fracture. Which statement would best represent a plan for this patient?

    a. Educate on a bone healthy lifestyle.
    b. Initiate an antiresorptive agent.
    c. Start an anabolic agent.
    d. Consider an antiresorptive and anabolic agent.

Answer a is correct.   The patient has a normal risk of major osteoporotic fracture and hip fracture over the next 10 years. The patient should be educated on preventative strategies, such as a bone healthy lifestyle.

Answers b, c, and d are incorrect.   As the patient has a normal risk of fractures, there is no need to initiate antiresorptive agent, an anabolic agent, or combination therapy.

25. Which regimen would be the best option for a postmenopausal female (10 years since her last menses) who is at risk of vertebral fractures and has a CrCl of 25 mL/min?

    a. Calcitonin
    b. Ibandronate
    c. Teriparatide
    d. Medroxyprogesterone

Answer a is correct. Calcitonin does not have any restrictions among patients with renal dysfunction. It is also a safe option for the treatment of postmenopausal osteoporosis.

Answer b is incorrect. Ibandronate is not appropriate as it is contraindicated, based on the patient's renal function.

Answer c is incorrect. Teriparatide cannot be prescribed to the patient due to her renal function below 30 mL/min.

Answer d is incorrect. Medroxyprogesterone is not used for the treatment of osteoporosis; it can significantly increase the risk of osteoporosis with long-term use.

---

26. Which medication is contraindicated in a patient with hypercalcemia?

    a. Calcitonin
    b. Alendronate
    c. Raloxifene
    d. Teriparatide

Answer d is correct. Teriparatide can elevate calcium levels and requires frequent monitoring of calcium levels during treatment.

Answers a and c are incorrect. There are no restrictions with these medications, based on calcium levels; however, it would be important to monitor calcium levels for a patient with osteopenia or osteoporosis.

Answer b is incorrect. Alendronate cannot be used in a patient with hypocalcemia.

CHAPTER 50 | Rheumatoid Arthritis

1. Patient GS, a 50-year-old Causasian female, presents to her primary care physician with a chief complaint of generalized fatigue and malaise over the past few months. She also describes having stiffness in her fingers each morning upon waking lasting at least 1 to 2 hours and notes that her fingers and toes (right and left) sometimes appear to be swollen. The physician orders tests including a basic metabolic panel, CBC, rheumatoid factor and X-rays of the hands and feet. Which of GS' complaints could lead the physician to a diagnosis of rheumatoid arthritis? Select all that apply.

    a. Complaints of morning stiffness
    b. Swelling in fingers
    c. Duration of symptoms
    d. Swelling in toes

Answers a, b, c, and d are correct. All of the above are consistent with classic signs and symptoms of rheumatoid arthritis, though only 60% to 70% of RA patients will test positive for rheumatoid factor. Radiological changes such as joint erosions or decalcification are other classic symptoms.

2. PT is a 38-year-old patient with a past medical history of rheumatoid arthritis. He is changing therapy at today's visit to an alternative agent. He had a sulfa allergic reaction 2 years ago. Which of the following DMARDs is contraindicated in a patient with a history of a sulfa allergy?

    a. Neoral
    b. Arava
    c. Rheumatrex
    d. Azulfidine
    e. Cytoxan

Answer d is correct. Azulfidine (sulfasalazine) is contraindicated in patients with history of hypersensitivity to medications containing sulfa.

Answer a is incorrect. Neoral (cyclosporine) is not contraindicated in patients with a sulfa allergy.

Answer b is incorrect. Arava (leflunomide) is not contraindicated in patients with a sulfa allergy.

Answer c is incorrect. Rheumatrex (methotrexate) is not contraindicated in patients with a sulfa allergy.

Answer e is incorrect. Cytoxan (cyclophosphamide) is not contraindicated in patients with a sulfa allergy.

---

3. JJ was diagnosed with RA with moderate disease activity and has been exhibiting symptoms for about 2 months. Which of the following medications are appropriate to consider in the initial medication regimen for JJ?

    a. Ibuprofen
    b. Prednisone
    c. Methotrexate
    d. Etanercept

Answer a is correct. NSAIDs such as ibuprofen possess analgesic and anti-inflammatory effects, which provide RA symptom relief. However, they do not affect the underlying disease process of RA, thus they should not be used as the *sole* treatment.

Answer b is correct. Corticosteroids like prednisone possess anti-inflammatory and immunosuppressive effects which improve symptoms in RA. They are recommended for "bridge therapy" to provide symptomatic relief until full onset of DMARD therapy or in short bursts for treatment of RA exacerbation. Additionally long-term, low-dose maintenance therapy may be used in patients refractive to DMARD or NSAID therapy. Long-term and high-dose corticosteroid treatment should be avoided due to risk of long-term side effects.

Answer c is correct. DMARDs reduce and prevent joint damage and preserve joint function. They should be initiated early, within the first 3 months of onset of symptoms. DMARDs take weeks to months for full onset of effect, thus NSAIDs and corticosteroids will be needed for symptom relief.

Answer d is incorrect. Biologic DMARDs should be used in patients who have moderate to severe RA and who have inadequate response to one or more DMARDs.

---

4. Which of the following nonpharmacologic therapies may be recommended to JJ? Select all that apply.

   a. Heat or cold therapy
   b. Physical therapy
   c. Weight reduction
   d. Cold therapy

Answers a, b, c, and d are correct. Nonpharmacologic therapy such as heat or cold therapy, physical therapy, and weight reduction as well as education, emotional support, rest, occupational therapy, and surgery (for severe cases) can be used to improve symptoms and maintain joint function in RA.

---

5. Which of the following is the correct mechanism of action for etanercept (Enbrel)?

   a. Monoclonal antibody which targets the CD20 antigen on B-lymphocytes
   b. TNF-α inhibitor
   c. Immunoglobulin protein which inhibits T-lymphocytes
   d. Dihydrofolate reductase inhibitor

Answer b is correct. Enbrel (etanercept) is a TNF-α inhibitor.

Answer a is incorrect. Rituximab is a monoclonal antibody that targets CD20 antigen on B-lymphocytes.

Answer c is incorrect. Abatacept is a T-cell inhibitor.

Answer d is incorrect. Methotrexate is a dihydrofolate reductase inhibitor.

---

6. Which of the following is a reason that DMARDs are preferred over non-DMARD for RA management?

   a. DMARD agents cause fewer adverse reactions than non-DMARDs.
   b. Non-DMARD agents are less cost-effective than DMARDs.
   c. DMARD agents may reduce or prevent joint damage and preserve joint function.
   d. Non-DMARD agents require close laboratory monitoring.

Answer c is correct. Unlike non-DMARD agents such as NSAIDs, aspirin, and COX-2 inhibitors, DMARDs reduce or prevent joint damage and preserve joint function and integrity.

Answer a is incorrect. Both DMARD and non-DMARD drug agents have associated adverse reactions and neither drug class is less likely to cause them than the other.

Answer b is incorrect. Though formulary restrictions may limit the availability of certain agents, drug costs are typically not a major factor in making therapeutic decisions.

Answer d is incorrect. Routine laboratory monitoring is recommended for patients on all types of rheumatoid arthritis medications.

---

7. Which brand/generic is correctly matched?

   a. Adalimumab/Enbrel
   b. Etanercept/Orencia
   c. Abatacept/Humira
   d. Infliximab/Remicade

Answer d is correct. Remicade is the brand name of infliximab.

Answer a is incorrect. Enbrel is the brand name of etanercept.

Answer b is incorrect. Orencia is the brand name of abatacept.

Answer c is incorrect. Humira is the brand name of adalimumab.

---

8. Which of the following agents is dosed weekly?

   a. Methotrexate
   b. Leflunomide
   c. Hydroxychloroquine
   d. Sulfasalazine

Answer a is correct. Methotrexate is dosed on a weekly basis and is available orally and for intramuscular, subcutaneous, and intravenous injection. Weekly dosing of the drug appears to cause less gastrointestinal toxicity (less damage to the mucosa) and fewer side effects than daily dosing. It is important to be vigilant when reviewing methotrexate prescriptions to verify proper dosing frequency. Emphasize to your patients that this medication is taken on a weekly, not daily, basis to minimize the risk of overdose.

Answer b is incorrect. Leflunomide is dosed daily.

Answer c is incorrect. Hydroxychloroquine is dosed daily.

Answer d is incorrect. Sulfasalazine is dosed bid or tid.

---

9. A physician prescribes Arava 100 mg as a loading dose for her patient who is newly diagnosed with RA. A correct maintenance dose for this medication would be:

   a. Methotrexate 20 mg daily
   b. Methotrexate 20 mg weekly
   c. Leflunomide 20 mg daily
   d. Leflunomide 20 mg weekly

Answer c is correct. Leflunomide is the generic name for Arava. After a loading dose of 100 mg daily given for 3 days, a standard maintenance dose of 20 mg daily thereafter may be used.

Answers a, b, and d are incorrect. Methotrexate is dosed on a weekly basis. Various branded methotrexate products are available, including Trexall, Otrexup, and Rheumatrex.

---

10. Which of the following monitoring parameters should be followed for patients receiving hydroxychloroquine?

    a. Tuberculin skin test at baseline due to the risk of serious infections.
    b. Hepatic function should be assessed at baseline, 6 months, and 12 months due to risk of hepatic toxicity.
    c. Renal function should be monitored every 6 months due to risk of renal impairment.
    d. Ophthalmological examination within 1 year of starting therapy due to the risk of retinal toxicity.

Answer d is correct. Hydroxychloroquine has been associated with various types of ocular toxicity including blurred vision, diminished visual acuity, abnormal color vision, and retinopathy. It appears that the toxicities are specific to the cornea and the macula of the eye. Retinal damage is dose-related and sometimes irreversible. Patients taking hydroxychloroquine are recommended to have an ophthalmology examination within 1 year following initiation of the drug. High-risk patients (those who take a daily dose >6.5 mg/kg, are renally impaired, have been taking the drug for more than 10 years, or have taken a cumulative dose of 200 g) should have the examination repeated every 6 to 12 months, while low-risk patients may repeat the examination approximately every 5 years.

Answer a is incorrect. Tuberculin skin tests are recommended prior to initiation of biologic agents; hydroxychloroquine is not a biologic agent.

Answer b is incorrect. Hydroxychloroquine does not commonly cause liver toxicity.

Answer c is incorrect. Hydroxychloroquine is not associated with kidney toxicity.

---

11. Which of the following are adverse reactions common to all biological DMARD agents? Select all that apply.

    a. Bone marrow suppression
    b. Heart failure exacerbation
    c. Increased susceptibility to infection
    d. Teratogenicity

Answer c is correct. All biological DMARD agents suppress the immune system by affecting various immunological components. Consequently, the body becomes more vulnerable to infection. Patients on biological DMARD therapy should be assessed regularly for any signs of infection. Localized signs may include unhealed skin wounds possibly leaking pus or other drainage, pain, swelling, or heat at the site of infection. Systemic infection symptoms include fever, chills, and other cold- or flu-like symptoms.

Answer a is incorrect. Bone marrow suppression is not an expected side effect of biological DMARD agents.

Answer b is incorrect. Anti-TNF-α agents (infliximab, etanercept, and adalimumab) are contraindicated in patients with New York Heart Association Class III or IV heart failure, but as a class biological DMARDs have not been shown to cause or exacerbate heart failure.

Answer d is incorrect. Biological agents have historically been assigned pregnancy category B and C by the U.S. Food and Drug Administration. Category B designation indicates that either animal reproduction studies have failed to demonstrate a risk to the fetus and there are no well-controlled studies in pregnant women or that animal studies have shown adverse effects but they have not been confirmed in controlled studies in pregnant women. Category C assignment means that animal reproduction studies have shown an adverse effect to the fetus and there are no adequate and well-controlled studies in humans, but the potential benefits may warrant use of the drug in pregnant women despite the potential risks.

---

12. Which of the following medications is an anti-TNF biologic DMARD?

    a. Tofacitinib
    b. Tocilizumab
    c. Rituximab
    d. Golimumab

Answer d is correct. Golimumab is an anti-TNF agent. It is a human IgG1 monoconal antibody specific for human TNF-α.

Answer a is incorrect. Tofacitinib is a nonbiologic DMARD which acts through the inhibition of janus kinase.

Answer b is incorrect. Tocilizumab is a humanized monoclonal antibody that selectively antagonizes interleukin-6 receptors.

Answer c is incorrect. Rituximab does not work by interfering with the actions of TNF-α. This drug is a monoclonal antibody that targets the CD20 antigen on B-lymphocytes.

---

13. Which of the following conditions would be a contraindication for receiving methotrexate?

    a. Slight renal impairment (CrCL = 50 mL/min)
    b. Mild thrombocytopenia (platelets = 100×10^9/L)
    c. Pregnancy
    d. Latent tuberculosis infection

Answer c is correct. Methotrexate is pregnancy category X and should be avoided in women who are pregnant or may become pregnant.

Answer a is incorrect. Methotrexate should be avoided in patients with very poor renal function (CrCL <30 mL/min), but there is no limit to its use in patients with mild or moderate impairment. Patients' serum creatinine should be measured regularly to screen for renal toxicity.

Answer b is incorrect. Patients with a platelet count of less than 50×10^9/L should not use methotrexate. A complete blood count should be measured at baseline, every 2 to 4 weeks after initiation of therapy for 3 months, and then periodically thereafter to monitor for signs of thrombocytopenia and bone marrow suppression.

Answer d is incorrect. Methotrexate should be avoided in patients with active tuberculosis, but there is not a contraindication to its use in patients latently infected. Patients with active bacterial infection, ongoing herpes zoster infection, or life-threatening fungal infection should not take methotrexate.

---

14. Why is folic acid 1 mg po daily often recommended along with methotrexate therapy?

    a. Folic acid can prevent renal toxicity caused by methotrexate.
    b. Folic acid can prevent gastrointestinal toxicity caused by methotrexate.
    c. Most people with rheumatoid arthritis have folic acid deficiencies.
    d. Folic acid will enhance the efficacy of methotrexate.

Answer b is correct. Folate (the naturally occurring form of folic acid, which is also known as vitamin B9) is necessary for the synthesis and maintenance of new cells. Methotrexate is a folic acid antagonist and will deplete the body's folate stores by inhibiting the enzyme dihydrofolate reductase. Since many fast-dividing cells (such as those that line the gastric mucosa) utilize folate during their replication, a deficiency of folic acid will inhibit their growth and proliferation. For this reason it is recommended that patients on methotrexate take 1 mg daily of folic acid.

Answer a is incorrect. Although methotrexate may cause renal toxicity, folic acid is not indicated to reduce the nephrotoxic effects of the drug.

Answer c is incorrect. Patients who have rheumatoid arthritis are not also likely to have a folate deficiency.

Answer d is incorrect. While folic acid has not been shown to decrease the efficacy of methotrexate, it will not enhance the efficacy of methotrexate.

---

15. A physician would like to add an anti-TNF agent which can be administered subcutaneously for a patient who has failed to respond adequately to methotrexate monotherapy after 3 months. Which of the following medications meets both of these criteria?

    a. Abatacept
    b. Cytoxan
    c. Cimzia
    d. Remicade
    e. Rituxan

Answer c is correct. Cimzia is an anti-TNF agent and is given as a SQ injection.

Answer a is incorrect. Abatacept is not an anti-TNF agent. It is an immunoglobulin protein agent that inhibits T-lymphocyte activation through the blockage of its stimulation by antigen-presenting cells. It is available both as an IV infusion and a SQ injection.

Answer b is incorrect. Cytoxan is a nonbiologic DMARD, not an anti-TNF agent. It is available orally and by IV injection.

Answer d is incorrect. Remicade is an anti-TNF agent, but it is not available as a subcutaneous injection. Remicade is available as an IV infusion given at weeks 0, 2, and 6 and then every 8 weeks thereafter.

Answer e is incorrect. Rituxan is not an anti-TNF agent. It is a monoclonal antibody that targets the CD20 antigen on B-lymphocytes. It is administered intravenously as two infusions 2 weeks apart.

---

16. Select the brand name for hydroxychloroquine.

    a. Arava
    b. Cytoxan
    c. Humira
    d. Plaquenil
    e. Rituxan

Answer d is correct. Plaquenil is the brand name for hydroxychloroquine.

Answer a is incorrect. Arava is the brand name for leflunomide.

Answer b is incorrect. Cytoxan is the brand name for cyclophosphamide.

Answer c is incorrect. Humira is the brand name for adalimumab.

Answer e is incorrect. Rituxan is the brand name for rituximab.

---

17. Which of the following is true about DMARD therapy?

    a. DMARDs reduce or prevent joint damage in RA.
    b. Onset of action is usually 1 to 2 weeks.
    c. Reserved for use in severe long-term RA.
    d. If a patient fails one DMARD, they will likely fail all DMARDs.

Answer a is correct.   Disease-modifying antirheumatic drugs (DMARDs) have been shown to slow or prevent disease progression.

Answer b is incorrect.   DMARDs have a typical onset of 1 to 6 months.

Answer c is incorrect.   It is recommended to initiate DMARDs within 3 months of the onset of symptoms. All RA patients are candidates for DMARD therapy.

Answer d is incorrect.   If one DMARD does not provide sufficient control of RA, the dose should be increased or additional DMARDs should be added or substituted.

---

18. AA is a 34-year-old woman who regularly picks up her Arava and Ortho Tri-Cyclen refills at your pharmacy. Today she arrives to pick up her Arava and states she will no longer need her Ortho Tri-Cyclen as she and her husband have decided to start trying to have a baby. Which of the following would be an appropriate response to this information?

    a. Continue Arava at a lower dose when she becomes pregnant, as rheumatoid arthritis typically improves during pregnancy.
    b. Change Arava to methotrexate during pregnancy.
    c. Discontinue Arava 2 to 3 weeks prior to trying to get pregnant.
    d. Undergo drug-elimination with cholestyramine prior to trying to get pregnant.

Answer d is correct.   Arava is pregnancy category X based on data suggesting increased risk for fetal death and teratogenic effects. Due to Arava's active metabolite and long half-life, patients wishing to become pregnant should undergo the drug elimination procedure with cholestyramine (8 g cholestyramine tid for 11 days; plasma levels M1 <0.02 mg/L must be verified on two separate occasions at least 14 days apart).

Answer a is incorrect.   RA symptoms may improve during pregnancy, but Arava is pregnancy category X and must be discontinued prior to conception.

Answer b is incorrect.   Both methotrexate and Arava are pregnancy category X.

Answer c is incorrect.   Arava must be discontinued approximately 3 months prior to conception to allow for a drug elimination and washout period.

---

19. Which of the following is true about rituximab? Select all that apply.

    a. It is available for administration intravenously.
    b. Premedication with corticosteroid, APAP, and antihistamine should be done prior to each dose.
    c. Dosing may be repeated every 7 days.
    d. It is available for administration subcutaneously.

Answer a is correct.   Rituximab is available only for IV administration.

Answer b is correct.   It is necessary to premedicate with a corticosteroid, acetaminophen, and an antihistamine prior to each dose of rituximab. The usual recommended dose is 1000 mg given by IV infusion. This medication should not be given as IV push or bolus dose. Infusion should be initiated at 50 mg/h, and may be increased to a maximum rate 400 mg/h (increasing by 50 mg/h every 30 minutes) if no infusion-related reaction develops. The next infusion may be initiated at 100 mg/h, and may be increased to a maximum rate of 400 mg/h.

Answer c is incorrect.   Dosing recommendations for rituximab indicated a repeat dose in 14 days. Subsequent courses may not be administered sooner than 16 weeks.

Answer d is incorrect.   Rituximab is not available for SQ administration.

---

20. DR is a 65-year-old female patient with RA which is being treated with methotrexate and Cimzia. It is November, and her doctor would like to know if DR can receive the flu vaccine. What would you recommend?

    a. DR should receive the Fluzone intramuscular vaccine.
    b. DR should receive the Flumist intranasal vaccine.
    c. DR should receive prophylactic oseltamivir.
    d. DR should not receive any vaccines while taking Cimzia for RA.

Answer a is correct.   Patients who are taking DMARDs (biologic or nonbiologic) should be vaccinated annually against influenza. Fluzone is an inactivated influenza vaccine, so it is safe to administer in patients taking biologic agents.

Answer b is incorrect.   The Flumist intranasal vaccine is a live attenuated vaccine (LAIV). Live attenuated vaccines are not recommended in patients on biologic DMARDs, like Cimzia, due to the risk of infection.

Answer c is incorrect.   Oseltamivir should not be administered to DR based upon the information provided. Vaccination is recommended to decrease the incidence of the influenza.

Answer d is incorrect.   Patients on biologic DMARDs should not receive live vaccines, but the inactivated influenza vaccine is recommended.

CHAPTER **51 | Osteoarthritis**

1. EM is a 63-year-old obese man with a history of increasing pain in his left knee. He presently cares for his 85-year-old mother who has had bilateral knee replacements secondary to OA. During his college years, he played on the intramural football team and suffered several knee injuries. During his career

as a radio announcer for sports, he maintained a sedentary lifestyle and does not presently exercise. Which of the following are risk factors for the development of OA in EM? Select all that apply.

a. Age
b. Genetics
c. Joint injury
d. Obesity

Answer a is correct. OA mainly affects adults >50 years old. This patient is over the age of 50.

Answer b is correct. OA can be inherited. This patient has a mother with a history of knee replacements secondary to OA.

Answer c is correct. Acute joint injury can place a patient at risk for OA. Tears of the meniscus as well as articular surface injury increases joint instability. This patient has a history of acute joint injury during his college years with sports participation which placed him at risk for injury.

Answer d is correct. Weight gain predisposes patients to development of OA secondary to overload of the knee. This patient is stated as being obese.

2. Which of the following is a sign or symptom of a patient with clinical presentation of OA?

a. Joint stiffness with rest
b. Normal range of motion with joint
c. Joint stability
d. Joint stiffness with movement
e. Frictionless joint movement

Answer a is correct. Patients will experience a stiffening of the joint at rest and improved mobility with increased movement.

Answer b is incorrect. Patients have a limited range of motion because of abnormal joint structure.

Answer c is incorrect. Patients will experience joint instability secondary to pathophysiological changes leading to abnormal anatomy.

Answer d is incorrect. OA patients will experience relief of stiffness with movement (gelling phenomenon) of the joint. Stiffness worsens with rest.

Answer e is incorrect. OA patients experience friction with movement as bone may move against bone secondary to cartilage destruction.

3. Which of the following are preventative measures for OA? Select all that apply.

a. Resistance exercise
b. Maintaining a healthy weight
c. Surgery
d. Joint rehabilitation

Answer a is correct. Building muscle strength with resistance exercise is a strategy for strengthening muscles, which could possibly prevent risk of OA later in life.

Answer b is correct. Avoiding obesity can decrease risk of OA development. Increased weight can increase load on joints and predispose them to damage.

Answer c is correct. Surgery may be needed for joint injuries to restore normal function. Surgery may assist with prevention of later life development of OA.

Answer d is correct. Rehabilitation of the joint may involve different types of exercise and regimen of rest to improve flexibility and proprioception (unconscious movement of the body with spatial awareness).

4. SL is a 62-year-old obese man with a history of degenerative joint disease in his left knee. Past medical history (PMH) is significant for dyslipidemia treated with gemfibrozil and diabetes with NPH 10 units bid and glipizide 10 mg bid. Blood sugar readings are not at goal with HgA1c of 8.5%. Current blood pressure is 130/80 mm Hg. He receives his second injection of 40 mg of Kenalog in his left knee today. Which side effect could cause a drug–disease state interaction in this patient?

a. Skin depigmentation
b. Adrenal insufficiency
c. Joint infection
d. Hyperglycemia

Answer d is correct. Patient is a diabetic. Glucocorticoid use is associated with carbohydrate intolerance and hyperglycemia. This would necessitate closer monitoring of his diabetes.

Answer a is incorrect. Skin depigmentation may occur with corticosteroids. However, this is not a disease drug state interaction this patient is at risk for. Increased pigmentation can be a sign associated with adrenal insufficiency.

Answer b is incorrect. Patient is not manifesting signs of hypotension, fever, or symptoms of weakness, anorexia, or myalgia associated with adrenal insufficiency. Adrenal insufficiency is a life-threatening situation.

Answer c is incorrect. He does not report any joint infection with symptoms of painful joint and abnormal white blood cell count.

5. What is the primary objective of pharmacologic therapy for OA?

a. Improve mobility
b. Weight loss
c. Pain relief
d. Improve muscle and joint strength

Answer c is correct. Pain relief is the primary objective of pharmacologic treatment.

Answer a is incorrect. Improvement of mobility without relief of pain may assist with increased movement; however, patients will not have improved quality of life. Improved mobility occurs as a result of pain relief.

Answer b is incorrect. Weight loss can improve signs and symptoms but will not provide acute pain relief. However, it is not the primary objective of medication therapy.

Answer d is incorrect. Improvement of muscle and joint strength can assist with support of the joint. However, this will not improve acute pain.

---

6. RT is a construction worker that presents to your clinic for knee pain. He is diagnosed with OA. He is currently obese and cannot take time off from work because of providing for his family. Additionally, he has a family history of OA. He would like to try nonpharmacologic therapy before starting a medication. Which of the following is(are) preventable risk factor(s) for developing OA in this patient? Select all that apply.

    a. Genetics
    b. Joint trauma history
    c. Repetitive movement
    d. Obesity

Answer d is correct. Weight loss is the most preventable risk factor for development of OA. Decrease of load on joints can prevent damage and possible malalignment.

Answer a is incorrect. Genetics is not modifiable.

Answer b is incorrect. History of joint trauma is not modifiable since it occurred in the past. Appropriate therapy at the time of trauma may assist to decrease development of future OA.

Answer c is incorrect. Repetitive movement is a risk factor for development of joint damage. Certain occupations may be associated with repetitive movements. This may not be easily modified unless measures are taken to address it.

---

7. Select the first-line pharmacologic agent for treating OA.

    a. Acetaminophen
    b. Intra-articular corticosteroids
    c. Tramadol
    d. Ibuprofen

Answer a is correct. Acetaminophen has been shown to be the most appropriate first-line agent to relieve pain and inflammation.

Answer b is incorrect. Intra-articular corticosteroids are appropriate for exacerbations of OA for patients who are not candidates for NSAIDs.

Answer c is incorrect. Tramadol is used for those with contraindications to nonselective NSAIDs and COX-2 inhibitors with failure on previous drug trials.

Answer d is incorrect. Nonselective NSAIDs is second-line therapy after acetaminophen.

---

8. Which of the following help to reduce NSAID-induced GI toxicity? Select all that apply.

    a. Nonacetylated salicylates
    b. COX-2 inhibitors
    c. Addition of misoprostol
    d. Addition of PPI

Answer a is correct. Nonacetylated salicylates are associated with decrease in GI toxicity.

Answer b is correct. Celecoxib demonstrated fewer GI ulcers when compared to traditional NSAIDs.

Answer c is correct. Misoprostol is protective for ulcers and potential GI complications.

Answer d is correct. PPIs reduce risk for GI ulcer development.

---

9. Which of the following are goals of OA management? Select all that apply.

    a. Teaching patient about the disease state
    b. Curing OA
    c. Providing pain relief
    d. Improving musculoskeletal movement
    e. Maintaining ability to perform activities of daily living

Answer a is correct. Patient education is a goal for OA treatment.

Answer c is correct. Pain relief is the primary goal for OA.

Answer d is correct. Improvement in musculoskeletal movement is a goal for OA treatment.

Answer e is correct. Patients should be able to perform activities of daily living even with OA.

Answer b is incorrect. At present, there is no cure for OA.

---

10. Place the following OA management options in the *correct* order in which treatment options for acute pain should be initiated?

Unordered Response	Ordered Response
COX-2 Inhibitor	Acetaminophen
Nonselective NSAID	Nonselective NSAID
Acetaminophen	COX-2 Inhibitor
Joint replacement	Tramadol/opioid analgesic
Tramadol/opioid analgesic	Joint replacement

Acetaminophen is the first-line pharmacologic agent to treat OA-induced acute pain. Nonselective NSAIDs or nonacetylated salicylates are the next viable option unless the patient has active or a PMH of GI bleeding. For patients with GI risk, NSAIDs + a GI protective agent or COX-2 inhibitors should be used. If all previous medications do not provide relief, tramadol can be trialed next. Opioids are last-line medications because of their addictive qualities and side effects (ie, respiratory depression).

11. AZ is a 72-year-old woman with a history of atrial fibrillation treated with warfarin. Her height is 5' 2", weight is 198 lb, blood pressure is 116/76 mm Hg, and SCr is 1.1. AZ is now complaining of pain and stiffness in her left knee. X-ray shows joint space narrowing and osteophytes at the joint. Which treatment should be initiated at this point? Select all that apply.

    a. Weight reduction
    b. Tylenol
    c. Celebrex
    d. Tramadol

Answer a is correct. Initiation of weight loss may assist with decreased load for the joint and possible symptom relief.

Answer b is correct. Acetaminophen is a first-line treatment for OA. Acetaminophen can potentiate the anticoagulant effect of warfarin therapy, but is an appropriate choice with monitoring of the patient.

Answer c is incorrect. Celecoxib is third-line treatment for OA and has demonstrated an increase in the anticoagulant effect of warfarin.

Answer d is incorrect. Tramadol is used for patients with contraindications to NSAIDs or have failed previous drug trials.

12. BY is a 65-year-old man with confirmed OA. He has been pain free on his current regimen of acetaminophen 650 mg every 6 hours for 2 years. PMH is significant for GI bleed 4 years ago and HTN. He now presents to your clinic with pain in his left hip. BY's medication regimen also consists of lisinopril 40 mg daily and hydrochlorothiazide 25 mg daily. What recommendation will you present to the physician?

    a. Increase acetaminophen to 1000 mg every 4 hours, reinforce fitness program.
    b. Add pantoprazole 40 mg daily to his regimen, reinforce fitness program.
    c. Stop acetaminophen, begin ibuprofen 400 mg tid, reinforce fitness program.
    d. Stop acetaminophen, begin Anaprox 250 mg bid, Protonix 40 mg daily, reinforce fitness program.
    e. Add celecoxib 200 mg daily, reinforce fitness program.

Answer d is correct. Naproxen is a member of the nonselective NSAID class. Increased CV disease may be higher in NSAIDs as a class. At this time, naproxen is the only nonselective drug studied that has a lower risk than ibuprofen or diclofenac. BY has a PMH of GI bleed, so a

GI protective agent such as pantoprazole should be added to his NSAID regimen. Reinforcing muscle-strengthening and range of motion exercises should be part of every OA treatment.

Answer a is incorrect. The maximum dose for acetaminophen is 4000 mg daily. This answer gives a daily dose of 6000 mg daily and increases the patient's risk for developing hepatotoxicity.

Answer b is incorrect. The addition of pantoprazole would provide some GI protection, but would not provide any more pain relief.

Answer c is incorrect. BY has HTN and is at high risk for CV disease. Though studies are not conclusive and all drugs in the nonselective NSAID class have not been studied, ibuprofen has shown some increased risk of MI, stroke, heart failure, and HTN.

Answer e is incorrect. Studies have shown that COX-2 inhibitors have an increased risk of MI, stroke, heart failure, and HTN. Celecoxib would not be an appropriate choice as BY has HTN and is high CV risk.

13. CK is a 58-year-old woman who presents to your pharmacotherapy clinic today with an international normalized ratio (INR) of 4.2 (she was previously stable for 6 months). She has a PMH of diabetes, atrial fibrillation, and HTN. The list of medications that she gives you from her pharmacy are as follows: metformin 1000 mg and glipizide 10 mg bid; warfarin 5 mg on Monday, Wednesday, and Friday and 2.5 mg on Sunday, Tuesday, Thursday, and Saturday; amlodipine 10 mg daily; potassium chloride 10 mEq daily; and hydrochlorothiazide 25 mg daily. CK has not had a warfarin dosage change in over 1 year. She tells you her right knee has been bothering her much more frequently than usual. Which of the following is the most likely reason for her INR fluctuation?

    a. CK took 5 mg warfarin tablets every day in the past week.
    b. After questioning CK about over-the-counter (OTC) use, she tells you she has been using Capsaicin-HP on her knee for the past week.
    c. After questioning CK about OTC use, she tells you she has been taking acetaminophen 650 mg every 6 hours to relieve her from knee pain for the past week.
    d. CK is not telling you about a herbal product she has begun taking.

Answer c is correct. A drug-drug interaction can occur between warfarin and acetaminophen. Acetaminophen may enhance the anticoagulant effect of warfarin. Acetaminophen is available OTC. Many patients do not consider an OTC drug as part of their medication list. Patients should always be asked what OTC medications they are taking.

Answer a is incorrect. Though this is a possibility, CK has been stabilized for 6 months. She is young and has not made this mistake previously.

Answer b is incorrect. Capsaicin-HP is a topical treatment and does not affect INR.

Answer d is incorrect. Though this is a possibility, CK has stated she is having knee pain. A proven drug interaction is seen between warfarin and acetaminophen. CK is most likely taking something for her pain, not a herbal product that is not labeled to help reduce pain.

---

14. DP is a 55-year-old man who has HTN and a positive family history of early CV disease. His medications include aspirin 81 mg daily and metoprolol 25 mg bid. DP's OA is no longer controlled with acetaminophen 650 mg every 6 hours. The physician wants to begin DP on a regimen including an NSAID. Which treatment do you recommend?

    a. Naproxen 250 mg bid
    b. Naproxen 500 mg tid
    c. Celebrex 200 mg daily
    d. Celebrex 800 mg daily

Answer a is correct. NSAIDs as a class are probably not the best option for a patient with high CV risk. In this situation, the physician will prescribe an NSAID regardless, so you should provide the option that will cause the least harm. Most nonselective NSAIDs have not been studied in regards to CV risk. But of those studied, naproxen seems to have less CV risk than others.

Answer b is incorrect. The frequency of naproxen is bid, not tid.

Answer c is incorrect. COX-2 inhibitors should be avoided in patients with high CV risk. This patient does not have any absolute contraindications to nonselective NSAIDs, so this therapy should be tried before COX-2 inhibitors.

Answer d is incorrect. This is an abnormal dose for OA treatment. In OA, dosages should begin at 200 mg daily or 100 mg bid.

---

15. The physician does not take your advice for DP in Question 14. She prescribes ibuprofen 800 mg three times per day. Which of the following do you need to counsel DP concerning?

    a. Do not take this medication, it might cause you harm.
    b. Take ibuprofen at least 30 minutes after aspirin or aspirin 8 hours after ibuprofen. Monitor your BP more often.
    c. Stop taking your aspirin. Do not take ibuprofen on an empty stomach.
    d. Stop taking your aspirin. Monitor your BP more often.

Answer b is correct. Ibuprofen may block the antiplatelet effect of aspirin. Ibuprofen may diminish the cardioprotective effect that aspirin is providing to this patient. Aspirin may decrease the effect of ibuprofen. To limit the interaction, the two drugs should be administered separately. The minimum time between these two drugs is ibuprofen at least 30 minutes after aspirin or aspirin 8 hours after ibuprofen. BP should be monitored because NSAIDs cause sodium and water retention, therefore, possibly raising BP.

Answer a is incorrect. The studies evaluating nonselective NSAIDs as a class are inconclusive. You should counsel the patient to monitor their BP more frequently, keep all appointments with their physician, and call the pharmacist or physician if any side effects are experienced.

Answer c is incorrect. This patient is a high-risk CV patient. Aspirin is being used for cardioprotection and should not be stopped. Ibuprofen should not be taken on an empty stomach.

Answer d is incorrect. BP should be monitored more often, but aspirin should not be discontinued without a physician's consent. The patient has a family history positive for CV disease.

---

16. A 44-year-old woman with a history of GI bleed presents to your community pharmacy. She tells you her pregnancy test from last night was positive. She presents refill bottles for her prescription of ibuprofen 400 mg every 8 hours and Cytotec 200 mcg bid and asks if these are okay for her to keep taking. You respond:

    a. Stop taking Cytotec. It is ok to continue ibuprofen.
    b. Stop taking ibuprofen. It is ok to continue Cytotec.
    c. Continue taking both medications. Call your physician as soon as you can.
    d. Continue taking both medications. Your pregnancy test may not be accurate.
    e. Stop taking both prescriptions. Let us call your physician together now to discuss your situation.

Answer e is correct. The patient should stop taking the medications immediately until the physician can be reached to assess pain control and pregnancy plans. NOTE: Misoprostol is a gastroprotective agent that prevents NSAID GI ulceration. However, it is a prostaglandin analog and is contraindicated in pregnancy and women of child bearing potential (unless a woman is capable of complying with effective contraception measures).

Answer a is incorrect. Ibuprofen has a C/D pregnancy rating. It has caused deformities and miscarriages in some cases.

Answer b is incorrect. Misoprostol has a pregnancy rating of X. It is an abortifacient.

Answer c is incorrect. Both medications should be stopped immediately if any chance of pregnancy exists. Then the physician should be called to prescribe alternative agents.

Answer d is incorrect. Pregnancy tests can have false-positives, but you should not take the risk of counseling the patient to continue an abortifacient.

---

17. Which of the following medications is contraindicated in patients with documented sulfa allergy?

    a. Ultram
    b. Toradol

c. Celebrex
d. Aspirin
e. HA

Answer c is correct. An allergy to sulfa is a contraindication to celecoxib.

Answer a is incorrect. Tramadol may be taken in patients with a history of sulfa allergy.

Answer b is incorrect. Toradol may be taken in patients with a history of sulfa allergy.

Answer d is incorrect. Aspirin is not contraindicated in patients with a sulfa allergy.

Answer e is incorrect. HA is not contraindicated in patients with a sulfa allergy.

18. AM is a 52-year-old woman whose medications include acetaminophen 500 mg four times per day, gabapentin 300 mg three times per day, gemfibrozil 600 mg twice daily, and fluoxetine 20 mg daily. At the direction of her physician, AM added ibuprofen 800 mg twice daily and capsaicin cream 0.025% three times per day as needed to her regimen. While putting on her contacts this morning, she experienced an immediate burning pain in her eyes. She immediately takes out her contacts, flushes her eyes, and calls you, her pharmacist. Which of the following is most likely causing her eye pain?

a. Capsaicin cream
b. Acetaminophen
c. Drug interaction between acetaminophen and gemfibrozil
d. Drug interaction between acetaminophen and gabapentin

Answer a is correct. Contact with the eyes should be avoided when using capsaicin because it causes a burning sensation and irritation. AM either did not wash her hands after applying the cream or did not wash the cream completely off of her hands before touching her contacts to her eyes.

Answer b is incorrect. Eye pain is not a side effect of acetaminophen.

Answer c is incorrect. There are no drug interactions between acetaminophen and gemfibrozil.

Answer d is incorrect. There are no drug interactions between acetaminophen and gabapentin.

19. KT is a 73-year-old woman with OA of the hand. Her medication list includes: salsalate 500 mg twice daily, Lantus 10 U at bedtime, hydrochlorothiazide 25 mg daily, and ibuprofen 400 mg as needed that was recently increased to 800 mg twice daily as needed because of pain. What recommendation(s) do you give to the physician during rounds? Select all that apply.

a. KT should not be on more than one NSAID at a time.
b. Ibuprofen should not be given as needed for OA.
c. Ibuprofen should be dosed three to four times daily.
d. Salsalate has a longer platelet effect than ibuprofen.

Answer a is correct. NSAIDs should not be used together as the anticoagulant effect is enhanced. The risk of bleeding increases. NOTE: patients may be on a baby aspirin for the anti-platelet effect and receive an NSAID for OA.

Answer b is correct. Agents being used to treat OA should be given round the clock. A drug will never be fully effective if used as needed.

Answer c is correct. The duration of ibuprofen is 4 to 6 hours. Its half-life is 2 to 4 hours in adults. Dosing this drug twice daily leaves 6 or more hours at which the patient is not experiencing any pain relief from the drug.

Answer d is incorrect. Salsalate is a nonacetylated salicylate and does not affect platelets like acetylated salicylates (aspirin) or NSAIDs.

20. GM is an 81-year-old woman with history of bilateral knee OA for 25 years. She has contraindications to surgery and has received one injection of HA (Synvisc One). She calls your clinic 2 days after the intra-articular injection and states that she has not felt any pain relief. You explain:

a. She will not experience pain relief at this point.
b. She may need concomitant administration of intra-articular glucocorticoid.
c. She should take glucosamine and chondroitin in addition to the use of HA.
d. She should stop NSAID therapy while Hyalgan is administered.

Answer a is correct. HA has a slow onset of action; therefore, the results of the medication are not evident immediately.

Answer b is incorrect. Patients should receive intra-articular corticosteroids for acute exacerbations and not as treatment for chronic inflammation.

Answer c is incorrect. Use of glucosamine and chondroitin in addition to HA will not improve patient response.

Answer d is incorrect. Patient should continue current NSAID treatment if she is receiving it. This will continue to decrease pain and inflammation for the patient.

21. A 59-year-old man with history of 2 months of joint pain in his knees with movement decides to treat with glucosamine chondroitin. He reports an allergy to shellfish. He asks for your recommendation. Which of the following counseling points do you discuss with the patient? Select all that apply.

a. No significant benefit is seen with use of glucosamine chondroitin as monotherapy.
b. Glucosamine chondroitin could be considered as an adjunct to other forms of therapy.
c. Glucosamine chondroitin is contraindicated in those with shellfish allergies.
d. GI symptoms of gas, bloating, and cramps may occur with use of glucosamine chondroitin.

Answer a is correct. Use of these agents as monotherapy did not show superiority to placebo.

Answer b is correct. Glucosamine chondroitin is not recommended and should not be used as monotherapy. It can be considered as an adjunct therapy for patients taking additional therapies.

Answer c is correct. Glucosamine is contraindicated with shellfish allergies.

Answer d is correct. GI symptoms are mild but may include gas, bloating, or cramps.

CHAPTER **52 | Parkinson Disease**

1. What is the primary neurotransmitter deficiency in PD?

    a. Acetylcholine
    b. Dopamine
    c. Norepinephrine
    d. Serotonin

Answer b is correct. The deficiency is caused by a loss of nigrostriatal neurons in the substantia nigra pars compacta.

Answer a is incorrect. There is a relative overactivity of acetylcholine in PD.

Answer c is incorrect. Adrenergic pathways may be affected by PD, but norepinephrine is not the primary neurotransmitter deficiency.

Answer d is incorrect. Serotonergic pathways may be affected by PD, but serotonin is not the primary neurotransmitter deficiency.

2. What is the primary goal of PD treatment?

    a. Cessation of disease progression
    b. Facilitate an increase in the storage capacity of dopamine
    c. Maintenance of functional ability
    d. Reversal of neuronal loss

Answer c is correct. The control of motor symptoms ultimately allows the PD patient to continue to function and perform normal activities of daily living. As there is no medication that stops disease progression, the goal is to maintain the patient's ability to function as long as possible.

Answer a is incorrect. There are currently no therapies that stop the progression of PD.

Answer b in incorrect. As PD progresses, additional neurons will cease to function and dopamine levels will continue to decrease. As there is no medication that stops disease progression, there is no medication that increases dopamine storage capacity.

Answer d is incorrect. There are no medications capable of reversing the loss of nigrostriatal neurons.

3. What is the role of carbidopa in the treatment of PD?

    a. It inhibits acetylcholine.
    b. It inhibits dopa decarboxylase.
    c. It inhibits COMT.
    d. It inhibits MAO.

Answer b is correct. Carbidopa inhibits dopa decarboxylase to prevent the conversion of levodopa to dopamine in the periphery allowing the drug to cross the blood brain barrier.

Answer a is incorrect. Anticholinergics (such as benztropine) inhibit acetylcholine.

Answer c is incorrect. COMT inhibitors (tolcapone and entacapone) inhibit COMT.

Answer d is incorrect. MAO inhibitors (selegiline and rasagiline) inhibit MAO.

4. KJ is a young-onset Parkinson disease patient who was started on therapy approximately 1 month ago. Her husband is on the phone to your clinic concerned about his wife's behavior. He claims that KJ has been shopping online almost continuously over the previous few weeks, and recently went out and purchased a new vehicle without his knowledge. Assuming this is a medication-induced phenomenon, which medication are you most likely to discover when you view KJ's medication profile? Select all that apply.

    a. Amantadine
    b. Pramipexole
    c. Rasagiline
    d. Rotigotine

Answer b is correct. Pramipexole is a DA, and has been associated with impulsive behaviors including gambling, shopping, and hypersexuality.

Answer d is correct. Rotigotine is a DA, and has been associated with impulsive behaviors including gambling, shopping, and hypersexuality.

Answer a is incorrect. Amantadine has not been associated with impulsive behavior.

Answer c is incorrect. Rasagiline has not been associated with impulsive behavior.

5. SP was diagnosed with PD 7 years ago. Originally, she was taking carbidopa/levodopa 25/100 mg po tid, which has since been increased to 50/250 mg po qid. Nonmotor symptoms include constipation and insomnia, and she also has arthritis for which she takes acetaminophen 650 mg po tid. Assuming another medication is to be added at this time, which medication would you suggest avoiding based on her history of present illness?

    a. Pramipexole
    b. Rasagiline
    c. Ropinirole
    d. Selegiline

Answer d is correct. Selegiline has an amphetamine metabolite, and has been associated with an increased incidence of insomnia. Doses should be given no later than early afternoon to help prevent this side effect in a patient for which it is indicated. In a patient with uncontrolled insomnia, the drug is best avoided.

Answer a is incorrect. The addition of a DA to supplement carbidopa/levodopa is a logical strategy. There appear to be no contraindications or concerns with the addition of this medication to SP's profile.

Answer b is incorrect. Rasagiline is a logical addition to SP's regimen. The drug inhibits MAO-B thereby increasing the amount of available dopamine in the brain. There appear to be no contraindications or concerns with the addition of this medication to SP's profile.

Answer c is incorrect. The addition of a DA to supplement carbidopa/levodopa is a logical strategy. There appear to be no contraindications or concerns with the addition of this medication to SP's profile.

---

6. For which PD symptom are anticholinergics primarily used?

   a. Bradykinesia
   b. Postural instability
   c. Rigidity
   d. Tremor

Answer d is correct. Anticholinergics help to correct the relative overactivity of acetylcholine that exists due to dopamine deficiency. It is this imbalance that is responsible for the tremor of PD.

Answer a is incorrect. Anticholinergics are not useful for patients with significant bradykinesia.

Answer b is incorrect. Anticholinergics do not help correct postural instability.

Answer c is incorrect. Anticholinergics are not useful for patients with significant rigidity.

---

7. AB is a long-term PD patient. His neurologist has written a new prescription for tolcapone 100 mg po tid. What laboratory values need to be monitored with the addition of this medication?

   a. Hematocrit
   b. Liver function tests
   c. Platelet count
   d. Serum glucose

Answer b is correct. Due to the emergence of several cases of fulminant liver failure in patients receiving tolcapone, monitoring of liver function tests is recommended at baseline, every 2 to 4 weeks for the next 6 months, and then periodically for the duration of therapy.

Answer a is incorrect. Routine monitoring of hematocrit is not required with tolcapone use.

Answer c is incorrect. Routine monitoring of platelet count is not required with tolcapone use.

Answer d is incorrect. Routine monitoring of serum glucose is not required with tolcapone use.

---

8. Which drug should be dosed simultaneously with levodopa?

   a. Amantadine
   b. Entacapone
   c. Pramipexole
   d. Rasagiline

Answer b is correct. Entacapone inhibits the action of COMT in the periphery to avoid the breakdown of levodopa and carbidopa before levodopa crosses the blood brain barrier. It must be present with levodopa to achieve this outcome.

Answer a is incorrect. Amantadine is typically dosed twice daily and may be administered to patients who are not receiving levodopa therapy.

Answer c is incorrect. Pramipexole stimulates dopamine receptors independent of levodopa and may be used as monotherapy.

Answer d is incorrect. Rasagiline inhibits the breakdown of dopamine in the brain and may be used as monotherapy without levodopa.

---

9. EF is a new patient at your clinic. He presents with tremor and rigidity, the onset of which he claims was "overnight." His symptoms appear to be parkinsonian in nature. In order to rule out drug-induced symptoms, his medication profile should be screened for which of the following? Select all that apply.

   a. Haloperidol
   b. Metoclopramide
   c. Prochlorperazine
   d. Risperidone

Answer a is correct. Haloperidol is an antipsychotic medication that has been associated with parkinsonism.

Answer b is correct. Metoclopramide is centrally acting and has been associated with parkinsonism.

Answer c is correct. Prochlorperazine is a phenothiazine antiemetic and has been associated with parkinsonism.

Answer d is correct. Risperidone is a second generation antipsychotic medication that has been associated with parkinsonism.

---

10. What is the mechanism of action of ropinirole?

    a. Direct replacement of dopamine in the CNS
    b. Direct stimulation of postsynaptic dopamine receptors

c. Inhibition of the enzymatic breakdown of dopamine in the CNS

d. Inhibition of the enzymatic breakdown of dopamine in the periphery

---

Answer b is correct. DAs bypass the nigrostriatal neurons and provide direct receptor stimulation exerting effects like dopamine.

Answer a is incorrect. Levodopa is converted to dopamine in the brain and serves to replace the neurotransmitter directly.

Answer c is incorrect. DAs do not inhibit the enzymatic breakdown of dopamine.

Answer D is incorrect. DAs do not inhibit the enzymatic breakdown of dopamine.

---

11. One of your long-term PD patients, WO, is complaining of hallucinations. She has experienced no recent additions to her medication regimen, or changes in medication doses. Her symptoms include visual hallucinations which are frightening to her, and the decision is made to initiate antipsychotic therapy. Which medication is the best initial choice for the treatment of PD associated psychosis?

a. Chlorpromazine
b. Haloperidol
c. Olanzapine
d. Pimavanserin

Answer d is correct. Pimavanserin exerts its activity at serotonergic receptors only. As such, it does not exacerbate symptoms of PD.

Answer a is incorrect. Chlorpromazine is an antidopaminergic antipsychotic and should be avoided in patients with PD.

Answer b is incorrect. Haloperidol is an antidopaminergic antipsychotic and should be avoided in patients with PD.

Answer c is incorrect. Olanzapine possesses antidopaminergic properties and has been known to increase symptoms of PD.

---

12. PY is a patient with PD who has a difficult time in swallowing medications. His family states he sometimes chokes on his medications and when he drinks more than just a sip of liquid. Which medication used for the treatment of PD is available in an oral formulation that might be a safer option for PY? Select all that apply.

a. Carbidopa/levodopa
b. Pramipexole
c. Selegiline
d. Trihexyphenidyl

Answer a is correct. Carbidopa/levodopa is available as an orally disintegrating tablet that may be taken without liquid.

Answer c is correct. Selegiline is available as an orally disintegrating tablet that may be taken without liquid.

Answer b is incorrect. There is no orally disintegrating formulation of pramipexole available.

Answer d is incorrect. There is no orally disintegrating formulation of trihexyphenidyl available.

---

13. Which medication can cause rebound PD symptoms, if stopped abruptly?

a. Amantadine
b. Carbidopa/levodopa
c. Pramipexole
d. Rasagiline

Answer a is correct. If amantadine is to be discontinued, it should be slowly tapered to avoid rebound symptoms.

Answer b is incorrect. Abrupt discontinuation of carbidopa/levodopa can lead to the development of neuroleptic malignant syndrome.

Answer c is incorrect. Abrupt discontinuation of pramipexole can lead to the development of neuroleptic malignant syndrome.

Answer d is incorrect. Rasagiline discontinuation does not require a taper.

---

14. GR was recently diagnosed with PD. His family practitioner initiated therapy with carbidopa/levodopa 10/100 mg three times daily. He has been taking the medication with meals, but he is experiencing significant nausea. GR has noticed very little difference in his symptoms. What is the most probable reason GR is experiencing such significant nausea?

a. Carbidopa/levodopa should be taken on an empty stomach.
b. Carbidopa/levodopa should be taken with a meal high in protein.
c. The levodopa component is being converted to dopamine in the periphery.
d. Carbidopa/levodopa always causes nausea.

Answer c is correct. The minimum daily dose of carbidopa necessary to prevent the peripheral conversion of levodopa to dopamine is 75 to 100 mg. The fact that GR has not noticed improvement in his symptoms supports the notion that levodopa is not crossing the blood brain barrier to be converted to dopamine.

Answer a is incorrect. It is true that the drug should be taken on an empty stomach for optimal absorption, but administration with food often helps to relieve nausea.

Answer b is incorrect. Amino acids compete with levodopa for transport into the brain. If carbidopa/levodopa is to be taken with food, a low-protein meal is recommended.

Answer d is incorrect. Though nausea is a frequent side effect associated with carbidopa/levodopa, it is not inevitable.

15. Comorbid conditions frequently present in persons with PD include which of the following? Select all that apply.

    a. Constipation
    b. Dementia
    c. Depression
    d. Hypotension

Answer a is correct. Neurological derangements in the gastrointestinal tract contribute to constipation in the PD patient.

Answer b is correct. Patients with PD are up to four times more likely to develop dementia than the non-PD population.

Answer c is correct. Depression is present in over half of patients with PD and may be part of the disease itself.

Answer d is correct. Hypotension in persons with PD may be disease related or drug induced.

16. You receive a communication from a pulmonologist about your patient, JL. JL has been experiencing shortness of breath upon exertion with increasing severity. The pulmonologist is inquiring as to JL's PD medications. Which is likely to be the cause of JL's symptoms?

    a. Bromocriptine
    b. Pramipexole
    c. Ropinirole
    d. Rotigotine

Answer a is correct. Bromocriptine is DA and an ergot derivative. Ergots are associated with the complication of pulmonary fibrosis.

Answer b is incorrect. Non-ergot DAs are significantly less likely to be associated with fibrotic complications.

Answer c is incorrect. Non-ergot DAs are significantly less likely to be associated with fibrotic complications.

Answer d is incorrect. Non-ergot DAs are significantly less likely to be associated with fibrotic complications.

17. What is the trade name of rasagiline?

    a. Azilect
    b. Comtan
    c. Mirapex
    d. Zelapar

Answer a is correct. The trade name of rasagiline is Azilect.

Answer c is correct. Mirapex is the trade name of pramipexole.

Answer d is correct. Zelapar is the trade name of the selegiline ODT formulation.

Answer b is incorrect. Comtan is the trade name of entacapone.

18. WR was diagnosed with PD 12 years ago. He has developed dementia which has progressively worsened over the last year. It has become difficult for his caregiver to administer oral medications as he is resistant to swallowing them, and frequently spits them out. Which DA is available in a dosage form that bypasses this problem?

    a. Bromocriptine
    b. Pramipexole
    c. Ropinirole
    d. Rotigotine

Answer d is correct. Rotigotine is available as a patch to be applied topically.

Answer a is incorrect. Bromocriptine is only available in oral formulations.

Answer b is incorrect. Pramipexole is only available in oral formulations.

Answer c is incorrect. Ropinirole is only available in oral formulations.

19. NE is a PD patient who is nonadherent with her medications because she has difficulty in remembering to take all but her morning doses. Which medications are available in formulations that might increase NE's success in taking her medications as prescribed? Select all that apply.

    a. Carbidopa/levodopa
    b. Pramipexole
    c. Rasagiline
    d. Rotigotine

Answer b is correct. Pramipexole is available in a once-daily formulation.

Answer c is correct. Rasagiline is available as a patch that is replaced once daily.

Answer d is correct. Rotigotine is available in a once-daily formulation.

Answer a is incorrect. Carbidopa/levodopa, despite being available in a controlled-release formulation, must still be dosed multiple times per day, and will necessitate more frequent dosing as the disease progresses.

20. MV has been taking carbidopa/levodopa for 6 years. He has begun to develop involuntary movements of his trunk and extremities which include tics and chorea. Which of the following is a true statement about the symptoms MV is experiencing? Select all that apply.

    a. The symptoms often appear when the cardinal motor symptoms of PD are under good control.
    b. Decreasing the dose of levodopa might alleviate the symptoms.

c. They rarely occur early in the disease process.

d. They are more likely to occur with DA monotherapy.

Answer a is correct. Dyskinesias in the Parkinson's patient frequently occur when disease symptoms are well controlled and dopamine receptors are adequately stimulated. For this reason, the term "peak dose" dyskinesia is often used.

Answer b is correct. Decreasing the levodopa dose may alleviate dyskinesias. However, symptom breakthrough often makes this difficult to achieve.

Answer c is correct. Dyskinesias are associated with levodopa use that has usually been continuous over several years with increasing doses.

Answer d is incorrect. DAs are less likely to induce dyskinesias compared to carbidopa/levodopa. For this reason, younger patients are often started on DAs first to delay carbidopa/levodopa exposure.

---

21. TS lives in a rural community where there is no neurology practice. For the last several years, he has been experiencing tremors, rigidity, and bradykinesia that began on his left side, but has since migrated and become bilateral, though his left side is still affected more than his right. He is diagnosed with PD and his motor symptoms are graded as moderate (tremor and bradykinesia), and moderate-severe (rigidity). What is the most appropriate order for the initiation and progression of treatment for his PD?

a. Benztropine, rasagiline, carbidopa/levodopa

b. Pramipexole, entacapone, carbidopa/levodopa

c. Ropinirole, levodopa/carbidopa, tolcapone

d. Carbidopa/levodopa, rotigotine, rasagiline

Answer d is correct. For patients with moderate-severe symptoms, carbidopa/levodopa is the preferred agent to initiate therapy. The addition of a DA is appropriate as second-line therapy. The addition of an MAO-B inhibitor will help prolong the effects of dopamine by minimizing it's metabolism by MAO.

Answer a is incorrect. An anticholinergic agent is used primarily for tremor, and since its effect on symptoms is mild, it is not indicated for someone with advanced disease. For patients with moderate-severe symptoms, carbidopa/levodopa is the preferred agent to initiate therapy.

Answer b is incorrect. For patients with moderate-severe symptoms, carbidopa/levodopa is the preferred agent to initiate therapy. Entacapone cannot be utilized until carbidopa/levodopa is part of the medication regimen.

Answer c is incorrect. For patients with moderate-severe symptoms, carbidopa/levodopa is the preferred agent to initiate therapy. DAs, while appropriate first-line therapy for milder symptoms, are not likely to control moderate-severe symptoms alone. Tolcapone should be reserved for use only after other agents have failed due to the risk of fulminant liver failure.

CHAPTER **53 | Epilepsy**

1. Select the treatable cause(s) of seizures. Select all that apply.

a. Hypoglycemia

b. Altered electrolytes

c. Infections

d. Genetic defects

Answers a, b, and c are correct. Hypoglycemia, altered electrolytes, and infections are treatable causes of seizures. A seizure produced by treatable causes does not represent epilepsy.

Note: medications that cause hypoglycemia and altered electrolytes could indirectly precipitate a seizure.

Answer d is incorrect. Genetic defects do not represent a treatable cause as they are not something modifiable.

Note: The underlying etiology of epilepsy is unknown in 80% of patients. The most common recognized causes of epilepsy are head trauma and stroke. Central nervous system tumors, infections, metabolic disturbances (hyponatremia and hypoglycemia), neurodegenerative diseases, and medications represent other causes.

---

2. WW is a 56-year-old hospitalized patient taking the following medications: cefepime, metoprolol succinate, levothyroxine, and acetaminophen. The patient developed seizures. Select the possible drug-induced cause(s) of seizures.

a. Levothyroxine

b. Acetaminophen

c. Cefepime

d. Metoprolol

Answer c is correct. Cefepime has been linked to seizures and nonconvulsive SE, a risk that is increased in patients with renal impairment and in patients with a history of a seizure disorder. Dosage adjustments are necessary. Other medications associated with development of seizures include tramadol, bupropion, theophylline, some antidepressants, some antipsychotics, amphetamines, cocaine, imipenem, lithium, excessive doses of penicillins or cephalosporins, sympathomimetics, and stimulants.

Answers a, b, and d are incorrect. None of these agents are associated with causing seizures.

---

3. JW is a 29-year-old woman presenting to the pharmacy with a new prescription for phenytoin. She is currently not taking any other medications. What should this patient be counseled about in relation to her new drug therapy? Select all that apply.

a. Avoid alcohol while taking this medication.

b. Use appropriate barrier methods of contraception.

c. Wear sunscreen. This medication is associated with increased photosensitivity.

d. Take this medication with food at the same time every day.

Answers a and b are correct. Alcohol should be avoided because it can inhibit the metabolism of phenytoin and increase CNS depression. Phenytoin can also interact with oral contraceptives and decrease their effect, so barrier methods of contraception are recommended. In general, all women of child-bearing age with a seizure disorder should be counseled about the risks of getting pregnant and the need for appropriate counseling and prenatal care if pregnancy is planned.

Answers c and d are incorrect. Phenytoin is not associated with increase sun sensitivity. Also, food can decrease phenytoin absorption and though it is important to take the medication every day, the timing of administration is not a factor in achieving therapeutic goals.

---

4. Select the goal therapeutic level for phenytoin in this patient.

   a. 4 to 12 mcg/mL
   b. 10 to 20 mcg/mL
   c. 50 to 100 mcg/mL
   d. No therapeutic drug monitoring is required with this drug.

Answer b is correct. Phenytoin's usual total serum concentration is 10 to 20 mg/L (10-20 mcg/mL).

Answer a is incorrect. Carbamazepine's usual serum concentration is 4 to 12 mg/L.

Answer c is incorrect. Valproic acid's usual serum concentration is 50 to 100 mg/L.

Answer d is incorrect. Serum concentrations of phenytoin should be monitored.

---

5. A year later, JW tells you that she wants to become pregnant and would like to change to a different AED that might be safer during pregnancy. What is important to discuss with her and her physician in regards to switching therapy?

   a. Her current medication should be stopped immediately in order to ensure that the current AED has been fully removed out of her system prior to getting pregnant.
   b. Her existing AED can be stopped abruptly and the new AED should be started at a low dose and titrated up to the target dose.
   c. Her new AED should be initiated at a low dose and titrated up to become minimally effective at which time the existing AED can be gradually tapered.
   d. She should avoid pregnancy altogether and remain on her current AED therapy.

Answer c is correct. Switching AEDs requires a titration process because abrupt discontinuation of an AED may lead to breakthrough seizures. The process requires starting the new AED at a low dose and titrating up to the minimal effective dose. Once the minimal effective dose is reached, the drug to be discontinued is gradually tapered, while the dose of the new AED continues to be increased to the target dose.

Answers a and b are incorrect. AEDs should not be abruptly discontinued as they can precipitate a seizure. Patients who are seizure-free may desire to discontinue their

medication. Factors favoring successful withdrawal of AEDs include a seizure-free period of 2 to 4 years, complete seizure control within 1 year of onset, an onset of seizures after age 2 but before age 35, and a normal neurologic examination and EEG. Withdrawal of AEDs is done slowly with a dose tapered over at least 3 months.

Answer d is incorrect. A patient that has a seizure disorder and desires to become pregnant should discuss the benefits and risks of drug therapy collaboratively with their healthcare provider to determine the best way to minimize risks to the patient and baby.

The following case pertains to questions 6 and 7.

6. A patient is admitted to the hospital with seizures that result in a sudden interruption of activities and a blank stare. What type of seizure disorder is this?

   a. Absence seizures
   b. Tonic-clonic
   c. Myoclonic
   d. Atonic

Answer a is correct. Absence seizures or petit mal result in sudden interruption of activities and a blank stare.

Answer b is incorrect. Tonic-clonic seizures or grand mal result in alternating muscle contractions and jerking.

Answer c is incorrect. Myoclonic seizures result in brief shock-like contractions of a muscle group.

Answer d is incorrect. Atonic seizures result in sudden loss of muscle tone ("drop attacks").

---

7. What is the recommended first-line treatment for this type of seizure disorder?

   a. Phenytoin
   b. Felbamate
   c. Levetiracetam
   d. Ethosuximide

Answer d is correct. Ethosuximide is the first-line treatment for absence seizures.

Answers a, b, and c are incorrect. None of these drugs treat absence seizures.

The following case pertains to questions 8 and 9.

8. BH is a 47-year-old man in SE in need of drug therapy. Intravenous dosing of phenytoin cannot be infused faster than 50 mg/min. Select the adverse reactions that are associated with infusions faster than 50 mg/min.

   a. Hypotension
   b. Gingival hyperplasia
   c. Anemia
   d. Rash

Answer a is correct. The dose cannot be infused faster than 50 mg/min due to the potential risks of hypotension and arrhythmias.

Answers b, c, and d are incorrect. Gingival hyperplasia, anemia, and rash are idiosyncratic reactions and not related to infusion rates or dose.

---

9. What is the water-soluble prodrug of phenytoin that is rapidly converted to phenytoin in the body and can be used as an alternate?

    a. Trileptal
    b. Tegretol
    c. Cerebyx
    d. Dilantin

Answer c is correct. Cerebyx is fosphenytoin, which is a prodrug of phenytoin. It is compatible with most intravenous solutions and is tolerated as an intramuscular injection. Fosphenytoin is dosed on PE, and it can be infused up to 150 mg PE/min. Although fosphenytoin has fewer cardiovascular side effects compared to phenytoin, blood pressure and ECG should still be monitored.

Answer a is incorrect. Trileptal is oxcarbazepine.

Answer b is incorrect. Tegretol is carbamazepine.

Answer d is incorrect. Dilantin is phenytoin.

---

10. GG is a 67-year-old woman on carbamazepine for her seizure disorder. Her family is worried about serious side effects because of her age. Which of the following are idiosyncratic adverse reaction(s) associated with use of carbamazepine?

    a. Aplastic anemia
    b. Hyponatremia
    c. Rash
    d. Colitis

Answers a, b, and c are correct. Aplastic anemia, hyponatremia, and rash are idiosyncratic reactions. Because idiosyncratic reactions may be life threatening, the AED may require discontinuation. Idiosyncratic reactions are associated with an immunologic reaction; therefore, cross-reactivity among AEDs is possible.

Answer d is incorrect. Carbamazepine is not associated with the development of colitis (eg, *Clostridium difficile* colitis).

---

11. Select the patient population or condition that often leads to fast titration of AEDs.

    a. Switching AEDs
    b. Discontinuing AEDs
    c. Children
    d. Women of child-bearing potential

Answer c is correct. Children require prompt control of seizures to avoid interference with development of the brain and cognition. AED doses are increased rapidly and frequent changes in the regimen are made to maximize control of seizures. Due to high metabolic rates in children, doses of AEDs are higher on a milligram per kilogram basis compared to adults.

Answer a is incorrect. Switching AEDs requires a titration process, because abrupt discontinuation of an AED may lead to breakthrough seizures. The process requires starting the new AED at a *low dose* and titrating up to the minimal effective dose. Once the minimal effective dose is reached, the drug to be discontinued is *gradually tapered*, while the dose of the new AED continues to be increased to the target dose.

Answer b is incorrect. Epilepsy is considered a lifelong disorder; however, patients who are seizure-free may desire to discontinue their medication. Withdrawal of AEDs is done slowly with a dose tapered over at least 3 months.

Answer d is incorrect. Women of child-bearing potential or who are pregnant have recommendations for AED management because several AEDs have been implicated in minor and serious birth defects. The majority of pregnant epileptic patients receiving AEDs produce a normal infant, but special recommendations must be followed. Recommendations include: use monotherapy when possible; *use lowest dose* possible to control seizures; monitor AED serum concentrations at the start of pregnancy and monthly thereafter; give supplemental folic acid 1 to 4 mg daily to all women of child-bearing potential; and administer supplemental vitamin K during the eighth month of pregnancy to women receiving enzyme-inducing AEDs.

The following case pertains to questions 12 and 13.

12. DD is an elderly man currently on phenytoin. He has begun experiencing confusion and nystagmus in the past week. His last serum creatinine was 3.6 mg/dL and albumin 2.4 g/dL. His only other medications are aspirin and omeprazole. What could this be a symptom of?

    a. Aura before seizure onset
    b. Lack of seizure control
    c. Phenytoin toxicity
    d. Normal side effects of the drug

Answer c is correct. Phenytoin is highly protein bound. The usual total (bound and unbound) concentration for phenytoin is 10 to 20 mcg/mL; however, the unbound (free) concentration is 1 to 2 mcg/mL. The unbound concentration is the component that produces seizure control and adverse reactions. Symptoms of phenytoin toxicity include confusion, nystagmus, blurred vision, diplopia, and slurred speech.

Answers a, b, and d are incorrect. The symptoms the patient is experiencing are not indicative of uncontrolled seizure disorder. Nystagmus is not a normal side effect from taking phenytoin but can be indicative of drug toxicity.

---

13. What could be contributing to the development of these symptoms? Select all that apply.

    a. Drug interaction
    b. Low albumin
    c. Renal impairment
    d. Not taking the medication

Answers b and c are correct. Low albumin and renal impairment can lead to more free (unbound drug) drug resulting in signs and symptoms of drug toxicity.

Answer a is incorrect. Neither aspirin nor omeprazole is known to increase the concentration of phenytoin.

Answer d is incorrect. The patient is experiencing symptoms of drug toxicity, not symptoms of uncontrolled seizure disorder.

---

14. A physician tells you that she would like to begin lamotrigine in a patient in order to avoid some drug interactions with other AEDs, but she would like to know if there are any other adverse effects she should educate the patient about. Which of the following should be addressed with the patient?

    a. Rash
    b. Edema
    c. Pancreatitis
    d. Alopecia

Answer a is correct. Rash is an idiosyncratic reaction associated with lamotrigine. Patients should be aware of the possibility of hypersensitivity reactions. If a patient experiences rash, the drug should be discontinued unless it was clearly caused by something else.

Answer b is incorrect. Gabapentin and pregabalin are associated with development of pedal edema.

Answers c and d are incorrect. Lamotrigine is not associated with development of pancreatitis or alopecia. Valproic acid has been linked to both of these effects.

The following case pertains to questions 15 and 16.

15. SB is a patient with newly diagnosed complex seizure disorder. His physician has noted that he is taking warfarin for atrial fibrillation and also has restless leg syndrome. For this reason, he would like to avoid an AED that is a substrate and inducer of the CYP-450 2C9. Which of the following should be avoided in this patient? Select all that apply.

    a. Phenytoin
    b. Phenobarbital
    c. Carbamazepine
    d. Primidone

Answers a, b, c, and d are correct. Phenytoin, phenobarbital, carbamazepine, and primidone are all substrates and inducers of the CYP-450 2C9.

---

16. Which of the following would be the best option for this patient based on the information presented?

    a. Gabapentin
    b. Levetiracetam
    c. Carbamazepine
    d. Ethosuximide

Answer a is correct. Gabapentin is renally eliminated and does not have interactions via the CYP-450 pathway. It can also be used to treat restless leg syndrome.

Answer b is incorrect. Though levetiracetam is renally eliminated, it is not the best option for this patient given the fact that gabapentin can also help to treat her other condition (restless leg).

Answer c is incorrect. Carbamazepine is a CYP-450 2C9 substrate and inducer which could decrease the effects of warfarin.

Answer d is incorrect. Ethosuximide is not indicated for treating complex seizures. It is indicated for treating absence seizures.

---

17. Select the dose-related adverse reaction(s) of AEDs. Select all that apply.

    a. Neutropenia
    b. Sedation
    c. Thrombocytopenia
    d. Ataxia

Answers b and d are correct. Sedation is a dose-dependent adverse reaction. Other dose-dependent adverse reactions include ataxia and diplopia.

Answer a is incorrect. Neutropenia (hematologic toxicity) is an idiosyncratic reaction and not related to dose or concentration.

Answer c is incorrect. Thrombocytopenia (hematologic toxicity) is an idiosyncratic reaction and not related to dose or concentration. Other idiosyncratic reactions include rash and hepatotoxicity.

---

18. Select the AED that is associated with the idiosyncratic adverse effect of gingival hyperplasia.

    a. Phenobarbital
    b. Primidone
    c. Tiagabine
    d. Phenytoin

Answer d is correct. Phenytoin is associated with gingival hyperplasia (gum overgrowth).

Answers a, b, and c are incorrect. These AEDs are not associated with gingival hyperplasia.

Note: Primidone is rarely used; however, it is important because it is metabolized to two active metabolites, one of which is phenobarbital.

---

19. Select the AED that is available in oral and parenteral formulations. Select all that apply.

    a. Neurontin
    b. Dilantin
    c. Keppra
    d. Trileptal

Answers b and c are correct. Phenytoin (Dilantin) and levetiracetam (Keppra) are available in oral and parenteral formulations.

Answers a and d are incorrect. They are available in oral formulations only.

---

20. Which drug(s) for SE can be given intramuscularly?

    a. Phenytoin
    b. Lamotrigine
    c. Diazepam
    d. Fosphenytoin

Answer d is correct. Fosphenytoin is a water-soluble, prodrug of phenytoin that is rapidly converted to phenytoin in the body. Unlike phenytoin, fosphenytoin is compatible with most intravenous solutions and is tolerated as an intramuscular injection.

Answer a is incorrect. Phenytoin cannot be administered intramuscularly. Phenytoin should not be administered via the intramuscular route due to alkaline nature.

Answer b is incorrect. Lamotrigine is not appropriate to use to treat SE.

Answer c is incorrect. Diazepam is recommended for treating SE but should be used intravenously. It is also available as a rectal preparation if no intravenous access exists.

---

21. You read a clinical study for a new antiepileptic medication that has strong data to support its efficacy against other AEDs. The treatment duration studied was 18 weeks. However, clinical studies have shown the following data related to safety:

Adverse Effect	Placebo %	New Drug %
Nausea	14	16
Diarrhea	12	11
Serious Arrhythmia	1	5

What is the number needed-to-harm (NNH) related to arrhythmia?

    a. 1
    b. 4

c. 20
d. 25

Answer d is correct. NNH is calculated as 1/risk difference. In this case, the difference in risk between placebo and the new drug is 5% − 1% = 4%. 1/0.04 = 25. This means that for every 25 patients treated with the new drug one will experience a serious arrhythmia over the course of 18 weeks of treatment.

Answers a, b, and c are incorrect.

The following case pertains to questions 22 and 23.

22. You get a call from a provider asking about the occurrence of vision loss with Sabril®. They tell you that they suspect this serious adverse drug event has occurred in a patient. Where should this event be reported?

    a. FDA MedWatch
    b. Centers for Disease Control
    c. PubMed
    d. National Library of Medicine

Answer a is correct. Serious adverse effects should be reported to FDA MedWatch.

Answers b, c, and d are incorrect. None of these would be appropriate for adverse drug event reporting.

---

23. You are asked to substitute the oral solution packets for the tablets because your patient has a hard time swallowing tablets. You look in the FDA Orange Book for information and this is what you find. What do you do based on this information?

Appl No	N022006	N020427
TE Code		
RLD	Yes	Yes
Active Ingredient	Vigabatrin	Vigabatrin
Dosage Form; Route	For solution; oral	Tablet; oral
Strength	500 mg/packet	500 mg
Proprietary Name	Sabril	Sabril
Applicant	Lundbeck LLC	Lundbeck LLC

    a. Substitute the product without calling the physician; the products are therapeutic equivalents.
    b. Call the physician to ask about switching products; they are not therapeutic equivalents.
    c. Substitute the product without calling the physician; the products are pharmaceutical equivalents.
    d. Call the physician to ask about switching products; they are therapeutic equivalents.

Answer b is correct. The physician would need to be called in order to make this switch because the products are not pharmaceutical or therapeutic equivalents.

Answers a, c, and d are incorrect. These products are not therapeutic equivalents because they are not pharmaceutical equivalents. In order for drugs to be therapeutic equivalents, they must be (a) approved as safe and effective, (b) be pharmaceutic equivalents, and (c) bioequivalent. In order for drugs to be pharmaceutic equivalents they must (a) contain identical amounts of the same active drug ingredient *in the same dosage form* and route of administration, and (b) meet compendial or other applicable standards of strength, quality, purity, and identity.

CHAPTER 54 | Headache

1. Which of the following plays a role in migraine pathogenesis? Select all that apply.

   a. Norepinephrine
   b. Serotonin
   c. Dopamine
   d. Substance P

Answers b and d are correct. Serotonin is a vasoactive neurotransmitter that is released by the brainstem nuclei of the trigeminovascular system. Plasma levels of serotonin are found to be deficient during a migraine attack. Drugs that affect serotonin are often effective in treatment of migraines.

Other agents discussed as playing an active role within the trigeminovascular system are the following neuropeptides: calcitonin gene-related peptide, substance P, and neurokinin A.

Answer a is incorrect. There are no data that supports involvement of norepinephrine with the pathophysiology of migraine.

Answer c is incorrect. Dopamine may also play a role in migraine headaches as dopamine receptor antagonists are effective treatments administered as monotherapy or with other antimigraine medications; however, there is a lack of clinical data to support this theory.

2. A patient presents to your community pharmacy complaining of a headache. She rates the headache as a 7 on a scale of 1 to 10, and the pulsating worsens as the headache progresses. She experiences nausea and sensitivity to light until the headache dissipates after about 12 hours. She is unable to function during the headache. Which of the following headache types is this patient experiencing?

   a. Migraine
   b. Tension
   c. Cluster
   d. Caffeine

Answer a is correct. The International Headache Society diagnostic criteria for migraine includes:

Headache lasts for 4 to 72 hours and

At least two of the following characteristics:

Unilateral location, Pulsating, Moderate to severe intensity, Aggravated by routine physical activity

At least one of the following: Nausea and/or vomiting, Photophobia, and phonophobia.

Answer b is incorrect. Tension headache would have a gripping/tightening quality, not aggravated by activity, no nausea or vomiting, photophobia and phonophobia are absent or one but not the other is present.

Answer c is incorrect. Cluster headache would last for no longer than 180 minutes and exhibits signs/symptoms of conjunctival injection, lacrimation, nasal congestion, rhinorrhea, sweating miosis, ptosis, or eyelid edema.

Answer d is incorrect. Caffeine is a trigger for headaches, not a type of headache.

3. Which of the following signs/symptoms are classified as red flags, indicating need for physician referral and diagnostic evaluation? Select all that apply.

   a. "Worst headache of my life"
   b. Acute headache that occurs after coughing/sneezing
   c. Headache onset age ≥40 years
   d. Blood pressure of 150/80 mm Hg

Answer a is correct. Headache associated with subarachnoid hemorrhage is often described by the patient as the "worst" headache.

Answer b is correct. Headache after coughing or sneezing could be benign. However, it can also be a sign of cranial mass lesion with cerebrospinal fluid path obstruction.

Answer c is correct. Headache at age ≥40 can be indicative of a new organic cause. Although it can also be benign, it requires physician evaluation.

Answer d is incorrect. A blood pressure reading of 150/80 mm Hg is not a red flag condition that would require physician referral for headache.

4. LK suffers from chronic migraines and is currently experiencing an acute attack. She calls your community pharmacy and asks your professional advice. In talking with her you learn that she stopped drinking regular coffee, joined a gym, and started a monophasic oral contraceptive in the past two weeks. She attended a wine and cheese party last night with friends she met at the gym. Which recommendation would be best to provide that may help prevent migraines in the future?

   a. Avoid intake of wine and cheese.
   b. She should resume drinking regular coffee.
   c. She may benefit from switching to a triphasic oral contraceptive.
   d. She should avoid physical activity.

Answer a is correct. Wine and cheese are tyramine containing foods which are known to be headache triggers. Other potential food triggers include alcohol, chocolate, citrus fruits, dairy, fermented foods, and foods containing additives such as monosodium glutamate, nitrites, saccharin, sulfites, or yeast. When trying to determine a trigger of a patient's headache, it is recommended that the patient eliminate all causative agents and then gradually add back in one item at a time.

Answer b is incorrect. Caffeine intake or withdrawal can be a trigger and so her recent discontinuation may have been a trigger for her current headache. However, since she has already cut regular coffee from her diet and future caffeine consumption could trigger additional migraines, it would be best for her to continue to limit regular coffee from her diet.

Answer c is incorrect. Estrogen or oral contraceptives are known triggers of migraine. A monophasic oral contraceptive would be preferred over a triphasic formulation because it provides a more consistent hormone level. It would not be appropriate to recommend changing to a triphasic contraceptive as this may trigger additional migraines.

Answer d is incorrect. Physical activity can be a trigger for some patients so it may be appropriate for LK to diary her headaches and physical activity to see if there is any correlation. Physical activity is very important for health, however, and it would not be appropriate to limit all physical activity.

---

5. Which of the following would be an absolute contraindication for receiving a selective 5-HT$_1$ receptor agonist (triptan)?

    a. Diabetes
    b. Ischemic heart disease
    c. Anemia
    d. Controlled hypertension

Answer b is correct. These medications are selective agonists for serotonin in the cranial arteries to cause vasoconstriction. Due to this constrictive nature, patients with ischemic heart disease or signs or symptoms of ischemic heart disease (including Prinzmetal angina, angina pectoris, myocardial infarction, or silent ischemia) should not take these medications.

Answer a is incorrect. There is no documentation of effect on blood glucose with these agents.

Answer c is incorrect. There is a 1% reported incidence of hemolytic anemia as an adverse effect. A diagnosis of anemia would not be a contraindication.

Answer d is incorrect. Uncontrolled hypertension, due to the information stated above, would be a contraindication. However, a patient with controlled hypertension would not be contraindicated if using for infrequent abortive treatment.

---

6. Which of the following is the brand name for rizatriptan?

    a. Imitrex
    b. Maxalt
    c. Amerge
    d. Frova

Answer b is correct. The generic name for Maxalt is risatriptan.

Answer a is incorrect. The generic name of Imitrex is sumatriptan.

Answer c is incorrect. The generic name for Amerge is naratriptan.

Answer d is incorrect. The generic name for Frova is frovatriptan.

---

7. A patient is taking Zomig ZMT. Which of the following is true regarding this medication? Select all that apply.

    a. It is a subcutaneous injection.
    b. Liquid is not required for administration.
    c. It is an orally disintegrating tablet.
    d. It is a transdermal patch.

Answers b and c are correct. Zomig ZMT is the orally disintegrating tablet dosage form of zolmitriptan. It does not require water for administration (answer b); this may be beneficial to those patients without access to water, requiring discrete administration, or who experience nausea with their headaches, where intake of large amounts of liquid with administration may aggravate this symptom. This medication is also available as a nasal spray solution and tablet.

Answer a is incorrect. Sumatriptan (Imitrex) is a selective serotonin agonist that is available as a subcutaneous injection. Zolmitriptan does not come in an injectable formulation.

Answer d is incorrect. Sumatriptan (Alsuma) is a selective serotonin agonist that is available as a transdermal patch. Zolmitriptan does not come as a transdermal patch.

---

8. A patient who currently takes oral sumatriptan often experiences headache recurrence, where the headache comes back within 24 hours after a positive response to the medication. Her physician would like a recommendation of a selective 5-HT$_1$ receptor agonist (triptan) with a longer half-life. Which of the following would you recommend?

    a. Frovatriptan
    b. Rizatriptan
    c. Zolmitriptan
    d. Almotriptan

Answer a is correct. Her current medication, sumatriptan (Imitrex) has an elimination half-life of 2.5 hours. Frovatriptan (Frova) has an elimination half-life of 26 hours. The longer half-life products may benefit a patient who is responsive to triptans but requires a longer-acting medication to last the duration of the headache.

Answer b is incorrect. Rizatriptan (Maxalt) has a similar elimination half-life of 2 to 3 hours.

Answer c is incorrect. Zolmitriptan (Zomig) has a similar elimination half-life of 3 hours.

Answer d is incorrect. Almotriptan (Axert) has a similar elimination half-life of 3.1 hours.

9. Which of the following are correct repeat dose instructions for the migraine medication?

   a. Zomig tablets: take one tablet now; may repeat in 2 hours
   b. Imitrex subcutaneous injection: use one injection now; may repeat in 30 minutes
   c. Amerge tablets: take one tablet now; may repeat in 2 hours
   d. Imitrex subcutaneous injection: use one injection now; may repeat in 30 minutes and then again at hour 2

Answer a is correct. Zomig (zolmitriptan) tablets may be repeated in 2 hours if needed, not to exceed two doses in 24 hours.

Answers b and d are incorrect. Imitrex (sumatriptan) subcutaneous injection can be repeated in 1 hour if the headache has not resolved, not to exceed two injections in 24 hours.

Answer c is incorrect. Amerge (naratriptan) tablets may be repeated in 4 hours if needed, not to exceed two doses in 24 hours.

10. Treximet is a combination headache medication made up of which of the following?

    a. Sumatriptan and naproxen
    b. Acetaminophen, aspirin, and caffeine
    c. Acetaminophen, isometheptene mucate, and dichloralphenazone
    d. Acetaminophen, butalbital, and caffeine

Answer a is correct. Treximet contains sumatriptan and naproxen.

Answer b is incorrect. Acetaminophen, aspirin, and caffeine are Excedrin Migraine.

Answer c is incorrect. Acetaminophen, isometheptene mucate, and dichloralphenazone are Midrin.

Answer d is incorrect. Acetaminophen, butalbital, and caffeine are Fioricet.

11. CJ is a 30-year-old patient admitted to the hospital with an unremitting migraine headache. She has tried two doses of naratriptan in the past 12 hours. She also takes lisinopril 10 mg once daily for her blood pressure and terbinafine for her onychomycosis. Her vital signs are BP 132/88 mm Hg, heart rate 70 beats/min, height 5 feet 5 inches, and weight 130 lb. The physician plans to administer dihydroergotamine. Which of the following are contraindications for CJ receiving this treatment?

    a. Uncontrolled hypertension
    b. Elevated heart rate

    c. Terbinafine
    d. Naratriptan

Answer d is correct. Administration of serotonin agonists within 24 hours of ergotamine medications should be avoided due to risk of increased vasoconstriction.

Answer a is incorrect. Although uncontrolled hypertension would be a contraindication, this patient's BP is <140/90 mm Hg and would be defined as controlled.

Answer b is incorrect. Heart rate is not currently elevated for this patient at 70 beats/min.

Answer c is incorrect. Ergotamine medications are contraindicated for use with potent inhibitors of CYP 3A4. Azole antifungals would be contraindicated. Terbinafine is a synthetic allylamine derivative used for treatment of onychomycosis of the toenail or fingernail. It is only a minor substrate of CYP 3A4. It has strong inhibition action on CYP 2D6 substrates.

12. Which of the following represent a severe adverse effect that may result from taking ergotamine tartrate? Select all that apply.

    a. Purple toe syndrome
    b. Ergotism
    c. Pruritus
    d. Nausea

Answer b is correct. Ergotism is intense ischemia that results in peripheral vascular ischemia and possible gangrene.

Answer a is incorrect. Purple toe syndrome is most commonly associated with warfarin therapy.

Answer c is incorrect. Pruritus is a side effect that can result from ergotamine; however, it is not commonly severe.

Answer d is incorrect. Nausea is a side effect that can result from ergotamine; however, it is not commonly severe.

13. JB is a 55-year-old woman who has suffered from migraines for many years. Her zolmitriptan 5 mg works well to abort her headaches when they occur. Over the past few months, her headaches have increased in frequency to one every 2 weeks. She also complains of difficulty sleeping. Her vital signs today upon physical examination are height 5 feet 6 inches, weight 140 lb, blood pressure 120/80 mm Hg, and heart rate 60 beats/min. Her physician would like to start her on prophylactic drug therapy. Which of the following drug therapy would be a best next step for prophylaxis for this patient? Select all that apply.

    a. Propranolol
    b. Botulinum toxin type A
    c. Amitriptyline
    d. Phenelzine

Answer b is correct. Botulinum toxin type A (Botox) is approved for migraine treatment and prophylaxis.

Answer c is correct. It is always best to treat comorbid conditions whenever possible. This patient complains of difficulty sleeping and amitriptyline is a medication that has an adverse effect of drowsiness. Amitriptyline is well established in the literature for effective prophylactic therapy. It is useful in patients with comorbid depression or insomnia. Nortriptyline would be a tricyclic antidepressant that would cause less drowsiness. Caution should be used with these medications in the elderly due to the side effects.

Answer a is incorrect. The patient has an HR of 60 beats/min and propranolol is a β-blocker which will slow the heart rate further.

Answer d is incorrect. Phenelzine (Nardil) is a monoamine oxidase inhibitors (MAOI). Significant lifestyle modifications regarding tyramine containing foods is necessary to avoid hypertensive crisis. This would not be an appropriate first choice for prophylactic medication for this reason.

---

14. Which of the following are prophylactic treatment options for migraine headache? Select all that apply.

    a. Verapamil
    b. Topiramate
    c. Valproic acid
    d. Ergotamine

Answer a is correct. Verapamil is a calcium channel blocker that is used for migraine prophylaxis. It would be useful for patients who cannot tolerate β-blockers or for patients with comorbid hypertension or angina.

Answer b is correct. Topiramate is an antiepileptic medication that was approved for use in migraines in 2004. It is dosed twice daily for migraine prevention. It would be useful for a patient with comorbid seizure disorder. It does have some more prominent cognitive side effects with >10% incidence, including memory difficulties, difficulty in concentrating, confusion, and speech difficulties.

Answer c is correct. Valproic acid is an antiepileptic medication also approved for migraine prophylaxis. It would be useful for those patients with comorbid seizure disorder or manic depressive illness.

Answer d is incorrect. Ergotamine is a medication that is only used for acute migraine treatment and should not be used for prophylaxis.

---

15. JJ is a 49-year-old man who experiences headache cycles two times a year, usually in the spring and fall. The headaches occur for about 3 to 4 weeks and he may have up to 5 headaches daily. The headaches are an unbearable type of pain that comes suddenly, located in his left eye, and stops within 1 to 2 hours. He experiences severe ocular and nasal symptoms, such as nasal stuffiness or rhinorrhea, ocular lacrimation, and ptosis. He tells you that in order to attempt to stop the pain, he sometimes rubs the areas of pain or even beats his head against objects.

Which of the following are appropriate abortive treatment options for this patient's headache?

    a. Oxygen
    b. Imitrex (sumatriptan) tablets
    c. Amitriptyline
    d. Topiramate

Answer a is correct. Oxygen administered at 5 to 10 L/min by non-rebreather facemask for approximately 15 minutes is a first-line abortive treatment for cluster headache. This patient exhibits primary symptoms of cluster headache as per the International Headache Society Diagnostic Criteria for Migraine:

Headache is unilateral, orbital in location, lasting for 15 to 180 minutes

Nasal congestion, rhinorrhea, ocular lacrimation, and ptosis are present

Frequency of headaches lasts from 7 days to 1 year

Answer b is incorrect. Due to the duration of cluster headache, sumatriptan tablets will not act quick enough to have an impact before the headache dissipates.

Answers c and d are incorrect. Amitriptyline and topiramate are prophylactic options for migraine and tension headache. There are no data to support its use as an abortive for cluster headache.

---

16. AB is a 25-year-old college student who has been having headaches 3 to 4 times a month that last for 12 to 24 hours for the past couple of months. He describes them as having a gripping quality with pressure on both sides of his head, as if someone is squeezing his head with a rubber band. He does not experience nausea or vomiting. His headaches do not stop him from going to class, but sometimes he finds himself having to turn off his radio when studying since he just can't handle any noise. Light does not bother him during his headaches. Which of the following abortive treatment options would be appropriate recommendations for AB's headache?

    a. NSAIDS
    b. Imitrex (sumatriptan)
    c. Amitriptyline
    d. Metoclopramide

Answer a is correct. NSAIDs and combination analgesic products are a primary abortive treatment for patients with tension headache. The patient presents with common symptoms of tension headache based on the International Headache Society Diagnostic Criteria for Tension headache:

Headache lasts for 30 minutes to 7 days

At least two of the following characteristics:

Pressing/tightening quality

Mild intensity

Bilateral location

Not aggravated by routine physical activity

No nausea/vomiting

Photophobia/Phonophobia absent or one but not the other is present

Other nonpharmacologic agents effective for treatment of tension headache include stress management, relaxation therapy, biofeedback, physical therapy.

Answer b is incorrect. The triptan class of medications has no documentation of efficacy in treatment of tension headache.

Answer c is incorrect. Amitriptyline is a prophylactic treatment option for migraine and tension headache. It would not have benefit as an abortive treatment.

Answer d is incorrect. Metoclopramide may be used as an adjunctive therapy for migraines that present with nausea and vomiting but would not be appropriate therapy to treat AB's tension headache.

17. DT is a 31-year-old woman who is 36 weeks pregnant. She currently has a headache with presentation most like a tension-type headache. She is requesting a recommendation for treatment. Which of the following is the best recommendation?

    a. Naproxen
    b. Ergotamine
    c. Acetaminophen
    d. Ibuprofen

Answer c is correct. Acetaminophen is a pregnancy category B. Although it does cross the placenta, it is believed to be safe for use during pregnancy at therapeutic doses for a short period of time. The patient may also find benefit in psychophysiologic therapy, such as stress management, relaxation therapy, and biofeedback, as well as physical therapy.

Answers a and d are incorrect. NSAIDs should be avoided late in the third trimester to prevent prostaglandin alterations that could lead to premature ductus arteriosus closure.

Answer b is incorrect. Ergotamine is a pregnancy category X. It may precipitate uterine contractions and ischemia leading to hypoxemia in the fetus.

18. MM presents to the emergency room (ER) with a severe migraine headache and nausea and vomiting. He has taken one dose of zolmitriptan 5 mg orally within the past 6 hours, but vomited within 10 minutes. Which of the following would be the most appropriate next step for treatment?

    a. Metoclopramide 10 mg IV
    b. Biofeedback
    c. Three days of inpatient dihydroergotamine IV
    d. Acetaminophen 650 mg per rectum (PR)

Answer a is correct. A single dose of antiemetic therapy administered 15 to 30 minutes prior to taking an abortive

migraine medication may assist with nausea and vomiting. Prochlorperazine and metoclopramide are commonly used. Metoclopramide may also be useful for the gastroparesis, is often associated with migraine, and improves medication absorption.

Answer b is incorrect. Biofeedback is a common nonpharmacologic treatment used for management of headache. Two types are available: electrophysiologic and thermal biofeedback. Although this may assist the patient in relaxation and minimize headache symptoms, this would not be appropriate as a primary strategy for a severe headache.

Answer c is incorrect. This patient has only had one dose of zolmitriptan and vomited after a short time. Following administration of an antiemetic agent and assuming the patient has had success in the past with serotonin receptor agonist treatment, a second dose of a triptan could be administered, either oral or subcutaneous. For intractable, severe migraine, inpatient treatment with dihydroergotamine may be an option, administered 0.5 to 1 mg every 8 hours for 3 days.

Answer d is incorrect. Acetaminophen has been found to be an ineffective sole treatment option for migraine. Treatment with acetaminophen for severe migraine is not an appropriate option.

19. A physician you work with at your ambulatory care practice site asks your advice. He would like to know which serotonin receptor agonist migraine medication(s) is available as a nasal spray. You respond: (Select all that apply)

    a. Sumatriptan
    b. Rizatriptan
    c. Zolmitriptan
    d. Naratriptan

Answer a is correct. Sumatriptan is available as Imitrex nasal spray.

Answer c is correct. Zolmitriptan is available as Zomig nasal spray.

Answers b is incorrect. Rizatriptan is available as Maxalt tablets and Maxalt MLT rapidly disintegrating tablets.

Answer d is incorrect. Naratriptan is available as Amerge oral tablets.

20. A patient is picking up a prescription for Migranal (dihydroergotamine) at your community pharmacy counter. She has not used this medication before. Which of the following is an important counseling point to provide?

    a. Remove the foil wrapper before inserting PR
    b. Once prepared, use within 8 hours
    c. Wear latex-free gloves to apply
    d. Take with a full glass of water

Answer b is correct. Migranal is a dihydroergotamine nasal spray. Once the spray applicator has been prepared, use within 8 hours and discard any remaining solution.

Answers a, c, and d are incorrect. It is not available as a suppository, topical product, or oral formulation.

---

21. Select the brand name for eletriptan.

    a. Maxalt
    b. Zomig
    c. Ergomar
    d. Relpax

Answer d is correct. Relpax is the brand name for eletriptan.

Answer a is incorrect. Maxalt is the brand name for rizatriptan.

Answer b is incorrect. Zomig is the brand name for zolmitriptan.

Answer c is incorrect. Ergomar is the brand name for ergotamine tartrate.

---

22. Which of the following herbal medications has evidence of support for the treatment of migraine?

    a. Glucosamine
    b. Black cohosh
    c. Feverfew
    d. Saw palmetto

Answer c is correct. Feverfew is used for fever, headaches, prevention of migraines, and menstrual irregularities. Clinical studies have used 50 to 100 mg of feverfew extract daily for migraine prophylaxis.

Answer a is incorrect. Glucosamine is commonly used for osteoarthritis, joint pain, back pain, and glaucoma.

Answer b is incorrect. Black cohosh has many uses, but it is most commonly used for symptoms of menopause, premenstrual syndrome, and dysmenorrhea. There is no claim regarding the use for treatment of migraine.

Answer d is incorrect. Saw palmetto is used in benign prostatic hypertrophy (although it is not recommended for routine use by the Urology guidelines).

---

23. A patient presents to pick up a new prescription for sumatriptan tablets. When verifying the prescription, the computer alerts you of a contraindication with a current prescription: Paxil 20 mg. Which of the following is the reason for this contraindication?

    a. Stevens-Johnson syndrome
    b. Serotonin syndrome
    c. Neuroleptic malignant syndrome
    d. Computer error—there is no contraindication

Answer b is correct. There is a potential increased risk of serotonin syndrome with administration of sumatriptan and paroxetine (Paxil).

Answer a is incorrect. There is no documentation of occurrence of these conditions with the concurrent administration of these agents.

Answer c is incorrect. There is no documentation of occurrence of these conditions with the concurrent administration of these agents.

Answer d is incorrect. There is a potential contraindication present.

CHAPTER **55 | Pain Management**

Use the following case for questions 1 and 2:

KK is a 65-year-old woman with a chief complaint of left arm, shoulder, and axillary pain. She underwent a left subtotal mastectomy, radiation, and chemotherapy for breast cancer. KK has currently no evidence of cancer, but complains of two types of pain. The first in her chest is a dull achy pain; the second is a burning and stinging pain down her left arm and nothing has worked well for this pain. She is also complaining of severe constipation. Her current medications are bupropion 150 mg bid, ibuprofen 600 mg one tablet tid, morphine sulfate extended release (ER) 30 mg bid, atenolol 50 mg every morning, and tamoxifen 10 mg bid. All medications are taken by mouth.

1. What is best therapeutic plan of this patient's analgesic regimen?

    a. Analgesic regimen should be discontinued, because long-acting opiate is not appropriate for this patient's pain.
    b. Increase morphine ER to 30 mg po every 4 hours since it is not providing adequate analgesia.
    c. Increase morphine ER to 60 mg po tid since it is not optimally controlling patient's pain.
    d. Add pain medication to focus on neuropathic symptoms.

Answer d is correct. Adding a medication to focus on the neuropathic pain would be appropriate (eg, TCA, gabapentin).

Answer a is incorrect. Based upon the patient's history, her pain is most likely moderate to severe; therefore, use of opioids would be appropriate—especially for the nociceptive pain in her chest. However, since the second pain is neuropathic, adjunctive pain medications like antidepressants or antiepileptics should be considered.

Answer b is incorrect. Large increases in dose or interval of opioids should be avoided to minimize risk of side effects (eg, respiratory depression). Also ineffective for the neuropathic pain.

Answer c is incorrect. The patient's pain is neuropathic; therefore, adding adjunctive therapy would be appropriate.

2. What is the best approach for the burning pain in this patient?

 a. Add amitriptyline low dose at bedtime and titrate
 b. Add duloxetine low dose at bedtime and titrate
 c. Add nortriptyline high dose at bedtime and titrate
 d. Add gabapentin low dose at bedtime and titrate

Answer d is correct. Gabapentin is often used for neuropathic pain (although only indicated for postherpetic neuralgia). Pregabalin is indicated for neuropathy (diabetic) and postherpetic neuralgia. Titration is necessary to reduce side effects.

Answer a is incorrect. The TCA amitriptyline is potentially effective in neuropathic pain; however, they are associated with a significant amount of side effects (especially in an elderly patient) and the patient is already receiving a stimulant antidepressant (bupropion).

Answer b is incorrect. Duloxetine is a serotonin-norepinephrine reuptake inhibitor (SNRI) and may be used in the treatment of neuropathic pain; however, since the patient is already receiving an antidepressant, this would not be the ideal therapy.

Answer c is incorrect. The TCA nortriptyline is potentially effective in neuropathic pain; however, they are associated with a significant amount of side effects (especially in an elderly patient) when started on high dose and the patient is already receiving a stimulant antidepressant (bupropion).

3. A patient with chronic pain from a long-standing back injury presents with worsening mild to moderate dull, achy, pressure like pain. The patient works many long and stressful hours. The patient currently takes ibuprofen 800 mg tid for his back pain. Which of the following recommendations would be least preferred?

 a. Increasing dose of ibuprofen
 b. Addition of scheduled acetaminophen
 c. Ensuring the patient is receiving adequate rest
 d. Ensuring the patient is receiving adequate emotional support

Answer a is correct. NSAIDs have a ceiling analgesic dose, thus increasing the dose is not likely to benefit the patient.

Answer b is incorrect. Adding an analgesic with a different mechanism could provide additional benefit for this patient's pain.

Answers c and d are incorrect. Adding nonpharmacological treatment modalities to pain treatment has been shown to be helpful—particularly with this patient since he works long and stressful hours.

4. TP is a 67-year-old man with newly diagnosed degenerative joint disease. He is prescribed an NSAID for management of the pain. TP has concerns about the NSAID causing side effects. Select the potential side effect(s) associated with using NSAIDs for pain management. Select all that apply.

 a. GI bleeding
 b. Antiplatelet effects
 c. Decreased renal function
 d. Fluid retention
 e. Somnolence

Answer a is correct. GI bleeding is a major disadvantage of the NSAIDs. GI bleeding will be less with COX-2 selective NSAIDs (eg, celecoxib), but it can still occur.

Answer b is correct. All NSAIDs have antiplatelet activity.

Answer c is correct. NSAIDs are common causes of renal dysfunction and kidney function should be monitored during therapy.

Answer d is correct. Fluid retention is caused by the NSAIDs ability to retain sodium and water. Therefore, NSAIDs may adversely affect blood pressure and systolic heart failure.

Answer e is incorrect. CNS side effects such as somnolence are not common with NSAIDs.

5. AO is a patient with osteoarthritis that presents to the orthopedic clinic. AO has a past medical history (PMH) of hypertension, chronic obstructive pulmonary disease, and reflux. Medications include lisinopril, as needed albuterol, metoprolol, chlorthalidone, meloxicam, and pantoprazole. The doctor at the clinic is worried about potential drug interactions. Select the medication(s) that AO is receiving that may have reduced effectiveness when used with their pain medication. Select all that apply.

 a. Lisinopril
 b. Albuterol
 c. Metoprolol
 d. Chlorthalidone

Answers a, c, and d are correct. NSAIDs (pain medication is meloxicam) may reduce the effectiveness of these blood pressure medications because of sodium and water retention.

Answer b is incorrect. NSAIDs are not expected to decrease the effectiveness of albuterol.

6. QP is a 71-year-old patient diagnosed with severe diabetic neuropathy. He is currently being treated with an α-blocker (terazosin) for an enlarged prostate. Terazosin has significantly improved the symptoms of the enlarged prostate, but the patient is having orthostatic hypotension episodes. Select the medication that would be most appropriate for QP's diabetic neuropathy.

 a. Naproxen
 b. Morphine

c. Nortriptyline
d. Gabapentin

Answer d is correct. Gabapentin is effective in the treatment of neuropathic pain and is not associated with orthostatic hypotension.

Answer a is incorrect. Neuropathic pain has a poor response to NSAIDs.

Answer b is incorrect. Neuropathic pain has a poor response to opioid analgesics.

Answer c is incorrect. Neuropathic pain responds to TCAs, but TCAs have a significant amount of side effects in older patients (>65).

7. HA is a 53-year-old patient with chronic pain from cancer. In addition to the cancer, HA has a PMH of gout, hypertension, and anemia. HA is currently taking desipramine, allopurinol, HCTZ, lisinopril, and iron. Select the potential side effect(s) associated with HA's pain medication. Select all that apply.

a. Drowsiness
b. Dry mouth
c. Constipation
d. Hyperkalemia

Answers a, b, and c are correct. TCAs are associated with anticholinergic side effects.

Answer d is incorrect. Hyperkalemia is not a side effect associated with TCAs.

8. Select the medication(s) that may cause CNS side effects. Select all that apply.

a. Gabapentin
b. Morphine
c. Amitriptyline
d. Duloxetine
e. Naproxen

Answers a, b, c, and d are correct. All pain medications have activity within the CNS and, therefore, are associated with CNS side effects.

Answer e is incorrect. NSAIDs are not commonly associated with CNS effects.

9. KL is a 69-year-old patient with a burning, stinging, and knife-like pain. KL's diagnoses include hypertension, diabetes mellitus II, multiple myeloma with recent chemotherapy, and depression. Which of the following is the most appropriate for the treatment of KL's pain?

a. Valproate
b. Pregabalin
c. Topiramate
d. Carbamazepine
e. Amitriptyline

Answer b is correct. Pregabalin is considered a first-line pain agent and the patient has no medical conditions that would prevent its use.

Answer a is incorrect. Valproate is considered a second-line neuropathic pain agent. It is a substrate, inhibitor, and inducer of the CYP-450 isoenzyme system; however, it is a weak inhibitor and inducer of the CYP-450 system.

Answer c is incorrect. Topiramate is considered a second-line neuropathic pain agent. It is an inhibitor and inducer of the CYP-450 system; however, it is a weak inhibitor and inducer.

Answer d is incorrect. Carbamazepine is considered a second-line neuropathic pain agent, unless it is trigeminal neuralgia. It is a substrate and strong inducer of the CYP-450 system; therefore, it is associated with significant drug interactions.

Answer e is incorrect. Amitriptyline is considered a second-line neuropathic pain agent due to its side effects; desipramine and nortriptyline are considered first-line agents in younger patients.

10. A patient presents to the pharmacy that has chronic neuropathic pain. The patient prefers to use a topical product for their pain. Select the best medication for this patient's pain.

a. Capsaicin
b. Amitriptyline
c. Carbamazepine
d. Topiramate

Answer a is correct. Capsaicin alters function of pain-sensitive nerve endings through substance-P depletion, helping with neuropathic pain and is the only topical product listed in the answer choices.

Answers b, c, and d are incorrect. These three agents are not commercially available in topical products.

11. VI is a 79-year-old female patient in the intensive care unit for sepsis. The cause of the sepsis is from a decubitus ulcer. The ulcer is very painful and the first year medical resident ordered meperidine for dressing changes. The patient has a PMH for hypertension, angina, chronic kidney disease, and osteoporosis. VI is anticipated to use the meperidine frequently. Select the potential side effect(s) associated with meperidine use in VI. Select all that apply.

a. Seizures
b. GI bleeding
c. Respiratory depression
d. Anemia

Answer a is correct. Normeperidine, the active metabolite of meperidine, may cause seizures in patients that are administered high doses or patients with renal dysfunction leading to decreased clearance of normeperidine.

Answer c is correct. Respiratory depression is associated with all opioids and is dose dependent.

Answer b is incorrect. GI bleeding is associated with NSAIDs.

Answer d is incorrect. Anemia is not expected from meperidine.

---

12. LD is a 62-year-old patient with chronic pain from an automobile accident several years ago. LD has chronic moderate to severe nociceptive pain. Additional PMH includes diabetes and CKD. The patient does not like to take pills or tablets. What is the BEST medication for LD's chronic pain?

    a. Morphine
    b. Oxycodone
    c. Meperidine
    d. Fentanyl

Answer d is correct. Fentanyl is available as a transdermal system (patch). It is also available as injection, lozenge, powder, and tablet. Good option for a patient with CKD.

Answers a, b, and c are incorrect. Opioids are available in multiple formulations including oral, solutions, ER, rectal and parenteral formulations, but these agents are not available in a patch formulation. CKD makes morphine and meperidine less than ideal options.

---

13. IT is a 74-year-old man with severe chronic nociceptive pain. He has been previously treated with scheduled acetaminophen, but is prescribed morphine today. The patient will be receiving morphine chronically. Select the medication that IT should receive in addition to the acetaminophen and morphine.

    a. Ibuprofen
    b. Gabapentin
    c. Capsaicin
    d. Bisacodyl

Answer d is correct. Patients receiving opioids, especially for chronic therapy, should receive a stimulant laxative because of the constipation. Examples of stimulant laxatives include sennosides, cascara, and bisacodyl.

Answer a is incorrect. IT has been receiving nonopioid analgesics in the past and they have not been effective. We are not given enough information to know if he has taken an NSAID; however, even if he had, that does not preclude use of an NSAID with an opioid. Combination analgesic therapy with an opioid and NSAID may produce better pain relief than an opioid alone; however, it is not required to use combination analgesics to treat pain.

Answer b is incorrect. Gabapentin is used for neuropathic types of pain. We are not given enough information about the type of pain to be able to make a recommendation for gabapentin or other medications that are effective against neuropathic pain.

Answer c is incorrect. Capsaicin is used for neuropathic types of pain. We are not given enough information about the type of pain to be able to make a recommendation for capsaicin or other medications that are effective against neuropathic pain.

---

14. SQ is a patient from a motor vehicle collision. She suffered a broken leg during the accident and was given opioids for pain management. SQ's pain has gone completely away but now has developed respiratory depression. Select the BEST medication to give SQ for her current symptoms.

    a. Flumazenil
    b. Naloxone
    c. Acetylcysteine
    d. Albuterol
    e. Ipratropium

Answer b is correct. Naloxone (Narcan) is an opioid antagonist that reverses respiratory depression.

Answer a is incorrect. Flumazenil (Romazicon) is a benzodiazepine antagonist and reverses the sedative effects of benzodiazepines used in conscious sedation and general anesthesia.

Answer c is incorrect. Acetylcysteine (Mucomyst) is an antidote for acetaminophen toxicity.

Answers d and e are incorrect. Both these agents are effective for shortness of breath related to respiratory disease not opioid related respiratory depression.

---

15. A patient is involved in a severe car accident and is going to require several surgeries to fix multiple broken bones. The patient is expected to have severe acute pain. Select the dosing method that should be employed for this patient.

    a. Intermittent
    b. Scheduled dosing
    c. Directly observed therapy
    d. As needed

Answer b is correct. Scheduled dosing or around the clock is the preferred method for controlling severe pain.

Answer a is incorrect. Intermittent, or as needed (prn), is used for patients on scheduled dosing of analgesics and experiencing breakthrough pain. For example, a patient receiving oxycodone 20 mg every 12 hours and is experiencing pain relief, but it does not last the entire dosing interval, may be prescribed a short-acting opioid for breakthrough pain on an as needed basis. Intermittent dosing can also be used for moderate intermittent pain, not severe constant pain.

Answer c is incorrect. Directly observed therapy is utilized in patients with tuberculosis and is not related to pain management.

Answer d is incorrect. As needed (prn) is used for patients on scheduled dosing of analgesics and experiencing breakthrough pain.

16. A patient presents with acute mild to moderate dull and achy pain from doing too much hard work. The patient is otherwise healthy and currently takes no medication. What is the best medication to treat the patient's pain?

    a. Naproxen
    b. Carbamazepine
    c. Oxycodone
    d. Capsaicin

Answer a is correct. Nonopioids are first line for mild to moderate nociceptive pain—options would be either acetaminophen or NSAIDs.

Answer b is incorrect. Not effective for nociceptive pain.

Answer c is incorrect. Oxycodone is more appropriate for moderate to severe nociceptive pain.

Answer d is incorrect. Capsaicin alters function of pain-sensitive nerve endings and can take weeks to work—not a good choice for acute pain.

17. Which of the following medications would be appropriate for a patient experiencing moderate to severe nociceptive pain that has high dose opioid requirements and cannot tolerate morphine due to side effects? Assume each of the medications used below will be used as monotherapy. Select all that apply.

    a. Fentanyl
    b. Diclofenac
    c. Hydromorphone
    d. Duloxetine

Answers a and c are correct. Both are opioids and helpful for moderate to severe nociceptive pain. Side effects does not preclude you from trying a different opioid.

Answer b is incorrect. NSAIDs are more beneficial for mild to moderate nociceptive pain.

Answer d is incorrect. Duloxetine is for neuropathic pain.

18. MS is a 32-year-old patient that presents to the doctor with new onset nociceptive back pain from playing backyard football. At times the pain feels like back spasms. MS has tried heat and ibuprofen with no success. Recommend a nonopioid for MS's back pain.

    a. Mexiletine
    b. Cyclobenzaprine
    c. Tapentadol
    d. Hydrocodone

Answer b is correct. Cyclobenzaprine is an option for acute back related pain, example of "muscle relaxant."

Answer a is incorrect. Used for neuropathic pain.

Answer c is incorrect. An opioid, so inappropriate since question is asking for nonopioid.

Answer d is incorrect. An opioid, so inappropriate since question is asking for nonopioid.

19. QY is a 41-year-old accountant with an acute pain issue. He would like to receive a medication that will not affect his ability to work, but will effectively treat his pain. Select the analgesic that is minimally associated with CNS side effects and does not slow intestinal motility.

    a. Naproxen
    b. Hydrocodone
    c. Meloxicam
    d. Amitriptyline

Answers a and c are correct. Naproxen and meloxicam are NSAIDs and exhibit minimal CNS side effects (especially compared to other analgesics) and are not associated with constipation.

Answer b is incorrect. Hydrocodone is an opioid and opioids are associated with CNS side effects and frequently cause constipation.

Answer d is incorrect. Amitriptyline is associated with CNS side effects and constipation.

20. A patient is experiencing a mild to moderate mixed nociceptive and neuropathic pain from acute shingles. The patient has no other significant PMH or other medications. Select the BEST pain medication for this patient.

    a. Ibuprofen
    b. Amitriptyline
    c. Carbamazepine
    d. Tramadol
    e. Morphine

Answer d is correct. Tramadol is effective for acute pain and based on its MAO it can help both nociceptive and neuropathic pain. Tramadol's analgesic properties are produced by binding to mu-opiate receptors causing inhibition of ascending pain pathways, altering the perception of pain. Tramadol also inhibits the reuptake of norepinephrine and serotonin.

Answer a is incorrect. NSAID's analgesic properties are produced by inhibition of prostaglandins and will help the neuropathic pain portion.

Answers b and c are incorrect. Amitriptyline and carbamazepine's analgesic effects are neuropathic only.

Answer e is incorrect. Morphine is more appropriate for moderate to severe nociceptive pain, not effective for neuropathic pain.

21. Rank the following opioid analgesics in order from least potent analgesic effect to most potent analgesic effect.

Unordered options	Ordered response
Hydrocodone	Codeine
Codeine	Hydrocodone
Hydromorphone	Hydromorphone
Fentanyl	Fentanyl

The least potent opioid analgesic in terms of analgesic effect is codeine. It is not used for the treatment of severe pain and has more utility as an antitussive. Hydrocodone has a potency that is equivalent to oral morphine. Hydromorphone is more potent than morphine. Fentanyl is the most potent of the opioids available, dosed in micrograms while all other opioids are dosed in milligrams.

CHAPTER 56 | Schizophrenia

1. Which of the following symptoms is/are associated with schizophrenia? Select all that apply.

   a. Tangentiality and disorganized speech
   b. Flat affect and alogia
   c. Impaired memory and attention
   d. Hallucinations and delusions

Answer a is correct. It describes positive symptoms associated with schizophrenia. Positive symptoms are symptoms that are added to normal functions. Positive symptoms commonly refer to hallucinations or delusions; however, there are also other positive symptoms which may be displayed by patients with schizophrenia. Disorganized speech, tangential thoughts, and tangential speech are other examples of positive symptoms.

Answer b is correct. It describes negative symptoms associated with schizophrenia. Negative symptoms are symptoms categorized as loss of normal functions. Alogia, which is a poverty of speech, is a negative symptom. Patients who present with a flat affect are unable to express emotion, which is also considered as a negative symptom. Avolition and anhedonia are other examples of negative symptoms.

Answer c is correct. It describes cognitive symptoms associated with schizophrenia. Impaired memory and attention are two common examples of cognitive symptoms that patients with schizophrenia may experience.

Answer d is correct. It describes positive symptoms associated with schizophrenia. Positive symptoms are symptoms that are added to normal functions.

2. Which of the following is/are accepted and reliable when diagnosing a patient with schizophrenia?

   a. Diagnosis can be confirmed by a laboratory measure such as a blood test.
   b. Diagnosis can be confirmed if the patient meets the Diagnostic and Statistical Manual-5 (DSM-5) criteria for schizophrenia.
   c. Diagnosis can be confirmed by conducting a brain imaging study on the patient.
   d. Diagnosis can be confirmed by a physical examination.

Answer b is correct. Using the DSM-5 criteria for diagnosing schizophrenia is the most reliable method of diagnosing patients with schizophrenia. In order for a patient to be diagnosed with schizophrenia, the patient must meet the diagnostic criteria stated in the DSM-5. This is currently the only accepted and reliable method for diagnosing schizophrenia.

Answer a is incorrect. Currently there are no laboratory measures that can be used to detect or confirm schizophrenia.

Answer c is incorrect. Currently brain imagining is not an accurate or accepted method for diagnosing schizophrenia.

Answer d is incorrect. A physical examination is not an appropriate method used to confirm a schizophrenia diagnosis.

3. Which of the following is the best way to reduce the risk of relapse?

   a. Acute treatment with antipsychotic therapy
   b. Acute treatment with nonpharmacologic therapy
   c. Maintenance treatment with nonpharmacologic therapy
   d. Maintenance treatment with antipsychotic therapy

Answer d is correct. Most patients with schizophrenia require life-long antipsychotic treatment to adequately manage symptoms. Long-term treatment with an antipsychotic will treat schizophrenia and will help prevent the patient from relapsing.

Answer a is incorrect. Acute treatment with antipsychotics temporarily treats and stabilizes the patient's symptoms, but, in most cases, it is not adequate to prevent relapse.

Answer b is incorrect. Non-pharmacologic therapy such as psychosocial support groups and programs may be useful when combined with antipsychotics; however, non-pharmacologic therapy by itself generally will not treat schizophrenia and prevent relapse. Acute treatment with non-pharmacologic therapy is not adequate to prevent relapse.

Answer c is incorrect. Non-pharmacologic therapy, such as psychosocial support groups and programs, may be useful when combined with antipsychotics; however, non-pharmacologic therapy by itself generally will not treat schizophrenia and prevent relapse. Maintenance treatment with nonpharmacologic therapy is not adequate to prevent relapse.

4. MY is a 27-year-old man who presents to his psychiatrist with symptoms associated with schizophrenia. MY reports to the psychiatrist that over the past several months he has experienced auditory hallucinations. During the evaluation the psychiatrist noted that MY also displays negative and cognitive symptoms. The psychiatrist would like to initiate MY on an antipsychotic in order to improve positive symptoms, negative symptoms, and cognitive symptoms. Which of the following is the best option for MY?

   a. Fluphenazine
   b. Haloperidol
   c. Perphenazine
   d. Paliperidone

Answer d is correct. Paliperidone is an SGA. SGAs are helpful for improving positive symptoms. This class of antipsychotics will also improve negative and cognitive symptoms.

Answers a, b, and c are incorrect. Haloperidol, Fluphenazine, and Perphenazine are FGAs. FGAs are beneficial for the improvement of positive symptoms only.

5. Which of the following antipsychotics exhibits a mechanism of action with greater affinity for D_2 receptors as compared to serotonin receptors? Select all that apply.

   a. Cariprazine
   b. Asenapine
   c. Haloperidol
   d. Fluphenazine

Answers c and d are correct. Haloperidol and Fluphenazine are FGAs. FGAs exhibit a mechanism of action with greater affinity toward D_2 receptors than toward serotonin receptors. FGAs generally exhibit high D_2 blockade and minimal affinity toward serotonergic receptors.

Answers a and b are incorrect. Cariprazine and Asenapine are SGAs. SGAs have more affinity toward serotonin receptors than D_2 receptors. SGAs generally exhibit moderate D_2 blockade and greater affinity toward serotonergic receptors.

6. Which of the following is the generic name for Rexulti®?

   a. Iloperidone
   b. Brexpiprazole
   c. Lurasidone
   d. Asenapine

Answer b is correct. Brexpiprazole is the generic name for Rexulti.

Answer a is incorrect. Iloperidone is the generic name for Fanapt.

Answer c is incorrect. Lurasidone is the generic name for Latuda.

Answer d is incorrect. Asenapine is the generic name for Saphris.

7. JL is a 34-year-old man who is admitted to the hospital for having visual and auditory hallucinations. JL has been experiencing these symptoms for several months. Upon admission, JL is diagnosed with schizophrenia. JL has no family history of psychiatric illnesses. JL does not have any other medical conditions and is not taking any medications. All of JL's labs are within normal limits. What is the best treatment for JL?

   a. Risperidone
   b. Clozapine
   c. Thiothixene
   d. Haloperidol

Answer a is correct. SGAs are first-line agents for treatment of schizophrenia. SGAs are considered as first-line agents, because they are effective and exhibit a decreased risk of movement disorders. All SGAs, with the exception of clozapine, may be used as first-line agents. The specific SGA chosen is based on several factors such as adverse effects, patient response, and cost.

Answer b is incorrect. Although clozapine is an SGA, it is not used as a first-line agent for the treatment of schizophrenia. Clozapine is an effective SGA; however, its adverse effect profile inhibits its use as a first-line treatment. Clozapine is used after a patient has failed therapy on SGAs and FGAs.

Answers c and d are incorrect. Haloperidol and Thiothixene are FGAs. FGAs are not considered as first-line treatment and generally are not used before trying an SGA. FGAs are an effective class of antipsychotics; however, because of the risk of movement disorders associated with FGAs, this class is generally not preferred over the SGAs.

8. YR is a 29-year-old woman newly diagnosed with schizophrenia. The treating psychiatrist has told YR that she will be started on an antipsychotic for the management of her schizophrenia. YR is having a very difficult time accepting her diagnosis and treatment and is seeking more information regarding her treatment. YR would like to know what adverse effects she can expect. YR should be counseled on which of the following adverse effects associated with antipsychotic use? Select all that apply.

   a. Dystonia
   b. Orthostasis
   c. Sedation
   d. Cholinergic effects

Answer a is correct. Dystonia is a type of EPS. EPS is a possible adverse effect with FGAs and SGAs; however, the risk of EPS is greater with FGAs.

Answer b is correct. Orthostasis is a possible adverse effect that may occur with FGAs and SGAs.

Answer c is correct. Sedation is a possible adverse effect that may occur with FGAs and SGAs.

Answer d is incorrect. Anticholinergic effects are a possibility with FGAs and SGAs.

---

9. AC is a 33-year-old woman with a 9-year history of schizophrenia. AC has a past medical history of asthma and chronic pain resulting from a motor vehicle accident. AC's current medications are an albuterol MDI and acetaminophen. GB has previously failed treatment with several SGAs and FGAs. The plan for AC is to initiate clozapine treatment. Which of the following parameter(s) are required to be monitored while AC is on clozapine? Select all that apply.

   a. Absolute neutrophil count
   b. Prolactin
   c. White blood cell
   d. Weight

Answers a is correct. Frequent ANC monitoring is required. Due to the risk of agranulocytosis, it is important to monitor ANC values. ANC values should be obtained on a weekly basis for the first 6 months of treatment. From 6 to 12 months, ANC values can be obtained every other week. Once the patient has been on clozapine treatment for 12 months, ANC values may be obtained on a monthly basis.

Answer d is correct. Clozapine is associated with weight gain. Patients on clozapine therapy should be monitored for weight gain.

Answer b is incorrect. It is not necessary to monitor prolactin levels while on clozapine treatment. Elevated prolactin levels are seen with risperidone, paliperidone and FGAs.

Answer c is incorrect. WBC monitoring is no longer needed with clozapine therapy. Current recommendations recommend monitoring ANC values.

---

10. CX is a 26-year-old man who has been diagnosed with schizophrenia. CX has a significant family history of schizophrenia. Family history includes father, paternal uncle, and brother diagnosed with schizophrenia. CX shows concerns regarding the use of antipsychotics, because his father has developed EPS while on antipsychotic treatment. CX would like to be educated on the types of EPS associated with antipsychotic use and should be counseled on movement disorders associated with the use of antipsychotics. Which of the following is a movement disorder that may occur with antipsychotic use? Select all that apply.

   a. Tardive dyskinesia
   b. Pseudoparkinsonism
   c. Akathisia
   d. Dystonia

Answer a is correct. Tardive dyskinesia is a type of extrapyramidal symptom. Patients with tardive dyskinesia experience involuntary abnormal movements. These movements may occur in many different areas of the body such as the facial area, extremities, or the spine. Tardive dyskinesia in many cases may be irreversible and generally develops after months or years of antipsychotic treatment.

Answer b is correct. Pseudoparkinsonism is a type of extrapyramidal symptom. Patients experiencing this type of EPS may present with symptoms such as bradykinesia, rigidity, and tremors. The onset of pseudoparkinsonism generally occurs 1 to 2 weeks after antipsychotic initiation.

Answer c is correct. Akathisia is a type of extrapyramidal symptom. Patients who experience akathisia may experience feelings of restlessness such as the inability to sit still or the need for constant movement. The onset of akathisia usually occurs days to weeks after antipsychotic initiation.

Answer d is correct. Dystonia is a type of extrapyramidal symptom. Dystonic reactions are described as muscle spasms. These muscle spasms, or contractions, usually occur in the neck, head, and trunk areas. The onset of dystonia occurs rapidly within the first few days following antipsychotic initiation.

---

11. LZ is a 31-year-old man with a 5-year history of schizophrenia. LZ has tried SGAs in the past; however, he has not had adequate response. LZ continues to present with severe positive symptoms such as delusions and auditory hallucinations. LZ was initiated on an FGA today. Which of the following adverse effects are most commonly associated with FGAs and should be discussed with LZ?

   a. Prolactin elevation and tardive dyskinesia
   b. Weight gain and hyperlipidemia
   c. Nephrotoxicity and toxic epidermal necrolysis
   d. Anxiety and depression

Answer a is correct. Prolactin elevation and tardive dyskinesia (a type of EPS) may occur with FGAs and are actually more likely to occur with the use of FGAs than with SGAs.

Answer b is incorrect. Metabolic abnormalities such as hyperlipidemia and weight gain are more likely to occur with SGAs. There is less risk of metabolic abnormalities and weight gain with FGAs.

Answer c is incorrect. Nephrotoxicity and Toxic Epidermal Necrolysis are not common adverse effects that occur with FGAs or SGAs.

Answer d is incorrect. Depression and anxiety are not common adverse effects that occur with FGAs or SGAs when used in the management of schizophrenia.

---

12. HN is a 33-year-old woman with a recent diagnosis of schizophrenia. She is refusing to take any antipsychotics, because she has read on the internet that these types of medications can cause weight gain and diabetes. After encouragement from the psychiatrist, she has agreed to try an antipsychotic. The attending psychiatrist would like to initiate HN on an antipsychotic that is least likely to cause weight gain and metabolic

disturbances. Which of the following is the best option for HN? Select all that apply.

a. Iloperidone
b. Olanzapine
c. Aripiprazole
d. Ziprasidone

Answers c and d are correct.   Aripiprazole and ziprasidone are the two SGAs associated with the lowest risk of weight gain and metabolic abnormalities. Lurasidone is also less likely to cause weight gain and metabolic effects. Clozapine and olanzapine are most likely to cause weight gain and metabolic abnormalities. Most of the other SGAs have moderate weight gain and metabolic effects.

Answer a is incorrect.   Iloperidone is not the best option because it is one of the SGAs with moderate effects on weight gain and metabolic effects. Aripiprazole and ziprasidone would be better options for this patient.

Answer b is incorrect.   Olanzapine is not a good option, because it is one of the SGAs associated with a greater risk of weight gain and metabolic abnormalities.

13. ZN is a 60-year-old man with a 25-year history of schizophrenia. He has a significant history of stopping his medications. ZN's reasons for non-adherence are that he does not like to take medications daily and he tends to skip his doses scheduled during the time that he is at work. ZN also has a history of not getting his antipsychotic medication refilled on time. Additionally, ZN has been hospitalized 4 times over the past 2 years as a result of nonadherence. Which of the following may be a potential option for ZN? Select all that apply.

a. Haloperidol decanoate.
b. Asenapine
c. Paliperidone palmitate
d. Aripiprazole lauroxil

Answers a, c, and d are correct.   Haloperidol decanoate, paliperidone palmitate, and aripiprazole lauroxil are all long-acting injections. Long-acting intramuscular injections are a good option for patients who are unable to adhere to antipsychotic treatment. This formulation allows the drug to be released slowly over a few weeks and is useful in patients who are unwilling to take medications on a daily basis. Other long-acting injections available include: Risperidone long-acting, fluphenazine decanoate, olanzapine pamoate, and aripiprazole monohydrate.

Answer b is incorrect.   This is not a long-acting formulation.

14. Rank the following antipsychotics from the highest likelihood of causing weight gain to the lowest likelihood of causing weight gain. Aripiprazole, Clozapine, Iloperidone, and Ziprasidone.

a. Aripiprazole < Clozapine < Iloperidone < Ziprasidone
b. Clozapine < Iloperidone < Ziprasidone < Aripiprazole

c. Iloperidone = Clozapine < Ziprasidone < Aripiprazole
d. Ziprasidone = Aripiprazole < Iloperidone < Clozapine

Answer d is correct.   Aripiprazole and ziprasidone are associated with minimal weight gain. The likelihood of iloperidone causing weight gain would be ranked in between clozapine and ziprasidone/aripiprazole. Significant weight gain is likely to occur with clozapine.

Answers a, b, and c are incorrect.

15. BC is a 31-year-old woman who presents to her psychiatrist today with negative and positive symptoms. Past medical history includes hypertension, seasonal allergies, and gastroesophageal reflux disease. Medications include atenolol, loratadine, and omeprazole. BC has been experiencing psychotic symptoms for several months now. Her psychiatrist has decided to start her on an SGA today. Which of the following should be monitored while BC is receiving treatment with an SGA? Select all that apply.

a. Fasting glucose
b. Blood pressure
c. Fasting plasma lipids
d. Weight

Answers a, b, c, and d are correct.   These are recommended monitoring parameters.

All of the answer choices should be monitored while receiving treatment with an SGA. SGAs may cause weight gain and metabolic abnormalities; therefore, it is recommended that patients receiving treatment should be monitored. Monitoring these parameters will allow early detection of adverse effects and metabolic abnormalities that may develop.

16. TM is a 34-year-old Caucasian man with a 3-year history of schizophrenia. TM has been on numerous antipsychotics in the past. One week ago, TM was admitted to the hospital due to worsening psychiatric symptoms while adherent to antipsychotic treatment. TM was started on clozapine treatment. It is now 1 week later and ANC values for TM have been drawn. The recommended ANC values during clozapine treatment should be:

a. ANC <2000/mm³
b. ANC >1000/mm³
c. ANC >1500/mm³
d. ANC >2000/mm³

Answer c is correct.   The patient's ANC should be in this range. Due to the risk of agranulocytosis which may occur with clozapine treatment, it is important that the ANC values do not fall below these parameters.

Answers a, b, and d are incorrect.   The correct laboratory values is ANC >1500/mm³.

17. SW is a 45-year-old woman with a 15-year history of schizophrenia. SW was on antipsychotic treatment; however, about 2 weeks ago she stopped taking her antipsychotic, because she lost her job and could not afford her medication. SW's psychiatrist has now prescribed haloperidol which she started taking 2 days ago. SW presents today with a stiff neck and muscle spasms. Her psychiatrist has identified this reaction as dystonia. Which of the following agents may be used to treat SW's EPS?

    a. Cyclobenzaprine
    b. Loxapine
    c. Benztropine
    d. Bromocriptine

Answer c is correct. Benztropine is an anticholinergic that can be used to treat dystonic reactions. Anticholinergics such as benztropine and diphenhydramine are usually the preferred drugs of choice for the treatment of this type of EPS.

Answer a is incorrect. Cyclobenzaprine is a muscle relaxant that is not recommended for the treatment of EPS.

Answer b is incorrect. Loxapine is an FGA.

Answer d is incorrect. Bromocriptine is a dopamine agonist used for Parkinson disease. It is not recommended for the treatment of dystonia.

18. NK was recently started on Paliperidone for the treatment of schizophrenia. He has been taking the Paliperidone for 3 days now and is not feeling well on this treatment. NK is experiencing muscle rigidity, hyperthermia, hypertension, and presents with an altered level of consciousness. Which of the following is NK experiencing?

    a. Tardive dyskinesia
    b. Dystonia
    c. Neuroleptic malignant syndrome
    d. Serotonin syndrome
    e. Hypertensive crisis

Answer c is correct. Neuroleptic malignant syndrome (NMS) may occur within the first 24 to 72 hours after antipsychotic treatment. NMS may occur with FGA and SGA treatment. Signs and symptoms associated with NMS include hyperthermia, hypertension, an altered level of consciousness, rigidity, and increased creatine kinase.

Answer a is incorrect. Tardive dyskinesia is a type of EPS and is described as abnormal involuntary movements that develop after months or years of antipsychotic treatment.

Answer b is incorrect. Dystonia is a type of EPS. Dystonic reactions are described as muscle spasms. These muscle spasms, or contractions, usually occur in the neck, head, and trunk areas. Dystonic reactions may occur within a few days of antipsychotic treatment.

Answer d is incorrect. Serotonin syndrome and NMS have *similar* presentations; however, serotonin syndrome usually occurs when two or more serotonergic drugs are combined. Serotonin syndrome encompasses a spectrum of symptoms. Mental status changes can include anxiety, agitated delirium, restlessness, and disorientation. Autonomic manifestations can include diaphoresis, tachycardia, hyperthermia, hypertension, vomiting, and diarrhea. Neuromuscular hyperactivity can manifest as tremor, muscle rigidity, myoclonus, and hyperreflexia. Hyperreflexia and clonus are particularly common.

Answer e is incorrect. A hypertensive crisis occurs when a monoamine oxidase inhibitor (MAOI) is combined with tyramine containing foods.

19. CJ is a 55-year-old man who was diagnosed with schizophrenia 30 years ago. Since his diagnosis, CJ has always been on an FGA; however, over the past several months, he has started to show signs of tardive dyskinesia. CJ's treating psychiatrist feels that it may be best for CJ to try an SGA at this point. CJ has a history of cardiac disease, and, therefore, his psychiatrist would like to avoid medications that may be associated with QTc prolongation. Which of the following antipsychotics should be avoided due to the risk of QTc prolongation?

    a. Cariprazine
    b. Brexpiprazole
    c. Ziprasidone
    d. Lurasidone

Answer c is correct. Ziprasidone has been associated with QTc prolongation.

Answer a is incorrect. There is a low risk of QTc prolongation with cariprazine.

Answer b is incorrect. There is a low risk of QTc prolongation with brexpiprazole.

Answer d is incorrect. There is a low risk of QTc prolongation with lurasidone.

20. The blockade of which of the following receptors is responsible for inducing EPS?

    a. Serotonin
    b. Dopamine-2 (D_2)
    c. Norepinephrine
    d. Histamine

Answer b is correct. D_2 blockade is responsible for alleviating positive symptoms; however, D_2 blockade is also responsible for inducing EPS. Both FGAs and SGAs block D_2 to some extent. FGAs block more D_2, making EPS more common with FGAs.

Answer a is incorrect. Serotonin blockade does not cause EPS.

Answer c is incorrect. Norepinephrine blockade does not cause EPS.

Answer d is incorrect. Histamine blockade does not cause EPS.

21. TL is a 39-year-old man with a 9-year history of schizophrenia who is being switched to an FGA. TL has tried asenapine, lurasidone, and aripiprazole in the past; however, his positive symptoms have been uncontrolled on these medications. The psychiatrist would now like to try TL on an FGA. TL has a history of unwanted side effects such as extreme dry mouth, constipation, and urinary incontinence. The treating psychiatrist would like to find a medication with the *least risk* of these adverse effects. Which of the following is the best option for TL?

    a. Haloperidol
    b. Chlorpromazine
    c. Loxapine
    d. Thioridazine

Answer a is correct. Haloperidol is the best option since it is a high-potency FGA. Highly potent FGAs, such as haloperidol, tend to exhibit less anticholinergic effects.

Answers b and d are incorrect. Chlorpromazine and thioridazine are not the best options because they are low-potency SGAs. Low-potency agents tend to have more anticholinergic adverse effects.

Answer c is incorrect. Loxapine is not the best option. Loxapine is a medium-potency FGA. Risk of anticholinergic side effects associated with a medium-potency FGA falls in between high- and low-potency agents.

22. TS is a 30-year-old woman with a 2-year history of schizophrenia. She has been on a few FGAs in the past, and they have all caused her prolactin levels to rise. The psychiatrist treating TS would like to avoid any agents likely to elevate prolactin levels. Which of the following agents should be avoided? Select all that apply.

    a. Aripiprazole
    b. Risperidone
    c. Ziprasidone
    d. Paliperidone

Answers b and d are correct. Risperidone and paliperidone should be avoided. Risperidone and paliperidone are associated with hyperprolactinemia. Risperidone and paliperidone, along with many of the FGAs, may cause prolactin elevation.

Answers a and c are incorrect. There is low risk of prolactin elevation with aripiprazole, and ziprasidone.

23. Which of the following is the brand name for lurasidone?

    a. Vraylar
    b. Latuda
    c. Fanapt
    d. Saphris

Answer b is correct. Latuda is the brand name for lurasidone.

Answer a is incorrect. Vraylar is the brand name for cariprazine.

Answer c is incorrect. Fanapt is the brand name for iloperidone.

Answer d is incorrect. Saphris is the brand name for asenapine.

24. Which of the following is commercially available in a long-acting injection formulation? Select all that apply.

    a. Risperidone
    b. Paliperidone
    c. Olanzapine
    d. Fluphenazine
    e. Aripiprazole

Answers a, b, c, d, and e are correct. Risperidone, paliperidone, olanzapine, fluphenazine, and aripiprazole are available in a long-injection formulation.

25. RI is a 34-year-old man who has an 8-year history of schizophrenia. RI has a history of medication nonadherence. RI was initiated on Invega Trinza® last month. How often should RI receive his Invega Trinza® injection?

    a. Every 2 weeks
    b. Monthly
    c. Every 6 weeks
    d. Every 3 months

Answer d is correct. Invega Trinza® should be administered once every 3 months. Patients are to be initiated on Invega Sustenna® and must remain on a stable dose for 4 months in order to be switched to Invega Trinza®.

Answer a is incorrect. Risperidone long-acting injection is administered every 2 weeks. Additionally, fluphenazine and lower doses of olanzapine pamoate may also be administered every 2 weeks.

Answer b is incorrect. Paliperidone palmitate (Invega Sustenna®) is administered monthly. Additionally, haloperidol, aripiprazole monohydrate, aripiprazole lauroxil and higher doses of olanzapine pamoate may be administered monthly.

Answer c is incorrect. Higher doses of aripiprazole lauroxil may be administered every 6 weeks.

26. BJ is a 39-year-old woman who has a 10-year history of schizophrenia. BJ over the past 10 years has tried many antipsychotics for the treatment of schizophrenia. BJ has no significant medical conditions and is not on any prescription medications. She does state that she uses acetaminophen on occasion for back pain and also uses loratadine during allergy season. BJ's psychiatrist would like to initiate her on cariprazine for the treatment of her schizophrenia. BJ is requesting additional information regarding adverse effects associated with this medication.

Which of the following adverse effect is most likely to occur with cariprazine?

a. Akathisia
b. Hyperprolactinemia
c. Increased risk of seizures
d. QTc prolongation

Answer a is correct.   Akathisia as well as EPS in general is an adverse effect associated with cariprazine. The risk of EPS and akathisia associated with cariprazine appears to be dose related.

Answer b is incorrect.   The risk of hyperprolactinemia associated with cariprazine is low. Hyperprolactinemia is generally associated with FGAs, risperidone, and paliperidone.

Answer c is incorrect.   The risk of seizures associated with cariprazine is low. Highest risk of seizures is seen with clozapine and chlorpromazine.

Answer d is incorrect.   The risk of QT prolongation is very low. Highest risk of QT prolongation is associated with ziprasidone, iloperidone, and thioridazine.

CHAPTER **57 | Anxiety Disorders**

Please use the following case for Questions 1 and 2.

A 27-year-old woman complains of excessive worrying, poor concentration, back and neck pain, and difficulty sleeping through the night. She constantly worries about losing her job as a data analyst despite the fact that she recently received a promotion. These symptoms have progressively worsened in the past 7 months and have negatively affected her relationship with her friends.

1. The psychiatrist is seeking a recommendation for this new diagnosis of generalized anxiety disorder. Which medication has an FDA indication for this disorder?

   a. Levomilnacipran
   b. Amitriptyline
   c. Bupropion
   d. Buspirone
   e. Fluvoxamine

Answer d is correct.   Buspirone has an FDA indication for generalized anxiety disorder.

Answer a is incorrect.   Levomilnacipram is only indicated for major depression.

Answer b is incorrect.   Amitriptyline is only indicated for depression.

Answer c is incorrect.   Bupropion is only indicated for depression, depression associated with seasonal affective disorder and smoking cessation.

Answer e is incorrect.   Fluvoxamine is only indicated for obsessive compulsive disorder.

2. The mechanism of action of buspirone is:

   a. Dopamine 2A partial agonist
   b. Selective serotonin reuptake inhibitor
   c. Serotonin and norepinephrine reuptake inhibitor
   d. Serotonin 1A partial agonist
   e. Serotonin and dopamine antagonist

Answer d is correct.   Buspirone works primarily by acting as a serotonin 1A partial agonist.

Answers a, b, c, and e are incorrect.   Buspirone has no action at dopamine or norepinephrine receptors and does not selectively inhibit the reuptake of serotonin.

3. Which of the following benzodiazepines has the longest duration of action at steady state?

   a. Alprazolam
   b. Oxazepam
   c. Diazepam
   d. Triazolam
   e. Lorazepam

Answer c is correct.   Diazepam has multiple metabolites which extends the half-life when administered in multiple doses.

Answers a and d are incorrect.   Alprazolam and triazolam have the shortest half-lives and do not have significant metabolites.

Answers b and e are incorrect.   Oxazepam and lorazepam have intermediate lengths of duration.

Please use the following case for Questions 4 and 5.

A 20-year-old man admits excessive anxiety when meeting new people or when he is in large crowds since middle school. While giving a speech for his college public speaking class, he fears being humiliated and worries when he will have to do it again. After 1 month, he dropped the class and avoids any future classes that involve oral presentations.

4. Which of the following antidepressants is the most appropriate initial treatment for this young man with newly diagnosed social anxiety disorder?

   a. Wellbutrin
   b. Cymbalta
   c. Remeron
   d. Oleptro
   e. Effexor XR

Answer e is correct.   Effexor XR is FDA indicated for social anxiety disorder and can be used first-line.

Answers a, b, c, and d are incorrect.   There is little evidence that they are as effective as first or second line use in social anxiety disorder. Wellbutrin may actually worsen anxiety.

5. The patient has had concerns with Effexor and side effects. The most significant dose-related adverse effect of Effexor is:

   a. Sedation
   b. Seizures
   c. Increased blood pressure
   d. Hepatotoxicity
   e. Renal dysfunction

Answer c is correct. At higher doses (>150 mg/d), Effexor has been associated with increased blood pressure.

Answer a is incorrect. While sedation may occur with all antidepressants, sedation is not dose-related. In fact, patients may experience insomnia and jitteriness with increased doses.

Answers b, d and e are incorrect. Seizures, hepatotoxicity, and renal dysfunction are not dose-dependent side effects of Effexor.

6. What is a significant concern for patients with panic disorder when starting an SSRI?

   a. Anxiety
   b. Bruxism
   c. Gastrointestinal upset
   d. Headache
   e. Sexual dysfunction

Answer a is correct. In patients with panic disorder, initiating a new SSRI can sometimes increase anxiety and precipitate a panic attack.

Answers b, c, d, and e are incorrect. Bruxism, gastrointestinal upset, headache, and sexual dysfunction are not increased in patients with panic disorder when compared to patients with other mood conditions.

7. Select the generic name for Cymbalta.

   a. Duloxetine
   b. Citalopram
   c. Mirtazapine
   d. Sertraline
   e. Venlafaxine

Answer a is correct. The brand name for duloxetine is Cymbalta.

Answer b is incorrect. The brand name is Celexa.

Answer c is incorrect. The brand name is Remeron.

Answer d is incorrect. The brand name is Zoloft.

Answer e is incorrect. The brand name is Effexor.

8. A 25-year-old woman presents to your community pharmacy explaining that she was recently diagnosed with obsessive-compulsive disorder. She has been consumed with disturbing thoughts that she will get the Zika virus. She has begun washing her hands after touching anything that is not her own property. This washing is so frequent that she cannot complete her tasks until she has washed her hands. Which of the following medications might be on her medication profile to help manage this issue? Select all that apply.

   a. Phenelzine
   b. Sertraline
   c. Clomipramine
   d. Paroxetine
   e. Clonazepam

Answers b, c, and d are correct. Sertraline, Clomipramine, and Paroxetine have an FDA indication for obsessive compulsive disorder.

Answer a is incorrect. Phenelzine is most effective for major depression, especially atypical depression.

Answer e is incorrect. While clonazepam is effective for many anxiety disorders, it has been most studied for use in panic disorder.

9. For the treatment of anxiety disorders, which of the following is an advantage of an SSRI compared to a tricyclic antidepressant? Select all that apply.

   a. Safer in overdose
   b. Can measure drug levels
   c. Lower seizure risk
   d. No gastrointestinal upset
   e. No sexual dysfunction

Answer a is correct. SSRIs are not associated with significant toxicity in overdose situations.

Answer b is incorrect. Drug levels are not available for SSRIs.

Answer c is correct. TCAs have the potential to lower seizure threshold, especially at high doses.

Answers d and e are incorrect. SSRIs and SNRIs are associated with gastrointestinal upset and sexual dysfunction.

10. The SSRIs are effective for treating which of the following anxiety disorders? Select all that apply.

    a. Generalized anxiety disorder
    b. Obsessive-compulsive disorder
    c. Post-traumatic stress disorder
    d. Panic disorder
    e. Social anxiety disorder

Answers a, b, c, d, and e are correct. SSRIs are effective for treating a variety of anxiety disorders, including GAD, OCD, PTSD, PD, and SAD.

11. A 50-year-old man with a history of alcohol abuse and cirrhosis presents to your clinic, and your attending physician wants to initiate a benzodiazepine for his panic attacks. Which of the following benzodiazepines would be most appropriate to minimize risk of adverse effects?

    a. Alprazolam, clonazepam, estazolam
    b. Chlordiazepoxide, clorazepate, diazepam
    c. Lorazepam, oxazepam, temazepam
    d. Lorazepam, clonazepam, triazolam
    e. Diazepam, clonazepam, lorazepam

Answer c is correct. Lorazepam, oxazepam, and temazepam are metabolized by glucuronidation pathways and are not affected by impaired hepatic function.

Answers a and b are incorrect. All benzodiazepines listed are metabolized by oxidative metabolism and are influenced by hepatic function.

Answer d is incorrect. Clonazepam and triazolam are both metabolized by CYP3A4.

Answer e is incorrect. Diazepam is metabolized by CYP3A4 and CYP2C19, and clonazepam is metabolized by CYP3A4.

12. A mother comes to pick up a new prescription for fluoxetine for her 10-year-old son who has been diagnosed with major depression and obsessive-compulsive disorder. Her son has never received an antidepressant. Along with medication counseling, what is the pharmacist required to provide? Select all that apply.

    a. Medication guide
    b. Package insert
    c. Brochure about depression
    d. List of educational websites for obsessive-compulsive disorder
    e. Depression Guideline

Answer a is correct. The FDA requires the provision of a medication guide on increased suicidality risk with all antidepressants among children and young adults.

Answers b, c, d, and e are incorrect. While these resources may be helpful, they are not required by the FDA.

13. A patient brings in a new prescription for alprazolam today and asks if it will interact with any of his medications. He is currently taking phenytoin and carbamazepine for seizures, citalopram for depression, acetaminophen with codeine for low back pain and warfarin for a recent DVT. Which of the following is most likely to have a clinically significant pharmacokinetic drug-drug interaction with the new prescription?

    a. Citalopram
    b. Carbamazepine
    c. Codeine
    d. Phenytoin
    e. Warfarin

Answer b is correct. Carbamazepine is a potent CYP3A4 inducer and can decrease the effects of alprazolam, which is a CYP3A4 substrate.

Answer a is incorrect. Citalopram does not have significant CYP enzyme inhibitory or inducing effects.

Answer c is incorrect. Codeine is metabolized by CYP2D6 and does not have appreciable CYP3A4 interactions.

Answer d is incorrect. Phenytoin is a potent CYP2C9 and 2C19 inducer; therefore, does not significantly affect alprazolam metabolism.

Answer e is incorrect. Warfarin is mostly metabolized by CYP2C9 and 2C19, so it does not have a significant interaction with alprazolam.

14. Which of the following benzodiazepines are available in orally disintegrating tablet formulation?

    a. Clonazepam
    b. Diazepam
    c. Oxazepam
    d. Lorazepam
    e. Alprazolam

Answers a and e are correct. Clonazepam and Alprazolam are available in ODT formulation.

Answers b, c, and d are incorrect. Diazepam is available in intravenous, rectal gel, solution, and tablet. Oxazepam is available as a capsule. Lorazepam is available in intravenous, solution and tablet formulations.

15. PP is a 38-year-old man with panic disorder who needs treatment. He also has a history of substance abuse with opioids and alcohol. Which of the following treatments is most appropriate for PP?

    a. Alprazolam
    b. Diazepam
    c. Imipramine
    d. Phenelzine
    e. Sertraline

Answer e is correct. Sertraline is effective in panic disorder and is safe in patients with a history of substance abuse.

Answers a and b are incorrect. While benzodiazepines (eg, alprazolam) are effective in the treatment of panic disorder, they are not ideal for use in patients with a history of substance abuse.

Answer c is incorrect. While imipramine has been well-studied for use in panic disorder, it is not well-tolerated compared to SSRIs. The risk of seizures with TCAs is concerning in a patient with a history of substance abuse.

Answer d is incorrect. Monoamine oxidase inhibitors should be considered as last line for use in panic disorder.

Please use the following case for Questions 16 and 17.

A 32-year-old pregnant woman in her first trimester presents with worsening of her obsessive-compulsive symptoms. Due to the potential risk of her compulsive behaviors on her fetus, she has agreed to start pharmacologic treatment.

16. Which of the following agents should be avoided?

    a. Citalopram
    b. Fluoxetine
    c. Fluvoxamine
    d. Paroxetine
    e. Sertraline

Answer d is correct. Paroxetine has been associated with cardiac malformations in the fetus when the drug is administered in the first trimester. Paroxetine is labeled as a Pregnancy Category D. The other SSRIs are in Pregnancy Category C.

Answers a, b, c, and e are incorrect. They can be used in first trimester without significant risk of causing fetal harm.

---

17. She was previously prescribed clonazepam at the start of her pregnancy, but it was discontinued. Which of the following was the reason for this discontinuation?

    a. Cleft palate
    b. Heart defects
    c. Limb abnormalities
    d. Pulmonary hypertension
    e. Renal defects

Answer a is correct. During the first trimester, benzodiazepines have been associated with cleft lip or cleft palate.

Answers b, c, d, and e are incorrect. Benzodiazepines are not associated with any of these malformations.

---

18. Which of the following medications has the lowest risk of causing serotonin syndrome when combined with sertraline?

    a. Clonazepam
    b. Fluoxetine
    c. Desipramine
    d. Phenelzine
    e. Desvenlafaxine

Answer a is correct. Clonazepam is a benzodiazepine and does not have appreciable serotonergic properties.

Answer b is incorrect. Fluoxetine is a selective serotonin reuptake inhibitor and will have increased risk of serotonin syndrome when combined with sertraline.

Answer c is incorrect. Desipramine is a tricyclic antidepressant and will have increased risk of serotonin syndrome when combined with sertraline.

Answer d is incorrect. Phenelzine is a monoamine oxidase inhibitor and will have increased risk of serotonin syndrome when combined with sertraline.

Answer e is incorrect. Desvenlafaxine is a serotonin norepinephrine reuptake inhibitor and will have increased risk of serotonin syndrome when combined with sertraline.

---

19. The brand name for escitalopram is:

    a. Celexa
    b. Effexor
    c. Lexapro
    d. Paxil
    e. Zoloft

Answer c is correct. The brand name for escitalopram is Lexapro.

Answer a is incorrect. The generic name is citalopram.

Answer b is incorrect. The generic name is venlafaxine.

Answer d is incorrect. The generic name is paroxetine.

Answer e is incorrect. The generic name is sertraline.

---

20. Place the following benzodiazepines in order of duration: alprazolam, oxazepam, triazolam, clonazepam. Start with the shortest duration and end with the longest duration.

    a. Alprazolam, oxazepam, triazolam, clonazepam
    b. Triazolam, alprazolam, oxazepam, clonazepam
    c. Clonazepam, triazolam, alprazolam, oxazepam
    d. Oxazepam, clonazepam, triazolam, alprazolam

Answer b is correct. Triazolam has a very short duration; Alprazolam has a short duration, Oxazepam has an intermediate duration, and Clonazepam has a long duration.

Answers a, c, and d are incorrect.

---

21. CD is a 34-year-old man experiencing frequent flashbacks and nightmares of a very traumatic event that occurred a few years ago. He feels constantly "on edge" and easily startled. His primary care provider diagnosed CD with PTSD. Which of the following medications should be avoided?

    a. Clonazepam
    b. Sertraline
    c. Prazosin
    d. Citalopram

Answer a is correct. Benzodiazepines should be avoided in PTSD as it is associated with worse outcomes.

Answers b, c, and d are incorrect. SSRIs are first-line for PTSD and Prazosin is used to treat nightmares associated with PTSD.

CHAPTER 58 | Bipolar Disorders

1. Which of the following are signs and symptoms of a manic episode? Select all that apply.

   a. Irritable mood
   b. Anhedonia
   c. Racing thoughts
   d. Psychomotor agitation
   e. Decreased need for sleep

Answer a is correct. Irritable mood is a symptom of mania. This may also be seen in a depressive episode, however.

Answer c is correct. Racing thoughts are a classic indication of mania.

Answer d is correct. Psychomotor agitation is a symptom of mania. This may also be seen in a depressive episode, however.

Answer e is correct. Decreased need for sleep is a classic symptom of mania. Depressed patients will not report a decreased need for sleep. They wish to sleep but cannot. Manic patients in an acutely manic episode may not wish to sleep and would rather engage in goal-directed activities and stay awake.

Answer b is incorrect. Anhedonia is the inability to feel pleasure while engaging in pleasurable and enjoyable activities. This is often seen as one of the signs of MDD (unipolar depression) and not a manic episode.

2. VV is a patient who was recently diagnosed with bipolar disorder before being discharged for a related hospitalization. VV reports a positive family history of mood disorders but denies hospitalizations of any family members. You explain to VV that it is possible that the family members were never hospitalized due to prominent symptoms of hypomania, characterized by which of the following?

   a. Multiple hospitalizations
   b. Psychotic episodes
   c. Impairment in social functioning
   d. Impairment in occupational functioning
   e. An inflated self-esteem

Answer e is correct. The symptoms of hypomania and mania are similar with respect to the target signs and symptoms. Hypomania is less severe than mania. Inflated self-esteem can still be detected in hypomania.

Answer a is incorrect. These patients are often able to function well; therefore, they do not require hospitalization.

Answer b is incorrect. There is no psychosis (eg, auditory and visual hallucinations, delusions) involved in hypomanic states.

Answer c is incorrect. There is no impairment in social functioning.

Answer d is incorrect. There is no impairment in occupational functioning.

3. The treatment team asks you, the clinical pharmacist, for a consult on a patient with bipolar disorder. There is a question regarding whether or not the patient meets criteria for rapid cycling. You explain to the team that there needs to be a confirmed history of _____ or more manic or depressive episodes within a _____ time period.

   a. two; 6-month
   b. two; 1-year
   c. three; 2-year
   d. four; 1-year
   e. four; 2-year

Answer d is correct. Rapid cycling is a term to describe when a patient experiences four or more episodes of depression or mania within a 12-month period. Rapid cycling is a specified term used in the DSM-IV-TR to describe the course of recurrent episodes. This term is used to specify bipolar disorder I and II but not depressive disorders such as MDD.

Answer a is incorrect. A 6-month period is not stated in the definition of rapid cycling.

Answer b is incorrect. The correct number of episodes required in a 12-month period is four, not two.

Answer c is incorrect. A 2-year period is not stated in the definition of rapid cycling; it is 1 year.

Answer e is incorrect. A 2-year period is not stated in the definition of rapid cycling; it is 1 year.

4. Patient LC requires treatment for bipolar disorder, and is currently in a depressive episode. The patient has a history of predominantly depressive episodes in the last 3 years. The patient refuses to take more than one medication at a time for management of symptoms and relapse prevention. Which medication will you recommend for LC, confident that it can be used as monotherapy for managing the associated symptoms? Select all that apply.

   a. Lithium
   b. Lamotrigine
   c. Olanzapine
   d. Quetiapine
   e. Citalopram

Answer a is correct. Lithium is the classic mood stabilizer often used alone to manage both phases of bipolar disorder: manic/hypomanic as well as depressive.

Answer b is correct. Lamotrigine is FDA-approved for bipolar disorder I and is often used as an alternative to lithium for bipolar depressive episodes and may be used as monotherapy if warranted.

Answer d is correct. Quetiapine is FDA-approved as monotherapy for managing bipolar depression.

Answer c is incorrect. Olanzapine is an AAP agent that is FDA-approved for the treatment of acute mania as well as maintenance treatment in bipolar disorder; however, it is not approved for managing bipolar depression monotherapy. Only when combined in the OFC (trade name Symbyax; fluoxetine is an SSRI antidepressant) is it approved for use in bipolar depression.

Answer e is incorrect. Citalopram is an SSRI that may be used in conjunction with a mood stabilizer (lithium, divalproex sodium, or an AAP agent) for the bipolar depressive episode, if lithium or lamotrigine is not used. An antidepressant should never be used as monotherapy, even in the depressive phase of BPD. It must always be used in conjunction with a mood stabilizing agent to prevent manic episodes (ie, antidepressant-induced manic switch).

---

5. JA is being transitioned from olanzapine to lithium for the management of bipolar disorder. You have been asked to provide a counseling session on medication adverse drug reactions after JA inquired about common and expected adverse drug reactions of lithium. Select the counseling point that should be discussed.

    a. Alopecia
    b. Increased urination
    c. Hyperammonemia
    d. Hyperthyroidism
    e. Diplopia

Answer b is correct. Lithium causes polyuria, which is a manifestation of nephrogenic diabetes insipidus. It also causes associated polydipsia, increased thirst.

Answer a is incorrect. Alopecia is most likely associated with valproate.

Answer c is incorrect. Hyperammonemia is associated with valproate.

Answer d is incorrect. Lithium is clearly associated with causing hypothyroidism, not hyperthyroidism; although there have been few paradoxical reports of hyperthyroidism and lithium.

Answer e is incorrect. Diplopia has been associated with CBZ.

---

6. You are asked to start a 24-year-old patient on lithium for the maintenance treatment of bipolar disorder. The patient's renal function is within normal limits and body mass index (BMI) is 22. What is the starting dose and frequency of lithium that you will recommend for this patient?

    a. 300 mg tid
    b. 15 mg qhs

    c. 200 mg bid
    d. 500 mg bid
    e. 50 mg every day

Answer a is correct. The recommended starting dose is 300 mg tid or less, depending on the patient's age and weight.

Answer b is incorrect. The recommended starting doses of 15 mg qhs is associated with olanzapine.

Answer c is incorrect. 200 mg bid is associated with CBZ.

Answer d is incorrect. 500 mg bid is a good starting dose for divalproex sodium.

Answer e is incorrect. 50 mg qd is a starting dose of lamotrigine if taken with CBZ.

---

7. Which of the following is the teratogenicity associated with lithium use in the first trimester of pregnancy?

    a. Cardiovascular
    b. Renal
    c. Hepatic
    d. Neuromuscular
    e. Dermatological

Answer a is correct. Lithium is associated with causing Ebstein anomaly, a cardiac abnormality. This is a condition in which the tricuspid valve is abnormal with secondary dilation of the right ventricular outflow tract.

Answer b is incorrect. Lithium can cause renal impairment to the person using lithium, but there is no association of renal-related birth defects in the newborn.

Answer c is incorrect. Lithium is not associated with causing liver damage.

Answer d is incorrect. CBZ and valproate are associated with causing spina bifida in pregnancy use.

Answer e is incorrect. Lithium can cause rash to the person taking it, but this would not be a teratogenic effect.

---

8. Which of the following are appropriate counseling points to mention to a patient starting lithium? Select all that apply.

    a. "You should avoid dehydration, so maintain your water intake."
    b. "Stop your medication if you experience persistent diarrhea."
    c. "Use caution while operating machinery or driving a car."
    d. "Ask your pharmacist before starting any new pain medications."
    e. "You should reduce your sodium intake while taking lithium."

Answer a is correct. This should be counseled to patients. Patients should maintain consistent levels of any caffeine intake and stay hydrated to avoid changes in lithium blood concentrations.

Answer b is correct. This should be counseled to patients. Although diarrhea is an expected adverse reaction of lithium, persistent diarrhea may be a sign of lithium toxicity. Patients are instructed to stop the lithium and call their doctor right away. The lithium dose may be stopped for 1 day until lithium blood levels can be obtained.

Answer c is correct. This should be counseled to patients. Lithium can cause fatigue and sedation; therefore, as with any central nervous system (CNS)-depressant medication, patients must be warned about lithium possibly impairing their ability to perform activities requiring mental alertness or intact physical coordination. These include operating machinery or driving a motor vehicle.

Answer d is correct. This should be counseled to patients. Patients taking lithium need caution about starting new pain medications such as ibuprofen or other nonsteroidal anti-inflammatory drugs (NSAIDs) that will increase the lithium blood concentration. Patients taking lithium may take sulindac (Clinoril), an NSAID that does not appear to increase lithium levels, aspirin, or acetaminophen.

Answer e is incorrect. This should *not* be counseled to patients. While on lithium, sodium intake should be maintained at consistent levels and not necessarily reduced. Reducing sodium intake may lead to lithium retention and higher blood concentrations and, therefore, toxicity.

---

9. A patient has been taking lithium for 3 years and has been stable on it without relapse of symptoms. There has been no change in renal function or other laboratory monitoring parameters. The patient is also being monitored by another health care professional. Together, you both agree that the patient's target therapeutic concentration should be which of the following ranges?

   a. 4 to 12 mcg/mL
   b. 4 to 12 mEq/L
   c. 50 to 125 mcg/mL
   d. 0.6 to 0.8 mEq/L
   e. 1 to 1.8 mEq/L

Answer d is correct. Three years of being on lithium is considered maintenance treatment, not acute treatment. Lithium is a cation; therefore the units are in mmol/L or milliequivalents per liter (mEq/L). Levels for maintenance treatment of lithium are generally between 0.6 and 0.8 mEq/L; however, it is suggested that for bipolar depressive episode treatment, higher levels may be needed. Some sources reference 0.6 to 1.0 mEq/L as the target level range.

Answer a is incorrect. Levels of 4 to 12 mcg/mL is associated with CBZ's target blood concentration in order to avoid toxicity.

Answer b is incorrect. The units are correct but the number value is incorrect. Levels >1.5 mEq/L is associated with toxicity; therefore, no patient will be maintained higher than 1.5 mEq/L.

Answer c is incorrect. Levels of 50 to 125 mcg/mL is associated with valproate target concentrations.

Answer e is incorrect. Levels >1.5 mEq/L is associated with toxicity; therefore, no patient will be maintained higher than 1.5 mEq/L.

---

10. Your 39-year-old patient with bipolar disorder is on several medications, reporting the following during your clinic visit:

    Aleve (naproxen sodium) 1 tablet twice daily for back pain when working, Motrin (ibuprofen) 400 mg 1 tablet every 8 hours as need for headache occurring three times per month, Cozaar (losartan) 50 mg 1 tablet bid, Glucophage (metformin) 850 mg 1 tablet bid. The patient smokes six to seven cigarettes per day, drinks alcohol occasionally, and has five large cups of coffee every morning except Fridays and Saturdays.

    Which of the following factors can affect the level of lithium when blood is drawn at the next clinic visit? Select all that apply.

    a. Aleve
    b. Cozaar
    c. Glucophage
    d. Smoking
    e. Coffee

Answer a is correct. Aleve (Naproxen sodium) is an over-the-counter NSAID that can increase lithium blood concentrations. Motrin is also implicated in this drug interaction. NSAIDs (except sulindac) decrease the renal clearance of lithium.

Answer b is correct. Cozaar (losartan) is an angiotensin-II receptor antagonist that is also associated with increasing lithium.

Answer e is correct. Caffeine in coffee will increase the elimination of lithium and may decrease lithium concentrations by 20%. Large amounts need to be consumed in order to see this effect clinically. This patient doesn't drink coffee on the weekends, which can further affect the levels of lithium.

Answer c is incorrect. Glucophage is metformin and no drug interaction has been reported between biguanides and lithium.

Answer d is incorrect. Smoking does not directly affect lithium concentrations. Lithium is not metabolized by CYP450 liver isoenzymes; therefore, smoking will not affect the elimination of lithium. Smoking can lower olanzapine serum concentrations.

---

11. The physician wants to know what extended-release preparations of lithium are available, if any. You advise that a prescription be written for which of the following?

    a. Lithium citrate
    b. Lithium carbonate tablets
    c. Lithium carbonate capsules
    d. Eskalith
    e. Lithobid

Answer e is correct. Lithobid is an extended-release, film-coated tablet.

Answer a is incorrect. Lithium citrate is the oral solution dosage form containing 8 mEq of lithium per teaspoon.

Answer b is incorrect. Lithium carbonate tablets or capsules and Eskalith are all the same regular release products.

Answer c is incorrect. Lithium carbonate tablets or capsules and Eskalith are all the same regular release products.

Answer d is incorrect. If the prescription were written for Eskalith CR specifically, this is an extended-release product.

---

12. A patient on the psychiatry ward is being considered for lithium treatment. You recommend which of the following laboratory parameters be checked prior to starting treatment? Select all that apply.

    a. Serum creatinine (SCr)
    b. Electrocardiogram (ECG)
    c. Thyroid function tests
    d. Liver enzyme tests
    e. Electrolytes

Answer a is correct. Scr as well as blood urea nitrogen (BUN) are markers of kidney function. These should be monitored in all lithium patients because lithium is cleared via the kidneys. Lithium can also cause renal impairment.

Answer b is correct. An ECG is recommended in patients who are already predisposed to cardiovascular disease and for those over the age of 40. Lithium can cause cardiac conduction abnormalities and worsen cardiac disease.

Answer c is correct. Hyperthyroidism can mimic manic states. This should be ruled out before a diagnosis of bipolar disorder is made. Moreover, lithium can cause hypothyroidism with long-term use, necessitating levothyroxine treatment.

Answer e is correct. Electrolytes should be monitored, because hyponatremic (low sodium) states can increase the risk of higher blood concentrations of lithium, causing lithium toxicity. Hyperkalemic (high potassium) can increase the risk of lithium-induced cardiac adverse events.

Answer d is incorrect. Lithium is not metabolized by the liver but is cleared almost exclusively by the kidneys. Liver functions tests are not required prior to starting lithium monotherapy.

---

13. PCOS has been associated with which of the following medications? Select all that apply.

    a. Cariprazine
    b. Divalproex sodium
    c. Lithium
    d. Lamotrigine
    e. Olanzapine

Answer b is correct. Divalproex sodium (valproate) is associated with causing polycystic ovaries in women.

Answer a is incorrect. The AAP, cariprazine, and others have not been associated with PCOS.

Answer c is incorrect. There is no clear relationship between lithium and PCOS.

Answer d is incorrect. There is no clear relationship between lamotrigine and PCOS.

Answer e is incorrect. The AAP, olanzapine, and others have not been associated with PCOS.

---

14. A patient was just admitted into the psychiatry emergency department for an acute manic episode presenting with a flight of ideas and hypersexuality toward staff, reporting "I am the best lover you will ever have in your entire life- that's what all of my partners say, and there are lots of them!" The patient is accompanied by a family member who reports a past medication history of divalproex sodium. What recommended loading dose (in kg/d) do you recommend for this individual?

    a. 5 mg
    b. 10 to 15 mg
    c. 20 to 30 mg
    d. 40 mg
    e. 50 to 55 mg

Answer c is correct. The recommended loading dose of divalproex sodium (Depakote) in inpatient settings for acute mania is 20 to 30 mg/kg/d in divided oral doses. The dose is usually divided into two to three doses if the calculated loading dose exceeds 2 g/d to improve tolerability.

Answer a is incorrect. This is not the recommended loading dose for Depakote. It is too low.

Answer b is incorrect. This is not the recommended loading dose for Depakote. It is too low.

Answer d is incorrect. This is not the recommended loading dose for Depakote. It is too high.

Answer e is incorrect. This is not the recommended loading dose for Depakote. It is too high.

---

15. A patient with bipolar disorder is concerned about using certain medications for her psychiatric condition. She heard that some medications are associated with causing a neural tube defect if taken during pregnancy. You confirm her suspicion and tell her that some agents are associated with causing this condition in the newborn when used by the mother during pregnancy. You proceed to counsel her about which of the following agent? Select all that apply.

    a. Lithium
    b. Divalproex sodium
    c. CBZ
    d. Paliperidone
    e. Risperidone

Answer b is correct. Valproate is associated with spina bifida. There is a 1% to 2% risk.

Answer c is correct. CBZ is associated with spina bifida. There is a 0.5% to 1% risk.

Answer a is incorrect. Lithium is associated mainly with causing rare instances of Ebstein anomaly.

Answer d is incorrect. To date, the AAPs, including paliperidone, have not been associated with causing any significantly greater structural birth defects compared to controls.

Answer e is incorrect. To date, the AAPs have not been associated with causing any significantly greater structural birth defects compared to controls. Risperidone has been reported as used during pregnancy without causing spina bifida.

---

16. It is recommended that the human leukocyte antigen type B, *HLA-B*1502*, allele is genotyped in Asian patients prior to taking which of the following medications? Select all that apply.

    a. Lithium
    b. CBZ
    c. Lorazepam
    d. Haloperidol
    e. Quetiapine

Answer b is correct. CBZ is associated with causing both SJS and TEN, two potentially fatal dermatologic reactions. The allelic variation of the *HLA-B gene*, *HLA-B*1502*, is associated with these serious dermatologic reactions, and it is recommended by the manufacturer that patient who are of ancestry in genetically at-risk populations be screened for the presence of this genetic marker. All medications can potentially cause a rash; however, there is a target genetic maker that has been linked specifically to CBZ. When a rash is seen with the use of lamotrigine, the medication should be discontinued.

Answer a is incorrect. There is no genetic marker linked with the rash induced by lithium.

Answer c is incorrect. There is no genetic marker linked with the rash induced by lorazepam.

Answer d is incorrect. There is no genetic marker linked with the rash induced by haloperidol.

Answer e is incorrect. There is no genetic marker linked with the rash induced by quetiapine.

---

17. You discover that a bipolar patient in the hospital ward has been "cheeking" medication for the past 4 days. You decide to recommend the same medication in an orally disintegrating tablet (ODT) formulation. Which of the following medications is available in an ODT dosage form?

    a. CBZ
    b. Haloperidol
    c. Lithium
    d. Quetiapine
    e. Risperidone

Answer e is correct. Risperidone is available in Risperdal-M Tab, an ODT dosage formulation. The other AAPs available in an ODT include olanzapine (Zyprexa Zydis), aripiprazole (Abilify Discmelt), and clozapine (Fazaclo). These are good alternatives to regular tablets in instances where the patient has difficulty swallowing or is suspected of cheeking his/her medication (ie, pretending to swallow the medication when in fact the patient is holding the medication between the gums of the teeth and cheek, only to later dispose of it in order to avoid taking the medication).

Answer a is incorrect. CBZ is available in an oral suspension, another viable dosage form options for "cheekers."

Answer b is incorrect. Haloperidol is available in an oral solution, which is another viable dosage form option for "cheekers."

Answer c is incorrect. Lithium is available in an oral solution, which is another viable dosage form option for "cheekers."

Answer d is incorrect. The only currently available dosage form of quetiapine is in a hard tablet formulation that must be swallowed.

---

18. Which of the following factors is likely to increase the risk of lamotrigine-related rash? Select all that apply.

    a. Coadministration with another anticonvulsant, valproate
    b. Coadministration with another anticonvulsant, CBZ
    c. Exceeding the recommended initial dose of lamotrigine
    d. Exceeding the recommended maximum dose of lamotrigine
    e. Exceeding the recommended dose escalation schedule of lamotrigine

---

Answer a is correct. This *will* increase the risk of rash. Valproate is known to increase lamotrigine almost double. Caution is advised when coadministering valproate and lamotrigine; their concomitant use is not contraindicated; rather, the dose of lamotrigine should be halved when used together.

Answer c is correct. This *will* increase the risk of rash.

Answer d is correct. This *will* increase the risk of rash.

Answer e is correct. This *will* increase the risk of rash. Following the careful and slow dose escalation recommendations of lamotrigine has resulted in fewer incidences of rash.

Answer b is incorrect. Coadministration with CBZ, a drug enzyme inducer, is likely to decrease the lamotrigine levels, not increase it. With lower lamotrigine blood levels, there is a lower risk of rash.

---

19. The psychiatric treatment team decides to start Risperdal Consta on a patient who has a history of nonadherence to the

current mood stabilizer for bipolar disorder in the past 6 years. They ask you, the clinical pharmacist, for the recommended starting dose and directions for administration. You reply with the following:

a. 2 mg tablet, 1 tab po bid
b. 3 mg ODT, 1 tab on top of the tongue everyday
c. 25 mg subcutaneously (SQ) every 2 weeks
d. 25 mg IM every 2 weeks
e. 50 mg IM every 2 weeks

Answer d is correct. Consta is the LAI formulation of risperidone. This dosage formulation is currently FDA-approved for monotherapy or adjunctive therapy to lithium or valproate for the maintenance treatment of bipolar I disorder. The recommended starting dose is usually 25 mg. A higher dose of 37.5 mg may be started if the patient was currently stable on a higher oral dose.

Answer a is incorrect. This is an oral dosage formulation, not the LAI formulation.

Answer b is incorrect. This is still an oral dosage formulation, not the LAI formulation. ODT is the oral disintegrating tablet placed on top of the tongue with dry hands.

Answer c is incorrect. Consta is administered IM, not SQ.

Answer e is incorrect. It is not recommended to start with a high dose of 50 mg. The dose can eventually be increased to 50 mg, however, over time.

20. Which agent is considered the safest option for treating a pregnant female with acute bipolar mania?

a. CBZ
b. Chlorpromazine
c. Haloperidol
d. Lithium
e. VPA

Answer c is correct. Pregnancy issues in bipolar disorder are complicated. The safest, established treatment option is a high-potency antipsychotic agent such as haloperidol.

Answer a is incorrect. As one of the three classic mood stabilizers, CBZ is generally considered unsafe to use during pregnancy, especially during the first trimester. It is pregnancy category D, meaning that there is evidence for risk to the fetus associated with their use; however, if used, CBZ should be used with caution and careful monitoring and concomitant administration of 4 to 5 mg/d of folic acid is recommended.

Answer b is incorrect. Low-potency antipsychotics, such as chlorpromazine (Thorazine), should generally be avoided during pregnancy.

Answer d is incorrect. As one of the three classic mood stabilizers, lithium is usually avoided during pregnancy, especially during the first trimester. During the first trimester, there is a greater risk of cardiac-related teratogenicity.

Lithium is pregnancy category D, meaning that there is evidence for risk to the fetus associated with its use; however, if lithium is to be used, caution with dosing and careful monitoring is advised.

Answer e is incorrect. The three classic mood stabilizers, lithium, CBZ, and divalproex sodium/VPA, are not safe to use during pregnancy, especially during the first trimester. They are all pregnancy category D, meaning that there is evidence for risk to the fetus associated with their use. Depakote has been associated with causing spina bifida; however, if VPA is to be used, concomitant administration of 4 to 5 mg/d of folic acid is recommended.

21. Symbyax is a combination product with several therapeutic indications. This product contains fixed doses of which of the following agents for treating bipolar depression?

a. Lithium + divalproex sodium
b. Risperidone + fluoxetine
c. Olanzapine + fluoxetine
d. Risperidone + sertraline
e. Lurasidone + sertraline

Answer c is correct. Symbyax is a combination product whose only indication is bipolar depression. It contains one AAP, olanzapine, plus one SSRI antidepressant, fluoxetine. The active ingredients include olanzapine and fluoxetine in the following milligram ratios: 3/25, 6/25, 6/50, 12/25, and 12/50. Patients are instructed to take it at bedtime: olanzapine is sedating and fluoxetine is activating. There are no other similar combination products currently available.

Answer a is incorrect. There is no such combination product commercially available containing these classic moods stabilizers, although they can be used together.

Answer b is incorrect. This antipsychotic and antidepressant combination is incorrect.

Answer d is incorrect. This antipsychotic and antidepressant combination is incorrect.

Answer e is incorrect. This antipsychotic and antidepressant (sertraline) combination is incorrect.

22. Which antidepressant is most likely to cause a switch into mania when used in a patient with bipolar disorder?

a. Amitriptyline
b. Bupropion
c. Citalopram
d. Escitalopram
e. Sertraline

Answer a is correct. Amitriptyline is the only agent on this list that is classified as a TCA. TCAs have classically been reported to be the class of antidepressants most likely to cause a switch to mania in bipolar patients.

Answer b is incorrect. Bupropion is a dopamine and norepinephrine reuptake inhibitor that is less likely to cause a switch into mania.

Answer c is incorrect. SSRIs, as a class, have a low probability of causing treatment-emergent mania. SSRIs include citalopram (Celexa), escitalopram, fluoxetine, fluvoxamine, paroxetine, and sertraline. The SSRIs are some of the most commonly used antidepressants in treating bipolar depression and are believed to be less likely to cause drug-induced mania.

Answer d is incorrect. SSRIs, as a class, have a low probability of causing treatment-emergent mania. Escitalopram (Lexapro) is an SSRI.

Answer e is incorrect. SSRIs, as a class, have a low probability of causing treatment-emergent mania. Sertraline (Zoloft) is an SSRI.

23. Which of the following medication classes can be used for a patient with bipolar disorder, even if some of them are used off-label? Select all that apply.

    a. ACE-Inhibitors
    b. Anticonvulsants
    c. Antidepressants
    d. Antipsychotics
    e. Calcium channel blockers

Answer b is correct. Anticonvulsants such as CBZ, valproate, and lamotrigine are FDA-approved for bipolar disorder treatment.

Answer c is correct. Although not FDA-approved for bipolar depression (except the combination product Symbyax that contains fluoxetine), antidepressants are often used in combination therapy for bipolar depressive episodes. They should not be used as monotherapy.

Answer d is correct. All of the AAPs (except clozapine) are FDA approved for various bipolar disorder mood episodes. Both oral and parenteral preparations are approved for use in bipolar disorder.

Answer e is correct. Although not commonly used, calcium channel blockers (ie, verapamil) have demonstrated mood-stabilizing properties, especially for acute mania.

Answer a is incorrect. ACE-inhibitors have no role in mood stabilization for bipolar disorders treatment.

24. You are providing a literature review grand rounds presentation of pharmacological treatments for bipolar disorder management. Which agent will you describe as effective for the treatment of bipolar I disorder and possibly more effective than lithium for bipolar depression?

    a. Dilantin
    b. Lamictal
    c. Lamisil
    d. Neurontin
    e. Trileptal

Answer b is correct. Lamictal is lamotrigine, an anticonvulsant that is FDA-approved for the treatment of bipolar I disorder. Whereas lithium may be more effective for manic episodes in bipolar disorder, no evidence exists to indicate that lamotrigine may be more effective for the depressive phase.

Answer a is incorrect. Dilantin (phenytoin) is an anticonvulsant that has shown some mood-stabilizing properties, but it not widely used for bipolar disorders treatment.

Answer c is incorrect. Lamisil is terbinafine, an antifungal agent. Do not confuse medications that sound and look like each other.

Answer d is incorrect. Neurontin (gabapentin) is an anticonvulsant that has shown some efficacy for mood stabilization. It has not, however, been shown to be more effective than lithium. It may be used as adjunctive treatment. It is not FDA-approved for mood disorders.

Answer e is incorrect. Trileptal (oxcarbazepine) is an anticonvulsant that may be used as a tertiary agent, if other mood stabilizers fail to control mood. Currently, it is not FDA-approved for the treatment of mood disorders; however, it is described in some of the bipolar disorder treatment guidelines as an alternative agent to CBZ for providing mood-stabilizing effects. Note: oxcarbazepine has been associated with causing hyponatremia.

25. You are the pharmacist on a Pharmacy and Therapeutic committee at your hospital. The committee has asked you to present on alternatives to lithium and lamotrigine for managing bipolar depression in patients with bipolar disorder. Which of the following agents will you present data on, based on their FDA-approved indication for this therapeutic use? Select all that apply.

    a. Asenapine
    b. Iloperidone
    c. Lurasidone
    d. Paliperidone
    e. Quetiapine

Answer c is correct. Lurasidone (Latuda) is an AAP that is FDA-approved for bipolar depression. Starting dose is 20 mg/d, and the dosing range for bipolar disorder is 20 to 120 mg/d.

Answer e is correct. Quetiapine (Seroquel) is an AAP that is indicated for use in bipolar depression. Starting dose is 50 mg once daily at bedtime and it may be increased up to 300 mg/d.

Answer a is incorrect. Asenapine (Saphris) is an AAP that has been studied for managing bipolar manic episodes.

Answer b is incorrect. Iloperidone (Fanpt) is an AAP only indicated for schizophrenia. It has limited use.

The manufacturer states, "In choosing among treatments, prescribers should consider the ability of iloperidone to prolong the QT interval and the use of other drugs first."

Answer d is incorrect. Paliperidone (Invega) is an AAP indicated for schizoaffective disorder. It has been studied in individuals with psychotic features combined with depressed or manic mood. It is currently not approved for bipolar depressive episodes in bipolar disorder.

---

26. Which of the following counseling points will you provide to a patient who is taking asenapine for managing a manic episode in bipolar disorder? Select all that apply.

    a. "Use this medication as directed, once daily at bedtime."
    b. "Inject all of the contents from the syringe to ensure the full dose."
    c. "Carefully and gently remove the tablet from its original package."
    d. "Do not eat or drink for 10 minutes after taking the dose."
    e. "Place tablet under tongue and allow it to dissolve completely."

Answer c is correct. Asenapine is sublingual tablet that must be removed very carefully from its original package. The manufacturer instructs for use: 'Do not remove tablet until you are ready to administer. Use dry hands when handling the tablet. Firmly press and hold thumb button, then pull out tablet pack. Do not push tablet through tablet pack. Do not cut or tear tablet pack. Peel back colored tab then gently remove the tablet.' (Quote adapted from Merck Sharp Dohme Corp. Whitehouse Station, NJ; Product information for Saphris [asenapine], updated on 01/2017).

Answer d is correct. Instructions for use explicitly state that one should not eat or drink for 10 minutes after taking the dose. Doing so may affect the bioavailability of the tablet dose form.

Answer e is correct. The route of administration of asenapine is sublingual (ie, *under* the tongue; not on top of the tongue such as ODT formulations that many of the AAPs are available in).

Answer a is incorrect. Asenapine is taken by mouth twice daily, not once daily.

Answer b is incorrect. Asenapine is not an injectable medication. It is an oral sublingual tablet.

---

27. You receive a prescription for cariprazine 1.5 mg po qd. You ask your pharmacy technician to fill which of the following products?

    a. Carbatrol
    b. Equetro
    c. Sinemet
    d. Tegretol
    e. Vraylar

Answer e is correct. Vraylar is the branded product of cariprazine. This is a relatively newer AAP indicated for acute mania or mixed episodes associated with bipolar I disorder.

Answer a is incorrect. Carbatrol is the branded product for CBZ.

Answer b is incorrect. Equetro is another branded product for CBZ.

Answer c is incorrect. Sinemet is the branded product of carbidopa/levodopa for Parkinson disease.

Answer d is incorrect. Tegretol is another branded product for CBZ.

CHAPTER **59** | Post-traumatic Stress Disorder

1. Which are core symptoms of PTSD? Select all that apply.

    a. Recurrent, intrusive, distressing memories of the trauma
    b. Ability to recall an important aspect of the trauma
    c. Avoidance of conversations about the trauma
    d. Hypervigilance

Answers a, c, and d are correct. Hypervigilance, recurrent memories of the trauma, avoidance of conversation, and *inability* to recall an important aspect of the trauma are all core symptoms of PTSD.

The following case pertains to questions 2 through 3.

LH is a 34-year-old woman who has experienced persistent flashbacks and nightmares after being robbed at gunpoint while leaving a restaurant several months ago. She finds it difficult to talk about the experience, and avoids situations that remind her of the event. She was recently diagnosed with PTSD.

2. Which agent should be used as a first-line treatment for PTSD in this patient?

    a. Phenelzine
    b. Paroxetine
    c. Amitriptyline
    d. Bupropion

Answer b is correct. Paroxetine is an SSRI and is a first-line agent.

Answer a is incorrect. Phenelzine is an MAOI and reserved for last-line treatment.

Answer c is incorrect. Amitriptyline is TCA and a third-line agent.

Answer d is incorrect. Bupropion is *not* effective in PTSD.

3. In addition to medication therapy, LH would like to receive some type of nonpharmacologic treatment. Which nonpharmacologic treatment for PTSD has the most evidence supporting its use and is often utilized in the management of PTSD?

   a. Group counseling
   b. Stress inoculation treatment
   c. Psychoeducation
   d. CBT

Answer d is correct. CBT is the most studied nonpharmacologic treatment in PTSD and is widely utilized in PTSD management.

Answers a, b, and c are incorrect. All others have data but they are still limited.

4. Which SSRIs is/are approved by the FDA for the treatment of PTSD? Select all that apply.

   a. Sertraline
   b. Fluoxiatine
   c. Paroxetine
   d. Citalopram

Answers a and c are correct. Sertraline and paroxetine are the only two agents that are FDA approved for PTSD.

Answers b and d are incorrect. While fluoxetine and citalopram have shown some benefits in treating this population, they are not FDA approved for PTSD.

5. TW is a 43-year-old man with PTSD. He has tried several medications in the past, including sertraline, escitalopram, and venlafaxine; however, he has not experienced significant improvement of symptoms with any of these agents. The physician wants to start alprazolam 1 mg twice daily and asks if this is appropriate. How do you correctly respond to the physician?

   a. Alprazolam is not effective in the treatment of PTSD and may worsen symptoms.
   b. Alprazolam is effective; however, dose should be started at 0.5 mg twice daily.
   c. Alprazolam is effective and dosing is appropriate.
   d. Alprazolam is not the most appropriate benzodiazepine to use. It is best to initiate clonazepam 0.5 mg twice daily.

Answer a is correct. Alprazolam is a benzodiazepine, which has not shown efficacy in clinical trials. Recent data show it may worsen symptoms.

Answers b, c, and d are incorrect. Benzodiazepines are not utilized in the management of PTSD.

6. RB is a 27-year-old male combat veteran who was diagnosed with PTSD 1 year ago. He was originally prescribed fluoxetine, but did not experience any improvement while taking the medication. He has been taking sertraline 200 mg daily for the past 2 months; however, he still experiences symptoms. His psychiatrist would like to change his medication regimen and asks for your

recommendation. Which medication(s) has demonstrated a favorable response in the management of PTSD? Select all that apply.

   a. Risperidone
   b. Venlafaxine
   c. Bupropion
   d. Prazosin

Answer a is correct. Risperidone may be used as adjunct for those with psychotic features.

Answer b is correct. Venlafaxine has shown benefits and is considered a first- or second-line agent.

Answer c is incorrect. Bupropion has not shown efficacy in clinical trials.

Answer d is correct. Prazosin may be used as adjunctive treatment in those complaining of nightmares.

7. What is the *correct* dosing range for sertraline recommended for the treatment of PTSD?

   a. 2 to 8 mg/d
   b. 20 to 60 mg/d
   c. 50 to 200 mg/d
   d. 200 to 800 mg/d

Answer c is correct. The correct dosing range for sertraline is 50 to 200 mg/d.

Answers a, b, and d are incorrect. All other doses are incorrect for sertraline in the treatment for PTSD.

8. Which of the following generic-brand name matches are correct?

   a. Sertraline—Zoloft
   b. Paroxetine—Prozac
   c. Citalopram—Celexa
   d. Imipramine—Tofranil

Answers a, c, and d are correct. The generic/brand name matches are correct for sertraline, citalopram, and imipramine.

Answer b is incorrect. The brand name for paroxetine is Paxil, while Prozac is the brand name for fluoxetine.

9. AB is a 32-year-old woman diagnosed with PTSD. She asks the pharmacist how long she needs to take the medication for the prevention of symptom recurrence. What is the goal for duration of treatment for PTSD?

   a. 1 month
   b. 6 months
   c. 12 months
   d. 5 years

Answer c is correct. Guidelines recommend that PTSD be treated for a minimum of 12 months.

Answers a, b, and d are incorrect. The goal length of duration for PTSD is at least 12 months. However, patient treatment needs to be individualized. Select patients may require a longer duration of treatment. There is no literature available for 5 years of treatment.

10. CR is a 42-year-old man who was diagnosed with PTSD. He was prescribed citalopram 20 mg daily. He returns for a refill 1 month later and states, "I feel somewhat better, but still have flashbacks." How would you counsel this patient?

    a. Call the MD to change the medication to another SSRI, such as paroxetine.
    b. Call the MD to change the medication to venlafaxine.
    c. Remind the patient, it may take 8 to 12 weeks for the medication to show full benefits.
    d. Advise the patient that according to Federal laws, it is not your responsibility to counsel.

Answer c is correct. Some response may be observed in 4 weeks; however, full clinical benefits may not be demonstrated until 8 to 12 weeks.

Answers a and b are incorrect. Clinical benefits of PTSD treatment may take several weeks. Changing therapy at this point can delay a treatment response and the alternative medication may not be as effective as the initial regimen. A patient needs to be treated for several weeks before consideration of changing to alternative regimen.

Answer d is incorrect. Pharmacists should be able to counsel all patients.

11. MN is a 23-year-old obese female diagnosed with PTSD after a car accident several years ago. Although MN has been treated with an SSRI and other agents, she still has recurrent, disturbing dreams of the event with minor daytime hallucinations. Her psychiatrist wants to prescribe a second generation antipsychotic for augmentation therapy and would like to avoid a medication with weight gain. Which agent do you *most* appropriately recommend as a pharmacist?

    a. Risperidone
    b. Olanzapine
    c. Quetiapine
    d. Haloperidol

Answer a is correct. Among the antipsychotics, risperidone carries the least amount of weight gain and has data to support its use in PTSD treatment.

Answer b is incorrect. Olanzapine is the antipsychotic with the highest propensity to cause weight gain/metabolic changes

Answer c is incorrect. Quetiapine also carries significant weight gain.

Answer d is incorrect. Second generation (atypical) neuroleptics are preferred for augmentation therapy.

12. PK is a 32-year-old woman diagnosed with PTSD. She would like to start a family soon, and plans on becoming pregnant

in the next year. Which of the following medications has a pregnancy rating of category D?

    a. Paroxetine
    b. Fluoxetine
    c. Citalopram
    d. Sertraline

Answer a is correct. Paroxetine is category D.

Answers b, c, and d are incorrect. All other SSRIs are pregnancy category C.

Category A

Adequate and well-controlled studies have failed to demonstrate a risk to the fetus in the first trimester of pregnancy (and there is no evidence of risk in later trimesters).

Category B

Animal reproduction studies have failed to demonstrate a risk to the fetus and there are no adequate and well-controlled studies in pregnant women.

Category C

Animal reproduction studies have shown an adverse effect on the fetus and there are no adequate and well-controlled studies in humans, but potential benefits may warrant use of the drug in pregnant women despite potential risks.

Category D

There is positive evidence of human fetal risk based on adverse reaction data from investigational or marketing experience or studies in humans, but potential benefits may warrant use of the drug in pregnant women despite potential risks.

Category X

Studies in animals or humans have demonstrated fetal abnormalities and/or there is positive evidence of human fetal risk based on adverse reaction data from investigational or marketing experience, and the risks involved in use of the drug in pregnant women clearly outweigh potential benefits

13. Which medication would you counsel a patient regarding drug-food interactions, especially avoiding tyramine containing foods?

    a. Prazosin
    b. Phenelzine
    c. Venlafaxine
    d. Zoloft

Answer b is correct. Phenelzine is an MAOI which can cause hypertensive crisis when taken concomitantly with tyramine containing foods (eg, red wine, aged cheeses).

Answers a, c, and d are incorrect. Those medications are not associated with tyramine drug interactions.

14. Which neurotransmitters are primarily implicated in PTSD? Select all that apply.

    a. Acetylcholine
    b. GABA

c. 5-HT

d. NE

Answers c and d are correct.   5-HT and NE are the primary neurotransmitters involved in PTSD.

Answers a is incorrect.   Acetylcholine does not appear to play a major role in PTSD

Answer b is incorrect.   GABA may play a minor indirect role in PTSD.

---

15. MR is a 14-year-old boy recently diagnosed with PTSD. Which medication has a Black Box Warning for increased risk of suicidal ideations in pediatrics, and if used in this patient, would require that the patient be monitored closely for this adverse effect? Select all that apply.

    a. Venlafaxine
    b. Lorazepam
    c. Sertraline
    d. Fluoxetine

Answers a, c, and d are correct.   SNRIs (eg, venlafaxine) and SSRIs (class wide) have a black box warning for suicidality.

Answer b is incorrect.   Lorazepam does not have the warning.

---

16. PT is a 57-year-old man with PTSD. He has not received any treatment for the disorder in the past. You are asked to provide a recommendation for initial medication therapy. Rank the following medication options in the order that they would be preferred.

Unordered Response	Ordered Response
Venlafaxine	Sertraline
Sertraline	Venlafaxine
Topiramate	Amitriptyline
Amitriptyline	Topiramate

SSRIs are the first-line treatment for PTSD. While venlafaxine is also considered to be a first-line agent, SSRIs may be preferred over venlafaxine since they appear to target more symptoms. Amitriptyline is a TCA, which are third-line agents. Topiramate is a mood stabilizer, which has limited evidence supporting its use in PTSD.

17. SB is a 23-year-old woman with PTSD and presents to the outpatient clinic with complaints of nightmares and difficulty in sleeping. She is currently on paroxetine 40 mg daily and cannot tolerate higher dosages. Which medication can be most appropriately used as adjunctive therapy?

    a. Olanzapine
    b. Prazosin
    c. Bupropion
    d. Alprazolam

Answer b is correct.   Prazosin has evidence to improve nightmare complaints in PTSD.

Answer a is incorrect.   Olanzapine is used as adjunct for psychotic symptoms.

Answers c and d are incorrect.   Bupropion and alprazolam are not effective in PTSD.

---

18. SSRIs have demonstrated effectiveness in which of the following core symptoms?

    a. Re-experiencing
    b. Numbing
    c. Avoidance
    d. Hyperarousal

Answers a, b, c, and d are correct.   Overall, SSRIs demonstrated effectiveness in reducing symptoms of re-experiencing, numbing, avoidance, and hyperarousal.

---

19. Which agent(s) is/are available in extended-release formulations? Select all that apply.

    a. Citalopram
    b. Venlafaxine
    c. Paroxetine
    d. Sertraline

Answers b and c are correct.   Venlafaxine and paroxetine are available in extended-release formulations.

Answers a and d are incorrect.   Citalopram and sertraline do not have extended-release formulations.

---

20. Place the SSRIs in order of maximum dose. Start with highest maximum dose.

Unordered Response	Ordered Response
Sertraline	Sertraline 200 mg
Escitalopram	Fluoxetine 80 mg
Paroxetine	Paroxetine 50 mg
Fluoxetine	Escitalopram 20 mg

CHAPTER **60 | Depression**

Use the following case to answer questions 1 through 5.

Sebastian W is a 30-year-old man with chronic neuropathic pain and just lost his job due to consistently missing deadlines. He presents to his physician with troubling symptoms of decreased appetite and sleep, increased feelings of guilt and worthlessness, impaired concentration, and decreased interest in his usual hobbies. Sebastian's mother was diagnosed with MDD when she was 30. Sebastian's physician diagnoses him with MDD.

1. The cause of Sebastian's MDD is most likely associated with which of the following? Select all that apply.

    a. Genetic factors
    b. Stress/environmental factors

c. Deficiency in neurotransmitters
d. Cultural factors

Answer a is correct. The occurrence of MDD exhibits a genetic pattern. First-degree relatives of MDD patients are more likely to develop MDD compared to first-degree relatives of control individuals.

Answer b is correct. Depression can occur in the absence or presence of major life and environmental stressors; however, there is an association between life stressors and depression. These stressors are also more likely to exacerbate an episode of MDD.

Answer c is correct. Classic views for the cause of MDD focus on the neurotransmitters such as NE, 5-HT, and DA. The neurotransmitter hypothesis asserts that depression is due to a deficiency of neurotransmitters. The supporting evidence for this hypothesis is that existing antidepressants increase neurotransmitters concentrations.

Answer d is incorrect. While rates of MDD may vary depending on gender and culture, these factors are not the cause of depressive episodes.

---

2. Which of the following neurotransmitter(s) may be involved in the pathophysiology of Sebastian's depression? Select all that apply.

   a. NE
   b. 5-HT
   c. DA
   d. Acetylcholine

Answer a is correct. NE is a neurotransmitter involved in the pathophysiology of depression. Select antidepressants inhibit the reuptake of NE (eg, TCAs and SNRIs). Antidepressants that inhibit the reuptake of NE may lead to the following effects: tremor, tachycardia, sweating, jitteriness, and increased blood pressure. TCAs can also cause severe cardiovascular complications in high dose/overdose because of a change in cardiac conduction.

Answer b is correct. 5-HT is a neurotransmitter involved in the pathophysiology of depression. Select antidepressants inhibit the reuptake of 5-HT (eg, SSRIs, SNRIs). Antidepressants that inhibit the reuptake of 5-HT may lead to the following effects: anxiety, insomnia, sexual dysfunction, and anorexia.

Answer c is correct. DA is a neurotransmitter involved in the pathophysiology of depression. Select antidepressants inhibit the reuptake of DA (eg, bupropion). Antidepressants that inhibit the reuptake of DA may lead to the following effects: euphoria, psychomotor activation, and aggravation of psychosis.

Answer d is incorrect. Acetylcholine is linked to several neurologic disorders, such as dementia and Alzheimer disease. However, acetylcholine is not believed to contribute to the onset of MDD.

3. What other symptom(s) of MDD would you ask Sebastian about? Select all that apply.

   a. Depressed mood
   b. Sleep duration and quality
   c. Suicidal thoughts or behaviors
   d. Psychomotor changes

Answer a is correct. Depressed mood is a symptom of MDD.

Answer b is correct. Impaired sleep duration and quality are symptoms of MDD.

Answer c is correct. Suicidal thoughts or behaviors is a symptom of MDD.

Answer d is correct. Psychomotor changes (whether agitation or retardation) are symptoms of MDD.

---

4. Sebastian's doctor decides to start him on a medication with dual neurotransmitter effects to target his neuropathic pain and MDD. Which of the following antidepressants inhibit the reuptake of both NE and 5-HT? Select all that apply.

   a. Desipramine
   b. Venlafaxine
   c. Escitalopram
   d. Phenelzine
   e. Bupropion

Answer a is correct. TCAs inhibit the reuptake of NE and 5-HT. All TCAs inhibit the reuptake of NE and 5-HT, but they may do so at different degrees. For example, amitriptyline inhibits the reuptake of 5-HT more than imipramine and imipramine inhibits the reuptake of NE more than amitriptyline. Therefore, TCAs have the same side effect profile based upon mechanism of action, but they may cause a particular side effect at different percentages.

Answer b is correct. SNRIs (venlafaxine, duloxetine, and levomilnacipran) inhibit the reuptake of NE and 5-HT. Venlafaxine inhibits 5-HT reuptake at low doses, with additional NE reuptake inhibition at higher doses. Duloxetine inhibits 5-HT and NE across all doses.

Answer c is incorrect. SSRIs inhibit the reuptake of 5-HT only.

Answer d is incorrect. MAOIs inhibit the reuptake of 5-HT, NE, and DA.

Answer e is incorrect. Bupropion inhibit the reuptake of NE and DA.

---

5. Three months later Sebastian returns to his doctor and mentions he is still having difficulty sleeping. Sebastian's doctor starts him on trazodone due to its sedating properties. Select the mechanism of action of trazodone that leads to the side effects of dizziness and sedation.

   a. 5-HT receptor antagonist
   b. 5-HT reuptake inhibitor

c. α$_1$-Adrenergic and histaminergic antagonism
d. Angiotension receptor blockade

Answer c is correct. α$_1$-Adrenergic receptor blockade and histaminergic antagonism may lead to dizziness and sedation. α$_1$-Adrenergic receptor blockade may lead to orthostatic hypotension, dizziness, and reflex tachycardia. Histaminergic antagonism may lead to sedation and weight gain.

Answer a is incorrect. 5-HT receptor antagonism may lead to increased rapid eye movement (REM) sleep, decreased sexual dysfunction (5-HT 2A receptor blockade), and increased appetite/weight gain (5-HT 2C receptor blockade).

Answer b is incorrect. 5-HT reuptake inhibition may lead to anxiety, insomnia, sexual dysfunction, and anorexia.

Answer d is incorrect. Trazodone does not block the angiotension receptor blocker.

6. Select the antidepressant that has a black box warning for rare cases of liver failure.

   a. Mirtazapine
   b. Bupropion
   c. Amitriptyline
   d. Nefazodone

Note: All antidepressants have the following black box warning: Antidepressants increase the risk of suicidal thinking and behavior in children, adolescents, and young adults (18-24 years of age) with MDD and other psychotic disorders.

Answer d is correct. The use of nefazodone as an antidepressant has declined after reports of hepatotoxicity. The FDA-approved nefazodone labeling includes a black box warning describing rare cases of liver failure. Because of the potential for hepatic injury associated with nefazodone use, treatment should not be initiated in individuals with active liver disease or with elevated baseline serum transaminases.

Answers a, b, and c are incorrect. None of these medications has a black box warning for hepatotoxicity.

7. Which of the following antidepressants is classified as a DA and NE reuptake inhibitor?

   a. Wellbutrin
   b. Elavil
   c. Viibryd
   d. Cymbalta

Answer a is correct. Bupropion (Wellbutrin) inhibits the reuptake of DA and NE.

Answer b is incorrect. Amitriptyline (Elavil) is a TCA that inhibits the reuptake of NE and 5-HT.

Answer c is incorrect. Vilazodone (Viibryd) inhibits the reuptake of 5-HT and a partial agonist at 5-HT1A.

Answer d is incorrect. Duloxetine (Cymbalta) is an SNRI that inhibits the reuptake of 5-HT and NE.

8. Utilization of which of the following medications would result in the highest risk of developing the side effect of hypertensive crisis?

   a. Phenelzine plus lisinopril
   b. Imipramine plus sertraline
   c. Tranylcypromine plus pseudoephedrine
   d. Venlafaxine plus lorazepam

Answer c is correct. The utilization of MAOIs and sympathomimetics leads to the pharmacodynamic interaction of hypertensive crisis.

Answer a is incorrect. Phenelzine is an MAOI and MAOIs are associated with hypertensive crisis reactions; however, the reaction is usually caused by a drug interaction of an MAOI and a sympathomimetic. Use of lisinopril will not cause this reaction.

Answer b is incorrect. Imipramine is a TCA and causes cardiovascular side effects (conduction abnormalities and orthostatic hypotension). When used with sertraline, patients are at risk of serotonin syndrome, not hypertensive crisis.

Answer d is incorrect. The utilization of SNRIs (like venlafaxine) and benzodiazepines do not cause hypertensive crisis.

9. Mia is a 49-year-old patient who suffered a myocardial infarction 1 week ago. Upon discharge, it was noted that Mia appeared depressed. At a follow-up visit with her physician a week later, Mia met criteria for a diagnosis of MDD. Her past medical history includes: treatment-refractory hypertension, diabetes mellitus (type II), and severe uncontrolled narrow angle glaucoma. Select the antidepressant that would be the safest and most effective pharmacotherapy option for Mia.

   a. Elavil
   b. Fetzima
   c. Zoloft
   d. Pamelor

Answer c is correct. Sertraline (Zoloft) is an SSRI antidepressant and lacks significant cardiovascular side effects due to the 5-HT-specific mechanism of action.

Answers a and d are incorrect. Amitriptyline (Elavil) and Nortriptyline (Pamelor) are TCA antidepressants and should not be used in patients in acute recovery of myocardial infarction. TCAs are associated with conduction abnormalities, QTc changes, and arrhythmias (if used in high doses) and should not be given to patients who are acutely postmyocardial infarction.

Answer b is incorrect. Levomilnacipran (Fetzima) is an SNRI antidepressant and should not be used in patients with uncontrolled narrow angle glaucoma or uncontrolled hypertension due to the risk of increasing both systolic and diastolic blood pressure.

10. A month later, Mia has fully recovered from her myocardial infarction and is feeling much better since initiation of her antidepressant 4 weeks ago. Mia presents for a follow-up today and states that while she is happy with the results of her antidepressant, she is concerned about her acquired sexual dysfunction. Which antidepressant can be administered to Mia to avoid a sexual dysfunction side effect?

    a. Wellbutrin
    b. Pamelor
    c. Prozac
    d. Cymbalta

Answer a is correct. Bupropion (Wellbutrin) is an antidepressant that inhibits the reuptake of DA and NE. This is a unique mechanism of action within the antidepressant class and is the least likely to cause sexual dysfunction.

Answer b is incorrect. Nortriptyline (Pamelor) is a TCA antidepressant that inhibits the reuptake of NE and 5-HT. 5-HT reuptake inhibition is associated with sexual dysfunction.

Answer c is incorrect. Fluoxetine (Prozac) is an SSRI antidepressant that inhibits the reuptake of 5-HT. 5-HT reuptake inhibition is associated with sexual dysfunction.

Answer d is incorrect. Duloxetine (Cymbalta) is an SNRI antidepressant that inhibits the reuptake of NE and 5-HT. 5-HT reuptake inhibition is associated with sexual dysfunction.

11. Harry is a 49-year-old patient diagnosed with major depressive disorder. His past medical history is significant for alcohol-induced liver damage (with increased liver function tests), hypertension, and hyperlipidemia. Which of the following antidepressants would be safe and appropriate for him? Select all that apply.

    a. Nefazodone
    b. Sertraline
    c. Vilazodone
    d. Duloxetine

Answer b is correct. Sertraline is an SSRI that undergoes significant hepatic metabolism. Caution should be used with sertraline in patients with hepatic damage and a lower dose may be utilized, but the medication is not contraindicated in hepatic impairment.

Answer c is correct. Vilazodone is an SSRI-like antidepressant with additional activity as a 5-HT1a partial agonist. Although vilazodone undergoes hepatic metabolism, the medication is not contraindicated in hepatic impairment and no adjustments are recommended when used in patients with hepatic impairment.

Answer a is incorrect. Nefazodone is associated with hepatic damage. Treatment should not be initiated in individuals with active liver disease or with elevated baseline serum transaminases.

Answer d is incorrect. Duloxetine is an SNRI that has demonstrated hepatotoxicity when used in patients with significant alcohol use and chronic hepatic disease. Duloxetine should not be used in the patient due to his alcohol-induced hepatic disease.

12. Felicia is a 44-year-old patient with a history of bulimia and multiple recent hospitalizations for electrolyte abnormalities that have caused seizures. Felicia has recently been diagnosed with MDD. Which of the following antidepressants is contraindicated in Felicia due to her comorbid condition?

    a. Wellbutrin
    b. Prozac
    c. Cymbalta
    d. Remeron

Answer a is correct. Bupropion (Wellbutrin) has a dose-dependent risk of seizures and the risk is increased in patients with a history of seizures and eating disorders. Bupropion is contraindicated in patients with anorexia/bulimia because they are at increased risk for electrolyte abnormalities and therefore prone to a higher risk of seizures.

Answers b, c, and d are incorrect. These medications are not contraindicated in Felicia.

13. On her most recent hospitalization, Felicia was found to have atrial fibrillation. Which of the following medications can be used safely in patients with cardiac conduction abnormalities and avoids alterations in the QTc interval? Select all that apply.

    a. Celexa
    b. Norpramin
    c. Zoloft
    d. Elavil

Answer c is correct. SSRI medications (like sertraline) are first-line therapy for the treatment of major depression. Sertraline (Zoloft) has been studied in patients with cardiac disease and found to be safe for use.

Answer a is incorrect. Although controversial, citalopram (Celexa) now has a warning for increased risk of QT prolongation with doses over 40 mg. It is not recommended for use in patients with certain electrolyte abnormalities, such as hypokalemia and hypomagnesemia. Given Felicia's recent hospitalizations for electrolyte abnormalities and seizures, this is not the safest option to treat her depression.

Answers b and d are incorrect. Due to the risk of QT changes and alterations in cardiac conductivity, desipramine (Norpramin) and amitriptyline (Elavil) is not the safest option for Felicia. SSRIs are first-line therapy for the treatment of depression and would be a safer option to try prior to discussing the use of a TCA.

14. Which of the following would cause a clinically significant drug interaction if taken with a TCA antidepressant?

   a. Alcohol
   b. Thioridazine
   c. Meperidine
   d. Fluoxetine

Answers a, b, c, and d are correct. Alcohol exhibits a pharmacodynamic interaction (additive sedation) with TCAs. Thioridazine alters cardiac conduction and would result in additive cardiac conduction abnormalities, increasing the patient's risk of arrhythmias. Meperidine exhibits a pharmacodynamic interaction (serotonin syndrome) with TCAs. Fluoxetine exhibits a pharmacokinetic interaction with TCAs.

Use the following case to answer questions 15 and 16.

15. Laura is a patient with MDD currently taking phenelzine. She has been experiencing painful sinus pressure, headaches, and congestion. She approaches your pharmacy and asks if she can take a decongestant for the congestion. You inform her that she cannot take the decongestant with her antidepressant medication due to the risk of what side effect?

   a. Serotonin syndrome
   b. Hypertensive crisis
   c. Sexual dysfunction
   d. Orthostatic hypotension

Answer b is correct. Hypertensive crisis is associated with concurrent use of MAOIs and sympathomimetics and tyramine-rich foods.

Answer a is incorrect. Serotonin syndrome is associated with concurrent use of MAOIs and serotonergic antidepressants, meperidine, dextromethorphan, and tramadol.

Answer c is incorrect. Sexual dysfunction is a side effect of antidepressants that have activity on 5-HT, but this dysfunction is unrelated to the combined use of antidepressants and decongestants.

Answer d is incorrect. Orthostatic hypotension is a common side effect of antidepressants that have α_1-adrenergic receptor blockade.

16. While Laura is at the pharmacy counter, you notice that she has been doing some grocery shopping before asking about the decongestant. Which of the following food items would result in a clinically significant interaction with her antidepressant? Select all that apply.

   a. Sauerkraut
   b. Eggs
   c. Blue cheese
   d. Whole milk

Answer a is correct. Sauerkraut is one of several foods that are contraindicated with MAOI medications. Sauerkraut

is high in tyramine content, increasing Laura's risk of experiencing hypertensive crisis.

Answer c is correct. Blue cheese is also a food product that is high in tyramine content and should be avoided in patients taking MAOIs. Other cheese products that must be avoided include cheddar, Gouda, Parmesan, provolone, and many others. Refer patients taking MAOIs to their physician or a trusted reference for further lists of dietary restrictions.

Answer b is incorrect. Eggs do not contain tyramine and are considered safe for consumption in patients taking MAOIs.

Answer d is incorrect. Milk products do not contain tyramine. Buttermilk may also be used in limited quantities, but there is no restriction on regular cow's milk, regardless of fat content.

17. Select the drug interaction(s) associated with Prozac. Select all that apply.

   a. Verapamil
   b. Carbamazepine
   c. Codeine
   d. Azithromycin

Answers a, b, and c are correct.

Verapamil is a CYP450 substrate of 1A2 (minor), 2B6 (minor), 2C9 (minor), 2C18 (minor), 2E1 (minor), and 3A4 (major). Verapamil is a CYP450 inhibitor of 1A2 (weak), 2C9 (weak), 2D6 (weak), and 3A4 (moderate). Fluoxetine may increase levels of verapamil and slightly increase levels of fluoxetine.

Carbamazepine is a CYP450 substrate of 2C8 (minor) and 3A4 (major). Carbamazepine is a CYP450 inducer of 1A2 (strong), 2B6 (strong), 2C8 (strong), 2C9 (strong), 2C19 (strong), and 3A4 (strong). Fluoxetine may slightly increase levels of carbamazepine, and carbamazepine will significantly decrease levels of fluoxetine.

Codeine is a CYP450 substrate of 2D6 (major). Codeine is a prodrug, which requires CYP2D6 to a more active opioid species. Fluoxetine will decrease levels of the more active metabolite, morphine.

Answer d is incorrect. Azithromycin lacks significant pharmacokinetic CYP450 drug interactions (which is unlike clarithromycin).

18. Select the brand name of paroxetine.

   a. Paxil
   b. Remeron
   c. Prozac
   d. Effexor

Answer a is correct. The brand name of paroxetine is Paxil.

Answer b is incorrect. The brand name of mirtazapine is Remeron.

Answer c is incorrect. The brand name of fluoxetine is Prozac.

Answer d is incorrect. The brand name of venlafaxine is Effexor.

19. Select the generic name of Pristiq.

    a. Desvenlafaxine
    b. Vortioxetine
    c. Duloxetine
    d. Vilazodone

Answer a is correct. Desvenlafaxine is the generic name for Pristiq.

Answer b is incorrect. Vortioxetine is the generic name for Trintellix.

Answer c is incorrect. Duloxetine is the generic name of Cymbalta.

Answer d is incorrect. Vilazodone is the generic name of Viibryd.

20. Which of the following antidepressants is available as a once-weekly formulation?

    a. Fluvoxamine
    b. Duloxetine
    c. Venlafaxine
    d. Fluoxetine

Answer d is correct. Fluoxetine is available as a tablet, capsule, oral solution, and a delayed-release capsule that is given once weekly.

Answer a is incorrect. Fluvoxamine is available as a tablet and extended-release capsule taken daily.

Answer b is incorrect. Duloxetine is only available as a delayed-release capsule taken daily.

Answer c is incorrect. Venlafaxine is available in tablet and capsule formulations taken daily or twice daily.

21. Mary Lou is a 76-year-old who has recently been diagnosed with depression. Mary Lou also has early stages of dementia and has difficulty swallowing tablets and capsules. Which of the following medications is available in a liquid formulation?

    a. Sertraline
    b. Venlafaxine
    c. Amitriptyline
    d. Duloxetine

Answer a is correct. Sertraline is available as a tablet and oral solution.

Answer b is incorrect. Venlafaxine is only available as an immediate-release and delayed-release capsule.

Answer c is incorrect. Amitriptyline is only available in a tablet formulation.

Answer d is incorrect. Duloxetine is only available as a delayed-release capsule.

22. Mary Lou's daughter returns to the doctor and asks for a new medication, saying Mary Lou doesn't like the taste of the liquid medication. The daughter would like to switch to a medication she can crush or open and put in applesauce. Which of the following medications can be crushed or opened due to its formulation or delivery mechanism? Select all that apply.

    a. Phenelzine
    b. Zoloft
    c. Cymbalta
    d. Paxil CR

Answer a is correct. Phenelzine tablets may be crushed for administration.

Answer b is correct. Zoloft is available as a liquid, but tablets may be crushed for administration.

Answer c is incorrect. Cymbalta capsules should not be opened or crushed per the manufacturer of the medication.

Answer d is incorrect. Paxil CR formulation cannot be crushed.

23. Two months later, Mary Lou presents with decreased appetite and weight loss and continues to have difficulty swallowing. Which of the following medications is available as an orally disintegrating tablet?

    a. Bupropion
    b. Duloxetine
    c. Mirtazapine
    d. Fluoxetine

Answer c is correct. Mirtazapine (Remeron) is available as an orally disintegrating tablet.

Answers a, b, and d is incorrect. Bupropion is available as IR, SR, and XL tablets. Duloxetine is available as delayed-release capsules. Fluoxetine is available as tablet, capsule, and oral solution.

24. Which of the following counseling point(s) apply to Wellbutrin SR? Select all that apply.

    a. Take this at bedtime because it can cause significant sedation.
    b. Do not take more than prescribed dose at once to minimize risk of seizure.
    c. This medication can cause significant sexual side effects.
    d. Improvement of depression symptoms may not occur for a few weeks, so it is important to continue to take the medication on a daily basis.

Answer b is correct. Bupropion has a dose-dependent risk of seizures.

Answer d is correct. Antidepressants, including bupropion, do not produce an immediate clinical response. Improvement in physical symptoms (sleep, appetite, energy) can occur within the first 2 weeks of treatment, but improvement in emotional symptoms may take 6 to 8 weeks for full effects.

Answer a is incorrect. Bupropion (Wellbutrin) should be avoided close to bedtime to minimize risk of insomnia.

Answer c is incorrect. Bupropion causes less sexual dysfunction than other antidepressants and can be used to treat sexual dysfunction caused by other antidepressants.

CHAPTER **61 | Diabetes Mellitus**

Use the following patient profile to answer questions 1 to 4.

JR is a 68-year-old African American man with a new diagnosis of T2DM. He was classified as having prediabetes (at risk for developing diabetes) 5 years before the diagnosis and has a strong family history of T2DM. JR's blood pressure was 150/92 mm Hg. His laboratory results revealed an A1c of 9.2%, glucose of 279 mg/dL, cholesterol panels renal/hepatic function were normal today.

Past Medical History:	Hypertension (diagnosed 4 years ago) Hyperlipidemia (diagnosed 2 years ago) Pancreatitis [idiopathic] (acute hospitalization 3 years ago)
Family History:	T2DM
Medication:	HCTZ 25 mg daily, Simvastatin 10 mg daily
Vitals:	BP: 150/92 mm Hg, P: 78 beats/min, RR: 12 Waist circumference 46 inches Weight: 267 lb Height: 5' 6" BMI: 43.1 kg/m²

1. What known risk factor(s) does JR display for the development of diabetes? Select all that apply.

    a. Obesity
    b. African American
    c. Family history of diabetes
    d. Prediabetes

Answers a, b, c, and d are correct. Obesity is a risk factor and should be used as a method to identify patients to be screened for diabetes. Obesity causes insulin resistance and along with other physiological mechanisms lead to abnormalities of glucose metabolism. Other uncontrolled risk factors can lead to prediabetes. If modifiable risk factors are not treated appropriately with lifestyle modifications or possibly drug therapy, the risk for diabetes increases and a diagnosis of diabetes may occur within 5 to 10 years. Non-modifiable risk factors such as minority populations (African American, Asian American, Latino, Native American, and Pacific Islanders) and known primary relatives with a history of T2DM can increase one's risk for developing T2DM.

2. Six weeks later, JR returns to obtain new labs results. He tests his blood glucose and blood pressures at home. Within the last 4 weeks he has started an exercise program 4 times per week consisting of cardio/resistant training for 40 minutes per session. JR indicates he is motivated to beat this and has reviewed a lot of educational material about diabetes.

Home blood pressure (mm Hg): [electronic cuff/sitting/right arm]	150/85, 161/74, 152/82, 148/83, 156/71, 150/74
Home fasting blood glucose readings (mg/dL)	278, 218, 219, 119, 156, 193

Today's Labs and Vitals

A1c → 8.1%	Fasting glucose → 176 mg/dL
Total cholesterol → 201 mg/dL	LDL cholesterol → 124 mg/dL
SCr → 0.98 mg/dL	Na → 138 mEq/L, K → 4.3 mEq/L
Albumin-to-creatinine ratio: 152 mg/g creatinine	
BP: 148/92 mm Hg	P: 75 beats/min

Due to elevated home and clinic blood pressure readings it has been decided a second blood pressure medication is needed. Which agent would be the best to start in order to achieve blood pressure control and prevent microvascular complications?

    a. Clonidine 0.1 mg twice daily
    b. Isosorbide mononitrate 60 mg daily
    c. Lisinopril 5 mg daily
    d. Terazosin 10 mg at bedtime

Answer c is correct. Lisinopril is an angiotensin-converting enzyme inhibitor and considered to be a drug of choice for renal protection in patients with diabetes with noted increase albumin excretion. ACEi and ARBs have demonstrated to reduce renal progression to overt proteinuria. African American's may not see the maximum effect of blood pressure lowering with ACEi due to a decrease amount of renin.

Answer a is incorrect. Clonidine does not have supporting data indicating renal protection for patients with diabetes. Dose provided would be an appropriate starting dose.

Answer b is incorrect. Isosorbide mononitrate is not typically used for hypertension; however, it may be used as an antianginal with blood pressure lower effects in specific populations with ischemic heart disease, uncontrolled, unstable/stable angina or heart failure.

Answer d is incorrect. Terazosin does not have data to indicate renal protective properties in patients with diabetes. Although terazosin should be dosed at night time due to possible adverse effects of nocturnal orthostatic hypotension, the starting dose of 10 mg is not recommended.

3. Today, JR's A1c value was an 8.1%, which is down from 6 weeks ago. Despite improvements in lifestyle choices, he has met the diagnosis for diabetes. As the clinical pharmacist in charge of

the diabetes management clinic, you provide him options of lifestyle, medications or both. He would like to start a drug therapy in addition to more stringent lifestyle modifications. Which drug therapy would be the best for JR to trial?

a. Pramlintide subcutaneously 15 mcg twice daily.
b. Liraglutide subcutaneously 0.6 mg daily for 1 week with an upward titration until glycemic goals have been met (do not exceed more than 1.8 mg daily).
c. Metformin 500 mg daily by mouth with an upward titration to 2000 mg/d (qd or bid) over several days to weeks.
d. Acarbose 100 mg three times daily by mouth with each meal.

Answer c is correct. Metformin is the drug of choice recommended for most patients with diabetes in addition to lifestyle modifications assuming no contraindications or intolerabilities are present upon evaluation. Metformin has also shown to provide positive weight neutral/loss effects in obese patients. It is crucial to know renal status of patients commencing metformin therapy to limit the risk of lactic acidosis (JR is without contraindication).

Answer a is incorrect. Pramlintide could be used for this patient as its weight loss abilities might help and his A1c is less than 9%; however, the ADA medical management of hyperglycemia guidelines does not mention this agent as a first-line agent. The dose indicated above is the starting dose for patients diagnosed with T1DM.

Answer b is incorrect. Liraglutide is a GLP-1 analog and has data to support an A1c reduction necessary to gain glycemic control and may assist with weight loss goals for this patient; however, JR has a past history of pancreatitis and GLP-1 analogs are not recommended due to this contraindication.

Answer d is incorrect. Although acarbose does have data to indicate its use in prediabetes, this agent is not recommended as first-line therapy by the ADA medical management of hyperglycemia. The starting dose provided above is not recommended due to the intolerability of gastrointestinal side effects. It is important to titrate this product up and educate the patient about appropriate administration with meals.

4. What preventative measures should JR be educated on to reduce the risk of complications associated with diabetes? Select all that apply.

a. Perform daily foot inspections.
b. See a dentist/dental hygienist routinely throughout the year.
c. Receive the pneumococcal vaccine yearly.
d. Assuming no contraindications, take an aspirin daily for cardioprotection.

Answers a, b, and d are correct. Patients should be encouraged to look at their feet daily to assess for signs of infection. Patients should be educated on these signs and when to follow-up with a health care provider. It is recommended for patients to have a physical examination/inspection of their feet and extremities with a health care provider yearly. Dental hygiene is important and patients are recommended to have their teeth cleaned twice a year and a yearly dentist appointment. Education on signs and symptoms of gingival disease and when to follow-up with a health care provider should also be provided. Aspirin therapy is recommended for cardioprevention in patients with diabetes; however, guidelines provide specific recommendations stratified by risk and age. It is also important to be aware of other disease states a patient may have (eg, s/p MI, CVA, or PAD) that may require aspirin at different dosages or durations.

Answer c is incorrect. It is recommended that all patients with diabetes (unless they have a contraindication) should receive the INFLUENZA vaccine yearly. Patients with diabetes are not candidates to receive the live-attenuated formulation. Patients with diabetes are at high risk for pneumococcal infections; however, they are recommended to obtain no more than 3 pneumococcal vaccinations per lifespan under the CDC recommendations.

5. What counseling information should a pharmacist provide to a patient taking a diuretic and ARB therapy in order to reduce the risk of side effects? Select all that apply.

a. Avoid/limit salt substitutes.
b. Stop exercising because these blood pressure medications will cause your blood pressure to drop significantly resulting in falls.
c. Stay hydrated.
d. Do not take an HMG-CoA Reductase inhibitor (statin) while on blood pressure medications.

Answers a and c are correct. Often times salt substitutes will replace NaCl with potassium salt supplements. Since ARB therapy may elevate potassium levels, it is recommended to limit or avoid salt substitutes that are known to add potassium salts. Due to the effect of sodium and water absorption, it is important for patients to stay well hydrated (assuming no contraindication to appropriate fluid replacement) to preserve the kidneys.

Answer b is incorrect. Although blood pressure medications can cause symptoms of hypotension, complete cessation of exercise is not recommended. It needs to be remembered that exercise clearance should come from the prescribing provider, but also that physical activity is recommended for wellness and disease states or disease complication prevention.

Answer d is incorrect. Here are no contraindications to use a statin therapy with a diuretic or ARB regimen. It is true that specific statins may have "contraindications for use" or "not to exceed" dosages if used in combination with particular antihypertensives (eg, amlodipine, verapamil), but alternative statin therapies or altering of antihypertensives regimens will allow treatment of both hyperlipidemia and hypertension.

Use the following patient profile for questions 6 and 7.

PT is a 58-year-old white woman with a BMI of 32 kg/m². She was recently referred to a dietitian for weight reduction and lost 40 lb over the past 8 months. She is very dedicated to getting her blood glucose under control. At this time she is not willing to go on insulin therapy. She tests her blood glucose at home: fasting blood glucose readings are all less than 130 mg/dL and her 2-hour postprandial glucose readings are in the range of 190 to 200 mg/dL. Her past medical history (PMH) is hypertension, hyperlipidemia, T2DM, sleep apnea, and depression; family history (FHx) is unknown (patient was adopted); and social history (SHx) is (+) tobacco use—1.5 packs per day for 42 years, (+) alcohol use—2 sifters (6 oz) of gin and tonic daily. Her medications are metformin 1000 mg twice daily, enalapril 10 mg twice daily, hydrochlorothiazide 25 mg daily, citalopram 40 mg daily, rosuvastatin 5 mg daily. Her laboratory results revealed normal electrolyte and cholesterol panels, normal renal and hepatic function A1c 7.9%

6. What therapy is the best option to help lower her A1c and improve glycemic control considering her specific patient profile concerns?

    a. Exenatide twice daily with meals
    b. Chlorpropamide 250 mg daily
    c. Increase metformin to 2000 mg twice daily
    d. Start insulin NPH 10 units at bedtime

Answer a is correct.   PT is having problems with her postprandial blood sugars which are not at goal (goal: <180 mg/dL 1-2 hours after a meal). Exenatide or any GLP-1 analog would be able to obtain her A1c goal of less than 7%, provide possible weight loss and is FDA approved to be used in combination with metformin therapy. At this time, there are no documented contraindications for use; however, it is important to assess for past pancreatitis cases and Self/Family History regarding thyroid cancers prior to selecting a GLP-1 analog. The present case indicates the lipid panel is normal without issues of hypertriglyceridemia; however, the patient does have daily alcohol usage which can increase risk of patient for pancreatitis in addition to the start of GLP-1 analog. Educate patient on the importance or risk of pancreatitis.

Answer b is incorrect.   PT has a history of daily alcohol use. Chlorpropamide is not recommended due to the disulfiram-like reaction and the increased risk of hypoglycemia. A second-generation agent would be a better consideration in this patient if a sulfonylurea is started.

Answer c is incorrect.   The maximum daily dose of metformin is 2550 mg; however, a plateau effect is noted at 2000 mg daily.

Answer d is incorrect.   Insulin is an option in this patient per the ADA medical management of hyperglycemia guidelines; however, the patient indicated she is not interested in taking insulin. Guidelines describe the importance of diabetes management to be patient centered, if the patient will not take the insulin, it does not help to prescribe it. Further understanding of why PT is psychologically resistant to insulin injection is needed to provide future education of possible insulin use as the disease progresses or if control declines. NPH may not be the recommended agent, as it is a basal insulin and her morning blood sugars are controlled. Therefore, a bolus insulin is a better recommendation.

7. Which of the following is/are common side effect(s) of glucophage?

    a. Weight gain
    b. Diarrhea
    c. Lactic acidosis
    d. Pancreatitis

Answer b is correct.   Diarrhea is the most common side effect with metformin use; however, it can be minimized with commencement of low doses and titrating slowly.

Answer a is incorrect.   Metformin is associated with 2 to 3 kg weight loss.

Answer c is incorrect.   Lactic acidosis is a *rare* side effect that may affect patients taking metformin. Lactic acidosis is associated in patients taking metformin who have hypoperfusion to the kidneys or increased lactic acid concentrations.

Answer d is incorrect.   Pancreatitis has not been reported with metformin use. Postmarketing surveillance indicates this side effect with DPP-IV inhibitors and GLP-1 analogs.

8. Commercially available Symlin should be administered by which route?

    a. Intravenously
    b. Intramuscularly
    c. Subcutaneously
    d. Via insulin pump

Answer c is correct.   Only FDA approved route of administration.

Answers a, b, and d are incorrect.   Not FDA approved for these routes of administration.

9. Which insulin can be mixed with insulin glargine in one syringe in order to decrease daily insulin injections?

    a. Insulin aspart
    b. Insulin regular
    c. Insulin detemir
    d. Insulin glargine cannot be mixed with any insulin in a given syringe/pen/insulin pump

Answer d is correct.   Insulin glargine is not FDA approved to mix with any insulin, even bolus insulin in a device.

Answer a is incorrect.   Insulin aspart should only be mixed with insulin NPH.

Answer b is incorrect. Insulin regular should only be mixed with insulin NPH.

Answer c is incorrect. Insulin detemir cannot be mixed with any insulins. Insulin detemir and glargine are both basal insulins.

---

10. Due to acarbose mechanism of action to lower blood glucose, what is the most appropriate way to treat a hypoglycemic reaction in a patient taking acarbose?

    a. 1 candy bar
    b. 3 to 4 glucose tablets
    c. 2-ounces of mash potatoes
    d. Inject 2 units of rapid-acting insulin at the time of episode

Answer b is correct. Due to the mechanism of action for acarbose, simple sugars are needed to treat a hypoglycemic reaction.

Answers a, c, and d are incorrect. The fat and carbohydrate content of a candy bar and mash potatoes will not be absorbed in a timely manner due to the mechanism of action for acarbose. Injecting insulin during the time of a hypoglycemic reaction would further lower blood glucose and cause harm.

---

11. Which drug would not be recommended for a patient with an ejection fraction of 32% and in symptomatic heart failure documented by a NYHA class III?

    a. Starlix
    b. Invokana
    c. Pioglitazone
    d. Victoza

Answer c is correct. Pioglitazone may cause or exacerbate heart failure. This is a class effect with both rosiglitazone and pioglitazone; therefore, TZD therapy is contraindicated in patients with NYHA III/IV heart failure. TZDs may be used in NYHA class I/II patient; however, follow-up assessing weight gain, edema, and other physical examination techniques would be recommended.

Answers a, b, and d are incorrect. There is no association of Liraglutide (Victoza), Canagliflozin (Invokana) and Nateglinide (Starlix) therapy and heart failure.

Use the following patient profile for questions 12 to 14.

EP is a 38-year-old female patient that comes in for diabetes education and management. She was diagnosed 12 years ago and states lately she is not able to control her diet although she continues a 1600 calorie diet with appropriate daily carbohydrate intake (per dietitian prescription) and walks 40 minutes every day of the week. She states compliance with all medications. She denies any history of hypoglycemia despite being able to identify signs and symptoms and describe appropriate treatment strategies.

PMH:	T2DM, HTN, obesity, depression, s/p thyroidectomy due to thyroid cancer
FHx:	Noncontributory
SHx:	(–) Smoking, alcohol use, past marijuana use while in high school
Medications:	Metformin 850 mg tid, Glipizide 20 mg bid, Lisinopril 20 mg daily, Sertraline 100 mg daily, Multivitamin daily
Vitals:	BP: 128/82 mg Hg, P: 72, BMI: 31 m/kg^2
Labs:	Na: 134 mEq/L, K: 5.4 mEq/L, Cl: 106 mEq/L, BUN: 16 mg/dL SCr: 0.89 mg/dL, Glucose: 128 mg/dL, A1c: 7.8%

12. In order to reduce the risk of side effects or to eliminate contraindications to therapy, what objective measure(s) of EP do you need to assess before you recommend canagliflozin? Select all that apply.

    a. Blood pressure
    b. CrCl or SCr
    c. Potassium concentration
    d. Sodium concentration

Answers a, b, c, and d are correct. SGLT2-inhibitors have been known to cause dehydration due to the mechanism of action and its effects on renal absorption of electrolytes and fluid status. It is important to know baseline sodium and potassium levels as SGLT2-inhibitors may cause hyponatremia or hyperkalemia. Baseline blood pressures would be beneficial to know in order to limit hypotension in patients taking an SGLT2-inhibitor. While the SGLT2-inhibitors can be used in renal insufficiency, each agent has their own renal restrictions or contraindications for use.

---

13. EP states that she is not ready to start insulin, but has heard about newer drug therapies that help limit weight gain or actually cause weight loss. Which drugs might EP be referring to? Select all that apply.

    a. Alogliptin
    b. Canagliflozin
    c. Exenatide once weekly
    d. Rosiglitazone

Answers a, b, and c are correct. Agents that act as incretin mimetics (DPP-IV inhibitors or GLP-1 analogs) have been known to be weight neutral or assist in weight loss, due to several mechanisms. SGLT2-inhibitors are known to have a weight loss effect.

Answer d is incorrect. The TZD, rosiglitazone is known to increase weight by mechanisms of edema and sodium/water retention.

---

14. Based on EP's profile above, which of the agents would be able to obtain an A1c goal of less than 7% with limited side effects projected to occur?

    a. Bydureon
    b. Farxiga

c. Januvia
d. Precose

Answer c is correct. Sitagliptin (Janvuia) is able to obtain an A1c goal of less than 7% based on clinical trials and currently the patient does not have any cautionary objective measures to not use this medication. DPP-IV inhibitors are weight neutral. DPP-IV inhibitors can be used in patients taking sulfonylureas; however, it may be recommended to reduce or stop the sulfonylurea dose.

Answer a is incorrect. Exenatide once weekly (Bydureon) has been able to demonstrate weight loss and decrease A1c% by 0.7% to 1.2% in clinical trials; however, it is contraindicated for EP due to the self-reported history of thyroid cancer.

Answer b is incorrect. Dapagliflozin (Farxiga) is contraindicated in this patient due to hyperkalemia which could be made worse by this drug. The package insert does not indicate a specific potassium concentration cutoff to no longer use this medication; however, there is another drug offered above that may be a better choice.

Answer d is incorrect. Precose may lower A1c less than 1% and may be associated with significant gastrointestinal side effects.

---

15. How many minutes before a meal should a patient administer glulisine insulin?

    a. 15 minutes before the start of a meal.
    b. 30 minutes before the start of a meal.
    c. 60 minutes before the start of a meal.
    d. Glulisine is a basal insulin and administration should be regardless of the mealtime.

Answer a is correct. Due to the rapid onset (0.25 hours), it is recommended to not take glulisine more than 15 minutes before the start of a meal.

Answer b is incorrect. If taken at 30 or more minutes before the start of a meal, hypoglycemia may occur because the onset of action occurs within 15 minutes.

Answer c is incorrect. If taken at 60 or more minutes before the start of a meal, hypoglycemia may occur because the onset of action occurs within 15 minutes.

Answer d is incorrect. Glulisine is a rapid-acting insulin and should be given to before a meal time to reduce the postprandial glucose levels.

---

16. Which of the following is true regarding the action of insulin?

    a. Enhances ketone production
    b. Stimulates glucose uptake in the periphery
    c. It activates peroxisome-proliferator-activated receptor-γ (PPAR-γ)
    d. Increases amylin production

Answer b is correct. Insulin stimulates glucose uptake into muscles and adipose tissue;

Stimulates hepatic glucose uptake;

Stimulates amino acid uptake and protein synthesis;

Inhibits hepatic glucose production;

Inhibits breakdown of triglycerides in adipose tissue;

Inhibits protein degradation.

Answer a is incorrect. Insulin inhibits ketone production.

Answer c is incorrect. This is a mechanism of action for TZDs.

Answer d is incorrect. Insulin does not increase amylin production.

---

17. Adjustments or selection of antihyperglycemic drug therapy should be based on which of the following concerns? Select all that apply.

    a. Blood glucose levels
    b. History of genital mycotic infections
    c. Frequency of hypoglycemic reactions
    d. Liver function tests if the patient is on a TZD

Answers a, b, c, and d are correct. TZDs are contraindicated in patients with ALT levels greater than 3 times upper limits of normal. SGLT2-inhibitors are known to cause mycotic infections in both male and females genitals. These infections are often treatable and therapy can be resumed; however, quality of life may be impacted. It is always crucial to adjust antihyperglycemic agents based on the patient's individual glucose levels and their risk for future hypoglycemic reactions.

---

18. Which of the following statements are true of repaglinide? Select all that apply.

    a. Dosage of repaglinide should be administered regardless of meal.
    b. Normal treatment of hypoglycemia is recommended for patients on repaglinide.
    c. Caution for hypoglycemic in concomitant therapy with gemfibrozil.
    d. Maximum dose of repaglinide is 16 mg daily (divided with meals).

Answer b is correct. Only α-glucosidase inhibitors have special treatment recommendation during a hypoglycemic reaction.

Answer c is correct. Gemfibrozil can increase blood level of repaglinide causing hypoglycemic reactions.

Answer d is correct. The maximum dosage regardless of baseline A1c is 16 mg daily divided with meals.

Answer a is incorrect. Repaglinide should be given approximately 30 minutes preprandial. However, it should only be administered if a meal is planned. If a patient does not eat, this medication should not be given.

19. Which drug therapy may mask the signs of hypoglycemia?

    a. Atenolol
    b. Valsartan
    c. Hydrochlorothiazide
    d. Pioglitazone

Answer a is correct. β Blockers have been known to mask signs or symptoms of hypoglycemia. The one sign that it may not mask is diaphoresis or sweaty palms.

Answer b is incorrect. Valsartan is not associated with masked hypoglycemia.

Answer c is incorrect. Hydrochlorothiazide is not noted to mask hypoglycemia; however, transiently may worsen glucose control.

Answer d is incorrect. Pioglitazone is not associated with masked hypoglycemia.

20. Place the following insulin products in order of onset. Start with the fastest onset.

Unordered Response	Ordered Response
NPH	Aspart
Detemir	Regular
Regular	NPH
Aspart	Detemir

CHAPTER 62 | Thyroid Disorders

1. BS is a 36-year-old woman who presents to her doctor with symptoms of anxiety, sleep disturbances, and recent weight loss. Her doctor suspects hyperthyroidism. Which of the following lab results would be consistent with overt hyperthyroidism?

    a. Increased TSH, increased thyroid hormones
    b. Decreased TSH, increased thyroid hormones
    c. Increased TSH, decreased thyroid hormones
    d. Decreased TSH, decreased thyroid hormones

Answer b is correct. Hyperthyroidism increased thyroid hormones that then decrease the amount of TSH needed by the thyroid gland.

Answer a is incorrect. Hyperthyroidism occurs when excess thyroid hormones are circulating in the body. As a result of the negative feedback system, increased concentrations of thyroid hormones will suppress the production of TSH so TSH levels will be decreased in hyperthyroidism.

Answer c is incorrect. Thyroid hormones are elevated in hyperthyroidism while TSH is suppressed. These lab results (increased TSH and decreased thyroid hormones) are typically found in hypothyroidism.

Answer d is incorrect. Thyroid hormones will be elevated in hyperthyroidism. TSH concentrations will be decreased.

2. MM is a pregnant 27-year-old woman who has just been diagnosed with hyperthyroidism. Which symptoms might MM be experiencing due to her diagnosis?

    a. Bradycardia and cold intolerance
    b. Tachycardia and heat intolerance
    c. Depression and cognition difficulties
    d. Weight gain and constipation

Answer b is correct. Tachycardia will occur due to increased adrenergic activity due to excess thyroid hormones. Heat intolerance and sweating are other common symptoms of hyperthyroidism due to increased metabolism.

Answer a is incorrect. Bradycardia and cold intolerance are typical symptoms of hypothyroidism.

Answer c is incorrect. Depression and cognition difficulties are typical symptoms of hypothyroidism.

Answer d is incorrect. Weight gain and constipation may occur due to her pregnancy but are more typical symptoms of hypothyroidism. Patients with hyperthyroidism may be more likely to experience frequent stools and weight loss instead.

3. MM is currently in first trimester of her pregnancy, but her doctor consults you for treatment options for hyperthyroidism throughout MM's pregnancy. Select all that apply.

    a. Surgery
    b. Radioactive iodine
    c. Methimazole
    d. Propylthiouracil

Answer d is correct. Propylthiouracil is the preferred treatment for hyperthyroidism in the first trimester of pregnancy. Due to significant adverse effects with propylthiouracil, use should be minimized, and the patient should be changed to methimazole in the second trimester.

Answer a is incorrect. Surgery is usually a last line option for the treatment of hyperthyroidism. Thyroidectomy requires precise surgical skills so that other glands around the thyroid are not damaged. Surgery should be avoided during pregnancy.

Answer b is incorrect. Radioactive iodine is contraindicated in pregnancy. It can cross the placenta and cause serious consequences in the fetus. Women should wait 6 to 12 months after treatment with radioactive iodine before trying to get pregnant.

Answer c is incorrect. Methimazole is the preferred antithyroid medication during the second and third trimesters of pregnancy to minimize the risk of hepatotoxicity associated with propylthiouracil. Methimazole should be avoided in the first trimester as it has been associated with more adverse effects in the fetus including aplasia cutis and gastrointestinal abnormalities.

4. Dr. M wants to know which antithyroid medication would be preferred in a nonpregnant patient with hyperthyroidism without thyroid storm and why. What is your response?

a. Propylthiouracil is preferred due to fewer side effects and less frequent dosing.
b. Methimazole is preferred due to fewer side effects and less frequent dosing.
c. Methimazole is preferred since it blocks the peripheral conversion of T_4 to T_3.
d. Propylthiouracil is preferred since it blocks the peripheral conversion of T_4 to T_3.

Answer b is correct. Methimazole does not produce side effects such as vasculitis and hepatotoxicity. Methimazole can also be dosed once daily.

Answer a is incorrect. Propylthiouracil has a higher incidence of serious side effects such as vasculitis and hepatotoxicity. Propylthiouracil must also be dosed multiple times a day.

Answer c is incorrect. Methimazole does not block the peripheral conversion of T_4 to T_3.

Answer d is incorrect. Propylthiouracil does block the peripheral conversion of T_4 to T_3 but this does not offer any additional benefit except in thyroid storm.

5. TS is a 35-year-old woman started on propylthiouracil for treatment of hyperthyroidism. Which of the following side effects might she experience that would require discontinuation of her medication? Select all that apply.

a. Agranulocytosis
b. Insomnia
c. Gastrointestinal upset
d. Hepatotoxicity

Answer a is correct. Agranulocytosis can occur with both methimazole and propylthiouracil. Diagnosis of agranulocytosis requires prompt treatment with broad spectrum antibiotics and discontinuation of the antithyroid drug. Cross-reactivity for agranulocytosis does occur between methimazole and propylthiouracil, so patients will need to be treated with radioactive iodine or surgery to correct the hyperthyroidism.

Answer d is correct. Development of hepatotoxicity warrants discontinuation of propylthiouracil.

Answer b is incorrect. Insomnia does not require discontinuation.

Answer c is incorrect. Gastrointestinal upset does not require discontinuation.

6. LR is a 32-year-old woman who is still experiencing symptoms of hyperthyroidism despite treatment with methimazole. Which medication can be added to provide additional symptomatic relief?

a. Nifedipine
b. Prednisone
c. Propranolol
d. Ibuprofen

Answer c is correct. β-Adrenergic blocking agents will slow the heart rate to help correct tachycardia and may improve other symptoms of hyperthyroidism including anxiety, palpitations, and tremor. These agents are added to antithyroid medications or around treatment with radioactive iodine for symptomatic relief only.

Answer a is incorrect. Certain calcium channel blockers (nondihyropyridine calcium channel blockers like verapamil and diltiazem) may be used to decrease the heart rate in patients with hyperthyroidism. Dihydropyridine calcium channel blockers like nifedipine, amlodipine, and felodipine do not slow the heart and may actually cause a reflex tachycardia, worsening hyperthyroidism symptoms.

Answer b is incorrect. Prednisone may be used to treat patients presenting in thyroid storm but has no additional symptomatic benefit for outpatient treatment of hyperthyroidism.

Answer d is incorrect. Ibuprofen will not provide symptomatic relief for the typical symptoms of hyperthyroidism.

7. YD presents to the emergency room in coma with fever and tachycardia. Based on results of his thyroid function tests, YD is diagnosed with thyroid storm. Which therapy would be preferred as initial treatment for YDs symptoms? Select all that apply.

a. Radioactive iodine
b. Propylthiouracil
c. Methimazole
d. Glucocorticoids

Answer b is correct. Propylthiouracil is the preferred treatment for patients presenting in thyroid storm. Not only will propylthiouracil block the formation of thyroid hormones, it also blocks the peripheral conversion of T_4 to the more potent T_3. Patients will need the multiple sites of action to help correct the symptoms of hyperthyroidism in thyroid storm.

Answer d is correct. Glucocorticoids are utilized in the treatment of thyroid storm.

Answer a is incorrect. Radioactive iodine will not immediately suppress production of thyroid hormones. Return to a euthyroid state generally takes 2 months. Due to the severe nature and high mortality associated with thyroid storm, the patient needs a more immediate reduction in thyroid hormone concentrations.

Answer c is incorrect. Methimazole only blocks the production of thyroid hormones, but does not affect the peripheral conversion of T_4 to T_3.

---

8. You are consulted by Dr. X to determine the plan for a patient's methimazole dose. She has been taking methimazole for 3 months. What is your response?

TSH	1.5	(0.4-4.0 mIU/L)
Free T$_4$	6.2	(4.5-11.2 mcg/dL)
Free T$_3$	125	(100-200 ng/dL)

   a. Begin reducing the dose of methimazole since thyroid function tests are within normal range.
   b. Stop methimazole now since thyroid function tests are within normal range.
   c. Methimazole will need to be continued indefinitely to maintain thyroid levels in the normal range.
   d. Gradually transition patient from methimazole to levothyroxine since the patient will become hypothyroid due to treatment from methimazole.

Answer a is correct. Antithyroid medications should be gradually reduced to maintain thyroid function tests within normal range. Treatment should continue for 12 to 18 months.

Answer b is incorrect. Methimazole should not be stopped suddenly, but gradually tapered off.

Answer c is incorrect. Treatment with antithyroid drugs should only continue for 12 to 18 months. Treatment for longer durations does not guarantee remission of hyperthyroidism.

Answer d is incorrect. Antithyroid medications do not typically induce hypothyroidism. Radioactive iodine typically induces hypothyroidism over time, and patients will require treatment with levothyroxine.

---

9. You have been asked to counsel a 72-year-old patient with a history of heart disease about her upcoming treatment with radioactive iodine. Which of the following should be included in your counseling recommendations? Select all that apply.

   a. The patient does not need to take any extra precautions due to exposure to radioactive iodine.
   b. The patient should be treated with methimazole up to 3 to 7 days prior to treatment with radioactive iodine to reduce the risk of cardiovascular events associated with post-treatment exacerbation of hyperthyroidism.
   c. Once the patient's thyroid function returns to normal after radioactive iodine therapy, she will no longer need to have her thyroid function monitored.
   d. The patient should anticipate a change to a hypothyroid state over time after treatment with radioactive iodine that will require treatment with levothyroxine.

Answer b is correct. Due to her age and past medical history, this patient is at risk for a cardiovascular event after treatment with radioactive iodine. She will need pretreatment with methimazole that should be resumed 3 to 5 days after iodine therapy. Treatment should be tapered over the next few weeks.

Answer d is correct. More often than not, radioactive iodine induces a hypothyroid state over time. Her thyroid function tests will need to be continually monitored. Once she becomes hypothyroid, she will need treatment with levothyroxine.

Answer a is incorrect. Patients need to take many precautions to minimize exposure of radioactive therapy to others.

Answer c is incorrect. More often than not, radioactive iodine induces a hypothyroid state over time. Her thyroid function tests will need to be continually monitored.

---

10. GB is a 55-year-old woman recently diagnosed with hypothyroidism. Which symptoms might she be experiencing?

   a. Bradycardia and cold intolerance
   b. Anxiety and nervousness
   c. Weight loss and insomnia
   d. Frequent bowel movements and edema

Answer a is correct. The decreased concentration of thyroid hormones in the body due to hypothyroidism decreases heart rate. Patients also present with cold intolerance due to a slower metabolism.

Answer b is incorrect. Anxiety and nervousness are common symptoms of hyperthyroidism that occur due to increased adrenergic activity.

Answer c is incorrect. Patients with hypothyroidism will typically gain weight due to a slower metabolism. Sleep disturbances are more likely to occur in hyperthyroidism, particularly insomnia. Patients with hypothyroidism may experience more fatigue.

Answer d is incorrect. Constipation is a more common problem with hypothyroidism while frequent bowel movements occur more often in hyperthyroidism. Edema does occur in hypothyroidism, but usually after a long history of hypothyroidism due to low cardiac output.

---

11. Which of the following lab results would indicate hypothyroidism in GB?

   a. Increased TSH, increased thyroid hormones
   b. Decreased TSH, increased thyroid hormones
   c. Increased TSH, decreased thyroid hormones
   d. Decreased TSH, decreased thyroid hormones

Answer c is correct. Hypothyroidism occurs when sufficient concentrations of thyroid hormones are not available in the body. As a result, TSH concentrations increase to compensate and produce more thyroid hormones.

Answer a is incorrect. TSH concentrations will increase in hypothyroidism due to insufficient concentrations of thyroid hormones, but thyroid hormone levels will be decreased.

Answer b is incorrect. These thyroid function test more accurately depict hyperthyroidism. TSH concentrations decrease in hyperthyroidism due to excess concentrations of thyroid hormones.

Answer d is incorrect. Thyroid hormones levels will be decreased in hypothyroidism, but TSH concentrations should increase to stimulate production of more thyroid hormones.

12. GBs doctor has been concerned about new trends in the treatment of hypothyroidism. He requests your recommendation for the most appropriate therapy for GB.

a. Desiccated thyroid hormone
b. Liothyronine
c. Levothyroxine
d. The combination of liothyronine and levothyroxine

Answer c is correct. Levothyroxine is the preferred thyroid replacement drug for hypothyroidism. Levothyroxine not only replaces T_4 concentrations but will then undergo peripheral conversion in the body to replace T_3.

Answer a is incorrect. Desiccated thyroid hormone was one of the first treatments available for hypothyroidism, but is rarely used due to the difficulty in standardizing concentrations and maintaining a euthyroid state for the patient. It contains a combination of T_4 and T_3 along with T_1 and T_2 derived from pigs' thyroids.

Answer b is incorrect. Liothyronine (T_3) does not replace T_4 concentrations.

Answer d is incorrect. The combination of levothyroxine and liothyronine has not proven to be significantly beneficial.

13. Which of the following patient counseling tips would be appropriate for GB? Select all that apply.

a. Levothyroxine will need to be continued lifelong.
b. Levothyroxine should be taken on an empty stomach to maximize absorption.
c. Levothyroxine should be taken with food to maximize absorption.
d. Levothyroxine produces immediate symptomatic relief of hypothyroidism.

Answer a is correct. Levothyroxine will need to be given lifelong to maintain a euthyroid state.

Answer b is correct. Due to the risk for decreased absorption with food or other medications, levothyroxine should be taken on an empty stomach.

Answer c is incorrect. Food will decrease the absorption of levothyroxine.

Answer d is incorrect. Due to the long half-life of levothyroxine, it may take 4 to 6 weeks to reach steady-state. Symptoms will not improve immediately.

14. As KM picks up her first prescription of levothyroxine, she asks you when she should have her thyroid function tests rechecked. What is your response?

a. 1 week
b. 1 month
c. 3 months
d. 6 months

Answer b is correct. The half-life of levothyroxine is 7 days. It may take 4 to 6 weeks to reach steady-state. Thyroid function tests should be checked 1 to 2 months after starting levothyroxine or any dose changes.

Answer a is incorrect. TSH concentrations may take 4 to 6 weeks to change after levothyroxine initiation or dose changes.

Answer c is incorrect. Thyroid function tests should be checked sooner to appropriately titrate the levothyroxine dose.

Answer d is incorrect. Thyroid function tests should be checked 4 to 6 weeks after starting levothyroxine or any dose changes.

15. Dr. Z in your clinic asks you what the most recent dosing recommendations are for initiating levothyroxine for the treatment of hypothyroidism. Which of the following responses are correct? Select all that apply.

a. Full treatment doses of levothyroxine may be started in some patients.
b. Levothyroxine must be started at low doses and titrated up slowly in all patients.
c. Patients with ischemic heart disease may begin levothyroxine at full treatment doses.
d. Full treatment doses of levothyroxine should be started only in younger healthy patients.

Answer a is correct. Caution should be used in patients over the age of 60 and those with ischemic heart disease as the positive chronotropic and inotropic effects of thyroid hormone may exacerbate myocardial ischemia. Levothyroxine should be started at 12.5 to 25 mcg daily and titrated up slowly every 4 to 6 weeks in certain patients. Otherwise, patients may be started with full treatment doses of 1.6 mcg/kg/d.

Answer d is correct. Only healthy patients should start full treatment doses of levothyroxine at 1.6 mcg/kg daily. The positive chronotropic and inotropic effects of thyroid hormone may exacerbate myocardial ischemia in patients with ischemic heart disease or those over the age of 60.

Answer b is incorrect. Starting all patients at a low dose and titrating up slowly prolongs recovery time. Healthy patients and those less than 60 years old may start full treatment doses safely.

Answer c is incorrect. Full treatment doses may exacerbate myocardial ischemia in patients with ischemic heart disease. These patients should start levothyroxine at 12.5 to 25 mcg daily, with a slow titration every 4 to 6 weeks.

---

16. Calculate an appropriate starting dose of levothyroxine in an otherwise healthy 42-year-old woman recently diagnosed with hypothyroidism. Her vitals are:

    Height 5′ 2″ Weight 235 lb

    Answer = _____

    Calculate based on ideal body weight (equals 50.1 kg) and starting dose of 1.6 mcg/kg/d since she is young and healthy. Round to nearest available tablet size.

Answer = 75 mcg daily

---

17. PR is a 35-year-old woman admitted for uncontrollable nausea and vomiting during the first trimester of her pregnancy. Her past medical history is significant for hypothyroidism and GERD. How should her hypothyroidism be managed during her hospitalization?

    a. Levothyroxine should be held until PR can restart her oral medication.
    b. Levothyroxine should be given intravenously until PR can restart her oral medication.
    c. Levothyroxine should be given orally at a lower dose to reduce nausea and vomiting.
    d. Levothyroxine should be changed to liothyronine to reduce nausea and vomiting.

Answer a is correct. PR may only miss a few doses while hospitalized until she gains control of her nausea and vomiting. Due to the long half-life of levothyroxine, PR will maintain her TSH concentration for several days even without receiving her levothyroxine dose.

Answer b is incorrect. Intravenous levothyroxine is generally reserved for treatment of myxedema coma or patients unable to take oral medications for an extended period of time. Additionally, the poor stability of reconstituted levothyroxine requires immediate administration.

Answer c is incorrect. Levothyroxine should not worsen nausea and vomiting unless she is receiving too much levothyroxine. In addition, most pregnant women require higher doses of levothyroxine.

Answer d is incorrect. Levothyroxine is the preferred thyroid replacement product for hypothyroidism and has been proven safe and effective in pregnancy. There is no medical reason to change PR to liothyronine.

---

18. FN is diagnosed with Hashimoto disease during the second trimester of her pregnancy. Which medication would be preferred for FN?

    a. Desiccated thyroid hormone
    b. Liothyronine alone

    c. Levothyroxine alone
    d. Levothyroxine in combination with liothyronine

Answer c is correct. Levothyroxine is the preferred thyroid replacement product. It provides T_4 that can be converted to T_3 in the peripheral tissues of the body. The risks of not treating hypothyroidism in pregnancy are much greater than the risk of treating with levothyroxine.

Answer a is incorrect. Desiccated thyroid hormone is not the preferred thyroid hormone replacement product used for hypothyroidism in general due to the difficulty in standardizing concentrations. Standardization is based on the iodine content instead of the hormonal content.

Answer b is incorrect. Generally, liothyronine is not used alone for the treatment of hypothyroidism. It does not replace T_4.

Answer d is incorrect. The combination of levothyroxine and liothyronine has not proven to be beneficial.

---

19. TC has been on amiodarone for 2 months and has now been diagnosed with amiodarone-induced hypothyroidism. What is the treatment of choice for amiodarone-induced hypothyroidism?

    a. Discontinuation of amiodarone
    b. Liothyronine alone
    c. Levothyroxine alone
    d. Levothyroxine in combination with liothyronine

Answer c is correct. Amiodarone-induced hypothyroidism responds to treatment with levothyroxine. Once amiodarone is discontinued, thyroid levels usually return to normal unless antithyroid antibodies have formed.

Answer a is incorrect. Amiodarone does not need to be discontinued, however, if stopped, thyroid levels should return to normal.

Answer b is incorrect. Generally, liothyronine is not used alone for the treatment of hypothyroidism. It does not replace T_4.

Answer d is incorrect. The combination of levothyroxine and liothyronine has not proven to be beneficial.

---

20. Which of the following is true?

    a. Radioactive iodine will adequately treat type 1 amiodarone-induced hyperthyroidism.
    b. Amiodarone must be discontinued to adequately treat type 1 amiodarone-induced hyperthyroidism.
    c. Amiodarone must be discontinued to adequately treat type 2 amiodarone-induced hyperthyroidism.
    d. Antithyroid medications may offer some benefit in type 2 amiodarone-induced hyperthyroidism.

Answer b is correct. Resumption of a euthyroid state requires the discontinuation of amiodarone.

Answer a is incorrect. Type 1 amiodarone-induced hyperthyroidism does not respond to radioactive iodine due to low radioiodine uptake with this form.

Answer c is incorrect. Type 2 amiodarone-induced hyperthyroidism is inflammatory in nature that may resolve after 1 to 3 months. Discontinuation of amiodarone may not be necessary.

Answer d is incorrect. Antithyroid medications only offer some benefit in type 1 amiodarone-induced hyperthyroidism. Corticosteroids may need to treat the inflammatory process associated with type 2 amiodarone-induced hyperthyroidism.

CHAPTER **63 | Contraception**

1. TK is a 23-year-old woman who comes to your pharmacy stating that she is taking the mini-pill and missed her dose yesterday. Based on this information, what is the best remedy in this situation?

    a. She should take two tablets today as soon as possible, no backup method is needed.
    b. She should start taking her tablets as scheduled and use a backup method for the next 48 hours.
    c. She should take two tablets today as soon as possible and use a backup method until she gets her period.
    d. She should start taking her tablets as scheduled and use a backup method until she gets her period.

Answer b is correct. Progestin-only oral contraceptives need to be taken at the same time every day. Missing a dose by more than 3 hours of its scheduled time is considered a missed dose and may alter the effectiveness of the medication. Therefore, a backup method is required for 48 hours.

Answer a is incorrect. Since this is a progestin-only oral contraceptive, its mechanism of action is very dependent on the timing of administration.

Answer c is incorrect. She does not need to use a backup method until her next period or double up on pills.

Answer d is incorrect. She does not need to use a backup method until her next period.

2. AC is a 26-year-old woman who presents to the pharmacy asking to buy emergency contraceptive (Plan B One-Step) and says she had unprotected intercourse 3 days ago. Based on the information, select the best statement as it relates to EC.

    a. EC will not be effective for AC because it has been longer than 24 hours since she has had unprotected sex.
    b. EC will not be effective for AC because it has been longer than 48 hours since she has had unprotected sex.
    c. EC cannot be provided to AC without a prescription from her doctor.
    d. EC may still work for AC because it is still within 72 hours since she has had unprotected sex.

    e. EC may still work for AC because it is still within 120 hours since she has had unprotected sex, but she will require a prescription.

Answer d is correct. EC is effective for up to 120 hours after unprotected intercourse.

Answer a is incorrect. EC is effective for up to 120 hours after unprotected intercourse.

Answer b is incorrect. EC is effective for up to 120 hours after unprotected intercourse.

Answer c is incorrect. Plan B One-Step does not require a prescription; there is no age restriction for Plan B One-Step.

Answer e is incorrect. EC is effective for up to 120 hours after unprotected intercourse but a prescription is not required.

3. Please select the appropriate ranked products based on EE content from highest to lowest.

    a. Contraceptive vaginal ring > contraceptive patch > oral combined contraceptive (30 mcg EE)
    b. Contraceptive patch > oral combined contraceptive (30 mcg EE) > contraceptive vaginal ring
    c. Oral combined contraceptive (30 mcg EE) > contraceptive vaginal ring > contraceptive patch
    d. All of the above provide the same amount of EE.

Answer b is correct. The contraceptive patch provides the most EE of choices provided. It provides 60% more EE than a 35 mcg oral formulation and the vaginal ring provides the least amount of EE, 15 mcg/d.

Answer a is incorrect. The contraceptive vaginal ring provides the least amount of estradiol, 15 mcg/d.

Answer c is incorrect. The COC provides 30 mcg of EE compared to the 15 mcg provided by the contraceptive vaginal ring and the contraceptive patch provides more than 35 mcg oral tablet.

Answer d is incorrect. The formulations offer varying amounts of EE.

4. GT is a 21-year-old woman who has a history of acne. Her acne has been refractory to doxycycline and topical agents. She is otherwise healthy. Her physician would like prescribe a hormonal treatment that has an FDA indication for acne. Which of the following could be recommended to GT? Select all that apply.

    a. Depo-Provera
    b. NuvaRing
    c. YAZ
    d. Estrostep

Answer c is correct. YAZ, Ortho Tri-Cyclen, Beyaz, and Estrostep are FDA approved for acne treatment.

Answer d is correct. YAZ, Ortho Tri-Cyclen, Beyaz, and Estrostep are FDA approved for acne treatment; although, most birth control pills will help relieve acne.

Answer a is incorrect. Depo-Provera is not FDA approved for acne treatment.

Answer b is incorrect. NuvaRing is not FDA approved for acne treatment.

5. JK is a 32-year-old woman who weighs 75 kg and is 5'1". Which of the following is best to avoid in overweight/obese patients due to the side effects of weight gain?
    a. Depo-Provera
    b. NuvaRing
    c. Xulane
    d. Yasmin

Answer a is correct. Depo-Provera is not the best agent to use in women who are overweight or obese since it may cause more weight gain.

Answer b is incorrect. NuvaRing has not been shown to cause a significant weight gain.

Answer c is incorrect. Xulane has not been shown to cause a significant weight gain but should be avoided due to decreased effectiveness in women weighing more than 198 lb.

Answer d is incorrect. Yasmin has not been shown to cause a significant weight gain.

6. How often is one NuvaRing inserted vaginally?
    a. 1 week
    b. 3 weeks
    c. 2 weeks
    d. 4 weeks

Answer b is correct. One vaginal contraceptive ring should be inserted for 3 weeks.

Answer a is incorrect. One vaginal contraceptive ring should be inserted for 3 weeks not for 1 week.

Answer c is incorrect. One vaginal contraceptive ring should be inserted for 3 weeks not for 2 weeks.

Answer d is incorrect. One vaginal contraceptive ring should be inserted for 3 weeks not for 4 weeks.

7. BD is a 28-year-old obese, woman who delivered a baby 1 week ago via C-section. She does not plan to breast-feed and would like to start a COC as soon as possible. When is the earliest she can start taking COCs without an increased risk of blood clots?
    a. Immediately
    b. 2 weeks postpartum
    c. 6 weeks postpartum
    d. 6 months postpartum

Answer c is correct. There is a higher risk of blood clots if COCs are taken less than 6 weeks postpartum. A woman may start COC/CHCs at 3 weeks postpartum if she has no risk factors for VTE and is not breastfeeding since COC/CHCs may affect breast milk in a woman with difficulty in producing milk. It is recommended to wait until 6 weeks postpartum if the patient has risk factors for VTE. BW recently had a C-section and is obese putting her at risk for a VTE; therefore, starting a COC/CHC at 6 weeks is the best recommendation.

Answer a is incorrect. There is a higher risk of blood clots if COCs are taken less than 3 to 6 weeks postpartum.

Answer b is incorrect. There is a higher risk of blood clots if COCs are taken less than 3 to 6 weeks postpartum. If BW takes COCs 2 weeks postpartum she may have an increased risk of clotting.

Answer d is incorrect. There is no need to wait for 6 months. The patient may start COC/CHCs as soon as 6 weeks postpartum if she chooses.

8. AJ is a 22-year-old woman who weighs 220 lb and would like to start hormonal contraception. Which of the following products would not be as effective in preventing pregnancy for AJ? Select all that apply.
    a. Depo-Provera
    b. NuvaRing
    c. Xulane
    d. Yasmin

Answer a is correct. There is no issue with effectiveness of Depo-Provera in women weighing more than 198 lb. However, it may increase weight gain.

Answer b is correct. At this time, there is no issue with effectiveness of NuvaRing in women weighing more than 198 lb.

Answer d is correct. There is no issue with effectiveness of Yasmin in women weighing more than 198 lb.

Answer c is incorrect. Xulane is not recommended in patients weighing 198 lb or more due to a higher failure rate in those women.

9. Which of the following products contains drospirenone and may increase potassium levels? Select all that apply.
    a. Safyral
    b. YAZ
    c. Cyclessa
    d. Nor-QD

Answer a is correct. Safyral contains drospirenone which is a derivative of spironolactone and may increase potassium levels.

Answer b is correct. YAZ contains drospirenone which is a derivative of spironolactone and may increase potassium levels.

Answer c is incorrect. Cyclessa does not contain drospirenone but contains desogestrel.

Answer d is incorrect. Nor-QD does not contain drospirenone. It is a progestin-only oral contraceptive.

---

10. RS just started a new COC 2 weeks ago and has had some mild nausea when she takes the pill. What is the best recommendation for RS with respect to changing products?

    a. Change the oral combined contraceptive to another agent this week
    b. Wait for 3 months to see if side effects improve, if not change products
    c. Wait for 2 months to see if side effects improve, if not change products
    d. Wait for 6 months to see if side effects improve, if not change products

Answer b is correct. It is recommended to try a COC for at least 3 months before changing products. For counseling, patients may be instructed to take COCs at bedtime to help decrease nausea.

Answer a is incorrect. It is recommended to try a COC for at least 3 months before changing products. Two weeks is not enough time for RS.

Answer c is incorrect. It is recommended to try a COC for at least 3 months before changing products. Two months is not enough time for RS.

Answer d is incorrect. It is recommended to try a COC for at least 3 months before changing products.

---

11. Select the name for levonorgestrel emergency contraceptive products. Select all that apply.

    a. Plan B One-Step
    b. Ortho Tri-Cyclen Lo
    c. My Way
    d. Xulane
    e. Next Choice One Dose

Answer a is correct. The generic name for Plan B One-Step is levonorgestrel. It contains one tablet of levonorgestrel 1.5 mg.

Answer c is correct. The generic name for My Way is levonorgestrel. It contains one tablet of levonorgestrel 1.5 mg.

Answer e is correct. The generic name of Next Choice One Dose is levonorgestrel. It contains one tablet of levonorgestrel 1.5 mg.

Answer b is incorrect. Ortho Tri-Cyclen Lo is EE and norgestimate. It is not marketed as an emergency contraceptive.

Answer d is incorrect. Xulane is a contraceptive patch that contains EE and norelgestromin. It is not marketed as an emergency contraceptive.

---

12. Select the contraceptive agent that is formulated as an injection.

    a. Desogen
    b. Mirena
    c. Estrostep
    d. Xulane
    e. Depo-Provera

Answer e is correct. Depo-Provera is an injectable progestin-only contraceptive available intramuscularly and subcutaneously.

Answer a is incorrect. Desogen is an oral combined contraceptive.

Answer b is incorrect. Mirena is an intrauterine system that provides progestin daily.

Answer c is incorrect. Estrostep is an oral combined contraceptive.

Answer d is incorrect. Xulane is a transdermal contraceptive patch.

---

13. JS is a 21-year-old man who comes to your pharmacy and states, "What can my girlfriend and I use to make sure she doesn't get pregnant and protect ourselves from, you know... diseases?" Select the best regimen to recommend from the following choices below.

    a. Water-based lubricant + male latex condom
    b. Oil-based lubricant + male latex condom
    c. Female condom + male latex condom
    d. Female condom + male lamb cecum condom
    e. Oil-based lubricant + male lamb cecum condom

Answer a is correct. Water-based lubricant is safe to use with latex condoms and do not comprise their ability to protect against STIs.

Answer b is incorrect. Oil-based lubricant is not safe to use with latex condoms since it comprises their ability to protect against STIs by breaking down the latex.

Answer c is incorrect. The female condom and male latex condom should not be used together. They may stick together, cause friction, and break.

Answer d is incorrect. The female condom and male lamb cecum condom should not be used together. They may stick together, cause friction, and break.

Answer e is incorrect. Oil-based and water-based lubricants may be used with male lamb cecum condoms; however, lamb cecum condoms themselves do not protect against all STIs.

---

14. Which of the following condoms conducts heat very well and protects against STIs? Select all that apply.

    a. Polyurethane
    b. Latex
    c. Lamb cecum
    d. Polyisoprene

Answer a is correct. Polyurethane condoms conduct heat better than latex condoms. They also protect against STIs; however, they may break easier than other condoms.

Answer d is correct. Polyisoprene condoms conduct heat better than latex condoms. They also protect against STIs; however, they may break easier than other condoms.

Answer b is incorrect. Latex condoms are best for protecting against STIs; however, they do not conduct heat as well as lamb cecum or polyurethane condoms.

Answer c is incorrect. Lamb cecum condoms conduct heat very well, but do not protect against all STIs.

---

15. QS is a 32-year-old woman who suffers from migraines without aura during her menses every time she takes the placebo pills in her oral contraceptive pack. The physician recommends that she switch to an extended cycle oral contraceptive to reduce the placebo pill weeks and number of menses to four per year. What is the appropriate number of active tablets contained in an extended cycle oral contraceptive product for QS to have four menses per year?

    a. 24
    b. 21
    c. 44
    d. 84
    e. 352

Answer d is correct. There are 84 active tablets in the product for an extended cycle regimen and marketed as such.

Answer a is incorrect. There are 24 active tablets in formulations such as YAZ and Loestrin 24.

Answer b is incorrect. There are 21 active tablets in most COC formulations, but not for an extended cycle product.

Answer c is incorrect. There are no formulations of COCs that have 44 active tablets.

Answer e is incorrect. There are extended regimen products that may allow one menses per year, but only 84 active with 7 placebo tablets will allow a woman to have four menses per year.

---

16. CS is a 36-year-old woman who admits to smoking one pack of cigarettes per day. She is getting married and would like to start hormonal contraception. Which of the following products is most appropriate for CS?

    a. NuvaRing
    b. Xulane
    c. Mircette
    d. Tri-Levlen
    e. Nor-QD

Answer e is correct. Nor-QD is a progestin-only oral contraceptive and is not contraindicated in women older than 35 years who smoke.

Answer a is incorrect. NuvaRing contains EE and etonogestrel. EE is contraindicated for use in women older than 35 years and who smoke more than 15 cigarettes per day. The risk of stroke and blood clots rises in this population.

Answer b is incorrect. Xulane contains EE and norgestrelomin. EE is contraindicated for use in women older than 35 years and who smoke more than 15 cigarettes per day. The risk of stroke and blood clots rises in this population.

Answer c is incorrect. Mircette contains EE and desogestrel. EE is contraindicated for use in women older than 35 years and who smoke more than 15 cigarettes per day. The risk of stroke and blood clots rises in this population.

Answer d is incorrect. Tri-Levlen contains EE and desogestrel. EE is contraindicated for use in women older than 35 years and who smoke more than 15 cigarettes per day. The risk of stroke and blood clots rises in this population.

---

17. Which of the following drugs may decrease the effectiveness of Ortho-Tri Cyclen? Select all that apply.

    a. Atorvastatin
    b. Carbamazepine
    c. Lamotrigine
    d. Acetaminophen
    e. Phenytoin

Answer b is correct. Carbamazepine induces the metabolism of EE and decreases its effectiveness.

Answer e is correct. Phenytoin induces the metabolism of EE and decreases its effectiveness.

Answer a is incorrect. Atorvastatin increases the levels of EE.

Answer c is incorrect. Lamotrigine may increase the levels of EE.

Answer d is incorrect. Acetaminophen does not affect the levels of EE or norgestimate.

---

18. DL is a 19-year-old woman who calls you and states that she forgot to take her Desogen (EE 30 mcg/0.15 mg desogestrel) tablets for the last 2 days. She says she is in her second week of the cycle. Select the following statement that is most appropriate for missed tablets.

    a. DL should take two tablets the next day and use a backup method for 7 days
    b. DL should continue taking her tablets as scheduled, one per day, no backup method is necessary
    c. DL should discard her pill pack and start a new one, use a backup method for 7 days
    d. DL should take two tablets for 2 days, no backup method is necessary

Answer a is correct. If two tablets of a COC are missed, the most recent missed dose should be taken and a backup method should be used for 7 days and EC may also be used if unprotected intercourse occurred within the last 5 days.

Answer b is incorrect. If two tablets of a COC are missed, a backup method should be used for 7 days and two tablets for 1 day should be taken. EC may also be used if unprotected intercourse occurred within the last 5 days.

Answer c is incorrect. DL does not need to start a new pack because she is in her second week of the cycle meaning she will have at least 7 days of active tablets remaining.

Answer d is incorrect. If two tablets of a COC are missed, the most recent dose should be taken with the regularly scheduled dose and a backup method should be used for 7 days. EC may also be used if unprotected intercourse occurred within the last 5 days.

19. Combined hormonal contraception is contraindicated in which of the following conditions? Select all that apply.

    a. History of DVT
    b. Migraine with aura
    c. Active liver disease
    d. Uncontrolled hypertension

Answers a, b, c, and d are correct. EE can increase the risk of blood clots. Therefore, CHCs are contraindicated in patients with a history of DVT. There is also a higher risk of stroke in patients who experience migraines with aura and take CHCs. Therefore, CHCs are contraindicated in patients with a history of migraines with aura. CHCs are metabolized through the liver and may also have side effects on the liver. Therefore, CHCs should not be used in patients with active liver disease. EE can increase blood pressure. Patients with uncontrolled hypertension may increase their risk of stroke if they use CHCs and have uncontrolled hypertension.

20. RR is a 26-year-old woman who has just been diagnosed with PMDD and is also seeking contraception. She is otherwise healthy and is not obese or overweight. Which of the following products is best to recommend for RR?

    a. YAZ
    b. Ortho Tri-Cyclen
    c. Estrostep
    d. Mircette
    e. Yasmin

Answer a is correct. YAZ is FDA approved for PMDD.

Answer b is incorrect. Ortho Tri-Cyclen is not FDA approved for PMDD, but is approved for acne treatment.

Answer c is incorrect. Estrostep is not FDA approved for PMDD, but is approved for acne treatment.

Answer d is incorrect. Mircette is not FDA approved for PMDD.

Answer e is incorrect. Yasmin is not FDA approved for PMDD.

CHAPTER **64 | Allergic Rhinitis**

1. Which of the following are classic symptoms of allergic rhinitis? Select all that apply.

   a. Rhinorrhea
   b. Congestion
   c. Sneezing
   d. Fever

Answers a, b, and c are correct. These are classic symptoms of allergic rhinitis.

Answer d is incorrect. Fever may be a sign of infection.

---

2. Which of the following is a potential adverse effect when using oral antihistamines for the management of allergic rhinitis in a 3-year-old child?

   a. HPA axis suppression
   b. Paradoxical agitation
   c. Rebound congestion
   d. Medication tolerance

Answer b is correct. This is a potential adverse effect of oral first-generation antihistamines in infants and young children.

Answer a is incorrect. HPA axis suppression is a potential adverse effect related to intranasal corticosteroids.

Answer c is incorrect. Rebound congestion is an adverse effect related to overuse of topical decongestants.

Answer d is incorrect. Medication tolerance is not a concern with the use of antihistamines.

---

3. MH is a 37-year-old man with a history of chronic nasal stuffiness. He reports symptoms all year round. His only other medical condition is high blood pressure. In addition to stuffiness, he has been sneezing a lot at work (which he finds very embarrassing). Also, his allergies have caused him to cancel park outings with his family. Which of the following best classifies MH's symptoms?

   a. Mild intermittent
   b. Moderate-to-severe intermittent
   c. Mild persistent
   d. Moderate-to-severe persistent

Answer d is correct. His symptoms are severe and chronic.

Answer a is incorrect. Since this patient's symptoms are affecting his quality of life, they are not mild. Also, since his symptoms are >4 d/wk and >4 consecutive weeks, they are persistent.

Answer b is incorrect. His symptoms are year round.

Answer c is incorrect. His symptoms affect his quality of life.

---

4. Which therapeutic option would be best for MH?

    a. Oral decongestant
    b. First-generation antihistamine
    c. Intranasal corticosteroid
    d. Intranasal decongestant

Answer c is correct. An intranasal corticosteroid is highly effective for congestion and sneezing.

Answer a is incorrect. This patient suffers from high blood pressure and an oral decongestant can cause blood pressure to increase. Also, decongestants are only useful for nasal congestion and not sneezing.

Answer b is incorrect. A first-generation antihistamine is not the best option due to its sedative and anticholinergic effects, but can be a good additional agent should the intranasal corticosteroid not provide significant relief of symptoms.

Answer d is incorrect. Since this patient has chronic symptoms, an intranasal decongestant is not indicated. Intranasal decongestants should not be used for more than a few days at a time. Also, these agents do not reduce the frequency of sneezing.

---

5. CF is a 25-year-old pregnant female (first trimester) who presents to the pharmacy complaining of constant sneezing, congestion, and a runny nose. Which therapeutic option would be best for CF?

    a. Intranasal corticosteroid
    b. Nonselective antihistamine
    c. Oral decongestant
    d. Mast cell stabilizer

Answer a is correct. An intranasal corticosteroid is highly effective since this patient has chronic symptoms. A good choice would be budesonide.

Answer b is incorrect. An antihistamine is not as effective for the nasal congestion.

Answer c is incorrect. This medication is not safe for use in the first trimester (associated with congenital malformations).

Answer d is incorrect. This option is not the most effective medication for the patient.

---

6. Select the brand name for levocetirizine.

    a. Clarinex
    b. Zaditor

c. Xyzal
d. Singulair

Answer c is correct. This is the brand name for levocetirizine.

Answer a is incorrect. This is the brand name for desloratadine.

Answer b is incorrect. This is the brand name for ketotifen fumarate.

Answer d is incorrect. This is the brand name for montelukast.

---

7. The use of pseudoephedrine is concerning in a patient with which of the following disease states? Select all that apply.

    a. Diabetes mellitus
    b. Chronic kidney disease
    c. Hypertension
    d. Osteoarthritis

Answer a is correct. Pseudoephedrine should be used with caution in patients with diabetes, since it may raise blood glucose.

Answer b is correct. Pseudoephedrine is renally eliminated and may accumulate in patients with chronic kidney disease, thereby increasing the risk of drug-related toxicity. Therefore, the drug should be used cautiously in patients with renal impairment.

Answer c is correct. Pseudoephedrine should be used with caution in controlled hypertension, as it may raise blood pressure. Its use should be avoided in patients with uncontrolled hypertension.

Answer d is incorrect. Pseudoephedrine does not have effects on osteoarthritis and can be used in patients with this disorder.

---

8. Which of the following antihistamines is available over-the-counter? Select all that apply.

    a. Desloratadine
    b. Diphenhydramine
    c. Ketotifen
    d. Levocetirizine

Answers b, c, and d are correct. Diphenhydramine, ketotifen, and levocetirizine are available over-the-counter.

Answer a is incorrect.

---

9. Which of the following classes of medication can be used for management of allergic rhinitis in pregnancy? Select all that apply.

    a. Oral antihistamines
    b. Intranasal corticosteroids

c. Oral decongestants
d. Topical decongestants

Answer a is correct. Oral antihistamines may be used in pregnancy (if approved by the health care provider), particularly cetirizine and levocetirizine.

Answer b is correct. Intranasal corticosteroids may be used during pregnancy. Budesonide may be preferred, based on safety data.

Answer c is correct. Decongestants may be used, but should not be given until after the first trimester, if the benefits outweigh the risks. Topical decongestants may be safer.

Answer d is correct. Topical decongestants are safe for use in pregnancy due to limited systemic absorption.

10. JS is a 23-year-old man with a history of seasonal allergic rhinitis. He complains of bothersome nasal stuffiness each year during the fall when ragweed pollen is prevalent. Which of the following medications is most appropriate to provide immediate relief of his nasal congestion?

a. Cetirizine
b. Chlorpheniramine
c. Fluticasone
d. Oxymetazoline

Answer d is correct. A topical decongestant can provide relief within minutes of application.

Answer a is incorrect. Oral antihistamines are better at preventing symptoms than treating them once they occur, and the onset is not immediate since they are oral formulations. Oral antihistamines are less effective at treating nasal congestion than intranasal corticosteroids and decongestants.

Answer b is incorrect. As above for cetirizine, chlorpheniramine will not provide adequate relief from nasal congestion.

Answer c is incorrect. Intranasal corticosteroids will provide some relief from nasal congestion 8 to 12 hours after administration, but may take up to 2 weeks for full effects to be realized.

11. Which of the following allergen avoidance techniques would be appropriate to help reduce JS's allergic symptoms caused by ragweed pollen?

a. Encase pillow and mattress in allergen-proof cover.
b. Keep windows closed and minimize outdoor activities.
c. Reduce indoor humidity to <50%.
d. Wash bedding in hot water.

Answer b is correct. This prevents pollen from entering the house and minimizes the subjects' exposure.

Answer a is incorrect. Pollen is an outdoor allergen and cannot be minimized through the use of allergen-proof covers on bedding.

Answer c is incorrect. This can help with indoor mold allergies, but does not assist with outdoor allergens such as pollen.

Answer d is incorrect. This can assist patients with indoor dust mite allergies, but does not assist with outdoor allergens such as pollen.

12. Which of the following medications would be beneficial to JS in reducing symptoms of seasonal allergic rhinitis when started prior to allergen exposure? Select all that apply.

a. Intranasal corticosteroid
b. Leukotriene antagonist
c. Oral antihistamine
d. Topical decongestant

Answers a, b, and c are correct. Intranasal corticosteroids, leukotriene antagonists, and antihistamines can be given prior to allergen exposure to minimize allergic rhinitis symptoms. Montelukast is most appropriate for patients that also have asthma. For maximal efficacy, these agents should be started prior to expected exposure to allergens.

Answer d is incorrect. Topical decongestants are used for patients who present with nasal congestion. They are not used prior to onset of symptoms or allergen exposure.

13. CW is an 8-year-old boy with seasonal allergic rhinitis and mild persistent asthma. Which of the following medications would be appropriate to manage symptoms of both his asthma and allergic rhinitis?

a. Intranasal beclomethasone
b. Intranasal cromolyn
c. Cetirizine
d. Montelukast

Answer d is correct. Montelukast is effective for management of both allergic rhinitis and asthma.

Answer a is incorrect. Intranasal corticosteroids are, at best, marginally efficacious for asthma and should not be substituted for inhaled corticosteroids and/or other methods of asthma management.

Answer b is incorrect. Although inhaled cromolyn sodium is used as an adjunct to asthma treatment, the intranasal cromolyn sodium is not indicated for management of asthma.

Answer c is incorrect. Oral antihistamines are not recommended for the treatment of asthma.

14. Sedation would most likely occur with which of the following antihistamines when used at recommended dosages for adult patients?

a. Desloratadine
b. Diphenhydramine
c. Fexofenadine
d. Olopatadine

Answer b is correct. Diphenhydramine is a first-generation antihistamine (nonselective) and can cause sedation at recommended doses. It is available in many over-the-counter sleep products.

Answer a is incorrect. Desloratadine is a second-generation antihistamine and has a low-sedation potential.

Answer c is incorrect. Fexofenadine is a second-generation antihistamine and has a low-sedation potential.

Answer d is incorrect. Olopatadine is an intranasal and ophthalmic antihistamine and has a low-sedation potential.

---

15. Which of the following antihistamines is available in an intranasal formulation?

    a. Azelastine
    b. Ketotifen
    c. Levocetirizine
    d. Loratadine

Answer a is correct. Azelastine is available as an intranasal formulation.

Answer b is incorrect. Ketotifen is available as an ophthalmic formulation.

Answer c is incorrect. Levocetirizine is available as an oral formulation.

Answer d is incorrect. Loratadine is available as an oral formulation.

---

16. Which of the following categories of allergic rhinitis medications is most likely to be associated with rhinitis medicamentosa (rebound nasal congestion) with prolonged use?

    a. Intranasal corticosteroid
    b. Intranasal decongestant
    c. Intranasal antihistamine
    d. Oral decongestant

Answer b is correct. Rebound nasal congestion can occur when patients use these agents for more than 3 to 5 days. If rhinitis medicamentosa occurs, patients must be weaned from the topical decongestant. The use of intranasal corticosteroids may be beneficial to manage symptoms during the weaning process.

Answer a is incorrect. Rebound nasal congestion is not an adverse effect related to intranasal corticosteroids. Intranasal corticosteroids are effective at managing nasal congestion associated with allergic rhinitis.

Answer c is incorrect. Rebound nasal congestion is not an adverse effect related to intranasal antihistamines.

Answer d is incorrect. Rebound nasal congestion is not an adverse effect related to oral decongestants, only topical decongestants.

---

17. Which of the following medications must be kept behind the pharmacy counter, since it may be used in the production of methamphetamine?

    a. Brompheniramine
    b. Chlorpheniramine
    c. Phenylephrine
    d. Pseudoephedrine

Answer d is correct. The Combat Methamphetamine Act of 2005 prohibited over-the-counter sales of pseudo-ephedrine. It also placed restrictions on the amounts of pseudoephedrine that could be purchased by individuals during a given month. Additional rules and restrictions apply in various states, including requiring photo identification for purchase of pseudoephedrine, maintenance of pseudo-ephedrine purchase logs, and, in some states, designation of pseudoephedrine as a Category V-controlled substance.

Answer a is incorrect. Brompheniramine has no sales restrictions.

Answer b is incorrect. Chlorpheniramine has no sales restrictions.

Answer c is incorrect. Phenylephrine has no sales restrictions and has replaced pseudoephedrine in many over-the-counter products.

---

18. NH is a 35-year-old woman who is taking a combination of cetirizine, intranasal fluticasone, pseudoephedrine, and montelukast to manage symptoms of persistent allergic rhinitis. She complains of feeling jittery and having palpitations after taking all of her medications in the morning. Which of the following medications is most likely causing her complaints?

    a. Cetirizine
    b. Fluticasone
    c. Montelukast
    d. Pseudoephedrine

Answer d is correct. Because of its sympathomimetic properties, pseudoephedrine is well known to cause anxiety, restlessness, tachycardia, and palpitations.

Answer a is incorrect. Oral antihistamines are infrequently associated with tachycardia or feelings of anxiety.

Answer b is incorrect. Fluticasone has minimal systemic absorption and is not associated with these adverse effects.

Answer c is incorrect. Montelukast has rarely been associated with feelings of anxiety and is not known to cause tachycardia.

---

19. TR is a 6-year-old boy with persistent allergic rhinitis. He is experiencing symptoms despite the use of an oral antihistamine, and the physician would like to add an intranasal corticosteroid. Which of the following is correct regarding the use of an intranasal corticosteroid for TR?

    a. Intranasal corticosteroids should not be combined with oral antihistamines in pediatric patients.

b. Growth may be slower in children while using intranasal corticosteroids.

c. The use of intranasal corticosteroids is contraindicated in children less than 12 years of age.

d. TR should obtain relief of his symptoms within minutes of using the intranasal corticosteroid.

Answer b is correct. Intranasal corticosteroids have been associated with growth suppression in children and growth may be slowed when children use these products.

Answer a is incorrect. Intranasal corticosteroids can be combined safely with oral antihistamines in pediatric patients.

Answer c is incorrect. Intranasal corticosteroids can be used in children as young as 2 years.

Answer d is incorrect. Intranasal corticosteroids do not provide immediate relief of symptoms. Partial relief may occur in several hours, but full effects may take 2 weeks to be achieved.

20. KW is a 45-year-old woman who experiences daily rhinorrhea despite the use of loratadine and intranasal fluticasone. Addition of which of the following medications would best target the symptoms of rhinorrhea?

a. Azelastine

b. Ipratropium

c. Oxymetazoline

d. Phenylephrine

Answer b is correct. Intranasal ipratropium specifically targets the symptom of rhinorrhea due to its antisecretory effects. Patients with problematic rhinorrhea despite existing drug therapy may benefit from addition of an intranasal anticholinergic agent such as ipratropium.

Answer a is incorrect. Since KW is already taking an oral antihistamine, addition of a topical antihistamine does not provide additional benefit.

Answer c is incorrect. Intranasal decongestants do not improve rhinorrhea, only nasal congestion.

Answer d is incorrect. Oral decongestants are best for congestion, not rhinorrhea.

CHAPTER **65 | Urology**

1. Which of the following is the brand name for dutasteride?

a. Hytrin®

b. Flomax®

c. Proscar®

d. Avodart®

e. Cardura®

Answer d is correct.

Answer a is incorrect. The generic name for Hytrin® is terazosin.

Answer b is incorrect. The generic name for Flomax® is tamsulosin.

Answer c is incorrect. The generic name for Proscar® is finasteride.

Answer e in incorrect. The generic name for Cardura® is doxazosin.

2. An 82-year-old patient, taking 2 mg of terazosin for BPH, comes into the pharmacy complaining of dizziness and generalized muscle weakness and persistent LUTS. What would you recommend to his physician?

a. Add finasteride 5 mg daily to his regimen

b. Switch his terazosin to doxazosin 4 mg

c. Switch his terazosin to tamsulosin 0.4 mg daily

d. Lower the dose of his terazosin to 1 mg

e. Add saw palmetto twice daily

Answer c is correct. Tamsulosin may afford better tolerability for this patient and would be expected to provide symptom relief relatively quickly, often within 1 week of therapy, as it does not require titration.

Answer a is incorrect. The patient is complaining of dizziness associated with his α-blocker therapy. Adding finasteride will not ameliorate this and, if a 5ARI were added, it may take several months to show benefit in symptom reduction.

Answer b is incorrect. Exchanging one long acting second generation agent for another would not be ideal and this patient may continue to experience the same side effects.

Answer d is incorrect. Lowering his dose of terazosin may improve tolerability; however, he still is experiencing symptoms of BPH. If his dose was lowered, he would likely continue to experience his symptoms.

Answer e is incorrect. Based on lack of clinical outcomes, phytotherapy is not recommended by the AUA for treatment of BPH.

3. What pregnancy category is finasteride?

a. A

b. B

c. C

d. D

e. X

Answer e is correct. 5ARIs are associated with male birth defects. 5ARI, including finasteride and dutasteride, should not be taken or handled by women who are pregnant or women of child-bearing age.

Answers a, b, c, and d are incorrect.

4. A patient reports that he has been taking his finasteride daily for the last 6 months for BPH. His last PSA was 2.6 ng/mL.

Today it is 1.3 ng/mL. This can be best explained by which of the following:

a. Finasteride stops the prostate from producing PSA.
b. Finasteride can cause erroneous results in laboratory testing for PSA.
c. PSA levels are often significantly decreased in patients taking 5ARI.
d. Finasteride has no effect on the PSA level.

Answer c is correct. As finasteride decreases the size of the prostate, there is less prostate volume to produce PSA. PSA levels can be expected to decrease as much as 50% after beginning therapy with either finasteride or dutasteride.

Answer a is incorrect. The prostate still produces PSA after patients begin taking 5ARI therapy.

Answer b is incorrect. The decrease in PSA is not an anomaly associated with erroneous laboratory testing for PSA.

Answer d is incorrect. Finasteride has a significant effect on the PSA level.

---

5. A patient planning on having cataract surgery next week presents with a prescription for tamsulosin. His symptoms are not bothersome but reports urinary hesitancy and straining. You decide to:

a. Fill the prescription and counsel the patient on risk of sexual side effects.
b. Call his physician and ophthalmologist and get his order changed to finasteride.
c. Call his physician and ophthalmologist to determine if treatment with tamsulosin should be deferred until after his cataract surgery.
d. Fill the prescription and counsel on risk of dizziness and orthostatic hypotension.
e. Call his physician and get his order changed to terazosin.

Answer c is correct. Use of tamsulosin prior to cataract surgery is associated with surgical complications. While these can be treated, it may be prudent to determine if treatment can be deferred until after his procedure. His physician and ophthalmologist should be made aware of his intention to start this medication prior to cataract surgery.

Answer a is incorrect. While tamsulosin can cause sexual side effects including ejaculatory disturbances, this is not the best answer.

Answer b is incorrect. Candidates for 5ARI include those with large prostate volume (typically greater than 40 g). Without this information, it would be difficult to recommend finasteride for this patient.

Answer d is incorrect. As stated above, use of tamsulosin prior to cataract surgery may increase risk for surgical complications that may be prevented by deferring treatment.

Answer e is incorrect. Surgical complications have been associated with all α-blockers. At this time, informing his

physician and discussing this issue with the patient is the best answer.

---

6. Which of the following is an advantage of tamsulosin when compared to doxazosin? Select all that apply.

a. Increased efficacy in reducing LUTS
b. Decreased orthostatic hypotension
c. Quicker onset of action in lowering symptoms
d. Decreased syncope

Answers b and d are correct. Tolerability is improved with use of tamsulosin as it specifically targets α_{1A}-receptors in the prostate. Discontinuation rates and cardiovascular side effects are reduced in patients taking tamsulosin versus other second generation α-blockers (doxazosin and terazosin).

Answer c is correct. As tamsulosin does not require titration to reach an effective dose, its effects are seen often within the first week of therapy.

Answer a is incorrect. Tamsulosin is not more efficacious than other α-blockers. Most α-blockers, including doxazosin, will lower the AUA Symptom Score 4-6 points.

---

7. Which of the following is responsible for increased prostate growth?

a. PSA
b. DHT
c. 5-α reductase
d. Testosterone

Answer b is correct. Androgens, specifically DHT, bind to androgen receptors and increase expression of genes that control prostate growth. For this reason, use of 5ARI, which inhibit the conversion of testosterone to DHT, are therapeutic targets to prevent this process.

Answer a is incorrect. As PSA is *produced* by the prostate, it may be high in patients with an enlarged prostate. However, it does not directly *cause* an increase in prostate growth.

Answer c is incorrect. While 5-α reductase facilitates the conversion of testosterone to DHT, it is simply the enzyme and is not directly responsible for increasing prostate growth. As stated above, by inhibiting 5-α reductase, production of DHT is reduced and the latter is what is directly responsible for prostate growth.

Answer d is incorrect. Testosterone binds to androgen receptors; however, it freely dissociates as well. DHT is the chief androgen involved in prostate growth and the target of 5ARI therapy.

---

8. Select the statement that correctly describes ED.

a. Individuals with diabetes are at higher risk.
b. It is uncommon in the United States.
c. It generally afflicts younger men.

d. Individuals with above normal blood pressure are protected.

e. Smokers are less likely to develop the condition.

Answer a is correct. Individuals with diabetes are three times more likely to develop ED. ED develops in diabetics because of the vascular and neurologic changes that may occur.

Answer b is incorrect. It is very common in the United States, with as many as 20 million men affected.

Answer c is incorrect. The prevalence of ED increases with increasing age. At 40 years of age, up to 5% of men are afflicted with complete to severe dysfunction. This increases to 15% to 25% in men over 65.

Answer d is incorrect. Hypertension is considered a risk factor for the development of ED.

Answer e is incorrect. Smoking increases the likelihood of ED.

---

9. Select a vascular cause of ED.

a. Depression
b. Parkinson disease
c. Hypogonadism
d. Anxiety
e. Dyslipidemia

Answer e is correct. Dyslipidemia can result in vascular changes that can result in ED.

Answer a is incorrect. The vascular component is an important cause of ED. Depression may have a psychological impact that could result in ED but does not affect the vascular system.

Answer b is incorrect. Parkinson disease can lead to ED because of its effect on the nervous system. It may also present as a psychological cause.

Answer c is incorrect. Decreased levels of testosterone may contribute to ED, but hypogonadism is not a vascular cause.

Answer d is incorrect. Performance anxiety may be a cause of ED. Generalized anxiety may be a psychological cause. The vascular system is not affected in anxiety.

---

10. Select the item that should be part of an evaluation of ED. Select all that apply.

a. A sexual history from the patient and partner
b. A medical history
c. A physical examination
d. A psychosocial assessment

Answers a, b, c, and d are correct. All of the above items are part of a comprehensive workup for ED.

---

11. KR is a 62-year-old Hispanic male with a history of hypertension. He complains of ED for which he seeks treatment. There is no identifiable organic cause for his ED. Select the statement that correctly describes the approach to treatment in this patient.

a. PDE5 inhibitors would not be the treatment of choice in this patient.
b. PDE5 inhibitors are less efficacious in Hispanics.
c. The use of a PDE5 inhibitor is not likely to be effective in this patient with hypertension.
d. A PDE5 inhibitor would exert its activity by enhancing the effect of nitric oxide.
e. He should not receive a PDE5 inhibitor because sexual intercourse would not be advisable because of his cardiac status.

Answer d is correct. PDE5 inhibitors exert their activity by enhancing the activity of nitric oxide.

Answer a is incorrect. PDE5 inhibitors are the treatment of choice in patients with ED that do not have an identifiable cause for their ED.

Answer b is incorrect. PDE5 inhibitors are effective in all ethnic groups.

Answer c is incorrect. PDE5 inhibitors are effective in patients with hypertension that develop ED.

Answer e is incorrect. There is no condition present in KR that would make sexual intercourse inadvisable.

---

12. DL is a 59-year-old Caucasian male with a history of BPH that is adequately managed with doxazosin who comes to the office with concerns about ED. His workup is unremarkable and a decision is made to start treatment with a PDE5 inhibitor. Select the statement that correctly describes treatment in this patient.

a. DL should be advised to take the medication immediately prior to sexual intercourse.
b. Use of a PDE5 inhibitor could lead to postural hypotension.
c. PDE5 inhibitors are contraindicated in patients with BPH.
d. The medication of choice would be sildenafil because of its greater efficacy.
e. The use of a PDE5 inhibitor is contraindicated in a patient receiving doxazosin.

Answer b is correct. PDE5 inhibitors cause some decrease in blood pressure in patients with normal blood pressure. Individuals that are also receiving α-blockers may have a more significant drop in blood pressure leading to postural hypotension or dizziness. Individuals on both medications should be cautioned about this potential drug interaction.

Answer a is incorrect. PDE5 inhibitors should be taken 30 to 60 minutes before anticipated intercourse.

Answer c in incorrect. PDE5 inhibitors are effective in patients with ED that have BPH.

Answer d is incorrect. There is no convincing evidence that one PDE5 inhibitor is more effective than another.

Answer e is incorrect. Taking the α-blocker doxazosin with a PDE5 inhibitor may lead to postural hypotension and dizziness but their use together is not contraindicated.

---

13. JC is a 72-year-old African-American male with ED and no contraindication to the use of a PDE5 inhibitor. Which of the following medications could potentially interact and lead to increased serum concentrations of the PDE5 inhibitor?

    a. Erythromycin
    b. Aspirin
    c. Ampicillin
    d. Haloperidol
    e. Influenza vaccine

Answer a is correct. Erythromycin inhibits the CYP3A4 enzyme system in the liver and impairs the metabolism of PDE5 inhibitors. The dose of the PDE5 inhibitor should be reduced.

Answer b is incorrect. Aspirin does not interact with PDE5 inhibitors.

Answer c is incorrect. Antibiotics are not known to interact with PDE5 inhibitors.

Answer d is incorrect. The use of antipsychotics may result in ED by causing hyperprolactinemia, but they do not affect the serum concentration of PDE5 inhibitors.

Answer e is incorrect. Vaccines do not interact with PDE5 inhibitors.

---

14. Select the brand name for tadalafil.

    a. Relenza®
    b. Viagra®
    c. Enzyte®
    d. Cialis®
    e. Levitra®

Answer d is correct.

Answer a is incorrect. The generic name of Relenza® is zanamivir.

Answer b is incorrect. The generic name of Viagra® is sildenafil.

Answer c is incorrect. Enzyte® is an over-the-counter product marketed for the treatment of ED.

Answer e is incorrect. The generic name of Levitra® is vardenafil.

---

15. Which statement best describes alprostadil?

    a. It should be the first agent tried for the treatment of ED.
    b. It is a nonspecific PDE5 inhibitor.
    c. It can be administered via a medicated transurethral suppository.
    d. Priapism has not been reported with the use of alprostadil.

    e. It exerts its activity by constricting smooth muscle in the penis.

Answer c is correct. A unique delivery system called Muse® places the drug into the urethra where it diffuses across the urethra into the body of the penis. The drug can also be administered by intracavernosal injection.

Answer a is incorrect. PDE5 inhibitors are the first-line choice for the treatment of ED unless there is a contraindication. Alprostadil is used when they are ineffective or cannot be tolerated.

Answer b is incorrect. Alprostadil works through its activity as a prostaglandin E_1 agonist. It causes vasodilation of the penile arteries by relaxing smooth muscle. Papaverine is a nonspecific phosphodiesterase inhibitor.

Answer d is incorrect. Priapism and prolonged erection can occur with the use of alprostadil.

Answer e is incorrect. The mechanism of action does not include vasoconstriction.

---

16. LT, a 75-year-old woman, has severe renal impairment (CrCl <30 mL/min). Which of the following are options for UUI? Select all that apply.

    a. Oxybutynin transdermal patch
    b. Tolterodine ER
    c. Solifenacin
    d. Oxybutynin IR
    e. Trospium chloride ER

Answer a is correct. Any delivery system of oxybutynin does not need to be renally adjusted in severe renal impairment.

Answer b is correct. Although it is cleared renally, the dose can be decreased and be used in patients with severe renal impairment.

Answer c is correct. Although it is cleared renally, the dose can be decreased and be used in patients with severe renal impairment.

Answer d is correct. Any delivery system of oxybutynin does not need to be renally adjusted in severe renal impairment.

Answer e is incorrect. The ER trospium chloride only comes in one dose for patients with CrCl >30 mL/min. It should not be used in severe impairment due to increased side effects.

---

17. Which subtype of muscarinic receptor is the primary target of antimuscarinics in patients with OAB?

    a. M_1
    b. M_2
    c. M_3
    d. M_4
    e. M_5

Answer c is correct. Antimuscarinics' therapeutic target is the M_3 receptors of the bladder.

Answer a is incorrect. A majority of the M_1 receptors are located in the CNS.

Answer b is incorrect. Although M_2 receptors can be found in the bladder, they are not clinically significant in UI.

Answers d and e are incorrect. M_4 and M_5 receptors are not clinically significant in UI.

18. TV, a 55-year-old woman, is postmenopausal. Along with UI, this patient is also suffering from symptoms of vaginal dryness, burning, and itching. Which of the following would be the best pharmacologic option for her?

    a. Oral estrogen
    b. Duloxetine
    c. OnabotulinumtoxinA
    d. Topical estrogen

Answer d is correct. The symptoms listed above describe vaginal atrophy. Micronized 17-β estradiol (Vagifem) is indicated for vaginal atrophy.

Answer a is incorrect. Studies have proven that postmeno-pausal women taking oral estrogen have an increased risk in UI.

Answer b is incorrect. Duloxetine is used in SUI.

Answer c is incorrect. Botulinum toxin is used for patients refractory or intolerant to antimuscarinics.

19. Which of the following are nonpharmacologic options for a patient with UI?

    a. Weight reduction
    b. Decrease fluid intake
    c. Increase intake of caffeine
    d. Pelvic floor exercises

Answer a is correct. Weight reduction is a suitable nonpharmacologic option for UI.

Answer b is correct. Decrease fluid intake is a suitable nonpharmacologic option.

Answer d is correct. Pelvic floor exercises are a suitable nonpharmacologic option.

Answer c is incorrect. A decrease in intake of caffeine is a suitable nonpharmacologic option for UI.

20. What type of incontinence can be described as having urinary urgency, frequency, and nocturia along with leakage during exercise?

    a. SUI
    b. UUI
    c. OI
    d. Mixed incontinence
    e. Functional incontinence

Answer d is correct. The above symptoms describe both OAB and SUI and therefore are defined as mixed inconti-nence because it is more than one type of UI.

Answer a is incorrect. The above symptoms are not SUI alone.

Answer b is incorrect. The above symptoms are not UUI alone.

Answer c in incorrect. The above symptoms are not OI alone.

Answer e is incorrect. The above symptoms are not caused by functional or cognitive impairments.

21. What is the brand name for mirabegron?

    a. Detrol LA
    b. Ditropan
    c. Myrbetriq
    d. Vesicare
    e. Sanctura XR

Answer c is correct.

Answer a is incorrect. The brand name is Tolterodine.

Answer b is incorrect. The brand name is oxybutynin.

Answer d is incorrect. The brand name is solifenacin.

Answer e is incorrect. The brand name is trospium chloride.

CHAPTER 66 | Vaccines and Immunizations

1. Which of the following can safely be given to a 6-month-old child who had an allergic reaction to the pertussis vaccine?

    a. DTaP
    b. Tdap
    c. Td
    d. DT

Answer d is correct. DT is indicated for the prevention of diphtheria and tetanus in children less than 7 years of age. It does not contain the pertussis vaccine. It should be used in children who have previously had an allergic reaction to the pertussis vaccine.

Answer a is incorrect. DTaP is indicated for the preven-tion of diphtheria, tetanus, and pertussis in children less than 7 years. However, it contains the pertussis vaccine and should not be used in a patient who has had an allergic reaction to the pertussis vaccine.

Answer b is incorrect. Tdap is FDA approved for use as a single booster dose in adolescents and adults between the ages of 11 and 64 years. ACIP recommends it for patients as young as 7 years and adults over the age of 65 years as a single booster dose due to the current pertussis outbreak. It also contains the pertussis vaccine. It should not be used in a 6-month-old who is allergic to the pertussis vaccine.

Answer c is incorrect. Even though Td does not contain the pertussis vaccine, it is indicated for use as a booster dose in adolescents and adults over the age of 7 years. It would not be appropriate to use this vaccine in a 6-month-old child.

2. KS, a 5-year-old girl, has an appointment today with her pediatrician to receive vaccines. Her vaccination record shows the following: Hep B at birth, 2 months, and 6 months; RV at 2, 4, and 6 months; DTaP at 2, 4, 6, and 15 months; Hib (ActHIB®) at 2, 4, 6, and 15 months; PCV at 2, 4, 6, and 15 months; IPV at 2, 4, and 6 months; MMR at 15 months; Varicella at 15 months; and Hep A at 15 months. She does not have any medical conditions and is not allergic to any medications or vaccines. What vaccines should KS receive today?

   a. DT, PPSV, IPV, MMR, MCV, and Hep A
   b. DTaP, IPV, MMR, Varicella, and Hep A
   c. Tdap, IPV, MMR, Varicella, and Hep A
   d. DTaP, PPSV, IPV, MMR, Varicella, and Hep A

Answer b is correct. KS has received four doses in the DTaP series already and therefore needs to receive the fifth and final DTaP dose. She has also received three doses of IPV and should receive the fourth dose today. KS received her first doses of the MMR and varicella vaccines at 15 months. She needs to receive the second dose of each today. Since KS only received one dose of the Hep A vaccine at 15 months, she needs to complete the two-dose series today. Even though it has been several years since the first dose, she does not need to start the series over again. She only needs one dose of the Hep A vaccine.

Answer a is incorrect. DT is indicated for children less than 7 years of age who have had an allergic reaction to the pertussis vaccine. KS has no vaccine allergies so DTaP should be used. PPSV should only be administered in high risk patients—KS does not have any conditions that would warrant administration of PPSV. It is recommended that adolescents receive the MCV at age 11 or 12 years. Children may receive it earlier if they are at high risk for meningococcal disease. Since KS is only 5 years old and does not have any risk factors for meningococcal disease, she should not receive MCV. Also, she needs to receive the second doses of MMR and Varicella.

Answer c is incorrect. Tdap should only be used as a single booster dose in patients at least 7 years of age. KS is too young to receive Tdap. Also, she will not need a booster until she has completed the five-dose series of DTaP.

Answer d is incorrect. PPSV should only be administered in high risk patients—KS does not have any conditions that would warrant administration of PPSV.

3. Which of the following vaccines is only given as a single dose?

   a. PCV
   b. Zoster
   c. RV
   d. Td

Answer b is correct. The zoster vaccine only requires one dose.

Answer a is incorrect. PCV requires four doses given at 2, 4, 6, and 12 to 15 months of age. Adults 19 years of age and older who are at high risk (cochlear implant, asplenia, cerebrospinal fluid leaks, immunocompromising condition, or immunosuppressive therapy) should receive one dose of PCV.

Answer c is incorrect. The RV vaccines require multiple doses. RotaTeq® requires three doses at 2, 4, and 6 months. Rotarix® requires two doses at 2 and 4 months of age.

Answer d is incorrect. Adults require a booster dose with Td every 10 years.

4. Which of the following pediatric vaccines is administered orally?

   a. IPV
   b. PCV
   c. RV
   d. Varicella

Answer c is correct. RV is the only vaccine listed that is administered orally.

Answer a is incorrect. IPV can be administered IM or SC. It cannot be administered orally.

Answer b is incorrect. PCV is administered IM, not orally.

Answer d is incorrect. The varicella vaccine is administered SC, not orally.

5. A 69-year-old man comes into your pharmacy after receiving a letter advertising your immunization program. He has diabetes and hypertension and smokes a pack of cigarettes a day. He does not have any medication or vaccine allergies. His vaccination record shows that he completed all of his childhood vaccinations (DTaP, Hib, PCV, IPV, and MMR) as well as the Hep B series, he had the chickenpox when he was 5 years old, and received his last Td booster 11 years ago. Which vaccines should this patient receive TODAY?

   a. Td, Zoster, PPSV, and Hep A
   b. Tdap, Varicella, and PPSV
   c. Td, Zoster, and PPSV
   d. Tdap, RZV, and PCV

Answer d is correct. This patient needs a tetanus-diphtheria-pertussis booster because it has been over 10 years since his last tetanus booster and ACIP now recommends use of Tdap in patients 65 years and older. He is a candidate for zoster because he is over the age of 60. He is a candidate for both the PCV and the PPSV vaccines because he is over 65.

He should receive the PCV vaccine first and receive PPSV in 12 months as this is the preferred spacing.

Answer a is incorrect. This patient needs a tetanus-diphtheria-pertussis booster because it has been over 10 years since his last tetanus booster and ACIP now recommends use of Tdap in patients 65 years and older. He is also a candidate for the zoster vaccine as well as the PCV and PPSV vaccine since he is over 60 and 65 years old, respectfully. He is not a candidate for Hep A vaccination because he is not a child and does not have any risk factors for Hep A infection.

Answer b is incorrect. This patient does need a tetanus-diphtheria-pertussis booster because it has been over 10 years since his last tetanus booster and ACIP now recommends use of Tdap in patients 65 years and older. Varicella is indicated in children greater than 12 months and adults without documented evidence of varicella immunity (eg, previous vaccination or documented case of chicken pox). Since he has had the chickenpox, he is not a candidate for varicella vaccination. He is a candidate for PPSV because he is over the age of 65; however, he should receive the PCV vaccine first.

Answer c is incorrect. This patient needs a tetanus-diphtheria-pertussis booster because it has been over 10 years since his last tetanus booster and ACIP now recommends use of Tdap in patients 65 years and older. He is a candidate for zoster and PPSV vaccines because he is over the age of 60 and 65, respectfully; however, he should receive the PCV vaccine first.

6. Which of the following diphtheria and tetanus vaccines should be used in adults as a one-time booster dose?

   a. Td
   b. DT
   c. Tdap
   d. DTaP

Answer c is correct. Adolescents and adults will require a booster dose of the pertussis vaccine once in their lifetime. It is recommended that one Td booster be replaced by a Tdap booster once in patients over the age of 7 years. Pregnant females are the only patients who receive repeat dosing of Tdap—they receive one dose in their third trimester with each pregnancy.

Answer a is incorrect. Adults will require a Td booster every 10 years.

Answer b is incorrect. DT is only indicated for children less than 7 years of age who have a contraindication to the pertussis vaccine.

Answer d is incorrect. DTaP is only indicated for children less than 7 years of age.

7. Which of the following adults under the age of 65 would require a PPSV? Select all that apply.

   a. Pregnant women
   b. Smokers

   c. Heart failure patients
   d. Hypertensive patients

Answer b is correct. Adults who smoke are considered to be at high risk for pneumococcal disease and therefore should receive PPSV.

Answer c is correct. Patients with chronic heart disease, such as heart failure, should receive PPSV.

Answer a is incorrect. Pregnant women are not considered to be at high risk for pneumococcal disease.

Answer d is incorrect. Patients with chronic heart disease should receive PPSV; however, patients who only have hypertension are not considered at high risk for invasive pneumococcal disease. It is not recommended to vaccinate hypertensive patients with PPSV.

8. How should the Hep B vaccine be administered?

   a. In the deltoid muscle at a 90° angle
   b. In the deltoid muscle at a 45° angle
   c. In the outer aspect of the triceps at a 45° angle
   d. In the anterolateral thigh at a 45° angle

Answer a is correct. The Hep B vaccine is administered IM and should be given in the deltoid muscle (for adults) and the anterolateral thigh (for infants) at a 90° angle.

Answer b is incorrect. Injections in the deltoid muscle should be given at a 90° angle.

Answer c is incorrect. Subcutaneous injections are given in the outer aspect of the triceps at a 45° angle. The Hep B vaccine is given IM.

Answer d is incorrect. Infants can receive intramuscular injections in the anterolateral thigh; however, it should be given at a 90° angle.

9. EP is pregnant and in her third trimester. Which of the following vaccines can EP receive? Select all that apply.

   a. HPV
   b. Hep B
   c. MMR
   d. Tdap

Answer b is correct. The Hep B vaccine can be administered to a pregnant female who has not received the vaccination before.

Answer d is correct. ACIP recommends that pregnant females in their third trimester receive one dose of Tdap with every pregnancy.

Answer a is incorrect. The HPV vaccine should not be administered to pregnant females because it is contraindicated in pregnancy.

Answer c is incorrect. The MMR vaccine is a live vaccine. Pregnant women should not receive live vaccines.

10. An 11-year-old woman fainted after receiving her 11 to 12-year-old routine vaccinations. Which of the following vaccines most likely caused her to faint?

    a. Tdap
    b. HPV
    c. MCV
    d. Hep B

Answer b is correct. The HPV vaccine has been associated with syncope after administration. It is recommended that patients remain seated or lie down for 15 minutes after receiving the vaccine.

Answer a is incorrect. Tdap has not been associated with syncope.

Answer c is incorrect. MCV has not been associated with syncope.

Answer d is incorrect. The Hep B vaccine has not been associated with syncope.

11. The live herpes zoster vaccine (ZVL) should be stored at what temperature?

    a. ≤5°F
    b. 6°F to 35°F
    c. 36°F to 46° F
    d. 47°F to 77° F

Answer a is correct. The herpes zoster vaccine needs to be kept frozen. Frozen vaccines should be stored in a freezer with a temperature less than 5°F.

Answer b is incorrect. Storing the herpes zoster vaccine at temperatures above 5°F can lead to loss of potency.

Answer c is incorrect. Vaccines that require refrigeration should be stored at temperatures between 36°F and 46°F. The herpes zoster vaccine should be kept frozen.

Answer d is incorrect. Temperatures between 47°F and 77°F are considered room temperature. The herpes zoster vaccine should be kept frozen.

12. JM, a 6-month-old infant is seeing his pediatrician today in order to receive his 6-month vaccinations. His vaccination records are as follows: Hep B at birth and 2 months; DTaP at 2 and 4 months; Hib (PedvaxHIB®) at 2 and 4 months; PCV at 2 and 4 months; and IPV at 2 and 4 months. JM does not have any medical conditions or allergies to medications or vaccines. Which vaccines should JM receive today?

    a. Hep B, RV, DTaP, Hib, PCV, and IPV
    b. Hep B, RV, DTaP, PCV, and IPV
    c. Hep B, DTaP, Hib, PCV, and IPV
    d. Hep B, DTaP, PCV, and IPV

Answer d is correct. At 6 months, JM will need his third dose of Hep B, DTaP, PCV, and IPV.

Answer a is incorrect. At 6 months, JM should receive the third dose of Hep B. He should not receive the RV vaccine because he is too old. The first dose of the RV vaccine needs to be administered by the age of 14 weeks 6 days. JM should receive the third dose of DTaP at 6 months. He does not need a third dose of the Hib vaccine because PedvaxHIB® is only a two-dose series and he does not need the booster dose until 12 to 15 months of age. JM should receive his third dose of PCV and IPV.

Answer b is incorrect. At 6 months, JM will need his third dose of Hep B, DTaP, PCV, and IPV. However, he should not receive the RV vaccine because he is too old. It is too late to start the series in JM.

Answer c is incorrect. At 6 months, JM will need his third dose of Hep B, DTaP, PCV, and IPV. Since he received his first two Hib vaccinations with PedvaxHIB®, he does not need a third dose.

13. A 68-year-old female patient calls your pharmacy complaining of a rash on the left side of her midsection. It wraps around her side; however, it doesn't cross her spine or belly button. She informs you that it doesn't itch; however, it is very painful. It started to appear 2 days ago. She thinks it is shingles and remembers having chickenpox as a child. She would like to know how she got this infection since she doesn't remember being around anyone recently who has had shingles. Which of the following statements should be included in your consultation with her regarding how she got the herpes zoster infection?

    a. The VZV causes shingles. It originally presents as the chickenpox rash, then lays dormant in the spine and can reemerge years later presenting as shingles.
    b. The VZV causes shingles. She had to have come into contact with someone who had an active case of shingles in order to get it herself.
    c. The VZV causes shingles. She had to have come into contact with someone who had an active case of chickenpox. She got shingles from it since she has already had chickenpox.
    d. The VZV only causes chickenpox. She had to have come into contact with another virus that causes shingles.

Answer a is correct. The VZV causes two conditions—chickenpox and shingles. Chickenpox is the primary infection. Once the infection has cleared, the VZV lies dormant in the sensory dorsal root ganglia of the spine. It reactivates years later to cause the shingles infection.

Answer b is incorrect. The VZV causes two conditions—chickenpox and shingles. Chickenpox is the primary infection. Once the infection has cleared, the VZV lies dormant in the sensory dorsal root ganglia of the spine. It reactivates years later to cause the shingles infection. Reactivation occurs because the patient's immunity to VZV decreases overtime, not because they came into contact with someone who had shingles.

Answer c is incorrect. The VZV causes two conditions—chickenpox and shingles. Chickenpox is the primary infection. Once the infection has cleared, the VZV lies dormant in the sensory dorsal root ganglia of the spine. It reactivates years later to cause the shingles infection. Reactivation occurs because the patient's immunity to VZV decreases overtime, not because they came into contact with someone who had chickenpox.

Answer d is incorrect. The VZV causes two conditions—chickenpox and shingles. Chickenpox is the primary infection. Once the infection has cleared, the VZV lies dormant in the sensory dorsal root ganglia of the spine. It reactivates years later to cause the shingles infection. Reactivation occurs because the patient's immunity to VZV decreases overtime, not because they came into contact with another, different, virus.

---

14. Which of the following patients can receive the Hib vaccine? Select all that apply.

   a. A 4-month-old child
   b. A 20-year-old smoker
   c. A 58-year-old man with leukemia
   d. A 26-year-old with asplenia

Answer a in correct. The Hib vaccine should be administered to children at 2, 4, and 12 to 15 months. An additional dose at 6 months is required if the child is vaccinated with ActHIB®.

Answer c is correct. A patient with leukemia may benefit from receiving the Hib vaccine.

Answer d is correct. A patient with functional or anatomical asplenia may benefit from receiving the Hib vaccine.

Answer b is incorrect. The Hib vaccine is generally not recommended in patients over the age of 5 years. However, administering one dose to patients with sickle cell disease, leukemia, Human Immunodeficiency Virus (HIV) infection, or who have had a splenectomy, is not contraindicated and should be considered. Smoking is not an indication to receive the Hib vaccine.

---

15. How should the live herpes zoster vaccine (ZVL) be administered?

   a. In the deltoid muscle at a 90° angle
   b. In the deltoid muscle at a 45° angle
   c. In the outer aspect of the triceps at a 45° angle
   d. In the anterolateral thigh at a 45° angle

Answer c is correct. The herpes zoster vaccine should be administered SC. Subcutaneous injections are given in the outer aspect of the triceps at a 45° angle.

Answer a is incorrect. The herpes zoster vaccine should be administered SC. Intramuscular injections are given in the deltoid muscle at a 90° angle.

Answer b is incorrect. The herpes zoster vaccine should be administered SC. Subcutaneous injections are given at a 45° angle; however, they are not given in the deltoid muscle.

Answer d is incorrect. The herpes zoster vaccine should be administered SC. Intramuscular injections are given to children in the anterolateral thigh at a 90° angle.

---

16. LM is an 18-year-old woman who is leaving for her first semester of college next month. She would like to know what vaccinations she needs before going to college. Her vaccination record shows the following: DTaP at 2, 4, 6, and 15 months, and 5 years; Hib (ActHIB®) at 2, 4, and 6 months; PCV at 2, 4, 6, and 15 months; IPV at 2, 4, and 6 months, and 5 years; MMR at 15 months and 5 years; Varicella at 15 months and 5 years; Hep A at 12 and 18 months; Hep B at 11 years, 11 years 2 months, and 11 years 6 months; and Tdap at 15 years. LM does not have any medical conditions and is not allergic to any medications or vaccines. What vaccines should LM receive today?

   a. MCV and HPV
   b. Tdap, MCV, and HPV
   c. Tdap and MCV
   d. PPSV and HPV

Answer a is correct. LM has not received the MCV or HPV vaccines. College freshman should receive the MCV vaccine if they have not previously been vaccinated. The HPV vaccine is recommended at age 11 to 12 years; however, it can be given in adult females up to the age of 26 who have not previously been vaccinated.

Answer b is incorrect. LM has completed her primary DTaP series and received a Tdap dose 3 years ago at the age of 15. She does not need another dose of Tdap. She will not need another Td booster for 7 years. LM does need the MCV and HPV vaccines.

Answer c is incorrect. LM has already received a Tdap booster and does not need another Td booster for 7 years. She does need to receive the MCV vaccine. She also needs the HPV vaccine because she has not previously received it.

Answer d is incorrect. LM does need to receive the HPV vaccine because she has not been vaccinated previously. She should also receive a meningococcal vaccine; however, the conjugate vaccine (MCV) is preferred over the polysaccharide vaccine (MPSV). If the MPSV vaccine is used, she would need to be revaccinated in 5 years with the MCV vaccine provided she remained at high risk for meningococcal disease.

---

17. TR, a 4-year-old girl, is in the doctor's office for her 4 to 6-year-old vaccinations. She has completed her Hep B, Hib, PCV, and Hep A series. She has no medical conditions and is not allergic

to any medications or vaccines. Five days ago she received the influenza vaccine. Which vaccines should TR receive today?

a. DTaP, IPV, MMR, and Varicella
b. DTaP, PPSV, IPV, and MMR
c. IPV only
d. DTaP and IPV

Answer a is correct. A 4-year-old girl who has completed her Hep B, Hib, PCV, and Hep A series would need to receive DTaP, IPV, MMR, and Varicella vaccinations. The fact that TR received an inactivated vaccine 5 days ago (the live attenuated influenza vaccine is currently not recommended) does not impact her ability to receive live or inactivated vaccines today.

Answer b is incorrect. PPSV should only be administered to children who have certain medical conditions (diabetes, asthma, cardiovascular disease, asplenia, or HIV infection). TR does not have any of these conditions.

Answer c is incorrect. TR needs the fifth dose of DTaP as well as the fourth dose of the IPV vaccine.

Answer d is incorrect. TR needs the fifth dose of DTaP, the fourth dose of the IPV vaccine, as well as the second doses of both MMR and Varicella.

18. When should the second dose of the Hep A vaccine be administered?

a. 28 days after the first dose
b. 2 months after the first dose
c. 6 months after the first dose
d. 30 days after the first dose

Answer c is correct. The two doses of the Hep A vaccine should be given 6 months apart.

Answers a, b, and d are incorrect.

19. Which of the following patients are at risk for Hep B infection and should be counseled to receive the Hep B vaccine to protect themselves? Select all that apply.

a. A 23-year-old man who has sex with men
b. A 58-year-old woman diabetic
c. A 63-year-old man with hypertension
d. A 34-year-old woman wound-care nurse

Answer a is correct. A man who has sex with men is considered at risk for Hep B infection and therefore should receive the Hep B vaccine.

Answer b is correct. ACIP now recommends diabetic patients aged 19 to 59 years of age receive the Hep B vaccine.

Answer d is correct. A wound-care nurse comes into contact with bodily fluids and is at risk for Hep B infection.

Answer c is incorrect. ACIP recommends that all infants receive the Hep B vaccine series starting at birth. Adolescents

previously unvaccinated should also receive the vaccine series. Adults at high risk who have not been previously vaccinated should also receive the vaccine series; hypertension is not considered a risk factor for Hep B infection.

20. Which of the following patients should receive the herpes zoster vaccine?

a. A 58-year-old diabetic
b. A 37-year-old without a spleen
c. A 68-year-old with hypertension
d. A 72-year-old allergic to neomycin

Answer c is correct. A 68-year-old with hypertension should receive the herpes zoster vaccine.

Answer a is incorrect. The herpes zoster vaccine is FDA approved for adults 50 years and older; however, ACIP still only recommends it for patients over the age of 60. A 58-year-old diabetic is too young to receive the vaccination, according to the current ACIP recommendations.

Answer b is incorrect. The herpes zoster vaccine should only be administered to adults over the age of 60, regardless of medical conditions.

Answer d is incorrect. The herpes zoster vaccine is a live vaccine and should not be administered to patients who are immunocompromised, pregnant, or allergic to gelatin or neomycin. This patient is 72 years old, but is also allergic to neomycin. He or she should not receive the herpes zoster vaccine.

CHAPTER 67 | Smoking Cessation

1. JT is a 47-year-old man who is interested in quitting smoking. He has smoked 1.5 packs per day for the last 17 years. He successfully quit cold turkey in the past that lasted for approximately 16 months, but went back to smoking after starting a new job. Based on the various components of nicotine dependence, which reason most likely caused JT to return to smoking?

a. Psychological dependence
b. Physiologic dependence
c. He did not use a pharmacologic aid to quit smoking.
d. Most persons will relapse within 24 months of a quit attempt.

Answer a is correct. While the physical addiction to nicotine resolves in 1 to 2 weeks after stopping smoking, the person will continue to have the cravings to perform the action of smoking. Because nicotine acts on the pleasure center and reward pathway in the brain, patients tend to equate smoking with pleasure and/or calming sensations. Since the body continues to achieve or recreate these sensations, the need to smoke persists indefinitely, but at diminished levels.

Answer b is incorrect. In the early weeks of tobacco cessation, patients will seek cigarettes to avoid withdrawal symptoms and the accompanying discomfort. These symptoms last for approximately 1 to 2 weeks. Since JT was abstinent from cigarettes for 16 months, the time period for physical withdrawal symptoms had passed.

Answer c is incorrect. The maintenance of a successful quit attempt is not altered by the modality in which a patient used to quit smoking. Since JT was able to quit cold turkey, his chances of relapsing are not increased.

Answer d is incorrect. While the risk of relapse back to smoking is continual and the number of patients who remain tobacco free dwindles with time, a patient cannot consider themselves without risk of relapse after 24 months.

Questions 2 and 3 are related to the same patient.

2. HN has decided that she would like to quit smoking, but is not comfortable quitting without supportive NRT. She decides that the gum will be her best choice because it is easily concealable among friends, family, and coworkers. She has smoked 1 to 1.5 packs per day for the last 13 years. What is the appropriate starting dose for the nicotine polacrilex gum for HN?

   a. 4-mg piece of gum; not to exceed 24 doses in 24 hours
   b. 4-mg piece of gum; not to exceed 20 doses in 24 hours
   c. 2-mg piece of gum; not to exceed 24 pieces in 24 hours
   d. Not enough information provided to determine the correct dosage strength for this patient

Answer d is correct. The recommended selection of dosage for this product is time to first cigarette. Since this case did not indicate if the patient has her first cigarette within the first 30 minutes after waking, then the clinician should specifically ask this question in order to select the most appropriate dosage.

Answers a, b, and c are incorrect. Nicotine gum and lozenges are dosed regarding their time to first cigarette. In the past, the gum was dosed based on numbers of cigarettes per day. However, the time to first cigarette provides a greater understanding and association with level of dependence.

3. Upon further consultation with HN, she indicates that she smokes within the 10 minutes after waking, when should HN reduce to the next dosage step/phase?

   a. She should not reduce the dosage formulation, but rather spread out the frequency of using the gum product.
   b. 8 weeks
   c. 6 weeks
   d. 4 weeks

Answer a is correct. When using the nicotine replacement products of the gum or lozenges, it is not recommended to alter dosage strengths.

Answers b, c, and d are incorrect. Since there is no reason for you to switch dosage strengths these answers would not make since. It is recommended for the patient to spread out the dosage schedule per the recommended package insert directions.

4. IO is 31 years old and starting a new job in a dental clinic. She wishes to quit smoking before she starts her new job because the clinic does not allow employees to smoke during their shift. However, she would also like to quit to preserve her lung health. She smokes approximately 15 cigarettes daily and has her first one in the car on the way to work (about 95 minutes after waking). She wishes to use the lozenges for her quit attempt. What product would you suggest that IO use?

   a. Nicotrol 4 mg
   b. Nicotrol 2 mg
   c. Commit 4 mg
   d. Commit 2 mg

Answer d is correct. IO's first cigarette is 95 minutes after waking in the morning, qualifying her to start with the 2-mg lozenge.

Answers a and b are incorrect. Nicotrol is not commercially available as a lozenge.

Answer c is incorrect. Just like the nicotine gum, nicotine lozenge dose is also based on the amount of time from waking in the morning to the person's first cigarette. If less than 30 minutes, then the dose is 4 mg. Being that IO's first cigarette of the day is approximately 95 minutes after waking, this dose would be too high.

5. Which condition can be made worse using nicotine polacrilex gum?

   a. TMJ disorder
   b. Gingival hyperplasia
   c. Oropharyngeal candidiasis
   d. Episodic epistaxis

Answer a is correct. TMJ disorder symptoms are worsened with repetitive chewing or chewing tough foods/items. Patients have to chew nicotine gum aggressively in order to use the nicotine gum; therefore, it may worsen TMJ symptoms.

Answer b is incorrect. While this condition may cause discomfort, its symptoms are not made worse with aggressive or repetitive chewing. The release and absorption of nicotine would not be affected.

Answer c is incorrect. Nicotine does not affect the immune function of the mouth and pharynx and will not increase the chances of a person developing oropharyngeal candidiasis.

Answer d is incorrect. The use of oral nicotine replacement products would not affect or be altered due to nasal irritation and nose bleedings.

6. JE is a 72-year-old man smoking one pack per day for the last 40 years smoking history. He has never attempted to quit smoking, but feels he must try after being hospitalized for pneumonia for 3 days. While he was in the hospital he was given a nicotine patch to wear and change daily until discharge. Upon discharge, he was not given the nicotine patch, but wants to continue using it to abstain from smoking. What dose of the patch should JE start?

    a. 21 mg/d patch

    b. 14 mg/d patch

    c. 7 mg/d patch

    d. He does not smoke enough to warrant NRT with a patch.

Answer a is correct. JE smokes approximately 20 cigarettes daily. The 21-mg nicotine patch is recommended for persons who smoke >10 cigarettes per day. He should continue this dose for approximately 6 weeks before decreasing to the 14-mg patch to maximize his chance of complete cessation.

Answer b is incorrect. A patient would only start on a 14-mg patch daily if he or she smoked <10 cigarettes per day *or* could not tolerate the adverse drug reactions (ADRs) associated with the 21-mg patch. If the patient were to start on the 14-mg patch, he or she should continue on this dose for approximately 6 weeks before decreasing the dose.

Answer c is incorrect. It is not recommended to start at a 7-mg patch daily unless the person requires NRT and cannot tolerate the 14-mg dose or 21-mg dose. If this dosage is selected, the patient may not be at the adequate dose to assist with the anticipated nicotine withdrawal symptoms and therefore the patient may indicate that after trying the 7-mg dose, this product was not effective and therefore may never try patch therapy again, if needed.

Answer d is incorrect. Since he smokes above 10 cigarettes per day he could use a nicotine patch in order to assist with cessation (per package inserts)

7. JE has been without a cigarette for 3 days with the help of the nicotine patch. On the fourth day, JE is under a great deal of stress and needs to go outside for a cigarette. Since he is still wearing the nicotine replacement patch, what adverse events will he most likely experience?

    a. Excess fatigue

    b. Lower extremity cramping

    c. Nausea, vomiting, and headache

    d. Tinnitus

Answer c is correct. Some of the most common signs and symptoms of nicotine toxicity include nausea, vomiting, headaches, increased blood pressure, and tachycardia. Since JE is already receiving a continuous supply of nicotine via the patch, the quick release of nicotine from the cigarette will only increase his chances of these side effects.

Answer a is incorrect. Most likely, JE will begin to experience symptoms consistent with anxiety and nervousness.

Answer b is incorrect. NRT while a patient is smoking appears to mimic a sympathetic overload. JE's lower extremities may feel anxious or overactive, but should not exhibit symptoms of traditional cramping.

Answer d is incorrect. Nicotine toxicity will not cause tinnitus and/or other hearing disturbances.

8. What would be a better choice for JE to use for breakthrough cravings while he is being treated with the nicotine patch?

    a. Nicorette gum

    b. Chantix 1 mg twice daily

    c. Zyban 150 mg twice daily

    d. He should not combine therapies for smoke tobacco cessation.

Answer a is correct. The nicotine patch will provide a basal release of nicotine to the patient over a 16- to 24-hour period. The Nicorette gum has the ability to provide the "quick fix" to help a person overcome a significant daytime craving. While the chances of developing nicotine toxicity increase when combining agents, the utility has proven to be better than any agent alone in resistant cases.

Answers b and c are incorrect. Each of the non-nicotine products that help patients quit smoking do not affect immediate craving issues. Varenicline will block nicotine receptor binding and gently stimulate the same receptors in an attempt to alleviate cravings all day. Bupropion will stabilize the dopaminergic response and reward pathway in the brain, but not provide instant relief.

Answer d is incorrect. In some patient cases, many of the best therapeutic options involve a combination of long-acting nicotine replacement product with an immediate release nicotine product.

Questions 9 through 11 are related to the same case.

9. OH is a 41-year-old woman with multiple psychiatric medical conditions. She started smoking approximately 5 years ago and has slowly increased her daily cigarette consumption to 2 packs per day. She started using Nicoderm CQ 21-mg patches, but has experienced various abnormal dreams, causing her to lose sleep over the last 3 nights. She will not continue using the patches if the dreams continue. What alternative(s) may OH trial to help combat this side effects?

    a. Nicoderm CQ 14 mg/d patch.

    b. Habitrol 21 mg/d patch

    c. Habitrol 14 mg/d patch

    d. Remove the Nicoderm CQ 21-mg patch prior to bed.

Answer d is correct. If the patient is already comfortable with the Nicoderm CQ 21-mg patch and already has a current supply of this formation at home, she can remove it prior to bedtime to see if this helps. If not, she could resort to answer a.

Answer a is incorrect. This would have a decrease in the nicotine replacement.

Answers b and c are incorrect. These agents are 24-hour formulations and (if left on) may cause excess adverse events in the evening and sleeping hours. Patients may always remove the 24-hour patch prior to bedtime.

---

10. OH decides not to use the nicotine patches and switches to the Commit nicotine lozenge. Which of the following administration scenarios alters the pharmacokinetics of the lozenge? Select all that apply.

    a. In the morning, immediately after waking
    b. In the afternoon, during her scheduled work break
    c. In the evening, after her dinner and coffee
    d. Before bedtime, watching the evening news

Answer c is correct. Products such as coffee, fruit juices, and certain foods can alter the pH of the mouth and either enhance or hinder drug absorption. An acidic product will decrease the pH of the mouth and lead to less transbuccal absorption of the nicotine product.

Answers a, b, and d are incorrect. Since a higher oral pH can affect the absorption of nicotine transbuccally, time of day has little to do with maximum (or minimum) absorption do to pharmacokinetics.

---

11. OH's provider also decides to use a prescription, non-nicotine, smoking cessation aid because she feels that using lozenges as needed will not be sufficient. Which of the following medications would be discouraged/contraindicated?

    a. Varenicline
    b. Bupropion
    c. Nortriptyline
    d. Clonidine

Answer a is correct. In 2007, the FDA issued a warning and requested a label change for varenicline that informed prescribers and customers of the agent's propensity to worsen depression and other neuropsychiatric conditions.

Answers b and c are incorrect. OH has a history significant for multiple psychiatric medical conditions. Bupropion and nortriptyline could both serve as primary or adjunct therapy for these neuropsychiatric conditions as well as help prevent cravings for nicotine.

Answer d is incorrect. While clonidine is not an ideal agent to choose, it does not have the warnings or precautions that the varenicline carries with it. The patient would need to be cautious of orthostatic hypotension, anticholinergic symptoms, or rebound cardiac symptoms (if stopped abruptly).

---

12. Which disease should be screened before starting varenicline? Select all that apply.

    a. Hypertension
    b. Diabetes
    c. Chronic obstructive lung disease
    d. Renal insufficiency
    e. Past medical history for mental health disease

Answer d is correct. Varenicline is metabolized and excreted via the kidneys. Patients with a creatinine clearance less than 30 mL/min, plasma drug concentrations were at least 2.1-fold greater than normal. These individuals should only receive up to 0.5 mg twice daily.

Answer e is correct. Since 2006, when varenicline was approved by the FDA, alarming numbers of adverse effects, including suicidal thoughts, erratic behavior, and aggressive behavior, have been reported. The large number of reports led to the release of a Public Health Advisory by the FDA in February 2008. The advisory stressed the importance of screening for any type of psychiatric illness or any behavior changes after starting varenicline. A boxed warning along with an update of the medication guide from the manufacturer was required by the FDA.

Answer a in incorrect. Varenicline does not have an effect on the sympathetic nervous system and only reports infrequent to rare cardiac adverse events.

Answer b is incorrect. No reports of new onset of diabetes or worsening glucose control have been associated with varenicline.

Answer c is incorrect. Chronic obstructive lung disease is not expected to have an impact on varenicline administration.

---

13. TY is a 40-year-old obese man with a medical history significant for hypertension and dyslipidemia. He also smokes cigarettes and has smoked 1.5 packs per day for the last 16 years. His most recent blood pressure was 161/94 mm Hg, which is consistent with his previous three readings. His physician is convinced that if TY were to lose weight and quit smoking, many of his medical issues would be easier to manage. TY requests assistance to quit smoking. Which of the following medications would be the best choice for TY?

    a. Bupropion
    b. Nicotine polacrilex gum
    c. Nicotine patch
    d. Varenicline

Answer d is correct. In this case, varenicline is the most appropriate choice because it would have the least negative impact on his other disease states and would increase his chances of quitting over quitting without pharmacologic assistance.

Answer a is incorrect. While bupropion is an acceptable agent to choose for tobacco cessation, the patient has concurrent uncontrolled hypertension. This is *not* a contraindication for therapy, but may worsen his hypertension or make it difficult to control. There are other options available that would not have this impact on his comorbidities.

Answers b and c are incorrect.   Since the patient has uncontrolled hypertension, choosing an agent that may worsen the condition should be avoided.

14. Insomnia and anxiety are common adverse events with bupropion, which of the following counseling points should be discussed with VX to minimize the side effects?

    a. Do not take the second dose after 5 o'clock in the evening.
    b. If the patient develops insomnia, omit the second dose of the day.
    c. Insomnia is a temporary adverse event and will resolve approximately 7 days after increasing the dose to twice daily.
    d. The insomnia and anxiety are most likely due to nicotine withdrawal and will resolve approximately 7 to 10 days after quitting smoking.

Answer a is correct.   In order for a patient to avoid such adverse events as insomnia and anxiety that interfere with restful sleep, the patient should avoid taking the second dose of the medication after 5 o'clock in the evening or 5 hours before a scheduled bedtime.

Answer b is incorrect.   While the patient may omit the second dose of the day to avoid evening and night adverse events, it also jeopardizes his or her ability to be able to deal with the withdrawal symptoms or cravings that the bupropion is attempting to alleviate.

Answer c is incorrect.   The insomnia is not a temporary effect and should be expected to continue throughout the course of therapy. If the patient is told to try and wait out the adverse event, the wakefulness and inability to sleep may lead to restarting smoking.

Answer d is incorrect.   Insomnia and irritability are signs and symptoms of nicotine withdrawal, but may also be attributed to the bupropion therapy. It is not appropriate to attribute these effects to the lack of nicotine and not appropriately address the adverse drug reaction.

15. Combination therapy is ideal for many patients attempting to quit smoking, which of the following combinations is/are appropriate? Select all that apply.

    a. Bupropion and nicotine polacrilex gum
    b. Nicotine patches and nicotine polacrilex gum
    c. Varenicline and nicotine polacrilex gum
    d. Nortriptyline and nicotine polacrilex gum

Answers a, b, and d are correct.   These three combinations use a long-acting agent in conjunction with a short-acting agent. The first agent listed will help diminish cravings and withdrawal symptoms while the nicotine polacrilex gum will help the user overcome cravings throughout the day and night.

Answer c is incorrect.   In this combination, the nicotine gum will be less effective at controlling cravings and more likely to cause adverse events such as nausea, vomiting,

and headache. Since the varenicline can block the nicotine receptors in the brain, the effect of the gum is blunted or blocked. However, varenicline also provides slight stimulation to the nicotine receptors and the nicotine from the gum, in conjunction with the varenicline, may mimic the symptoms of nicotine toxicity.

16. LK is a 62-year-old woman with osteoporosis, chronic allergic rhinitis, and a 50-pack-year history of smoking cigarettes. At a recent trip to the dentist, she was told that due to poor oral hygiene and tooth decay, she needs her teeth removed and fitted for dentures. He also recommends that she quit smoking during this time period as it most likely contributed to her current predicament. Which agent listed below would be the best agent for LK to choose?

    a. Nicotine polacrilex gum
    b. Nicotine lozenge
    c. Nicotine nasal inhaler
    d. Nicotine transdermal patch

Answer d is correct.   Since the other three options for therapy were not appropriate given the woman's medical conditions and limitations, she could be tried on the nicotine patch. The first dose would be used for approximately 6 weeks and then she would begin to step down with her therapy. If she started with the 21-mg patch, then she would follow-up with 2 weeks of the 14-mg patch and 2 weeks of the 7-mg patch. If she started with the 14-mg patch, she would only need to follow up with the 7-mg patch for 2 weeks.

Answer a is incorrect.   Since the patient is having her teeth extracted and fitted to dentures, the use of nicotine gum is not ideal. The gum may stick to the dentures and pull them out of place during the day.

Answer b is incorrect.   While the lozenge offers the benefits of the gum without the need to chew, it also increases the chance of nicotine toxicity in this situation. If LK used the nicotine lozenge immediately after her procedure or during the healing process, there is a chance that she will absorb too much, too quickly, given the inflamed state of her mouth and gums.

Answer c is incorrect.   Since the patient has a history of chronic allergic rhinitis, the nicotine nasal spray may cause unacceptable local side effects to the patient causing irritation to the nasal passage.

17. AI is a 28-year-old woman with a past medical history significant for polycystic ovarian syndrome (PCOS), hypertriglyceridemia, epilepsy, hyperthyroidism, and tobacco abuse for the last 9 years. Which of her medical conditions is considered a precaution for using bupropion therapy?

    a. PCOS
    b. Hypertriglyceridemia
    c. Epilepsy
    d. Hyperthyroidism

Answer c is correct. Epilepsy or seizures is a precaution for bupropion use. The use of this medication will decrease the seizure threshold and may make it easier for a person to experience a seizure. Using the medication concurrently with other medications that have the same effect on the seizure threshold further increases the risk of seizure.

Answer a is incorrect. Bupropion will not have an effect on PCOS.

Answer b is incorrect. Using bupropion has not demonstrated a change in serum triglyceride levels and would not affect this woman's free fatty acid levels.

Answer d is incorrect. While bupropion may worsen some of the symptoms of hyperthyroidism, it is not a contraindication. Persons with overt hyperthyroidism exhibiting symptoms should most likely not start tobacco cessation therapy with bupropion, but may consider after surgery or medical management.

---

18. What is the brand name of clonidine?

    a. Chantix
    b. Pamelor
    c. Aventyl
    d. Catapres

Answer d is correct. The brand name of clonidine is Catapres.

Answer a is incorrect. The brand name of varenicline is Chantix.

Answers b and c are incorrect. The brand name of nortriptyline is Pamelor and Aventyl.

---

19. Which of the following formulations is/are NRT available? Select all that apply.

    a. Patch
    b. Nasal inhaler
    c. Oral inhaler
    d. Lozenge

Answers a, b, c, and d are correct. NRT is available in multiple dosage forms and delivery devices, allowing for various cessation strategies. Additionally, NRT is available as a gum.

---

20. RI is a 54-year-old man on oral therapy for smoking cessation. He has been attempting to quit smoking for several years with no success. He is currently receiving second line therapy for smoking cessation. RI feels the current therapy is helping; however, he is having dry mouth, sedation, and blurred vision. Additionally, he has been having difficulty in urinating. He went to his urologist because of the urination problem (he has a past medical history of benign prostatic hypertrophy); however, the urologist said his prostate specific antigen is within the reference range and was not causing his difficulty in urinating. RI presents to your pharmacy seeking guidance on his current symptoms. Which of the following medications could be contributing to RI's symptoms? Select all that apply.

    a. Nicoderm
    b. Aventyl
    c. Seroquel
    d. Pamelor
    e. Chantix

Answers b and d are correct. Nortriptyline has two possible brand names (Aventyl and Pamelor). Nortriptyline is a tricyclic antidepressant (TCA) that is also an oral second line option for smoking cessation. The most common side effects associated with TCAs are those related to the anticholinergic activity of these medicines. The anticholinergic effects are common and may lead to drug discontinuation. Anticholinergic effects include: dry mouth, blurry vision, constipation, drowsiness, sedation, hallucinations, memory impairment, and difficulty in urinating. Although anticholinergics have side effects, they are also used therapeutically in gastrointestinal disorders (eg, diarrhea, overactive bladder); chronic obstructive pulmonary disease; dizziness and motion sickness; poisoning caused by toxins such as organophosphates or muscarine (which may be found in insecticides and poisonous mushrooms); and symptoms of neuroleptic induced side effects.

Answer a is incorrect. Nicoderm is a nicotine patch and is used first line for smoking cessation. The patient was receiving oral second line therapy.

Answer c is incorrect. Quetiapine (Seroquel) is a second generation neuroleptic that is used for schizophrenia. It is also used for depression augmentation therapy. Although quetiapine does have anticholinergic side effects, the medication is not commonly utilized or recommended for smoking cessation.

Answer e is incorrect. Varenicline (Chantix) is an oral medication utilized for smoking cessation. However, varenicline is not commonly associated with RI's symptoms.

CHAPTER 68 | Ocular Pharmacology

Questions 1 to 5 pertain to the following case.

KM is a 44-year-old African American female with decreased peripheral vision and a blind spot on the left side. She was in a motor vehicle accident because she did not see the car in the left lane. She complains of brow ache and headaches that have become worse over the past 2 weeks. Intraocular pressure measures 28 in the right eye and 26 in the left eye. She is on a fixed income and buying medications is often difficult. She works odd jobs with varying shifts. Blood pressure was 140/95.

Diagnosis: POAG, Hypertension, and Insomnia

Medications: Amlodipine 5 mg daily, Pilocarpine 2% both eyes four times daily, Tylenol PM® 2 at bedtime.

Allergies: Sulfa. Blue eyes turned brown on Xalatan® and she refused treatment.

1. Which of the following are true about KM? Select all that apply.

   a. She has at least three risk factors for glaucoma
   b. Pilocar® is first-line therapy for POAG
   c. She could have drug induced glaucoma
   d. Diphenhydramine may worsen glaucoma
   e. Amlodipine may worsen glaucoma

Answer a is correct. KM risks for glaucoma include age more than 40 years, African American, elevated IOP and family history.

Answers c and d are correct. She is taking the antihistamine diphenhydramine (Tylenol PM), which can worsen glaucoma.

Answer b is incorrect. Pilocarpine is last line therapy due to side effects.

Answer e is incorrect. Amlodipine does not worsen glaucoma.

---

2. Which of the following could affect KM's glaucoma therapy? Select all that apply.

   a. Titration of the blood pressure medication can affect intraocular pressures.
   b. Adherence may be an issue
   c. Pilocarpine causes systemic side effects and NLO education could help
   d. Acetaminophen may increase intraocular pressure

Answer a is correct. Changes in blood pressure affect intraocular pressure.

Answer b is correct. Adherence may be an issue because of financial issues or KM's work schedule. Additionally, adherence has been shown to be a contributing factor into glaucoma outcomes.

Answer c is correct. NLO will help decrease risk of side effects and improve efficacy of the eye drops.

Answer d is incorrect. Acetaminophen does not affect the intraocular pressure.

---

3. Which glaucoma medication is contraindicated for KM?

   a. Timolol
   b. Iopidine
   c. Brimonidine
   d. Dorzolamide
   e. Tafluprost

Answer d is correct. Dorzolamide is a carbonic anhydrase inhibitor which contains sulfa. KM has a sulfa allergy.

Answers a, b, c, and e are incorrect. KM does not have contraindications to those medications.

---

4. Which medication may be causing KM to have brow aches?

   a. Amlodipine
   b. Acetaminophen
   c. Diphenhydramine
   d. Pilocarpine
   e. Latanoprost

Answer d is correct. Older centrally acting agents such as pilocarpine can cause brow aches.

Answers a, b, c, and e are incorrect. They are not associated with causing brow aches.

---

5. Rank the following pharmacist recommendations by order of importance for KM's glaucoma therapy? Start with the most important. All options must be used.

Unordered Response	Ordered Response
Assess Refill histories every 3-6 mo and provide adherence education as needed	Discontinue Tylenol PM
Discontinue Pilocarpine and start timolol XE if intraocular pressures remain high	Discontinue Pilocarpine and start timolol XE if intraocular pressures remain high
Review eye drop technique and educate about nasolacrimal occlusion	Review eye drop technique and educate about nasolacrimal occlusion
Discontinue Tylenol PM	Assess Refill histories every 3-6 months and provide adherence education as needed

6. Which class of medications is associated with darker, thicker, and longer eye lashes? Select all that apply.

   a. Prostaglandin analogs
   b. Carbonic anhydrase inhibitors
   c. α-Blockers
   d. Sympathomimetics
   e. β-Blockers

Answer a is correct. Prostaglandin analogs cause hyperpigmentation and hypertrichosis of the eye lashes.

Answers b, c, d, and e are incorrect. They are not associated with darker, thicker, and longer eye lashes.

---

7. Which of the following medications can cause drug-induced Glaucoma? Select all that apply.

   a. Corticosteroids
   b. Antihistamines
   c. Cimetidine
   d. Benazepril
   e. Aspirin

Answers a, b, and c are correct. Corticosteroids, antihistamines, and cimetidine are medications that can worsen glaucoma. Corticosteroids and antihistamines have a high risk and cimetidine has a low risk.

Answers d and e are incorrect.   Benazepril and aspirin are not associated with causing glaucoma.

8. Which of the following are true regarding counseling about Nasolacrimal Occlusion? Select all that apply.

   a. Medication effectiveness
   b. Decrease side effects
   c. Increase systemic absorption of eye drops
   d. Increase the need for multiple eye drops
   e. Increase the cost of therapy

Answers a and b are correct.   NLO enhances eye drop absorption to improve efficacy and decrease all side effects.

Answers c, d, and e are incorrect.   NLO may decrease systemic absorption, need for multiple eye drops and the cost of therapy.

9. Rank the medication categories from highest to lowest ability to lower intraocular pressure (potency). All options must be used.

Unordered Response	Ordered Response
Brinzolamide	Latanoprost
Timolol	Timolol
Latanoprost	Brinzolaminde
Brimonidine	Brimonidine

Note: Latanoprost lowers intraocular pressure up to 36%, Timolol by up to 34%, Brinzolaminde 26%, and finally Brimonidine up to 16%.

10. Select the brand name for Latanoprost.

   a. Lumigan
   b. Xalatan
   c. Zioptan
   d. Alphagan

Answer b is correct.   Xalatan is the brand name for Latanoprost.

Answer a is incorrect.   Lumigan is the brand name for Bimatoprost.

Answer c is incorrect.   Zioptan is the brand name for Tafluprost.

Answer d is incorrect.   Alphagan is the brand name for Brimonidine.

11. Rank the following β-adrenergic blocking agents in order of percent strength. Start with the lowest percent strength.

Unordered Response	Ordered Response
Metipranolol	Betaxolol (Betoptic-S) 0.25%
Carteolol	Metipranolol (Optipranolol) 0.3%
Betaxolol	Carteolol (Cartrol) 1%

12. Which of the following topical β-blockers utilized for the treatment of glaucoma are nonselective β-blockers? Select all that apply.

   a. Timolol
   b. Metipranolol
   c. Carbachol
   d. Levobunolol

Answers a, b, and d are correct.   They are nonselective β-blockers.

Answer c is incorrect.   Carbachol is a direct-acting cholinergic agonist.

13. Which of the following products contains timolol? Select all that apply.

   a. Combigan
   b. Timoptic
   c. Azopt
   d. Xalatan

Answer a is correct.   Combigan is a combination product consisting of timolol and brimonidine.

Answer b is correct.   Timoptic is the brand name for timolol.

Answer c is incorrect.   Azopt is the brand name of brinzolamisde.

Answer d is incorrect.   Xalatan is the brand name for latanoprost.

14. Place the following topical antibiotics in order based upon formulation strength. Start with the lowest percent strength.

Unordered Response	Ordered Response
Azithromycin	Ofloxacin 0.3% solution
Moxifloxacin	Moxifloxacin 0.5% solution
Ofloxacin	Azitrhomycin 1% solution

15. Which of the following are topical fluoroquinolones used for the treatment of conjunctivitis? Select all that apply.

   a. Quixin
   b. Vigamox
   c. Ocuflox
   d. Ciloxan

Answers a, b, c, and d are correct.   Quixin is the brand name for levofloxacin; Vigamox is the brand name for moxifloxacin; Ocuflox is the brand name for ofloxacin; and Ciloxan is the brand name for ciprofloxacin. Additionally, the four agents may be utilized for conjunctivitis management.

16. Which of the following aminoglycoside antibiotics are formulated in a solution and ointment for ophthalmic use? Select all that apply.

   a. Tobramycin
   b. Azithromycin

c. Gentamicin
d. Erythromycin

Answers a and c are correct. Tobramycin (Tobrex, others) and gentamicin (Garamycin) are aminoglycoside antibiotics for ophthalmic use formulated in a 0.3% solution and ointment.

Answers b and d are incorrect. Azithromycin (Azasite) and Erythromycin (Ilotycin, others) are macrolide antibiotics. Azithromycin is available in a 1% solution and erythromycin is available in a 0.5% ointment.

17. Which of the following antiviral agents is commercially available as a topical solution for ophthalmic use?

    a. Trifluridine
    b. Valacyclovir
    c. Famciclovir
    d. Foscarnet

Answer a is correct. Trifluridine is available as a 1% topical solution for the treatment of herpes simplex keratitis.

Answers b, c, and d are incorrect. Valacyclovir and famciclovir are commercially available as oral tablets and foscarnet is for parenteral use.

18. Rank the following antiviral medications based upon their lowest commercially available mg tablet dose. Start with the lowest mg.

Unordered Response	Ordered Response
Acyclovir	Famciclovir 125 mg
Famciclovir	Acyclovir 400 mg
Valacyclovir	Valacyclovir 500 mg

Note: Acyclovir is also available in 200 mg capsules.

19. Which of the following antiviral agents is available in parenteral and oral formulations?

    a. Valganciclovir
    b. Ganciclovir
    c. Valacyclovir
    d. Acyclovir

Answer d is correct. Acyclovir is available as tablets and capsules and intravenous medication.

Answer a is incorrect. Valganciclovir is available orally.

Answer b is incorrect. Ganciclovir is utilized for the treatment of cytomegalovirus retinitis and is available as intravenous medication.

Answer c is incorrect. Valacyclovir is available as tablets.

20. Which of the following antifungals agents is commercially available as a 5% topical suspension? Select all that apply.

    a. Amphotericin b
    b. Natamycin

c. Fluconazole
d. Itraconazole

Answer b is correct. Natamycin is available as a 5% topical suspension.

Answers a, c, and d are incorrect. The only currently available topical ophthalmic antifungal preparation is natamycin. Other antifungal agents may be compounded for topical, subconjunctival, or intravitreal routes of administration.

CHAPTER 69 | Pregnancy and Lactation: Therapeutic Considerations

The following case pertains to questions 1 through 3.

SB is a 30-year-old woman who wants to start vitamins before she becomes pregnant. She wants to try to become pregnant sometime this year. She takes acetaminophen for headaches, her vaccines are current, and she consumes about 600 mg of caffeine per day.

1. Which component of a multivitamin is most important for SB to decrease the risk of NTDs?

    a. Calcium
    b. Iron
    c. Vitamin D
    d. Folic acid

Answer d is correct. Adequate intake of folic acid decreases the incidence of NTDs by 50% to 70%. Neural tube defects can occur in the first 4 weeks of development. It is important that all women of childbearing age take 400 mcg of folic acid daily. Some women with a higher risk of a pregnancy affected by NTDs may require 4 mg daily.

Answer a is incorrect. Calcium plays an important role in bone health. A fetus will require 30 grams of calcium for a full term pregnancy. Recommended daily calcium intake is 1300 mg for ages 14 to 18 years and 1000 mg for women 19 to 50 years.

Answer b is incorrect. Iron is important to support the increase in red cell mass, expanded plasma volume, and the growth of the fetal-placental unit. The CDC recommends 27 to 30 mg of elemental iron daily.

Answer c is incorrect. Adequate vitamin D is important for maintaining the proper amount of calcium and phosphorus for healthy bones and teeth.

2. If SB does become pregnant, which vaccines are safe to administer during pregnancy?

    a. Varicella and MMR
    b. Influenza (inactivated) and Tdap
    c. Tdap and HPV
    d. Influenza (inactivated) and MMR

Answer b is correct.   Influenza is associated with a high morbidity and mortality. The vaccine is available as inactivated virus and has no reports of harm to the fetus. The CDC recommends pregnant women receive the vaccine in any trimester. Tdap is recommended with each pregnancy and is safe to administer. During pregnancy it is best to administer between 27 and 36 weeks gestation to reduce the transmission of pertussis which can result in death.

Answer a is incorrect.   Varicella and MMR are live vaccines. Due to the theoretical risk of disease transmission to the fetus, live vaccines should be avoided during pregnancy unless the benefit of receiving the vaccines outweighs the risk.

Answer c is incorrect.   Tdap should be given with each pregnancy. The CDC does not recommend HPV vaccine during pregnancy. If a woman becomes pregnant during the HPV vaccine series, the series should be delayed until after delivery. If the vaccine is given during pregnancy, no intervention is needed.

Answer d is incorrect.   Inactivated influenza vaccine is safe during all trimesters, but MMR is a live vaccine and should be avoided during pregnancy unless the benefit of receiving the vaccine outweighs the risk.

---

3. Which statement is correct concerning SB's caffeine consumption?

   a. No change is necessary
   b. Caffeine is a known teratogen and she should avoid any consumption
   c. She should limit caffeine consumption to <200 mg daily
   d. She may safely consume caffeine up to 1000 mg daily

Answer c is correct.   Consumption of caffeine <200 to 300 mg daily has not been associated with an increased risk of miscarriage.

Answer a is incorrect.   Infertility, miscarriage, and low birth weight may be associated with caffeine consumption. Current research suggests a dose-response between the risk of miscarriage and caffeine. Low to moderate consumption, <200 to 300 mg daily, has not been associated with an increased risk of miscarriage.

Answer b is incorrect.   Studies are inconsistent with pregnancy outcomes associated with caffeine consumption. Many studies are retrospective and have confounding bias. Caffeine does cross the placenta and could affect the fetus by causing tachycardia, tremors, tachypnea, and more wakeful hours after birth.

Answer d is incorrect.   Based on current studies, low to moderate consumption of caffeine appears to be safe (<200-300 mg/d).

---

4. JW comes to the clinic today for a follow-up on her epilepsy. She would like to become pregnant within the next 12 months. Her current medications include prenatal vitamin, valproic acid, budesonide, albuterol, and acetaminophen. Which of her medications is of most concern in pregnancy?

   a. Valproic acid
   b. Acetaminophen
   c. Budesonide inhaler
   d. Prenatal vitamin

Answer a is correct.   Valproic acid is associated with neural tube defects, cardiovascular defects, facial and limb anomalies, growth restriction, hepatotoxicity, neonatal withdrawal, and developmental disorders.

Answer b is incorrect.   Acetaminophen is considered safe during pregnancy and is the recommended pain reliever.

Answer c is incorrect.   Budesonide is considered safe during pregnancy and is the drug of choice for asthma.

Answer d is incorrect.   Prenatal vitamins are recommended to assist in maintaining proper intake of vitamins and minerals during pregnancy. The vitamins will ensure adequate doses of folic acid, iron, and calcium. It is best to initiate a vitamin at least 1 month prior to conception.

---

5. Which of the following medications may be dispensed to a pregnant patient? Select all that apply.

   a. Cephalexin
   b. Enoxaparin
   c. Isotretinoin
   d. Levothyroxine

Answer a is correct.   An increased risk of teratogenic effects has not been observed.

Answer b is correct.   Enoxaparin does not cross the placenta and is recommended over unfractionated heparin for the treatment of venous thromboembolism.

Answer d is correct.   Levothyroxine does not significantly cross the placenta and has not been shown to increase the risk of congenital abnormalities.

Answer c is incorrect.   Isotretinoin is contraindicated in pregnancy. Isotretinoin labeling contains a black box warning concerning birth defects. Due to the high possibility of birth defects, patients, prescribers, wholesalers, and dispensing pharmacists must be registered in the REMS program.

---

6. Which of the following are strategies for minimizing teratogenicity of drug exposure during pregnancy? Select all that apply.

   a. Use monotherapy for the shortest duration
   b. Use a medication with a long history of safety
   c. Choose a drug with a high molecular weight
   d. Choose a drug with weak ionization

Answer a is correct.   Multiple drugs given together may increase the risk of adverse outcomes. Monotherapy for the shortest duration possible reduces the risk of exposure.

Answer b is correct. Drugs with a long history of safety have more evidence of the benefit versus risk to the fetus than drugs with less documented exposure during pregnancy.

Answer c is correct. Drugs with a high molecular weight are not likely to cross the placenta due to size.

Answer d is incorrect. Drugs with strong ionization are less likely to cross the placenta by passive diffusion versus those with weak ionization.

7. Which of the following is a pharmacokinetic parameter that should be considered when calculating an appropriate dosing regimen for a pregnant patient?

   a. Decreased renal clearance
   b. Increased absorption
   c. Increased plasma volume
   d. Increased protein binding

Answer c is correct. Plasma volume is increased by about 50% in pregnancy, and may result in an increased apparent volume of distribution for drugs.

Answer a is incorrect. Renal blood flow and glomerular filtration are increased during pregnancy, thereby enhancing the renal clearance of medications. Medications that are predominantly renally excreted as unchanged drug may require an increase in dosage.

Answer b is incorrect. Absorption of most drugs is not significantly altered in pregnancy.

Answer d is incorrect. Albumin concentrations decrease during the second trimester, resulting in reduced protein binding.

8. A patient who is 28-weeks gestation is prescribed cefuroxime for an upper respiratory tract infection. Cefuroxime is largely excreted unchanged in the urine. Which is correct regarding the use of cefuroxime in this patient?

   a. A reduction in dosage may be needed to adequately treat the infection.
   b. Antibiotics such as cefuroxime should be avoided in pregnancy.
   c. The maximum concentration (C_{max}) of cefuroxime may be increased.
   d. The volume of distribution of cefuroxime may be increased.

Answer d is correct. Plasma volume is increased by about 50% in pregnancy, and may result in an increased apparent volume of distribution for drugs.

Answer a is incorrect. Renal blood flow and glomerular filtration are increased during pregnancy, thereby enhancing the renal clearance of medications. Medications that are predominantly renally excreted as unchanged drug (such as cefuroxime) may require an increase in dosage.

Answer b is incorrect. Cefuroxime may be used in pregnancy if indicated.

Answer c is incorrect. Because the volume of distribution may be increased in pregnancy, the C_{max} may be reduced (not increased).

9. Which best summarizes changes in hepatic metabolism that occur during pregnancy?

   a. Decreased activity of cytochrome P450 isoenzymes
   b. Increased activity of cytochrome P450 isoenzymes
   c. No change in activity of cytochrome P450 isoenzymes
   d. Variable effects on activity of cytochrome P450 isoenzymes

Answer d is correct. The activity of CYP3A4, CYP2C9, and CYP2D6, as well as select UGT isoenzymes is increased, whereas the activity of CYP1A2 and CYP2C19 isoenzymes is diminished.

Answers a, b, and c are incorrect. Effects on hepatic metabolism in pregnancy are variable, with some cytochrome P450 isoenzymes showing enhanced activity, and others showing less activity.

10. A 36-year-old woman has gestational diabetes that is inadequately controlled with diet. Which medication would be best to initiate?

    a. Canagliflozin
    b. Glipizide
    c. Insulin
    d. Pioglitazone

Answer c is correct. Insulin is the preferred therapy for the management of gestational diabetes. Metformin and glyburide are alternatives.

Answer a is incorrect. There are no adequate and well-controlled studies with canagliflozin in pregnancy, and it is not a recommended therapy for the management of gestational diabetes.

Answer b is incorrect. Glipizide has less data in pregnancy than glyburide, and it is not a preferred therapy for the management of gestational diabetes.

Answer d is incorrect. There are no adequate and well-controlled studies with pioglitazone in pregnancy, and it is not a preferred therapy for the management of gestational diabetes.

11. Which of the following is appropriate for the management of gestational hypertension? Select all that apply.

    a. Captopril
    b. Labetalol
    c. Losartan
    d. Methyldopa

Answer b is correct.   Labetalol is a preferred therapy for gestational hypertension.

Answer d is correct.   Methyldopa is a preferred therapy for hypertension in pregnancy due to its long history of safety.

Answer a is incorrect.   ACE inhibitors such as captopril should be avoided in pregnancy due to the potential for teratogenic effects.

Answer c is incorrect.   Angiotensin receptor blockers such as losartan should be avoided in pregnancy due to the potential for teratogenic effects.

12. A 27-year-old woman who is 36-weeks gestation has a positive screening test for colonization with Group B *Streptococcus*. She displays no acute symptoms and has no known drug allergies. Which of the following therapies is most appropriate during labor and delivery?

    a. Intravenous cefazolin
    b. Intravenous penicillin G
    c. Oral ampicillin
    d. No therapy is warranted since she is afebrile

Answer b is correct.   Intravenous penicillin G administered from the time of membrane rupture through delivery is the preferred therapy for Group B *Streptococcus*.

Answer a is incorrect.   Intravenous cefazolin is an alternative to penicillin G in penicillin-allergic patients who do not have a history of severe allergic reaction to penicillin.

Answer c is incorrect.   Although ampicillin is an alternative to penicillin G for Group B *Streptococcus*, oral therapy is not indicated in this situation.

Answer d is incorrect.   Women who have a positive screening test for Group B *Streptococcus* should be treated regardless of symptoms.

13. A patient who is 24-weeks gestation is suffering from occasional mild heartburn. Which of the following is the most appropriate therapy?

    a. Antacid containing calcium carbonate
    b. Famotidine
    c. Omeprazole sodium bicarbonate
    d. Pantoprazole

Answer a is correct.   Antacids that contain calcium are first-line therapy for mild heartburn symptoms in pregnancy. They have the added benefit of providing calcium supplementation that may be needed in pregnancy.

Answer b is incorrect.   Although famotidine may be used for the management of heartburn symptoms in pregnancy, it should only be used if the patient does not obtain relief with first-line antacids.

Answer c is incorrect.   Proton pump inhibitors (PPIs) such as omeprazole may be used in pregnancy. However, they are best used for moderate to severe symptoms not relieved by antacids. Also, sodium bicarbonate should be avoided, since the sodium can exacerbate water retention in pregnancy.

Answer d is incorrect.   PPIs such as pantoprazole may be used in pregnancy. However, they are best used for moderate to severe symptoms not relieved by antacids.

14. A 32-year-old who is 30 weeks gestation requires treatment for a urinary tract infection. She has no known drug allergies. Assuming that the infecting organism is sensitive to the following antibiotics, which is an appropriate choice? Select all that apply.

    a. Cephalexin
    b. Ciprofloxacin
    c. Nitrofurantoin
    d. Sulfamethoxazole/trimethoprim

Answer a is correct.   Cephalexin is a recommended therapy for management of urinary tract infection in pregnancy.

Answer c is correct.   Nitrofurantoin is a recommended therapy for management of urinary tract infection in pregnancy. However, nitrofurantoin is contraindicated in late pregnancy (38-42 weeks gestation), as it has the potential to induce hemolytic anemia in the neonate. Since this patient is only 30 weeks gestation, nitrofurantoin could be used.

Answer b is incorrect.   Fluoroquinolones such as ciprofloxacin should generally be avoided in pregnancy. Although impaired joint formation has not been noted in available data, the safety of these drugs is less studied than other agents.

Answer d is incorrect.   Sulfamethoxazole/trimethoprim is pregnancy category D. Other drugs with better risk profiles should be used. Note: Use of sulfonamides should be avoided in late pregnancy, as they can displace bilirubin and contribute to newborn kernicterus.

15. Which describes appropriate pharmacotherapy of a chronic medical condition in pregnancy?

    a. Diabetes—exenatide
    b. Dyslipidemia—rosuvastatin
    c. Hypothyroidism—levothyroxine
    d. Venous thromboembolism—warfarin

Answer c is correct.   It is important to correct hypothyroidism in pregnancy, as it may result in impaired neurological development in the fetus.

Answer a is incorrect.   Insulin is the preferred therapy for the management of diabetes in pregnancy. Metformin and glyburide are alternatives for type 2 diabetes.

Answer b is incorrect.   Statins should not be administered in pregnancy due to the potential for teratogenic effects. Bile acid resins are an alternative.

Answer d is incorrect. Warfarin should be avoided in pregnancy (with the exception of high risk women with mechanical heart valves) due to the potential for teratogenic effects. Low-molecular-weight heparin is preferred, and unfractionated heparin is an alternative.

16. EH is a 27-year-old woman who is breastfeeding her 6-week-old infant every 4 hours without difficulty. Her current medications include multivitamin. She is suffering from a cold and would like to take a decongestant. Which of the following recommendations is best?

    a. Phenylephrine 15 mg po q6h
    b. Pseudoephedrine 30 mg po q6h
    c. Oxymetazoline 2 sprays each nostril q12h for 3 days
    d. No decongestant is safe for use while breastfeeding

Answer c is correct. Oxymetazoline is a topical decongestant that will not adversely affect the milk supply. It is recommended for the treatment of congestion for 3 to 4 days in a mother who is breastfeeding.

Answer a is incorrect. Phenylephrine is not recommended because it may result in a decrease in milk supply. This is especially important in mothers where breastfeeding is not established.

Answer b is incorrect. Pseudoephedrine may also result in a decrease in milk supply and is not recommended.

Answer d is incorrect. Mothers that are breastfeeding may safely use oxymetazoline for a short duration.

17. Which of the following references would be an appropriate comprehensive resource for drug information in a patient that is breastfeeding? Select all that apply.

    a. Clinical Pharmacology
    b. Drugs in Pregnancy and Lactation: A Reference Guide to Fetal and Neonatal Risk
    c. LactMed
    d. Up to Date

Answer b is correct. Drugs in Pregnancy and Lactation: A Reference Guide to Fetal and Neonatal Risk is a well-known resource for drug information pertaining to pregnancy and lactation. The information includes clinical evidence found in the literature.

Answer c is correct. LactMed is a online reference specific to breastfeeding. It provides extensive information on drug use during lactation.

Answer a is incorrect. Clinical Pharmacology includes a lactation section for each drug, but it may not provide enough information to fully support a recommendation.

Answer d is incorrect. Up to Date may provide information for pregnancy and lactation, but it is not a comprehensive resource and may not provide enough information to make a recommendation.

18. PB is a 32-year-old woman presenting with a decrease in milk production. She has been breastfeeding her daughter for 4 months. Her medications include prenatal vitamin, ibuprofen, and calcium carbonate. She also recently started drospirenone/ethinyl estradiol for contraception. Which of the following medications is likely affecting her milk supply?

    a. Calcium carbonate
    b. Drospirenone/ethinyl estradiol
    c. Ibuprofen
    d. Prenatal vitamin

Answer b is correct. Drospirenone/ethinyl estradiol may decrease the milk supply because it contains estrogen. Progestin-only methods of birth control are preferred in women who are breastfeeding. In a mother with an established milk supply, a combination oral contraceptive with ethinyl estradiol (<35 mcg/d) may be considered if the patient is at least 4 weeks postpartum.

Answer a is incorrect. Calcium carbonate is compatible with breastfeeding.

Answer c is incorrect. Ibuprofen is compatible with breastfeeding.

Answer d is incorrect. Prenatal vitamins do not adversely affect the milk supply. Prenatal vitamins should continue during breastfeeding to support adequate intake of vitamins and minerals.

19. Which of the following medications is a galactagogue?

    a. Metoprolol
    b. Diphenhydramine
    c. Metoclopramide
    d. Warfarin

Answer c is correct. Metoclopramide is a drug that may increase milk supply. Before initiating metoclopramide, the lactating mother should try to increase supply by breastfeeding her infant more frequently. If the infant is fed more often, the demand may increase the supply.

Answer a is incorrect. Metoprolol does not adversely affect the milk supply.

Answer b is incorrect. Diphenhydramine may have no effect or may slightly decrease milk supply.

Answer d is incorrect. Warfarin does not adversely affect the milk supply.

20. Which of the following are strategies for minimizing drug exposure to the breastfeeding infant? Select all that apply.

    a. Choose an alternate route of administration
    b. Choose an alternate drug
    c. Take medication before the infant's longest sleep period
    d. Prescribe low doses of medication more frequently

Answer a is correct. Routes that decrease the systemic absorption of the drug minimize the exposure to the infant. An example would be an inhaled corticosteroid.

Answer b is correct. An alternate drug may a safer alternative.

Answer c is correct. This ensures the longest period between feedings and allows more of the drug to be eliminated before the next feeding.

Answer d is incorrect. Medications prescribed should be of the appropriate dose for the indication and the nursing mother. Once-daily dosing is optimal, as it allows the dose to be given before the longest infant sleep period to reduce the risk of exposure.

21. Which of the following is the brand name for the prescription product extended-release doxylamine/pyridoxine?

    a. Bonjesta
    b. Diclegis
    c. Fragmin
    d. Unisom

Answer a is correct. Bonjesta is an extended-release combination product containing doxylamine/pyridoxine.

Answer b is incorrect. Diclegis is a delayed-release combination product containing doxylamine/pyridoxine.

Answer c is incorrect. Fragmin is the brand name for the low-molecular-weight heparin dalteparin.

Answer d is incorrect. Unisom is the brand name for the over-the-counter sleep product containing doxylamine.

CHAPTER **70 | Pharmacoeconomics**

1. Which of the following parameters is evaluated by a pharmacoeconomic analysis?

    a. Cost
    b. Outcomes
    c. Cost and outcomes
    d. Side effects
    e. Side effects and number needed to harm

Answer c is correct. A pharmacoeconomic analysis measures cost and outcomes. Outcomes research is defined as an attempt to identify, measure, and evaluate the end results of health care services. It may include not only clinical and economic consequences, but also outcomes, such as patient health status and satisfaction with their health care. Pharmacoeconomics is a type of outcomes research, but not all outcomes research is pharmacoeconomic research.

Answers a, b, d, and e are incorrect. If only cost is measured without regard for outcomes, this is a cost analysis. If

only an outcome is measured without regard to costs, this is a clinical or outcome study.

2. What type of pharmacoeconomic analysis assumes the outcomes are equal?

    a. Epidemiologic study
    b. Retrospective study
    c. Cost-minimization
    d. Parametric analysis

Answer c is correct. A cost minimization analysis measures cost in dollars and outcomes are assumed to be equivalent.

Answers a, b, and d are incorrect.

3. A study is evaluating the cost associated with emergency room visits. What type of cost would emergency room visits represent? Select all that apply.

    a. Direct medical
    b. Direct nonmedical
    c. Indirect
    d. Intangible

Answer a is correct. Direct medical costs are the medically-related inputs used *directly* in providing the treatment. Examples of direct medical costs include costs associated with pharmaceutical products, physician visits, emergency room visits, and hospitalizations.

Answers b, c, and d are incorrect. The example above represents a direct medical cost; however, studies of an illness may include all four types of costs. For example, the cost of a procedure would include the direct medical costs of the procedure (medication, laboratory tests, and physician services), direct nonmedical costs (travel and lodging, if required), indirect costs (cost due to the patient missing work), and intangible costs (fear about procedure).

4. A study is evaluating the cost associated with hotel and meal expenses for a patient traveling to see a subspecialist. What type of cost would hotel and meal expenses represent?

    a. Direct medical
    b. Direct nonmedical
    c. Indirect
    d. Intangible

Answer b is correct. Direct nonmedical costs are not medical in nature, but are directly associated with treatment. Examples include the cost of traveling to and from the physician's office or hospital, babysitting for the children of a patient, and food and lodging required for patients and their families during out-of-town treatment.

Answers a, c, and d are incorrect. Most studies only report the direct medical costs. This may be appropriate depending on the objective of the study or the perspective of the study. However, an illness may (and most likely does) include all four types of costs. It depends upon the perspective as to which costs will be evaluated.

5. A study is evaluating the cost associated with missing work due to an illness. What type of cost would missing work represent?

   a. Direct medical
   b. Direct nonmedical
   c. Indirect
   d. Intangible

Answer c is correct. Indirect costs result from the loss of productivity due to illness or death.

Answers a, b, and d are incorrect.

6. A study is evaluating the cost associated with anxiety due to an illness. What type of cost would anxiety represent?

   a. Direct medical
   b. Direct nonmedical
   c. Indirect
   d. Intangible

Answer d is correct. Intangible costs include the costs of pain, suffering, anxiety, or fatigue that occur because of an illness or the treatment of an illness. It is difficult to measure or assign values to intangible costs.

Answers a, b, and c are incorrect.

7. A pharmacoeconomic analysis is to be conducted between simvastatin and atorvastatin. While these medications have different lowering of LDL (percentage points), they are considered equivalent in terms of decreasing primary cardiovascular mortality and safety per discussion with your attending physician. He wants you to conduct an analysis comparing the two agents. Which type of analysis would be utilized?

   a. CMA
   b. CBA
   c. CEA
   d. CUA

Answer a is correct. A CMA measures cost in dollars and outcomes are assumed to be equivalent. The outcomes (eg, efficacy, incidence of adverse drug interactions) are expected to be equal, but the costs are not.

Answers b, c, and d are incorrect. This example is a CMA. The advantage of a CMA is that it is simple compared to the other types of analyses because outcomes need not be measured. The disadvantage of this type of analysis is that it can only be used when outcomes are assumed to be identical.

8. The pharmacy director at an academic medical center has been allotted on full time equivalent (FTE) to hire a clinical

pharmacy specialist. He requested three FTEs in the area of cardiology, critical care, and infectious diseases. Now he has to decide which type of specialist he should hire. Instead of make a gut call, he has decided to include the economist faculty member from the College of Pharmacy to assist. What type of analysis should be conducted to evaluate which position should be hired?

   a. CMA
   b. CBA
   c. CEA
   d. CUA

Answer b is correct. A CBA measures inputs and outcomes in monetary terms.

Answers a, c, and d are incorrect. The example above is best conducted using a CBA. One advantage to using a CBA is that alternatives with different outcomes can be compared, because each outcome is converted to the same unit (dollars). For example, the costs (inputs) of providing a pharmacokinetic service versus a diabetes clinic can be compared with the cost savings (outcomes) associated with each service, even though different types of outcomes are expected for each alternative. CBAs are performed to determine how institutions can best spend their resources to produce monetary benefits.

9. A medical center located in the Northeast part of the United States is dealing with resistant bacterial organisms at their institution. Specifically, they are over whelmed with cases of extended spectrum β-lactamase gram-negative rods. The medical center director charges pharmacy service with comparing different types of treatment to optimize clinical cure outcomes. Which of the following types of pharmacoeconomic evaluations should be conducted?

   a. CMA
   b. CBA
   c. CEA
   d. CUA

Answer c is correct. CEA evaluates the costs that are measured in natural units (eg, cures, years of life, blood pressure).

Answers a, b, and d are incorrect. The example represents a CEA. A CEA is the most common type of pharmacoeconomic analysis and it measures costs in dollars and outcomes in natural health units. An advantage of using a CEA is that health units are common outcomes practitioners can readily understand and these outcomes do not need to be converted to monetary values.

10. Which of the following pharmacoeconomic models evaluated adjusted life years?

   a. CMA
   b. CBA
   c. CEA
   d. CUA

Answer d is correct.   A CUA takes patient preferences into account when measuring health consequences. The most common unit used in conducting CUAs is QALYs.

Answers a, b, and c are incorrect.   This example represents CUA. A QALY is a health-utility measure combining quality and quantity of life, as determined by some valuations process. The advantage of using this method is that different types of health outcomes can be compared using one common unit (QALYs) without placing a monetary value on these health outcomes (like CBA). The disadvantage of this method is that it is difficult to determine an accurate QALY value.

CHAPTER **71 | Statistics**

1. Which of the following is the outcome variable for a study? Select all that apply.

    a. DV
    b. IV
    c. Confounder
    d. Population

Answer a is correct.   There are three types of variables: dependent (DV), independent (IV), and confounding. The DV is the response or outcome variable for a study.

Answers b and c are incorrect.   The IV is a variable that is manipulated and a confounding variable is any variable that has an effect on the DV over and above the effect of the IV, but is not of specific research interest.

Answer d is incorrect.   A population refers to all objects of a similar type in the universe, while a sample is a fraction of the population chosen to be representative of the specific population of interest. Thus, samples are chosen to make generalizations about the population of interest.

2. Which of the following represent scales of measurement? Select all that apply.

    a. Nominal
    b. Ordinal
    c. Interval
    d. Ratio scales

Answers a, b, c, and d are correct.   There are four levels of measurement: nominal, ordinal, interval, and ratio scales. The scale of measurement is an important consideration when determining the appropriate statistical test to answer the research question and hypothesis.

3. A pharmacy resident in South Carolina is charged with evaluating daptomycin as her research project for the year. She is evaluating all patients within 18 months and comparing them to vancomycin. The primary outcome is clinical response as defined by clearance of bacteremia within 5 days. Her data

collection sheet has two boxes for the primary outcome (yes and no). What type of measurement scale is the resident collecting?

    a. Nominal
    b. Ordinal
    c. Interval
    d. Ratio scales

Answer a is correct.   A nominal scale consists of categories that have no implied rank or order (male versus female; or absence versus presence). The patient can fit into only one category; that is, the data points are mutually exclusive.

Answers b, c, and d are incorrect.   An ordinal scale has all of the characteristics of a nominal variable; however, the data are placed into rank-ordered categories. Interval scales increase the information provided by an ordinal scale by allowing researchers to quantify a meaningful distance between two units (eg, temperature). Ratio scales differ from interval scales in that they have an absolute zero (eg, blood pressure).

4. The pharmacy resident in question number 3 completed her study and demonstrated that vancomycin has a higher cure rate of bacteremia at 5 days as compared to daptomycin. She was concerned that she had introduced error into her study because of a low sample size (17 daptomycin patients and 34 vancomycin patients). Additionally, she was concerned that measuring the outcome as yes/no impacted the results. She is going to repeat the study and make two modifications: (1) she has recruited other pharmacy residents to participate to increase the sample size and (2) she has changed the primary outcome to days bacteremic. She will record the number of days until the patient has a negative blood culture. What type of measurement scale is the resident now collecting?

    a. Nominal
    b. Ordinal
    c. Interval
    d. Ratio scales

Answer d is correct.   Ratio scales differ from interval scales in that they have an absolute zero (eg, blood pressure).

Answers a, b, and c are incorrect.   Although researchers should not confuse absolute and arbitrary zero points, this difference is nonessential as interval and ratio scales are analyzed by identical statistical procedures.

5. The pharmacy resident is also measuring the impact of obesity on the clinical outcomes. She is recording each patient's weight, height, and BMI. What type of variables is she recording?

    a. Continuous
    b. Discrete
    c. Categorical
    d. Dichotomous

Answer a is correct. Continuous variables consist of data measured on interval or ratio scales. Examples of continuous variables include age, BMI, uncategorized lab values (eg, a blood pressure of 160/95 as opposed to high blood pressure).

Answers b, c, and d are incorrect. Discrete variables consist of data measured on nominal or ordinal scales. Discrete variables are often termed nominal or categorical, or, if a variable is measured on a nominal scale with only two levels (eg, male versus female), it may be termed dichotomous.

---

6. The resident is compiling the data of the repeat daptomycin study. A fellow resident collected the same variables she collected; however, instead of recording actual BMI, she categorized patients based on the World Health Organization's (WHO) classification of obesity. What type of variable is she recording by using the WHO system? Select all that apply.

    a. Continuous
    b. Discrete
    c. Categorical
    d. Dichotomous

Answers b and c are correct. Discrete variables consist of data measured on nominal or ordinal scales. This example represents ordinal.

Answer a is incorrect. Examples of continuous variables include age, BMI, and **uncategorized** outcomes.

Answer d is incorrect. If a variable is measured on a nominal scale with only two levels (eg, male versus female), it may be termed dichotomous. The WHO obesity categorization has several categories.

---

7. Which of the following are measures of central tendency? Select all that apply.

    a. Mean
    b. Median
    c. Mode
    d. Average

Answers a, b, c, and d are correct. Measures of central tendency are helpful in identifying the distribution of the data numerically. Common measures of central tendency are the mean (aka average), median, and mode. The appropriate measure of central tendency depends on the scale of measurement for the variable being studied.

---

8. Which of the following measures of central tendency is calculated by summing all data for a variable and dividing by the total number of patients? Select all that apply.

    a. Mean
    b. Median
    c. Mode
    d. 50th percentile

Answer a is correct. The mean is the most common and appropriate measure of central tendency for normally distributed data measured on an interval or ratio scale. It is best described as the average numerical value for data within a variable. The mean is calculated by summing all data for a variable and dividing by the total number of patients (total sample size or simply n).

Answers b, c, and d are incorrect.

---

9. The pharmacy resident from question number 3 is writing her residency report about her study (the first study). She has to report measures of central tendency as appropriate. What measure of central tendency should she utilize for her primary outcome? Select all that apply.

    a. Mean
    b. Median
    c. Mode
    d. Average

Answer c is correct. The mode is the most appropriate measure of central tendency for nominal data. The mode is the most frequently occurring value or category within a variable. Further, a variable could have two, three, or more modes; thus, a variable with two modes is referred to as bimodal, with three modes, trimodal.

Answers a, b, and d are incorrect.

---

10. The pharmacy resident has completed her study report and is not analyzing the second study. She has decided to utilize BMI as categorized by the WHO. What measure of central tendency should be utilized? Select all that apply.

    a. Mean
    b. Median
    c. Mode
    d. 50th percentile

Answers b and d are correct. The median is most appropriate for data measured on an ordinal scale; however, it can also be presented for continuous variables to assist in describing the variable distribution. The median is the absolute middle value in the data (exactly at the 50th percentile); that is, half of the data points fall above and half below the median. It is important to note that outliers (ie, data points that are disconnected from the other data points) can significantly affect the mean, but not the median. Therefore, a comparison of the mean and median can give insight into whether outliers influenced the mean and overall distribution of the data points within a variable.

Answers a and c are incorrect.

---

11. Which of the following are measures of variability? Select all that apply.

    a. SD
    b. Range

c. IQR
d. Variance

Answers a, b, c, and d are correct. The most common measures of variability (or dispersion) are the range, IQR, variance, and SD. Measures of variability are useful in indicating the spread of data for a variable. These measures are also useful in association with measures of central tendency to assess how scattered the data are around the mean or median.

12. Which of the following are measures of variability?

a. Mean
b. SD
c. Student paired t test
d. Nominal data

Answer b is correct. The most common measures of variability (or dispersion) are the range, IQR, variance, and SD. Measures of variability are useful in indicating the spread of data for a variable. These measures are also useful in association with measures of central tendency to assess how scattered the data are around the mean or median. SD is a measure of the dispersion of a set of data from its mean. It is calculated as the square root of variance by determining the variation between each data point relative to the mean. If the data points are further from the mean, there is higher deviation within the data set.

Answer a is incorrect. The mean is the average of the numbers: a calculated "central" value of a set of numbers. To calculate: just add up all the numbers, then divide by how many numbers there are.

Answer c is incorrect. A paired t-test is used to compare two population means where you have two samples in which observations in one sample can be paired with observations in the other sample.

Answer d is incorrect. There are four measurement scales (or types of data): nominal, ordinal, interval and ratio. These are simply ways to categorize different types of variables. Nominal scales are used for labeling variables, without any quantitative value. Nominal scales could simply be called labels.

13. Which of the following terms describes variability around the median?

a. SD
b. IQR
c. Ordinal data
d. ANOVA

Answer b is correct. The IQR is a measure of dispersion used to describe data measured on ordinal, interval, or ratio scales. The IQR is a measure of variability directly related to

the median. The IQR is the difference between the 75th and 25th percentile.

Answer a is incorrect. Statistics plays a vital role in biomedical research. It helps present data precisely and draws the meaningful conclusions. While reviewing data, be aware of using adequate statistical measures. In biomedical journals, SEM and SD are used interchangeably to express the variability, though they measure different parameters. SEM quantifies uncertainty in estimate of the mean whereas **SD indicates dispersion of the data from mean**. As readers are generally interested in knowing the variability within sample, descriptive mean data should be precisely summarized with SD.

Answer c is incorrect. Ordinal data is data which is placed into some kind of order or scale. This is easy to remember because ordinal sounds like order. An example of ordinal data is rating happiness on a scale of 1-10.

Answer d is incorrect. The ANOVA is used to determine whether there are any statistically significant differences between the means of three or more independent (unrelated) groups.

14. Which of the following statements identifies properties of a normal distribution (Gaussian distribution) regarding the central tendency, variability, and shape? Select all that apply.

a. Primary shape is a bell curve
b. Mean, median, and mode are identical
c. The distribution is symmetrical
d. Skewness and kurtosis are zero

Answers a, b, c, and d are correct. The normal distribution, also called Gaussian distribution, is one of the most important density curves. This distribution is the most commonly used distribution in statistics. It is very important to know whether a variable is distributed normally in the population, or whether the variable distribution approaches normal. The distribution of the DV is of primary importance when determining which statistical test to employ. A normal curve has several easily identifiable properties uncovered by analyzing the numerical measures of central tendency, variability, and shape (Fig. 74-1). Specifically, this includes the following characteristics: (1) the primary shape is a bell-curve; (2) the mean, median, and mode are identical; (3) the curve is symmetric around the mean; that is, the distribution is symmetrical and reflects itself perfectly when folded in half; and (4) skewness and kurtosis are zero.

15. What type of distribution is utilized for nominal data?

a. Gaussian
b. Binomial
c. Positive skew
d. Negative skew

Answer b is correct. Many discrete outcomes or events can be dichotomized into one of two mutually exclusive groups. The binomial distribution, also termed the Bernoulli distribution, is appropriate for this type of event or outcome (ie, DV), and calculates the exact probability of the event or outcome. Note the binomial distribution approximates the normal distribution when n is large and the probability of the outcome is 0.50 (ie, 50/50).

Answer a is incorrect.   The normal distribution, also known as the Gaussian or standard normal distribution, is the probability distribution that plots all of its values in a symmetrical fashion, and most of the results are situated around the probability's mean. Values are equally likely to plot either above or below the mean.

Answers c and d are incorrect.   Skewed distributions are asymmetrical and have data that clusters toward one end. A distribution is said to be skewed when the data points cluster more toward one side of the scale than the other, creating a curve that is not symmetrical. In other words, the right and the left side of the distribution are shaped differently from each other. There are two types of skewed distributions. A distribution is positively skewed if the scores fall toward the lower side of the scale and there are very few higher scores. Positively skewed data is also referred to as skewed to the right because that is the direction of the "long tail end" of the chart. A distribution is negatively skewed if the scores fall toward the higher side of the scale and there are very few low scores.

16. A case-control study of 2300 participants looked at the association between acetaminophen and renal disease. The study included 537 cases. There were 224 cases and 130 controls taking acetaminophen. The 2 × 2 table has been filled in.

Acetaminophen	Renal Disease	No Renal Disease	
Exposed	224	130	354
Unexposed	313	1633	1946
	537	**1763**	**2300**

What is the odds ratio of this study?

a. OR = (224/354)/(313/1946) = 3.93
b. OR = (224/313)/(130/1633) = 8.99
c. OR = (224/2300) = 0.097

Answer b is correct.   In a case-control study, the odds ratio is calculated by dividing the odds that cases were exposed to the risk (ie, A/C) by the odds that the controls were exposed (ie, B/D).

Answer a is incorrect.   This is a relative risk calculation.

Answer c is incorrect.   This is a proportion of exposed cases out of the total sample.

17. What is an example of a nonparametric test?

a. Student's t test
b. z test

c. ANOVA
d. Fisher's exact test

Answer d is correct.   The test can only be applied to 2 × 2 contingency tables; however, it is most useful when the sample size is small. Conceptually, Fisher;s exact test is identical to the chi square test, in that, the two variables being compared must be discrete and have mutually exclusive categories.

Answers a, b, and c are incorrect.   All are parametric tests.

18. Which of the following statement(s) is true about statistical power? Select all that apply.

a. Power increases when Type 1 error increases
b. Power increases when sample size decreases
c. Power increases when effect size increases
d. Power is unaffected by error variance

Answers a and c are correct.   Statistical power can be increased by increasing alpha (not advised) and effect size.

Answers b and d are incorrect.   Statistical power is influenced by four factors: alpha (the probability value at which the null hypothesis is rejected), effect size (the size of the treatment effect), error variance (the precision of the measurement instrument), and the sample size. Statistical power can be increased by increasing sample size as well as deceasing error variance.

19. Azithromycin was compared to amoxicillin and levofloxacin in a retrospective, observational pharmacoepidemiology study. The study used a national cohort of patients from an insurance claims database. The research question was: does azithromycin have a higher risk of all causes of death compared to a control antibiotic group? The hypothesis from the research group was that azithromycin will have a higher rate of all causes of death. The study produced the following study results:

Hazard Ratio (95% CIs) for Multiple Comparisons of All Causes of Death

Antibiotic	Amoxicillin
Azithromycin	1.48 (1.05-2.09)
Levofloxacin	2.49 (1.70-3.64)

Based upon the results of the study, select the statement that accurately describes the azithromycin and amoxicillin contrast.

a. Amoxicillin has a 48% increased risk of death compared to azithromycin.
b. Azithromycin has a 48% increased risk of death compared to amoxicillin.
c. There is no statistical significance among the results of azithromycin compared to azithromycin.
d. Levofloxacin has a 2.49-fold increased risk of death compared to amoxicillin.

Answer b is correct. Azithromycin has a 48% increased risk of death compared to amoxicillin. The results demonstrate a point estimate of 1.48 and a 95% CI (1.05-2.09). Therefore, the hazard ratio is interpreted that azithromycin has a 48% higher risk.

Answer a is incorrect. The dependent variable is azithromycin because of the way the research question was asked and because of the way the antibiotics are listed in the table.

Answer c is incorrect. In retrospective studies, if the CI crosses one, there is no statistical significance. However, the CI from this study does not cross one; therefore, the observation is statistically significant. You can determine statistical significance by looking at the CI or *p* value. This study did not give a *p* value.

Answer d is incorrect. The statement is correct; however, the question asked about azithromycin and not levofloxacin.

---

20. Azithromycin was compared to amoxicillin and levofloxacin in a retrospective, observational pharmacoepidemiology study. The study used a national cohort of patients from an insurance claims database. The research question was: does azithromycin have a higher risk of arrhythmia compared to a control antibiotic group? The hypothesis from the research group was that azithromycin will have a higher rate of arrhythmia. The study produced the following study results:

Hazard Ratio (95% CIs) for Multiple Comparisons Arrhythmia

Antibiotic	Amoxicillin	Azithromycin	Levofloxacin
Amoxicillin	1	0.56 (0.38-0.83)	0.41 (0.26-0.64)
Azithromycin	1.77 (1.20-2.62)	1	0.73 (0.47-1.13)
Levofloxacin	2.43 (1.56-3.79)	1.37 (0.88-2.13)	1

Based upon the results of the study, select the statement that accurately describes the azithromycin and amoxicillin contrast(s).

a. Amoxicillin has a 77% increased risk of arrhythmia compared to azithromycin.
b. There is not statistical difference in arrhythmia risk between azithromycin and amoxicillin.
c. Amoxicillin has a 56% lower risk of arrhythmia compared to azithromycin.
d. Amoxicillin has a 44% lower risk of arrhythmia compared to azithromycin.

Answer d is correct. The point estimate of 0.56 demonstrates that amoxicillin has a lower risk (because it is less than 1). However, when the point estimate is less than one for hazard ratio, odds ratio, you subtract the number from one to find the risk. You read the data as: for the contrast of amoxicillin compared to azithromycin, the point estimate is 0.56 with a 95% CI of 0.38 to 0.83. Therefore, the point estimate reveals that amoxicillin has a 44% lower risk of arrhythmia and the 95% CI demonstrates that the risk is also lower and ranges from 17% to 62% lower risk (subtract the CI values from 1).

Answer a is incorrect. The point estimate reveals that azithromycin has a 77% increased risk of arrhythmia compared to amoxicillin.

Answer b is incorrect. Both contrasts [0.56 (0.38-0.83) and 1.77 (1.20-2.62)] do not cross one; therefore, there is statistical significance.

Answer c is incorrect. When the point estimate for a retrospective study is less than one, subtract the number from one.

---

21. Which of the following CIs indicates the results are statistically significant? Select all that apply.

Hazard Ratio (95% CIs) for Multiple Comparisons Arrhythmia

Antibiotic	Amoxicillin	Azithromycin	Levofloxacin
Amoxicillin	1	0.56 (0.38-0.83)	0.41 (0.26-0.64)
Azithromycin	1.77 (1.20-2.62)	1	0.73 (0.47-1.13)
Levofloxacin	2.43 (1.56-3.79)	1.37 (0.88-2.13)	1

a. The amoxicillin to amoxicillin contrast
b. The amoxicillin to levofloxacin contrast
c. The levofloxacin to amoxicillin contrast
d. The azithromycin to amoxicillin contrast
e. The azithromycin to levofloxacin contrast

Answer b is correct. The amoxicillin to levofloxacin contrast has a point estimate of 0.41 and a 95% CI of 0.26 to 0.64. Since the CI does not cross 1 (retrospective, observational study), the result is statistically significant. Therefore, this result indicates that amoxicillin has a 59% (1—point estimate) lower risk of arrhythmia compared to levofloxacin and the CI demonstrates that the LOWER risk is between 36% lower up to a 74% lower risk (the CI values subtracted from one).

Answer c is correct. The levofloxacin to amoxicillin contrast has a point estimate of 2.43 and a 95% CI of 1.56 to 3.79. Since the CI does not cross 1, the result is statistically significant. Therefore, this result indicates that levofloxacin has a 2.43-fold increased risk of arrhythmia compared to amoxicillin and the CI demonstrates that the HIGHER risk is between 56% higher up to a 3.79-fold higher risk.

Answer d is correct. The azithromycin to amoxicillin contrast has a point estimate of 1.77 and a 95% CI of 1.20 to 2.62. Since the CI does not cross 1 (retrospective study), the result is statistically significant. Therefore, the result indicated that azithromycin has a 77% increased risk of arrhythmia compared to amoxicillin and the CI demonstrates that the HIGHER risk is between 20% higher up to a 2.62-fold higher risk.

Answer a is incorrect. Amoxicillin compared to itself is 1, because it is identical (refer to the equation for calculations of ratios). This is the only time you will see a perfect 1. You may see number close, but there is usually some variation, hence a CI will be given.

Answer e is incorrect. The azithromycin to levofloxacin contrast has a point estimate of 0.73 and a 95% CI of 0.47 to 1.13. Since the CI crosses 1 (retrospective study), the result is not statistically significant. Therefore, you would fail to reject the null hypothesis (the null hypothesis would be the risk of arrhythmia would be the same between azithromycin and levofloxacin). I personally like the term fail to reject the null hypothesis as compared to accepting the null. If you accept the null, you will state the antibiotics are equal, but the study showed they are not equal. The point estimate demonstrates that azithromycin has a 27% lower risk of arrhythmia compared to levofloxacin and that is not the same. However, the CI demonstrates that the risk may be 53% lower or up to 13% higher (1—the CI numbers). Since a drug cannot be lower and higher risk, it is not statistically significant. In summary, this study result demonstrates (point estimate) that azithromycin has a 27% lower risk of arrhythmia. However, if the study were to be repeated, it is very possible that azithromycin could have a higher risk of arrhythmia compared to levofloxacin (because of the CI data).

---

22. Which of the following definitions describes ITT?

    a. A design where the independent variable typically involves participants randomized into fixed levels of treatment (or arms), with each arm indicating a different treatment or comparison (eg, placebo, active control)
    b. A design which has the primary purpose of having a participant serve as his or her own control
    c. A design that implements changes (or adaptations) in the design or endpoint analyses based on the results of a predetermined (ie, prior to initiation of the study) set of interim analyses
    d. The analysis includes all participants in the arm to which they were randomized originally
    e. Evaluates only compliant participants with complete data

---

Answer d is correct. ITT requires the analysis to include all participants in the arm to which they were randomized originally. The ITT approach is often employed in the presence of violations to protocol and patients being lost to follow-up, and is the approach most often used in the literature. Note: there have been some modifications of this term over time. Some individuals may define ITT as randomized and received one dose of medication, although the exact correct definition is randomized (irrespective of mediation receipt). Several literature examples are using an mITT (modified intention to treat). I *personally* do not think mITT exists because it can be modified by several mechanisms. I think mITT becomes per protocol.

Answer a is incorrect. That is the definition for Parallel-Groups Design. The most common RCT is a parallel-groups design.

Answer b is incorrect. That is the definition for crossover design. The second most common RCT employs a crossover design. The purpose of the crossover design is to study treatment effects using the participant as his or her own control.

Answer c is incorrect. That is an adaptive design.

Answer e is incorrect. That is the definition for per protocol. Although this analysis is straightforward analytically and allows researchers to evaluate a more accurate treatment effect, it has substantial limitations, primarily, reduced statistical power compared to an ITT approach, because participants with incomplete data are not considered in the analysis, and results in an inflated Type I error rate.

---

23. A study was evaluating the mortality of a new medication for acute coronary syndrome compared to the standard of care. The outcome of interest (mortality) was recorded as yes or no at the end of the 3-year study period. Patients were randomized to treatment groups and the results were reported as ITT. What would be the statistical test that can evaluate the outcome of interest?

    a. Pearson's chi square test
    b. Cochran-Mantel-Haenszel test
    c. Independent samples t test
    d. Student's t test
    e. Analysis of covariance

Answer a is correct. Pearson's chi square test (or simply the chi square test) is one of the most common statistical tests used in the biomedical sciences. It is used to assess for significant differences between two or more mutually exclusive groups for two variables measured on nominal, dichotomous, or categorical scales.

Answer b is incorrect. The Mantel-Haenszel chi square test (or Cochran-Mantel-Haenszel test or Mantel-Haenszel test) measures the association of three discrete variables, which usually consists of two dichotomous IVs and one categorical confounding variable or covariate.

Answers c and d are incorrect. The independent samples t test (also referred to as Student's t test) is used to assess for a statistically significant difference between the means of the two mutually exclusive (ie, independent) groups.

Answer e is incorrect. ANCOVA is an extension of ANOVA where main effects and interactions are assessed after statistically adjusting for one (or more) confounding variables called covariates. That is, ANCOVA adjusts all group means to create the situation as if all participants scored identically on the covariate.

---

24. A study was evaluating the cholesterol values of a new medication for dyslipidemia compared to the standard of care. The outcome of interest (mean total cholesterol level) was recorded as a continuous variable (ie, ratio data). Patients were randomized to treatment groups and the results were reported as ITT. The total cholesterol values for the study represented a normal distribution. What would be the statistical test that can evaluate the outcome of interest?

    a. Paired t test
    b. ANOVA
    c. T test
    d. Mann-Whitney

Answer c is correct. The independent samples t test (also referred to as Student's t test) is used to assess for a statistically significant difference between the means of the two mutually exclusive (ie, independent) groups. However, the data must be normally distributed.

Answer a is incorrect. The paired samples t test (also known as the matched t test or nested t test) is used when one group of participants is measured on the dependent variable twice, or two groups of participants are matched on specific characteristics.

Answer b is incorrect. A one-way repeated measures ANOVA (or simply repeated measures ANOVA) is an extension of the paired samples t test to situations where the DV is measured three or more times. This can occur when the same participants are measured repeatedly or when three or more matched groups are measured once.

Answer d is incorrect. The Mann-Whitney test is the nonparametric alternative to the independent samples t test and is one of the most powerful nonparametric tests. It is used when the distribution of a continuous DV is not normal (the data in this study was normally distributed) or when the DV is measured on an ordinal scale. The Mann-Whitney test is based on ranked data. That is, instead of using the actual values of the DV, as an independent samples t test does, each participant's DV value is ranked with the highest value receiving the highest rank and the lowest value receiving the lowest rank. The ranks within each group are then summed, and the test assesses whether the difference in ranked sums between groups is statistically significant.

25. A study was evaluating the mean blood pressure values of a new medication for hypertension compared to the standard of care. The outcome of interest (mean blood pressure) was recorded as a continuous variable (ie, ratio data). Each patient served as their own control. The results were reported as ITT. The mean blood pressure values for the study had mean and median that were very different. What would be the statistical test that can evaluate the outcome of interest?

    a. Paired t test
    b. Wilcoxon signed-rank test
    c. Kruskal-Wallis One-Way ANOVA
    d. Fisher's exact test

Answer b is correct. The Wilcoxon signed-rank test (or simply signed-rank test) is the nonparametric alternative to a paired samples t test. The test is used typically when the distribution of the DV is not normal (this study has data that is not normally distributed because the mean and the median are different; recall that a normal distribution occurs when the mean = median = mode) or when the DV is measured on an ordinal scale to assess for differences between two repeated measurements (or two matched groups).

Answer a is incorrect. Normally, this would be the correct test as the paired samples t test (also known as the matched t test or nested t test) is used when one group of participants is

measured on the DV twice, or two groups of participants are matched on specific characteristics. However, the data are not normally distributed.

Answer c is incorrect. The Kruskal-Wallis one-way ANOVA by ranks (or simply, the Kruskal-Wallis test) is the nonparametric alternative to the one-way ANOVA. The test is an extension of the Mann-Whitney test to assess group differences between three or more mutually exclusive groups. The Kruskal-Wallis test is typically used when the distribution of a continuous DV is not normal or when the DV is measured on an ordinal scale.

Answer d is incorrect. Fisher's exact test is ubiquitous in the biomedical literature. The test can only be applied to 2 × 2 contingency tables; however, it is most useful when the sample size is small. Conceptually, Fisher's exact test is identical to the chi square test, in that, the two variables being compared must be discrete and have mutually exclusive categories.

CHAPTER 72 | Pharmacy Math I

1. Identify the Roman numeral with a value of 50.

    a. X
    b. M
    c. I
    d. L

Answer d is correct. L = 50.

Answer a is incorrect. X = 10.

Answer b is incorrect. M = 1000.

Answer c is incorrect. I = 1.

2. Identify the Arabic value of DCXXIV.

    a. 624
    b. 626
    c. 1024
    d. 1026

Answer a is correct. D = 500, C = 100, X = 10, I = −1, V = 5 (500 + 100 + 10 + 10 −1 +5 = 624).

Answer b is incorrect. The Roman numeral for 626 would be DCXXVI.

Answer c is incorrect. The Roman numeral for 1024 would be MXXIV.

Answer d is incorrect. The Roman numeral for 1026 would be MXXVI.

3. If 120 mL of a cough syrup contains 0.4 g of dextromethorphan, how many milligrams are contained in 1 teaspoonful?

    a. 0.016 mg
    b. 16 mg

c. 160 mg
d. 1.6 mg

Answer b is correct.

$$\frac{0.4\text{ g}}{120\text{ mL}} = \frac{x\text{ g}}{5\text{ mL}}\ x = 0.016\text{ g} = 16\text{ mg}$$

Answers a, c, and d are incorrect.

4. Interferon injection contains 5 million U/mL. How many units are in 0.65 mL?

   a. 3,250 U
   b. 32,500 U
   c. 325,000 U
   d. 3,250,000 U

Answer d is correct.

$$\frac{5,000,000\text{ units}}{1\text{ mL}} = \frac{x\text{ units}}{0.65\text{ mL}}$$

$$x = 3,250,000\text{ units}$$

Answers a, b, and c are incorrect.

5. An inhalant solution contains 0.025% w/v of a drug in 5 mL. Calculate the number of milligrams in this solution.

   a. 0.125 mg
   b. 1.25 mg
   c. 12.5 mg
   d. 0.0125 mg

Answer b is correct. 0.025 % w/v = 0.025 g/100 mL. Convert this percent w/v to mg/mL= 25 mg/100 mL.

$$\frac{25\text{ mg}}{100\text{ mL}} = \frac{x\text{ mg}}{5\text{ mL}}\ x = 1.25\text{ mg}$$

Answers a, c, and d are incorrect.

6. How many milligrams of a drug would be contained in a 10 mL container of a 0.65% w/v solution of a drug?

   a. 0.65 mg
   b. 6.5 mg
   c. 65 mg
   d. 650 mg

Answer c is correct. 0.65% w/v = 0.65 g/100 mL Converted to milligrams, this equals 650 mg/100 mL.

$$\frac{650\text{ mg}}{100\text{ mL}} = \frac{x\text{ mg}}{10\text{ mL}}\ x = 65\text{ mg}$$

Answers a, b, and d are incorrect.

7. How many milliequivalents of potassium chloride are in 240 mL of a 10% solution of KCl? The gram molecular weight is 74.5 g (K 39 atomic weight; Cl 35.5 atomic weight).

   a. 24 mEq
   b. 0.0745 mEq
   c. 2.4 mEq
   d. 322 mEq

Answer d is correct. The atomic weight of K is 39 and the atomic weight of Cl is 35; therefore, the molecular weight of KCl is 74.5.

- 74.5 = 1 molecular weight for KCl
- 74.5 g = 1 equivalent weight
- 74.5 mg = 1 milliequivalent weight (0.0745 g)

$$\frac{10\text{ g}}{100\text{ mL}} = \frac{x\text{ g}}{240\text{ mL}}\ \ x = 24\text{ g KCl}$$

$$\frac{0.0745\text{ g}}{1\text{ mEq}} = \frac{24\text{ g}}{x\text{ mEq}}\ \ x = 322.2\text{ mEq}$$

Answers a, b, and c are incorrect.

8. How many milliosmoles (mOsmol) of sodium chloride are there in 1 L of a 0.9% solution of normal saline solution? Molecular weight of NaCl = 58.5.

   a. 58.5 mOsmol
   b. 308 mOsmol
   c. 1 mOsmol
   d. 9000 mOsmol

Answer b is correct.

- Molecular weight of NaCl = 58.5 1 mole = 58.5 g
- 1 millimole = 58.5 mg = 2 milliosmoles, since NaCl dissociates into 2 particles

- $$\frac{900\text{ mg}}{100\text{ mL}} = \frac{x\text{ mg}}{1000\text{ mL}}$$

  $$x = 9000\text{ mg of NaCl in a liter (1000 mL)}$$

- $$\frac{58.5\text{ mg}}{2\text{ mOsmol}} = \frac{9000\text{ mg}}{x\text{ mOsmol}}$$

  $$x = 308\text{ mOsmol}$$

Answers a, c, and d are incorrect.

9. What is the percentage concentration (w/v) of a 250 mL solution containing 100 mEq of ammonium chloride? Molecular weight of NH_4Cl is 53.5.

   a. 53.5%
   b. 5.35%
   c. 2.14%
   d. 21.4%

Answer c is correct.

- Molecular weight of NH_4 = is 53.5
- 1 equivalent weight = 53.5 g
- 1 mEq = 53.5 mg

$$\frac{53.5\text{ mg}}{1\text{ mEq}} = \frac{x\text{ mg}}{100\text{ mEq}}\ \ x = 5350\text{ mg or 5.35 g}$$

$$\frac{5.35\text{ g}}{250\text{ mL}} = \frac{x}{100}\ \ x = 2.14\%$$

Answers a, b, and d are incorrect.

10. How many millimoles of HCl are contained in 130 mL of a 10% solution? Molecular weight = 36.5.

    a. 356 mmol
    b. 34 mmol
    c. 36.5 mmol
    d. 13 mmol

Answer a is correct.

- Molecular weight of HCl = 36.5
- 1 mole = 36.5 g
- 1 millimole = 36.5 g/1000 = 0.0365 g = 36.5 mg

$$\frac{10\ g}{100\ mL} = \frac{x\ g}{130\ mL} \quad x = 13\ g\ HCl$$

$$\frac{0.0365\ g}{1\ mmol} = \frac{13\ g\ HCl}{x\ mmol} \quad x = 356\ mmol$$

11. How many 60 mg tablets of codeine sulfate should be used to make this cough syrup?

    $Rx:$ Codeine SO_4 30 mg/teaspoon
         Cherry Syrup qs ad 150 mL

    Sig: 1 teaspoonful every 6 hours as needed for cough

    a. 7
    b. 15
    c. 20
    d. 24

Answer b is correct.

- 1 teaspoon = 5 mL

$$\frac{30\ mg}{5\ mL} = \frac{x\ mg}{150\ mL} \quad x = 900\ mg$$

$$\frac{60\ mg}{1\ tab} = \frac{900\ mg}{x\ tab} \quad x = 15\ tablets$$

Answers a, c, and d are incorrect.

12. How many milliliters of a 17% solution of benzalonium chloride is required to prepare 350 mL of a 1:750 w/v solution?

    a. 2.75 mL
    b. 0.275 mL
    c. 27.5 mL
    d. 275 mL

Answer a is correct.

$$\frac{1\ g}{750\ mL} = \frac{x\ g}{350\ mL} \quad x = 0.47\ g$$

$$\frac{17\ g}{100\ mL} = \frac{0.47\ g}{x\ mL} \quad x = 2.75\ mL$$

Answers b, c, and d are incorrect.

13. If 7 mL of a diluent is added to an injectable containing 0.5 g of a drug with a final volume of 7.3 mL, what is the final concentration of the parenteral solution in mg/mL?

    a. 6.85 mg/mL
    b. 0.069 mg/mL
    c. 685 mg/mL
    d. 68.5 mg/mL

Answer d is correct.

$$\frac{500\ mg}{7.3\ mL} = \frac{x\ mg}{1\ mL} \quad x = 68.5\ mg$$

Therefore, the final concentration in mg/mL is 68.5 mg/mL.

Answers a, b, and c are incorrect.

14. A medication order of a drug calls for a dose of 0.6 mg/kg to be administered to a child weighing 31 lb. The drug is to be supplied from a solution containing 0.25 g in 50 mL bottles. How many milliliters of this solution are required to fill this order?

    a. 8.45 mL
    b. 0.00845 mL
    c. 1.69 mL
    d. 0.25 mL

Answer c is correct.

$$\frac{1\ kg}{2.2\ lb} = \frac{x\ kg}{31\ lb} \quad x = 14\ kg$$

$$\frac{0.6\ mg}{1\ kg} = \frac{x\ mg}{14\ kg} \quad x = 8.45\ mg\ or\ 0.00845\ g$$

$$\frac{0.25\ g}{50\ mL} = \frac{0.00845\ g}{x\ mL} \quad x = 1.69\ mL$$

Or, solving by dimensional analysis:

$$31\ lb \times 1\ kg/2.2\ lb \times 0.6\ mg/kg \times 1\ g/1000\ mg \\ \times 50\ mL/0.25\ g = 1.69\ mL$$

Answers a, b, and d are incorrect.

15. A solution contains 2 mEq of KCl/mL. If a TPN order calls for the addition of 180 mg of K^+, how many milliliters of this solution should be used to provide the potassium required. Atomic weight of K = 39 and the atomic weight of Cl = 35.5.

    a. 343.85 mL
    b. 2.3 mL
    c. 39 mL
    d. 74.5 mL

Answer b is correct.

Answers a, c, and d are incorrect.

$$\frac{1\ \text{mEq KCL}}{74.5\ \text{mg KCL}} = \frac{2\ \text{mEq KCL}}{x\ \text{mg KCl}} \quad x = 149\ \text{mg KCL}$$

$$\frac{39\ \text{mg K}}{74.5\ \text{mg KCl}} = \frac{x\ \text{mg K}}{149\ \text{mg KCl}} \quad x = 78\ \text{mg K}$$

$$\frac{78\ \text{mg K}}{149\ \text{mg KCl}} = \frac{180\ \text{mg K}}{x\ \text{mg KCl}} \quad x = 343.85\ \text{mg KCl}$$

$$\frac{149\ \text{mg KCl}}{1\ \text{mL}} = \frac{343.85\ \text{mg KCl}}{x\ \text{mL}} \quad x = 2.3\ \text{mL}$$

16. A TPN solution contains 750 mL of D5W. If each gram of dextrose provides 3.4 kcal, how many kcal would the TPN solution provide?

    a. 127.5 kcal
    b. 37.5 kcal
    c. 34 kcal
    d. 75 kcal

Answer a is correct.

$$\frac{5\ \text{g dextrose}}{100\ \text{mL}} = \frac{x\ \text{g}}{750\ \text{mL}} \quad x = 37.5\ \text{g}$$

$$\frac{3.4\ \text{kcal}}{1\ \text{g}} = \frac{x\ \text{kcal}}{37.5} \quad x = 127.5\ \text{kcal}$$

Answers b, c, and d are incorrect.

17. Select the definition of specific gravity.

    a. Ratio of the weight of a material to the weight of the same volume of standard material.
    b. The mixing of solutions or solids possessing different percentage strengths.
    c. The expression of two ratios which are equal.
    d. Grams of ingredient in 100 g of product; assumed for mixtures of solids and semisolids.

Answer a is correct. Specific gravity is defined as ratio of the weight of a material to the weight of the same volume of standard material.

Answer b is incorrect. Alligation: The mixing of solutions or solids possessing different percentage strengths presents a calculation problem which may be solved using an arithmetic method called alligation.

Answer c is incorrect. A proportion is the expression of two ratios which are equal. It is usually written in one of two ways: two equal fractions (a/b = c/d) or using a colon (a:b = c:d).

Answer d is incorrect. Percent weight-in-weight: % (w/w) = grams of ingredient in 100 g of product; assumed for mixtures of solids and semisolids.

18. Select the apothecary measure of volume.

    a. Grain
    b. Scruple
    c. Dram
    d. Minim

Answer d is correct. A minim is an apothecary measure of volume.

Answers a, b, and c are incorrect. Grain, scruple, and dram are an apothecary measure of weight.

19. 480 minims equals:

    i. 8 fluidrams
    ii. 1 fl oz
    iii. 1 gallon

    a. i and ii
    b. i and iii
    c. ii and iii
    d. All of the above

Answer a is correct. 480 minims = 8 fluidrams and 1 fl oz 1 gallon = 61440 minims.

20. 437.5 grains equal how many ounces?

    a. 1 oz
    b. 16 oz
    c. 30 oz
    d. 38 oz

Answer a is correct. 437.5 grains = 1 oz

21. What should be the flow rate of the medication in milliliters per hour if 100 mg of medication is added to 250 mL of NS and the desired rate of delivery is 5 mg/h?

    Solution:

$$\frac{250\ \text{mL}}{100\ \text{mg}} \times \frac{5\ \text{mg}}{1\ \text{h}} = 12.5\ \text{mL/h}$$

CHAPTER 73 | Clinical Toxicology

The following case pertains to questions 1 to 3.

1. RC is a 40-year-old, 170 lb man. He reports a toothache for which he has been taking four 500-mg acetaminophen tablets every 3 to 4 hours for the last 3 days without relief. Additionally, he complains of nausea and new onset of right upper quadrant pain. His last dose of acetaminophen was 2 hours prior to physical examination. Which of the following would be considered factors that would increase the risk of hepatotoxicity in RC? Select all that apply.

    a. Chronic alcohol use
    b. Concurrent isoniazid therapy
    c. Acquired immunodeficiency syndrome
    d. >40 years of age

Answer a is correct. Chronic alcohol use is recognized as a factor for increased risk of hepatotoxicity due to (1) potential induction of CYP2E1 and resulting increase in the hepatotoxic acetaminophen metabolite NAPQI, (2) depleted glutathione stores due to poor nutrition frequently associated with alcoholism, (3) pre-existing liver dysfunction associated with chronic alcohol abuse.

Answer b is correct. Isoniazid is an inducer of CYP2E1 and recognized as a factor for potential increased risk of hepatotoxicity due to resulting increase in the hepatotoxicity acetaminophen metabolite NAPQI.

Answer c is correct. Acquired Immunodeficiency Syndrome (AIDS) is associated with depleted glutathione stores.

Answer d is incorrect. Patient age is not currently recognized as a factor that would increase risk of hepatotoxicity.

2. Which of the following would be an appropriate measure in the evaluation/treatment of RC?

   a. Acetaminophen level should be plotted on the Rumack-Matthew nomogram to determine if antidote therapy is indicated.
   b. Antidote therapy should be initiated immediately.
   c. Acetaminophen level should be ordered to determine need for antidote therapy.
   d. Activated charcoal should be administered and acetaminophen level should be ordered to determine need for antidote therapy.

Answer b is correct. In adult patients reporting repeated supratherapeutic doses of acetaminophen with evidence of acetaminophen toxicity (nausea, vomiting, malaise, diaphoresis, abdominal pain), acetaminophen antidote should be initiated as soon as possible to prevent additional toxicity.

Answer a is incorrect. The Rumack-Matthew nomogram is only appropriate to determine risk of acetaminophen-induced hepatic toxicity for acute ingestions of acetaminophen. It is not appropriate to use the nomogram for chronic ingestions, ingestions of extended release acetaminophen preparations, and acute ingestions with unknown time of ingestion.

Answer c is incorrect. In asymptomatic patients, acetaminophen levels in conjunction with other factors (AST, comorbid conditions, history) are utilized in determining relative risk and need for antidote therapy in repeated supratherapeutic cases, but in the symptomatic patient, intervention to prevent ongoing toxicity should be initiated as early as possible.

Answer d is incorrect. Activated charcoal would not be expected to have a high benefit-to-risk ratio 2 hours post ingestion of 2 g of acetaminophen in a patient with complaints of nausea and effective antidote available.

3. The decision is made to treat RC with the antidote for acetaminophen. Which of the following is a form of acetylcysteine that could be given intravenously as antidote therapy in acetaminophen poisoning? Select all that apply.

   a. Acetylcysteine solution 20%
   b. Acetadote injection
   c. Acetylcysteine solution 10%
   d. Acetylcysteine injection

Answer a is correct. Acetylcysteine solution is available in 10% and 20% concentrations. While not approved by the FDA for intravenous administration and not recommended unless (1) acetylcysteine injection formulation is unavailable and (2) intravenous route is deemed medically necessary, the solution formulation has been utilized in patients requiring intravenous administration (intractable vomiting, pregnancy) for treatment of acetaminophen poisoning. If acetylcysteine solution is given intravenously, it should be diluted appropriately in D5W and administered through a 0.2 micron Millipore filter.

Answer b is correct. Acetadote is a brand of acetylcysteine injection and FDA-approved for intravenous administration.

Answer c is correct. Acetylcysteine 10% solution is not FDA approved for intravenous administration but has been administered intravenously in specific scenarios of acetaminophen overdose (see **Answer a** comment for more complete explanation).

Answer d is correct. Acetylcysteine injection is an FDA-approved generic formulation of Acetadote injection.

4. MP is a 40-year-old, 107-lb woman brought to the emergency department by EMS after collapsing at a concert. On physical examination, MP is noted to be responsive only to painful stimuli, has a respiratory rate of 6, and constricted pupils. Which of the following agent(s) would be most likely associated with these physical findings?

   a. Methylphenidate
   b. Amitriptyline
   c. Donepezil
   d. Hydromorphone

Answer d is correct. Opioid toxicity is associated with the "opiate triad" of CNS depression, respiratory depression, and miosis.

Answer a is incorrect. Methylphenidate produces sympathomimetic excess in overdose, the symptoms of which can be extremely similar to anticholinergic syndrome clinically. The deviating clinical finding will often be the fact that adrenergic toxicity is associated with diaphoresis.

Answer b is incorrect. Amitriptyline has strong anticholinergic properties. The mnemonic is reflective of the altered mental status, mydriasis with loss of accommodation, flushed skin, hyperthermia, and dry skin and mucous membranes associated with anticholinergic toxicity.

Answer c is incorrect. Donepezil inhibits cholinesterases resulting in increased cholinergic tone. Symptoms of cholinergic excess are associated with the mnemonic SLUDGE (salivation, lacrimation, urination, defecation, GI distress, and emesis) or DUMBBELS (diarrhea and diaphoresis, urination, miosis, bronchorrhea/bronchospasm, bradycardia, emesis, lacrimation, lethargy, salivation).

---

5. ZW presents to the emergency department with a chief complaint of tinnitus and five episodes of emesis. She reports ingestion of #50 enteric coated aspirin tablets 90 minutes prior to arrival. On physical examination, her heart rate is 92 beats/min, blood pressure 115/80, respiratory rate is 32, and she is diaphoretic. If ZW's history is accurate, arterial blood gases will most likely indicate which of the following acid-base derangements?

    a. Metabolic acidosis
    b. Respiratory alkalosis
    c. Partially compensated metabolic acidosis
    d. Partially compensated respiratory acidosis

Answer b is correct. Salicylates directly stimulate the respiratory center. Early in the course of toxicity, this stimulation leads to an increased respiratory rate. Hyperventilation reduces systemic CO_2 levels. The effect on pH by this reduction in "respiratory acid" is an increase in systemic pH due to a respiratory alkalosis. As the course of salicylate toxicity progresses, a mixed acid-base picture develops as the initial respiratory alkalosis continues, but a metabolic acidosis that is not purely compensatory develops. This acidosis is due to increased salicylate level concentrations which are weak acids, uncoupling of oxidative phosphorylation and resultant lactic acid production, increased free fatty acid metabolism and impaired renal function, and accumulation of other organic acids.

Answers a, c, and d are incorrect.

---

6. How much aspirin equivalent is contained in 5 mL of the topical analgesic, oil of wintergreen (100% methyl salicylate)?

    a. 140 mg
    b. 500 mg
    c. 1400 mg
    d. 7 g

Answer d is correct. Methyl salicylate has an aspirin equivalent factor of 1.4, meaning it is 1.4 times more potent compared to aspirin. With the given variables, 100% methyl salicylate would equate to 100 g of methyl salicylate per 100 mL of oil of wintergreen, or stated in different units 1000 mg of methyl salicylate per 1 mL of oil of wintergreen. When this is converted to aspirin equivalents by multiplying the 1000 mg/mL by 1.4 it is determined that each 1 mL of oil of wintergreen contains 1400 mg of aspirin equivalent. Adjusting for a volume of 5 mL would give the correct answer of 7 g of aspirin equivalent per 5 mL of 100% oil of

wintergreen product. This highlights the potential toxicity of methyl salicylate products as 1 mL of this product would almost meet the minimum toxic dose of 150 mg/kg for a 10 kg child, and 5 mL, theoretically, could prove fatal.

Answers a, b, and c are incorrect.

---

7. Which toxin antidote combination pairing is correct? Select all that apply.

    a. Butorphanol and naloxone
    b. Cyanide and hydroxocobalamin
    c. Fomepizole and isopropyl alcohol
    d. Pyridoxine and isoniazid
    e. Deferoxamine and iron

Answer a is correct. Butorphanol is a synthetic mixed agonist-antagonist opioid analgesic. Excessive dose would be expected to produce general opioid toxicity, and treatment with naloxone should be considered in the management of overdose.

Answer b is correct. Cyanide is a rapid-acting toxin that inhibits mitochondrial cytochrome a3 forcing a shift to cellular anaerobic respiration lactate production, metabolic acidosis, and cellular hypoxia. Death can result in minutes. Hydroxocobalamin binds cyanide molecules by substituting a hydroxo-linked ligand to the trivalent cobalt ion to form cyanocobalamin (vitamin B_{12}) which is then eliminated in the urine.

Answer d is correct. Pyridoxine is the antidote for significant isoniazid (INH) toxicity. Significant INH poisoning is classically characterized as seizures that are refractory to standard therapy (benzodiazepines, barbiturates), coma, and metabolic acidosis. INH alters the metabolism and creates a functional depletion of pyridoxine. This state of pyridoxine deficiency impairs the synthesis and metabolism of gamma aminobutyric acid (GABA), the major inhibitory neurotransmitter in the CNS, resulting in seizure activity. Pyridoxine as an INH antidote should be administered intravenously at a dose that is equivalent to the dose of INH ingested up to a maximum of 5 g. If the dose is unknown, 5 g should be given empirically. Pyridoxine doses utilized in treatment of INH toxicity may deplete hospital stock.

Answer e is correct. Deferoxamine chelates free iron following iron overdose. The chelate complex ferrioxamine is then eliminated in the urine. Urine color may be a "vin-rose" (red-brown) color following deferoxamine administration, indicating presence of ferrioxamine in the urine; however, color change is not always seen. Adverse effects associated with administration of deferoxamine in acute iron poisoning include: infusion rate-related hypotension, pulmonary toxicity for patients treated for longer than 24 hours, and infection.

Answer c is incorrect. Fomepizole is a competitive antagonist of alcohol dehydrogenase (ADH) and is most commonly used in ethylene glycol and methanol poisonings. While isopropyl alcohol is metabolized via ADH, fomepizole is not utilized for blocking metabolism as the major metabolite is acetone.

The following case pertains to questions 8 and 9.

8. GL is a 58-year-old woman with history of congestive heart failure treated with digoxin. She presents to the emergency department with a history of ingesting #60 digoxin 0.25-mg tablets 6 hours ago. Her electrocardiogram revealed high-degree heart block with a ventricular rate of 40 to 50 beats/min, a potassium level of 5.8 mEq/L and a digoxin concentration of 12 ng/mL. Which of the following should GL's medical record be evaluated as a precaution, should digoxin immune Fab fragments' administration be necessary. Select all that apply.

   a. Papaya or papain allergy
   b. Patients treated previously with digoxin immune Fab fragments
   c. Sheep protein allergy
   d. Latex allergy

Answer a is correct.   Papain is used to segment whole antibody in the production of digoxin immune Fab fragments. Caution is warranted for patients with papain, papaya extract, or the pineapple enzyme bromelain.

Answer b is correct.   By design, the Fab fragment lacks the antigenic determinants of the Fc fragment and is associated with significantly reduced potential of anaphylactoid reaction compared to intact immunoglobulin; however, patient previously treated with digoxin immune Fab fragment are at increased risk of immunogenic reaction.

Answer c is correct.   Patients with known sheep protein allergy are at increased risk of immunogenic reaction as the manufacturer of digoxin immune Fab fragments utilizes sheep (ovine) immunized with a digoxin derivative to form the anti-digoxin antibodies.

Answer d is correct.   Certain latex and dust mite allergens share antigenic structures with papain and patients with these allergies may be allergic to papain.

---

9. Digoxin immune Fab fragments in an appropriate dose for the given ingestion was initiated. Within 60 minutes, the patient's clinical status improved, but a repeat digoxin concentration 6 hours after Fab administration returned at 19 ng/mL. What is the best answer to explain the increase in GL's digoxin concentration?

   a. Continued absorption of digoxin.
   b. The time frame of ingestion was incorrect, and ingestion was closer to time of presentation.
   c. Administration of digoxin immune Fab fragment has increased serum levels of total digoxin.
   d. Endogenous digoxin-like immunoreactive substance.

Answer c is correct.   Digoxin serum levels can be determined as both free and total digoxin. Digoxin levels reported

as the more frequent total digoxin value can rise dramatically following administration of digoxin immune Fab fragments. This is due to the Fab binding of circulation plasma digoxin and establishing a concentration gradient that favors redistribution of digoxin from tissue back into the plasma; however, the digoxin will almost all be bound and not able to interact with receptors. This would explain GL's digoxin level increase following Fab administration. Total digoxin levels will remain elevated and be clinically misleading until Fab fragments are eliminated from the body.

Answer a is incorrect.   Digoxin is associated with a biphasic distribution pattern in which it is absorbed into the plasma compartment and then slowly redistributed to the tissue. This delay in steady-state plasma concentrations results in misleadingly high plasma concentrations (two- to threefold) early after ingestion (<4-6 hours) compared to more reliable steady state levels drawn 6 or more hours after ingestion. This is the opposite of what was seen with GL and as such **Answer a** is not the correct answer.

Answer b is incorrect.   Due to the same biphasic distribution properties discussed for **Answer a**, the digoxin level following acute overdose would be expected to be higher in the first 4 to 6 hours than it would be after 6 hours of ingestion. As such, if the ingestion had been closer to the time of presentation, the level would be expected to be higher than it would be 6 or more hours post-ingestion when the follow-up digoxin serum level was drawn.

Answer d is incorrect.   Endogenous digoxin-like immunoreactive substance (EDLIS) is a naturally occurring substance chemically and functionally similar to exogenous digoxin. It has been noted in neonates and patients with several other conditions including renal and hepatic dysfunction, pregnancy, congestive heart failure, type 1 diabetes mellitus, and post-strenuous exercise. EDLIS can cross-react with digoxin assays if present EDLIS is not expected to increase digoxin levels by more than 2 ng/mL and clinical implications are unknown. Additionally, naturally occurring digitalis glycosides from plants and animals may cross-react with the digoxin assay if ingested.

---

10. The administration of which of the following agents would be indicated in the setting of tricyclic antidepressant overdose associated with seizures or QRS interval more than 115 ms?

    a. Sodium bicarbonate
    b. Flumazenil
    c. Physostigmine
    d. Procainamide

Answer a is correct.   Serum alkalinization with a goal of establishing a systemic pH between 7.45 and 7.55 is indicated in the setting of tricyclic antidepressant (TCAD) toxicity with evidence of widening QRS interval and/or seizure activity. Mechanisms by which sodium bicarbonate administration may provide benefit are as follows:

1. Increased systemic sodium levels may overcome blocked sodium channels and/or increased systemic pH results in increased non-ionized TCAD, decreasing ligand receptor interaction between ionized TCAD and the sodium channel.

2. Wide complex dysrhythmia and hypotension can be reversed by administration of sodium bicarbonate in sufficient doses. Seizures will not respond to this sodium bicarbonate therapy, and should be treated with standard measures, but if seizures occur in the setting of TCAD overdose sodium bicarbonate therapy is warranted because they indicate significant toxicity.

3. Other potential therapies could include administration of hypertonic 3% saline to increase systemic sodium levels or hyperventilation to increase systemic pH; however, these have not been found to provide the same level benefit as treatment with sodium bicarbonate.

Answer b is incorrect. Administration of flumazenil may precipitate generalized seizures in the setting of TCAD overdose and is contraindicated.

Answer c is incorrect. Physostigmine is a cholinesterase inhibitor and can reverse some anticholinergic symptoms of TCAD poisoning. Historically, it has been utilized to treat TCAD-induced antimuscarinic symptoms; however, use has been abandoned as physostigmine is associated with increased incidence of dysrhythmia, bradycardia, asystole, and seizures.

Answer d is incorrect. Procainamide is a class IA antidysrhythmic agent and has a mechanism of action that blocks cardiac fast sodium channels. These are the same channels antagonized in TCAD poisoning leading to QRS prolongation, and utilization may worsen cardiac toxicity. As such, administration of agents with sodium channel-blocking properties (class IA and IC antidysrhythmics) is an absolute contraindication in TCAD poisoning.

---

11. Which vasopressor would be the best choice for hypotension due to tricyclic antidepressant toxicity that is refractory to fluid and sodium bicarbonate support?

    a. Norepinephrine
    b. Epinephrine
    c. Dopamine
    d. Dobutamine

Answer a is correct. Hypotension in the setting of tricyclic antidepressant toxicity is largely due to alpha-adrenergic blockade. For this reason, a direct-acting alpha-adrenergic agonist (norepinephrine, phenylephrine) is the preferred vasopressor.

Answer b is incorrect. Epinephrine acts as an agonist at β_1, β_2, and α_1 adrenergic receptor effects. Due to this mixed agonist action, α-adrenergic receptor-induced vasoconstriction is often cancelled out by the β_2 adrenergic receptor vasodilation and, as such, is not a preferred vasopressor.

Answer c is incorrect. Dopamine is an indirect-acting agent with a mixed mechanism of action depending on the dose administered. At lower doses (1-5 mcg/kg/min) dopamine acts on renal and mesenteric dopamine receptors, resulting in selective vasodilation. At intermediate doses (5-15 mcg/kg/min), dopaminergic and β_1 adrenergic receptors are stimulated, but there is minimal increase in systolic or diastolic pressures. It is not until higher doses (>15 mcg/kg/min) that a direct alpha-adrenergic agonist effect resulting in more significant vasoconstriction is demonstrated from dopamine. Additionally, it is possible that blockade of endogenous norepinephrine and dopamine reuptake by TCAD mechanism of action could result in catecholamine depletion, blunting the indirect action of dopamine and further reducing potential benefit as a vasopressor. If dopamine is utilized in the setting of TCAD, induced hypotension doses should be in the higher range in attempt to counter the alpha-receptor blockade.

Answer d is incorrect. Dobutamine is an inotrope and not a vasopressor. Due to significant β_1 stimulation resulting in increased cardiac output, reflex vasodilation and hypotension occur with dobutamine administration.

---

12. Which of the following are differences between calcium gluconate and calcium chloride parenteral preparations?

    a. The mechanism of action of calcium chloride is superior in calcium channel blocker poisoning.
    b. The mechanism of action of calcium gluconate is superior in calcium channel blocker poisoning.
    c. Calcium chloride provides three times more cation compared to calcium gluconate on an equal volume basis.
    d. Calcium gluconate is more irritating when given intravenously than calcium chloride.

Answer c is correct. Calcium chloride contains 13.6 mEq of calcium per gram compared to calcium gluconate, which provides 4.65 mEq of calcium per gram. Both products are commercially available as 10% solutions, making calcium chloride three times more potent per equivalent volume of calcium gluconate.

Answer a is incorrect. Administration of either of the calcium salts in appropriate dose provides the body with increased cation levels to attempt to overcome competitive blockade imposed by calcium channel blockers.

Answer b is incorrect. See explanation above.

Answer d is incorrect. Calcium chloride is significantly more irritating when given intravenously compared to calcium gluconate.

The following case pertains to questions 13 and 14.

13. RF, a 47-year-old, 205 lb man presents to the emergency department and states that he took an overdose of his "heart medication" 3 hours ago. He now feels lethargic and nauseated. His vitals reveal a heart rate of 45 beats/min and blood pressure of 85/40 mm Hg. The ED staff contacts the patient's pharmacy and is told the patient has prescriptions for atenolol, amlodipine, and digoxin. Which of the following agents should not be administered prior to return of digoxin serum concentration determination?

    a. Atropine
    b. Fluid bolus
    c. Calcium salt
    d. Glucagon

Answer c is correct. Administration of calcium salts is appropriate in the treatment of calcium channel blocker toxicity and may be effective in β-blocker toxicity but should not be utilized in the setting of bradycardia and hypotension where digoxin cannot be ruled out as a cause or confounding factor. Administration of calcium salts in the setting of digoxin poisoning theoretically may worsen toxicity by increasing intracellular calcium levels and could precipitate asystole.

Answer a is incorrect. Atropine is a first-line agent in the treatment of bradycardia due to β-blocker, calcium channel blocker, or digoxin toxicity.

Answer b is incorrect. Appropriate fluid bolus is a first-line therapy for hypotension due to β-blocker or calcium channel blocker toxicity and would not be expected to adversely affect a patient with concomitant digoxin.

Answer d is incorrect. Administration of glucagon is appropriate in the treatment of β-blocker toxicity and may be effective in calcium channel blocker toxicity. Glucagon is not a therapy utilized to treat digoxin toxicity, but it would not be contraindicated to use in settings of mixed agent poisoning.

14. Administration of intravenous 0.9% saline, atropine, calcium chloride, dopamine, and norepinephrine does not result in adequate improvement in RF's clinical status, and the physician orders the initiation of hyperinsulinemia-euglycemia therapy. At an infusion rate of 0.5 U/kg/h, how much regular insulin would be administered to RF in the first 30 minutes at this rate?

    a. 23 Units
    b. 47 Units
    c. 51 Units
    d. 103 Units

Answer a is correct. RF's weight of 205 lb divided by 2.2 to yield kilograms results in a weight of 93 kg. At a weight of 93 kg and a dose of 0.5 Units/kg/h would result in a total hourly dose of 47 Units/h. This hourly dose of 47 Units then divided by 60 would result in a per minute infusion rate of 0.78 units/min, multiplied by 30 would then give the final answer of 23 total Units of insulin administered during the first 30 minutes of the infusion.

Answer b is incorrect. 47 Units would be the total for 60 minutes of infusion for RF at a rate of 0.5 Unit/kg/h.

Answer c is incorrect. 51 Units would be the total for 30 minutes of infusion at a rate of 0.5 Unit/Pound/h.

Answer d is incorrect. 103 Units would be the total for 60 minutes of infusion at a rate of 0.5/Pound/h.

15. KR is a 39-year-old man brought to the emergency department by his wife. She states that he has been vomiting for the last 2 hours and acting abnormal following an argument approximately 4 hours ago. Initial laboratory data results include: sodium of 144 mEq/L, potassium 3.8 mEq/L, bicarbonate 8 mEq/L, chloride 98 mEq/L, BUN 23 mg/dL, creatinine 0.7 mg/dL, glucose 93 mg/dL, calcium 9.6 mg/dL, and albumin 4 g/dL. Arterial blood gas values on room air were determined to be: pH 7.34, Pco_2 11 mm Hg, Po_2 93 mm Hg. What is the calculated anion gap for this patient?

    a. 23
    b. −49.8
    c. 147
    d. 38

Answer d is correct. Conventionally, the anion gap is calculated using the formula of subtracting the sum of serum chloride and bicarbonate values from the serum sodium level (for this case ([144 Na^+ − (98 Cl^- + 8 HCO_3^-) = 38]). There is a degree of variance depending on method of measurement in establishing a "normal" range for anion gap with some methods setting a normal value of 12 (+/−4) and others 7 (+/−4). In patients with hypoalbuminemia, a correction factor should be accounted for in determining the anion gap as it decreases approximately 3 mEq/L per 1 g/dL decrease in the serum albumin. In the setting of a metabolic acidosis, determination of the presence of a high anion gap can aid in narrowing the differential diagnosis. The mnemonic MUDPILES (methanol, uremia, diabetic ketoacidosis, phenothiazines/paraldehyde, isoniazid/iron, lactic acidosis, ethylene glycol/ethanol, salicylates) represents frequent causes of metabolic acidosis associated with a high anion gap.

16. Which opioid is associated with both proconvulsant activities in overdose?

    a. Meperidine
    b. Methadone
    c. Hydrocodone
    d. Heroin

Answer a is correct. Seizures are associated with accumulation of the meperidine metabolite normeperidine.

Answer b is incorrect. Methadone is associated with prodysrhythmic properties even in therapeutic levels as it can prolong QT/QTc interval, potentially precipitating torsades de pointes; however, seizures are not a frequent adverse effect.

Answer c is incorrect. Hydrocodone is not commonly associated with intrinsic proconvulsant or prodysrhythmic activity in overdose.

Answer d is incorrect. Heroin is not commonly associated with intrinsic proconvulsant or prodysrhythmic activity in overdose.

17. ES is an 84 year-old, 200 lb man that presents to the emergency department after accidentally taking four of his metoprolol 200 mg tablets due to an error involving his weekly pill organizer. Which of the following is a first-line agent in the management of metoprolol toxicity associated with a high incidence of nausea and vomiting?

    a. Atropine
    b. Calcium gluconate
    c. Glucagon
    d. Milrinone

Answer c is correct. Glucagon is the agent of choice for β-blocker toxicity not responsive to atropine and fluid administration. β-Adrenergic receptors and glucagon are both coupled to G proteins that, upon stimulation, result in increased adenyl cyclase and resultant cAMP. This provides the positive inotropic and chronotropic effects of $β_1$-receptor stimulation. In β-blocker poisoning, administration of glucagon provides an effective bypass of antagonized β-receptors. Glucagon should initially be given as a 3 to 5 mg intravenous bolus and repeated until response, upon which time a continuous infusion should be initiated at the cumulative response dose per hour. Nausea and vomiting are frequent adverse effects following administration of the higher doses utilized to treat β-blocker toxicity, and close attention should be paid to the risk of aspiration or obstruction following emesis in patients with decreased levels of consciousness. Additionally, patients should be observed for hypoglycemia or hyperglycemia and hypokalemia. Glucagon has a short duration of action compared to that of the majority of β-antagonist. This combined with higher dose therapy may deplete entire hospital supplies following significant overdose.

Answer a is incorrect. Atropine is utilized as a first-line agent for bradycardia due to β receptor antagonism. In the majority of moderate to severe β-blocker poisonings, atropine will fail to significantly increase heart rate, and inotropic therapy is necessary. Effects from atropine administration would be anticholinergic in nature and not nausea and vomiting.

Answer b is incorrect. Calcium salt administration may improve blood pressure but not heart rate in the setting of β-blocker poisoning and is not considered a first-line therapy.

Answer d is incorrect. Milrinone is a phosphodiesterase inhibitor (PDI) and decreases the breakdown of cAMP allowing for increased intracellular cAMP levels and improved myocardial function. PDI will increase cardiac output as evidence of their utility in the treatment of advanced cardiac failure, but use of PDI in the management of β-blocker toxicity is reserved for patients failing more proven therapies. Hypotension and difficulty in titration and long half-life are properties that significantly limit PDI use.

18. JD is a 39-year-old woman that presents to the emergency department at 3:00 pm and reports an acute ingestion of 10 g of acetaminophen 1 hour prior to arrival. On physical examination, she is emotional and upset but without other physical complaint. She reports a past medical history of depression treated with fluoxetine. What is the earliest time that an acetaminophen level can be drawn and plotted on the Rumack-Matthew nomogram to appropriately determine potential hepatotoxic risk and need for antidote administration for JD?

    a. Immediately on presentation to the emergency department
    b. 4:00 pm
    c. 6:00 pm
    d. 10:00 pm

Answer c is correct. The time to peak concentration following therapeutic dose of acetaminophen can range from 10 to 90 minutes depending on formulation, presence of food, or other coingestants (anticholinergics, opiates). Following acute overdose, complete absorption and peak acetaminophen levels can take longer. In order to reasonably assure complete absorption, the Rumack-Matthew nomogram was developed and validated utilizing a 4-hour post-ingestion time as the earliest point to evaluate acetaminophen levels and determine potential hepatotoxicity. Levels drawn prior to 4 hours post-ingestion cannot be used to determine potential risk unless the level returns as "non-detectable". Levels drawn after 4 hours can be plotted on the nomogram up to 24 hours post-ingestion; however, there is some concern that the levels closer to 24 hours may not be as accurate in determining hepatotoxic risk compared to levels closer to 4 hours post-ingestion. In the case, JD presented to the emergency room at 3:00 pm, which was reported to be 1 hour after here ingestion (ie, ingestion time at 2:00 pm). As such the earliest the Rumack-Matthew nomogram can be utilized would be 6:00 pm (4 hours after the ingestion time of 2:00 pm).

19. ZM is a 44-year-old, 170 lb man who was found unresponsive in the middle of a city. He is noted to have a blood pressure of 115/60 mm Hg, a heart rate of 61 beats/min, and a respiratory rate of 6 breaths/min; his ECG reveals a normal sinus rhythm. He is afebrile, has no apparent trauma, and is noted to have an odor of alcohol on his breath. Prescription bottles for methadone and clonazepam were found in his shirt pocket. Which of these agents would be appropriate to administer with ZM's history? Select all that apply.

    a. Flumazenil
    b. Naloxone
    c. Thiamine
    d. Dextrose

Answer b is correct. Naloxone is routinely used in the setting of undifferentiated coma. While use may precipitate withdrawal, opioid withdrawal compared to benzodiazepine, ethanol, or other withdrawal syndromes is not life-threatening. In order to prevent withdrawal, dosing should be initiated at a lower dose and titrated to effect or total dose of 10 mg.

Answer c is correct. Thiamine along with dextrose is routinely used in the setting of undifferentiated coma. Thiamine is administered in this setting due to potential thiamine deficiency and concerns of Wernicke's encephalopathy. In general, it should be given prior to administration of dextrose, but dextrose should not be held if thiamine administration would cause delay. The 100 mg intravenous dose is well-tolerated and potential benefit outweighs risk. Need for thiamine in children would be atypical and is not routinely performed in the setting of undifferentiated coma in this population.

Answer d is correct. Dextrose is routinely used in the setting of undifferentiated coma unless rapid bedside glucose determination can be made. Adults should be given 25 g (50 mL) of 50% dextrose and children 0.5 to 2 g/kg of not more than 25% dextrose intravenously.

Answer a is incorrect. Flumazenil is an antagonist of benzodiazepine receptors but has limited utility as an antidote. It should not be used in the setting of an undifferentiated comatose patient. Risk of precipitating withdrawal seizures at which point benzodiazepines would be rendered of limited therapeutic benefit is one concern. Additionally, in the setting of mixed overdose presence, a benzodiazepine may be providing some therapeutic seizure protection, and administration of flumazenil could unmask toxicity of other agents leading to more significant toxicity.

20. Which of the following are requirements of The Poison Prevention and Packaging Act (PPPA) of 1970? Select all that apply.

    a. Limits the quantity of flavored "children's" aspirin tablets to #36, 81 mg tablets.
    b. With limited exceptions, requires pharmacists to dispense oral prescription drugs in child-resistant packaging unless the patient or prescribing practitioner requests non-child-resistant packaging.
    c. Allows manufactures of over-the-counter medications and certain household substances to package a single size, which does not comply with the PPPA if (1) it also supplies the substance in packages that do comply and (2) the packages of such substances bear conspicuous labeling that states "This package for households without young children."
    d. Requires child-resistant packaging for iron-containing over-the-counter and dietary supplements that contain a total of 250 mg or more of elemental iron per package.

Answers a, b, c, and d are correct. All presented answers are mandates of the PPPA. The PPPA requires child-resistant packaging for some hazardous household products as well as most oral prescription and over-the-counter medications. Additionally, certain specific products have dosage unit or total container quantity limit restrictions per the PPPA. Child-resistant packaging must be designed to be significantly difficult for children under 5 years of age to open within a reasonable time and not difficult for normal adults. For those who might have difficulty opening such containers, the PPPA allows manufactures one non-complying size product provided it carries a warning that it is not recommended for use in households with children and requires that the product is also supplied in child-resistant packages of the same size. Regulated prescription drugs may be dispensed in non-child-resistant packaging upon the specific request of the prescribing doctor or the patient. There has been significant reduction in child deaths from ingestion of household products and medications following enactment of the PPPA.

CHAPTER 74 | All Hazards Preparedness

1. Preparedness is achieved and maintained by which of the following? Select all that apply.

    a. Planning
    b. Organizing
    c. Training
    d. Exercising

Answers a, b, c, and d are correct. Preparedness is achieved and maintained through a continuous cycle of planning, organizing, training, equipping, exercising, evaluating, and taking corrective action. Organization at the local or state level will vary, but virtually all plans will be based on the NIMS. NIMS provides a systematic, proactive approach to guide departments and agencies at all levels of government, nongovernmental organizations, and the private sector. The guide allows agencies to work seamlessly to prevent, protect against, respond to, recover from, and mitigate the effects of incidents, regardless of cause, size, location, or complexity, in order to reduce the loss of life and property and harm to the environment.

2. Virtually all disaster plans are based on what national system?

    a. National Planning System (NPS)
    b. National Incidence Management System (NIMS)
    c. Federal Incidence Bureau System (FIBS)
    d. Strategic National Planning System (SNPS)

Answer b is correct. Organization at the local or state level will vary, but virtually all plans will be based on the NIMS. NIMS provides a systematic, proactive approach to guide departments and agencies at all levels of government, nongovernmental organizations, and the private sector.

Answers a, c, and d are incorrect.

3. The SNS provides what during an incidence of national significance?

a. Highly trained medical personal from around the country to disseminate supplies
b. Pharmaceuticals only to the state
c. Active military medical personnel to support the public
d. Pharmaceuticals and medical supplies to the state in need

Answer d is correct. The CDC SNS has large quantities of medicine and medical supplies to protect the American public if there is a public health emergency (terrorist attack, flu outbreak, earthquake) severe enough to cause local supplies to run out. Once Federal and local authorities agree that the SNS is needed, medicines will be delivered to any state in the United States in time for them to be effective. Each state has plans to receive and distribute SNS medicine and medical supplies to local communities as quickly as possible.

Answer a is incorrect. The state is responsible for dissemination.

Answer b is incorrect. The SNS supplies not only pharmaceuticals but also supplies and equipment.

Answer c is incorrect. Active military medical personnel are to support the armed forces. However, the governor may call up his state's National Guard to assist in the disaster.

4. Which government official must request the SNS?

a. President of the United States
b. Director of Health and Human Services
c. Governor
d. Speaker of the House

Answer c is correct. The governor of the afflicted state must request for the SNS. If the request is granted, the material will be on site within 12 hours, hence they are often referred to as 12-Hour Push Packs. It is the requesting states' responsibility to manage the housing, dissemination, and administration of the material once it is received. However, this response time is inadequate for a nerve agent event, as treatment must be accomplished in less than 12 hours.

Answers a, b, and d are incorrect.

5. The CHEMPACK Program stores nerve agent antidotes with participating local or state entities. What are the antidotes provided by this program? Select all that apply.

a. Atropine
b. Pyridoxine
c. Pralidoxime
d. Diazepam

Answers a, c, and d are correct. As a result of the rapid onset of severe signs and symptoms, nerve agents are stored and shipped differently than other treatments found in the SNS. They are stored under CHEMPACK. CHEMPACK is a voluntary program of the SNS operated by the CDC for the benefit of the US civilian population. Its mission is to provide state and local governments a sustainable nerve agent antidote cache. The CHEMPACK contains materials for a nerve agent exposure and does not contain other materials.

In the event of an OP poisoning, three agents need to be readily available (atropine, pralidoxime, and diazepam). Atropine will be used to counter the muscarinic effects commonly seen. However, it has little affinity for nicotinic receptors and will not reverse respiratory paralysis, fasciculation, or general muscle weakness. Pralidoxime will be used to reverse the binding of the OP to the acetylcholinesterase as long as aging has not occurred. Aging is the process by which the OP covalently binds the acetylcholinesterase rending it useless. Aging can occur in less than 12 hours with some of the militarized Ops; this is the principal reason for the CHEMPACK. Diazepam will be used to prevent or treat seizures.

Answer b is incorrect. Pyridoxine, vitamin B_6, is required by your body for utilization of energy in the foods you eat, production of red blood cells, and proper functioning of nerves. It is used to treat and prevent vitamin B_6 deficiency resulting from poor diet, certain medications, and some medical conditions.

6. Which of the following is considered a Category A threat agent? Select all that apply.

a. Smallpox
b. Novel H1N1
c. Anthrax
d. Botulism

Answer a is correct. Smallpox is definitely considered a Category A threat. The orthopoxvirus variola (smallpox) causes an acute febrile illness with a corresponding rash that develops into small, pus-filled blisters.

Answer c is correct. Anthrax is definitely considered a Category A threat. *B. anthracis* is an encapsulated, aerobic, gram-positive, spore-forming, rod-shaped bacterium. The bacterium is known to cause cutaneous, gastrointestinal, respiratory, and oropharyngeal infections.

Answer d is correct. *C. botulinum* is an anaerobic, gram-positive, spore-forming rod that produces a potent neurotoxin. The spores are heat-resistant and can survive in foods that are incorrectly or minimally processed. Seven types (A, B, C, D, E, F, and G) of botulism are recognized, based on the antigenic specificity of the toxin produced by each strain. Types A, B, E, and F cause human botulism naturally, human cases of other types would be suggestive of an act of terrorism. Types C and D cause most cases of botulism in animals. Animals most commonly affected are wild fowl and poultry, cattle, horses, and some species of fish. Botulinum-infected patients with extensive muscle weakness, ptosis, dysphagia, great frequency of gastrointestinal effects, and urinary retention are at a greater risk of developing respiratory failure. Mechanical ventilation may be required.

Answer b is incorrect. H1N1 (formerly known as swine flu) is not a Category A threat, although it could result in the SNS being activated. An influenza pandemic is a global disease outbreak that occurs when a new influenza A virus emerges for which there is little or no immunity in the human population. Since immunity is low, the virus can spread quickly. In late March and early April 2009, novel swine influenza A (properly called 2009 H1N1) was detected in the United States for the first time.

7. Which agent is found in the SNS and is indicated for postexposure prophylaxis to inhaled *B. anthracis*?

  a. Dapsone
  b. Daptomycin
  c. Doxycycline
  d. Dicloxacillin

Answer c is correct. Doxycycline is one of the two antibiotics (ciprofloxacin is the other) that is stored by the government to combat some of the threat agents. Ciprofloxacin or doxycycline is indicated as initial therapy for postexposure prophylaxis to prevent inhalational anthrax from inhaled spores. There is presently no evidence to support either agent over the other for prophylaxis. Therefore, a patient's individual history will be the determining factor.

Answer a is incorrect. Dapsone is used or treatment of leprosy or prophylaxis of toxoplasmosis or pneumocystis in immunocompromised patients.

Answer b is incorrect. Daptomycin is used for the treatment of gram positive infections, for example, methicillin resistant Staphylococcus aureus (MRSA) and vancomycin resistant Enterococcus (VRE).

Answer d is incorrect. Dicloxacillin is a penicillin antibiotic used for the treatment of skin and soft tissue infections caused by penicillinase producing strains of Staphylococci (eg MSSA).

8. Antibiotic therapy for postexposure prophylaxis to inhaled *B. anthracis* should last for how many days?

  a. 30
  b. 40
  c. 60
  d. 90

Answer c is correct. The optimal duration of prophylaxis is uncertain; however, 60 days was recommended, primarily on the basis of animal studies of anthrax deaths and spore clearance after exposure.

Answers a and b are incorrect. In one human case during the Sverdlovsk outbreak (former Soviet Union, 1979), anthrax developed 43 days after spores were released into the atmosphere (time of exposure unknown). Therefore, 30 and 40 days of therapy appears inadequate.

Answer d is incorrect. The optimal duration of prophylaxis is uncertain; however, 60 days was recommended, primarily on the basis of animal studies of anthrax deaths and spore clearance after exposure. The possible need for longer prophylaxis and vaccine use was discussed. The Department of Health and Human Services has additional options for prophylaxis of inhalational anthrax for persons who wish to take extra precautions, especially those whose exposure may have been high. Three options are now offered: (1) 60 days of antibiotic prophylaxis; (2) 100 days of antibiotic prophylaxis, and (3) 100 days of antibiotic prophylaxis, plus anthrax vaccine as investigational postexposure treatment.

9. An 18-year-old patient has been diagnosed with a pneumonic form of *Y. pestis*. What is the best course of action for the individual(s) exposed to the patient?

  a. Start ciprofloxacin 500 mg every 12 hours once symptoms appear.
  b. Start doxycycline 100 mg every 12 hours for 7 days in all individuals exposed during the patient's clinical course.
  c. Await the patient's culture and sensitivity results and start the most appropriate antibiotic as prophylaxis in the exposed individuals.
  d. Prophylaxis is not beneficial.

Answer b is correct. Doxycycline 100 mg every 12 hours for 7 days in an 18-year-old is an appropriate regimen.

Answer a is incorrect. Ciprofloxacin is an appropriate antibiotic choice, but waiting for symptoms to appear is wrong. All patients suspected to have an exposure should be treated as soon as possible regardless of signs and symptoms.

Answer c is incorrect. Awaiting cultures and sensitivity with an invasive organism such as *Y. pestis* is inappropriate, when an exposure is known.

Answer d is incorrect. Prophylaxis can be beneficial for exposed patients.

10. A pharmacist working in local retail pharmacy receives a call during a bioterrorism drill from an emergency department physician. He states they have a confirmed case of pneumonic tularemia. The patient states a former coworker threatened everyone in the workplace. Upon questioning from the police, it was determined the coworker had released *F. tularensis* into the air ducts of his former workplace approximately 3 days prior. There are six individuals in that area and he has written them each a prescription for ciprofloxacin 500 mg every 12 hours for 7 days as prophylaxis. However, the air duct system is shared with a daycare and eight children have been potentially exposed. All of the children are <30 kg. The physician asks for an antibiotic recommendation. Which of the following is the best treatment recommendation for all of the children?

  a. Doxycycline 50 mg every 12 hours for 7 days
  b. Doxycycline 2.2 mg/kg every 12 hours for 7 days
  c. Ciprofloxacin 500 mg once daily for 7 days
  d. Ciprofloxacin 25 mg/kg every 12 hours for 7 days

Answer b is correct. Doxycycline 2.2 mg/kg every 12 hours for 7 days is an appropriate dose for children <30 kg.

Answer a is incorrect. The dose of doxycycline is potentially too high in some and to low in others. Weight based dosing of doxycycline should be utilized.

Answer c is incorrect. Ciprofloxacin is an appropriate antibiotic choice, but the dose is too high for children 30 kg or less. The dose should be Ciprofloxacin 10 to 15 mg/kg every 12 hours for 7 days.

Answer d is incorrect. Ciprofloxacin 25 mg/kg every 12 hours is an excessive dose for children 30 kg or less. The dose should be ciprofloxacin 10 to 15 mg/kg every 12 hours for 7 days.

---

11. Which of the following botulism types can be treated with an antitoxin obtained from the CDC? Select all that apply.

    a. Type A
    b. Type B
    c. Type C
    d. Type E

Answers a, b, and d are correct. There is a bivalent antitoxin preparation containing types A and B, and a monovalent antitoxin preparation type E (suggestive of contaminated seafood) for treatment of botulism caused by the aforementioned toxins.

Answer c is incorrect. *Experimentally the military* has an antitoxin for all types including G.

---

12. Twelve patients with type G botulism have been diagnosed in the United States in the past 24 hours. All had recently flown through Toronto Pearson International Airport in the last 72 hours from various destinations. All are experiencing a rapid descending paralysis. What is the most likely reason for the outbreak?

    a. Contaminated seafood at an airport vendor
    b. Deliberate release of toxin within the airport
    c. Person to person contamination
    d. Serendipity

Answer b is correct. Type G is unusual in humans. Multiple cases of type G infection with a single source of contact (airport) is a deliberate release until otherwise ruled out.

Answer a is incorrect. Although a food vendor could be implicated, the seafood suggests type E.

Answer c is incorrect. Botulism is not spread from person to person contamination.

Answer d is incorrect. A virtual statistical impossibility considering it is type G.

---

13. What is presently the best course of treatment for Ebola?

    a. Fluid replacement, ventilation, and additional supportive care as needed
    b. High dose ribavirin
    c. Cryotherapy to drop the core temperature to <95°F
    d. A cocktail of acyclovir, protease inhibitor, and interferon

---

Answer a is correct. Although some data may support the use of an experimental serum that destroys infected cells. Supportive care including fluid replacement, oxygenation, and ventilation is presently the best course of treatment.

Answer b is incorrect. Ribavirin can be used for other types of hemorrhagic fever. It is ineffective for Ebola.

Answer c is incorrect. Nothing to support dropping the core temperature.

Answer d is incorrect. No evidence to support this.

---

14. A person with smallpox is no longer considered infectious when what event occurs?

    a. Defervescence
    b. The last pustule scabs over
    c. Sloughing of the last pustule scab
    d. When the rash turns to pustules

Answer c is correct. The sloughing of the last scab is considered the point where a patient is no longer infectious.

Answer a is incorrect. An afebrile patient could be infectious.

Answer b is incorrect. Although it is probably positive in the clinical course; the patient is still considered infectious.

Answer d is incorrect. A patient at this stage is highly infectious.

---

15. Which of the following signs and symptoms are considered clinically significant control with atropine in a postexposure OP patient?

    a. Miosis, salivation, and muscle twitching
    b. Mydriasis, dry mucous membranes, flushing, and tachycardia
    c. Tachycardia, bronchorrhea, and salivation
    d. Decreased bronchial secretions and increased ease of ventilation

---

Answer d is correct. A patient can still have miosis and other symptoms, but adequate atropine is based on increased ease of ventilation and decreased bronchial secretions. The patient does not have to be dry, but secretions should be reduced.

Answer a is incorrect. This would signal marked cholinergic syndrome.

Answer b is incorrect. This would signal anticholinergic syndrome and the patient has most likely received excessive atropine.

Answer c is incorrect. This patient has been inadequately treated and needs additional atropine based on the bronchorrhea.

---

16. An adult patient with sarin poisoning has been decontaminated and is now in the triage area. He has small pupils, sweating, and copious salivation and nasal secretions. He begins having a seizure almost immediately after being brought to the triage area. Which is the best course of treatment?

    a. Administer diazepam 10 mg, followed by a 2 mg bolus of atropine, and then pralidoxime 2 g in 100 cc of NS infused over 30 minutes.
    b. A 2 mg bolus of atropine and repeat as needed, then pralidoxime 2 g in 100 cc of NS infused over 30 minutes. If the seizure activity has not abated post pralidoxime, then give 5 mg of diazepam.
    c. Administer 10 mg of diazepam for the seizure then no additional therapy as the other signs and symptoms are not concerning.
    d. Administer 5 g of pralidoxime via intravenous pyelography (IVP) since it will replenish gamma-aminobutyric acid (GABA), then give atropine 2 g prn until bronchorrhea decreases.

Answer a is correct. An attempt to immediately control the seizure should be made. This patient is having significant cholinergic signs and symptoms so atropine and 2-pam should be given.

Answer b is incorrect. Delaying seizure treatment for 30 minutes is inappropriate.

Answer c is incorrect. The diazepam is correct, but withholding atropine and 2-pam is inappropriate.

Answer d is incorrect. Pyridoxine (vitamin B_6), not pralidoxime, is the GABA precursor. A benzodiazepine is needed in this patient.

---

17. A 3-year-old child and her 65-year-old grandmother were riding in car that was involved in a three-vehicle accident at 3 am. They have only minor injuries, but one of the other vehicles was carrying I131 for use as an imaging agent. The I131 container was not properly stored or sealed and it entered the side window of the vehicle with the child and grandmother. Many of the compounded I131 capsules were ruptured and dispersed throughout the car. They are 20 minutes postaccident and no one is answering the phone at the nuclear pharmacy; there is no paperwork with the I131 product and the delivery driver is unconscious. Which is the best advice for the grandmother and child?

    a. Treat both with KI.
    b. Treat the grandmother with KI and leave the child untreated.
    c. Treat the child with KI and leave the grandmother untreated.
    d. Treat both with Prussian blue.

Answer c is correct. There are too many unknowns in this case. An argument could be made to withhold KI if the dose was known. However, the dose is not known and the product

was inadequately stored, the child was definitely exposed and given children's sensitivity to I131 treating is the appropriate course for the child. Grandmother is older than 40 years of age. Her risk of thyroid disease secondary to the exposure is virtually nil.

Answer a is incorrect. The grandmother is in no danger from a small I131exposure. Treating the child can be debated. See Answer c.

Answer b is incorrect.

Answer d is incorrect. Prussian blue is not indicated for I131.

---

18. The first case of novel H1N1 was reported in the United States in late March-early April 2009. By the end of June, reported cases topped 1 million US residents. The logical reason for rapid dissemination of the disease is most likely which of the following?

    a. The seasonal flu vaccine weakened the immune system.
    b. The wet spring months are better for viral survival.
    c. The population lacks immunity.
    d. Antivirals are infective.

Answer c is correct. A pandemic outbreak occurs because the population lacks immunity.

Answers a, b, and d are incorrect.

---

19. Select the brand name for doxycycline.

    a. Vibramycin
    b. Zosyn
    c. Zovirax
    d. Valtrex

Answer a is correct. Brand names for doxycycline include: Doryx, Doxy, Monodox, Vibramycin, and Vibra-Tabs.

Answer b is incorrect. Zosyn is the brand name for piperacillin/tazobactam.

Answer c is incorrect. Zovirax is the brand name for acyclovir.

Answer d is incorrect. Valtrex is the brand name for valacyclovir.

---

20. Select the brand name for ciprofloxacin.

    a. Levaquin
    b. Cipro
    c. Avelox
    d. Flagyl

Answer b is correct. Cipro is the brand name for ciprofloxacin.

Answer a is incorrect. Levaquin is the brand name for levofloxacin.

Answer c is incorrect. Avelox is the brand name for moxifloxacin.

Answer d is incorrect. Flagyl is the brand name for metronidazole.

CHAPTER 75 | Herbal and Nonherbal Dietary Supplements

1. Which product affects circadian rhythm and also functions as a hormone to aid in ovulation and sexual maturity?

   a. Saw palmetto
   b. St. John's wort
   c. Black cohosh
   d. Melatonin

Answer d is correct. Due to this effect on the body, melatonin is commonly used for insomnia and is not recommended for use in adolescents.

Answer a is incorrect. Saw palmetto inhibits 5-α-reductase, dihydrotestosterone receptors, and has some anti-inflammatory activity.

Answer b is incorrect. St. John's wort works in neural synapses to influence reuptake of neurotransmitters and also has some GABA antagonism.

Answer c is incorrect. Black cohosh affects the vasovagal system and may have some estrogenic effects.

2. Which product can be utilized for postmenopausal symptoms, primarily hot flushes?

   a. Saw palmetto
   b. Kava
   c. Black cohosh
   d. RYR

Answer c is correct. This is due to black cohosh's effects on the vasovagal system.

Answer a is incorrect. Saw palmetto is primarily used for BPH.

Answer b is incorrect. Kava is primarily utilized for anxiety and insomnia.

Answer d is incorrect. RYR can be used for hyperlipidemia.

3. A 42-year-old woman visits your pharmacy with complaints of increased sensitivity to the sun after starting a new natural product. Which of the following is most likely to cause this side effect?

   a. Garlic
   b. Kava
   c. Echinacea

   d. Chondroitin
   e. St. John's wort

Answer e is correct. Increased photosensitivity is well-documented effect; patients should be educated to wear sunscreen.

Answers a, b, c, and d are incorrect. These products are not associated with sun sensitivity as a side effect.

4. What should be taken into consideration when a patient starts a new natural supplement? Select all that apply.

   a. The cheapest product
   b. Quality considerations
   c. Efficacy of the product
   d. How the supplement works
   e. The natural product must be more effective than the alternative prescription medication

Answer b is correct. Utilize reliable quality information available for natural products. Some supplements, as seen with kava, may have harmful contaminants. This information may be hard to come by since the Food and Drug Administration (FDA) does not regulate natural products. A resource such as ConsumerLab can be utilized to determine the quality of natural supplements.

Answer c is correct. Similar to quality considerations, utilize high-quality, available information and studies regarding efficacy when recommending products. This may also be limited depending on the product.

Answer d is correct. This information can be useful to determine interactions or additive effects but this may be limited or extrapolated from in vitro or animal studies.

Answer a is incorrect. The cheapest product may not be the most effective or may have quality issues, compared to a product that has verified quality but may be higher in price.

Answer e is incorrect. Usually natural products are not as effective as prescription products. This does not need to be a requirement for a patient to take a natural product instead of the alternative prescription product; the severity of the medical condition and the patient's expectations should be considered.

5. A 78-year-old man with a history of BPH, hypertension, and depression wants to try saw palmetto for his BPH. Which of the following is/are true regarding saw palmetto? Select all that apply.

   a. It is usually well tolerated but increased bleeding time has been reported.
   b. Saw palmetto has been shown to decrease prostate size.
   c. It is not safe to use in pregnancy.
   d. Can have additive effects with blood pressure medications.
   e. This patient should not utilize saw palmetto due to known interactions with antidepressants.

Answer a is correct. Combination with antiplatelet/anticoagulant medications needs to be closely monitored.

Answer c is correct. It is contraindicated in pregnancy and lactation due to hormonal effects.

Answer b is incorrect. This has not been shown with saw palmetto. Benefit may only be seen with reduction of some symptoms related to BPH.

Answer d is incorrect. This effect has not been observed with use of saw palmetto.

Answer e is incorrect. Few interactions have been reported with saw palmetto including estrogens, contraceptives, and antiplatelet/anticoagulant medications. The patient should be advised to monitor for any changes in depression symptoms or antidepressant side effects if he begins saw palmetto therapy.

---

6. A 55-year-old man with a history of hypertension and BPH was recently informed he has high cholesterol. He wants to try a natural product first before taking a "statin." Which of the following could he try for hypercholesterolemia? Select all that apply.

   a. RYR
   b. Garlic
   c. Kava
   d. Glucosamine sulfate
   e. Fish oil

Answer a is correct. RYR contains a "statin" analog, which contributes to its cholesterol-lowering effects. The patient should be educated on this fact, which may affect his desire to use the product.

Answer b is correct. Garlic is usually utilized for high blood pressure and cholesterol, but effect sizes may be small. It may or may not be an appropriate choice for the patient.

Answer e is correct. Fish oil is most effective for high triglyceride reduction, but is also used for cardiovascular health and for small effects on other lipids. It may or may not be an appropriate choice for the patient.

Answer c is incorrect. Kava is primarily used for anxiety and insomnia.

Answer d is incorrect. Glucosamine is usually used for OA and joint health.

---

7. A 24-year-old woman wants to start taking St. John's wort for depression. She has a history of insomnia, anxiety, and asthma. Which of the following is/are true regarding St. John's wort? Select all that apply.

   a. St. John's wort is a potent CYP3A4 inducer.
   b. Drowsiness is a side effect of this product so it may help her insomnia.
   c. St. John's wort has drug-drug interactions with oral contraceptives, immunosuppressive agents, and serotonergic agents.

d. St. John's wort may help with lowering blood pressure.
   e. St. John's wort use should be limited to mild to moderate depression, not severe.

Answer a is correct. This interaction has been seen with case reports and human studies.

Answer c is correct. This is mediated by the CYP3A4 and p-glycoprotein interactions and the serotonergic effects of St. John's wort.

Answer e is correct. This supplement may not be effective for severe or refractory depression.

Answer b is incorrect. Insomnia has been reported with St. John's wort.

Answer d is incorrect. Blood pressure lowering has not been reported with St. John's wort.

---

8. A patient is being discharged from the hospital on warfarin. Before leaving the hospital, you look over his prescriptions and natural products. Which natural products could increase his risk of bleeding with concomitant warfarin use due to the supplement's antiplatelet/anticoagulant properties? Select all that apply.

   a. Chondroitin and glucosamine sulfate
   b. Evening primrose oil
   c. Black cohosh
   d. Garlic
   e. High doses of fish oil

Answers a, b, d, and e are correct. These products have theoretical cautions or case reports to this effect.

Answer c is incorrect. This risk has not been reported for black cohosh.

---

9. Which of the following statement(s) is/are true about garlic? Select all that apply.

   a. Garlic does NOT have GI side effects.
   b. Medicinal doses of garlic are safe in pregnancy.
   c. This product may be utilized for the treatment of acne.
   d. It is safe to use with prescription medications since it does not interact with any drugs.
   e. Garlic may need to be avoided in patients with low blood pressure.

Answer e is correct. This is due to the supplement's possible antihypertensive effects.

Answer a is incorrect. Nausea, vomiting, and heartburn have been reported, especially with higher doses.

Answer b is incorrect. Although there are no clinical reports of garlic's adversely affecting pregnancy, other evidence suggests there is a risk when medicinal amounts are ingested.

Answer c is incorrect. This supplement is not usually taken for acne and has no information to support this use.

Answer d is incorrect. Garlic has several interactions with medications, especially those metabolized by CYP3A4.

10. A 60-year-old man wants to start glucosamine and chondroitin. He has a history of depression, hyperlipidemia, and OA and he's allergic to PCN (rash). He currently takes citalopram, atorvastatin, and ibuprofen as needed. Which of the following statements is NOT true in regard to glucosamine and chondroitin?

    a. The most common side effects include GI-related symptoms.
    b. There are different forms of glucosamine available.
    c. Glucosamine and chondroitin are contraindicated with atorvastatin.
    d. The mechanisms of these products are related to synthesis of cartilage or prevention of cartilage degradation.

Answer c is correct. A drug interaction with atorvastatin has not been reported for glucosamine or chondroitin.

Answer a is incorrect. Most common adverse effects include GI upset, nausea, constipation and diarrhea.

Answer b is incorrect. Glucosamine sulfate and hydrochloride are available.

Answer d is incorrect. Chondroitin and glucosamine both serve as building blocks for cartilage production; chondrocytes are stimulated and matrix metalloproteinase is inhibited.

11. Which of the following is/are true regarding safety and side effects of fish oil? Select all that apply.

    a. Common side effects may include belching, bad breath, and nausea.
    b. Common interactions with fish oil include antivirals and antibiotics.
    c. Keeping fish oil capsules in the freezer or taking enteric-coated capsules can decrease some side effects.
    d. It is known that fish oil inhibits several CYP enzymes.

Answer a is correct. These are well-known side effects of fish oil.

Answer c is correct. This can reduce the fishy taste or "fish burps."

Answer b is incorrect. These interactions have not been reported with fish oil.

Answer d is incorrect. CYP interactions have not been reported.

12. Which of the following is considered an appropriate dose in regard for the mentioned supplement?

    a. 2 grams of fish oil by mouth daily
    b. 400 mg of melatonin by mouth 30 minutes prior to HS
    c. 40 mg by mouth daily in divided doses of RYR
    d. 100 mcg by mouth bid of black cohosh

    e. 10 mg glucosamine sulfate with 5 mg chondroitin sulfate by mouth tid

Answer a is correct. Usual dosing for fish oil is 1 to 4 grams daily.

Answer b is incorrect. Though higher and lower doses have been, melatonin is commonly dosed at 0.3 to 5 mg.

Answer c is incorrect. Usual doses of RYR are 1.2 to 2.4 g/d, but doses as low as 600 mg daily have been used.

Answer d is incorrect. A typical dose of black cohosh is 20 mg of standardized extract bid.

Answer e is incorrect. For OA, the glucosamine sulfate typical dose is 1500 mg daily while the chondroitin dose is 1200 mg daily, both given in divided doses.

13. A 23-year-old woman comes to your pharmacy stating she was exposed to the flu less than 24 hours ago. She has been feeling fine overall except for a runny nose. She would like to take a natural product for possible flu prevention. Which product do you recommend for her?

    a. Evening primrose oil
    b. Saw palmetto
    c. Kava
    d. Echinacea

Answer d is correct. This can be used to prevent and treat symptoms of upper respiratory infection.

Answers a, b, and c are incorrect. None of these are usually used for prevention of infection or illness. Kava should not be recommended due to safety concerns.

14. Which of the following side effect(s) is/are associated with oral evening primrose oil use?

    a. Weight loss
    b. Kidney stone formation
    c. Hair loss
    d. Overall, evening primrose oil is well tolerated with some GI side effects

Answer d is correct. Evening primrose oil can cause abdominal pain, nausea, diarrhea, vomiting, dyspepsia, flatulence, and distension but can resolve with continued use.

Answers a, b, and c are incorrect. These side effects have not been reported with evening primrose oil use.

15. A patient comes to your pharmacy with a medication list containing efavirenz, tenofovir, emtricitabine, melatonin, and amlodipine. Which of the following natural products should NOT be recommended for this patient, considering the MAJOR interactions between the herbal product and their prescriptions?

    a. Saw palmetto
    b. St. John's wort

c. Kava

d. Glucosamine and chondroitin

Answer b is correct. St. John's wort is known to induce CYP3A4 and P-glycoprotein transporter, both of which affect the metabolism of amlodipine and efavirenz (Non-nucleoside reverse-transcriptase inhibitors [NNRTI]).

Answer a is incorrect. Saw palmetto is not known to interact with HIV regimens, melatonin, or amlodipine.

Answer c is incorrect. Kava should not be recommended do to hepatotoxicity concerns. The available evidence is contradictory or theoretical regarding CYP and P-glycoprotein interactions.

Answer d is incorrect. Glucosamine and chondroitin are not known to have interactions with *human immunodeficiency virus* (HIV) regimens, melatonin, or amlodipine.

---

16. Which of the following should NOT be recommended in patients with chronic liver damage or liver failure?

a. Melatonin

b. Evening primrose oil

c. Fish oil

d. Black cohosh

Answer d is correct. Though not well documented, there is some concern that black cohosh may exacerbate liver problems in patients with chronic liver issues such as hepatitis or that there may be additive effects with hepatotoxic medications.

Answer a is incorrect. Melatonin has not been reported to cause liver damage or increase risk of liver damage.

Answer b is incorrect. Evening primrose oil has not been reported to cause liver damage or increase risk of liver damage.

Answer c is incorrect. Fish oil has not been reported to cause liver damage or increase risk of liver damage.

---

17. Which education points are appropriate to relay to a patient who is considering starting kava? Select all that apply.

a. Kava should not currently be recommended to patients.

b. Keep your healthcare providers updated on all prescription, OTC, and herbal products you are taking.

c. Kava has evidence to support efficacy for anxiety.

d. It is essential to monitor kidney function while taking kava.

Answer a is correct. Due to safety concerns related to possible hepatotoxicity.

Answer b is correct. This is crucial for any patient, especially those taking herbal products since the safety and efficacy is not as well-established as prescription and OTC products.

Answer c is correct. Kava is also used for insomnia, but that evidence is minimal and is more conflicting than evidence for anxiety.

Answer d is incorrect. Liver function will need to be monitored as kava can cause hepatoxicity. No kidney effects have been reported.

---

18. Which of the following is true in regards to melatonin therapy? Select all that apply.

a. This is an endogenous substance naturally produced by the body.

b. Melatonin can be utilized for jet lag.

c. Glomerular filtration rate (GFR) and creatinine clearance (CrCl) need to be monitored if used chronically.

d. Melatonin may decrease adverse effects associated with radiation or chemotherapy.

e. Melatonin interacts with anticoagulant/antiplatelet medications due to increased risk of bleeding with concomitant use.

Answer a is correct. Melatonin is utilized by the body to control circadian rhythm but also functions as a hormone to help with ovulation and sexual maturity.

Answer b is correct. Melatonin may also be used for insomnia.

Answer d is correct. Limited evidence is available supporting reduced toxicity of chemotherapy/radiation with concomitant melatonin. Melatonin acts as an antioxidant in this case but it may interact with other therapies and should be thoroughly discussed with the patient's oncologist before starting the concomitant therapy.

Answer c is incorrect. This substance is not known to cause renal toxicity so renal monitoring is not necessary during melatonin therapy.

Answer e is incorrect. Anticoagulant activity has not been associated with melatonin therapy.

---

19. A 70-year-old female patient of yours wants to take glucosamine sulfate and chondroitin for her OA. She has taken Tylenol® in the past but it has not totally relieved her pain. She currently takes metformin, glimepiride, lisinopril, low dose aspirin (81 mg), and hydrochlorothiazide. She has a history of hypertension, diabetes, and chronic kidney disease. She is allergic to cephalexin. Which of the following statements is an appropriate assessment regarding utilization of glucosamine/chondroitin for OA therapy in this patient?

a. This patient should NOT take glucosamine/chondroitin because of its drug-disease interaction with diabetes.

b. This patient doesn't need the combination of glucosamine/chondroitin; she could safely take glucosamine hydrochloride as monotherapy for her OA.

c. This patient should NOT add glucosamine/chondroitin due to the increased risk of renal toxicity from the supplement.

d. This patient could try glucosamine/chondroitin but needs to have her kidney function closely monitored to prevent progression of her chronic kidney disease (CKD).

e. This patient could try glucosamine/chondroitin but needs to monitor for bleeding due to the increased risk from concomitant low-dose aspirin.

Answer e is correct. Bleeding and increased INR have been reported with glucosamine/chondroitin, thus this natural product may have some antiplatelet/anticoagulant effects. It is critical for this patient to monitor for signs of bleeding such as easy bruising; if this occurs, glucosamine/chondroitin therapy will need to be stopped.

Answer a is incorrect. Glucosamine/chondroitin does not have a contraindication for use in diabetic patients; however, closer monitoring of glucose during the first few weeks of therapy is advisable.

Answer b is incorrect. Glucosamine hydrochloride is not recommended as monotherapy. This form of glucosamine is only recommended with chondroitin sulfate.

Answer c is incorrect. Glucosamine/chondroitin is not known to cause renal toxicity, either monotherapy or in combination with other medications.

Answer d is incorrect. Glucosamine/chondroitin is not known to have any renal effects to warrant renal monitoring.

20. Which of the following medications may interact with medicinal doses of garlic? Select all that apply.

a. Metoprolol
b. Oral contraceptives
c. Rilpivirine
d. Metformin
e. Fentanyl

Answer a is correct. Garlic has some antihypertensive effects and may be additive when combined with other blood pressure medications.

Answer b is correct. This is due to CYP3A4 induction by garlic, which can cause increased metabolism of oral contraceptives.

Answer c is correct. Rilpivirine is an NNRTI and its metabolism may be increased by the CYP3A4 induction by garlic.

Answer e is correct. This is due to CYP3A4 induction by garlic, which can cause increased metabolism of fentanyl.

Answer d is incorrect. Metformin is not metabolized by the CYP enzymes with which garlic is known to interact.

21. A 35-year-old woman wants to start taking oral evening primrose oil for "breathing and wheezing" in addition to her other medications. Upon review of her medical history, you find she has seasonal asthma, history of *deep vein thrombosis* (DVT), and high blood pressure. Her current medications include Xarelto®, Proair® inhaler PRN, enalapril, and metoprolol. Which of the following statements is the BEST assessment regarding starting oral evening primrose oil therapy for this patient?

a. Evening primrose oil could be considered in this patient since limited adverse events have been reported and this is an overall well-tolerated supplement.

b. Evening primrose oil should NOT be considered for this patient due to the CYP interaction with Xarelto, increasing the metabolism and clearance of Xarelto.

c. Evening primrose oil should be cautiously considered in this patient due to the antihypertensive effects of the supplement.

d. Evening primrose oil should NOT be recommended for this patient since it has not shown to be efficacious for asthma and it increases her risk of adverse bleeding if combined with Xarelto.

Answer d is correct. Evidence suggests this may not be effective for asthma. It could be considered for a trial use in this patient if there were no safety concern regarding the interaction with Xarelto. The potential benefit does not seem to outweigh the risk of the supplement in this patient.

Answer a is incorrect. It is true that evening primrose oil is well-tolerated by patients but for this particular patient, the interaction with Xarelto is concerning and may increase her risk of bleeding.

Answer b is incorrect. Evening primrose oil is not known to interact with CYP enzymes so this would not be a concern in this patient.

Answer c is incorrect. Evening primrose oil is not known to have antihypertensive effects.

22. A 43-year-old man with OA is interested in adding glucosamine/chondroitin to his medication/herbal product regimen to decrease pain and increase mobility since he maintain a very active lifestyle. He is interested in this route before trying a prescription product. He currently takes fluticasone nasal spray for seasonal allergies, propranolol for blood pressure and heart rate, bupropion XL for mood, and valacyclovir for cold sores. He is severely allergic to shellfish (anaphylaxis), and carries an EpiPen. Which of the following statements is the BEST assessment regarding glucosamine/chondroitin for this patient?

a. Glucosamine/chondroitin should be safe for this patient to try from a safety/interactions standpoint.

b. Due to the patient's allergy, glucosamine/chondroitin could be started in this patient with proper education and monitoring.

c. Glucosamine/chondroitin should NOT be started in this patient since glucosamine is usually produced from shellfish chitin.

d. Glucosamine/chondroitin should NOT be started in this patient due to the MAJOR drug-disease interactions with depression and cold sores.

e. Glucosamine/chondroitin interacts with valacyclovir but since the patient only takes this PRN for cold sores, it would be safe to be taken together.

Answer c is correct. Chondroitin monotherapy may be considered as an alternative.

Answers a and b are incorrect. There is a significant safety concern in this patient since he has a severe allergic reaction to shellfish. Since there is a chance for the glucosamine product to contain shellfish, this natural product is contraindicated for this patient. However, patients with more mild reactions to shellfish may be able to try the product after some education, especially regarding self-monitoring for allergic reactions.

Answers d and e are incorrect. Glucosamine/chondroitin do not have these known drug-disease/drug-drug interactions.

CHAPTER **76** | **Sterile Compounding Regulations and Best Practices for Sterile Compounding per USP 797**

1. What is the proper order of gowning and hand hygiene when preparing to enter the clean room?

   a. Don on shoe covers, mask, hair cover, facial hair cover, gown, perform hand hygiene
   b. Don on hair cover, mask, facial hair cover, gown, shoe covers, perform hand hygiene
   c. Don on shoe covers, hair cover, mask, facial hair cover, perform hand hygiene, gown
   d. Perform hand hygiene, don on shoe covers, hair cover, face mask, facial hair cover, gown

---

Answer c is correct. Gowned from cleanest to dirtiest, perform hand hygiene, and then put on gown.

Answer a is incorrect. Gown on after hand hygiene.

Answer b is incorrect. Must start from dirties parts and continue to the cleanest.

Answer d is incorrect. Cannot do hand hygiene before covering dirtiest parts.

---

2. When cleaning positive air pressure horizontal LAFW, the correct order of cleaning surfaces and the motion to clean is:

   a. Top using side to side motion from inside out, IV hanging pole using gripping motion, bottom using back to front motion going from one side to the other, sides using up, and down motion working from inside out.
   b. Bottom using side to side motion from inside out, top using side to side motion from inside out, IV hanging pole using gripping motion, sides using up, and down motion from inside out.

   c. Top using side to side motion from inside out, hanging pole using gripping motion, sides using top to bottom motion from inside out, bottom using side to side motion from inside out.
   d. Top using front to back motion from one side to the other, hanging pole using gripping motion, sides using side to side motion from top to bottom, bottom from side to side inside out.

Answer c is correct. Always clean from cleanest to dirtiest, motion perpendicular to the air flow.

Answer a is incorrect. Bottom of the LAFW is the last part to be cleaned.

Answer b is incorrect. Order completely incorrect.

Answer d is incorrect. Order of surfaces is right but the motion is not—top should be side to side from inside out, side should be perpendicular to air flow.

---

3. When referring to laminar air flow in the LAFW, we are talking about:

   a. Horizontal flow of air coming from HEPA filter in the LAFW
   b. Vertical flow of air coming from the HEPA filter in the BSC
   c. Unidirectional flow of air coming from HEPA filter
   d. Turbulent flow of air produced by HEPA filter

Answer c is correct. Unidirectional air flow as laminar is not specifically horizontal or vertical direction.

Answer a is incorrect. Laminar refers to air flow in one direction.

Answer b is incorrect. Laminar refers to air flow in one direction.

Answer d is incorrect. Turbulent is the opposite of laminar.

---

4. Which of the statements regarding media fill testing is correct?

   a. It is used to assess personnel's ability to don on sterile gloves.
   b. It is used to test SECs performance.
   c. It is used to test performance of the cleaning and sanitizing agents.
   d. It is used for assessment of aseptic technique of compounding personnel.

Answer d is correct. Media fill testing can be used as an assessment tool for compounders and it should mimic the most complex compounding activity of the compounder.

Answer a is incorrect. Sterile fingertip testing is used to assess gloving technique.

Answer b is incorrect. Environmental monitoring and viable and nonviable particle testing is used for SECs performance.

Answer c is incorrect. Media fill testing alone cannot detect failure of cleaning agents.

5. A pharmacy technician prepared TPN (from sterile components only) for one patient inside of ISO class 5 LAFW that was inside of the ISO class 7 compliant buffer room. What is the appropriate BUD for this product?

    a. 9 days if refrigerated
    b. 48 hours if refrigerated
    c. 14 days if refrigerated
    d. 3 days if refrigerated

Answer a is correct. Medium risk level product has 9 days BUD in refrigerated environment.

Answer b is incorrect. No product according to the USP chart has 48 hour refrigerated BUD.

Answer c is incorrect. Only low risk products have 14 days BUD refrigerated, but TPN is more complex preparation.

Answer d is incorrect. High-risk products have 3 days BUD; this TPN preparation is medium risk.

6. Adenosine injection was prepared as a STAT dose in the emergency room at bedside by withdrawing liquid from one vial into a syringe but without access to LAFW or buffer room. What would be the correct BUD for this preparation?

    a. 24 hours refrigerated
    b. 24 hours at room temperature
    c. 1 hour at room temperature
    d. Cannot determine BUD, insufficient amount of information provided

Answer c is correct. BUD of immediate use preparation is 1 hour in room temperature.

Answer a is incorrect. It is immediate use preparation.

Answer b is incorrect. It is immediate use preparation.

Answer d is incorrect. There is sufficient information to determine BUD as per Chapter 797.

7. If turned off, for a minimum of how long should a BSC and horizontal positive air flow LAFW run prior to use?

    a. The BSC should run for at least 4 minutes and the horizontal LAFW should run for at least 30 minutes.
    b. The BSC should run for at least 30 minutes and the horizontal LAFW should run for at least 10 minutes.
    c. The BSC should run for at least 30 minutes and the horizontal LAFW should run for at least 1 hour.
    d. Both should run for at least 30 minutes.

Answer a is correct. It only takes 4 minutes to purge BSC due to negative air pressure of the PEC as opposed to positive air pressure LAFW.

Answer b is incorrect. BSC does not need 30 minutes to purge.

Answer c is incorrect. BSC does not need 30 minutes to purge, LAFW does not need 1 hour.

Answer d is incorrect. BSC only needs 4 minutes to purge.

8. When entering a vial with a needle, which is appropriate technique to use?

    a. Enter the vial at a 90° angle, bevel down.
    b. Enter the vial at a 90° angle, bevel up.
    c. Enter the vial at a 45° angle, bevel down.
    d. Enter the vial at a 45° angle, bevel up.

Answer d is correct. Best practice to avoid coring.

Answer a is incorrect. 90° angle can cause coring.

Answer b is incorrect. 90° angle can cause coring.

Answer c is incorrect. Bevel down can increase chance of coring.

9. What is the appropriate BUD for a Minibag Plus® product assembled in the LAFW under proper conditions as a part of batch?

    a. 45 days if frozen
    b. BUD does not apply as with proprietary products expiration date is assigned based on manufacturer's recommendations.
    c. 9 days in refrigerator
    d. Unable to determine, as not sufficient amount of information is provided.

Answer b is correct. Follow manufacturer's recommendations.

Answer a is incorrect. This product follows manufacturer's recommendations not BUD.

Answer c is incorrect. It is not medium risk preparation.

Answer d in incorrect. Information needed is provided.

10. Which of the following is an example of a primary engineering control?

    a. Buffer room
    b. BSC
    c. Ante room
    d. SEC

Answer b is correct. PEC

Answer a is incorrect. SEC

Answer c is incorrect. SEC

Answer d is incorrect. Not a USP 797 defined space, possibly SEC

11. Which of the following statements discussing the term "critical site" are correct? Select all that apply.

    a. Hub of the needle as well as the shaft are considered critical sites of the needle.
    b. Critical sites should be exposed to first air at all times.

c. Critical sites must not be contaminated by microorganisms but it is acceptable to expose them to physical contaminants, if sterility is preserved.

d. If critical site is touched and contamination is suspected, it must be wiped with sterile 70% IPA to prevent contamination.

Answers a, b, and d are correct. The hub of the needle as well as the shaft are considered critical sites of the needle. Critical sites should be exposed to first air at all times. If critical site is touched and contamination is suspected, it must be wiped with sterile 70% IPA to prevent contamination. However, one would not wipe a needle (critical site), if contamination were suspected.

Answer c is incorrect. Physical contamination is still a concern and the preparation is not considered sterile.

12. According to USP Chapter 797, minimum frequency of cleaning floors in the buffer room is:

   a. Hourly
   b. Daily
   c. Weekly
   d. Monthly

Answer b is correct. Per USP 797

Answer a is incorrect. Too frequent

Answer c is incorrect. Not frequent enough per US 797

Answer d is incorrect. Not frequent enough

13. Which of the following statements is true regarding proper hand hygiene prior to entering buffer room?

   a. Wash your arms from the wrists toward the finger tips making sure your gown stays dry.
   b. Jewelry, such as rings, is allowed as long as it is properly cleaned with 70% IPA.
   c. Wash your hands all the way up to your elbows with antimicrobial soap for 30 seconds.
   d. You can use waterless sanitizer in place of thorough hand wash.

Answer c is correct. Must wash up to elbows for a minimum of 30 seconds.

Answer a is incorrect. Must wash arms up to the elbows.

Answer b is incorrect. Cannot wear any jewelry.

Answer d is incorrect. Waterless sanitizer is insufficient to remove physical and chemical contaminants and hands must be washed with soap and water.

14. Which of the following PECs should NOT be used to prepare hazardous medications?

   a. BSC
   b. Compounding aseptic containment isolator

c. Horizontal positive LAFW
d. All of the above are appropriate to prepare hazardous medications.

Answer c is correct. Positive LAFW should never be used to compound hazardous preparations.

Answer a is incorrect. BSC should be used for hazardous drug compounding.

Answer b is incorrect. CACI should be used for hazardous drug compounding.

Answer d is incorrect. Not all three should be used for hazardous drug compounding.

15. Which of the following statements regarding hazardous drug compounding per USP 797 is correct? Select all that apply.

   a. Personnel needs additional training when handling hazardous medications.
   b. CSTDs can be used in place of PECs and SECS, as they provide sufficient amount of protection to the compounder.
   c. Proper PPE must be worn when unpacking shipment of chemotherapeutic agents.
   d. When gowning for hazardous drug compounding, one must use impervious gown to avoid/limit any exposure.

Answers a, c, and d are correct. Personnel needs additional training when handling hazardous medications and proper PPE must be worn when unpacking shipment of chemotherapeutic agents. Additionally, when gowning for hazardous drug compounding, one must use impervious gown to avoid/limit any exposure.

Answer b is incorrect. CSTDs do not replace the use of PECs and SECs; only further reduce chance of exposure.

16. Label instructions on a pharmacy bulk package of 10 g of vancomycin HCl state that when 95 mL of SWFI are added to the powder, the resultant solution will have concentration of 500 mg per 5 mL. How many milliliters of SWFI should the pharmacist add to the dry powder to prepare the concentration of 1000 mg per 5 mL?

Solution:

Step 1: What is the final volume when reconstituted the vial?

10,000 mg/X = 500 mg/5 mL, solve for X, X = 100 mL

Step 2: Determine the powder volume

100 mL – 95 mL = 5 mL powder volume

Step 3: Calculate new dilution volume

10,000 mg/X = 1000 mg/5 mL, solve for X, X = 50 mL

Step 4: determine the volume added

50 mL – PV = **45 mL**

17. Due to national drug shortage, you need to prepare 250 mL NS bags using 23.4% NaCl vial and sterile water. How many milliliters of 23.4% NaCl solution will you need to prepare 10 bags of 250 mL NS?

Solution:

V1 × C1 = V2 × C2

V1 × 23.4% = 250 mL × 0.9%

V1 = 9.615 mL

To make 10 bags: 10 × 9.615 mL = **96.15 mL** of 23.4% NaCl is needed

18. How many milliliters of injection containing 40 mg of gentamicin in each 1 mL should be used in filling a medication order calling for 85 mg of gentamicin to be administered IV in a 100 mL NS small volume parenteral IV bag?

Solution:

40 mg per 1 mL = 85 mg per X mL

Solve for X = **2.125** mL of 40 mg per 1 mL

19. A pharmacist received a medication order to add 50,000 units of heparin to 1 L of D5W for a 175 lb patient. The rate of infusion was prescribed as 5000 units/h. What is the dose of heparin received by the patient on a unit/kg/min basis?

Solution:

Convert 175 lb to kg: 79.55 kg

Dimensional analysis: Patient receives 5000 units/h, thus 5000 units/79.55 kg/60 min = **1.05 units/kg/min**

20. A physician prescribed continuous heparin infusion of 18 units/kg/h for a patient with VTE. It is to be prepared in 250 mL IV NS and it is to run over next 6 hours for a patient who weighs 91 kg. How many mL of 10,000 units per 10 mL heparin do you need to add to the IV bag?

Solution:

18 U × 91 kg × 6 hours = 9828 Units, thus **0.9828 mL** of heparin

Index

Note: f and t indicate figures and tables, respectively.

THE TOP 100 INJECTABLE DRUGS

Generic	Brand	Generic	Brand
Acetylcysteine	Acetadote	Ganciclovir	Cytovene
Acyclovir	Zovirax	Gentamicin	Garamycin
Alteplase	Activase	Granisetron	Kytril
Amiodarone	Cordarone	Haloperidol	Haldol
Amphotericin B	Fungizone, Amphocin	Heparin	N/A
Ampicillin sodium	Principen	Hydralazine	Apresoline
Ampicillin + sulbactam	Unasyn	Hydrocortisone	A-Hydrocort, Solu-Cortef
Atropine	AtroPen	Hydromorphone	Dilaudid
Azithromycin	Zithromax	Imipenem/Cilastatin	Primaxin
Aztreonam	Azactam	Infliximab	Remicade
Bumetanide	Bumex	Iron sucrose	Venofer
Butorphanol	Stadol	Ketorolac	Toradol
Caspofungin	Cancidas	Labetalol	Normodyne, Trandate
Cefazolin	Ancef	Levothyroxine	Synthroid, Levoxyl
Cefepime	Maxipime	Lidocaine	Xylocaine
Cefotaxime	Claforan	Linezolid	Zyvox
Ceftriaxone	Rocephin	Lorazepam	Ativan
Cefuroxime	Zinacef	Mannitol	Osmitrol
Chlorpromazine	Thorazine	Meperidine	Demerol
Ciprofloxacin	Cipro	Meropenem	Merrem
Cisplatin	Platinol	Methotrexate	Rheumatrex, Trexall
Clindamycin	Cleocin	Methylprednisolone	Solu-Medrol, A-Methapred
Dantrolene	Dantrium	Metoclopramide	Reglan
Daptomycin	Cubicin	Metoprolol	Lopressor
Darbepoetin alfa	Aranesp	Metronidazole	Flagyl
Dexamethasone	Decadron	Micafungin	Mycamine
Diazepam	Valium	Midazolam	Versed
Digoxin	Lanoxin	Milrinone	Primacor
Diphenhydramine	Benadryl	Morphine	Duramorph, Astramorphe PF
Dobutamine	Dobutrex	Nafcillin sodium	Unipen
Dopamine	Intropin	Nalbuphine	Nubain
Droperidol	Inapsine	Naloxone	Narcan
Enoxaparin	Lovenox	Norepinephrine	Levophed
Epinephrine	Epipen, Adrenalin	Ondansetron	Zofran
Epoetin alfa	Epogen, Procrit	Oxytocin	Pitocin
Ertapenem	Invanz	Palonosetron	Aloxi
Esomeprazole	Nexium	Pamidronate	Aredia
Fentanyl	Sublimaze	Pantoprazole	Protonix
Filgrastim	Neupogen	Pentobarbital	Luminal
Fluconazole	Diflucan	Phenylephrine	Neosynephrine
Fosphenytoin	Cerebyx	Phenytoin sodium	Dilantin
Furosemide	Lasix	Piperacillin	Pipracil

(Continued)